Postgraduate Haematology

Postgraduate Haematology

EDITED BY

A. Victor Hoffbrand MA, DM, FRCP, FRCPath, FRCP (Edin), DSc, FMedSci

Emeritus Professor of Haematology, Royal Free and University College Medical School, and Honorary Consultant Haematologist, Royal Free Hospital, London, UK

Daniel Catovsky MD, DSc (Med), FRCPath, FRCP, FMedSci

Emeritus Professor of Haematology, Institute of Cancer Research, Sutton, Surrey, UK

Edward G.D. Tuddenham MD, FRCP, FRCPath

Professor of Haemostasis, MRC Haemostasis Research Group, Imperial College School of Medicine, Hammersmith Hospital, London, UK

Fifth edition

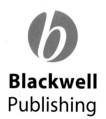

Blackwell
Publishing

© 2005 by Blackwell Publishing Ltd
Blackwell Publishing Inc., 350 Main Street, Malden, Massachusetts 02148-5020, USA
Blackwell Publishing Ltd, 9600 Garsington Road, Oxford OX4 2DQ, UK
Blackwell Publishing Asia Pty Ltd, 550 Swanston Street, Carlton, Victoria 3053, Australia

First published as *Tutorials in Postgraduate Haematology* © William Heinemann Ltd 1972
Reprinted 1975
Second edition 1981 published © Butterworth Ltd
Reprinted 1983, 1986
Third edition 1989 published © Butterworth Ltd
Reprinted 1992
Fourth edition 1999 published © Butterworth-Heinmann Ltd
Revised and reprinted 2001 by Arnold
Fifth edition 2005
3   2007

Library of Congress Cataloging-in-Publication Data
Postgraduate haematology / edited by A. Victor Hoffbrand, Daniel
Catovsky, Edward G.D. Tuddenham.–5th ed.
    p.; cm.
Includes bibliographical references and index.
ISBN 978-1-4051-0821-8
1. Blood–Diseases.   2. Hematology.
[DNLM: 1. Blood.   2. Hematologic Diseases. WH 100 P857 2004]
I. Hoffbrand, A. V.   II. Catovsky, D. (Daniel)   III. Tuddenham, Edward G. D.

RC633.P67 2004
616.1'5–dc22

2004015936

ISBN 978-1-4051-0821-8

A catalogue record for this title is available from the British Library

Set in 9.5/12pt Minion by Graphicraft Limited, Hong Kong
Printed and bound In India by Replika Press Pvt. Ltd

Commissioning Editor: Maria Khan
Development Editor: Rebecca Huxley
Production Controller: Kate Charman

For further information on Blackwell Publishing, visit our website:
http://www.blackwellpublishing.com

Contents

Contributors

Irit Avivi
Department of Haematology and Bone Marrow
Transplantation
Ramban Medical Center
Haifa
Israel

Barbara J Bain
Department of Haematology
St Mary's Hospital
London
UK

John A Barbara
National Blood Service
North London Centre
London
UK

Imelda Bates
Senior Clinical Lecturer in Tropical Haematology
Liverpool School of Tropical Medicine
Liverpool
UK

Anthony J Bench
Senior Scientist
Department of Haematology
Addenbrookes Hospital
Cambridge
UK

Malcolm K Brenner
Center for Cell and Gene Therapy
Baylor College of Medicine
Houston, TX
USA

Alan K Burnett
Department of Haematology
University Hospital of Wales, College of Medicine
Cardiff
UK

James B Bussell
New York Hospital
New York, NY
USA

Jenny L Byrne
Department of Haematology
City Hospital
Nottingham
UK

Peter J Campbell
Department of Haematology
Cambridge Institute for Medical Research
Addenbrookes Hospital
Cambridge
UK

Daniel Catovsky
Emeritus Professor of Haematology
Institute of Cancer Research
Sutton
Surrey
UK

Ronjon Chakraverty
Royal Free and University College Medical School
London
UK

April Chiu
New York Hospital
New York, NY
USA

Doug Cines
Department of Pathology and Laboratory
Medicine
University of Pennsylvania
Philadelphia, PA
USA

Hannah Cohen
Consultant in Haematology
Department of Haematology
University College Hospitals NHS Foundation
Trust
London
UK

Marcela Contreras
National Blood Service
North London Centre
London
UK

Christine Costello
Department of Haematology
Chelsea and Westminster Hospital
London
UK

Charles Craddock
Leukaemia Unit
Department of Haematology
Queen Elizabeth Hospital
Birmingham
UK

Geoff Daniels
Blood Group Unit
Bristol Institute for Transfusion Sciences
Bristol
UK

Inderjeet S Dokal
Department of Haematology
Hammersmith Hospital
London
UK

J Peter Donnelly
Department of Haematology
University Hospital Nijmegen
Nijmegen
The Netherlands

Mark T Drayson
Department of Immunology
University of Birmingham Medical School
Birmingham
UK

Ivy Ekem
Lecturer and Acting Head
Department of Haematology

University of Ghana Medical School
Accra
Ghana

Letizia Foroni

Department of Haematology
Royal Free and University College Medical School
London
UK

Paula M Gameiro

Centre of Molecular Pathology
Haemato-oncology Unit
Portuguese Intitute of Oncology Francisco Gentil
Lisboa
Portugal

Nicola Gökbuget

JW Goethe University Hospital
Medical Clinic II
Frankfurt
Germany

John M Goldman

Department of Haematology
Imperial College School of Medicine
Hammersmith Hospital
London
UK

Anthony H Goldstone

Department of Haematology
University College London
London
UK

Hugh JB Goodman

National Amyloidosis Centre
Royal Free and University College Medical School
Royal Free Hospital
London
UK

Myrtle Gordon

Department of Haematology
Imperial College School of Medicine
London
UK

Edward C Gordon-Smith

Department of Haematology
St George's Hospital Medical School
London
UK

Peter J Grant

Academic Unit of Molecular Vascular Medicine
University of Leeds

Leeds General Infirmary
Leeds
UK

Michael Greaves

Department of Medicine and Therapeutics
University of Aberdeen
Aberdeen
UK

Anthony R Green

Department of Haematology
Cambridge Institute for Medical Research
Addenbrookes Hospital
Cambridge
UK

Ralph Green

University of California
Davis Medical Center
Sacramento, CA
USA

Christine J Harrison

Leukaemia Research Fund
Cytogenetics Group
Cancer Sciences Division
University of Southampton
Southampton
UK

Paul Harrison

Oxford Haemophilia Centre
The Churchill Hospital
Headington
Oxford
UK

Philip N Hawkins

National Amyloidosis Centre
Royal Free and University College Medical School
Royal Free Hospital
London
UK

Douglas R Higgs

Professor of Molecular Haematology
Weatherall Institute of Molecular Medicine
John Radcliffe Hospital
Oxford
UK

Dieter Hoelzer

Professor of Internal Medicine
JW Goethe University Hospital
Medical Clinic II
Frankfurt
Germany

A Victor Hoffbrand

Emeritus Professor of Haematology
Royal Free and University College Medical School
and Honorary Consultant Haematologist
Royal Free Hospital
London
UK

Ronald Hoffman

University of Illinois, College of Medicine
Chicago, IL
USA

Derralynn A Hughes

Lecturer in Haematology
Department of Academic Haematology
Royal Free and University College Medical School
London
UK

Beverley J Hunt

Department of Haematology
Guy's St Thomas' Trust
St Thomas' Hospital
London
UK

Peter G Isaacson

Department of Histopathology
University College London Medical School
London
UK

Geoffrey Kemball-Cook

Haemostasis Group
MRC Clinical Sciences Centre
Faculty of Medicine, Imperial College
London
UK

Sally B Killick

Department of Haematology and Oncology
Royal Bournemouth Hospital
Bournemouth
Dorset
UK

Michael A Laffan

Department of Haematology, Faculty of Medicine
Imperial College School of Medicine
Hammersmith Hospital
London
UK

Ashutosh Lal

Hematology/Oncology
Children's Hospital and Research Center at Oakland
Oakland, CA
USA

Christine A Lee
Katharine Dormandy Haemophilia Centre and
Haemostasis Unit
Royal Free Hospital
London
UK

Ollivier Legrand
Department of Haematology and Medical
Oncology
Hôtel-Dieu of Paris
Paris
France

S Mitchell Lewis
Department of Haematology
Faculty of Medicine
Imperial College of Science, Technology and
Medicine
Hammersmith Hospital
London
UK

Der-Cherng Liang
Pediatric Hematology–Oncology
Mackay Memorial Hospital
Taipei
Taiwan

Ri Liesner
Consultant in Paediatric Haemostasis and
Thrombosis
Great Ormond Street Hospital
London
UK

David Linch
Royal Free and University College Medical School
University College London
Department of Haematology
London
UK

Ann-Margaret Little
The Anthony Nolan Research Institute
Royal Free Hospital
London
UK

Lucio Luzzatto
Scientific Director
Istituto Nazionale per la Ricerca sul Cancro
Istituto Scientifico per lo Studio e la Cura dei
Tumori
Genova
Italy

Samuel J Machin
Professor of Haematology
Department of Haematology
University College Hospitals NHS Foundation
Trust
London
UK

Stephen Mackinnon
Department of Haematology
Royal Free and University College Medical School
London
UK

John H McVey
Haemostasis Group
MRC Clinical Sciences Centre
Faculty of Medicine, Imperial College
London
UK

J Alejandro Madrigal
The Anthony Nolan Research Institute
Royal Free Hospital
London
UK

Pier M Manucci
Professor and Chairman of Internal Medicine
The University of Milan and IRCCS Maggiore
Hospital
Milan
Italy

Maurizio Margaglione
Genetica Medica
Universita' Degli Studi di Foggia
Foggia
Italy

Jean-Pierre Marie
Department of Haematology–Oncology
Hôtel-Dieu of Paris
Paris
France

Judith C W Marsh
Department of Haematology
St George's Hospital Medical School
London
UK

Steven G E Marsh
The Anthony Nolan Research Institute
Royal Free Hospital
London
UK

Stephen P Marso
St Luke's Hospital
Mid-American Heart Institute
Kansas City, MO
USA

Estella Matutes
Academic Department of Haematology
Royal Marsden Hospital
London
UK

Atul B Mehta
Department of Haematology
Royal Free Hospital
London
UK

Paul A H Moss
Moseley
Birmingham
West Midlands
UK

Tariq I Mughal
University of Massachusetts Medical Center
Division of Haematology and Oncology
Worcester, MA
USA

Michael J Nash
Research Fellow/Specialist Registrar
Department of Haematology
University College London
London
UK

Rosario Notaro
Human Genetics
Istituto Nazionale per la Ricera sul Cancro
Genova
Italy

David G Oscier
Department of Haematology and Oncology
Royal Bournemouth Hospital
Bournemouth
UK

Flora Peyvandi
Associate Professor of Internal Medicine
The University of Milan and IRCCS Maggiore
Hospital
Milan
Italy

Michael Potter
Department of Haematology
Royal Marsden Hospital
London
UK

Archibald G Prentice
Haematology Department
Derriford Hospital
Plymouth
UK

Ching-Hon Pui
Lymphoid Disease Program
St Jude Chilen's Research Hospital
Memphis, TN
USA

Amin Rahemtulla
Department of Hematology
Faculty of Medicine, Imperial College London
Hammersmith Hospital
London
UK

Farhad Ravandi
Department of Leukemia
University of Texas – MD Anderson Cancer
Center
Houston, TX
USA

Irene A G Roberts
Professor of Paediatric Haematology
Department of Haematology, Faculty of Medicine
Imperial College of Science, Technology and
Medicine
Hammersmith Hospital
London
UK

Raphaël F Rousseau
Center of Cell and Gene Therapy
Texas Children's Cancer Center
Baylor College of Medicine
Houston, TX
USA

Nigel H Russell
Department of Haematology
City Hospital
Nottingham
UK

Sam Schulman
Department of Haematology, Coagulation Unit
Karolinska University Hospital
Stockholm
Sweden
and Department of Medicine
HHS General Hospital
Hamilton
Ontario
Canada

Lucinda K M Summers
Academic Unit of Molecular Vascular Medicine,
University of Leeds
Leeds General Infirmary
Leeds
UK

Wayne Tam
New York Hospital
New York, NY
USA

Clare P F Taylor
Royal Free Hospital
London
UK

Evangelos Terpos
Department of Haematology
Faculty of Medicine, Imperial College London
Hammersmith Hospital
London
UK

Kirsty J Thomson
Department of Haematology
University College Hospital
London
UK

Edward G D Tuddenham
Professor of Haemostasis
MRC Haemostasis Research Group
Imperial College School of Medicine
Hammersmith Hospital
London
UK

George Vassiliou
Department of Haematology
University of Cambridge
Cambridge Institute for Medical Research
Cambridge
UK

Elliott P Vichinsky
Hematology/Oncology
Children's Hospital and Research Center at
Oakland
Oakland, CA
USA

Isobel D Walker
Consultant Haematologist
Department of Haematology
Glasgow Royal Infirmary and Princess Royal
Maternity
Glasgow
UK

Stephen P Watson
BHF Chair in Cardiovascular Sceinces and Cellular
Pharmacology
Centre for Cardiovascular Sciences
Institute of Biomedical Research
Division of Medical Sciences
University of Birmingham
Birmingham
UK

David J Weatherall
Weatherall Institute of Molecular Medicine
John Radcliffe Hospital
Oxford
UK

A David B Webster
Department of Clinical Immunology
Royal Free Hospital School of Medicine
London
UK

William G Wood
Professor in Haematology
Weatherall Institute of Molecular Medicine
John Radcliffe Hospital
Oxford
UK

Mark Worwood
Department of Haematology
University Hospital of Wales, College of Medicine
Cardiff
UK

Lynny Yung
Clinical Lymphoma Research Trust Fellow
British National Lymphoma Investigation
London
UK

Preface to the fifth edition

Major changes for this new edition have occurred in the editorship, publishing and style of *Postgraduate Haematology* since the 4th edition was published 6 years ago. Mitchell Lewis, who played a major role in the design and writing of the first edition, which appeared in 1972, and was co-editor for the first four editions, has stepped down from this role. We are delighted that he has, nevertheless, contributed two chapters to this volume, one on the spleen and the other on laboratory practice. Daniel Catovsky has joined as co-editor to oversee particularly the section of the book dealing with malignant haematological disorders.

We are also pleased to welcome Blackwell Publishing Ltd, well respected for its impressive list of haematological books and journals, as publishers for this 5th edition. We are particularly grateful to Rebecca Huxley, who has taken on the publishing process, and to Jane Fallows, who has drawn all the scientific diagrams.

For the 5th edition, *Postgraduate Haematology* has been divided into smaller chapters. This has enabled us to bring in many younger authors with knowledge and expertise in particular areas. It has also facilitated the incorporation of the new information on mechanisms of disease, laboratory investigation and clinical management that has been gained over the last 6 years. Although the book has expanded to over 1000 pages, it is still aimed at providing haematologists in training and consultants with a text that is up to date and easy to read and that gives ready access to the information on diagnosis and treatment needed in the laboratory and clinic.

Microscopic appearances of the blood diseases are illustrated throughout the book. These illustrations are mainly reproduced from the 4th edition but we wish to thank Elsevier Inc. for permission to reproduce figures from the 3rd edition of the *Color Atlas of Clinical Haematology*, edited by A.V. Hoffbrand and J.E. Pettit and published by Harcourt Publishers Ltd.

Finally we wish to thank Megan Evans and Wanda Malinowski for their expert secretarial help throughout the preparation of this new edition.

AVH, DC, EGDT
2005

Preface to the first edition

In this book the authors combine an account of the physiological and biochemical basis of haematological processes with descriptions of the clinical and laboratory features and management of blood disorders. Within this framework, each author has dealt with the individual subjects as he or she thought appropriate. Because this book is intended to provide a foundation for the study of haematology and is not intended to be a reference book, it reflects, to some extent, the views of the individual authors rather than providing comprehensive detail and a full bibliography. For these the reader is referred to the selected reading given at the end of each chapter. It is hoped that the book will prove of particular value to students taking either the Primary or the Final Part of the examination for Membership of the Royal College of Pathologists and the Diplomas of Clinical Pathology. It should also prove useful to physicians wishing to gain special knowledge of haematology and to technicians taking the Advanced Diploma in Haematology of the Institute of Medical Laboratory Technology, or the Higher National Certificate in Medical Laboratory subjects.

We wish to acknowledge kind permission from the editors and publishers of the *British Journal of Haematology*, the *Journal of the Royal College of Physicians of London* and the *Quarterly Journal of Medicine* for permission to reproduce figures 4.1, 4.5, 4.10, 4.11, 4.12, 9.4 and 9.10, also the publishers of *Progress in Haematology* for figure 7.2, and many other publishers who, together with the authors, have been acknowledged in the text. We are particularly grateful to Professor J.V. Dacie for providing material which formed the basis of many of the original illustrations in Chapters 4–8. We are greatly indebted to Mrs T. Charalambos, Mrs J. Cope and Mrs D. Haysome for secretarial assistance and to Mrs P. Schilling and the Department of Medical Illustration for photomicrography, art work and general photography.

Finally, we are grateful for the invaluable help and forbearance we have received from Mr R. Emery and William Heinemann Medical Books.

London, 1972   AVH
                                                                                                        SML

CHAPTER 1

Stem cells and haemopoiesis

Myrtle Gordon

1

Introduction

The lifelong production of blood cells occurs in haemopoietic tissue. This involves a very high level of cell turnover, demanded by the need to replace mature circulating blood cells at a rapid rate, and is necessitated by the limited lifespan of the mature cells. Granulocytes survive for only a few hours and erythrocytes for a few months, so that some 10^{13} new cells must be replaced each day to maintain steady-state blood counts. This is equivalent to an annual number of cells approximating the total body weight, but the total bone marrow of an adult human contains around 10^{12} cells, 10-fold less than daily needs. From these estimates it is clear that the blood cells required for lifelong haemopoiesis cannot be preformed in the body.

The bone marrow, which is the major site of haemopoiesis in adult humans, contains cells that represent the stages in the development of the different types of blood cells (Figure 1.1). The later stages are recognizable as belonging to the major lineages of haemopoiesis (granulocytes, erythrocytes, monocyte/macrophages, megakaryocytes, eosinophils, basophils, and T and B lymphocytes). They are the myelocytes, metamyelocytes, erythroblasts, reticulocytes, etc. Earlier stages of development become progressively less morphologically distinct in their lineage affiliation and fewer in number, whereas the least frequent cells, which cannot be discriminated morphologically, are the committed progenitor cell populations and the stem cells.

The stem cells are the most important cells in haemopoietic cell production. They are ultimately responsible for regenerating haemopoiesis following damage to the haemopoietic system by myelotoxic chemotherapy or after stem cell transplantation. This is accomplished by stem cell division, producing new stem cells to maintain the stem cell pool (stem cell renewal) and differentiating cells that are the progenitor cells of each of the blood cell lineages. Estimates of stem cell frequency in human bone marrow are about one stem cell per 20 million nucleated cells.

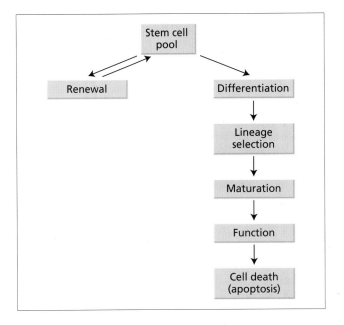

Figure 1.1 Stages in haemopoietic cell development.

They are very difficult to measure, although various assays for candidate human stem cells have been developed. These include both *in vitro* and *in vivo* assays such as long-term bone marrow culture (LT-BMC), cobblestone-area colony (CAFC) formation and the NOD/SCID mouse repopulating assay.

Haemopoiesis is regulated by soluble factors that were discovered when immobilization of bone marrow cells in a semisolid matrix containing medium 'conditioned' by the growth of a cell line in culture resulted in the growth of clonal colonies of granulocytes and macrophages. Identification of the active factors in the conditioned medium led eventually to cloning, production of recombinant protein and clinical use of cytokines in the therapy of haematological disease.

In addition to the haemopoietic system, the bone marrow contains stromal stem cells (mesenchymal stem cells), which are important for constructing the haemopoietic microenvironment. The microenvironment provides more than simply mechanical support and has been shown to be an essential component of the long-term bone marrow culture system. Moreover, damage to the microenvironment, for example by chemotherapy, has been implicated in haemopoietic insufficiency after treatment.

Studies in haemopoietic stem cell biology have now expanded to embrace the concepts of stem cell plasticity. This term refers to the ability of haemopoietic and stromal (mesenchymal) stem cells to produce cells associated with other tissues, such as liver, lung and muscle. Although this area remains highly controversial, the therapeutic applications of haemopoietic stem cell plasticity are obvious as it would provide an easily accessible source of cells that could be redirected to repair a variety of damaged tissues.

Sites of haemopoiesis

The development of the haemopoietic system is associated with the development of suitable microenvironments, which are colonized by migrating stem cells. The migration of stem cells from site to site must require mechanisms for their entry, transit and exit. These processes probably involve specific recognition and adhesive interactions between the stem cells and cells of the various microenvironments. Extracellular matrix-degrading enzymes such as the metalloproteinases have been implicated in the reversal of adhesion and exit from tissues.

There has been a long-accepted dogma that the adult haemopoietic system originates in the embryonic yolk sac. The mesenchyme of the yolk sac differentiates into endothelial cells, on the one hand, and haemopoietic stem cells on the other. At this stage, haemopoiesis consists of blood islands, consisting of primitive primordial cells (haemocytoblasts) and erythroblastoid cells surrounded by endothelial cells. The observation that endothelial and haemopoietic cell development occur in close proximity led to the hypothesis that these two cell types are derived from a common precursor, the haemangioblast, which represents the origin of the circulatory system as well as the blood cells. Following the development of the circulation, stem cells can migrate into the embryo where they sequentially seed the liver, spleen and bone marrow.

Challenging the yolk sac origin of adult haemopoiesis, embryografting experiments in birds revealed that adult haemopoiesis is derived from an intraembryonic source. This is the aorta–gonad–mesonephros (AGM) region, located in the para-aortic splanchnopleure. It is not overtly erythropoietic, unlike yolk sac haemopoiesis, but contains a spectrum of lymphoid and myeloid stem and progenitor cells. Similarly, active haemopoiesis is found in the AGM region of embryo mice. It is thought that a second wave of fetal liver colonization, originating in the AGM region, supplies stem cells for the eventual development of the adult haemopoietic system, in contrast with the primitive and temporary haemopoiesis derived from the yolk sac.

Primitive erythropoiesis persists as the major visible haemopoietic activity in the fetal blood vessels, liver and spleen but large numbers of granulocytes can be found in the connective tissue, outside the organs, for most of intrauterine life. Granulocytic cells are not produced in large numbers until haemopoiesis is established in the bone marrow. This occurs at different times in different bones and coincides with the process of ossification. Large numbers of stem cells are found in umbilical cord blood as well as in the fetal circulation, and this has led to the use of cord blood as an alternative to bone marrow as a source of cells for transplantation. At birth, haemopoietic activity is distributed throughout the human skeleton but it gradually recedes with time so that in normal adult life haemopoiesis is found mainly in the sternum and pelvis, with small amounts in other bones like the ribs, skull and vertebrae.

A small number of stem cells are present in the circulation of normal adult humans. This number increases physiologically in some circumstances, such as following exercise and during infections, and may be increased pharmacologically by administration of haemopoietic growth factors and/or cytotoxic chemotherapy. This phenomenon has been exploited to provide large numbers of circulating stem cells, which can then be collected by leucapheresis and used as a source of cells for stem cell transplantation.

The stromal microenvironment

The documentation of haemopoiesis migrating from site to site suggested that there might be specialized conditions that determine the sequence of colonization. Geiger *et al.* (1998) demonstrated the influence of the embryonic and fetal liver microenvironments by injecting adult marrow stem cells into blastocysts and finding they resumed the adult and fetal programmes of haemopoietic cell development. In contrast, when haemopoietic stem cells from fetal liver are injected into adults they develop along adult lines. Indeed, fetal liver has been used as a source of haemopoietic stem cells for clinical transplantation in some circumstances. Charbord and colleagues characterized a cell type in early-gestation fetal liver, but not in late-gestation fetal liver, with mixed endodermal and mesodermal features that supported haemopoietic cell proliferation *in vitro*. Thus, these fetal stromal cells were only present during the haemopoietic phase of liver development.

Early *in vivo* studies in adult mice demonstrated that the microenvironment in the spleen induced erythropoietic differentiation of transplanted bone marrow cells, whereas the microenvironment in the marrow induced granulopoietic differentiation, demonstrating quite clearly that different microenvironmental conditions can determine lineage expression. *In vitro*, adult bone marrow stromal cells form adherent layers that are believed to represent the haemopoietic microenvironment and provide support for haemopoietic activity in long-term bone marrow cultures. The stromal cells consist of several cell types, namely macrophages, endothelial cells, fibroblasts and fat cells, together with their extracellular matrix, consisting of collagen, fibronectin and proteoglycan constituents.

Stem cell trafficking

The ability of stem cells to traffic around the body and to search out sites suitable for haemopoiesis is well demonstrated by (a) the 'homing' of transplanted stem cells to the bone marrow and (b) the chemotherapy and cytokine-induced 'mobilization' of stem cells into the circulation. Homing involves transendothelial migration from the bloodstream into the marrow microenvironment, whereas mobilization involves detachment from the microenvironment and transendothelial migration in the reverse direction. Together, these processes may provide a paradigm for stem cell trafficking in general (Figure 1.2). They are likely to involve multifactorial processes involving chemokines, cytokines, adhesion molecules and matrix-degrading enzymes.

In vitro experiments have shown that stromal cell-derived chemokine gradients across an endothelial barrier induce stem cells to migrate from one side to the other. Chemokines are cytokines with direct chemotactic effects on receptor-expressing target cells. However, stromal cell-derived factor 1 (SDF-1) is the only chemokine that acts on haemopoietic stem and progenitor cells. Once the stem cells have gained the extravascular spaces in the bone marrow, the stromal cells provide a plethora of potential sites for recognition by stem cells, including cell surface and extracellular matrix ligands for adhesion molecules (CAMs) on the stem cell surface. Haemopoietic stem and progenitor cells express a wide variety of cell adhesion molecules of different classes (e.g. selectins and integrins), but they are not specific for stem cells as they are also expressed by mature leucocytes.

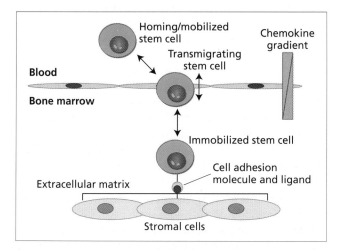

Figure 1.2 Stages in the homing and mobilization of stem cells.

Cytokines and cytokine receptors may also act in cytoadhesion as stem cell factor (SCF; c-Kit ligand) is expressed on the cell surface by stromal cells and its receptor, c-Kit, is expressed by stem cells. Similarly, the Notch ligand, Jagged, is expressed by stromal cells, whereas Notch is expressed by stem cells.

Clearly, cytokines play a role in the release of stem cells from the marrow microenvironment as cytokine administration is used to induce stem cell mobilization into the peripheral blood. Cytokines increase metalloproteinase expression, release stem cell factor from the stromal cell surface and induce stem cell migration through the endothelial barrier. Thus, stem cell trafficking may be a dynamic and continuous process, depending on the prevailing haemopoietic activity.

Organization of haemopoiesis

The haemopoietic system is a hierarchy of cells in which multipotent haemopoietic stem cells give rise to lineage-committed progenitor cells, which divide to generate the maturing and mature blood cells (Figure 1.3).

Stem cells

Assays for stem cells

Stem cells are found at a very low frequency in haemopoietic tissue and cannot be recognized in stained smears of bone marrow. In animal models, the best assay for stem cells is a repopulating assay, which tests the ability of the cells to engraft and restore haemopoiesis in a myeloablated host. For human stem cells, a variety of *in vitro* assay systems have been used, but the most widely accepted is the long-term bone marrow culture system (LT-BMC). This method reproduces the microenvironment of the bone marrow *in vitro* by growing a feeder layer of stromal cells. When haemopoietic long-term culture-initiating cells (LT-CICs) are seeded onto the stromal layer, they are induced to proliferate and produce progenitor cells that can be measured in the clonogenic assays detailed below. However, the endpoint of this assay is indirect, in that committed colony-forming cells produced by the LT-CICs are enumerated. Consequently, limiting dilution analysis is necessary to determine LT-CIC numbers. However, limiting dilution is statistically based and the procedure is very cumbersome.

A variety of clonal assays for candidate stem cells have also been used. The cobblestone area-forming cell (CAFC) assay resembles the long-term culture assay in that haemopoietic cells are seeded onto stromal layers. In this case, however, the formation of colonies containing cells of a cobblestone-like morphology is observed. The blast colony-forming cell (Bl-CFC) assay and high proliferative potential colony-forming cell assay (HPP-CFC) detect cells that share certain characteristics with stem cells but are generally considered to be less primitive than stem cells.

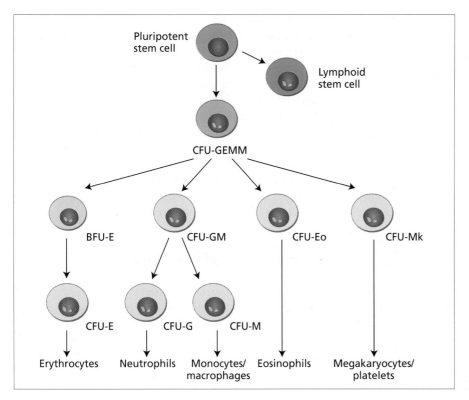

Figure 1.3 Hierarchical organization of haemopoiesis.

Stem cell properties, phenotype and purification

Morphologically, haemopoietic stem cells are undifferentiated and resemble small lymphocytes. Normally, a large fraction is quiescent, in G_0 phase of the cell cycle, which protects them from the action of cell cycle-dependent drugs such as 5′-fluorouracil, and S-phase-specific agents such as cytosine arabinoside and hydroxyurea. The quiescent state of stem cells is maintained by transforming growth factor β (TGF-β). The activity of TGF-β is mediated by p53, a tumour suppressor that regulates cell proliferation and targets the cyclin-dependent kinase inhibitor p21. The cyclin-dependent kinase inhibitors regulate the activities of cyclin–cyclin-dependent kinase (CDK) complexes. Inhibition of the cyclin–CDK complexes prevents phosphorylation of the retinoblastoma proteins that remain bound to transcription factors belonging to the E2F family. As a consequence, genes required for progression of the cell cycle are not transcribed and cells remain quiescent (Figure 1.4). Stromal cells express TGF-β, which is involved in maintaining stem cell quiescence in the bone marrow microenvironment.

The immunophenotype of haemopoietic stem cells is summarized in Table 1.1 and consists of the presence of markers that are expressed by stem cells (CD34, Thy-1) and those that are absent (CD33, CD38, HLA-DR and lineage-specific (lin) markers). CD34 is the best-known marker of human stem and progenitor cells. It is a member of the sialomucin family of glycoproteins, which are heavily glycosylated molecules with potential adhesion and signalling capabilities. CD34 has been

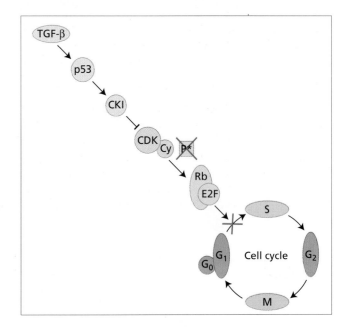

Figure 1.4 Maintenance of stem cell quiescence.

implicated in the binding together of cells from the KG1a line and of primary human CD34$^+$ progenitor cells.

The importance, interest and rarity of stem cells have led to extensive efforts to purify them, based on stem cell characteristics that distinguish them from other cells in the haemopoietic

Table 1.1 Basic immunophenotype of haemopoietic stem cells.

Positive	Negative
CD34	CD33
Thy-1	CD38
AC133	Lineage markers
c-Kit	HLA-DR

system. The resistance of stem cells to cell cycle-dependent drugs, particularly to 5′-fluorouracil, has been used as one of the stages in stem cell purification. Fluorescence-activated cell sorting of cells labelled by monoclonal antibodies to phenotypic markers is a widely used strategy for stem cell purification, as is magnetic bead sorting. Despite efforts to purify stem cells to phenotypic homogeneity, the resulting populations are not functionally homogeneous.

Stem cell renewal and differentiation

Stem cells are capable of self-renewal and differentiation when they divide and are responsible for producing all the mature blood cells throughout life. This means that when steady-state stem cells divide, only 50% of the daughter cells, on average, differentiate, the remaining 50% do not differentiate, but maintain stem cell numbers. This could be accomplished by asymmetric cell division, so that each dividing stem cell forms one new stem cell and one differentiated cell (Figure 1.5a). Alternatively, balanced numbers of stem cells could divide symmetrically to form either two new stem cells or two differentiated cells (Figure 1.5b). Clearly, the asymmetric model does not allow for regeneration of the stem cell population but, by altering the proportions of renewing and differentiating stem cells, the symmetric division model can account for stem cell recovery (Figure 1.5c) because it permits an increase in the proportions of symmetrical self-renewing divisions and a reduction in the proportion of differentiating divisions. The symmetrical model of stem cell division means that self-renewal and differentiation are likely to be properties of the stem cell population at large, rather

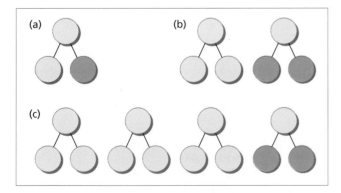

Figure 1.5 Models of stem cell self-renewal and differentiation.

than characteristics of each individual stem cell. However, this mechanism is accompanied by extinction of the differentiating stem cells because the clones they produce will not contain any stem cells.

Regulation of self-renewal

Control of haemopoietic stem cell proliferation kinetics is critically important for the regulation of haemopoietic cell production. Nonetheless, information about the control of stem cell renewal versus differentiation, and how this might be manipulated to improve haemopoietic cell regeneration, is still incomplete. Control mechanisms could be intrinsic or extrinsic to the stem cells, or a combination of both.

Extrinsic factors

Extrinsic control would mean that self-renewal and differentiation can be controlled by external factors, such as cell–cell interactions in the haemopoietic microenvironment or cytokines, and thereby be responsive to demands for increased haemopoietic cell production. Regulation in the bone marrow microenvironment, and in the stromal layers of long-term bone marrow cultures, may be mediated by adjacent cells or local cytokine production. SCF is produced by stromal cells and occurs as a transmembrane protein as well as a soluble protein. It binds to its receptor, c-Kit, expressed by haemopoietic stem cells and is essential for normal blood cell production. Flt3 ligand is also a transmembrane protein and is widely expressed in human tissues. It binds to Flt3 on haemopoietic cells and is important for cell survival and cytokine responsiveness. TGF-β reduces stem cell cycling and maintains stem cell multipotency.

The Notch-1–Jagged pathway may serve to integrate extracellular signals with intracellular signalling and cell cycle control. Notch-1 is a surface receptor on haemopoietic stem cells that binds to its ligand, Jagged, on stromal cells. This results in cleavage of the cytoplasmic portion of Notch-1, which can then act as a transcription factor. c-Kit, the receptor for SCF, and receptors for TGF-β and tumour necrosis factor α (TNF-α) may also act in this way.

Intrinsic factors

The expression of several transcription factors has been shown to be essential for haemopoietic cell development from the earliest stages. SCL (stem cell leukaemia haemopoietic transcription factor) and GATA-2 are required for the development of haemopoiesis in the yolk sac, whereas absence of AML-1 results in failure of fetal liver haemopoiesis, although erythropoiesis in the yolk sac is not affected. Candidate genes that are targeted by these transcription factors include c-Kit, the receptor for granulocyte colony-stimulating factor (G-CSF), globin genes and myeloperoxidase.

There is evidence from murine studies that haemopoietic progenitor cells from different inbred mouse strains vary widely in number and proliferative activity. These observations indicate that genetically determined constitutional variation in human haemopoiesis is also likely to exist. This view is supported by the fact that parameters such as clonogenic cell frequency and numbers, proliferation ability and capacities for mobilization and expansion vary widely among individuals in the general human population. Associations have been reported between genetic markers and the frequency and activity of stem cells in mouse strains. De Haan and colleagues (2002) concluded that the expression levels of a large number of genes may be responsible for controlling stem cell behaviour. These collections of genes may be analogous to those responsible for the interindividual behaviour of human haemopoietic stem cells.

In contrast to the genetic basis for constitutional variation, certain specific genes have been demonstrated to influence haemopoietic cell kinetics. Growing evidence implicates gene products involved in cell cycle control, such as the cyclin-dependent kinase inhibitors (CKIs) p16, p21 and p27 (Figure 1.4) and the maintenance of stem cell quiescence. They have been shown to enhance proliferation and repopulating efficiency of bone marrow cells in gene knockout, knockin and gene transfer models. Loss of CKIs increases clonal expansion by haemopoietic progenitor cells and the size of the stem cell pool; the Fas and Fas ligand genes, which generally are associated with the process of cell death by apoptosis, also influence haemopoiesis as part of a mechanism suppressing progenitor cell proliferation.

Finally, lessons can be learned from studies of disease pathogenesis. Many cell cycle control genes and genes promoting cell death by apoptosis are tumour-suppressor genes that have been found to be deleted or mutated in leukaemia and other cancers. Fanconi's anaemia is an autosomal recessive bone marrow failure syndrome associated with an increased tendency for spontaneous chromosome breaks. The disease can be caused by mutations in at least seven different genes. The genes *FANCA*, *FANCC*, *FANCD1*, *FANCD2*, *FANCE* and *FANCF* have been cloned, and the corresponding proteins play important roles in DNA repair. In dyskeratosis congenita mutations have been identified in the *DKC1* gene, which encodes dyskerin. Dyskerin is a component of small nucleolar ribonuclear protein particles and the telomerase complex, indicating that the disease is due to defective telomerase.

Overall, intrinsic and extrinsic control mechanisms may be considered separately, but a picture is emerging of the integration of extracellular signalling, signal transduction, transcription factors and cell cycle control in the determination of stem cell fate.

Stem cell lineage selection

The 50% of daughter stem cells that differentiate supply cells that are destined to form all of the eight blood cell lineages. The mechanisms determining the blood cell lineages selected by the differentiating progeny of stem cells probably involve aspects of the transcriptional control of lineage-specific genes. Greaves and colleagues proposed that several lineage-specific genes are accessible to transcription factors or 'primed' in uncommitted

cells. Accordingly, individual primitive cells were found to exhibit low levels of transcription of lineage-affiliated genes. Moreover, single stem cells expressed low levels of several of these genes, indicating that final lineage selection had not yet occurred. The multilineage 'priming' of stem cells is supported experimentally by the results of replating colonies composed of blast cells. This revealed that the blast cells themselves were bipotent or oligopotent progenitors for various lineages of blood cell development, and that the combinations of lineages found within individual colonies appeared to be randomly distributed, although some combinations are more common than others.

It is likely that differences in the expression levels of transcription factors determine the lineage affiliation of a differentiating cell (Figure 1.6). The transcription factors PU1 and GATA-1 have been implicated in myeloid and erythroid/megakaryocyte lineage specifications respectively. The common precursors of the myeloid, erythroid and megakaryocytic lineages coexpress PU1 and GATA-1, but GATA-1 is downregulated during myeloid cell development and PU1 during erythroid/megakaryocytic cell development. The decision of bipotent granulocyte/monocyte precursors to proceed along the granulocytic or monocyte macrophage lines of differentiation is influenced by C/EBP-α, which is required for granulocytic cell development.

Stem cell plasticity

Reports that transplanted bone marrow cells can contribute to the repair and regeneration of a spectrum of tissue types including brain, muscle, lung, liver, gut epithelium and skin have

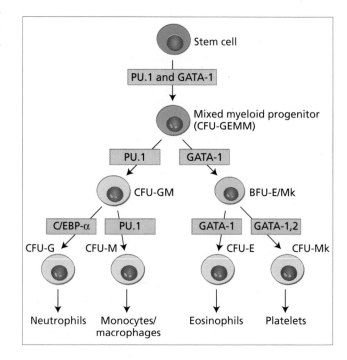

Figure 1.6 Transcription factors involved in lineage selection by haemopoietic stem and progenitor cells.

attracted considerable attention. The important implication of these observations is that haemopoietic stem cells could be used clinically for tissue replacement therapies. The multipotential nature of haemopoietic stem cells appears to be well suited to a wider role in tissue repair as they already demonstrate the capacity to make renewal, differentiation and lineage choices. Moreover, cultured blood cells can transdifferentiate from one lineage to another. Cell fusion is an alternative mechanism accounting for the contribution of bone marrow cells to tissue repair (e.g. after myocardial infarction), possibly involving the macrophage component of the marrow infusion.

A second bone marrow stem cell population with tissue-regenerating potential, the multipotent adult progenitor cells (MAPCs), representing a subpopulation of mesenchymal (stromal) stem cells, was isolated by Verfaillie and colleagues. The MAPCs develop over a period of time in culture, during which they seem to lose tissue-restricted gene expression and become able to differentiate into mesenchymal cell types (osteoblasts, chondrocytes, adipocytes and sketetal myoblasts) endothelium, neuroectoderm and hepatocytes.

Progenitor cells

The progenitor cells are the progeny of stem cells, and it is likely that some of the candidate stem cells measured in the assays mentioned above are in fact intermediate between stem and progenitor cells. As haemopoietic cell development proceeds from stem cells to progenitor cells, the probability of renewal decreases and that of differentiation increases commensurately. Thus, although the probability of self-renewal is highest within the stem cell population, it is by no means a property of stem cells alone. This has been amply demonstrated by replating progenitor cell-derived colonies grown *in vitro* and observing secondary colony formation. It is uncertain at what stage the capacity for self-renewal is lost completely. Indeed, early kinetic studies revealed that even promyelocytes divide two or three times before they differentiate into myelocytes.

Beginning in the 1960s, *in vitro* colony assays have been developed for the enumeration of clonogenic progenitor cells in haemopoietic tissue. The availability of different assays has allowed the investigation of distinct cell populations at different stages of haemopoietic cell development. The mixed lineage colony-forming cells (CFU-mix) consist of combinations of granulocytes, eosinophils, monocytes, erythrocytes and megakaryocytes and are the most primitive cells in this class. Granulocyte–macrophage colony-forming cells (CFU-GM) are bipotential and succeeded by single-lineage CFU-G and CFU-M. The erythroid lineage is represented by the burst-forming unit erythroid (BFU-E) and colony-forming unit erythroid (CFU-E), whereas separate assays exist for megakarocyte precursors (CFU-Mk).

Colony formation *in vitro* is stimulated by haemopoietic growth factors and cytokines. Some of the growth factors are named after their target cells, such as granulocyte–macrophage colony-stimulating factor (GM-CSF) and G-CSF. Others indicate which cell types they act on, such as erythropoietin (erythropoiesis), thrombopoietin (megakaryopoiesis) and SCF.

Maturing and mature cells

The maturing and mature haemopoietic cells are recognizable on stained smears of blood or bone marrow. During maturation, the cells maintain some capacity for division that can influence the blood count because each additional division would double the blood count. Eventually, however, the capacity for cell division is lost because of expulsion of the nucleus (red cells), fragmentation (platelets) or nuclear distortion (polymorphonuclear granulocytes). In contrast, mature lymphocytes have a monomorphic nucleus and retain the ability to divide. The end-products of haemopoietic cell development are cells that are highly specialized for their different functions in the body.

Cell death (apoptosis)

The final stage in the life of a blood cell is death and disposal by apoptosis. Apoptotic cell death is a mechanism for disposing of unwanted or excess cells, and it occurs widely in biological systems. It ensures the destruction of cells without releasing any lysosomal or granule contents that would cause an inflammatory reaction. Apoptosis involves a complex series of events that culminate in the activation of the caspase proteases, fragmentation of DNA and phagocytosis of apoptotic bodies by macrophages.

In haemopoiesis, apoptosis is used to dispose of mature end cells once they have fulfilled their function. In addition, it has also been proposed as a mechanism for negative regulation of cell production. Accordingly, a reduction in cell death could account for an increase in haemopoietic stem and progenitor cell numbers. However, this mechanism presupposes that substantial numbers of stem and progenitors are lost by apoptosis in steady-state haemopoiesis. Haemopoietic cytokines and growth factors act as survival factors for haemopoietic progenitor cells and prevent the death of factor-dependent cell lines *in vitro*. Also, components of the apoptotic machinery have been implicated in the feedback negative regulation of erythropoiesis and myelopoiesis, cell cycle regulation and cell differentiation. These observations suggest that the apoptotic pathways may have regulatory functions that do not culminate in cell death.

Haemopoietic growth factors and receptors

The haemopoietic growth factors and cytokines are the soluble regulators of blood cell production and are produced by several cell types in different sites in the body. They are glycoproteins

Table 1.2 Haemopoietic cytokines and their target cells.

Cytokine	Target cell(s)
IL-3	CFU-GEMM, HPP-CFC, CFU-GM, CFU-Eo, CFU-Baso, BFU-E, CFU-Mk
GM-CSF	HPP-CFC, CFU-GEMM, CFU-GM, CFU-Eo, CFU-Baso, CFU-Mk, BFU-E, CFU-M, CFU-G, dendritic cells
G-CSF	HPP-CFC, CFU-GEMM, CFU-GM, CFU-G
M-CSF (c-Fms ligand)	HPP-CFC, CFU-GEMM, CFU-M
Epo	CFU-E
SCF (c-Kit ligand)	HPP-CFC, CFU-GEMM, CFU-GM, CFU-Baso, BFU-E
IL-1	HPP-CFC
IL-4	CFU-GM, CFU-Baso, BFU-E, dendritic cells
IL-5	CFU-Eo
IL-6	HPP-CFC, CFU-GM, BFU-E
IL-11	CFU-Mk, CFU-GM, BFU-E
Thrombopoietin	CFU-Mk
Flt3 ligand	LT-CIC, CFU-GEMM, CFU-GM, dendritic cells
Fibroblast growth factor (FGF2 and FGF4)	CFU-GM, BFU-E, stromal cells
Leukaemia inhibitory factor (LIF)	CFU-Mk, BFU-E

References and further details will be found in Garland *et al.* (1997) and Thomson and Lotze (2003).
Baso, basophil; BFU-E, burst-forming unit erythroid; CFU, colony-forming unit; Eo, eosinophil; GEMM, granulocyte, erythrocyte, monocyte, megakaryocyte; GM, granulocyte–macrophage; HPP-CFC, high proliferative potential colony-forming cell; LT-CIC, long-term culture-initiating cell; Mk, megakaryocyte.

with little primary amino acid homology, although molecular modelling of secondary structure suggests that they possess similar structural features, such as bundles of anti-parallel α-helices joined by loops and β-sheets. Different sequences have been identified by deletional mutagenesis, which are required for secretion, biological activity and receptor binding. Some cytokines, such as SCF, exist in membrane-bound form as well as a soluble form because they lack the signal sequence responsible for release from the cell as a result of alternative splicing.

Cytokine responses and signal transduction

The responses of haemopoietic cells to cytokines include survival, proliferation, differentiation and stimulation of mature cell function. Once cytokines have bound to their receptors on the cell surface, they activate signal transduction pathways that transmit the signal to the nucleus and ultimately stimulate the transcription of regulatory genes. Haemopoietic progenitors require multiple cytokines for their optimal growth and development (Table 1.2). These growth factors act in concert to coordinate the various cellular functions that are necessary for the cell division and progressive differentiation required for the formation of mature functioning end cells. There are many examples of cytokines acting in synergy when the outcome is greater than expected from the sum of the individual cytokines acting alone. Also, cytokines are pleiotropic in their actions, and several cytokines are known to share the same functions. This

level of complexity is very difficult to rationalize, but it is becoming apparent that intracellular coordination is achieved by co-localization of sequentially acting signalling proteins, or by binding interactions with adaptor complexes, cytoskeletal structures or molecular targets, for the selective activation of downstream targets. Outside the cell, haemopoietic cell responses may be modulated by controlled access of cytokines to target cell receptors, as discussed below.

Many haemopoietic growth factor and cytokine receptors belong to the haematopoietin receptor superfamily (Figure 1.7). These are type 1 transmembrane glycoproteins with modular extracellular domains. All members dimerize when they bind their ligand. G-CSF and erythropoietin (Epo) receptors homo-dimerize, whereas the β-chains of the interleukin (IL) 3, IL-5 and GM-CSF receptors dimerize with a common beta (β_c) chain to form a high-affinity receptor. Other members of the haematopoietin receptor superfamily (IL-6, IL-11, IL-12 and leukaemia inhibitory factor, LIF) require the presence of a transmembrane protein, gp130, to transduce a signal.

A separate group of receptors has intrinsic tyrosine kinase activity and contains receptors for SCF, hepatocyte growth factor (HGF) and Flt3 ligand (FL). It is evident that cytokine receptor systems not only act in a linear-independent manner, but also influence the activity of other cell-surface receptor systems. Biochemical studies have revealed interactions between haemopoietic cytokine receptors, including interactions of β_c with Epo and G-CSF receptors. However, it is not established

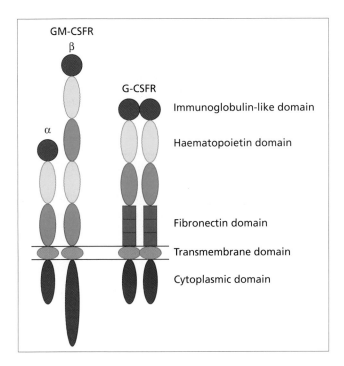

Figure 1.7 Representation of the modular structures of the haematopoietin receptor superfamily, exemplified by the receptors for GM-CSF and G-CSF (after Lewis and Gordon, 2003).

that these biochemically documented phenomena, such as receptor transmodulation, transphosphorylation and physical interaction, are biologically significant.

Cytokines regulate a variety of haemopoietic cell functions through the activation of multiple signal transduction pathways (Figure 1.8). The major pathways relevant to cell proliferation

and differentiation are the Janus kinase (Jak)/signal transducers and activators of transcription (STATs), the mitogen-activated protein (MAP) kinase and the phosphatidylinositol (PI) 3-kinase pathways. Jaks function upstream of STATs, which are activated by phosphorylation, and then dimerize and migrate to the nucleus, where they bind to specific DNA motifs. Thus, the Jak–STAT pathway represents the most direct pathway for transmitting a signal from the cytokine receptor to DNA. Ras regulates the best-characterized MAPK cascade, which consists of Raf isoforms MEK1/2 and ERK1/2 and controls proliferation. PI3 kinases phosphorylate inositol lipids, which, in turn, activate downstream targets (Akt, Erk, p70s6k, vav–rac) and influence many different cellular processes. These include cell survival, cell cycle progression, proliferation and reorganization of the actin cytoskeleton. The Jak–STAT pathway is implicated in IL-3, IL-6, Epo and G-CSF signalling, the MAP kinase pathway in Epo, GM-CSF, G-CSF and IL-3 signalling, and the PI3 kinase pathway in IL-6, Epo, GM-CSF, G-CSF and M-CSF signalling.

Thus, all of the haemopoietic growth factors appear to be capable of activating all of the major signal transduction pathways simultaneously. The several pathways that have been identified and the multiple responses, pleiotropism and redundancy that are well-known features of haemopoietic cytokines raise the possibility that a particular cytokine may have different effects in different cell types and possibly utilize different signal transduction pathways for specific functions. Moreover, combinations of cytokines may cooperate to activate further signal transduction pathways that are not activated when cytokines are used individually. Such interactions among receptor-mediated signals provide a mechanism for merging the activities of different ligand–receptor systems and achieving novel cellular outcomes.

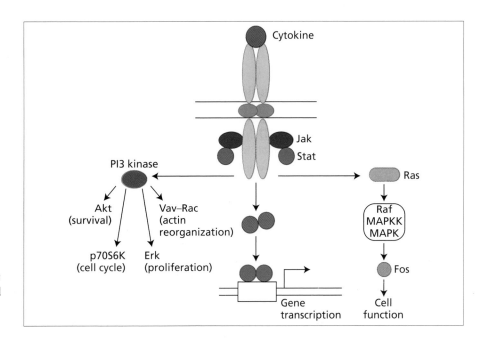

Figure 1.8 Generalized diagram of the signal transduction pathways activated by cytokines and their receptors in haemopoietic cells.

Physiology of the cytokine response

Colony formation *in vitro* is a simple model of haemopoietic regulation by cytokines, which involves the interaction of soluble proteins with specific receptors on the surface of the target cells. In culture, the cytokines are freely available at a uniform concentration and any cell which expresses the corresponding receptor will be able to respond. However, this is unlikely to be the situation *in vivo* where stem and progenitor cells are located in the haemopoietic microenvironment and there is a need to control haemopoietic cell production more precisely.

Several mechanisms have the potential to control the access of cytokines to their target cells and are likely to be physiologically important. The first mechanism is the localization of the stem and progenitor cells. The fact that these cells are found predominantly in the haemopoietic microenvironment rather than freely distributed in the bloodstream and tissues indicates that there is a mechanism to retain them there, and it has been extensively demonstrated that stem and progenitor cells express cell adhesion molecules that bind them to proteins expressed by the stromal cells of the marrow microenvironment. Cytokines can also bind to components of the microenvironment, in this case to extracellular matrix proteins produced by the microenvironmental stromal cells, and this may act to direct the cytokine to the appropriate target cell and modify the concentration or duration of exposure. Several cytokines are produced in membrane-bound or soluble forms, which can have different activities. For example, soluble SCF is active for only a short time, whereas membrane-bound SCF is more durable. In the circulation, cytokines can bind to soluble proteins, including soluble receptors, and these interactions may function as carriers for transport of the cytokine in an inactive form from its site of production to its site of action, protect the cytokine from proteolytic degradation or, in some circumstances, inactivate it.

Negative regulation of haemopoiesis

Like all homeostatic systems, haemopoiesis is regulated by a balance of positive and negative influences. They include cytokines such as the macrophage inflammatory protein, MIP-1α, and TGF-β. As well as directly inhibitory factors, a variety of other mechanisms with the potential to block cytokine action have been described. Interleukin 1α and IL-1β have an endogenous receptor agonist that blocks IL-1 binding to its receptor; several cytokines (TNF, IL-2, IL-4) are blocked by soluble receptors that compete with cell-surface receptors and some cytokines inhibit the activities of others.

The location of haemopoiesis in the marrow microenvironment, represented *in vitro* by stromal cell cultures, and the predominantly quiescent nature of the haemopoietic stem cell population indicate a negative role of the microenvironment in suppressing stem cell activity. Early studies of haemopoiesis in long-term bone marrow cultures, in which stromal cells support haemopoiesis for a prolonged period of time *in vitro*, revealed periodic oscillations in the cell cycle activity of stem cells that could be related to the presence of positive and negative cytokines implicated in maintaining homeostasis of the haemopoietic system.

Clinical applications of stem cell research

Stem cell research has provided the growth points for several clinical activities as well as for advances in experimental haematology.

Stem cell transplantation

Bone marrow and stem cell transplantation is the most obvious application of stem cell research. It originated in early studies of the haematological reconstitution of mice whose bone marrow had been ablated by ionizing radiation. It soon became apparent that haematological rescue of these animals required infusion of syngeneic marrow because transplantation of cells from a different strain resulted in a wasting condition called 'secondary disease', which is now known as graft-versus-host disease (GvHD). Both the transplantation of stem cells into mice and the recognition of the importance of histocompatibility in the murine system were important contributions to modern clinical transplantation. The identification of the stem cell immunophenotype and the development of cell separation technologies facilitated the development of graft engineering to improve the results of clinical transplantation. One application of cell separation was to deplete the graft of T lymphocytes, either by removing T cells or purifying CD34$^+$ cells. However, it soon became apparent that a graft-versus-leukaemia activity (GvL) was removed, along with the potential for GvHD, and efforts to isolate GvL from GvHD continue today.

Haemopoietic growth factors

Haemopoietic growth factors such as G-CSF, GM-CSF and erythropoietin are administered to cytopenic patients to stimulate cell production. They were originally identified by their colony-stimulating activity *in vitro*.

Stem cell mobilization

G-CSF, in particular, is widely used to mobilize stem cells (peripheral blood progenitor cells, PBPCs) into the peripheral blood from where they can be harvested by leucapheresis and used as a source of stem cells for transplantation. Initially the procedure was used for autografting but mobilization of PBPCs from allogeneic donors is practised at present.

Stem cell expansion

In cases when insufficient stem cells are available for successful engraftment, it would be advantageous to be able to increase the number of stem cells during a period of *in vitro* culture. For this, 'stem cell expansion' is conducted in the presence of combinations of cytokines, with the aim of inducing stem cell renewal and population growth. A large number of studies have investigated a variety of culture conditions and combinations of cytokines. Frequently used cytokines include Flt3 ligand, thrombopoietin, IL-3 and stem cell factor. Although large increases in numbers of colony-forming progenitor cells have been reported, there is little evidence for expansion of long-term repopulating stem cells.

Gene therapy

The self-renewal and expansion capacities of haemopoietic stem cells make them the ideal vehicle for gene therapy of genetic disorders. The transduced genes will be expressed for long periods of time in the stem cell population and in their differentiating and mature descendants (see Chapter 27).

Selected bibliography

Almeida-Porada G, Porada CD, Chamberlain J et al. (2004) Formation of human hepatocytes by human hematopoietic stem cells in sheep. *Blood* 104: 2582–90.

Bacigalupo A (2004) Mesenchymal stem cells and haematopoietic stem cell transplantation. *Clinical Haematology* 17: 387–99.

Bailey AS, Jiang S, Afentoulis M et al. (2004) Transplanted adult hematopoietic stem cells differentiate into functional endothelial cells. *Blood* 103: 13–19.

Chagrui J, Lepage-Noll A, Anjo A et al. (2003) Fetal liver stroma consists of cells in epithelial-to-mesenchymal transition. *Blood* 101: 2973–82.

Charbord P (2001) Mediators involved in the control of hematopoiesis by the microenvironment. In: *Hematopoiesis: A Developmental Approach* (LI Zon, ed.), pp. 702–17. Oxford University Press, New York.

de Haan G, Bystrykh LV, Weesing E et al. (2002) A genetic and genomic analysis identifies a cluster of genes associated with hematopoietic cell turnover. *Blood* 100: 2056–62.

Dieterlen-Lievre F, Pardanaud L, Caprioli A et al. (2001) Non-yolk sac hematopoietic stem cells: The avian paradigm. In: *Hematopoiesis: A Developmental Approach* (LI Zon, ed.), pp. 201–8. Oxford University Press, New York.

Dzierzak E, Oostendorp R (2001) Hematopoietic stem cell development in mammals. In: *Hematopoiesis: a Developmental Approach* (LI Zon, ed.), pp. 209–17. Oxford University Press, New York.

Garland JM, Quesenberry PJ, Hilton DJ (eds) (1997) *Colony-stimulating Factors*. Marcel Dekker, New York.

Geiger H, Sick S, Bonifer C et al. (1998) Globin gene expression is reprogrammed in chimeras generated by injecting adult hematopoietic stem cells into mouse blastocysts. Cell 93: 1055–65.

Gordon MY (1993) Hemopoietic growth factors and receptors: Bound and free. *Cancer Cells* 3: 127–33.

Gordon MY (1993) Human haemopoietic stem cell assays. *Blood Reviews* 7: 190–7.

Gordon MY, Marley SB, Davidson RJ et al. (2000) Contact-mediated inhibition of human haematopoietic progenitor cell proliferation may be conferred by stem cell antigen, CD34. *The Hematology J* 1: 77–86.

Graf T (2002) Differentiation plasticity of hematopoietic cells. *Blood* 99: 3069–101.

Heissig B, Hattori K, Dias S et al. (2002) Recruitment of stem and progenitor cells from the bone marrow niche requires MMP-9 mediated release of kit-ligand. *Cell* 109: 625–37.

Herzog EL, Chai L, Krause DS (2003) Plasticity of marrow-derived stem cells. *Blood* 102: 3483–92.

Hilton DJ (1997) Receptors for hematopoietic regulators. In: *Colony-stimulating Factors*, 2nd edn (JM Garland, PJ Quesenberry, DJ Hilton, eds), pp. 49–70. Marcel Dekker, New York.

Jiang Y, Jahagirdar BN, Reinhardt RL et al. (2002) Pluripotency of mesenchymal stem cells derived from adult marrow. *Nature* 418: 41–9.

Jordan JD, Landau EM, Iyengar Y (2000) Signaling networks: The origins of cellular multitasking. *Cell* 103: 193–200.

Karanu FN, Murdoch B, Galacher L et al. (2000) The Notch ligand Jagged-1 represents a novel growth factor of human hematopoietic stem cells. *Journal of Experimental Medicine* 192: 1365–72.

Körbling M, Estrov Z (2003) Adult stem cells for tissue repair – a new therapeutic concept? *New England Journal of Medicine* 349: 570–82.

Krause DS, Fackler MJ, Civin CI et al. (1996) CD34 structure, biology and clinical utility. *Blood* 87: 1.

Krug U, Ganser A, Koeffler HP (2002) Tumor suppressor genes in normal and malignant hematopoiesis. *Oncogene* 13: 3475–95.

Lemischka I (2002) A few thoughts about the plasticity of stem cells. *Experimental Hematology* 30: 848–52.

Lewis JL, Gordon MY (2003) Haemopoietic cytokines. In: *The Cytokine Handbook*, 4th edn (EAW Thompson, MT Lotze, eds), pp. 1255–77. Elsevier Science, London.

Lyman SD, McKenna HJ (2003) Flt3 ligand. In: *The Cytokine Handbook*, 4th edn (AW Thompson, MT Lotze, eds), pp. 989–1010. Elsevier Science, London.

Marrone A, Mason PJ (2002) Dyskeratosis congenita. *Cellular and Molecular Life Sciences* 60: 507–17.

Martin-Rendon E, Watt SM (2003) Stem cell plasticity. *British Journal of Haematology* 122: 877–91.

May G, Enver T (2001) The lineage commitment and self-renewal of blood stem cells. In: *Hematopoiesis: a Developmental Approach* (LI Zon, ed.), pp. 61–81. Oxford University Press, New York.

McNiece IK, Briddell RA (2003) Stem cell factor. *The Cytokine Handbook*, 4th edn (AW Thompson, MT Lotze, eds), pp. 1011–16. Elsevier Science, London.

Medvinsky A, Smith A (2003) Fusion brings down barriers. *Nature* 422: 823–5.

Mohle R, Bautz F, Rafii S et al. (1999) Regulation of transendothelial migration of hematopoietic progenitor cells. *Annals of the New York Academy of Sciences* 872: 176–86.

Moore MAS, Han W, Ye Q (2001) Notch signalling during hematopoiesis. In: *Hematopoiesis: A Developmental Approach* (LI Zon, ed.), pp. 323–36. Oxford University Press, New York.

Orkin SH (2001) Transcriptional control during erythroid and megakaryocytic development. In: *Hematopoiesis: A Developmental Approach* (LI Zon, ed.), pp. 348–54. Oxford University Press, New York.

Schwartz RE, Reyes M, Koodie L *et al.* (2002) Multipotent adult progenitor cells from bone marrow differentiate into functional hepatocyte-like cells. *Journal of Clinical Investigation* **109**: 1291–302.

Teruel MN, Meyer T (2000) Translocation and reversible localization of signaling proteins: a dynamic future for signal transduction. *Cell* **103**: 181–4.

Thomson AW, Lotze MT (eds) (2003) *The Cytokine Handbook*, 4th edn, pp. 1255–77. Elsevier Science, London.

Tischkowitz MD, Hodgson SV (2003) Fanconi anaemia. *Journal of Medical Genetics* **40**: 1–10.

Verfaillie CM (2001) *Ex vivo* expansion of stem cells. In: *Hematopoiesis: A Developmental Approach* (LI Zon, ed.), pp. 119–29. Oxford University Press, New York.

Young PR (1998) Pharmacological modulation of cytokine action and production through signaling pathways. *Cytokine and Growth Factor Reviews* **9**: 239–57.

Zhu J, Emerson SG (2002) Hematopoietic cytokines, transcription factors and lineage commitment. *Oncogene* **21**: 3295–313.

CHAPTER 2

Erythropoiesis

Douglas R Higgs and William G Wood

2

Introduction

The process of erythropoiesis includes all steps of haemopoiesis, starting with the initial specification of haemopoietic stem cells (HSCs) from mesoderm during embryogenesis. This continues with the decisions of these cells to undergo self-renewal or differentiation, through the process of lineage specification and proliferation to form committed erythroid progenitors. Finally, erythroblasts undergo terminal differentiation and post-mitotic maturation as they develop into red blood cells.

In a normal adult, the numbers of circulating red blood cells and their precursors remain more or less constant with a balance between the continuous loss of mature cells by senescence and new red cell production in the marrow. This balance is maintained by an oxygen-sensing system that is affected by the red cell mass and responds via the production of erythropoietin (Epo), which, in turn, controls red cell production by binding and signalling to committed erythroid progenitors. Many other cytokines, growth factors and hormones also influence erythroid proliferation, differentiation and maturation.

Over the past 10 years, key transcription factors controlling the internal programmes of erythroid progenitors have been identified and some insights into their roles in lineage specification and erythroid differentiation have been discovered. Understanding the basic biology of erythropoiesis provides a logical basis for the diagnosis and treatment of the inherited and acquired anaemias that are so frequently encountered in clinical practice.

The origins of blood during development

Primitive haemopoiesis in man (predominantly erythropoiesis) first appears in the blood islands of the extraembryonic yolk sac at around day 21 of gestation. About 1 week later (days 28–40), definitive haemopoietic stem cells emerge from the vitelline artery and the ventral wall of the embryonic aorta within the aorta–gonad–mesonephros (AGM) region. Both primitive (embryonic) and definitive (fetal/adult) haemopoietic stem cells arise in close association with endothelial cells. Several lines of evidence now suggest that haemopoietic and endothelial cells may emerge from a common progenitor, the haemangioblast, giving rise to both blood cells and blood vessels (see Chapter 1). At about 30–40 days, definitive haemopoiesis starts to occur in the fetal liver and definitive erythroid cells are released into the circulation at about 60 days. By 10–12 weeks, haemopoiesis starts to migrate to the bone marrow, where eventually erythropoiesis is established during the last 3 months of fetal life (Figure 2.1).

Primitive and definitive erythropoietic cells are distinguished by their cellular morphology, cell-surface markers, cytokine responsiveness, growth kinetics, transcription factor programmes and more general patterns of gene expression. In particular, the types of haemoglobin produced are quite distinct in embryonic (Hb Gower I $\zeta_2\varepsilon_2$, Gower II $\alpha_2\varepsilon_2$ and Hb Portland $\zeta_2\gamma_2$), fetal (HbF $\alpha_2\gamma_2$) and adult (HbA $\alpha_2\beta_2$ and HbA$_2$ $\alpha_2\delta_2$) erythroid cells. These specific patterns of globin expression have provided critical markers for identifying the developmental stages of erythropoiesis. Nevertheless, it is still not clear whether primitive and definitive haemopoiesis in mammals have entirely separate origins or if they are both derived from common stem cells that arise during early development. Accurately defining the embryological origins of these cells continues be of considerable importance for understanding the normal mechanisms that establish and maintain haemopoietic stem cells and how these programmes are subverted in common haematological disorders.

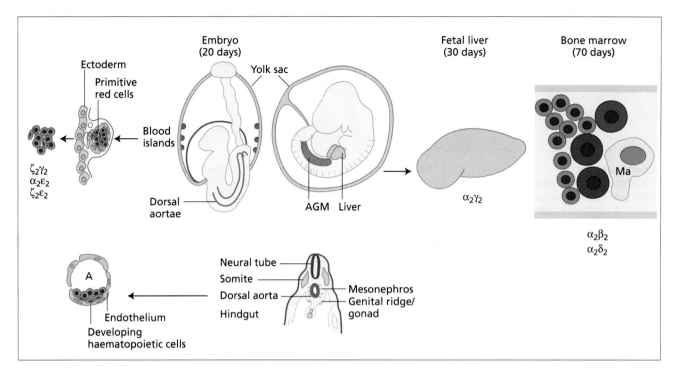

Figure 2.1 An outline of the origin and development of erythropoiesis during embryogenesis. Although both primitive (blood islands) and definitive (AGM, liver and bone marrow) haemopoiesis are derived from mesoderm, probably via a haemangioblast, the true origin of these early cells is not yet clear. The figure shows the formation of embryonic blood islands in the extraembryonic yolk sac and the formation of definitive haemopoiesis initially in the aorta–gonad–mesonephros region, with subsequent migration to the liver and bone marrow. 'A' denotes a magnified image of the early embryonic aortic region. Ma denotes a macrophage. The specific types of haemoglobin formed at each stage of erythropoiesis are indicated. The approximate times at which CD34$^+$ cells first appear at each site are given in days of gestation (adapted from Dzierzak *et al.* (1998) *Immunology Today* **19**: 228–36).

Differentiation of haemopoietic stem cells to form erythroid progenitors

At all stages of development there is a continuous need to renew senescent blood cells that are ultimately lost from the peripheral blood days, weeks or months after undergoing terminal differentiation. For example, throughout adult life approximately 10^{11} senescent red cells must be replaced every day, and there are similar requirements for other mature blood cells (e.g. granulocytes). To prevent depletion of the haemopoietic cells requires a system that not only maintains a self-renewing stem cell pool, but also has the potential to differentiate into all types of highly specialized mature blood cells through a process referred to as lineage specification.

At present, the mechanisms underlying self-renewal and the early events committing multipotential haemopoietic stem cells (HSCs) to an increasingly restricted repertoire of lineage(s) are not fully understood. A popular interpretation is that commitment of multipotential haemopoietic cells to one or another lineage is a stochastic process. The probability of commitment to any particular lineage may be influenced by a complex interplay between the internal transcriptional programmes and epigenetic patterns (e.g. changes in nuclear position, replication timing, chromatin modification, DNA methylation) with external signals from the microenvironment (e.g. cytokines, growth factors and cell–cell interactions).

It is of interest that microarray analyses of haemopoietic stem cells and their progeny consistently show a very wide range of gene expression in the earliest cell populations. Furthermore, many of the genes that are specific to individual lineages (e.g. erythroid, myeloid or lymphoid) are already transcribed, albeit at low levels, in HSCs. In other words, HSCs appear to show 'multilineage priming' and, as their progeny become committed to one pathway of differentiation, that lineage-specific gene expression programme becomes reinforced, whereas those of other lineages are suppressed.

In human adult bone marrow, approximately 1 per 10^4–10^6 nucleated cells are long-lived, multipotential HSCs that can be enriched on the basis of their cell-surface markers (e.g. CD33$^+$ and CD34$^+$ and lack of lineage-specific markers; see Figures 2.2 and 2.3), but such markers do not exclusively select stem cells (see Chapter 1). The only rigorous assay for *bona fide* HSCs is to

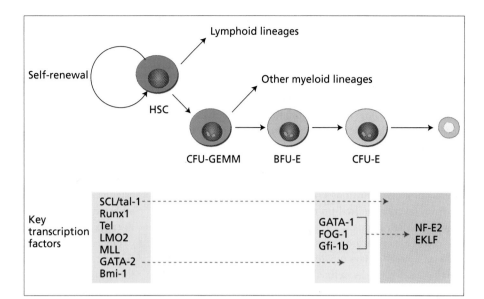

Figure 2.2 Summary of some steps in self-renewal, lineage specification and differentiation of haemopoietic stem cells to red cells. Some of the key transcription factors involved in this process are summarized underneath.

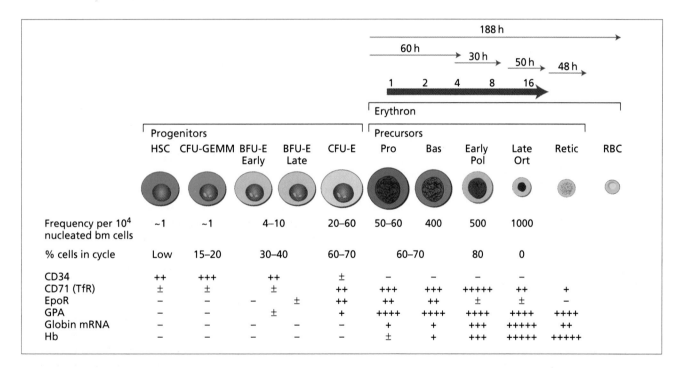

	Progenitors				Precursors					
	HSC	CFU-GEMM	BFU-E Early	BFU-E Late	CFU-E	Pro	Bas	Early Pol	Late Ort	Retic	RBC
Frequency per 10⁴ nucleated bm cells	~1	~1	4–10		20–60	50–60	400	500	1000		
% cells in cycle	Low	15–20	30–40		60–70	60–70		80	0		
CD34	++	+++	++		±	–	–	–	–		
CD71 (TfR)	±	±	±		++	+++	+++	+++++	++	+	
EpoR	–	–	–	±	++	++	++	±	±	–	
GPA	–	–	±		+	++++	++++	++++	++++	++++	
Globin mRNA	–	–	–	–	–	+	+	+++	+++++	++	
Hb	–	–	–	–	–	±	+	+++	+++++	+++++	

Figure 2.3 The specification and terminal differentiation of erythroid cells from haemopoietic stem cells. Above, the estimated times for maturation of terminally differentiating cells are shown. The abbreviations are as follows; pronormoblasts (Pro), basophilic erythroblasts (Bas), polychromatic erythroblasts (Pol), orthochromatic erythroblasts (Ort), reticulocytes (retic), mature red blood cells (RBCs). The number of divisions from pronormoblasts to orthochromatic normoblasts (1–16) are also shown. Some examples of the expression patterns of key cell-surface markers are shown below.

measure their ability to contribute, throughout life, to all haemopoietic lineages *in vivo*. This has been amply demonstrated in mice, and the repeated, predictable success of human bone marrow transplantation clearly demonstrates the existence of such cells in man.

As stem cells differentiate, they form multipotential progenitor cells that have short-term repopulating ability but have lost long-term repopulating ability. Such cells can be assayed *in vitro* by their ability to form 'cobblestone' areas under stromal cells in long-term marrow cultures. Further differentiation progressively restricts the lineage potential of these cells as well as reducing their proliferative capacity, resulting in tri-, bi- and unipotential progenitors. These progenitor cells are functionally defined by their ability to produce clonal colonies in semisolid medium supplemented with a cocktail of haemopoietic cell growth factors permissive for the growth of all lineages.

Erythroid cells are found in multilineage colonies (CFU-GEMM), which include granulocytes, macrophages and megakaryocytes, and in bipotential colonies with megakaryocytes (CFU-E/Mk). The earliest progenitors that are restricted to the erythroid lineage produce large colonies *in vitro*, consisting of several subunits, known as erythroid bursts (BFU-E, containing from several hundred up to 30 000 cells) after 12–14 days of growth. Their frequency in bone marrow is ~4–10/10^4 nucleated cells. Late erythroid progenitors form colonies (CFU-E) of 8–64 cells after ~7 days *in vitro* and constitute 20–60/10^4 bone marrow cells. CFU-Es defined in these culture systems most closely correspond *in vivo* to pronormoblasts (also known as proerythroblasts), the earliest recognizable erythroid precursor in the bone marrow. Once formed, these cells are destined to undergo terminal differentiation to form mature red cells as discussed later.

Although erythroid progenitors and their progeny can be grown effectively in supplemented culture systems, erythroid differentiation and maturation within the adult bone marrow *in vivo* are dependent on the microenvironment provided by the stromal cells (fibroblasts, fat cells, endothelial cells, macrophages and smooth muscle cells). There are also immunoregulatory cells (monocytes, macrophages and lymphocytes) that contribute to local cytokine production. Erythroblasts are not randomly distributed in the bone marrow but are organized into erythroblastic islands containing one or two central macrophages, surrounded by layers of erythroblasts at different stages of maturation (Figure 2.1).

The transcription factor programme underlying erythropoiesis

As discussed above in the stochastic model of cell differentiation, many factors must be integrated for a cell to make the decision to undergo self-renewal or differentiation, become quiescent, proliferate or undergo apoptosis. Over the past few years, it has emerged that key transcription factors play a major role in regulating the formation, survival, proliferation and differentiation of multipotent stem cells as they undergo the transition to erythroid cells. These transcription factors may operate on their own or as members of multicomponent complexes involved in activation and/or repression. Many of the key transcription factors were originally identified because they are associated with chromosomal translocations found in leukaemia. This supports a model in which dysregulation of the normal transcriptional programme plays a causal role in haematological malignancies.

At present, the key transcription factors known to be involved in specifying haemopoietic stem cells as they develop during embryogenesis and in maintaining them throughout life include Runx1 (AML-1), SCL (tal-1), LMO2 (rhombotin), Tel (ETV6), MLL and GATA-2 (Figure 2.2). In addition, the homeobox (Hox) genes and proteins that modify their expression (e.g. Bmi-1) have also been shown to play a role in haemopoiesis. However, it is of interest to point out here that many of these factors (e.g. SCL, Runx1) appear to act quite differently in primitive as opposed to definitive haemopoiesis. Furthermore, not only is their importance in early definitive progenitors well established, but also many of these transcription factors play additional roles, later in differentiation, in specific haemopoietic lineages, including erythropoiesis.

Once progenitor cells have been committed to become erythroid cells, the most important transcription factors that enable them to proceed through terminal differentiation are GATA-1 and its cofactor FOG-1 (friend of GATA-1). GATA-1 was first identified by its ability to bind functionally important regulatory sequences in the globin genes. Since then, GATA-binding motifs have been found in the promoters and/or enhancers of virtually all erythroid-specific genes studied, including haem biosynthetic enzymes, red cell membrane proteins (including blood group antigens) and erythroid transcription factors (e.g. erythroid Kruppel-like factor, EKLF and GATA-1 itself). GATA-1 expression is restricted to erythroid, megakaryocytic, eosinophilic, mast cells and multipotential progenitors of the haemopoietic, system. However, GATA-1 expression is highly upregulated in pronormoblasts and basophilic erythroblasts (Figures 2.2 and 2.3).

Gene targeting studies in mice have shown that GATA-1 is essential for normal erythropoiesis. Mice that produce no GATA-1 die from severe anaemia. Although they produce adequate numbers of erythroid colonies (CFU-E), there is an arrest in erythroid maturation at the pronormoblast stage of differentiation. *In vitro* differentiated mouse embryonic stem (ES) cells lacking GATA-1 also fail to mature past the pronormoblast stage and undergo rapid apoptosis, indicating a role for GATA-1 in survival and maturation of erythroblasts.

GATA-1 may protect mature erythroblasts from apoptosis by directly or indirectly inducing expression of the anti-apoptotic protein Bcl-X$_L$. GATA-1 almost certainly regulates gene expression working as part of a multiprotein complex interacting, for example, with FOG-1, LMO2, SCL and a variety of ubiquitously expressed transcription factors. FOG-1 is a protein containing multiple zinc fingers, four of which interact with GATA-1. Like GATA-1, FOG-1 is expressed in erythroid and megakaryocytic cells and is coexpressed and directly interacts with GATA-1 during development. Genetically modified mice that express no FOG-1 also die in mid-gestation as a result of severe anaemia with arrest in erythroid maturation at the pronormoblast stage.

GATA-2 is a second member of the GATA family of proteins that is involved in haemopoiesis. Both GATA-1 and GATA-2 are particularly relevant for erythropoiesis. Both are expressed in multipotent progenitors, although GATA-2 appears to be more important than GATA-1 at this stage, when GATA-2 plays an important role in the expansion and maintenance of haemopoietic progenitors. During erythroid differentiation the level of GATA-2 declines as GATA-1 increases. In mouse embryos lacking GATA-2, erythrocytes are present, but in severely reduced numbers. There appears to be some overlap and redundancy between the roles of GATA-1 and GATA-2; in the absence of GATA-1 increased levels of GATA-2 may fulfil some, but not all, of the normal roles of GATA-1. Furthermore, there is evidence that the level of GATA-2 is regulated by the level of GATA-1. During normal erythroid development, it has been suggested that GATA-2 may initiate the erythroid programme in early erythroid progenitors to be replaced later by GATA-1 during terminal erythroid maturation.

Expression of the two related zinc-finger DNA-binding proteins Gfi-1 and Gfi-1b is restricted to haemopoietic cells. Gfi-1b is expressed only in multipotent progenitors, megakaryocytes and erythroblasts, in which its pattern of expression mimics that of GATA-1. Gfi-1b-deficient mouse embryos die with a failure to produce mature red cells, although early precursors are formed normally. This is very similar to the phenotype observed in GATA-1-deficient embryos. However, from *in vitro* colony assays in which Gfi-1b is overexpressed, it appears that its effect is not on erythroid commitment, but rather it promotes the proliferation of erythroid progenitors as they undergo the transition from late BFU-Es to CFU-Es.

Erythroid Kruppel-like factor (EKLF) is a zinc finger-like protein of the Kruppel family, which binds the consensus sequence 5′-NCNCNCCCN-3′ and is mainly restricted to erythroid cells. These binding sites are found in the regulatory elements of several erythroid-specific genes, including the β-globin gene. Disruption of binding at this site gives rise to β-thalassaemia. Mice in which EKLF is absent die from severe anaemia at the fetal liver stage caused in part by β-thalassaemia, but also due to the failure to synthesize correctly other EKLF-regulated proteins (e.g. the red cell membrane protein Band3 and the α-globin-stabilizing protein AHSP) required for red cell maturation. Therefore, EKLF may play a wider role than originally predicted in coordinating erythroid cell maturation and globin gene regulation.

Sequence motifs of the general class (T/C)GCTGA(G/C)TCA(T/C), called Maf recognition elements (MAREs), have been found in the enhancers of many erythroid-specific genes (e.g. globins, haem synthesis enzymes), and it was shown that they bind the transcription factor NF-E2. Purification of NF-E2 revealed that it consists of two subunits, p45NF-E2 and p18NF-E2 (now known as MafK). Both proteins contain basic zipper (b-zip) domains through which they form heterodimers and bind DNA. p45 is expressed mainly in erythroid cells, whereas p18 is widely expressed, although it is the predominant small Maf family member in erythroid cells. Furthermore, it is now known that both p45 and p18 are members of larger groups of proteins with overlapping functions. Other p45-like molecules include Nrf1, 2 and 3 and Bach1 and 2. All of these proteins bind as obligate heterodimers with Maf proteins. It seems likely that binding to MARE elements is an important aspect of erythroid-specific activation, but it is not clear which proteins in this family bind the key sites or whether there is redundancy in the need for specific members of this family.

At present it is not fully understood how these transcription factors combine to commit cells to the erythroid lineage and terminal erythroid differentiation. However, this could involve the presence or absence of specific transcription factors, changes in the levels of the proteins and/or protein modification. One principle that seems to be emerging is that factors affiliated with different lineages such as GATA-1 (erythroid) and PU1 (lymphocytes and granulocytes) are both present in uncommitted progenitors, reflecting the potential to develop along alternative different pathways (so-called multilineage priming). It is now known that GATA-1 and PU1 interact and cross-antagonize each other. Therefore, as cells differentiate, reinforcement of the transcriptional programme of one lineage may actively suppress an alternative lineage.

Terminal maturation of committed erythroid cells

After the erythroid programme has been specified, the final phase of erythropoiesis involves the maturation of committed erythroid progenitors to fully differentiated red cells. The earliest recognizable erythroid precursor cell in the bone marrow is the pronormoblast (Figure 2.4a, i) – which, as discussed above, corresponds to the CFU-Es identified *in vitro*. The pronormoblast is a relatively large cell (12–20 microns) with a non-granular, deep-blue cytoplasm and a large nucleus occupying about three-quarters of the cell, having a finely stippled chromatin pattern that contains one or more prominent nucleoli. On electron microscopy, there appears to be relatively little heterochromatin in these cells.

The cytoplasm contains numerous ribosomes, several mitochondria, centrioles, a prominent Golgi apparatus and a few strands of rough endoplasmic reticulum. Division of these cells leads to smaller (10–16 microns) basophilic normoblasts (Figure 2.4a, ii). Again, the cytoplasm stains deep blue and the nucleus occupies a large proportion of the cell but has a coarser reticular chromatin pattern with a few small masses of condensed chromatin adjacent to the nuclear membrane. Further divisions form early polychromatic and late polychromatic normoblasts (10–12 microns), with increasing development of a pink cytoplasm and condensed (6 microns) nuclei (Figure 2.4a, iii). Late polychromatic/orthochromatic normoblasts (Figure 2.4a, iv) are non-dividing cells with deeply staining structureless nuclei.

As the cell proceeds through terminal differentiation, nucleoli disappear and the nucleus condenses further and is eventually extruded. Such nuclei are phagocytosed and degraded by the macrophages of the bone marrow. Ultrastructural studies have shown that nuclear extrusion usually occurs outside the sinusoids of the bone marrow, and that newly formed reticulocytes usually pass through pre-existing gaps in the walls of these sinusoids by diapedesis. Thus, the mature reticulocyte has no nucleus but has a few mitochondria and ribosomes and its cytoplasm stains predominantly pink because of the high concentration of haemoglobin. The cytoplasm still has a greyish tint due to the presence of ribosomes. When stained supravitally, the ribosomes precipitate into basophilic granules or a reticulum. Reticulocytes continue to synthesize haemoglobin for 24–48 h after release from the bone marrow. On average, these cells are about 20% larger than mature red cells, which are circular flat, biconcave discs with a mean diameter of 8.5 microns.

It has been estimated that, on average, four divisions occur within the morphologically recognizable proliferating precursor pool, so that each newly formed pronormoblast develops into 16 red cells (Figure 2.3). As a small amount of cell death (ineffective erythropoiesis) normally occurs, the average amplification is slightly less than 16-fold. The majority (60–80%) of pronormoblasts, basophilic normoblasts and early polychromatic normoblasts are in cell cycle, mostly in S-phase, with G_1 and G_2 stages lasting for only a few hours. At any time, about 3% pronormoblasts, 5% basophilic erythroblasts and 6% polychromatic normoblasts are undergoing mitosis, which has been variously estimated to last for between 60 and 100 min. Erythroid cells eventually exit from the cell cycle and, consistent with this, late polychromatic/orthochromatic erythroblasts are postmitotic, non-dividing cells.

Changes in the cell surface phenotype that accompany erythroid differentiation and maturation

The cell-surface phenotypes of erythroid progenitors and precursors are quite distinctive, reflecting the different signalling programmes of the cells as they differentiate. These markers are also of value in the analysis of erythroid progenitors and precursors as they can be used to identify and purify subpopulations of cells. CD34 is present on nearly all multipotent progenitors and committed BFU-E but is lost on later erythroid progenitors (CFU-E) and all precursors.

A similar pattern of expression is shown for the receptor c-Kit. Epo receptor (EpoR, see below) first appears in small numbers (20–50 copies per cell) on late BFU-Es, increases in CFU-Es and pronormoblasts (~1000 copies per cell) and subsequently declines and disappears in later erythroid precursors. CD71 (transferrin receptor, TfR) allows transferrin-bound iron to be taken into the cell and is present on early haemopoietic cells but is considerably upregulated on cells that are actively synthesizing haemoglobin, reaching a peak of 800 000 molecules

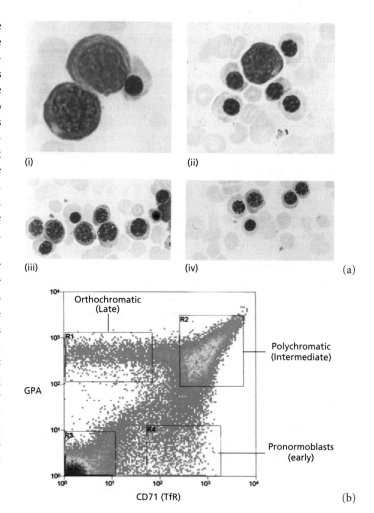

Figure 2.4 (a) Examples of pronormoblasts (i), basophilic and polychromatic erythroblasts (ii) and polychromatic and orthochromatic erythroblasts (iii and iv). All of these different cell types can also be conveniently viewed at: http://hsc.virginia.edu/medicine/clinical/pathology/educ/innes/text/nh/mature.html. (b) An example of early (pronormoblasts), intermediate (polychromatic erythroblasts) and late (orthochromatic erythroblasts) separated on the basis of their cell-surface markers (CD71 and GPA).

per cell on polychromatic normoblasts. CD71 levels diminish in the late phase of terminal differentiation and the receptor is not detectable on mature erythrocytes. Glycophorin A (GPA) is a membrane sialoglycoprotein whose expression is highly upregulated as erythroid progenitors mature from pronormoblasts. Combinations of these cell-surface markers can be used to distinguish early, intermediate and late erythroid precursors (Figure 2.4b). Developing erythroid cells express cell-surface adhesion molecules that interact with the extracellular matrix; these include ICAM-1 (a member of the immunoglobulin superfamily) and integrin $\alpha_4\beta_1$ VLA4 (CD29, CD49d), which interacts with fibronectin. These adhesion molecules are most highly expressed in the early precursors and lost as maturation proceeds, freeing erythroid cells to exit the bone marrow.

Changes in gene expression in erythroid differentiation and maturation

As cells go through the final divisions of erythropoiesis and post-mitotic maturation there is progressive condensation of chromatin accompanied by complex changes in gene expression. When assessed by microarray analysis, many mRNAs are downregulated as multipotent progenitors enter terminal differentiation, reflecting the commitment of multipotent cells to a single specialized lineage. A subset of general mRNAs associated with proliferation, replication and cell cycle control show alterations as the growth characteristics of the cells change. mRNAs encoding proteins that characterize the red cell phenotype are, in general, upregulated. Examples include blood group antigens, red cell membrane proteins (e.g. spectrin, ankyrin, actin, protein 4.1), red cell glycolytic pathway enzymes, carbonic anhydrase and enzymes of the haem synthesis pathway (e.g. δ-aminolaevulinic acid synthase, ALA synthase). A full catalogue of these changes in gene expression can be found at http://hembase.niddk.nih.gov.

The main purpose of erythropoiesis is to synthesize large amounts of haemoglobin (Figures 2.3–2.5). Globin mRNA sequences are first expressed in pronormoblasts and early basophilic erythroblasts. Globin chain synthesis parallels accumulation of globin mRNA, increasing at the polychromatophilic and orthochromatic stages. The amount of globin mRNA reaches 20 000 molecules per cell in late polychromatic orthochromatic erythroblasts. During the later stages of erythroid cell maturation, the amount of RNA per cell and the rate of total protein synthesis declines, but the relative stability of globin mRNA ensures that globin becomes the predominant polypeptide made in late erythroblasts and reticulocytes.

The individual components of the haemoglobin synthetic pathway (iron, free porphyrins, haem and monomeric globin chains) are all extremely toxic to the cell, and consequently many positive and negative feedback loops have evolved and been incorporated into this process. The synthesis of globin must be very accurately matched with the synthesis of haem in which some steps take place in the cytoplasm and others occur in the mitochondria (Figure 2.5). mRNAs encoding many components of the haem biosynthetic pathway (e.g. ALA synthase and porphobilinogen deaminase, PBGD) are coordinately upregulated in terminal erythroid differentiation and their genes contain similar cis-regulatory elements.

Continued translation of globin chains from mRNA only occurs in the presence of adequate haem. Reduced levels of haem rapidly trigger the formation of the 'haem regulated inhibitor' (HRI), a kinase that interacts with the translation initiating factor eIF-2α and prevents translation of α- and β-globin mRNA. The synthesis of haem itself is also regulated at many points and is particularly sensitive to the levels of available iron. Via a well-characterized pathway involving the iron-regulatory proteins (IRP1 and IRP2), binding to iron response elements (IREs) in the mRNA transcripts of ferritin, TfR and ALA synthase, the level of intracellular iron thus controls the

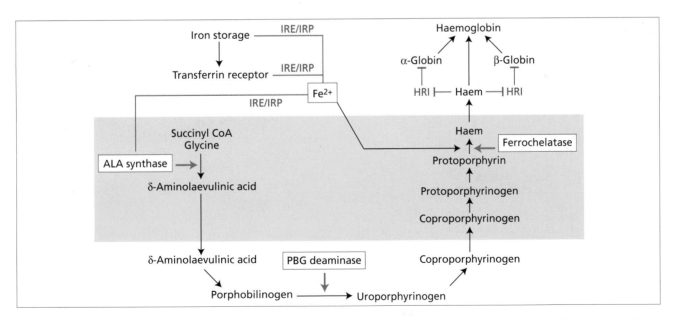

Figure 2.5 The coordination of globin synthesis, haem synthesis and iron regulation. Blue lines indicate some of the known regulatory feedback systems. The red shaded box indicates reactions occurring in the mitochondria. Rate-limiting controls of haem synthesis are shown in black boxes.

translation of RNAs involved in iron storage, iron transport and haem synthesis (see Chapter 3). The recent discovery of hepcidin, which controls the uptake of iron from the gut, iron transport across the placenta and iron release from macrophages, adds another level of control to this complex system (see Chapter 3). Not surprisingly, diseases affecting the supply of iron (iron deficiency and the anaemia of chronic disease), the synthesis of haem (sideroblastic anaemia, lead poisoning, alcohol ingestion) or the synthesis of globin (thalassaemia) have inter-related effects on globin synthesis, haem synthesis and iron metabolism (Figure 2.5).

No mechanistic connection between haemoglobin synthesis and erythroid proliferation or differentiation has yet been established. However, it has been postulated that haemoglobin content and/or haemoglobin concentration *per se* may be a negative regulator of cell division. When haemoglobin synthesis is reduced or delayed, as in iron deficiency, the cells may undergo an extra division, yielding smaller hypochromic cells. Alternatively, when haemoglobin synthesis exceeds DNA synthesis, as in megaloblastic anaemias, the cells may skip a division and nuclear extrusion may occur early, resulting in macrocytosis. Although plausible, these hypotheses remain unproven.

The regulation of erythropoiesis by signalling pathways

The normal red cell lifespan is 120 days and therefore, to maintain equilibrium, approximately 1% of the circulating red cell pool must be replaced daily. For a total of ~3×10^{13} circulating erythrocytes and a lifespan of 120 days, the erythrocyte production rate needs to be maintained at ~10^{10}/h in the steady state.

Erythropoiesis accounts for about 20% of the nucleated cells in a normal bone marrow reflected in the myeloid–erythroid ratio (usually ~4:1). As committed erythroid cells become late BFU-E and CFU-E, they upregulate expression of the receptor for erythropoietin (EpoR). Signalling through this receptor is thought to prevent apoptosis and may also stimulate proliferation. Therefore, at the late BFU-E and CFU-E stages there is considerable potential for controlling the overall level of erythropoiesis. Soon after reaching the CFU-E stage, erythroid cells enter the phase of terminal differentiation, after which there is only limited potential for further expansion. The two major components regulating erythropoiesis include sensing hypoxia and regulating the supply of erythroid precursors, mainly by controlling the numbers of erythroid progenitors via the Epo–EpoR signalling pathway.

Sensing hypoxia

Tissue hypoxia induces a variety of physiological responses in addition to activation of the Epo–EpoR pathway (see below). Parallel responses include the stimulation of new blood vessels by vascular endothelial growth factor (VEGF) and metabolic changes (e.g. in glycolytic pathway enzymes) that enable continued energy production despite inadequate oxygen availability. In addition, expression of the transferrin receptor is upregulated. Over the past few years the mechanisms by which cells sense hypoxia and orchestrate their response have been discovered. It has been shown that the most important mediator of this cellular response is a transcription factor called HIF (hypoxia-inducible factor), which activates the genes that influence the adaptive responses to hypoxia including those encoding Epo, glycolytic pathway enzymes, transferrin receptor and VEGF (Figure 2.6).

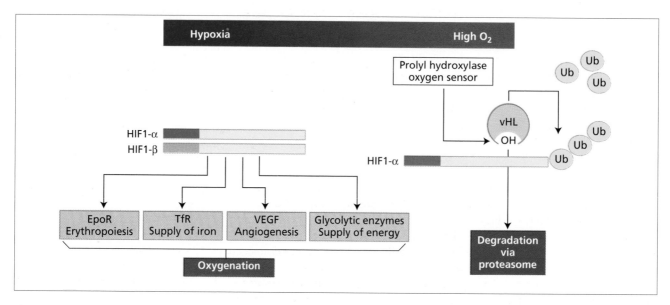

Figure 2.6 The oxygen-sensing system. vHL indicates the von Hippel–Lindau protein. Ub indicates ubiquitination.

HIF is a heterodimer constituting one of three α-subunits (HIF1-α, HIF2-α or HIF3-α) bound to the aryl hydrocarbon receptor nuclear translocator (ARNT), also known as HIF1-β. HIF1-α is a member of the basic helix–loop–helix (bHLH) family of transcription factors in which the HLH domains mediate subunit dimerization, whereas the basic domains bind DNA HIF binds to hypoxia-response elements (HREs, 5′-TACGTG-3′) located in the regulatory regions of hypoxia-inducible genes such as the gene encoding Epo (see below). Whereas changes in oxygen levels do not affect the levels of HIF1-β, which is expressed constitutively, hypoxia elevates the levels of HIF1-α subunits by increasing protein stability.

The oxygen sensor is probably a ferrous iron prolyl hydroxylase that requires molecular oxygen as a cosubstrate to hydroxylate specific proline residues in the α-subunits of HIF. Once hydroxylated, HIF1-α subunits become targets for ubiquitination by the widely expressed von Hippel–Lindau (vHL) protein and are thus targeted for proteosomal degradation. Under normal circumstances the α-subunits are undetectable, but, when cells are exposed to hypoxic stimuli, the oxygen sensor can no longer hydroxylate the α-subunits of HIF. In this situation, α-subunits accumulate as they are no longer polyubiquitinated and degraded. This allows the α-subunits to heterodimerize with HIF1-β and activate the hypoxia-response genes. If the vHL protein is mutated (vHL syndrome), there is prolonged stimulation by HIF, leading to the development of polycythaemia (Epo stimulation) and vascular tumours (VEGF stimulation).

Erythropoietin and the erythropoietin receptor

The Epo gene contains a hypoxia-response element at its 3′-end. Increased levels of the HIF heterodimer upregulate transcription of the Epo gene, increasing serum levels of the protein. The binding of Epo to the erythropoietin receptor (EpoR) results in signal transduction to the nucleus, and this constitutes the most important pathway for controlling definitive erythropoiesis. Careful clinical and haematological studies together with the analysis of experimental animal models have been important in establishing exactly which aspects of erythropoiesis are regulated by the Epo–EpoR system. Fetal livers of genetically modified mice, in which Epo or EpoR has been deleted, are devoid of late erythroid cells but contain normal numbers of BFU-E, demonstrating that this signalling system is not required for lineage specification but is essential for proliferation and differentiation of erythroid precursors into mature cells.

When tissue oxygenation is compromised owing to reduced ambient oxygen tension, blood loss, shortened red cell survival or any uncompensated need for increased oxygen delivery, the level of Epo rises, stimulating red cell production. Late BFU-E and particularly CFU-E are the key targets for Epo activity. When circulating Epo increases, apoptosis of these erythroid progenitors decreases and CFU-Es rapidly respond by proliferating and differentiating. Therefore, the most important effect of Epo is to increase the number of progenitor cells that develop into viable pronormoblasts. It has also been suggested that Epo is able to speed up the rate of terminal differentiation by shortening the cell cycle and maturation times of erythroblasts, thereby explaining the macrocytosis that often accompanies 'stress' erythropoiesis; this remains to be confirmed.

The erythropoietin signalling system is relatively well understood. Erythropoietin is a heavily glycosylated, 34-kDa protein. The level of Epo is controlled via the oxygen tension in the kidney. There are no preformed stores of Epo and it has a short plasma half-life of 6–9 h, allowing relatively rapid responses to changes in tissue oxygenation. Normally, 90% of the hormone is produced in the peritubular complex of the kidney and 10% in the liver and elsewhere.

The Epo receptor belongs to the cytokine receptor superfamily. Like other members of this family (growth hormone, prolactin and G-CSF), Epo was thought to induce dimerization of cell-surface receptors (EpoRs), triggering autophosphorylation and activation of the Janus family of protein tyrosine kinases (JAK2). More recent data suggest an alternative model in which unliganded EpoR dimers exist in a conformation that prevents activation of JAK2, but the receptor may undergo a ligand-induced conformational change that allows JAK2 to be activated. JAK2 and/or other kinases then phosphorylate specific tyrosine residues in the EpoR, creating docking sites for the SH2 domains of several signal transduction proteins, which eventually results in the activation of at least three signal transduction pathways: STAT5, Ras/MAP kinase and PI3 kinase (Figures 2.7 and 2.8).

Considerable interest has concentrated on the JAK2–STAT5 pathway. JAK2 is essential for erythropoiesis, and genetically modified mice in which JAK2 expression has been eliminated die as embryos, with a phenotype similar to mice deficient in Epo or EpoR. However, the numbers of erythroid progenitors are more severely diminished, suggesting that JAK2 is required earlier in erythropoiesis than Epo–EpoR. JAK2 is rapidly phosphorylated in response to Epo stimulation. Dimerization or conformational changes of the EpoR brings the associated JAK2 molecules into close proximity, enabling them to transphosphorylate and activate each other (Figures 2.7 and 2.8). STAT5 is phosphorylated and activated by EpoR. Phosphorylated STAT5 dissociates from the receptor, dimerizes and moves to the nucleus, where it activates gene expression and is thought to be important as an anti-apoptotic signal. Both fetal and adult mice defective in STAT5 have a defect in regulating survival of early erythroblasts, leading to a persistent anaemia.

Activation of the PI3 kinase and Ras–MAP kinase pathway (Figure 2.8) may be sufficient for normal erythroid differentiation, although they may not be essential as other pathways can compensate for loss of signalling through PI3 kinase. Therefore, in erythroid cells, activation of several, apparently redundant

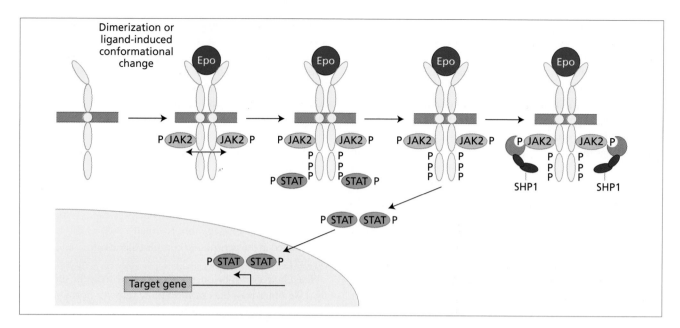

Figure 2.7 A summary of signalling via the Epo receptor as described in the text. P denotes regions of phosphorylation. The diagram shows Epo-induced dimerization or conformational change with transphosphorylation of JAK2, followed by phosphorylation of the Epo receptor. This is followed by binding and phosphorylation of STAT5. Binding of SHP1 (far right) to the Epo receptor activates its phosphatase activity, which can then dephosphorylate JAK2 and terminate signalling.

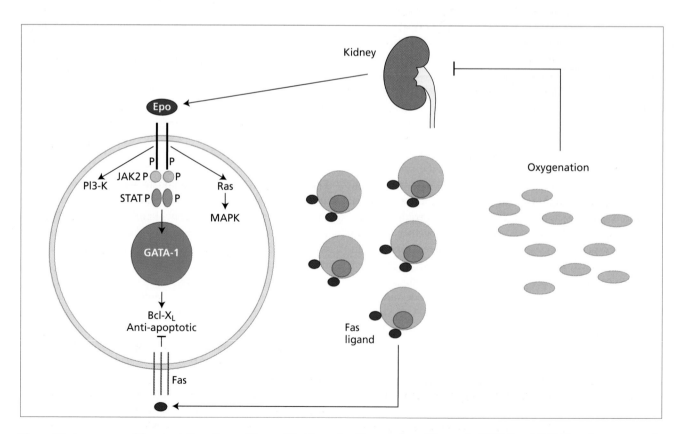

Figure 2.8 A summary of the apoptotic pathways (Epo and Fas) in erythroid progenitors. These cells (BFU-E and CFU-E) undergo apoptosis in the absence of Epo signalling or in the presence of Fas signalling. Bcl-X_L may be the key pathway through which these effects are mediated.

intracellular signalling pathways can support differentiation. Nevertheless, it is thought at present that these pathways may converge by activating a few, important anti-apoptotic proteins, including Bcl-2, Bcl-X_L and protein kinase B (also known as Akt) (Figure 2.8).

The full control of this system is complex and it should be noted that the EpoR pathway can also be activated by other mechanisms. For example, activation of c-Kit by its ligand, stem cell factor (SCF), causes tyrosine phosphorylation of the EpoR and a functional interaction between the two receptors is essential for normal erythropoiesis.

Mechanisms for switching off the Epo–EpoR signalling pathway also exist. Specific phosphorylated tyrosines that occur on the Epo-stimulated dimerized EpoR provide docking sites for the SH2 domains of protein tyrosine phosphatases such as SHP1. Binding activates the phosphatase, which removes the activating phosphates from JAK2, terminating the positive signal from this pathway (Figure 2.7).

Other signalling pathways

Erythropoiesis is also influenced by pathways other than Epo–EpoR. Erythroid progenitors express receptors for Epo, SCF, insulin-like growth factor (IGF-1) and insulin. After Epo, the second most important signalling system for erythropoiesis involves SCF (Kit ligand) and its receptor (c-Kit). Activation by SCF induces tyrosine phosphorylation of its own receptor. SCF was originally identified by its ability to stimulate proliferation of multipotent haemopoietic progenitors, but it is also effective in supporting growth of committed progenitors, including erythroid progenitors, acting synergistically with Epo.

In addition to SCF and Epo, recent observations have shown that stimulation of the nuclear hormone receptors for dexamethasone (glucocorticoid receptor) and oestrogen (oestrogen receptor) produces sustained proliferation of erythroid progenitors. Furthermore, the nuclear hormone receptors for thyroid hormone (c-ErbA/thyroid hormone receptor), all-*trans* retinoic acid (retinoic acid receptor) and 9-*cis*-RA (RXR) were found to promote erythroid differentiation. Such observations are consistent with previous reports showing that patients with a wide range of endocrine disorders (hypothyroidism, hypopituitarism, Addison's disease and male hypogonadism) all have variable degrees of normochromic normocytic anaemia. It appears, therefore, that many hormones of the endocrine system can modify erythropoiesis.

Apoptosis during normal erythropoiesis

Programmed cell death (apoptosis) plays an important role in normal erythropoiesis (Figure 2.8), helping to regulate the accumulation of erythroid precursors to match the need for new mature red cells. Excess erythroid precursors are removed by apoptosis, and at least two pathways seem to be involved. First, it appears that late BFU-E, CFU-E and pronormoblasts may all require continuous signalling via the erythropoietin receptor, which is highly expressed on the surface of these cells, to prevent apoptosis. In the absence of Epo, these cells rapidly undergo programmed cell death in culture. It has been shown that, in part, this reflects a need for signals from the EpoR, via the JAK2–STAT 5 pathway, to induce or stabilize expression of the anti-apoptotic protein Bcl-X_L.

Apoptosis of erythroid precursors may also occur as a result of activation of the Fas receptor (FasR, known as CD95) that is present on both early and late erythroid precursors, although its activating ligand (FasL, known as CD95L) appears only on late erythroblasts. Binding of FasL to FasR activates proteolytic caspases that cleave intracellular proteins, possibly including the erythroid transcription factor GATA-1, with subsequent loss of Bcl-X_L. This regulation of erythropoiesis by negative feedback is thought to take place in the erythropoietic islands of the bone marrow, where the number of mature erythroblasts may control the expansion and differentiation of their less mature precursors.

As well as extracellular anti-apoptotic signals, erythroblasts also use internal programmes to ensure their own survival. The transcription factor GATA-1 is essential for maturation of erythroblasts; the absence of GATA-1 leads to apoptosis and a block in maturation. Some of the target genes regulated by GATA-1 are likely to be important for cell survival. Although many of the targets are unknown, it is clear that GATA-1 strongly induces expression of Bcl-X_L and may therefore cooperate with EpoR signalling. In this way, Epo signalling, Fas-mediated signalling and GATA-1 converge on Bcl-X_L, which represents a key target of the erythroid cell survival programme.

Erythropoiesis in clinical practice

Erythropoiesis is disturbed to a greater or lesser extent in almost all multisystem diseases and so the reader is referred to other chapters and references for specific examples. The aim of this chapter is to provide a framework for thinking about the process of erythropoiesis in clinical practice. The first stage involves the production of committed erythroid progenitors. The second involves controlling red cell production, which is mainly achieved via the oxygen sensor influencing the level of Epo, which, in turn, controls the numbers of late BFU-Es and CFU-Es, although many other hormones cytokines and growth factors may modify the response. The third phase requires terminal erythroid differentiation to mature red cells containing large amounts of specific proteins such as haemoglobin. This phase makes significant demands on a variety of nutritional factors and cofactors, particularly iron, vitamin B_{12} and folate, but also manganese, cobalt, vitamin C, vitamin E, vitamin B_6

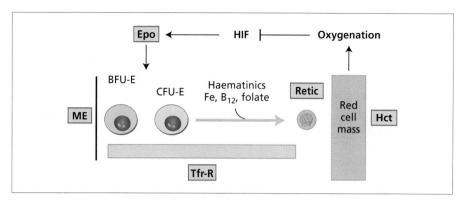

Figure 2.9 Summary of the regulation of erythropoiesis with the key points for assessment boxed in blue. ME denotes assessment of the M/E ratio in the bone marrow.

(pyridoxine), thiamine, riboflavin, pantothenic acid and amino acids. Absolute or relative deficiencies of these cofactors can negatively regulate erythropoiesis. The output from this process (red cell mass) is required to meet the demands for adequate tissue oxygenation, which, itself, has a major influence on the production of erythropoietin, thus completing the regulatory loop (Figure 2.9).

Simple diagnostic tools are available to test the circuit in a logical manner (also see Chapter 6). First, one can evaluate the overall level of erythropoiesis by estimating the ratio of myeloid precursors–erythroid precursors in the marrow (normally ~4:1, but with a very broad normal range). Total erythropoiesis can be measured accurately using radioactive (^{59}Fe) ferrokinetic assays. The plasma iron turnover measures the total (i.e. effective and ineffective) amount of erythropoiesis, whereas the red cell iron utilization assay measures effective erythropoiesis. To a large extent, these two parameters can now be assessed much more easily by measuring the levels of soluble transferrin receptor (sTfR) and the reticulocyte count. Soluble sTfR is a truncated form of the receptor which circulates in a complex with transferrin. The erythroblasts rather than the reticulocytes are the main source of sTfR and, when iron stores are adequate and available, measuring the level of sTfR (NR 5.0 ± 1.0 mg/mL) is a good guide to the total level of erythropoiesis. STfR levels are increased when erythropoiesis is stimulated and decreased when diminished. The interpretation of sTFR levels is complicated in iron deficiency as this condition independently raises the level of sTfR. The reticulocyte count (0.5–2.0% or 25–75 × 10^9/L) is raised in proportion to the degree of anaemia when erythropoiesis is effective (e.g. uncomplicated response to bleeding), but is relatively low when erythropoiesis is ineffective (e.g. β-thalassaemia) or an abnormality prevents a normal response (e.g. nutritional deficiency).

The output of the system, the red cell mass, can be accurately measured by radioactive dilution techniques using ^{51}Cr, but can often be reliably estimated from the haematocrit or concentration of haemoglobin. Changes in red cell size, shape and haemoglobin content, often reflected in the red cell morphology, may provide important guides to specific abnormalities in red cell maturation (e.g. haemoglobinopathies, thalassaemia,

nutritional deficiencies). If the red cell mass is appropriate to meet the demands for oxygenation then Epo production will be suppressed and the serum level will be in the normal range of (~25–50 mU/mL in cord blood and ~10–30 mU/mL in adults). If there is inadequate oxygenation, the level of Epo will, in general, be raised in proportion to the degree of anaemia (e.g. up to 3–10 U/mL after severe blood loss) unless there is some impediment to Epo production (e.g. chronic renal failure, anaemia of chronic diseases). For any given degree of anaemia the level of Epo in the blood may vary depending on the underlying conditions. For example, the levels tend to be very high in aplastic anaemia and less than anticipated in thalassaemia. This may reflect the different numbers of precursors in the marrow that are able to bind available Epo molecules, thus altering the number of free Epo molecules that are measured.

These apparently straightforward assessments may be more difficult to interpret when there are multiple causes of abnormal erythropoiesis, and in particular when complicated by nutritional deficiencies, which should always be evaluated in parallel with these studies. In addition to the common nutritional anaemias, the vast number of specific diagnostic tests to determine the inherited or acquired disorders that may perturb each phase of erythropoiesis are described elsewhere in this book.

Proper oxygen delivery to the tissues requires sufficient circulating mature red cells, and any appropriate therapy should be aimed at correcting this. An important caveat is that excessive red cells may cause a sluggish circulation that can cause ischaemia, leading to serious complications (e.g. myocardial infarction and stroke). The simplified circuit presented here to describe the process of erythropoiesis (Figure 2.9) indicates three potential routes for therapeutic intervention. The first is to correct nutritional deficiencies, usually iron and less commonly folate or vitamin B_{12}. The recent discovery of the role of the iron-regulatory peptide hepcidin in the anaemias of chronic disorders suggests that some remaining common forms of anaemia related to this class (caused by inability to use stored iron) may be amenable to rational treatment in the not too distant future. A second frequently used approach is to correct anaemia, of any cause, with red cell transfusion, and the criteria for such treatment are set out in other sections of this book. The final approach is to increase erythropoiesis by administering recombinant human erythropoietin (rHuEpo). Following its considerable benefit to patients with the anaemia of chronic renal failure who are not capable of making normal levels of Epo, rHuEpo has been assessed in a wide range of disorders (e.g. aplastic anaemia, red cell aplasia, thalassaemia intermedia, cancer of all types, haematological malignancy, myelodysplastic syndrome, rheumatoid arthritis, autologous blood donors, after stem cell transplantation and more). A review of its effectiveness in these situations is beyond the scope of this chapter, but the considerable expense involved in treating patients, often over relatively long periods of time, with a hormone that does not always directly address the known pathophysiology of the anaemia requires careful consideration.

Finally, there are some conditions in which hormonal deficiency is known to contribute to anaemia (e.g. hypothyroidism, Addison's disease). In these cases appropriate correction of the hormonal deficiency logically helps correct the anaemia. Some rare forms of anaemia respond to a variety of therapies for unexplained reasons. For example, some cases of Diamond–Blackfan anaemia (DBA) respond to corticosteroids, and some cases of congenital dyserythropoietic anaemia (CDA) respond to α-interferon, suggesting that there are still many unknown aspects to this clinically important and intellectually fascinating process of erythropoiesis.

Selected bibliography

Erythropoiesis in the context of general haemopoiesis

Cross MA, Enver T (1997) The lineage commitment of haemopoietic progenitor cells. *Current Opinion in Genetics Development* 7: 609–13.

Dzierzak E (2003) Ontogenic emergence of definitive hematopoietic stem cells. *Current Opinions in Hematology* 10: 229–34.

Joshi C, Enver T (2003) Molecular complexities of stem cells. *Current Opinions in Hematology* 10: 220–8.

Marshall CJ, Thrasher AJ (2001) The embryonic origins of human haemopoiesis. *British Journal of Haematology* 112: 838–50.

Orkin SH (2000) Diversification of haemopoietic stem cells to specific lineages. *Nature Review of Genetics* 1: 57–64.

Tavian M, Hallais M-F, Péault B (1999) Emergence of intraembryonic hematopoietic precursors in the pre-liver human embryo. *Development* 126: 793–803.

Wickramasinghe SN (1975) Erythropoiesis. In: *Human Bone Marrow* (SN Wickramasinghe, ed.), pp. 162–232. Blackwell Scientific Publications, Oxford.

Regulation and differentiation of erythroid cells

Beguin Y (2003) Soluble transferrin receptor for the evaluation of erythropoiesis and iron status. *Clinica Chimica Acta* 329: 9–22.

Constantinescu SN, Ghaffari S, Lodish HF (1999) The erythropoietin receptor: structure, activation and intracellular signal transduction. *Trends in Endocrinology and Metabolism* 10: 18–23.

De Maria R, Zeuner A, Eramo A et al. (1999) Negative regulation of erythropoiesis by caspase-mediated cleavage of GATA-1. *Nature* 401: 489–93.

Panzenbock B, Bartunek P, Mapara MY et al. (1998) Growth and differentiation of human stem cell factor/erythropoietin-dependent erythroid progenitor cells in vitro. *Blood* 92: 3658–68.

Safran M, Kaelin WG Jr. (2003) HIF hydroxylation and the mammalian oxygen-sensing pathway. *Journal of Clinical Investigation* 111: 779–83.

Transcription factors controlling erythropoiesis

Bungert J, Engel JD (1996) The role of transcription factors in erythroid development. *Annals of Medicine* 28: 47–55.

Cantor AB, Orkin SH (2002) Transcriptional regulation of erythropoiesis: an affair involving multiple partners. *Oncogene* 21: 3368–76.

Gubin AN, Njoroge JM, Bouffard GG et al. (1999) Gene expression in proliferating human erythroid cells. *Genomics* 59: 168–77.

Shivdasani RA, Orkin SH (1996) The transcriptional control of hematopoiesis. *Blood* 87: 4025–39.

Sieweke MH, Graf T (1998) A transcriptional factor party during blood cell differentiation. *Current Opinions in Genetic Development* 8: 545–51.

Erythropoiesis in clinical practice

Beguin Y (2003) Soluble transferrin receptor for the evaluation of erythropoiesis and iron status. *Clinica Chimica Acta* 329: 9–22.

Eschbach JW (2000) Current concepts of anaemia management in chronic renal failure: impact of NKF-DOQI. *Seminars in Nephrology* 20: 320–9.

Muirhead N, Bargman JA, Burgess E et al. (1995) Evidence-based recommendations for the clinical use of recombinant human erythropoietin. *American Journal of Kidney Disease* 26: S1–24.

Samol J, Littlewood TJ (2003) The efficacy of rHuEPO in cancer-related anaemia. *British Journal of Haematology* 121: 3–11.

CHAPTER 3

Iron metabolism, iron deficiency and disorders of haem synthesis

3

Mark Worwood and A Victor Hoffbrand

Introduction

Iron (atomic weight = 55.85) is essential for many metabolic processes. It shares with other transition metals two properties of particular importance in biology – the ability to exist in more than one relatively stable oxidation state and the ability to form many complexes. Its ability to exist in both ferric and ferrous states underlies its role in critical enzyme reactions concerned with oxygen and electron transport and the cellular production of energy. As well as physiologically active iron compounds, many of which are haem proteins, there are also specialized proteins of iron transport and storage. The latter are necessary to enable iron to remain in solution at neutral pH, at which ferric iron is insoluble, and to limit the potential toxicity of this reactive metal. The insolubility of ferric iron also means that, although the earth's crust contains approximately 4% iron, and iron may be plentiful in the diet, much of this is unavailable. As a result, the body is limited in the adjustments it can make to excessive loss of iron, which frequently occurs due to haemorrhage, and iron deficiency is the most common cause of anaemia throughout the world. The general need to conserve the metal is reflected in the absence of any physiological mechanism for excretion of iron, control of iron balance being at the level of iron absorption. This is important in the rarer but potentially fatal disorders of iron overload.

Distribution of body iron

The concentration of iron in the adult human body is normally about 50 mg/kg in males and 40 mg/kg in females. The largest component is circulating haemoglobin, with 450 mL (1 unit) of whole blood containing about 200 mg of iron (Figure 3.1). Much of the remainder is contained in the storage proteins, ferritin and haemosiderin. These are found mainly in the reticuloendothelial (RE) cells of the liver, spleen and bone marrow (which gain iron from breaking down red cells), and in parenchymal liver cells (which normally gain most of their iron from the plasma iron-transporting protein, transferrin).

Functional iron-containing proteins

Haemoglobin (molecular weight = 64 500) contains four haem groups linked to four globin chains, and can bind four molecules of oxygen. Myoglobin (mol. wt = 17 000) accounts for 4–5% of body iron and has a single haem group attached to its one polypeptide chain. It has a higher affinity for oxygen than haemoglobin and behaves as an oxygen reserve in muscles. The mitochondria contain a series of haem and non-haem iron proteins (including the cytochromes *a*, *b* and *c*, succinate dehydrogenase and cytochrome oxidase) that form an electron transport pathway responsible for the oxidation of intracellular

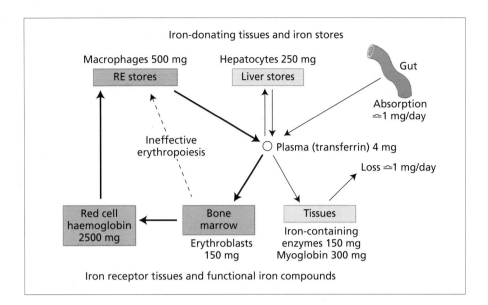

Figure 3.1 The major compartments of iron in a 70-kg man. Iron supply for erythropoiesis and release of iron from senescent red cells dominate internal iron exchange.

substrates and the simultaneous production of adenosine triphosphate. Haem is an essential component of microsomal and mitochondrial cytochrome P450, which is concerned with hydroxylation reactions (including drug detoxification by the liver), and of cyclo-oxygenase, involved in prostaglandin synthesis. Other haem proteins include the enzymes catalase and lactoperoxidase, which are concerned with peroxide breakdown, and tryptophan pyrrolase, involved in the oxidation of tryptophan to formylkynurenine. There is a smaller group of iron sulphur proteins (e.g. xanthine oxidase, reduced nicotinamide adenine dinucleotide dehydrogenase and aconitase). Iron is also necessary for the function of ribonucleotide reductase, a key enzyme in DNA synthesis.

Ferritin and haemosiderin

Ferritin is the primary iron storage protein and provides a reserve of iron. It consists of an approximately spherical apoprotein shell (mol. wt = 480 000) enclosing a core of ferric hydroxyphosphate (up to 4000 iron atoms). Human ferritin is made up from 24 subunits (mol. wt *c.* 20 000) of two immunologically distinct types: H and L. These are coded by genes on chromosomes 11 and 19 respectively. There are multiple gene copies, many of which are presumably pseudogenes, on 12 different chromosomes. An intronless gene on chromosome 5 (q23.1) codes for mitochondrial ferritin – a novel H-type ferritin. The internal cavity of the ferritin molecule communicates with the exterior via six channels, through which ferrous iron may enter (to interact with a ferroxidase centre on the ferritin H subunit) or leave (after reduction, e.g. by dihydroflavins or ascorbic acid).

The way in which ferritin iron is mobilized is poorly understood, and a process in which the entire ferritin molecule is degraded within lysosomes prior to iron release has also been suggested. Variation in the proportion of H to L subunits explains the heterogeneity of ferritin from different tissues on isoelectric focusing: L-rich ferritins (from spleen and liver) are more basic than H-rich ferritins (from heart and red cells). There may be functional differences between different isoferritins (e.g. in iron storage or intracellular iron transport) but this is not established. The small amount of ferritin normally present in serum contains little iron and consists almost exclusively of L subunits. It is also heterogeneous, owing to glycosylation. This glycosylation and the direct relationship of serum concentration to storage iron in macrophages suggest that serum ferritin is secreted by macrophages in response to changing iron levels.

Haemosiderin, unlike ferritin, is a water-*in*soluble crystalline, protein–iron complex, visible by light microscopy when stained by the Prussian blue (Perls') reaction. It has an amorphous structure, with a higher iron–protein ratio than ferritin, and is probably formed by the partial digestion of ferritin aggregates by lysosomal enzymes. In normal subjects, the majority of storage iron is present as ferritin, and haemosiderin is predominantly found in macrophages rather than hepatocytes. In iron overload, the proportion present as haemosiderin increases considerably in both cell types.

Transferrin and transferrin receptors

Transferrin is a single chain polypeptide (mol. wt = 79 500) present in plasma (1.8–2.6 g/L) and extravascular fluid (Table 3.1). It has a plasma half life of 8–11 days. The protein is synthesized predominantly by the liver, synthesis being inversely related to iron stores. Two atoms of ferric iron bind to each molecule. Although transferrin contains only about 4 mg of body iron at any time, it is vital to iron transport, with over 30 mg iron passing through this compartment each day (Figure 3.1). The binding sites (N-terminus and C-terminus) contain three tyrosine

Table 3.1 Iron transport proteins, oxidoreductases, storage proteins and regulators.

Gene (protein)	Chromosome location	Tissue expression	Structure	Function	Regulation	Mutations and disease
DcytB (duodenal cytochrome b1)	–	Enterocyte +	TMP, 6TMD	Ferric reductase	Fe (hepcidin)	–
DMT1 (SLC11A2)	12q13	Widespread	TMP, 568 aa	Fe uptake	Fe (3′ IRE)	Mk mouse, Belgrade rat
Hemojuvelin (HJV)	1q21	Liver, heart, muscle	Membrane bound receptor or secreted protein	Regulator of hepcidin synthesis	?	Juvenile haemochromatosis
Ferroportin 1 (SLC11A3)	2q32	Liver, spleen, enterocyte	TMP, 571 aa 9TMD	Fe export	Fe (5′ IRE)	Human HC autosomal dominant
Hepcidin (HAMP)	19q13	Plasma (liver)	20–25 aa peptide	Regulator of iron transport	Fe (HFE)	Juvenile HC (digenic HC)
Hephaestin	Xq11–q12	Enterocyte	TMP, 1TMD copper protein with homology to caeruloplasmin	Fe^{2+} oxidase	–	Sla mouse
HFE	6p21.3	Widespread	HLA class I heavy chain	Regulates Tf iron uptake and hepcidin expression	?	Human HC autosomal recessive
Transferrin receptor (TFRC)	3q26.2–qter	Widespread – highest number in erythroblasts	TMP dimer of 90 000 kDa polypeptide	Binds transferrin	Fe (IRE)	(Lethal in knockout mouse)
Transferrin receptor (TFR2)	7q22	Widespread	60% similarity in extracellular domain to TFRC	Binds transferrin, iron haemostasis, regulator of hepcidin synthesis	No IRE	Human HC autosomal recessive
Transferrin	3	Plasma, extravascular space	Single chain polypeptide, glycoprotein	Iron transport	Iron stores	Atransferrinaemia
Ferritin heavy chain (FTH1)	11q13	Widespread, cytosolic	Subunit of ferritin	Iron storage (catalytic subunit for iron incorporation)	Fe (IRE)	Autosomal dominant Fe overload (very rare)
Ferritin light chain (FTL)	19q13.3–q13.4	Widespread, cytosolic	Subunit of ferritin	Iron storage	Fe (IRE)	Hyperferritinaemia and cataract syndrome
IRP1	9p22–p13	Widespread	Cytoplasmic, mol. wt 98 000 with 4Fe–4S cluster	Regulation of synthesis of FTH, FTL, TFRC, DMT1, ferroportin 1, ALAS2	Iron stores	Not known
IRP2	15	Widespread	Cytoplasmic, mol. wt 105 000. No 4Fe–4S cluster	As IRP1	Iron stores	Not known

aa, amino acid; HC, haemochromatosis; IRE, iron response element; IRP, iron regulatory protein; TMD, transmembrane domain; TMP, transmembrane protein.

and two histidine residues and an arginine group. The binding of iron involves simultaneous attachment of an anion, usually bicarbonate. The uptake of iron from transferrin requires that the protein is attached to specific receptors on the cell surface. The transferrin receptor gene (TFRC) codes for a transmembrane protein (mol. wt = 185 000), each of two subunits being able to bind one transferrin molecule. The human transferrin receptor can be identified with anti-CD71 antibodies. A second receptor, TFR2, also binds transferrin (Table 3.1); it may act as the homeostatic iron sensor, regulating hepcidin synthesis in response to diferric transferrin concentration (Fig. 3.2).

Lactoferrin is a glycoprotein (mol. wt = 77 000) that is structurally related to transferrin. It is found in milk and other secretions and in neutrophils. It is thought to have a bacteriostatic action at secreting surfaces by depriving micro-organisms of the iron needed for their growth.

Intracellular transit iron and plasma non-transferrin-bound iron

It is thought that there is a transit pool of 'metabolically active', or 'labile' iron both within and outside cells, which receives iron from degraded haem or ferritin, exchanges with transferrin and is incorporated into newly synthesized iron-containing proteins. It is also a major source of iron chelated by desferrioxamine (Chapter 4). Within cells, low-molecular-weight chelates (e.g. with citrate) may be present. Within plasma in iron overload, it may also exist as oligomeric iron oxide, either free or bound to albumin. Low-molecular-weight chelates are likely to be the form of iron sensed by the regulatory mechanisms of iron homeostasis and which is particularly toxic in iron overload conditions (Chapter 4). The detection of labile iron is difficult and relies on scavenging of the iron by chelators, followed by detection of the chelate. Fluorescent iron-scavenging molecules provide the best detection systems at present.

Cellular iron homeostasis

Synthesis of several of the proteins involved in iron metabolism is regulated at the level of RNA translation by two cytoplasmic iron-dependent proteins, namely IRP1 and IRP2 (Table 3.1). These are capable of binding to mRNAs that contain a sequence forming a stem and loop structure called an *iron-responsive element* or IRE (Figure 3.2). IRP1 (mol. wt = 98 000) contains an iron–sulphur (4Fe–4S) cluster and functions as a cytoplasmic aconitase with low affinity for the IRE when intracellular iron is abundant. When iron is scarce, however, the iron–sulphur cluster is no longer present and IRP1 binds to the IRE with high affinity. IRP2 (mol. wt = 105 000) is expressed ubiquitously but is less abundant than IRP1. There is in IRP2 an extra stretch of 73 amino acids between amino acids 37 and 38 of IRP1. This stretch is rich in proline, serine and cysteine and mediates

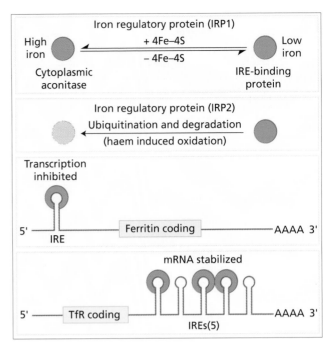

Figure 3.2 Coordinate regulation of expression of ferritin and transferrin receptor: the role of the iron response element (IRE)–IRP mechanism. When cellular iron levels are low, IRP binds to the IRE stem and loop structures of mRNA to inhibit translation of ferritin, but increase translation of transferrin receptors (TfR) by preventing degradation of the mRNA. When iron levels are high, the IRP functions as a cytoplasmic aconitase and no longer binds to the IREs. Ferritin synthesis can thus proceed, while TfR synthesis is reduced. IRP2 binds to IREs when iron levels are low, but is degraded after ubiquitination (initiated by haem-induced oxidation) when iron levels are high. The IRPs therefore provide two ways of sensing iron requirements either involving Fe–S proteins or haem proteins.

IRP2 degradation in iron-replete cells. Activation of IRP2 requires accumulation of the protein as a result of new synthesis. Degradation takes place after the addition of iron. IRP2 knockout mice exhibit disturbances of iron metabolism in the intestinal mucosa and the central nervous system.

The 3′-untranslated region (3′-UTR) of transferrin receptor mRNA contains five IREs, whereas the 5′-UTR region of ferritin mRNA contains a single IRE. Binding of IRP when there are low levels of intracellular iron protects the transferrin receptor mRNA from cytoplasmic degradation but inhibits translation of ferritin mRNA by interfering with the binding of initiation factors. In contrast, when intracellular iron is increased, the opposite effects occur. Thus, coordinated regulation of the two iron proteins acts to maintain a constant intracellular iron content over the short term by balancing cellular iron uptake and storage.

Erythroid δ-aminolaevulinic acid synthase (ALAS2) mRNA also has an IRE in its 5′-UTR region, whereas 'housekeeping'

Group (age, years)	Daily loss (mg)		Requirement for growth (mg)	Total (mg)
	Urine, skin, faeces, etc.	Menses		
Children				
0.5–1	0.17	–	0.55	0.72
1–3	0.19	–	0.27	0.46
4–6	0.27	–	0.23	0.50
7–10	0.39	–	0.32	0.71
Males				
11–14	0.62		0.55	1.17
15–17	0.90	–	0.60	1.50
18+	1.05	–	–	1.05
Females				
11–14*	0.65	–	0.55	1.20
11–14	0.65	0.48[†]	0.55	1.68
15–17	0.79	0.48[†]	0.35	1.62
18+	0.87	0.48[†]	–	1.35
Post menopause	0.87	–	–	0.87
Lactating[‡]	1.15	–	–	1.15

Table 3.2 Daily iron losses and requirements (WHO 2001).

*Non-menstruating.

[†]Median loss.

[‡]**Average dietary requirement during pregnancy is 3–4 mg.**

ALAS1 mRNA does not. This suggests that the IRP–IRE system may be involved in matching iron supply to haem synthesis, with repression of protoporphyrin synthesis in iron-deficient erythroblasts (p. 33). Mitochondrial aconitase interconverts citrate and isocitrate and has a putative IRE at the 5′-UTR of its mRNA. In the liver, its activity decreases in iron deficiency, suggesting a role in iron metabolism perhaps related to a role for citrate as an intracellular iron carrier. DMT1 has a 3′-IRE and ferroportin 1 has a 5′-IRE (Table 3.1) but binding of IRP is weak compared with the TFRC and ferritin IREs.

Normal iron balance

The amount of iron in the body at birth depends on the blood volume and haemoglobin concentration, the birth weight (which determines blood volume) being particularly important. Delay in clamping the cord leads to an increased red cell mass by placental transfusion. The level of maternal iron stores has little effect on fetal iron. The newborn contains about 80 mg/kg at full term. Neonatal iron reserves are utilized for growth, and from 6 months to 2 years virtually no iron stores are present. Thereafter, iron stores gradually accumulate during childhood to around 5 mg/kg. In men, there is a further increase between 15 and 30 years to about 10–12 mg/kg (total up to approximately 1 g), whereas iron stores remain lower in women (average 300 mg)

until the menopause. It would take 4 years or more for a man to deplete body iron stores and develop iron deficiency anaemia solely due to lack of dietary intake or malabsorption.

Requirements are higher in menstruating women and during periods of rapid growth in infancy and adolescence (Table 3.2). Menstrual loss has a median value of 30 mL, but the 95th centile value is 118 mL blood per month (equivalent to 1.9 mg iron per day), which has been found to be significantly associated with iron deficiency. Requirements are highest of all in pregnancy.

Iron absorption

Iron absorption depends not only on the amount of iron in the diet, but also, and more importantly, on the bioavailability of that iron, as well as the body's needs for iron. A normal Western diet provides approximately 15 mg of iron daily. Of that iron, digestion within the gut lumen releases about one-half in a soluble form, from which about 3 mg may be taken up by mucosal cells and only about 1 mg (or 5–10% of dietary iron) transferred to the portal blood in a healthy man. Iron absorption can thus be influenced at several different stages.

Dietary and luminal factors

Much of dietary iron is non-haem iron derived from cereals

Table 3.3 Iron absorption.

Favoured by	Reduced by
Dietary factors	
Increased haem iron	Decreased haem iron
Increased animal foods	Decreased animal foods
Ferrous iron salts	Ferric iron salts
Luminal factors	
Acid pH (e.g. gastric HCl)	Alkalis (e.g. pancreatic secretions)
Low-molecular-weight soluble chelates (e.g. vitamin C, sugars, amino acids)	Insoluble iron complexes (phytates, tannates in tea, bran)
Ligand in meat (unidentified)	
Systemic factors	
Iron deficiency	Iron overload
Increased erythropoiesis (e.g. after haemorrhage)	Decreased erythropoiesis
Ineffective erythropoiesis	Inflammatory disorders (Hepcidin)
Pregnancy	
Hypoxia	

(commonly fortified with additional iron in the UK), with a lesser component of haem iron from meat and fish. Even in iron deficiency, the maximum iron absorption from a mixed Western diet is no more than 3–4 mg daily. This figure is much less with the predominantly vegetarian, cereal-based diets of most of the world's population.

Iron is released from protein complexes by acid and proteolytic enzymes in the stomach and small intestine, and haem is liberated from haemoglobin and myoglobin. Iron is maximally absorbed from the duodenum and less well from the jejunum, probably because the increasingly alkaline environment leads to the formation of insoluble ferric hydroxide complexes. Luminal factors enhancing or inhibiting absorption are listed in Table 3.3. Therapeutic ferrous iron salts are well absorbed on an empty stomach, but when taken with a meal, absorption is reduced as a result of the same ligand-binding processes that affect dietary non-haem iron.

Mucosal factors: molecular aspects of iron absorption and its regulation

A variety of mechanisms for the binding of non-haem iron to the mucosal membrane have been described. Both specific, saturable and receptor-mediated mechanism, and passive diffusion at higher doses may occur.

Recently discovered membrane transport proteins, regulatory proteins and associated oxidoreductases involved in iron transport through the intestinal cell are listed in Table 3.1. The proposed process is illustrated in Figure 3.3. Non-haem iron is released from food as Fe^{3+} and reduced by Dcytb to Fe^{2+}. This is transported across the brush border membrane by DMT1. It is assumed that iron enters the labile pool and some may be incorporated into ferritin and lost when the cells are exfoliated. Iron destined for retention by the body is transported across the serosal membrane by ferroportin 1 before uptake by transferrin as Fe^{3+}. Hephaestin is a copper-containing ferroxidase (Table 3.1) expressed predominantly in villous cells of the small intestine. It is implicated in conversion of Fe^{2+} to Fe^{3+} in the basolateral transfer step of iron absorption, which is impaired in mice with a defective hephaestin gene. Hephaestin appears to be located intracellularly, with a perinuclear distribution, however, and its role as a ferroxidase in basolateral iron release is still unclear.

Haem iron is initially bound by haem receptors at the brush border membrane and released intracellularly by haem oxygenase

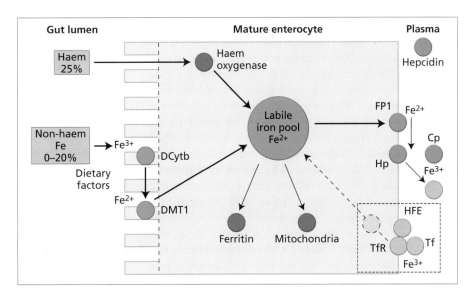

Figure 3.3 Molecular pathways of iron absorption. The area enclosed in the dotted box refers to the uptake of iron from the plasma in the developing enterocyte in the intestinal crypt. Otherwise, the diagram refers to iron absorption by the villous epithelial cell. Cp, caeruloplasmin; FP1, ferroportin 1; Hp, hephaestin; Tf, transferrin; TfR, transferrin receptor. For further details see text and Table 3.1.

before entering the labile iron pool and following a common pathway with iron of non-haem origin.

Regulation of iron absorption

Iron absorption may be regulated both at the stage of mucosal uptake and at the stage of transfer to the blood. How each of these factors listed in Table 3.3 inform the mucosal cells of how much iron to take up or to transfer to the plasma is becoming clearer. It has been assumed that as epithelial cells develop in the crypts of Lieberkühn, their iron status reflects that of the plasma (transferrin saturation), and this programmes the cells to absorb iron appropriately as they differentiate along the villus. There are situations when this does not apply, however. In genetic haemochromatosis transferrin, saturation is high yet iron absorption is increased. One hypothesis concerning the transfer stage suggests that each of the iron-donating tissues (macrophages, liver and gut: see Figure 3.1) supplies iron to plasma transferrin in proportion to the amount of available iron in those tissues, the iron being transported to satisfy the needs of the main receptor tissue, the erythroid marrow. Within this framework, the amount of iron to be supplied by the intestinal cells would be dependent on the output from other donor tissues, being increased when there is tissue iron deficiency. Furthermore, when there is a rise in plasma iron turnover owing to increased erythron demands for iron, output from all the donor tissues, including the gut, might be expected to increase.

Hepcidin

There is now convincing evidence of a more direct regulation of iron absorption by hepcidin. This product of the *HAMP* gene (Table 3.1) is a small peptide (20–25 amino acids) with several isoforms released from a large prepropeptide of 84 amino acids. It is predominantly expressed in the liver and is downregulated when iron stores are reduced and upregulated when iron stores are increased or by inflammation. Hepcidin is the predominant negative regulator of iron absorption in the small intestine, iron transport across the placenta and iron release from macrophages, probably by binding to ferroportin and acclerating its destruction. The key role of hepcidin is confirmed by the presence of nonsense mutations in the hepcidin gene, homozygous in the affected members, in several families with severe juvenile haemochromatosis (Chapter 4). A deficient hepcidin response to iron loading may contribute to iron overload in HFE-linked and other genetic haemochromatosis (Chapter 4). In anaemia of inflammation, hepcidin production is increased up to 100-fold, and this may account for the defining feature of this condition, sequestration of iron in macrophages. HFE and transferrin receptor 2 and hemojuvelin probably have indirect roles in the control of iron absorption through the regulation of hepcidin synthesis. Also, in conditions of increased erythroid turnover, serum hepcidin levels are low in those with increased iron absorption.

Hemojuvelin

Juvenile haemochromatosis (Chapter 4) is most frequently associated with mutations in the hemojuvelin gene (Table 3.1). Mutations in this gene produce a phenotype very similar to that resulting from mutations in the HAMP gene. It has been suggested that both hemojuvelin and HFE may act by regulating hepcidin synthesis.

Internal iron exchange

Iron uptake by erythroid cells

The fate of iron bound to plasma transferrin has been studied by injecting a trace amount of radioactive ^{59}Fe bound to transferrin. About 85% of the ^{59}Fe normally enters developing red cells for incorporation into haemoglobin. This tissue distribution of transferrin-bound iron reflects the expression of transferrin receptors, which are present in high concentration on cells with a high iron requirement. The latter includes any rapidly dividing cells but is normally dominated by the cells of the erythron.

The expression of surface transferrin receptors is increased if cells have inadequate iron, and reduced if they are iron replete (p. 29). Cell transferrin receptors have the highest affinity for diferric transferrin. The transferrin–receptor complex is taken up by a process of receptor-mediated endocytosis (Figure 3.4). The iron is released at the low pH of the endosome, before the apotransferrin and receptor are recycled to the plasma and the

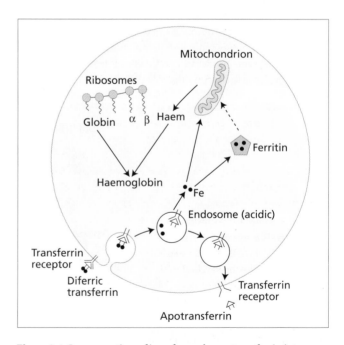

Figure 3.4 Incorporation of iron from plasma transferrin into haemoglobin in developing red cells. Uptake of transferrin iron is by receptor-mediated endocytosis.

cell membrane respectively. Iron release from the endosome is via DMT1 (Table 3.1) and the iron enters the mitochondria or ferritin. Direct transfer of storage iron from macrophages to erythroblasts (rhopheocytosis) is now thought to be of little physiological significance. A soluble, truncated form of the receptor derived from these cell surfaces is detectable in serum. It is bound to transferrin and increased concentrations provide an early indication of an impaired iron supply to the tissues (p. 36). In the absence of iron deficiency, the serum transferrin receptor concentrations reflect erythroid activity.

Breakdown of haemoglobin iron

After phagocytosis by macrophages, haem from senescent red cells is broken down by haem oxygenase (HMOX1) to release iron. As ferrous iron, it can then either enter ferritin (where it is oxidized to ferric iron by the ferritin protein) or be released into plasma (via ferroportin 1), where its binding to transferrin (also as the ferric form) may be facilitated by a plasma ferrous oxidase (e.g. caeruloplasmin). The release of macrophage iron is controlled by hepcidin, with high levels, as in inflammation or iron overload, reducing iron release. Changes in the release of iron from macrophages are thought to account for the diurnal rhythm of serum iron concentration, which is highest in the morning and lowest in the evening.

Role of liver

Hepatocytes have an important role in iron metabolism (Figure 3.1), being capable of taking up extra iron when the transferrin iron saturation (and thus the proportion of diferric transferrin) is increased, and of releasing iron from stores when there is greater need in other tissues for iron. An increased percentage saturation of the plasma transferrin (iron-binding capacity) is the earliest indication of a risk of parenchymal iron overload in hereditary haemochromatosis and the iron-loading anaemias. Through the iron-regulated synthesis of hepcidin, the liver also directly controls iron absorption from the intestine (p. 31).

Some 5–10% of haemoglobin from senescent red cells is normally released intravascularly and bound by haptoglobin prior to its removal by macrophages. An increase in this pathway is seen in haemolytic and dyserythropoietic anaemias, and may provide a further route by which the liver accumulates excess iron in such disorders, in addition to the uptake of transferrin iron and any free (non-transferrin-bound) iron from the plasma. Large particles of colloidal iron, including therapeutic parenteral iron preparations, are also removed from the circulation by macrophages of the RE system.

Fate of iron in the erythroid cell

Some 80–90% of iron taken into developing erythroblasts is converted to haem within 1 h. Any iron taken up in excess of the requirement for haem synthesis is incorporated in ferritin (Figure 3.4). The red cell ferritin content is therefore increased when haemoglobin synthesis is impaired, as in thalassaemia syndromes or sideroblastic anaemia. Excess iron may be seen in the cytoplasm of mature red cells as one or more siderotic granules. These are composed of haemosiderin and stain blue with Perls' reaction and purplish blue with Romanowsky stains, when they are called Pappenheimer bodies. The spleen removes these granules by its pitting action.

Haem synthesis

Haem consists of a protoporphyrin ring with an iron atom at its centre. Haem is synthesized from the precursors succinyl CoA and glycine, which condense to form δ-aminolaevulinic acid (ALA) under the action of ALA synthase (ALAS), with pyridoxal phosphate as a coenzyme (p. 19). 'Housekeeping' ALAS (ALAS1) is coded by a gene on chromosome 3, but, in erythroid cells erythroid-specific ALAS2 predominates and is coded on the X chromosome. ALA can be utilized for the formation of both purines and haem. Four molecules of porphobilinogen condense under the influence of porphobilinogen deaminase (PBGD) and uroporphyrinogen cosynthase to form the tetrapyrrole ring compound uroporphyrinogen III. The latter is converted to protoporphyrin IX. Finally, iron in the ferrous form is incorporated under the influence of the enzyme ferrochelatase. Iron in haem has six coordinating valencies: four link the iron to nitrogen atoms in each pyrrole ring, whereas the remaining two link haem to histidine residues in the globin chain, the distal bond being unstable and easily replaced by oxygen to form oxyhaemoglobin.

The mitochondria play a major role in haem synthesis as they contain ALAS, coproporphyrinogen oxidase and ferrochelatase, the enzyme sequence from ALA to coproporphyrinogen being situated in the cytoplasm. The mitochondria are also the site of the citric acid cycle, which supplies succinate. The mature red cell, which lacks mitochondria, is therefore unable to synthesize haem.

A number of porphyrins are formed by side reactions during the synthesis of protoporphyrin. In the porphyrias (p. 39), many of these compounds accumulate in the major sites of haem synthesis, the liver and the red cells.

Control mechanisms in haem synthesis

As well as the developmental regulation of haem formation during erythroid differentiation, synthesis of haem and globin is coordinated so that there is no significant excess of either. Moreover, the entry of iron into the cell and its incorporation into haem are regulated so that the normal cell obtains sufficient iron for its needs, but not more. ALAS2 is rate limiting in the erythroid–haem biosynthetic pathway. Its activity reaches a peak in the polychromatic normoblast and then diminishes so that no activity is present in the mature cell. Interleukin 3 and erythropoietin act as inducers for transcription of mRNA for ALAS2 and PBGD, and this may be most important in the developmental regulation of haem production during erythroid differentiation. The coordination of haem and globin synthesis is further discussed in Chapter 2.

Diagnostic methods for investigating iron metabolism

The large amount of iron present as haemoglobin means that the degree of any anaemia must always be considered in assessing iron status. Reduced amounts of haemoglobin accompany an overall reduction in body iron in iron deficiency anaemia or after acute blood loss. In other anaemias, including the anaemia of chronic disease and the megaloblastic anaemias, iron is redistributed from the red cells to macrophage iron stores, with a corresponding increase in marrow-stainable iron and serum ferritin. The various measurements of iron status are listed in Table 3.4 and described below in more detail. No single measurement is ideal for all clinical circumstances, as all are affected by confounding factors (Table 3.4) and changes may develop sequentially (as in progressive negative iron balance) or may affect particular body iron compartments. Reference ranges for

haemoglobin and the various measures of iron status are given in Appendix 1. Table 3.5 summarizes the changes in measures of iron status accompanying various types of hypochromic anaemia. The assessment of *iron overload* is discussed in Chapter 4.

Storage iron

Serum ferritin

In healthy subjects, the serum ferritin concentration correlates with iron stores, as assessed by quantitative phlebotomy or tissue biopsy. This has led to the widespread use of immunoassays for serum ferritin as a convenient, non-invasive measure of iron stores. Normal concentrations of serum ferritin range from about 15 to 300 μg/L, and are higher in men (median about 90 μg/L) than in premenopausal women (median 30 μg/L). In women, after the menopause, serum ferritin concentrations increase but remain below levels in men. In neonates, the concentration in cord blood (median approximately 100 μg/L) rises further over the first 2 months of life as fetal haemoglobin is broken down, and thereafter falls to low levels (median 20–30 μg/L) throughout childhood and adolescence.

Values for serum ferritin concentration below 15 μg/L are virtually specific for storage iron depletion, but normal values do not exclude this and values above 300 μg/L do not necessarily, or even usually, indicate iron overload. This is because ferritin synthesis is influenced by factors other than iron (in

Table 3.4 Potential confounding factors in the interpretation of measures of iron status.

Measurement	Confounding factors
Iron stores	
Serum ferritin	Increased: as an acute-phase protein (e.g. in infection, inflammation or malignancy) and by release of tissue ferritins by damage, especially to iron-rich organs (e.g. with hepatic necrosis, chronic liver disease, splenic or bone marrow infarction in sickle cell disease) Decreased: by ascorbate deficiency
Tissue iron supply	
Serum iron and transferrin saturation	Labile measures: normal short-term fluctuations mean that a single value may not reflect iron supply over a longer period
Serum transferrin receptor	Directly related to extent of erythroid activity as well as being inversely related to iron supply to cells
Red cell protoporphyrin/red cell ferritin/% hypochromic red cells	Stable measures: reduced iron supply at time of red cell formation leads to increases in protoporphyrin and hypochromic red cells, and reduced red cell ferritin. However, values may not reflect current iron supply. May be increased by other causes of impaired iron incorporation into haem (e.g. lead poisoning, sideroblastic anaemias)
Functional iron	
Hb concentration	Other causes for anaemia besides iron deficiency; a reciprocal relationship with iron stores should be expected in all anaemias except in iron deficiency anaemia
Red cell MCV, MCH	May be reduced in other disorders of haemoglobin synthesis (e.g. thalassaemia, sideroblastic anaemias) in addition to iron deficiency

MCH, mean corpuscular haemoglobin; MCV, mean corpuscular volume.

Table 3.5 Differential diagnosis of hypochromic anaemia.

	Iron deficiency	Chronic disease	Thalassaemia trait (α or β)	Sideroblastic anaemia
MCV/MCH	↓	↓ or N	↓	↓ (congenital), ↑N (acquired)
Serum iron	↓	↓	N	↑
TIBC	↑	↓ or N	N	N
Transferrin saturation	↓	↓	N	↑
Serum ferritin	↓	N or ↑	N	↑
Serum TfR	↑	N	N	N or ↑
Bone marrow iron stores	↓	N or ↑	N	N or ↑
Erythroblast iron	↓	↓	N	Ring forms

N, Normal; TfR, transferrin receptor.

particular, it behaves as an acute-phase reactant in many inflammatory diseases). For this reason, serum ferritin concentrations of < 50 µg/L may be associated with a lack of storage iron in patients with the anaemia of chronic disease. A ferritin concentration of > 100 µg/L suggests the presence of storage iron. Algorithms designed to predict storage iron levels from serum ferritin concentration and an indicator of inflammation or infection (erythrocyte sedimentation rate or C-reactive protein) have not proved to be useful. Damage to tissues (particularly the liver) can release large amounts of tissue ferritin into the plasma.

There is a rare autosomal dominant genetic abnormality of ferritin synthesis (hereditary hyperferritinaemia with cataract syndrome) in which excess synthesis of ferritin L-chain is associated with high serum ferritin concentrations (in the absence of iron overload) and with cataracts. The latter are due to deposition of L-type ferritin (with little iron) in the lens. Over 20 point mutations and deletions of the IRE loop of L-ferritin mRNA, which prevent its interaction with IRP, have been described. There is no overall increase in body iron.

Bone marrow aspiration

Staining the bone marrow for iron gives an indication of RE iron stores as well as erythroblast iron (Figure 3.5a). In iron deficiency anaemia, RE iron and erythroblast iron are absent (Figure 3.5b).

Iron supply to the tissues

Serum iron and iron-binding capacity

The serum iron and, more particularly, the saturation of the total iron-binding capacity of transferrin (TIBC) give a measure of the iron supply to the tissues. In normal subjects, the serum iron shows a diurnal rhythm, with values being lower in the morning than in the evening. In iron deficiency and iron overload, however, values stabilize at low or high levels respectively. A serum transferrin saturation (serum iron/TIBC × 100) that is persistently less than 15% is insufficient to support normal erythropoiesis. A rise in TIBC is characteristic of iron deficiency (i.e. an absence of storage iron). A reduced serum iron concentration with a normal or reduced TIBC is a characteristic response to infection and inflammation. A sustained increase in transferrin saturation to more than 50% is an early change in the development of parenchymal iron loading (Chapter 4).

Serum transferrin receptors

Plasma concentrations reflect both the number of erythroid precursors and iron supply to the bone marrow. In clinical practice, these two factors must be considered in interpreting transferrin receptor levels. Increased erythropoiesis from any cause results in high serum concentrations so the assay has been used as a replacement for ferrokinetic procedures as a means of identifying increased erythropoiesis. In the anaemia of chronic diseases, the assay provides a valuable indicator of deficiency of body iron stores. Serum transferrin receptor levels only increase in this situation in the absence of storage iron. Further improvement in sensitivity and specificity has been described using various ferritin–transferrin receptor ratios. At the moment, several units and reference ranges are in use and the assay is therefore method specific. In general hospital practice, some consider that the serum transferrin receptor assay adds little to the diagnostic information provided by the ferritin assay.

Red cell protoporphyrin

When iron supply to the erythron is limited, iron incorporation into haem is restricted, leading to accumulation of the immediate precursor, protoporphyrin IX. This is lost only slowly from circulating red cells; concentrations greater than the normal upper limit of 80 µmol/mol haemoglobin therefore indicate that a reduction in iron supply has been present over the previous few weeks. Protoporphyrin levels may also increase in patients with side-roblastic anaemias and lead poisoning. Convenient analysers measure zinc protoporphyrin – the form in which most of the protoporphyrin exists in iron deficiency.

Red cell ferritin

The ferritin in the circulating erythrocyte is but a tiny residue of that present in its nucleated precursors in the bone marrow

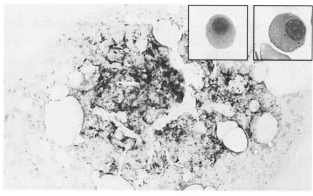

(a)

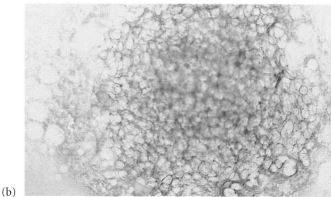

(b)

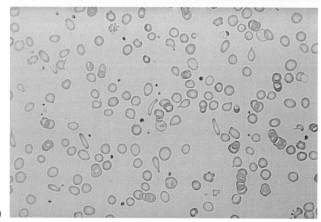

(c)

Figure 3.5 (a) Normal bone marrow showing plentiful iron in macrophages (Perls' stain) with iron granules in erythroblasts (insets). (b) Iron deficiency: bone marrow showing absence of stainable iron (Perls' stain). (c) Iron deficiency: peripheral blood film showing hypochromic microcytic red cells.

and only about 10 ag/cell (10^{-18} g/cell) remains in the erythrocyte. In general, red cell ferritin levels reflect the iron supply to the erythroid marrow and tend to vary inversely with red cell protoporphyrin levels. Despite some advantages over serum ferritin as a measure of storage iron (e.g. not affected by release of ferritin from damaged liver cells) the assay of red cell ferritin has seen little routine application. This is largely because it is

necessary to prepare red cells free of white cells (which have much higher levels of ferritin).

Percentage of hypochromic red cells

As iron supply to the erythron diminishes, the new red cells produced are increasingly hypochromic. Assessment of the haemoglobin content of individual red cells, which is possible using some automated cell counters, allows measurement of the percentage of hypochromic cells. Values rising to above 6% may help in the early identification of impaired iron supply in patients with chronic renal failure who are receiving treatment with recombinant erythropoietin, when associated inflammatory disease means that other measures of iron status can be misleading.

Iron deficiency anaemia

Sequence of events

Depletion of iron stores

When the body is in a state of negative iron balance, the first event is depletion of body stores, which are mobilized for haemoglobin production. Iron absorption is increased when stores are reduced, before anaemia develops and even when the serum iron level is still normal, although the serum ferritin will have already fallen.

Iron-deficient erythropoiesis

With further iron depletion, when the serum ferritin is below 15 µg/L, the serum transferrin saturation falls to less than 15% due to a rise in transferrin concentration and a fall in serum iron. This leads to the development of iron-deficient erythropoiesis and increasing concentrations of serum transferrin receptor and red cell protoporphyrin. At this stage, the haemoglobin, mean corpuscular volume (MCV) and mean corpuscular haemoglobin (MCH) may still be within the reference range, although they may rise significantly when iron therapy is given.

Iron deficiency anaemia

If the negative balance continues, frank iron deficiency anaemia develops. The red cells become obviously microcytic and hypochromic (Figure 3.5c), and poikilocytosis becomes more marked. The MCV and MCH are reduced, and target cells may be present. The reticulocyte count is low for the degree of anaemia. The serum TIBC rises and the serum iron falls, so that the percentage saturation of the TIBC is usually less than 10%.

The number of erythroblasts containing cytoplasmic iron (sideroblasts) is reduced at an early stage in the development of deficiency, and siderotic granules are entirely absent from these cells when iron deficiency anaemia is established. The erythroblasts have a ragged, vacuolated cytoplasm and relatively pyknotic nuclei. The bone marrow macrophages show a total absence of iron, except where very rapid blood loss outstrips the ability to mobilize the storage iron. Platelets are frequently increased.

Tissue effects of iron deficiency

When iron deficiency is severe and chronic, widespread tissue changes may be present, including koilonychia (ridged nails, breaking easily), angular stomatitis (especially in those with badly fitting dentures), glossitis (hair thinning) and pharyngeal webs (Paterson–Kelly syndrome). Partial villous atrophy, with minor degrees of malabsorption of xylose and fat, reversible by iron therapy, has been described in infants suffering from iron deficiency, but not in adults. There is a higher incidence of atrophic gastritis and histamine-fast achlorhydria in iron-deficient patients than in control subjects, and acid secretion may increase with iron therapy in some of these patients. Gastric atrophy may also predispose to iron deficiency. Pica is some-times present; in some who eat clay or chalk, this may be the cause rather than the result of iron deficiency.

Iron-dependent enzymes in the tissues are usually better pre-served than other iron-containing compounds. In severe iron deficiency, however, these enzymes are not inviolate and their levels may fall. This may be partly responsible for the general tis-sue changes, with mitochondrial swelling in many different cells (including, in the experimental animal, hepatic and myocar-dial cells), poor lymphocyte transformation and diminished cell-mediated immunity, and impaired intracellular killing of bacteria by neutrophils.

A particular concern has been the finding that infants with iron deficiency anaemia may have impaired mental develop-ment and function, and that this deficit may not be completely restored by iron therapy. There is recent evidence that pre-mature labour is more frequent in mothers with iron deficiency anaemia. It remains controversial whether impaired work performance seen in adults results from the anaemia or from depletion of mitochondrial iron-containing enzymes. It is also unclear to what extent some of the other tissue effects of iron deficiency can occur even in the absence of anaemia.

Causes of iron deficiency (Table 3.4)

Diet

Defective intake of iron is rarely the sole or major cause of iron deficiency in adults in Western communities. The diet may con-tain insufficient or poorly available iron as a result of poverty, religious tenets or food faddism. Iron deficiency is more likely to develop in subjects taking a largely vegetarian diet – the majority of the world's population – who also have increased physiolo-gical demands for iron.

Increased physiological iron requirements

Iron deficiency is common in infancy, when demands for growth may be greater than dietary supplies. It is aggravated by prema-turity, infections and delay in mixed feeding. It is also frequent in adolescence, in females and in pregnancy (Table 3.1). The fetus acquires about 280 mg of iron and a further 400–500 mg is required for the temporary expansion of the maternal red cell mass. Another 200 mg of iron is lost with the placenta and with the bleeding at delivery. Although iron absorption increases throughout pregnancy and increased requirements are partly offset by amenorrhoea, this may not be sufficient to meet the resultant net maternal outlay of over 600 mg iron.

Blood loss

Blood loss is the most common cause of iron deficiency in adults. A loss of more than about 6–8 mL of blood (3–4 mg of iron) daily becomes of importance, as this equals the maximum amount of iron that can be absorbed from a normal diet. The loss is usually from the genital tract in women or from the gas-trointestinal tract in either sex. The most common cause on a world basis is infestation with hookworm, in which anaemia is related to the degree of infestation. In the UK, menorrhagia, haemorrhoids and peptic ulceration are common, as well as gastric bleeding because of salicylates or other non-steroidal anti-inflammatory drugs, hiatus hernia, colonic diverticulosis and bowel tumours (Table 3.6). Some unusual causes of blood loss deserve mention. Cow's milk intolerance in infants may lead to gastrointestinal haemorrhage. Self-induced haemorrhage may occur as an unusual form of Munchausen syndrome. Chronic intravascular haemolysis, such as that in paroxysmal nocturnal haemoglobinuria or mechanical haemolytic anaemia, may be a serious source of urinary iron loss.

Malabsorption

Malabsorption may be the primary cause of iron deficiency or it may prevent the body adjusting to iron deficiency from other causes. Dietary iron is poorly absorbed in gluten-induced enteropathy, in both children and adults, although patients with this disease often show a response, albeit sluggish, to oral ther-apy with inorganic iron.

Management of iron deficiency

Management entails (i) identification and treatment of the underlying cause and (ii) correction of the deficiency by therapy with inorganic iron. Iron deficiency is commonly due to blood loss and, wherever possible, the site of this must be identified and the lesion treated.

Oral therapy

In most patients, body stores of iron can be restored by oral iron therapy. Iron is equally well absorbed from several simple fer-rous iron salts, and, as ferrous sulphate is the cheapest, this is the

Table 3.6 Causes of iron deficiency.

Blood loss	
Uterine	Menorrhagia, post-menopausal bleeding, parturition
Gastrointestinal	Oesophageal varices, hiatus hernia, peptic ulcer, aspirin ingestion, hookworm, hereditary telangiectasia, carcinoma of the stomach, caecum or colon, ulcerative colitis, angiodysplasia, Meckel's diverticulum, diverticulosis, haemorrhoids, etc.
Renal tract	Haematuria (e.g. renal or bladder lesion), haemoglobinuria (e.g. paroxysmal nocturnal haemoglobinuria)
Pulmonary tract	Overt haemoptysis, idiopathic pulmonary haemosiderosis
Widespread bleeding disorders	
Self-inflicted	
Malabsorption	Gluten-induced enteropathy (child or adult), gastrectomy, atrophic gastritis, chronic inflammation, clay eating, etc.
Dietary	Especially vegetarian diet

drug of first choice; 200 mg of ferrous sulphate contains 67 mg of iron. Where smaller doses are required, 300 mg of ferrous gluconate provides 36 mg of iron. It is usual to give 100–200 mg of elemental iron each day to adults and about 3 mg/kg per day as a liquid iron preparation to infants and children. The side-effects of oral iron, such as nausea, epigastric pain, diarrhoea and constipation, are related to the amount of available iron they contain. If iron causes gastrointestinal symptoms, these can usually be ameliorated by reducing the dose, or taking the iron with food, but this also reduces the amount absorbed. Enteric-coated and sustained-release preparations should not be used, as much of the iron is carried past the duodenum to sites of poor absorption. Iron reduces absorption of tetracyclines (and vice versa) and of ciprofloxacin.

The minimum rate of response should be a 20 g/L rise in haemoglobin every 3 weeks, and the usual rate is 1.5–2.0 g/L daily. This will be slower when the dose tolerated is less than 100 mg per day, but this is seldom of clinical importance. It is usually necessary to give iron for 3–6 months to correct the deficit of iron in circulating haemoglobin and in stores (shown by a rise in serum ferritin to normal).

Failure to respond to oral iron is most commonly due to the patient not taking it, although there may be continued haemorrhage or malabsorption. It is important to reassess the diagnosis as other causes of microcytic anaemia include many of the iron-loading anaemias. For instance, many patients with thalassaemia trait, sideroblastic anaemia or other anaemias have been treated with iron before haemoglobin studies, bone marrow examination or other tests have revealed the correct diagnosis. A poor response may also be obtained if the patient has an infection, renal or hepatic failure, an underlying malignant disease or any other cause of anaemia in addition to iron deficiency.

Parenteral iron therapy

This is usually unnecessary, but it may be given if subjects genuinely cannot tolerate oral iron, particularly if gastrointestinal disease, such as inflammatory bowel disease, is present. It is also occasionally necessary in gluten-induced enteropathy and when it is essential to replete body stores rapidly (e.g. where severe iron deficiency anaemia is first diagnosed in late pregnancy), or when oral iron cannot keep pace with continuing haemorrhage (e.g. in patients with hereditary haemorrhagic telangiectasia). Patients with chronic renal failure who are being treated with recombinant erythropoietin are also likely to require parenteral iron therapy. In this situation, the demand for iron by the expanded erythron may outstrip the ability to mobilize iron from stores, leading to a 'functional' iron deficiency. Increased red cell loss at dialysis contributes to iron needs and oral iron therapy is usually inadequate to prevent an impaired response to erythropoietin. The use of '% hypochromic cells' for detection of functional iron deficiency is discussed on p. 36.

From all parenteral preparations, the iron complex is taken up by macrophages of the reticuloendothelial system, from which iron is released to circulating transferrin, which then takes it to the marrow. In the UK, three preparations are available. Iron sorbitol (Jectofer®) is given deep (to avoid skin staining) by intramuscular (i.m.) injection (50–100 mg of iron per day) but not intravenously. Iron dextran (CosmoFer®) is given intravenously by slow injection or infusion. An iron–sucrose complex, Venofer®, is given by slow intravenous infusion or injection and is now considered to be the safest form. The deficit in body iron should be calculated from the degree of anaemia; it is usually 1–2 g. In patients receiving erythropoietin treatment in chronic renal failure, smaller intravenous doses of Venofer® (25–150 mg/week) may be used, with regular monitoring of serum ferritin to avoid iron overload. With iron sorbitol, some low-molecular-weight iron is released into the circulation and about 20% is excreted in the urine; this may exacerbate urinary tract infection. Parenteral iron should not be used if there is a history of allergy as anaphylaxis occasionally occurs. For iron dextran, a test dose should therefore be given slowly, followed by close medical supervision of the rest of the infusion. Flushing, nausea, urticaria, shivering, general aches and pains, dyspnoea

Table 3.7 Human porphyrias.

Form	Inheritance	Enzyme defect	Clinical features*
Hepatic			
Acute intermittent porphyria	Autosomal dominant	Porphobilinogen deaminase	A
Hereditary coproporphyria	Autosomal dominant	Coproporphyrinogen oxidase	A + P
Porphyria variegate	Autosomal dominant	Protoporphyrinogen oxidase	A + P
Porphyria cutanea tarda	Acquired or (rare) autosomal dominant	Uroporphyrinogen decarboxylase	P
Erythropoietic			
Congenital erythropoietic porphyria	Autosomal recessive	Uroporphyrinogen cosynthase	P
Erythropoietic protoporphyria	Autosomal dominant	Ferrochelatase	P

*Acute attacks (A) of gastrointestinal and/or nervous system are related to the accumulation of porphyrin precursors (ALA and PBG). Photosensitive skin lesions (P) are seen when the level of the enzyme defect in the haem synthetic pathway leads to the accumulation of formed porphyrins.

and syncope are possible immediate adverse effects. Delayed reactions, including arthralgia, fever and lymphadenopathy, are well described and can persist for several days. An exacerbation of rheumatoid arthritis may also be precipitated.

Pathological alterations in haem synthesis

Porphyrias

These are a group of inherited or acquired diseases, each characterized by a partial defect in one of the enzymes of haem synthesis (Chapter 2). Increased amounts of the intermediates of haem synthesis accumulate, the disorders being classified by whether the effects are predominantly in the liver or the erythron (Table 3.7). A full discussion of these disorders is beyond the scope of this chapter, but those with a particular haematological overlap will be mentioned briefly.

Congenital erythropoietic porphyria

This is a very rare autosomal recessive disorder that is due to reduced uroporphyrinogen III synthase activity. Most patients are heteroallelic for mutations in the uroporphyrinogen III synthase gene. Large amounts of porphyrinogens accumulate, and their conversion by spontaneous oxidation to photoactive porphyrins leads to severe, and disfiguring, cutaneous photosensitivity and dermatitis, as well as a haemolytic anaemia with splenomegaly. Increased amounts of uroporphyrin and coproporphyrin, mainly type I, are found in bone marrow, red cells, plasma, urine and faeces. Ring sideroblasts have been found in the marrow in some cases but rarely in large numbers. The age of onset and clinical severity of the disease are highly variable, ranging from non-immune hydrops fetalis to a later onset in which there are only cutaneous lesions. Treatment, including avoidance of sunlight and splenectomy to improve red cell sur-

vival, is only partially effective. High-level blood transfusions to suppress erythropoiesis (combined with iron chelation therapy) have been used to reduce porphyrin production sufficiently to abolish the clinical symptoms. Allogeneic bone marrow transplantation has been successful.

Erythropoietic protoporphyria

This is the most common erythropoietic porphyria and is usually caused by an autosomal dominant inherited deficiency of ferrochelatase, which results in increased free (not Zn) protoporphyrin concentrations in bone marrow, red cells, plasma and bile. Bone marrow reticulocytes are the primary source of the excess protoporphyrin. This leaks from cells and is excreted in the bile and faeces. Molecular analysis of the ferrochelatase gene has revealed a variety of missense, nonsense and slicing mutations as well as deletions and insertions. The onset of the disease is usually in childhood. Expression of the gene is variable, and photosensitivity and dermatitis range from mild or absent to moderate in degree. There is little haemolysis, but a mild hypochromic anaemia may occur, and accumulation of protoporphyrins can occasionally lead to severe liver disease. Treatment is by the avoidance of sunlight; β-carotene may also diminish photosensitivity. Iron deficiency should be avoided as this may increase the amount of free protoporphyrin.

Porphyria cutanea tarda

This is the most common of the hepatic porphyrias and occurs worldwide. The incidence in the UK has been estimated at 2–5 per million. Type I or 'sporadic' porphyria cutanea tarda (PCT) accounts for 80% of cases of PCT. The underlying metabolic abnormality is decreased activity of uroporphyrinogen decarboxylase (UROD) in the liver. Type II disease is an autosomal dominant disorder caused by mutations in the UROD gene. Type III disease is a rare familial form and appears to result from unknown inherited defects that affect hepatic UROD activity.

Table 3.8 Sideroblastic anaemias.

Hereditary	
X-linked	Mutations of erythroid-specific ALAS2 (Xp11.21), associated with spinocerebellar ataxia – ABC7 mutations (Xq13.3)
Mitochondrial	DNA deletions (e.g. Pearson and Kearns–Sayre syndromes)
Autosomal	Thiamine responsive, mutations in THTR-1 (DIDMOAD), other
Acquired	
Primary	Refractory anaemia with ring sideroblasts in FAB classification of myelodysplasia
Secondary	Abnormal pyridoxine metabolism: pyridoxine antagonists (isoniazid, penicillamine), alcohol, pyridoxine deficiency
	Mitochondrial toxicity: chloramphenicol, lead poisoning
	Other diseases: e.g. rheumatoid arthritis, myxoedema, carcinomatosis

DIDMOAD, diabetes insipidus, diabetes mellitus, optic atrophy and deafness.

There is a marked increase in porphyrins in liver, plasma, urine and faeces. In the urine, uroporphyrin and heptacarboxyl porphyrin predominate with lesser amounts of coproporphyrin and penta- and hexacarboxylporphyrin. The disease is characterized by photosensitivity and dermatitis. It is precipitated in middle or later life, more often in men than women, by factors such as liver disease, alcohol excess or oestrogen therapy. A modest increase in liver iron is a common feature.

Either the homozygous or heterozygous presence of the *HFE* C282Y and H63D mutations may predispose to the development of PCT. Prevalence of the C282Y mutation is increased in both sporadic (type I) and familial (type II) PCT. In the UK, only homozygosity for C282Y (found in about 25% of patients) is significantly more common than in the general population (0.7%). In southern Europe, where C282Y is much less common, the H63D mutation is associated with PCT. Iron is known to inhibit uroporphyrinogen decarboxylase. Removal of the iron by repeated phlebotomy is standard treatment, usually leading to remission.

Lead poisoning

Chronic ingestion of lead in humans causes an anaemia that is usually normochromic or slightly hypochromic. Red cell lifespan is shortened and there is a mild rise in reticulocytes, but jaundice is rare. Basophilic stippling is a characteristic, although not universal, finding and it is thought to be due to precipitation of RNA, resulting from inhibition of the enzyme pyrimidine 5'-nucleotidase. Siderotic granules, and occasionally Cabot rings, are found in circulating red cells. The bone marrow shows increased sideroblasts, in some patients with ring sideroblasts. Red cell protoporphyrin and coproporphyrin are raised, as are urinary excretion of ALA, coproporphyrin III and uroporphyrin I.

The cause of the anaemia appears to be multifactorial. Haemolysis, probably due to the blocking of sulphydryl groups, with consequent denaturation of structural proteins, and damage to mitochondria with defective haemoglobin production due to inhibition of the enzymes of haem synthesis, are the major factors.

Sideroblastic anaemia

The sideroblastic anaemias comprise a group of refractory anaemias (Table 3.8), in which there are variable numbers of hypochromic cells in the peripheral blood, with an excess of iron in the bone marrow, many of the developing erythroblasts containing iron granules arranged in a ring around the nucleus (Figure 3.6). These ring sideroblasts (more than four perinuclear granules per cell and covering one-third or more of the nuclear circumference) are the diagnostic feature of the anaemia and, although they may form a small percentage of the erythroblasts in a wide variety of clinical disorders, they are present in large numbers (> 15% erythroblasts) in primary sideroblastic anaemias. The various types of sideroblast that may be seen in the marrow are classified in Table 3.9.

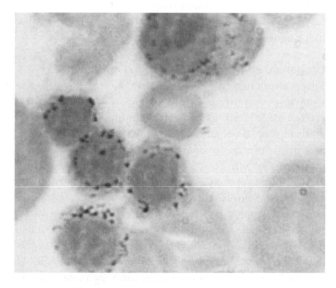

Figure 3.6 Sideroblastic anaemia. Erythroblasts showing perinuclear rings of iron (Perls' stain).

Table 3.9 Siderocytes and sideroblasts.

Siderocyte	Mature red cell containing one or more siderotic granules (Pappenheimer bodies)
Normal sideroblast	Nucleated red cell containing one or more siderotic granules, granules few, difficult to see, randomly distributed in the cytoplasm, reduced proportion of sideroblasts in iron deficiency and anaemia of chronic disorders
Abnormal sideroblasts	Cytoplasmic iron deposits (ferritin aggregates): increased granulation, granules larger and more numerous than normal, easily visible and randomly distributed, proportion of sideroblasts usually parallels the percentage saturation of transferrin (e.g. haemolytic anaemia, megaloblastic anaemia, iron overload, thalassaemia disorders) Mitochondrial iron deposits (non-ferritin iron): ring sideroblasts in inherited and acquired sideroblastic anaemias

Inherited sideroblastic anaemias

These are rare disorders manifesting mainly in males, usually in childhood or adolescence, but occasionally presenting late in life, when they need to be distinguished from the more common acquired 'refractory anaemia with ring sideroblasts'.

X-linked sideroblastic anaemia

In most reported families, inheritance has followed an X-linked pattern. More than 25 different mutations of erythroid-specific ALAS2, located at Xp11.2l, have been identified. All have been single-base substitutions. Most lead to changes in protein structure, causing instability or loss of function. They are found scattered over the seven exons (out of 11) encoding the C-terminal, catalytically active part of the protein. Mutations affecting the promoter have also been shown to cause disease. Function may be rescued to a variable degree by administration of pyridoxal phosphate – the essential cofactor for ALAS2 – the best responses occurring when the mutation affects the pyridoxal phosphate-binding domain of the enzyme. The response is better if iron overload is reduced by phlebotomy or chelation.

A rare form of X-linked sideroblastic anaemia (ASAT), refractory to pyridoxine, is caused by abnormalities in the ATP-binding cassette transporter gene (ABC7) at Xq13.3. This form is associated with early-onset, non-progressive cerebellar ataxia. A useful diagnostic distinction is the presence within the red cells of increased zinc protoporphyrin, despite adequate iron stores, rather than the low/normal levels found in patients with abnormalities in ALAS2. The anaemia is mild to moderately severe. Three abnormalities of protein structure have been described, and these lie within 34 amino acids of one another at the C-terminal end of the transmembrane domain.

Female carriers of X-linked sideroblastic anaemia may show partial haematological expression, usually with only mild or no anaemia, although, rarely, with a severe dimorphic anaemia. This may depend on variation in the severity of the defect, as well as the degree of lyonization of the affected X-chromosome. Late onset in some patients suggests that the degree of lyonization may change with age. Iron loading may also aggravate the defect in haem synthesis in both males and females with sideroblastic anaemia.

Patients with X-linked sideroblastic anaemia show a hypochromic, often microcytic, anaemia. There may be a few circulating siderocytes, normoblasts and cells with punctate basophilia, but these features become pronounced only if the spleen has been removed. The bone marrow shows erythroid hyperplasia and the erythroblasts tend to be microcytic with a vacuolated cytoplasm. There are many (> 15%) ringed sideroblasts. The ineffective erythropoiesis is not usually accompanied by bone deformities, but some bossing of the skull and enlargement of the facial bones may result from the erythroid expansion. The spleen may be enlarged. Patients may present with severe iron overload even when the anaemia is relatively mild, but the rate of iron loading is accelerated if red cell transfusions are needed. Iron loading, however, aggravates the anaemia.

Mitochondrial DNA mutations

Deletions of mitochondrial DNA, sometimes associated with duplications, are known to be the cause of Pearson marrow–pancreas syndrome, typically consisting of sideroblastic anaemia, pancreatic exocrine dysfunction and lactic acidosis. This is a severe disorder of early onset, presenting usually with failure to thrive, persistent diarrhoea and lactic acidosis. All haemopoietic cell lineages can be affected, and the anaemia is typically macrocytic with prominent vacuoles in cells of both myeloid and erythroid lineages.

Mitochondrial DNA has its own genetic code and encodes mitochondrial tRNA and ribosomal RNA as well as several mitochondrial proteins. In Pearson's syndrome, deletions may encompass tRNA as well as mitochondrial genes and therefore have an effect on the function of all mitochondrion-encoded proteins, causing a considerable loss of mitochondrial function. The presence of many different mitochondria within nucleated cells enable the coexistence of normal and abnormal species, the proportion of which is likely to vary within different tissues, a phenomenon known as *heteroplasmy*. The extent to which different tissues are affected depends to some extent on this proportion and detection often requires the study of different tissues. Inheritance is difficult to determine for the same reason and most cases are described as of 'sporadic' occurrence.

Abnormalities of a high-affinity transporter of thiamine

A gene (*SLC19A2*) encoding a putative thiamine transporter (THTR-1) that is widely and variably expressed has now been mapped to the long arm of chromosome 1 (1q23.3). Abnormalities in this gene are responsible for the thiamine-responsive megaloblastic anaemia (TRMA), or Roger's syndrome. This syndrome is inherited in an autosomal recessive manner and combines diabetes insipidus, diabetes mellitus, optic atrophy and deafness (DIDMOAD), which respond in varying degrees to pharmacological doses of thiamine (vitamin B_1). Ring sideroblasts in varying numbers are typically present and onset is usually in childhood, although some symptoms may be present in infancy. A direct link between the presence of the mutation and mitochondrial iron loading has yet to be demonstrated.

There are still a substantial number of cases of inherited sideroblastic anaemias in which the exact underlying genetic defect remains obscure. These cases may or may not show sex-linked inheritance and often show a macrocytic or dimorphic picture.

Acquired sideroblastic anaemias

Primary acquired sideroblastic anaemia (refractory anaemia with ring sideroblasts)

This is a form of myelodysplasia (refractory anaemia with ring sideroblasts), and arises as a clonal disorder of haemopoiesis. The anaemia is often macrocytic with raised red cell protoporphyrin concentrations, in contrast to X-linked sideroblastic anaemia. Marked erythroid hyperplasia may be present, together with increased iron stores. In these patients, abnormalities in the white cell or platelet precursors are usually absent and the risk of transformation to acute myeloid leukaemia appears less than in other myelodysplastic disorders. Smaller numbers (< 15%) of ring sideroblasts may be present in patients with any of the other myelodysplastic and myeloproliferative diseases. Recent data suggest that acquired defects of mitochondrial DNA may underlie iron transport abnormalities in primary acquired sideroblastic anaemia.

Secondary sideroblastic anaemias

Sideroblastic anaemia associated with pyridoxine deficiency has been described, although not completely documented, in a few patients with gluten-induced enteropathy, in pregnancy, and with haemolytic anaemias, such as sickle cell disease and mechanical or autoimmune haemolytic anaemia. Sideroblastic anaemia may be found as a complication of antituberculous chemotherapy, particularly with isoniazid and cycloserine (pyridoxine antagonists). Sideroblastic anaemia occurs in alcoholism if there is associated malnutrition and folate deficiency. Suggested mechanisms include interference with haem formation and pyridoxine metabolism. The anaemia rapidly reverses with abstinence from alcohol, a normal diet and pyridoxine therapy. Chloramphenicol inhibits mitochondrial protein synthesis and in some patients causes ring sideroblast formation,

presumably as a result of impaired haem formation in the mitochondria. Lead inhibits several enzymes concerned in haem synthesis and may damage structural mitochondrial proteins. In some cases, ring sideroblasts are visible in the marrow.

Treatment

Pyridoxine

Some patients with X-linked sideroblastic anaemia respond to pyridoxine, given initially in doses of 100–200 mg per day. The response is usually partial. Some patients require only small doses (less than 10 mg per day) to maintain a higher haemoglobin concentration.

Pyridoxine therapy is almost always ineffective in primary acquired sideroblastic anaemias. Some secondary sideroblastic anaemias may, however, be completely reversed by pyridoxine therapy. This has been described in alcoholism, haemolytic anaemia and gluten-induced enteropathy, as well as in patients receiving antituberculous chemotherapy, in whom the drugs have been stopped and pyridoxine administered.

Other forms of treatment

Folic acid may benefit patients with secondary anaemia. For refractory patients, the anaemia may remain stable and, if the patient is transfusion independent, no treatment is needed. Patients requiring regular red cell transfusions require iron chelation therapy. Iron loading may aggravate the anaemia and, in some patients, improvement in the anaemia has followed iron removal by phlebotomy or iron chelation therapy. Splenectomy should usually be avoided, as it does not benefit the anaemia and leads to persistently high platelet counts postoperatively, with a high incidence of thromboembolism.

Selected bibliography

Anderson KE, Sassa S, Bishop DF, Desnick RJ (2001) Disorders of heme biosynthesis: X-linked sideroblastic anaemia and the porphyrias. In: *The Metabolic and Molecular Basis of Inherited Disease*, 8th edn (CR Scriver, AL Beaudet, WS Sly, D Valle, B Childs, KW Kinzler, B Vogelstein, eds), pp. 2991–3062. McGraw-Hill, New York.

Andrews NC (2002) A genetic view of iron homeostasis. *Seminars in Hematology* 39: 227–34.

Babcock M, de Silva D, Oaks R *et al.* (1997) Regulation of mitochondrial iron accumulation by. YFH1p, a putative homolog of frataxin. *Science* 276: 1709–11.

Barrett TG, Bundey S, Macleod AF (1995) Neurodegeneration and diabetes: UK nationwide study of Weifrom (DIDMOAD) syndrome. *Lancet* 346: 1458–63.

Beguin Y (2003) Soluble transferrin receptor for the evaluation of erythropoiesis and iron status. *Clinica Chimica Acta* 329: 9–22.

British Nutrition Foundation's Task Force (1995) Iron: *Nutritional and Physiological Significance*. Chapman & Hall, London.

Cairo G, Pietrangelo A (2000) Iron regulatory proteins in pathobiology. *Biochemical Journal* 352: 241–50.

Cazzola M (2002) Hereditary hyperferritinaemia/cataract syndrome. *Clinical Haematology* 15: 385–98.

Cazzola M, Dezza L, Bergamaschi G *et al.* (1983) Biologic and clinical significance of red cell ferritin. *Blood* 62: 1078–87.

Drtieko TB, Bárány P, Cazzola M *et al.* (1997) Management of iron deficiency in renal anaemia: guidelines for the optimal therapeutic approach in erythropoietin-treated patients. *Clinical Nephrology* 48: 1–8.

Drysdale J, Arosio P, Invernizzi R *et al.* (2002) Mitochondrial ferritin: a new player in iron metabolism. *Blood Cells, Molecules and Diseases* 29: 376–83.

Ganz T (2003) Hepcidin, a key regulator of iron metabolism and mediator of anemia of inflammation. *Blood* 102: 783–8.

Harrison PM, Arosio P (1996) Ferritins: molecular properties, iron storage function and cellular regulation. *Bba-Bioenergetics* 1275: 161–203.

Hentz MW, Muckenthaler MU, Andrew NC (2004) Balancing acts: molecular control of mammalian iron metabolism. *Cell* 117: 285–97.

Hider RC (2002) Nature of nontransferrin-bound iron. *European Journal of Clinical Investigation* 32: 50–4.

Lebay V, Ras T, Baran D *et al.* (1999) Mutations in SCL19AZ cause thiamine-responsive megaloblastic anaemia associated with diabetes mellitus and deafness. *Nature Genetics* 22: 300–4.

Locatelli F, Aljama P, Bárány P *et al.* (2004) Revised European best practice guidelines for the management of anaemia in patients with chronic renal failure. *Nephrology Dialysis Transplantation* 19, Supplement 2.

Lozoff B, De Andraca I, Castillo M *et al.* (2003) Behavioral and developmental effects of preventing iron-deficiency anemia in healthy full-term infants. *Pediatrics* 112: 846–54.

May A, Bishop DF (1998) The molecular biology and pyridoxine-responsiveness of X-linked sideroblastic anaemia. *Haematologica* 83: 56–76.

Nemeth E, Tuttle MS, Powelson J *et al.* (2004) Hepcidin regulates iron efflux by binding to ferroportin and inducing its internalization. *Science* (in press).

OMIM (Online Mendelian Inheritance in Man) www.ncbi.nlm.nih.gov/OMIM/ (*knowledge base of human genes and genetic disorders*).

Roy C, Andrews NC (2001) Recent advances in disorders of iron metabolism: mutations, mechanisms and modifiers. *Human Molecular Genetics* 10: 2181–6.

Srai SKS, Bomford A, McArdle HJ (2002) Iron transport across cell membranes: molecular understanding of duodenal and placental iron transport. *Clinical Haematology* 15: 243–60.

WHO (2001) *Iron Deficiency Anaemia. Assessment, Prevention and Control. A Guide for Programme Managers.* WHO, Geneva.

Worwood M (2001) Iron deficiency anaemia and iron overload. In: *Dacie and Lewis Practical Haematology: Laboratory Methods, Ferritin, Serum Iron and TIBC, Serum Transferrin Receptor* (SM Lewis, BJ Bain, I Bates, eds), pp. 115–128. Churchill Livingstone, London.

CHAPTER 4

Iron overload

A Victor Hoffbrand and Mark Worwood

4

Introduction

Excessive iron accumulation may eventually lead to tissue damage. Iron overload of the parenchymal cells of the liver commonly arises when there is excessive iron absorption, whereas iron administered parenterally (e.g. as multiple transfusions) is first taken up in senescent red cells by macrophages. There is no absolute distinction, however, between the two sources of iron loading, as iron in macrophages is slowly released to transferrin, from which it can be taken up by parenchymal cells. A classification of iron overload is shown in Table 4.1. Severe iron overload, arbitrarily defined as more than a 5-g excess, is confined to the genetic haemochromatosis, together with the iron-loading anaemias and sub-Saharan (African) dietary iron overload.

Genetic haemochromatosis

Classification

Genetic haemochromatosis (GH) is now being classified according to the genetic defect causing iron overload (Table 4.2). The vast majority of cases are of type 1 – involving the *HFE* gene (Chapter 3). In populations of northern European origin about 90% of patients with GH are homozygous for the *HFE* Cys282Tyr mutation (C282Y). In southern Europe, homozygosity for C282Y is found in only about 60% of patients with GH. Types 1, 2 and 3 are autosomal recessive disorders, but type 4 haemochromatosis is inherited as a dominant condition. In type 4, mutations in the ferroportin 1 gene are associated with iron accumulation in macrophages with a raised serum ferritin concentration. The transferrin saturation may be normal.

Table 4.1 Causes of iron overload.

Severe iron overload (> 5 g excess)

Excess iron absorption	Hereditary haemochromatosis
	Massive ineffective erythropoiesis (e.g. β-thalassaemia intermedia, sideroblastic anaemia, congenital dyserythropoietic anaemia)
Increased iron intake	Sub-Saharan dietary iron overload (in combination with a genetic determinant of increased absorption)
	Excess parenteral iron therapy
Repeated red cell transfusions	Congenital anaemias (e.g. β-thalassaemia major, red cell aplasia)
	Acquired refractory anaemias (e.g. myelodysplasia and aplastic anaemia)

Modest iron overload (< 5 g excess)

	Chronic liver disease (e.g. alcoholic cirrhosis)
	Porphyria cutanea tarda
	Rare genetic disorders of iron metabolism (e.g. atransferrinaemia, aceruloplasminaemia)

Focal iron overload*

	Pulmonary haemorrhage, idiopathic pulmonary haemosiderosis
	Chronic haemoglobinuria (e.g. paroxysmal nocturnal haemoglobinuria)

*May occur in association with general body iron deficiency.

Table 4.2 Classification of genetic haemochromatosis.

Type	Gene	Inheritance and phenotype	Severity	Incidence
1	HFE	AR parenchymal, iron overload	Highly variable	Common
	Digenic (HFE, HAMP, HJN)	AR parenchymal, iron overload	Unknown	Rare
2 (juvenile)	Hemojuvelin	AR parenchymal, iron overload	Severe	Rare
	HAMP	AR parenchymal, iron overload	Severe	Rare
3	TFR2	AR parenchymal, iron overload	Severe	Rare
4	Ferroportin 1	AD RE iron	Variable	Rare

AD, autosomal dominant; AR, autosomal recessive.
For gene symbols see Table 3.1.

Type 1 haemochromatosis

Inherited as an autosomal recessive trait, this is one of the most common genetic conditions found in populations of northern European origin. In the UK, about one in eight people are carriers of the C282Y mutation of the HFE gene, and about 1 in 200 are homozygous for this mutation. Homozygosity is strongly associated with GH, with about 90% of patients with genetic iron overload having this genotype. Digenetic disease has been described – patients being heterozygous for HFE C282Y and a mutation in the HAMP (hepcidin) gene. In homozygotes, there is a gradual accumulation of iron, leading to tissue damage, which may present as cirrhosis of the liver, diabetes, hypogonadism, arthritis and a slate-grey skin pigmentation. Hepatocellular carcinoma develops in 25% of established cases with cirrhosis. Most patients present between the ages of 40 and 60 years, but the clinical penetrance is low (see p. 48). Full phenotypic expression of the disorder is dependent upon other factors, including dietary iron intake, blood loss and probably other genetic factors modifying the genotype. Menstrual losses account for a lower frequency and generally delayed onset in women.

Nature of the defect

A defect in the regulation of intestinal iron absorption, at the stage of either mucosal iron uptake or mucosal transfer, is probable, but the molecular basis of the disorder is only now beginning to be understood. The responsible gene is known to be located on the short arm of chromosome 6, close to the human leucocyte antigen A locus (HLA-A), and association with HLA-A3 and, to a lesser extent, B7 suggested a founder mutation in a chromosome carrying the A3, B7 haplotype. Subsequent linkage analyses using multiple genetic markers have supported this suggestion, and positional cloning led to the identification of a novel MHC class I-like gene, 4 Mb telomeric to the HLA A locus. The gene, *HFE*, contains seven exons, and in over 80% of patients there is homozygosity for a missense mutation. This mutation, G to A at nucleotide 845, results in a cysteine to tyrosine substitution at amino acid 282 (C282Y) in exon 4. A second variant in exon 2 (187C→G) results in a histidine to aspartic acid substitution at amino acid 63 (His63Asp or H63D). This is carried by about 20% of the general population. In the UK, about 90% of patients presenting with haemochromatosis are homozygous for HFE C282Y, and another 4% are compound heterozygotes for the two mutations. *HFE* was therefore a strong candidate for the haemochromatosis gene and this was confirmed by the demonstration that HFE knockout mice and mice homozygous for the C282Y mutation develop iron overload.

How this abnormality might give rise to the iron loading has been the subject of much debate. After the demonstration that in some cell lines the normal HFE protein binds to the transferrin receptor and reduces iron uptake from transferrin, it was speculated that this would be the mechanism leading to increased iron absorption. It was difficult to explain, however, how increased iron uptake from transferrin in developing intestinal epithelial cells, as a result of the failure of expression of the mutated HFE protein, causes increased iron absorption. Moreover, duodenal mucosal iron levels in haemochromatosis are normal or reduced. More recently, it has been shown that hepcidin release from the liver requires expression of HFE and that in mice lacking HFE or expressing the C282Y protein hepcidin expression is low (Chapter 3). Hepcidin is a negative regulator of iron absorption possibly by binding ferroportin and causing its internalization. Lack of hepcidin upregulates expression of a number of iron transport proteins in the intestinal mucosa, thus increasing iron uptake and absorption. Hepcidin also controls iron release from macrophages. This explains the findings in the early stages of haemochromatosis – increased iron absorption, a raised serum iron and a paucity of iron in macrophages. Most recent data suggest that HFE, transferrin receptor 2 and hemojuvelin defects result in reduced hepcidin secretion.

HFE mutation frequencies worldwide

Genotypes have been reported for over 50 000 subjects throughout the world. The C282Y mutation is confined to populations of European origin and within Europe is most frequent in the north. The highest frequencies for the allele are found in Ireland,

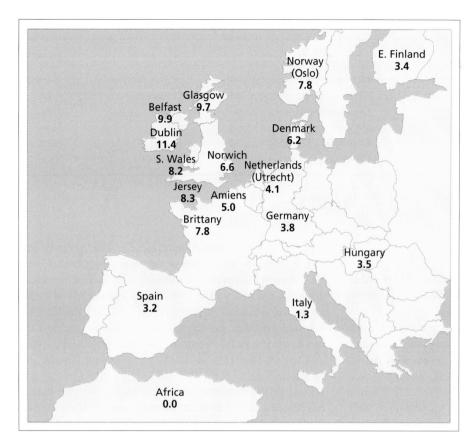

Figure 4.1 Frequency of chromosomes carrying the C282Y mutation in regions of Europe (from Worwood 2004 with permission).

Scotland, Wales, Brittany and Scandinavia (Figure 4.1) and the lowest frequencies in southern Italy and Greece. The H63D mutation is found throughout the world but is most common in Europe, where allele frequencies vary from 10% to 20% with a mean of 15%. The only other variant found throughout Europe is Ser65Cys (S65C), which has a frequency of about 2%. Other *HFE* gene mutations associated with iron accumulation have been described – mostly in individual families.

HFE mutations and iron status

The haemochromatosis gene may have increased in frequency because of a selective advantage for heterozygotes – protection against iron deficiency anaemia. Homozygotes would be unlikely to suffer the effects of iron overload before reproducing. About 25% of heterozygotes, identified by HLA typing of family members of haemochromatosis patients, have either a raised transferrin saturation or a raised serum ferritin. Coexistent disease may be the explanation for raised ferritin concentrations in many heterozygotes for *HFE* C282Y. In population surveys, slight but significantly higher values for serum iron and transferrin saturation have been found in heterozygotes for either C282Y or H63D compared with subjects lacking these mutations. The differences in ferritin levels are smaller and not significant. In compound heterozygotes, and those homozygous for H63D, there are greater differences in both transferrin saturation and serum ferritin although significantion accumulation is rare. In heterozygotes for C282Y or H63D, haemoglobin levels are slightly higher than in subjects lacking mutations, but it has not been clearly demonstrated that this leads to a lower prevalence of anaemia among women carrying either mutation. There is little information about S65C, but in combination with C282Y or H63D it may be associated with mild iron accumulation.

HFE mutations and morbidity

Although advanced haemochromatosis is characterized by diabetes, arthritis and cirrhosis, there is little evidence that possession of HFE mutations is a risk factor for these conditions except through iron overload. The frequency of homozygosity or heterozygosity for C282Y or H63D mutations is not generally increased in patients with arthritis, diabetes and heart disease. Homozygosity for C282Y is more frequent in patients with cirrhosis and hepatoma than in the general population. In one study, homozygosity for C282Y was increased in patients with type 1, late-onset diabetes. Alcohol is a definite risk factor for the development of cirrhosis in patients homozygous for C282Y. The significance of other genetic modifiers remains uncertain.

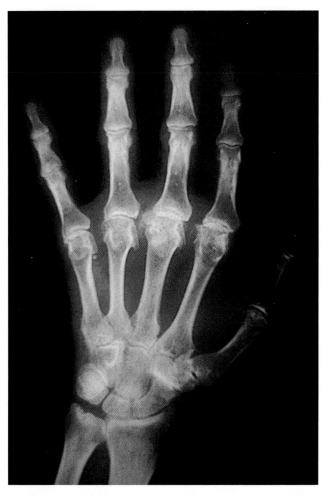

Figure 4.2 Radiograph of hand – patient with haemochromatosis showing loss of joint space and erosion of cartilage at the metacarpophalangeal joints.

Diagnosis: clinical

The variety of clinical presentations and their lack of specificity for haemochromatosis means that a high degree of clinical suspicion is needed. Fatigue, diabetes mellitus, gonadal failure and arthritis may be present for several years before the diagnosis is made. Arthritis particularly affects the second and third metacarpophalangeal joints (Figure 4.2), and destructive arthropathy of hip and knee joints occurs in 10% of patients. There is chondrocalcinosis with pyrophosphate deposition in the joints. Abdominal pain may result from hepatic enlargement or hepatocellular carcinoma. Grey skin pigmentation results from excess melanin deposition.

Diagnosis: iron status

Transferrin saturation and serum ferritin

In asymptomatic subjects, iron accumulation is indicated by a raised transferrin saturation (> 55% for men and > 50% for women). Most men and about 50% of women who are homozygous for *HFE* C282Y will have a raised transferrin saturation. As iron accumulates, the serum ferritin concentration rises, and values of > 200 μg/L (women) and 300 μg/L (men) suggest iron overload. Serum ferritin concentrations largely reflect iron turnover in phagocytic cells and do not provide an early indication of iron accumulation in liver parenchymal cells. Thus, measurement of transferrin saturation is essential for early detection of iron loading. In patients with infection, inflammation or malignancy, or undergoing surgery, transferrin saturation may, however, be depressed and the serum ferritin concentration elevated. In most cases, genotyping will confirm the diagnosis of GH.

Liver biopsy

In patients homozygous for C282Y with normal serum transaminase activity, serum ferritin concentration < 1000 μg/L and without hepatomegaly there is no need for a liver biopsy in order to make a diagnosis of GH. A liver biopsy is essential to assess tissue damage in patients with evidence of liver disease or a serum ferritin concentration > 1000 μg/L. In patients with an unexplained raised transferrin saturation and serum ferritin, who are not homozygous for C282Y, a liver biopsy may be required to confirm iron overload (Figure 4.3a and b).

Part of the liver biopsy should be washed to remove extraneous blood before wrapping in aluminium foil and drying to constant weight for chemical measurement of iron concentration. Values in excess of 80 μmol/g dry weight (4.5 mg/g dry weight) indicate iron overload. In the differential diagnosis of GH, where there is a progressive increase in iron with age, it is useful to express the result as the 'hepatic iron index' (μmol iron/g dry weight divided by age in years). An elevated index (> 2.0) generally separates patients with homozygous GH from heterozygotes or those with alcoholic liver disease. The hepatic iron index may be helpful in distinguishing iron overload due to GH from the more modest iron overload that can occur secondary to chronic liver disease (usually alcoholic). As alcohol is one of the factors that may enhance the phenotypic expression of GH, this diagnostic distinction is important.

Desferrioxamine-induced iron excretion

The measurement of urine iron excretion following a single i.m. injection of 0.5 g of desferrioxamine (DFX) is still occasionally useful in the assessment of possible iron overload, particularly when clinical considerations rule out the more definitive liver biopsy. Urinary excretion of iron greater than 2 mg in 24 h indicates increased iron stores. A number of other factors influence iron chelation by DFX (p. 54) and, although hepatocytes are an important site of action of the drug, reticuloendothelial iron is also a major source of urine iron excretion in response to the drug. The value of the test as a measure of parenchymal iron overload is therefore limited.

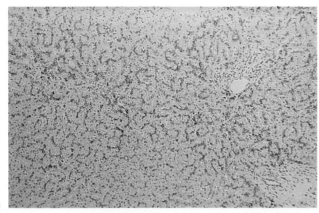

(a)

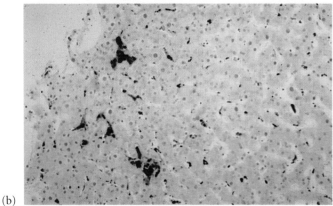

(b)

Figure 4.3 Liver histology (Perls' stain). (a) Liver biopsy for a patient with type 1 haemochromatosis, showing staining predominantly in parenchymal cells. (b) Liver biopsy for a patient with type 4 haemochromatosis, showing iron staining predominantly in Kupffer cells.

Mobilization of iron by phlebotomy to calculate iron stores

This is carried out by once-weekly venesection (450 mL of blood) until the serum ferritin concentration is < 20 μg/L and transferrin saturation is < 16%. Haemoglobin (Hb) levels should be measured weekly and the rate of venesection reduced if anaemia develops. Serum ferritin should be monitored monthly. The transferrin saturation should be measured weekly when the ferritin concentration drops below 50 μg/L. Once storage iron has been removed the serum ferritin concentration will be less than 15 μg/L, the transferrin saturation < 16% and anaemia will develop. The amount of iron removed at each venesection is calculated by weighing the blood bag before and after venesection (density of blood is 1.05 g/mL) and assuming that 450 mL of blood (Hb concentration = 13.5 g/dL) contains 200 mg of iron. Iron absorption should be allowed for at a rate of 3 mg per day (20 mg per week). With these assumptions, 25 weekly venesections will remove 4.5 g of iron. The amount of storage iron measured by the technique in normal adults has been shown to be about 750 mg in men and 250 mg in women.

Non-invasive methods (see also p. 51)

The superconducting quantum interface device (SQUID) bio-susceptometry technique is sensitive, accurate and reproducible. It depends on the paramagnetic properties of haemosiderin and ferritin. Unlike magnetic resonance imaging (MRI), it does not distinguish parenchymal from reticuloendothelial iron, but the result closely correlates with chemical estimation of liver iron, except when fibrosis is present. Machines are expensive to build and run and at present there are only four worldwide (none in the UK).

Although MRI techniques are being increasingly used as indirect measures of both liver and heart iron (see p. 52), they require special analytical skills and have not been generally applied to type 1 haemochromatosis.

Treatment

Removal of excess iron by regular phlebotomy greatly reduces the mortality from cardiac and hepatic failure, although hepatocellular carcinoma accounts for a substantial proportion of deaths in those with established disease. Early diagnosis is therefore a priority, as patients identified and treated before the onset of cirrhosis of the liver have a normal life expectancy.

Phlebotomy should be at a rate of 450 mL of blood each week, but the rate may need to be reduced if anaemia develops. Weekly phlebotomy will need to be continued for at least 6 months to remove a total iron excess, which is usually greater than 5 g in established symptomatic disease but may be more than 20 g. The amount of iron removed before anaemia develops should be calculated (see above). Since the advent of genetic testing, confirmation of iron overload by liver biopsy is not necessary in the absence of liver damage and quantitative phlebotomy provides the only practical way of confirming the presence of iron overload.

When iron stores are exhausted, the frequency of phlebotomy should be reduced to two to four units each year, to continue indefinitely. The aim is to maintain a normal transferrin saturation (< 50%) and a serum ferritin in the low normal range (< 50 μg/L).

Fatigue and transaminase elevation usually reverse on venesection. In some patients, diabetes mellitus, hypogonadism and arthralgia improve, but cirrhosis and arthritis are not reversible.

Iron chelation with DFX given as a continuous intravenous infusion (see below) may have a limited role in the short-term management of patients with life-threatening cardiac failure.

Clinical penetrance

Before the discovery of the *HFE* gene, it was assumed that every family member who was homozygous for haemochromatosis would eventually accumulate sufficient iron to cause tissue damage. Recent studies, in which subjects homozygous for *HFE* C282Y have been compared with 'wild-type' subjects, have shown that the frequencies of lethargy, arthralgia and diabetes are the same. There is, however, a small but significant increase in the percentage of subjects with either raised serum transaminase activity or fibrosis/cirrhosis in the C282Y homozygous group. Furthermore, population surveys have shown that less than 5% of subjects homozygous for C282Y ever receive a diagnosis of haemochromatosis. Despite much debate about ascertainment bias in family and population surveys, it is becoming clear that most men who are homozygous for C282Y will have a raised transferrin saturation before the age of 30 years; a proportion will have an elevated serum ferritin concentration, but only a minority will eventually develop fibrosis and cirrhosis of the liver. Only about 50% of homozygous women have a raised transferrin saturation, and progression through iron accumulation and tissue damage is usually, but not always, slower. In one population study in the USA, the clinical penetrance was estimated to be as low as 1%.

Family testing

Physicians should discuss with the patient the desirability of testing all first-degree relatives over the age of consent in order to identify those at risk. Transferrin saturation and serum ferritin concentration should be measured along with *HFE* genotyping. Genetic testing may identify other family members homozygous for *HFE* C282Y. If the serum ferritin concentration is normal and there is no evidence of liver disease, transferrin saturation and serum ferritin should be measured at yearly intervals and treatment instituted if necessary. Compound heterozygotes are at lesser risk of iron overload but should also be tested by measuring transferrin saturation and serum ferritin – perhaps at 3-yearly intervals. For heterozygotes, iron status should be determined and, if normal, reassessed after 5 years to ensure that no other iron-loading genes are present. About 25% of heterozygotes for C282Y show minor abnormalities of iron metabolism, e.g. a raised transferrin saturation or serum ferritin concentration. Raised ferritin concentration may relate to chronic disease rather than increased iron stores. Iron accumulation similar to that in C282Y homozygotes is rarely seen.

Associations with other conditions

The *HFE* C282Y mutation is relatively common; heterozygosity, and even homozygosity, may occur with other haematological conditions, including inherited sideroblastic anaemia. The occasional presence of iron overload in patients with haematological disorders such as congenital spherocytosis, in whom it is otherwise uncommon, may be due to a combined effect on iron absorption of increased eythropoiesis and coincidental inheritance of the heterozygous state for GH. Porphyria cutanea tarda is discussed in Chapter 3.

Population screening

Widespread population screening on the basis of measures of iron status or by genetic testing has been proposed. Genetic testing of the whole population would, however, be premature, as the precise level of risk for a C282Y homozygote developing iron overload is not yet known. Once the factors that convey a high risk of developing significant iron overload and tissue damage have been identified, it may be appropriate to reconsider this question.

Type 2 (juvenile) haemochromatosis

Juvenile haemochromatosis is a rare autosomal recessive disease, with clinical symptoms appearing in the second and third decades of life, characterized by cardiomyopathy and hypogonadism. The hemojuvelin locus has been mapped to chromosome 1q21. Iron absorption is greater than in type 1 haemochromatosis. Mutations were found in Greek, Canadian and French families with G320V, accounting for two-thirds of these mutations. Like *HFE*, hemojuvelin modulates hepcidin expression and serum hepcidin is low in homozygous affected individuals with hemojuvelin mutations.

Mutations in the hepcidin (HAMP) gene (see Chapter 3) have been described in several families with a type of juvenile haemochromatosis not linked to chromosome 1. Affected subjects were homozygous for the mutation in each case.

Type 3 haemochromatosis

Haemochromatosis type 3 is phenotypically similar to *HFE*-associated haemochromatosis but is due to mutations in the transferrin receptor 2 gene (Table 4.2). TFR2 shows moderate homology to TFR, may bind transferrin but is not iron-regulated. Hepcidin levels are low in type 3, suggesting TFR2 has a role in hepcidin synthesis (see Table 3.1).

Type 4 haemochromatosis

Haemochromatosis type 4 has peculiar genetic and clinical features compared with the other forms. First, it is inherited as an autosomal dominant trait. Second, patients have increased serum ferritin levels, but may have a normal transferrin saturation. Third, at liver biopsy iron is increased in the reticuloendothelial cells, as well as in hepatocytes. These features suggest a different pathophysiology of the disease. Haemochromatosis type 4 is now known to be due to heterozygous mutations in the iron exporter, ferroportin 1, coded for on chromosome 2q32 (Figure 4.4). Along with missense mutations, a deletion of valine at amino acid 162 has been found in families from the UK, France, Italy and Australia, suggesting that this may be a relatively common cause of iron accumulation. The phenotype is similar to that found in the anaemia of chronic disease, and it is unlikely that a ferroportin 1 mutation would be suspected unless there was significant iron overload and a clear familial association. Figure 4.3 illustrates the difference between the parenchymal iron overload found in most cases of GH and the predominantly

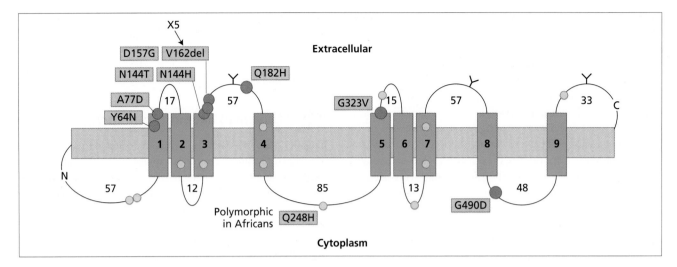

Figure 4.4 Iron-loading mutations in the ferroportin 1 gene. The nine predicted transmembrane helices (1–9) are shown in relation to the lipid bilayer, with the mutations marked (red circles). The 12 Cys residues are marked with yellow circles and three putative exposed N-linked oligosaccharide sites (Y) are shown. The N- and C-termini are denoted (N and C). The residue lengths of the loops are denoted by numbers adjacent to each loop. Mutations are clustered at either end of TM helices 1 and 3 or at the extracellular loop at the C-terminal end of the helix (from Worwood 2004 with permission).

reticuloendothelial distribution in a case of type 4 haemochromatosis due to the valine 162 deletion. In one family, weekly venesection rapidly caused anaemia, and venesection with erythropoietin therapy was successful in reducing iron stores. It is not yet clear whether the degree of tissue damage at a given serum ferritin level is similar to type 1 haemochromatosis or whether the reticuloendothelial distribution is less toxic. In people of African origin, Gln248His in ferroportin 1 is a common variant that may be associated with a tendency to iron loading and mild anaemia.

Neonatal haemochromatosis

This is a condition that is recognized at birth but may occur *in utero*. It is characterized by heavy parenchymal iron deposition in several organs and irreversible liver failure. The only therapeutic option used to be liver transplantation. Neonatal haemochromatosis has been linked in some cases to the presence of a maternal factor, e.g. an antiribonuclear factor antibody. Infusions of gammaglobulin in pregnancy appear to reduce the severity of the condition and it has been proposed that the disease is due to an alloantibody (as rhesus incompatibility) but the target antigen is unknown. No mutations in the *HFE* gene are reported and chromosome 1q linkage has been excluded.

Increased iron intake

African iron overload (Bantu siderosis) results from the combination of a dietary component (a traditional beer that contains iron) and an unknown susceptibility gene. Mutations in the *HFE* gene have been excluded but mutations of the ferroportin gene may play a role (see above). Iron deposition, as in type 4 haemochromatosis, occurs both in hepatocytes and in reticuloendothelial cells. Serum ferritin is usually elevated, but transferrin saturation may be normal. The condition occurs in sub-Saharan Africa. It is a cause of hepatic fibrosis and cirrhosis, and associations with diabetes mellitus, peritonitis, scurvy and osteoporosis have been described. The iron overload is associated with a poor outcome in tuberculosis, an infection that is highly prevalent in sub-Saharan Africa.

Other causes of iron overload

Atransferrinaemia

This is a rare recessive genetic disorder associated with a severe hypochromic anaemia with, in some cases, excessive iron deposition in the reticuloendothelial cells. In all cases tested, some iron–transferrin has been detected by iron-binding ability or immunologically. Complete absence of transferrin would presumably lead to fetal death.

Iron and neurodegeneration

Aceruloplasminaemia

This is also a rare recessive disorder in which there is a deficiency of ferroxidase activity as a consequence of mutations in the ceruloplasmin gene on chromosome 3q. Clinically, the condition presents in middle age, with progressive degeneration of the retina and basal ganglia and with diabetes mellitus. Iron accumulates in the liver, pancreas and brain with smaller amounts in the heart, kidneys, thyroid, spleen and retina. The serum iron is low. The total iron-binding capacity of transferrin (TIBC) is normal and ferritin is normal or raised. Interestingly, there is evidence that iron chelation with DFX may decrease brain iron stores and halt the progression of the neurological degeneration.

Hallervorden–Spatz syndrome

This is an autosomal recessive neurodegenerative disorder associated with iron accumulation in the brain. Clinical features include extrapyramidal dysfunction, onset in childhood and a relentlessly progressive course. Histological study reveals iron deposits in the basal ganglia. Hallervorden–Spatz syndrome is caused by a defect in a novel pantothenate kinase gene that causes accumulation of cysteine. Iron binding by cysteine may cause iron accumulation and oxidative stress which is a likely explanation for the pathophysiology of the disease.

Neuroferritinopathy

A previously unknown, dominantly inherited, late-onset basal ganglia disease, variably presenting with extrapyramidal features similar to those of Huntington's disease or Parkinsonism also shows iron accumulation in the forebrain and cerebellum. The disorder was mapped 19q13.3, which contains the gene for ferritin light-chain polypeptide (FTL). An adenine insertion at position 460–461 was found that was predicted to alter carboxy-terminal residues of the gene product. Abnormal aggregates of ferritin and iron in the brain contrasted with low serum ferritin levels.

These diseases may serve as a model for complex neurodegenerative diseases, such as Parkinson's disease, Alzheimer's disease, and Huntington's disease, in which accumulation of iron in the brain is also observed. Possession of the C282Y mutation of the *HFE* gene does not appear to be a risk factor for these conditions.

Friedrich's ataxia

This is a neurodegenerative disease characterized by loss of sensory neurones in the spinal cord and dorsal root ganglia. There is mitochondrial iron overload and a loss of activity of iron–sulphur cluster-containing enzymes. Patients frequently die from cardiomyopathy. The majority of Friedrich's ataxia (FRDA) cases result from the expansion of triple nucleotide repeats within an intron of the *FRDA* gene (human chromosome 9q13), leading to reduced expression of frataxin mRNA and protein. Point mutations have also been identified in a small number of cases. Frataxin is found in the mitochondrion where, in FRDA, there is increased oxidative stress and decreased activity of iron–sulphur proteins. Oxidative damage following iron accumulation is thought to precipitate the neurone loss in FRDA. This is confirmed by experiments in yeast that show that iron is redistributed to the mitochondria of Yfh (yeast frataxin homologue)-deficient yeast and that this iron accumulation precedes oxidative damage. Frataxin shows structural similarity

to ferritin, suggesting that frataxin may regulate mitochondrial iron homeostasis by storing excess iron.

Iron loading anaemias

Removal of iron is essential in patients with transfusion-dependent anaemias, such as thalassaemia major, to prevent death from iron overload, usually due to cardiac failure or arrythmia. Intake of iron ranges from 0.32 to 0.64 mg/kg of body weight daily in splenectomized thalassaemia major patients, derived from 100–200 mL of pure red cells per kg per year. The iron content of each transfusion is: volume (mL) × haematocrit × 1.16 mg. Patients with anaemias associated with increased iron absorption, e.g. thalassaemia intermedia, who are too anaemic to be venesected to remove iron, may also require iron chelation therapy, although the rate of iron loading is considerably lower at about 0.1 mg/kg per day. The only iron-chelating drug widely available is desferrioxamine (DFX). This is orally inactive and given by slow subcutaneous or intravenous infusion. Deferiprone, an orally active iron chelator, first used clinically in 1987, is now licensed for DFX 'failures' in over 40 countries, whereas a third drug, ICL670, is undergoing phase III clinical trials (Table 4.3 and Figure 4.7).

Iron chelation therapy is monitored by:
1 tests of body iron burden (Table 4.4);
2 tests of function of the organs sensitive to iron overload (Table 4.5);
3 tests to detect potential side-effects of the particular chelating drug being used.

Tests (1) and (2) are discussed first. The results and side-effects with the individual iron-chelating drugs are then described.

Tests of body iron burden

Serum ferritin

Serum ferritin is useful in monitoring changes in body iron, although the absolute level is an imprecise measure of total body iron. There is a wide range of liver iron at any given serum ferritin level. This is partly because serum ferritin mainly reflects reticuloendothelial iron and partly because inflammation, e.g. hepatitis C infection, raises the level, whereas vitamin C deficiency, frequent in iron overload, lowers it. The Thalassaemia International Federation (TIF) guidelines recommend maintaining the level < 1000 μg/L in thalassaemia major. One study found that if two-thirds were at levels below 2500 μg/L, cardiac complications were infrequent. Others have found a level consistently less than 1500 μg/L to be associated with few complications.

Liver iron

Liver iron may be measured chemically after liver biopsy, by MRI or, in a few specialized units, by SQUID (see p. 48).

Table 4.3 Characteristics of desferrioxamine, deferiprone and ICL 670.

	Desferrioxamine	*Deferiprone*	*ICL 670 (Deferasirox)*
Structure	Hexadentate	Bidentate	Tridentate
Molecular weight	560	139	373
Iron–chelator complex	1:1	1:3	1:2
Plasma clearance $T^{1/2}$	20 min	53–166 min	1–16 h
Absorption	Negligible	Peak 45 min	Peak 1–2.9 h
Iron excretion	Urine + faecal	Urine	Faecal
Therapeutic daily dose	40 mg/kg	75 mg/kg	20 mg/kg
Route	Parenteral	Oral	Oral
Clinical experience	30 years	18 years	1–2 years
Side-effects	Ototoxicity, retinal toxicity, growth defect, cartilage and bone abnormalities	Agranulocytosis, arthropathy, gastrointestinal disturbance, transient transaminitis, zinc deficiency	Skin rashes, gastrointestinal disturbance

Table 4.4 Tests of body iron burden.

1	Serum ferritin		
2	Serum iron and % saturation of iron-binding capacity		
3	Serum non-transferrin-bound iron		
4	Liver iron	Chemical estimation SQUID MRI CT	
5	Cardiac iron	MRI (Indirect)	Gradient-echo T2* Spin-echo
6	Urine iron in response to standard dose of chelator (desferrioxamine or deferiprone)		

CT, computerized tomography; MRI, magnetic resonance imaging; SQUID, superconducting quantum interface device.

Chemical estimation is the gold standard but can be inaccurate if fibrosis is present. Levels > 15 mg/g dry weight have been associated in DFX-treated patients with a high risk of cardiac disease, liver fibrosis and cirrhosis. Levels between 7 and 15 mg/g dry weight are associated with liver damage only if there is also hepatitis C infection and have been considered relatively safe from cardiac disease but associated with damage to the endocrine organs. Levels less than 7 mg/g are found in carriers of haemochromatosis.

MRI techniques are being increasingly used as indirect measures of liver and cardiac iron. They have the advantage of being non-invasive and are more widely available than SQUID (which is suitable for liver but not cardiac iron). MRI is also the only practical method of performing sequential studies of iron in the heart, pituitary or other endocrine organs. Different MRI techniques have been used. They all rely on a shortening of relaxation time and thus reduction in signal intensity with iron overload. Gradient-echo imaging with the calculation of the T2* has a short total imaging time, reducing movement artefacts. It also is extremely sensitive and reproducible. The spin-echo technique is less sensitive to iron in the form of haemosiderin and ferritin and requires a longer imaging time, allowing greater movement artefacts. It is improved by comparing the signal with that of a tissue (skeletal muscle) that does not develop iron load. Both methods show a close correlation between signal intensity and chemically estimated liver iron but have yet to be calibrated directly against chemically estimated heart iron.

Cardiac iron

As cardiac failure or arrhythmia is the usual cause of death in transfusional iron overload, it is essential to monitor cardiac iron. Iron is deposited in myocytes and interstitial fibrosis develops. Direct measurement of cardiac iron by endomyocardial biopsy is inappropriate as the technique is highly invasive

Table 4.5 Monitoring for iron-induced tissue damage organ.

1	Cardiac function		ECG ± exercise
			24-h monitor
			Echocardiography, MUGA ± stress tissue, Doppler echography, MRI
2	Liver structure and function	Liver function tests Liver histology	
3	Bone	Osteoporosis	Bone density (Dexa scan)
4	Endocrine system	Diabetes	Urine glucose
			HbAIC
			Glucose tolerance test
			IGF-1
		Growth and sexual development	Sitting and standing height
			Tanner staging
			Radiography for bone age
			Testosterone, oestradiol
			LH, FSH
			SHBG
			Pulsatile GNRH release
			Sperm tests
		Thyroid	T_4, TSH
		Parathyroid	Calcium, phosphate
			PTH

ECG, electrocardiogram; FSH, follicle-stimulating hormone; GNRH, gonadotrophin-releasing hormone; HbAIC, glycated haemoglobin; IGF, insulin-like growth factor; LH, luteinizing hormone; MRI, magnetic resonance imaging; MUGA, multigated acquisition scan; PTH, parathyroid hormone; SHBG, sex hormone-binding globulin; TSH, thyroid-stimulating hormone.

and inaccurate as iron localizes mainly in the ventricular myo- and epicardium. MRI offers a reproducible, sensitive, albeit indirect measure: the lower the T2* value, the greater cardiac iron. The T2* technique appears to be most sensitive (Figure 4.5). A T2* value of < 20 ms correlates with the presence of cardiac dysfunction detected by echocardiography or 24-h rhythm monitoring or the need for cardiac therapy (Figure 4.6). Using this and the spin-echo technique, poor correlation has been found between derived myocardial iron and liver iron (MRI derived) or serum ferritin in patients receiving DFX. Others using the spin-echo technique have found a positive relation between MRI-determined liver iron and urine iron excretion after chelator administration in non-thalassaemic patients.

Urine iron excretion

Iron excretion after a single infusion of a standard dose DFX or oral dose of deferiprone is related to body iron. Urine iron is derived from the labile iron pool chelated mainly extracellularly with DFX and probably intracellularly with deferiprone. With DFX (but not deferiprone) urine iron excretion is increased by ascorbate and is proportionately higher if the haemoglobin is lower. The test is useful when commencing therapy with

deferiprone, with which iron excretion is highly dose related, and for monitoring therapy, in some studies correlating closely with liver and cardiac iron. Several estimations must be performed at any given dose, however, in view of the variability found.

Non-transferrin-bound iron

This is present in plasma in patients with gross iron overload. It is highly toxic, promoting the formation of free radicals causing peroxidation of membrane lipids. Part of the early improvement in liver and cardiac function with chelation therapy may be due to removal of this fraction, even before iron burden is substantially lowered. Its clearance by DFX is short lived as it reappears in plasma within hours of stopping an infusion. This provides a rationale for using 24-h continuous infusions in patients with iron-induced cardiomyopathy. Non-transferrin-bound iron is absent from plasma of well-chelated patients.

Tests of organ function

The tests that are usually needed are listed in Table 4.4. Heart function is best tested by measurement of left ventricular ejection

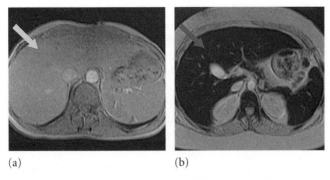

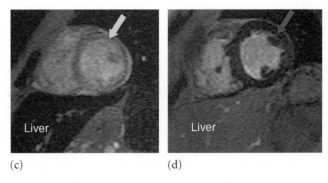

(a)   (b)   (c)   (d)

Figure 4.5 Magnetic resonance imaging T2* technique. Tissue appearances of liver and spleen: (a) normal; (b) tissue iron overload; (c) severe liver iron overload with normal cardiac iron;

(d) severe cardiac iron deposition with minimal liver iron deposition (reproduced from Anderson *et al.* 2001 with permission).

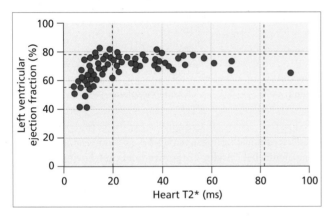

Figure 4.6 Relationships of myocardial T2* and left ventricular ejection fraction in patients with thalassaemia major and iron overload (reproduced from Anderson *et al.* 2001 with permission).

fraction and by tests for rhythm disturbance. Liver function assessment requires routine liver function tests as well as liver biopsy to assess liver structure and liver iron burden (histologically and chemically). The endocrine system is also damaged by iron and appropriate tests are listed in Table 4.4. The anterior pituitary is particularly sensitive, with damage resulting in reduced growth and impaired sexual maturation. Direct damage to the ovaries or testes may also occur but is usually less important. Hypogonadic hypogonadism, defects of growth hormone secretion and in its receptor, and deficiency of insulin-like growth factor mainly account for growth failure; DFX may also cause this. Diabetes mellitus and pre-diabetes, due to iron deposition in the pancreatic islets, are frequent, especially in patients with genetic susceptibility. Hypothyroidism and hypoparathyroidism are also common in poorly chelated patients. Osteoporosis is well recognized in iron-overloaded thalassaemia patients; it is due to multiple factors and is detected by bone density studies.

Iron chelation therapy

Desferrioxamine

Pharmacokinetics

Desferrioxamine mesylate (DFX) is the main agent licensed in all countries in clinical use at present. It is not absorbed orally and, after parenteral injection, it is rapidly cleared from the plasma, being excreted in the urine, taken up by hepatocytes or metabolized in the tissues (Table 4.3). This accounts for the much greater mobilization of iron by continuous intravenous (i.v.) or slow subcutaneous (s.c.) infusions, which allow more prolonged exposure of the drug to the chelatable iron than with i.m. injection.

DFX is a trihydroxamic acid (hexadendate) (Figure 4.7), one molecule binding covalently to all six oxygen sites on one ferric ion to form the red chelate, ferrioxamine. This is excreted in urine and bile. Faecal iron is derived from hepatocytes. Urine iron also derives, at least in part, from hepatocytes, although other body sources, especially iron released from macrophages, contribute. Urinary iron excretion tends to level off at higher doses, but this does not occur with bile excretion, which increases linearly with the dose. Bile iron may therefore predominate at high doses, and this is also the major route of excretion when total body iron has been reduced to relatively low levels. Urine iron excretion tends to be less immediately after blood transfusions, but this is accompanied by a reciprocal increase in faecal iron excretion. Increased erythropoiesis, as in haemolytic anaemias, is associated with an increase in urine iron excretion in relation to body iron stores.

Clinical studies

Therapy with DFX is expensive and inconvenient. Its use should, therefore, be restricted to those patients in whom iron overload is the main threat to life. Most studies have been with thalassaemia major, but patients with other inherited anaemias, e.g.

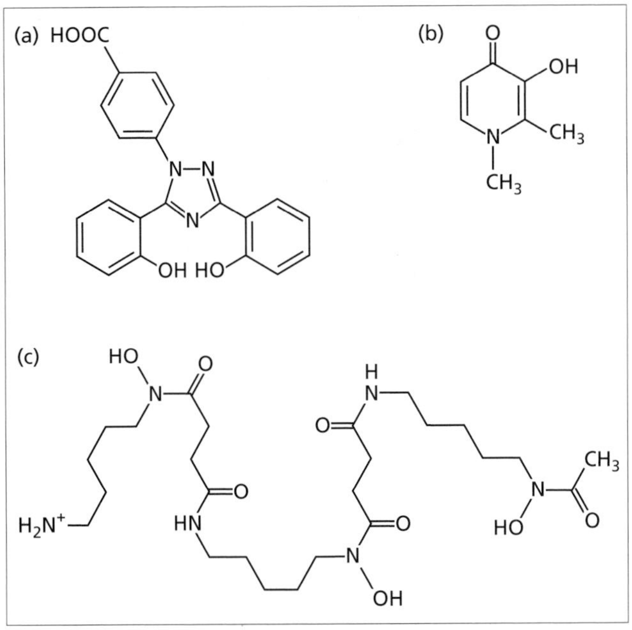

Figure 4.7 Chemical structures of three iron chelators. (a) ICL 670. (b) Deferiprone. (c) Desferrioxamine.

Diamond–Blackfan, Fanconi, sickle cell, sideroblastic anaemia or acquired disorders, especially myelodysplasia, myelofibrosis red cell aplasia or aplastic anaemia, may require iron chelation therapy. In elderly patients with acquired, transfusion-dependent, refractory anaemias, the prognosis of the underlying haematological disease may not justify the inconvenience of s.c. DFX therapy. In children, tissue damage from iron may be present from very early life; regular iron chelation should begin in thalassaemia major after transfusion of about 12 units of blood or when the serum ferritin exceeds 1000 µg/L. In young children, treatment should be started at 20 mg/kg to prevent tissue damage due to iron without causing toxicity due to excess DFX. A local anaesthetic cream (e.g. EMLA) reduces pain from the needle insertion.

The standard adult dose is 40 mg/kg, given as an 8- to 12-h infusion s.c. or at least 5 days each week. DFX may also be given intravenously via a separate line at the time of blood transfusion. To avoid toxic effects, the dose should be restricted to a maximum of 1 g with each unit of blood.

Repletion of ascorbic acid deficiency, which sometimes accompanies iron overload, or ascorbate therapy even in those with normal tissue levels of ascorbate, increases urinary iron excretion but has no effect on bile iron excretion. Supplements of vitamin C should be 100–200 mg per day. In some less severely anaemic patients with chronic ineffective erythropoiesis and iron loading from the gut (e.g. with thalassaemia intermedia or sideroblastic anaemia), cautious phlebotomy may be used instead of or added to regular s.c. DFX to produce a rate of iron mobilization similar to that achieved in the treatment of hereditary haemochromatosis.

In patients unable to comply with s.c. DFX or those with iron-induced cardiomyopathy, continuous intravenous (i.v.) DFX may be given via an indwelling catheter (e.g. Hickman) or Port-a-Cath chamber. Removal of liver iron is more rapid than removal of cardiac iron with this intensive chelation regime. Continuous s.c. DFX can also be administered using a disposable balloon infuser system with pre-prepared DFX solution (e.g. 4 g of DFX to be infused over 48 h) rather than using a battery-operated infusion pump. Continuous infusion avoids the reappearance of toxic NTBI in plasma. Twice-daily i.m. injections of DFX produce significant iron excretion, but these are painful and the long-term efficacy of this approach is unproven. Trials of DFX bound to starch to prolong its action are in progress.

Body iron stores can be restricted to 5–10 times normal in well-chelated, regularly transfused patients. There is improved cardiac function and survival in patients who comply with the rigorous therapy. Iron-induced cardiomyopathy can be reversed in some, but not all, patients with continuous DFX therapy. Growth and pubertal development are improved in many, but not all, patients; diabetes and other endocrine abnormalities still occur frequently. Serum ferritin levels in well-chelated thalassaemia major patients usually plateau between 1500 and 2500 µg/L. Unfortunately, through lack of compliance, premature deaths usually from iron-induced cardiac damage occur in a substantial proportion of thalassaemia major patients. In Turin, 95% of compliant (250 or more DFX infusions per year) patients were alive at 30 years compared with only 12% of non-compliant patients. In the UK, only 50% of thalassaemia major patients were alive at 35 years, deaths being largely due to failure of compliance with DFX.

Side-effects

The adverse effects possible with DFX include rare generalized sensitivity reactions, local soreness related to the site of injection (usually due to the needle being inserted too superficially) and exacerbation of some infections, notably of the urinary tract and precipitation of *Yersinia enterocolitis*. Auditory (high-tone sensorineural hearing loss) and visual neurotoxicity (night blindness, visual field loss, retinal pigmentation and changes on electrical tests) are relatively frequent. Growth and bone defects may also occur. The spine may be affected, with sitting height reduced; rickets-like bone lesions, genu valgum and metaphysical changes are described, especially in children (Figure 4.8).

Auditory, visual and growth side-effects of DFX occur mainly if the body iron burden is low and doses of DFX high, and particularly in children. A therapeutic index = mean daily dose (mg/kg)/current serum ferritin (µg/L) can be calculated. If this is below 0.025 at all times, these side-effects of DFX do not occur.

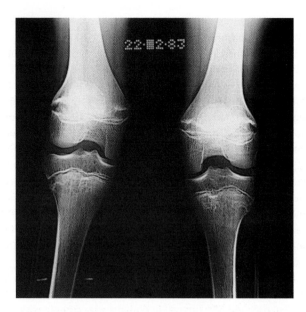

Figure 4.8 Bone and cartilage defects due to DFX.

Deferiprone

Pharmacokinetics

Deferiprone is rapidly absorbed, appearing in plasma within 15 min of ingestion, with a peak plasma level within 45–60 min (Table 4.3). It forms a 3:1 chelator–iron complex, which is excreted with the free drug and glucuronide derivative in urine. Only 4% of a single oral dose of the drug is excreted bound to iron, even in heavily iron-loaded patients. Its iron chelation site is inactivated by glucuronidation, the speed of which varies from patient to patient. This explains much of the individual variation in response, the area under the curve of the concentration of free drug in plasma being related to amount of iron excreted.

Deferiprone mobilizes iron from parenchymal and RE pools and from transferrin, ferritin and haemosiderin. Unlike DFX, it

is also capable of chelating iron from intact red cells *in vitro* and *in vivo*, shown in patients with sickle cell anaemia and thalassaemia intermedia. The enhanced ability of deferiprone to cross cell membranes may underlie what is emerging as its superior ability compared with DFX to protect the heart from iron and also the 'shuttle effect' for iron when the two drugs are given simultaneously (see later and Figure 4.9). Few balance studies have been performed. These suggest that on average deferiprone at 75 mg/kg is about 60% as effective as DFX at 60 mg/kg, but may be as effective as DFX 40 mg/kg. However, wide individual variations occur, especially with deferiprone. Moreover, it is easier for patients to comply with deferiprone than DFX on all 7 days each week.

Clinical studies

The usual dose used in most trials has been 75 mg/kg daily. Long-term studies show that serum ferritin levels tend to fall in those starting with the highest levels (> 3000 μg/L), but, in patients with lower levels, tend to remain unchanged or to increase so that levels usually plateau around 2000–2500 μg/L. The effect on liver iron is variable, but in studies of previously poorly chelated thalassaemia major patients from 10% to 30% show liver iron levels above 15 mg/g dry weight, i.e. in the so-called 'danger' zone. More and longer-term trials are needed to document this more exactly. MRI studies have also suggested that liver iron may on average be higher in patients treated with deferiprone (75 mg/kg 7 days per week) compared with those treated with DFX (40 mg/kg 5 days per week).

In the liver, DFX has the advantage of facilitated transport into cells by an active mechanism. Deferiprone, on the other hand, may have greater penetration of myocardial cells because of its lower molecular weight and because it is lipophilic. Retrospective studies have suggested, on the basis of T2* studies, echocardiography, clinical incidence of cardiac disease and need for cardiac therapy, that deferiprone 75 mg/kg is more effective at protecting the heart from iron-induced cardiomyopathy in routine clinical practice over 3–6 years than DFX. Prospective

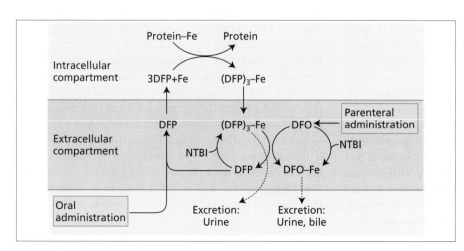

Figure 4.9 The concept of combination therapy: DFO, desferrioxamine; DFP, deferiprone; NTBI, non-transferrin-bound iron (modified from Liu *et al.* 2002).

randomized studies are now in progress, comparing the efficacy of the two chelators.

For patients inadequately chelated by DFX, efforts at increased compliance with DFX are first needed. The use of deferiprone at the dose of 75 mg/kg for those inadequately chelated is now licensed in 43 countries. Increasing the dose of deferiprone to 100 mg/kg daily has been shown to improve iron status, and longer-term trials at this higher dose are in progress to establish whether it results in increased side-effects. An alternative to raising the dose of deferiprone for those inadequately chelated by 75 mg/kg per day is to combine DFX and deferiprone therapy, and this approach is discussed below.

Side-effects

The complications of deferiprone therapy are now well established. The most severe is agranulocytosis (neutrophils $< 0.5 \times 10^9$/L), with an estimated incidence of around 0.5–1.0%. Lesser degrees of neutropenia (0.5–1.5×10^9/L) are more frequent, around 3%, occurring more frequently in non-splenectomized patients. Agranulocytosis and neutropenia spontaneously recover when the drug is discontinued, usually within 4–28 days but, occasionally, are more prolonged, e.g. up to 124 days. The mechanism appears to be idiosyncratic, more common in females, with no definite evidence of an immune mechanism established. Patients should be monitored by blood counts every week for at least the first 8–12 weeks of therapy and every 2 weeks thereafter for 2 years. There are no data to show agranulocytosis is more frequent in patients with stem cell or progenitor cell defects, e.g. aplastic anaemia, Diamond–Blackfan syndrome or myelodysplasia, but it seems sensible to monitor these patients particularly closely.

Painful joints, especially the knees, have been reported at around 5–10% in most large series. Some but not all studies show that this complication is most frequent in the most iron-loaded patients and with higher doses of deferiprone. It usually, but not invariably, resolves with withdrawal of the drug and it is often possible to reintroduce the drug, commencing with lower doses. There is no evidence for any immune abnormality induced by deferiprone underlying the arthropathy.

Gastrointestinal side-effects, e.g. nausea and abdominal pain, occur in about 8% of patients. In most the drug can be reintroduced long term, initially at a lower dose. Zinc deficiency has been described in diabetic and pre-diabetic patients. Rarely, it can lead to clinical features, e.g. skin rashes and hair loss. It is easily treated by oral zinc therapy. Liver fibrosis was suggested as a complication of deferiprone therapy in one study, but larger studies show that liver fibrosis in multiply transfused patients is not a direct consequence of deferiprone. Nevertheless, transient increases in liver enzymes have been associated with deferiprone therapy and a few patients have been withdrawn from therapy because of a persistent rise in liver enzyme levels. There have been no definite reports of renal, cardiac or neurological side-effects. Although immunological changes and systemic lupus syndrome were suggested to occur in a few patients, these have not been confirmed as side-effects in large studies.

Combination therapy

Urine iron excretion when the two drugs DFX and deferiprone are given simultaneously is equivalent to the sum of the excretion when the drugs are given on separate days. There is evidence for a 'shuttle' effect in which deferiprone enters cells, chelates iron and then returns to plasma, where the iron is transferred to DFX for excretion in urine or bile (Figure 4.9). All studies of combination therapy, e.g. deferiprone on 7 days a week, DFX on 2 days, have shown a significant fall in serum ferritin levels over 6–18 months. Toxicities are also reduced by avoiding the necessity for high doses of either drug. The combination may also be effective at removing both cardiac and liver iron. Longer-term studies are needed, however, to establish that there are no increased side-effects when the two are used together. Alternating therapy has also been studied, e.g. 4 days of deferiprone and 2 days of DFX each week, with improved compliance and improved iron status in previously poorly compliant (with DFX) children over 6–12 months of therapy.

ICL 670 (bishydroxylphenylthiazole, Deferasirox, Exjade)

This compound, (4-[3,5-bis(2-hydroxyphenyl)-1,2,4-triazol-1-yl]benzoic acid (Figure 4.4), forms a 2:1 chelator–iron complex and increases predominantly faecal iron excretion. After a single oral dose, only 6% of iron excretion occurs in the urine (Table 4.3). It is highly selective for iron, rapidly absorbed and circulates for several hours. Peak plasma concentration after a single oral dose occurs at about 2 h, and the drug is still detectable in plasma in almost all patients at 24 h, with a mean elimination half-life of between 11 and 16 h after multiple-dose administration. At the dose of 20 mg/kg used in early studies, total body iron excretion ranged from 7.7 to 28.5 mg iron per day in thalassaemia major patients, and short-term trials suggest that it may be able to reduce liver iron to the same extent as s.c. DFX 40 mg/kg on 5 days per week over 12 months of therapy. Side-effects of ICL 670 in short-term trials include gastrointestinal symptoms and skin rashes.

Other potential iron chelators

GT56-252 (Deferitrin), a desferrithiocin derivative, is in phase I clinical trials at present. It is a 2:1 chelator with iron, with dominant faecal excretion. It has a half-life in plasma of several hours and is well tolerated in short-term trials. Pyridoxal isonicotinoyl hydrazone (PIH) is a tridentate iron chelator. It increases urine and faecal iron excretion but, in the main trial so far, was not sufficiently effective to produce a negative iron balance in thalassaemia major. Many derivatives of PIH await further studies. Other iron chelators that have been found too toxic, or not sufficiently effective, for clinical use include desferrithiocin, a tridentate chelator, and HBED (N,N'-bis(2-hydroxybenzyl)-ethylenediamine-N,N'-diacetic acid), a hexadentate chelator. GT56-252, a desferrithiocin derivative, is in phase I clinical trials at present.

Thalassaemia intermedia

For these patients, and other severely anaemic patients who are not transfusion dependent or only need a few transfusions each year, iron loading occurs mainly through increased iron absorption. The anaemia may be too severe for venesections. DFX can be used to chelate iron but care must be taken to avoid side-effects of the drug in these moderately iron-loaded patients. Oral iron chelation with deferiprone has also been shown effective in 'de-ironing' such patients, potentially reducing serum ferritin and liver iron to normal. A rise in haemoglobin level may occur. This may be due to removing iron from the renal oxygen sensor, augmenting the effect of hypoxia and increasing erythropoietin secretion from the kidney. The role in haemoglobin may also result from deferiprone directly removing iron from erythroblasts and mature red cells, reducing ineffective erythropoiesis and haemolysis. Improved haemopoiesis has also been described in myelodysplasia after chelation with DFX.

Acute iron poisoning

Acute oral iron poisoning produces a severe necrotizing gastritis and enteritis, followed by metabolic acidosis and, after a day or two, cardiovascular collapse and evidence of liver damage. DFX should be given both orally and parenterally. The instillation of 5 g into the stomach after a 1% sodium bicarbonate gastric lavage (to reduce further absorption) and an injection of 1–2 g i.m. may be tried. If a large number of tablets have been taken, an i.v. DFX infusion up to a maximum dose of 80 mg/kg in 24 h should be used. Deferiprone has not yet been used in this setting.

Selected bibliography

Ajioka RS, Kushner JP (2002) Hereditary hemochromatosis. *Seminars in Hematology* **39**: 235–41.

Ajioka RS, Kushner JP, Beutler E (2003) Debate: clinical consequences of iron overload in hemochromatosis homozygotes. *Blood* **101**: 3347–58 (four papers).

Anderson LJ, Holden S, Davis B *et al.* (2001) Cardiovascular T2-star (T2*) magnetic resonance for the early diagnosis of myocardial iron overload. *European Heart Journal* **22**: 2171–9.

Anderson LJ, Wonke B, Prescott E *et al.* (2002) Improved myocardial iron levels and ventricular function with oral deferiprone compared with subcutaneous desferrioxamine in thalassaemia. *Lancet* **360**: 516–20.

Barman Balfour JA, Foster RH (1999) Deferiprone: a review of its clinical potential in iron overload in beta thalassemia major and other transfusion-dependent diseases. *Drug* **3**: 553–78.

Beutler E, Felitti VJ, Koziol JA *et al.* (2002) Penetrance of 845G→A (C282Y) HFE hereditary haemochromatosis mutation in the USA. *Lancet* **359**: 211–18.

Breuer W, Empers MJJ, Pootrakul P *et al.* (2001) Deferoxamine-chelatable iron, a component of serum non-transferrin-bound iron used for assessing chelating therapy. *Blood* **97**: 792–8.

Camaschella C, Roetto Q, Gobbi MD (2002) Genetic haemochromatosis: genes and mutations associated with iron loading. *Best Practice and Research in Clinical Haematology* **15**: 261–76.

Dooley JS (2002) Diagnosis and management of genetic haemochromatosis. *Best Practice and Research in Clinical Haematology* **15**: 277–94.

Feder JN, Gnirke A, Thomas W *et al.* (1996) A novel MHC Class I-like gene is mutated in patients with hereditary hemochromasosis. *Nature Genetics* **13**: 399–408.

Fischer R, Longo F, Nielsen P *et al.* (2002) Monitoring long-term efficacy of iron chelation therapy by deferiprone and desferrioxamine in patients with β-thalassaemia major: application of SQUID biomagnetic liver susceptometry. *British Journal of Haematology* **121**: 938–48.

Gabutti V, Piga A (1996) Results of long-term iron chelating therapy. *Acta Haematologica* **95**: 26–36.

Gordeuk VR (2002) African iron overload. *Seminars in Hematology* **39**: 263–9.

Gordeuk VR, Caleffi A, Corradini E (2003) Iron overload in Africans and African-Americans and a common mutation in the SCL40A1 (ferroportin 1) gene. *Blood Cells, Molecules and Diseases* **31**: 299–304.

Guidelines on the diagnosis and therapy of Genetic Haemochromatosis (http://www.bcshguidelines.com/).

Hoffbrand AV, Cohen A, Hershko C (2003) Role of deferiprone in chelation therapy for transfusional iron overload. *Blood* **102**: 17–24.

Jackson HA, Carter K, Darke C, Guttridge MG, Ravine D, Hutton RD, Napier JA *et al.* (2001) HFE mutations, iron deficiency and overload in 10 500 blood donors. *British Journal of Haematology* **114**: 474–84.

Ke Y, Qian ZM (2003) Iron misregulation in the brain: a primary cause of neurodegenerative disorders. *Lancet Neurology* **2**: 246–53.

Liu DY, Liu ZD, Hider RC (2002) Oral iron chelators – development and application. *Clinical Haematology* **15**: 369–84.

Modell B, Khan M, Darlison M (2000) Survival in beta-thalassaemia major in the United Kingdom: data from the UK Thalassaemia Register. *Lancet* **3**: 2051–2.

Muckenthaler M, Roy CN, Custodio AO *et al.* (2003) Regulatory defects in liver and intestine implicate abnormal hepcidin and Cybrd1 expression in mouse hemochromatosis. *Nature Genetics* **34**: 102–7.

Niderau C, Stremmel W, Strohmeyor GWW (1994) Clinical spectrum and management of haemochromatosis. *Clinical Haematology* **7**: 881–901.

Olivieri NF, Brittenham GM (1997) Iron chelating therapy and the treatment of thalassemia. *Blood* **89**: 739–61.

Papanikolaou G, Samuels ME, Ludwig EH *et al.* (2003) Mutations in HFE2 cause iron overload in chromosome 1q-linked juvenile hemochromatosis. *Nature Genetics*, advance online publication.

Piga A, Gaglioti C, Fogliacco E, Tricta F (2003) Comparative effects of deferriprone and deferoxamine on survival and cardiac disease in patients with thalassemia major: a retrospective analysis. *Haematologica* **88**: 489–96.

Ponka P (2001) Rare causes of iron overload. *Seminars in Hematology* **39**: 249–62.

Pootrakul PS, Sirankapracha P, Sankote J *et al.* (2003) Clinical trial of deferiprone iron chelation therapy on β-thalassaemia/haemoglobin E patients in Thailand. *British Journal of Haematology* **122**: 305–10.

Porter JB (2001) Practical management of iron overload. *British Journal of Haematology* **115**: 239–52.

Porter JB, Davis B (2002) Monitoring chelation therapy to achieve optimal outcome in the treatment of thalassaemia. *Best Practice and Research in Clinical Haematology* **15**: 329–68.

Richardson DR, Ponka P (1998) Pyridoxal isonicotinoyl hydrazone and its analogs: potential orally effective iron-chelating agents for the treatment of iron overload disease. *Journal of Laboratory and Clinical Medicine* **131**: 306–14.

Whittington PF, Hibband JU (2004) High-dose immunoglobulin during pregnancy for recurrent neonatal haemochromatosis. (In preparation.)

Worwood M (2004) Haemochromatosis – genetic testing in diagnosis and management. *Blood Reviews* (in press).

CHAPTER 5

Megaloblastic anaemia

5

A Victor Hoffbrand and Ralph Green

Introduction

The megaloblastic anaemias are a group of disorders characterized by the presence of distinctive morphological appearances of the developing red cells in the bone marrow. The cause is usually deficiency of either cobalamin (vitamin B_{12}) or folate, but megaloblastic anaemia may arise because of genetic or acquired abnormalities affecting the function or metabolism of these vitamins or because of defects in DNA synthesis not related to cobalamin or folate (Table 5.1).

Underlying basic science

Biochemical basis of megaloblastic anaemia

The common feature of all megaloblastic anaemias is a defect in DNA synthesis that affects rapidly dividing cells in the bone marrow and other tissues. All conditions that give rise to megaloblastic changes share in common a disparity in the rate of synthesis or availability of the four immediate precursors of DNA: the deoxyribonucleoside triphosphates (dNTPs), dA(adenine)TP and dG(guanine)TP (purines) and dT(thymine)TP and

Table 5.1 Causes of megaloblastic anaemia.

Cobalamin deficiency or abnormalities of cobalamin metabolism (Table 5.4)
Folate deficiency or abnormalities of folate metabolism (Table 5.8)
Therapy with antifolate drugs (e.g. methotrexate)
Independent of either cobalamin or folate deficiency and refractory to cobalamin and folate therapy:
  Some cases of acute myeloid leukaemia, myelodysplasia*
  Therapy with drugs interfering with synthesis of DNA
    (e.g. cytosine arabinoside, hydroxyurea, 6-mercaptopurine, azidothymidine (AZT))
  Orotic aciduria (responds to uridine)
  Lesch–Nyhan syndrome (? responds to adenine)

*Folate deficiency also occurs frequently in these diseases.

dC(cytosine)TP (pyrimidines) required for ordered DNA replication during the S-phase of the cell cycle (Figure 5.1). In deficiencies of either folate or cobalamin, the defect in DNA synthesis is caused by a failure to convert adequate amounts of deoxyuridine monophosphate (dUMP) to thymidine monophosphate (dTMP). This is because folate is needed as the

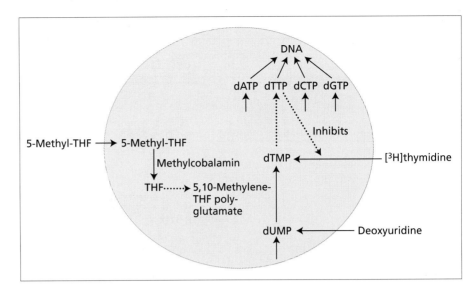

Figure 5.1 Deoxyuridine suppression test. The circle represents a bone marrow or other haemopoietic cell. THF, tetrahydrofolate; MP, monophosphate; TP, triphosphate; d, deoxyribose; A, adenine; T, thymine; C, cytosine; G, guanine.

coenzyme 5,10-methylene tetrahydrofolate polyglutamate for conversion of dUMP to dTMP and the availability of this coenzyme is reduced in either cobalamin or folate deficiencies.

Synthesis of new strands of DNA during the S-phase of the cell cycle commences with separation of the two parent strands from each other at many points along the chromosome. At a number of points of origin, RNA primers are synthesized first and new DNA strands are then synthesized bidirectionally using the parent strands as templates, with A pairing with T and G with C. The RNA primer is ultimately hydrolysed and the gap filled with DNA. The small pieces of DNA (Okazaki fragments) are then joined up to make complete new chromosomal DNA.

The reduced supply of dTTP in megaloblastic anaemia owing to folate or cobalamin deficiency appears to slow elongation of newly originated replicating segments. Thus, small fragments accumulate, single-stranded areas become points of weakness, where mechanical or enzymatic breakage may occur, and the failure to form bulk DNA may impair contraction of newly replicated lengths of DNA, thus leaving the chromosomes elongated, despirilled and with random breaks. Late-replicating DNA is particularly affected, many of the gross defects in DNA appearing in late replication. Indeed, some cells become arrested and die at this stage. Apoptosis occurs particularly at the late stage of erythroblast differentiation and can be prevented by thymidine. Surprisingly, measurements of dTTP concentration in megaloblasts have not shown a deficiency. This may be because the overall cell concentration masks a localized deficiency at the multienzyme complex directly concerned with DNA replication.

An alternative theory for megaloblastic anaemia in cobalamin or folate deficiency is the misincorporation of uracil into DNA because of a build-up of deoxyuridine triphosphate (dUTP) at the replication fork in consequence of the block in conversion of dUMP to dTMP (Figure 5.1). As dUTP does not normally occur in DNA, there is a mechanism for recognition of this aberrant material for excision and repair, but as long as dTTP remains in short supply this may not be possible. Repeated cycles of futile excision and misrepair may occur with disruption of the normal programme of DNA synthesis leading to apoptotic cell death. Data on this theory are conflicting. It does not explain megaloblastic anaemia due to defects of DNA synthesis at sites other than thymidylate synthesis (e.g. with drugs such as hydroxyurea, cytosine arabinoside or 6-mercaptopurine, or with enzyme deficiencies such as orotic aciduria or thiamine-responsive megaloblastic anaemia; see below). A reduced supply of one of three other deoxyribonucleoside triphosphates or malfunction of DNA polymerase is the likely cause of these megaloblastic anaemias.

Cobalamin–folate relationship

Folate is required for many other reactions in mammalian tissues, including two in purine synthesis (Table 5.2), but impairment of these is far less important clinically.

Only two reactions in the body are known to require cobalamin (Figure 5.2). Methylmalonyl CoA isomerization, which requires deoxyadenosyl(ado)-cobalamin, is discussed later. The methylation of homocysteine to methionine requires both 5-methyltetrahydrofolate (THF) as methyl donor and methylcobalamin as coenzyme (Figure 5.3). This reaction, which is almost completely irreversible, is the first step in the pathway by which methyl-THF, which enters bone marrow and other cells from plasma, is converted into all the intracellular folate coenzymes (Figure 5.3). The coenzymes are all polyglutamated (the larger size aiding retention in the cell), but the enzyme folate polyglutamate synthase cannot use methyl-THF as substrate. Tetrahydrofolate is needed as substrate for synthesis of folate polyglutamates. In cobalamin deficiency, methyl-THF

Table 5.2 Biochemical reactions of folate coenzymes of folate coenzymes.

Reaction	Coenzyme form of folate involved	Single carbon unit transferred	Importance
Formate activation	THF	$-CHO$	Generation of 10-formyl-THF
Purine synthesis			
Formation of glycinamide ribonucleotide	5,10-Methenyl-THF	$-CHO$	Formation of purines needed for DNA, RNA synthesis, but reactions probably not rate limiting
Formylation of amino-imidazole-carboxamide-ribotide (AICAR)	10-Formyl-THF	$-CHO$	
Pyrimidine synthesis			
Methylation of deoxyurine monophosphate (dUMP) to thymidine monophosphate (dTMP)	5,10-Methenyl-THF	$-CH_3$	Rate limiting in DNA synthesis Oxidizes THF to DHF Some breakdown of folate at the C-9–N-10 bond
Amino acid interconversion			
Serine–glycine interconversion	THF	$=CH_2$	Entry of single carbon units into active pool
Homocysteine to methionine	5-Methyl-THF	$-CH_3$	Demethylation of 5-methyl THF to THF; also requires cobalamin, flavine adenine dinucleotide, ATP and adenosylmethionine
Forminoglutamic acid to glutamic acid in histidine catabolism	THF	$-HN-CH=$	Basis of the Figlu test (now obsolete)

DHF, dihydrofolate; THF, tetrahydrofolate.

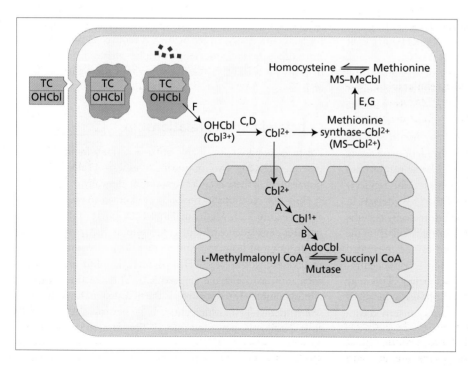

Figure 5.2 Intracellular cobalamin metabolism. Cbl^{1+}, Cbl^{2+}, Cbl^{3+} refer to the oxidation state of the central cobalt atom of cobalamin. A–G refer to the sites of blocks that have been identified by complementation analysis in infants with metabolic defects. AdoCbl, adenosylcobalamin; MeCbl, methylcobalamin; TC, transcobalamin. The mitochondrial lysosomal and cytoplasmic compartments are indicated (reproduced with permission from *Paediatric Haematology*, eds JS Lilleyman, IM Hann and VS Blanchette, 2nd edn, 1999, Churchill Livingstone).

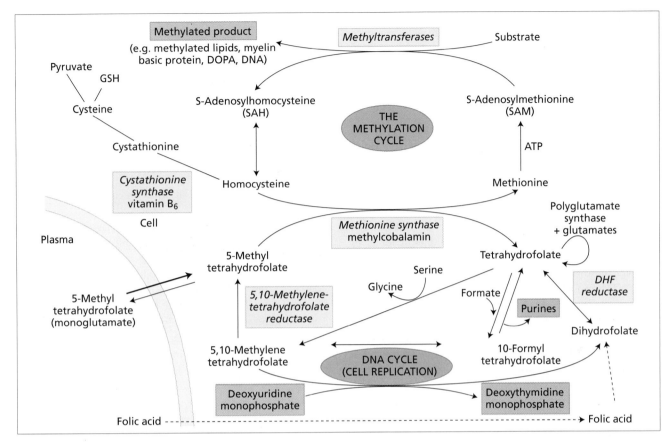

Figure 5.3 The role of folates in DNA synthesis and in formation on S-adenosylmethionine (SAM), which is involved in numerous methylation reactions. Enzymes are shown in yellow boxes (figure prepared in conjunction with Professor John Scott).

accumulates in the plasma, while intracellular folate concentrations fall due to failure of formation of intracellular folate polyglutamates because of 'THF starvation' or 'methylfolate trapping'.

This theory explains the abnormalities of folate metabolism, which occur in cobalamin deficiency (high serum folate, low cell folate, positive purine precursor AICAR excretion; Table 5.2) and also why the anaemia that occurs in cobalamin deficiency will respond to folic acid in large doses. The explanation of why the serum cobalamin falls in folate deficiency may also be related to impairment of the homocysteine–methionine reaction, with reduced formation of methylcobalamin, the main form of cobalamin in plasma, but other mechanisms may be responsible.

Clinical features

Many symptomless patients are detected through the finding of a raised mean corpuscular volume (MCV) on a routine blood count. The main clinical features in more severe cases are those of anaemia. Anorexia is usually marked and there may be weight loss, diarrhoea or constipation. Other particular features include glossitis, angular cheilosis, a mild fever in the more severely anaemic patients, jaundice (unconjugated) and reversible melanin skin hyperpigmentation, which may occur with either deficiency. Thrombocytopenia sometimes leads to bruising (and this may be aggravated by vitamin C deficiency in malnourished patients. The (anaemia and) low leucocyte count may predispose to infections, particularly of the respiratory or urinary tracts. Cobalamin deficiency has also been associated with impaired bactericidal function of phagocytes.

General tissue effects of cobalamin and folate deficiencies

Epithelial surfaces

These deficiencies, when severe, affect all rapidly growing (DNA-synthesizing) tissues. After the marrow, the next most affected tissues are the epithelial cell surfaces of the mouth, stomach, small intestine, respiratory, urinary and female genital tracts. The cells show macrocytosis, with increased numbers of multinucleate and dying cells. The deficiencies may cause cervical smear abnormalities.

Complications of pregnancy

The gonads are also affected and infertility is common in both men and women with either deficiency. Maternal folate deficiency has been implicated as a cause of prematurity and both folate and cobalamin deficiency have been implicated in recurrent fetal loss.

Neural tube defects

Folic acid supplements at the time of conception and in the first 12 weeks of pregnancy reduce by about 70% the incidence of neural tube defects (NTDs) (anencephaly, meningomyelocele, encephalocele and spina bifida) in the fetus. Most of this protective effect can be achieved by taking folic acid, 0.4 mg daily. The incidence of cleft palate and harelip can also be reduced by prophylactic folic acid. There is no clear simple relationship between maternal folate status and these fetal abnormalities, although the lower the maternal folate, the greater the risk to the fetus. NTDs can also be caused by antifolate and anti-epileptic drugs.

An underlying maternal folate metabolic abnormality has also been postulated. One abnormality has been identified: reduced activity of the enzyme 5,10-methylenetetrahydrofolate reductase (MTHFR) (Figure 5.3) caused by a common 677C-T polymorphism in the *MTHFR* gene. The prevalence of the homozygous state in the general population varies from 5% to 15% in various populations. In one study, the prevalence of this polymorphism was found to be higher in the parents of NTD fetuses and in the fetuses themselves – homozygosity for the TT mutation was found in 13% compared with 5% in control subjects. The polymorphism codes for a thermolabile form of MTHFR. The homozygous state results in a lower mean serum and red cell folate compared with control subjects, as well as significantly higher serum homocysteine levels. Tests for mutations in other enzymes possibly associated with NTDs, e.g. methionine synthase or serine–glycine hydroxymethylase, have been negative. Autoantibodies to folate receptors (see p. 77) have, however, recently been detected in 9 out of 12 women who were or had been pregnant with a fetus with a NTD, but in only 2 out of 20 control women. Antiserum to folate receptors results in resorption or multiple developmental abnormalities in mouse embryos. It is possible, therefore, that the association of antibodies to maternal folate receptors and NTDs reflects a causal relation.

Cardiovascular disease

Children with severe homocystinuria (blood levels of 100 μmol/L or more) due to deficiency of one of three enzymes, methionine synthase, MHTFR or cystathionine synthase (Figure 5.3), suffer from vascular disease, e.g. ischaemic heart disease, cerebrovascular disease or pulmonary embolus as teenagers or in young adulthood. Lesser degrees of raised serum homocysteine and low levels of serum folate have been found to be associated with cerebrovascular, peripheral vascular and coronary heart disease and predisposition to deep vein thrombosis.

Meta-analysis shows a significant association between serum homocysteine (normal range 5–15 μmol/L) and ischaemic heart disease, stroke, deep vein thrombosis and pulmonary embolism. The odds ratios for a 5 μmol/L increase in serum homocysteine were 1.42 in 72 genetic (MHTFR) studies and 1.32 in 20 prospective studies of serum homocysteine, 1.60 for deep vein thrombosis with or without pulmonary embolism in genetic studies, and for stroke 1.65 in genetic studies and 1.59 in prospective studies. As the genetic and prospective studies do not share the same potential sources of error but both yield highly significant results, the authors considered the results strong evidence of a causal association between homocysteine and cardiovascular disease.

Heterozygosity for the C677T mutation has also been shown to increase the risk of thrombosis in subjects heterozygous for factor V Leiden. Men who consume relatively large amounts of folate have a significantly reduced risk of developing ischaemic (but not haemorrhagic) stroke. It remains possible that homocysteine levels may be high as a consequence of the vascular damage or may merely be a marker for some other underlying factor that is responsible for both the vascular damage and the raised homocysteine. Folate deficiency, for example, may be such a factor. Folate levels have been found in various studies to be lower in patients with myocardial infarct and carotid artery disease than control subjects. There are some reports of prevention of arterial disease recurrence or progression by prophylactic folic acid or cobalamin. In one study, combined folic acid, cobalamin and pyridoxine daily for 1 year was associated with increased patency of coronary arteries compared with placebo in patients who had undergone coronary angioplasty and stenting. Data from large multicentre prospective trials of folic acid in prevention of cardiovascular disease are needed. Extremely high levels of homocysteine (> 50 μmol/L) are toxic to endothelia. When homocysteine levels are only mildly (15–25 μmol/L) or moderately (25–50 μmol/L) elevated then another mechanism needs to be invoked to explain vascular damage or increased risk of thrombosis. Several mechanisms have been proposed, including oxidant damage through the generation of peroxide produced during thiol oxidation to form disulphides and interaction of free reduced homocysteine with cysteine residues on coagulation factors, platelets, adhesion molecules or endothelial cells. Promotion of vascular wall inflammation through the generation of proinflammatory cytokines and interference with key methylation reactions are also possible mechanisms.

Malignancy

Prophylactic folic acid in pregnancy has been found to reduce the subsequent incidence of acute lymphoblastic leukaemia (ALL) in childhood. A significant negative association has also been found with the *MTHFR* 677(CT) polymorphism and leukaemias with *MLL* translocations, but a positive association with hyperdiploidy in infants with ALL or acute myeloid leukaemia or with childhood ALL. A second polymorphism in the *MHTFR* gene, A1298C, is also strongly associated with hyperdiploid leukaemia. Neither polymorphism is associated with the TEL–AML1 fusion. There are various positive and negative associations between polymorphisms in folate-dependent enzymes and the incidence of adult ALL.

The C677T polymorphism is thought to lead to increased thymidine pools and 'better quality' of DNA synthesis by shunting one-carbon groups towards thymidine and purine synthesis. This may also explain its reported association with a lower risk for colorectal cancer. The incidence of colon cancer was also lower in subjects taking vitamin supplements containing folic acid and with higher folate intake compared with control subjects in the Nurses Health Study. Other tumours that have been associated with folate polymorphisms or status include follicular lymphoma, breast cancer and gastric cancer.

Other tissues

Folate deficiency causes reduced regeneration of cirrhotic liver. Patients with gluten-induced enteropathy and those with sickle cell anaemia have also been reported to show stunted growth, which has been improved coincidentally with commencement of folic acid therapy, but it is not certain how much the growth improvement in these children was due to folic acid and how much to other, simultaneously administered vitamins. In the fragile X syndrome, sister chromatid exchange and DNA breaks are increased *in vitro* in a folate-deficient medium, apparently at the Xq28 site. No *in vivo* abnormality of folate metabolism can be detected.

Neurological manifestations

Cobalamin deficiency may cause bilateral peripheral neuropathy or degeneration (demyelination) of the posterior and pyramidal tracts of the spinal cord and, less frequently, optic atrophy or cerebral symptoms.

The patient classically presents with paraesthesiae, muscle weakness or difficulty in walking and sometimes dementia, psychotic disturbances or visual impairment. Long-term nutritional cobalamin deficiency in infancy leads to poor brain development and impaired intellectual development. Folate deficiency may cause mental changes such as depression and slowness and has been suggested to cause organic nervous disease, but this is uncertain. Methotrexate injected into the cerebrospinal fluid may, however, cause brain or spinal cord damage. Neural tube defects in the fetus are discussed above.

The biochemical basis for cobalamin neuropathy, however, remains obscure. Its occurrence in the absence of methylmalonic aciduria in transcobalamin (TC) deficiency, and in monkeys given nitrous oxide, suggests that the neuropathy is related to the defect in homocysteine–methionine conversion. Accumulation of S-adenosylhomocysteine in the brain, resulting in inhibition of transmethylation reactions, has been suggested. Measurements of methylation of arginine in myelin basic protein in fruit bats with cobalamin neuropathy, or in rats exposed to N_2O, however, show no defect of methylation.

Psychiatric disturbance is common in both folate and cobalamin deficiencies. This, like the neuropathy, has been attributed to a failure of the synthesis of S-adenosylmethionine (SAM), due to reduced conversion of homocysteine to methionine. SAM is needed in methylation of biogenic amines (e.g. dopamine), as well as of proteins, phospholipids and neurotransmitters in the brain (Figure 5.3). A reduced ratio of SAM to S-adenosylhomocysteine is postulated to result in reduced methylation. In cobalamin deficiency there is an intriguing inverse correlation between the degree of anaemia, on the one hand, and the severity of the myeloneuropathy on the other hand. Moreover, although pernicious anaemia is more frequent in women, the neuropathy is more frequent in men.

Plasma homocysteine is a risk factor for dementia and Alzheimer's disease, shown in a median follow-up period of 8 years in one study of 1092 subjects. Studies showing an association between lower serum levels of folate or cobalamin and higher homocysteine levels with Alzheimer's disease have been reported, subjects with the vitamin deficiencies being more likely to develop Alzheimer's disease in subsequent years than control subjects.

Haematological findings

Peripheral blood

Oval macrocytes, usually with considerable anisocytosis and poikilocytosis, are the main feature (Figure 5.4a). The MCV is usually > 100 fL unless a cause of microcytosis (e.g. iron deficiency or thalassaemia trait) is present, when there is a raised red cell distribution width (RDW) and the film is dimorphic. In other cases, the MCV may be normal owing to excess fragmentation of red cells. Some of the neutrophils are hypersegmented (more than five nuclear lobes). Both macrocytosis and hypersegmented neutrophils may also occur in other situations (Table 5.3). Together, however, they strongly suggest megaloblastic haemopoiesis. There may be leucopenia due to a reduction in granulocytes and lymphocytes, but this is not usually less than 1.5×10^9/L; the platelet count may be moderately reduced, rarely to less than 40×10^9/L. Occasionally, a leucoerythroblastic blood picture is seen. The severity of all these changes parallels the degree of anaemia (provided no other cause of anaemia is present): in the non-anaemic patient, the presence of a few macrocytes and hypersegmented neutrophils in the peripheral blood may be the only indication of the underlying disorder.

Bone marrow

In the severely anaemic patient, the marrow is hypercellular and there is an accumulation of primitive cells due to selective death

Macrocytosis	Alcohol
	Liver disease (especially alcoholic)
	Reticulocytosis (haemolysis or haemorrhage)
	Aplastic anaemia or red cell aplasia
	Hypothyroidism
	Myelodysplasia
	Myeloma and macroglobulinaemia
	Leucoerythroblastic anaemia
	Myeloproliferative disease
	Pregnancy
	Newborn
	Congenital dyserythropoietic anaemia (type II)
	? Chronic respiratory failure
Hypersegmented neutrophils	Renal failure
	Congenital (familial)
	? Iron deficiency

Table 5.3 Conditions in which macrocytosis or hypersegmented neutrophils may occur in the absence of megaloblastic anaemia.

Note: Falsely high MCV recorded when cold agglutinins, paraproteins or marked leucocytosis are present.

of more mature forms. The most characteristic finding is dissociation between nuclear and cytoplasmic development in the erythroblasts, with the nucleus maintaining a primitive appearance despite maturation and haemoglobinization of the cytoplasm; fully haemoglobinized (orthochromatic) erythroblasts, which retain nuclei, may be seen. The nucleus of the megaloblast has an open, fine, lacy appearance; the cells are larger than normoblasts and an increased number of cells with eccentric lobulated nuclei or nuclear fragments may be present (Figure 5.4b). Mitoses and dying cells are more frequent than normal. Giant and abnormally shaped metamyelocytes and enlarged hyperpolyploid megakaryocytes are characteristic. Severe florid megaloblastic changes may be confused with erythroleukaemia (acute myeloid leukaemia, FAB M6). Rarely, the marrow may be hypocellular or red cell precursors are lost almost completely from the marrow and a mistaken diagnosis of myeloid leukaemia may be made. Iron staining shows increase in both reticuloendothelial stores and in the developing megaloblasts.

In less anaemic patients, the changes in the marrow may be difficult to recognize. The terms 'intermediate', 'mild' and 'early' have been used to describe megaloblastic changes that are not so florid as those seen in the severely anaemic, uncomplicated case. The changes may be mild and difficult to recognize, even in a severely anaemic patient, if the anaemia is largely due to other factors (e.g. iron deficiency, infection, malignant disease, haemolysis) and the megaloblastosis is an incidental phenomenon. The term 'megaloblastoid' has several different connotations including the dysplastic changes seen in the myelodysplastic syndromes and is best avoided.

Chromosomes

Bone marrow cells, transformed lymphocytes and other proliferating cells in the body show a variety of changes including random breaks, reduced contraction, spreading of the centromere, and exaggeration of secondary chromosomal constrictions and overprominent satellites. Similar abnormalities may be produced by antimetabolite drugs (e.g. cytosine arabinoside, hydroxyurea and methotrexate) that either interfere with DNA replication or folate metabolism and that also cause megaloblastic appearances.

Ineffective haemopoiesis

There is an accumulation of unconjugated bilirubin in plasma due to the death of nucleated red cells in the marrow (ineffective erythropoiesis). Other evidence for this includes raised urine urobilinogen, reduced haptoglobins and positive urine haemosiderin, raised serum lactate dehydrogenase to values of between 1000 and 10 000 IU/dL and raised serum iron, non-transferrin-bound iron and ferritin levels. Carbon monoxide production is also increased. The serum lysozyme may also be raised, suggesting ineffective granulopoiesis.

In rare patients, ineffective haemopoiesis is associated with features of disseminated intravascular coagulation, with raised serum fibrin degradation products. Thrombocytopenia, when it occurs, is usually caused by ineffective megakaryopoiesis. A weakly positive direct antiglobulin test due to complement can lead to a false diagnosis of autoimmune haemolytic anaemia.

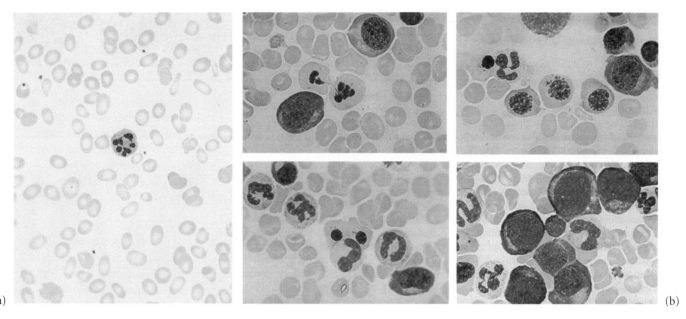

(a)

(b)

Figure 5.4 (a) The peripheral blood in severe megaloblastic anaemia. (b) The bone marrow in severe megaloblastic anaemia.

Cobalamin

Cobalamin (vitamin B_{12}) exists in a number of different chemical forms. The molecule consists of two halves: a 'planar group' and 'nucleotide' set at right angles to it (Figure 5.5). The planar group is a corrin ring and the nucleotide consists of the base, 5,6-dimethylbenziminazole, and a phosphorylated sugar, ribose-s-phosphate. In nature, the vitamin is mainly in the 5′-deoxyadenosyl (ado) form. This is the main form in human tissues and is located in the mitochondria. It serves as the cofactor for the enzyme methylmalonyl CoA mutase. The other major natural cobalamin is methylcobalamin, the main form in human plasma, as well as the cytosolic form in cells. It serves as the cofactor for the enzyme methionine synthase. There are also minor amounts of hydroxocobalamin, which is the form to which methyl- and ado-cobalamin are rapidly converted by exposure to light, hydroxocobalamin having its cobalt atom in the fully oxidized Cbl^{3+} state, whereas the cobalt exists as reduced Cbl^{1+} in the methyl- and ado-cobalamin forms (Figure 5.2). A glutathionyl cobalamin form has also been identified.

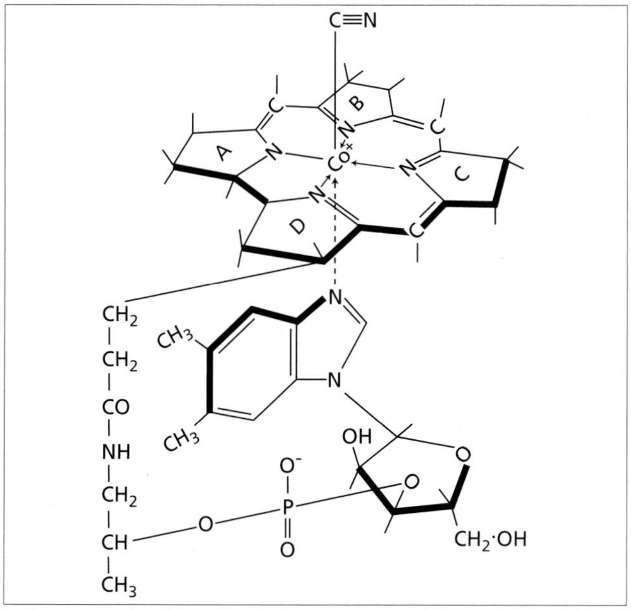

Dietary sources and requirements

Cobalamin is synthesized solely by micro-organisms. Ruminants obtain cobalamin from the foregut but the only source for humans is food of animal origin. The highest amounts are found in liver and kidney (up to 100 μg/100 g) but it is also present in shellfish, organ and muscle meats, fish, chicken and dairy products – eggs, cheese and milk – which contain small amounts (6 μg/L). Vegetables, fruits and all other foods of non-animal origin are free from cobalamin unless they are contaminated by bacteria. Cooking does not usually destroy cobalamin.

A normal Western diet contains between 5 and 30 μg of cobalamin daily. Adult daily losses (mainly in the urine and faeces) are between 1 and 3 μg (about 0.1% of body stores) and, as the body does not have the ability to degrade cobalamin, daily requirements are also about 1–3 μg. Body stores are of the order of 2–3 mg and are sufficient for 3–4 years if supplies are completely cut off.

Figure 5.5 The structure of vitamin B_{12} (cyanocobalamin).

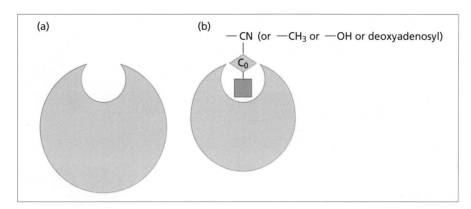

(a)

(b)

— CN (or —CH$_3$ or —OH or deoxyadenosyl)

C$_0$

Figure 5.6 (a) Intrinsic factor; (b) intrinsic factor–cobalamin complex. Intrinsic factor has been estimated to have a molecular radius of 3.6 nm, vitamin B$_{12}$ 0.8 nm and the complex 3.2 nm.

Absorption

Two mechanisms exist for cobalamin absorption. One is passive, occurring equally through the duodenum and the ileum; it is rapid but extremely inefficient as less than 1% of an oral dose can be absorbed by this process. Passive absorption of cobalamin can occur through other mucous membranes such as the sublingual and nasal mucosae. Recently, oral, sublingual and intranasal preparations of cobalamin have become popular as an alternative to intramuscular (i.m.) injections for treatment of cobalamin deficiency and long-term maintenance of cobalamin status. The other mechanism is active; it occurs through the ileum in humans and is efficient for small (a few micrograms) oral doses of cobalamin. This is the normal mechanism by which the body acquires cobalamin and is mediated by gastric intrinsic factor (IF).

Dietary cobalamin is released from protein complexes by enzymes in the stomach, duodenum and jejunum; it combines rapidly with a salivary glycoprotein (R binder) related to plasma transcobalamin I (TCI). These belong to the family of cobalamin-binding proteins known as haptocorrins (HCs). Subsequently, the R binder is digested by pancreatic trypsin and the cobalamin transferred to IF. Binding of cobalamin to IF is favoured by an alkaline pH; it binds one molecule for one molecule. All forms of cobalamin are absorbed by the same IF mechanism. The nucleotide portion of cobalamin fits into a pit on the surface of the protein, whereas the –CN, –OH, –CH$_3$ or deoxyadenosyl group is opposite the site of attachment (Figure 5.6). Pseudo-cobalamin compounds, in which the 5,6-dimethylbenzimidazole nucleotide is replaced by other nucleotides that may attach to the R binder, do not attach to IF and therefore remain unabsorbed through the active physiological mechanism.

Intrinsic factor is a glycoprotein with a molecular weight of 45 000. It is produced in the microsomes or endoplasmic reticulum of the gastric parietal cells in the fundus and body of the stomach of humans. The IF–cobalamin complex, in contrast with free IF, is resistant to enzyme digestion. IF–cobalamin has a smaller molecular radius (3.2 nm) than free IF (3.6 nm) (Figure

5.6), and some peptide bonds that are open to attack by proteolytic enzymes when IF is free are protected in the complex.

The IF–cobalamin complex passes to the ileum, where IF attaches to a specific receptor (cubilin, mol. wt 460 000) on the microvillus membrane of the brush border surface of the ileal absorptive cells. Cubilin is also present in yolk sac and renal proximal tubular epithelium. The attachment of the IF–cobalamin complex requires calcium ions and a pH around neutral. It is probably a physical process, not requiring energy. Cubulin appears to traffic by means of amnionless (AMN), a 600 000-Da endocytic receptor protein that mediates the uptake of a number of ligands. Cubulin and AMN appear to be subunits of a novel complex in which AMN binds tightly to the amino-terminal third of cubulin and directs sublocalization and endocytosis of cubulin with its ligand (IF–cobalamin complex). Defects in cubulin and AMN are implicated in autosomal recessive megaloblastic anaemia, characterized by intestinal malabsorption of cobalamin (see p. 72).

Cobalamin then enters the ileal cell, but the exact fate of the IF is unknown. Intrinsic factor does not enter the bloodstream as such, as after a delay of about 6 h, absorbed cobalamin appears in portal blood, attached to transcobalamin (II) which is probably synthesized in the ileum, either by mucosal cells or by venous endothelial cells in the submucosa.

The ileum has a restricted capacity to absorb cobalamin because of limited receptor sites and, although 50% or more of a single dose of 1 μg of cobalamin may be absorbed, with doses above 2 μg the proportion absorbed falls rapidly. Moreover, after one dose of IF–cobalamin complex has been presented, the ileal cells become refractory to further doses for about 6 h.

Enterohepatic circulation

Between 0.5 and 5.0 μg of cobalamin enter the bile each day. This binds to IF and a portion of biliary cobalamin is normally reabsorbed together with cobalamin derived from sloughed intestinal cells. Bile may enhance cobalamin absorption. Because of the appreciable amount of cobalamin undergoing enterohepatic circulation, cobalamin deficiency develops more rapidly in individuals who malabsorb cobalamin than it does in vegans, who ingest no cobalamin, but in whom reabsorption of biliary cobalamin is intact.

Transport

Two main cobalamin transport proteins exist in human plasma; they both bind cobalamin one molecule for one molecule (Figure 5.7). One HC, also known as TCI, is a glycoprotein. It is closely related to other HCs (so-called 'R') cobalamin-binding proteins in milk, gastric juice, bile, saliva and other fluids. These HCs differ from each other only in the carbohydrate moiety of the molecule. TCIII was a name used to describe a minor isoprotein of TCI in plasma, which differs from TCI by its composition of sugars and cobalamin content. TCI and TCIII are derived primarily from the specific granules in neutrophils. Overall, HCs are normally about two-thirds saturated with cobalamin, which they bind tightly. HCs do not enhance cobalamin entry into tissues. Glycoprotein receptors on liver cells are concerned in the removal of HCs from plasma, and TCI may have a role in the transport of cobalamin analogues to the liver for excretion in bile.

The other major cobalamin transport protein in plasma is transcobalamin (TC, also known as transcobalamin II). TC is a β-globulin (mol. wt 38 000) synthesized by liver, and by other tissues including macrophages, ileum and endothelium. It normally carries only 20–60 ng of cobalamin per litre of plasma and

readily gives up cobalamin to marrow, placenta and other tissues, which it enters by receptor-mediated endocytosis; TC is not re-utilized. It has a 20% amino acid homology and more than 50% nucleotide homology with human HC and with rat IF. The regions of homology of HC, TC and IF are probably involved in cobalamin binding. Five different inherited isoproteins of TC, separated by polyacrylamide gel electrophoresis, have been described; all are functionally active. Recent evidence suggests that common polymorphisms in the TC gene may affect predisposition to cobalamin deficiency. TC occurs in cerebrospinal fluid and bind cobalamin (approximately 10 ng/L) there. Alterations may occur in the TC and HC levels in a variety of disease states (Table 5.4). In general, an increase in HC causes an increase in serum cobalamin, whereas an increase in TC does not.

Cobalamin analogues

Cobalamin analogues are corrinoids, which may be cobamides (which contain substitutions in the place of ribose, e.g. adenoside) or cobinamides (which have no nucleotide at all). The analogues are relatively inert for the microbiological assay organisms *Euglena gracilis* and *Lactobacillus leichmannii*. In competitive binding assays that use HC but not pure IF as the binding protein, cobalamin analogues lead to falsely high serum cobalamin levels. HC may carry analogues to the liver for excretion in the bile. It is unclear whether they are inert or inhibit cobalamin-dependent reactions. The proportion of analogues derived from diet, gut bacteria or endogenous breakdown of cobalamins is unknown. They are present in fetal blood and tissues.

Causes of cobalamin deficiency

Cobalamin deficiency is usually due to malabsorption. The only other cause is inadequate dietary intake. Cobalamin deficiency due to excess degradation occurs as a result of exposure to the anaesthetic gas nitrous oxide (N_2O). N_2O causes irreversible oxidation of the active Cbl^{1+} during catalytic shunting of labile methyl groups in the methionine synthase reaction (see p. 61).

Inadequate dietary intake

Adults

Dietary cobalamin deficiency arises in vegans who omit meat, fish, eggs, cheese and other animal products from their diet. The largest group in the world consists of Hindus, and it is likely that many millions of Indians are at risk for deficiency of cobalamin on a nutritional basis. Not all vegans, however, develop cobalamin deficiency of sufficient severity to cause anaemia or neuropathy, even though subnormal cobalamin levels have

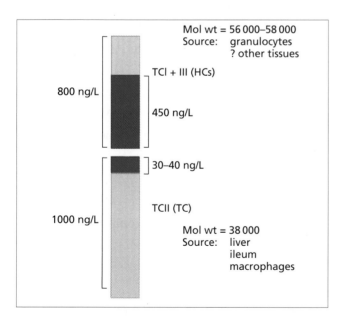

Figure 5.7 The serum cobalamin-binding proteins (TCs, transcobalamins). Dark blue rectangles, endogenous serum cobalamin; light blue rectangles, unsaturated cobalamin-binding protein; HCs, haptocorrins.

Haptocorrin	Increased (usually with elevated serum cobalamin)
	Myeloproliferative diseases, especially chronic myeloid leukaemia, myelosclerosis, polycythaemia vera
	Hepatoma
	Increased granulocyte production (e.g. inflammatory bowel disease, liver abscess)
	Eosinophilia due to hypereosinophilic syndrome
	Congenital absence: low total serum cobalamin; no clear clinical abnormality
Transcobalamin (II)	Increased (sometimes with no elevation of serum cobalamin)
	Liver disease
	Gaucher's disease
	Autoimmune disease
	Long-continued hydroxocobalamin therapy
	Congenital absence: normal or decreased total serum cobalamin; megaloblastic anaemia or pancytopenia within a few weeks of birth; impaired cobalamin absorption, may be associated with defective cellular and humoral immunity

Table 5.4 Alteration in plasma cobalamin-binding proteins in disease.

been found in up to 50% of randomly selected, young, adult Indian vegans. Explanations of why nutritional cobalamin deficiency may not progress to megaloblastic anaemia include the following:

1 The diet of most vegans is probably not totally lacking cobalamin. The serum cobalamin level may not be an accurate measure of their body stores.

2 The enterohepatic circulation of cobalamin is still intact in vegans and thus losses are less than in conditions of malabsorption.

3 Daily losses of cobalamin are thought to be related to body stores; therefore, as the body stores become depleted, daily losses become smaller and the amount of cobalamin needed to maintain the status quo may also become smaller. There is, however, no evidence that the daily requirement for cobalamin changes.

Dietary cobalamin deficiency may also arise rarely in non-vegetarian subjects who exist on grossly inadequate diets because of poverty or psychiatric disturbance.

Infants

Cobalamin deficiency has been described in infants born to severely cobalamin-deficient mothers. These infants develop megaloblastic anaemia about 3–6 months of age, presumably because they are born with low stores of cobalamin and because they are fed breast milk of low cobalamin content. This occurs most commonly in Indian vegans, but a similar condition has also been described in unrecognized maternal pernicious anaemia and in strict practitioners of veganism living in Western countries whose offspring have shown growth retardation, impaired psychomotor development and other neurological sequelae.

Table 5.5 Causes of cobalamin deficiency causing megaloblastic anaemia.

Nutritional	Vegans
Malabsorption	Pernicious anaemia
Gastric causes	Congenital IF absence or functional abnormality
	Total or partial gastrectomy
Intestinal causes	Intestinal stagnant loop syndrome: jejunal diverticulosis, ileocolic fistula, anatomical blind loop, intestinal stricture, etc.
	Ileal resection and Crohn's disease
	Selective malabsorption with proteinuria
	Tropical sprue
	Transcobalamin deficiency
	Fish tapeworm

Gastric causes of cobalamin malabsorption
(Tables 5.5 and 5.6)

Pernicious anaemia

Pernicious anaemia (PA) may be defined as a severe lack of intrinsic factor due to gastric atrophy. It is a common disease in north Europeans but it occurs in all countries and ethnic groups. The overall incidence is about 120 per 100 000 population in the UK, but there is wide variation between one area and the next. The prevalence rate in Western countries may be as high as 2–3%. The ratio of incidence in men and women is approximately 1:1.6 and the peak age of onset is 60 years, with only 10%

Table 5.6 Malabsorption of cobalamin may occur in the following conditions but is not usually sufficiently severe and prolonged to cause megaloblastic anaemia.

Gastric causes
Simple atrophic gastritis (food cobalamin malabsorption)
Zollinger–Ellison syndrome
Gastric bypass surgery
Use of proton pump inhibitors

Intestinal causes
Gluten-induced enteropathy
Severe pancreatitis
HIV infection
Radiotherapy
Graft-versus-host disease

Deficiencies of cobalamin, folate, protein, ?riboflavin, ?nicotinic acid

Therapy with colchicine, para-aminosalicylate, neomycin, slow-release potassium chloride, anticonvulsant drugs, metformin, phenformin, cytotoxic drugs

Alcohol

of patients presenting being less than 40 years of age. In some ethnic groups, notably black people and Latin Americans, the age of onset of PA is generally lower. The disease occurs more commonly than by chance in close relatives, in subjects with other organ-specific autoimmune diseases (see below), in those with premature greying, blue eyes and vitiligo, and in persons of blood group A. An association with human leucocyte antigen (HLA) 3 has been reported in some but not all series and in those with endocrine disease, with HLA-B8, -B12 and -BW15. The life expectancy is normal in women once regular treatment has begun. Men have a slightly subnormal life expectancy as a result of a higher incidence of carcinoma of the stomach than in control subjects.

Diagnosis
This is usually suspected from the clinical picture and the findings of megaloblastic anaemia due to cobalamin deficiency. A lack of IF may be demonstrated by cobalamin absorption studies. Tests for circulating gastric autoantibodies are also important.

Tests of gastric secretion
Direct measurements on gastric juice following pentagastrin stimulation are now rarely performed. Hydrochloric acid or pepsin production and intrinsic factor output were previously measured.

Serum assays
The serum gastrin level is usually raised in PA (> 200 μg/L), the hormone coming from endocrine cells in the gastric fundus.

Raised serum gastrin also occurs in simple atrophic gastritis. Serum pepsinogen I levels are low (below 30 μg/L) in over 90% of those affected.

Gastric biopsy
This usually shows atrophy of all layers of the body and also fundal atrophy, with loss of glandular elements, an absence of parietal and chief cells and replacement by mucous cells, a mixed inflammatory cell infiltrate and perhaps intestinal metaplasia. The infiltrate of plasma cells and lymphocytes contains an excess of CD4 cells. The antral mucosa is usually well preserved. *Helicobacter pylori* infection is infrequent in pernicious anaemia, but it has been suggested that *H. pylori* gastritis may represent an early phase of atrophic gastritis, which is gradually replaced, in some individuals, by an immune process with disappearance of *H. pylori* infection.

Immune phenomena
In addition to the appearance of gastric mucosa, there is a large body of evidence that suggests that immune mechanisms play an important role in the pathogenesis of PA. This aspect of the disease is discussed next under four main headings.

Antibodies to gastric antigens
IF antibodies. Two types of IF antibody may be found in the sera of patients with PA: both are immunoglobulin (Ig) G. One, the 'blocking' or 'type I' antibody, prevents the combination of IF and cobalamin, whereas the other, the 'binding' 'type II' or 'precipitating' antibody, which attaches to IF whether joined to cobalamin or not, prevents attachment of IF to ileal mucosa. The blocking antibody occurs in the serum of about 55% of patients and the binding antibody in 35%. IF antibodies cross the placenta and cause temporary IF deficiency in the newborn infant. Pernicious anaemia patients also show cell-mediated immunity to IF. An increased CD4/CD8 lymphocyte ratio in blood has been described in PA patients with IF antibodies.

IF antibodies are rarely found in conditions other than PA. Type I antibody has been detected rarely in the sera of patients without PA but with thyrotoxicosis, myxoedema, Hashimoto's disease or diabetes mellitus, and in relatives of PA patients. IF antibodies have also been detected in gastric juice in about 80% of PA patients. These antibodies may reduce absorption of dietary cobalamin by combining with small amounts of remaining IF in the gastric juice. Achlorhydria favours the formation of this antigen–antibody complex.

Parietal cell and gastrin receptor antibodies. Parietal cell antibody is present in the sera of almost 90% of adult patients with PA, but it is frequently present in other subjects. Thus, it occurs in as many as 16% of randomly selected female subjects aged over 60 years and in a smaller proportion of younger control subjects; it is found more frequently than in control subjects in relatives of

PA patients. These antibodies are also found more frequently in patients with simple atrophic gastritis, chronic active hepatitis and thyroid disorders and their relatives, as well as in Addison's disease, rheumatoid arthritis and other conditions. The parietal cell antibody is directed against the α- and β-subunits of the gastric proton pump (H^+,K^+-ATPase). The sera of PA patients may also contain an autoantibody to the gastrin receptor, although this test is not used clinically.

Association with other 'autoimmune' diseases
There is a clinical association between PA and thyroid diseases, vitiligo, hypoparathyroidism and Addison's disease. These diseases are often found in close relatives of patients with overt disease due to one of these conditions.

Response to steroid therapy
Steroid therapy improves the gastric lesion, at least temporarily, in a proportion of patients with PA. There may be regeneration of the mucosa with a return of secretion of acid and IF, and an improvement in cobalamin absorption. When steroid therapy is withdrawn, there is a relapse within a few weeks. These findings suggest that an autoimmune process is continuously damaging the gastric mucosa in PA and preventing regeneration. Temporary remission of neurological symptoms has been observed in PA, erroneously diagnosed as multiple sclerosis and treated with steroids.

Hypogammaglobulinaemia
PA is found more often than by chance in patients with a deficiency of IgA or with complete hypogammaglobulinaemia. These subjects resemble others with PA, except that they often present relatively early (before the age of 40 years), they have a lower incidence of serum IF and parietal cell antibodies, and they may show intestinal malabsorption. They may also have a history of recurrent infections. The gastric lesion is similar to that in other causes, except that plasma cells are absent from the inflammatory cell infiltrate and the antrum is involved. Serum gastrin levels are normal.

Juvenile pernicious anaemia
This usually occurs in older children and resembles PA of adults. Gastric atrophy, achlorhydria and serum IF antibodies are all present, although parietal cell antibodies are usually absent. About one-half of these patients show an associated endocrinopathy such as autoimmune thyroiditis, Addison's disease or hypoparathyroidism; in some, mucocutaneous candidiasis occurs.

Congenital intrinsic factor deficiency or functional abnormality
The affected child usually shows no demonstrable IF but has a normal gastric mucosa and normal secretion of acid. The inheritance is autosomally recessive. These patients usually present with megaloblastic anaemia in the first, second or third year of life when stores of cobalamin accumulated from the mother *in utero* are used up; a few have presented as late as the second decade. Parietal cell and IF antibodies are absent. Variants have been described in which the child is born with IF that can be detected immunologically but is unstable or functionally inactive, being unable either to bind cobalamin or to facilitate its uptake by the ileum.

Gastrectomy
Following total gastrectomy, cobalamin deficiency is inevitable and prophylactic cobalamin therapy should be commenced immediately following the operation. After partial gastrectomy, 10–15% of patients also develop this deficiency. This usually manifests 4 years or more following the operation, but may occur sooner. The exact incidence and time of onset is most influenced by the size of the resection and the pre-existing size of the cobalamin body store.

Simple atrophic gastritis (food cobalamin malabsorption)
For the normal IF-mediated mechanism of cobalamin absorption, certain requirements in the gastrointestinal lumen must be met. These include adequate gastric output of acid and pepsin to ensure the release of food cobalamin. Failure of this mechanism is believed to be responsible for a condition more common in the elderly known as *food cobalamin malabsorption*, but there is no definitive proof of this. This is associated with low serum cobalamin levels, with or without evidence of cobalamin deficiency, such as raised serum levels of methylmalonic acid and homocysteine, and abnormal deoxyuridine suppression. Few show clinically important cobalamin deficiency and, typically, these patients have normal cobalamin absorption as measured by the standard Schilling test, which measures absorption of crystalline cobalamin. A modified test using food-bound cobalamin must be used to demonstrate the malabsorption. Some patients with food cobalamin malabsorption may go on to develop clinically significant cobalamin deficiency, but the frequency of occurrence and reasons for this progression are not clear.

Intestinal causes of cobalamin malabsorption

Intestinal stagnant loop syndrome
Malabsorption of cobalamin occurs in a variety of intestinal lesions in which there is colonization of the upper small intestine by faecal organisms. This may occur in patients with jejunal diverticulosis, enteroanastomosis, intestinal stricture or fistula, or with an anatomical blood loop due to Crohn's disease, tuberculosis or an operative procedure. It is not known with certainty which organisms are responsible for the consumption of cobalamin. Bacterial overgrowth in the small intestine may also cause spurious elevation of serum methylmalonate (see below). Some bacteria produce copious quantities of propionate, the immediate precursor of methylmalonate.

Ileal resection

Removal of 1.2 m or more of terminal ileum causes malabsorption of cobalamin. In some patients, following ileal resection, particularly if the ileocaecal valve is incompetent, colonic bacteria may contribute further to the onset of cobalamin deficiency.

Selective malabsorption of cobalamin with proteinuria (Imerslund syndrome: Imerslund–Gräsbeck syndrome: congenital cobalamin malabsorption: autosomal recessive megaloblastic anaemia MGA1)

This autosomally recessive disease is the most common cause of megaloblastic anaemia due to cobalamin deficiency in infancy in Western countries. More than 200 cases have been reported, with familial clusters in Finland, Norway, the Middle East and North Africa. The patients usually present with megaloblastic anaemia between the ages of 1 and 5 years, secrete normal amounts of IF and gastric acid, but are unable to absorb cobalamin due to a congenital defect of the ileum. In some cases, e.g. in Finland, impaired synthesis, processing or ligand binding of cubilin due to inherited mutations have been implicated. In others, e.g. in Norway, mutation of the gene for *AMN* has been reported. Other tests of intestinal absorption are normal. Over 90% of these patients show non-specific proteinuria but renal function is otherwise normal and renal biopsy has not shown any consistent renal defect. A few of these patients have shown aminoaciduria and congenital renal abnormalities, such as duplication of the renal pelvis.

Tropical sprue

Nearly all patients with acute and subacute tropical sprue show malabsorption of cobalamin; this may persist as the principal abnormality in the chronic form of the disease, when the patient may present with megaloblastic anaemia or neuropathy due to cobalamin deficiency. Absorption of cobalamin usually improves after antibiotic therapy and, in the early stages, after folic acid therapy.

Fish tapeworm infestation

The fish tapeworm (*Diphyllobothrium latum*) lives in the small intestine of humans and accumulates cobalamin from food, rendering this unavailable for absorption. People acquire the worm by eating raw or partly cooked fish. Infestation is common around the lakes of Scandinavia, Germany, Japan, North America and Russia. Megaloblastic anaemia or cobalamin neuropathy occurs only in those with a heavy infestation, with the worm high in the small intestine. Many carriers have no cobalamin deficiency.

Gluten-induced enteropathy

Malabsorption of cobalamin occurs in about 30% of untreated patients (presumably those in whom the disease extends to the ileum) and correlates with the degree of steatorrhoea. Cobalamin deficiency is not usually severe in these patients and is probably never the cause of megaloblastic anaemia unless another lesion causing malabsorption of cobalamin (e.g. the stagnant loop syndrome) is present. The absorption improves when these patients are treated with a gluten-free diet.

Severe chronic pancreatitis

In this condition, lack of trypsin is thought to cause dietary cobalamin attached to gastric non-IF (R) binder to be unavailable for absorption. It has also been proposed that in pancreatitis, the concentration of calcium ions in the ileum falls below the level needed to maintain normal cobalamin absorption.

HIV infection

Serum cobalamin levels tend to fall in patients with HIV infection and are subnormal in 10–35% of those with AIDS. Increased levels of apoTC, possibly derived from macrophages, are usual. Malabsorption of crystalline cobalamin not corrected by IF has been shown in some, but not all, patients with subnormal serum cobalamin levels. Food cobalamin absorption studies have not been reported. Cobalamin deficiency sufficiently severe to cause megaloblastic anaemia or neuropathy is rare.

Zollinger–Ellison syndrome

Malabsorption of cobalamin has been reported in the Zollinger–Ellison syndrome. It is thought that there is a failure to release cobalamin from R binding protein due to inactivation of pancreatic trypsin by high acidity, as well as interference with IF binding of cobalamin.

Radiotherapy

Both total body irradiation and local radiotherapy to the ileum (e.g. as a complication of radiotherapy for carcinoma of the cervix) may cause malabsorption of cobalamin.

Graft-versus-host disease

This commonly affects the small intestine. Malabsorption of cobalamin due to abnormal gut flora, as well as damage to ileal mucosa, is frequent.

Drugs

Neomycin, colchicine, phenytoin (dephenylhydantoin), para-aminosalicylate, phenformin, metformin, slow-release potassium chloride and alcohol have all been reported to cause malabsoption of cobalamin and, rarely, megaloblastic anaemia due to cobalamin deficiency has been reported with phenformin therapy. The use of H_2-blockers for treatment of peptic ulcer disease causes a decrease in cobalamin absorption, and continued use may lead to lowering the serum cobalamin level.

Cobalamin and folate deficiencies

Both severe cobalamin and folate deficiencies affect the function of the small intestine; malabsorption of cobalamin due to ileal dysfunction may be found in patients with either deficiency. It may take several weeks of cobalamin therapy to correct the ileal absorptive defect in patients with PA. Deficiencies of protein, riboflavin and pyridoxine have also been reported to cause malabsorption of cobalamin.

Abnormalities of cobalamin metabolism

Congenital TC (transcobalamin II) deficiency or abnormality

Infants with TC deficiency usually present with megaloblastic anaemia within a few weeks of birth. Serum cobalamin and folate levels are normal but the anaemia responds to massive (e.g. 1 mg three times weekly) injections of cobalamin, which cause free cobalamin to enter marrow cells by passive diffusion in the absence of functional TC. Some cases show neurological complications. In some cases, the protein is present in normal amounts but is unable to bind cobalamin or to attach to the cell surface and so is functionally inert. Genetic abnormalities so far found include nutations of an intra-exonic cryptic splice site, extensive deletion, single nucleotide deletion, nonsense mutation and an RNA editing defect. These infants do not show methylmalonic aciduria, but malabsorption of cobalamin occurs in all cases and reduced immunoglobulins occurs in some. Less severe cases present later in childhood. Failure to institute adequate cobalamin therapy or treatment with folic acid may lead to neurological damage.

Congenital methylmalonic acidaemia and aciduria

The infants with this abnormality are ill from birth with vomiting, failure to thrive, severe metabolic acidosis, ketosis and mental retardation. Anaemia, if present, is normocytic and normoblastic. The condition may arise as a result of a functional defect in either the mitochondrial methylmalonyl coenzyme A (CoA) mutase or its cofactor ado-cobalamin (Figure 5.2). Mutations in the methylmalonyl CoA mutase are not responsive, or only poorly responsive, to treatment with cobalamin. Two disorders result in cobalamin-responsive methylmalonic acidaemia. In Cb (cobalamin) 1A disease, there is failure of reduction of Cob(III) (Cbl^{3+}) alamin or Cob(II) (Cbl^{2+}) alamin to Cob(I) (Cbl^{1+}) alamin in mitochondria; in Cb1B disease there is a defect of an adenosyltransferase required for synthesis of ado-cobalamin (Figure 5.2). A proportion of the infants with CbIA and Cb1B respond to cobalamin in large doses, whereas the others are unresponsive. In those who do not respond to cobalamin, the enzyme methylmalonyl CoA mutase is lacking (mut^0) or defective (mut^-). Some children have combined methylmalonic aciduria and homocystinuria due to defective formation of both cobalamin coenzymes. The defects are in the transfer of cobalamin from the endocytic compartment to lysosomes to the cytoplasm (Cb1F) or in reduction of cobalamin after transfer to the cytoplasm from the Cob(III)alamin to the Cob(I)alamin state (Cb1C and Cb1D diseases). Over 100 cases of

the Cb1C disease have been described. It usually presents in the first year of life with feeding difficulties, developmental delay, microcephaly, seizures, hypotonia and megaloblastic anaemia.

Some patients have homocystinuria and megaloblastic anaemia, often with neurological defects but without methylmalonic aciduria. There is a selective deficiency of methyl cobalamin. These conditions have been termed Cb1E and Cb1G disease (lack of association of methyl cobalamin with methionine synthase).

Acquired abnormality of cobalamin metabolism: nitrous oxide inhalation

Nitrous oxide irreversibly oxidizes methyl cobalamin from its active, fully reduced CobI state to an inactive precursor with the CobII state. This has been shown to inactivate methylcobalamin and methionine synthase. This occurs in both humans and experimental animals and is of importance in the megaloblastic anaemia that occurs in patients undergoing prolonged N_2O anaesthesia (e.g. in intensive care units). A neuropathy resembling cobalamin neuropathy has been described in dentists and anaesthetists who are repeatedly exposed to N_2O and in monkeys exposed to the gas for many months. In patients with low cobalamin stores, megaloblastic anaemia or cobalamin neuropathy may be precipitated after shorter exposure to N_2O. Recovery from N_2O exposure requires regeneration of methionine synthase, as this protein is damaged by active oxygen derived from the N_2O–cobalamin reaction. Methylmalonic aciduria does not occur at first as ado-cobalamin is not inactivated by N_2O. Later, however, after generalized depletion of cobalamin, methylmalonate levels in serum, urine and cerebrospinal fluid rise.

Diagnosis of cobalamin deficiency

The diagnosis of cobalamin or folate deficiency has traditionally depended on the recognition of the relevant abnormalities in the peripheral blood and/or bone marrow and subsequent analysis of the blood levels of the vitamins. Other causes of macrocytosis and hypersegmented neutrophils are listed in Table 5.3. Assays of serum methylmalonic acid and homocysteine (see below) have, however, shown these to be raised in some subjects without haematological abnormalities, including a proportion with normal levels of serum cobalamin and folate in whom, nevertheless, the levels of the metabolites fall to normal with cobalamin and/or folate therapy. The significance of these biochemical changes remains controversial. They may imply functional cobalamin or folate deficiency, not reflected by subnormal levels of the vitamins or by disturbed haemopoiesis. If so, it would imply that the accepted normal serum and red cell levels of the vitamins reflect body stores which are sufficiently high to prevent haematological changes but in some subjects may not be optimal for prevention of other complications of the deficiencies including thrombosis and vascular disease and neural tube defect in the fetus.

Deoxyuridine suppression test

In normal bone marrow, deoxyuridine (dU) considerably suppresses the uptake of radioactive thymidine into DNA. This is thought to be due to conversion of dU to thymidine triphosphate (dTTO) via dU monophosphate (dUMP), which inhibits thymidine kinase, on which thymidine uptake depends (Figure 5.1). Deoxyuridine suppresses radioactive thymidine incorporation less effectively in megaloblastic anaemia due to folate or cobalamin deficiency because of the block in dUMP methylation to dTMP. In cobalamin deficiency, the test can be corrected with cobalamin or 5-formyltetrahydrofolate (5-formyl-THF, folinic acid) but not with 5-methyl-THF, whereas, in folate deficiency, both the folate analogues, but not cobalamin, correct the test. In refractory megaloblastic anaemia (e.g. of sideroblastic anaemia, erythroleukaemia, or due to antimetabolite drugs which inhibit DNA synthesis at a separate point from thymidylate synthesis), the test gives results as in a normoblastic marrow. Performance of the dU suppression test is laborious and the test is rarely performed other than in specialized laboratories.

Measurement of the serum cobalamin

Serum cobalamin is usually measured by one of a number of radioisotope dilution, or enzyme-linked immunosorbent assays. These are frequently automated. Normal serum cobalamin levels range from 160 to 200 ng/L to about 1000 ng/L (ng × 0.738 = pmol, so 200 ng/L = 148 pmol/L). In patients with megaloblastic anaemia due to cobalamin deficiency, the level is usually less than 100 ng/L. In general, the more severe the deficiency, the lower the serum cobalamin level. In patients with spinal cord damage due to the deficiency, levels are very low even in the absence of anaemia. Values of between 100 and 200 ng/L are regarded as borderline. They may occur, for instance, in pregnancy, in patients with megaloblastic anaemia due to folate deficiency and in patients with HC deficiency. The relative concentrations of HC and TC also influence the total serum cobalamin level. Raised serum cobalamin levels (if not due to recent therapy) are usually due to a rise in HC (Table 5.4), or to liver or renal disease with increased saturation of HC and TC.

The serum cobalamin level is still generally considered to be sufficiently robust, cost-effective and most convenient to rule out cobalamin deficiency in the vast majority of patients suspected of having this problem. The reliability of the serum cobalamin assay was established with microbiological assays. Using the newer assays, normal levels have been reported in patients responsive to cobalamin therapy.

Serum holotranscobalamin (HoloTCII; Holo TC)

Since TC is the plasma cobalamin transport protein that is responsible for cellular uptake and delivery of cobalamin, the notion was put forward that measurement of circulating cobalamin that was bound to TC (HoloTC), would provide a more meaningful measure of cobalamin status than total serum cobalamin. Since HoloTC represents only 20–30% of the total serum cobalamin, there have been formidable problems in establishing a HoloTC assay. Such an assay has been produced and recently became available in Europe. Validation of the clinical usefulness and limitations of this test indicate that it may, in conjunction with the serum cobalamin level, provide improved sensitivity for detection of cobalamin deficiency. Additionally, it may be useful as a confirmatory test to establish true cobalamin deficiency in patients with low serum cobalamin.

Serum methylmalonate and homocysteine levels

Deoxyadenosyl cobalamin is required as a coenzyme in the isomerization of methylmalonyl CoA to succinyl CoA. In patients with cobalamin deficiency sufficient to cause anaemia or neuropathy, the serum methylmalonate (MMA) level is raised. Sensitive methods for measuring MMA and homocysteine in serum have been introduced and recommended for the early diagnosis of cobalamin deficiency, even in the absence of haematological abnormalities or subnormal levels of serum cobalamin or folate. Serum MMA fluctuates, however, in patients with renal failure. Mildly elevated serum MMA and/or homocysteine levels occur in up to 30% of apparently healthy volunteers, with serum cobalamin levels up to 350 ng/L and normal serum folate levels; 15% of elderly subjects, even with cobalamin levels > 350 ng/L, have this pattern of raised metabolite levels. These findings bring into question the exact cut-off points for normal MMA and homocysteine levels. It is also unclear at present whether these mildly raised metabolite levels have clinical consequences and how many of the subjects will progress to clinically overt cobalamin deficiency. When cobalamin supplies to the cell are suboptimal, there may be preferential use as methylcobalamin for methionine synthesis compared with ado-cobalamin for MMA metabolism. Urine MMA excretion may also be used to screen for cobalamin deficiency but this also is increased in aminoaciduria (e.g. Fanconi's syndrome).

Homocysteine exists in plasma as single molecules, as two molecules linked together (homocystine) and as mixed homocysteine–cysteine disulphides. Serum homocysteine levels are raised in both early cobalamin and folate deficiency, but they may be raised in other conditions, e.g. chronic renal disease, alcoholism, smoking, pyridoxine deficiency, hypothyroidism therapy with steroids, cyclosporin and other drugs. Levels are also higher in serum than in plasma, in men than in pre-menopausal women, women taking hormone replacement therapy or oral contraceptive users and in elderly subjects and patients with several inborn errors of metabolism affecting enzymes in trans-sulphuration pathways of homocysteine metabolism. Thus, homocysteine levels are not widely used for diagnosis of cobalamin or folate deficiency. Homocysteine levels are useful, however, in thrombophilia screening and in assessing for cardiovascular risk factors (see Chapter 58).

Tests for the cause of cobalamin deficiency

The principal methods used in diagnosing the cause of cobalamin deficiency are listed in Table 5.7. Many of these tests are mentioned elsewhere in this chapter, and others are described in texts of gastroenterology. Studies of cobalamin absorption are, however, of particular importance.

Cobalamin absorption

This is usually assessed by one of two different techniques: whole-body counting or urinary excretion (Schilling test). Hepatic uptake, faecal excretion and plasma radioactivity have also been measured but are not now used routinely. Whole-body counting is available at only a few specialized centres.

Table 5.7 Tests for the cause of cobalamin deficiency.

Clinical history: diet, drugs, operations, etc.
Cobalamin absorption using radioactive cobalamin: Alone; with food; with IF; after a course of antibiotics
Tests for tissue-specific antibodies in serum (e.g. IF, parietal, cell, thyroid, gliadin, endomysial, transglutaminase
Endoscopy with gastric biopsy
Measurement of IF in gastric juice after maximal stimulation (e.g. with pentagastrin); this test is rarely performed now
Small intestinal studies
Examination of urine for proteinuria
Stools for fish tapeworm ova

Cyanocobalamin labelled with the isotopes [57]Co or [58]Co is used clinically. The patient is fasted overnight. The test is performed giving radioactive cyanocobalamin (1 μg) orally. A 24-h urine specimen is collected for determination of radioactivity excreted alone. Then, 2 h later an i.m. injection of cyanocobalamin or hydroxocobalamin (1 mg) is given ('flushing dose'); if this shows malabsorption, the dose is given again after 48 h with IF. The results distinguish between gastric and intestinal causes of cobalamin malabsorption. If intestinal malabsorption is present, the test may be repeated after antibiotic therapy to reduce possible bacterial interference with cobalamin absorption. As the Schilling test involves the injection of 1 mg of non-radioactive hydroxocobalamin (or cyanocobalamin), this will also treat the patient. A combined test (Dicopac) is available, in which two isotopes of cyanocobalamin are given simultaneously, one alone and one attached to IF. The excretion of the two isotopes is compared in the same 24-h urine. The results are less clear-cut than when the two tests are performed separately because of some exchange of isotopes attached to IF. It is a useful test, however, when incomplete urine collections are likely.

The standard test is performed using crystalline radioactive cyanocobalamin. Tests using food-bound (e.g. egg ovalbumin) radioactive cyanocobalamin have been devised to parallel normal dietary cobalamin more closely. Such tests may detect malabsorption of cobalamin in some patients, for example those with atropic gastritis and low serum cobalamin levels, but with normal absorption of crystalline cyanocobalamin. Because of concerns with radioisotope use and disposal, Schilling tests are being used less frequently.

Folate

Dietary folate

Folic acid (pteroylglutamic acid) is a yellow, crystalline, water-soluble substance (mol. wt 441). It is the parent compound of a large family of folate compounds. Pteroylglutamic acid consists of three parts: pteridine, *para*-aminobenzoate and L-glutamic acid (Figure 5.8). It is only a minor component of normal food folates (probably less than 1%), which differ from it in three respects (Figure 5.8): (i) they are partly or completely reduced at

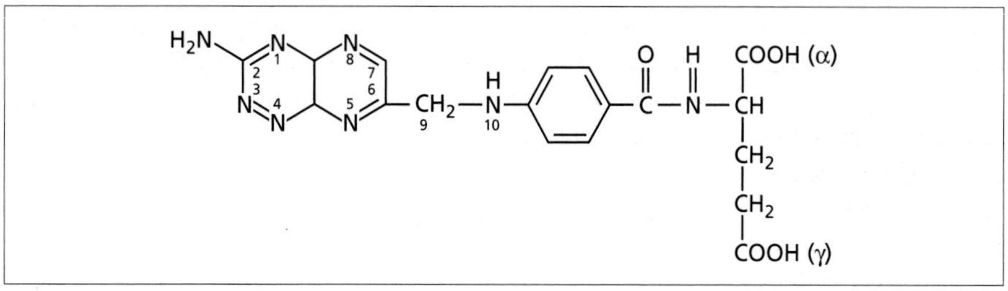

Figure 5.8 The structure of folic acid (pteroylglutamic acid).

positions 4, 5, 7 and 8 in the pteridine portion to di- or tetrahydrofolate (THF) derivatives; (ii) they usually contain a single carbon unit of varying degrees of reduction, such as a methyl group at N-5 or N-10; and (iii) 70–90% of natural folates contain a chain of three or more glutamate residues linked to each other by the unusual γ-peptide bond and are called pteroyl- or folate-polyglutamates. In human cells, four, five and six glutamate residues are usual.

Most foods contain some folate. The highest concentrations are found in liver and yeast (> 200 μg/100 g), spinach, other greens and nuts (> 100 μg/100 g). The total folate content of an average Western diet is about 250 μg daily, but the amount varies widely according to the type of food eaten and the method of cooking. Folate is easily destroyed by heating, particularly in large volumes of water; over 90% may be lost.

Body stores and requirements

Total body folate in the adult is about 10 mg, the liver containing the largest store. Daily adult requirements are about 100 μg. Up to 13 μg of folate is lost as such in the urine each day, but breakdown products of folate are also lost in urine. Losses of folate also occur in sweat and skin; faecal folate is largely derived from colonic bacteria. Stores are only sufficient for about 4 months in normal adults, so severe folate deficiency may develop rapidly.

Absorption

The principal site of folate absorption is the upper small intestine, and there is a steep fall-off in absorptive capacity in the lower jejunum and ileum. The absorption of all forms tested is rapid, a rise in blood level occurring within 15–20 min of ingestion.

The small intestine has a tremendous capacity to absorb folate monoglutamates, as about 90% of a single dose is absorbed regardless of whether this is small (100 μg) or large (15 mg). Absorption of pteroylglutamic acid occurs by a saturable process, although it is unclear whether an active mechanism or facilitated diffusion is involved. The existence of patients with a specific defect in absorption of folates, including pteroylglutamic acid itself, however, does suggest that a special mechanism exists.

The absorption of folate polyglutamates with higher numbers of glutamate residues is reduced. This may be due to the limited capacity of the small intestine to hydrolyse these compounds or to their limited transfer in the mucosal cell. On average, about 50% of food folates is absorbed.

Polyglutamate forms are hydrolysed by pteroylpolyglutamate hydrolase (PPH, also known as folylpoly-gamma-glutamate carboxypeptidase) to the monoglutamate derivatives, either in the lumen of the intestine or within the mucosa; they do not enter portal blood intact. The exact intracellular site of hydrolysis of dietary pteroylpolyglutamates in the enterocytes is unknown, although PPH has been shown to be concentrated in the lysosomes of the cells and is also present on the brush border. Mono- or polyglutamate forms of dietary folate, which are already partly or completely reduced, are converted to 5-methyltetrahydrofolate within the small intestinal mucosa before entering the portal plasma. The monoglutamates are actively transported across the enterocyte by a carrier-mediated mechanism. Pteroylglutamic acid at doses greater than 400 μg is absorbed largely unchanged and converted to natural folates in the liver. Lower doses are converted to 5-methyltetrahydrofolate during absorption through the intestine.

Enterohepatic circulation

About 60–90 μg of folate enters the bile each day and is excreted into the small intestine. Loss of this folate, together with the folate of sloughed intestinal cells, accelerates the speed with which folate deficiency develops in malabsorption conditions.

Transport

Folate is transported in plasma; about one-third is loosely bound to albumin and two-thirds is unbound. In all body fluids (plasma, cerebrospinal fluid, milk, bile) folate is largely, if not entirely, 5-methyl-THF in the monoglutamate form. A carrier-mediated active process is involved in the entry of folate into cells, the rate of uptake being linked to the rate of folate polyglutamate synthesis in the cell, which in replicating cells is related to the rate of DNA synthesis. Reduced folates are more rapidly taken up than oxidized folates. In most cells, folates are retained with tight binding to folate-binding proteins, three of which are enzymes involved in methyl group metabolism, sarcosine dehydrogenase, dimethylglycine dehydrogenase and glycine N-methyltransferase, until the cell dies. Intact liver cells can release folate. Two types of folate-binding protein are involved in entry of methyl-THF into cells. A high-affinity folate receptor takes folate into cells internalized in a vesicle (caveola), which is then acidified, releasing folate into the vesicle lumen. Folate is then carried by the membrane folate transporter into the cytoplasm; the caveola recycles to the cell surface, where its high-affinity receptors are re-utilized. The high-affinity receptor is attached to the outer surface of the cell membrane by glycosyl phosphatidylinositol linkages. They may be involved in transport of oxidized folates and folate breakdown products to the liver for excretion in bile. The congenital disease of folate-specific malabsorption, in which there is also a transport defect, may be a defect of a specific folate-binding protein, but this has yet to be established.

Biochemical functions

Folates (as the intracellular polyglutamate derivatives) act as coenzymes in the transfer of single-carbon units from one compound to another (Figure 5.3 and Table 5.2). Two of these reactions are involved in purine and one in pyrimidine synthesis necessary for DNA and RNA replication. Folate is coenzyme in another reaction, methionine synthesis, in which cobalamin is also involved and THF is regenerated. THF is the acceptor of single carbon units newly entering the active pool via conversion of serine to glycine. Methionine, the other product of the methionine synthase reaction, is the precursor for *S*-adenosylmethionine (SAM), the universal methyl donor involved in over 100 methyltransferase reactions.

During thymidylate synthesis, 5,10-methylene-THF is converted to DHF (dihydrofolate) (Figure 5.3). The enzyme DHF reductase converts this to THF. The drugs methotrexate, pyrimethamine and, mainly in bacteria, trimethoprim inhibit DHF reductase, and this prevents formation of the active folate coenzymes from DHF. A small fraction of the folate coenzyme is not recycled during thymidylate synthesis but is degraded at the C-9–N-10 bond.

Causes of folate deficiency (Table 5.8)

Nutritional

Dietary folate deficiency is common. Indeed, in most patients with folate deficiency a nutritional element is present. Certain individuals are particularly prone to have diets containing inadequate amounts of folate, including the old, edentulous, poor, alcoholic and psychiatrically disturbed, and patients after gastric operations. In relation to the size of the total body folate stores, which are in the order of 15–25 mg, the daily requirement of 100–200 mg is large. Consequently, with total cessation of intake or absorption, depletion of stores will occur in 3–6 months. In the

Table 5.8 Causes of folate deficiency.

Dietary
Particularly in: old age, infancy, poverty, alcoholism, chronic invalids and the psychiatrically disturbed; may be associated with scurvy or kwashiorkor

Malabsorption
Major causes of deficiency
Tropical sprue, gluten-induced enteropathy in children and adults, and in association with dermatitis herpetiformis, specific malabsorption of folate, intestinal megaloblastosis caused by severe cobalamin or folate deficiency

Minor causes of deficiency
Extensive jejunal resection, Crohn's disease, partial gastrectomy, congestive heart failure, Whipple's disease, scleroderma, amyloid, diabetic enteropathy, systemic bacterial infection, lymphoma, salazopyrine

Excess utilization or loss
Physiological
Pregnancy and lactation, prematurity

Pathological
Haematological diseases: chronic haemolytic anaemias, sickle cell anaemia, thalassaemia major, myelofibrosis
Malignant diseases: carcinoma, lymphoma, leukaemia, myeloma
Inflammatory diseases: tuberculosis, Crohn's disease, psoriasis, exfoliative dermatitis, malaria
Metabolic disease: homocystinuria
Excess urinary loss: congestive heart failure, active liver disease
Haemodialysis, peritoneal dialysis

Antifolate drugs
Anticonvulsant drugs (dephenylhydantoin, primidone, barbiturates), sulphasalazine
Nitrofurantoin, tetracycline, anti-tuberculosis (less well documented)

Mixed causes
Liver diseases, alcoholism, intensive care units

Note: In severely folate-deficient patients with causes other than those listed under Dietary, poor dietary intake is often present.

USA and other countries where fortification of the diet with folic acid has been adopted to reduce the incidence of neural tube defects, the prevalence of folate deficiency has dropped dramatically and is now almost restricted to high-risk groups with increased folate needs. Nutritional folate deficiency occurs in kwashiorkor and scurvy, and in infants with repeated infections or who are fed solely on goats' milk, which has a low folate content (6 µg/L) compared with human or cows' milk (50 µg/L), as well as high concentrations of a high-affinity folate-binding protein.

Malabsorption

Malabsorption of dietary folate occurs in tropical sprue, in gluten-induced enteropathy in children and in adults, when it is associated with dermatitis herpetiformis. In the rare congenital syndrome of selective malabsorption of folate, there is an associated defect of folate transport into the cerebrospinal fluid, and these patients show megaloblastic anaemia, responding to physiological doses of folic acid given parenterally but not orally. These patients also show mental retardation, convulsions and other central nervous system abnormalities. Minor degrees of malabsorption may also occur following jejunal resection or partial gastrectomy, in Crohn's disease and in systemic infections but, in these conditions, if severe deficiency occurs, it is usually largely due to poor nutrition.

Malabsorption of folate has been described in patients receiving salazopyrine, cholestyramine and triamterene. It has also been associated with anticonvulsant drug therapy, alcohol abuse and folate deficiency, but these relationships are less well established. In the intestinal stagnant loop syndrome, the predominant effect of the small intestinal bacteria is to cause a rise in serum, red cell and urinary folate by synthesizing folate, which is then absorbed.

Excess utilization or loss

Pregnancy

Folate requirements are increased by 200–300 µg to about 400 µg daily in a normal pregnancy, partly because of transfer of the vitamin to the fetus, but mainly because of increased folate catabolism due to cleavage of folate coenzymes in rapidly proliferating tissues at the C-9–N-10 bond. Megaloblastic anaemia due to this deficiency is now largely prevented by prophylactic folic acid therapy. It occurred in 0.5% of pregnancies in the UK and other Western countries, but the incidence is much higher in countries where the general nutritional status is poor. The anaemia is more common in twin pregnancies, is most likely to occur in the last trimester, especially in the late winter and early spring months (in the UK), and may also present in the early post-partum period during lactation. The deficiency is more common in pregnant women who also suffer from iron deficiency, probably because these patients have a poor diet.

The usual presentation of the anaemia is similar to that of other megaloblastic anaemias, but occasionally, when there is an associated infection, acute arrest of haemopoiesis with pancytopenia may occur; this resembles aplastic anaemia, except that the marrow shows obvious megaloblastic changes.

A number of consequences of folate deficiency in pregnancy have been described, including antenatal and post-partum haemorrhages, prematurity and congenital malabsorption in the fetus. These have not been fully established, but several studies have shown that prophylactic folic acid therapy reduces the incidence of neural tube defects (see p. 64).

Prematurity

The newborn infant, whether full term or premature, has higher serum and red cell folate concentrations than the adult, but the newborn infant's demand for folate has been estimated to be up to 10 times that of adults on a weight basis and the neonatal folate level falls rapidly to the lowest values at about 6 weeks of age. The falls are steepest and are liable to reach subnormal levels in premature babies, a number of whom develop megaloblastic anaemia responsive to folic acid at about 4–6 weeks of age. This occurs particularly in the smallest babies (< 1500 g birth weight) and in those who have feeding difficulties or infections, or who have undergone multiple exchange transfusions. In these babies, prophylactic folic acid should be given.

Haematological disorders

Folate deficiency frequently occurs in chronic haemolytic anaemia, particularly in sickle cell disease, autoimmune haemolytic anaemia and congenital spherocytosis. In these and other conditions of increased cell turnover, folate deficiency arises because it is not completely re-utilized after performing coenzyme functions, and it is partly lost as pteridines in the urine due to cleavage at the C-9–N-10 bond. Patients with chronic myelofibrosis may develop folate deficiency at some stage of the illness. There is also a high incidence of mild folate deficiency in patients with leukaemia, lymphoma, myeloma or carcinoma, although it is unusual for this to progress to megaloblastic anaemia. Treatment with folic acid should be avoided (as it may 'feed' the tumour) unless severe megaloblastic anaemia due to folate deficiency is clinically important.

Inflammatory conditions

Chronic inflammatory diseases, such as tuberculosis, rheumatoid arthritis, Crohn's disease, psoriasis, exfoliative dermatitis, bacterial endocarditis and chronic bacterial infections, cause deficiency by reducing the appetite and by increasing the demand for folate. Systemic infections may also cause malabsorption of folate. Severe deficiency is virtually confined to the patients with the most active disease and the poorest diet. Fever per se has also been suggested to interfere with folate metabolism by inhibiting temperature-dependent folate enzymes. In patients with subclinical folate deficiency from causes other than infections, intercurrent infections often precipitate severe megaloblastic anaemia.

Homocystinuria

This is a rare metabolic defect in the conversion of homocysteine to cystathionine. Folate deficiency occurring in most of these patients may be due to excessive utilization because of compensatory increased conversion of homocysteine to methionine.

Long-term dialysis

As folate is only loosely bound to plasma proteins, it is easily removed from plasma by haemodialysis or peritoneal dialysis (in contrast, cobalamin is not removed from plasma by dialysis as it is firmly protein bound). The amount of body folate that can be removed in this way is relatively small. Nevertheless, in patients with anorexia, vomiting, infections and haemolysis, folate stores may become depleted and megaloblastic anaemia can supervene. Routine folate prophylaxis is now given.

Congestive heart failure, liver disease

Excess urinary folate losses of more than 100 μg per day may occur in some of these patients. The explanation appears to be release of folate from damaged liver cells.

Antifolate drugs

A large number of epileptics who are receiving long-term therapy with diphenylhydantoin (phenytoin, Dilantin) or primidone (Mysoline®), with or without barbiturates, develop low serum and red cell folate levels. In some of these patients, megaloblastic anaemia supervenes. A number of mechanisms have been suggested: inhibition of folate absorption, inhibition of the action of or synthesis of folate-dependent enzymes, displacement of folate from its plasma transport protein and induction of folate-utilizing enzymes. None of these theories has been established. A dietary element is present in the patients with the severest deficiencies.

Alcohol may also be a folate antagonist, as patients who are drinking spirits may develop megaloblastic anaemia that will respond to normal quantities of dietary folate or to physiological doses of folic acid only if the alcohol is withdrawn. Macrocytosis is associated with chronic alcohol intake even when folate levels are normal. Resumption of alcohol intake rapidly inhibits the haematological response to small doses of folate. The mechanism is unknown. Inadequate folate intake is the major factor in the development of deficiency in spirit-drinking alcoholics. Beer is relatively folate-rich in some countries, depending on the technique used for brewing.

The drugs that inhibit dihydrofolate reductase include methotrexate, pyrimethamine and trimethoprim. Methotrexate has the most powerful action against the human enzyme, whereas trimethoprim is most active against the bacterial enzyme and is only likely to cause megaloblastic anaemia when used in conjunction with sulphamethoxazole in patients with pre-existing folate or cobalamin deficiency. The activity of pyrimethamine is intermediate. The antidote to these drugs is folinic acid (5-formyl-THF).

Congenital abnormalities of folate metabolism

A number of infants have been described with congenital defects of folate enzymes (e.g. cyclohydrolase or methionine synthase). Some had megaloblastic anaemia.

Diagnosis of folate deficiency

Serum folate

This may be measured microbiologically with *Lactobacillus casei*, by radioassay or by an enzyme-linked immunosorbence assay (ELISA) technique. The serum folate level is low in all folate-deficient patients. In most laboratories, the normal range is quoted as from 2.0 μg/L (11 nmol/L) to about 15 μg/L. The serum folate is markedly affected by recent diet; inadequate intake for as little as 1 week may cause the level to become subnormal. Because of this, the serum folate assay is a very sensitive test and may show a low result before there is haematological or other biochemical evidence of deficiency.

The serum folate level rises in severe cobalamin deficiency because of blockage in conversion of methyl THF, the major circulating form, to THF; raised levels have also been reported in the intestinal stagnant loop syndrome, acute renal failure and active liver damage. (High levels are also obtained when the patient is receiving folic acid therapy, when the serum is contaminated with folate or folate-producing bacteria or, if a sample is haemolysed, because of the high concentration of folate in red cells.)

Red cell folate

The red cell folate assay is a valuable test of body folate stores. It is less affected by recent diet and traces of haemolysis than is the serum assay. In normal adults, concentrations range from 160 to 640 μg/L of packed red cells. Subnormal levels occur in patients with megaloblastic anaemia due to folate deficiency but also occur in nearly two-thirds of patients with megaloblastic anaemia due to cobalamin deficiency. If cobalamin deficiency is excluded, however, a low red cell folate can be used as an indication that severe folate deficiency is present and warrants full investigation and treatment. False normal results may occur if the folate-deficient patient has received a recent blood transfusion (as the folate content of the transfused red cells will be measured) or if the patient has a raised reticulocyte count (e.g. due to haemorrhage or haemolytic anaemia).

Serum homocysteine (see p. 75)

General management of megaloblastic anaemia

It is usually possible to establish which of the two deficiencies, folate or cobalamin, is the cause of the anaemia and to treat only with the appropriate vitamin. In patients who enter hospital severely ill, however, it may be necessary to treat with both vitamins in large doses once blood samples have been taken for cobalamin and folate assay and a bone marrow has been performed (if deemed necessary). Transfusion is usually unnecessary and inadvisable. If it is essential, packed red cells should be given slowly and one or two units will be ample. Exchange transfusion, as well as the usual treatment for heart failure, should be considered in patients with extreme anaemia and congestive heart failure. Platelet concentrates are of value in reducing spontaneous bleeding in the rare patients with severe thrombocytopenia. Potassium supplements have been recommended to obviate the danger of the hypokalaemia that has been recorded in some patients during the initial haematological response.

Treatment of cobalamin deficiency

It is usually necessary to treat patients who have developed cobalamin deficiency with lifelong regular cobalamin therapy. In the UK, the form used is hydroxocobalamin; in the USA cyanocobalamin is used. In a few instances, the underlying cause of cobalamin deficiency can be permanently corrected, for instance the fish tapeworm, tropical sprue or an intestinal stagnant loop that is amenable to surgery.

The indications for starting cobalamin therapy are a well-documented megaloblastic anaemia or neuropathy due to the deficiency. It is also necessary to treat any patients with haematological abnormalities due to cobalamin deficiency, even in the absence of anaemia (e.g. hypersegmented neutrophils or megaloblastic erythropoiesis). Patients with borderline serum cobalamin levels but no haematological or other abnormality should be followed, for example, at yearly intervals to make sure that the cobalamin deficiency does not progress. If malabsorption of cobalamin or rises in serum MMA levels have also been demonstrated, they should also be given regular maintenance cobalamin therapy. Cobalamin should be given routinely to all patients who have had a total gastrectomy or ileal resection. Patients who have undergone gastric reduction for control of obesity or who are receiving long-term treatment with proton pump inhibitors should be screened and, as necessary, given cobalamin replacement.

Replenishment of body stores should be complete with six 1000-μg i.m. injections of *hydroxocobalamin* given at 3–7 day intervals. More frequent doses are usually used in patients with cobalamin neuropathy, but there is no evidence that these produce a better response. For maintenance therapy, 1000 μg of hydroxocobalamin i.m. once every 3 months is satisfactory. Hydroxocobalamin is the preferred form. In the USA, hydroxocobalamin has not yet been approved and marketed for purposes of routine cobalamin replacement. Because of the poorer retention of cyanocobalamin maintenance treatment, protocols generally use higher and more frequent doses (1000 μg i.m., monthly). Toxic reactions are extremely rare and are usually due to contamination in its preparation rather than to cobalamin itself. Because a small fraction of cobalamin can be absorbed passively through mucous membranes even when there is complete failure of the physiological IF-dependent mechanism, large daily oral doses (1000–2000 μg) of cyanocobalamin can be used for replacement and maintenance of normal cobalamin status. Sublingual therapy has also been proposed for those in whom injections are difficult because of a bleeding tendency and may not tolerate oral therapy. If this approach is used, it is important to monitor compliance, particularly with elderly, forgetful patients.

Treatment of folate deficiency

There is probably never any need to give folic acid parenterally, except in patients receiving parenteral nutrition who cannot swallow tablets. Oral doses of 5–15 mg folic acid daily are satisfactory, as sufficient folate is absorbed from these extremely large doses even in patients with severe malabsorption. The length of time therapy must be continued depends on the underlying disease. It is customary to continue therapy for about 4 months, when all folate-deficient red cells will have been eliminated and replaced by a few folate-replete populations.

Before large doses of folic acid are given, cobalamin deficiency must be excluded and, if present, corrected, otherwise cobalamin neuropathy may develop, despite a response of the anaemia of cobalamin deficiency to folate therapy. This applies particularly in the USA and other countries where folic acid fortification of the diet or widespread use of folic acid supplements occur. Recent studies, however, suggest that there is no increase in the proportion of subjects with low serum cobalamin levels and no anaemia since fortification of the diet.

Long-term folic acid therapy is required when the underlying cause of the deficiency cannot be corrected and the deficiency is likely to recur, for instance in chronic haemolytic anaemias such as thalassaemia major and sickle cell anaemia, and in chronic myelofibrosis. It may also be necessary in gluten-induced enteropathy if this does not respond to a gluten-free diet. Where mild but chronic folate deficiency occurs, it is preferable to encourage any improvement in the diet after correcting the deficiency with a short course of folic acid. In any patient receiving long-term folic acid therapy, it is important to measure the serum cobalamin level at regular (e.g. once yearly) intervals to exclude the coincidental development of cobalamin deficiency.

Folinic acid (5-formyltetrahydrofolate)

This is a stable form of fully reduced folate. It is given orally or parenterally to overcome the toxic effects of methotrexate or other dihydrofolate reductase inhibitors.

Prophylactic folic acid

In many countries, food is fortified with folic acid (in grain or flour) to prevent neural tube defects. Prophylactic folic acid is being increasingly used to reduce homocysteine levels to prevent cardiovascular disease. As yet there is no definite proof of this benefit, although circumstantial evidence does support this approach (see p. 64).

Pregnancy

Folic acid, 400 µg daily, should be given as a supplement throughout pregnancy. In women who have had a previous fetus with a neural tube defect, 5 mg daily is recommended when pregnancy is contemplated and throughout the subsequent pregnancy. In women of childbearing age, a supplementary intake of folic acid of 400 µg daily is recommended, so that this extra intake will be present from conception. Combined iron and folic acid preparations are generally satisfactory, except that they are usually expensive and, if the patient cannot tolerate the iron and stops taking the tablets, folic acid therapy will also be discontinued.

Prematurity

The incidence of folate deficiency is so high in the smallest premature babies during the first 6 weeks of life that folic acid (e.g. 1 mg daily) should be given routinely to babies weighing less than 1500 g at birth and to larger premature babies who require exchange transfusions or develop feeding difficulties, infections or vomiting and diarrhoea.

Haemolytic anaemia and dialysis

Prophylactic folic acid is usually also given to patients with chronic haemolytic anaemia or those who are undergoing long-term haemodialysis.

Megaloblastic anaemia not due to cobalamin or folate deficiency or altered metabolism

This may occur with many antimetabolic drugs (e.g. hydroxyurea, cytosine arabinoside, 6-mercaptopurine) that inhibit DNA replication at a particular point in the supply of precursor or by inhibiting DNA polymerase. In the rare disease orotic aciduria, two consecutive enzymes in purine synthesis are defective. The condition responds to therapy with uridine, which bypasses the block. In thiamine-responsive megaloblastic anaemia, there is a genetic defect in the high-affinity thiamine transport (*SLC19A2*) gene. This causes defective RNA ribose synthesis through impaired activity of transketolase, a thiamine-dependent enzyme in the pentose cycle. This leads to reduced nucleic acid production and consequent induction of cell cycle arrest or apoptosis. It may be associated with diabetes mellitus and deafness and the presence of many ringed sideroblasts in the marrow (p. 41). The explanation is unclear for megaloblastic changes in the marrow in patients with acute myeloid leukaemia (AML), especially $FABM_6$, and other leukaemias and myelodysplasia. When assessed by the dU suppression test (p. 75), the fault is not at the thymidylate synthase reaction.

Other nutritional anaemias

Protein deficiency

Anaemia is usual in children and adults with severe protein deficiency (kwashiorkor). The anaemia, which may be partly masked by haemoconcentration, is usually normoblastic, but megaloblastic changes have been described in 10–60% of patients in different series. Hypoplasia, or even aplasia, of the marrow has also been reported. The mechanism by which protein deficiency causes anaemia is not completely understood. Lack of protein does not seem to reduce haemoglobin synthesis directly. Studies on experimental animals suggest that the major faction is diminution or erythropoietin secretion. This is probably due to a reduction in general tissue metabolism and therefore oxygen consumption, with a consequent reduced stimulus for erythropoietin secretion. In most patients, other factors contribute to the anaemia. These include infections, deficiencies of folate and iron, and also, possibly, deficiencies of vitamins C, E and B_{12} and other trace substances. Riboflavin deficiency may also contribute to the anaemia and become apparent only during the response to protein.

Scurvy

There is usually a moderate or severe normocytic, normochromic anaemia in scurvy because of external haemorrhage and haemorrhage into tissues, and from impaired erythropoiesis. In some patients, the anaemia is megaloblastic, which appears to be partly due to associated nutritional folate deficiency and partly due to impairment of folate metabolism caused by vitamin C deficiency. Vitamin C is not established, however, as playing a role in normal folate metabolism.

Other deficiencies

Deficiencies of nicotinic acid and panthothenic acid cause anaemia in experimental animals but have not been shown to do so in humans. However, riboflavin deficiency may cause anaemia in humans, resembling the anaemia of protein deficiency. Copper is essential for haemopoiesis and normal iron metabolism. A deficiency of copper causes an anaemia resembling that in iron deficiency in experimental animals. Anaemia due to copper deficiency, however, has never been documented in humans. Copper excess (as in Wilson's disease) causes a haemolytic anaemia.

Selected bibliography

Blount BC, Mack NM, Wehr CM *et al.* (1997) Folate deficiency causes uracil misincorporation into human DNA and chromosome breakage: implications for cancer and neuronal damage. *Proceedings of the National Academy of Sciences of the USA* 94: 3290–5.

Boros LG, Steinkamp MP, Fleming JC *et al.* (2003) Defective RNA ribose synthesis in fibroblasts from patients with thiamine-responsive megaloblastic anemia (TRMA) *Blood* 102: 3556–61.

Carmel R (1995) Malabsorption of food cobalamin. *Baillière's Clinical Haematology* 8: 639–55.

Chanarin I, Metz J (1997) Diagnosis of cobalamin deficiency: the old and the new. *British Journal of Haematology* 97: 695–700.

Christensen EI, Birn H (2002) Megalin and cubilin: Multifunctional endocytic receptors. *National Review of Molecular and Cellular Biology* 3: 258–68A.

Clarke R, Smith AD, Jobst KA *et al.* (1998) Folate, vitamin B$_{12}$ and serum total homocysteine levels in confirmed Alzheimer's disease. *Archives of Neurology* 55: 1449–55.

Creizel AE, Dudas I (1992) Prevention of the first occurrence of neural tube defects by periconceptual vitamin supplementation. *New England Journal of Medicine* 327: 1832–5.

D'Angelo A, Selhub J (1997) Homocysteine and thrombotic disease. *Blood* 90: 1–11.

Delpre G, Stark P, Niv Y (1999) Sublingual therapy for cobalamin deficiency as an alternative to oral and parenteral cobalamin supplementation. *Lancet* 354: 740–1.

Frosst P, Blom HJ, Milos R *et al.* (1995) A candidate genetic risk factor for vascular disease: a common mutation in methylenetetrahydrofolate reductase. *Nature Genetics* 10: 111–13.

Fyfe JC, Madsen M, Hojrup P *et al.* (2004) The functional cobalamin (vitamin B$_{12}$) intrinsic factor receptor is a novel complex of cubulin and aminonless. *Blood* 103: 1573–9.

Giovannucci E, Stamfer MJ, Colditz GA *et al.* (1998) Multivitamin use, folate and colon cancer in women in the Nurses Health Study. *Annals of Internal Medicine* 129: 517–24.

Green R (1995) Metabolite assays in cobalamin and folate deficiency. *Baillière's Clinical Haematology* 8: 533–66.

Green R, Miller JW (1999) Folate deficiency beyond megaloblastic anemia: hyperhomocysteinemia and other manifestations of dysfunctional folate status. *Seminars in Hematology* 36: 47–64.

He K, Anwar M, Rimm E *et al.* (2004) Folate, vitamin B$_6$ and B$_{12}$ intakes in relation to risk of stroke among men. *Stroke* 35: 169–74.

Healton EB, Savage DG, Brust JC *et al.* (1991) Neurologic aspects of cobalamin deficiency. *Medicine (Baltimore)* 70: 229–245.

Herzlich B, Herbert V (1988) Depletion of serum holotranscobalamin II An early sign of negative vitamin B12 balance. *Laboratory Investigations* 58: 332–7.

Koury MJ, Horne DW, Brown ZA *et al.* (1997) Apoptosis of late-stage erythroblasts in megaloblastic anemia: association with DNA damage and macrocyte production. *Blood* 89: 4617–23.

Kozyraki R, Kristiansen M, Silahtraroglu A *et al.* (1998) The human intrinsic-factor-vitamin B$_{12}$ receptor: molecular characterization and chromosomal mapping of the gene to 10p within the autosomal megaloblastic anemia (MAI) region. *Blood* 91: 3593–600.

Lincz L, Scorgie FE, Kerridge I *et al.* (2003) Methionine synthase genetic polymorphs in MSA27569 alters susceptibility to follicular but not diffuse large B-cell non-Hodgkin's lymphoma or multiple myeloma. *British Journal of Haematology* 120: 1051–4.

Lucock M (2004) Is folic acid the ultimate functional food component for disease prevention. *British Medical Journal* 328: 211–14.

Miller JW, Ramos MI, Garrod MG *et al.* (2002) Transcobalamin II 775G> C polymorphism and indices of vitamin B12 status in healthy older adults. *Blood* 100: 718–20.

Mills JL, McPartlin JM, Kirke PN *et al.* (1995) Homocysteine metabolism in pregnancies complicated by neural tube defects. *Lancet* 345: 149–51.

Mills JL, VonKohirin I, Conley MR *et al.* (2003) Low vitamin B$_{12}$ concentrations in patients without anemia: the effect of folic acid fortification of grain. *American Journal of Clinical Nutrition* 77: 1474–7.

MRC Vitamin Study Research Group (1991) Prevention of neural tube defects: results of the Medical Research Council Vitamin Study. *Lancet* 338: 131–7.

Rosenblatt DS, Whitehead VM (1999) Cobalamin and folate deficiency: acquired and hereditary disorders in children. *Seminars in Hematology* 36: 19–34.

Rothenberg SP, daCosta MP, Sequeira JM *et al.* (2004) Auto-antibodies against folate receptors in women with a pregnancy complicated by a neural tube defect. *New England Journal of Medicine* 350: 134–42.

Savage DG, Lindebaum, J (1995) Neurological complications of acquired cobalamin deficiency: clinical aspects. *Clinical Haematology* 8: 657–78.

Schnyder G, Roffi M, Pin R *et al.* (2001) Decreased rate of coronary restenosis after lowering of plasma homocysteine levels. *New England Journal of Medicine* 345: 1593–1600.

Seshadri S, Beiser A, Selhub J *et al.* (2002) Plasma homocysteine as a risk factor for dementia and Alzheimer's disease. *New England Journal of Medicine* 346: 476–83.

Shaw GM, Lammer EJ, Wasserman CR *et al.* (1995) Risks of facial clefts in children born to women using multi-vitamins containing folic acid periconceptually. *Lancet* 346: 393–6.

Skibola CF, Smith MT, Kane E *et al.* (1999) Polymorphisms in the methylenetetrahydrofolate reductase gene are associated with susceptibility to acute leukaemia in adults. *Proceedings of the National Academy of Sciences of the USA* 62: 1044–51.

Solomon LR (2005) Cobalamin-responsive disorders in the ambulatory case setting: unreliability of cobalamin, methylmalonic acid and homocysteine testing. *Blood* (in press).

Stopack A (2000) Links between *Helicobacter pylori* infection, cobalamin deficiency and pernicius anemia. *Archives of Internal Medicine* **160**: 1229–30.

Tanner SM, Aminoff M, Wright FA *et al.* (2003) Amnionless, essential for mouse gastrulation, is mutated in recessive hereditary megaloblastic anemia. *Nature Genetics* **33**: 426–9.

Toh M-H, Van Driel IR, Gleeson PA (1997) Pernicious anemia. *New England Journal of Medicine* **337**: 1441–8.

Van der Put MMJ, Steegers-Theunissen PM, Frosst P *et al.* (1995) Mutated methylenetetrahydrofolate reductase as a risk factor for spina bifida. *Lancet* **346**: 1070–1.

Wald DS, Low M, Morris JK (2002) Homocysteine and cardiovascular disease: evidence of causality from a meta-analysis. *British Medical Journal* **325**: 1202–6.

Ward M, McNulty H, McPartlin J *et al.* (1997) Plasma homocysteine, a risk factor for cardiovascular disease, is lowered by physiological amounts of folic acid. *Quarterly Journal of Medicine* **90**: 1–6.

Weir DG, Scott JM (1995) The biochemical basis of the neuropathy in cobalamin deficiency. *Clinical Haematology* **8**: 479–98.

Welch GN, Loscalzo J (1998) Homocysteine and artherothrombosis. *New England Journal of Medicine* **338**: 1042–50.

Wickramasinghe SN (ed.) (1995) Megaloblastic anaemia. *Clinical Haematology* **8**: 441–703.

Wickramasinghe SN (1995) Morphology, biology and biochemistry of cobalamin and folate deficient bone marrow cells. *Clinical Haematology* **8**: 441–59.

CHAPTER 6

Haemoglobin and the inherited disorders of globin synthesis

David J Weatherall

6

Introduction

The inherited diseases of haemoglobin are the commonest single-gene disorders; the World Health Organization estimates that about 7% of the world population are carriers. In many developing countries, where there is a very high neonatal and childhood mortality from infection and malnutrition, these conditions are not yet recognized as an important public health problem. However, once economic conditions improve and infant death rates fall, the genetic disorders of haemoglobin start to place a major burden on the health services, a phenomenon that has already been observed in many parts of the world. As a result of migrations of populations, these conditions are being seen with increasing frequency in many countries in which they had not been recognized previously. Some of them, particularly sickle cell anaemia and the more severe forms of thalassaemia, cause life-threatening medical emergencies, chronic disability and distress for families and are a major drain on health resources.

The structure, genetic control and synthesis of haemoglobin

Structure and function

Different haemoglobins are synthesized in the embryo, fetus and adult, each adapted to their particular oxygen requirements. They all have a tetrameric structure made up of two different pairs of globin chains, each attached to one haem molecule (Figure 6.1). Adult and fetal haemoglobins have α-chains combined with β-chains (HbA, $\alpha_2\beta_2$), δ-chains (HbA$_2$, $\alpha_2\delta_2$) and

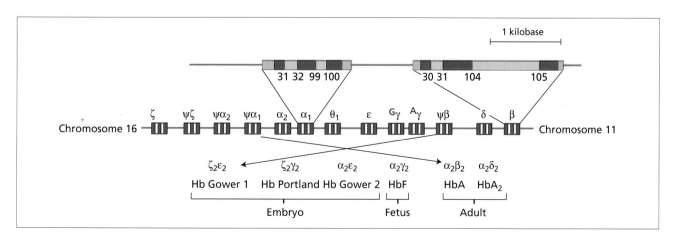

Figure 6.1 The genetic control of haemoglobin.

γ-chains (HbF, $\alpha_2\gamma_2$). In embryos, α-like chains called ζ-chains combine with γ-chains to produce Hb Portland ($\zeta_2\gamma_2$), or with ε-chains to make Hb Gower 1 ($\zeta_2\varepsilon_2$), and α- and ε-chains combine to form Hb Gower 2 ($\alpha_2\varepsilon_2$). Fetal haemoglobin is itself heterogeneous. There are two kinds of γ-chains that differ in their amino acid composition at position 136, where they have either glycine or alanine; those with glycine are called $^G\gamma$-chains and those with alanine $^A\gamma$-chains. The $^G\gamma$- and $^A\gamma$-chains are the products of separate ($^G\gamma$ and $^A\gamma$) loci.

The sigmoid shape of the oxygen dissociation curve, which reflects the allosteric properties of haemoglobin, ensures that oxygen is rapidly taken up at the high oxygen tensions found in the lungs and is released readily at the low tensions encountered in the tissues. It is quite different to myoglobin, a molecule that consists of a single globin chain with haem attached to it and which has a hyperbolic dissociation curve. The transition from a hyperbolic to a sigmoid curve reflects cooperativity between the four haem molecules. When one haem takes on oxygen, the affinity for oxygen of the remaining haems of the tetramer increases markedly. This is because haemoglobin can exist in two configurations, deoxy(T) and oxy(R) (T and R stand for tight and relaxed states respectively). The T form has a lower affinity than the R form for ligands such as oxygen. At some point during the sequential addition of oxygen to the four haems, transition from the T to R configuration occurs and the oxygen affinity of the partially liganded molecule increases dramatically. The oxygen dissociation curve, which reflects these changes, can be modified in several ways. First, oxygen affinity is decreased with increasing CO_2 tensions – the Bohr effect. This facilitates oxygen loading to the tissues, where a drop in pH due to CO_2 influx lowers oxygen affinity. In contrast, in the lungs, efflux of CO_2 and an increase in intracellular pH increases oxygen affinity and hence uptake. Oxygen affinity is also modified by the level of 2,3-biphosphoglycerate (2,3-BPG) in the red cell. Increasing concentrations shift the oxygen dissociation curve to the right, i.e. reduce oxygen affinity, whereas diminishing concentrations have the opposite effect. The clinical relevance of the allosteric properties of haemoglobin and the factors that modify its oxygen dissociation curve are considered together with the pathological haemoglobins in later sections and in Chapter 7.

Genetic control, regulation and synthesis

Globin genes

The arrangement of the two main families of globin genes is illustrated in Figure 6.1. The β-like globin genes form a linked cluster on chromosome 11, which is spread over approximately 60 kb (kb = kilobase or 1000 nucleotide bases); they are arranged in the order 5′-ε-$^G\gamma$-$^A\gamma$-ψβ-δ-β-3′. The α-like globin genes also form a linked cluster, in this case on chromosome 16, in the order 5′-ζ-ψζ-ψα1-α2-α1-3′. The ψβ, ψζ and ψα genes are pseudogenes, that is they have sequences that resemble the β-,

ζ- or α-genes but contain mutations that prevent them from synthesizing any products. They may be 'burnt out' remnants of genes that were functional at an earlier stage of evolution. Like most mammalian genes, the globin genes have one or more noncoding inserts called intervening sequences (IVS) or introns at the same position along their length (Figure 6.2). The non-α-globin genes contain two introns of 122–130 and 850–900 basepairs between codons 30 and 31 and 104 and 105 respectively. Similar, although smaller, introns are found in the α- and ζ-globin genes. At the 5′ non-coding (flanking) regions of the globin genes, there are blocks of nucleotide homology that are found in analogous positions in many species. The first, the ATA box, is about 30 bases upstream from the initiation codon. The second, the CCAAT box, is about 70 basepairs upstream from the 5′ end of the genes. About 80–100 bases upstream, there is the sequence GGGG^{T}G, or C^{A}CCC, which may be inverted or duplicated. These promoter elements are involved in the initiation of transcription and hence play an important role in the regulation of the structural genes. At the 3′ non-coding regions of all the globin genes, there is the sequence AATAAA, which is the signal for cleavage and poly-A addition to RNA transcripts (see below).

Regulation

The globin gene clusters contain several types of regulatory elements that interact to promote erythroid-specific gene expression and to coordinate changes in globin gene activity during development. They include promoter elements, enhancers, i.e. regulatory elements that increase gene expression despite being located at a variable distance from the genes, and, in the case of the β-globin gene cluster, a master sequence called the 'locus control region' (LCR), or 'locus activating region' (LAR), which lies upstream from the cluster. The α-gene cluster has a homologous upstream sequence designated HS40 (HS stands for DNase 1 *hypersensitive site*, which is characteristic of these regions). Each of these sequences has a modular structure made up of an array of short motifs that represent the binding sites for transcriptional activators or repressors.

The regulation of globin gene expression is mediated at several levels; although most occurs at the transcriptional level, there is some fine-tuning during and after translation. Most DNA that is not involved in gene transcription is tightly packaged into a compact, chemically modified form that is inaccessible to transcription factors and polymerases and which is heavily methylated. Activity is associated with a change in the structure of the chromatin surrounding a gene, which can be identified by enhanced sensitivity to nucleases. Erythroid lineage-specific nuclease hypersensitive sites are found at several locations in the β-globin gene cluster. Four are distributed over a 20-kb region upstream from the ε-globin gene in the region of the β-globin LCR. This key regulatory region establishes a transcriptionally active domain spanning the entire β-globin gene cluster. Several enhancer sequences have been identified in this cluster. All

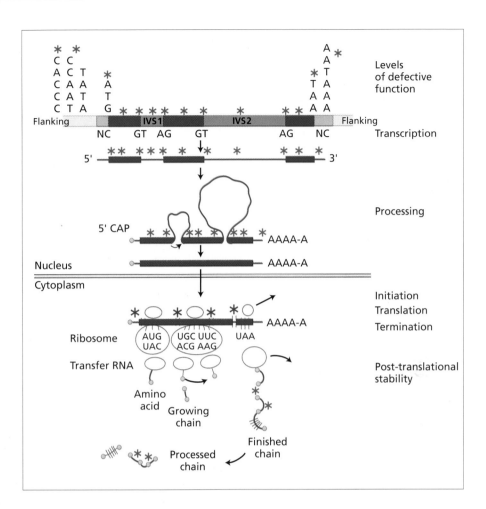

Figure 6.2 The genetic control of the synthesis of a globin chain. *Levels of action of mutations.

of these regulatory regions bind a number of erythroid-specific transcription factors, notably GATA-1 and NF-E2, as well as factors that are more ubiquitous in their tissue distribution (see Chapter 2).

The binding of haemopoietic-specific factors activates the LCR, which renders the entire β-globin gene cluster transcriptionally active. Transcription factors also bind to enhancer and promoter sequences, which work in tandem to regulate the expression of the individual genes in the clusters. Some of the transcription factors are developmental stage specific and may be involved in the (still poorly understood) differential expression of the embryonic, fetal and adult globin genes.

Transcription and processing

When a globin gene is transcribed, messenger RNA (mRNA) is synthesized from one of its strands by the action of RNA polymerase II. This process involves the interaction of a number of transcription factors, other proteins and, possibly, the LCR to form an initiation complex. The primary transcript is a large mRNA precursor that contains both introns and exons. While in the nucleus, it undergoes a number of modifications (Figure 6.2). First, the introns are removed and the exons are spliced together.

This too is a complex, multistep process involving several different proteins that constitute the spliceosome. The exon–intron junctions always have the sequence GT at their 5′ end, and AG and their 3′ end; if there is a mutation at these sites, normal splicing cannot occur. The mRNAs are modified at their 5′ end by the addition of a CAP structure, and at their 3′ end by the addition of a string of adenylic acid residues (poly-A). The processed mRNA now moves into the cytoplasm to act as a template for globin chain production.

Translation

Amino acids are transported to the mRNA template on carriers called transfer RNAs; there are specific transfer RNAs for each amino acid. The order of amino acids in a globin chain is determined by a triplet code, i.e. three bases (codons) code for a particular amino acid. The transfer RNAs also contain three bases, anticodons, which are complementary to mRNA codons for particular amino acids. The transfer RNAs carry amino acids to the template, where they find the right position by codon–anticodon basepairing. The mRNA is translated from the 5′ to the 3′ end (left to right). The transfer RNAs are held in appropriate steric conformation with the mRNA by the two subunits that make up the ribosomes. There are specific initiation (AUG) and termination (UAA, UAG, UGA) codons. When the ribosomes reach the termination codon translation ceases, the completed globin chain is released, and the ribosomal subunits fall apart and are recycled. Individual globin chains combine with haem, which is synthesized through a separate pathway, and with themselves to form definitive haemoglobin molecules.

Classification of the disorders of haemoglobin

The genetic disorders of haemoglobin are divided into those in which there is a reduced rate of production of one or more of the globin chains, the thalassaemias, and those in which there is a structural change in a globin chain leading to instability or abnormal oxygen transport. In addition, there is a harmless group of mutations which interfere with the normal switching of fetal to adult haemoglobin production, known collectively as hereditary persistence of fetal haemoglobin; in many cases, these can be regarded as well-compensated forms of thalassaemia. Like all classifications, this way of splitting up the haemoglobin disorders is not entirely satisfactory; some structural variants, HbE for example, are synthesized in reduced amounts and hence produce the clinical picture of thalassaemia.

The thalassaemias and related disorders

The thalassaemias are the commonest single-gene disorders. The condition was first recognized in 1925 by a Detroit physician,

Thomas B. Cooley, who described a series of infants who became profoundly anaemic and developed splenomegaly over the first year of life. In 1936, Whipple and Bradford, in describing the pathological changes of the condition for the first time, recognized that many of their patients came from the Mediterranean region, and hence invented the word 'thalassaemia' from the Greek θαλασσα, meaning 'the sea'. More recently, it has become clear that thalassaemia occurs widely throughout the world and that its clinical picture can result from the interaction of many different mutations. The high frequency reflects heterozygote protection against malaria.

Definition and classification

The thalassaemias are a heterogeneous group of genetic disorders of haemoglobin synthesis, all of which result from a reduced rate of production of one or more of the globin chains of haemoglobin (Table 6.1). They are divided into the α-, β-, $\delta\beta$- or $\gamma\delta\beta$-thalassaemias, according to which globin chain is produced in reduced amounts. In some thalassaemias, no globin chain is synthesized at all, and these are called α^0- or β^0-thalassaemias; in others, designated α^+- or β^+-thalassaemias, the globin chain is produced at a reduced rate. The $\delta\beta$-thalassaemias are subdivided in the same way. Because thalassaemia occurs in populations in which structural haemoglobin variants are common, it is not unusual to receive a thalassaemia gene from one parent and a gene for a structural haemoglobin variant from the other. Furthermore, both α- and β-thalassaemia occur commonly in some countries, and hence individuals may receive genes for both types. These different interactions produce a clinically diverse family of genetic disorders that range in

Table 6.1 The thalassaemias and related disorders.

α-Thalassaemia	α^0	
	α^+	
	Deletion (-α)	
	Non-deletion (α^T)	
β-Thalassaemia	β^0	
	β^+	
	Normal HbA$_2$	
	'Silent'	
$\delta\beta$-Thalassaemia	$(\delta\beta)^0$	
	$(^A\gamma\delta\beta)^0$	
	$(\delta\beta)^+$	
γ-Thalassaemia		
δ-Thalassaemia	δ^0	
	δ^+	
$\epsilon\gamma\delta\beta$-Thalassaemia		
Hereditary persistence of fetal haemoglobin	Deletion	$(\delta\beta)^0$ $(^A\gamma\delta\beta)^0$
	Non-deletion	Linked to β-globin genes $^G\gamma\beta^+$ $^A\gamma\beta^+$
		Unlinked to β-globin genes

severity from death *in utero* to extremely mild, symptomless hypochromic anaemias.

Most thalassaemias are inherited in a Mendelian recessive fashion. Heterozygotes are usually symptomless, although usually they can be recognized by simple haematological analysis. More severely affected patients are either homozygotes for α- or β-thalassaemia or compound heterozygotes for different molecular forms of α- or β-thalassaemia or for one or other form of thalassaemia and a gene for a structural haemoglobin variant. Clinically, the thalassaemias are classified according to their severity into major, intermediate and minor forms. *Thalassaemia major* is a severe, transfusion-dependent disorder. *Thalassaemia intermedia* is characterized by anaemia and splenomegaly, though not of such severity as to require regular transfusion. *Thalassaemia minor* is the symptomless carrier state.

β-Thalassaemias

The β-thalassaemias are the most important types of thalassaemia because they are so common and usually produce severe anaemia in their homozygous and compound heterozygous states.

Distribution

The β-thalassaemias occur widely in a broad belt, ranging from the Mediterranean and parts of North and West Africa through the Middle East and Indian subcontinent to South-East Asia. The high-incidence zone stretches north through the former Yugoslavia and Romania and the southern parts of the former USSR and includes the southern regions of China. The disease is particularly common in South-East Asia, where it occurs in a line starting in southern China and stretching down through Thailand and the Malay peninsula and Indonesia to some of the Pacific island populations. In this region, and in some of the Mediterranean island and mainland countries, gene frequencies range between 2% and 30%. It should be remembered that β-thalassaemia is not confined entirely to these high-incidence regions and it occurs sporadically in every racial group.

Table 6.2 The different classes of β-thalassaemia mutations.

Transcription	Deletions
	Promoters
Processing of mRNA	Splice junction
	Consensus sequence
	Internal IVS
	Cryptic splice sites in exons
	Cleavage and polyadenylation site
	CAP site
Translation	Nonsense
	Frameshift
	Initiation site
Post-translational instability	Exon 3 mutations
	Other unstable β-chains

Molecular pathology

The main classes of mutations that cause β-thalassaemia are summarized in Table 6.2 and in Figure 6.3. They may involve any step in globin chain production: transcription, translation or the post-translational stability of the globin gene product.

Transcription

The mutations that involve transcription include deletions and point mutations involving the globin gene promoter regions. With the exception of a deletion of about 600 bases at the 3′ end of the β-globin gene, which is restricted to certain Indian populations, major deletions are uncommon. A large number of point mutations involve the promoters or adjacent regions, most of which downregulate the β-globin gene to a varying degree and hence cause relatively mild forms of β-thalassaemia.

Processing

A wide variety of mutations interfere with processing of the primary mRNA transcript. Those within introns or exons, or at

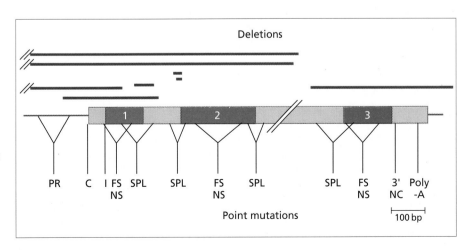

Figure 6.3 The classes of mutations that underlie β-thalassaemia. PR, promoter; C, CAP site; I, initiation codon; FS, frameshift; NS, nonsense mutation; SPL, splicing mutation; Poly-A, poly-A addition site mutation.

their junctions, interfere with the mechanism of *splicing* the exons together after the introns have been removed. Single-base substitutions at the invariant GT or AG sequences at intron–exon junctions prevent splicing altogether and cause β^0-thalassaemia. The sequences adjacent to the GT in the introns are also relatively conserved, so-called *consensus sequences*. Several β-thalassaemia mutations involve this region or other parts of the introns and are associated with variable degrees of defective β-globin production; alternative splicing sites are produced so that both normal and abnormal mRNA species are synthesized. An incorrectly spliced mRNA is not functional because it contains intron sequences; in some cases a nonsense mutation or frameshift is generated.

In exons, there are also sequences that resemble the consensus sequences at the intron–exon junctions. Mutations may activate these 'cryptic' sites, again leading to abnormal splicing.

Translation

Mutations that involve translation of β-globin mRNA fall into two groups. First, there are *nonsense mutations*, that is single-base changes that produce stop codons in the middle of the coding part of the mRNA. Mutations of this type would cause premature termination of globin chain synthesis but, as part of the surveillance mechanism that is active in quality control of the processed mRNA, it appears that message that contains mutations of this type is not transferred to the cell cytoplasm, a phenomenon called *nonsense-mediated decay*. Other exon mutations result in *frameshifts*, that is one or more bases are lost or inserted and the reading frame for the genetic code is thrown out of phase.

Post-translational stability

Finally, some forms of thalassaemia result from instability of the β-globin gene product. For example, it appears that nonsense mutations in exon 3 are not subjected to nonsense-mediated decay and hence abnormal mRNA is transported to the cytoplasm and translated. The result may be long, unstable β-globin gene products that form inclusion bodies in the red cell precursor. This is the basis for dominant β-thalassaemia. In other cases, highly unstable β-chains may be produced, which, although they form a viable haemoglobin molecule, are rapidly destroyed in the circulation, leading to a chronic haemolytic anaemia (see later in chapter).

Pathophysiology

The molecular defects in β-thalassaemia result in absent or reduced β-chain production. α-Chain synthesis is unaffected and hence there is imbalanced globin chain production, leading to an excess of α-chains. In the absence of their partners, they are unstable and precipitate in the red cell precursors, giving rise to large intracellular inclusions that interfere with red cell maturation. Hence there is a variable degree of intramedullary destruction of red cell precursors, i.e. ineffective erythropoiesis. Those red cells which mature and enter the circulation contain α-chain

inclusions that interfere with their passage through the micro-circulation, particularly in the spleen. However, the damage to the red cell precursors and their progeny in β-thalassaemia is not entirely mechanical. The degradation products of excess α-chains, particularly haem and iron, produce a wide range of deleterious effects on red cell membrane proteins and lipids, which are manifest by marked abnormalities of electrolyte homeostasis and membrane deformability. The end result is an extremely rigid red cell with a shortened survival.

Thus, the anaemia of β-thalassaemia results from both ineffective erythropoiesis and haemolysis. It stimulates erythropoietin production, which causes expansion of the bone marrow and may lead to serious deformities of the skull and long bones. Because the spleen is being constantly bombarded with abnormal red cells, it hypertrophies. The resulting splenomegaly, together with bone marrow expansion, causes a major increase in the plasma volume, which also contributes to the anaemia.

As mentioned previously, HbF production almost ceases after birth. However, some adult red cell precursors (F cells) retain the ability to produce a variable number of γ-chains. Because the latter can combine with excess α-chains to form HbF, cells which make relatively more γ-chains in the bone marrow of β-thalassaemics are partly protected against the deleterious effect of α-chain precipitation. Hence, they come under selection in the marrow and peripheral blood and thus relatively large amounts of HbF are found in the red cells. It is possible that there may also be a genuine increase in HbF production as well as selection of F cells; the mechanism is not understood. Because δ-chain synthesis is unaffected, the disorder is characterized by a relative or absolute increase in HbA_2 $(\alpha_2\delta_2)$ production. These interactions are summarized in Figure 6.4.

It follows, therefore, that if the anaemia is corrected with blood transfusion, erythropoietin drive is shut off, growth and development are normal, bone deformities do not occur and splenomegaly is less marked. On the other hand, each unit of blood contains 200 mg of iron; with regular transfusion there is steady accumulation of iron in the liver, endocrine glands and myocardium. Thus, although well-transfused thalassaemic children grow and develop normally, they die of iron overload unless steps are taken to remove iron.

Phenotype–genotype relationships

The β-thalassaemias show remarkable phenotypic variability, ranging from severe life-threatening anaemia to an extremely mild condition that may be identified only by chance. The molecular basis for this diversity is at least partly understood (Figure 6.5).

The genetic modifiers of the β-thalassaemia phenotype can be divided into primary, secondary and tertiary. Primary modifiers are the different mutations which, because of their variable effects on β-globin gene expression, may affect the output of β-globin chains, ranging from zero to a very mild reduction. Secondary modifiers are those that reduce the degree of imbal-

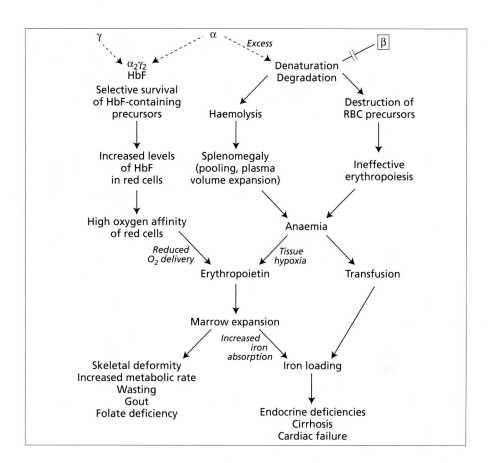

Figure 6.4 The pathophysiology of β-thalassaemia.

ance of globin chain synthesis. They include the co-inheritance of α-thalassaemia and a variety of ill-understood genetic modifiers of γ-chain production in adult life. Although several genes with the latter property have been identified, it seems likely that many remain to be discovered. Tertiary modifiers are those that affect the complications of disease; the severity of bone disease, iron loading and jaundice may be affected by polymorphisms of genes involved in the metabolic pathways concerned with these complications. Similarly, it seems very likely that the propensity to infection is modified by polymorphisms involving the immune system and its regulation. Finally, it should be remembered that environmental factors, long neglected, may also play an important role in modifying the β-thalassaemic phenotype.

Clinical findings

Most severe forms of β-thalassaemia present within the first year of life with failure to thrive, poor feeding, intermittent bouts of infection and general malaise; the infant is pale, and in many cases splenomegaly is already established. There are no other specific clinical signs and the diagnosis depends on the haematological changes outlined below. If the infant receives regular blood transfusion, early development is normal and further symptoms do not occur until puberty, when the effects of iron loading start to appear. If, on the other hand, the infant is not adequately

transfused, the typical clinical picture of β-thalassaemia major develops.

In the well-transfused child, early growth and development are normal and splenomegaly is minimal. However, without adequate iron chelation therapy, there is a gradual accumulation of iron and the effects of tissue siderosis start to appear by the end of the first decade. The adolescent growth spurt fails to occur and hepatic, endocrine and cardiac complications of iron overloading produce a variety of complications, including diabetes, hypoparathyroidism, adrenal insufficiency and progressive liver failure. Secondary sexual development is delayed, or does not occur at all. The short stature and lack of sexual development may lead to serious psychological problems. By far the commonest cause of death, which usually occurs towards the end of the second or early in the third decade, is progressive cardiac damage. Ultimately, these patients die either in protracted cardiac failure or suddenly due to an acute arrhythmia, often precipitated by infection.

The clinical picture in children who are inadequately transfused is quite different. Early childhood is interspersed with a series of distressing complications and the rates of growth and development are retarded. There is progressive splenomegaly, and hypersplenism may cause a worsening of the anaemia, sometimes associated with thrombocytopenia and a bleeding

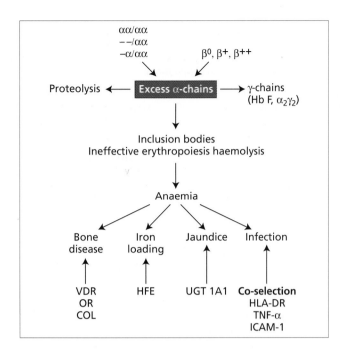

Figure 6.5 The modification of the β-thalassaemia phenotype. The different levels of genetic modification are shown; primary modifiers involve different β-thalassaemia alleles, secondary modifiers involve the reduction of globin chain imbalance due to either increased HbF production or the co-inheritance of α-thalassaemia, and the tertiary modifiers affect the different complications of the disease. UGT1A1, UDP glucuronsyltransferase; VDR, vitamin D receptor; OR, oestrogen receptor; Col, collagen genes; TNF, tumour necrosis factor; ICAM1, intercellular adhesion molecule 1.

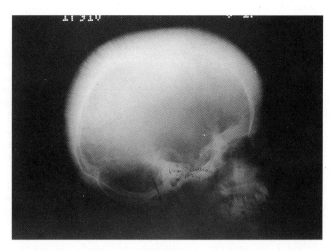

Figure 6.6 The skull in β-thalassaemia.

formed teeth and malocclusion, and inadequate drainage of the sinuses and middle ear may lead to chronic sinus infection and deafness. If these children survive to puberty, they develop the same complications of iron loading as the well-transfused patients. In this case, iron accumulation results from an increased rate of gastrointestinal absorption as well as the inadequate transfusion regimen.

Children who are adequately transfused and chelated may grow and develop normally although, presumably reflecting the extreme sensitivity of the endocrine system to even mild iron overload, there may still be problems with growth, sexual maturation and osteoporosis. Regardless of how they are managed they are prone to blood-borne infection, notably hepatitis B and C, HIV and malaria.

Haematological changes

Haemoglobin values on presentation range from 2 to 8 g/dL. The red cells show marked hypochromia and variation in shape and size, and many hypochromic macrocytes and misshapen microcytes, some of which are mere fragments of cells (Figure 6.7). There is moderate anisochromia and basophilic stippling. There are always some nucleated red cells in the peripheral blood, after splenectomy they appear in large numbers. There is a slight elevation in the reticulocyte count. The white cell and platelet counts are normal unless there is hypersplenism. The bone marrow shows marked erythroid hyperplasia with a myeloid–erythroid (M/E) ratio of unity or less. Many of the red cell precursors show ragged inclusions after incubation of the marrow with methyl violet; similar inclusions are found in the peripheral blood cells after splenectomy.

The bilirubin level is usually elevated and haptoglobins are absent. The ^{51}Cr-labelled red cell survival is shortened. The serum iron level rises progressively and most transfusion-dependent children have a totally saturated iron-binding capacity. This change is mirrored by a high plasma ferritin level, and liver

tendency. Because of bone marrow expansion, there may be deformities of the skull with marked bossing and overgrowth of the zygomata, giving rise to the classical 'mongoloid facies' of β-thalassaemia. These signs are associated with radiological changes, which include a lacy, trabecular pattern of the long bones and phalanges and a typical 'hair on end' appearance of the skull (Figure 6.6).

These bone changes may be accompanied by recurrent fractures. There is increased proneness to infection that may cause a catastrophic drop in the haemoglobin level. Because of the massive marrow expansion resulting from the chronic anaemia, these children are hypermetabolic and develop intermittent fevers and fail to thrive. They have increased requirements for folic acid and may become acutely folate depleted with worsening of their anaemia. Because of the increased turnover of red cell precursors, hyperuricaemia and secondary gout occur occasionally. There is a bleeding tendency which, although partly due to thrombocytopenia secondary to hypersplenism, may also be exacerbated by liver damage. Because of the deformities of the skull, there may be distressing dental complications, with poorly

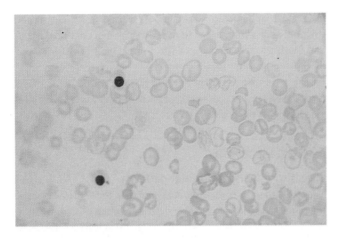

Figure 6.7 The peripheral blood appearances in β-thalassaemia (×750).

biopsies show an increase of iron in both the reticuloendothelial and parenchymal cells.

Haemoglobin changes

The HbF level is always elevated and it is heterogeneously distributed among the red cells. In β^0-thalassaemia, there is no HbA, whereas in β^+-thalassaemia the level of HbF ranges from 30% to 90%. The HbA_2 level is of no diagnostic value, reflecting the heterogeneity of the cell populations in the blood; those with high levels of HbF have low levels of HbA_2, whereas those which contain predominantly HbA have much higher levels; the measured level of HbA_2 represents an average value that is often in the normal range.

Heterozygous β-thalassaemia

Carriers for β-thalassaemia are usually symptom free except in periods of stress such as pregnancy, when they may become more anaemic. Splenomegaly is rare. Haemoglobin values are in the 9–11 g/dL range. The red cells show hypochromia and microcytosis with characteristically low values. The reticulocyte count is normal. The bone marrow shows moderate erythroid hyperplasia.

The characteristic finding is an elevated HbA_2 level in the 4–6% range. There is a slight elevation of HbF in the 1–3% range in about 50% of cases.

β-Thalassaemia in association with haemoglobin variants

In many populations, because there is a high incidence of β-thalassaemia and various haemoglobin variants; it is quite common for an individual to inherit a β-thalassaemia gene from one parent and a gene for a structural haemoglobin variant from the other. Although numerous interactions of this type have been described, only three are common: sickle cell β-thalassaemia, HbC β-thalassaemia and HbE β-thalassaemia.

The clinical manifestations of *sickle cell β-thalassaemia* vary from race to race. In African populations, extremely mild forms of β^+-thalassaemia occur, which, when they interact with the sickle cell gene, produce a condition characterized by mild anaemia and few sickling crises. The condition is compatible with normal survival and is often ascertained by chance haematological examination. On the other hand, in Mediterranean populations, and less commonly in Africans, individuals may inherit a β^0- or severe β^+-thalassaemia determinant. The phenotype of sickle cell β^0 or severe β^+-thalassaemia is often indistinguishable from sickle cell anaemia (see Chapter 7). The diagnosis can be confirmed by haemoglobin electrophoresis, which in sickle cell β^+-thalassaemia shows HbS together with 5–30% HbA and an elevated HbA_2 value. In sickle cell β^0-thalassaemia, the haemoglobin consists of HbS with an elevated level of HbF and HbA_2. One parent has the sickle cell trait and the other has the β-thalassaemia trait.

HbC β-thalassaemia is restricted to West Africans and some North African and southern Mediterranean populations. It is characterized by a mild haemolytic anaemia associated with splenomegaly. The peripheral blood film shows numerous target cells and thalassaemic red cell changes with a moderately elevated reticulocyte count. Haemoglobin electrophoresis shows a preponderance of HbC. The diagnosis is confirmed by finding the HbC trait in one parent and the β-thalassaemia trait in the other.

HbE β-thalassaemia is the commonest severe form of thalassaemia in South-East Asia and parts of the Indian subcontinent. HbE is inefficiently synthesized and hence, when it is inherited together with β^0-thalassaemia, there is a marked deficiency of β-chain production. The clinical and haematological changes are variable. There is usually severe anaemia and splenomegaly with typical thalassaemic bone changes. Although not always transfusion dependent, haemoglobin values are in the 4–9 g/dL range, with an average of 6–7 g/dL. There are thalassaemic red cell changes and the bone marrow shows marked erythroid hyperplasia with α-chain inclusions in many of the red cell precursors.

Although very little is known about the natural history of this disorder, it is clear that in many parts of South-East Asia and India it causes a very high mortality in early life. Complications include a marked proneness to infection, secondary hypersplenism, progressive iron loading, neurological lesions due to masses of extramedullary erythropoietic tissue extending in from the inner tables of the skull or vertebrae, folate deficiency, leg ulcers and recurrent pathological fractures. On the other hand, some patients grow and develop normally with few complications.

The diagnosis is confirmed by finding only HbE and HbF on haemoglobin electrophoresis and by demonstrating the HbE trait in one parent and the β-thalassaemia trait in the other. In cases of HbE β^+-thalassaemia, small quantities of HbA are present.

Variant forms of β-thalassaemia

Although most β-thalassaemia heterozygotes have HbA_2 levels in the 4–5% range, there is a subgroup with higher levels, in excess of 8% of the total haemoglobin. This condition results from small deletions which involve the 5′ end of the β-globin gene including its promoter region. Otherwise, the clinical and haematological pictures are identical to the common forms of β-thalassaemia. Some β-thalassaemia heterozygotes have normal HbA_2 levels. In most cases, this is due to the co-inheritance of δ-thalassaemia. There is an extremely mild form of β-thalassaemia that is completely silent in heterozygotes and is only identified when it is co-inherited with a common form of β-thalassaemia.

β-Thalassaemia occasionally follows a dominant pattern of inheritance, that is it is symptomatic in heterozygotes. The clinical picture is characterized by a moderate degree of anaemia and splenomegaly with marked thalassaemic changes of the red cells, and ineffective erythropoiesis with intracellular inclusion bodies. Although not usually transfusion dependent, such individuals load iron and may develop liver or endocrine damage. As described earlier most of these patients have mutations involving exon 3 of the β-globin gene.

δβ-Thalassaemias

Classification and molecular genetics

These disorders are much less common than the β-thalassaemias. In some cases, they result from deletions of the β- and δ-globin genes (Figure 6.8), whereas in others there appears to have been

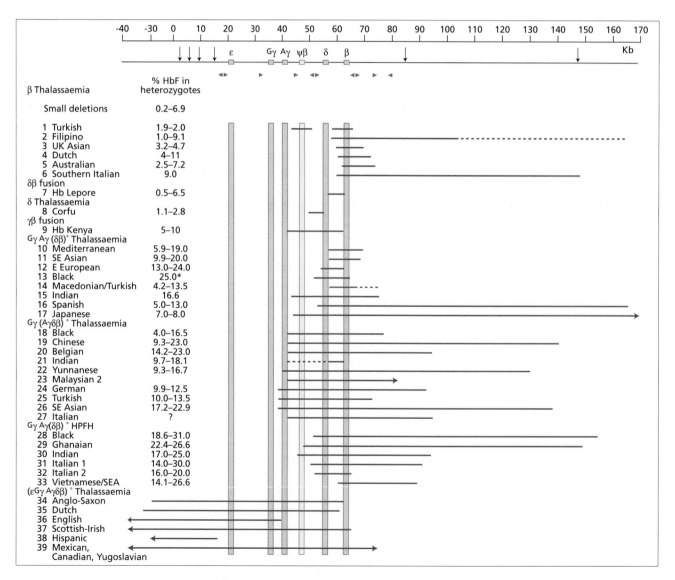

Figure 6.8 The deletions that underlie δβ-thalassaemia and hereditary persistence of fetal haemoglobin. The upper arrows represent DNase I-hypersensitive sites (from Weatherall and Clegg 2001 with permission).

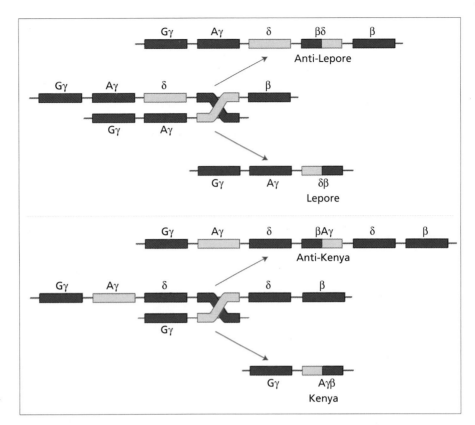

Figure 6.9 The mechanisms for the production of haemoglobin Lepore and related variants.

mispaired synapsis and unequal crossing over between the δ- and β-globin gene loci, with the production of δβ fusion genes (Figure 6.9). The latter produce δβ fusion chains, which combine with α-chains to form haemoglobin variants called the *Lepore haemoglobins* (Lepore was the family name of the first patient to be recognized with this disorder). Hence it is usual to classify this group of conditions into the $(\delta\beta)^0$ *thalassaemias* and the *Hb Lepore* $(\delta\beta)^+$ *thalassaemias*.

The $(\delta\beta)^0$ thalassaemias result from different length deletions of the β-globin gene cluster. In some cases these leave both the $^G\gamma$ and $^A\gamma$ genes intact, whereas in others the $^A\gamma$ genes are also involved, leaving only the $^G\gamma$ genes. Hence the disorders are called $(\delta\beta)^0$ or $(^A\gamma\delta\beta)^0$ thalassaemias (Figure 6.8). The deletions leave the γ-globin genes active in adult life and, although their output is not as high as in the fetus, it is usually sufficient to make these conditions relatively mild. The Lepore haemoglobins are also heterogeneous, depending on the precise site of the abnormal crossover event and hence the structure of the δβ fusion variant (Figure 6.9). γ-Chain production is not as high in these conditions and hence there is a more severe clinical phenotype.

Clinical and haematological changes

In homozygous δβ-thalassaemia there is mild anaemia and splenomegaly, with haemoglobin values of 8–10 g/dL and 100% HbF. Heterozygotes have thalassaemic blood pictures, elevated levels of HbF of 5–20% and normal levels of HbA_2. Homozygotes for Hb Lepore are usually similar to those for β-thalassaemia, although the disorder may be milder and non-transfusion dependent; the haemoglobin consists of F and Lepore only. Carriers have thalassaemic blood pictures associated with about 5–15% Hb Lepore.

Hereditary persistence of fetal haemoglobin

This is a heterogeneous group of conditions in which there is persistent fetal haemoglobin production in adult life in the absence of major haematological abnormalities. Although of little clinical importance, it may modify the phenotype of the β-haemoglobinopathies.

Some forms of hereditary persistence of fetal haemoglobin (HPFH) result from long deletions of the β-globin gene cluster, similar to those that cause δβ-thalassaemia (Figure 6.8). Homozygotes, with 100% HbF, have a mild thalassaemia-like blood picture and are mildly polycythaemic, reflecting the high oxygen affinity of HbF. Heterozygotes have no haematological abnormalities but have 20–30% HbF.

Another type of HPFH results from point mutations in the promoter regions upstream from either the $^G\gamma$ or $^A\gamma$-globin genes, which allow the γ-globin genes to be active in adult life; the linked β-globin genes also remain active. Hence they are called $^G\gamma\beta^+$ and $^A\gamma\beta^+$ HPFH. Heterozygotes have elevated levels of HbF in the 10–15% range; this consists either of $^{G}\gamma$ or $^{A}\gamma$ HbF, depending on the particular mutation involved.

There is a third type of HPFH in which there are low levels of HbF, in the 1–5% range. It was first recognized in Switzerland and is sometimes called Swiss HPFH, although it is now clear that it is a heterogeneous condition. Genetic evidence suggests that the determinant is, at least in some cases, unlinked to the β-globin gene cluster, in one case on chromosome 6. The importance of this type of HPFH is that, when inherited with β-thalassaemia or sickle cell anaemia, it causes an unusually high level of HbF production and hence reduces the severity of the phenotype.

εγδβ-Thalassaemias

These rare conditions result from long deletions of the β-globin gene cluster, which involve the β-globin LCR (Figure 6.8). There is no output from the globin genes of the cluster. Clearly, the homozygous state would not be compatible with survival. Heterozygotes have severe haemolytic disease of the newborn, with anaemia and hyperbilirubinaemia. If they survive the neonatal period, they grow and develop normally; in adult life they have the haematological picture of heterozygous β-thalassaemia, with mild anaemia, hypochromic microcytic red cells and a haemoglobin pattern of normal HbA_2 β-thalassaemia.

α-Thalassaemias

Distribution

The α-thalassaemias occur widely throughout sub-Saharan Africa, the Mediterranean region, the Middle East, the Indian subcontinent and South-East Asia in a line stretching from southern China through Thailand, the Malay peninsula and Indonesia, to the Pacific island populations.

Classification and inheritance

Because both HbA and HbF have α-chains, genetic disorders of α-chain synthesis result in defective fetal and adult haemoglobin production. In the fetus, a deficiency of α-chains leads to the production of excess γ-chains, which form γ_4-tetramers, or Hb Bart's; in adults, excess of β-chains form β_4-tetramers or HbH.

There are two α-globin genes on chromosome 16 (Figure 6.1) and hence there are two main types of α-thalassaemia: α^0-thalassaemia, in which both genes are inactivated ($-/\alpha\alpha$), and α^+-thalassaemia, in which only one of the pair is affected ($-\alpha/\alpha\alpha$). There are two important clinical disorders caused by α-thalassaemia, the Hb Bart's hydrops syndrome and HbH disease. The former results from the homozygous inheritance of α^0-thalassaemia ($-/-$). HbH disease usually results from the co-inheritance of both α^0 and α^+-thalassaemia ($-\alpha/-$). These interactions are summarized in Figure 6.10.

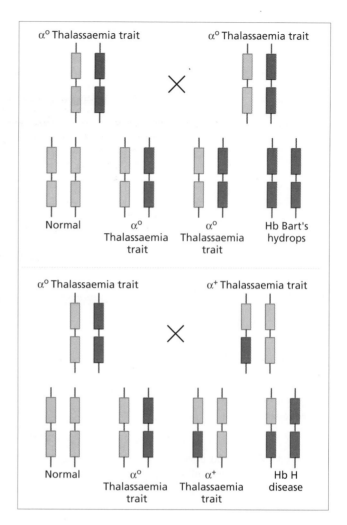

Figure 6.10 The genetics of α-thalassaemia.

Molecular pathology

The α^0-thalassaemias result from deletions of both α-globin genes. There are many different-sized deletions; however, one is particularly common in South-East Asia and another occurs mainly in Mediterranean populations (Figure 6.11). α^0-Thalassaemia may also result from deletions about 40 kb upstream from the α-globin gene cluster, which involve the HS40 region.

The molecular basis of the α^+-thalassaemias is more complicated. In some cases, they result from deletions that remove one of the linked pairs of α-globin genes, leaving the other one intact ($-\alpha/\alpha\alpha$). In others, both α-globin genes are intact but one of them has a mutation that either partially or completely inactivates it ($\alpha^T\alpha/\alpha\alpha$).

Each α-gene lies within a boundary of homology approximately 4 kb long. These regions were generated by a duplication, and subsequently were subdivided, presumably by insertions and deletions, to give three homologous subsegments that are

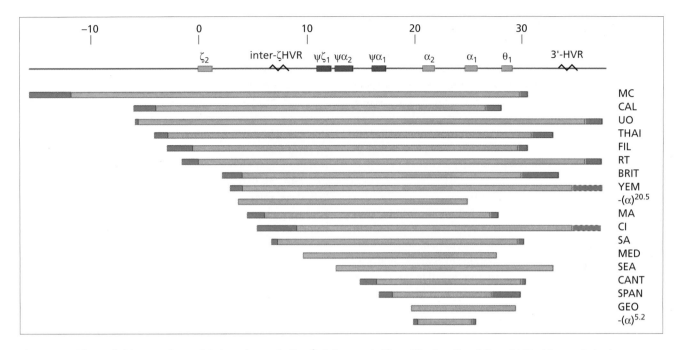

Figure 6.11 The α-globin gene cluster deletions that underlie α⁰-thalassaemia (from Weatherall and Clegg 2001 with permission).

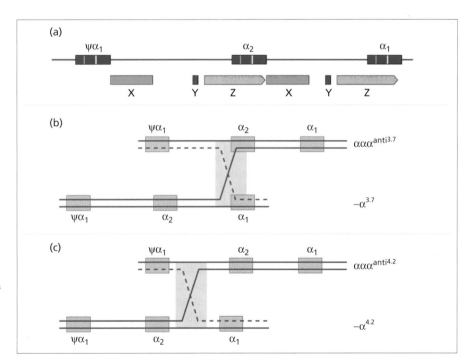

Figure 6.12 The molecular mechanisms that underlie the deletion forms of α⁺-thalassaemia. (a) Normal cluster showing X, Y and Z homology boxes; (b) 3.7-kb deletion; (c) 4.2-kb deletion.

designated X, Y and Z (Figure 6.12). The duplicated Z boxes are 3.7 kb apart and the X boxes are 4.2 kb apart. Misalignment and reciprocal crossover between these segments at meiosis produces a chromosome with either single ($-\alpha$) or triplicated ($\alpha\alpha\alpha$) α-globin genes. If the crossover occurs between the Z boxes, 3.7 kb of DNA is lost, an event that is described as a *right-ward deletion*, written as $-\alpha^{3.7}$. A crossover between the two X boxes deletes 4.2 kb, the *leftward deletion*, $-\alpha^{4.2}$. There are at least three different subtypes of the 3.7-kb deletion.

In the non-deletion forms of α-thalassaemia, the α-globin genes are intact but one of them is inactivated by a mutation, many of which are similar to those that cause β-thalassaemia.

One particularly common form, found in South-East Asia, results from a single-base change in the chain termination codon UAA, which changes to CAA. The latter is the codeword for the amino acid glutamine. Hence, when the ribosomes reach this point, instead of the chain terminating, mRNA that is not normally transcribed is read through until another stop codon is reached. Thus, an elongated α-globin chain is produced, which is synthesized at a reduced rate. The resulting variant is called *Hb Constant Spring*. Because the termination codon can change in other ways, there is a family of variants of this kind.

Genotype–phenotype relationships

As the Hb Bart's hydrops syndrome follows the homozygous inheritance of α^0-thalassaemia, this condition occurs only in populations in which α^0-thalassaemia is common, notably those of South-East Asia and the Mediterranean islands. Similarly, because most forms of HbH disease are due to the co-inheritance of α^0- and α^+-thalassaemia, it is also restricted mainly to these regions. In South-East Asia, it may be due to the inheritance of α^0- and α^+-thalassaemia, or α^0-thalassaemia and Hb Constant Spring.

The homozygous states for the non-deletion forms of α^+-thalassaemia often have a more severe phenotype than those for the deletion forms and may result in HbH disease. Those homozygous for $(-\alpha/-\alpha)$ deletion forms have a mild hypochromic anaemia, very similar to the heterozygous state for α^0-thalassaemia; the results of having only two out of the normal four α-genes seem to be the same whether the two genes are missing from the *same* chromosome or *opposite pairs* of homologous chromosomes.

Pathophysiology

The pathophysiology of α-thalassaemia is different to that of β-thalassaemia. A deficiency of α-chains leads to the production of excess γ- or β-chains, which form Hb Bart's and HbH respectively. These soluble tetramers do not precipitate extensively in the bone marrow and hence erythropoiesis is more effective than in β-thalassaemia. However, HbH is unstable and precipitates in red cells as they age. The inclusion bodies produced in this way are trapped in the spleen and other parts of the microcirculation, leading, together with membrane damage mediated by haem and iron, to a shortened red cell survival. Furthermore, both Hb Bart's and HbH have a very high oxygen affinity and their oxygen dissociation curves resemble myoglobin. Thus, the severe forms of α-thalassaemia are due to defective haemoglobin production, the synthesis of homotetramers that are physiologically useless and a haemolytic component.

The haemoglobin Bart's hydrops syndrome

This is a common cause of fetal loss throughout South-East Asia and is also encountered in the Mediterranean region. There is no production of α-chains and hence neither fetal nor adult haemoglobin. The fetus is usually stillborn between 28 and 40 weeks, or, if liveborn, takes a few gasping respirations and then expires within the first hour after birth. Affected neonates show the typical picture of hydrops fetalis, with gross pallor, generalized oedema and massive hepatosplenomegaly. There is an increased frequency of congenital abnormalities and a very large friable placenta. All these findings are due to severe intrauterine anaemia. The haemoglobin is in the 6–8 g/dL range and there are gross thalassaemic changes of the red cells, with many nucleated forms in the blood. The haemoglobin consists of approximately 80% Hb Bart's and 20% Hb Portland ($\zeta_2\gamma_2$). It is believed that these infants survive to term because they continue to produce embryonic haemoglobin. Apart from fetal death, this syndrome is characterized by a high incidence of toxaemia of pregnancy and obstetric complications due to the large placenta.

Haemoglobin H disease

This condition is characterized by a variable degree of anaemia and splenomegaly but it is unusual to find severe thalassaemic bone changes or growth retardation. Patients usually survive into adult life, although the course may be interspersed with severe episodes of haemolysis associated with infection or worsening of the anaemia due to progressive hypersplenism. In addition, oxidant drugs may increase the rate of precipitation of HbH and exacerbate the anaemia. Haemoglobin values range from 7 to 10 g/dL and the blood film shows typical thalassaemic changes. There is a moderate reticulocytosis and, on incubation of the red cells with brilliant cresyl blue, numerous inclusion bodies are generated by precipitation of the HbH under the redox action of the dye. After splenectomy large, preformed inclusions can be demonstrated on incubation of blood with methyl violet. Haemoglobin analysis reveals 5–40% HbH, together with HbA and a normal or reduced level of HbA_2.

α-Thalassaemia traits

α^0-Thalassaemia trait is characterized by a mild hypochromic anaemia with red cell indices similar to those of the β-thalassaemia trait; the HbA_2 level is normal. There are no diagnostic tests with which to identify this condition with certainty except DNA analysis. Deletional α^+-thalassaemia carriers have near-normal haematological findings. The heterozygous states for the non-deletion forms of α^+-thalassaemia are sometimes associated with very mild hypochromic anaemia; the type associated with Hb Constant Spring can be identified by the presence of trace amounts of the variant on haemoglobin electrophoresis at an alkaline pH.

α^0-Thalassaemia carriers can be identified with more certainty in the neonatal period, when they have 5–10% Hb Bart's, which disappears over the first few months of life and is not replaced by HbH. Some α^+-thalassaemia carriers have slightly increased levels of Hb Bart's, in the 1–3% range, but its absence does not exclude the diagnosis.

Other forms of α-thalassaemia

There are several other forms of α-thalassaemia that are completely unrelated in their pathogenesis and distribution through the conditions described in the previous sections. They comprise the α-thalassaemia mental retardation syndromes and the association of α-thalassaemia with myelodysplasia.

There are two forms of α-thalassaemia associated with mental retardation, one encoded on chromosome 16 (ATR-16), the other on the X chromosome (ATRX). ATR-16 results from the loss of approximately two megabases from the subtelomeric end of the short arm of chromosome 16, as a result of either simple deletion or chromosomal translocations. Affected children usually have a relatively mild degree of mental retardation and no dysmorphic features. On the other hand, ATR-X, which because of its mode of inheritance affects boys, is associated with widespread dysmorphic features and severe mental retardation. It results from many different mutations of the *ATR-X* gene, the product of which has many features in common with DNA helicases, transcription factors that are involved in the modelling of chromatin, and gene regulation. The product of this gene appears to play an important role in the transcription of the α-globin genes and, undoubtedly, many other genes during early development.

An α-thalassaemic phenotype is also found in association with forms of myelodysplasia in elderly patients. Recently, it has been found that this condition is also caused by mutations of the *ATR-X* gene. The blood films of such patients show dimorphic features, with populations of red cells containing HbH inclusion bodies and a variable level of HbH in peripheral blood. The relationship of the mutations of *ATR-X* to the neoplastic phenotype remains to be determined.

Thalassaemia intermedia

Definition and molecular pathology

The term *thalassaemia intermedia* is used to describe patients with the clinical picture of thalassaemia which, although not transfusion dependent, is associated with a much more severe degree of anaemia than is found in carriers for α- or β-thalassaemia. Many conditions follow this clinical course, e.g. HbC or HbE thalassaemia, the δβ-thalassaemias, and the wide variety of disorders that result from the interactions of the different β- and δβ-thalassaemia determinants (Table 6.3). However, many children with thalassaemia intermedia have parents who are typical β-thalassaemia carriers. The mechanisms that underlie the phenotypic diversity of this condition were discussed earlier.

Clinical and haematological changes

At one end of the spectrum are individuals who, except for mild anaemia, are symptom free. At the other, there are patients who have haemoglobin values in the 5–7 g/dL range and who develop marked splenomegaly, severe skeletal deformities due to expansion of bone marrow, and, as they get older, become heavily iron loaded because of increased intestinal absorption of iron. Recurrent leg ulceration, arthritis, folate deficiency, symptoms due to extramedullary haemopoietic tumour masses in the chest and skull, gallstones and a marked proneness to infection are particularly characteristic of this group of thalassaemias. Because

Table 6.3 β-Thalassaemia intermedia.

Mild forms of β-thalassaemia
 Homozygosity for mild β⁺-thalassaemia alleles
 Compound heterozygosity for two mild β⁺-thalassaemia alleles
 Compound heterozygosity for a mild and more severe β-thalassaemia allele

Inheritance of α- and β-thalassaemia
 β⁺-thalassaemia with α⁰-thalassaemia (––/αα) or α⁺-thalassaemia (–α/αα or –α/–α)
 β⁺-thalassaemia with genotype of HbH disease (––/–α)

β-Thalassaemia with elevated γ-chain synthesis
 Homozygous β-thalassaemia with heterocellular HPFH
 Homozygous β-thalassaemia with Gγ or Aγ promoter mutations
 Compound heterozygosity for β-thalassaemia and deletion forms of HPFH

Compound heterozygosity for β-thalassaemia and β-chain variants
 HbE/β-thalassaemia
 Other interactions with rare β-chain variants

Heterozygous β-thalassaemia with triplicated α-chain genes (ααα)

Dominant forms of β-thalassaemia

Interactions of β and (δβ)⁺ or (δβ)⁰-thalassaemia

99

of the heterogeneity of these disorders, it is possible to determine the course that is likely to evolve in an individual patient only by following the patient very carefully from early childhood. The haemoglobin constitution of the intermediate forms of β-thalassaemia is similar to that found in the major forms.

Prevention and treatment

Thalassaemia produces a severe public health problem and a serious drain on medical resources in many populations. Apart from marrow transplantation, there is no definitive treatment, and most countries in which the disease is common are putting a major effort into programmes for its prevention.

Prevention

There are two major routes to the prevention of the thalassaemias. As the carrier states for the β-thalassaemias can be easily recognized, it is possible to screen populations and provide genetic counselling about the choice of marriage partners. There is very little information about the effect of this approach on the frequency of births of affected babies, and such that is available is not encouraging. Hence, most countries are developing screening programmes at antenatal clinics. When heterozygous carrier mothers are found, their husbands are tested and, if they are also carriers, the couple are offered the possibility of prenatal diagnosis and termination of pregnancies carrying fetuses with severe forms of thalassaemia.

Prenatal diagnosis should be offered only to couples at risk for having children with severe disease. Termination of pregnancies at risk for milder forms of thalassaemia is undertaken, but should be considered only after very careful counselling of the parents; some children with intermediate forms of thalassaemia are symptom free and develop normally; others have more severe anaemia and bone deformity.

Prenatal diagnosis of thalassaemia can be made by globin-chain synthesis studies of fetal blood samples obtained by fetoscopy at 18–20 weeks' gestation, or by fetal DNA analysis on amniotic fluid cells obtained by amniocentesis earlier in the second trimester. These approaches have now been largely replaced by direct analysis of fetal DNA obtained by chorionic villus sampling between the 9th and 13th weeks of gestation.

Low error rates, less than 1%, have been reported from most laboratories using fetal DNA analysis. Potential pitfalls include maternal contamination of fetal DNA, non-paternity and technical problems with DNA analysis. Details of the DNA technology used in prenatal diagnosis are given in the Selected bibliography at the end of this chapter.

Bone marrow transplantation

The place of marrow transplantation for the treatment of β-thalassaemia is now much clearer. In centres with broad experience of the procedure, and if it is carried out within the first few years of life and before there is iron loading (provided that there

is a good HLA match for the donor), the success rate appears to be close to 90%. It is lower if there is already iron loading of the liver or if the transplant is carried out in older patients. The main complications are severe infection during the period of transplantation and either acute or chronic graft-versus-host disease. So far, after over 15 years of surveillance, there have been no reports of secondary bone marrow malignancies in children treated in this way. A number of approaches are being tried to overcome the problem of lack of matched donors. In a few cases, HLA typing has been carried out after *in vitro* fertilization to attempt to obtain an HLA-matching sibling, although there is still considerable ethical concern about this approach. It is still too early to determine the role of haemopoietic stem cell therapy for the treatment of this disease.

Symptomatic treatment

The symptomatic management of severe β-thalassaemia involves regular blood transfusion, the judicious use of splenectomy if hypersplenism develops, and the administration of chelating agents to attempt to deal with the problem of iron overload from regular blood transfusion. When the diagnosis of severe β-thalassaemia is suspected during the first year of life, the infant should be followed for several weeks to make sure that the haemoglobin is falling to a level at which regular transfusion will be necessary, particularly important if he or she has presented with infection that may cause the haemoglobin level to fall. It is difficult to be dogmatic about exactly when transfusions should be started, but if the infant is severely anaemic and is feeding poorly or otherwise failing to thrive, transfusion will almost certainly be necessary. The object is to maintain the pre-transfusion haemoglobin level above 9 g/dL, and this usually requires transfusion every 4 weeks. Either washed or frozen red cells should be used, but whole blood should be avoided because of the danger of sensitization to serum or white cell components. A full blood group genotype should be obtained before the first transfusion. A careful check on the pre- and post-transfusion haemoglobin level should be kept and the transfusion requirements carefully plotted. It is vital that body iron status is assessed regularly in these children. Although this may be achieved in part by serum ferritin estimations, there is good evidence that this does not provide a completely accurate reflection of body iron, which is much better assessed by measuring the hepatic iron concentration. Whenever possible, these children should undergo regular liver biopsies, ideally annually but at least every 2–3 years; in experienced hands, this has a very low morbidity and provides a much better guide to the effectiveness of iron chelation therapy. Non-invasive approaches to assessing body iron load are discussed in Chapter 4.

The gold standard for iron chelation therapy is desferrioxamine. There is extensive evidence that if this drug is given at adequate doses, and if compliance is satisfactory, patients may be maintained indefinitely at safe body iron loads and may grow and develop normally. At present, it is recommended that the drug is started at a dose of 25–35 mg/kg, given by an 8- to 12-h subcutaneous infusion overnight, approximately 1 year after the start of regular transfusion. The usual dose in older children and adults is 40 mg/kg. Patients should receive up to 200 mg of ascorbate on the day of infusion, approximately 30 min before it is started. Intolerance to desferrioxamine is extremely rare but, particularly at high doses, there may be ocular changes, including cataracts and retinal damage, or acoustic nerve impairment. Other complications, particularly if the drug is given to patients with low body iron levels, include reduction in linear growth, sometimes associated with evidence of cartilaginous dysplasia of the long bones and spine. Infection with *Yersinia enterocolitica* is a rare but well-documented complication. But these complications are rare in children who are kept under careful surveillance and the main problem posed by desferrioxamine is non-compliance; much can be done by intensive support by doctors, dedicated nursing staff and families. However, for this reason the search continues for an effective oral chelating agent. The place of these agents at present for the prevention and management of iron overload is discussed in Chapter 4.

If there is a marked increase in blood requirement, hypersplenism should be suspected. Any thalassaemic child with an easily palpable spleen probably has some degree of hypersplenism. Splenectomy should be carried out as late as is feasible and, if possible, not in the first 5 years because the incidence of postsplenectomy infection seems to be particularly high in early childhood. Apart from increased transfusion requirements, the presence of neutropenia or thrombocytopenia is a useful guide to the presence of hypersplenism. Pneumococcal vaccine should be administered before surgery, and after the operation children should be maintained on prophylactic penicillin indefinitely and the parents warned about the danger of overwhelming infection. Because of this risk it is becoming customary to also immunize these children against *Streptococcus pneumoniae* and *Haemophilus influenzae*.

Well-transfused children maintained on a good diet do not usually develop important vitamin deficiency states. However, folic acid deficiency occurs in poorly transfused children or in those with thalassaemia intermedia, and it is probably better to maintain these patients on regular folate supplements. In those who develop iron loading with end-organ failure, endocrine replacement therapy may be necessary to improve growth and secondary sexual development and, if necessary, to treat diabetes mellitus. These children require expert endocrinological assessment before treatment. Because the occurrence of osteoporosis is also likely to be due to hypogonadism, similar precautions should be followed. In those who develop cardiac abnormalities, intensive chelation therapy may improve cardiac function.

However well children are managed there is a serious risk of blood-borne infection, particularly hepatitis B and C, HIV and, in tropical countries, malaria. Much can be achieved by adequate screening of blood products, but the possibility of these complications should be constantly borne in mind and viral infec-

tions treated with appropriate antiviral agents. In some tropical countries, particularly where screening of the blood is difficult, prophylactic antimalarial therapy is given after transfusion.

The role at present for more experimental forms of therapy, notably attempts to reactivate higher levels of fetal haemoglobin production, which, except in a few rare cases, have not been successful for the treatment of thalassaemia, is discussed in Chapter 7, and the current status of research into somatic gene therapy is reviewed in Chapter 26.

Structural haemoglobin variants related to thalassaemia

The unstable haemoglobin disorders

The unstable haemoglobin disorders are a rare group of inherited haemolytic anaemias that result from structural changes in the haemoglobin molecule, which cause its intracellular precipitation with the formation of Heinz bodies. Their true incidence is not known and there have been several well-documented instances in which patients with one of these variants have had no affected relatives, suggesting that they have arisen by a new mutation.

Molecular pathology and pathogenesis
Most of the unstable haemoglobins result from single amino acid substitutions or small deletions. For example, substitutions in or around the haem pocket can disrupt its anatomy and allow in water, with subsequent oxidative damage to haem, which leads to precipitation of haemoglobin. Some substitutions, such as those involving proline residues, cause a marked disturbance of the secondary structure of globin chains. A few variants result from deletions of either single amino acids or several residues. For example, in Hb Gun Hill, five amino acids are missing, including the haem binding site. As the unstable haemoglobins precipitate in the red cells or their precursors, they produce intracellular inclusions, or Heinz bodies, which, together with oxidant damage to their membranes, make the cells more rigid and hence cause their premature destruction in the microcirculation.

Clinical features
All these conditions are characterized by a haemolytic anaemia of varying severity, and splenomegaly. There may be a history of the passage of dark urine, particularly during episodes of infection. Like all chronic haemolytic anaemias, there is an increased incidence of pigment gallstones with their associated complications. The condition may become worse during periods of intercurrent infection and, in the more severe forms, such episodes are associated with life-threatening anaemia. There is a high risk of haemolytic episodes after the administration of oxidant drugs. Apart from intermittent icterus and splenomegaly, there are no characteristic physical findings.

Laboratory diagnosis

The peripheral blood film shows typical features of haemolysis but the red cell morphology may be normal. Occasionally, there is mild hypochromia and microcytosis. Heinz bodies are present in the peripheral blood after splenectomy. The most characteristic feature of the unstable haemoglobins is their heat instability. If a dilute haemoglobin solution is heated at 50°C for 15 min, the unstable haemoglobins precipitate as a dense cloud. A similar effect can be induced by isopropanalol. Some of these variants can be seen on haemoglobin electrophoresis but others, because they result from a neutral amino acid substitution, produce no electrophoretic changes and can be demonstrated only by the heat precipitation test.

Treatment

Because these haemoglobins are so rare there has been very little experience of the effects of splenectomy. From the information that is available, and from the author's personal experience, it appears that if a child has had several life-threatening episodes of anaemia or is running a steady-state haemoglobin level that is impairing development or well-being, splenectomy should be undertaken.

High-oxygen-affinity haemoglobin variants

We saw earlier how homozygotes for hereditary persistence of HbF are mildly polycythaemic because of the high oxygen affinity of fetal haemoglobin. There is a family of rare haemoglobin variants that produce the same effect.

Molecular pathology

The high-oxygen-affinity haemoglobin variants result from single amino acid substitutions at critical parts of the haemoglobin molecule which are involved in the configurational changes that underlie haem–haem interaction and the production of a sigmoid oxygen dissociation curve at the junctions between the α- and β-subunits. Others involve the amino acids that are involved with the binding of 2,3-biphosphoglycerate (2,3-BPG) to haemoglobin. As mentioned earlier, increasing concentrations of 2,3-BPG tend to push the oxygen dissociation curve to the right; fetal haemoglobin has a high oxygen affinity (left-shifted curve) because it cannot interact with 2,3-DPG; mutations of the DPG binding sites have a similar effect.

All the high oxygen affinity variants have a left-shifted oxygen dissociation curve with a reduced P_{50}. Thus, the haemoglobin holds on to oxygen more avidly than normal. This leads to tissue hypoxia, which, in turn, causes an increased output of erythropoietin and an elevated red cell mass.

Clinical features

Most affected persons are completely healthy and are identified only when a routine haematological examination shows an unusually high haemoglobin level or packed cell volume.

There have been one or two reports of arterial or venous occlusive disease. There is no splenomegaly and, apart from a raised red cell mass, there are no associated haematological findings. Although it might be expected that a high-oxygen-affinity haemoglobin would cause defective oxygenation of the fetus, none of the reported families has had a history of frequent stillbirths.

Diagnosis

The condition should be suspected in any patient with a pure red cell polycythaemia associated with a left-shifted oxygen dissociation curve. The diagnosis can be confirmed by haemoglobin analysis.

Treatment

In asymptomatic persons, no treatment is necessary. The difficulty arises if there is associated vascular disease with symptoms of coronary or cerebral artery insufficiency. There is insufficient published information to determine how this complication should be managed. As these patients require a high haemoglobin level for oxygen transport, venesection should be carried out with great caution.

Low-oxygen-affinity haemoglobin variants

At least six haemoglobin variants with reduced oxygen affinity have been reported. The first to be described, Hb Kansas, was found in a mother and son with unexplained cyanosis. The subjects were asymptomatic and had normal haemoglobin levels without any evidence of haemolysis. Like many of the high-affinity variants, the amino acid substitution in this variant was at the interface between the α- and β-globin chains. For reasons that are not clear, some substitutions in this region give rise to variants with a relatively low oxygen affinity. This condition should be thought of in any patient with an unexplained congenital cyanosis.

Congenital methaemoglobinaemia due to haemoglobin variants

Several α- and β-globin variants associated with methaemoglobinaemia have been discovered. These disorders, unlike the genetic methaemoglobinaemias due to enzyme defects, follow a dominant pattern of inheritance.

Selected bibliography

Jessup M, Manno CS (1998) Diagnosis and management of iron-induced heart disease in Cooley's anemia. *Annals of New York Academy of Sciences* **850**: 242–50.

Olivieri NF (1998) Thalassaemia: clinical management. *Clinical Haematology* **11**: 147–62.

Porter JB (2001) Practical management of iron overload. *British Journal of Haematology* **115**: 239–52.

Steinberg MH, Forget BG, Higgs DR, Nagel RL (2001) *Disorders of Hemoglobin*. Cambridge University Press, Cambridge.

Weatherall DJ (2001) Phenotype–genotype relationships in monogenic disease: lessons from the thalassaemias. *Nature Review of Genetics* **2**: 245–55.

Weatherall DJ, Clegg JB (2001) Inherited haemoglobin disorders: an increasing global health problem. *Bulletin of the World Health Organization* **79**: 704–11.

Weatherall DJ, Clegg JB (2001) *The Thalassaemia Syndromes*, 4th edn. Blackwell Science, Oxford.

Weatherall DJ, Letsky EA (2000) Genetic haematological disorders. In: *Antenatal and Neonatal Screening* (N Wald, I Leck eds), 2nd edn, pp. 243–81. Oxford University Press, Oxford.

CHAPTER 7

Sickle cell disease

Ashutosh Lal and Elliott P Vichinsky

Introduction

Sickle cell disease is an inherited chronic haemolytic anaemia whose clinical manifestations arise from the tendency of the haemoglobin (HbS or sickle haemoglobin) to polymerize and deform red blood cells into the characteristic sickle shape. This property is due to a single nucleotide change in the β-globin gene leading to substitution of valine for glutamic acid at position 6 of the β-globin chain ($\beta^{6glu \rightarrow val}$ or β^s). The homozygous state (HbSS or sickle cell anaemia) is the most common form of sickle cell disease, but interaction of HbS with thalassaemia and certain variant haemoglobins also leads to sickling. The term sickle cell disease (SCD) is used to denote all entities associated with sickling of haemoglobin within red cells (Table 7.1).

Geographic distribution of sickle mutation

Several distinct β-globin gene haplotypes are associated with the sickle mutation, and their distribution provides evidence for origin of the mutation in several locations within Africa (the Senegal, Benin and Bantu haplotypes) and Asia (the Arab–Indian haplotype). The sickle trait bestows survival benefit in areas endemic for falciparum malaria, and the distribution of SCD historically paralleled this disease. The sickle haemoglobin-containing red cells inhibit proliferation of *Plasmodium falciparum*, and are more likely to become deformed and removed from the circulation. In recent times, the dissemination of the sickle mutation in different areas of the world took place from the movement of populations via trade routes and the slave trade (Table 7.2). Prevalence of SCD varies tremendously among ethnic and tribal groups within a geographic area. The disease is observed occasionally among the white population –10% of patients with HbSS identified by the California newborn screening programme are not of African descent.

Pathophysiology

Molecular basis of sickling

Deoxygenation of HbS leads to a conformational change that exposes a hydrophobic patch on the surface of the β^s-globin chain at the site of β^6 valine (Figure 7.1). Binding of this site to a complementary hydrophobic site on a β-subunit of another haemoglobin tetramer triggers the formation of large polymers. The polymers consist of staggered haemoglobin tetramers that aggregate into 21-nm-diameter helical fibres, with one inner and six peripheral double strands. The polymerization proceeds after a delay, the length of which is extremely sensitive to the intracellular deoxy-HbS concentration. Even a small increase in deoxy-HbS concentration, such as might occur with cellular dehydration, profoundly shortens the delay time and augments sickling. The process of polymerization is highly cooperative and its kinetics are best explained by the double nucleation model.

Table 7.1 The sickling syndromes.

Genotype	Mean haemoglobin (g/dL)	MCV	Haemoglobin electrophoresis (%)				
			S	A	F	A_2	Other
SS	8.1	N	80–95	–	2–20	N	–
SS $-\alpha/\alpha\alpha$, SS $-\alpha/-\alpha$	8.6, 9.2	↓, ↓	80–90, 80–90	–, –	2–20, 2–20	3.3–3.8, 3.3–3.8	–, –
SC	11.0	↓	40–50	–	1–4		C: 40–50
S-β^0-thalassaemia	8.8	↓	75–90	–	2–20	4–6	–
S-β^+-thalassaemia	11.5	↓	50–85	5–30	2–20	4–6	–
SD Punjab	8.2	N	40	–	2.5–5	2–3	D Punjab: 50
SO Arab	8.1	N	45	–	4–7		O-Arab: 45
S Lepore	11.0	↓	75	–	3.5–40	2	Lepore: 10
SE	13.0	↓	60	–	4		E: 30–35
SHPFH	13.7	N or ↓	60–70	–	25–35	1.5–2.5	–
AS*	N	N	30–45	50–65	2–5	N	–

*Sickle cell trait is asymptomatic.

Table 7.2 Areas of high prevalence of sickle mutation.

Geographic region		Heterozygote rate (%)
Africa	Northern	1–2
	Western	10–30
	Central	7–37
	Southern	0–5
Mediterranean	Northern Greece Southern Italy	1–27
Americas	United States: African ancestry	8
	Caribbean: African ancestry	10
	Brazil: non-white	7
Asia	Saudi Arabia: south-west	5
	Saudi Arabia: eastern province	25
	India: central India – tribal population	20–30

The haemoglobin tetramers first aggregate into a nucleus, which rapidly expands into a fibre (homogeneous nucleation). The newly formed fibre provides nuclei on its surface for aggregation of haemoglobin tetramers to form several more fibres (heterogeneous nucleation).

The polymerization of HbS in the circulating red cells is influenced by the oxygenation status, the intracellular haemoglobin concentration and the presence of non-sickle haemoglobins. Acidosis and elevated level of 2,3-diphosphoglycerate (2,3-DPG) promote polymer formation by reducing the oxygen affinity of haemoglobin. The presence of HbA within the red cells, as in sickle trait, inhibits polymerization by diluting HbS. The inhibitory effect of HbF on polymerization of HbS is more profound owing to the greater amino acid disparity between the β^s- and γ-globin chains.

Effect on erythrocytes

Red cells acquire the sickle or elongated shape upon deoxygenation as a result of intracellular polymerization of HbS, a phenomenon that is reversible upon reoxygenation. Even in the normally shaped red cells, however, the presence of HbS polymer reduces deformability, with consequent increase in blood viscosity. Repeated or prolonged sickling progressively damages the red cell membrane, which is a phenomenon of primary importance in the pathophysiology of SCD. Membrane damage causes movement of potassium ions and water out of the cell by the Gardos pathway and potassium–chloride co-transport, leading to dehydration of red cells. The intracellular haemoglobin concentration rises (producing dense cells), which shortens the delay time to sickle polymer formation. A

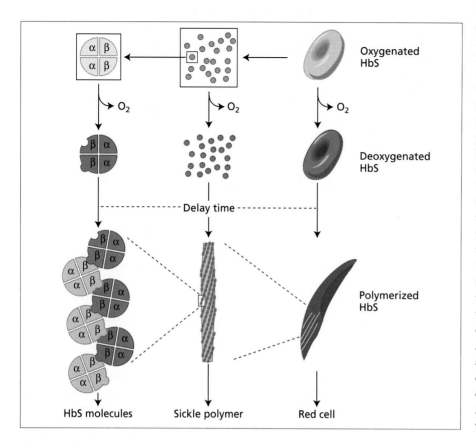

Figure 7.1 Induction of red cell sickling. As red cells traverse the microcirculation, oxygen is released from oxy-HbS (red circles), generating deoxy-HbS (purple circles). Conformational change exposes a hydrophobic patch at the site of the β^6-valine replacement, shown as a projection (left column), which can bind to a complementary hydrophobic site on a subunit of another haemoglobin tetramer, shown as an indentation. Only one of the two β^6-valine sites in each HbS tetramer makes this contact. The middle column shows the assembly of deoxy-HbS into a helical 14-strand fibre, shown as a twisted rope-like structure. The delay time is inversely proportional to the intracellular haemoglobin concentration raised to the 15th power. As deoxy-HbS polymerizes and fibres align, the red cell is distorted into an elongated banana or 'sickle' shape (right column) (from Bunn, HF, 1997, *New England Journal of Medicine* 337: 762, with permission).

second key consequence of membrane damage is alteration of the chemistry of the red cell membrane. Perturbation of lipid organization causes negatively charged phosphatidylserine to appear on the red cell surface instead of its normal location in the inner monolayer. In addition, the red cells become abnormally adherent to the vascular endothelium through vascular cell adhesion molecule 1 (VCAM-1), thrombospondin and fibronectin.

Vaso-occlusion

Several processes contribute to development of vaso-occlusion in SCD. Slowing of blood flow arises from abnormal regulation of vascular tone as a result of diminished nitric oxide-induced vasodilatation. This is aggravated by increase in blood viscosity, resulting from less deformable red cells, a phenomenon called abnormal rheology. Vaso-occlusion is initiated by adhesion of young, deformable red cells to the vascular endothelium, and is followed by trapping of rigid, irreversibly sickled cells (Figure 7.2). Adhesion occurs in the post-capillary venules and is promoted by leucocytosis, platelet activation and inflammatory cytokines. Genetic influences independent of the sickle mutation probably modulate the tendency for vaso-occlusion in individuals and account for phenotypic variation seen in this disease.

Haemolysis

SCD is characterized by chronic intravascular and extravascular haemolysis. Sickling-induced membrane fragmentation and complement-mediated lysis cause intravascular destruction of red cells. Membrane damage also leads to extravascular haemolysis through entrapment of poorly deformable cells or uptake by macrophages. The red cell survival measured by ^{51}Cr assay is 4–25 days, with dense cells surviving for a considerably shorter time than red cells containing some HbF (F cells). Patients have greatly expanded bone marrow space, but the serum erythropoietin level is lower than expected for the extent of anaemia owing to decreased oxygen affinity of HbS. Individuals with concomitant deletion of one or two α-globin genes, or the Senegal or Arab–India haplotypes, have higher baseline haemoglobin levels.

Clinical manifestations

Clinical symptoms vary tremendously between patients with SCD for several reasons. The disease is more severe in patients with HbSS or HbS β^0-thalassaemia than in those with HbS β^+-thalassaemia or HbSC disease. The Arab–Indian haplotype produces a less severe disease than the African haplotypes. The

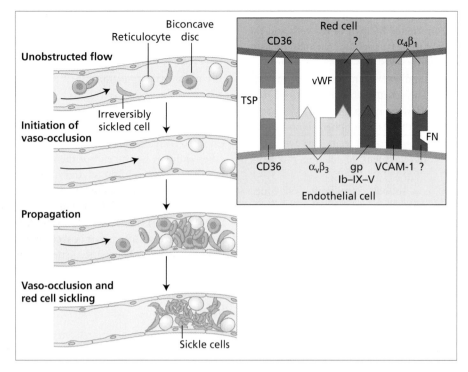

Figure 7.2 Endothelial red cell adhesion and vaso-occlusion in sickle cell disease. Adhesive sickle reticulocytes initiate vaso-occlusion by becoming attached to the endothelium of vessel walls. Thereafter, poorly deformable red cells begin to accumulate behind the site of adhesion, ultimately resulting in an occluded vascular segment containing many sickled red cells. The inset shows the site of red cell attachment to an endothelial cell and several adhesion mechanisms that could participate in the vaso-occlusive process. On the red cell, the relevant adhesion receptors include CD36, which binds thrombospondin (TSP), and integrin $\alpha_4\beta_1$, which binds both fibronectin (FN) and vascular cell adhesion molecule 1 (VCAM-1). On the endothelial cell, the receptors include CD36; integrin $\alpha_v\beta_3$; the complex of glycoproteins Ib, IX, and V (gp Ib–IX–V), which binds von Willebrand factor (vWF); and VCAM-1. Question marks indicate unidentified receptors (from Hebbel RP, 2000, *New England Journal of Medicine* **342**: 1910, with permission).

co-inheritance of one or two α-gene deletions also modifies the clinical picture. The high HbF level observed in hereditary persistence of fetal haemoglobin (HPFH) is associated with very mild disease. However, for poorly recognized reasons, the disease severity varies enormously even within the subgroup of patients with HbSS.

In countries with inadequate healthcare, SCD is associated with high mortality in the first 3 years of life as a result of sepsis and splenic sequestration. In the developed world, the typical patient with SCD has moderately severe anaemia, leads a relatively normal life interrupted by 'crises' as a result of vaso-occlusion, and has a life expectancy of over 45 years.

Anaemia

The underlying β-globin genotype primarily determines the baseline haemoglobin value in SCD, but exacerbation of anaemia can occur for numerous reasons. Patients with more severe anaemia at baseline have a greater probability of developing stroke and renal dysfunction. On the other hand, a higher haemoglobin level is associated with higher incidence of painful episodes, avascular necrosis and acute chest syndrome. Infants with SCD have lower than normal haemoglobin levels after the neonatal period, and the decline continues until it reaches a nadir between 12 and 15 months of age. Boys are slightly more anaemic than girls in the first decade, whereas adult men have higher haemoglobin values than women. Gradual exacerbation of anaemia is observed in both sexes beginning in the fifth decade.

A gradual decrease in haemoglobin level from the baseline value may indicate an underlying folate or iron deficiency. In older patients, however, inadequate erythropoietin production due to chronic renal insufficiency is the most important aetiology of worsening anaemia. Many such patients will become transfusion dependent, although recombinant human erythropoietin therapy can improve the anaemia.

Acute exacerbations of anaemia are observed with aplastic crises and splenic sequestration. The transient arrest of erythropoiesis and the resultant reticulocytopenia in aplastic crisis is most often due to parvovirus B19 infection. Severe anaemia is the consequence of the shortened lifespan of red cells and the course is similar to other chronic haemolytic anaemias. Aplastic crisis is typically preceded by fever and upper respiratory or gastrointestinal symptoms, and several family members may fall ill over a period of days. The reticulocytopenia begins 5 days after exposure, lasts for 7–10 days and is followed by recovery with reticulocytosis and normoblasts in peripheral blood. Blood transfusion is often required in the short term. Parvovirus B19 infection is followed by development of lifelong protective immunity.

Splenic sequestration is a serious complication in young children whose spleen has not yet undergone fibrosis due to recurrent vaso-occlusion. The peak incidence of first episode of sequestration is between 6 and 12 months of age and it affects 30% of all patients. Approximately 15% of patients die during the acute episode and the condition recurs in one-half of the survivors. Episodes may be triggered by a viral illness and the rapid acute enlargement of the spleen traps a significant proportion of the blood volume. Clinically, the child presents with acutely worsening anaemia (> 2 g/dL fall in haemoglobin), reticulocytosis, enlarging spleen and hypovolaemic shock. Prompt restoration of the blood volume and correction of anaemia is required. Splenectomy is recommended following a sequestration crisis due to the risk of recurrences. Chronic transfusion therapy or partial splenectomy is sometimes used in infants with life-threatening anaemic episodes. Parent education to detect splenic enlargement and seek early medical attention significantly reduces the risk of death from sequestration crisis.

Acute painful episode

Acute episode of pain due to vaso-occlusion is the most frequent symptom for which patients with SCD seek medical attention. More frequent painful episodes are observed in patients with HbSS, low HbF level, α-thalassaemia and higher baseline haemoglobin levels. Painful episodes are more common in young adults and tend to diminish in older patients. One-third of the patients with SCD rarely experience pain, whereas a small subgroup of patients suffer from recurrent episodes. When patients maintain a pain diary, painful events are noted on up to half of the days but are not severe enough to require visit to a physician. Painful episodes vary in intensity and generally last for a few days. The majority of the episodes have no identifiable cause, although some attacks are precipitated by cold, dehydration, infection, stress or menses.

In young children, initial pain episode typically presents as dactylitis or hand–foot syndrome, with swelling over dorsal surface of hands and feet. It arises from bone infarction affecting the small bones and the swelling subsides over 1–2 weeks. The radiographs show thinning of cortex and destructive changes of the affected small bones several weeks after onset. In older children and adults, the common sites of pain are the back, chest,

extremities and abdomen. Chest pain is of special significance as it can precede development of acute chest syndrome. Frequent, incapacitating painful episodes that are inadequately managed have adverse psychosocial consequences and stress the physician–patient relationship.

Growth and development

Children with SCD are born with normal weight but fall behind other children by the end of the first year. The weight deficit persists through adulthood and imparts a thin habitus to the typical patient, although obesity is seen in some cases. The rate of growth is lower than normal in SCD patients, and the pubertal growth spurt is delayed by 1–2 years, but the final adult height is normal. Delays also occur in skeletal maturation and onset of puberty, and female patients achieve menarche 1–2 years later than their peers.

Infections

Early loss of splenic function from recurrent vaso-occlusion and the inability to make specific immunoglobulin G (IgG) antibodies to polysaccharide antigens increases the risk of fulminant sepsis. Pneumococcal infection is a serious problem in SCD, particularly in children under 3 years (Figure 7.3a–c). Meningitis can accompany pneumococcal sepsis, and the overall mortality rate is 20–50%. Patients who have had previous pneumococcal sepsis are at increased risk for recurrent episodes and must remain on lifelong penicillin prophylaxis. *Haemophilus influenzae* type B is the next most common organism and affects older children. There is considerable variation in the relative incidence of bacterial organisms causing sepsis in young children with SCD in various regions of the world. In Africa, *Salmonella* spp., *Klebsiella* spp., *Escherichia coli* and *Staphylococcus* spp. are more commonly isolated from the blood of febrile children than *Streptococcus pneumoniae*. Pneumococcal infections are particularly infrequent in the eastern province of Saudi Arabia and Nigeria. Furthermore, the incidence of pneumococcal and *H. influenzae* sepsis has declined owing to penicillin prophylaxis and vaccination of infants. The risk of death during septic episodes has decreased considerably owing to empirical use of antibiotics to treat fever in SCD.

Of the other infections, pneumonia is particularly common in SCD and can be difficult to differentiate from non-infective causes of acute chest syndrome. The most frequent organisms responsible for pneumonia are *Mycoplasma pneumoniae*, *Chlamydia pneumoniae*, *S. pneumoniae* and *H. influenzae*. Lung infections can also arise due to respiratory viruses. In adults, bacteraemia and urinary tract infections due to *E. coli* and other Gram-negative organisms are more frequent. Patients with SCD are susceptible to osteomyelitis owing to bone infarction resulting from vaso-occlusion. The infection is typically due to *Salmonella* spp. or *Staphylococcus aureus*.

Neurological complications

Neurological complications are an important cause of morbidity in SCD. Transient ischaemic attacks or stroke due to cerebral infarction or haemorrhage occur in 25% of patients with SCD (Figure 7.4a). The risk of stroke is increased with lower baseline haemoglobin, low HbF level, high leucocyte count or high systolic blood pressure. Vascular damage results from elevated cerebral blood flow velocities and interaction of rigid or adherent sickle cells with the vessel wall. Angiography demonstrates stenosis or occlusion of vessels in the circle of Willis and internal carotid arteries, sometimes with aneurysm formation or development of moya moya disease (Figure 7.4b). Increased blood flow velocity due to stenosis can be detected by transcranial Doppler ultrasonography in asymptomatic patients, and flow rates of > 200 cm/s correlate with a high risk of stroke.

Stroke due to infarction is more frequent in younger children and those over 30 years, whereas haemorrhage is more common between 20 and 30 years. Stroke is rare in infants, increases to 1 in 100 patients per year between 2 and 9 years, and then diminishes to half of that incidence in older patients. Focal seizures or transient ischaemic attacks (TIAs) are common presenting symptoms of stroke, followed by hemiparesis, coma, speech or visual disturbances. The site of bleeding in haemorrhagic stroke is frequently subarachnoid, and these patients present with severe headache, vomiting and coma. Death can occur during the acute event, particularly with haemorrhagic stroke. Patients with neurological symptoms should be evaluated by computerized tomography (CT) or magnetic resonance imaging (MRI) to distinguish thrombosis from haemorrhage. Immediate exchange transfusion to lower HbS level to < 30% is required. Patients with haemorrhage may require surgical intervention to ligate accessible aneurysms.

As stroke recurs in two-thirds of the survivors within 3 years, all such patients should be maintained on regular transfusions to lower HbS level for several years. Development of first stroke in children at risk, who are identified by elevated cerebral Doppler blood flow velocity, can be prevented effectively through regular transfusions. Even in the absence of overt stroke, silent cerebral infarcts are commonly observed on MRI in SCD and are linked to progressive neuropsychiatric and neurological damage, and poor school performance. Early detection and treatment is important in preventing further neurocognitive impairment.

Pulmonary complications

Acute and chronic pulmonary complications are the leading cause of death in older patients. The acute chest syndrome is characterized by hypoxia, tachypnoea, fever, chest pain and pulmonary infiltrate on chest radiographs (Figure 7.4c). Acute chest syndrome often follows a painful event, particularly in adults (Table 7.3). The pathogenesis of acute chest syndrome involves vaso-occlusion, infection or both. Infections due to *Mycoplasma*,

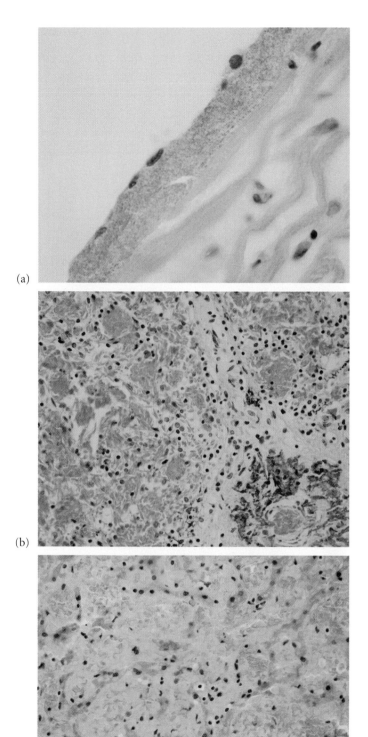

(a)

(b)

(c)

Figure 7.3 Overwhelming pneumococcal sepsis in 7-year-old child. (a) Numerous bacteria in the blood adjacent to the right ventricular wall. Massive sequestration of the spleen (b) and the liver (c).

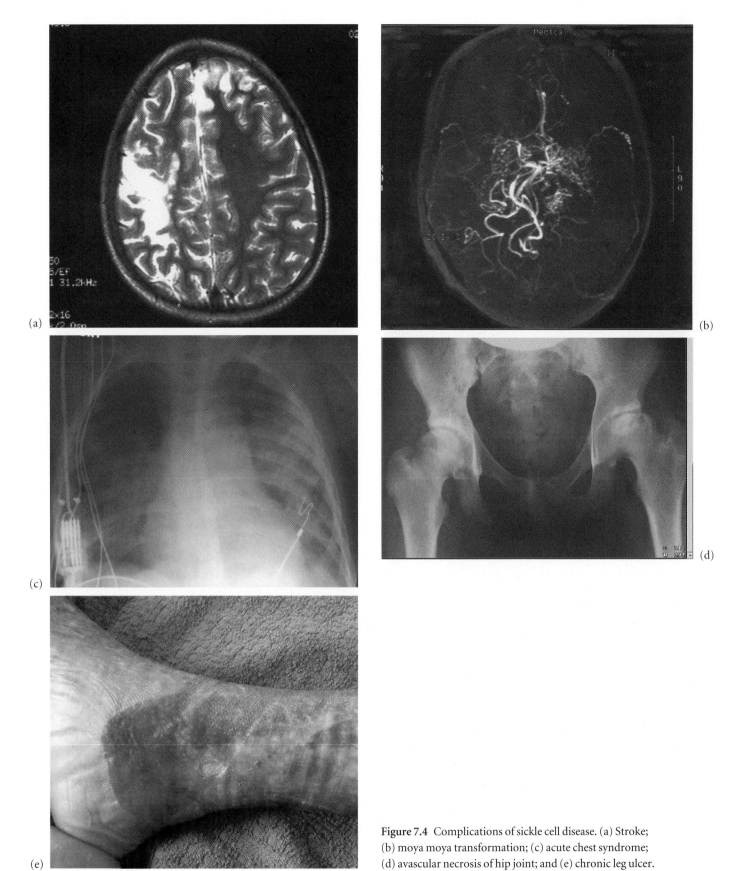

Figure 7.4 Complications of sickle cell disease. (a) Stroke; (b) moya moya transformation; (c) acute chest syndrome; (d) avascular necrosis of hip joint; and (e) chronic leg ulcer.

Table 7.3 Presenting symptoms of acute chest syndrome.

Symptom	Children (%)	Adults (%)
Fever	86	70
Shortness of breath	31	58
Chest pain	27	55
Extremity pain	22	58
Rib pain	14	30

Adults are more likely than children to have pain preceding the onset of pulmonary symptoms.

Chlamydia, Legionella, pneumococcus, *H. influenzae* and viruses are more likely in children. Fat-laden pulmonary macrophages in the airways due to fat embolization from the bone marrow are present in one-half of the cases. Hypoxia due to acute chest syndrome can result in widespread sickling and vaso-occlusion, with risk of multiorgan failure. Patients should receive supplemental oxygen, incentive spirometry and antibiotic therapy directed towards the common organisms. One commonly used regimen consists of cefuroxime and erythromycin, although antibiotics should be guided by local experience. Most patients have a bronchoreactive component and should receive bronchodilator therapy. Recent data suggest that early transfusion may prevent the progression of pneumonia. Urgent blood transfusion is always required for persistent hypoxia or worsening lung consolidation. Partial exchange transfusion and mechanical ventilation is sometimes needed in rapidly progressive cases. Nitric oxide and steroids may be beneficial in life-threatening cases.

Chronic pulmonary problems seen in SCD are restrictive and obstructive lung disease, hypoxaemia and pulmonary hypertension. Chronic complications are more frequent in patients with a history of acute chest syndrome. The prognosis for severe pulmonary hypertension is poor and no satisfactory management is available. Hydroxyurea, regular transfusions, vasodilators, anticoagulation and oxygen inhalation have been tried in some patients. Early treatment with transfusion therapy is being evaluated in asymptomatic patients with early pulmonary hypertension.

Hepatobiliary complications

The liver can be affected by intrahepatic trapping of sickle cells, transfusion-acquired infection and transfusional haemosiderosis. Episodes of cholestasis due to intrahepatic sickling can lead to liver failure in rare instances. Pigmented gallstones are seen in two-thirds of patients, particularly those with HbSS, and can occur in young children. Patients with abdominal symptoms attributable to gallstones should undergo cholecystectomy, although the management of asymptomatic gallstones is less clear. Laparoscopic cholecystectomy can be safely performed, but associated common duct bile stones first require endoscopic retrograde cholangiopancreatography.

Pregnancy

The steady-state haemoglobin level falls in SCD during pregnancy, similar to the decline in haemoglobin observed in normal pregnant women. Folate deficiency can exacerbate the anaemia and supplements should be provided throughout pregnancy. Painful episodes become more common in the last trimester. The incidence of pre-eclampsia is higher than normal in SCD patients and there is a slight increase in maternal mortality. Risk to the fetus from abortion, stillbirth, low birth weight and neonatal death is also increased. Prophylactic transfusions during pregnancy or the type of delivery do not alter the outcome for mother or newborn. It is safe to use oral contraceptives for birth control in SCD.

Renal complications

The hypoxic, acidotic and hypertonic renal medulla favours vaso-occlusion, leading to destruction of the vasa recta and hyposthenuria in the first year of life. It presents clinically as enuresis or nocturia, and patients are susceptible to dehydration in hot weather. Haematuria as a result of papillary necrosis usually originates from the left kidney. Management is generally by bed rest and hydration, although sometimes blood transfusion and ε-aminocaproic acid are required. Proteinuria due to glomerular injury precedes development of nephrotic syndrome and chronic renal insufficiency in the third or fourth decade. The progression to renal failure can be delayed by angiotensin-converting enzyme inhibitors. Careful control of blood pressure, avoidance of non-steroidal anti-inflammatory drugs and aggressive treatment of urinary tract infection and anaemia are important objectives for patients with chronic renal insufficiency. Patients with end-stage renal disease are treated with dialysis and renal transplantation. Some renal complications, such as hyposthenuria and haematuria, are also observed in individuals with sickle trait.

Priapism

Priapism occurs in two-thirds of males with SCD, with a peak incidence in the second and third decades. It is caused by vaso-occlusion leading to obstruction of venous drainage from the penis. It typically affects the corpora cavernosa alone, resulting in a hard penis with a soft glans. Episodes can be brief (stuttering) or prolonged, when they last for longer than 3 h. Recurrent priapism leads to fibrosis and eventual impotence. Young boys require explanation of symptoms and the need to seek early help for priapism. At the onset of priapism, patients should drink extra fluids and attempt to urinate. Persistent priapism requires intravenous hydration and analgesia. Partial exchange transfusion, aspiration of the cavernosa or the creation of fistula between glans and corpora cavernosa (Winter procedure) are performed for resistant cases. Agents used to prevent recurrences of priapism include etilefrine, gonadotropin-releasing hormone analogues, stilbestrol and pseudoephedrine.

Ocular complications

Vaso-occlusion of retinal and other vascular beds in the eye can lead to grave complications. Patients with SCD can develop abnormal (comma-shaped) conjunctival vessels, iris atrophy, retinal pigmentary changes and retinal haemorrhages. Much more serious, however, is neovascularization causing proliferative retinopathy appearing as a 'sea fan' with its potential for vitreous haemorrhage and retinal detachment. Such patients are treated with laser photocoagulation or vitrectomy. The incidence of proliferative changes is substantially higher in HbSC and S-β^+-thalassaemia patients than in HbSS. All patients with SCD should have annual ophthalmological evaluation, beginning in the second decade.

Sudden change in vision in a patient with SCD is an ocular emergency. Central retinal artery occlusion requires immediate treatment with hyperoxygenation and reduction of intraocular pressure, but the prognosis for vision is poor. Hyphaema, which can arise after minor trauma, leads to glaucoma due to sickling of blood in the anterior chamber. The elevated intraocular pressure causes ischaemic optic atrophy and retinal artery occlusion. Individuals with sickle trait are also vulnerable to this complication. Urgent surgical attention is required to wash out blood from the anterior chamber.

Bone complications

The chronic haemolytic process results in expansion of the medullary space, although the resultant bony changes are less pronounced than in thalassaemia. Bone infarction due to vaso-occlusion produces tenderness, warmth and swelling, which can be difficult to distinguish from osteomyelitis. In such cases, cultures from blood and direct aspiration are negative and radiographs later show patchy sclerosis and cortical thickening. Collapse of vertebral end plates due to infarction produces the codfish appearance. Patients are managed with analgesia and hydration until resolution of symptoms.

Avascular necrosis of the femoral head is a serious complication that is difficult to treat and leads to chronic disability and pain (Figure 7.4d). Patients with coexisting α-thalassaemia have a higher incidence of osteonecrosis at a younger age. The condition also affects the humeral head but with less functional consequences. The outcome is better in young patients with immature capital epiphysis, who should be treated with analgesics and avoidance of weight bearing for 3–6 months. In older adolescents and adults the condition is more likely to progress

to degenerative arthritis with conservative management. Core decompression and osteotomy have been tried, but hip arthroplasty is required for patients with severe symptoms.

Leg ulcers

Chronic leg ulcers are frequent in adult patients with SCD, particularly affecting males with HbSS genotype (Figure 7.4e). Ulcers arise near the medial or lateral malleolus and may be single or multiple. Occlusion of skin microvasculature from sickle red cells predisposes to ulcers, which are made worse by trauma, infection or warm climate. Ulcers are always colonized with pathogenic bacteria (*Pseudomonas aeruginosa*, *S. aureus*, and *Streptococcus* spp.) and acute infection can occur. The ulcers are painful and resistant to healing and, although bed rest and elevation of the leg are efficacious, they may not be practical owing to the chronic nature of the problem. Treatment requires debridement, elastic dressings, zinc sulphate and, in some cases, red cell transfusions and skin grafting.

Variant sickle cell syndromes

Sickle cell trait

Sickle cell trait (HbAS) is a benign condition that has no haematological manifestations and is associated with normal growth and life expectancy. Sickle cell trait affects 8–10% of African–Americans and up to 25–30% of the population in West Africa. Upon electrophoresis, the ratio of HbA–HbS is 60:40, owing to the greater affinity of α-globin chains for β^A-globin chains. Impaired urine-concentrating ability and haematuria can occur, and an increased incidence of urinary tract infection is observed in pregnant women with sickle cell trait. A slight risk of sudden death during military training has been reported, and splenic infarction is possible at very high altitudes. Genetic counselling should be provided to individuals with sickle cell trait.

HbSC disease

HbC is found among individuals of African descent and the compound heterozygote state HbSC accounts for 25–50% of patients with SCD. The vaso-occlusive complications seen in patients with HbSC resemble those of HbSS but are less severe. Splenomegaly and the risk of sequestration can persist into adult life. Of particular note is the higher incidence of proliferative retinopathy in HbSC beginning in the second decade. The haemoglobin level (10–12 g/dL) is higher than in HbSS, and the red cells are relatively microcytic with a higher mean cell haemoglobin content (MCHC). Peripheral blood smear reveals frequent target cells, intraerythrocytic crystals and rare sickle cells. The pathogenesis of sickling in HbSC involves membrane damage with resultant water and cation loss and increase in intraerythrocytic concentration of HbS. Equal amounts of HbS and HbC are present in the red cells and the solubility test for sickle haemoglobin is positive. The electrophoretic appearance of HbSC, HbSE and HbSO-Arab at pH 8.4 is similar, but a distinction can be made based upon ethnicity and by performing isoelectric focusing or agar gel electrophoresis at pH 6.5.

Sickle cell–β-thalassaemia

Sickle cell–β-thalassaemia compound heterozygotes account for less than 10% of patients with sickle syndromes. The majority of these patients have the β^+-phenotype, with the proportion of HbA ranging from 3% to 25%. The clinical phenotype is mild and disease severity correlates with the amount of HbA present. The clinical manifestations of less frequent HbS-β^0 genotype are similar in severity to those of HbSS. The red cells are microcytic and hypochromic, and variable number of target cells and sickle cells are observed. Reticulocytosis (10–20%) is present and the level of HbA_2 is elevated.

Sickle cell anaemia with coexistent α-thalassaemia

Co-inheritance of α-thalassaemia ($-\alpha/\alpha\alpha$ or $-\alpha/-\alpha$) with SCD is common, and such patients have less severe anaemia and demonstrate hypochromia and microcytosis. In general, the clinical severity is similar to that seen in HbSS patients with a normal complement of α-globin genes.

Sickle cell–HPFH

Approximately 1 out of 100 patients with HbSS has an elevated HbF level due to deletional or non-deletional mutations that maintain γ-globin gene expression after birth. Such individuals have 20–30% HbF and < 2.5% HbA_2. The haemoglobin level is normal with microcytosis, and target cells are observed in peripheral smear. The clinical course is benign, and vaso-occlusive complications are rare because of the inhibition of sickling by elevated HbF.

Other sickling syndromes

Sickle cell–Hb Lepore disease
Co-inheritance of Hb Lepore with sickle cell mutation produces a clinical picture similar to that of S-β-thalassaemia but with a low HbA_2 level.

Sickle cell–HbD disease
Of all the D or G haemoglobins, HbD Punjab (D Los Angeles) alone interacts with HbS to produce moderately severe haemolytic anaemia in compound heterozygotes. Target cells and irreversibly sickled cells (ISCs) are observed in the peripheral smear, and the clinical manifestations resemble mild sickle cell anaemia.

Sickle cell–HbO Arab disease
HbO Arab resembles HbC on alkaline electrophoresis and produces a moderately severe haemolytic anaemia in association with HbS. The disease is more severe than HbSC, and numerous sickled erythrocytes are observed on peripheral smear.

Sickle cell–HbE disease
HbSE disease causes mild haemolysis and no remarkable abnormality of red blood cell morphology. HbE makes up only 30% of the total haemoglobin because of the thalassaemic nature of the mutation. Patients are generally asymptomatic, although occasionally significant vaso-occlusive complications and anaemia have been observed.

Diagnosis

Peripheral blood findings

The peripheral blood picture depends upon the type of sickle cell syndrome. The haemoglobin level is normal in the newborn period, but anaemia develops and sickle or cigar-shaped ISCs can be observed in the peripheral blood by 3–4 months of age as HbF declines. In HbSS disease, the red cells are normocytic and normochromic, with polychromasia, many ISCs and fewer target cells (Figure 7.5a). The average reticulocyte count is 10% (4–20%) and normoblasts may be observed. Red cells are microcytic in the presence of coexisting α-thalassaemia or iron deficiency. In S-β-thalassaemia ISCs, target cells and hypochromic microcytic red cells are prominent. The red cell morphology in HbSC disease is characterized by predominant target cells and rare ISCs. The occasional Howell–Jolly body, indicative of loss of splenic function in SCD, may be observed. The white cell count is elevated ($12–20 \times 10^9$/L) as a result of an increase in mature neutrophils. The platelet count is also elevated to $300–500 \times 10^9$/L as a result of decreased splenic function.

Other laboratory tests

The measurement of clotting factors in SCD indicates mild ongoing activation of the coagulation system, even in the steady state. The erythrocyte sedimentation rate is consistently low. The serum levels of unconjugated bilirubin and lactate dehydrogenase are elevated, and haptoglobin is decreased.

Haemoglobin electrophoresis

HbS can be identified by cellulose acetate electrophoresis at pH 8.4 (Table 7.1 and Figure 7.5b). HbD and HbG have the same electrophoretic mobility with this method, but can be distinguished using citrate agar electrophoresis at pH 6.2 or thin-layer isoelectric focusing. Distinction cannot be made between HbSS and HbS β^0-thalassaemia on electrophoresis. The diagnosis of

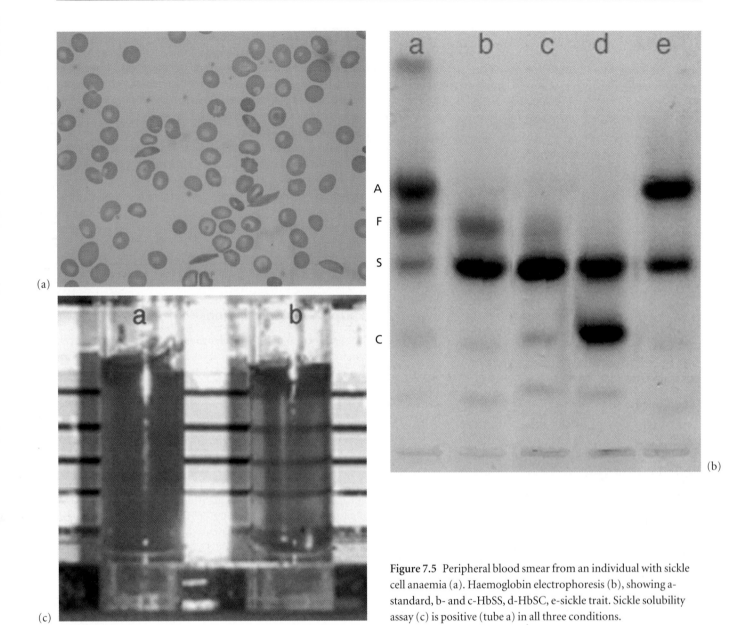

Figure 7.5 Peripheral blood smear from an individual with sickle cell anaemia (a). Haemoglobin electrophoresis (b), showing a-standard, b- and c-HbSS, d-HbSC, e-sickle trait. Sickle solubility assay (c) is positive (tube a) in all three conditions.

S-β^0-thalassaemia is suggested by microcytosis and elevated HbA$_2$, and confirmed by finding β-thalassaemia trait in one of the parents. HbA and HbS are observed upon electrophoresis in both sickle cell trait and HbS β^+-thalassaemia; however, the HbA fraction is greater than 50% in the former, but ranges from 5% to 30% in the latter. The level of HbF is variably elevated with higher levels observed in patients with the Arab–Indian and Senegal haplotypes.

Other tests to detect sickle haemoglobin

Sickling of red cells can be induced by sealing a drop of blood under a coverslip to exclude oxygen or by adding 2% sodium metabisulphite. The solubility test for HbS utilizes a reducing agent such as sodium dithionite, which is added to the haemolysate. The deoxy-HbS is insoluble and renders the solution turbid (Figure 7.5c). Both these tests are unable to distinguish sickle cell trait from sickle cell anaemia and cannot be used for primary diagnosis. They are useful to aid in the identification of an abnormal electrophoretic band as HbS and for identifying sickle cell trait in units of red cells prior to transfusion.

Newborn screening

Universal newborn screening is recommended to identify SCD in the neonatal period. The efficacy of penicillin prophylaxis in preventing death from early sepsis in SCD provided the rationale for development of screening programmes. Blood samples obtained by heel prick are spotted onto filter paper and tested by electrophoresis or chromatography. Neonates with HbSS disease and HbS β^0-thalassaemia have an FS pattern (the order of haemoglobins indicates their relative abundance in the sample). In sickle cell trait, the haemoglobin pattern is FAS, whereas newborns with HbS β^+-thalassaemia have an FSA pattern. Finally, the presence of the FSC pattern suggests HbSC disease. Family studies help to make the definitive diagnosis and, when both parents are unavailable, DNA-based testing is useful.

Prenatal diagnosis

Prenatal diagnosis is available through direct detection of the GAG → GTG mutation responsible for SCD in the fetal cells. Genetic counselling is difficult owing to the marked variability in clinical manifestations within the same genotype, and the lack of ability at present to predict individual phenotype. Preimplantation diagnosis and selection of healthy embryos may offer a solution to this ethical problem.

Therapy

This section discusses general issues in management of sickle cell disease. The treatment of specific complications is addressed under clinical manifestations.

Routine health care

The majority of children with SCD can be managed by paediatricians or community physicians in coordination with a haematologist. Adults with SCD should also continue to have routine office visits. Patients who suffer from more severe complications or need therapy to modify the course of SCD require specialized care at experienced centres.

The level of healthcare available to patients with SCD varies tremendously in different countries. Where resources are limited, the primary focus should be on penicillin prophylaxis, vaccination, education and analgesia for painful episodes. Where comprehensive care is available, both medical and psychosocial needs should receive attention (Figure 7.6). Sickle cell centres should have specialists in several fields, who are available to address complications that may affect different organs.

In cases when diagnosis is made on newborn screening, the infant should be seen within 1–2 months to instruct parents about infections and splenic enlargement. Routine immunization should include pneumococcal, *H. influenzae*, hepatitis B and influenza vaccines. All children receive prophylactic penicillin (penicillin V orally twice daily or benzathine penicillin by

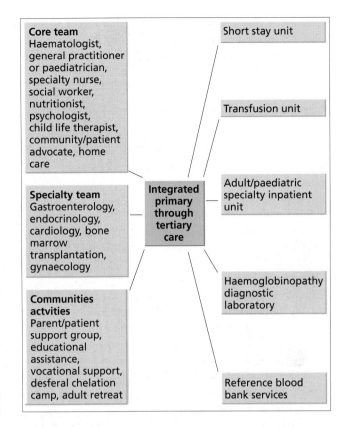

Figure 7.6 Comprehensive care of patients with sickle cell disease.

i.m. injection once per month), which may be stopped after the age of 5 years in the absence of any episode of pneumococcal sepsis or splenectomy. Folic acid supplementation (1 mg per day) is recommended. Evaluation of cerebral blood flow by transcranial Doppler should be performed on all children after 2 years to identify those at risk for stroke. Annual retinal examination is begun at 10 years. Sexually active women should have routine pelvic examinations and receive instructions about birth control.

Infections

Fever in children with SCD requires urgent attention in the office or emergency room. A complete blood count (CBC), blood and urine cultures and chest radiographs should be obtained, and lumbar puncture should be performed if meningitis is suspected. Very young children with fever or older children who appear septic should be hospitalized for intravenous antibiotics. The choice of antibiotics depends upon causative agents prevalent locally and the pattern of resistance. In the USA, cefuroxime or ceftriaxone are preferred, whereas high-dose penicillin is used in several other countries. Many patients older than 2 years who do not look septic or seriously ill can be managed at home after receiving ceftriaxone in the emergency department. Antibiotics should continue for 1 week when bacteraemia is documented.

In the presence of pneumonia, a macrolide should be added to cover *Mycoplasma* or *Chlamydia*. Antibiotics for osteomyelitis should provide coverage for *Salmonella* and *S. aureus* and are given for a period of 4–6 weeks.

Transfusion therapy

Blood transfusion in SCD is used to treat severe anaemia or to reduce the amount of circulating sickle haemoglobin. Only sickle-negative blood, which can be identified by negative sickle solubility test, is used for transfusions. The blood should also be leucodepleted, and matched for common minor E, C and Kell antigens. A simple transfusion is used to treat severe anaemia that is often associated with aplastic crisis and splenic sequestration. Older patients with renal failure may also need transfusions for declining haemoglobin level.

Dilution of circulating sickle haemoglobin can be accomplished by simple transfusion if the baseline haemoglobin level is low. Exchange transfusion or erythrocytopheresis is required to prevent hyperviscosity from the significant rise in haemoglobin when the patient has high baseline haemoglobin or when a greater reduction in HbS is desired. The final haemoglobin level should not exceed 12 g/dL after simple or exchange transfusion. Conditions in which a reduction in the proportion of HbS is required are stroke, progressive acute chest syndrome, persistent priapism or preparation for general anaesthesia. Longer-term reduction in HbS through regular transfusions is advocated to prevent recurrence of stroke and sequestration, and in selected patients with leg ulcers or chronic pain. Routine blood transfusion is not needed for pain episodes, infections, minor surgery or uncomplicated pregnancy.

It is possible to eliminate most complications of SCD with the use of chronic transfusions to suppress endogenous sickle haemoglobin production. However, alloimmunization, iron overload and transmission of viruses are significant risks that limit the use of transfusions to the management of severe complications. In addition, because of the limited availability and decreased safety of blood, criteria for transfusion are more stringent in less developed countries. The high incidence of alloimmunization from minor blood group incompatibility (Rh, Kell, Duffy and Kidd) between donors and recipients can be avoided by use of phenotypically matched units. Patients on long-term transfusions develop iron overload, which requires chelation with desferrioxamine. Liver biopsies are usually necessary to measure iron burden because the serum ferritin is unreliable. As iron accumulation can be reduced or prevented by erythrocytopheresis, this technique is now preferred when venous access is available.

Pain management

Prompt management of pain is essential, given its frequent occurrence and potential adverse psychological consequences.

Patients with recurrent pain are best managed in a familiar ambulatory setting rather than the emergency ward. The patient should be evaluated for potential infectious, traumatic or surgical causes of pain. Pain assessment tools are available for young patients and are also helpful in older patients to follow the response to therapy. Adequate hydration should be provided along with analgesia with narcotics and non-steroidal anti-inflammatory agents. Several narcotic agents are available for oral and parenteral use and the choice of medicine depends upon local experience as well as the patient's preference. The use of incentive spirometry reduces the potential for developing hypoxia and acute chest syndrome secondary to hypoventilation. Undertreatment of pain can be avoided by using patient-controlled analgesia, which has the added benefit of reducing apparent drug-seeking behaviour. Narcotic addiction is no more frequent in sickle cell patients than in others requiring analgesia. Non-steroidal anti-inflammatory agents improve pain control with or without narcotics. Providing psychosocial support and reassurance, and allaying anxiety are important goals. Chronic pain is rare in SCD and may require long-acting narcotics for management.

Hydroxyurea

Hydroxyurea (HU) is a tremendously important drug in the management of patients with SCD who have severe clinical manifestations. HU inhibits ribonucleotide reductase, leading to S-phase arrest of replicating cells, and is used in SCD because of its ability to stimulate production of HbF. HU increases HbF as a result of stress erythropoiesis induced by its myelosuppressive effect. Patients show variable response in the degree of rise in HbF, and some experience no change from the baseline value. Other biological effects of HU play an equally significant role in the beneficial clinical effects observed during HU therapy. Erythrocytes of patients on HU have increased water content and deformability and decreased adherence to vascular endothelium. There is elevation of the haemoglobin level, mean cell volume (MCV), HbF and F cells, whereas total white cell and neutrophil count, reticulocyte count and the number of dense sickle cells decrease. Patients on HU experience 50% reduction in the incidence of acute painful episodes and acute chest syndrome. The transfusion needs and the risk of death are also decreased, but the incidence of stroke remains unaffected.

HU therapy is offered to patients (adults and children over 6 years) with frequent pain episodes or acute chest syndrome. Use of HU in very young children should carefully balance the anticipated benefit with potential unknown risks in this age group. HU is started at a dose of 15 mg/kg per day and increased to 25 mg/kg per day provided that there are no side-effects. Patients require frequent monitoring of blood counts, as well as renal and hepatic function. Myelosuppression is the most commonly encountered side-effect and temporary cessation of therapy and dose reduction is required for neutropenia,

Table 7.4 Advances in the management of sickle cell disease.

Category	Intervention
1 Newborn screening	Counselling
	Comprehensive care
2 Infection	Prophylactic penicillin
3 Brain injury prevention	Screening with TCD, MRI
	Neurocognitive testing
4 Transfusion safety and iron overload prevention	Phenotypically matched RBC
	Erythrocytopheresis
5 Lung injury prevention	Incentive spirometry
	Antibiotics (including macrolides)
	Transfusion
	Nitric oxide
	Prevention with hydroxyurea
6 Surgery/anaesthesia	Preoperative transfusion
7 Avascular necrosis of the hip	Decompression coring
8 Priapism	Adrenergic agonist
	Anti-androgen therapy
9 Pain	Prevention with hydroxyurea
	Patient-controlled analgesic devices
	Non-steroidal anti-inflammatory drugs
10 Renal	ACE inhibitors for proteinuria
	Improved renal transplantation
11 Gall bladder disease	Laparoscopic cholecystectomy
12 Severe disease	Allogeneic bone marrow transplantation
	Chronic transfusions
	Hydroxyurea

ACE, angiotensin-converting enzyme; MRI, magnetic resonance imaging; TCD, transcranial Doppler.

thrombocytopenia, reticulocytopenia or fall in haemoglobin. Dose modification is necessary for patients with renal failure. Skin pigmentation affecting the nails, palms and soles is commonly observed. Despite concerns about the leukaemogenic and teratogenic effects of HU, no convincing increase has been reported in SCD so far.

New therapeutic modalities

A better appreciation of the pathophysiology of SCD will make it possible to exploit new therapeutic mechanisms (Table 7.4). Agents under development include membrane-active chemicals that improve hydration of sickle cells by blocking Gardos channels and potassium–chloride co-transport, or inhibit red cell adherence to endothelium. Decreased availability of nitric oxide (NO) has an important role in vaso-occlusion in SCD, and agents that correct NO deficiency may have significant therapeutic benefit. Newer agents to induce HbF synthesis that are being studied include orally effective butyrate compounds and analogues of azacytidine.

Bone marrow transplantation

Allogeneic bone marrow transplantation (BMT) from matched sibling donor cures 85% of children with SCD less than 16 years of age. However, 5–10% of patients die of complications related to BMT and another 10% experience graft rejection with the return of SCD (Figure 7.7). Additional long-term risks after BMT are infertility and second malignancy. Selection of candidates for BMT is complex owing to the uncertain long-term course of the disease. Although it is clear that high-risk patients benefit from this treatment, the role of BMT in asymptomatic children is not defined. Indications accepted at present to consider transplantation include stroke, recurrent acute chest syndrome or recurrent vaso-occlusive episodes in patients under 16 years old who have an HLA-matched sibling.

Gene therapy

Correction of SCD by gene therapy requires efficient insertion of a gene into repopulating haemopoietic cells and regulated

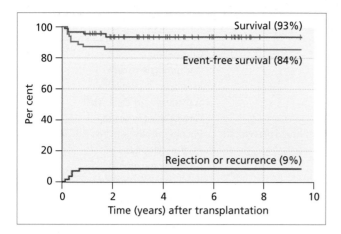

Figure 7.7 Outcome after transplantation for 59 children with advanced, symptomatic sickle cell disease. Kaplan–Meier estimates for survival and event-free survival following marrow transplantation are shown. An event is defined as death, graft rejection or recurrence of sickle cell disease. A cumulative incidence curve for graft rejection and return of sickle cell disease is also depicted (from Walters *et al.*, 2001, *Biology of Blood and Marrow Transplantation* 7: 665, with permission).

expression in erythropoietic lineage. An anti-sickling haemoglobin, constituting 20–30% of the total haemoglobin, would be enough to produce clinical response. Mouse models of sickle cell disease have considerably helped in the effort to develop gene therapy, and correction of sickling phenotype has been demonstrated in such animals.

Psychosocial issues

Recurrent pain and the unpredictable course of the illness place SCD patients at higher risk of depression and poor family relationships. Despite this, with integrated medical care and social support most patients with SCD are well adjusted. Addiction to narcotics is an uncommon phenomenon and is the result of

social influences rather than analgesic therapy. Attention to psychological well-being as well as educational and vocational support are important components of the care provided to SCD patients.

Selected bibliography

Adams RJ, McKie VC, Hsu L *et al.* (1998) Prevention of a first stroke by transfusions in children with sickle cell anemia and abnormal results on transcranial Doppler ultrasonography. *New England Journal of Medicine* **339**: 5–11.

Charache S, Terrin ML, Moore RD *et al.* (1995) Effect of hydroxyurea on the frequency of painful crises in sickle cell anemia. Investigators of the Multicenter Study of Hydroxyurea in Sickle Cell Anemia. *New England Journal of Medicine* **332**: 1317–22.

Embury SH, Vichinsky, EP (2000) Sickle cell disease. In: *Hematology: Basic Principles and Practice* (R Hoffman, EJ Benz Jr, SJ Shattil *et al.* eds), 3rd edn. Churchill Livingstone, Philadelphia.

Hebbel RP (1997) Perspectives series: cell adhesion in vascular biology. Adhesive interactions of sickle erythrocytes with endothelium. *Journal of Clinical Investigation* **99**: 2561–4.

Section on Hematology/Oncology Committee on Genetics. American Academy of Pediatrics (2002) Health supervision for children with sickle cell disease. *Pediatrics* **109**: 526–35.

Sergeant GR, Sergeant BE (2001) *Sickle Cell Disease*, 3rd edn. Oxford University Press, Oxford.

Shafer FE, Lorey F, Cunningham GC *et al.* (1996) Newborn screening for sickle cell disease: 4 years of experience from California's newborn screening programme. *American Journal of Pediatric Hematology/Oncology* **18**: 36–41.

Vichinsky E (2002) New therapies in sickle cell disease. *Lancet* **360**: 629–31.

Vichinsky EP, Neumayr LD, Earles AN *et al.* (2000) Causes and outcomes of the acute chest syndrome in sickle cell disease. National Acute Chest Syndrome Study Group. *New England Journal of Medicine* **342**: 1855–65.

Walters MC, Storb R, Patience M *et al.* (2000) Impact of bone marrow transplantation for symptomatic sickle cell disease: an interim report. Multicenter investigation of bone marrow transplantation for sickle cell disease. *Blood* **95**: 1918–24.

CHAPTER 8

Hereditary disorders of the red cell membrane

8

Edward C Gordon-Smith

Introduction

This chapter and the next deal with genetically determined disorders of the red cell, other than those of haemoglobin, which cause its premature destruction. In this chapter, genetic changes that affect the structure and function of the red cell membrane are described. Chapter 9 describes the inherited defects in red cell metabolism that shorten red cell survival.

Whereas the primary genetic changes underlying these disorders are quite heterogeneous, many of the manifestations are similar, as they result mainly from the increased rate of red cell destruction and from the consequent hyperactivity of the erythroid component of the bone marrow. Therefore, the description of individual conditions will be prefaced with a brief consideration of the pathophysiology of haemolysis.

Haemolysis

Definitions

Haemolysis means that the destruction of red cells is accelerated. Normally, in adults, the bone marrow output is well below its maximal capacity. Red cell production can be increased about sixfold in the adult by increasing the cellularity of existing haemopoietic marrow, as well as by expansion of haemopoietic marrow into the long bones. In the newborn, and during infancy, marrow expansion depends on expanding the medullary cavity of bones, leading to thinning of cortical bone. These bony changes are most extreme in the β-thalassaemia syndromes, but some skeletal changes, usually some bossing of the frontal bones, may be seen in more extreme hereditary haemolytic anaemias of other causes.

Increased red cell destruction is often completely matched by increased production, resulting in compensated haemolysis. When the rate of haemolysis exceeds the maximum erythropoietic capacity of the bone marrow, or when the latter is limited (e.g. because of inadequate supply of iron or folate or by ineffective erythropoiesis), the result is haemolytic anaemia. As in any haemolytic disorder, with or without anaemia, the consequences of haemolysis are always present and, as the same underlying pathogenetic process may cause at different times, even in the same patient, either a compensated haemolytic disorder or haemolytic anaemia, the two terms are often used, somewhat loosely, as though they are interchangeable.

General features of haemolysis

The clinical and laboratory aspects of haemolysis depend on the consequences of increased red cell destruction and production as well as the main process by which destruction takes place. Increased red cell destruction leads to an increase in unconjugated bilirubin from increased haemoglobin turnover. Unconjugated bilirubin does not appear in the urine, although there will be an increase in urinary urobilinogen. The bilirubin level is usually not more than two to three times normal because the normal liver is able to increase excretion to compensate for at least some of the increased production. Jaundice is usually mild in hereditary haemolytic anaemias although there are important exceptions.

In the neonate, particularly premature infants, liver function is not fully developed and more severe jaundice requiring urgent therapeutic intervention may occur. A rare but potentially confusing problem is the co-inheritance of Gilbert's syndrome, which comprises a group of congenital liver enzyme deficiencies that impair bilirubin conjugation. On its own, Gilbert's

Table 8.1 Main features of haemolytic anaemia.

Increased red cell destruction		Unconjugated hyperbilirubinaemia	Mild jaundice
			Increased risk of gallstones
		Increased urinary and faecal urobilinogen	
		Decreased serum haptoglobin and haemopexin	
	Extravascular	Increased iron stores	
		Splenomegaly	
	Intravascular	Haemoglobinaemia and haemoglobinuria	
		Haemosiderinuria	
		Methaemalbuminaemia	
		Decreased iron stores	
Increased red cell production		Marrow expansion	·Bone changes
		Increased erythropoiesis ↓M:E ratio	
		Reticulocytosis	Polychromasia
		Increased folate requirements	Macrocytosis

syndrome does not produce clinical jaundice except when there is inadequate calorie intake, but in conjunction with haemolytic anaemia the hyperbilirubinaemia may be considerable. The increased bilirubin of haemolysis does increase the risk of gall-stones and cholecystitis, which in turn may lead to an increase in serum bilirubin.

In the degradation of haemoglobin, the molecule is broken down to two $\alpha\beta$ subunits, which are bound to haptoglobin, the complex being rapidly internalized in the hepatocyte after binding to the haptoglobin complex receptor. In the presence of haemolysis, serum haptoglobin levels are greatly reduced or absent. Haptoglobin is, however, an acute-phase protein and levels will increase in the presence of inflammation. Haemopexin is another haem-binding protein produced by the liver, which is decreased in haemolysis. Chronic haemolytic anaemia may increase iron content of the body through increased iron absorption as a result of anaemia coupled to the retention of the haem iron following binding to haptoglobin and haemopexin. In rare cases of inherited haemolytic anaemia, this iron overload may be sufficient to produce clinically important effects, particularly if there is co-inheritance of a haemochromatosis gene. In most haemolytic anaemias, owing to membrane defects, the destruction of red cells takes place extravascularly in the reticulo-endothelial system and the iron is retained as described. When destruction is intravascular, free haemoglobin will be released into the plasma, producing haemoglobinaemia and methaemal-binaemia, and will pass through the glomerulus to produce haemoglobinuria and haemosiderinuria. Iron deficiency is thus more likely than overload in intravascular haemolysis.

Increased red cell production leads to expansion of the red cell precursor compartment of the bone marrow as described above. There are also changes in the structure of the marrow as a consequence of the chronic anaemia, which allows the early release of reticulocytes and, in more marked cases, of haemolytic anaemia

nucleated red cells and even myelocytes. In the peripheral blood, the polychromasia and macrocytosis of reticulocytosis are the result of this increased throughput and release. The increased cell production requires an increased supply of folate, which, at least theoretically, can produce folate deficiency unless supplements are given. It is usual to give folic acid (e.g. 400 µg daily or 5 mg once weekly) daily to people with chronic haemolytic anaemia. The main features of haemolytic anaemia are summarized in Table 8.1.

Classification

Because of the unique structural and functional specialization of the mature red cell, the impact on it of a wide range of exogenous or endogenous changes is relatively uniform: the cell will be destroyed prematurely. According to the site of the primary change, haemolytic disorders have been traditionally classified as being due either to intracorpuscular or to extracorpuscular causes. According to the nature of the primary change, haemolytic disorders have also been classified as inherited or acquired. These two classifications correlate almost completely with each other, in that extracorpuscular causes are usually acquired, whereas intracorpuscular causes are usually inherited. One notable exception is paroxysmal nocturnal haemoglobinuria, a disease in which an intracorpuscular defect is acquired as a result of a somatic mutation (see Chapter 11).

Although in every cell all molecules and organelles are naturally interdependent, it is convenient to consider the red cell as a conveyance for a large amount of haemoglobin contained in a plasma membrane, the stability of which is maintained by an appropriate metabolic machinery. Unfavourable genetic changes in any of these components may cause haemolysis. Accordingly, inherited haemolytic disorders can be classified into three major groups: (i) genetic disorders of haemoglobin (see Chapter 6); (ii) abnormal membrane (including the cytoskeleton); and (iii) abnormal metabolism (enzymopathies) (see Chapter 9).

Red cell metabolism

The details of red cell metabolism are considered in Chapter 9. Suffice to say in this chapter that the red cell membrane requires a supply of both ATP and reducing power to maintain its proper integrity. The way in which energy is supplied to the membrane is intimately related to its structure. The main pathway for metabolizing ATP in the membrane is via Na^+,K^+-ATPase. The enzyme glyceraldehyde-3-phosphate dehydrogenase (Ga3PD) is closely associated with the inner layer of the membrane. It catalyses the conversion of Ga3P to 1,3-diphosphoglycerate (1,3-DPG), with the production of NADH. ATP is produced in the next step of the glycolytic pathway, the conversion of 1,3-DPG to phosphoglycerate, which occurs in intimate contact with the membrane.

The red cell membrane

The red cell membrane, like all other cell membranes, consists of a lipid bilayer that is stabilized and given specific properties by the proteins, glycolipids and other specialized molecules and structures with which it is associated.

The lipid bilayer consists of approximately equal molar quantities of phospholipids and cholesterol molecules. The charged phosphatidyl groups of the phospholipids are hydrophilic and form the outer and inner surfaces of the bilayer. The interior of the membrane is formed by hydrophobic bonding of the acyl chains and cholesterol, which form the internal parts of the two leaflets (Figure 8.1). The arrangement is energy efficient but the two leaflets are not symmetrical. The outer leaflet consists mainly of phosphatidylcholine and sphingomyelin, inner leaflet phosphatidylethanolamine and phosphatidylserine (Figure 8.2). The maintenance of the asymmetry and the proper function of the membrane requires energy. In the mature red cells; this is provided by ATP from the glycolytic pathway and reducing power mainly in the form of glutathione.

The normal biconcave shape and function of the red cell membrane are determined by the membrane proteins and their interactions with the lipid bilayer and with each other. There are two main sorts of protein–membrane associations. The integral proteins have strong hydrophobic domains that associate with the hydrophobic part of the bilayer. Many of these integral proteins span the membrane and provide channels between the plasma and cytosolic compartments. The cytostolic, inner domains of these proteins interact with each other and with the second main group, the proteins of the cytoskeleton. The integral proteins that provide the links between the plasma surface and the cytoskeleton have conveniently been referred to as 'vertical con-

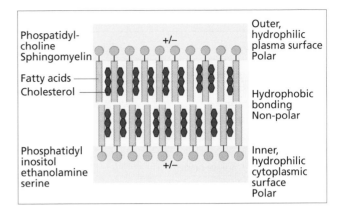

Figure 8.1 Arrangement of membrane lipids. The acyl chains of the diacyl phosphatidyl glycerides are hydrophobic non-polar domains and they form hydrophobic bonds with the acyl groups of the opposite layer. Cholesterol is present in roughly equimolar amounts and determines the fluidity of the membranes.

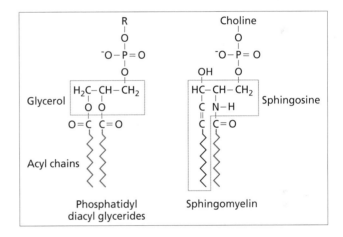

Figure 8.2 Main lipids of the red cell membrane. The outer, plasma layer, contains most of the neutral lipids sphingomyelin and phosphatidylcholine (lecithin). The inner, cytoplasmic layer, contains mostly acidic groups, phosphatidylserine, ethanolamine and inositol. 'R' may be choline, serine, ethanolamine or inositol.

nections', whereas the proteins of the cytoskeleton that make up the inner network of the cell membrane are characterized as 'horizontal connections'. Genetic abnormalities that produce spherocytes mainly have mutations affecting the vertical connections. Mutations of the horizontal system usually produce elliptocytosis or more bizarre-shaped changes. The main proteins are listed in Table 8.2, and their arrangement is shown schematically in Figure 8.3.

In addition to the compartments mentioned so far, there are numerous surface proteins that provide the main interface with the plasma, including the blood group systems and other

Table 8.2 Proteins of the red cell membrane.

Band*	Protein	Gene location	Function	Associated haemolytic anaemias
1	α-Spectrin	SPTA1, 1q21	Cytoskeleton network	HE, HS
2	β-Spectrin	SPTB, 14q22–q23	Cytoskeleton network	HPP
2.1	Ankyrin	ANK1, 8p11.2	Vertical contact	HS
2.9	Adducin ADD1, ADD2	α chain 10q24.2–q24.3, β-chain 4p16.3	Promotes spectrin binding to actin, binds Ca^+/calmodulin	(HS, HE in mice)
3	Band 3. Solute carrier family 4 (anion exchanger) member 1	EPB3 (SLC4A1), 17q21–q22	Anion exchange channel, ii blood groups, binds glycolytic enzymes	HS, SAO, HAC
4.1	Protein 4.1	EPB41, 1p36.2–p34	Stabilizes spectrin–actin contact	HE
4.2	Protein 4.2 (pallidin)	EPB42(PLDN), 15q15	Spectrin–ankyrin complex	HS (Japan)
5	β-Actin	ACTB, 7p22–p12	Spectrin network junction	?
6	Ga3PD	12p13.31–p13.1	Links ATP production to membrane	?
PAS†-1	Glycophorin A	4q28.2–q31.1	MN blood groups	?
PAS-2	Glycophorin C	2q14–q21	Gerbich blood groups	HE
PAS-3	Glycophorin B	4q28–q31	Ss blood groups	?

HAC, hereditary acanthocytosis; HE, hereditary elliptocytosis; HS, hereditary spherocytosis; HPP, hereditary pyropoikilocytosis; SAO, South-East Asia ovalocytosis; Ga3PD, gyceraldehyde-3-phosphate dehydrogenase.
*The band numbers refer to the position on SDS-PAGE electrophoresis.
†Periodic acid–Schiff stain – bands seen only on PAS-stained gels.

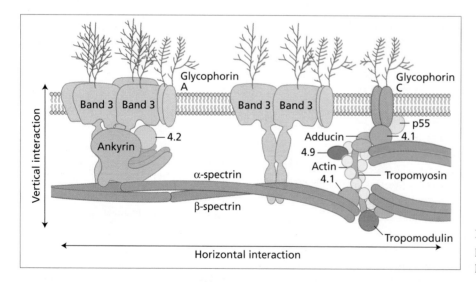

Figure 8.3 Arrangement of membrane proteins (after Tse & Lux, 1999, with permission).

receptors. Many of these molecules are heavily glycosylated, as are the integral proteins the glycophorins. Sialic acid, which is the main side-chain of the glycophorins, contributes the most part to the negative surface change of the erythrocyte. Many of these surface proteins are linked to the membrane by the glycosyl phosphatidylinositol (GPI) anchor, which provides the hydrophobic domain required for association with the inner hydrophobic part of the membrane. Somatic mutations in the gene phosphatidylinositol glycan A (PIG-A) leads to a failure to produce the anchor and to paroxysmal nocturnal haemoglobinuria (PNH), as discussed in Chapter 11.

The integral proteins and vertical interaction

The two major integral proteins that span the lipid bilayer are band 3 (the anion channel protein) and the glycophorins

A, B and C. Band 3 and associated molecules, 4.2 (pallidin) and ankyrin (2.1), form one major vertical interactive pathway with binding to the β-chain of the spectrin tetramer through ankyrin. Glycophorin C and protein 4.1 also provide a vertical interaction but the association with spectrin is through a link with actin, which is a key part of the horizontal network.

The band 3–4.2–ankyrin–spectrin complex is a central part of the organization of the lipid bilayer and loss of part of this complex leads to loss of lipid from the outer leaflet of the bilayer, reducing the surface area–volume ratio of the red cell and leading to the characteristic spherocytes of the phenotype hereditary spherocytosis.

The main protein of the cytoskeleton is spectrin. Spectrin consists of two subunits, α and β, which associate side by side to produce a heterodimer. The dimers associate head to head to form tetramers about 200 nm long. The tail end of the dimer makes contact with the specialized domain in the actin molecule, a contact stabilized by protein 4.1. The actin molecule has binding domains for a number of spectrin dimers, which produce the more or less hexagonal network of spectrin tetramers on the inner surface of the membrane associated with the lipid bilayer. Spectrin–actin–4.1 interactions provide much of the flexibility of the red cell membrane. Deficiencies of spectrin that affect these horizontal interactions tend to induce a loss of flexibility in the membrane and elliptocytosis.

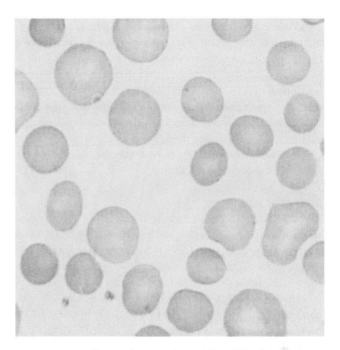

Figure 8.4 Hereditary spherocytosis, peripheral blood. Small spherocytic red cells lack area of central pallor. Large polychromatic red cells (reticulocytes) result in normal MCV, although MCHC may be increased.

The clinical phenotypes of hereditary membrane disorders

Mutations in the genes that control the proteins of the membrane and their interaction mainly produce changes in the shape of the red cells, which is characteristic in any individual. Many of the conditions are inherited as an autosomal dominant disorder, homozygosity for major defects mainly being lethal. Severe, bizarre or unexpected red cell morphology is often produced by double heterozygosity or inheritance of more than one defect of the membrane proteins. The mutations affecting the red cell membrane are many and heterogeneous, but the effect on the phenotype can be classified in five main categories. These are: (i) hereditary spherocytosis (HS); (ii) hereditary elliptocytosis (HE) and hereditary pyropoikilocytosis (HPP); (iii) South-East Asian ovalocytosis (SAO); (iv) hereditary acanthocytosis; and (v) hereditary stomatocytosis (HSt).

Hereditary spherocytosis

As the name implies, hereditary spherocytosis (HS) is a genetically determined haemolytic anaemia characterized by the spherical shape of the affected red cells. The spherical shape produces a characteristic appearance in the stained blood film of round cells with smaller than normal diameter, which lack the area of central pallor of the normal biconcave discs (Figure 8.4). The old name, 'familial acholuric jaundice', emphasizes the presence of jaundice in the absence of bile in the urine, distinguishing this jaundice from that caused by hepatobiliary problems. The disorder is generally inherited as a dominant condition with a wide spectrum of severity. The usual clinical picture is of mild to moderate haemolytic anaemia but varies from severe neonatal haemolysis with kernicterus (rare) to clinically silent and asymptomatic (usual) haemolysis. Autosomal recessive inheritance occurs in a few mutations, often producing severe haemolysis.

In Caucasian populations, HS is one of the most common haemolytic anaemias due to membrane defects, with a prevalence of clinically apparent disease of 200–300 per million of the population. The occurrence of clinically silent cases probably means that the overall prevalence is slightly higher.

Clinical features

The commonest forms of HS present as mild anaemia and jaundice, with a modestly enlarged spleen. However, the genetic heterogeneity of HS (see below) is reflected in the clinical presentation. As the main site of increased red cell destruction in HS is the spleen, it is not surprising that the size of the spleen tends to reflect the severity of the haemolysis, although splenomegaly is rarely marked – enlargement below the umbilicus being very uncommon. When HS presents in adolescence or adult life, it needs to be distinguished from other causes of microspherocytosis, particularly warm autoimmune haemolytic anaemia.

HS may present at birth. The functions of the spleen become mature only after birth, so severe anaemia *in utero* is rare. Erythropoiesis is highly active before birth but enters a phase of reduced activity in the neonatal period. Severe anaemia, developing over 5–30 days post delivery and requiring transfusion, may result from this double physiological development of reduced production and increased destruction, but the anaemia may greatly reduce during the first year of life as compensatory erythropoiesis develops. Decisions about splenectomy do not need to be taken during this time.

Molecular pathology

About 60% of HS cases result from a defect in the ankyrin–spectrin complex, with both α and β (genes *SPTA1*, *SPTB*) of the spectrin dimer or ankyrin (*ANK1*) being implicated in different genetic types (Table 8.2). A further 25% involve deficiency in band 3, the anion channel. In the remainder of the dominantly inherited HS families there is a deficiency of protein 4.2 or no abnormality has yet been identified. Deficiency of protein 4.2 is particularly common in Japanese families with HS (Table 8.2). These defects involving spectrin–ankyrin–band 3 interactions affect the 'vertical interactions' described by Jiri Palek and colleagues.

It will be appreciated that the genetic defect that produces the dominant form of HS affects only one of a pair of genes. The presence of one abnormal protein influences the protein–protein interactions of these complexes, leading to partial deficiency of several proteins, even if they are not genetically disturbed. This is particularly true of spectrin. Complete loss of complex function is probably not viable, so homozygous children are not found. Double heterozygosity or inheritance of separate membrane defects does occur and is associated with usually severe haemolytic anaemia. Other recessive forms of HS are also seen in which the inheritance of one defective gene involving the spectrin subunit produces no clinical effect, whereas homozygosity produces a severe defect and haemolysis.

Laboratory diagnosis

The typical findings of extravascular haemolysis are present in HS (Table 8.1). The diagnosis is usually made on the basis of morphology of the blood, backed up where possible with a family history. The mean cell haemoglobin concentration (MCHC) is often increased above 35 g/L in HS, but the presence of macrocytic reticulocytes usually results in a low normal mean cell volume (MCV) rather than true microcytosis. These changes result not only from the reduction of surface area–volume ratio but also from the slight dehydration of HS cells. A number of variants of the typical HS features have been described, usually the more severe forms that may have denser and less perfectly round cells in the peripheral blood. In infancy, the morphology may be more difficult to interpret. The effect of immature splenic function and the macrocytosis and anisocytosis of infancy combine with the HS phenotype to produce red cell appearances not typical of the developing HS. Family studies may assist in the diagnosis.

Osmotic fragility test

The osmotic fragility test measures the sensitivity of red cells to lysis *in vitro* to swelling caused by incubation in increasingly hypotonic saline solutions. Red cells are able to swell with increasing volume until the pressure disrupts the unstretchable membrane and lysis occurs. In normal red cells with the biconcave disc shape, 50% lysis occurs when the saline solution reaches about 0.5% sodium chloride. The more rigid HS cells have less ability to swell and so lyse at higher concentrations – a right-shifted osmotic fragility curve. One of two patterns may be seen in HS, a generally right-shifted curve, which is the more common finding, and one where there appears to be a 'tail' of lysis-sensitive cells. Incubation of blood for 24 h at 37°C accentuates the fragility (Figure 8.5).

The acidified glycerol lysis test (AGLT) uses glycerol to slow the entry of water into the cells *in vitro*. The time taken for lysis to occur is a function of the osmotic resistance of the cells. HS cells lyse more rapidly than normal cells. The test is easier to perform than the osmotic fragility test.

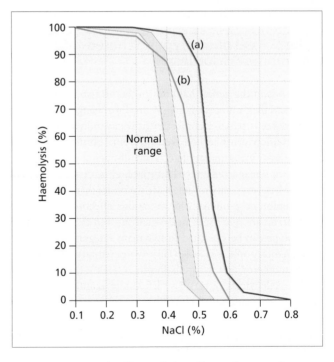

Figure 8.5 Osmotic fragility test in hereditary spherocytosis. Osmotic fragility is increased in the microspherocytes (right shift), but there is also a small population of resistant cells due to increased reticulocytes. After splenectomy, the microspherocytes remain but the proportion of reticulocytes is reduced to normal values and the resistant cells are not seen.

Autohaemolysis test

The autohaemolysis test examined the ability of red cells to withstand metabolic deprivation by incubation *in vitro* for 24 h with and without the addition of glucose. It is a crude, insensitive test which has generally been abandoned.

Identification of protein abnormalities or gene defects

Methods that identify the defective gene or its product are the most specific for membrane defects but are beyond the scope of most routine haematology laboratories. The original identification of membrane proteins using sodium dodecyl sulphate-solubilized polyacrylamide gel (SDS-PAGE) electrophoresis has led to the classification according to the banding system indicated in Table 8.2. The identification of specific genetic abnormalities may be important in compound haemolytic syndromes but requires specialist laboratories.

One screening test for HS makes use of the binding of eosin-labelled maleimide, in the form of eosin-5 maleimide, to lysin 430 in band 3 and cysteine molecules in surface proteins, particularly rhesus blood groups. In about 25% of HS patients there is a deficiency of band 3 and a loss of surface proteins caused by the instability of the lipid bilayer. HS red cells bind eosin-5 maleimide less than normal cells, by about 25–30%. Even when the main defect is not in band 3, there may be sufficient loss of eosin-5 maleimide binding to indicate HS. The screening test has to be used in conjunction with morphology because South-East Asian ovalocytosis, congenital dyserythropoietic anaemia type II and cryohydrocytosis also give reduced fluorescence.

Clinical course and complications

In most kindred, the course of the disorder is similar in affected members although, as with most inherited defects, there is some variable penetrance and it is not rare to find a very mildly affected parent with more severely affected offspring.

As with all congenital haemolytic anaemias, the anaemia may be aggravated by environmental factors. This may be consequent on an increase in the red cell destruction or a decrease in production. Increased jaundice may occur during viral infections or bacterial sepsis, the anaemia also being aggravated by a decrease in production consequence on the effects of the acute-phase response or the inhibition of erythropoiesis by interferon gamma (IFN-γ).

Primary infection with parvovirus 19 produces a specific and marked inhibition of erythropoiesis, often characterized as an aplastic crisis. In patients with a shortened red cell survival, severe anaemia may be produced by the inhibition, which lasts for some 4–7 days. In normal individuals with a red cell lifespan of 120 days, such an inhibition produces no clinical effect. The anaemia associated with parvovirus infection in HS may require urgent transfusion. The diagnosis is made by finding absent parvovirus antibodies with subsequent appearance of IgM antibodies. The presence of IgG antibodies at the time of the anaemia excludes the diagnosis.

Acute anaemia due to splenic sequestration is a relatively uncommon complication of HS in childhood. The pathogenesis is probably increased splenic size and activity leading to increased trapping of HS cells within the spleen. This complication may also require urgent transfusion.

Malnutrition may increase anaemia because of folate deficiency but also from increased jaundice through the effect of low-calorie input on unconjugated bilirubin levels in the blood.

The anaemia of pregnancy may aggravate a haemolytic anaemia and hence bring the condition to the attention of clinicians and patients. Classical HS is not a risk to mother or child in pregnancy.

Gallstones are an expected complication in HS as in other chronic haemolytic anaemias. Silent gallstones require no intervention. Recurrent cholecystitis or biliary colic may require cholecystectomy accompanied by splenectomy (see below). Leg ulcers are a rare but well-recognized complication of HS, as with other chronic haemolytic anaemias. Extramedullary haemopoietic masses, usually paravertebral, occur rarely in more severe HS.

Management

Patients with well-compensated haemolysis and no transfusion requirements need no treatment other than reassurance and folic acid supplements (e.g. 400 µg daily or 5 mg weekly). For people with a well-balanced and adequate diet, folic acid supplements are probably unnecessary, but custom dictates the practice should be continued. Radiolucent gallstones, if detected by chance on ultrasound, are common and need no treatment unless complications arise. Gallstones without recurrent inflammation are not a risk factor for a carcinoma of the gall bladder. Recurrent cholecystitis or obstruction would be an indication for cholecystectomy, which would also be an indication for splenectomy.

Splenectomy

For the great majority of patients with autosomal dominant forms of HS, and most patients with *de novo* disease, splenectomy restores the lifespan of the red cells to normal and hence cures the haemolysis and hyperbilirubinaemia. In HS, the spleen is responsible for the removal of the older red cells that have lost the most surface through lipid loss from the outer layer. This removal of damaged but functional cells shortens the lifespan and causes jaundice and reticulocytosis. However, splenectomy carries short- and long-term risks that must be weighed against the benefits in any individual patient. Post splenectomy, the blood film continues to show spherocytosis together with changes of a splenectomy film. The osmotic fragility remains increased.

Risks of splenectomy (see also Chapter 21)

The immediate risks associated with splenectomy include those of any abdominal operation together with an increased risk of thrombosis, associated with a marked rise in platelet count that occurs promptly after splenectomy. In HS, in which the erythropoietic drive returns to normal following splenectomy, the platelet count also returns to normal and the risk diminishes. In conditions in which haemolysis persists, the platelet count remains elevated, sometimes markedly, and the increased risk of thrombosis continues.

The major hazard of splenectomy is the long-term susceptibility to severe infection, the so-called overwhelming postsplenectomy infection (OPSI) (see also Chapter 21). The spleen plays an important role in filtering and phagocytosing bacteria, and removing parasitized red cells from the blood. The spleen is the major source for mounting the rapid, specific immunoglobulin M (IgM) response to organisms that enter through the gut. The main organisms of this class are the encapsulated organisms, *Streptococcus pneumoniae*, *Haemophilus influenzae* type B and *Neisseria meningitidis*. Pneumococcal infection is responsible for about 70% of OPSI and has a 60% mortality. Lack of a spleen greatly increases the virulence of the infection, with progression from the first feeling of fever and non-specific flu-like symptoms to irreversible endotoxic shock occurring in a matter of hours. Patients may present with purpura, evidence of disseminated intravascular coagulation (DIC), multiorgan failure, hypotension and peripheral limb ischaemia. Diarrhoea and vomiting are common prodromes. It is this speed of progression that makes the prophylaxis of this fortunately uncommon complication so important. Prophylaxis depends on education and awareness for the patient, specific measures to reduce the risk from particular organisms and the provision of information concerning the splenectomy for healthcare workers (Table 8.3). There is no direct evidence that phenoxymethylpenicillin (e.g. 250 mg twice daily) reduces the risk of OPSI in splenectomized patients, but good evidence that it does so in homozygous sickle cell patients who have functionally inactive spleens. It is on this evidence that such antibiotic prophylaxis (or erythromycin 250 mg b.d. for those sensitive to penicillin) is recommended (see also Chapter 21). The actual incidence of OPSI is difficult to calculate. The overall risk has been stated as 0.04 per hundred patient-years for patients without added immunosuppression, but considerably higher for those immunocompromised by malignancy or chemotherapy. The risk is greatest in the first 2 years post splenectomy but continues lifelong. Children under the age of 5 years are particularly susceptible and splenectomy should be avoided in this group if at all possible.

Indications for splenectomy

Patients with marked haemolysis producing symptoms or requiring transfusion should be splenectomized, although preferably not before the age of 5 years (later if possible). Recurrent aplastic crises are also an indication. Attacks of cholecystitis or biliary colic warrant cholecystectomy and splenectomy, but symptomless gallstones are not a necessary indication.

Table 8.3 Guidelines for prevention and management of infection for the splenectomized patient*.

All patients receive polyvalent, pneumococcal immunization, preferably 2 weeks prior to splenectomy, with a booster dose every 5–10 years

Any unimmunized patient should receive *Haemophilus influenzae* type B vaccine

Meningococcal immunization (types A and C) are not routinely recommended but should be given to travellers to countries where meningitis is possible, and during outbreaks in the UK

Influenza immunization may be beneficial and should be given

Lifelong, prophylactic antibiotics (oral phenoxymethyl penicillin or an alternative)

Awareness of risks of malaria and scrupulous prophylaxis if at risk

Animal, particularly dog and tick bites, may be dangerous

Leaflet card for patients to alert health professionals to risk of OPSI

Patients developing infection despite measures should receive systemic antibiotics and be admitted urgently to hospital

*After 'Guidelines from British Committee for Standards in Haematology' (1996), *British Medical Journal* 312: 430–4.

Hereditary elliptocytosis and hereditary pyropoikilocytosis

Deficiency of spectrin tetramers, the horizontal links of the cytoskeleton, produces a wide spectrum of disease from fully compensated haemolysis with mildly elliptocytic red cells to severe and life-threatening anaemia with grossly distorted cells. When the morphological characteristic is a relatively uniform elliptical shape, the condition is referred to as hereditary elliptocytosis (HE). Haemolytic anaemia associated with the more distorted forms, which are also heat labile, is called hereditary pyropoikilocytosis (HPP). Within a family, HE and HPP may both be present, the more severely affected individuals having both a total spectrin deficiency as well as a relative deficiency of spectrin tetramers. This may be caused by co-inheritance of a low-expression allele for α-spectrin, compound heterozygosity for two HE alleles or HE homozygosity. A number of families have been described in which mutations involving the initiation codon of the protein 4.1 gene result in failure to produce the protein. In heterozygotes with this variant, elliptocytosis occurs without haemolysis; in homozygotes, there is a severe haemolysis with pyropoikilocytosis.

Clinical features

As mentioned above, the HE/HPP group of haemolytic anaemias has a heterogeneous clinical presentation and molecular basis. Heterogeneity is amplified by the not uncommon co-inheritance of a mutated gene *in trans* (see below) with the HE gene, usually resulting in more marked heterotetramer deficiency.

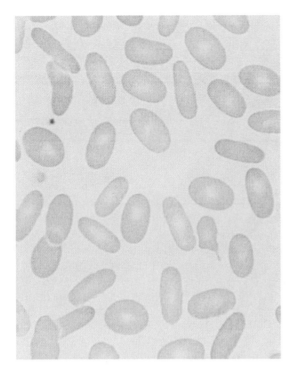

Figure 8.6 Hereditary elliptocytosis, peripheral blood. Characteristic elliptocytes of mild common HE.

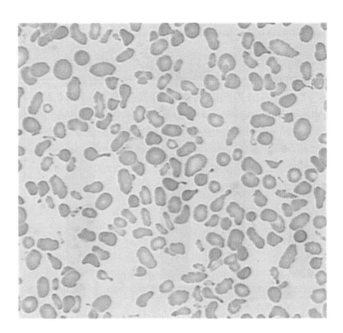

Figure 8.7 Hereditary pyropoikiloctosis, peripheral blood. Marked anisocytosis and poikilocytosis in the film from a child with homozygous hereditary elliptocytosis.

Mild common hereditary elliptocytosis

Frequently, HE is discovered by chance from a blood film (Figure 8.6) or the presence of marginally raised bilirubin. Some affected people have no evidence of shortened red cell survival, whereas others have a well-compensated haemolytic anaemia. No treatment is required, although the blood film of partners should be examined if there is consanguinity, making homozygosity in offspring possible. For patients with mild haemolysis, anaemia may increase during infections, in pregnancy, with folate deficiency or with other conditions that are likely to enhance anaemia.

Silent carriers: low-expression genes

Mutations that produce low expression (LE) of α-spectrin, may lead to no haematological abnormality because of the normal overexpression of α-spectrin in red cells when compared with β-spectrin. However, when these defects are inherited *in trans*, on the other allele from an HE gene, HPP may result. Several mutations have been described, particularly commonly in codon 28, which produces LE genes. A common polymorphism, intron 45 C → T, is spectrin α^{LELY}, standing for 'low-expression allele Lyon'.

Hereditary elliptocytosis and poikilocytosis in the neonate

In the neonate, the manifestations of HE may be a more marked pyropoikilocytosis resembling HPP, with more fragmented red

cells. These red cells are susceptible to fragmentation above 40°C, whereas normal cells only fragment above 50°C. The morphological changes and haemolysis gradually decrease over the first year until the typical picture of mild HE remains. Treatment of neonatal pyropoikilocytosis is required only if the anaemia is such as to warrant transfusion.

Spherocytic hereditary elliptocytosis

In rare Caucasian families with HE, haemolysis with modest splenomegaly is found with a blood film that has a low proportion of abnormally shaped cells, ranging from spherocytes to elliptocytes. Splenectomy is not usually indicated.

Hereditary pyropoikilocytosis

The characteristics of hereditary pyropoikilocytosis (HPP) are densely contracted and fragmented cells (Figure 8.7), moderate to severe haemolysis and heterogeneity of manifestations within a family. In general, patients with HPP have spectrin deficiency in addition to the abnormalities of spectrin–spectrin contacts that produce the heterotetramer deficiency of HE. One parent of an HE propositus may have normal haematology but carry a mutation *in trans*, which leads to spectrin deficiency. The affected cells show thermal lability and fragmentation at lower temperatures than normal. HPP is more common in black people.

Hereditary elliptocytosis in Africa

In some parts of West Africa, a high incidence (up to 1.6% of the population) of HE has been found. Interestingly, there is a considerable molecular heterogeneity for the basis of the condition in this area. *In vitro, Plasmodium falciparum* is less able to parasitize HE cells that have mutations in α-spectrin, glycophorin C or protein 4.1. Invasion is reduced in red cells from homozygous patients, and intracellular multiplication reduced, particularly in homozygous 4.1(–) red cells. It seems possible that the varieties of HE offer some protection against the clinical manifestations of falciparum malaria.

Laboratory investigation

The standard approach to the diagnosis of HE/HPP is the identification of haemolysis, coupled to a careful examination of the blood film of the patient and as many first-degree relatives as possible. Examples of blood films are shown in Figures 8.6 and 8.7. Other acquired causes of elliptocytic or fragmented red cells need to be excluded, including iron, folate or vitamin B_{12} deficiency, and the microangiopathic haemolytic anaemias. Congenital dyserythropoietic anaemia and thalassaemia intermedia also need to be excluded.

As with the investigation of HS, SDS-PAGE may reveal protein abnormalities, although more specific identification requires a sophisticated approach beyond the abilities of most haematology laboratories.

Treatment

Patients with chronic haemolysis should be given folate supplements. Splenectomy is indicated for severe haemolytic anaemia in patients with HPP or homozygous HE. Response in HPP may not be complete, but the anaemia is usually markedly alleviated. There may be a theoretical risk of increased thrombotic tendency due to remaining high platelet count, but the risk is small. The precautions against OPSI are the same as for HS.

Hereditary stomatocytosis and related disorders

Stomatocytes are so called from the mouth-like slit or 'stoma' that appears on blood films (Figure 8.8). The appearance seems to be produced by folding of cells during preparation. Stomatocytes are leaky to cations. There are other variations with Na^+ or K^+ leaks that are clinically similar to stomatocytosis without the obvious morphological changes.

All of these conditions are inherited in autosomal dominant fashion, they mostly produce moderate haemolytic anaemia, with haemoglobin of 10 g/dL or above, and they have macrocytosis. There are two main variants: overhydrated HSt, in which the MCHC is low, and dehydrated HSt, with an increased MCHC.

The blood film may show stomatocytosis but, more commonly, the film is unremarkable, apart from macrocytosis and polychromasia. The group is rare, estimates suggesting 1 in 10 000 to 100 000 of the population being affected. Associated

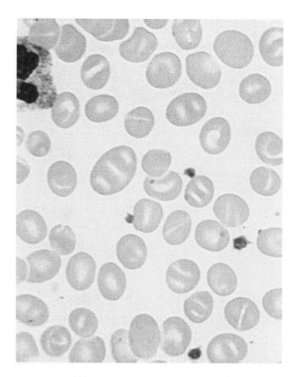

Figure 8.8 Hereditary stomatocytosis, peripheral blood.

features, however, make the conditions important beyond their rarity (Table 8.4). Pseudohyperkalaemia may occur because K^+ leaks rapidly from the red cells at room temperature. In some individuals, there is no evidence of haemolysis, only macrocytosis and pseudohyperkalaemia. Unless the cause of the apparent hyperkalaemia is diagnosed, unnecessary, and even dangerous, investigation and treatment may be undertaken. In some families, the K^+ leak is greatly increased *in vitro* by cold (cryohydrocytosis). In dehydrated HSt, there may be marked perinatal ascites that resolves spontaneously over the first year of life, but which again can lead to extensive unnecessary investigation. The third problem with HSt, both over- and dehydrated varieties, is that splenectomy is followed by very marked thrombotic tendencies such that splenectomy should not be performed.

Laboratory investigations

Tests for haemolysis and examination of the blood film of the patient and close relatives are the first steps in diagnosis. The finding of a raised serum potassium, together with macrocytosis, especially with some evidence of haemolysis, indicates the pseudohyperkalaemia of dehydrated HSt.

The definitive studies involve the measurement of intracellular $[Na^+]$ or $[K^+]$ and their flux through the membrane at different temperatures. Four subgroups have been defined according to the intracellular sodium concentration (normal values 5–10 mmol/L). Patients with pseudohyperkalaemia may have normal or slightly high values in dehydrated HSt sodium

Table 8.4 Features of hereditary stomatocytosis and related disorders.

Characteristic	Expression	Group affected
Haemolytic anaemia	Mild to moderate	All variants
	Absent	H pseudohyperkalaemia
Morphology	Macrocytosis	All variants
	Stomatocytosis	Variable
MCHC	Decreased	Overhydrated HSt (hydrocytosis)
	Increased	Dehydrated HSt (H xerocytosis, desiccocytosis)
Serum [K$^+$]	Raised *in vitro*	Pseudohyperkalaemia
		Dehydrated HSV
		Cryohydrocytosis
Thrombotic tendency	Post splenectomy	All variants
Fluid balance	Perinatal oedema	Dehydrated HSt

concentration 12–18 mmol/L, in families with cryohydrocytosis (temperature-sensitive leak) 20–50 mmol/L and in overhydrated HSt 60 mmol/L or more.

Treatment

There is rarely a need for measures to raise the haemoglobin and splenectomy should be avoided because of the risk of thrombosis, including hepatic and portal vein thrombosis. If splenectomy is necessary lifelong, anticoagulation should be introduced.

Rh$_{null}$ syndrome

The Rh system forms a large complex traversing the lipid bilayer several times, containing extracellular thiol groups. In the Rh$_{null}$ phenotype, the complex is absent. The condition is very rare and is inherited as a recessive disorder. Patients have mild to moderate haemolytic anaemia that may respond to splenectomy, and the blood film shows occasional stomatocytes. The Rh complex involves two genes, one encoding for the D polypeptide, the other for the Cc and Ee polypeptide, depending on post-translational splicing. Mutation of one or other of the genes encoding these proteins is the molecular basis underlying Rh$_{null}$ phenotype.

South-East Asian ovalocytosis

A dominantly inherited ovalocytosis is found in parts of South-East Asia, where falciparum malaria is common, particularly in Papua New Guinea, Borneo and the Philippines. The red cell morphology is ovalo-rather than elliptocytic. Stoma-like slits may be present and transverse banding in the red cells is seen (Figure 8.9). Most individuals have no haemolysis, but, in a few, mild anaemia may be present. Cells have increased rigidity, unlike HE in which rigidity is decreased. The molecular defect is a deletion of nine amino acids at the transmembrane cytosol junction of band 3, a defect that possibly limits the mobility of band 3 within the membrane. Homozygosity is not found and is presumably lethal *in utero*.

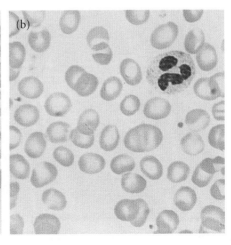

Figure 8.9 South-East Asian ovalocytosis, peripheral blood films. Mild ovalocytosis and some stomatocytosis. Some cells have apparent transverse ridge.

Abnormalities of membrane lipids

Acanthocytosis

Acanthocytes, or spur cells, show prominent, somewhat regular projections on the surface, best demonstrated by scanning electron microscopy. They are formed when the outer lipid layer of the membrane acquires additional lipid. Acanthocytosis is an acquired characteristic of severe liver disease, usually end stage, and the result of interaction of altered plasma lipids.

A-β-lipoproteinaemia

A-β-lipoproteinaemia is a rare inherited defect with absent β-apolipoprotein, which results in low serum cholesterol but increased sphingomyelin, which enters the cell membrane and produces the acanthocytes. The main clinical features are retinitis pigmentosa, fat malabsorption and hepatic encephalopathy.

McLeod phenotype

In the McLeod phenotype, acanthocytosis occurs (Figure 8.10), together with decreased expression of the Kell antigen. The defective gene is on the X chromosome, Xp21, close to genes for Duchenne muscular dystrophy and retinitis pigmentosa, conditions with which the phenotype has been linked. The gene codes for the Kx protein that carries the Kell blood group protein. There may be mild anaemia.

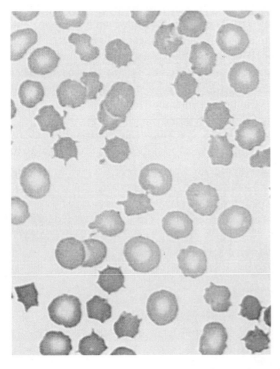

Figure 8.10 McLeod syndrome, peripheral blood. Note the marked acanthocytosis.

Selected bibliography

Reviews

Chu X, Thompson D, Yee LJ, Sung LA (2000) Genomic organization of mouse and human erythrocyte tropomodulin genes encoding the pointed end capping protein for the actin filaments. *Gene* **256**: 271–81.

Davies KA, Lux SE (1989) Hereditary disorders of the red cell membrane skeleton. *Trends in Genetics* **5**: 222–7.

Delaunay J (2002) Molecular basis of red cell membrane disorders. *Acta Haematologica* **108**: 210–8.

Delaunay J, Dhermy D (1993) Mutations involving the spectrin heterodimer contact site: clinical expression and alterations in specific function. *Seminars in Hematology* **30**: 21–33.

Elgsaeter A, Stokke BT, Mikkelsen A, Branton D (1986) The molecular basis of erythrocyte shape. *Science* **234**: 1217–23.

Gilligan DM, Bennett V (1993) The junctional complex of the membrane skeleton. *Seminars in Hematology* **30**: 74–83.

McKusick VA (1973) Phenotypic diversity of genetic disease resulting from allelic series. *American Journal of Human Genetics* **25**: 446–56.

Palek J, Jarolin P (1993) Clinical expression and laboratory detection of red blood cell membrane protein mutations. *Seminars in Hematology* **30**: 249–83.

Pawloski JR, Hess DT, Stamler JS (2001) Export by red blood cells of nitric oxide bioactivity. *Nature* **409**: 622–6.

Tanner, MJA (1993) Molecular and cellular biology of the erythrocyte anion exchanger (AE1) *Seminars in Hematology* **30**: 34–57.

Tse WT, Lux SE (1999) Red cell membrane disorders. *British Journal of Haematology* **104**: 2–13.

Hereditary spherocytosis

Agre P, Asimos A, Casella JF, McMillan C (1986) Inheritance pattern and clinical response to splenectomy as a reflection of erythrocyte spectrin deficiency in hereditary spherocytosis. *New England Journal of Medicine* **315**: 1579–83.

Barry M, Scheuer PJ, Sherlock S, Ross CF, Williams R (1968) Hereditary spherocytosis with secondary haemochromatosis. *Lancet* **ii**: 481–5.

Bolton-Maggs PHB, Stevens RF, Dodd NJ *et al.* Guidelines for the diagnosis and management of hereditary spherocytosis. *Submitted.*

Bruce LJ, Ghosh S, King MJ *et al.* (2002) Absence of CD47 in protein 4.2-deficient hereditary spherocytosis in man: an interaction between the Rh complex and band 3 complex. *Blood* **100**: 1878–85.

Delhommeau F, Cynober T, Schischmanoff PO *et al.* (2000) Natural history of hereditary spherocytosis during the first year of life *Blood* **95**: 393–7.

Dhermy D, Galand C, Bournier O *et al.* (1997) Heterogenous band 3 deficiency in hereditary spherocytosis related to different band 3 gene defects. *British Journal of Haematology* **98**: 32–40.

Eber SW, Gonzalez JM, Lux ML *et al.* (1996) Ankyrin-1 mutations are a major cause of dominant and recessive hereditary spherocytosis. *Nature Genetics* **13**: 214–18.

Gallagher PG, Forget BG (1998) Hematologically important mutations: spectrin and ankyrin variants in hereditary spherocytosis. *Blood Cells, Molecules and Diseases* **24**: 539–43.

Gallagher PG, Ferreira JDS, Costa FF et al. (2000) A recurrent frameshift mutation of the ankyrin gene associated with severe hereditary spherocytosis. British Journal of Haematology 111: 1190–3.

Hanspal M, Yoon S-H, Yu H et al. (1991) Molecular basis of spectrin and ankyrin deficiencies in severe hereditary spherocytosis: evidence implicating a primary defect of ankyrin. Blood 77: 165–73.

Ideguchi H, Nishimura J, Nawata H et al. (1990) Genetic defect of erythrocyte band 4.2 protein associated with hereditary spherocytosis. British Journal of Haematology 74: 347–53.

Iwamoto S, Kajii E, Omi T et al. (1993) Point mutation in the band 4.2 gene associated with autosomal recessively inherited erythrocyte band 4.2 deficiency. European Journal of Haematology 50: 286–91.

Jacob HS, Jandl JH (1964) Increased cell membrane permeability in the pathogenesis of hereditary spherocytosis. Journal of Clinical Investigation 43: 1704–20.

King MJ, Behrens J, Rogers C et al. (2000) Rapid flow cytometric test for the diagnosis of membrane cytoskeleton-associated haemolytic anaemia. British Journal of Haematology 111: 924–33.

Korsgren C, Lawler J, Lambert S et al. (1990) Complete amino acid sequence and homologies of human erythrocyte membrane protein band 4.2. Proceedings of the National Academy of Sciences of the USA 87: 613–17.

Lefrere JJ, Courouce A-M, Girot R et al. (1986) Six cases of hereditary spherocytosis revealed by human parvovirus infection. British Journal of Haematology 62: 653–8.

Miraglia del Giudice E, Perrotta S, Pinto L et al. (1992) Hereditary spherocytosis characterized by increased spectrin/band 3 ratio. British Journal of Haematology 80: 133–6.

Miraglia del Giudice E, Francese M, Nobili B et al. (1998) High frequency of de novo mutations in ankyrin gene (ANK1) in children with hereditary spherocytosis. Journal of Pediatrics 132: 117–20.

Miraglia del Giudice E, Perrotta S, Nobili B et al. (1999) Coinheritance of Gilbert syndrome increases risk for developing gallstones in patients with hereditary spherocytosis. Blood 94: 2259–62.

Miraglia del Giudice E, Nobili B, Francese M et al. (2001) Clinical and molecular evaluation of non-dominant hereditary spherocytosis. British Journal of Haematology 112: 42–7.

Okamoto N, Wada Y, Nakamura Y et al. (1995) Hereditary spherocytic anemia with deletion of the short arm of chromosome 8. American Journal of Medical Genetics 58: 225–9.

Reinhart WH, Wyss EJ, Arnold D et al. (1994) Hereditary spherocytosis associated with protein band 3 defect in a Swiss kindred. British Journal of Haematology 86: 147–55.

Rybicki AC, Heath R, Wolf JL et al. (1988) Deficiency of protein 4.2 in erythrocytes from a patient with a Coombs negative hemolytic anemia: evidence for a role of protein 4.2 in stabilizing ankyrin on the membrane. Journal of Clinical Investigation 81: 893–901.

Splenectomy

Anon (1985) Splenectomy – a long term risk of infection. Lancet ii: 928–9 [Editorial].

Anon (1998) The place of pneumococcal vaccination. Drug and Therapeutics Bulletin 36: 73–6 [Editorial].

McMullin M, Johnston G (1993) Long term management of patients after splenectomy. British Medical Journal 307: 1371–2 [Editorial].

Working Party of the British Committee for Standards in Haematology Clinical Haematology Work Force (1996) Guidelines for the prevention and treatment of infection in patients with an absent or dysfunctional spleen. British Medical Journal 312: 430–4.

Hereditary elliptocytosis

Gallagher PG, Forget BG (1996) Hematologically important mutations: spectrin variants in hereditary elliptocytosis and hereditary pyropoikilocytosis. Blood Cells and Molecular Diseases 22: 254–8.

Glele-Kakai C, Garbarz M, Lecomte MC et al. (1996) Epidemiological studies of spectrin mutations related to hereditary elliptocytosis and spectrin polymorphisms in Benin. British Journal of Haematology 95: 57–66.

Marchesi SL, Letsinger JT, Speicher DW et al. (1987) Mutant forms of spectrin alpha-subunits in hereditary elliptocytosis. Journal of Clinical Investigation 80: 191–8.

Randon J, Boulanger L, Marechal J et al. (1994) A variant of spectrin low-expression allele alpha-LELY carrying a hereditary elliptocytosis mutation in codon 28. British Journal of Haematology 88: 534–40.

Hereditary pyropoikilocytosis

Agre P, Orringer EP, Chui DHK et al. (1981) A molecular defect in two families with hemolytic poikilocytic anemia: reduction of high affinity membrane binding sites for ankyrin. Journal of Clinical Investigation 68: 1566–76.

Gallagher PG, Petruzzi MJ, Weed SA et al. (1997) Mutation of a highly conserved residue of beta-1 spectrin associated with fatal and near-fatal neonatal hemolytic anemia. Journal of Clinical Investigation 99: 267–77.

Goel VK, Li X, Chen H et al. (2003) Band 3 is a host receptor binding merozoite surface protein 1 during the Plasmodium falciparum invasion of erythrocytes. Proceedings of the National Academy of Sciences of the USA 100: 5164–9.

Liu S-C, Palek J, Prchal J et al. (1981) Altered spectrin dimer–dimer association and instability of erythrocyte membrane skeletons in hereditary pyropoikilocytosis. Journal of Clinical Investigation 68: 597–605.

Hereditary stomatocytosis, pseudohyperkalaemia

Delaunay J, Stewart G, Iolascon A (1999) Hereditary dehydrated and overhydrated stomatocytosis: recent advances. Current Opinion in Hematology 6: 110–14.

Grootenboer S, Schischmanoff PO, Cynober T et al. (1998) A genetic syndrome associating dehydrated hereditary stomatocytosis, pseudohyperkalaemia and perinatal oedema. British Journal of Haematology 103: 383–6.

Grootenboer S, Schischmanoff PO, Laurendeau I et al. (2000) Pleiotropic syndrome of dehydrated hereditary stomatocytosis, pseudohyperkalemia, and perinatal edema maps to 16q23–q24. Blood 96: 2599–605.

Stewart GW, Turner EJ (1999) The hereditary stomatocytoses and allied disorders: congenital disorders of erythrocyte membrane permeability to Na and K. *Baillière's Best Practice in Clinical Haematology* 12: 707–27.

Stewart GW, Corrall RJ, Fyffe JA *et al.* (1979) Familial pseudohyperkalaemia. A new syndrome. *Lancet* ii: 175–7.

Stewart GW, Amess JA, Eber SW *et al.* (1996) Thrombo-embolic disease after splenectomy for hereditary stomatocytosis. *British Journal of Haematology* 96: 303–10.

South-East Asian ovalocytosis and malaria

Goel VK, Li X, Chen H *et al.* (2003) Band 3 is a host receptor binding merozoite surface protein 1 during the *Plasmodium falciparum* invasion of erythrocytes. *Proceedings of the National Academy of Sciences of the USA* 100: 5164–9.

Hadley T, Saul A, Lamont G *et al.* (1983) Resistance of Melanesian elliptocytes (ovalocytes) to invasion by *Plasmodium knowlesii* and *Plasmodium falciparum* malaria parasites *in vitro*. *Journal of Clinical Investigation* 71: 780–2.

Liu S-C, Zhai S, Palek J *et al.* (1990) Molecular defect of the band 3 protein in South-East Asian ovalocytosis. *New England Journal of Medicine* 323: 1530–8.

CHAPTER 9

Disorders of red cell metabolism

Edward C Gordon-Smith

9

Introduction

The main function of the red cell is to carry haemoglobin (Hb) around the circulation in high concentration and in a functional state so that gas exchange may occur efficiently in the lungs and in the tissue capillaries. Oxygen is thus taken up in the lungs in exchange for carbon dioxide and delivered to the tissues at physiological pH and gas pressure. The structure and function of Hb is discussed in Chapter 6. In order to fulfil its function, the red cell needs a supply of energy in the form of ATP and a source of reducing power. A mature red cell has no DNA or RNA and hence is incapable of protein synthesis, and the mitochondria that are present in reticulocytes have been lost during maturation, so that the only source of energy as ATP is derived from anaerobic glycolysis and the linked reducing system of the hexose monophosphate shunt (pentose phosphate pathway) and the glutathione cycle. ATP is required to maintain the membrane in its deformable state, with asymmetric lipid layers, and to regulate ion and water exchange.

Reducing power is required to reduce methaemoglobin (MetHb) back to its functional state of deoxyhaemoglobin and to counteract the strong oxidative stresses that a cell carrying molecular oxygen around the circulation is likely to encounter. The main process that reduces MetHb utilizes reduced nicotine adenine dinucleotide (NADH), reduced from nicotine adenine dinucleotide (NAD$^+$) by the glycolytic pathway. Reduction and detoxification of free oxygen radicals and hydrogen peroxide produced during reactions to infection is provided by reduced nicotine adenine dinucleotide phosphate (NADPH) generated by the first steps of the pentose phosphate pathway, catalysed by glucose-6-phosphate dehydrogenase (G6PD) and the linked enzyme 6-phosphogluconate dehydrogenase. NADPH drives the glutathione cycle, glutathione (GSH) being the major reducing agent within the red cell.

The lack of protein synthesis in the mature red cell means that none of the enzymes in the metabolic pathways can be replaced during the red cell lifespan. Over the 120 days of normal red cell survival, enzyme activities decline at variable but predictable rates. This decline probably contributes to the ageing process of the red cell. Many of the mutations that affect red cell metabolism and provoke haemolytic anaemia cause instability and premature inactivation of the enzyme; other mutations directly affect the catalytic activity.

The glycolytic pathway (Embden–Meyerhof pathway)

Glycolysis (or, more correctly, glucolysis) is the process by which glucose is converted to pyruvate through a number of steps, with a net gain of two moles of ATP generated for each mole of glucose metabolized by the pathway. Glucose is derived from the plasma by a facilitated transfer through the membrane. Pyruvate and lactic acid are in equilibrium as determined by the redox potential of the cell (NAD$^+$/NADH) and can diffuse out. The internal milieu of the cell, with its high K$^+$ concentration and presence of other cations, such as magnesium, necessary for efficient glycolysis, is maintained through the activity of various ion and cation channels in the membrane, with energy linked by appropriate ATPases. The glycolytic pathway also provides the redox reaction to convert MetHb to deoxyhaemoglobin through utilizing NADH, in a reaction catalysed by MetHb-NADH reductase (cytochrome b_3). The various products and functions of the glucose metabolism are shown schematically in Figure 9.1 and in more detail in Figure 9.2.

The Rapoport–Luebering shunt

One of the essential roles of metabolism in the red cell is to provide sufficient 2,3-diphosphoglycerate (2,3-DPG) to regulate

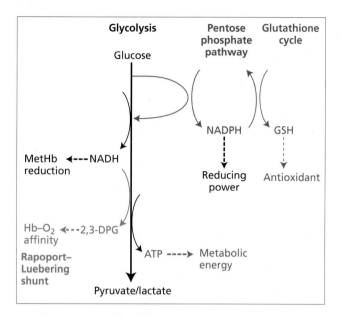

Figure 9.1 Principal pathways of energy production in the mature red cell. The glycolytic pathway provides energy in the form of ATP. Under normal conditions, MetHb is reduced by the coupled reaction with NADH⁺. The Rapoport–Luebering shunt provides 2,3-DPG for control of Hb oxygen affinity. Reducing power is produced by the pentose phosphate pathway and is linked to redox reactions through the glutathione cycle.

the oxygen affinity of Hb. 2,3-DPG is produced from 1,3-DPG under the influence of the enzyme diphosphoglycerate mutase in linked reactions that form the Rapoport–Luebering shunt (Figure 9.2). 2,3-DPG is broken down to 3-phosphoglycerate by a phosphatase and thus re-enters the glycolytic pathway. It should be noted that, when metabolism takes place by the Rapoport–Luebering shunt, there is a bypass of the stage of ATP production. The shunt thus not only provides the 2,3-DPG for interaction with the Hb tetramer but also acts as an energy control mechanism for glycolysis.

Disorders of the glycolytic pathway

Mutations of most of the enzymes in the glycolytic pathway have been described in association with congenital non-spherocytic haemolytic anaemia (CNSHA). However, deficiency of pyruvate kinase (PK) is far and away the most common defect. The haemolysis is the result of a failure to produce sufficient ATP.

Pyruvate kinase

PK catalyses the final steps of the glycolytic pathway with the conversion of phosphoenolpyruvate (PEP) to pyruvate, with the concomitant phosphorylation of ADP to ATP, leading to overall net gain of ATP from this pathway. There are four types of PK

in different tissues derived from two separate genes. The *PKM* gene, on chromosome 15, produces PKM1 and PKM2 through differences in post-transcriptional splicing. PKM1 is present in skeletal muscles, PKM2 in leucocytes, kidneys, adipose tissue and lungs. The second PK gene, on chromosome 1, gives rise to PKL in the liver and PKR in red cells. The isoenzymes are transcribed differently through the influence of tissue-specific promoters. The active enzymes are homotetramers. PKM2, PKR and PKL all demonstrate marked allosteric reactions with several ligands. PKM1, on the other hand, has no allosteric interactions.

The main ligands that are involved in the allosteric control of PKR in the erythrocyte are shown in Figure 9.3. PK is one of the dominant controlling steps in glucose metabolism (together with hexokinase), exerting its effect through major feedback loops, especially through the requirement of activation by fructose 1,6-diphosphate.

Pyruvate kinase deficiency

PK deficiency leads to a chronic CNSHA with extravascular haemolysis.

Molecular biology

PK deficiency is the commonest of the enzymopathies of the glycolytic pathway, at least 300 times more common than any other. Best estimates based on gene frequency in the white population suggest a prevalence of about 50 per million. Well over 100 different mutations have been described in PK deficiency, the majority involving point mutations or deletions in the transcribed gene, but a substantial number involving the promoter region. Haemolytic anaemia due to PK deficiency is an autosomal recessive disorder. Many individuals are compound heterozygotes. Not surprisingly, there is enormous genetic heterogeneity between affected individuals reflected in the multiplicity of quantitative and kinetic defects detected (Figure 9.3). Because PKR is a homotetramer composed of four chains derived from the products of the two alleles, enzyme kinetic variations are many and genotype/phenotype correlates are not predictable. Within families, however, the severity of the haemolysis tends to be similar in affected individuals. PK catalyses the ultimate step in the glycolytic pathway. Deficient activity leads to accumulation of substrates further up the pathway, including 2,3-DPG. The increased concentration of 2,3-DPG in PK-deficient red cells shifts the oxygen dissociation curve to the right, indicating low oxygen affinity. Patients with PK deficiency tolerate apparent anaemia well because the lower Hb content will deliver the same amount of oxygen to tissues as the normal Hb, at least under normal conditions, although oxygen reserve would be limited.

Reticulocytes have alternative means of producing energy in the form of ATP, through oxidative respiratory pathway of the remaining mitochondria. They can also synthesize enzyme in those defects where lack of stability is the major cause of enzyme deficiency in the mature cell. Reticulocytes thus have a metabolic advantage over mature red cells in PK deficiency.

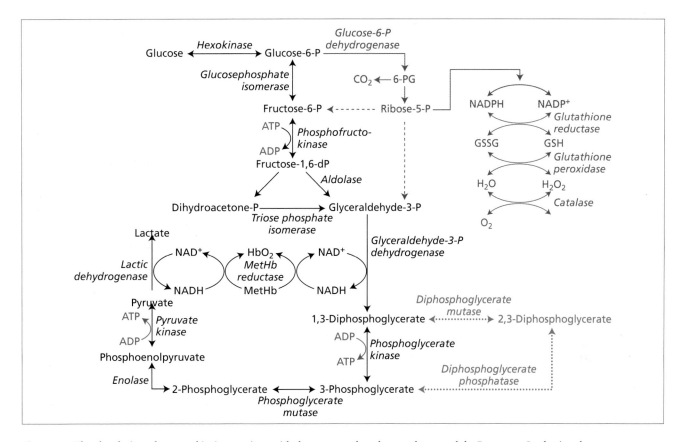

Figure 9.2 The glycolytic pathway and its interactions with the pentose phosphate pathway and the Rapoport–Luebering shunt.

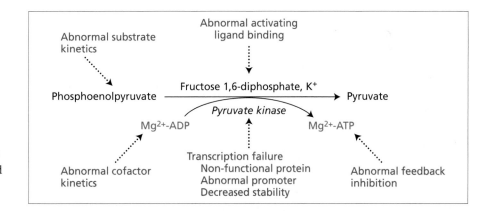

Figure 9.3 The reactions of pyruvate kinase, showing the main ligands that influence activity and the sites affected by various mutations encountered in PK deficiency.

Clinical features

The genetic heterogeneity is reflected in the wide variation of the phenotype. The presenting features may vary from severe neonatal jaundice and anaemia (Figure 9.4), rarely even presenting with hydrops fetalis, severe CNSHA requiring repeated transfusions, moderate haemolysis with exacerbation during infections or pregnancy, to symptomless compensated haemolysis with only a minor apparent anaemia. The majority of reported cases

have presented in childhood. PK deficiency does not usually have an adverse effect on the outcome of pregnancy, although occasionally transfusion may be required to compensate for the added dilutional anaemia (Figure 9.5).

Jaundice, as with other congenital haemolytic anaemias, may be exacerbated by co-inheritance of other genes, for example, of Gilbert's syndrome. The haemolysis is nearly always extravascular, although rare examples with some intravascular haemolysis

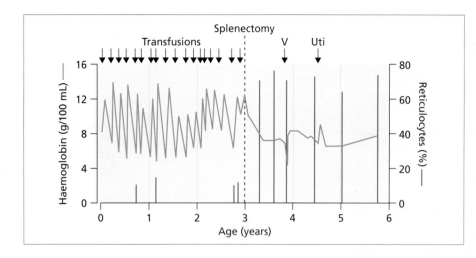

Figure 9.4 Effect of splenectomy in a child with severe CNSHA due to PK deficiency. Splenectomy was delayed until the child was 3 years old. Note the marked reticulocytosis post splenectomy (V, viral infection; Uti, urinary tract infection). The child grew normally despite Hb of around 8 g/dL (see text).

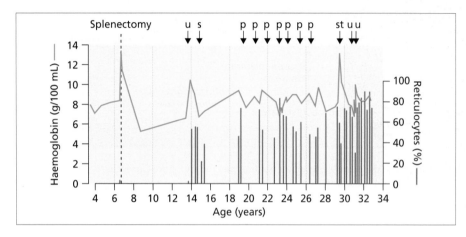

Figure 9.5 Multiple successful pregnancies in a splenectomized patient with PK deficiency. Transfusion was required during pregnancy (p) and before surgery (st, sterilization) and during infection (u, urinary tract infection; s, sepsis).

have been detected. Gallstones are common in PK deficiency and may lead to bouts of cholecystitis and biliary colic (Figure 9.6). Jaundice may also be increased by administration of drugs that affect bile excretion. As with other cases of congenital haemolytic anaemias with extravascular haemolysis, excess iron accumulation may occasionally develop even in the absence of transfusion or co-inheritance of a haemochromatosis gene.

The spleen is usually palpable in cases where there is significant haemolysis, although in milder cases, it may be evident only by using ultrasound or other imaging techniques.

Pyruvate kinase deficiency is not associated with abnormalities of other tissues, as the deficient enzyme is unique to the red cells, but occasionally individuals are seen with associated abnormalities due to deletions within chromosome 1, close to the PK gene.

Laboratory diagnosis
The blood count reveals a normochromic anaemia with reticulocytosis, sometimes producing a slight macrocytosis. An increased mean cell Hb concentration (MCHC) is occasion-

ally seen in severe cases as a result of dehydration brought about by ATP deficiency. This dehydration also produces the characteristic spur cells or acanthocytes seen on the blood film (Figure 9.7a and b). Apart from the spur cells (which are not specific) and the very large reticulocytosis post splenectomy (Figure 9.7c), there is nothing to distinguish PK deficiency from other causes of CNSHA.

The autohaemolysis test, involving the incubation of defibrinated red cells with and without glucose for 48 h at 37°C, has traditionally been used for screening tests. The haemolysis in the unfortified aliquot is uncorrected by the addition of glucose (type II). The test is not specific and has mainly been abandoned in favour of the enzyme assay.

The definitive diagnosis depends on the analysis of enzyme activity and kinetics, although the finding of an elevated 2,3-DPG level (2–3 times normal) may be a useful pointer. Characterization of the enzyme requires measurement of maximal activation under optimal conditions (V_{max}), kinetic studies to determine substrate(s) concentration at which the enzyme shows 50% V_{max} (K_m), thermal stability, pH optimum and

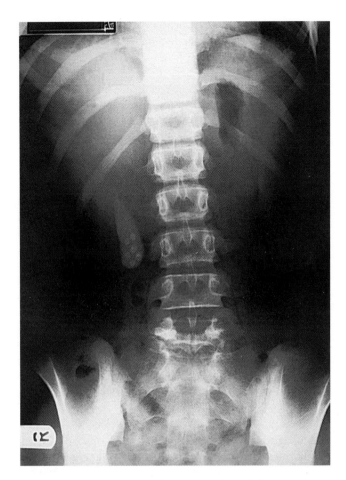

Figure 9.6 Plain radiograph of a patient with PK deficiency, showing a calcified gall bladder with mixed calcified pigment stones as a result of repeated attacks of inflammatory cholecystitis.

electrophoretic mobility. Meaningful enzyme levels can be achieved only after the total removal of leucocytes, which have up to 300 times the PK activity of red cells. The effect of reticulocytes also has to be taken into account. International guidelines for investigation of PK deficiency have been published. Typically, homozygotes have about 25% of the normal V_{max} activity, allowing for the age of the red cells and heterozygotes 50–60%, but the range is great and there is much overlap in the V_{max} between the groups, emphasizing the need for kinetic and other studies (Figure 9.8).

Management

The mainstay of management of patients who have severe enough haemolysis to warrant treatment is splenectomy. Assessment of the need for splenectomy should take into account the symptoms of the patient, not the Hb level. The low Hb (even as low as 7.0 g/dL) may be well tolerated because of the right-shifted oxygen dissociation curve. Indications for splenectomy include severe neonatal haemolysis and chronic transfusion

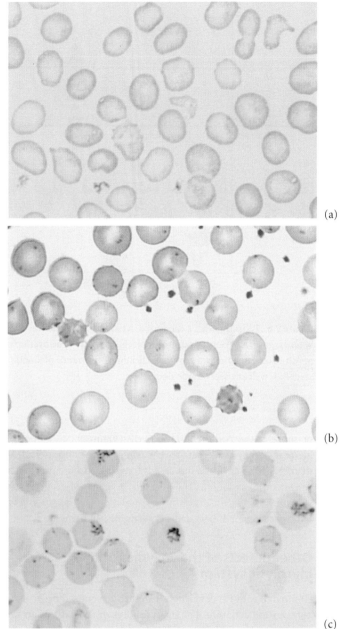

Figure 9.7 PK deficiency, peripheral blood. (a) Red cell anisocytosis and poikilocytosis presplenectomy. (b) Postsplenectomy showing acanthocytes or 'prickle' cells. (c) Gross reticulocytosis post splenectomy (supravital new methylene blue stain).

requirements. The dangers of splenectomy, particularly the risk of overwhelming sepsis, are discussed in Chapters 8 and 21. Splenectomy raises the effective Hb so that transfusion is not required but does not prevent hyperbilirubinaemia, so biliary complications may still arise after splenectomy.

Following splenectomy for PK deficiency, there is a huge elevation of the reticulocyte count, which may reach 80%

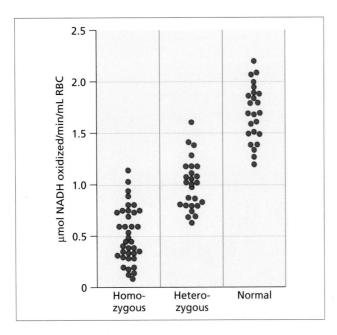

Figure 9.8 PK activity V_{max} measured in patients, obligate heterozygotes and normal control subjects. Note the wide overlap of values between the two groups, indicating importance of kinetic studies as well as effect of reticulocytosis.

or more of the peripheral blood cells (Figure 9.7c). Although pregnancy may exacerbate this anaemia, there is no indication that PK deficiency itself has an adverse effect on the pregnancy or outcome, as long as the anaemia is managed as necessary (Figure 9.5). As with all chronic haemolytic anaemias, folic acid, 5 mg per week or 400 μg daily, is a sensible supplement.

Other defects of the enzymes of the glycolytic system

Compared with PK deficiency, the other defects of the glycolytic pathway are very rare. The main features of these disorders are summarized in Table 9.1.

Hexokinase

Hexokinase (HK1) catalyses the phosphorylation of glucose to G6P, the first step in the glycolytic pathway. The enzyme in the red cell differs from that in nucleated cells, which have oxidative respiration, by lacking a porin-binding domain that links the enzyme to the mitochondrial membrane. The red cell enzyme is derived from alternative splicing of the gene product. The enzyme provides a major rate-limiting step in glycolysis and has extensive allosteric interactions, being highly pH sensitive and regulated in its activity by its products, G6P, P_i, 2,3-DPG and disulphide compounds. The enzyme activity decays predictably with age of the normal red cell, and may be used as a comparator

for other enzyme activities, when absolute levels may be difficult to interpret because of the age distribution of the red cells.

Hexokinase deficiency

Hexokinase deficiency has been recorded in fewer than 30 cases but, even within this small number, there is evidence of molecular and phenotypic heterogeneity. Complete hexokinase deficiency is probably lethal. Most patients have moderately reduced activity for the age of the red cell and, in the majority of cases, it is the stability of the enzyme that is affected by the mutation. Combined heterozygosity for complete gene deletion and a nonsense mutation affecting activity has been recorded as a typical example of compound genetic inheritance. In most recorded cases, the activity of the enzyme is reduced to between 10% and 20% of normal. As with other glycolytic enzyme deficiencies, there is variable non-spherocytic haemolytic anaemia, in this case mostly relatively mild. Obligate heterozygotes have reduced levels of the enzyme, but assays of the activity in patients with haemolytic anaemia due to hexokinase deficiency may be difficult to interpret because of the higher activity in reticulocytes and in young cells. Typically, the reduced hexokinase activity is associated with a fall in the concentration of 2,3-DPG within the cells. Patients have less exercise tolerance for a given level of Hb than would be expected because of the left shift in the oxygen dissociation curve.

Glucosephosphate isomerase

Glucosephosphate isomerase (GPI) catalyses the second step of the Embden–Meyerhof pathway, the interconversion of G6P to fructose 6-phosphate (F6P). The enzyme is also known as phosphohexose isomerase, phosphoglucose isomerase, autocrine motility factor and neuroleukin (NLK). The names 'autocrine motility factor' and 'neuroleukin' indicate that the protein has other actions in other cells. The interconversion of the hexose phosphates is driven towards F6P by the rapid metabolism of that product along the metabolic pathway, so that the concentration of F6P in the red cell is low and drives the reaction towards its formation.

Glucosephosphate isomerase deficiency

Deficiency of GPI is one of the commonest causes of CNSHA after G6PD deficiency and PK deficiency. It is about as equally common as pyrimidine 5′-nucleotidase deficiency (see later). The mutations that give rise to GPI deficiency are very heterogeneous – out of the 20 characterized mutations, 14 appear in only a single family and 11 out of the 20 occur in compound heterozygotes. The clinical picture perhaps reflects this genetic heterogeneity. Most reported cases are of mild to moderate haemolytic anaemia, but in one Indian family stillbirths and hydrops occurred in several siblings before early delivery and exchange transfusion for hydrops allowed survival. The mutations described mainly affect the stability of GPI, which is perhaps why no associated anomalies are found in nucleated cells. In T lymphocytes, GPI

Table 9.1 Main features of glycolytic enzyme deficiencies.

Enzyme	Genetics (chromosome/inheritance)	Haematology	Other systems affected	Comment
Hexokinase (HKI)	10q11.2 AR	CNSHA High O_2 affinity	None directly*	Very rare, occasional AD
Glucose phosphate isomerase (GPI)	19cen–q12 AR	CNSHA	None directly*	Most common after PK deficiency
Phosphofructokinase (PFK)	1(M) and 21(L) Complex	Erythrocytosis Minimal haemolysis	Dominated by myopathy	Tarui's disease, subunit genes
Fructose diphosphate aldolase (ALDOA)	16q22–q24 AR	CNSHA Intermittent HA	Dysmorphism, myopathy	Very rare (three families)
Triose phosphate isomerase (TPI)	12p13 AR	CNSHA Infections	Neuromuscular, cardiac	Neuromuscular defects dominate, sudden death, Splx not helpful
Phosphoglycerate kinase (PGK)	Xq13 X-linked	CNSHA	CNS, myopathy, rhabdomyolysis	Rare (28 families), variable systems involved
Diphosphoglycerate mutase (DPG mutase)	7q23–q34 AR	Erythrocytosis	None	Very rare, low 2,3-DPG
Glyceraldehyde-3-P-dehydrogenase	12p13 AD	None	None	Membrane protein band 6, associated with HS, gene syntenic with TPI
Pyruvate kinase (PK)	1q21–q22 (PKLR) AR rarely AD	CNSHA	None	Commonest CNSHA

AD, autosomal dominant; AR, autosomal recessive; CNSHA, congenital non-spherocytic haemolytic anaemia; Splx, splenectomy.
*Neurological signs may be secondary to hypoxia or ischaemia.

acts as NLK, a lymphokine that induces the formation of antibody-secreting cells. It is also present in neutrophils, but there is no increase in infections in deficient subjects. In some severely deficient patients, neurological retardation has been thought to be related to hypoxia or ischaemia *in utero* rather than to direct metabolic effects.

Phosphofructokinase

Phosphofructokinase (PFK) catalyses a reaction in which F6P is phosphorylated to fructose-1,6-diphosphate, ATP being the donor of the phosphate group. Under normal physiological conditions, this may be the major rate-limiting step in glycolysis in the red cell. PFK is a tetramer, which in the red cell is a heterote-

tramer made up from M or L subunits. Two separate genes code for the two subunits. In muscle, PFK is a homotetramer (M_4) and in liver a homotetramer (L_4). In the red cell, there may be five isoenzymes composed of different numbers of L- and M-type subunits. A third subunit is found in platelets.

Phosphofructokinase deficiency

Deficiency of the M subunit leads to glycogen storage disease type 7 (Tarui's disease). It is characterized by muscle cramps and myoglobinuria on exertion. Shortened red cell viability may be a minor component of this disease. Evidence of haemolysis may be accompanied by mild erythrocytosis as a result of the decreased production of 2,3-DPG.

Fructose diphosphate aldolase A (ALDOA)

Fructose-1,6-diphosphate aldolase catalyses the conversion of fructose 1,6-diphosphate to glyceraldehyde 3-phosphate (Ga3P) and dihydroxyacetone phosphate (DHAP). There are three aldolases in human tissues (A, B and C), of which only A is expressed in the red cell. ALDOA is produced in the developing embryo and forms also the bulk of the enzyme in muscle, where it may be as much as 5% of the total cellular protein. In the red cell, the reaction catalysed by the enzyme is for all intents and purposes irreversible.

Fructose diphosphate aldolase A deficiency

The condition is extremely rare, with only three families having been definitely identified as having ALDOA deficiency. Two families have been described in which the propositus presented with CNSHA, mental retardation and dysmorphic features that are similar in the two families. In at least one family, the mutation produced an unstable enzyme. In a third patient, symptoms were mainly of myopathy, with weakness and premature fatigue. Anaemia and jaundice were intermittent and rhabdomyolysis occurred. There was severe deficiency of both muscle and red cell enzyme activity.

Triose phosphate isomerase

Triose phosphate isomerase (TPI) catalyses the interconversion of DHAP and Ga3P. In the glycolytic pathway of the red cell, all DHAP is converted to Ga3P, which is then metabolized down the glycolytic pathway, providing the ultimate two molecules of ATP for each molecule of glucose metabolized by that pathway. The enzyme is a homodimer, present in all tissues. In tissues other than the red blood cell, DHAP is an important precursor for the biosynthesis of ether glycerolipids (plasmalogens).

Triose phosphate isomerase deficiency

Triose phosphate isomerase deficiency produces a severe syndrome present from birth, consisting of CNSHA, a progressive neurological disorder with spasticity and CNS degeneration. Cardiac failure and sudden death due to arrhythmias are also features. Death occurs usually about 5 years of age. There is, as usual, some variation, and haemolysis without neurological degeneration, and the opposite, have been described. Splenectomy does not appear to be effective in modifying the haemolysis and does not influence the neurological complications. The diagnosis is made based on clinical suspicion, together with the appropriate enzyme assay. A number of point mutations that lead to the syndrome have been identified, but far and away the most predominant is Glu104Asp, a mutation linked by common haplotypes, suggesting descent from a common ancestor.

Phosphoglycerate kinase

Phosphoglycerate kinase (PGK) catalyses the reversible conversion of 1,3-DPG to 3-phosphoglycerate, generating one molecule of ATP for each molecule of 1,3-DPG metabolized by this pathway. It should be noted that two molecules of the 1,3-DPG are produced for each molecule of glucose metabolized by this pathway. PGKA, the active enzyme in the red blood cell, is the product of a gene on the X chromosome. The enzyme is monomeric and is expressed in all tissues (a testis has an additional PGKB gene coded on an autosome).

Phosphoglycerate kinase deficiency

In total, 28 families with PGK deficiency have been reported, and sequencing data are available for 16 families. Overall, 15 different *PGK1* gene mutations have been identified. CNSHA occurred in 17 out of the 28 families, CNS disorders in 13 and myopathy with or without rhabdomyolysis in 13. All three systems were involved in only one of the families. Anaemia, when present, is usually well tolerated because of the increased concentration of 2,3-DPG produced by the increased flow of 1,3-DPG to 2,3-DPG via the Rapaport–Leubering shunt in the presence of the mutated PGK deficiency. Splenectomy has been effective in some cases of severe anaemia, but less so in others.

Defence against oxidative stress – the production of reducing power

As with all cells, but perhaps more urgently, the red blood cell needs to be protected against the effects of free radicals, hydrogen peroxide and other highly oxidative material in order to maintain the membrane integrity and functional activity. In addition, Hb has to be maintained in its functional state, and the steady production of MetHb reversed back to deoxyhaemoglobin, which is able to combine reversibly with oxygen. The major generator of reducing power within the red cell is the pentose phosphate pathway (hexose monophosphate shunt), which generates reducing power in the form of NADPH from NADP+ coupled to the oxidation of G6P to 6-phosphogluconate and the subsequent oxidation of that compound to ribose 5-phosphate, the two reactions catalysed by the enzyme G6PD and 6-phosphogluconate dehydrogenase (6PGD) (Figure 9.9).

Glutathione (GSH) is important for the protection of cells from oxidative damage by these free radicals, protection against the effects of infection, the maintenance of protein sulphydryl groups in the reduced state and the maintenance of membrane transport. A constant supply of GSH is provided by the glutathione cycle, linked to the pentose phosphate pathway through the action of glutathione reductase (Figure 9.10).

An excess of oxidative stress over the reducing power of the red cell leads to intravascular haemolysis following denaturation of the Hb and precipitation as Heinz bodies and peroxidation of the red cell membrane. Methaemoglobinaemia may occur. The clinical features that emerge, acute intravascular haemolysis, Heinz body haemolytic anaemia or methaemoglobinaemia, depend upon the nature of the oxidative stress and the size of the imbalance between the stress and the redox potential.

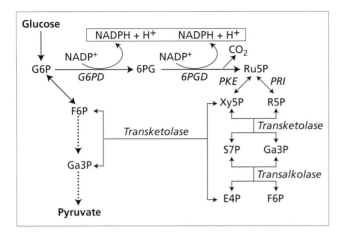

Figure 9.9 The pentose phosphate pathway. Substrates: G6P, glucose-6-phosphate; 6PG, 6-phosphogluconate; Ru5P, ribulose-5-phosphate; R5P, ribose-5-phosphate; Ga3P, glyceraldehye-3-phosphate; F6P, fructose-6-phosphate; Xy5P, xylose-5-phosphate; S7P, septulose-7-phosphate; E4P, erythrothrose-4-phosphate. Enzymes: G6PD, glucose-6-phosphate dehydrogenase; 6PGD, 6-phosphogluconate dehydrogenase; PKE, phosphoketoepimerase; PRI, phosphoribose isomerase.

Pentose phosphate pathway (hexose monophosphate shunt)

The reactions of the pentose phosphate pathway are shown schematically in Figure 9.2 and in more detail in Figure 9.9. In most cells, the pentose phosphate pathway is an essential pathway for the production of ribose and incorporation into RNA. In the red cell, its only function is the production of reducing power in the form of NADPH. The first step of the pathway, catalysed by G6PD, utilizes G6P as the substrate. G6P is also a substrate for the glycolytic pathway. Under normal circumstances, about 10% of glucose is metabolized by the pentose phosphate pathway, the activity of that pathway being determined by the availability of NAD^+ and feedback inhibition by ATP. Under conditions of oxidative stress, the flux through the pentose phosphate pathway can be greatly increased. The products of the pathway re-enter the glycolytic pathway through F6P or Ga3P.

From the point of view of haematological disorders, G6PD deficiency is by far the most important step in the pathway. However, other enzymes of the pathway can be important in acquired disorders, some steps being inhibited by drugs, including oestrogen–progesterone contraceptive pills.

Glucose-6-phosphate dehydrogenase

G6PD catalyses the first step of the pentose phosphate pathway and is the enzyme controlling flux through that pathway. The activity is controlled by the availability of $NADP^+$. Conversion of G6P to 6PG is accompanied by the reduction of $NADP^+$ to NADPH, and the second step in the pathway, the oxidation of 6PG to ribose 5-phosphate, produces a second molecule of NADPH.

The gene for G6P is located on the X chromosome at Xq28. The gene has 13 exons and 12 introns. The gene is transcribed as

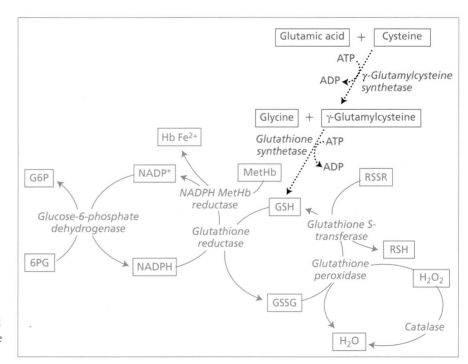

Figure 9.10 The glutathione cycle and synthetic pathways. GSH is synthesized in two linked steps. The redox control is exercised by the glutathione cycle linked to the NADPH of the pentose phosphate pathway by glutathione reductase.

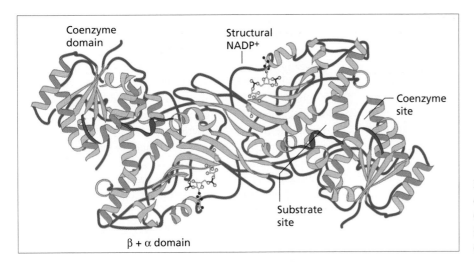

Figure 9.11 Structure of G6PD in dimer form, showing active sites for G6P and NADP⁺. Mutations that affect interactions of the monomers lead to CNSHA.

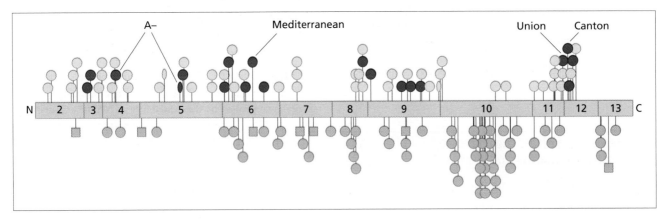

Figure 9.12 G6PD gene map showing mutation sites (courtesy of Tom Vulliamy, Hammersmith Campus, Imperial College, London). Numbered boxes refer to the location of *G6PD* exons: yellow circles, class I and II variants; yellow ellipses, class IV variants; red circles, polymorphic variants; green circles and squares, class I variants caused by amino acid substitutions and small in-frame deletions, respectively.

a monomer of 514 amino acids that come together to produce an equilibrium of dimers and tetramers (Figure 9.11). Each monomer has an NADP⁺-binding domain and a large domain, with the active site between the two. The gene is a household gene, active in all cells, with an essential role in the production of RNA in nucleated cells. Not surprisingly, the gene is highly conserved in evolutionary history. Complete inactivity of the enzyme in nucleated cells would not be compatible with life. The clinical consequences of G6PD deficiency are virtually confined to the red blood cell, with occasional evidence of leucocyte malfunction in some variants. The majority of mutations affect the stability of the transcribed enzyme so that there is a rapid decline in activity in the mature enucleate red cell as it ages.

In the red blood cell, G6PD catalyses the first reaction of the pentose phosphate pathway, the conversion of G6P to 6-phosphogluconate through the reduction of NADP⁺ to NADPH (Figure 9.9). The availability of NADP⁺ is determined by the activity of the glutathione cycle, which is linked to the pentose phosphate pathway through the activity of the enzyme glutathione reductase (Figure 9.12). The availability of NADP⁺ is the major rate-limiting step for the pentose phosphate pathway.

Glucose-6-phosphate dehydrogenase deficiency

G6PD deficiency is the commonest genetically determined enzyme deficiency in the world population, with an estimated 400 million people being affected. At least 127 different variants associated with deficient enzyme activity have been described, as well as a number of polymorphisms that do not affect the enzyme activity. The G6PD variants have been classified into four groups according to their activity relative to the 'wild-type' G6PD type B (Table 9.2). In Africa, the variant G6PD A⁻ is the predominant polymorphism with equivalent activity to G6PD type B.

Table 9.2 Classification of G6PD deficiency (WHO).

Class	Enzyme activity (% normal)	Examples	Clinical Effects
I	Severe (usually < 20)	Santiago de Cuba (Gly447Arg)	CNSHA, acute exacerbations
II	< 10	Mediterranean (Ser188Phe)	Favism
		Canton (Arg459Leu)	AIVHA (drug induced)
		Orissa (Ala44Gly)	Neonatal jaundice
III	Moderate (> 10, < 60)	A⁻ (Val68Met; Aas126Asp)	AIVHA (drug induced), neonatal jaundice
IV	100	B⁻ (wild type)	None
		A (Asn126Asp)	None

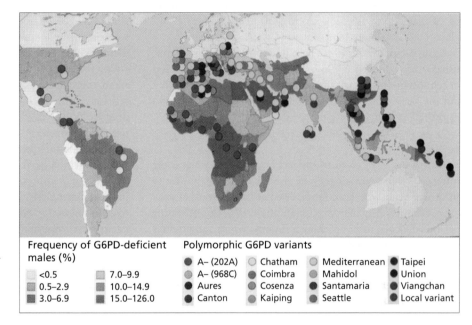

Figure 9.13 Global distribution of *G6PD* gene variants causing G6PD deficiency. Shaded areas indicate the prevalence of G6PD deficiency. The coloured dots depict the distribution of 14 of the most common variants (from Luzzatto & Notaro, 2001, *Science* 293: 442, with permission).

Frequency of G6PD-deficient males (%)
- <0.5
- 0.5–2.9
- 3.0–6.9
- 7.0–9.9
- 10.0–14.9
- 15.0–126.0

Polymorphic G6PD variants
- A– (202A)
- A– (968C)
- Aures
- Canton
- Chatham
- Coimbra
- Cosenza
- Kaiping
- Mediterranean
- Mahidol
- Santamaria
- Seattle
- Taipei
- Union
- Viangchan
- Local variant

Epidemiology

G6PD deficiency is widely disseminated throughout Africa, the Mediterranean basin, the Middle East, South-East Asia, and indigenous populations of the Indian subcontinent. G6PD A⁻ is common in Africa (it has a second mutation in the G6PD A⁻ gene – see Figure 9.12), the Mediterranean variant in southern Italy, Sardinia and other places around the Mediterranean basin, and G6PD Canton in southern China. These variants are only the most common amongst many different mutations in these areas and throughout the rest of the affected world (Figure 9.13). This distribution of the deficiency equates with areas where *Plasmodium falciparum* malaria is common, and this is thought to be the evolutionary drive that produced such widespread polymorphisms (Figure 9.13). It has subsequently been confirmed that G6PD deficiency does indeed protect against lethal falciparum malaria, particularly in childhood, and this protection, especially in hyperendemic areas, more than outweighs the haematological problems associated with deficiency.

Clinical features

There are four main syndromes associated with G6PD deficiency. In all four syndromes, haemolysis is aggravated or promoted by exposure to oxidative stress through infection or ingestion of oxidative foods or drugs, but the clinical presentations differ. Age always modifies the clinical effects although not always as might be expected. The four syndromes are neonatal jaundice, favism, CNSHA and drug-induced haemolytic anaemia. The neonatal jaundice syndrome has been described in class I, II and III variants: favism in mainly, although not exclusively, class II, CNHSA in class I and the drug-induced haemolysis mainly class III. Although G6PD deficiency is most common in males, the prevalence of the gene in many parts of the world (Figure 9.13) means that female homozygotes are not uncommon, and heterozygous females are often susceptible to oxidative stress because of the effects of X-inactivation and marked lyonization in leaving a significant population of deficient red cells.

Neonatal jaundice and G6PD deficiency in infancy

Neonatal jaundice is a severe manifestation of G6PD deficiency and is a major source of potential morbidity from kernicterus. Most common variants have been associated with the syndrome, including the A⁻ and Mediterranean variants. In parts of the world where the mutations are common, the deficiency is the most prevalent cause of neonatal jaundice. The jaundice probably starts *in utero* in the perinatal period, but the clinical problem becomes apparent only about the second or third day after birth. Between 10% and 50% of deficient infants are affected. Phototherapy or exchange transfusion may be required to prevent neurological sequelae. Anaemia is not a feature, and it is thought that this is a manifestation of liver enzyme deficiency, coupled perhaps to the physiological underdevelopment of neonatal liver function or the co-inheritance of UDP-glucuronyl transferase 1 deficiency of Gilbert's syndrome.

Acute haemolytic crises may occur in G6PD-deficient infants, usually through exposure to oxidative stress, including nitrites or nitrates in water or the ingestion of fava beans by the mother but, in some cases of severe acute haemolysis, even fatal, no cause has been obvious.

Favism

Favism is the term given to the G6PD syndrome when acute intravascular haemolysis may be precipitated by exposure to the broad bean *Vicia fava*. Fresh, dried or frozen beans or even exposure to pollen may precipitate the crisis. The offending agent is divicine, or its aglycone isouramil, which can produce free oxygen radicals on autoxidation. Divicine is not present in peas or beans of other types, which may be eaten without effect. The amount of haemolysis is dose related, which may explain the marked variation in susceptibility not only between children and adults, but also in the same individual at different times. There is variation in divicine content between different cultivars; some fungi can break down the compound and the amount may vary in different seasonal environments. In children, acute haemolysis, sometimes life-threatening, is common, but renal failure is uncommon although there may be systemic symptoms of fever and loin pain. Renal failure occurs more often in adults, possibly because of comorbidity. Favism is usual in class II variants, for example Mediterranean and Canton, but may occur in others, including the African A⁻ variant. Although fava beans give the syndrome its name, some other compounds with which affected individuals may come in contact can cause acute haemolysis, including topical henna and some of the pulses used to make up local sweetmeats.

In between attacks of favism or exposure to oxidizing substance, the blood count is normal, with no evidence of haemolysis. The coincidence of infection, which promotes the formation of hydrogen peroxide following the oxygen burst in neutrophils and macrophages, with ingestion of oxidizing substances, even mild ones such as chloramphenicol, may promote haemolysis even although the drug on its own does not.

Chronic non-spherocytic haemolytic anaemia

Sporadic cases in virtually all populations of CNHSA are found with underlying G6PD deficiency. Many of the mutations that cause CNHSA occur on exon 10 and affect the formation of dimers or tetramers (Figures 9.11 and 9.12). The haemolysis is extravascular, although additional oxidative stress may provoke an acute intravascular episode.

Drug-induced acute haemolysis

The introduction of primaquine and its derivative pamaquine as antimalarials to replace quinine during the Pacific phase of the Second World War and the later Korean War revealed that a portion of men exposed, particularly in the black population, suffered from sever acute intravascular haemolysis. Intensive studies by Carson and others from the University of Chicago, working at the Statesville Penitentiary Malaria Project, finally identified the problem as G6PD deficiency and identified that young red cells and reticulocytes had sufficient activity to withstand the oxidative stress so that haemolysis lessened as the reticulocyte level rose. It became apparent that many other drugs could also produce haemolysis, but mostly fava beans did not. The common A⁻ variant of Africa is the main example of class III mutations producing this type of haemolysis.

The haemolysis is dose related and may be self-limiting. Although it is important to recognize which drugs are likely to produce haemolysis (Table 9.3), it is also important to realize that the disease for which the drugs may be needed, for example falciparum malaria, may be fatal and the haemolysis is a lesser problem.

Laboratory diagnosis

The acute intravascular haemolysis raises the suspicion of G6PD deficiency. The blood film shows red cells with contracted Hb in 'ghost' membrane (Figure 9.14). Haemoglobinuria may be gross, producing almost black urine without red cells in the centrifuge deposit.

Several screening tests have been devised to identify G6PD deficiency in red blood cells. The most widely used tests have been the brilliant Cresyl blue decolorization test, the MetHb reduction test and an ultraviolet spot test. These tests can reliably distinguish between deficient or not deficient individuals, but are not reliably quantitative. Hemizygous deficient males and homozygous deficient females will be identified, the threshold being a G6PD activity of about 30% of normal.

If a screening test indicates deficiency or is doubtful, the ideal follow-up test for definitive diagnosis is quantification of G6PD activity by spectrophotometric assay. Standardized methods have been published. There are two clinical situations in which quantification is especially important. First, during a haemolytic attack, the oldest red cells (with the least G6PD activity) are destroyed selectively, and therefore the surviving red cells have a relatively higher (but still deficient) G6PD activity. This increases further as the reticulocyte response sets in over the

Table 9.3 Drugs to be avoided in G6PD deficiency*.

Antimalarials	Analgesics
Primaquine (can be given at reduced dosage, 15 mg daily or 45 mg twice weekly under survelliance)	Acetylsalicylic acid (aspirin); moderate doses can be used
Pamaquine	Acetophenetidin (phenacetin); safe alternative, paracetamol
Sulphonamides and sulphones	*Antihelminthics*
Sulphanilamide	β-Naphthol
Sulphapyridine	Stibophan
Sulphadimidine	Niridazole
Sulphacetamide (Albucid)	
Salicylazosulphapyridine (Salazopyrin)	*Miscellaneous*
Dapsone†	Vitamin K analogues (1 mg menaphthone can be given to babies)
Sulphoxone†	Naphthalene (mothballs)†
Glucosulphone sodium (Promin)	Probenecid
Septrin	Dimercaprol (BAL)
	Methylene blue
Other antibacterial compounds	Toluidine blue
Nitrofurans	
Nitrofurantoin	
Furazolidone	
Nitrofurazone	
Nalidixic acid	

*This list is compiled on the basis of data available for patients with the 'A⁻' variant of G6PD deficiency. It can be generally assumed to be applicable to patients from Africa and of African descent. For patients with the Mediterranean type of G6PD deficiency, with an unknown variant, or with CNSHA, the following should also be added: acetanilide, chloramphenicol, chloroquine (may be used under surveillance when required for prophylaxis or treatment of malaria), mepacrine, p-amino salicylic acid and thiazosulphone. Many other drugs may produce haemolysis in particular individuals.
†These drugs may cause haemolysis in normal individuals if taken in large doses.

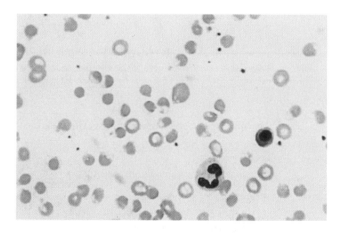

Figure 9.14 G6PD deficiency. Peripheral blood film following acute oxidant drug-induced haemolysis shows an erythroblast and damaged red cells, including 'blister' and 'bite' cells.

following days. During this time, a screening test might yield a false-normal result and, rarely, even a quantitative test might do so. In such cases, the best counsel is to repeat the test a couple of weeks later. Alternatively, the oldest remaining cells can be isolated by differential centrifugation and they can be shown to have a low G6PD activity. The diagnosis of heterozygous females can be especially difficult; in extreme cases, it can only be done by family studies. However, from the practical point of view, it must be borne in mind that the probability of clinically significant haemolysis in a heterozygote roughly correlates with the proportion of G6PD-deficient red cells in her blood. Therefore, if a normal level of G6PD activity is found in a heterozygote, she is unlikely to be at risk of G6PD-related haemolysis. In regions where G6PD has a high prevalence and the main variants are known, DNA analysis is the most effective way of identifying heterozygotes.

Management
Mostly, management is dictated by the symptoms and signs in

Table 9.4 Association between G6PD deficiency and jaundice in male newborns.

Groups of newborns	n	G6PD deficiency %
Normal	500	22.5
Mild jaundice (bilirubin 150–200)	38	45
Severe jaundice (bilirubin >230)	70	60
Admitted with kernicterus	20	78

Data collected in Ibadan, Nigeria.
Bilirubin values in μmol/L.

the patient, although education in the avoidance of oxidizing substances is important (Table 9.3). In many populations, the condition is well known and the need for avoidance recognized. Neonatal jaundice may need urgent therapy to prevent neurological damage (Table 9.4). Extreme hyperbilirubinaemia can be prevented by administration of Sn-mesoporphyrin if the diagnosis is known at birth. Acute intravascular haemolysis may require transfusion but the anaemia is often self-limiting (Table 9.5). High fluid intake should be encouraged to prevent renal damage. CNSHA may be severe enough to warrant active treatment and splenectomy may be helpful.

Glutathione

Glutathione (GSH) is the major intracellular thiol in aerobic cells and is equally important in the red blood cell. It is thought to have a number of critical functions: protecting cells against oxidative damage, participation in detoxification of foreign compounds, maintenance of protein sulphydryl groups in a reduced state and, possibly, transport of amino acids. In the red cell, its main function is as an antioxidant. GSH is synthesized from glutamate, cysteine and glycine by the link reactions of two enzymes; γ-glutamylcysteine synthetase and glutathione synthetase (Figure 9.10). GSH exerts its function in preserving thiol groups and reducing hydrogen peroxide and free oxygen radicals through reactions catalysed by the enzymes glutathione peroxidase and glutathione-S-transferase respectively. The oxidized glutathione (GSSG) is reduced back to GSH by the action of glutathione reductase, the hydrogen donor being NADPH (Figure 9.10). Failure to maintain the GSH level as a result of deficiency in the synthetic pathways or deficiency in the recycling process leads to chronic haemolytic anaemia and increased susceptibility to oxidative stress.

Glutathione deficiency

Complete loss of GSH synthesis is probably lethal. Severe deficiency leads to 5-oxoprolinuria, metabolic acidosis and mental retardation. A milder deficiency limited to red cells is associated with haemolytic anaemia aggravated by oxidative stress. Low levels of GSH caused by γ-glutamylcysteine synthetase or glutathione synthetase deficiency, with CNSHA, have been described. Haemolytic anaemia due to glutathione reductase and glutathione peroxidase deficiency have also been reported (Table 9.6).

Nucleotide metabolism

Adenosine nucleotides, ATP (85–90%), ADP (10–12%) and AMP (1–3%), constitute the main nucleotide pool in the mature red cell. The cell has no mechanism for making nucleotides once the RNA of the reticulocytes has been degraded. The cell does have an effective salvage mechanism for maintenance of the adenine pool, with the enzymes adenosine deaminase (ADA)

Table 9.5 Characteristic features of haemolytic attack in G6PD deficiency.

Phase	Clinical	Laboratory
Acute	Abrupt onset	
	Malaise, prostration	
	Pallor	Anaemia; Heinz bodies; reticulocytosis; G6PD deficient
	(Abdominal pain)	
	Fever	Leucocytosis
	Dark urine	Haemoglobinuria; haptoglobin absent
	Haemoglobinaemia	
	Methaemalbuminaemia	
	Jaundice	Hyperbilirubinaemia
	(Renal failure)	↑Urea ↑creatinine
Recovery	Gradual but rapid cessation of haemolysis	Reticulocytes peak days 5–8
	Urine clears in few days	G6PD increases but rarely to normal range
	Jaundice clears in 1–2 weeks	

Table 9.6 Enzymopathies of the glutathione cycle and synthetic pathways.

Enzyme	Genetics	Haematology	Other systems	Comments
Glutathione synthetase	20q11.2, AR	CNSHA, Heinz bodies, oxidative HA	Neurological, metabolic acidosis	5-Oxoprolinaemia/uria, RBC deficiency, may have no neurological disease, nine families
γ-Glutamylcysteine synthetase	6p12 GLCLC, C 1p21 GLCLR, AR	CNSHA, oxidative HA, basophilic stippling	Neurological	Variable neurological features, five families
Glutathione reductase	8p21, AR	Favism	None	Most reports due to FAD deficiency, one family
Glutathione peroxidase (GPx1)	3p21.3, AR	HDN, acute IVHA	None	Self-limited neonatal jaundice, one Japanese family

AR, autosomal recessive; FAD, flavine adenine dinucleotide; HDN, haemolytic disease of the newborn; IVHA, intravascular haemolytic anaemia.

and adenylate kinase involved in the regulation. Deficiency of the enzymes in the salvage pathway does not lead to haemolysis. ADA deficiency is associated with severe combined immune deficiency and excess activity is found in Diamond–Blackfan anaemia. During maturation of reticulocytes, the RNA is broken down to pyrimidine and purine nucleotides, which are dephosphorylated to nucleosides that can diffuse out of the cell. The purine nucleotides enter the salvage pathway. Deficiency of pyrimidine 5′-nucleotidase leads to accumulation of pyrimidine nucleotides, which interferes with the adenine nucleotide pool, producing haemolysis.

Pyrimidine 5′-nucleotidase

Pyrimidine 5′-nucleotidase (P5N1), also called pyrimidine 5′-monophosphate hydrolase, catalyses the dephosphorylation of the pyrimidine 5′-monophosphates, uridine monophosphate (UMP) and cytodine monophosphate (CMP), to the corresponding nucleosides (Figure 9.15). In red blood cells, there are two isoforms of P5N, type 1 (P5N1), which has a high affinity for UMP and CMP, and type 2 (P5N2), which hydrolyses deoxypyrimidine nucleotide monophosphates. It is deficiency of P5N1 that leads to haemolytic anaemia. The gene (P5′N1)

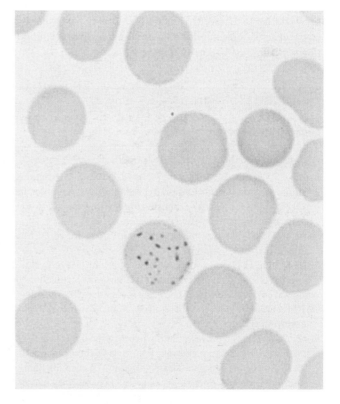

Figure 9.16 Peripheral blood film from P5N1-deficient patient, showing basophilic stippling (a similar appearance is seen in chronic lead poisoning).

is localized on chromosome 7p15–14. The gene consists of 10 exons, with alternative splicing at exon 2, which gives rise to isoforms with 286 and 297 amino acids. The 286 protein has the characteristics of P5′N1. The enzyme is strongly inhibited by lead.

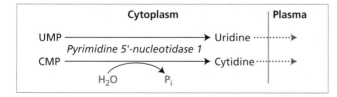

Figure 9.15 Pyrimidine nucleotide catabolism in the reticulocyte. P5N1 converts the nucleotides to monophosphates, which diffuse out of the cell.

Pyrimidine 5′-nucleotidase deficiency

Pyrimidine 5′-nucleotidase deficiency is not uncommon, although only some 40 or 50 families have been reported in the literature. It is probably the third most common enzyme deficiency causing haemolytic anaemia, perhaps equal to GPI deficiency. Nearly all reported cases have shown homozygosity for the mutation, and the mutation has been specific for individual families. There is, however, a suggestion that certain mutations (Del G576 and INS GG743) might be more prevalent in southern Italy or southern Mediterranean regions. One compound heterozygote was found in this region.

Deficiency of P5N1 is associated with a recessively inherited haemolytic anaemia characterized by marked basophilic stippling in the red cells (Figure 9.16) and accumulation of high concentrations of pyrimidine nucleotides. The haemolysis is usually mild to moderate, although more severe cases have been reported. Splenectomy is usually of little value, though benefit has been reported in some cases. The appearance of the blood film is similar to that seen in lead poisoning, and the mechanism of the anaemia in lead poisoning certainly involves the inhibition of pyrimidine 5′-nucleotidase.

Selected bibliography

General and reviews

Arya R, Layton DM, Bellingham AJ (1995) Hereditary red cell enzymopathies. *Blood Reviews* 9: 165–75.

Beutler E, Blume KG, Kaplan JC *et al.* (1979) International Committee for Standardization in Haematology: recommended screening test for glucose-6-phosphate dehydrogenase (G-6-PD) deficiency. *British Journal of Haematology* 43: 465–7.

Dacie JV (1999) *The Haemolytic Anaemias*, Vol. 1, 3rd edn. Churchill Livingstone, London.

Miwa S, Fujii H (1996) Molecular basis of erythroenzymopathies associated with hereditary haemolytic anaemia: tabulation of mutant enzymes. *American Journal of Hematology* 51: 122–32.

OMIM. Online Mendelian Inheritance in Man (www.ncbi.nih.gov/entrez/query).

Roper D, Layton M, Lewis SM (2001) Investigation of the hereditary haemolytic anaemias: membrane and enzyme abnormalities. In: *Dacie and Lewis, Practical Haematology* (SM Lewis, BJ Bain, I Bates, eds), 9th edn, pp. 167–98. Churchill Livingstone, London.

Enzyme deficiencies of the Embden–Meyerhof pathway

Pyruvate kinase deficiency

Baronciani L, Bianchi P, Zanella A (1996) Hematologically important mutations: red cell pyruvate kinase. *Blood Cells Molecules and Diseases* 22: 85–9.

Beutler E, Baronciani L (1996) Mutations in pyruvate kinase. *Human Mutation* 7: 1–6.

Beutler E, Gelbart T (2000) PK deficiency prevalence and the limitations of a population-based survey [Letter]. *Blood* 96: 4005–6.

Bianchi P, Zappa M, Bredi E *et al.* (1999) A case of complete adenylate kinase deficiency due to a nonsense mutation in AK-1 gene (Arg 107→Stop, CGA→TGA) associated with chronic haemolytic anaemia. *British Journal of Haematology* 105: 75–9.

Carey PJ, Chandler J, Hendrick A *et al.* (2000) Prevalence of pyruvate kinase deficiency in a northern European population in the north of England [Letter]. *Blood* 96: 4005.

Gilsanz F, Vega MA, Gomez-Castillo E *et al.* (1993) Fetal anemia due to pyruvate kinase deficiency. *Archive of Diseases of Childhood* 69: 523–4.

Kugler W, Laspe P, Stahl M *et al.* (1999) Identification of a novel promoter mutation in the human pyruvate kinase (PK) LR gene of a patient with severe haemolytic anaemia. *British Journal of Haematology* 105: 596–8.

Manco L, Bento C, Ribeiro ML *et al.* (2002) Consequences at mRNA level of the PKLR gene splicing mutations IVS10(+1)G→C and IVS8(+2)T→G causing pyruvate kinase deficiency. *British Journal of Haematology* 118: 927–8.

Marshall SR, Saunders PWG, Hamilton PJ *et al.* (2000) The dangers of iron overload in pyruvate kinase deficiency. *British Journal of Haematology* 120: 1090–1.

Miwa S, Fujii H (1996) Molecular basis of erythroenzymopathies associated with hereditary hemolytic anemia: tabulation of mutant enzymes. *American Journal of Hematology* 51: 122–32.

Zanella A, Bianchi P, Fermo E *et al.* (2001) Molecular characterization of the PK-LR gene in sixteen pyruvate kinase-deficient patients. *British Journal of Haematology* 113: 43–8.

Other enzymes of the Embden–Meyerhof pathway

Beutler E, West C, Britton HA *et al.* (1997) Glucose phosphate isomerase (GPI) deficiency mutations associated with hereditary nonspherocytic haemolytic anemia (HNSHA). *Blood cells, Molecules and Diseases* 23: 402–9.

Kreuder J, Borkhardt A, Repp R *et al.* (1996) Brief report: inherited metabolic myopathy and hemolysis due to a mutation in aldolase A. *New England Journal of Medicine* 334: 1101–4.

McCann SR, Finkel B, Cadman S *et al.* (1976) Study of a kindred with hereditary spherocytosis and glyceraldehyde-3-phosphate dehydrogenase deficiency. *Blood* 47: 171–81.

Morimoto A, Ueda I, Hirashima Y *et al.* (2003) A novel missense mutation (1060G→C) in the phosphoglycerate kinase gene in a Japanese boy with chronic haemolytic anaemia, developmental delay and rhadomyolysis. *British Journal of Haematology* 122: 1009–13.

Murakmi K, Kanno H, Tancabelic J *et al.* (2002) Gene expression and biological significance of hexokinase in erythroid cells. *Acta Haematologica* 108: 204–9.

Tani K, Fujii H, Takegawa S *et al.* (1983) Two cases of phosphofructokinase deficiency associated with congenital hemolytic anaemia found in Japan. *American Journal of Hematology* 14: 165–79.

Valentin C, Pissard S, Martin J *et al.* (2000) Triose phosphate isomerase deficiency in three French families: two novel null alleles, a frameshift mutation (TPI Alfortville), and an alteration in the initiation codon (TPI Paris). *Blood* 96: 1130–5.

Vora S, Corash L, Engel WK *et al.* (1980) The molecular mechanisms of the inherited phosphofructokinase deficiency associated with haemolysis and myopathy. *Blood* 69: 629–35.

Vora S, DiMauro S, Spear D et al. (1987) Characterisation of the enzyme defect in late-onset muscle phosphofructokinase deficiency: new subtype of glycogen storage disease type 7. *Journal of Clinical Investigation* **80**: 1479–85.

Waterbury L, Frenkel EP (1972) Hereditary nonspherocytic haemolysis with erythrocyte phosphofructokinase deficiency. *Blood* **39**: 315–425.

Glucose-6-phosphate dehydrogenase deficiency

Reviews

Beutler E (1993) Study of glucose-6-phosphate dehydrogenase: history and molecular biology *American Journal of Hematology* **42**: 53–8.

Beutler E (1994) G6PD deficiency. *Blood* **84**: 3613–36.

Kwok CJ, Martin ACR, Au SWN et al. (2002) G6PDdb, an integrated database of glucose-6-phosphate dehydrogenase (G6PD) mutations. *Human Mutation* **19**: 217–24.

Mason, PJ (1996) New insights into G6PD deficiency [Annotation]. *British Journal of Haematology* **94**: 585–91.

Glucose-6-phosphate dehydrogenase deficiency, evolution and malaria

Cappadoro M, Giribaldi G, O'Brien E et al. (1998) Early phagocytosis of glucose-6-phosphate dehydrogenase (G6PD)-deficient erythrocytes parasitized by *Plasmodium falciparum* may explain malaria protection in G6PD deficiency. *Blood* **92**: 2527–34.

Ganczakowski M, Town M, Bowden DK et al. (1995) Multiple glucose 6-phosphate dehydrogenase-deficient variants correlate with malaria endemicity in the Vanuatu archipelago (southwestern Pacific). *American Journal of Human Genetics* **5**: 294–301.

Luzzatto L, Notaro R (2001) Malaria. Protecting against bad air. *Science* **293**: 442–3.

Luzzatto L, Usanga EA, Reddy S (1969) Glucose-6-phosphate dehydrogenase deficient red cells: resistance to infection by malarial parasites. *Science* **164**: 839–42.

Notaro R, Afolayan A, Luzzatto L (2000) Human mutations in glucose 6-phosphate dehydrogenase reflect evolutionary history. *FASEB J* **14**: 485–94.

Ruwende C, Khoo SC, Snow RW et al. Natural selection of hemi- and heterozygotes for G6PD deficiency in Africa by resistance to severe malaria. *Nature* **376**: 246–9.

Tishkoff, SA, Varkonyi R, Cahinhinan N et al. (2001) Haplotype diversity and linkage disequilibrium at human G6PD: recent origin of alleles that confer malarial resistance. *Science* **293**: 455–62.

Town M, Bautista JM, Mason PJ et al. (1992) Both mutations in G6PD A- are necessary to produce the G6PD deficient phenotype. *Human Molecular Genetics* **1**: 171–4.

Vulliamy TJ, Othman A, Town M et al. (1991) Polymorphic sites in the African population detected by sequence analysis of the glucose-6-phosphate dehydrogenase gene outline the evolution of the variants A and A⁻. *Proceedings of the National Academy of Sciences of the USA* **88**: 8568–71.

Glucose-6-phosphate dehydrogenase deficiency in newborn

Kappas A, Drummond GS, Valaes TA (2001) Single dose of Sn-mesoporphyrin prevents development of severe hyperbilirubine-mia in glucose-6-phosphate dehydrogenase-deficient newborns. *Pediatrics* **108**: 25–30.

Molecular pathology

Beutler E, Kuhl W, Gelbart T et al. (1991) DNA sequence abnormalities of human glucose-6-phosphate dehydrogenase variants. *Journal of Biological Chemistry* **266**: 4145–50.

Beutler E, Westwood B, Prchal JT et al. (1992) New glucose-6-phosphate dehydrogenase mutations from various ethnic groups. *Blood* **80**: 255–6.

Carson PE, Flanagan CL, Ickes CE et al. (1956) Enzymatic deficiency in primaquine-sensitive erythrocytes. *Science* **124**: 484–5.

Maeda M, Constantoulakis P, Chen C-S et al. (1992) Molecular abnormalities of a human glucose-6-phosphate dehydrogenase variant associated with undetectable enzyme activity and immunologically cross-reacting material. *American Journal of Human Genetics* **51**: 386–95.

MacDonald D, Town M, Mason P et al. (1991) Deficiency in red blood cells [Letter]. *Nature* **350**: 115.

PubMed ID: (2005)960.

PubMed ID: 1353664.

Stevens DJ, Wanachiwanawin W, Mason PJ et al. (1990) G6PD Canton: a common deficient variant in South East Asia caused by a 459 arg-to-leu mutation. *Nucleic Acids Research* **18**: 7190.

Vulliamy TJ, D'Urso M, Battistuzzi G et al. (1988) Diverse point mutations in the human glucose-6-phosphate dehydrogenase gene cause enzyme deficiency and mild or severe hemolytic anemia. *Proceedings of the National Academy of Sciences of the USA* **85**: 5171–5.

Vulliamy T, Beutler E, Luzzatto L (1993) Variants of glucose-6-phosphate dehydrogenase are due to missense mutations spread throughout the coding region of the gene. *Human Mutation* **2**: 159–67.

Susceptibility to infection

Costa E, Vasconcelos J, Santos E et al. (2002) Neutrophil dysfunction in a case of glucose-6-phosphate dehydrogenase deficiency. *Journal of Pediatric Hematology/Oncology* **24**: 164–5.

Mallouh AA, Abu-Osba YK (1987) Bacterial infections in children with glucose-6-phosphate dehydrogenase deficiency. *Journal of Pediatrics* **111**: 850–2.

Mamlok RJ, Mamlok V, Mills GC et al. (1987) Glucose-6-phosphate dehydrogenase deficiency, neutrophil dysfunction and *Chromobacterium violaceum* sepsis. *Journal of Pediatrics* **111**: 852–4.

van Bruggen R, Bautista JM, Petropoulou T et al. (2002) Deletion of leucine 61 in glucose-6-phosphate dehydrogenase leads to chronic nonspherocytic anemia, granulocyte dysfunction, and increased susceptibility to infections. *Blood* **100**: 1026–30.

Epidemiology

Kaeda JS, Chhotray GP, Ranjit MR et al. (1995) A new glucose-6-phosphate dehydrogenase variant, G6PD Orissa (44 ala-gly), is the major polymorphic variant in tribal populations in India. *American Journal of Human Genetics* **57**: 1335–41.

Assays

Beutler E (1984) *Red Cell Metabolism. A Manual of Biochemical Methods*, 2nd edn. Grune and Stratton, Orlando.

Beutler E, Blume KG, Kaplan JC *et al.* (1979) International Committee for Standardization in Haematology. Recommended screening test for glucose-6-phosphate (G-6-PD) dehydrogenase deficiency. *British Journal of Haematology* **43**: 465–7.

Roper D, Layton M, Lewis SM (2001) Investigation of the hereditary haemolytic anaemias: membrane and enzyme abnormalities. In: *Dacie and Lewis, Practical Haematology* (SM Lewis, BJ Bain, I Bates, eds), 9th edn, pp. 167–198. Churchill Livingstone, London.

World Health Organization Scientific Group (1967) Standardization of procedures for the study of glucose 6 phosphate dehydrogenase. WHO Tech Rep Ser 366.

World Health Organization Scientific Group on Glucose-6-Phosphate Dehydrogenase (1990) *Bulletin of the World Health Organization* **67**: 601–11.

Clinical

Raupp P, Hassan J Ali, Varughese M *et al.* (2001) Henna causes life threatening haemolysis in glucose-6-phosphate dehydrogenase deficiency. *Archives of Disease in Childhood* **85**: 411–12.

Pyrimidine 5′-nucleotidase deficiency

Bianchi P, Fermo E, Alfinito F *et al.* (2003) Molecular characterization of six unrelated Italian patients affected by pyrimidine 5-prime-nucleotidase deficiency. *British Journal of Haematology* **122**: 847–51.

McMahon JN, Lieberman JE, Gordon-Smith EC *et al.* (1981) Hereditary haemolytic anaemia due to red cell pyrimidine 5′-nucleotidase deficiency in two Irish families with a note on the benefit of splenectomy. *Clinical and Laboratory Haematology* **3**: 27–34.

Rees DC, Duley JA, Marinaki AM (2003) Pyrimidine 5′-nucelotidase deficiency. *British Journal of Haematology* **120**: 375–83.

Vives-Corrons JL (2000) Chronic non-spherocytic anaemia due to congenital pyrimidine 5′-nucleotidase deficiency: 25 years later. *Baillière's Best Practice and Research in Clinical Haematology* **13**: 103–18.

CHAPTER 10

Acquired haemolytic anaemias

10

Edward C Gordon-Smith and Judith CW Marsh

Introduction

Acquired haemolytic anaemias are usually divided into two main categories depending on the mechanism by which the premature destruction of red blood cells is produced. In the immune haemolytic anaemias, antibodies are the main agents of destruction. The non-immune-acquired haemolytic anaemias include diverse causes and mechanisms of haemolysis. In most anaemias, there is some shortening of the red cell survival, but in the haemolytic anaemias this shortening of red cell lifespan is the major cause of the anaemia and produces the classical features of haemolysis.

Immune haemolytic anaemias

Antibody-mediated haemolysis is an important cause of acquired haemolytic anaemia. Antibodies may be autoantibodies produced by the patient's own immune system and directed against epitopes of his/her own red cell antigens or they may be alloantibodies. Alloantibodies may be produced by the patient and directed against antigens not present on that person's own red cells, but either introduced as foreign red cell antigens by blood transfusion or are secondarily acquired by the patient's red cells, as in drug-induced haemolysis. Alloantibodies directed against the patient's red cell antigens might also be introduced from outside the patient, most notably from the mother in haemolytic disease of the newborn. A simple classification of immune haemolytic anaemias is given in Table 10.1. Typically, the immune haemolytic anaemias are distinguished from the non-immune by detecting antibody on the surface of the red cells by the direct antiglobulin test (DAT), also known as the Coombs test. The DAT is an essential investigation required

in identifying the cause in any case of acquired haemolytic anaemia.

Autoimmune haemolytic anaemia

The site and severity of red cell destruction depend on structural and functional characteristics of the antibody and efficiency of the mechanism of destruction. The degree of anaemia depends on the rate and acuteness of the destruction and the capacity of the bone marrow to compensate.

Antibody characteristics

Antibody characteristics that influence the site and intensity of red cell destruction in autoimmune haemolytic anaemia (AIHA) can be evaluated using the DAT. The thermal range of antibody binding also characterizes the antibody.

Immunoglobulin class

Monospecific antihuman globulin reagents for the DAT are routinely available for the detection of immunoglobulin G (IgG), IgM, IgA and for complement components C3c and C3d. Multispecific reagents are also available, as are reagents specific for IgG subclasses, but the latter are difficult to standardize and are not in routine use.

Warm-acting antibodies

Warm-acting antibodies are most active *in vitro* at 37°C. The antibodies are polyclonal, and IgG antibodies predominate. Where the specificity of the antibody can be determined, it is most commonly in the rhesus blood group complex. The most frequent patterns detected by the DAT on the red cell surface ar: IgG alone; IgG and complement; and complement alone. Antibodies may be detected in the serum at 37°C by the indirect antiglobulin test in about 50–60% of patients; this will rise

Table 10.1 Classification of immune haemolytic anaemias.

Autoimmune haemolytic anaemia	Warm antibody type	Primary – idiopathic	
		Secondary – associated with:	Autoimmune disease
			Lymphoproliferative disorders
			Infections
			Ovarian cysts
			Some cancers
			Drugs
	Cold antibody type	Cold haemagglutinin disease	
		Cold antibody syndromes associated with:	Infections
			Lymphoproliferative disorders
	Paroxysmal cold haemoglobinuria	Post viral	
		Syphilis	
Alloimmune haemolytic anaemia	Induced by red cell antigens	Haemolytic transfusion reactions	
		Haemolytic disease of the newborn	
		Post-stem cell allografts	
	Drug dependent	Antibody/macrophage mediated	
		Antibody/complement mediated	

to > 90% when the red cell membrane of the reagent cells is modified with papain or another proteolytic enzyme. Antibody may also be eluted from the red cell membrane in a majority of cases and the specificity determined. A subtype of warm AIHA has been defined in which both warm- and cold-type antibodies are found. Both tend to be lytic, and this 'mixed type' AIHA tends to produce severe haemolysis with an intravascular component. It is most commonly associated with systemic lupus erythematosus (SLE) or lymphoproliferative disease.

Cold-acting antibodies

Cold-acting antibodies are predominantly IgM and are most actively bound to antigen in the cold (4°C). Cold antibodies act as both agglutinins and lysins *in vitro*; the two functions may have different thermal ranges. The higher the titre and range of the lysin, the greater the propensity to produce haemolysis as well as agglutination. Cold agglutinin titres may reach very high levels (> 10^{24} at 4°C), but are not necessarily associated with active haemolysis. The IgM antibodies have specificity mainly for the I antigen, although 'i' specificity may be found in Epstein–Barr virus (EBV)-associated antibodies and some cases of lymphoproliferative disease. Rarely, anti-P activity is found. *In vitro*, the IgM antibodies elute off the red cell membrane, usually leaving bound complement to be detected by anti-C3d in the DAT. In cold haemagglutinin disease and most cases associated with lymphoproliferative disease, the cold antibodies are monoclonal. Those associated with infection are polyclonal.

The antibodies in paroxysmal cold haemoglobinuria (PCH) are IgG in type and bind to antigen below 20°C. When the temperature is raised to 37°C in the presence of complement, lysis occurs. This biphasic reaction is the basis of the Donath–Landsteiner reaction.

Complement activation

Autoantibodies against red cell antigens may activate complement on the red cell membrane. Antibody binding to two adjacent sites on the red cell membrane is required to activate the Cl complement component by the classical pathway. IgM molecules are pentameric and a single molecule can bind adjacent sites; IgG molecules will activate complement if they form a 'doublet': IgG1, IgG2 and IgG3 can activate complement, whereas IgG4 and IgA do not. In AIHA, complement activation usually stops at the C3 stage, where C3b is bound to the membrane and further proteolysed to form the inactive component C3d, which is detected by the appropriate DAT. Complement beyond the C3 stage may lead to the formation of the membrane attack complex and intravascular haemolysis. Autoimmune haemolytic anaemia due to IgG_2 alone is very rare, and that due to IgG4 or IgA alone is uncommon. It is interesting that in the rare case of IgA AIHA, complement does become activated on the cell surface. In general, when there is more than one class or subclass of antibody on the cell surface the haemolysis is more intense and may be intravascular.

Specificity of red cell autoantibodies

Warm-type autoimmune haemolytic anaemia
In most cases, the antibody detected in the patient's serum is pan reacting with all cells in a routine group O panel. Some 10–15%

of antibodies show specificity for rhesus antigens, particularly anti-e, anti-D or anti-c. A greater proportion show specificity by reacting with all cells except −/− Rh[null] cells. Other rare specificities against high-frequency antigens include anti-En[a], anti-Wr[b] or anti-U. Usually, autoantibodies show reactivity against a number of antigens and are not as specific as alloantibodies.

Cold-type autoimmune haemolytic anaemia

In cold agglutinin syndrome, anti-i specificity is usually seen. Occasionally, there is specificity for anti-I, and even more rarely for anti-Pr, anti-P, anti-M or anti-N, and even cold-reacting anti-A or anti-B. In PCH, the specificity is anti-P.

Effector mechanisms for immune red cell destruction *in vivo*

Two main effector mechanisms exist *in vivo*: (i) cell-mediated, predominantly extravascular, immune destruction and (ii) complement-mediated intravascular haemolysis.

Cell-mediated immune red cell destruction

Human macrophages and monocytes have cell-surface receptors for the Fc portion of IgG and for antigenic determinants present on activated C3. Cellular immune destruction is mediated through these receptors. Neutrophils and lymphocytes also have these receptors, but macrophages of the reticuloendothelial system within the spleen, liver and bone marrow are the main site of destruction *in vivo*.

Fc receptor mechanism

Macrophages have Fc receptors for IgG1, and IgG3 molecules, but not for IgG2, IgG4, IgM or IgA. Only IgG-coated red cells are destroyed in this way, but, in warm AIHA, this is clinically important, as 70–75% of autoantibodies are IgG. Phagocytosis and antibody-dependent cell-mediated cytotoxicity are the major Fc receptor-dependent modes of antibody-coated cell destruction.

The role of the spleen

The splenic vasculature is adapted to make the spleen an efficient filter for such particles as effete red cells, bacteria and immune complexes. As blood passes through the central arteries towards the red pulp, the branches of the central artery have a plasma-skimming effect, which raises the haematocrit of the blood within the central artery as they pass towards the splenic cords. There, red cells come into close contact with the splenic macrophages. The low plasma content and the relative lack of free plasma IgG molecules allow the red cell-bound IgG to interact preferentially with the macrophage Fc receptors, leading to phagocytosis of the coated red cells. When phagocytosis is partial, so that only portions of the cell membrane are removed, the remaining circulating red cell becomes spherocytic, although the somewhat rigid spherocytes may themselves be trapped in the splenic sinusoids and destroyed.

The spleen is thus most commonly the major site of red cell destruction when IgG alone is the main Fc binding protein on the red cell surface (see Chapter 21).

The role of the liver

Kupffer cells are macrophages that are present in the liver sinusoids and which express Fc receptors on their surface. The blood flow through the sinusoids is rapid compared with the spleen and there is no plasma-skimming effect. IgG-coated red cells are not preferentially destroyed in this situation, where there is competition for Fc receptors from circulating IgG. Here, red cell destruction is more dependent on cells being coated with C3.

C3 receptor mechanisms

Two types of C3 receptor have been identified on macrophages, CR_1 and CR_3. CR_1 is specific for an antigenic site in the C3c region of activated C3b which is not exposed on native C3. The breakdown product of C3b ($_iC3b$) is also a major ligand for the CR_1 receptor and is the only ligand for CR_3. Immune adherence of C3b-coated red cells to macrophages occurs mainly through the CR_1 receptor, whereas CR_3 receptor binding triggers phagocytosis. The largest concentration of C3b-binding macrophages is found in the liver sinusoids so that the liver becomes the major site for trapping and phagocytosing C3b-coated red cells. There is no competition for complement receptor sites from non-activated C3 in the plasma. If the spleen is very large, this too becomes an important site of cell destruction.

In cold AIHA, the IgM agglutinins bind most avidly to red cells in the peripheral circulation, where the temperature may be as low as 10–20°C. Complement activation occurs and leads to C3b and $_iC3d$ expression on the red cell membrane. Macrophage destruction of red cells is the main mechanism of haemolysis in IgM cold antibody-coated cells and also occurs in warm AIHA as a result of complement fixing IgG and IgM antibodies.

Complement-mediated intravascular haemolysis

Intravascular complement-mediated haemolysis is a minor mechanism for red cell destruction in most patients with AIHA. In a small proportion of patients, such a mechanism may predominate and produce severe intravascular haemolysis. Complement-induced intravascular haemolysis in warm AIHA is most likely to occur when more than one class or subclass of Ig is present on the red cell surface. Intravascular haemolysis has been reported with IgA-coated red cells, although the mechanism is obscure, as IgA does not itself fix complement.

In cold AIHA syndromes, intravascular haemolysis may be precipitated by exposure to cold. In such cases, lytic as well as agglutinating antibodies with a high thermal range may be demonstrated *in vitro*. This pattern is not uncommon in cold AIHA associated with *Mycoplasma pneumoniae*. Acute intravascular haemolysis is the usual presentation in paroxymal cold haemoglobinuria, where the antibody is IgG in type.

Other factors influencing red cell destruction and production

Bone marrow function

The ability of the marrow to increase erythropoiesis may be impaired. Autoantibodies may be produced, which act against reticulocytes and erythroblasts, as well as mature red cells. Red cell production may also be reduced by folate deficiency secondary to the increased demand. Lymphoproliferative diseases may impair production through infiltration of the marrow.

Reticuloendothelial function

The severity of cellular immune red cell destruction depends overall on macrophage function. Reticuloendothelial function may be reduced in SLE by the clearance of immune complexes, a process known as reticuloendothelial blockade. In methyldopa-induced AIHA, the drug has been shown to reduce reticuloendothelial clearance of IgG-coated red cells, which might explain why many patients with a strongly positive DAT due to methyldopa have little or no haemolysis.

Hypocomplementaemia

Partial protection from complement-mediated lysis may occur in patients with chronic cold haemagglutinin disease (CHAD), in which continuous complement activation may lead to relative complement deficiency. Hypocomplementaemia is common in SLE and may also be caused by chronic activation of the complement pathway. In addition, there is a strong association between SLE and the occurrence of null alleles for the C_2 and C_4 genes, which causes a genetically determined complement deficiency.

Warm-type autoimmune haemolytic anaemias

Clinical features

Presentation is variable and depends upon the speed with which anaemia develops, the capacity of the bone marrow to compensate and the effects of any associated disease. Most commonly, the onset is insidious, with the gradual awareness of symptoms of anaemia or the observation of pallor or icterus by friends or relatives. Occasionally, the onset is acute, with rapidly developing anaemia and, in older patients, the risk of heart failure. If there is an acute onset with intravascular haemolysis, haemoglobinuria may be noticed. Mild jaundice is present. More marked icterus (bilirubin > 90 μmol/L) suggests coexisting liver disease or biliary tract obstruction due to pigment gallstones or biliary sludge. Splenomegaly is common, but rarely at more than 2–3 cm below the costal margin at presentation. Marked splenomegaly suggests the possibility of a lymphoproliferative disease. The peripheral blood film is characterized

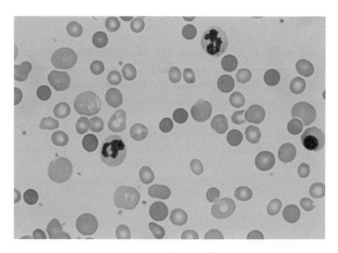

Figure 10.1 Warm autoimmune haemolytic anaemia. Blood film showing spherocytosis, polychromasia and nucleated red blood cell (×40).

by spherocytosis and polychromasia (Figure 10.1), circulating nucleated red cells, and, in some cases, red cell agglutination. Rarely, there may be reticulocytopenia associated with a positive DAT. There is a moderate increase in bilirubin, which is unconjugated, so bilirubin does not appear in the urine, which contains excess urobilinogen. There is an increase in lactate dehydrogenase (LDH) due to lysis of red cells, but other liver function tests are normal unless there is associated liver or biliary tract disease. The DAT is positive except in very rare cases where the amount of antibody remaining on the red cell surface is insufficient to be detected by the conventional DAT.

Idiopathic warm AIHA

In approximately 30% of patients with a DAT-positive haemolytic anaemia, no associated disorder is found. Idiopathic AIHA may occur at any age. There is a peak incidence during infancy and early childhood, a second rise during the third decade, with the majority of cases occurring after the fifth decade. There is a preponderance of female patients in both idiopathic and secondary AIHA. A careful drug history should always be taken to exclude drug-induced AIHA, and chemical exposure at work or in the domestic environment must be assessed. In girls, AIHA may precede clinical or immunological evidence of SLE, so that negative serology for SLE does not exclude that disease at a later date. As mentioned above, the presentation may vary from the gradual onset of anaemia to an acute haemolytic process. Systemic symptoms are rare other than those of anaemia. Pallor and jaundice are present. The spleen is nearly always enlarged, usually to between one and a half to five times its normal size. Enlargement to the umbilicus or below is not a feature of idiopathic AIHA and suggests a secondary AIHA.

Evans syndrome

A small subgroup of patients with idiopathic AIHA also have immune thrombocytopenia (ITP). The thrombocytopenia may coincide with the haemolysis or may arise as separate episodes. This is known as Evans's syndrome. The platelet and red cell antibodies are distinct and do not cross-react. The diagnosis is important because there appears to be a higher incidence of underlying illness such as immunodeficiency or autoimmune lymphoproliferative disease in children and SLE and T-cell lymphoma in adults. Management is as for warm AIHA or immune thrombocytopenic purpura (see Chapter 56) but patients with Evans's syndrome tend to be more resistant to initial therapy with prednisolone. Episodes of immune neutropenia or pancytopenia have also been described in association with a positive DAT.

Warm autoimmune haemolytic anaemia in infancy and childhood

AIHA of unknown cause occurs in infancy and in young children. In infancy, the onset is often acute and anaemia may be profound and difficult to control. The majority of cases in children are transient, although the onset may also be acute. It is interesting that in this group the sex difference is reversed, with more boys being affected. In childhood, the haemolytic episode is frequently precipitated by infection. IgG antibodies may be transferred from a mother with AIHA across the placenta to produce haemolysis in the newborn.

Warm autoimmune haemolytic anaemia associated with other autoimmune diseases

AIHA is often associated with SLE, especially in young women. Autoantibodies are usually IgG, and both IgG and C3d are found on the red cell surface. Occasionally, the DAT may be positive owing to immune complexes absorbed on to the red cell surface. The spleen is important for clearing such coated cells and splenectomy should be avoided if possible. Otherwise, treatment is as for idiopathic AIHA (see below). This condition is also described with other autoimmune, or presumed autoimmune, diseases notably rheumatoid arthritis, Sjögren's syndrome and ulcerative colitis; AIHA is also part of the spectrum of autoimmune diseases associated with agammaglobulinaemia.

Warm autoimmune haemolytic anaemia in lymphoproliferative diseases

The most common association is with B-cell chronic lymphocytic leukaemia (CLL), low-grade B-cell non-Hodgkin's lymphoma or Hodgkin's disease. The antibodies are polyclonal and have no distinct pattern of antibody type or specificity. The formation of antibodies in this group is thought to be due to immune dysregulation rather than direct production by the malignant clone. The AIHA may precede the diagnosis of lymphoma, sometimes by months or years. On other occasions, the presentations may be simultaneous or the AIHA may be delayed.

Warm autoimmune haemolytic anaemia due to drugs

Warm AIHA has most frequently been associated with methyldopa. Mefenamic acid, L-dopa and procainamide have also been reported to provoke this condition. About 20% of patients receiving methyldopa develop a positive DAT, but only 1–2% develop haemolytic anaemia. IgG is always present on the red cell surface, and antibodies usually show rhesus specificity, most commonly anti-e or anti-c. The other drugs are more likely to produce clinically important haemolysis. The mechanism by which AIHA is produced by exposure to drugs is not known. Alteration to the red cell membrane or modulation of the immune response by the drug have both been suggested. Treatment of patients with CLL with fludarabine and other purine analogues may provoke a very severe and life-threatening acute autoimmune haemolytic anaemia and, less commonly, other autoimmune cytopenias. The mechanism may be related to a decrease in autoregulatory T cells caused by treatment with fludarabine.

Warm autoimmune haemolytic anaemia and carcinoma

AIHA has been recorded with a number of malignancies, but it is not clear that there is a true association. It may be associated with ovarian cysts, with the cyst fluid containing the agglutinin. It has been suggested that there is also an association with ovarian carcinoma.

Warm autoimmune haemolytic anaemia and viral infections

In children, but rarely in adults, AIHA may follow a viral infection. Haemolysis is usually brisk but self-limiting. It is possible that the virus alters the red cell membrane, which provokes 'auto' antibodies against the altered antigens or that antiviral antibodies cross-react with membrane antigens. A third possibility is that immune complexes form between the virus and specific antibodies are secondarily absorbed onto the red cell surface, leading to immune destruction.

Treatment

Corticosteroids

First-line treatment of warm AIHA is with corticosteroids. The initial dose should be prednisolone 1–2 mg per kg of body weight per day. The dose may be given once daily if tolerated. A proton pump inhibitor or H$_2$ antagonist should be given at the same time as the steroids to reduce the risk of gastric erosions. High doses of corticosteroid should be continued for 10–14 days, according to response. In patients who respond, the dose should then be reduced steadily, down to one-half of the starting dose over the next 2 weeks and more gradually thereafter. In practice, the reduction in the dose is tailored to individual patients and their response. It is important not to stop the steroids too quickly and allow relapse. For patients who do not respond or who require unacceptably high doses of prednisolone to maintain a reasonable haemoglobin, other measures should be tried.

Cytotoxic immunosuppressive drugs

Azathioprine, 1.5–2.0 mg/kg per day, may be given to patients who respond poorly to prednisolone. On its own, azathioprine is mostly ineffective and is given for its steroid-sparing action. It should be continued for at least 3 months to assess its value, as response is not usually seen for 4–6 weeks. Cyclophosphamide 1.5–2.0 mg/kg per day may also be used in this way. It should be emphasized that there are no controlled trials to prove the worth of the use of these cytotoxic drugs and that their use is not without hazard, particularly bone marrow depression. Mycophenolate mofetil is an alternative immunosuppressive agent that is currently being assessed in refractory AIHA and ITP.

Cyclosporin

Oral cyclosporin has been used in steroid-resistant cases. No randomized clinical trials have been conducted but there are single case reports of success. A starting schedule of 5 mg/kg per day in two divided doses is appropriate. Close monitoring of renal and hepatic function is necessary and trough plasma levels of 100–200 mg/L must be maintained. The dose should be reduced if there is marked jaundice. Response may not be seen for 2–3 months.

Intravenous immunoglobulin

Intravenous immunoglobulin has been used in AIHA, particularly when IgG is the main component on the red cell surface. The dose used is the same as for ITP, 0.4 mg/kg per day for 4 5 days. AIHA responds less frequently to intravenous immunoglobulin than does ITP.

Splenectomy

Splenectomy is considered if there is no response to corticosteroids after 3 months' trial. Patients with predominantly IgG on the red cell surface respond best, and those with complement often respond poorly. Out of selected patients, about one-third achieve a complete remission and do not require steroids, one-third have a significantly reduced steroid requirement and the remainder show no or only transient response. There is no certain way to determine who will respond to splenectomy, although isotope studies may help in coming to a decision. The problems of splenectomy are dealt with in more detail in Chapter 8.

Monoclonal antibody therapy

The use of the monoclonal antibodies Campath-1H (anti-CD52) and rituximab (anti-CD20) for refractory AIHA is being explored at present for both warm and cold types of AIHA. Rituximab has produced remissions in some cases of warm AIHA but also in about 50% of patients with CHAD. Anecdotal success with Campath-1H in warm AIHA is also recorded. The success rate for AIHA does not seem to be as high as for ITP (rituximab) or immune neutropenia (Campath 1H).

Blood transfusion

Blood transfusion must be given if the clinical situation demands it, despite the impossibility of achieving a satisfactory cross-match in the presence of a positive DAT. The least incompatible, grouped blood should be used and transfused slowly. Some authors recommend the use of blood lacking antigens to which the autoantibodies react, but others point out that specificity is rarely absolute and that there is the risk of provoking an alloantibody response.

Prognosis

The prognosis in warm AIHA depends on a number of variables, including age, associated diseases and severity of haemolysis. In all patients, AIHA should be considered a serious and potentially life-threatening disease. Estimates of mortality of idiopathic AIHA in adults vary from 10% at 5 years to 40% at 7 years. The higher figures are mainly in patients aged over 50 years. Most deaths occur in the first 2 years after diagnosis. In children, mortality is much lower, probably about 5%, with the majority of patients recovering completely. Apart from death, AIHA may carry considerable morbidity, particularly from prolonged high-dose steroid therapy.

Cold-type autoimmune haemolytic anaemias

The clinical features of the cold haemagglutinin syndromes vary with the pathogenesis of the disorder. Serological tests are useful in identifying the cause and in determining treatment. The serological characteristics of the antibodies found in these syndromes are shown in Table 10.2.

Clinical features

Idiopathic cold haemagglutinin disease

Cold haemagglutinin disease is mainly seen in older people and runs a chronic course. Although the condition is mostly benign, the clinical features may be very distressing and disabling. Purplish skin discoloration, maximal over the extremities (acrocyanosis), may be present in cold weather. Acrocyanosis is due to stasis in the peripheral circulation secondary to red cell agglutination. On warming the skin, the colour returns to normal or there is transient erythema. This sequence distinguishes acrocyanosis from Raynaud's syndrome. Haemolysis is usually present and the patient may be mildly icteric. Occasionally, haemolysis dominates the clinical picture, depending on the ability of the antibody to activate complement on the red cell surface. The cold agglutinins are monoclonal IgM_K, but serum

Table 10.2 Serological characteristics of cold acting antibodies in the cold agglutinin syndromes.

Disorder		Specificity		
		Anti-I	Anti-i	Anti-P
Idiopathic (CHAD)		Mono IgMκ		Mono (rare)
Secondary to:	Lymphoproliferative disease	Mono IgMκ/λ (IgG)	Mono	
	Mycoplasma pneumoniae	Poly		
	Infectious mononucleosis	Poly	Poly	
Paroxysmal cold haemoglobinuria				Poly

Mono, monoclonal; poly, polyclonal.

electrophoresis may not reveal a monoclonal band because the concentration of the protein is too low. Cold haemagglutinin disease may be thought of as a pre-malignant B-cell disorder, which only presents clinically because of the specificity of the antibody for red cell surface antigens.

In the laboratory, spontaneous agglutination of red cells is frequently observed, both macroscopically and on the peripheral blood film if made at room temperature (Figure 10.2). Automated blood cell counters detect the agglutinates and record erroneously high mean corpuscular volume and low Hb values, unless the sample is tested at 37°C. The DAT shows only C3d on the red cell surface; IgM cold agglutinins are not detected because they elute from the cell surface *in vitro*.

Cold agglutinin syndromes and lymphoproliferative disorders

Occasionally, the cold agglutinin syndrome accompanies or precedes a B-cell lymphoma or CLL. In these cases, the antibody is monoclonal and is a product of the malignant clone. The serological specificity is either anti-I or anti-i. Haemolysis is often more troublesome than symptoms of agglutination. The prognosis is usually that of the underlying lymphoproliferative disease.

Cold agglutinin syndromes and infections

Haemolysis due to cold agglutinins may follow infections, almost always due to *M. pneumoniae*, or infectious mononucleosis. Rare cases following *Listeria* or *Toxoplasma* infections have been reported. The antibodies are mostly polyclonal IgM in type but occasional IgG cold antibodies are found. The antibodies develop in response to the infecting organism and cross-react with the red cell antigens. Haemolysis appears 2–3 weeks after the infection and is usually mild and self-limiting. Occasionally, very severe and even fatal acute intravascular haemolysis develops after *M. pneumoniae* infection. Blood transfusion through a blood warmer may be urgently required.

Treatment

General

Management of cold haemagglutinin syndromes is difficult. All patients should avoid exposure to cold, and electrically heated gloves and socks are available for use in winter. Wintering in a warm climate is a pleasant alternative. Folic acid supplements should be given to patients with chronic haemolysis.

Alkylating agents

Chlorambucil may be effective in reducing antibody production. Intermittent regimens such as 10 mg/day for 14 days every 4 weeks or continuous treatment of 2–4 mg/day are both effective. Long-term treatment carries the risk of marrow suppression and the development of myelodysplasia and acute myeloid leukaemia. Chlorambucil is most effective when there is an underlying B-cell neoplasm and may be less so in the idiopathic CHAD.

Corticosteroids

Corticosteroids are rarely of use in cold haemagglutinin

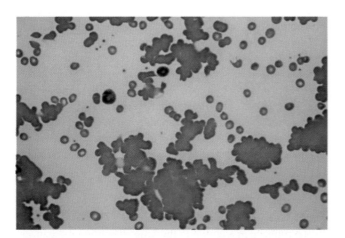

Figure 10.2 Cold haemagglutinin disease. Blood film showing gross haemagglutination (×20).

syndromes. They should be used only in exceptional circumstances when the antibodies are present in low titres and have a high thermal range. Their use should be avoided in other cases.

Splenectomy

Removal of the spleen is rarely of any use. The cells are coated with C3b and destruction occurs mainly in the liver.

Blood transfusion

Blood transfusions should be given with due regard to the difficulty in cross-matching in the presence of cold haemagglutinins. Blood should be given through an in-line blood warmer. The patient should be in a warm environment, preferably at 37°C. Special precautions are needed for surgical procedures to keep the patient warm.

Plasma exchange

The titre of cold agglutinin may be lowered temporarily by plasma exchange. The procedure may be useful in the control of severe symptoms.

Monoclonal antibody therapy

Both rituximab and Campath-1H monoclonal antibodies have been used anecdotally in the treatment of refractory cold-type AIHA. Rituximab is particularly appealing for idiopathic cold haemagglutinin disease and cold agglutinin syndromes with associated B-lymphoproliferative disorders because the antibody targets the CD20 molecule present on mature B-cells, which proliferate in low-grade lymphoproliferative disease, and are the precursors of autoantibody-producing plasma cells in autoimmune cytopenias associated with underlying malignancy as well as in idiopathic autoimmune cytopenia.

Paroxysmal cold haemoglobinuria

The rare syndrome usually occurs in children following acute viral infections. The original cases were described by Donath, Landsteiner and Ehrlich in congenital and tertiary syphilis but such cases are no longer encountered. A history of cold exposure is not always present and presentation is with sudden intravascular haemolysis, haemoglobinuria, abdominal pain, pallor and prostration.

The cold antibody is IgG, which is biphasic, reacting with red cells below 20°C in the peripheral circulation and causing lysis by complement activation as the red cells are warmed to 37°C in the central vessels. The antibody has specificity for the P antigen.

Treatment depends on keeping the patient warm, preferably at 37°C ambient temperature and giving transfusion, as required. The rare pp cells are not usually available and transfusion of ABO and rhesus compatible, P-positive blood should be given through a blood warmer.

Alloimmune haemolytic anaemia

Drug-induced immune haemolytic anaemia

Features and diagnosis

Immune haemolytic anaemia produced by drugs is rare but, in some cases, it may be very severe and even life-threatening. There are three main mechanisms by which red cell destruction is increased by antibodies bound to the red cell surface. Autoimmune haemolytic anaemia induced by methyldopa has been described in the previous section. Immune antibodies which require the presence of the drug to produce a positive DAT may react with red cells when the drug is bound to the red cell surface (drug adsorption mechanism) or when immune complexes are produced between the drug and the antibody, which is absorbed on to the red cell surface where complement is fixed and activated, leading to acute intravascular haemolysis.

The diagnosis of drug-induced immune haemolytic anaemia should be made in three stages: (i) diagnosis of a DAT-positive haemolytic anaemia; (ii) careful drug history; and (iii) serological demonstration of drug-specific antibody, which interacts with red cells.

Pathogenesis

Drug adsorption (hapten) mechanism

Penicillin is the prototype drug, although cephalosporins and other penicillin derivatives have also been implicated. Drugs in this group readily form hapten–carrier complexes with plasma proteins, which enhance drug-specific antibody production. It has been estimated that 90% of individuals receiving penicillin produce clinically insignificant IgM antipenicillin antibodies. When high-dose intravenous penicillin is administered, the drug is absorbed on to the red cell surface, where it becomes non-specifically attached to red cell surface proteins. A minority of patients on high-dose intravenous penicillin therapy (> 1 Mu daily) develop high-titre IgG antipenicillin antibodies that attach to the drug bound to the red cell surface and cause predominantly extravascular haemolysis. The clinical picture is usually of mild to moderate haemolysis but, if it is unrecognized, so that large doses of the drug are continued in the presence of increasing antibody levels, complement fixation and acute intravascular haemolysis may occur. The DAT becomes positive after some weeks of treatment and is due to IgG only on the red cell surface. When the drug is stopped, the DAT rapidly becomes negative and haemolysis stops. Antibody in the patient's serum or eluate from the red cells will react with normal red cells only in the presence of the drug. The clinical and serological features are shown in Table 10.3.

Membrane modification mechanism

Cephalosporin, in addition to the drug absorption mechanism, can cause a positive DAT by modifying red cell membrane components. Cisplatin and carboplatin have also been reported

Table 10.3 Drug-induced immune haemolytic anaemias: clinical and serological features.

	Drug absorption	Mechanism	
		Immune complex	Autoimmune
Examples	Penicillin	Many Few cases each	Methyldopa Mefenamic acid
Dose/duration	Large therapeutic doses Prolonged	Very low dose Short	Usually about 6 weeks
Haemolysis	Extravascular Subacute	Intravascular Acute	Extravascular Minimal/subacute
DAGT	IgG or IgG + C′	C′ only	IgG only
Serum antibody reaction	To drug-treated cells	Reacts only in presence of drug or metabolite	To normal red cells
Eluate reaction	To drug-treated cells	Non-reactive	To normal red cells

to cause immune haemolytic anaemia by this mechanism. As a result, a variety of plasma proteins, including immunoglobulin and complement, may attach through a non-immune mechanism to the red cell membrane. This may result in the finding of a positive DAT but rarely causes immune haemolytic anaemia.

Immune complex innocent bystander mechanism

Several drugs have been reported to cause immune haemolytic anaemia by this mechanism. Those most frequently reported are rifampicin, phenacetin, quinine, quinidine, nomifensine, hydrochlorothiazide and chlorpropramide and, more recently, intravenous cephalosporins and diclofenac (see below). Hapten–carrier complexes are formed between these drugs and plasma proteins, leading to the production of drug-specific antibodies. Once drug antibodies are present, reintroduction of the drug causes immune complexes to form, which are absorbed on to the red cell membrane and complement is activated.

Classically, haemolysis occurs on the second or subsequent exposure to the drug and may develop within minutes or hours of drug ingestion. Severe intravascular haemolysis may occur with fever, rigors or nausea and, in extreme cases, acute renal failure. Several groups have reported fatal immune haemolysis with the third-generation cephalosporin ceftriaxone, and cefotaxime and ceftazidime have also been reported to cause immune haemolytic anaemia. Second-generation cephalosporins have also been implicated, although there are fewer reports with them than with third-generation antibiotics. Diclofenac can also cause an immune haemolytic anaemia with intravascular haemolysis, and this is thought to be mediated by both immune complex and drug adsorption mechanisms.

Autoimmune mechanism

Methyldopa is the paradigm drug in autoimmune drug-induced haemolytic anaemia. Typically, the DAT becomes positive about

6 weeks after the drug is started and is strongly positive due to IgG on the red cell surface. Haemolysis is usually absent or trivial, although this is not true with some other drugs that produce haemolysis by this route, notably mefenamic acid (Ponstan®). The antibodies usually show no Rh specificity when tested against Rh_{null} cells. It should be noted that some drugs may produce haemolysis by both the immune complex and autoimmune mechanisms, depending on the circumstances.

Serological diagnosis of drug-induced haemolytic anaemia

Drug absorption and membrane modification mechanisms

The DAT is usually positive with IgG1, or IgG and C3 on the red cell surface. The red cell eluate and serum do not react against normal or enzyme-modified red cells. Warm-reacting drug-specific antibody in the eluate and serum is only detected after preincubation of the test red cells with the appropriate drug.

Immune complex mechanism

The DAT is usually positive but may be negative if performed immediately after a brisk 'episode' of haemolysis. The red cell eluate is not reactive even in the presence of the drug. The drug-specific antibody is best detected by preincubating the patient's serum with the drug in solution to allow immune complexes to form. The preincubated serum is then tested against normal and enzyme-modified groups of cells in the presence of fresh complement. In some cases (e.g. nomifensine), the antibodies may be specific for metabolites rather than for the parent drug. Drug metabolite antibodies may be detected by preincubating drug metabolite obtained from the serum or urine of a volunteer (who has taken the drug) with the patient's serum. A simplified summary of the serological investigation of a patient with suspected drug-induced immune haemolysis is shown in Table 10.3.

Table 10.4 Non-immune acquired haemolytic anaemias.

Cause	Examples	Mechanisms
Infections	Falciparum malaria	Intracellular organisms
	Babesiosis	
	Bartonella	
	Meningococcal sepsis	Endotoxin-induced DIC
	Pneumococcal sepsis	
	Gram-negative sepsis	
	Atypical mycobacterial infections	Haemophagocytic syndromes
	Viruses	
	Clostridium perfringens	Enzyme toxins
	Snake, spider bites	
Chemical and physical agents	Drugs	Oxidative damage
	Industrial/domestic substances	
	Burns	Heat, osmotic lysis (freshwater)
	Drowning	
	Lead poisoning	Dehydration of RBC (salt)
	Copper (Wilson's disease)	Enzyme inhibition
Fragmentation (mechanical) haemolysis	Cardiac haemolysis	Lysis on prosthetic surfaces
	Microangiopathic haemolytic anaemia (MAHA)	Vasculitis, endothelial cell swelling, fibrin shear
	March haemoglobinuria	
Acquired membrane disorders	Liver disease	Lipid/cholesterol changes
	Paroxysmal nocturnal haemoglobinuria	Somatic mutation

The non-immune acquired haemolytic anaemias

Haemolysis and haemolytic anaemia may be the consequence of a wide variety of acquired conditions that do not lend themselves to a precise and logical classification. Classification tends to be based on causes rather than mechanisms, although there are some common pathogenetic mechanisms that lead to red cell destruction. The main groups of agents causing haemolysis are infections, vascular disorders (mechanical disorders), chemical and physical agents, and disorders affecting the red cell membrane. A classification is shown in Table 10.4.

Infections causing haemolytic anaemia

A variety of infections may produce haemolysis through several different pathways. Haemolysis may be a consequence of direct invasion of the red cell by a micro-organism or may arise from alterations in the microcirculation, leading to mechanical haemolysis. The intracellular organisms tend to produce the more severe haemolysis.

Malaria

Some degree of haemolysis is seen in all types of malarial infection, but the most severe abnormalities are found in *Plasmodium falciparum* infection. *P. falciparum* infection is one of the most common causes of anaemia in the world. Many factors may contribute to the anaemia, including marrow suppression, dyserythropoiesis, folate deficiency, hypersplenism and red cell sequestration, as well as haemolysis. The condition has two main components: extravascular destruction of parasitized cells in the reticuloendothelial system, particularly the spleen, and intravascular lysis when the sporozoites break out of the red cells in the circulation. In most patients, the systemic symptoms of malaria dominate the clinical picture but, occasionally, acute intravascular haemolysis is the presenting emergency problem. Haemolysis in malaria is often associated with a positive Coombs test.

Blackwater fever

Acute intravascular haemolysis leading to the passing of black or dark-red urine is an uncommon but well described and feared complication of falciparum malaria. The syndrome usually occurs after a few days of typical malaria fever. The appearance of black urine is usually accompanied by further fever and often back pain in the renal angle. Oliguric renal failure may ensue, particularly if the patient becomes hypotensive and hypovolaemic from dehydration. Pulmonary and cerebral symptoms may develop. The condition was first described in white people, most of whom had been treated with quinine, and the importance of this association was stressed. However, the condition is seen in all populations in endemic areas and certainly does not seem to be confined to non-immune individuals. In these indigenous populations, glucose-6-phosphate dehydrogenase (G6PD) deficiency may play a part in the pathogenesis as well as quinine exposure. The spread of chloroquine-resistant malaria in the Far East has led to an increased use of quinine and an increase in the incidence of blackwater fever.

The degree of parasitaemia is very variable. In about one-half of the cases the parasite count may be high, whereas in others the count may be low, perhaps because of the intense intravascular haemolysis. The red cell count may fall to 1×10^{12}/L within 24 h of the start of the haemoglobinuria. There is usually a rise in fibrin degradation products in the serum, but this rise is not often marked and is compatible with a degree of renal failure. Intravascular coagulation does not seem to play a major role in pathogenesis.

Immediate treatment is directed towards correction of the fluid and electrolyte loss, counteracting the anaemia, and eradication of the parasite. Renal dialysis may be required and may have to be continued for 1 month or more before renal function returns. Subsequent attacks of falciparum malaria are likely to produce further episodes of blackwater fever in susceptible individuals, so scrupulous prophylaxis should be followed.

Babesiosis

Infection with the intracellular protozoan *Babesia* is uncommon and symptomatic disease is mostly confined to splenectomized patients, at least in the European variety. *Babesia* is a tick-borne organism, the tick in Europe being *Ixodes vicinus*, associated with cattle, and in America, *Ixodes dammini*, carried by rodents and deer.

In splenectomized patients, the disease has an acute onset and is often fatal. There is a 1- to 3-day period of malaise, sometimes with vomiting and diarrhoea, followed by high fever, rigors, jaundice, acute intravascular haemolysis, haemoglobinuria, renal failure and death. In North America, unsplenectomized patients may experience a milder self-limiting disease, although intravascular haemolysis does occur.

The diagnosis is made from the peripheral blood film, where the parasites, looking very similar to *P. falciparum*, are seen in the red cells. There may be a history of tick bite or of exposure to potential vectors. Treatment is difficult. Clindamycin may be effective and imidocarb diproprionate, a drug used in veterinary practice, 0.6 mg/kg i.m. 12-hourly for four doses, proved effective in one desperate case. Exchange transfusion and renal support may be required in severely affected patients.

Bartonella (Oroya fever)

Infection with *Bartonella bacilliformis* is found only in the western Andes of Peru and neighbouring countries. The diagnosis is made from the peripheral blood film. The organism is an intracellular, Gram-negative rod during the acute attack, becoming coccoid in recovery. In non-immune individuals, there may be intense haemolysis, partly intravascular, partly through erythrophagocytosis. The organism is rapidly killed by chloramphenicol, tetracyclines, penicillin or aminoglycosides.

Clostridium perfringens

Clostridium perfringens septicaemia causes an intense intravascular haemolysis with prominent microspherocytosis. The spherocytosis is the result of membrane destruction by lipases and proteases produced by the organism. Although the organism is sensitive to a variety of antibiotics, the appearance of intravascular haemolysis is usually a harbinger of death because of the toxaemia.

Toxoplasmosis

Infection with *Toxoplasma gondii* acquired *in utero* may produce haemolysis and a syndrome similar to haemolytic disease of the newborn. In adults, toxoplasmosis is not associated with haemolysis, except perhaps in the immunocompromised host.

Bacterial infections

Intravascular coagulation produced by bacterial infection may be accompanied by some degree of intravascular haemolysis with fragmentation of red cells. Septicaemia from meningococcal or pneumococcal infection may show evidence of haemolysis, but such features are not clinically significant compared with the other effects of the septicaemia.

Haemorrhagic fevers

Haemorrhagic fevers may be accompanied by haemolysis. Dengue fever is widespread in many parts of the world and may cause intravascular haemolysis. Other haemorrhagic fevers, for example, yellow fever and West African haemorrhagic fevers, may also produce haemolysis.

Haemophagocytic syndrome

The haemophagocytic syndrome (HPS) is characterized by proliferation of macrophages in the bone marrow, spleen, liver and lymph nodes, with inappropriate phagocytosis of erythroid precursors, granulocytes and platelets. In some variations, the skin may be involved. It may occur in severe systemic infections such as cytomegalovirus (CMV), fungal infection and tuberculosis. Clinically, the patient presents with persistent fever, pancytopenia, jaundice and evidence of liver dysfunction, often with a coagulopathy. The manifestations may be acute or subacute, with the patient exhibiting severe malaise, weight loss and rapidly developing pancytopenia. The jaundice in part is the result of the destruction of red cells and their precursors in the marrow, spleen or liver, usually associated with a marked rise in lactic dehydrogenase. There is an acute-phase response, with elevated serum ferritin levels and increases in interferon-γ and tumour necrosis factor α with variable changes in other cytokines. The syndrome seems to associated with an abnormal T-cell activation, which triggers the macrophage response and which may be the consequence of a T-cell lymphoma or may be unmasked by a variety of infections. The two main subdivisions of the syndrome are infection-associated HPS (IAHPS) and malignant HPS (MHPS). Clinically, the distinction may be very difficult because in the lymphomas the proliferation may be trivial, the syndrome being derived from the release of cytokines, and, in MHPS, superadded infection is common. Likewise, in IAHPS it may be impossible to identify the underlying infection. In children, IAHPS seems to be more common, whereas, in adults, the majority of cases are associated with lymphoma.

Fragmentation haemolysis – mechanical haemolytic anaemias

The relationship between the vascular endothelium, the cellular elements of the blood and the mechanisms of haemostasis and fibrinolysis is clearly intricate and complex. The integrity of the red blood cell may be destroyed by contact with abnormal endothelial surfaces, although not all abnormalities of vessels cause haemolysis. It may be that some adherence between the red cell and the abnormal vessel wall is necessary for fragmentation of the red cell to occur, and that this usually happens in the context of abnormal flow as well as an altered endothelium. The situations in which fragmentation haemolysis may occur are the presence of prosthetic material and altered flow following cardiovascular surgery, the trapping or adherence of red cells in arteriovenous malformations, and the destruction of red cells

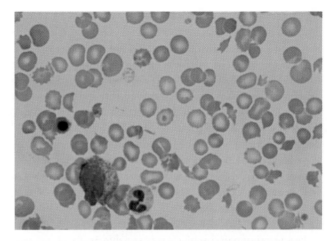

Figure 10.3 Microangiopathic haemolytic anaemia. Blood film from a patient with carcinoma and bone marrow metastases. Note fragmentation of red cells, leucoerythroblastic changes with nucleated red cell and metamyelocyte and low platelets suggesting possible DIC (×40).

in pathologically altered small blood vessels (microangiopathic haemolytic anaemia).

The characteristic features of fragmentation haemolysis are the appearance of the blood film (Figure 10.3) and the presence of intravascular haemolysis. Depending on the underlying vascular pathology, there may be a reduction in the platelet count and evidence of disseminated intravascular coagulation (DIC). The rate of red cell destruction also varies according to the pathogenesis, so the signs of intravascular haemolysis vary from absence of haptoglobin, elevated LDH and minimal haemosideriuria, to acute intravascular destruction with haemoglobinaemia and haemoglobinuria. The major causes of fragmentation haemolysis are shown in Table 10.5.

Vascular origin	Pathogenesis	Platelets
Cardiac haemolysis	Prosthetic heart valves	Normal
	Patches, grafts	
	Paraprosthetic or perivalvular leaks	
Arteriovenous malformations	Kasabach–Merritt syndrome	Very low
	Malignant haemangioendotheliomas	
Microangiopathic	TTP-HUS	Low
	Malignant disease	Normal/low
	Vasculitis	Normal/low
	Pre-eclampsia, HELLP	Low
	Renal vascular disorders	Normal/low
	Disseminated intravascular coagulation	Low

Table 10.5 Mechanical anaemias – fragmentation haemolysis: classification.

TTP, thrombotic thrombocytopenic purpura; HUS, haemolytic uraemic syndrome; HELLP, haemolysis with elevated liver function tests and low platelets.

Cardiac haemolytic anaemia

This syndrome was so called because it mainly occurred after cardiac surgery in which prosthetic valves, patches or grafts were inserted. Haemolysis usually becomes significant only when there is turbulent flow that brings the circulating red cells into intimate contact with the prosthetic material. There are certain situations in which the haemolysis may be of considerable clinical importance.

Periprosthetic or perivalvular leaks

If after insertion of a prosthesis or repair of a heart valve a leak occurs around the valve or through a suture track, there may be severe intravascular haemolysis without any evidence of haemodynamic distress. A difficulty may be that fragmentation of red cells is not always prominent, although spherocytes may be present. However, once autoimmune haemolysis is ruled out, the diagnosis can scarcely be anything other than cardiac haemolysis in a patient who has had cardiac surgery. The haemolysis can be cured only by further surgery.

Ambulatory haemolysis

A patient who has undergone valve replacement may show only slight evidence of haemolysis while in hospital but produce significant anaemia after discharge. This is thought to occur because the higher cardiac output associated with the greater exercise as an outpatient produces more turbulence and hence greater opportunity for red cell fragmentation. A similar mechanism is thought to operate if the patient becomes iron deficient as a result of chronic intravascular haemolysis. Iron replacement and advice about the level of exercise may prevent or delay the need for further surgery.

Cardiopulmonary post-perfusion syndrome

Acute intravascular haemolysis may occur in patients who have undergone cardiopulmonary bypass surgery. The haemolysis may be accompanied by neutropenia and pulmonary distress. The syndrome does not strictly belong in this section, as the haemolysis seems to be caused by complement activation and binding of the membrane attack complex to the red cell surface. The blood film shows ghost red cells rather than fragmentation. The condition is self-limiting and the patient requires only supportive care.

Arteriovenous malformation

Fragmentation of red cells may be seen in the Kasabach–Merritt syndrome, in which platelets are trapped in the vascular network of giant arteriovenous malformations, sometimes with evidence of a consumption coagulopathy. The bleeding disorder is of greater significance than the haemolysis in these patients. A similar picture, usually with clear evidence of a consumptive coagulopathy with evidence of DIC, may be seen in malignant haemangio-endothelioma, in which the tumour tends to invade and grow along veins.

Microangiopathic haemolytic anaemias

This term is used to describe intravascular haemolysis with fragmentation of red cells caused by their destruction in an abnormal microcirculation. Proof of microangiopathy may be lacking in those not subjected to a post-mortem, and MAHA should be considered a clinical syndrome. The three main pathological lesions that give rise to microangiopathic haemolytic anaemias (MAHA) are deposition of fibrin strands, often associated with DIC; platelet adherence and aggregation; and vasculitis. The vessel abnormalities may be generalized or confined to particular sites or organs. In most cases, the haemolysis is of less consequence than the underlying cause of the microangiopathy, but the fragmentation of red cells may be important in pointing to the diagnosis. Some of the disorders producing MAHA are given in Table 10.6. Only well-defined clinical syndromes will be described here in detail.

Microangiopathic haemolytic anaemia and malignant disease

Fragmentation of red cells with chronic intravascular haemolysis may occur in malignant disease. Clinically significant anaemia may occur, especially when there is invasion of the tumour into a large blood vessel (as in haemangiopericytoma), but, more commonly, the haemolysis is trivial or well compensated. The fragmentation may simply be noted on the blood film. A blood film that shows evidence of MAHA together with leuco-erythroblastic changes is virtually diagnostic of malignant disease with secondary deposits in the bone marrow (Figure 10.3). Mucin-secreting tumours are most likely to produce MAHA.

In acute leukaemia, particularly, but not exclusively, promyelocytic (M3), there may be intense intravascular coagulation that may be accompanied by MAHA. The coagulation changes dominate the clinical picture.

Microangiopathic haemolytic anaemia and infection

Infections, particularly septicaemia, may provoke intravascular coagulation and MAHA. Generally, the coagulation changes and septic shock overshadow the mild fragmentation but, occasionally, infections produce a chronic state of partially compensated intravascular and marked red cell fragmentation.

Thrombotic thrombocytopenic purpura

Thrombotic thrombocytopenic purpura (TTP) (see also Chapter 52) is an acute syndrome characterized by fever, neurological signs, haemolytic anaemia with fragmented red cells and thrombocytopenia. Mild proteinuria is common but major renal impairment is less usual. Two main categories exist: congenital and acquired. The underlying pathological process is of abnormal platelet aggregation in small blood vessels. The congenital TTP is mainly due to mutations in the gene *ADAMTS 13*, which encodes for a metalloprotease of the ADAMTS family, which specifically degrades von Willebrand factor (vWF). The mutations lead to deficiency of the protease ADAMTS 13, persistence

Disease	Microangiography
Haemolytic-uraemic syndrome	Endothelial cell swelling, microthrombi in renal vessels
Thrombotic thrombocytopenic purpura	Platelet plugs, micro-aneurysms, small vessel thrombi
Renal cortical necrosis	Necrotizing arteritis
Acute glomerular nephritis	
Malignant hypertension	
Pre-eclampsia	Fibrinoid necrosis
HELLP	
Polyarteritic nodosa	Vasculitis
Wegener's granulomatosis	
Systemic lupus erythematosus	
Homograft rejection	Microthrombi in transplanted organ
Mitomycin C	Uncertain
Cyclosporin	Renal vessel anomalies
Carcinomatosis	Abnormal tumour vessels, intravascular coagulation, disseminated or localized
Primary pulmonary hypertension	Abnormal vasculature
Cavernous haemangioma(Kasabach-Merritt)	Local vascular changes, thrombosis

Table 10.6 Causes of microangiopathic haemolytic anaemia.

HELLP, haemolysis with elevated liver function tests and low platelets.

of unusually large vWF (ULvWF) multimers, which, in turn, can induce platelet aggregation and the formation of platelet VWF plugs in small blood vessels. The acquired form, which is also associated with low levels of ADAMTS 13, is the result of the formation of autoantibodies to the metalloproteinase. Although the association of ADAMTS 13 deficiency with TTP has clarified much of the pathogenesis, it should be remembered that not all cases show this association and other pathways will certainly be described.

Epidemiology
TTP is a rare condition. In the USA the incidence is about 3–4 cases per million. Acquired cases are much more common than congenital. Affected families may be found with autosomal recessive inheritance. The acquired disease has the age and sex distribution seen in most antibody-mediated autoimmune diseases. Women are more frequently affected than men; the disease may occur at any age but is more common between 20 and 50 years. The female preponderance is enhanced by the association of TTP with pregnancy. The most common course is of a single episode, which may be fatal but relapsing and chronic subacute forms exist, particularly, but not exclusively, in the familial or congenital cases.

Clinical features
The typical presentation is of an acute illness presenting with neurological signs, fever and a blood film showing fragmented red cells and thrombocytopenia. Frequently, the presentation is not typical but more insidious, with episodes of headache, personality change or vague neurological disturbances. These disturbances may be sensory or motor deficits, seizures or even coma. Often the neurological signs fluctuate considerably. Renal impairment is demonstrated by proteinuria but frank renal failure is not a feature at presentation.

Gastrointestinal involvement may present as diarrhoea. Pallor and icterus may indicate haemolysis but frank haemorrhagic signs are rare. Chest pain due to cardiac ischaemia may occur.

Laboratory findings
The diagnosis is made on the basis of the clinical presentation and the evidence for haemolytic anaemia with fragmented red cells and thrombocytopenia. Bilirubin is elevated, as is the serum LDH, indicating intravascular haemolysis. LDH is a useful marker for measuring the activity of the microangiopathic process. Coagulation abnormalities are not a consistent feature, in contrast to MAHA associated with DIC. The presence of ULvWF may be demonstrated at presentation. More specific diagnosis showing ADAMTS deficiency and or autoantibodies requires specialist laboratories. At post-mortem, platelet plugs and fibrin plugs may be found in capillaries (Figure 10.4a and b). The pathophysiology is discussed further in Chapter 52.

Treatment
Plasmapheresis
Until the introduction of repeated plasmapheresis, the mortality of TTP was about 80%, death usually being caused by myocardial

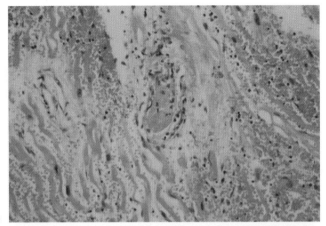

(a)

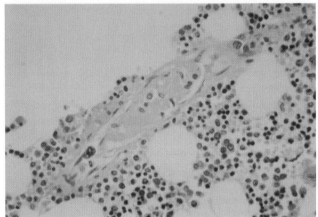

(b)

Figure 10.4 Thrombotic thrombocytopenic purpura. Microthrombi in capillaries. (a) Section from the myocardium; (b) thrombus in a bone marrow capillary (haemotoxylin and eosin, ×100) (courtesy of Dr Margaret Burke).

infarction (Figure 10.4). Removal of antibody in the patient's plasma and replacement of the metalloproteinase by fresh-frozen plasma has reduced the mortality to less than 15%. Presentation in coma or a very low platelet count is a poor prognostic sign. Treatment should be started with plasmapheresis as an emergency as soon as the diagnosis is made. The initial procedure for an adult aims for a 1 to 1.5 plasma volume exchange. Replacement fluid is mainly virally inactivated fresh-frozen plasma, with cryosupernatant being preferred or added in some centres as it lacks the highest vWF multimers. As very large volumes of plasma are used virally inactivated product should be used where possible. The plasmapheresis needs to be repeated daily for up to 20 days and sometimes longer. Treatment effect is monitored by examination of the blood film for fragments, by platelet count and LDH. Remission is judged to have occurred when the platelet count is within the normal range for three successive days and the LDH is normal. Plasmapheresis may then

be reduced in frequency, but relapse is not uncommon if it is stopped early.

Plasma infusion
Infusion of FFP alone may achieve remission in congenital cases with primary deficiency of ADAMTS 13 but is not as effective as plasma exchange in acquired disease.

Immunosuppression
During the acute management, corticosteroids are not usually of benefit, and indeed there is little evidence from randomized trials of their efficacy at any time. However, they may have a role in resistant or relapsing disease. Likewise, vincristine has been advocated in resistant cases. It should be noted that there are overlaps between TTP, ITP and the antiphospholipid syndrome, which make the use of such measures reasonable in some cases. Cyclosporin may have a place in maintaining remission in chronically relapsing disease.

Antibiotics
Many cases present with features suggesting infection and infections may precipitate relapse. The possibility of occult infection, particularly a Gram-negative urinary tract infection, should be considered and appropriate antibiotics given if there is a suspicion of infection. Plasma exchange itself provides a portal for infection and antibiotics, including Gram-positive cover, administered if fever returns during treatment.

Splenectomy
Splenectomy has been used for many years in resistant cases, but there are no proper studies to support this. However, stable long-term remissions may be achieved in some patients with both resistant and relapsed disease.

Antiplatelet and antithrombotic treatment
Aspirin and dipyridamole are both used in conjunction with plasma exchange in many series. There is some soft evidence to support their use. Clopidogrel and ticlopidine have each been associated with promoting TTP and so are not recommended. Defibrotide is an antithrombotic agent of unknown action which has been used with some success in refractory cases, but it is not a licensed treatment.

Haemolytic uraemic syndrome
Haemolytic uraemic syndrome (HUS) has some of the features of TTP, but the kidney is the main organ targeted rather than the CNS. Some cases may be associated with ADAMTS 13 deficiency but the majority are not. Infants, young children and the elderly are mainly afflicted. HUS may be caused by infection with *Escherichia coli* O157, a strain that produces a verotoxin. Haemolysis is less marked than in TTP, and coagulation abnormalities are more prominent. The role of plasma exchange in

management is less certain. The syndrome is discussed further in Chapter 52.

March haemoglobinuria

Haemoglobinuria following running has been documented for about 100 years. Its origin is mechanical, with destruction of red cells occurring in the feet. It can be cured by wearing soft shoes or running on soft ground. The disorder may arise in joggers and is benign except that it may lead to extensive invasive investigations unless recognized. The blood film does not show any red cell fragmentation or consistent abnormality. Occasionally, haemoglobinuria after running is accompanied by nausea, abdominal cramps and aching legs, and enthusiastic athletes with this condition may exhibit mild splenomegaly and jaundice.

Chemical and physical agents

Oxidative haemolysis

Oxidative substances may cause haemolysis in people with normal red cell metabolism and normal HbA if the oxidative stimulus is large enough. The major causes of oxidative haemolysis in normal subjects are shown in Table 10.7. The clinical features of this condition are dependent on the main sites of oxidative attack, whether on the membrane of the red cell, the globin chains or the haem group.

Chronic intravascular haemolysis with Heinz bodies

Dapsone and Salazopyrin (salicylazosulphapyridine) will cause oxidative intravascular haemolysis in normal subjects if taken in high enough dosage. Red cells show the 'bite' abnormality of the chemically damaged cell (Figure 10.5). Heinz bodies may be absent or scanty in patients with an intact spleen. Dapsone is used in the treatment of G6PD-deficient subjects with leprosy and in the treatment of dermatitis herpetiformis, in which functional hyposplenism occurs; Heinz bodies appear in the latter case, acute intravascular haemolysis in the former.

Haemosiderinuria may be detected in patients taking these drugs, and there may be polychromasia and macrocytosis. Haemolysis is usually well compensated and there is no need to

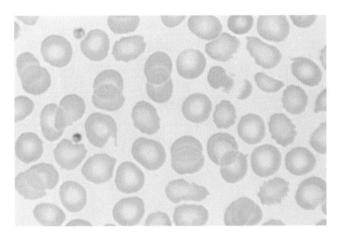

Figure 10.5 Oxidative haemolysis caused by drug (phenacetin). Note red cells with contracted haemoglobin.

stop the treatment unless the anaemia is severe. A dose reduction may sometimes be needed.

Methaemoglobinaemia is uncommon unless the patient is partially deficient in NADH methaemoglobin reductase. The gene for this abnormality may not be very uncommon, and it may account for some people becoming cyanosed after taking dapsone-containing antimalarial preparations.

Methaemoglobinaemia with or without haemolysis

Nitrites in water or vegetable juices may cause methaemoglobinaemia in infants who have a physiological impairment of the reducing systems. Well water that comes from land with an excess of nitrites and which is used to reconstitute artificial feeds has produced cyanosis in infants. Cases have also been described following the enthusiastic feeding of juice from carrots grown on organically fertilized land and of spinach juice (spinach has a high concentration of nitrogen-fixing bacteria on its leaves).

Nitrate drugs, for example amyl nitrate, also produce methaemoglobinaemia and have proved fatal when taken in high enough dosage for 'recreational' purposes.

Table 10.7 Substances causing oxidative haemolysis and/or methaemoglobinaemia in normal people.

Substance	Use	Remarks
Dapsone	Leprosy; dermatitis herpetiformis	Chronic haemolysis; slow acetylators more susceptible
Maloprim	Antimalarial	Methaemoglobinaemia in NADH-MetHb reductase-depleted subjects
Salazopyrine	Ulcerative colitis	Chronic intravascular haemolysis
Phenazopyridine	Analgesic in urinary tract infections	Methaemoglobinaemia
Menadiol	Water-soluble vitamin K analogue	Haemolysis/kernicterus in infants
Nitrites	Fertilizer; present in well water and some vegetable juices	Methaemoglobinaemia in infants
Nitrates, 30 g	Amyl nitrate, butyryl nitrite; abused recreationally	Acute i.v. haemolysis; renal failure; fatal
Arsine	Gas produced in smelting and other industrial processes	Acute i.v. haemolysis; renal failure

Water-soluble analogues of vitamin K (menadiol sodium diphosphate) cause haemolysis with or without methaemoglobinaemia in infants and *in utero* if given to the mother during the third trimester. Fat-soluble vitamin K preparations must be used if required in these situations.

Methaemoglobinaemia due to oxidative drugs may be treated with intravenous methylene blue in doses of 1–2 mg/kg. Ascorbic acid by mouth may also be used. These measures are ineffective in G6PD-deficient patients and when very strong oxidant substances are implicated. In these circumstances, methylene blue should be avoided because it acts as an oxidant and makes the condition worse.

Acute intravascular haemolysis, methaemoglobinaemia and renal failure

These conditions occur following exposure to strong oxidizing substances that are found mainly in industrial or horticultural pursuits, e.g. sodium chlorate is a popular weed killer and arsine is a gas that is produced in various industrial settings. Acute intravascular haemolysis and haemoglobinuria develop. The serum becomes brown, often very dark, so that blood cells cannot be seen in anticoagulated preparations, due to the presence of methaemalbumin, methaemoglobin and free haemoglobin. Oliguric renal failure usually develops over about 24 h. The blood film shows microspherocytosis and bizarre forms.

Plasma exchange and renal dialysis are the mainstays of treatment, methylene blue being ineffective. Poisoning with arsine is usually reversible with these measures. Chlorate poisoning is more difficult, 30 g being a generally fatal dose. It is mostly ingested deliberately in suicide attempts.

Thermal injury

Normal red cells when heated *in vitro* show no changes when heated to 46°C for 1 h but show temperature- and duration-dependent changes above 47–50°C. Some hereditary membrane defects produce red cells that have increased thermal fragility (see Chapter 8).

Haemolysis following burns

Severe burns may be accompanied by intravascular haemolysis with haemoglobinuria. The intravascular haemolysis is related to the extent and severity of the burns. The gross haemoglobinuria occurs over the first 24 h after the burns and ceases thereafter. The blood film shows spherocytosis and schistocytes, the morphological abnormalities reflecting the thermal damage and the amount of lysis. Prolonged anaemia post burning is related to inflammation, occult blood loss and infection rather than haemolysis.

Acquired disorders of the red cell membrane

The mature red cell does not have the capacity for the repair of its membrane. The lipids of the membrane are in equilibrium with the lipids of the plasma and changes in the ratio of free cholesterol to phospholipids in plasma may affect the red cell shape and, in some instances, lead to haemolysis. This is most commonly seen in liver disease, but other inherited lipid disorders may affect the red cell secondarily.

Liver disease

Some degree of shortening of the red cell survival occurs in most cases of acute hepatitis, cirrhosis and Gilbert's disease, but anaemia is not present and there is only a slight rise in reticulocytes, which may not be detectable. Biliary obstruction is associated with the appearance of target cells and fulminant hepatitis with acanthocytosis, both consequent on changes in the plasma lipid composition.

Zieve's syndrome is an uncommon disorder, seen mainly in alcoholics. It comprises intravascular haemolysis and acute abdominal pain. These patients usually have cirrhosis and jaundice. The cause is unknown but is probably related to lipid changes in the blood. Spherocytes are seen in the peripheral blood.

Wilson's disease may present as acute intravascular haemolysis. This is probably not a membrane disorder but is consequent on the high levels of copper ions in the blood. The haemolysis may antedate the development of hepatic or neurological features, but Keyser–Fleischer rings are usually present. The blood film may show spherocytosis. The diagnosis is made once the condition is suspected. Apart from caeruloplasmin deficiency, patients have a specific aminoaciduria.

Hereditary acanthocytosis (a-β-lipoproteinaemia)

This rare inherited deficiency of low-density lipoproteins is characterized by retinitis pigmentosa, steatorrhoea, ataxia and mental retardation. The haemolysis that occurs is of minor importance to such patients, but the blood film may indicate the diagnosis, with the red cells showing marked acanthocytosis.

Vitamin E deficiency

Deficiency of vitamin E may occur in infants who are fed a diet rich in polyunsaturated fatty acids. There is haemolysis with contracted cells and a thrombocytosis. Oedema may be present. Vitamin E is an antioxidant, and oxidative damage to the red cell membrane is thought to be the cause of the haemolysis.

Selected bibliography

Acquired haemolytic anaemia – general

Dacie JV (1992) *The Haemolytic Anemias*, Vol. 3. *The Autoimmune Haemolytic Anaemias*, 3rd edn. Churchill Livingstone, Edinburgh.

Dacie JV (1995) *The Haemolytic Anaemias*, Vol. 4. *Secondary or Symptomatic Haemolytic Anaemias*, 3rd edn. Churchill Livingstone, Edinburgh.

Autoimmune haemolytic anaemia

Ekvall H (2003) Malaria and anemia. *Current Opinion in Hematology* 10: 108–14.

Gharib M, Poynton C (2002) Complete, long-term remission of refractoryidiopathic cold haemagglutinin disease after Mabthera. *British Journal of Haematology* 117: 247–8.

Hall GW (2001) Kassabach–Merritt syndrome: pathogenesis and management. *British Journal of Haematology* 112: 851–62.

Iannitto E, Ammatuna E, Marino C *et al.* (2002) Sustained response of refractory chronic lymphocytic leukaemia complicated by acute haemolytic anaemia to anti-CD20 monoclonal antibody. *Blood* 99: 1096–7.

Jeffries LC (1994) Transfusion therapy in autoimmune hemolytic anemia. *Hematology–Oncology Clinics of North America* 8: 1087–104.

Marani TM, Trich MB, Armstrong PM (1996) Carboplatin induced immune hemolytic anaemia. *Transfusion* 36: 1016–18.

Myint H, Copplestone JA, Orchard J *et al.* (1995) Fludarabine-related autoimmune haemolytic anaemia in patients with chronic lymphocytic leukaemia. *British Journal of Haematology* 91: 341–4.

Petz LD (1993) Drug-induced autoimmune hemolytic anemia. *Transfusion Medicine Review* 7: 242–54.

Salama A, Kroll H, Wittmann G *et al.* (1996) Diclof enac-induced immune haemolytic anaemia: simultaneous occurence of red blood cell autoantibodies and drug dependent antibodies. *British Journal of Haematology* 95: 640–4.

Treon SP and Anderson KC (2000) The use of rituximab in the treatment of malignant and non-malignant plasma cell disorders. *Seminars in Oncology* 27: 79–85.

Mechanical haemolytic anaemias

Aqui NA, Stein SH, Konkle BA *et al.* (2003) Role of splenectomy in patients with refractory or relapsed thrombotic thrombocytopenic purpura. *Journal of Clinical Apheresis* 18: 51–4.

Davidson RJL (1969) March or exertional haemoglobinuria. *Seminars in Hematology* 6: 150.

Fontana S, Kremer Hovinga JA, Studt J-D *et al.* (2004) Plasma therapy in thrombotic thrombocytopenic purpura: review of the literature and the Bern experience in a subgroup of patients with severe acquired ADAMTS-13 deficiency. *Seminars in Hematology* 41: 48–59.

Levy GC, Nichols WC, Lian EC *et al.* (2001) Mutations in a member of the ADAMTS gene family cause thrombotic thrombocytopenic purpura. *Nature* 413: 488–94.

Rock GA, Shumack, Buskard NA *et al.* (1991) Comparison of plasma exchange with plasma infusion in the treatment of thrombotic thrombocytopenic purpura. The Canadian Apheresis Study Group. *New England Journal of Medicine* 325: 393–7.

Yarranton H, Machin SJ (2003) An update on the pathogenesis and management of acquired thrombotic thrombocytopenic purpura. *Current Opinion in Neurology* 16: 367–73.

CHAPTER 11

Paroxysmal nocturnal haemoglobinuria

Lucio Luzzatto and Rosario Notaro

Introduction

Paroxysmal nocturnal haemoglobinuria (PNH) is an acquired chronic haemolytic anaemia in which haemolysis is largely intravascular. In addition to haemolytic anaemia, the patient may have thrombosis and pancytopenia. This triad, when present, is highly characteristic of PNH.

PNH is a rare disorder (estimated prevalence of less than 1 in 100 000) that can occur anywhere in the world. There is no evidence of family clustering and PNH has been observed at all ages from 1 to 72 years; however, it is most common in young adults.

Clinical features

The commonest initial complaint in PNH is fatigue, due to anaemia, which may range from mild to very severe. Sometimes the patient reports that one morning he or she passed very dark urine (e.g. 'it looked like Coca-Cola'; or 'it looked like blood rather than urine'). This 'classical' presentation occurs in only a minority of patients. However, if specific questions are asked, or if serial urine specimens are collected and inspected (Figure 11.1), haemoglobinuria can be documented at some time in virtually all patients.

Apart from pallor and mild jaundice, there may be no *physical findings* in a patient with PNH in the *steady state*. In some patients, one may elicit on deep palpation abdominal tenderness (usually on the midline above the umbilicus). Enlargement of the spleen is rare, and it suggests there has been thrombosis in the splenic or in the portal vein. Liver enlargement is also relatively rare, and it suggests hepatic vein thrombosis, which may present abruptly, giving the clinical picture of a full-blown Budd–Chiari syndrome, including ascites. On questioning, it is not unusual to elicit a history of attacks of abdominal pain,

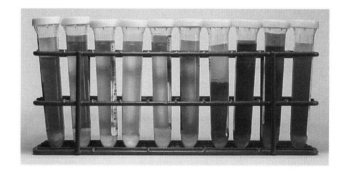

Figure 11.1 Consecutive urine samples from a patient with PNH. The patient had stated that she had had haemoglobinuria in the past, but not at the moment. The figure illustrates the marked variability in haemoglobinuria over a short time interval and that subjective self-assessment of haemoglobinuria may be deceptive. After this test, the same patient's assessment of her haemoglobinuria became more reliable.

which may last from hours to several days, may be associated with either diarrhoea or constipation, and perhaps with more intense haemoglobinuria. Recurrent dysphagia and erectile dysfunction may also occur.

The natural history of PNH is that of a very chronic disorder that may afflict the patient continuously for decades, although in many cases a good quality of life is possible. Without treatment, the median survival is estimated to be about 10 years. In some cases, after many years, full spontaneous recovery may take place. Not infrequently, at some stage in the disease, the anaemia may be associated with other cytopenias; indeed, when a PNH patient becomes less haemolytic and more pancytopenic he or she becomes very similar to a patient with aplastic anaemia (AA). Conversely, a patient with AA may subsequently develop PNH: the term 'PNH-AA syndrome' has been used to designate

Table 11.1 Diagnosis of dark urine.

Different sorts of dark urine	Causes	Additional tests	Possible diagnosis
Haematuria	Many	Clears on centrifugation	Mostly urinary tract pathology
Myoglobinuria	Rhabdomyolysis	Ultrafiltration, spectroscopy	March myoglobinuria
Haemoglobinuria	Intravascular haemolysis	Serology after blood transfusion	Incompatible blood transfusion
		Donath–Landsteiner antibody	Paroxysmal cold haemoglobinuria
		G6PD activity	G6PD deficiency
		Blood film for malaria parasites	'Blackwater fever'
		Blood culture	*Clostridium welchii* septicaemia
		History of marching	March haemoglobinuria
		History of heart prosthetic valve	Microangiopathic haemolytic anaemia
		Ham, flow cytometry for CD59	PNH

Modified from Luzzatto L, Notaro R (2003). Paroxysmal nocturnal hemoglobinuria. In: *Blood: Principles and Practice of Hematology* (RI Handin, SE Lux, TP Stossel, eds), 2nd edn, pp. 319–334. Lippincott Williams & Wilkins, Philadelphia.

these patients. Several lines of evidence (see below) suggest that in fact there is a component of AA (bone marrow failure) in every PNH patient.

There may be also some overlap between PNH and MDS: however, this is difficult to assess in an individual case, because the bone marrow morphology of PNH has in itself features of myelodysplastic syndrome (MDS). Unlike MDS, however, it is very rare that PNH evolves to AML; the estimated frequency is less than 2%.

Laboratory findings and diagnosis

The anaemia may be normocytic, but it is often macrocytic on account of an absolute reticulocytosis, which may be quite high (200×10^9/L or even higher). If the mean corpuscular volume (MCV) is normal rather than high, there probably is superimposed iron deficiency. Apart from polychromasia, the red cell morphology is not characteristic. The neutrophils may range from normal to below 1.0×10^9/L; the platelets may range from normal to below 20×10^9/L; the lymphocytes are usually normal, but there may be lymphopenia and there may be an increase in large granular lymphocytes. The bilirubin level is usually only moderately increased, in striking contrast to lactate dehydrogenase (LDH), which is often in the thousands (U/L), while haptoglobin is markedly decreased. The serum iron and transferrin saturation index (TSI) may be decreased, indicating secondary iron deficiency, even when the serum ferritin is normal. The bone marrow aspirate will usually yield a cellular marrow with erythroid hyperplasia, which may be very marked. As stated above, there may be MDS-like changes in one or more cell lineages. The bone marrow trephine usually confirms erythroid hyperplasia, but it proves often to be less cellular than might have been expected from the aspirate.

In many cases, the telltale sign of PNH is haemoglobinuria (which, of course, must be differentiated from haematuria, by simply centrifuging the urine – Table 11.1). Haemoglobinuria by itself, and especially if combined with some other features, must lead to the suspicion of PNH (Table 11.2). The definitive diagnosis of PNH is carried out by either the Ham test (still highly reliable) or by flow cytometry with appropriate antibodies. The Ham test gives no false-negative results; it can give rise to false-positive results only in congenital dyserythropoietic anaemia type II (but not if the patient's serum is used), or if the patient's red cells are already coated with a lytic antibody. Therefore, direct Coombs' test ought to be carried out always in parallel to a Ham test: when the former is positive, the latter becomes unreliable (and the likely diagnosis is autoimmune haemolytic anaemia rather than PNH).

Flow cytometry is now regarded as the gold standard; it provides an accurate quantification of the size of the PNH cell population and the best antibody in our hands is anti-CD59 (Figure 11.2). In contrast to conventional 'phenotyping' of

Table 11.2 When PNH should be suspected.

1. Haemoglobinuria due to intravascular haemolysis (see Table 11.1)
2. Haemolytic anaemia with a low platelet and/or low neutrophil count
3. Haemolytic anaemia and recurrent abdominal pain with or without blood in the stool
4. Hepatic vein thrombosis (Budd–Chiari syndrome)
5. Any venous thrombosis anywhere in young adult with low platelet and/or the neutrophil counts
6. Idiopathic pancytopenia (IAA)

leukaemic cells, one is looking for a CD59⁻ cell population, and it is important to see a bimodal distribution in both red cells and granulocytes (a 'tail' of negative cells is not diagnostic and could be a technical artifact). In a typical patient there may be, for instance, 30% CD59⁻ red cells and 90% CD59⁻ granulocytes. Flow cytometry is, of course, very sensitive, and therefore very small PNH cell populations can be detected, and they are detected (especially in granulocytes), particularly in patients with non-severe aplastic anaemia. This raises the issue of what size of PNH cell population should be regarded as diagnostic of PNH. Any cut-off point is bound to be arbitrary, but we have never seen appreciable haemolytic anaemia in a patient in whom less than 5% red cells are of the PNH type. It does not seem sensible to change the diagnosis from, for example, non-severe aplastic anaemia to PNH just because 3% of the granulocytes have the PNH phenotype (in jargon this situation is sometimes referred to as 'lab PNH'), because it should not affect clinical decisions.

Pathogenesis and pathophysiology

Haemolytic anaemia

Haemolytic anaemia in PNH is a due to an intracorpuscular abnormality of the red cell. In this respect, PNH is similar to inherited haemolytic anaemias, such as those caused by an enzyme defect. However, PNH is an acquired disorder, and there is no evidence that it is inherited. The abnormality of red cells in PNH is indeed an enzyme defect, but it is caused by a somatic mutation rather than by an inherited mutation. This explains the 'mosaicism' found in the blood of PNH patients, whereby cells belonging to the PNH clone, which have arisen through a somatic mutation, coexist with the remaining qualitatively normal cells.

We now know that the somatic mutation is in an X-linked gene that has been called *PIG-A*, for phosphatidylinositol glycan complementation group A. *PIG-A* encodes one of the subunits

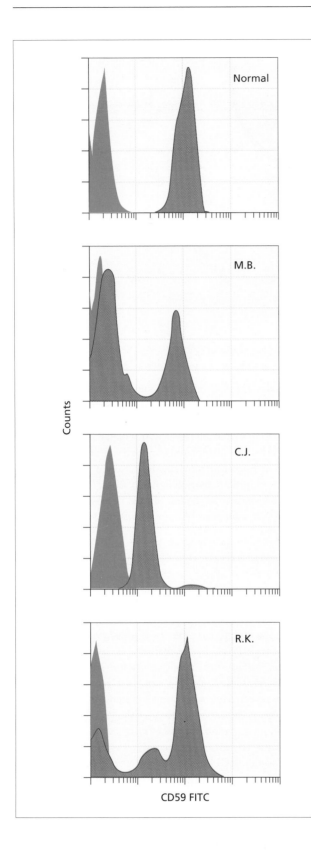

Figure 11.2 (*left*) Different patterns of PNH red cells populations in several PNH patients. The top panel is from a normal individual. Patient MB has 57% red cells that lack CD59 completely (PNH III red cells). Patient CJ has only 4% normal red cells; 96% of her red cells have a partial deficiency of CD59 (PNH II red cells), indicating that virtually her entire haemopoiesis is supported by a PNH clone with a missense mutation of *PIG-A*. The trimodal distribution of red cells in patient RK indicates the coexistence, along with normal red cells, of a PNH III clone (22%) and a PNH II clone (12%) (modified from Dacie JV, Lewis SM, Luzzatto L *et al.* (1995) Laboratory methods used in the investigation of paroxysmal nocturnal haemoglobinuria (PNH). In: *Practical Haematology* (JV Dacie, SM Lewis, eds), 8th edn, pp. 287–96. Churchill Livingstone, London).

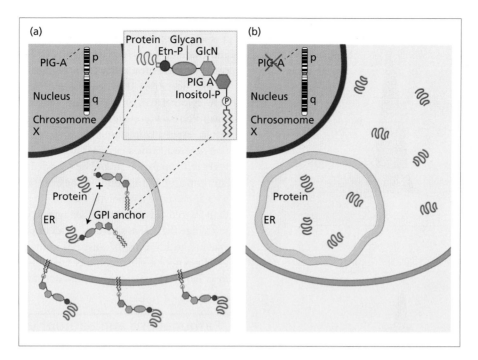

Figure 11.3 The molecular basis of the cellular abnormality in PNH. In a normal cell (a) a complex biosynthetic pathway produces in the endoplasmic reticulum (ER) a glycophospholipid molecule (see inset) called glycosylphosphatidylinositol (GPI). An early step in the biosynthetic pathway is catalysed by an acetylglucosaminyl transferase; one of the subunits of this enzyme is encoded by the gene *PIG-A*, located on the short arm of the X chromosome (band Xp22). A number of cellular proteins become covalently linked to the GPI molecule, which serves to convey and anchor them as extracellular surface proteins to the cell membrane. The PNH cell (b) has a mutation in the *PIG-A* gene, causing a serious defect in the acetylglucosaminyl transferase. This in turn causes a total or partial block in the synthesis of the GPI molecule. As a result, the proteins that require a GPI anchor are unable to become membrane bound and will be lacking from the cell surface (modified from Luzzatto L, Notaro, R. (2003) Paroxysmal nocturnal hemoglobinuria. In: *Blood: Principles and Practice of Hematology* (RI Handin, SE Lux, TP Stossel, eds), 2nd edn, pp. 319–34. Lippincott Williams & Wilkins, Philadelphia).

of the enzyme responsible for the transfer of *N*-acetylglucosamine (GlcNAc) onto phosphatidylinositol. This is the first step of the complex biosynthetic pathway that in the end produces the glycosylphosphatidylinositol (GPI) anchor required for anchoring many proteins to the cell membrane (Figure 11.3 and Table 11.3). One of these proteins, CD59 or membrane inhibitor of reactive lysis (MIRL), normally protects the red cell from being lysed by the membrane attack complex (C5–C8) that forms when complement (C) is activated. In essence, the hypersusceptibility to C of PNH red cells is the consequence of CD59 deficiency. Chronic intravascular haemolysis in PNH is probably explained by activation of C through the 'alternative' pathway, which goes on at a low rate all the time, whereas the dramatic exacerbation of haemolysis that is characteristically associated with intercurrent viral or bacterial infection in patients with PNH is probably explained by brisk activation of C by an antigen–antibody reaction (i.e. through the 'classical' pathway).

Molecular analysis

More than 180 mutations in the *PIG-A* gene have been identified in patients with PNH. In the majority of cases (about 75%), these mutations are such (small insertion/deletions producing frameshifts, nonsense mutations, only two large deletions) that they can be expected to cause complete absence of the product of the *PIG-A* gene, thus, they account for the PNH III phenotype. The remaining mutations are either missense or, in a few cases, small in-frame deletions; these may account for PNH cases with partial deficiency of GPI-anchored proteins (PNH II). In almost every patient with PNH, the *PIG-A* mutation underlying the PNH phenotype is different, which is not surprising as we are dealing not with inherited mutations, but with somatic mutations that take place *de novo* in haemopoietic stem cells. In fact, when PNH cells are investigated in detail, it is not at all rare to find that more than one PNH clone may be present in the same PNH patient, either simultaneously or in sequence.

Table 11.3 Some GPI-linked molecules on human haemopoietic cells.

	RBC	PMN	Mono	Plts	Lymph	HSC
Complement regulators						
CD55 (DAF)	+	+	+	+	+	
CD59 (MIRL)	+	+	+	+	+	+
Adhesion molecules						
CD48		+	+		+	
CD58 (LFA-3)	+	†	†	†	†	
CD66b and CD66c		+				
Enzymes						
Acetylcholinesterase	+					
Leucocyte alkaline phosphatase		+				
CD157		+	+			
Receptors						
CD14			+			
CD16 (FcγRIII)		+	*‡		+ (1)	
CD87 (u-PAR)		+	+		+ (2)	
Others						
CD52			+		+	
CD90					*(2)	+
Prion protein	+	+	+	+	+	

*Expressed only upon 'activation' or only in a subset of cells.
†Present in both GPI-linked and transmembrane form.
‡Present only in transmembrane form in this cell type.
The GPI-linked form is present only in B cells (1), only on T lymphocytes (2).
CD52, target of alemtuzumab (Campath-1H); CD157, ectoenzyme of the family of cyclic ADP-ribose-generating cyclases; DAF, decay accelerating factor: may cooperate with CD59 in protecting against C-mediated lysis; HSC, haemopoietic stem cells; LFA-3, leucocytes functional antigen-3; lymph, lymphocytes; MIRL, membrane inhibitor of reactive lysis; Mono, monocytes; Plts, platelets; PMN, granulocytes; RBC, red blood cells; u-PAR, urokinase plasminogen activator receptor.

Thrombosis

Thrombosis is one of the most immediately life-threatening complications of PNH, and yet one of the least understood in its pathogenesis. It could be due to impaired fibrinolysis, because the urokinase plasminogen activator receptor (uPAR) is a GPI-linked protein; alternatively, C activation could cause hypercoagulability or hyperactivity of platelets, or both. For instance, it could be speculated that deficiency of CD59 on the PNH platelet could lead to abnormal insertion of the C5b–9 complex in the platelet membrane, as is the case with the red cell. Although all of these three factors may play a role in producing a thrombophilic state in PNH, it seems very likely that the primary cause lies in the PNH platelets, which are abnormal precisely because they belong to the PNH clone. This notion is supported by the occurrence of cerebral infarction in a patient who did not have PNH, but who had congenital CD59 deficiency and chronic haemolysis.

Bone marrow failure and relationship between paroxysmal nocturnal haemoglobinuria and acquired aplastic anaemia (AAA)

PNH has an intimate link with AAA, for several reasons. As stated above, sometimes a patient with PNH becomes 'less haemolytic' and more pancytopenic and ultimately evolves to frank AAA. In terms of pathogenesis, it is believed that AAA is essentially an organ-specific autoimmune disease that is mediated by 'activated' cytotoxic (CD8+) T lymphocytes, which are able to inhibit haemopoietic stem cells. Recently, skewing of the T-cell repertoire indicating the presence of abnormally expanded T-cell clones has been observed also in PNH. Most importantly, intensive immunosuppressive treatment is standard of care in AAA, and a beneficial response to the same treatment can be obtained also in PNH (see below).

In view of these facts, it seems that an element of BMF in PNH is the rule rather than the exception; an extreme view is that

PNH is a form of AAA in which BMF is masked by the enormous expansion of the PNH clone that populates the patient's bone marrow. In other words, it appears that two different mechanisms cooperate in producing PNH: autoimmune damage to stem cells and a somatic mutation in the *PIG-A* gene. This notion is supported by two further lines of evidence. Using targeted inactivation of the *PIG-A* gene in mouse embryonic stem cells, one can produce mice with a PNH cell population. However, this population does not grow further, as it does in PNH patients. Using refined flow cytometry technology, PNH cells harbouring *PIG-A* mutations can be demonstrated in normal people at a frequency of the order of 10 per million. Both of these findings indicate that some other factor is required in addition to a somatic mutation in the *PIG-A* gene in order to cause PNH. Most likely, the same cytotoxic damage to stem cells that would otherwise cause PNH spares the PNH stem cells, thus allowing the PNH clone to grow to the size when it gives clinical PNH. The mechanism whereby the PNH cells escape damage is not yet known.

Management of paroxysmal nocturnal haemoglobinuria

In dealing with a patient with PNH, we must always consider that, unlike other acquired haemolytic anaemias, PNH may be lifelong. In addition, we must keep in mind the triad that defines the disease, namely haemolysis, BMF and the tendency to thrombosis. At the same time, we must consider, for each individual patient and upon discussion with the patient, whether to be content with supportive treatment or whether to aim for radical treatment.

Supportive treatment

Supportive treatment, supervised by somebody who has experience of PNH, can help the patient to 'live with PNH' for years, sometimes for decades, and often with good quality of life. The increased rate of erythropoiesis consequent on haemolysis requires supplements of folic acid (at least 3 mg per day) inde-

finitely. Whenever there is evidence of iron deficiency, it is equally important to provide iron supplementation, until the iron status is normalized. Blood transfusion of filtered red cells should be given whenever necessary. Some patients may require blood transfusion at bimonthly or even monthly intervals. Compared with other conditions requiring periodic blood transfusion, one advantage in PNH is that iron overload is not a problem in most cases, because it is prevented by iron loss through the urine. Prednisone is credited with controlling episodes of massive haemoglobinuria and, when this is associated with intercurrent infection, a short course of prednisone may sometimes appear helpful. However, the haemoglobinuria usually subsides anyway when the infection is controlled.

On the other hand, long-term administration of prednisone, even at a low dosage, is always *contraindicated*, in view of the serious potential side-effects. Any patient who has had deep vein thrombosis at any one site in the abdomen or in a limb should be on regular anticoagulant prophylaxis. During an episode of abdominal vein thrombosis, *thrombolytic therapy* with tissue plasminogen activator (tPA) must be seriously considered because, although it is not free of risk (especially if the patient is thrombocytopenic), it may be highly effective and it may prevent irreversible damage (Figure 11.4). Unlike with arterial thrombosis, tPA is worth a trial, even several days from the clinical onset of the thrombotic event.

Bone marrow transplantation and immunosuppressive treatment

At the moment, the only form of treatment that can provide a cure for PNH is *allogeneic bone marrow transplantation* (BMT); when an HLA-identical sibling is available, BMT should be offered to any young patient with PNH, especially if there is severe pancytopenia. Results similar to those for AA can be expected, with long-term disease-free survival ranging from 60% to 100% in the few series that have been published. Recently, BMT from unrelated donors in PNH has been also successful. The majority of patients will not have a potential sibling donor, and some of those who do may not wish to undergo BMT. Given the common pathogenesis of PNH and

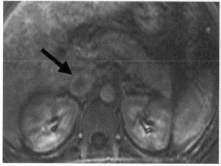
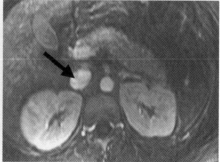

(a)   (b)

Figure 11.4 Successful thrombolytic therapy in PNH. (a) Magnetic resonance venography in a 29-year-old woman who presented with acute Budd–Chiari syndrome, and who also had a thrombus partially occluding the inferior vena cava. (b) Repeat study after a 48-h infusion of tissue plasminogen activator (from R Thertulien *et al.*, unpublished).

AA, a logical alternative is immunosuppressive treatment with ALG (ATG) and cyclosporin A. Although no formal trial has ever been conducted, this approach has helped particularly to relieve severe thrombocytopenia and/or neutropenia in patients in whom these were the main problem(s): by contrast, there is often little beneficial effect on the haemolysis itself.

A new approach to controlling haemolysis

One of the most frustrating aspects of the management of PNH has been, until now, the absence of an effective way to control haemolysis. Eculizumab, a humanized antibody against complement protein C5 that inhibits the activation of terminal components of complement, has been tested in a small group of transfusion-dependent PNH patients. The results thus far appear very promising; indeed, reduced intravascular haemolysis and less haemoglobinuria have been documented, as well as a marked decrease in transfusion requirement in most patients.

Selected bibliography

Araten D, Nafa K, Pakdeesuwan K et al. (1999) Clonal populations of hematopoietic cells with paroxysmal nocturnal hemoglobinuria genotype and phenotype are present in normal individuals. *Proceedings of the National Academy of Sciences of the USA* **96**: 5209–14.

Bessler M, Mason PJ, Hillmen P et al. (1994) Paroxysmal nocturnal haemoglobinuria (PNH) is caused by somatic mutations in the PIG-A gene. *EMBO Journal* **13**: 110–17.

Bessler M, Schaefer A, Keller P (2001) Paroxysmal nocturnal hemoglobinuria: insights from recent advances in molecular biology. *Transfusion Medicine Review* **15**: 255–67.

Ham TH (1937) Chronic hemolytic anemia with paroxysmal nocturnal hemoglobinuria. A study of the mechanism of hemolysis in relation to acid-base equilibrium. *New England Journal of Medicine* **217**: 915–18.

Hillmen P, Lewis SM, Bessler M et al. (1995) Natural history of paryxysmal nocturnal hemoglobinuria. *New England Journal of Medicine* **333**: 1253–8.

Hillmen P, Hall C, Marsh JC et al. (2004) Effect of eculizumab on hemolysis and transfusion requirements in patients with paroxysmal nocturnal hemoglobinuria. *New England Journal of Medicine* **350**: 552–9.

Karadimitris A, Manavalan JS, Thaler HT et al. (2000) Abnormal T-cell repertoire is consistent with immune process underlying the pathogenesis of paroxysmal nocturnal hemoglobinuria. *Blood* **96**: 2613–20.

Karadimitris A, Luzzatto L (2001) The cellular pathogenesis of paroxysmal nocturnal haemoglobinuria. *Leukemia* **15**: 1148–52.

Lewis SM, Dacie JV (1967) The aplastic anaemia–paroxysmal nocturnal haemoglobinuria syndrome. *British Journal of Haematology* **13**: 236–51.

Luzzatto L, Bessler M (1996) The dual pathogenesis of paroxysmal nocturnal hemoglobinuria. *Current Opinion in Hematology* **3**: 101–10.

Luzzatto L, Notaro R (2003) Paroxysmal nocturnal hemoglobinuria. In: *Blood: Principles and Practice of Hematology* (RI Handlin, SE Lux, TP Stossel, eds), 2nd edn, pp. 319–34. Lippincott Williams & Wilkins, Philadelphia.

Miyata T, Takeda J, Iida J et al. (1993) The cloning of PIG-A, a component in the early step of GPI-anchor biosynthesis. *Science* **259**: 1318–20.

Omine M, Kinoshita T (ed.) (2003) *Paroxysmal Nocturnal Hemoglobinuria and Related Disorders – Molecular Aspects and Pathogenesis*, p. 285. Springer-Verlag, Tokyo.

Oni SB, Osunkoya BO, Luzzatto L (1970) Paroxysmal nocturnal hemoglobinuria: evidence for monoclonal origin of abnormal red cells. *Blood* **36**: 145–52.

Raiola AM, Van Lint MT, Lamparelli T et al. (2000) Bone marrow transplantation for paroxysmal nocturnal hemoglobinuria. *Haematologica* **85**(1): 59–62.

Rosse WF (1986) The control of complement activation by the blood cells in paroxysmal nocturnal haemoglobinuria. *Blood* **67**: 268–9.

Rosse WF, Dacie JV (1966) Immune lysis of normal human and paroxysmal nocturnal hemoglobinuria (PNH) red blood cells. I The sensitivity of PNH red cells to lysis by complement and specific antibody. *Journal of Clinical Investigation* **45**: 736–48.

Rotoli B, Luzzatto L (1989) Paroxysmal nocturnal hemoglobinuria. *Seminars in Hematology* **26**: 201–7.

Shichishima T, Saitoh Y, Terasawa T et al. (1999) Complement sensitivity of erythrocytes in a patient with inherited complete deficiency of CD59 or with the Inab phenotype. *British Journal of Haematology* **104**: 303–6.

Watanabe R, Inoue N, Westfall B et al. (1998) The first step of glycosylphosphatidylinositol biosynthesis is mediated by a complex of PIG-A, PIG-H, PIG-C and GPI1. *EMBO Journal* **17**: 877–85.

Wiedmer T, Hall SE, Ortel TL et al. (1993) Complement-induced vesiculation and exposure of membrane prothrombinase sites in platelets of paroxysmal nocturnal hemoglobinuria. *Blood* **82**: 1192–6.

Young NS, Moss, J (ed.) (2000) *Paroxysmal Nocturnal Hemoglobinuria and the GPI-linked Proteins*, p. 279. Academic Press, New York.

Zoumbos NC, Gascon P, Djeu JY et al. (1985) Circulating activated suppressor T lymphocytes in aplastic anemia. *New England Journal of Medicine* **312**: 257–65.

CHAPTER 12

Inherited aplastic anaemia/bone marrow failure syndromes

12

Inderjeet S Dokal

Introduction

A number of inherited (constitutional/genetic) disorders are characterized by aplastic anaemia (AA)/bone marrow (BM) failure, usually in association with one or more somatic abnormalities (Table 12.1). The features of some of these are summarized in Table 12.2. The precise incidence/prevalence of these remains unclear but, collectively, they represent approximately 10–20% of patients presenting with AA and constitute a significant clinical burden, as many are associated with premature

Table 12.1 The inherited bone marrow failure syndromes.

Pancytopenia
Fanconi anaemia (FA)
Dyskeratosis congenita (DC)
Shwachman–Diamond syndrome (SDS)
Reticular dysgenesis
Pearson syndrome (PS)
Familial aplastic anaemia (autosomal and X-linked forms)
Myelodysplasia
Non-haematological syndromes (Down, Dubowitz syndromes)

Single cytopenia (usually)
Anaemia (Diamond–Blackfan anaemia, DBA)
Neutropenia (severe congenital neutropenia, SCN, including
    Kostmann syndrome)
Thrombocytopenia (congenital amegakaryocytic
    thrombocytopenia, CAMT, amegakaryocytic
    thrombocytopenia with absent radii, TAR)

mortality. The BM failure may present at birth or at a variable time thereafter, including in adulthood in some cases. The BM failure may involve all or a single lineage; in some cases it may initially be associated with a single cytopenia and then progress to pancytopenia. Scientifically, they constitute an important group of diseases as recent advances in understanding the genetics of some of these are not only beginning to unravel their pathophysiology but are also providing important insights into normal haemopoiesis.

The two syndromes that are frequently associated with generalized BM failure/aplastic anaemia (AA) are Fanconi anaemia (FA) and dyskeratosis congenita (DC). These two syndromes are now also two of the best characterized and will be discussed in some detail in this chapter [followed by sections on Shwachman–Diamond syndrome (SDS), Diamond–Blackfan anaemia (DBA), congenital neutropenia, thrombocytopenia with absent radii (TAR) and congenital amegakaryocytic thrombocytopenia (CAMT)] to demonstrate their clinical and genetic heterogeneity, management and possible impact on our understanding of the pathophysiology of the more common 'idiopathic aplastic anaemia'. Indeed, both FA and DC patients can sometimes present with AA alone as their initial manifestation and can thus pose a diagnostic/management challenge.

Fanconi anaemia

Clinical features

Since the first description by Fanconi in 1927, FA has become to be recognized as an autosomal recessive disorder in which there is progressive BM failure and an increased predisposition

Table 12.2 Characteristics of the bone marrow failure syndromes.

	FA	DC	SDS	DBA	TAR	SCN	IAA
Inheritance pattern	AR	XLR, AR, AD	AR	AD and AR	AR	AD, AR	?
Somatic abnormalities	Yes	Yes	Yes	Yes	Yes	Rare	? None
Bone marrow failure	AA (> 90%)	AA (~80%)	AA (20%)	RCA	Megs	Neutropenia	Yes (100%)
Short telomeres	Yes	Yes	Yes	?	?	?	Yes
Malignancy	Yes	Yes	Yes	Yes	? No	Yes	Yes
Chromosome instability	Yes	Yes	Yes	?	?	?	Yes
Number of genes	At least 7	At least 3	?1	At least three	?	?	?
Genes identified	7	2	1	1	No	1	?

AA, aplastic anaemia; AD, autosomal dominant; AR, autosomal recessive; DBA, Diamond–Blackfan anaemia; DC, dyskeratosis congenita; FA, Fanconi anaemia; IAA, idiopathic AA; Megs, low megakaryocytes; RCA, red cell aplasia; SCN, severe congenital neutropenia; SDS, Shwachman–Diamond syndrome; TAR, thrombocytopenia with absent radii; XLR, X-linked recessive.

to malignancy, especially acute myeloid leukaemia. Most, but not all, affected individuals also have one or more somatic abnormalities including skin (café-au-lait spots), skeletal (absent thumbs, radial hypoplasia, scoliosis), genitourinary (under-developed gonads, horseshoe kidneys), gastrointestinal, cardiac and neurological anomalies (Table 12.3). Some of these somatic abnormalities are shown in Figure 12.1. The course of the disease and the pattern of somatic abnormalities show considerable variation, with approximately one-third of patients having no somatic abnormalities. This makes diagnosis based on clinical criteria alone difficult and unreliable.

Table 12.3 Somatic abnormalities in FA (modified from Auerbach *et al.* 1998).

Abnormality	Percentage of patients
Skeletal (radial ray, hip, vertebral, scoliosis, rib)	71
Skin pigmentation (café-au-lait, hyper- and hypopigmentation)	64
Short stature	63
Eyes (microphthalmia)	38
Renal and urinary tract	34
Male genital	20
Mental retardation	16
Gastrointestinal (e.g. anorectal, duodenal atresia)	14
Heart	13
Hearing	11
Central nervous system (e.g. hydrocephalus, septum pellucidum)	8
No abnormalities	30

The cumulative incidence of BM failure by the age of 40 years is 90%. At birth the blood count is usually normal. Pancytopenia develops insidiously and presents in most cases between the ages of 5 and 10 years (median age 7 years). However, in some cases the pancytopenia develops in adolescence or even in adult life. The haemoglobin (Hb) and platelet count are usually first to fall; the granulocytes are usually well preserved in the early stages. As the pancytopenia develops, the BM becomes progressively hypocellular. There is often a marked increase in macrophage activity with evidence of haemophagocytosis. BM failure leading to fatal haemorrhage or infection is the main cause of death in FA patients. In a recent analysis from the International Fanconi Anemia Registry (IFAR), the median survival time was 24 years.

FA is associated with an increased risk of leukaemia and other malignancies. The leukaemias are usually of the acute myeloid type, particularly FAB types M4 (myelomonocytic) and M5 (monocytic). In some cases, leukaemia may be the initial event leading to the diagnosis of FA. The cumulative incidence of haematological malignancy by the age of 40 years is 33%. Besides these haematological malignancies, there is a significant risk of hepatic tumours and squamous cell carcinoma, including squamous cell carcinomas of the vulva, oesophagus, head and neck. The cumulative incidence of solid tumours is calculated to be 28% by the age of 40 years. The impression is that malignancies occur mainly in patients with late-onset BM failure and longer survival, with a median age of 13 years for leukaemia and 25 years for solid tumours. Furthermore, long-term follow-up in FA patients who have been treated by haemopoietic stem cell transplantation (SCT) is showing a higher incidence of non-haematological malignancies in patients with FA than patients with other types of BM failure who underwent SCT, again emphasizing the predisposition to malignancy.

(a) (b) (c)

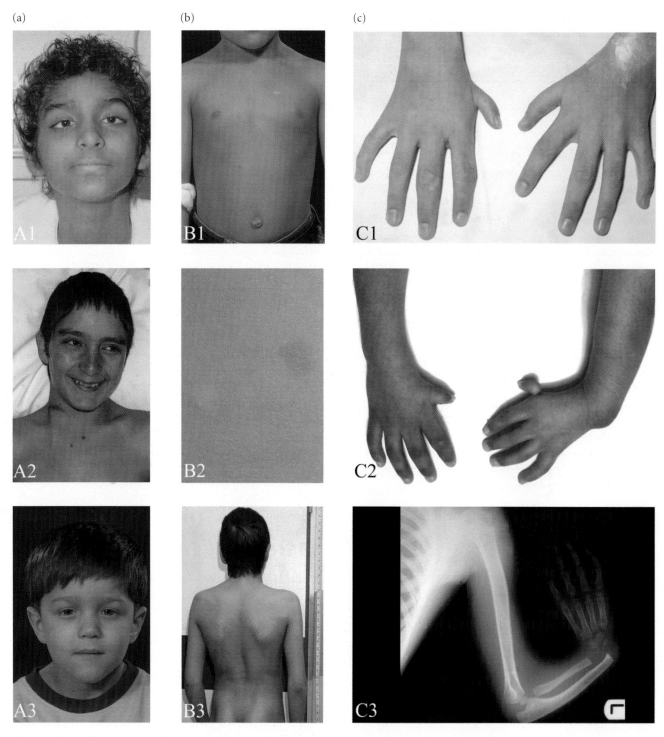

Figure 12.1 (a) Photographs of FA patients (A1–A3) with small mouth and chin ('Fanconi facies'). (b) Abnormalities of pigmentation (hyper- and hypopigmentation) on the abdomen (B1) with a close-up (B2) of a café-au-lait spot and a hypopigmented patch. The bottom photograph (B3) shows the back of a FA patient, demonstrating lumbar scoliosis. (c) Hands/forearms of FA children showing hypoplastic thumbs (C1), rudimentary ('dangling') thumbs (C2) and a radiograph (C3) showing rudimentary thumb (skeletal) development.

(a)

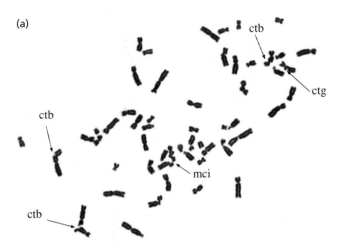

(b)

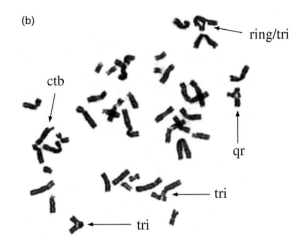

Figure 12.2 (a and b) Chromosomal abnormalities seen in FA lymphocytes following incubation with diepoxybutane. ctb, chromatid break; ctg, chromatid gap; mci, multiple chromatid interchanges (complex rearrangement); tri, triradial; qr, quadriradial (courtesy of Nicola Foot, Cytogenetics Section, Hammersmith Hospital).

Cell and molecular biology

Cells from FA patients show an abnormally high frequency of spontaneous chromosomal breakage and hypersensitivity to the clastogenic effect of DNA cross-linking agents such as diepoxybutane (DEB) and mitomycin C (MMC). A laboratory test is available for FA. This is based on the increased chromosomal breakage seen in FA cells compared with normal control subjects after exposure to low concentrations of DEB or MMC ('DEB/MMC stress test') (Figure 12.2). Other features of the FA cell phenotype include abnormal cell cycle kinetics (prolonged G_2 phase), hypersensitivity to oxygen, increased apoptosis and accelerated telomere shortening.

There is considerable genetic heterogeneity in FA. Complementation analysis of somatic cell hybrids has provided evidence for eight complementation groups (FA-A, FA-B, FA-C, FA-D1, FA-D2, FA-E, FA-F and FA-G), suggesting that there are several FA genes. Table 12.4 shows the approximate prevalence of the different FA subgroups and shows that a large number of FA mutations have been identified. Thus, although it is now possible to undertake molecular analysis in FA patients (including the use of retroviral complementation with cloned FA cDNAs and immunoblots for FA proteins), the considerable molecular heterogeneity means that the DEB/MMC stress test remains the front-line diagnostic test.

Identification of the first five FA genes (FANCA, FANCC, FANCE, FANCF and FANCG) provided no immediate clues to their function as they showed no significant homology to each other or to other known genes in the databases. Subsequent studies have demonstrated that the FANCA, FANCC, FANCE, FANCF and FANCG proteins encoded by these genes interact with each other and are part of a larger nuclear complex. The

Table 12.4 FA complementation groups/genetic subtypes.

Complementation group/gene	Approximate percentage of FA patients	Chromosome location	Protein(amino acids)	Mutations identified
A (FANCA)	65–70	16q24.3	1455	> 120
B (FANCB*)	< 2	?	?	?
C (FANCC)	5–10	9q22.3	558	10
D1 (FANCD1*)	< 2	13q12–13	3417	9
D2 (FANCD2)	< 2	3p25.3	1451	5
E (FANCE)	2–5	6p21.3	536	3
F (FANCF)	< 2	11p15	374	6
G (FANCG)	10–15	9p13	622	21

*FANCD1, and possibly FANCB, were recently shown to be BRCA2.

The percentages of the different subgroups refer to the EUFAR (European Fanconi Anaemia Registry) data.

identification of the *FANCD2* gene provided an important link between the FA proteins and DNA repair. The nuclear complex containing the FA proteins (A/C/E/F/G) is required for the activation of the FANCD2 protein to a mono-ubiquitinated (a post-translational modification of a protein by the addition of a single ubiquitin molecule) isoform (FANCD2-Ub). In normal (non-FA) cells, FANCD2 is mono-ubiquitinated at lysine 561 in response to DNA damage (e.g. MMC) and is targeted to discrete nuclear foci.

Activated FANCD2 protein collocalizes and co-purifies with the breast cancer susceptibility protein, BRCA1, a protein that is important in many DNA damage-response pathways. These nuclear foci appear in cells after DNA damage and in those cells undergoing DNA replication. Proteins such as the recombination molecule RAD51, and those in the RAD50–NBS1–MRE11 DNA repair pathway are also present in BRCA1-containing foci (NBS1, complex Nijmegen breakage syndrome 1; MRE11, meiotic recombination 11). In cells from A, C, E, F or G patients, FANCD2 ubiquitination is not observed and it is not targeted to nuclear foci. ATM (ataxia telangiectasia mutated) can phosphorylate both FANCD2 and BRCA1. The ATM-dependent phosphorylation of FANCD2 (at serine 222) occurs in response to ionizing radiation. Therefore, this puts FANCD2 in a central position in signalling DNA damage; double-strand DNA breaks caused by ionizing radiation result in ATM-dependent phosphorylation of FANCD2 at serine 222, whereas interstrand DNA cross-links caused by MMC produce mono-ubiquitination of FANCD2 at lysine 561 via the FA nuclear complex.

Recently, it has been shown that cell lines derived from FA-D1 (and possibly FA-B) patients have biallelic mutations in *BRCA2*. This finding now links the cloned FA genes (*FANCA*, *FANCC*, *FANCD2*, *FANCE*, *FANCF*, *FANCG*) with *BRCA1* and *BRCA2* in a common pathway. BRCA2 protein is important in the repair of DNA damage by homologous recombination, in part by regulating the activity of RAD51. Cells lacking BRCA2 inaccurately repair damaged DNA and are hypersensitive to DNA cross-linking agents. These recent scientific developments therefore suggest that BRCA2 and other FA proteins cooperate in a common DNA damage response pathway, 'the FA/BRCA pathway'. A schematic representation of the FA/BRCA pathway is given in Figure 12.3. The precise functions of BRCA1 and BRCA2 in this pathway remain to be elucidated. It is also possible that the FA proteins have other functions in addition to their role in this pathway.

In vitro gene transfer studies have demonstrated that introduction of the appropriate wild-type FA gene into FA human lymphoid and haemopoietic cells markedly enhances their growth and normalizes their response to MMC; and in lymphoid lines, cell kinetics (G_2 phase) and chromosomal breakage are normalized. Thus, the transfer of the wild-type FA genes corrects the extreme sensitivity to DNA cross-linking agents, the hallmark of the FA cell phenotype. These studies provide the rationale for haemopoietic gene therapy (discussed below).

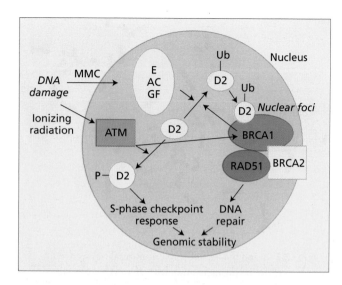

Figure 12.3 Schematic representation of the FA/BRCA pathway. In response to DNA damage (MMC) the FA protein complex (A/C/E/F/G complex) is formed and results in mono-ubiquitination of FANCD2 (D2). Mono-ubiquitination targets D2 to DNA repair nuclear foci containing BRCA1, BRCA2, and RAD51, which are important in maintaining genomic stability by promoting homologous recombination repair. D2 phosphorylation by ATM in response to DNA damage induced by ionizing radiation is important in S-phase checkpoint response.

Murine mouse models of FA have shown that haemopoietic progenitors are hypersensitive to tumour necrosis factor α (TNF-α) and interferon-γ. This differential hypersensitivity to interferon-γ is thought to be mediated by *fas*-induced apoptosis and may turn out to be an important mechanism in the development of progressive BM failure in FA. It is noteworthy that patients with idiopathic AA usually have raised interferon-γ levels, thus providing a possible link in the pathophysiology of BM failure in both idiopathic and FA-associated AA. The presence of short telomeres in cells from both FA and idiopathic AA patients can also be expected to be important in the pathophysiology of BM failure in both diseases. This issue is discussed further in relation to DC.

Treatment

The main cause of premature mortality in FA patients is the development of BM failure. Until the advent of haemopoietic SCT, treatment consisted largely of supportive care and attempts to stabilize and improve haemopoietic function by administrating androgens (oxymetholone) and corticosteroids (prednisolone). Although oxymetholone treatment can produce useful, trilineage responses in more than 50% of patients the majority will become refractory. Oxymetholone is associated with side-effects, including liver dysfunction and increased risk of hepatic tumours. It is a very good holding treatment until more definitive treatment can be planned using haemopoietic SCT, which has now become the treatment of choice. From the *in vitro* and *in vivo* studies it has become clear that cells from FA patients are hypersensitive to agents such as cyclophosphamide and high-dose irradiation compared with non-FA patients. Therefore, SCT conditioning regimens have been modified by reducing the dose of cyclophosphamide and radiation. Using the low-dose cyclophosphamide (20 mg/kg) and 4.5–6 Gy of thoracoabdominal irradiation, the actuarial survival for patients transplanted using HLA-identical sibling donors is around 70% at 2 years. The results using unrelated donors have been less good, with 2-year survival between 20% and 40%. In order to improve these results, the role of conditioning protocols using fludarabine is being investigated. Additionally, long-term follow-up of patients who have survived after SCT shows a much higher incidence of malignancies, particularly of the head and neck, usually 8–10 years after the transplant. This in part relates to the inherent predisposition of FA patients to malignancy (which can perhaps now be explained given the link to BRCA1 and BRCA2) and in part to factors such as the use of radiotherapy in the conditioning. Some groups are therefore exploring low-dose cyclophosphamide (20–40 mg/kg) SCT protocols that avoid the use of radiotherapy. Preliminary results using fludarabine (120–150 mg/m^2) in association with low-dose cyclophosphamide are very encouraging for both sibling and unrelated stem cell transplants. Longer follow-up is necessary to determine if such protocols will be associated with a lower risk of malignancy.

In addition to SCT, alternative treatment strategies are being explored. The identification of the FA genes, combined with the *in vitro* gene transfer data that show that FA haemopoietic stem cells rescued by gene therapy should have a *selective growth advantage* within the hypoplastic BM environment, has resulted in clinical studies of retroviral-mediated gene therapy for FA patients. The pilot study on FA-C patients was associated with no serious side-effects but efficacy was limited. Further studies on this approach are needed.

The identification of FA *mosaic* patients strengthens the case for future trials of gene therapy. In such cases, the DEB/MMC test may be negative or only demonstrate chromosomal instability in a subgroup of cells. Somatic mosaicism is due to reversion of a pathogenic allele to 'wild' type in a single haemopoietic (somatic) cell. The mechanism of how this occurs can vary, but in each case it generates one 'normal' FA allele and the resulting cell effectively becomes a 'heterozygous cell', which would be expected to have a growth/survival advantage in the background of FA cells. These mosaic patients can have an improvement in their haematological profile, suggesting that a single pluripotent stem cell may be sufficient to restore adequate haemopoiesis. FA patients with somatic mosaicism can thus be regarded as having undergone 'natural haemopoietic gene therapy'.

Dyskeratosis congenita

Clinical features

Classical dyskeratosis congenita (DC) is an inherited disease characterized by the triad of abnormal skin pigmentation, nail dystrophy and mucosal leucoplakia (Figure 12.4). Since its first description in 1906 by Zinsser, a variety of non-cutaneous

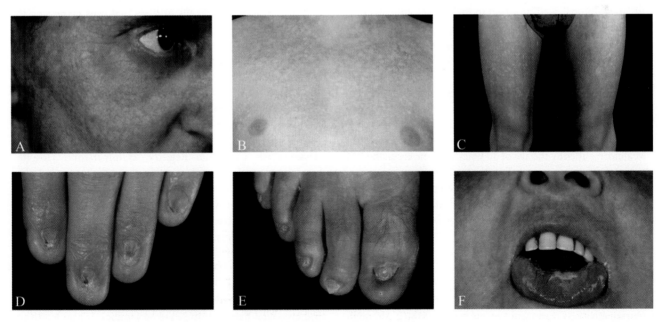

Figure 12.4 Photographs of DC patients showing abnormal skin pigmentation (A, B, C), nail dystrophy (D, E) and leucoplakia of tongue (F).

Table 12.5 Somatic abnormalities in dyskeratosis congenita.

Abnormality	Percentage of patients
Abnormal skin pigmentation	89
Nail dystrophy	88
Bone marrow failure	85.5
Leucoplakia	78
Epiphora	30.5
Learning difficulties/developmental delay/mental retardation	25.4
Pulmonary disease	20.3
Short stature	19.5
Extensive dental caries/loss	16.9
Oesophageal stricture	16.9
Premature hair loss/greying/sparse eyelashes	16.1
Hyperhiderosis	15.3
Malignancy	9.8
Intrauterine growth retardation	7.6
Liver disease/peptic ulceration/enteropathy	7.3
Ataxia/cerebellar hypoplasia	6.8
Hypogonadism/undescended testes	5.9
Microcephaly	5.9
Urethral stricture/phimosis	5.1
Osteoporosis/aseptic necrosis/scoliosis	5.1
Deafness	0.8

(dental, gastrointestinal, genitourinary, neurological, ophthalmic, pulmonary and skeletal) abnormalities have also been reported (Table 12.5). BM failure is the principal cause of early mortality, with an additional predisposition to malignancy and fatal pulmonary complications. X-linked recessive, autosomal dominant and autosomal recessive forms of the disease are recognized. It is therefore now acknowledged that DC is a very heterogeneous disorder, both clinically and genetically.

Clinical manifestations in DC often appear during childhood. The skin pigmentation and nail changes typically appear first, usually by the age of 10 years. BM failure usually develops below the age of 20 years; 80–90% of patients will have developed BM abnormalities by the age of 30 years. In some cases, the BM abnormalities may appear before the mucocutaneous manifestations and the patients may be categorized to have 'idiopathic aplastic anaemia'. The main causes of death are BM failure/immunodeficiency (~60–70%), pulmonary complications (~10–15%) and malignancy (~10%).

Cell and molecular biology

DC has many features in common with FA, in which cells display hypersensitivity to clastogenic agents such as MMC. Although the occasional DC patient may show some evidence of chromosome breakage, in general there is no significant difference in chromosomal breakage between DC and normal lymphocytes with or without the use of bleomycin, DEB, MMC and γ-irradiation. This observation enables DC patients to be distinguished from FA.

Primary DC skin fibroblasts are abnormal both in morphology and in growth rate. Furthermore, they show unbalanced chromosomal rearrangements (dicentrics, tricentrics, translocations) in the absence of any clastogenic agents. In addition, peripheral blood (PB) and BM metaphases from some patients show numerous unbalanced chromosomal rearrangements in the absence of any clastogenic agents. These studies provide evidence for a defect that predisposes DC cells to developing chromosomal rearrangements. DC, like FA, may thus be regarded as a chromosomal instability disorder but with a predisposition principally to chromosomal rearrangements rather than the gaps and breaks seen in FA.

Haemopoietic progenitor studies have shown reduced numbers of all progenitors compared with control subjects and there is usually a downward decline with time. The degree to which the progenitors are reduced can vary from patient to patient and they can be reduced even when the PB count is normal. The demonstration of abnormalities of growth and chromosomal rearrangements in fibroblasts suggests that the BM failure is likely to be a consequence of abnormalities in both haemopoietic stem cells and stromal cells.

X-chromosome inactivation patterns (XCIPs) have been studied in PB cells of women from X-linked DC families by investigating a methylation-sensitive restriction enzyme site in the polymorphic human androgen receptor locus (HUMARA) at Xq11.2–Xq12. All carriers of X-linked DC showed complete skewing in XCIP. The presence of the extremely skewed pattern of X-inactivation in PB cells suggests that cells expressing the defective gene have a growth/survival disadvantage over those expressing the normal allele. Furthermore, a skewed XCIP provides important information about carrier status for use in the counselling of families at risk of DC. In addition, XCIPs data allow us to distinguish an inherited mutation from a de novo event in sporadic male DC cases, as well as autosomal from X-linked forms of the disease.

The majority of DC patients recruited on the DCR (Dyskeratosis Congenita Registry, Hammersmith Hospital, London) are male. This observation suggests that the X-linked recessive form of DC represents a major subset of cases. Initially, through linkage analysis in one large family with only affected males, it was possible to map the gene for the X-linked form to Xq28. The availability of polymorphic genetic markers from the Xq28 and additional X-linked families facilitated positional cloning of the gene (DKC1) that is mutated in X-linked DC. The identification of the DKC1 gene in 1998 made available a genetic test that can be used to confirm diagnosis in suspected cases and antenatal diagnosis in X-linked families. It also led to the demonstration that another rare syndrome, the Hoyeraal–

Hreidarsson (HH) syndrome, is due to mutations in the *DKC1* gene. HH is a severe multisystem disorder characterized by severe growth failure, abnormalities of brain development (usually cerebellar hypoplasia), aplastic anaemia and immunodeficiency (T$^+$ B$^-$ NK$^-$ severe combined immunodeficiency). The recognition that HH is a severe variant of DC has further highlighted the considerable variability of the DC phenotype.

In addition to providing an accurate diagnostic test, this genetic advance has provided insights into the pathogenesis of DC. The *DKC1* gene is expressed in all tissues of the body, indicating that it has a vital 'housekeeping function' in the human cell. This correlates well with the multisystem phenotype of DC. The *DKC1* gene and its encoded protein, dyskerin, are highly conserved throughout evolution. Dyskerin is a nucleolar protein that is associated with the H/ACA class of small nucleolar RNAs (snoRNAs) and is involved in pseudo-uridylation of specific residues of ribosomal RNA (rRNA). This step is essential for ribosome biogenesis and therefore initially suggested that DC arises largely because of defective ribosome biogenesis.

Subsequent studies have shown that dyskerin also associates with the RNA component of telomerase (hTR), which also contains an H/ACA consensus sequence. Telomerase is an enzyme complex that is important in maintaining the telomeres of chromosomes. The precise composition of the telomerase complex is unknown, but two essential components, the RNA component (hTR) and the catalytic reverse transcriptase (hTERT), have been well characterized. Telomerase activity can be reconstituted *in vitro* using just the hTR and hTERT. In patients with X-linked DC, it was initially demonstrated that the level of hTR was reduced and that telomere lengths were much shorter than in age-matched normal control subjects. Subsequently, it was found that telomeres are also shorter in cells from patients with autosomal forms of DC. This therefore suggested that DC might principally be a disease of telomere maintenance rather than of ribosomal biogenesis. Further clarification came from linkage analysis in one large DC family, which showed that the gene for autosomal dominant DC is on chromosome 3q, in the same area where the gene for *hTR* had been previously mapped. This led to *hTR* mutation analysis in this and other DC families and the demonstration that autosomal dominant DC is due to mutations in the *hTR* gene.

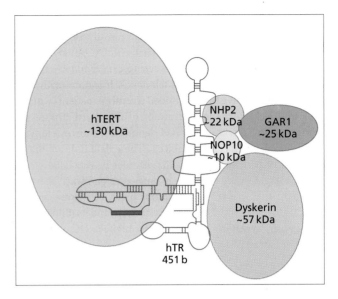

Figure 12.5 Putative associations between dyskerin and hTR (human telomerase RNA) in the telomerase complex. hTERT represents human telomerase reverse transcriptase. GAR1, NHP2 and NOP10 are ribo-nucleoproteins (RNPs) that are known to associate with dyskerin and the H/ACA class of small nucleolar RNAs (snoRNAs).

As the *DKC1*-encoded protein dyskerin and hTR are both components of the telomerase complex (Figure 12.5), it now appears that DC arises principally from an abnormality in telomerase activity. Affected tissues are those that need constant renewal, consistent with a basic deficiency in stem cell activity due to defective telomerase activity. The demonstration of *DKC1* and *hTR* mutations in DC families provides an accurate diagnostic test, including antenatal diagnosis, in a significant subset of cases (Table 12.6). For DC patients, this now also provides the basis for designing new treatments. For the wider community it provides the first direct genetic link between a human disease that is characterized by features of premature ageing (premature grey hair/hair loss, early dental loss, abnormalities of skin pigmentation, nail dystrophy, bone marrow failure,

Table 12.6 Dyskeratosis congenita genetic subtypes.

DC subtype	Approximate percentage of DC patients	Chromosome location	Gene product	Mutations identified
X-linked recessive	40	Xq28	Dyskerin	30
Autosomal dominant	5	3q21–3q28	hTR	6
Autosomal recessive*	50	?	?	?

*The genetic basis of this subtype is unknown and may represent more than one genetic locus.
Data are based on the DCR registry.

increased predisposition to malignancy) and short telomeres. Therefore, unravelling the biology of this rare disease has important implications not only for patients with DC but also for the more common disorders, such as ageing, cancer and AA, that are also associated with abnormal telomeres. It is noteworthy *that* hTR mutations have been identified recently in patients with AA but who lacked diagnostic features of DC. Furthermore, AA patients with *hTR* mutations had significantly shorter telomeres than age-matched control subjects. These data indicate that in a subset of patients with AA the disorder is associated with a genetic lesion in the telomere maintenance pathway. They also highlight the diverse manifestations of DC: its severe variant form as the HH syndrome, its classical form and its mildest form as ' aplastic anaemia'. The similarities between DC and AA are given in Table 12.2.

Treatment

As in FA, the anabolic steroid oxymetholone can produce an improvement in haemopoietic function in many (> 50%) patients for a variable period of time. Transient successful responses to granulocyte–macrophage colony-stimulating factor (GM-CSF), granulocyte colony-stimulating factor (G-CSF) and erythropoietin have also been reported. The use of oxymetholone and growth factors may be synergistic in some patients. The main treatment for severe BM failure, however, is allogeneic SCT, and there is some experience using both sibling and alternative stem cell donors. Unfortunately, because of early and late fatal pulmonary/vascular complications after SCT, the results of conventional transplants have been less successful than in FA. The presence of pulmonary disease in a significant proportion of DC patients perhaps now explains the high incidence of fatal pulmonary complications in the setting of SCT. It also highlights the need to avoid agents (such as busulphan and radiotherapy) that are associated with pulmonary toxicity. As BM failure is the main cause of premature death in DC patients and SCT is the only curative option for the BM failure at present, SCT should continue to be performed on carefully selected patients. Perhaps the best candidates for SCT are patients with no pre-existing pulmonary disease and who have sibling donors. SCT using fludarabine-based protocols that avoid radiotherapy and busulphan appears to be giving encouraging preliminary results.

DC is theoretically a good candidate for haemopoietic gene therapy. In any given patient, DC is a single-gene disorder and the cells that need to be targeted (haemopoietic stem cells) are accessible. Furthermore, there is evidence from fibroblast culture studies and from skewed XCIPs in X-linked DC carriers that cells transfected with the normal gene would have growth/survival advantage compared with the uncorrected cells. Such an advantage would also be predicted from the role of dyskerin and hTR in telomere maintenance.

Shwachman–Diamond syndrome

Clinical features

Shwachman and Bodian and their colleagues first reported this disease independently in 1964. It is now recognized as an autosomal recessive disorder characterized by exocrine pancreatic insufficiency (100%), bone marrow dysfunction (100%) and other somatic abnormalities (particularly involving the skeletal system). Signs of pancreatic insufficiency (malabsorption, failure to thrive) are apparent early in infancy (note that the pancreatic function can improve in a subset of Shwachman–Diamond syndrome (SDS) patients by 4 years of age). Other common somatic abnormalities include short stature (~70%), protuberant abdomen and an ichthyotic skin rash (~60%). Metaphyseal dysostosis is seen on radiographs in ~75% of patients. Other abnormalities include hepatomegaly, rib/thoracic cage abnormalities, hypertelorism, syndactyly, cleft palate, dental dysplasia, ptosis and skin pigmentation.

The spectrum of haematological abnormalities includes neutropenia (~60%), other cytopenias (approximately 20% have pancytopenia), myelodysplasia and leukaemic transformation (~25%). The age at which leukaemia develops varies widely from 1 to 43 years. Acute myeloid leukaemia is the commonest category and there is an unexplained preponderance of cases of leukaemia in males (M/F ratio = ~9:1).

Exocrine pancreatic insufficiency and haematological abnormalities are also seen in Pearson's syndrome (PS), and this is therefore an important differential diagnosis. In PS, the anaemia is usually more prominent than neutropenia and the marrow usually shows ringed sideroblasts along with vacuolation of myeloid and erythroid precursors. In addition, acidosis, abnormalities of liver function and mitochondrial DNA rearrangements are seen in PS. PS has a worse prognosis than SDS, with many patients dying before the age of 5 years from liver or marrow failure. Other differential diagnoses to be excluded are cartilage hair syndrome and cystic fibrosis.

The SDS gene (*SBDS*) on 7q11 was identified in 2003. The majority (> 90%) of SDS patients have been found to have mutations in this gene. Its precise function is unknown but, based on the function of its homologues, it is predicted to have an important role in RNA metabolism and/or ribosome biogenesis. Several abnormalities in SDS cells have been observed, including haemopoietic stem and stromal defects, increased rates of apoptosis and short telomeres. It will be now interesting to see how mutations in the *SBDS* gene lead to all these cell defects, the increased frequency of isochromosome 7q[i(7q)] and the clinical abnormalities characteristic of SDS. More immediately, this advance provides a genetic test that will facilitate diagnosis in difficult cases. It will also enable researchers to determine the role of the *SBDS* gene in AA, myelodysplastic syndrome (MDS) and leukaemia in general.

Treatment

The malabsorption in SDS responds to treatment with oral pancreatic enzymes. For those with neutropenia, G-CSF may produce an improvement in the neutrophil count. Some patients with anaemia and/or thrombocytopenia may achieve haematological responses with oxymetholone treatment. As in other cases of bone marrow failure, supportive treatment with red cell and platelet transfusions and antibiotics is very important. The main causes of death are infection or bleeding.

Recent analysis of SDS patients has showed that the incidence of myelodysplasia and transformation to acute myeloid leukaemia (~15–25%) is higher than reported previously. The development of leukaemia, often with features of myelodysplasia, usually has a poor prognosis. SDS patients with leukaemia treated with conventional courses of chemotherapy usually fail to regenerate normal haemopoiesis. As this is a constitutional disorder all somatic cells, including haemopoietic stem cells, are abnormal. In addition, the haemopoietic stem cells may have accumulated secondary abnormalities as suggested by complex karyotypes (especially involving chromosome 7) often observed in the BM from such patients. Therefore, for those who develop leukaemia the only approach likely to be successful is allogeneic SCT, perhaps in the future using low-intensity conditioning regimens that include fludarabine. The similarities between SDS and the other common inherited bone marrow failure syndromes emphasize that SDS should be regarded as a disorder with high propensity to develop both AA and leukaemic transformation, particularly acute myeloid leukaemia with erythroid differentiation (AML-M6). As these complications may not develop until adult life, it is important to continue close haematological follow-up throughout life.

Diamond–Blackfan anaemia

Clinical features

Red cell aplasia was first reported in 1936 by Josephs. In 1938, Diamond reported on four children with hypoplastic anaemia, and this has now come to be recognized as Diamond–Blackfan anaemia (DBA) or congenital pure red cell aplasia. DBA usually presents in early infancy, with symptoms of anaemia such as pallor or failure to thrive. The hallmark of classical DBA is a selective decrease in erythroid precursors and normochromic macrocytic anaemia associated with a variable number of somatic abnormalities such as craniofacial, thumb, cardiac and urogenital malformations. Hitherto the diagnostic criteria for DBA have been (i) normochromic, usually macrocytic, but occasionally normocytic anaemia developing in early childhood; (ii) reticulocytopenia; (iii) normocellular BM with selective deficiency of erythroid precursors (erythroblasts < 5%); (iv) normal or slightly decreased leucocyte counts; and (v) normal or often increased platelet counts.

There is considerable heterogeneity in the associated somatic abnormalities, pattern of inheritance and response to therapy. Analysis of 350 cases recruited to the DBA Registry of North America (DBAR) has confirmed previous findings as well as highlighting new features. The annual incidence of DBA is ~5 per million live births. The median age at presentation was 8 weeks and 93% of patients presented in the first year of life. In total, 82% were initially responsive to steroids, 16% were non-responsive and 1.6% were never treated with steroids; 36% of patients were receiving transfusions at analysis. The actuarial survival rates at older than 40 years were 100% for those in sustained remission, 88% for steroid-maintained patients and 58% for transfusion-dependent patients. The 23 deaths reported to the registry included severe AA (1), infections (4), complications of iron overload (2), vascular access-related death (1), malignancy (6) and transplant-related toxicity (9).

In the DBAR, 7% of families had more than one affected individual. Most of the familial cases displayed autosomal dominant pattern of inheritance. Somatic anomalies, excluding short stature, were found in 47% of patients. Of these, 50% were of the face and head (high-arched palate, cleft lip, hypertelorism and flat nasal bridge), 38% were upper limb and hand (flat thenar eminence, triphalangeal thumb), 39% genitourinary and 30% cardiac. Height was below the third centile for age in ~30%.

MDS and AML have been reported in a few patients with DBA, suggesting an increased predisposition to haematological malignancies. There are also cases that have evolved into AA; neutropenia and thrombocytopenia are relatively common after the first decade. Giri and colleagues (2000) reported on moderate to severe BM hypocellularity in 21 out of 28 (75%) patients with steroid-refractory DBA; marrow hypoplasia correlated with the development of neutropenia (9 out of 21; 43%) and/or thrombocytopenia (6 out of 21; 29%). Furthermore, using *in vitro* long-term culture-initiating cell (LTC-IC) assay, they provided evidence for a trilineage haemopoietic defect in patients with refractory DBA. Thus, although DBA has been regarded classically as a pure red cell aplasia, a more global haemopoietic defect is likely to be present, and this may be seen more frequently in the future as patients are surviving longer due to improved medical care.

Cell and molecular biology

The classical haematological profile in DBA patients consists of normochromic macrocytic anaemia, reticulocytopenia and a normocellular marrow with selective deficiency of red cell precursors. A number of different defects of *in vitro* erythroid progenitor proliferation, differentiation and cytokine responsiveness have been reported but have not clarified the mechanism of *in vivo* erythroid failure. For many years, based on the typical selective deficiency in red cell precursors, many researchers believed that DBA is due to an intrinsic problem with erythroid proliferation/differentiation. On the other hand, the observation of a wide range of somatic abnormalities in a significant proportion of patients and case reports of thrombocytopenia, neutropenia and AA, together with the recent evidence for a trilineage haemopoietic defect, suggest that the primary problem in DBA is not confined to the erythroid lineage.

The establishment of DBA registries, recent advances in genetics and the identification of a female with a balanced X;19 translocation has facilitated a change in research strategy in DBA. Genetic mapping studies localized a gene responsible for DBA to a 1-Mb region on 19q13 on the basis of (i) the identification of a *de novo* balanced reciprocal X;19 translocation breakpoint in a girl with DBA; (ii) linkage analysis in multiplex DBA families; and (iii) *de novo* microdeletions associated with the disease. Cloning of the chromosome 19q13 breakpoint demonstrated that this breakpoint interrupts the gene (*RPS19*) encoding ribosomal protein S19. The subsequent finding of *RPS19* mutations in 10 out of 40 unrelated DBA patients provided good evidence for the primary role of this gene in the pathogenesis of DBA in approximately 25% of DBA cases.

Further analysis of 172 DBA families (190 patients) by the DBA Working Group of the European Society of Paediatric Haematology and Immunology (ESPHI) has demonstrated heterozygosity for mutations affecting the *RPS19* gene in 42 out of 172 index patients (24.4%), thus confirming the genetic heterogeneity of DBA. Interestingly, mutations in the *RPS19* gene were also found in some apparently unaffected individuals from DBA families presenting only with an isolated elevation of erythrocyte adenosine deaminase activity (eADA). The lack of a genotype–phenotype correlation implies that other factors modulate the phenotypic expression of the primary genetic defect in families with *RPS19* mutations.

Further linkage analysis in DBA families has identified a second DBA locus on chromosome 8p23.2–23.1 to which ~40% of DBA families map; however, a significant proportion of families map to neither the locus on chromosome 8 nor the locus on chromosome 19. This suggests that there are likely to be at least three DBA genes.

The *RPS19* gene shows a ubiquitous expression profile and encodes a 145-amino-acid protein with a predicted molecular weight of 16 kDa. This protein has significant homologies with proteins from diverse species. It is one of many ribosomal proteins that constitute a major component of cellular proteins, but their functions, apart from being part of the ribosome, are unknown.

The demonstration of *RPS19* mutations in ~25% of DBA families now makes it possible to confirm the diagnosis in a subset of DBA patients. This is useful when counselling families. However, the observed poor genotype–phenotype correlations

means that predictions about prognosis are not easy. Functional assays would be useful and may become available in the future. Furthermore, identification of the other DBA genes may now follow more rapidly.

Treatment

The first line of treatment for DBA remains corticosteroids. Once a maximal Hb response has been achieved, the dose of prednisolone should be tapered slowly until the patient is on the lowest dose possible on an alternate-day regimen. The dose required to achieve this can vary considerably from patient to patient. For those patients who fail to respond or become refractory to steroids, blood transfusion is the mainstay of treatment. As in thalassaemia, the major complication from transfusions is iron overload, and chelation of iron with desferrioxamine should therefore be commenced as soon as patients have increased iron stores. Splenectomy may be indicated in the event of an increased transfusion requirement secondary to hypersplenism. For patients who are transfusion dependent and who have a compatible sibling donor, haemopoietic SCT may be appropriate and is potentially curative. A recent pilot study reported on haematological response in three out of nine patients who were treated with metoclopramide. This observation suggests an alternative therapy for steroid-resistant patients. It also suggests a role for prolactin in erythropoiesis as metoclopramide is known to release prolactin from the pituitary.

Congenital and cyclical neutropenias

Congenital neutropenia is a heterogeneous disorder. It includes Kostmann's syndrome, which was first described in 1954. Although the original description by Kostmann was of an autosomal recessive disorder, other congenital neutropenia subtypes (both sporadic and autosomal dominant) have been included subsequently in this category. The neutropenia is usually recognized at birth and the neutrophil count is often $< 0.2 \times 10^9$/L. The Hb and platelet count are usually normal and the bone marrow shows a 'promyelocyte maturation arrest' with abundant promyelocytes but with a selective reduction in myelocytes, metamyelocytes and neutrophils.

The neutropenias are associated with severe infections and early death. No patient has developed AA but myeloid leukaemias (~10%) can occur. The availability of G-CSF has revolutionized the outcome of these children and probably has no aetological role in the evolution to leukaemia. However, somatic mutations in the gene that encodes the G-CSF receptor have been documented during the evolution to leukaemia in some neutropenic patients receiving G-CSF. For patients who become refractory to G-CSF or who develop leukaemia, SCT may be appropriate and curative.

Table 12.7 Laboratory tests useful in the investigation of patients with bone marrow failure.

Test		Diagnostic value
Peripheral blood		
Fetal haemoglobin		High level suggestive of generalized BM failure
DEB/MMC-chromosomal breakage		Increased in FA
Mutation analysis of specific genes	*FANCA to FANCG*	Mutated in FA
	DKC1 and *hTR*	Mutated in X-linked and autosomal dominant DC
	SBDS	Mutated in SDS
	RPS19	Mutated in ~25% of DBA
	ELA2	Mutated in congenital and cyclic neutropenia
	c-mpl	Mutated in CAMT
Mitochondrial DNA analysis		Deletions seen in Pearson syndrome
X-Chromosome inactivation patterns		Skewed in carriers of X-linked DC
Ham's (CD59 analysis)		Abnormal in paroxysmal nocturnal haemoglobinuria
Telomere length		Short in AA patients including DC, FA, SDS
Constitutional karyotype		Abnormality suggestive of constitutional AA
Other investigations		
To identify somatic abnormalities	Skeletal survey	Presence of somatic abnormalities in association
	Ultrasound of abdomen	with AA is suggestive of constitutional AA
	Pulmonary function tests	
	Echocardiogram	
Exocrine pancreatic function		Abnormal in SDS and PS
Neutrophil chemotaxis		Abnormal in SDS
Fibroblast cultures		Abnormalities seen in DC

Cyclical neutropenia is characterized by a neutrophil count that usually reaches a nadir with a 21-day periodicity. Around the nadir, patients may develop fever and mouth ulcers. In cyclical neutropenia, the pattern of inheritance is usually autosomal dominant. Linkage analysis in affected families resulted in the localization of the disease to 19p13.3. Subsequent studies identified mutations in the gene encoding neutrophil elastase (*ELA2*). An extraordinary twist to the story was the identification of *ELA2* mutations also in many patients with congenital neutropenia. In cyclical neutropenia, the mutations are usually clustered around the active site of the molecule, whereas the opposite face of the molecule tends to be mutated in congenital neutropenia patients. Neutrophil elastase is a serine protease that is synthesized predominantly at the promyelocytic stage and can be expected to be important in neutrophil development. Further studies are needed to understand the precise mechanism of how *ELA2* mutations result in neutropenia and to identify the genetic defects in other congenital neutropenic patients who lack *ELA2* mutations.

Thrombocytopenia with absent radii

Thrombocytopenia with absent radii (TAR) is an autosomal recessive disorder characterized by hypomegakaryocytic thrombocytopenia and bilateral radial aplasia. Babies with TAR often have haemorrhagic manifestations at birth when the diagnosis is usually made, owing to the characteristic physical appearance combined with thrombocytopenia. Additional skeletal (absent ulnae, absent humeri, clinodactyly) and other somatic (microcephaly, hypertelorism, strabismus, heart defects) abnormalities may be seen in some patients.

The platelet count is usually below 50×10^9/L. The leucocyte count can be normal or raised, sometimes up to 100×10^9/L ('leukaemoid reaction'). BM cellularity is normal and myeloid and erythroid lineages are normal or increased. Megakaryocytes are absent or decreased. Most patients bleed in infancy and then improve after the first year. The mainstay of management is prophylactic and therapeutic use of platelet transfusions. TAR patients have a very good prognosis after infancy. There have been no reports of AA or leukaemia.

The pathophysiology of TAR is unknown. Thrombopoietin levels are usually elevated and thrombopoietin receptor expression on the surface of TAR platelets is normal. Therefore, defective megakaryocytopoiesis/thrombocytopoiesis does not appear to be caused by a defect in thrombopoietin production. There is some evidence that it may be due to a lack of response to thrombopoietin in the signal transduction pathway of the thrombopoietin receptor (*c-mpl*).

Congenital amegakaryocytic thrombocytopenia

Congenital amegakaryocytic thrombocytopenia (CAMT) is a rare disorder that usually presents in infancy and is characterized by isolated thrombocytopenia and reduction/absence of megakaryocytes in the bone marrow, usually with no somatic abnormalities. It is genetically heterogeneous with autosomal recessive and X-linked subtypes. Approximately 50% of patients will develop AA usually by the age of 5 years. For patients with severe thrombocytopenia or AA, the treatment of choice is SCT if a compatible donor is available.

In a subgroup of CAMT patients, mutations in the gene encoding for the thrombopoietin receptor (c-Mpl) have been identified. As patients with *c-mpl* mutations can also have abnormalities in the leucocyte count, Hb level and CNS abnormalities (e.g. cerebral and cerebellar hypoplasia), this study highlights the important role of the c-Mpl receptor in haemopoiesis in general and in CNS development. It also substantiates the genetic heterogeneity of CAMT.

Conclusion

Since the identification of the first FA gene (*FANCC*) in 1992, there have been significant advances in our understanding of FA, DC and other BM failure syndromes. This is already facilitating diagnosis, as highlighted in Table 12.7. It can be anticipated that a further understanding of the pathophysiology of these disorders is likely to lead to a better knowledge of normal haemopoiesis and how this becomes defective in many patients presenting with the more common forms of aplastic anaemia. Indeed, recent studies have already established a link between DC and AA and, in turn, to defective telomerase. These advances also suggest that new treatment strategies, based on correction of the primary defect in each syndrome, may now emerge.

Selected bibliography

All inherited bone marrow failure syndromes
Alter BP, Young NS (1998) The bone marrow failure syndromes. In: *Hematology of Infancy and Childhood* (DG Nathan, HS Orkin, eds), pp. 237–335. WB Saunders, Philadelphia.

Fanconi anaemia
Auerbach AD, Buchwald M, Joenje H (2001) Fanconi anemia. In: *The Metabolic and Molecular Basis Of Inherited Disease* (CR Scriver *et al.*, eds), pp. 753–68. McGraw-Hill, New York.
Guardiola P, Socie G, Pasquini R *et al.* (1998) Allogeneic stem cell transplantation for Fanconi anaemia. *Bone Marrow Transplant* (1998); 21 (Suppl. 2): 24–7.
Guardiola Ph, Pasquini R, Dokal I *et al.* (2000) Outcome of 69 allogeneic stem transplantations for Fanconi anemia using HLA-matched unrelated donors: a study on behalf of the European Group for Blood and Marrow Transplantation. *Blood* 95: 422–9.
Howlett NG, Taniguchi T, Olson S *et al.* (2002) Biallelic inactivation of *BRCA2* in Fanconi anemia. *Science* 297: 606–9.
Joenje H, Patel KJ (2001) The emerging genetic and molecular basis of Fanconi anaemia. *Nature Review of Genetics* 2: 446–57.
Liu JM, Kim S, Read EJ *et al.* (1999) Engraftment of hematopoietic progenitor cells transduced with the Fanconi anemia group C gene (*FANCC*). *Human Gene Therapy* 10: 2337–46.
Taniguchi T, Garcia-Higuera I, Xu B *et al.* (2002) Convergence of the Fanconi anemia and ataxia telangiectasia signalling pathways. *Cell* 109: 459–72.
Waisfisz Q, Morgan NV, Savino M *et al.* (1999) Spontaneous functional correction of homozygous Fanconi anaemia alleles reveals novel mechanistic basis for reverse mosaicism. *Nature Genetics* 22: 379–83.

Dyskeratosis congenita
Dokal I (2000) Dyskeratosis congenita in all its forms. *British Journal of Haematology* 110: 768–79.
Heiss NS, Knight SW, Vulliamy TJ *et al.* (1998) X-linked dyskeratosis congenita is caused by mutations in a highly conserved gene with putative nucleolar functions. *Nature Genetics* 19: 32–8.
Knight SW, Heiss NS, Vulliamy TJ *et al.* (1999) Unexplained aplastic anaemia, immunodeficiency, and cerebellar hypoplasia (Hoyeraal–Hreidarsson syndrome) due to mutations in the dyskeratosis congenita gene, DKC1. *British Journal of Haematology* 107: 335–9.
Mitchell JR, Wood E, Collins K (1999) A telomerase component is defective in the human disease dyskeratosis congenita. *Nature* 402: 551–5.
Vulliamy T, Marrone A, Goldman F *et al.* (2001) The RNA component of telomerase is mutated in autosomal dominant dyskeratosis congenita. *Nature* 413: 432–5.
Vulliamy T, Marrone A, Dokal I *et al.* (2002) Association between aplastic anaemia and mutations in telomerase RNA. *Lancet* 359: 2168–70.

Shwachman–Diamond syndrome
Boocock GRB, Morrison JA, Popovic M *et al.* (2003) Mutations in *SBDS* are associated with Shwachman–Diamond syndrome. *Nature Genetics* 33: 97–101.
Dror Y, Freedman MH (2002) Shwachman–Diamond syndrome. *British Journal of Haematology* 118: 701–13.

Diamond–Blackfan anaemia
Draptchinskaia N, Gustavsson P, Andersson B *et al.* (1999) The gene encoding ribosomal protein S19 is mutated in Diamond–Blackfan anaemia. *Nature Genetics* 21: 169–75.
Vlachos A, Klein GW, Lipton JM (2001) The Diamond Blackfan anemia registry: tool for investigating the epidemiology and biology of Diamond–Blackfan anemia. *Journal of Pediatric Hematology/Oncology* 23: 377–82.
Willig T-N, Dratchinskaia N, Dianzani I *et al.* (1999) Mutations in ribosomal protein S19 and Diamond Blackfan anemia: wide variations in phenotypic expression. *Blood* 94: 4294–306.

Congenital and cyclical neutropenia

Dale DC, Person RE, Bolyard A *et al.* (2000) Mutations in the gene encoding neutrophil elastase in congenital and cyclic neutropenia. *Blood* **96**: 2317–22.

Congenital amegakaryocytic thrombocytopenia

Ihara K, Ishii E, Eguchi M *et al.* (1999) Identification of mutations in the c-mpl gene in congenital amegakaryocytic thrombocytopenia. *Proceedings of the National Academy of Science USA* **96**: 3132–6.

CHAPTER 13

Acquired aplastic anaemia, other acquired bone marrow failure disorders and dyserythropoiesis

13

Edward C Gordon-Smith and Judith CW Marsh

Introduction – bone marrow failure

Bone marrow failure implies that peripheral blood cytopenia has arisen primarily as a result of a specific failure of bone marrow precursor cells to produce mature cells, rather than the production of abnormal cells that have a shortened survival or the production of normal cells that are subjected to an abnormal environment. In bone marrow failure, the remaining cells in the marrow appear morphologically normal, or near normal, reflecting only minor changes produced by 'marrow stress', including a mild increase in dyserythropoietic forms, often with some macrocytosis of red cells. The stroma of the marrow does not appear to be disturbed. These observations distinguish the true marrow failures from myelodysplastic and myeloproliferative syndromes.

There are two major groups of bone marrow failure: the aplastic anaemias, in which the failure lies in the pluripotent stem cell, and the single-cell cytopenias, in which the failure lies in one of the committed cell lines. There is overlap between these groups, for single-cell failure may occasionally progress to total marrow failure, and, following partial recovery, aplastic anaemia may continue with a prolonged period of single-cell deficiency. It is convenient to consider the two groups separately.

Aplastic anaemias

Aplastic anaemia is defined as the presence of pancytopenia in the peripheral blood and a hypocellular marrow in which normal haemopoietic marrow is replaced by fat cells. The diagnosis of aplastic anaemia requires at least two of the following in addition to a hypocellular marrow: (i) haemoglobin < 10 g/dL; (ii) platelet count < 100×10^9/L; and (iii) neutrophil count < 1.5 $\times 10^9$/L. Abnormal cells are not found in either the peripheral blood or the bone marrow. The diagnosis is based on the absence of cells, not the presence of any characteristic feature.

There are a variety of ways in which this haematological pattern can be produced, as indicated in Table 13.1. Distinguishing between these forms of aplastic anaemia is a matter of awareness, careful observation of haematological material, particularly the granulocyte and megakaryocyte morphology, history and physical examination.

Inevitable aplastic anaemia

Most cytotoxic drugs, penetrating ionizing radiation and radioactive substances concentrated in the marrow are capable of producing aplastic anaemia through their effects on actively dividing cells. The timing and duration of the aplasia and the order in which cell lines recover depend to some extent on the nature of the cytotoxic agent and the dose. Recovery is usual, with the exception of marrow rendered aplastic by whole-body irradiation given in a critical dose that destroys the haemopoietic system without killing the patient from additional toxicity. Although, in general, the development and recovery of aplasia following exposure to cytotoxic drugs are predictable, there are exceptions. Repeated or prolonged exposure to small doses of alkylating agents, particularly busulphan, may lead to a prolonged and unpredictable aplasia, even when given for myeloproliferative disorders such as chronic myeloid leukaemia, essential thrombocythaemia or myelofibrosis.

Table 13.1 The aplastic anaemias.

Aetiology	Examples	Clinical course
Inevitable	Ionizing radiation Cytotoxic drugs	Predictable Recovery usual
Idiosyncratic	Idiopathic Drug induced Viral Commercial solvents	Prolonged Unpredictable recovery Clonal evolution
Inherited	Fanconi anaemia Dyskeratosis congenita Others	Usually progressive Increased malignancy
Industrial	Benzene	Dose dependent Proliferative disorders more common
Immune	Drug induced Viruses (e.g. Epstein–Barr virus) Systemic lupus erythematosus	Usually recovers spontaneously or with treatment of primary disorder
Malignant	Acute lymphoblastic leukaemia Hypoplastic acute myeloid leukaemia Hypoplastic myelodysplastic syndrome	Usually but not exclusively in children

Idiosyncratic acquired aplastic anaemia

Acquired aplastic anaemia may occur spontaneously or appear following exposure to drugs or viruses that do not produce marrow failure in the great majority of persons exposed to these agents. The disease is characterized by its unpredictable onset and prolonged course, death usually occurring as a result of a deficiency of granulocytes or platelets and a failure in support measures.

Incidence

In Western countries, the incidence is about 2–3 per million of the population per year. Higher figures given in the past were probably the result of including cases of pancytopenia that were not aplastic by strict criteria but included cases of myelodysplasia. In the East, the incidence appears to be 5- to 10-fold higher, the reason apparently lying in the environment rather than in genetic factors, as people who move from the East to the West have the same incidence as the local population.

Aetiology

In about one-third of the patients with acquired aplastic anaemia, suspicion may be directed to a particular agent, usually a drug, chemical or virus. Thus, in at least two-thirds of patients, no aetiological agent can be identified (idiopathic aplastic anaemia).

Drugs

The list of drugs recorded as 'causing' aplastic anaemia is long, but mostly only a single or a few cases have been reported for each drug, and it is not profitable to detail them all because the evidence against many of these drugs is slim. Some of the more commonly implicated drugs are listed in Table 13.2. A difficulty in determining the role of drug exposure to the development of aplastic anaemia is the delay between exposure to the drug and the identification of marrow damage. Typically, there is a delay of 2–3 months between first exposure and the onset of pancytopenia. This delay may be longer, although an exposure that took place for a short period 6 months to a year previously weakens the association, and exposure more than 1 year earlier makes the association unlikely.

Perhaps most attention has been given to chloramphenicol. It is estimated that somewhere between 1:25 000 and 1:40 000 people exposed to oral chloramphenicol will develop aplastic anaemia. The evidence is purely epidemiological, as there are no tests to demonstrate that chloramphenicol is responsible for aplastic anaemia in any particular case The aplasia is unpredictable and prolonged. Chloramphenicol also causes a dose-dependent suppression of haemopoiesis, particularly affecting erythropoiesis, through its action on mitochondrial DNA, but this suppression is not related to the development of prolonged aplastic anaemia. The majority of patients who develop aplastic anaemia following chloramphenicol have been on standard therapeutic doses and received the drug for an appropriate length of time. Some of the early reports concerned patients who had received prolonged treatment. Subsequently, reports appeared of only patients who had been exposed to the drug for 1 day, giving credence to the idea that this adverse reaction was not dose dependent. There have been only 24 reported cases of aplastic anaemia following exposure to chloramphenicol eye

Table 13.2 Drugs associated with idiosyncratic acquired aplastic anaemia.

Class	Examples
Antibiotics	Chloramphenicol
	Sulphonamides
	Cotrimoxazole
Antimalarials	Chloroquine
Anti-inflammatories	Phenylbutazone
	Indomethacin
	Naproxen
	Diclofenac
	Ibuprofen
	Piroxicam
Antirheumatics	Gold salts
	D-Penicillamine
Antithyroids	Carbimazole
	Methylthiouracil
	Propylthiouracil
Psychotropic/antidepressants	Phenothiazines
	Mianserin
	Dothiepin
Anticonvulsants	Carbamazepine
	Phenytoin
Antidiabetics	Chlorpropamide
Carbonic anhydrase inhibitors	Acetazolamide

drops in the 45 years since the drug was first introduced, which suggests that the association is no greater than background and that eye drops are not a hazard.

Sulphonamides have also been thought to cause aplastic anaemia, and there are several reports of aplasia following cotrimoxazole administration. Again, it is difficult to be sure of the strength of the association, especially as the antibiotics may be given for an infection that is the first marker of an undetected marrow dyscrasia. The association of co-trimoxazole with neutropenia and aplastic anaemia may not be due to the sulphonamide moiety, as trimethoprim alone has a similar adverse event profile.

A few case reports have appeared associated with other antibiotics, but there is no clear evidence that this is not a chance association in most instances. Most are more likely to produce single cytopenias, mainly through antibody-mediated peripheral destruction.

Non-steroidal anti-inflammatory drugs (NSAIDs) have been incriminated in causing aplastic anaemia. The pyrazalone derivatives, phenylbutazone and oxyphenbutazone, have the highest incidence of aplasia in this group, but the indole derivatives,

indomethacin and sulindac, have both been reported in association with aplastic anaemia. Other NSAIDs that have been linked to the cause of aplastic anaemia are listed in Table 13.2. It seems possible that the development of aplastic anaemia in response to NSAIDs is, at least in some respects, a class effect in that there have been cases of relapse of aplastic anaemia, which followed exposure to one NSAID when the patient was subsequently given another, chemically unrelated NSAID. This group of drugs illustrates well the difficulties in establishing causal relationships with aplastic anaemia. They are widely used by patients with an underlying disease that may have an autoimmune basis (e.g. rheumatoid arthritis) and who might have an increased risk of developing blood dyscrasias as a result of their disease.

Gold salts deserve a special mention. Neutropenia and eosinophilia are common with their use. Gold-induced auto-immune thrombocytopenia may also occur; the autoantibody targets platelet glycoprotein V. Persistence with gold injections in the face of a falling neutrophil count may lead to aplasia or aplasia may appear without warning. Gold salts are one of the few drugs for which careful monitoring of blood counts may prevent the development of aplasia. Gold may be removed from the body by chelation with dimercaprol (British anti-Lewisite, BAL), which is usually given by intramuscular injection, which makes it difficult to administer to patients with aplastic anaemia. There is no evidence that removal of gold in this way accelerates recovery, and it is possible to detect gold in the marrow of patients who have recovered from gold-induced aplasia more than 1 year after recovery.

Aminosalicylates are used in the management of ulcerative colitis and rheumatoid arthritis. Sulphasalazine (Salazopyrin®) has long been known to be associated with blood dyscrasias, including aplastic anaemia. It was thought that the haemopoietic toxicity was due to the sulphonamide moiety, but cases of aplastic anaemia following exposure to mesalazine (5-aminosalicylic acid) and osalazine have also been reported.

Industrial and domestic chemicals have also been implicated. Solvents have long been linked to aplastic anaemia. Benzene is a myelotoxin. Exposure to sufficient levels leads inevitably to marrow damage but there seems to be wide variation between individuals in the dose required, and it is doubtful whether it produces aplasia of the idiosyncratic variety (see below). Insecticides, in particular lindane (γ-hexachlorocyclohexane), pentachlorophenols and DDT, have each been debated in this regard. Self-reported house treatment for woodworm has recently been strongly associated with risk of aplastic anaemia, along with exposure to radiation in the workplace.

Viruses

Hepatitis, presumably of viral origin, is a precursor of aplastic anaemia in about 5–10% of cases in the West; it is perhaps double that in the Far East. In the majority of patients, no specific hepatitis virus can be identified and the association is based on clinical grounds and the presence of abnormal liver function tests. In most cases, no identifiable virus is found, although occasionally it occurs following hepatitis A, B or C or Epstein–Barr virus infection. The delay between the clinical hepatitis and the onset of pancytopenia is of the order of 2–3 months, a similar period to that between drug exposure and aplasia. Further evidence to support the association is a finding that 28% of patients who underwent orthotopic liver transplantation for fulminant liver failure following viral hepatitis developed aplastic anaemia, whereas patients transplanted for other reasons had no marrow failure. A recent study from the European Blood and Marrow Transplantation (EBMT) Severe Aplastic Anaemia Working Party has shown that the outcome of treatment of post-hepatitic aplastic anaemia compared with idiopathic aplastic anaemia is similar whether treated with bone marrow transplantation or immunosuppressive therapy.

Parvovirus B19 infection in non-immune individuals may lead to a transient pure red cell aplasia of clinical importance to people with haemolytic anaemia (see below). The virus specifically infects the erythroid burst-forming units (BFU-E) and is not associated with true aplastic anaemia.

Epstein–Barr virus infection is commonly accompanied by neutropenia or thrombocytopenia, probably of an immune origin. Rarely, there may be true marrow aplasia, which behaves like other cases of acquired disease, although within this group there are some patients who have transient aplasia with spontaneous recovery in 4–6 weeks. Human immunodeficiency virus (HIV) is often accompanied by cytopenias; pancytopenia with a hypocellular marrow occurs in some cases.

Other causes of aplastic anaemia

Aplastic anaemia may occasionally occur in association with systemic autoimmune disorders such as systemic lupus erythematosus (SLE). As well as producing a hypocellular bone marrow, SLE may also be associated with a truly autoimmune pancytopenia with a cellular bone marrow. Aplastic anaemia can present in pregnancy, although this may be due to chance, and other possible causes listed above should also be sought. The disease may remit spontaneously after termination, whether spontaneous or therapeutic, and after delivery, but not in all cases, and much support may be needed. Aplastic anaemia often progresses during pregnancy, but not always.

Pathogenesis

The pathogenesis of aplastic anaemia remains unclear, but an autoimmune mechanism appears to be important. There may also be an as yet unidentified underlying genetic predisposition. There is some association of human leucocyte antigen (HLA) DR2, specifically the DR15 split, with acquired aplastic anaemia. There is debate about whether the primary defect is in the haemopoietic stem cell itself or is the result of environmental factors, particularly immunological attack, on the cell. There is evidence of both quantitative and qualitative stem cell defects in aplastic anaemia and increased apoptosis of remaining early

haemopoietic progenitor cells. Not only do cytotoxic suppressor T lymphocytes release cytokines, such as interferon-γ and tumour necrosis factor α (TNF-α), that are inhibitory to haemopoietic progenitor cells, but TNF-α also upregulates Fas antigen expression on CD34$^+$ cells, which may be one of the possible mechanisms for the reduced survival of aplastic anaemia marrow progenitor cells. However, the most persuasive evidence for the autoimmune pathogenesis for aplastic anaemia remains the clinical response to antilymphocyte globulin (ALG) in about two-thirds of patients.

Telomere shortening

Prolonged survival of patients with aplastic anaemia has provided the opportunity to study the effects of increased proliferative demand on remaining stem cells over time, both during the aplastic phase and following remission. Somatic cells show progressive shortening of the terminal restriction fragments (TRFs) of chromosomes with age. Haemopoietic stem cells show this age-related shortening as measured in the TRF length of their progeny, the circulating leucocytes. The telomere length is determined by the number of divisions that a cell undergoes, modified by the capacity of the enzyme telomerase to replace the fragments. Patients with acquired aplastic anaemia show increased TRF loss in leucocytes compared with age-matched control subjects, and the extent of the loss correlates with the duration of disease. In patients who make a full haemopoietic recovery, the rate of TRF loss returns to normal for ageing. Telomeres, which are complex structures located at the ends of eukaryotic chromosomes, have a role in preventing aberrant recombination at the chromosome ends. It is at least theoretically plausible that the accelerated TRF loss in aplastic anaemia provides the background for the increased risk of transformation to myelodysplastic syndrome (MDS) or acute leukaemia with cytogenetic anomalies.

In the inherited disorder dyskeratosis congenita, in which aplastic anaemia usually develops in the second or third decade, the underlying genetic defects affect the telomerase complex, which has both RNA and protein components. In the X-linked form of the disease there are mutations in the gene *DKC1*, which codes for the protein dyskerin. In the autosomal dominant form there is a mutation that leads to a large deletion in telomerase RNA. Stem cells from patients with both types have markedly short telomeres. Although the phenomenon of telomere shortening is different in acquired AA compared with age-matched control subjects, it is intriguing to speculate that perturbation in telomere turnover might be related to the pathogenesis of bone marrow failure in both types.

Haematology

The peripheral blood film shows pancytopenia without gross morphological abnormalities in the circulating cells. There may be some macrocytosis of remaining red cells, usually with an absolute reticulocytopenia. A relative reticulocytosis should always raise the possibility of associated paroxysmal nocturnal haemoglobinuria (PNH). Granulocytes often show increased staining of granules, the so-called toxic granulation of neutropenia. Monocytes are usually reduced in proportion to the granulocytes. Platelets are reduced and of small and uniform size. There is a variable reduction in the lymphocyte count between individuals; the count is sometimes normal or even increased so that the total white cell count is normal or near normal but, more commonly, the lymphocyte count is reduced. Abnormal cells are not seen. The bone marrow aspirate is normally easily obtained, typically with many fragments, which appear hypocellular (Figure 13.1a). The cell trails are hypocellular, with a relative increase in lymphocytes and plasma cells and other non-haemopoietic forms. Remaining haemopoietic precursors are normal in appearance.

In the early stages of aplastic anaemia, haemophagocytosis may be prominent. In a high proportion of cases, the hypocellularity of the marrow is patchy, with quite extensive areas of cellular marrow remaining. The bone marrow aspirate may, under these circumstances, be misleadingly cellular. A trephine biopsy (sometimes more than one) is necessary to assess cellularity properly.

The bone marrow trephine shows the fat replacement of marrow with or without the remaining islands of cellularity (Figure 13.1b and c). Non-haemopoietic cells remain, sometimes giving the impression of a chronic inflammatory infiltrate. Reticulin is not increased. The most common mistake in the diagnosis of aplastic anaemia is to make the diagnosis on the basis of a bone marrow aspirate in the presence of pancytopenia without obtaining adequate trephine specimen. Other conditions that can also present with pancytopenia and a hypocellular bone marrow include hypocellular myelodysplastic syndrome, hypocellular acute myeloid leukaemia, hypocellular acute lymphoblastic leukaemia, hairy cell leukaemia, lymphoma, myelofibrosis, mycobacterial infections and anorexia nervosa or prolonged starvation, emphasizing the importance of careful examination of not only the bone marrow but also a well-stained peripheral blood film.

Cytogenetic analysis of the bone marrow should be performed, although it is often difficult to obtain sufficient metaphases in a very hypocellular bone marrow. Abnormal cytogenetic clones occur in up to 11% of patients with otherwise typical aplastic anaemia, and their presence does not necessarily indicate a diagnosis of myelodysplastic syndrome. The most frequently observed abnormalities include trisomy 8, trisomy 6, 5q– and anomalies of chromosomes 7 and 13. Often the abnormal clone is small, constituting only a small proportion of total metaphases, and not infrequently it may be transient and disappear spontaneously or after haematological response to immunosuppressive therapy.

Peripheral blood lymphocytes should also be examined cytogenetically in all patients under the age of 35 years for spontaneous and di-epoxybutane (or mitomycin C)-induced increase

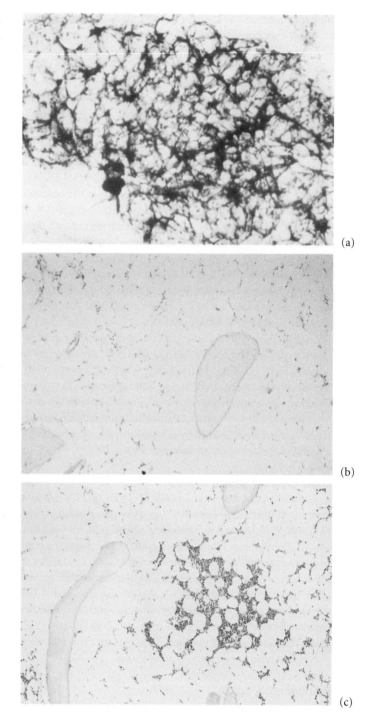

(a)

(b)

(c)

Figure 13.1 Aplastic anaemia. (a) Bone marrow aspirate showing fragments with typical lacy appearance and fatty hypocellular trails (×80). (b) Bone marrow trephine biopsy showing absence of haemopoietic tissue and its replacement by fat (×40). (c) Trephine biopsy showing island of preserved cellularity ('hot spot', ×40).

in chromosome breakages and aberrations characteristic of Fanconi anaemia, an inherited from of aplastic anaemia (see Chapter 12).

Paroxysmal nocturnal haemoglobinuria (PNH) should be excluded by performing a Ham test and/or flow cytometry. Analysis of phosphatidylinositol glycan (PIG)-anchored proteins such as CD55 and CD59 by flow cytometry is the much more sensitive test for PNH. Small PNH clones occur in around 25% of patients with aplastic anaemia, but the clinical significance of a small PNH clone is uncertain. Such clones can remain stable, diminish in size, disappear or increase. What is clinically important is the presence of a significant PNH clone with clinical or laboratory evidence of haemolysis, which will be detected by the Ham test. Urine should also be examined for haemosiderin to exclude intravascular haemolysis, which is a constant feature of haemolytic PNH. Evidence of haemolysis associated with PNH should be quantified with the reticulocyte count, serum bilirubin, serum transaminases and lactate dehydrogenase (see Chapter 11).

Special tests may be of interest in the diagnosis and prognosis of aplastic anaemia. Short-term clonogenic cultures of bone marrow show a uniform reduction in aplastic anaemia in both committed and multipotent progenitor cells. The more primitive long-term culture initiating cells are markedly reduced or absent. Stroma from aplastic marrow may be difficult to grow to confluence *in vitro*, but aplastic stroma is able to support haemopoiesis from normal stem cells but normal stroma is unable to reverse the defect in colony formation from AA stem cells.

Clinical presentation

The clinical features derive from the decrease in peripheral blood cells and are non-specific. The patient may be feeling completely well at the time when easy bruising or petechiae appear or may have a more or less prolonged period of feeling tired from anaemia. Sometimes infection is the presenting feature, but this is less common in idiosyncratic aplastic anaemia than bleeding manifestations. The spleen, liver and lymph nodes are not enlarged and jaundice is only a feature in those patients with post-hepatitis aplasia who have a prolonged cholestatic phase after the infection.

At presentation, it is necessary to take a detailed drug, occupational and symptomatic history to try to establish any aetiological agent so that this may be avoided in the future. Unfortunately, this is not always easy. It is difficult to dissuade someone who may have been exposed to industrial chemicals, for example, to give up work on the possibility that the chemicals just might be involved in the cause of the disease.

Clinical course

The clinical course is modified by the transfusion support and antibiotic therapy that the patient receives. There are some events that may interrupt the clinical course, apart from the catastrophes associated with the low platelet count and neu-

Table 13.3 Definition of disease severity of aplastic anaemia (AA).

Severe AA	BM cellularity < 25%, or 25–50% with < 30% residual haemopoietic cells
	Two out of three of the following: neutrophils < 0.5×10^9/L, platelets < 20×10^9/L, reticulocytes < 20×10^9/L
Very severe AA	As for severe AA but neutrophils < 0.2×10^9/L
Non-severe AA	Patients not fulfilling the criteria for severe or very severe AA
	With a hypocellular marrow, with two out of three of the following: neutrophils < 1.5×10^9/L, platelets < 100×10^9/L, haemoglobin < 10 g/dL

tropenia. The proliferative capacity of the marrow is greatly reduced, but the marrow also appears to be unstable in that abnormal clones of cells, PNH, myelodysplasia or leukaemia, may appear during the disease, sometimes all three in the same individual. In patients who have a remission or partial response, about 25–40% will develop a clonal disorder or relapse within 5–10 years, although this is not necessarily associated with a poor prognosis. The degree of aplasia may vary. In an attempt to categorize aplastic anaemia according to its severity and prognosis, Camitta and colleagues devised a system for scoring the disease in individual patients into severe aplastic anaemia (SAA) and non-severe aplastic anaemia (NSAA). Subsequently, as support and treatment improved, a third category of very severe aplastic anaemia (VSAA) was added (Table 13.3). One of the most important attributes of this scoring system is the ability it gives to compare different treatments for similar degrees of severity at all ages.

The initial assessment will characterize the severity of the condition at that time but will not indicate the course in a particular patient. SAA or VSAA tends not to improve without definitive treatment. NSAA may remain stable or slowly worsen with time, even without the development of abnormal clones.

Treatment

The treatment of aplastic anaemia depends first on providing total support for the patient while awaiting bone marrow recovery and, second, on attempts to accelerate that recovery. It should be emphasized that support and encouragement may be required for months or years before some sort of remission occurs and that disappointment and anxiety bedevil the management of aplastic anaemia. Patients, relatives and staff all need help in maintaining morale.

Support for the aplastic anaemia patient

This consists of providing blood product support and protecting patients from infection by isolating them from sources of infection as far as possible and in the use of antibiotics, both prophylactic and therapeutic.

Blood product support is mainly with packed red cells and platelet transfusions, to maintain a safe blood count. Patients are usually transfused with packed cells as required; in non-bleeding patients this is about 1 unit per week, given as three or four units every 3 or 4 weeks. Prophylactic platelet transfusions should be given when the platelet count is $< 10 \times 10^9$/L (or $< 20 \times 10^9$/L in the presence of fever), rather than giving platelets only in response to bleeding. Prediction of bleeding is difficult in an individual patient. Fatal haemorrhage, usually cerebral, is more common in patients who have $< 10 \times 10^9$/L platelets, retinal haemorrhages, buccal haemorrhages or rapidly spreading purpura. However, cerebral haemorrhage may be the first major bleed in patients who have none of these other bleeding manifestations. A proportion of patients will become sensitized to platelet transfusions if random donors are used. Those who are sensitized will have to receive HLA-matched platelets. Family members should be avoided unless bone marrow transplantation has been ruled out as treatment. Platelets given twice per week are usually sufficient to prevent bleeding.

Antibiotics may be used prophylactically, particularly in patients with severe neutropenia ($< 0.2 \times 10^9$/L). These patients may acquire infection from the gastrointestinal tract (particularly aerobic pathogens) or from the upper respiratory passages. Good mouth care with chlorhexidine mouthwash is of benefit. Patients should be in reverse-barrier isolation while in hospital. Measures to decrease potential intestinal pathogens include the use of non-absorbable antibiotics and antifungal agents, and the provision of low-bacterial food. When fever or signs of infection develop, fevers should be treated immediately in severely neutropenic patients, that is, with the prompt administration of broad-spectrum intravenous antibiotics, particularly those active against Gram-negative organisms. Treatment should be started after taking appropriate samples for microbiology but before the results are available. The antibiotics should be continued until at least 72 h of normal temperature has been achieved, but, unfortunately, in the severely neutropenic patient, infection is rarely eradicated and all too frequently fever returns after stopping the therapy.

Staphylococcus epidermidis is a common cause of bacteraemia in patients who have a central line in place. If fever in the neutropenic patient does not resolve within 24 h, vancomycin or teicoplanin (or other antibiotic active against *S. epidermidis*) should be added to the Gram-negative antibiotic regimen. Failure of the fever to resolve after this in the absence of a positive blood culture suggests the possibility of a fungal infection and intravenous amphotericin should be added early to the regimen. Granulocyte colony-stimulating factor (G-CSF) may raise the neutrophil count and improve their function, and may have a role to play in the eradication of infection in aplastic patients, although no formal trials have been conducted. G-CSF tends to have the weakest effect in the most severely aplastic patients.

Restoration of marrow activity

Spontaneous remission of aplastic anaemia may occur, but this may not happen for several months or even years and the majority of patients with SAA die from the complications of neutropenia or thrombocytopenia before this can occur. Bone marrow transplantation is a therapeutic option open to younger patients who have an HLA-matched sibling donor and is discussed in detail below.

Immunosuppressive therapy

Immunosuppressive therapy with ALG and/or cyclosporin has proved to be effective in increasing the remission rate in aplastic anaemia. There is no role for the use of corticosteroids in the treatment of aplastic anaemia, other than a short course when used with ALG to help prevent serum sickness. Coticosteroids are ineffective in the treatment of aplastic anaemia; they encourage bacterial and fungal colonization and can precipitate serious gastrointestinal haemorrhage in the presence of severe thrombocytopenia.

Antilymphocyte globulin

The use of ALG in the treatment of aplastic anaemia was pioneered by George Mathé and his colleagues in Paris in the 1960s and developed by Bruno Speck in Basle. The benefit of ALG in promoting marrow recovery in aplastic anaemia was later confirmed in randomized trials conducted in the USA.

Preparations. Antilymphocyte globulin is available from a number of commercial companies. The antihuman lymphocyte globulin is raised either in horses or in rabbits. A variety of immunogens are used in the preparation of the spectrum of polyclonal antibodies, which make up the various preparations of ALG. In many preparations, the immunogen is a thymocyte-derived cell line or thymocytes obtained from thymuses removed during cardiac surgery in children. These preparations are usually called antithymocyte globulin (ATG). The main combinations used in the preparation of ALG or ATG and the range of antibodies obtained are shown in Table 13.4. During preparation, unwanted antihuman antibodies are removed by absorption with specific tissues, but most preparations still have some antiplatelet activity. Although, clearly, there is not biological equivalence between preparations, no proper comparative studies have been carried out to identify essential characteristics or antibody components. Most preparations have been developed for the prevention of graft rejection in cardiac or renal transplants, but it is not evident that the same antibody profile is needed for the treatment of aplastic anaemia.

Administration. Antilymphocyte globulin is a highly immunosuppressive drug. It should be prescribed only by physicians familiar with using the drug. It must be given only as an inpatient therapy, and patients should be nursed in isolation facilities with reverse-barrier nursing. Prophylactic antibiotics

Table 13.4 Antilymphocyte (ALG) and antithymocyte globulin (ATG) preparations. Variations in animal origin, immunogens and antibody content.

Animal	Immunogens used	Range of antibodies from different preparations
Horse	Lymphocytes	CD3 (< 0.03–0.58)
	Thymocytes	CD5 (0–12.2)
	Lymphocytes + thymocytes	CD11a (3.15–20.3)
	T lymphoblasts	CD18 (18.7–269)
	B lymphoblasts	CD45 (0.16–4.01)
		β_2-Microglobulin (0.8–12.5)
Rabbit	T lymphoblasts	
	Thymocytes	

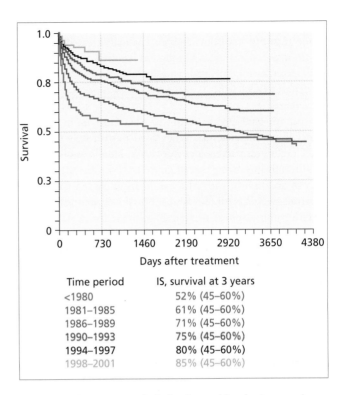

Time period	IS, survival at 3 years
<1980	52% (45–60%)
1981–1985	61% (45–60%)
1986–1989	71% (45–60%)
1990–1993	75% (45–60%)
1994–1997	80% (45–60%)
1998–2001	85% (45–60%)

Figure 13.2 Response survival of patients with aplastic anaemia treated with immunosuppressive therapy (ALG with or without cyclosporin). Data from EBMTR SAA working party showing improved survival with time (with permission).

and antifungal therapy should be used routinely. It is sclerosing to veins and should be given through a central line. A test dose of the preparation should be given before starting the full dosage, to test for anaphylaxis. A test dose (10 mg in 100 mL of saline) intravenously over half an hour must be given beforehand. Providing that the patient does not show evidence of anaphylaxis to the test dose, the full dose may be administered, starting on the same day as the test dose. Because of the anti-platelet activity of ALG, platelets should be given before and after the infusion, although not during the administration of the ALG. The full dose is given over 12–18 h.

Reactions are common. Fever, rigors, rashes, hypotension or hypertension are usual on the first day of treatment but become less troublesome as the therapy continues. These effects can usually be ameliorated by slowing the rate of infusion and giving corticosteroids, antihistamine (e.g. Piriton®) and pethidine. Although the test should exclude patients with anaphylaxis, pulmonary haemorrhage and capillary leak have been seen occasionally during the first day of administration of the full dose.

The treatment schedule is by no means established on the basis of clinical trials. The original European trials used administration of ALG daily for 5 days. This is the most widely followed regimen, but other schedules have been described, so far without any clear superiority over the 5-day course. The dosage varies from preparation to preparation, and the instructions of the manufacturers should be followed.

Serum sickness. Serum sickness occurs in about three-quarters of the patients given ALG. Some 7–10 days after its administration, fever, rash and severe joint pains may appear. Proteinuria may be seen, but frank renal failure has not yet been reported. The syndrome is self-limiting, but symptoms may respond to corticosteroids, requiring high doses for about 7 days. Prophylactic prednisolone (1 mg/kg per day) should be given to

help prevent or ameliorate serum sickness. Ideally, patients should be kept under observation as an inpatient until the risk of serum sickness is over; this is usually 2–3 weeks from the start of ALG treatment.

Response. Response to ALG is delayed, with improvement in marrow function rarely being seen before 6 weeks. Approximately 50% of patients respond by 3 months and up to 67% by 6 months (Figure 13.2). Patients with severe aplastic anaemia respond less well than non-severe patients, particularly if the neutrophil count is $< 0.2 \times 10^9$/L. Age does not seem to be a factor in response.

Further treatment. If there is no response to ALG after 4–6 months, a second course may be tried, either rabbit ATG if horse ALG has been used in the first instance, or a second course of horse ALG. In responding patients, the marrow does not usually return entirely to normal and some degree of cytopenia may persist for several years, although the patient may not require transfusion support.

Relapse occurs in 25–40% of responders over 10 years. Relapse does not always indicate a return to transfusion dependence but may herald the development of PNH, myelodysplastic syndrome or acute myeloid leukaemia (AML). Even when a stable recovery has been observed, patients treated with immunosuppression should be followed regularly for many years with screening for PNH and cytogenetic studies.

Cyclosporin

Cyclosporin has been used both with ALG and alone in the treatment of aplastic anaemia. When used immediately following ALG, cyclosporin accelerates recovery in blood counts without significantly improving overall survival. However, the combination of cyclosporin with ALG results in improved failure-free survival, meaning that fewer patients require a second course of ALG for non-response or relapse, compared with ALG alone, and the combination delays the onset of relapse after ALG. A significant proportion of patients are dependent on continued cyclosporin long-term after ALG. For patients with NSAA, the use of cyclosporin alone is associated with a significantly lower response rate and failure-free survival than the combination of ALG and cyclosporin. Nevertheless, cyclosporin may be used on its own if there are contraindications to using ALG in a particular patient. An appropriate starting dose of cyclosporin is 5 mg/kg per day in divided doses, the dose being adjusted according to blood pressure, renal function tests and blood levels of the drug.

Haemopoietic growth factors

Circulating levels of haemopoietic growth factors are markedly elevated in most patients with aplastic anaemia. They should not be used on their own in newly diagnosed patients in the mistaken belief that they may cure the disease. G-CSF will raise the neutrophil count in patients with aplastic anaemia, although the smallest benefit is seen in those with the most severely affected marrow. One study from Europe showed that G-CSF given after a course of ALG and cyclosporin appears to reduce the risk of severe infections after ALG, but does not improve the response rate and survival. Other growth factors, including erythropoietin, granulocyte–macrophage colony-stimulating factor (GM-CSF), interleukin 3 (IL-3), IL-6 and stem cell factor have proved to be largely ineffective and/or toxic to patients with aplastic anaemia. Trials with thrombopoietin in aplastic anaemia have not been reported, but it is not yet known whether it will be effective in the presence of already high plasma levels of the growth factor in aplastic anaemia, and there is potential concern about the development of anti-thrombopoietin antibodies.

Androgens

Historically androgens, or anabolic steroids, were the first specific form of therapy used in aplastic anaemia. They have a temporary benefit in the management of Fanconi anaemia and appeared to be effective in some cases of acquired aplastic anaemia, with some patients being androgen dependent. A European trial demonstrated that the addition of oxymetholone to ALG resulted in improved response compared with ALG alone, although their use has diminished since the introduction of cyclosporin to immunosuppressive protocols for treatment of aplastic anaemia. The androgens are usually given in high doses (for example, oxymetholone 2.5 mg/kg per day), starting after the period of serum sickness. Side-effects include virilization (and so are often unacceptable to female patients), prostatic enlargement, salt retention and hepatotoxicity, including the development of peliosis hepatitis and/or hepatocellular carcinoma after prolonged usage. If there is no response after 6 months, the androgens should be stopped. If there is a response, androgens should be slowly reduced, first to an alternate day therapy and then increasing the interval between doses.

Other treatments

The use of high-dose cyclophosphamide without stem cell support has been advocated as an alternative treatment for aplastic anaemia on account of its highly immunosuppressive qualities and the observation that autologous haematological recovery may occur following graft rejection after allogeneic bone marrow transplantation (BMT) in aplastic anaemia patients. Its use in this manner is generally not recommended, however, because of the perhaps predictably prolonged delayed neutrophil and platelet recovery and high risk of serious infective, particularly fungal, infections that are often fatal when the drug is administered at high doses without stem cell support. Furthermore, its use does not prevent the later onset of clonal disorders such as PNH or myelodysplasia. Mycophenolate mofetil is an immunosuppressive drug that inhibits proliferation of B and T lymphocytes and has been used in refractory aplastic anaemia in a recent European pilot study but found to be ineffective.

Allogeneic bone marrow transplantation for severe aplastic anaemia

Allogeneic bone marrow transplantation (BMT) for aplastic anaemia was first introduced by E Donnall Thomas and Rainer Storb and colleagues in 1969. BMT or peripheral blood stem cell (PBSC) transfusion is the treatment of choice for young patients with SAA who have an HLA-identical sibling donor. The age at which transplantation is no longer the treatment of choice depends upon the severity of the disease, the general health of the patient and the nature of the presenting symptoms. The results of BMT collected by the European Blood and Marrow Transplant Registry (EBMTR) are shown in Figure 13.3. Overall survival is around 75–90%. There is a marked age effect, most notably with poor outcome for patient over the age of 40 years compared with younger patients. BMT has a better long-term survival than immunosuppressive treatment once the graft is firmly established and the patient is off immunosuppressive treatment. Patients are not at increased risk of later clonal disorders following a successful transplant. This has to be weighed against the increased risk of transplant-related mortality in the early post-transplant period and the poor quality of life if

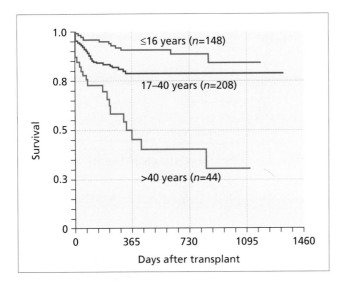

Figure 13.3 Survival following HLA-matched sibling donor stem cell transplantation. Data from EBMTR SAA working party, showing effect of age on outcome (with permission). The groups are not strictly similar, the oldest age group being transplanted significantly later than the youngest.

the patient develops chronic graft-versus-host disease (GvHD) Early and late graft failure occur in 10–15% of patients. For patients over the age of 40 years, transplantation using a 'low-intensity' conditioning regimen may be reserved for those who fail to respond to ALG and have an HLA-identical sibling donor.

Bone marrow is the preferred source of stem cells rather than G-CSF-mobilized PBSCs due to a worse survival and higher incidence of chronic GvHD with PBSC. At least 3×10^8/kg of body weight of the recipient nucleated marrow cells (3×10^6 CD34$^+$ cells) should be given; a lower stem cell dose increases the risk of graft failure.

The main causes of failure of BMT for aplastic anaemia are graft failure and post-graft infections. Patients with aplastic anaemia are immunocompetent apart from the neutropenia and indeed may be immunostimulated by infections and blood transfusions. Infection may be present before the transplant and become unmanageable afterwards. Chronic GvHD occurs in about 25% of successful transplants. Improvements in survival since 1969 may be attributed mainly to a reduction in graft failure and better support for the patient.

Conditioning for bone marrow transplantation

The most widely used regimen includes cyclophosphamide alone. High-dose irradiation was too toxic and low-dose total body or total lymphoid irradiation, although reducing the risks of rejection, did not improve overall survival. More recent schedules include ALG or Campath-1H with cyclophosphamide or low cyclophosphamide with fludarabine.

Cyclophosphamide

Cyclophosphamide, at a dose of 50 mg/kg per day intravenously for 4 days, has been used alone in the immunosuppression of patients with aplastic anaemia, although the rejection rate with this regimen is high unless additional post-graft immunosuppression is given, especially in multiply transfused patients (see below).

Cyclophosphamide is given intravenously, usually in 250–500 mL of saline over 0.5–1.0 h. Side-effects include nausea and vomiting (usually relatively mild), haemorrhagic cystitis, cardiomyopathy, fluid retention and alopecia. The haemorrhagic cystitis may be prevented or greatly modified by giving mesna (2-mercapto-ethane sulphonate) intravenously to neutralize the effects of metabolites of cyclophosphamide in the urine. Mesna (40% of the daily cyclophosphamide dose) is given intravenously 30 min before each cyclophosphamide infusion and the same dose is given at 3, 6, 9, 12, 16 and 20 h after each cyclophosphamide dose. This regimen is repeated on each day that the cyclophosphamide is given and the day after the last dose. The cardiotoxicity of cyclophosphamide is not usually a problem at the doses quoted unless there is already cardiac damage. Late haemorrhagic cystitis (after 20 days) may occur in transplant patients but is usually caused by virus infections (particularly adenovirus) rather than cyclophosphamide.

Antilymphocyte globulin

Additional immunosuppression is given with cyclophosphamide to help reduce graft failure. It is given daily on the first 4 days of cyclophosphamide.

For patients over the age of 40 years, in whom HLA identical sibling BMT is being considered, a 'mini' or reduced-intensity conditioning regimen is now recommended, similar to that for matched unrelated donor BMT (see later).

Irradiation

There is now no role for the use of irradiation in BMT for aplastic anaemia. Total body irradiation (TBI) or total lymphoid irradiation (TLI) were previously used in an attempt to reduce graft failure because of their immunosuppressive properties. Their use did reduce graft failure but at the expense of increasing GvHD, interstitial pneumonitis and the later risk of solid tumours, as well as developmental delay and sterility.

Cyclosporin

Cyclosporin was introduced into BMT regimens for aplastic anaemia both to reduce graft failure and to minimize GvHD. Results of BMT for aplastic anaemia have improved considerably since its introduction, mainly because of the reduction in graft failure. It was recognized early in the use of cyclosporin that graft failure may follow if the drug is stopped early and it is usual to continue cyclosporin for a year post transplantation for aplastic anaemia. The dose is adjusted to keep the blood level between 250 and 300 µg/L.

Methotrexate

Methotrexate is added to cyclosporin to reduce GvHD at a dose of 10 mg/m^2 intravenously on day 1, then 8 mg/m^2 on days 3, 6 and 11. There is an increase in mucositis and liver toxicity with this drug.

Results of allogeneic transplant

Figure 13.3 shows the survival of patients who received allogeneic BMT for severe aplastic anaemia. Patients who have successful transplants without chronic GvHD have a good quality of life. Children grow normally and have normal endocrine function. Males and females remain fertile and there seems to be no increased risk of congenital abnormalities or miscarriages compared with the normal population. Fertility returns rapidly after the transplant and patients may become pregnant within 3 months while still on cyclosporin. They should be warned of this possibility, although it should be noted that cyclosporin is not teratogenic. Chronic GvHD is the main problem in long-term follow-up, with about 25% of patients being affected.

There are two main types of graft failure seen in aplastic anaemia transplantation. Primary failure is probably related to the disease in that these patients never show any evidence of engraftment. No neutrophils or reticulocytes are seen in the peripheral blood post graft. These patients have a poor outlook and second transplants are usually unsuccessful. Secondary failure occurs after some evidence of engraftment and is probably a true immunological rejection event, although it should be remembered that reactivation of cytomegalovirus infection will also lead to a fall in blood counts. Autologous recovery may still take place, providing that the patient is kept fully supported. Second transplants from the same or another sibling donor have a success rate of about 25%.

Bone marrow transplantation from donors other than HLA-matched siblings

BMT from unrelated volunteer donors and mismatched family donors has been carried out for severe aplastic anaemia. Until fairly recently, the major problems encountered have been increases in graft failure, GvHD and infection. The overall survival in collected series was very poor, with only about 30% disease free survival (Figure 13.4). Better survival has been reported over the last few years, probably due to better matching using DNA high-resolution HLA typing and avoiding any degree of mis-match and improved conditioning regimens as well as improved supportive care. The EBMT has recently proposed a low-intensity conditioning regimen of cyclophosphamide 300 mg/m^2 for 4 days, fludarabine 30 mg/m^2 for 4 days and ALG for 4 days, with cyclosporin starting earlier on day −6 instead of day −1, along with methotrexate.

Benzene-induced aplastic anaemia

Benzene is a carcinogen. Chronic exposure to benzene used as a

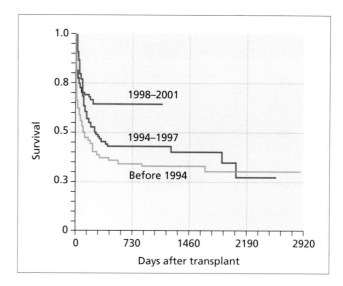

Figure 13.4 Survival following stem cell transplant from matched unrelated volunteer donors, showing improved outcome with time. Data from the EBMTR SAA working party (with permission). These results were obtained with full dose conditioning.

solvent produces pancytopenia associated with a hyperplastic or dysplastic marrow, which may later become leukaemic or, more rarely, be associated with aplastic anaemia. In China, the incidence of aplastic anaemia in workers chronically exposed to high concentrations of benzene has been reported as 9 cases out of 74 828 that were exposed. Benzene has been used experimentally to produce aplastic anaemia in rabbits. Benzene itself is now rarely used as a solvent, having been replaced by non-aromatic organic solvents, but it is still encountered in the petroleum industry and benzene derivatives are ubiquitous in occupations such as photographic development. However, the evidence that these compounds produce aplastic anaemia at the very low concentrations permitted by industrial safety guidelines (1 p.p.m.) is lacking, although there is some evidence that low doses (10 p.p.m.) may have an effect on erythropoiesis.

Malignant aplastic anaemia

Acute leukaemia

Acute lymphoblastic leukaemia (ALL) may present as aplastic anaemia, particularly, although not exclusively, in childhood. The aplasia is not distinguishable from true aplastic anaemia on haematological grounds, but there are some clinical observations which raise the possibility that the aplasia is a prodrome of ALL. Fever and documented infection are more common presentations than in aplastic anaemia. The platelets tend to be relatively better preserved than neutrophils compared with acquired aplasia. The spleen is frequently enlarged, although it may be only just palpable or evident only on ultrasound. The aplasia usually lasts 3–6 weeks, when spontaneous or corticosteroid induced 'remission' occurs. The ALL usually follows after a period of apparently normal haemopoiesis, often 1–3 months after recovery. The phenotype of the ALL does not differ from primary ALL and the prognosis is not affected.

AML may present in a similar way to ALL in childhood, with a period of aplasia, but this is much less common. Rarely, AML may present with a relatively stable degree of aplasia, which may persist for several months before the blood becomes frankly leukaemic. In these patients, suspicion may be aroused by finding occasional circulating blasts in the peripheral blood or in a buffy coat preparation, by a low neutrophil alkaline phosphatase, and by the presence of an excess of myeloblasts in the cells remaining in the bone marrow. It is important to be aware of this possibility in the differential diagnosis of aplastic anaemia because these patients are probably best treated by early bone marrow transplantation when an HLA identical sibling donor is available, using TBI and some additional chemotherapy. Patients without a donor may be supported with blood transfusion until they become frankly leukaemic. Attempts to produce remission are often, but not always, unsuccessful because the aplastic marrow remains aplastic.

Hypoplastic myelodysplastic syndrome

Some patients with MDS may present with a hypoplastic marrow. The remaining haemopoietic cells usually show the changes of MDS with hypogranular neutrophils and micromegakaryocytes, and there may be an increase in reticulin in the bone marrow. Dyserythropoiesis is not a useful feature to confirm MDS as it is also a common feature in aplastic anaemia. Cytogenetic analysis of the bone marrow may reveal abnormalities more suggestive of MDS, such as monosomy 7, but cytogenetic abnormalities can occur in around 11% of patients with otherwise typical aplastic anaemia. There have been some therapeutic studies that suggest that ALG (ATG) may be effective in producing at least partial remission in hypoplastic MDS and possibly in refractory anaemias.

Single lineage acquired bone marrow failure syndromes

Acquired pure red cell aplasia

Failure of erythropoiesis may be inherited or acquired (Table 13.5). The acquired disorder may be primary or secondary and may be transient or chronic. Whatever the cause, pure red cell aplasia (PRCA) is characterized by anaemia and reticulocytopenia, with reduction of red cell precursors in the marrow. The marrow usually shows a complete absence of red cell precursors, but some forms of either the inherited or acquired disease may be associated with the absence of the late forms of erythropoietic precursors: a picture of maturation arrest. Granulocyte and megakaryocyte series are normal or increased.

Failure of erythropoiesis may occur as a primary acquired event or may be associated with other disorders. The condition presents as anaemia with reticulocytopenia and bone marrow with either a total lack of erythrocyte precursors or a maturation arrest with a lack of late erythroid precursors.

Primary acquired pure red cell aplasia

The majority of patients with this rare condition are aged between 20 and 50 years. They have the symptoms of a slowly progressive anaemia. There are no additional physical findings. The Coombs' test may be weakly positive but it is not normally possible to demonstrate a humoral inhibitor to erythropoiesis in the peripheral blood or cellular inhibition in the marrow. The bone marrow is cellular, with an absence of red cell precursors. In some, there is an increase in reticulin. It is important to exclude other causes of red cell aplasia (see below).

Secondary acquired pure red cell aplasia

Pure red cell aplasia is a well known association with thymoma. About 5% of thymomas are associated with PRCA and about 10–20% of patients with PRCA have a thymoma. The majority of tumours show spindle cell morphology but some are

Table 13.5 Clinical classification of pure red cell aplasia.

Congenital	Diamond–Blackfan anaemia	
Acquired paediatric	Transient erythroblastopenia of childhood	Systemic lupus erythematosus, rheumatoid arthritis
	Parvovirus-induced aplastic crisis	Chronic lymphocytic leukaemia, lymphoma
Adult	Idiopathic	T-large granular lymphocytosis
	Primary autoimmune	Thymoma
	Secondary	Myelodysplastic syndrome
		Hypogammaglobulinaemia
		Drugs: azathioprine, isoniazid, phenytoin, rHuEPO
		Hepatitis, Epstein–Barr virus, parvovirus
		Others: major ABO mis-match BMT, pregnancy

lymphomas. The tumour may usually be diagnosed on plain radiography but tomography or computerized tomography scanning may be required. There may be associated abnormalities of other systems linked to the thymoma, for example myasthenia gravis. The response to thymectomy is unpredictable. About one-half of the patients respond to surgery but some relapse later. Some patients develop PRCA only after removal of the thymoma and some show no response. For patients who fail to respond to thymectomy, immunosuppressive treatment is used (see below).

Pure red cell aplasia may be associated with a variety of lymphoid disorders including B- and T-cell lymphomas and particularly T-large granular lymphocytosis. The main conditions are shown in Table 13.5. The PRCA may precede the appearance of the lymphoma but the latter may be identified in some patients at the time of diagnosis of the PRCA by immunoglobulin or T-cell receptor gene rearrangement studies. The anaemia usually, but not always, responds to treatment of the lymphoma.

Pure red cell aplasia is associated with a number of autoimmune disorders. There may be a positive direct antiglobulin test (DAT) that indicates the nature of the aplasia. It occurs in patients with agammaglobulinaemia, and may also be associated with systemic lupus erythematosus, Sjögren's syndrome or rheumatoid arthritis. The majority of these anaemias will respond to treatment with corticosteroids, with or without azathioprine. The response may be steroid-dependent or there may be a relapsing and remitting course.

A long list of drugs have been incriminated in the aetiology of PRCA, but the association is very rare and mostly there is only a single case for each drug. Exceptions are azathioprine, phenytoin, procainamide and isoniazid, for which several cases each have been reported. More recently, recombinant human erythropoietin (rHuEpo), when used predominantly in chronic renal failure patients, has been reported to cause PRCA associated with anti-erythropoietin antibodies, resulting in a sudden and severe anaemia that is unresponsive to increased dose of rHuEpo. In this situation the rHuEpo must be discontinued immediately and regular blood transfusional support given; immunosuppressive therapy may be required for the PRCA.

Treatment of acquired pure red cell aplasia

Any drugs that have been implicated in pure red cell aplasia being given to the patient should be discontinued. Prednisolone is the initial treatment of choice at a dose of 1 mg/kg daily for 4 weeks. If response occurs, the dose is slowly tapered and discontinued. For non-responders, remission may be induced by azathioprine, or cyclosporin with or without ALG, and there have been anecdotal reports of response with cyclophosphamide and vincristine. There is increasing interest in the use of monoclonal antibody therapy with, for example, Campath-1H (anti-CD52) or rituximab (anti-CD20) in the treatment of refractory PRCA and other autoimmune cytopenias.

Transient red cell aplasias

Parvovirus B19 aplastic crisis

Infection with parvovirus 19, the wild-type human virus, produces the syndrome of fifth disease (fever, rash, arthralgia) in non-immune subjects. B19 specifically infects and lyses erythroid precursor cells. The cellular receptor is the blood group P antigen, globoside, which is expressed on some colony-forming unit erythroid (CFU-E) and all pro-erythroblasts and subsequent erythroid cells. Viral DNA can be identified not only in serum but also in bone marrow erythroid precursors by *in situ* PCR, as well as in proliferating CFU-E. Erythropoiesis virtually ceases for the duration of acute infection, which is some 5–10 days. This is unimportant in patients who have a normal red cell survival but produces an acute, and sometimes life-threatening fall in haemoglobin in patients with haemolytic anaemia. Recovery begins with the emergence of immunoglobulin M (IgM) antibodies to the virus. At this time, the marrow may contain giant pro-erythroblasts with marked vacuolation. Immunosuppressed patients or those with immunodeficiency may develop prolonged PRCA and patients with PRCA should be checked for IgG antibodies to the virus. Absence of the antibody raises the possibility of parvovirus-induced PRCA, which can be confirmed by PCR for viral DNA.

Transient erythroblastopenia of childhood

This syndrome is characterized in children by the development of normocytic, normochromic anaemia with reticulocytopenia and absent erythroid precursors in the marrow. There is nearly always a prodromal viral illness. The red cell aplasia lasts a few weeks and recovers spontaneously. There are no associated physical anomalies. The differential diagnosis is from Diamond–Blackfan anaemia.

Amegakaryocytic thrombocytopenias

Thrombocytopenia with absent megakaryocytes may be congenital or acquired. Acquired amegakaryocytic thrombocytopenia may develop at any age and result in a prolonged thrombocytopenia. The condition may remain stable for many years or may progress to total aplasia, a myelodysplastic syndrome or AML. The marrow in the early stages is normo- or hypercellular, with absent megakaryocytes. Treatment is supportive, although isolated case reports have suggested an improvement with ALG or cyclosporin.

Dyserythropoiesis

Dyserythropoiesis is caused by defects in erythropoiesis, which lead to the production of abnormal erythroid cells; some of these cells are destroyed within the marrow during maturation, whereas those that reach maturity and enter the circulation may show morphological abnormalities and are liable to have a shortened lifespan. Conditions that may be referred to as dyserythropoiesis include a wide range of diseases that primarily affect either the nucleus or the cytoplasm. Examples affecting the nucleus are cobalamin and folate deficiencies (see Chapter 4), where there is a defect in DNA production due to enzymatic abnormalities in the pathways of pyrimidine and purine synthesis.

Disorders that primarily involve cytoplasm include disturbances in haemoglobin production that may be due to impaired availability of any component of the haemoglobin molecule. The most common cause is iron deficiency. When there is an adequate amount of iron available but it is not utilized, sideroblastic anaemia may occur: there is failure of mitochondrial synthesis of protophorphyrin with accumulation of iron within the mitochondria, which is seen as ring sideroblasts (see Chapter 3). Impairment in globin synthesis results in thalassaemic syndromes. It is apparent that dyserythropoiesis is a very common phenomenon and is associated primarily or secondarily with a large number of different diseases that seem to have little in common with each other to justify their inclusion in a single category. The term is, however, a useful one, as it suggests an important aspect of the pathogenesis of the anaemias, and indicates the fact that there is an inter-relationship of the various aspects of the erythropoietic mechanism, whereby a defect at any stage will lead to a similar end result.

Morphological features

These include: binuclearity and multinuclearity, asynchrony between nuclear and cytoplasmic maturation, and premature nuclear extrusion; nuclear budding, fragmentation and degeneration (karyorrhexis); and various abnormalities of mitosis. There is also persistence of intercellular connection by cytoplasm and abnormalities of the cytoplasm itself, such as vacuolation, basophilic stippling and the presence of an excessive amount of siderotic granules. The extent to which these abnormalities are apparent in a bone marrow varies considerably between cases, but all the features can be seen readily in certain conditions (e.g. megaloblastic anaemias, AML M6 or myelodysplasia). The morphology of megaloblastic anaemia demonstrates the effect of uncoupling of nuclear and cytoplasmic maturation including the immature open nuclear chromatin in the megaloblasts.

Other indications of dyserythropoiesis

Ferrokinetic studies show an accelerated clearance of plasma iron with decreased erythrocyte incorporation of the order of 25–50%, increased plasma iron turnover and an accumulation and retention of the iron in the bone marrow. A useful parameter of ineffective erythropoiesis is the serum bilirubin. An unconjugated hyperbilirubinaemia is observed in many dyserythropoietic conditions; this is evidence of increased haemoglobin catabolism. Intramedullary destruction of progenitor cells results in the liberation of various enzymes, notably lactic dehydrogenase

and aldolase, and destruction of nuclear material leads to an increased level of uric acid. Red cell survival is usually reduced.

Congenital dyserythropoietic anaemias

In addition to the non-specific phenomenon of dyserythropoiesis described above, there is a group of disorders of variable severity with recessive inheritance, known as congenital dyserythropoietic anaemias (CDA). They are characterized by chronic anaemia with a relatively low reticulocyte count, jaundice and haemosiderosis. Peripheral blood films show anisocytosis, poikilocytosis and irregularly crenated and contracted cells. The marrow shows one of three patterns:

Type I. Megaloblastic changes, macrocytosis, internuclear chromatin bridges, but binuclearity not prominent; proerythroblasts and basophilic erythroblasts especially affected (Figure 13.5).

Type II. Binuclearity, especially of late erythroblasts, multinuclearity, pluripolar mitoses, karyorrhexis (Figure 13.6).

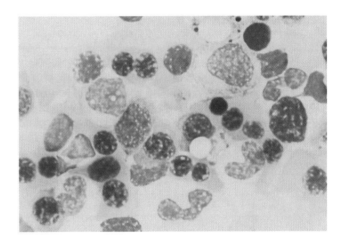

Figure 13.5 CDA type I. Bone marrow aspirate showing internucleur bridging in normoblasts.

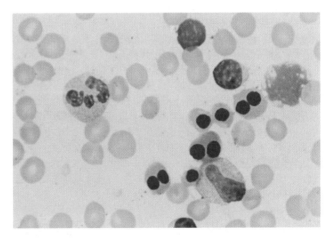

Figure 13.6 CDA type II (HEMPAS). Bone marrow aspirate showing typical multinuclearity.

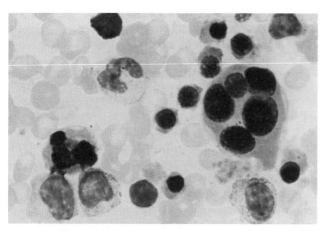

Figure 13.7 CDA type III. Giant multinucleated erythroblast from the marrow.

Type III. Multinuclearity with up to 12 nuclei, gigantoblasts, macrocytosis (Figure 13.7).

There is an overlap between types I and II and there are variants of each type. There are also a number of reports of congenital ineffective erythropoiesis, which do not fit into any of the three categories given.

CDA type II

Type II will be described first as it is the most common type of CDA. It is transmitted as an autosomal recessive disease; the geographical distribution of the earlier recorded cases suggests a particularly high frequency in north-west Europe, in Italy and in North Africa. It is usually diagnosed in the first few years of life.

Some cases have presented with anaemia and/or jaundice at birth, and this should be considered in the evaluation of non-immune hydrops fetalis. The clinical manifestations include a variable degree of jaundice, hepatomegaly and splenomegaly, cirrhosis, and diabetes, even in patients who have neither been transfused nor treated with iron. A few patients have been mentally retarded. The serum iron and transferrin saturations are increased.

Type II has an eponym, 'Hempas' – hereditary erythroblast multinuclearity with positive acidified serum – because of the unique feature that the red cells are haemolysed by some acidified normal sera but not by the patient's own serum, unlike PNH. In Hempas, there is a specific antigen on the erythrocytes, which reacts with an IgM anti-Hempas antibody present in the sera of about 30% of normal people in sufficient amounts to cause lysis. This susceptibility to lysis is probably due to abnormal complement control resulting from a defect in the complement-regulating protein glycophorin A (see below).

In common with other types of dyserythropoiesis, there is enhanced I and i antigen activity, demonstrated *in vitro* by increased agglutination and by a positive cold-antibody (anti-I) lysis test.

Type II shows the abnormal features described above. In addition, there is a characteristic peripheral arrangement of endoplasmic reticulum giving the appearance of a 'double membrane' (Figure 13.8).

Pathogenesis appears to be an enzymatic defect in the glycosylation pathway leading to abnormalities in glycoprotein bands 3 and 5.5 and glycophorin A. Two different enzyme defects have been identified, namely deficiency of alpha-mannosidase II and *N*-acetylglucosaminyl transferase II.

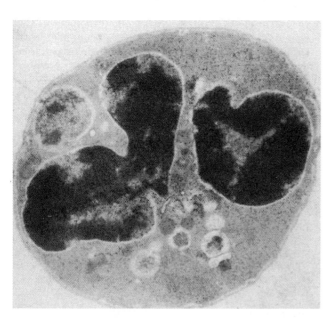
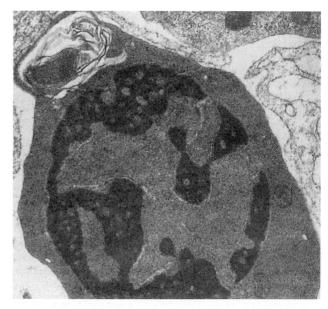

Figure 13.8 CDA type II. Electron micrographs of erythroblast, showing peripheral arrangement of endoplasmic reticulum with 'double membrane' appearance.

CDA type I

Type I has been identified far less frequently than CDA II. It has an autosomally recessive inheritance; no method is available to identify heterozygous subjects. Clinical features are similar to those of CDAII. Most patients present with splenomegaly and mild to moderate macrocytic anaemia. Two cases have been reported with skeletal defects in fingers and toes resembling the features seen in congenital aplastic anaemias. Haematologically, it differs from type II by its bone marrow morphological appearance, and electron microscopy shows a high proportion of cells with a 'Swiss cheese' nuclear abnormality. Serological reactions are negative, especially in the acidified serum lysis test. It has been suggested that the primary defect is in the nucleoprotein or the nuclear membrane, with various secondary effects, including failure of protein synthesis and altered globin chain synthesis.

CDA type III

Type III is the rarest form. It is notable for the multinuclearity and gigantoblasts in the bone marrow. Indeed, the erythroblasts are especially remarkable for being present with up to 12 nuclei in a cell (Figure 13.7). Morphologically, the condition is more likely to be confused with erythroleukaemia than with other types of CDA, but the clinical picture is of a mild anaemia with a good prognosis, and there is no granulocytopenia or thrombocytopenia.

As with other types of CDA, there is ineffective erythropoiesis. In the few cases studied, the red cells have been strongly haemolysed by both anti-I and anti-i sera, but the acidified serum lysis test has been negative. In a few reported cases, it appears to have been inherited as an autosomal recessive, but in one Swedish family it appears to be an autosomal dominant trait, and the abnormal gene has been localized to chromosome 15q21–q25.

Management

Patients with only mild anaemia require no intervention. Even if anaemia is more severe, blood transfusion should be kept to a minimum because of the predisposition of the patients to develop iron overload and secondary haemochromatosis. If regular transfusions are necessary the patients should be monitored for evidence of iron overload and desferrioxamine therapy should be given careful consideration. Splenectomy may be of benefit in CDAII, especially in cases with severe anaemia, when it is likely to reduce transfusion requirements. The benefit of splenectomy in CDAI is more problematic.

There have been two reports of the effectiveness of interferon-α in cases of CDAI with severe anaemia: after several weeks of treatment (e.g. 3 million units 2–3 times per week), the haemoglobin became normal and there was substantial reduction in the extent of ineffective erythropoiesis; the haemoglobin level fell when treatment was discontinued or when the dose was reduced, and it recovered when treatment at the previous dose

level was resumed. There is insufficient evidence on the effects of long-term continuous treatment.

Selected bibliography

Acquired aplastic anaemia

Bacigalupo A, Chaple M, Hows J et al. (1993) Treatment of aplastic anaemia (AA) with antilymphocyte globulin (ALG) and methylprednisolone (Mpred) with or without androgens: a randomized trial from the EBMT SAA Working Party. *British Journal of Haematology* 83: 145–51.

Bacigalupo A, Brand R, Oneto R et al. (2000) Treatment of acquired severe aplastic anaemia: bone marrow transplantation compared with immunosuppressive therapy – The European Group for Blood and Marrow Transplantation experience. *Seminars in Hematology* 37: 69–80.

Ball SE, Gibson FM, Rizzo S et al. (1998) Progressive telomere shortening in aplastic anaemia. *Blood* 91: 3582–92.

Baumelou E, Guiguet M, Mary JY and the French Cooperative Group for Epidemiological Study of Aplastic Anaemia (1993) Epidemiology of aplastic anaemia in France: a case control study. 1. Medical history and medication use. *Blood* 81: 1471–8.

Brown KE, Tisdale J, Barrett AJ et al. (1997) Hepatitis-associated aplastic anaemia. *New England Journal of Medicine* 336: 1059–64.

Camitta BM (2000) What is the definition of cure for aplastic anemia? *Acta Hematologica* 103: 16–18.

Camitta BM, Thomas ED, Nathan DG et al. (1976) Severe aplastic anaemia; a prospective study of the effect of early marrow transplantation on acute mortality. *Blood* 48: 63–9.

Deeg HJ, Leisenring W, Storb R et al. (1998) Long term outcome after marrow transplantation for severe aplastic anaemia. *Blood* 91: 3637–45.

Deeg HJ, Seidel K, Casper J et al. (1999) Marrow transplantation from unrelated donors for patients with severe aplastic anemia who have failed immunosuppressive therapy. *Biology of Blood and Marrow Transplantation* 5: 243–52.

Elebute MO, Ball SE, Gordon-Smith EC et al. (2002) Autologous recovery following non-myeloablative unrelated donor bone marrow transplantation for severe aplastic anaemia. *Annals of Haematology* 81: 378–81.

Frickhof en N, Heimpel H, Kaltwasser JP et al. (2003) for the German Aplastic Anaemia Study Group. Antithymocyte globulin with or without cyclosporin A: 11-year follow-up of a randomized trial comparing treatments of aplastic anaemia. *Blood* 101: 1236–42.

Gluckman E, Rokicka-Milewska R et al. (2002) Results and follow-up of a phase III randomized study of recombinant human-granulocyte stimulating factor as support for immunosuppressive therapy in patients with severe aplastic anaemia. *British Journal of Haematology* 119: 1075–82.

International Agranulocytosis and Aplastic Anaemia Study (1987) Incidence of aplastic anaemia: relevance of diagnosis criteria. *Blood* 70: 1718–21.

Kernan NA, Bartscg G, Ash RC et al. (1993) Analysis of 462 transplantations from unrelated donors facilitated by the National

Marrow Donor ProgrAmerican. *New England Journal of Medicine* **328**: 593–602.

Killick SB, Marsh JCW (2000) Aplastic anaemia: management. *Blood Reviews* **14**: 157–71.

Lewis SM, Bain BJ, Bates I (eds) (2001) *Dacie and Lewis, Practical Haematology*, 9th edn, pp. 219–25. Churchill Livingstone, London.

Locascuilli A, Arcese W, Locatelli F *et al.* and Italian Aplastic Anaemia Study Group (2001) Treatment of aplastic anaemia with granulocyte colony stimulating factor and risks of malignancy. *Lancet* **357**: 43–4.

Marsh JCW (2000) Hematopoietic growth factors in the pathogenesis and for the treatment of aplastic anemia. *Seminars in Hematology* **37**: 81–90.

Marsh JC, Ball SE, Darbyshire P *et al.* for the British Committee for Standards in Haematology (2004) Guidelines for the diagnosis and management of acquired aplastic anaemia. *British Journal of Haematology* **123**: 782–801.

Marsh J, Schrezenmeier H, Marin P *et al.* (1999) A prospective randomized multicentre study comparing cyclosporin alone versus the combination of antithymocyte globulin and cyclosporin for treatment of patients with non-severe aplastic anaemia: a report from the European Blood and Marrow Transplant (EBMT) Severe Aplastic Anaemia Working Party. *Blood* **93**: 2191–5.

Muir KR, Chilvers CED, Harriss C *et al.* (2003) The role of occupational and environmental exposures in the aetiology of acquired severe aplastic anaemia: a case control investigation. *British Journal of Haematology* **123**: 906–10.

Sanders JE, Hawley J, Levy W *et al.* (1996) Pregnancies following high dose cyclophosphamide with or without high dose busulphan or total body irradiation and bone marrow transplantation. *Blood* **87**: 3045–52.

Schrezenmeier H, Bacigalupo A (eds) (2000) *Aplastic Anaemia, Pathophysiology and Treatment*. Cambridge University Press, Cambridge.

Smith MT (1996) Overview of benzene-induced aplastic anaemia. *European Journal of Haematology* **57** (suppl): 107–11.

Socie G, Rosenfeld S, Frickhofen N *et al.* (2000) Late clonal diseases of treated aplastic anaemia. *Seminars in Hematology* **37**: 91–101.

Storb R, Leisenning W, Anasetti C *et al.* (1997) Long term follow up of allogeneic marrow transplants in patients with aplastic anaemia conditioned with cyclophosphamide with antithymocyte globulin. *Blood* **89**: 3890–901.

Tichelli A, Socie G, Marsh J *et al.* (2002), on behalf of the European Group for Blood and Marrow Transplantation (EBMT) Severe Aplastic Anemia Working Party. Outcome of pregnancy and disease outcome among women with aplastic anemia treated with immunosuppression. *Annals of Internal Medicine* **137**: 164–72.

Tisdale JF, Dunn DE, Geller N *et al.* (2000) High dose cyclophosphamide in severe aplastic anaemia: a randomized trial. *Lancet* **356**: 1554–7.

Vassiliou GS, Webb DK, Pamphilon D *et al.* (2001) Improved outcome of alternative donor bone marrow transplantation in children with severe aplastic anaemia using a conditioning regimen containing low-dose total body irradiation, cyclophosphamide and Campath. *British Journal of Haematology* **114**: 701–5.

Vulliamy T, Marrone A, Goldman F *et al.* (2001) The RNA component of telomerase is mutated in autosomal dominant dyskeratosis congenital. *Nature* **413**: 432–5.

Young NS, Alter BP (eds) (1994) *Aplastic Anaemia: Acquired and Congenital*. WB Saunders, Philadelphia.

Acquired pure red cell aplasia

Casadevall N, Nataf J, Viron B *et al.* (2002) Pure red cell aplasia and Anti-erythropoietin antibodies in patients treated with recombinant erythropoietin. *New England Journal of Medicine* **346**: 469–75.

Charles RJ, Sabo KM, Kidd PG *et al.* (1996) The pathophysiology of pure red cell aplasia: Implications for therapy. *Blood*; **87**: 4831–8.

Dessypris EN (2002) Pure red cell aplasia. In: *Hematology, Basic Principles and Practice*, 3rd edn (R Hoffman, EJ Benz, SJ Shattil *et al.*, eds). Successful treament of pure red cell aplasia with rituximab in patients with chronic lymphocytic leukaemia. *Blood* **99**: 1092–4.

Lacy MQ, Kurtin PJ, Tefferi A (1996) Pure red cell aplasia: association with large granular lymphocyte leukaemia and the prognostic value of cytogenetic abnormalities. *Blood* **87**: 3000–6.

Willis F, Marsh JCW, Bevan DH *et al.* (2001) The effect of treatment with Campath-1H in patients with autoimmune cytopenias. *British Journal of Haematology* **114**: 891–8.

Dyserythropoiesis

Fukada MN, Papayannopoulou T, Gordon-Smith EC *et al.* (1984) Defect in glycosylation of erythrocyte membrane proteins in congenital dyserythropoietic anaemia type II (HEMPAS). *British Journal of Haematology* **56**: 55–68.

Marks PW, Mitus AJ (1996) Congenital dyserythropoietic anemias. *American Journal of Haematology* **51**: 55–63.

Tomita A, Parker CJ (1994) Aberrant regulation of complement by the erythrocytes of hereditary erythroblastic multinuclearity with a positive acidified serum lysis test (HEMPAS). *Blood* **83**: 250–9.

Wickramasinge SN (1997) Response of CDA type I to alpha-interferon. *European Journal of Haematology* **58**: 121–3.

Red cell immunohaematology: introduction

14

Marcela Contreras and Geoff Daniels

Introduction

The primary purpose of transfusion medicine is to provide 'safe' blood when the clinician requires it. However, blood groups and immunohaematological problems of blood transfusion and transplantation are extremely interesting in their own right and their solutions have much to offer to haematology in general.

Blood group serology or immunohaematology includes the study of antigenic molecules present on the various cellular and soluble components of whole blood, together with study of the antibodies and lectins that recognize them and their interactions. However, in practice, the term blood group serology generally is restricted to red cell surface antigens and their interactions with specific antibodies. In this narrower sense, the complexities of HLA, granulocyte, platelet and plasma protein determinants do not normally fall within the blood group serologist's realm, even though all are likewise genetically polymorphic and play a role in blood transfusion.

The narrower definition of blood group serology encompasses the following: (i) the determination of the phenotype of red cells with antibodies and reagents of known specificity; (ii) the search for and identification of antibodies with red cells of known phenotype; and (iii) compatibility testing of patients' sera against cell samples from donor units of the same ABO and RhD groups. At present, more than 2 million units of red cells are transfused to patients each year in the UK alone.

The aim of this chapter is to provide an introduction to blood group serology and to include aspects of immunology and biochemistry that contribute to our understanding of blood group antigens, antibodies and antigen–antibody reactions.

The red cell membrane and chemistry of blood group antigens

The red cell membrane is composed of about 40% (w/w) lipids and up to 10% carbohydrates, the remainder being proteins. The exact arrangement of its components is still unresolved, but a rough model is shown in Figure 14.1.

The lipids of the red cell membrane can be subdivided into 60% (w/w) phospholipids, 30% (w/w) neutral lipids (mainly cholesterol) and 10% (w/w) glycolipids. The phospholipids and glycolipids play a role in the structure of the membrane and are thought to be important in the maintenance of red cell shape. These lipids have a molecular arrangement reminiscent of a tuning fork, with the hydrophobic fatty acids forming the 'prongs' and the polar group the 'handle'. They are arranged in a bilayer with the 'prongs' pointing inwards and the hydrophilic 'handle' pointing out towards the plasma or towards the cytoplasmic surface of the membrane. Cholesterol is inserted between the other lipids. This arrangement allows the interior of the membrane to be in a semifluid state and the whole membrane to be very flexible. The lipid bilayer does not allow the passive transfer of ions.

The carbohydrates are attached to the lipids and proteins, and occur only on the external surface of the membrane. They are

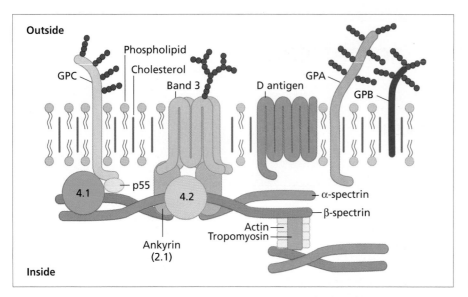

Figure 14.1 Diagrammatic representation of red cell membrane.

composed of chains of monosaccharides, the majority of which are hexoses.

About 20–40% of the proteins of the membrane are released relatively easily (e.g. by changing the ionic strength of the medium) and are therefore not very firmly attached (peripheral proteins). The remaining 60–80% are released only after drastic treatment with detergents or bile salts; these integral proteins penetrate the lipid bilayer and, in some cases, are bound to the cytoskeleton. After red cell membranes have been treated with the detergent sodium dodecyl sulphate, the proteins can be separated electrophoretically on a polyacrylamide gel according to their molecular mass. If the gel is stained for protein, up to eight bands are seen, as shown in Figure 14.2. Bands 1 and 2 are proteins that are easily released by a low-ionic-strength medium. They are monomers and dimers of the contractile protein spectrin, which form a network of tetramers on the inner surface of the membrane, contributing to the maintenance of the red cell shape. Band 5 (actin) links the spectrin tetramers together. Band 3, the anion exchanger, exists in the membrane as dimers and higher oligomers linked to the cytoskeleton through ankyrin (band 2.1), band 4.2 and band 4.1.

If the polyacrylamide gel is stained for sialic acid with periodic acid–Schiff (PAS) stain, four or five bands are seen (Figure 14.2). These bands contain four sialic acid-rich glycoproteins called glycophorins, and their dimers. The genetically related glycophorins (GP), GPA and GPB, exist as monomers, dimers and as a heterodimer of GPA and GPB. Additional bands represent the minor glycophorins, GPC and its truncated isoform, GPD. The genes for all these glycophorins have been cloned and sequenced, and the amino acid sequence deduced. All of the carbohydrate of these molecules (60%, w/w) is located on the external domains, which extend far beyond the lipid bilayer, allowing charged groups to extend some distance into

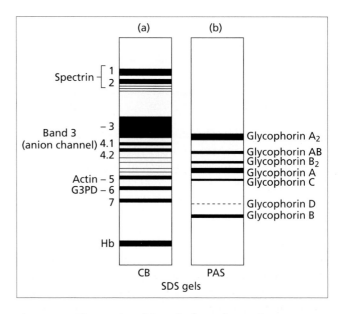

Figure 14.2 The proteins of the red cell membrane after separation by electrophoresis in sodium dodecyl sulphate (SDS) gels. (a) Stained for protein (Coomassie blue, CB); (b) stained for carbohydrate (periodic acid–Schiff reagent, PAS).

the plasma. The molecules cross the lipid bilayer once. GPA, GPC and GPD extend well into the cytosol and appear to interact with the cytoskeleton, whereas GPB extends only a short distance into the cytosol (Figure 14.1).

Blood group antigens have been found in the polypeptide and carbohydrate moieties of membrane glycoproteins and in the carbohydrate moieties of glycolipids (Table 14.1). Most blood groups represent amino acid sequence changes in glycoproteins,

Table 14.1 Blood group active proteins.

Protein	Blood group	Mol. wt (kDa)*	Copies per cell (×10³)	Function
Band 3 (CD233)	Diego; ABH†	100	1000	Anion transport; cytoskeletal attachment
UT-B1	Kidd, ABH†	46–60	14	Urea transport
Aquaporin 1	Colton, ABH†	40–60	200	Water channel
Aquaporin 3	GIL	45		Glycerol and water channel
GLUT-1	ABH†	55	500	Glucose transport
RhD and RhCcEe proteins (CD240D and CE)	Rh	30–34	100–200	Involved in NH_3^+ or CO_2 transport?
RhAG (CD241)	Duclos, ABH†	35–100	100–200	Involved in NH_3^+ or CO_2 transport?
Kx protein	Kx	37		Neurotransmitter transport?
Duffy gp (CD234)	Duffy	40–50	6–12	Chemokine receptor
Lutheran gp (CD239)	Lutheran	78 and 85	2–4	Adhesion (to laminin)
ICAM-4	LW	37–47	3–5	Adhesion
CD44	Indian	80	6–10	Adhesion (to hyaluronan)
Xg and CD99 gps	Xg	23–28 and 32	1–10	Adhesion?
ERMAP	Scianna	60–68		Adhesion?
EMMPRIN (CD147)	Ok	35–68		Signal transduction?
CDw108	JMH	76	1–3	Adhesion?
Kell gp (CD238)	Kell	93	4–8	Endopeptidase
Acetylcholinesterase	Yt	72	7–10	Acetylcholinesterase
Dombrock gp	Dombrock	47–57		ADP-ribosyltransferase
DAF (CD55)	Cromer	70	6–14	Complement regulation
CR1 (CD35)	Knops	190	0.2–1	Complement regulation
Glycophorin A (CD235A)	MN	43	1000	Sialic acid carrier
Glycophorin B (CD235B)	Ss	25	250	Sialic acid carrier
Glycophorins C and D (CD236)	Gerbich	40 and 30	143 and 82	Sialic acid carrier; cytoskeletal attachment

*Apparent molecular weight determined by electrophoresis.
†Carbohydrate antigens.
gp, glycoprotein.

although the Rh antigens are non-glycosylated proteins containing two or three molecules of palmitic acid. ABH and Ii antigens are found predominantly on the carbohydrate moieties of the major red cell glycoproteins band 3 (anion exchanger) and on GLUT-1, the glucose transporter, although they are also present on some other minor glycoproteins and on the carbohydrate portions of membrane glycolipids. P, P1 and P^K antigens are expressed on the carbohydrate of glycolipids. The M and N antigens arise from interactions between the carbohydrate and polypeptide in the glycoprotein GPA. In addition to the antigens on integral membrane components, some are adsorbed passively from plasma (e.g. Lewis, Chido/Rogers). Structural details of selected antigens are given in Chapter 15.

Antigens

Originally, an antigen was defined as the part of a molecule that is bound by a specific antibody. More recently, it has become customary to define an antigen as a substance that can stimulate an immune response (immunogenicity). Immune responses can be either positive or negative. Positive responses lead to the production of antibodies (humoral immunity) and/or proliferation of immunocompetent cells (cellular immunity) that can bind and eliminate their stimulatory antigen. In negative responses, the cells that mediate humoral and cellular immune responses are rendered non-responsive. This state is described as acquired immunological tolerance and is important in preventing autoimmune disease, as well as in establishing the 'take' or acceptance of transplanted syngeneic and allogeneic tissues.

The hallmark of the adaptive immune response is its specificity: specific immunocompetent cells and/or antibodies are produced, which can distinguish molecules that differ only by two or three atoms (e.g. TNP versus DNP). As described later, even the difference between the A and B antigens is minimal. However, antibodies can often react with antigens similar to, but not identical to, the stimulatory antigen (cross-reactivity). As far as is known, specific immune responses to human red cells are mediated by antibodies only; *specific* cell-mediated immunity to red cell alloantigens or autoantigens has not been described.

The parts of an antigen that bind antibodies or cellular receptors are called antigenic determinants or epitopes, and those parts of the antibodies that bind to them are called paratopes. Most antigens that occur naturally are of high molecular weight, and each antigenic molecule may have several different or several identical epitopes. As antibodies are specific for the individual epitopes and not for the antigen as a whole, antisera will usually be a collection of antibodies specific for different regions of the antigen in question, arising from different clones of immunocompetent cells (polyclonal antibodies); such antibodies can sometimes be distinguished serologically by anti-idiotype reagents (see below).

The biological significance of blood group antigens

The functions of several red cell membrane protein structures bearing blood group antigenic determinants are known, or can be deduced from their structure (Table 14.1). Some are membrane transporters, facilitating the transport of biologically important molecules through the lipid bilayer: band 3 membrane glycoprotein, the Diego antigen, provides an anion exchange channel for HCO_3^- and Cl^- ions; the Kidd glycoprotein is a urea transporter; the Colton glycoprotein is aquaporin 1, a water channel; the GIL-antigen is aquaporin 3, a glycerol transporter; and the Rh protein complex might function as an ammonium transporter or a CO_2 channel. The Lutheran, LW, and Indian (CD44) glycoproteins are adhesion molecules, possibly serving their functions during erythropoiesis. The Duffy glycoprotein is a chemokine receptor and might function as a 'sink' or scavenger for unwanted chemokines. The Cromer and Knops antigens are markers for decay accelerating factor and complement receptor 1, respectively, which protect the cells from destruction by autologous complement. Some blood group glycoproteins have enzyme activity: the Yt antigen is acetylcholinesterase and the Kell antigen is an endopeptidase with the ability to cleave a biologically inactive peptide to produce the vasoconstrictor endothelin-3. The C-terminal domains of the Gerbich antigens, GPC and GPD, and the N-terminal domain of the Diego glycoprotein, band 3, are attached to components of the cytoskeleton and function to anchor the membrane to it skeleton. The carbohydrate moieties of the membrane glycoproteins and glycolipids, especially those of the most abundant glycoproteins, band 3 and GPA, constitute the glycocalyx, an extracellular coat that protects the cell from mechanical damage and microbial attack.

The difference between allelic red cell antigens (e.g. A and B, K and k, Fy^a and Fy^b) is small, often being just one monosaccharide or one amino acid. The biological importance of these differences is unknown and there is little evidence to suggest that one antigen confers any significant advantage over another. Most blood group systems have a null phenotype in which the whole blood group protein is absent from the red cells or any other cells. These usually result from homozygosity for gene deletions or inactivating mutations within the genes. In most cases, individuals with these null phenotypes are apparently healthy, suggesting that, whatever the precise function of the missing structure may be, some other structure must be able to substitute in its absence. However, there are exceptions; 15% of Caucasians lack the D protein of the Rh system with no ill effect, but those rare individuals who lack both D and CcEe Rh proteins have chronic haemolysis, which may be compensated by increased red cell production, but may require splenectomy for stabilization. Absence of the Kx protein causes weakness of expression all Kell system antigens, as a result linkage between the two proteins in the membrane, but is also associated with acanthocytosis and neurological and muscular disorders. Individuals lacking the Diego antigen, the anion transporter, can only survive with extreme medical intervention, and no person with Yt-null phenotype and absence of the neurotransmitter acetylcholinesterase has been found. People with the rare Bombay phenotype lack ABH antigens from all tissues, with no apparent ill effect or red cell abnormality.

Some blood group antigens are exploited by pathological micro-organisms as receptors for attaching and entering cells. Consequently, in some cases absence of antigens can be beneficial. The Duffy glycoprotein, expressing Fy^a or Fy^b, is used by *Plasmodium vivax* to penetrate red cells. The Fy(a–b–) phenotype is common in Africans and confers resistance *P. vivax* malaria. Fy(a–b–) in Africans results from homozygosity for a mutation in an erythroid-specific transcription factor binding site, meaning that the Duffy glycoprotein is absent from red cells but is expressed in other tissues. It is likely that interaction between cell surface molecules and pathological micro-organisms has been a major factor in the evolution of blood group polymorphism.

Antibodies

Antibodies are immunoglobulins (Ig) produced by the B lymphocytes of the adaptive immune system in response to an antigen for which they exhibit specific binding.

Depending on the origin of the antigenic stimulus, antibodies can be termed: (i) alloantibodies, when produced by an individual against epitopes present in another individual of the same species; (ii) autoantibodies, when reactive with determinants present on the individual's own antigens; and (iii) heteroantibodies (or xenoantibodies), when produced against antigenic determinants present on the cells of another species. The first two are the antibodies encountered routinely in the blood bank; heteroantibodies can be used as antiglobulin sera or typing reagents when raised in animals against human antigens and are often present in reagents as monoclonal antibodies.

There are five classes of immunoglobulins: IgM, IgG, IgA, IgD and IgE. Antibodies with specificity for blood group antigens are

Table 14.2 Effector functions of the immunoglobulin isotypes*.

	IgG1	IgG2	IgG3	IgG4	IgA1	IgA2	Se IgA	IgM	IgE
Complement fixation: classical pathway§	+	(+)	++	−	−	−	−	++++	−
Complement fixation: alternative pathway	−	−	−	−	+†	++	−	−	−†
Placental transfer	++	+	+	+	−	−	−	−	−
Lymphocyte/macrophage FcR binding	++	−	+++	−	−	−	−	−	?‡
Mast cell binding	−	−	−	(?)	−	−	−	−	+++
Binding to *Staphylococcus aureus* protein A	+	+	−	+	−	−	−	−	−

*No biological function has been ascribed to IgD, but it might be intimately involved in maturation of B cells into competent effector cells and/or memory cells.

†Aggregated molecules can activate the alternative pathway.

‡Human IgE has been reported to bind to macrophages.

§IgG molecules fix complement only up to C3.

Se IgA, secretory IgA.

found only in the IgG, IgM and, rarely, IgA classes. IgA antibodies play a minor role in blood group serology as they only appear as alloantibodies together with IgM and/or IgG. Some of the biochemical and biophysical differences between IgG, IgM and IgA are listed in Table 14.2.

Biochemistry of immunoglobulins

Figure 14.3 shows a diagram of the basic immunoglobulin molecule. This consists of four polypeptide chains arranged as two L (light) chains and two identical H (heavy) chains. The

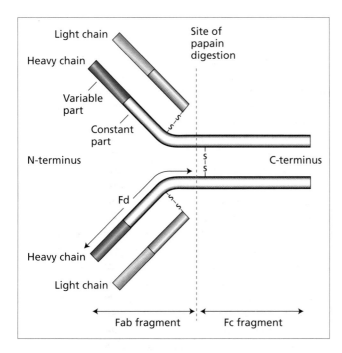

Figure 14.3 Structure of the basic immunoglobulin molecule.

light and heavy chains are usually held together by disulphide (S–S) bonds. IgG and serum IgA molecules are mainly monomers of this basic immunoglobulin structure; secretory IgA is mainly dimeric. IgM molecules are pentamers, with the basic immunoglobulin molecules held together by S–S bonds and a J (joining) chain (Figure 14.4).

There are two distinct types of light chain, kappa (κ) and lambda (λ). These are common to all immunoglobulins. Either of these chains may combine with any heavy chain, but in any one immunoglobulin both light chains are of the same type and are identical. Kappa chains occur in about 65% and lambda chains in about 35% of the normal immunoglobulins in each class. Each class has an immunologically distinct heavy chain: γ for IgG, μ for IgM, α for IgA, δ for IgD and ε for IgE (Figure 14.4). There are four subclasses of human IgG (IgGI, IgG2, IgG3 and IgG4, with γ1, γ2, γ3 and γ4 heavy chains), and two IgA subclasses (IgA1 and IgA2, with α1 and α2 chains).

Analyses of various light chains from different sources show that the amino acid sequence differs in one-half of the chain (variable region), whereas in the other half the sequence remains remarkably constant (constant region) between light chains of the appropriate kappa or lambda groups. Similarly, in the corresponding heavy chain, there is a variable region and a constant region when different chains are analysed.

Papain can split the basic Ig molecule into three fragments at a site near the S–S bonds that hold the heavy chains together (Figure 14.3). One fragment contains the C-termini of the heavy chains and is called the Fc fragment. The other two are called Fab fragments, each of which consists of the N-terminus of the heavy chain (Fd portion) and the whole of the light chain, and contains the antigen binding site of the molecule.

Repetition of amino acid sequences within the heavy chain constant regions indicates that there are either three (for IgG and IgA) or four (for IgM, IgD, IgE) constant region domains for H chains. These are designated C_H1, C_H2, C_H3 and C_H4. In

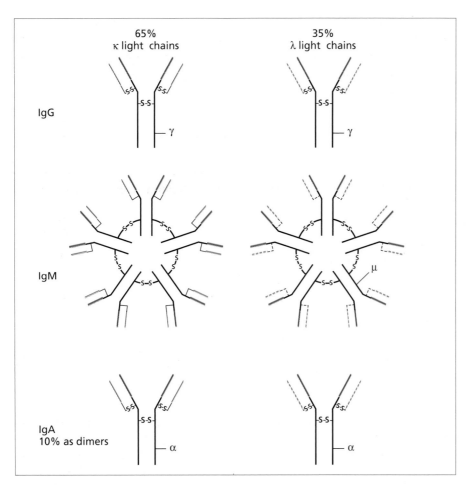

Figure 14.4 Structure of IgG, IgM and IgA molecules.

contrast, there is only one constant region domain for light chains and only one variable region domain for heavy and light chains. The segment between the C_H1 and C_H2 is called the *hinge region*. This area imparts flexibility to the immunoglobulin molecule so that antigen binding sites can span varying distances.

The vast majority of the differences between antibodies of various specificities occur in three or four short amino acid sequences in the L- and H-chain variable regions. These hypervariable sequences contact the antigen on binding and provide the basis of antibody specificity.

The remaining sequences within the variable region are known as the framework determinants. These are believed to provide the general skeleton of the antigen-recognizing region, within which variations in and between hypervariable sequences generate specificity for the different epitopes bound by different antibodies.

Amino acid sequences within framework and hypervariable segments can sometimes be recognized by specific antisera, usually from another species, raised by deliberate immunization with a particular antibody. The sequences recognized are referred to as idiotopes, and the sera that define them are called anti-idiotypes.

The idiotype of the particular immunoglobulin molecule represents the sum of all the idiotopes of all its framework and hypervariable sequences.

The binding of anti-idiotype sera that recognize idiotopes within hypervariable sequences of the immunizing immunoglobulin can be inhibited by the specific hapten recognized by that immunizing antibody. This is because contact between the hapten and the hypervariable sequences blocks access of the idiotype-specific antibody. In contrast, binding of anti-idiotypes to framework determinants of the immunizing antibody is usually not blocked by the binding of the hapten recognized by that antibody.

The great diversity in the repertoire of antibodies generated by the immune system in response to the immense variety of antigens that it encounters is a direct reflection of the immune system's ability to generate variations within the three hypervariable sequences. This ability is partly genetic in origin and arises from the random selection and joining of several separate genetic elements that produce a single intact variable region gene coding for the final variable region amino acid sequence.

The variable region genes comprise: (i) genes coding for a

large number of V-region sequences, with approximately 150 κ-chain, 125 λ-chain and 500 or so H-chain variable region genes; each of these genes is arranged in three exons, the random joining of which provides the variations that generate the first and second hypervariable sequences; (ii) in H chains only, approximately 10–20 D ('diversity') genes; and (iii) in both H and L chains, five or six J ('joining') genes.

The random joining of numerous choices, in a variety of combinations of V–J genes in L chains and V–D–J genes in H chains, during ontogeny of the immune response, generates the third hypervariable sequence and provides an additional somatic contribution for increasing the repertoire of the immune system. Following V–J/V–D–J joining, which is achieved by splicing together of certain DNA sequences and deletion of others during B-cell maturation, a further increase in antibody diversity is achieved by mutation in the spliced V gene DNA of mature B cells, during their proliferation in an ongoing immune response.

Biological and physical properties of immunoglobulins

Immunoglobulins are essentially multifunctional; not only do they bind antigen, but they also perform various other functions depending on the Ig class. Most of these additional functions reside in the Fc fragment and are listed in Table 14.2. The most important include: (i) complement fixation (lgM > IgG3 > lgG1 > IgG2); IgA does not bind complement in the classical pathway; (ii) binding to Fc receptors of mononuclear phagocytic cells, in particular monocytes and macrophages (IgG3 » IgG1); and (iii) transplacental passage; there is preferential active transport of IgG1 relative to the other IgG subclasses.

Some functions can be ascribed to particular domains. For example, C_H2 or C_H2/C_H3 for complement (Clq) binding and control of catabolic rate; the hinge region for binding to the Fc receptors of macrophages and monocytes; $C_H2 + C_H3$ for binding to staphylococcal protein A (IgG3 does not bind) and to the Fc receptors on placental syncytial trophoblasts and lymphocytes.

For blood group-specific antibodies, these class-dependent biological functions contribute to their clinical significance. In the majority of cases, antigen–antibody binding does not cause red cell destruction per se; immune-mediated red cell destruction is usually a consequence of these secondary effector functions.

As only IgG passes the placental barrier, only IgG blood group antibodies can cause haemolytic disease of the fetus and the newborn, although only IgGl and IgG3 will mediate significant immune red cell destruction. The IgG level in cord blood will be much the same as the level in the mother. The passively transferred maternal IgG gradually disappears from the infant after birth and is almost gone by 3 months of age. The serum of newborn infants contains a small amount of IgM of fetal origin but almost no IgA; the production of IgA and IgG starts at about 1–2 months of age.

There are many ways of separating IgG and IgM molecules by physical methods (e.g. gel filtration and affinity chromatography). In routine serology, IgG is easily distinguishable from IgM by treating sera with mild reducing agents such as 2-mercaptoethanol or dithiothreitol (DTT) at low concentrations. These agents split the S–S bonds of the J chains, which link the IgM subunits, thereby rendering them non-agglutinating; IgA is either slightly affected or not affected by such reducing agents.

Blood group antibodies

There are several terms that have been used in the past and are still sometimes used to describe different types of blood group antibodies. These are 'naturally occurring' and 'immune' antibodies, 'cold' and 'warm' antibodies, and IgM, 'complete' (or saline) and IgG, 'incomplete' antibodies. They are described below and an attempt is made to correlate these terms with the class of immunoglobulin involved.

Naturally occurring and immune antibodies

Antibodies are naturally occurring when they are produced without any obvious immunizing stimulus such as pregnancy, transfusion or injection of blood. These antibodies are not present at birth and, in the case of anti-A and anti-B, start to appear in the serum of children with the appropriate ABO groups at about 3–6 months of age. ABO antibodies are probably produced in response to antigens of bacteria, viruses and other substances that are inhaled or ingested; many Gram-negative organisms have antigens that are structurally similar to the A and B antigens. Despite this probable antigenic stimulus, the term 'naturally occurring' is retained for these 'non-red cell-induced' antibodies. 'Immune' blood group antibodies are only produced after pregnancy or following transfusion or injection of blood or blood group substances.

Cold and warm antibodies

Cold antibodies give higher agglutination titres at low temperatures (0–4°C) and many of them will not agglutinate red cells at 37°C. Most naturally occurring antibodies are cold reacting. Some, such as naturally occurring anti-A and -B, have a wide thermal range and will still react at 37°C, at which temperature they will activate complement and lyse red cells, but the titre will be much higher at 0–4°C. Cold antibodies that fail to react above 30°C are of no clinical significance and can be ignored for blood transfusion purposes.

The thermal optimum of warm antibodies is 37°C and this implies that higher titres are obtained at this temperature. Immune antibodies are warm reacting. Any red cell antibody reacting above 30°C should be considered potentially capable of destroying red cells *in vivo*.

IgM and IgG antibodies

IgM or 'complete' antibodies agglutinate red cells when they are suspended in saline. They are often called saline or directly agglutinating antibodies in laboratory parlance. Conversely, 'incomplete', IgG antibodies will not agglutinate saline-suspended red cells. However, lack of agglutination does not mean that the antibodies have not bound to their antigen, and it can be shown that they have reacted by using antiglobulin reagents, which facilitate agglutination (see below). Most naturally occurring antibodies are cold reacting, complete, IgM. Immune antibodies are always warm reacting; most are partly IgG, but some may be IgM. Exceptionally, IgG complete antibodies are found.

Monoclonal antibodies

Animal sera have, in general, been a poor source of blood grouping reagents. Deliberate immunization of laboratory animals to produce blood group-specific heteroantibodies has had limited success as only a few polyclonal specificities have been made in rabbits, goats and chickens. The most useful reagents have been anti-A, -B, -M, -N, -P1, -Le^a, -Le^b and -LW.

The advent of monoclonal antibody technologies has increased the repertoire of blood grouping reagents. By fusing the spleen cells of immunized mice or rats with drug-sensitive myeloma cells and selecting for drug-resistant hybrids, it has been possible to establish permanently growing cloned cell lines in tissue culture that secrete antibodies of desired specificities. Several murine hybrids secreting human blood group-specific monoclonal antibodies have now been established, many of which were raised using immunogens other than intact red cells (e.g. anti-A, -B, -Le^a, -Le^b, -M and -N).

Attempts to produce human monoclonal antibodies by the cell fusion approach have been of limited success due to the lack of suitable human myelomas. Nevertheless, human monoclonal antibodies specific for RhD, C, c, E and e, the ABO blood group antigens, and several other antigens including Jk^a and Jk^b have been obtained by the alternative approach of transforming isolated peripheral blood lymphocytes from immunized individuals with Epstein–Barr virus. Monoclonal antibodies of murine and human origin have widely replaced polyclonal blood grouping reagents in everyday ABO and D grouping.

The future of antibody reagent production may lie in recombinant DNA technology, but a useful blood grouping reagent is still to be produced by these methods.

Lectins

Lectins are sugar-binding proteins, mostly extracted from plants and lower vertebrate animals. They are useful tools for routine and experimental blood group serology. They combine with simple sugars (e.g. fucose, galactose, N-acetylgalactosamine) present on the glycolipids and glycoproteins of cell membranes and body fluids. Most lectins agglutinate red cells irrespective of target cell phenotype; hence only a handful are used with any regularity in blood group serology. The three most commonly used blood group-specific lectins are extracts from *Dolichos biflorus* (the hyacinth bean), *Vicia graminea* (horse gram) and *Ulex europaeus* (common gorse), which have anti-A$_1$, anti-N and anti-H specificities respectively. Several other lectins have proven valuable in investigating red cell polyagglutinability (see Chapter 15). In addition to blood grouping, lectins are also used for determining ABH secretor status, separating mixtures of red cells, and for partially purifying and identifying blood group active membrane glycoproteins.

Lectins are not immunoglobulins. They are not produced as a result of a specific immune response and do not possess the uniform molecular structure of immunoglobulins. Some exist as simple monomers (e.g. *Ulex*), whereas others are polymers (e.g. *Dolichos*). The lectins used in blood grouping are highly specific for monosaccharides. For example, *U. europaeus* and *D. biflorus* lectins recognize L-fucose and N-acetyl-D-galactosamine respectively. This specificity does not depend solely upon the presence of the particular sugar, but is also influenced by its orientation and conformation, the nature of the carrier molecule, and the number and distribution of reactive molecules in the red cell membrane. There are only seven monosaccharides on the red cell membrane, in various combinations with each other and their lipid and protein carriers; the similarities in these combinations lead to cross-reactivity of many lectins.

Complement

Complement consists of a series of proteins, mainly enzymes present in fresh plasma as inactive precursors, which react sequentially with each other to form products that are important in the immune destruction of cells, including bacteria. In complement activation, there are two stages of relevance. The first stage is the generation of the active form of the third component, C3b, which leads to the coating, or opsonization, of the cell with a large amount of protein. There are two pathways by which active C3b may be generated: the classical and alternative pathways (Figure 14.5). The second stage is the lytic stage: activation of the proteins of the membrane attack complex (MAC), components C5 through to C9, which leads to the destruction of red cells in the circulation.

In general terms, the complement cascade is analogous to the clotting sequence. Activation of one component or group of components leads to the generation of enzyme activity for activation of the next components. However, to lead to haemolysis, the activated components in the plasma must bind to the red cell membrane (except Cl, which binds only to a specific binding site on the antibody); they do this with varying degrees of efficiency. Moreover, some activated components, for example Cl, C4 and

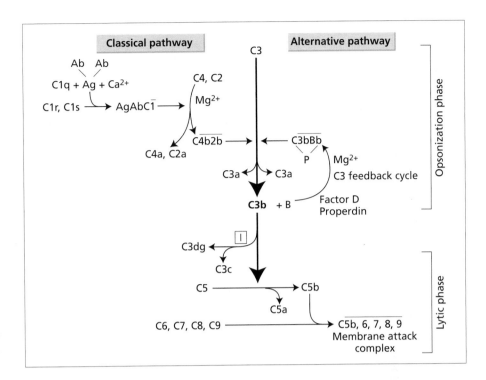

Figure 14.5 The complement cascade. Component C3b plays a central role in the classical and alternative pathways.

C3, have specific inactivators in the plasma as well as (for C3b and C4b) in the red cell membrane itself, and, even though these components bind to the red cell membrane, their active life may be very short (half-life, $T_{1/2}$, of 2–25 min). As a consequence, and as happens with several IgG blood group antibodies such as anti-Jk^a and -Fy^a, the whole sequence is not completed and there is no intravascular haemolysis; in these cases, early components can be detected on the red cell surface with suitable antiglobulin reagents.

Complement components in the classical pathway are called C1 to C9 in their native form. Apart from C4, which is activated before C2 and C3, the components are activated sequentially according to their numerical order. Complement components in the alternative pathway include factor B, factor D and properdin. In the activation of the 'classical' components, small-molecular-weight fragments, C4a, C3a, C5a, are released, which have important chemotactic and anaphylactic activity. C3a and C5a, as well as the release of vasoactive amines and cytokines, lead to most of the signs and symptoms observed in severe haemolytic transfusion reactions and also in febrile non-haemolytic transfusion reactions.

The opsonization phase of the complement sequence (Figure 14.5)

The classical pathway

The classical pathway can be activated by many factors, including antigen–antibody complexes, enzymes (trypsin, plasmin, lysosomal enzymes), endotoxins and low-ionic-strength media.

Only one molecule of IgM on a cell membrane is necessary to activate the complement system, although at least two out of the five IgM subunits must attach to the cell membrane for activation to occur. At least two IgG molecules must combine with antigen sites very close together on the cell membrane to bring about complement activation.

The first component of complement is a complex of three protein molecules Clq, Clr and Cls. After complement-fixing antibodies have bound to their red cell antigens (EA is often used to denote the resulting erythrocyte–antibody complex), C1 binding sites are exposed on the Fc fragments. If two such sites are sufficiently close together (approximately 25–40 nm), the Cl complex is fixed through its Clq subunits. Clq is a complex molecule with six immunoglobulin binding sites. Binding of Clq activates Clr, which, in turn, cleaves the third molecule, Cls, yielding the active enzyme form of the Cl complex, which is held together by calcium. In the presence of EDTA or other chelating agents, the complex falls apart and the whole process of complement fixation will not occur.

Cls can now activate sequentially C4 and C2 in the presence of magnesium, generating a second enzyme, $\overline{C4b2b}$, called C3 convertase.

The cell-bound $\overline{C4b2b}$ can optimally activate several thousand C3 molecules. As C3 is present in large amounts (100–150 mg/dL) in the serum, the fixation of C3 can considerably increase the globulin coating of the red cells. Although C3b is still intact, opsonized red cells will adhere to monocytes and macrophages through their C3b receptors and may then be phagocytosed. C3b has a short half-life and there is no free C3b in plasma.

Hence, C3b coating of IgG-sensitized cells neutralizes the inhibitory effect of free plasma IgG on macrophage immune adherence and amplifies erythrophagocytosis 100-fold. Thus, C3b-coated, IgG-sensitized cells are destroyed mainly in the liver, where there are numerous phagocytic cells with receptors able to bind cells coated with IgG and C3b. The active phase of C3 is transient because it is rapidly degraded by an enzyme (C3b inactivator, C3bINA or factor I) and its accelerator (βIH or factor H) so that only C3dg remains on the red cell surface. C3dg is an end-product of the complement sequence and, by occupying the C3 sites, can prevent further binding of C3b and therefore haemolysis of the red cell. C3dg, unlike C3b, is not capable of adhering to receptors on macrophages and monocytes, so that cells coated with C3dg may return to the circulation and will be resistant to further lysis. This explains the existence of a population of C3dg-coated cells refractory to lysis in chronic cold haemagglutinin disease. C3dg-coated cells can be detected by anticomplement in the antiglobulin test.

C4b2b3b will 'trigger' the fixation of C5, C6, C7, C8 and C9 leading to the membrane attack complex on normal red cells and bringing about their lysis.

The alternative pathway

The alternative pathway does not necessarily involve antibody and represents non-specific 'innate' immunity. The proteins of the alternative pathway form a feedback loop for the conversion of C3 to C3b; the latter is both a product and reactant of this loop.

The alternative pathway can be activated by aggregated IgA, zymosan, bacterial cells or lipopolysaccharides. Initiation of the alternative pathway is a two-step process: (i) binding of C3b to an activator and (ii) interaction of bound C3b with neighbouring surface structures. Initially, spontaneously generated fluid-phase C3b interacts with factor B to form a complex. Factor B is activated through cleavage by the protease factor D, releasing a fragment Ba into the plasma and yielding a transient alternative C3 convertase, C3bBb. The latter can be stabilized by properdin, which is essential for preventing the dissociation of C3bBb by factor H.

The alternative C3 convertase splits serum C3 into C3a and C3b. C3b attaches to the cell surface and can then combine with more factor B and D, thereby restarting the feedback loop. The amount of C3b deposited by the alternative pathway is low owing to the small amount of convertase generated and to the inefficient deposition of C3b from plasma. This contrasts with the vast numbers of C3b molecules generated by the classical pathway. The two sources of C3b are indistinguishable; both act on C5 to start the lytic phase.

The classical and alternative pathways cannot be separated from each other *in vivo*. The alternative pathway amplifies the classical pathway because, when C3b is generated, factors B and D may be activated and complexed with it to generate further C3b.

The lytic phase of the complement sequence
(Figure 14.5)

The lytic phase starts with the activation of C5 by C3b, yielding membrane-bound C5b and fluid-phase C5a. This step is followed by non-enzymatic interaction of C5b with C6, C7, C8 and C9. These molecules adhere to each other to form the MAC and insert themselves into the lipid bilayer of the red cell membrane. C8 catalysed by C9 produces protein-lined cylinders in the red cell membrane and are about 10 nm in diameter. They form pores through which ions and water can enter. The osmotic pressure exerted by haemoglobin draws water into the cell until it swells and bursts.

Optimum temperature and pH for complement lysis

Many of the active complement components are enzymes and as such are very sensitive to changes in pH and temperature. The optimum pH for haemolysis to occur is 6.8 and the optimum temperature is 32–37°C. At temperatures below 15°C, the red cell cannot be haemolysed by complement and it is assumed that the last stages of complement fixation do not occur. However, the early stages of complement fixation can occur at 15°C and the components can be detected on the red cell surface with anti-complement reagents.

The ability of the antibody to bind complement

Why some antibody molecules bind complement easily and others do not is not fully understood, but several factors seem to be important.

1 The immunoglobulin class and subclass of the antibody, as discussed later.

2 At least two Clq binding sites properly aligned and close together are necessary for complement fixation. One molecule of IgM antibody carries several Clq binding sites, whereas one molecule of IgG carries only one, and will therefore need another molecule of IgG alongside it (IgG doublet) in order to fix Clq. Therefore, for IgG antibodies to cause lysis by complement, there must be many more molecules available. It has been shown that only one molecule of IgM anti-sheep red cell antibody is needed to lyse a sheep red cell, but at least 700–1000 molecules of IgG antibodies are needed to ensure that the two IgG molecules are aligned so that the whole process of the complement cascade can start.

3 If the antigen site density is low or moderate, it may be difficult for two IgG molecules to be properly aligned however much antibody is available. This may partly explain the poor performance of IgG antibody molecules in complement fixation when compared with IgM.

4 Flexibility at the hinge region is important; the wider the angle at the Y junction, the greater the ability of the IgG antibody to fix complement.

In red cell destruction caused by complement-fixing lytic antibodies, the number of red cells that can be rapidly destroyed is limited only by the amount of antibody and complement available. In ABO-incompatible transfusions, there may be no surviving A or B red cells in the circulation within 1 h of transfusion. However, if antibodies are only weakly or partially able to fix complement (most anti-Jk^a, -K and -Fy^a), red cell destruction will be extravascular and will proceed more slowly. Anti-Le^a will destroy only a proportion of transfused Le(a+) red cells intravascularly; the remaining cells will become Le(a−) and will have normal survival (see Chapter 15). This explains the two-component red cell survival curves seen when labelled Le(a+) cells are injected into subjects with anti-Le^a.

Clinical significance of red cell antibodies

The clinical significance of different red cell antibodies depends partly on their destructive capacity and partly on their frequency. For example, anti-PP1P^K (anti-Tj^a) is a very potent haemolysin, but it is of minimal importance in blood transfusion practice owing to its great rarity. Conversely, ABO and D antibodies are by far the most significant, due to their high frequency and destructive capacity.

Several factors influence immune red cell destruction *in vivo*. These include:

1 *Plasma concentration and avidity of the antibody.*
2 *Thermal amplitude of the antibody.*
3 *Immunoglobulin class and subclass.* The complement-fixing ability of most warm-reacting IgM antibodies makes them clinically significant. Of the IgG subclasses, IgG1 and IgG3 have clinical importance because of the ability of some to fix complement and their avidity for the Fc receptors of mononuclear phagocytic cells, the effector cells of *in vivo* extravascular immune red cell destruction.
4 *Antibody specificity.* Several warm-reacting antibodies are incapable of causing *in vivo* red cell destruction (e.g. anti-Ch, -Rg, -Cs^a, -Kn^a, -Xg^a and most examples of anti-Yt^a).
5 *Antigen density on the red cell membrane.* The likelihood and degree of sensitization of a red cell with antibody and complement increases with the number of antigen sites on the surface.
6 *Volume of incompatible red cells transfused.* A small volume of incompatible red cells will be destroyed more rapidly than a large volume from the same donor. Larger volumes of cells may exhaust the circulating antibody available and saturate the mononuclear phagocytic system (MPS). This difference is important in interpreting ^{51}Cr survival tests, which employ small volumes of red cells and therefore might overestimate the destruction of larger volumes.
7 *Presence of antigen in donor plasma.* Lewis antigens (Le^a and Le^b) and the Chido and Rogers antigens are primarily in plasma and are only secondarily adsorbed onto red cells. The free antigen in plasma, especially when whole blood is transfused, will react with the antibody and inhibit its binding to red cells. In addition, group A and B cells have less Le antigens than group O red cells used in antibody screening and identification. Hence, cross match-compatible blood unscreened for Lewis phenotype is transfused to patients with Lewis antibodies. Furthermore, when Lewis-positive blood is transfused to patients with antibodies, the cells lose their Lewis antigens and become Le(a−b−). For this reason, Lewis antibodies are unable to cause delayed haemolytic transfusion reactions.
8 *Activity of cells of the mononuclear phagocyte system.* The ability of macrophages to remove sensitized red cells varies between individuals. Splenectomy and drugs such as corticosteroids will decrease the clearance of IgG-sensitized cells.
9 *Sensitivity of red cells to complement.* Resulting from absence of cell bound complement regulators, patients with paroxysmal nocturnal haemoglobinuria have red cells that are highly sensitive to lysis by complement activation.
10 *Extent of complement activation.* Some antibodies regularly bind complement and others do so rarely or not at all. Of the complement-binding antibodies, IgM (e.g. anti-A, -B, -PP1P^K) will activate the complement cascade through to C9, but for most (e.g. IgG anti-Fy^a, -Jk^a, -K) the cascade is interrupted at the C3 stage. Red cells coated with IgG and C3b will be destroyed extravascularly in the liver. As a rule, Rh antibodies do not fix complement.

Blood group antigen–antibody reactions

In blood group serology, the interaction between the antigen sites on the cells and the corresponding antibody is normally detected by observing agglutination of the cells concerned. Agglutination is the result of the cross-linking of individual red cells by antibody molecules and can be thought of as occurring in two stages. The first stage is the fundamental reaction, i.e. the combination of the antibody molecules with their specific antigen sites. The second stage is the actual linkage of the individual antibody-coated red cells.

First stage of agglutination: combination of antibody with antigen

The combination of antigen with antibody cannot be observed directly; it arises from the fit of the antigen into a structurally complementary site within the antibody molecule. The resulting complex is then stabilized by various short-range forces between the chemical groups of the antigen-binding site in the antibody and the antigenic determinant itself. These weak, short-range forces include ionic attraction (e.g. between COO$^-$ and NH$_3^+$), hydrogen bonding (e.g. between -OH, -NH$_2$ and -CO), van der Waals' forces and hydrophobic interactions. Individually, these forces are weak; however, when in close apposition, the simultaneous formation of a large number of bonds stabilizes antigen binding. The greater the interface between antigen and antibody, the stronger are the binding forces generated and the greater the affinity of the antibody for its specific antigen.

The association of antigen (Ag) with antibody (Ab) is reversible and obeys the law of mass action so that, at equilibrium:

$$(Ag) + (Ab) \underset{k_2}{\overset{k_1}{\rightleftharpoons}} (AgAb)$$

where k_1 and k_2 are rate constants of association and dissociation respectively. Hence, at equilibrium:

$$K = \frac{k_1}{k_2} = \frac{(AgAb)}{(Ag)(Ab)}$$

where K is the equilibrium constant for the reaction and reflects the strength of association between antigen and antibody. The greater the value of K, the greater the amount of antigen–antibody complex formed.

Factors affecting the first stage of agglutination

Factors that affect the equilibrium constant include pH, ionic strength and temperature.

pH

Most antibodies are not affected by changes in pH within the range 5.5–8.5. However, this is not true for all antibodies, and, in order to make one day's work similar to the next, routine serology should be carried out with saline buffered to pH 7.0–7.4. Below pH 4 and above pH 9, antigen–antibody complexes are largely dissociated and the antibody can be recovered in the supernatant. This is the basis of some elution techniques.

The ionic strength of the medium

In saline of normal ionic strength, the ionized groups of both antigen and antibody are partially neutralized by oppositely charged ions in the medium. By lowering the ionic strength while maintaining tonicity, the ions become exposed and theoretically there should be an increase in attraction. Decreasing the ionic strength increases the rate of association (k_1) of antigen with antibody but has little effect on their rate of dissociation (k_2). For example, a 1000-fold increase in k_1 with a threefold fall in k_2 has been observed for anti-D by reducing the ionic strength to 0.03 mol/L. Low-ionic-strength solutions (LISS) containing 0.03 mol/L NaCl in a solution of sodium glycinate are used routinely in some blood banks to increase the speed and sensitivity of pretransfusion tests. Regrettably, LISS can lead to a failure in detection of some clinically important antibodies, in particular anti-K.

Low-ionic-strength solutions are also used to coat red cells with complement components via the alternative pathway. A few drops of fresh whole blood can be taken into 1–2 mL of 10% sucrose, incubated for 10 min at 37°C and washed, to provide control cells coated with C3 and C4 for the antiglobulin test. For this reason, the use of LISS under uncontrolled conditions can lead to unwanted positive direct and indirect antiglobulin tests.

The temperature of the reaction

The effect of temperature on antigen–antibody reactions includes: (i) an alteration in the equilibrium constant of the antibody and (ii) an alteration of the rate of encounter. With warm antibodies, the equilibrium constant is not changed by variations in temperature, but decreasing the temperature from 37°C to 4°C slows the rate of reaction 20-fold. With cold antibodies, there is an increase in the equilibrium constant with decreasing temperature and, even though the rate is reduced, stronger reactions and higher titres are found at lower temperatures.

Second, or 'visual', stage of agglutination

Factors that affect the second stage of agglutination

These include the degree of contact of the antibody-coated red cells with each other, the span of the antibody molecules, the electrical charge of the red cells, the location and density of the antigen sites on the red cells and the capacity of the antibody to bind complement after reacting with the antigen.

The degree of contact of antibody coated cells

It is obvious that the antibody molecules cannot form bridges between individual cells until the cells are close together. This contact can be achieved by allowing the cells to settle by gravity; full settling does not occur in a saline serum medium until 1–2 h have elapsed. Settling can always be accelerated by centrifugation. However, as red cell drifts mimicking agglutination may be formed, it is best to centrifuge at quite low speeds for not more than 1 min.

In a colloidal medium (e.g. albumin), settling of the red cells occurs after 3–6 h of incubation of serum and cells. However, if albumin is added to the mixture after centrifugation, incubation times can be reduced to 1 h.

The electrical charge of the red cells

Red cells suspended in 9 g/L of NaCl are negatively charged; because of this charge and the repulsive force that it generates, there is always a gap between individual red cells. The minimum distance of approach of unsensitized cells is approximately 18 nm between their actual membranes. This is considerably greater than the maximum distance between the two arms (valencies) of an IgG molecule (12 nm). IgM molecules, with a greater distance (approximately 30 nm) between the antigen-combining sites, are able to bridge this gap and thus cause agglutination of appropriate cells suspended in saline. Conversely, IgG anti-D cannot cross-link two D-positive cells in saline. Cells coated in this way approach each other to within 6 nm between the Fc ends of the coating IgG. Agglutination of IgG-coated cells can then be brought about by various agents that bring them closer together or by molecules that cross-link coating IgG.

The treatment of cells with proteases (trypsin, papain, bromelin, ficin) or neuraminidase removes negatively charged neuraminic acid from the red cell membrane. Proteases, but not neuraminidase, also remove hydrophobic membrane glycoproteins, thus enabling enzyme-treated cells to come sufficiently close together to allow agglutination by IgG antibodies.

The span of the antibody molecule
The span of an IgG molecule can be increased by mild reduction and alkylation, which opens up the hinge region by cleaving S–S bonds. Antibodies treated in this way can be used as direct agglutinins and are available as 'saline' reagents from commercial companies.

The location and density of antigen sites
The fourth factor that affects the second stage of agglutination is the number of antigen sites on each red cell and, therefore, the number of possible sites for antibody combination. IgG anti-A, -B, -M and -N may agglutinate the appropriate red cells in saline; this may be due to the comparatively high number of the corresponding antigen sites (see Chapter 15 and Table 14.1). For those antigens that protrude from the cell surface (e.g. ABO, MN, I, i), agglutination by the corresponding antibodies will occur more readily than for antigens embedded in the membrane (e.g. Rh).

The number of antigen sites is, for some blood group systems, a reflection of the genotype; *MM* cells will carry twice the number of M antigens as *MN* cells and will be more readily agglutinated by the appropriate antibody (dosage effect). In other systems (e.g. ABO, D), dosage is not apparent.

The capacity of the antibody to bind complement
The last factor that affects the second stage of agglutination is the ability of antibody to bind complement after reacting with its antigen. Here it should be remembered that if an antibody binds complement there might be no agglutination. The simplest explanation of this absence of agglutination is that the added presence of complement molecules, close to the antibody, prevents the antibody molecules from linking up individual cells. This lack of agglutination can be very important. For instance, in grouping or compatibility tests, anti-A and -B in a patient's fresh serum may cause partial lysis of the red cells and no agglutination of the unlysed cells. If this lysis is not noticed, the test may be read as negative and grossly incompatible blood might be regarded as compatible.

The use of enzyme-treated red cells

Several proteases (papain from papaya, trypsin from calf spleen, bromelin from pineapple, ficin from figs) are used under strictly standardized conditions to treat red cells and potentiate agglutination.

Whether or not enzyme treatment of the red cells enhances agglutination by an antibody depends on the nature of the appropriate antigen. Agglutination by Rh, Lewis, P1, Kidd, I and i antibodies is enhanced regardless of whether the antibodies are

IgM or IgG. Agglutination by most examples of anti-K is not enhanced with enzyme-treated cells. Some protein antigens are destroyed by protease treatment of intact red cells. These include M, N, S, Fy^a, Fy^b, Xg^a, In^a, In^b, Yt^a, Ch, Rg, Pr and Tn (see Chapter 15).

Detection of red cell antigen–antibody reactions

Principles of agglutination techniques

There are various ways of detecting antigen–antibody reactions *in vitro*. In manual methods, tubes, microplates or gels can be used. The most widely used methods employ the following techniques.

Direct agglutination
Most IgM antibodies will directly agglutinate the appropriate red cells suspended in saline. This method is used routinely for ABO and RhD grouping using monoclonal antibodies.

Indirect agglutination
Apart from ABO, antibodies against most blood group antigens are IgG and generally will not bring about direct agglutination of red cells. Such antibodies can be detected with the aid of agents that enhance agglutination, for example, proteases, albumin and other colloids, and aggregating agents such as polybrene. When proteases are used, more reproducible and reliable tests are achieved if the cells are enzyme-treated before incubation with the relevant serum.

The antiglobulin or Coombs' test
The antiglobulin test is used to detect IgG antibodies that do not cause direct agglutination of red cells carrying the corresponding antigen when suspended in saline. The technique can be used to test directly, with an antiglobulin reagent, for the presence of antibodies or complement components that have been bound to the red cells *in vivo* – the direct antiglobulin test (DAT). Second, the test can be used to detect IgG antibodies in a patient's serum by adding the appropriate test red cells and then, after incubation and thorough washing of the cells, adding an antiglobulin reagent that will agglutinate cells coated *in vitro* with antibody or complement components. This is the indirect antiglobulin test (IAT).

Whereas this was mainly carried out in tubes, the use of microplates and microcolumns containing a matrix of either a gel or glass beads is becoming increasingly popular. With columns, the wash phase, as described below, has been eliminated. IATs are also used with many reagent antibodies for determining blood group phenotypes. If an IAT is undertaken with red cells suspended in normal ionic strength saline (NISS), maximum antibody uptake, and hence maximum sensitivity, is achieved within a 60- to 90-min incubation period. However, the incubation phase for IATs can be reduced to 10–15 min by using low-ionic-strength solutions (LISS). LISS IATs may be performed by either suspending the test red cells in LISS before adding the patient's serum or by adding LISS to the red cell–serum mixture. LISS IAT is less sensitive than NISS IAT for the detection of some examples of anti-K if the incubation time is reduced below 15 min. A further disadvantage of LISS IAT is that, if used in the cold, clinically insignificant antibodies such as anti-P1 and anti-Le^a may be detected more readily because of their increased uptake under low-ionic-strength conditions. In view of the many LISS preparations available, it is important that the manufacturer's instructions are followed strictly.

When the DAT and IAT are performed in tubes, it is essential that the red cells are washed three or four times with a large volume of saline before adding the antiglobulin reagent, as any free IgG or complement will neutralize the anti-IgG or anti-complement reagent and lead to false-negative reactions.

Antihuman globulin (AHG) serum was originally made by injecting animals, usually rabbits, sheep or goats, with human serum. The animal's immune system is able to differentiate very well between the large collection of foreign proteins that make up human serum, and, under optimum conditions, an animal can make distinct antibodies against a wide variety of serum proteins. Of particular relevance to the antiglobulin test are antibodies against IgG and complement, which should always be present in polyspecific AHG serum. The anti-IgG component is essential for pretransfusion antibody screening and cross-matching, as the vast majority of clinically significant antibodies, apart from anti-A and -B, are IgG. The anti-complement component is needed for the detection of occasional examples of weak complement-binding antibodies (e.g. some anti-Jk^a) and for the detection of in vivo complement coating of red cells (i.e. in the DAT). Antiglobulin reagents are now generally produced from monoclonal antibodies to C3d and polyclonal antibodies to IgG.

The basic composition of a polyspecific reagent is a blend of anti-IgG and -C3d. Anti-C4d should be avoided and antibodies against IgA and IgM are not necessarily always present in polyspecific reagents. Pure anti-IgG, anti-IgA and -IgM serum can be made in animals by injecting the appropriate purified immunoglobulin and removing any antibody against L chains by absorption.

Most IgM blood group antibodies can be detected readily by direct agglutination. On those occasions when it is desirable to detect subagglutinating amounts of IgM active at 37°C, the lack of anti-IgM in polyspecific reagents can be offset by the ability of the IgM antibody to fix complement in the presence of fresh serum. Moreover, as only a few molecules of IgM are needed to start the complement sequence and can then lead to the binding of many hundreds of molecules of C3, the agglutination of complement-coated cells by anti-complement sera can be a very sensitive method of detecting IgM antibodies. Some

anti-IgG preparations will agglutinate red cells coated with sub-agglutinating quantities of IgM owing to the presence of anti-L-chain activity. Of course, complement-fixing IgG antibodies will also be detected with anti-complement sera but, in most cases, they can be detected effectively by anti-IgG. However, there are exceptional examples of complement-fixing IgG red cell alloantibodies (e.g. anti-Jk^a), that are not detectable with anti-IgG, and anti-complement is essential for their identification.

Polyspecific antiglobulin reagents composed of anti-IgG and anti-C3d are perfectly suitable for pretransfusion testing, including the cross-match. For those rare cases of autoimmune haemolytic anaemia in which the test with polyspecific AHG is negative, it is necessary to test with anti-IgA and anti-IgM, which are now available ready for use in gel microcolumns. Polyclonal and monoclonal reagents against the four human IgG subclasses are commercially available and are generally used in research for characterizing clinically significant red cell alloantibodies.

Standardization of anti-human globulin reagents

All antiglobulin reagents available at present, monospecific or polyspecific, are standardized by the producer and issued pre-diluted for immediate use or within the gel or bead matrix of a microcolumn.

Antiglobulin reagents standardized for use in haemagglutination tests should not agglutinate red cells, regardless of their ABO type, after incubation with compatible serum (i.e. they should be free of unwanted antibodies, especially anti-species). The antiglobulin reagent should not agglutinate washed red cells taken from units of blood intended for transfusion when they are nearing the end of their shelf-life. The final dilution of the anti-IgG component should be sufficient to allow the optimal detection of weak examples of incomplete non-complement-fixing IgG alloantibodies (e.g. anti-D, -c) coated on single antigen dose (heterozygous) target cells (e.g. D/d or C/c). The anti-C3d component should be optimized so that complement bound to the cells will be detected but not so strong that stored cells, with traces of bound C3d and C4d, react non-specifically. As plasma is now used by most laboratories for pretransfusion testing, alloantibodies that theoretically might only react with the anti-C3 in an AHG reagent will be missed. However, there is no evidence that significant antibodies are not being detected.

When new batches of an AHG reagent or IAT microcolumns are acquired by a laboratory, they should be subjected to a minimum verification with several IgG antibodies of different specificities to ensure that all are detectable. Laboratories should confirm that, on each day of use, the AHG reagent is reacting according to the manufacturer's specifications, with control red cells coated weakly with IgG. The control IgG-coated cells are the same cells as those used to check the validity of negative antiglobulin tests when a washing step is part of the process; the weakly coated cells are added to each tube giving a negative result, followed by repeat centrifugation and reading. Agglutination of these cells confirms that the AHG reagent in the tube had not been neutralized by residual unbound IgG that was not removed during washing of the original test cells.

Agents that enhance agglutination
Various agents may be added to serological mixtures to enhance the agglutinability of red cells. These include albumin and LISS, as described above, as well as polybrene and polyethylene glycol (PEG). Whereas albumin and LISS work by reducing interfacial red cell surface tension and increasing electrostatic attraction, respectively, the mode of action of polybrene and PEG is not so clear. Polybrene is the bromide salt of polymerized hexadimethrine and, as a quaternary amine, is thought to interact with negatively charged sialic acid groups. Hence, polybrene appears to enhance agglutinability by cross-linking red cells via their glycophorins.

In the polybrene test, red cells are first incubated briefly with serum in a low-ionic medium; polybrene is then added and, after a brief incubation, centrifuged and the supernatant decanted. A resuspending solution composed of a mixture of dextrose and citrate (to neutralize excess polybrene) is then added, and the red cell pellet gently agitated and assessed for agglutination. Polybrene will have aggregated the red cells non-specifically; red cells coated with antibody will persist as agglutinates, whereas uncoated cells will readily disperse on agitation due to neutralization by citrate. Polybrene tests can subsequently be processed for an indirect antiglobulin test (IAT) if so desired (see below).

Polyethylene glycol is relatively easier to use than polybrene. A 20% solution of PEG (M_r 3350) in phosphate-buffered saline (PBS) is added to a red cell–serum mixture, which is then treated as for a standard IAT. It is essential to use anti-IgG as the AHG agent in PEG IAT in order to prevent false-positive results owing to non-specific binding of complement to the red cells. A few clinically significant antibodies that have caused red cell haemolysis (e.g. anti-Jk^a) were detected only by PEG IAT.

Inhibition of agglutination
Expected agglutination reactions with known antigens and antibodies can be neutralized by soluble antigens of the appropriate specificity. For example, the saliva of group A secretors inhibits the agglutination of group A cells by anti-A. Hydatid cyst fluid with P1P^K activity can be used to confirm the presence of anti-P1 in sera. Soluble antigens produced by recombinant DNA technology will become useful in reference laboratories as aids to sorting out complex serological problems.

Haemolysis
Red cell lysis indicates a positive antigen–antibody reaction mediated by complement-fixing antibodies. A pink or red coloured supernatant after settling or centrifugation of red cell–antibody mixtures is an indication of red cell lysis.

Absorption and elution tests
Specific antibodies can be removed from serum by absorption with red cells carrying the corresponding antigen. Bound antibodies can be subsequently recovered from the washed sensitized red cells by elution with heat treatment, freeze–thawing, low pH or chloroquine treatment.

Specialized methods
These include radiolabelling, flow cytometry and enzyme-linked immunosorbent assays (ELISAs) used for the estimation of the number of antigen sites on red cells and when more sensitive antiglobulin techniques are required. The essence of these approaches is the use of a labelled antiglobulin: for radiometric assays, ^{125}I is usually used to 'tag' the antiglobulin molecules; in flow cytometry, fluorescent anti-IgG is used (or antibodies can be directly coupled with a fluorescent dye); in the case of ELISA, enzymes are attached covalently (i.e. conjugated) to the antiglobulin.

The execution of these assays requires antibody-coated cells or particles to be incubated with the labelled antiglobulin reagent. After incubation, excess unbound antiglobulin is washed away and bound, labelled antiglobulin is then measured. For radiometric assays, this is achieved by simply counting radioactivity in a gamma counter. For flow cytometry, a cytofluorimeter is used to measure fluorescence of each cell. For ELISA tests, the bound enzyme conjugate is detected through the enzyme's ability to modify, and usually effect a colour change, in its substrate (Figure 14.6). The colour intensity of the modified substrate can then be measured with a spectrophotometer.

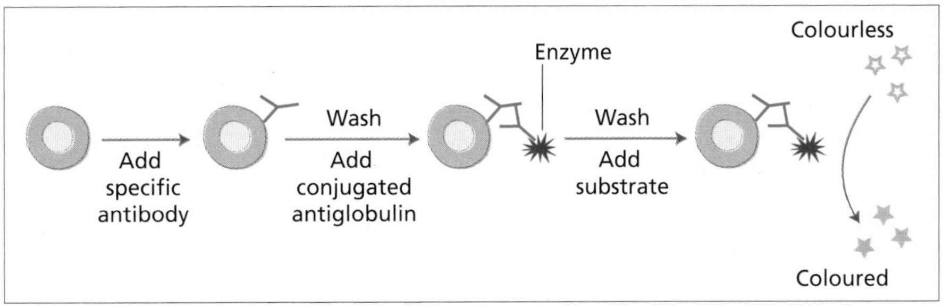

Figure 14.6 The enzyme-linked immunosorbent assay (ELISA) for cell-bound antibodies. Enzyme substrate is represented by open and closed stars, for colourless and coloured derivatives respectively.

Microcolumn tests (gel and beads)

The principle of microcolumn tests is the separation of agglutinated from non-agglutinated red cells by centrifugation through a miniature filtration column. For blood grouping, red cells are layered on microcolumns impregnated with blood grouping sera; for antibody screening and identification, phenotyped panel red cells are mixed with patients' sera within the incubation chamber of the microcolumn. After centrifugation, agglutinated red cells are retained towards the top of the microcolumn because the agglutinates are trapped by the column matrix, whereas unagglutinated red cells form a button at the bottom of the column.

Positive and negative results are discriminated by the appearance of cells trapped within the matrix or at the bottom of the microcolumn respectively. Antiglobulin tests can be accomplished by centrifuging the mixture of red cells and patient's serum through a column impregnated with anti-IgG or polyspecific AHG. Any red cells coated with IgG antibody will be agglutinated by the free anti-IgG in the matrix of the column, giving a positive result. No washing of sensitized cells is required as IgG in the serum does not penetrate the column and so does not neutralize the anti-IgG in the column. The advantages of microcolumn techniques are the ease of reading and reproducibility, and the fact that the tests can be stored for later examination or checking. In the Diamed ID system, Sephadex gels are used. The Ortho Biovue system uses glass beads rather than gels. Both systems can be automated and the agglutination results evaluated by image analysis.

Microplate techniques

Semi-automated blood grouping and antibody screening can be performed in microtitre plates, which can also be used for extended phenotyping of red cells, antibody identification and large-scale screening for rare red cells and antibodies. A single microplate is equivalent to 96 short test tubes and the same basic principles of discrete analysis of agglutination apply. The advantages of these techniques include enhanced sensitivity, speed of performance, reduced reagent requirements, simplicity and reduced requirements for laboratory space and expensive equipment. Several commercial microplate-based blood grouping systems are now available (e.g. IBG system). These incorporate the use of bar codes to identify samples, automated liquid handling of samples and reagents, and plate readers linked to computers for easy and accurate record-keeping.

Microplates containing red cells adhered to the surface of the plastic, solid-phase systems help to reduce the variability between tests that is inherent in liquid-phase systems when undertaken by different operators, and easily lend themselves to automated reading of results. Blood grouping (e.g. for ABO and D groups) by solid phase can be accomplished by the use of U-shaped microplate wells coated with the relevant antibody (e.g. anti-A, -B, -D); suspensions of patients' or donors' red cells are added to the wells and then centrifuged. Positive results appear as a carpet of cells coated over the bottom of the well. Negative results appear as a tight pinhead of unattached cells in the centre of the well.

Antibody screening and identification by a solid-phase technique can be achieved with microplates coated with a panel of phenotyped red cell ghosts, following chemical activation of the plastic. The wells are incubated with patient serum and LISS, washed and then anti-IgG is added. Anti-IgG will bind to those wells where the patient's IgG red cell antibody has bound to the relevant red cell ghost of the phenotyped panel; the presence of bound anti-IgG is then easily detected by adding indicator red cells coated with IgG (e.g. D+ cells coated with anti-D), followed by brief centrifugation, as described above.

Automated techniques

Fully automated blood grouping and antibody screening are carried out in transfusion centres where large numbers of donor samples are tested daily and increasingly in hospital transfusion laboratories using microcolumn techniques or microplates as described above. In automated systems such as the Olympus PK, test samples are mixed with typing sera and screening cells in individual wells of a special microplate, which are constructed to have a terraced surface at the bottom of the well. After incubation and settling of the red cells in the reaction mixtures, agglutination patterns are distinguished either on the basis of light transmission (model 7100) or through image analysis with the aid of a computer-controlled CCD camera (model 7200).

Other automated systems are available for use with microcolumns (e.g. Diamed's Gel-Station and Ortho AutoVue systems). These are fully automated, walk-away, systems using bar codes to identify both samples, reagents and test cards. Each has a pipetting (liquid handling) station, incubator, centrifuge and reader linked to a computer to maintain the identity of the sample being tested throughout the entire testing process. Similar walk-away systems are available for use with solid-phase microplate systems, e.g. Biotest's Tango, Immucor's Galileo.

In another automated system, reactions take place in small cuvettes and reactions are read by the principles of changes in light scatter properties utilized in aggregometry to detect agglutinates (e.g. Menarini Boss system).

A continuous flow analyser is commonly used for quantification of anti-D or -c, especially in antenatal serology, and for antibody detection. There are several different methods to quantify the anti-D concentration in samples from antenatal patients and immunized volunteers, as well as in plasma pools used for the manufacture of anti-D immunoglobulin.

Manual titration, the most common method, is simple, but provides only a fairly crude semi-quantitative estimate of the concentration of anti-D. Radioisotope methods give more accurate estimates and do not require standards, but their sensitivity is poor and they are too laborious for routine use.

Quantitative haemagglutination methods using continuous-flow automated analysers and appropriate anti-D/c international standards are sensitive (e.g. down to 0.02 IU anti-D/mL), relatively simple, objective, rapid, of acceptable reproducibility, and amenable to routine use and standardization. The method involves the agglutination of D+ red cells by the anti-D to be quantified, in the presence of an agglutination enhancer, while being pumped through a series of coils at set temperatures to allow the desired incubation of the segments of reactants. The agglutinates are sedimented and removed, whereas the remaining unagglutinated red cells are haemolysed by a detergent. The absorbance of the haemolysate is proportional to the amount of haemoglobin and is thus inversely proportional to the number of agglutinated cells removed. This reflects the antibody concentration, which can be calculated using the values obtained from the standard, run in parallel, in iu/mL.

Blood grouping reagents

To avoid potential fatalities due to errors in ABO and D grouping, it is essential that the chosen ABO typing reagents have suitable potency and comply with the European Directive on *in vitro* diagnostic devices and the associated Common Technical Specifications and carry the 'CE' mark to show they are in conformance.

Blood grouping reagents prepared from polyclonal antisera should be free of unwanted antibodies and should have been exhaustively tested with an extensive panel of cells to exclude common and rare specificities (e.g. anti-Bg (HLA), -Vw, -Wr^a), before they are issued for routine use. Unwanted contaminating antibodies are generally not a problem with monoclonal reagents as they have to be extensively tested before being placed on the market. Good IgM monoclonal reagents are now available for ABO, Rh and K typing.

Strict adherence to the manufacturer's instructions for each reagent is essential. Standard operating procedures should include writing out the worksheet prior to testing, labelling all tubes, microplates, or gels, recording results immediately after reading, repeating discrepancies and using adequate controls. Any other equipment used in an investigation (centrifuge, incubator) must be calibrated and in range at the time that the investigation is undertaken.

ABO grouping has an in-built control in the reverse grouping (serum check, see Chapter 15). However, controls for D typing must always be used in order to prevent a D-negative patient being mistyped as D-positive. At least two potent anti-D reagents should be used in Rh typing.

Antibody screening and identification

Patients' sera should be screened against unpooled group O cells from selected individuals known to carry the following antigens between them: D, C, E, c, e, M, N, S, s, P1, Le^a, Le^b, K, k, Fy^a, Fy^b,

Jk^a and Jk^b. Ideally, one cell sample should be R$_1$R$_1$ (DCe/DCe) and the other R$_2$R$_2$ (DcE/DcE), and a minimum homozygous expression of Fy^a and Jk^a should be present on one of the red cell samples. It is generally possible to meet these requirements with two cells but, if more antigens are required with homozygous expression, it might be necessary to use three cells.

The techniques employed for antibody screening need only include a well-controlled IAT, commonly now using microcolumn techniques. For antibody identification, a second sensitive technique, in addition to the IAT, such as the use of enzyme-treated cells, PEG or the manual polybrene tests, should be used. Saline tests are not essential and all incubations should be performed at 37°C; antibodies reacting at lower temperatures are of no clinical importance.

It is recommended that an autologous control be used by incubating the patient's serum with the patient's cells, by the methods used for antibody identification. All tests must follow a written standard operating procedure. Blood bankers should not forget that the main aim of blood group serology is to provide hazard-free transfusions.

Molecular techniques for blood grouping

Almost all the genes for human blood groups have now been cloned and the molecular bases for most of the blood group polymorphisms have been determined. Consequently, it is now possible to predict blood group phenotypes from DNA with a high degree of accuracy. The usual requirement for such tests is the determination of fetal blood groups. When a pregnant woman has a blood group antibody with the potential to cause haemolytic disease of the newborn (HDN, see Chapter 16) it is beneficial to be able to determine whether her fetus has the corresponding antigen and, consequently, whether it is at risk from HDN. Such tests usually involve D typing, but may also involve typing for c and K antigens, and, rarely, other blood group antigens. The usual source of fetal DNA is amniocytes, obtained by amniocentesis, an invasive procedure with a small risk of spontaneous abortion and a 20% risk of transplacental haemorrhage, which could boost the mother's antibody. Non-invasive tests for D are now being introduced, from 16 weeks' gestation onwards, in which fetal D type is predicted from the small quantity of free fetal DNA present in the maternal plasma.

The other use of molecular methods for blood grouping is for regularly transfused patients, where serological methods are not possible because of the presence of transfused red cells that are always present in the patient's blood. If genotypes can be determined for all clinically important blood group polymorphisms in transfusion-dependent patients then matched blood can be provided to prevent the patient from making multiple antibodies to blood group antigens. Tests are carried out on DNA that is isolated from whole blood from the transfused patient, and accurate results can be obtained despite the potential for contamination with DNA from the donors.

Five types of tests are commonly used in blood group genotyping, all involving the polymerase chain reaction (PCR).

1 Amplification of a portion of a blood group gene to determine whether it is present. This only applies to *RHD* of the Rh system. Presence of the amplified product is usually detected by gel electrophoresis, although monitoring of the amplification by the use of a fluorescent probe in a 'real-time' system is the usual method for detecting fetal *RHD* in maternal plasma.

2 Amplification of a portion of a gene followed by detection of the polymorphism with restriction endonucleases (see Chapter 15).

3 Selective amplification of a specific allele by the use of an allele-specific primer (see Chapter 15).

4 Amplification of a portion of a gene followed by direct sequence of the amplified product.

5 Allelic discrimination by real time quantitative PCR, in which relative quantities of a pair of alleles are measured.

It is unlikely that molecular genetics will be used for routine ABO and Rh typing of donors and patients, at least in the near future. However, there may be other roles for molecular blood grouping in the future. One such function could be genotyping large numbers of blood donors for multiple blood groups in order to establish a database of donors typed for all clinically significant blood groups. This would be valuable for the treatment of transfusion-dependent patients, as it would facilitate the provision of compatible blood for those patients who have made blood group antibodies and matched blood for those who have not. To perform such testing, high throughput methods will be required. Many techniques for detecting DNA polymorphisms are now available, and some are being developed for blood group testing.

Selected bibliography

General

Mollison PL, Engelfriet CP, Contreras M (1997) *Blood Transfusion in Clinical Medicine*, l0th edn. Blackwell Science, Oxford.

Immunology

Abbas AK, Lichtman AH, Pober IS (2000) *Cellular and Molecular Immunology*, 4th edn. Saunders, Philadelphia, PA.

Janeway CA, Travers P, Walport M *et al.* (2001) *Immunobiology*, 5th edn. Garland Publishing, New York.

Roitt IM, Brostoff J, Male, DK (2001) *Immunology*, 5th edn. Mosby, London.

Red cell membrane

Cartron JP, Ratinel C (1992) Human erythrocyte glycophorins: protein and gene structure analysis. *Transfusion Medicine Review* 6: 63–92.

Daniels G (1999) Functional aspects of red cell antigens. *Blood Review* 13: 14–35.

Daniels G (2002) *Human Blood Groups*, 2nd edn. Blackwell Science, Oxford.

Issitt PD, Anstee DJ (1998) *Applied Blood Group Serology*, 4th edn. Montgomery Scientific Publications, Durham, NC.

Antigen–antibody reactions

Bell CA (1982) *Seminar on Antigen–Antibody Reactions Revisited*. American Association of Blood Banks, Arlington VA.

International Forum (1995) What is the best technique for the detection of red cell alloantibodies? *Vox Sanguinis* 69: 292–300.

Knight RC, de Silva M (1996) New technologies for red cell serology. *Blood Reviews* 10: 101–10.

Sinor LT (1990) Advances in solid phase red cell adherence methods and transfusion serology. *Transfusion Medicine Review* 6: 26–31.

Blood grouping methods

American Association of Blood Banks (2002) *American Association of Blood Banks Technical Manual*, 14th edn. AABB, Bethesda, MD.

BCSH Blood Transfusion Task Force (1996) Guidelines for pretransfusion compatibility procedures in blood transfusion laboratories. *Transfusion Medicine* 6: 273–83.

Guidelines for the Blood Transfusion Services in the United Kingdom (2002) The Stationery Office, London (www.the-stationery-office.co.uk/nbs/rdbk(2001)/guidelines.htm).

van der Schoot CE, Tax GHM, Rijnders RJP, de Haas M, Christaens GCML (2003) Prenatal typing of Rh and Kell blood group antigens: the edge of a watershed. *Transfusion Medicine Review* 17: 32–44.

CHAPTER 15

Antigens in human blood

Marcela Contreras and Geoff Daniels

15

Introduction

The main topic of this chapter is red cell antigens and their antibodies. However, in human blood there are many other antigenic structures that stimulate the production of antibodies in recipients of blood transfusions. Leucocyte antibodies are an important cause of febrile transfusion reactions in patients who have had previous transfusions or pregnancies. Lymphocytotoxic antibodies and, rarely, platelet antibodies may be a cause of failure of the platelet count to rise after platelet transfusions. Thus, a description of granulocyte and platelet antigens and antibodies is also included. The HLA system is covered in Chapter 23. Antibodies against proteins present in plasma may lead to urticarial or anaphylactic transfusion reactions; these will be considered briefly.

Approximately 280 red cell antigens have now been recognized and authenticated by the International Society of Blood Transfusion; of these, 245 belong to one of 29 blood group systems (Table 15.1). Each system represents a single gene locus, or two or more very closely linked loci of homologous genes, and each system is genetically discrete from all the others. In addition, there are about 40 antigens that have not been included in systems. Most blood groups are inherited as mendelian characters, although environmental factors may occasionally affect blood group expression. The genes representing the 29 systems have been located on a specific chromosome (Table 15.1). All are autosomal except *XG* and *XK*, which are X-borne, and *MIC2*, which is on both the X and Y chromosomes. All the genes have been cloned, with the exception of *P1*.

Blood group antigens may be integral proteins or glycoproteins of the red cell membrane, or they may be membrane glycolipids. In proteins and glycoproteins blood group polymorphisms and variants may represent differences in the amino acid sequence (e.g. Rh and Kell antigens). In glycoproteins and glycolipids, the blood group activity may reside in the carbohydrate moiety and polymorphism is associated with difference in oligosaccharide sequence (e.g. ABO). In some glycoproteins, blood group polymorphism may be caused by amino acid substitutions, but antigen expression is also dependent on glycosylation of the polypeptide.

The ABO system

The clinical importance of a blood group system in blood transfusion lies in the frequency of its antibodies and in the possibility that such antibodies will destroy incompatible cells *in vivo*. The ABO system was the first to be recognized and remains the most important in transfusion and transplantation (histo-blood group system). The reason for this is that almost everybody over the age of about 6 months has clinically significant anti-A and/or

Table 15.1 Human blood group systems.

No.	Name	Symbol	No. of antigens	Gene name(s)	Chromosome
001	ABO	ABO	4	ABO	9
002	MNS	MNS	43	GYPA, GYPB, GYPE	4
003	P	P1	1	P1	22
004	Rh	RH	49	RHD, RHCE	1
005	Lutheran	LU	20	LU	19
006	Kell	KEL	25	KEL	7
007	Lewis	LE	6	FUT3	19
008	Duffy	FY	6	FY	1
009	Kidd	JK	3	SLC14A1	18
010	Diego	DI	21	SLC4AE1 (AE1)	17
011	Yt	YT	2	ACHE	7
012	Xg	XG	2	XG, MIC2	X/Y
013	Scianna	SC	5	SC	1
014	Dombrock	DO	5	DO	12
015	Colton	CO	3	AQP1	7
016	Landsteiner–Wiener	LW	3	LW	19
017	Chido–Rodgers	CH/RG	9	C4A, C4B	6
018	H	H	1	FUT1	19
019	Kx	XK	1	XK	X
020	Gerbich	GE	8	GYPC	2
021	Cromer	CROM	12	DAF	1
022	Knops	KN	8	CR1	1
023	Indian	IN	2	CD44	11
024	Ok	OK	1	CD147	19
025	Raph	RAPH	1	CD55	11
026	John Milton Hagen	JMH	1	SEMA7A	15
027	I	I	1	GCNT2	6
028	Globoside	GLOB	1	B3GALT3	3
029	Gill	GIL-	1	AQP3	9

anti-B in their serum if they lack the corresponding antigens on their red cells. Thus, if we consider the incidence of ABO blood groups in the UK (Table 15.2), transfusions given without regard to ABO groups would result in a major incompatibility (patient has the antibody and the antigen is in the transfused red cells) about once in every three cases.

The antigens of the ABO system

The vast majority of human bloods can be grouped into six main ABO phenotypes (Table 15.3), although several other rare weak variants can be distinguished serologically. The incidence of ABO groups varies very markedly in different parts of the world and in different races. Even in the UK, there is some variation between north and south, and cities in some areas with large immigrant populations will reflect racial differences. In such areas, the blood groups of the patient population do not reflect those of the predominantly white blood donors.

Table 15.2 Incidence of ABO groups in southern England.

Phenotype	Frequency (%)	
O	44.9	
A_1	30.8	41.1
A_2	10.3	
B	10.1	
A_1B	2.7	3.9
A_2B	1.2	

A_1 and A_2 subgroups

The distinction between the A_1 and A_2 subgroups is usually made by using anti-A_1, which will agglutinate A_1, but not A_2, red cells. Anti-A_1 can be obtained in several ways: (i) it can be made by absorbing anti-A (from group B people) with A_2 red cells; (ii)

Table 15.3 ABO grouping.

Agglutination of test cells with				Agglutination by test serum of			ABO group of test sample	Possible genotype
Anti-A	Anti-A$_1$	Anti-B	Anti-A,B*	A cells	B cells	O cells		
−	−	−	−	+	+	−	O	O/O
+	+	−	+†	−	+	−†	A$_1$	A^1/A^1, A^1/O, A^1/A^2
+	−	−	+	−/+‡	+	−	A$_2$	A^2/A^2, A^2/O
−	−	+	+	+	−	−	B	B/B, B/O
+	+	+	+	−	−	−†	A$_1$B	A^1/B
+	−	+	+	−/+‡	−	−	A$_2$B	A^2/B

*Anti-A,B (group O serum) is not generally used in routine laboratories.

†Some group A$_1$ and A$_1$B individuals may have weak anti-H in their plasma.

‡Serum from a proportion of A$_2$ (1–8%) and A$_2$B (22–35%) individuals will contain anti-A$_1$.

it is found in the serum of some A$_2$ and A$_2$B persons (Table 15.3); (iii) it can be made from a saline extract of the seeds of the hyacinth bean, *Dolichos biflorus*; and (iv) mouse monoclonal anti-A$_1$. Anti-A$_1$ is not used routinely as it is not necessary to distinguish group A$_1$ from group A$_2$ blood for most transfusion recipients. There is no specific antibody for A$_2$ red cells; if anti-A is absorbed with A$_1$ cells, all the antibody is removed. Group B serum can therefore be thought of as containing two antibodies: anti-A, which agglutinates both A$_1$ and A$_2$ red cells, and anti-A$_1$, which agglutinates only A$_1$ red cells. The anti-A component of group O serum also has both antibodies.

The presence of the A^2 allele in the presence of A^1 cannot be determined by serology. Among people who are genotypically *A/O* or *A/B*, approximately three possess the A^1 gene for every one who possesses A^2 (Table 15.2).

The difference between the A$_1$ and A$_2$ subgroups is partly quantitative: the red cells of A$_1$ and A$_1$B subjects have more A antigen sites than A$_2$ and A$_2$B subjects respectively (Table 15.4). There is also good evidence for a qualitative difference between A$_1$ and A$_2$. Relatively low abundance A-active oligosaccharide structures, called repetitive type 3A and type 4A (see p. 230) are present on A$_1$, but not A$_2$ red cells. This qualitative difference must be very subtle, because A$_2$ red cells can absorb all the anti-A from group B serum if the absorption is carried out at 0–4°C for sufficient time.

For practical purposes, A$_2$ can be regarded as a weaker form of A. Table 15.4 shows quantitative differences in the number of A antigen sites on A$_1$ and A$_2$ red cells. The table also shows that when both the A and B antigens are present, there are less sites for each than when either is present alone. The practical importance of this lies in the fact that the A antigen of A$_2$B red cells may give an extremely weak reaction with anti-A, which could be missed in routine grouping tests if reagents of inadequate potency are used. Moreover, if the same person's serum contains anti-A$_1$ and is tested in the reverse grouping only with A$_1$ and not A$_2$ red cells, they will be grouped as B. For this reason, potent anti-A reagents reacting with A$_2$B cells should be used in routine blood grouping.

The H antigen

Group O cells have no antigens in the ABO system (Table 15.3). However, they do possess H antigen, the precursor upon which the products of the *ABO* genes act. The H gene (called *FUT1*) segregates independently from *ABO* and is on a different chromosome: *ABO* on chromosome 9, *FUT1* on chromosome 19. The H antigen is present to some extent on almost all red cells, regardless of the ABO group, but the amount of H antigen varies with the ABO group as follows: O > A$_2$ > A$_2$B > B > A$_1$ > A$_1$B.

Individuals with the rare Bombay phenotype are homozygous for inactive H genes (*h/h*). Their red cells are not agglutinated by anti-A or -B, regardless of *ABO* genotype, but are not group O as they are also not agglutinated by anti-H. The serum of Bombay subjects contains anti-H, anti-A and/or anti-B. Parents and offspring of Bombay individuals, who are heterozygous for the

Table 15.4 Numbers of A and B antigen sites on red cells of various ABO groups.

Blood group of red cell	Approx. no. of A antigen sites	Approx. no. of B antigen sites
A$_1$ adult	1 000 000	−
A$_1$ cord	300 000	−
A$_1$B adult	500 000	−
A$_1$B cord	220 000	−
A$_2$ adult	250 000	−
A$_2$ cord	140 000	−
A$_2$B adult	120 000	400 000
B adult	−	700 000

inactive H allele (*H/h*), have H and red cells of normal ABO phenotype.

Development of the A, B and H antigens

The A and B antigens can be detected on the red cells of very young fetuses, but their reactions are weaker than those of adults. Table 15.4 shows that there are fewer A and B antigen sites on cord than on adult red cells. Similarly, the H antigen is less well developed at birth than in adult life. After birth, the expression of the A, B and H antigens increases until about 3 years of age, and thereafter, in health, remains stable throughout life.

Distribution of the A, B and H antigens

ABH antigens are often referred to as histo-blood group antigens because they are widely distributed in the body. They are therefore very important in transplantation. They are present on white cells, platelets and epidermal and other tissue cells. They are also present in an alcohol-soluble form in the plasma of people of suitable ABO groups, whether they are secretors or non-secretors of A, B or H, and in the saliva and other secretions of ABH secretors (see later).

Rare ABO variants

Rare ABO variants are usually disclosed because an expected ABO antibody is missing. A sample typed as group O that has anti-B but no anti-A will usually prove to be a weak A variant. The presence of weak A or B antigens can be demonstrated either by using potent antisera or by absorption and elution.

Rare ABO variants can arise from:

1 *Rare* ABO *genes*. These include A_3, A_x, A_{end}, A_m and A_{el} variants. All are extremely rare and are usually recognized by their variable reactions with anti-A and/or anti-A,B sera. Similarly, subgroups of B have been described; all are very rare.
2 *Genes segregating independently of* ABO. These rare variants are the H-deficiency or Bombay phenotypes described on p. 231.
3 *Environmental effects*. Weakening of the A antigen can occur in various types of leukaemia (usually acute myeloid). The A antigen may revert to almost normal in remission. Similar weakening of B, H, I and RhD has been described. B-like antigens may be acquired by group A individuals who are suffering from bowel infections, usually associated with carcinoma or strictures of the large bowel. Red cells with an acquired B antigen are agglutinated by some anti-B, including some monoclonal anti-B, but not by the patient's own anti-B. Bacterial deacetylases convert *N*-acetylgalactosamine, the immunodominant sugar of the A antigen, into galactosamine, a structure similar to galactose, the immunodominant sugar of the B antigen (see p. 230). In some cases, acquired B may also be associated with polyagglutination (see p. 243).

Antibodies of the ABO system

Anti-A, -B and -A,B

Sera taken from people over the age of about 6 months which do not contain the expected A and B antibodies (Table 15.3) are very rare. They should always be investigated thoroughly; often, some interesting explanation will be found, for example a rare subgroup of A, a blood group chimera or congenital absence of IgM.

It is likely that ABO antibodies arise in response to A- and B-like antigens present on bacterial, viral or animal molecules. Titres of ABO antibodies vary considerably with age, reaching a peak in young adults and then declining in old age. Titres vary depending on the techniques used; normal adult sera can have anti-A titres, by direct agglutination in saline medium, in the range 16–1024 and anti-B titres in the range 4–256, but most have saline titres below 100. The anti-A and anti-B titres of group O subjects are much higher than in group B or A subjects respectively.

Naturally occurring anti-A and -B are antibodies that react better at lower temperatures than at 37°C. The antibodies always have some IgM component and, in group A and B persons, they are almost entirely IgM. However, the antibodies from group O individuals, even before immunization, usually have some IgG anti-A,B, an antibody that cross-reacts with both A and B structures.

Immune anti-A and -B can be produced by persons of the appropriate ABO group after immunization with red cells or blood group substances. Immune anti-A and anti-B can also arise after various vaccinations and inoculations for the prophylaxis of infections. Here, the A-like antigens come from the hog pepsin digest used in their preparation.

Following immunization, the thermal characteristics of the antibodies change, but group A and B subjects continue to produce antibodies that are mainly IgM. Most group O persons, however, will produce IgG as readily as IgM anti-A,B. This correlates with the fact that mothers of children with ABO haemolytic disease of the newborn (HDN) are almost always group O. Immune anti-A,B are mainly IgG2, which does not cause HDN because there are no Fc receptors for IgG2 on the cells of the mononuclear phagocyte system. When the maternal serum contains potent IgG1 and/or IgG3 ABO antibodies, HDN may occur, although this is usually mild compared with Rh HDN. Some IgA anti-A or -B is produced following immunization with A or B substances. Some differences in the serological properties of immune and naturally occurring anti-A and -B are shown in Table 15.5, which also gives an indication to ways of detecting IgG anti-A or -B in the presence of IgM anti-A or -B, which has relevance to ABO HDN, as discussed in Chapter 17.

Dangerous 'universal' donors

Good practice in pretransfusion testing requires compatibility testing, which consists of incubating the patient's serum with the

Table 15.5 Some properties of immune and naturally occurring anti-A and -B.

	Naturally occurring IgM	Immune IgM	IgG
Complement binding (at 37°C)	++/+++	+++	++
Agglutination of appropriate cells	+++	+++	+++
Cross the placenta	−	−	+++
Enhanced by anti-IgG	−	−	+++
Inhibited by soluble A or B substances (e.g. saliva)	+++	+++	−*
2-ME or DTT sensitive	+++	+++	−

*IgG ABO antibodies are usually inhibited only by large amounts of specific substance.
2-ME, 2-mercaptoethanol; DTT, dithiothreitol.

donors' red cells. Group O red cells can be given to A, B or AB recipients and group O donors were formerly, inappropriately called 'universal donors'. Group O donors have anti-A, -B and -A,B in their plasma, which will react with the recipient's A or B cells. Normally, if group A, B or AB recipients are transfused with a relatively small number of group O units of whole blood, the anti-A or -B that is transfused will be diluted out and neutralized by the plasma of the adult recipient, especially if plasma-reduced blood is used. However, if the transfused units contain potent immune haemolytic antibodies, this neutralization and dilution effect may be insufficient and the antibodies may cause a marked destruction of the A or B red cells of the recipient, leading to a severe acute haemolytic transfusion reaction (HTR). For this reason, the practice of transfusing group O blood to non-O recipients should be strongly discouraged.

Moreover, there is usually a shortage of group O blood, and not infrequently a surplus of group A blood. In the vast majority of cases, including emergencies, there is enough time to perform a rapid ABO group on the patient's cells, which will allow the transfusion of group-specific blood. If there is no time to do an ABO group before transfusion, red cells in optimal additive solution, devoid of plasma, should be given until the patient's blood group is known. The practice of transfusing group O platelets to non-O patients should be discouraged, as the dose of adult platelets will contain at least 300 mL of plasma, unless part of it has been replaced by platelet-additive solution. Group O fresh-frozen plasma (FFP) and cyroprecipitate should only be given to group O recipients. This matter is discussed again in Chapter 17.

Anti-A$_1$

Anti-A$_1$, reactive at room temperature (18–22°C), can be found in the serum of 1–8% of group A$_2$ and 22–35% of group A$_2$B persons. Most of these antibodies are more of a nuisance in compatibility tests than of clinical importance because they often do not agglutinate A$_1$ red cells at 30°C and above, and so are unable to cause increased *in vivo* red cell destruction. Very rarely, anti-A$_1$ able to agglutinate A$_1$ red cells at 37°C may lead to significant

destruction of A$_1$ red cells *in vivo*. The appropriate group A$_2$ or A$_2$B red cells should be cross-matched in these rare instances.

Anti-H

Several forms of anti-H exist.

1 *Clinically significant 'true' anti-H* occurs in the serum of persons with Bombay phenotype and is very rare. When it does occur, it is very important from the point of view of selecting blood for transfusion; as the antibody is active at 37°C, only Bombay phenotype blood may be transfused.

2 *Anti-H and anti-HI*, commonly found in the serum of group A$_1$, B and A$_1$B persons, react much more strongly with adult than with cord red cells. Anti-H is inhibited by secretor saliva; anti-HI is not. Although these antibodies agglutinate O red cells at 20°C, they do not usually agglutinate them at temperatures above 30°C. Very occasionally, anti-H/-HI may cause rapid destruction of at least some of the transfused O red cells *in vivo*. However, these antibodies will not interfere with the survival of transfused cells if ABO identical units, i.e. A$_1$, B or A$_1$B donor units are chosen for A$_1$, B or A$_1$B recipients respectively.

ABH secretor status

About 80% of the UK population are ABH secretors as they have H antigen, plus A or B according to their ABO genotype, in a water-soluble form in their body secretions. The remaining 20% are non-secretors and have no secreted ABH antigens, regardless of ABO genotype.

Biochemistry and biosynthesis of ABH antigens

ABH antigens

A, B and H antigens on red cells are predominantly glycoproteins, the majority being on the N-glycans of the anion exchanger (band 3) and the glucose transporter. ABH antigens on red cells are also expressed on glycosphingolipids, which include paraglobosides (Table 15.6). Soluble ABH antigens are

Table 15.6 Some glycolipids of the red cell surface expressing H, A, B, P1, P^K, P and LKE activity.

Structure	Antigen	Name
Paragloboside series		
Galβ1→4GlcNAcβ1→3Galβ1→4Glc–Cer	–	Paragloboside
Fucα1→2Galβ1→4GlcNAcβ1→3Galβ1→4Glc–Cer	Type 2 H	
Fucα1→2Galβ1→4GlcNAcβ1→3Galβ1→4Glc–Cer 3 ↑ 1 GalNAc	Type 2 A	
Fucα1→2Galβ1→4GlcNAcβ1→3Galβ1→4Glc–Cer 3 ↑ 1 Gal	Type 2 B	
Galα1→4Galβ1→4GlcNAcβ1→3Galβ1→4Glc–Cer	P1	
Globoside series		
Galβ1→4Glc–Cer	–	Lactosylceramide, Gb2
Galα1→4Galβ1→4Glc–Cer	P^K	Globotriosylceramide, Gb3
GalNAcβ1→3Galα1→4Galβ1→4Glc–Cer	P	Globoside, Gb4
NeuAcα2→3Galβ1→3GalNAcβ1→3Galα1→4Galβ1→4Glc–Cer	LKE	Sialosylgalactosylgloboside
Fucα1→2Galβ1→3GalNAcβ1→3Galα1→4Galβ1→4Glc–Cer	Type 4 H	Globo-H

Cer, ceramide; Fuc, fucose; Gal, galactose; GalNAc, *N*-acetylgalactosamine; Glc, glucose; GlcNAc, *N*-acetylglucosamine.

glycoproteins. Differences in the terminal sugars of the glycoproteins and glycolipids determine the specificity of these antigens: L-fucose (Fuc) for H; L-fucose + *N*-acetyl-D-galactosamine (GalNAc) for A; and L-fucose + D-galactose (Gal) for B.

Two major types of carbohydrate chain endings serve as acceptors for the fucosyltransferases that synthesize H antigen. Type 1 and type 2 chains have Gal joined to *N*-acetylglucosamine (GlcNAc) through 1→3 and 1→4 linkages respectively. A- and B-transferases synthesize the transfer of Ga1NAc

and Gal, respectively, from their donor substrates UDP-GalNAc and UDP-Gal, to the terminal galactosyl residue of type IH and type 2H, creating A and B epitopes and masking H specificity (Figure 15.1).

Secretory glycoproteins possess both type 1 and type 2 linkages, whereas red cells synthesize type 2 chains only. Plasma glycolipids, passively adsorbed onto the red cells have only type 1 chains; these also carry Lewis antigens (see p. 231). Other chains, called type 3 and 4, are also present in low numbers on

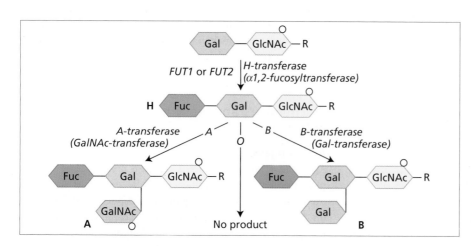

Figure 15.1 Biosynthetic pathway of H antigen from its precursor, and of A and B antigens from H. H remains unconverted in the absence of *A* or *B* gene products. R, remainder of molecule.

red cells, but probably only on glycolipids. Type 3, 4 and 6 chains are found in heart and kidney tissues, and may be target epitopes for the rejection of transplanted organs.

ABO genes

The *ABO* gene is located on the long arm of chromosome 9, comprises seven exons and encodes proteins with a structure characteristic of glycosyltransferases. Products of the *A* and *B* alleles differ by four amino acids encoded by exon 7, two of which determine whether the enzyme product has GalNAc-transferase (A) or Gal-transferase (B) activity.

The majority of *O* alleles (called O^1) resemble *A*, but have a single base deletion in exon 6, which creates a shift in the reading frame and scrambles the amino acid sequence after the first quarter of the transferase polypeptide; introduction of a premature stop codon truncates any putative polypeptide. About 3% of *O* alleles (called O^2) have a single nucleotide polymorphism (SNP) that changes one of the vital amino acids in the catalytic site, inactivating the enzyme.

The A^2 allele has a single base deletion immediately before the usual termination codon, creating a reading frameshift and abolition of this stop codon. This creates an A-transferase with an extraneous 21 amino acids on its C-terminus, which accounts for its reduced efficiency as a GalNAc-transferase. A^1, A^2, B, O^1 and O^2 genotypes can be identified by polymerase chain reaction (PCR) with allele-specific primers or followed by analysis with restriction enzymes.

Gene sequences for many variants of *A*, *B*, and *O* alleles have been determined and, in most cases, there is heterogeneity, with more than one mutation accounting for the same phenotype.

H genes

At least two genes, *FUT1* and *FUT2*, are responsible for production of H antigen. Both encode α1,2-fucosyltransferases that catalyse the transfer of fucose to the terminal galactose residue of the H precursor chain (Figure 15.1). *FUT1* is active in mesodermally derived tissues, including haemopoietic tissues, and is responsible for H expression on red cells. Homozygosity for inactivating mutations in *FUT1* gives rise to Bombay and related phenotypes. *FUT2* is responsible for the expression of H antigen in endodermally derived tissues, including those responsible for secretions, and hence is the gene responsible for ABH secretion. Secretors are homozygous or heterozygous for an active allele (*Se*) at *FUT2*; non-secretors are homozygous for an inactive allele (*se*).

The Lewis system

Antigens of the Lewis system and their biosynthesis

The Lewis system differs from all other blood group systems in that it is primarily a system of soluble antigens present in secre-

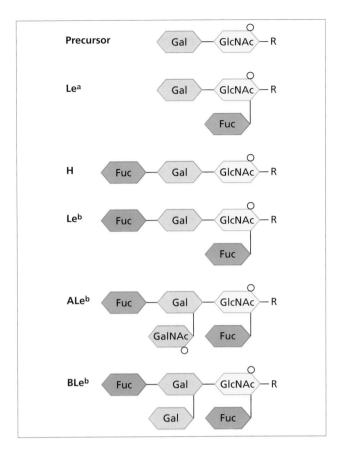

Figure 15.2 Diagrammatic representation of H and Lewis antigens. Le^a requires the action of the Lewis α1,4-fucosyltransferase, H the action of the H α1,2-fucosyltransferase, Le^b the action of both Lewis and H fucosyltransferases, and ALe^b and BLe^b the action of Lewis and H fucosyltransferases and the A or B glycosyltransferases.

tions and in plasma. The Lewis antigens on red cells are adsorbed passively from the plasma, and the constant presence of plasma is needed to maintain Lewis antigen on the red cells. There are two basic Lewis antigens; Le^a and Le^b. Expression of either requires the presence of an active Lewis gene, but Lewis phenotypes are also governed by the gene controlling H secretion (*FUT2*). Lewis antigens in saliva and plasma are glycoproteins and glycolipids respectively.

The Lewis gene, *FUT3*, encodes an α1,4-fucosyltransferase that catalyses the addition of L-fucose in 1→4 linkage to the subterminal *N*-acetylglucosamine of type 1 chains (Figure 15.2). If the type 1 core structure has been unmodified, Le^a antigen is produced. If the secretor α1,2-fucosyltransferase has already modified the type 1 chains to produce type 1H, the action of the Le-transferase leads to the formation of Le^b. In a white population, 75% have active Lewis and secretor genes and hence, Le(a−b+) red cells, 20% have an active Lewis gene, but are H non-secretors and have Le(a+b−) red cells, and 5% are homozygous for Lewis genes with inactivating mutations and are

Table 15.7 The Lewis system and secretion of ABH.

Genotype		Antigens in Saliva			Plasma/red cells*	
FUT2 (Secretor)	FUT3 (Lewis)	Le^a	Le^b	ABH	Le^a	Le^b
Se/Se, Se/Se^w or Se/se	Le/Le or Le/le	+	++	++	w/−	++
Se/Se, Se/Se^w or Se/se	le/le	−	−	++	−	−
Se^w/Se^w or Se^w/se	Le/Le or Le/le	++	++	++	++	++
Se^w/Se^w or Se^w/se	le/le	−	−	++	−	−
se/se	Le/Le or Le/le	+++	−	−	++	−
se/se	le/le	−	−	−	−	−

*Le^a and Le^b on red cells are passively adsorbed from plasma.

Le, active allele at FUT3 locus; le, inactive allele; Se, active allele at FUT2 locus; Se^w, weakly active allele; se, inactive allele; w, weak.

Le(a−b−) (Table 15.7). In Oriental populations there is a low incidence of non-secretors, but a high incidence of a weak secretor allele of FUT2. Competition between the Lewis and weak-secretor transferases leads to the Le(a+b+) red cell phenotype.

Adsorption of the Lewis substances by red cells

Le(a+b−) and Le(a−b+) red cells incubated in Le(a−b−) plasma lose their Lewis antigens into the plasma. Similarly, if Le(a+b−) or Le(a−b+) red cells are transfused to an Le(a−b−) person, the transfused cells will gradually lose the Le^a or Le^b antigens and will group as Le(a−b−) within 1 week of transfusion. So, if the patient has anti-Le^a or -Le^b, the red cells that were not destroyed in the first few days, will not be haemolysed once they become Le(a−b−).

Development of Lewis antigens on red cells

The Lewis antigens are poorly developed at birth and red cells from cord blood are usually Le(a−b−). Thereafter, Le^a develops first, followed by Le^b if the relevant Lewis and secretor genes are present. The cells of children between the ages of 6 months to 4 years often type as Le(a+b+) if they are destined to become Le(a−b+). The definitive adult Lewis phenotype may not be reached until the age of 4–5 years.

Antibodies of the Lewis system

Lewis antibodies are generally made only by individuals with the Le(a−b−) red cell phenotype. Anti-Le^a occurs fairly frequently. As only 5% of the UK population are Le(a−b−), approximately 20% of individuals potentially able to make anti-Le^a appear to make the antibody. The incidence of Le(a−b−) is much higher in people of African origin and Lewis antibodies detectable at 22°C or above may be found in up to 10% of random serum samples from black people.

Anti-Le^b commonly accompanies anti-Le^a. Pure anti-Le^b is uncommon and is made by people who are non-secretors and whose red cells are Le(a−b−). Very rarely, anti-Le^b can be made by Le(a+b−) individuals.

Serological characteristics of Lewis antibodies

Lewis antibodies are predominantly IgM, even after deliberate stimulation. They usually agglutinate the appropriate cells at 20°C. All Lewis antibodies bind complement and may lyse the appropriate cells. Usually, Lewis antibodies do not agglutinate red cells in saline at 37°C, but can be detected with anticomplement in an indirect antiglobulin test (IAT).

Clinical significance of Lewis antibodies

Some patients may have Lewis antibodies reacting at 37°C. Anti-Le^a is usually more haemolytic than anti-Le^b, and there are some anti-Le^{a+b} that can be very potent, leading to increased intravascular red cell destruction in the initial stages of transfusion. However, all Lewis antibodies lead to two-component survival curves of transfused incompatible red cells; i.e. the first cells are destroyed at an accelerated rate and the remainder will have a normal survival. The red cells that survive normally have been stripped of their adsorbed Lewis antigens and have become Le(a−b−), the same as the recipient.

It is therefore recommended that, for patients with Lewis antibodies reacting at 37°C, ABO identical red cells compatible in an IAT cross-match at 37°C should be transfused. It is important to choose ABO identical cells as group A, B and AB cells carry less Lewis antigens than any group O cell routinely used in antibody screening. This is because the A and B transferases compete with the Lewis transferase for the same precursor substrate. The provision of pre-typed Le(a−b−) blood for patients with Lewis antibodies is not necessary, as it is always easy to find cross match-compatible red cells at 37°C.

Lewis antibodies do not cause HDN as they are almost always IgM and newborn infants have Le(a−b−) red cells.

P blood groups

P1 was discovered by Landsteiner and Levine, who used suitably absorbed sera of rabbits injected with human red cells.

About 75% of subjects tested were positive for P1, which is inherited as a mendelian dominant character. P1 frequency varies in different populations and the P1-negative phenotype is called P_2. P1 is weakly expressed at birth and its strength varies considerably in adults. For this reason, identification of anti-P1 can be difficult, as panel cells will have varying expression of the antigen.

Anti-P1 is a naturally occurring antibody commonly found in the serum of P_2 individuals. Unlike anti-A and -B, anti-P1 rarely causes transfusion reactions because it is usually a cold-reacting IgM antibody, often not reactive above 30°C. Potent anti-P1 can be found in patients with hydatid disease and can be inhibited by hydatid cyst fluid.

P1 is a structure in the paragloboside series of glycolipids. The *P1* gene is probably an $\alpha1,4$-galactosyltransferase that adds galactose to the P1-precursor, paragloboside, although the biosynthetic pathway has not been fully elucidated (see Table 15.6). A precursor of paragloboside is lactosylceramide, which is converted to the P^K antigen by $\alpha1,4$-galactosyltransferase-1. In most people, almost all P^K is further converted to P antigen (globoside) by $\beta1,3$-*N*-acetylgalactosaminyltransferase-1. The very rare p phenotype results from deficiency of $\alpha1,4$-galactosyltransferase-1 and leads not only to absence of P^K and P, but also P1, giving rise to suggestions that $\alpha1,4$-galactosyltransferase-1 might also be the enzyme responsible for P1 synthesis. Deficiency of $\beta1,3$-*N*-acetylgalactosaminyltransferase-1 causes the P^K phenotype, in which the red cells express P^K antigen strongly, but no P (globoside). P^K red cells may be P_1 or P_2.

Anti-PP1P^K and anti-P invariably occur in the sera of the very rare individuals with p and P^K phenotypes respectively. Anti-PP1P^K react with all red cells except those of the p phenotype; anti-P react with all red cells except those of the P^K and p phenotypes. They are usually strong IgM antibodies, are often lytic at 37°C, and can cause severe transfusion reactions if incompatible red cells are transfused. Occasionally, IgG anti-P or anti-PPl P^K are found and have been associated with spontaneous early abortion. The biphasic Donath–Landsteiner antibody is found in the sera of patients suffering from paroxysmal cold haemoglobinuria. It is always IgG, usually has anti-P specificity and is an autoantibody.

I and i antigens

The antigens I and i are not controlled by allelic genes: i is the biosynthetic precursor of I. I and i antigens are carbohydrates and are on the interior structures of the complex oligosaccharides that carry ABO, H and Lewis antigens. The i antigen represents linear structures that are converted to I-active branched structures by the product of the I gene (*GCNT2*), a $\beta1,6$-*N*-acetylglucosaminyltransferase. This enzyme is not active in newborn infants. Consequently, red cells of most adults are agglutinated strongly by anti-I and only weakly by anti-i, whereas red cells from cord blood give the opposite result. The agglutinability of an infant's red cells with anti-I increases, and with anti-i decreases, with maturity; at about 18 months of age the red cells give the reactions of adult cells. Adults who are homozygous for rare inactivating mutations in *GCNT2* have the adult i phenotype; their red cells react weakly with anti-I and strongly with anti-i, and their serum contains anti-I.

In haematological disorders such as thalassaemia, megaloblastic anaemia, sideroblastic anaemia, hereditary spherocytosis, paroxysmal nocturnal haemoglobinuria and some aplastic and dyserythropoietic anaemias, agglutinability by anti-i is increased without a reciprocal decrease in the agglutinability by anti-I.

Anti-I

Autoanti-I that agglutinates the patient's own and other adult ABO-compatible red cells at 20°C, but not at 30°C, occurs in a variety of disorders and after blood transfusions. These patients' red cells give a negative direct antiglobulin test. A transient increase in strength, titre and thermal range of anti-I regularly occurs after infections with *Mycoplasma pneumoniae* and occasionally leads to acute haemolysis; red cells of such patients give a positive direct antiglobulin test, as do those of patients suffering from chronic cold haemagglutinin disease (CHAD). In CHAD, the autoantibody is nearly always monoclonal and usually has anti-I specificity. All anti-I in CHAD are IgM and complement binding.

Anti-i

Autoanti-i is found transitorily in many patients suffering from infectious mononucleosis. Very occasionally, the titre and thermal range of this antibody may lead to acute haemolysis, particularly if the patient's red cells are more agglutinable than normal with anti-i. Red cells of these patients give a positive direct antiglobulin test.

Autoanti-i may occasionally be the antibody specificity in chronic CHAD. Such patients often have an underlying lymphoma.

The Rh system

The Rh blood group system, the fourth system to be discovered, is the second most important in blood transfusion. This is not because Rh antibodies are usually present when the Rh antigen is absent, but because anti-RhD is formed readily when RhD-positive blood is transfused to an RhD-negative person. Moreover, as these immune antibodies are normally IgG, they are able to cross the placenta and cause HDN. The Rh system now contains a total of 49 antigens, but D (RH1), because of its high immunogenicity, is by far the most important. This is due to the ability of anti-D to cause severe HDN and HTRs.

The Rh antigens

The D antigen (RH1)

In 1939, Levine and Stetson reported that a patient, who had delivered a stillborn infant and then suffered a severe reaction to transfusion of her husband's blood, had an antibody that agglutinated the red cells of 85% of ABO-compatible donors. In 1940, Landsteiner and Wiener found that guinea pigs and rabbits injected with rhesus monkey red cells made an antibody that not only agglutinated rhesus monkey red cells, but also the red cells of 85% of people of European origin. The human and animal antibodies were originally thought to be the same, and the human antibody was called anti-Rhesus.

Many years later, it was realized that the human antibody (now called anti-D of the Rh system) does not identify the same antigen as the rabbit and guinea pig rhesus antibody, the error arising out of a phenotypic association between the antigens. As it was now too late to change the name of the whole system, Levine suggested that the antigen defined by the original rhesus antibody should be called LW in honour of Landsteiner and Wiener. The blood group system originally identified by the human antibody is now called the Rh system.

For clinical purposes, individuals can be classified as Rh-positive (have the D antigen) and Rh-negative (lack the D antigen).

The expansion to include C, E, c and e (RH2 to RH5)

By the end of 1943, four antisera detecting genetically related antigens were available to Fisher and Race, who noticed that two of them appeared to give antithetical results. They proposed that the antigens recognized by these two antisera were allelic and called them C and c. They gave further letters, D (the original Rh antigen) and E, to the antigens recognized by the other two antisera and postulated that each had an alternative, which they called d and e. Anti-e was found in 1945. Anti-d has never been found as no d antigen exists. Fisher and Race proposed that the Rh antigens were controlled by three closely linked genes, giving rise to eight gene complexes or haplotypes: *CDe*, *cDE*, *cDe*, *CDE*, *cde*, *Cde*, *cdE* and *CdE*. At about the same time, Wiener proposed that there was only one Rh gene, controlling a number of blood factors, equivalent to C, c, D, E and e.

Molecular genetics has shown that there are two Rh genes, one encoding D, the other encoding the Cc and Ee antigens. However, as the Cc and Ee polymorphisms are determined by separate regions of a single gene, the CDE terminology of Fisher and Race is still suitable for understanding Rh at most levels (although the Wiener terminology is often used as a shorthand – Table 15.8). The approximate frequencies of the Rh gene complexes in three populations are shown in Table 15.8. In a white population, the first three complexes form 94% of the total and combinations of these three will give the most common genotypes (Table 15.9). Genotype frequencies vary considerably in different parts of the world. For instance, *dce/dce* varies from about 35% in Basques to 0.3% in Japanese and Chinese.

Numerous variants of e are known, generally found only in people of African origin.

Probable Rh genotype

When a person's Rh phenotype is known, the probable genotype can be discerned and its likelihood calculated from known genotype frequencies within the same population. In people of white European origin, the phenotype is usually determined initially with anti-D, -C, -c and -E. If there is no agglutination with anti-E, homozygosity for *e* is assumed. If there is agglutination with anti-E, anti-e is used to distinguish between *E/E* and *E/e*. Phenotype determinations and the genotypes that they most commonly represent are shown in Table 15.10. When probable genotype determinations are carried out, it is very important that the ethnic origin of the person is known; figures for one population will not apply to people of other populations. For example, in Caucasian populations, *dce* is 15 times more common than *Dce*, whereas in African populations *Dce* has a

Table 15.8 Eight Rh haplotypes and their frequencies in English, Nigerian and Hong Kong Chinese populations.

Haplotype			Frequencies (%)		
CDE	Rh-Hr	Numerical	English	Nigerian	Chinese
DCe	R^1	RH 1,2,–3,–4,5	42	6	73
dce	r	RH –1,–2,–3,4,5	39	20	2
DcE	R^2	RH 1,–2,3,4,–5	14	12	19
Dce	R^0	RH 1,–2,–3,4,5	3	59	3
dcE	r″	RH –1,–2,3,4,–5	1	Very rare	Very rare
dCe	r′	RH –1,2,–3,–4,5	1	3	2
DCE	R^z	RH 1,2,3,–4,–5	Rare	Very rare	Rare
dCE	r^y	RH –1,2,3,–4,–5	Very rare	Very rare	Rare

Results of testing with anti-D, -C, -c, -E and -e, red cells from 2000 English donors, 274 Yoruba of Nigeria and 4648 Cantonese from Hong Kong.

Table 15.9 The most common Rh genotypes in the UK population.

Genotype		Frequency (%)
DCe/dce	R^1r	31
DCe/DCe	R^1R^1	16
dce/dce	rr	15
DCe/DcE	R^1R^2	13
DcE/dce	R^2r	13
DcE/DcE	R^2R^2	3

slightly higher frequency than *dce*. Consequently, the phenotype D+C+c+E−e+ represents a probable genotype of DCe/dce in a white person, but of DCe/Dce in a black person.

Variations in antigen strength and site density with phenotype

Red cells of a person who is homozygous for the allele producing a red cell antigen will often react more strongly with the appropriate antisera than red cells of a person who is heterozygous at the same locus. For example, red cells of persons who are homozygous for the gene producing the C antigen (i.e. genotypically *C/C*), give stronger reactions with anti-C than the red cells of persons who are heterozygous for the same gene (*C/c*). Similarly, this dosage effect occurs with the c, E and e antigens, but is not clearly apparent for D. Table 15.10 shows the number of D antigen sites on red cells of different phenotypes as estimated by the use of ^{125}I-labelled anti-IgG to quantify bound IgG

anti-D. D antigen expression is affected by the presence of other Rh antigens on the red cells. The *DcE* haplotype produces high levels of D expression and, for reasons still to be explained, *C* causes depression of D antigen produced by the Rh haplotype on the opposite chromosome.

Molecular genetics of Rh

Rh genes and proteins

Rh antigens are encoded by two, closely linked genes, with 92% homology. *RHD* encodes the D antigen and *RHCE* encodes the Cc and Ee antigens. Each consists of 10 exons and, unusually for homologous genes, the two genes are in opposite conformation on the chromosome (Figure 15.3). The two genes are separated by an unrelated gene, *SMP1*. Each gene encodes a 416-amino-acid polypeptide (M_r 30–32 kDa), which is palmitoylated but not glycosylated. The polypeptides encoded by *RHD* and *RHCE* differ by 31–35 amino acids, depending on the *RHCE* genotype.

There is substantial evidence that the Rh polypeptides traverse the lipid bilayer 12 times, with both termini in the cytoplasm and six extracellular loops that provide the putative sites for antigenic activity (Figure 15.3). Rh antigen activity is very dependent on the conformation of the proteins within the membrane and may involve interactions between two or more of the extracellular loops. Removal of the proteins from the membrane generally ablates all antigenic activity.

D, C/c and E/e polymorphisms

In white people, the D-negative phenotype results from homozygosity for a complete deletion of the *RHD* gene. Consequently,

Table 15.10 Determining probable Rh genotype in the UK population and the number of D antigen sites on red cells of those phenotypes.

Reactions with anti-					Common genotypes	Genotype incidence (%) for each phenotype		No. of D antigen sites
D	C	c	E	e		Unselected persons	Fathers of infants with anti-D HDN	
+	+	+	−	+	DCe/dce*	94	79	9900–14 600
					DCe/Dce	6	21	
+	+	−	−	+	DCe/DCe*	96	99	14 500–19 300
					DCe/dCe	4	1	
+	−	+	+	+	DcE/dce*	94	79	14 000–16 000
					DcE/Dce	6	21	
+	−	+	+	−	DcE/DcE*	86	96	15 800–33 000
					DcE/dcE	14	4	
+	+	+	+	+	DCe/DcE*	90	97	23 000–31 000
					DCE/dce			
					DcE/dCe	10	3	
					DCe/dcE			
					DCE/Dce			
−	−	+	−	+	dce/dce	100	0	0

*Probable genotype.

235

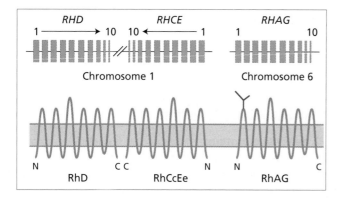

Figure 15.3 Rh and related genes and the polypeptides they encode, showing the 10 exons of *RHD* and *RHCE* in reverse orientation on chromosome 1 and of *RHAG* on chromosome 6, and the RhD and RhCcEe polypeptides and RhAG glycoprotein crossing the membrane 12 times.

D-negative represents the absence of the whole RhD protein from the membrane and anti-D can detect epitopes on any of the external loops of the RhD protein. D-positive people may be homozygous or hemizygous for the presence of *RHD*. Most D-negative black Africans, however, have an inactive *RHD*, called the *RHD*-pseudogene (*RHDψ*), that contains a 37-basepair duplication in exon 4 and a translation stop codon in exon 6.

The Cc polymorphism is associated with three or four amino acid substitutions encoded by exons 1 and 2 of *RHCE*, although the definitive change is Ser103 for C and Pro103 for c in the second extracellular loop of the RhCcEe protein. E and e are associated with Pro226 and Ala226, respectively, in the fourth extracellular loop.

The Rh molecular complex

The two Rh proteins are closely associated in the red cell membrane with a glycoprotein, the Rh-associated glycoprotein (RhAG). RhAG is homologous to the Rh proteins and has a similar conformation in the membrane, spanning the membrane 12 times, but is glycosylated on the first extracellular loop (Figure 15.3). Unlike *RHD* and *RHCE*, which are on chromosome 1, the gene encoding RhAG is on chromosome 6. The complex of Rh proteins and RhAG is probably also associated with several other red cell membrane proteins – the LW glycoprotein (ICAM-4), band 3 (the anion exchanger and Diego blood group antigen), CD47, the Duffy glycoprotein and glycophorin B – to form the Rh molecular complex.

The function of the Rh complex is unknown, although evidence exists that RhAG might function as an ammonium transporter or a CO_2 channel. The Rh proteins are only present on erythroid cells, but RhAG and related proteins are more widely distributed and homologues are found throughout the animal and plant kingdoms.

Variants of D

Weak D (D^u)

Cells that have the weak D phenotype (previously known as D^u) should, for most transfusion purposes, be regarded as D-positive. Weak D red cells have fewer D sites per cell than normal D-positive red cells. In a white population, the gene for weak D is commonly accompanied by *RHCE* encoding C or E antigen (*D^uCe* or *D^ucE*), and *D^uce* is rare. Weak D is more common in Africans and is usually produced by *D^uce*. It is important that anti-D typing reagents should detect most weak D phenotypes, especially in blood donors. However, very weak forms of D will be typed as D-negative. The weakest form of weak D, named DEL, can only be detected serologically by absorption and elution tests.

In the UK, the recommended method for D typing of patients requires direct agglutination tests, in duplicate, with potent IgM monoclonal anti-D reagents. An antiglobulin test is not required. This means that very weak D red cells will be typed as D-negative. This is not important, as the patient will be harmlessly transfused with D-negative red cells. Donors are not typed any longer for D by an antiglobulin test, as this is not necessary because it is unlikely that transfusion of very weak D red cells to a D-negative patient will result in immunization of the patient. One point in favour of abolishing the antiglobulin test in D-typing is that it might lead to the dangerous misclassification of a D-negative mother or blood transfusion recipient whose red cells give a positive direct antiglobulin test as D-positive.

By definition, individuals with weak D phenotype cannot make anti-D, as they have low levels of a complete D antigen on their red cells. However, in a few cases the boundaries between weak D and partial D (see below) have been blurred, and a few individuals with a phenotype previously considered to be weak D have in fact been weak partial D and have produced anti-D.

Weak D results from missense mutations in *RHD* that encode amino acid changes in the cytoplasmic or membrane-spanning domains of the D protein, but not in any of the loops exposed to the exterior of the cells. Based on molecular genotype, over 20 different types of weak D have been identified. Most weak D antigens represent three types: type 1, 70%, Val270Gly; type 2, 18%, Gly385Ala; and type 3, 5%, Ser3Cys.

Partial D

The D antigen comprises a mosaic of many epitopes. Most D-positive individuals have normal D antigens with all epitopes present, but there are some persons with rare D-positive red cells in which some D epitopes are missing. If immunized with normal D-positive red cells, individuals with partial D can make antibody to those D epitopes which they lack. This antibody will not react with their own cells, or with partial D red cells of the same type, but will behave as anti-D when tested with red cells of common Rh phenotypes. In some cases, the D epitopes of a partial D antigen will be expressed weakly, and the term partial weak D applies. Over 20 different types of partial D have been recognized and the classification of these D variants can only be made by a few specialized reference laboratories. About 30 D epitopes have been defined by using monoclonal antibodies.

In the UK, it is recommended that anti-D reagents for typing patients should not detect DVI, the most commonly encountered partial D antigen associated with anti-D production. Consequently, DVI patients will be transfused with D-negative red cells and DVI pregnant women will be given anti-D prophylaxis. Ideally, one of the anti-D reagents used for typing donor red cells should detect DVI.

Most partial D antigens are produced by *RHD*, part of which has been replaced by the equivalent segment of an *RHCE* gene. For example, the common form of DVI is produced by an *RHD–CE–D* hybrid gene in which exons 4–6 have the nucleotide sequence of *RHCE*, and external loops 3 and 4 of the encoded hybrid protein have the amino acid sequence of an RhCe protein. Consequently, a protein is produced with a sequence similar enough to *RHD* to be stable in the membrane, but different enough to lack many epitopes of D. Some partial D antigens result from a single nucleotide change in an external loop of the RhD protein.

Other Rh antigens

Table 15.11 lists the antigens of the Rh system recognized by the International Society of Blood Transfusion. A few of these are described below.

C^w and C^x antigens (RH8 and RH9)

C^w and C^x occur in about 2% and 0.2% of white people, respectively, although substantially higher frequencies are found in Finns. They appear to have an allelic relationship, although C^w and C^x represent Gln41Arg and Ala36Thr substitutions in an RhCcEe protein respectively. Anti-C^w and anti-C^x have caused HDN but, on the rare occasions on which this occurs, it is usually mild.

G antigen (RH12)

With only rare exceptions, G is expressed when either D or C, or both, are present. Anti-G, therefore, recognizes a determinant common to the products of *RHD* and the C allele of *RHCE*. Anti-G usually occurs with anti-D (see p. 238) and it is essential

Table 15.11 Antigens of the Rh system.

Number	Alternative names	Frequency*	Number	Alternative names	Frequency*
RH1	D	Polymorphic	RH31	hr^B	Polymorphic
RH2	C	Polymorphic	RH32	R^N	Low
RH3	E	Polymorphic	RH33	Har	Low
RH4	c	Polymorphic	RH34	Hr^B	High
RH5	e	Polymorphic	RH35	R^N-like	Low
RH6	ce, f	Polymorphic	RH36	Be^a	Low
RH7	Ce	Polymorphic	RH37	Evans	Low
RH8	C^w	Polymorphic	RH39	C-like	Polymorphic
RH9	C^x	Low	RH40	Tar	Low
RH10	V	Polymorphic†	RH41	Ce-like	Polymorphic
RH11	E^w	Low	RH42	Cce^s	Polymorphic†
RH12	G	Polymorphic	RH43	Crawford	Low
RH17	Hr$_o$	High	RH44	Nou	High
RH18	Hr	High	RH45	Riv	Low
RH19	hr^s	Polymorphic	RH46	Sec	High
RH20	VS	Polymorphic†	RH47	Dav	High
RH21	C^G	Polymorphic	RH48	JAL	Low
RH22	CE	Low	RH49	STEM	Low
RH23	D^w	Low	RH50	FPTT	Low
RH26	c-like	Polymorphic	RH51	MAR	High
RH27	cE	Polymorphic	RH52	BARC	Low
RH28	hr^H	Polymorphic†	RH53	JAHK	Low
RH29	Total Rh	High	RH54	DAK	Low
RH30	Go^a	Low	RH55	LOCR	Low
			RH56	CENR	Low

*Polymorphic => 1%, < 99% in at least one major population.
†Only polymorphic in black people, low in other populations.

that anti-D typing reagents do not contain anti-G, which could lead to mistyping of Cde/cde women of childbearing age as D-positive.

VS and V antigens (RH20 and RH10)
VS and V have frequencies of about 40% and 10%, respectively, in Africans, but are rare in other ethnic groups. Both are associated with an *RHCE* mutation encoding Leu245Val, but only VS is expressed when a Gly336Cys mutation is also present. Neither anti-VS nor anti-V have caused HDN or an HTR.

Compound antigens
Antibodies to the compound antigens, anti-ce (-f, -RH6), -Ce (-RH7), -cE (-RH27) and -CE (-RH22), define pairs of CcEe antigens only when they are encoded by the same *RHCE* gene. For example, anti-Ce and -cE, will react with D+C+c+E+e+ cells of *DCe/DcE* genotype, but not *DCE/dce*, whereas the reverse applies to anti-ce and -CE.

Rh$_{null}$, Rh$_{mod}$ and D--

Rh$_{null}$ and Rh$_{mod}$
Rh$_{null}$ red cells lack all antigens of the Rh system and people with this rare phenotype can make an antibody, antiRh29, which reacts with all red cells except those of the Rh$_{null}$ phenotype. They also lack LW antigens, RhAG and Fy5 of the Duffy system, and have weakened expression of CD47 and of S, s and U antigens on glycophorin B. Rh$_{null}$ subjects have a chronic haemolytic stomatocytic anaemia, which is usually compensated but may require splenectomy, and probably arises from the CD47 deficiency.

There are two modes of inheritance of the Rh$_{null}$ phenotype.
1 The amorph type, the rarer of the two, results from homozygosity for a deletion of *RHD* (characteristic of most D-negatives) plus homozygosity for an inactivating mutation (frameshift or splice site) in *RHCE*. Consequently, neither Rh protein is produced. Both parents are heterozygous for the mutations and possess only one-half of the usual quantity of Rh antigens.
2 The regulator type arises from homozygosity for inactivating mutations (frameshift, splice site, missense) in *RHAG*, the gene encoding RhAG. In the absence of RhAG, no Rh antigens are expressed, despite the presence of normal Rh genes. Consequently, individuals with the regulator type of Rh$_{null}$ inherit normal Rh genes from their parents and pass them on to their offspring. These parents and offspring are heterozygous for the *RHAG* mutation and have apparently normal Rh antigens, although there may be some weakening of expression. The parents of both types of Rh$_{null}$ individuals are usually consanguineous.

Rh$_{mod}$ is similar to Rh$_{null}$ of the regulator type, but there is only partial inactivation of *RHAG*, caused by missense mutations, encoding single amino acid substitutions, and resulting in weakened expression of all Rh antigens. Rh$_{mod}$ individuals cannot make anti-Rh29.

D-- and related phenotypes
Homozygosity for a rearranged *RHCE* gene, together with an active *RHD*, results in a series of phenotypes, called D--, D••, Dc- and DC^w-, in which no E or e antigens and, in the case of D-- and D••, no C or c, is produced. These phenotypes are very rare and have enhanced expression of D. If transfused, individuals with these phenotypes produce anti-Hr$_o$ (-RH17), an antibody that reacts with all red cells except for Rh$_{null}$ cells and cells with D-- and related phenotypes.

Antibodies of the Rh system

Naturally occurring antibodies
Generally, Rh antibodies are only produced following immunization by red cells. However, anti-E is often naturally occurring; about one-half may occur without a history of pregnancy or transfusion. Rarely, naturally occurring anti-D and anti-C^w are found and such antibodies react optimally with enzyme-treated cells.

Immune antibodies
The clinical importance of the Rh system lies in the readiness with which anti-D arises after stimulation with D-positive red cells by pregnancy or transfusion. Prophylaxis of Rh immunization with anti-D immunoglobulin has led to a significant decrease in the incidence of anti-D, but it still remains the most common immune antibody of clinical relevance detected in a routine blood transfusion laboratory. D is considerably more immunogenic than the other Rh antigens, which have the following order of immunogenicity: c > E > e > C.

About 20–30% of anti-D sera also appear to contain anti-C. Usually, this anti-C is not a separable antibody and is probably more correctly called anti-G (see p. 237). About 1–2% of anti-D sera also contain anti-E. Anti-C (and anti-G) in the absence of anti-D is very uncommon.

The incidence of other Rh antibodies is much lower, but together they are more common than the antibodies against K (Kell), which is the most immunogenic antigen after D. In routine screening, pure anti-E is the most common, followed by anti-c, although anti-c is a more common cause of HDN, which can be severe. This is probably because about one-half of the examples of anti-E are weak, naturally occurring antibodies. Anti-e, like anti-C, is very rare. The vast majority of Rh antibodies are IgG and do not fix complement. Anti-D may occasionally be partly IgA. IgM anti-D is very rare.

D immunization
The realization that D-negative women without anti-D who had just delivered a D-positive child could be protected from forming anti-D by the injection of IgG anti-D soon after delivery has been a powerful stimulus for experimental work on D-negative volunteers. About 90% of D-negative people will make anti-D after the transfusion of a large volume of D-positive

cells, and 70% will respond to repeated small volumes. Responders to D can usually be identified from survival curves after a single injection of ^{51}Cr-labelled D-positive cells. Serological methods are relatively insensitive for detecting very low levels of anti-D.

ABO-incompatible D-positive red cells are less likely to stimulate the production of anti-D than ABO compatible D-positive cells when injected into a D-negative recipient. Two explanations have been offered for this protection. First, it might be due to competition for the antigens so that the red cells are taken up by anti-A or anti-B-forming cells and are thus unavailable for anti-D-forming cells. Second, it might be that anti-A and -B bring about intravascular lysis with sequestration of the red cell stroma predominantly in the liver, which is an unfavourable site for antibody formation. Neither of these explanations is very satisfactory and the reason for the protection afforded by ABO-incompatible red cells remains uncertain. This protection is the basis of the lower incidence of maternal Rh sensitization when mother and infant are ABO incompatible.

It has been shown that 20 μg (100 IU) of anti-D immunoglobulin given intramuscularly will give complete protection from 1 mL of concentrated D-positive red cells (approximately 2 mL of blood). This figure is the basis for the standard dose of 100 μg (500 IU) anti-D Ig given post partum in the UK, as it will cover the vast majority of transplacental haemorrhages (TPH). A dose of 3.2–4.0 mg of anti-D Ig given intravenously will protect a D-negative recipient against the consequences of inadvertently transfusing a unit of D-positive whole blood (c. 200 mL of red cells).

The mechanism of protection by anti-D immunoglobulin is not really known. Two explanations have been suggested. The first is that the passively administered antibody leads to phagocytosis of antibody-coated red cells and their rapid destruction by macrophages in the spleen before they can combine with receptors of immunologically competent cells. The second is a central mechanism by which the Fc fragment of the antibody combined to antigen might give a suppressive or inactivating signal to the immunocompetent cells. It has been calculated that the amount of passive antibody needed to protect the recipient from antibody formation is less than that needed to cover all the D antigen sites on the injected Rh-positive cells.

Prior to the advent of Rh immunoprophylaxis, the first ABO-compatible, D-incompatible infant resulted in the primary immunization of about 17% of D-negative women. In about one-half of these women, the antibodies appeared within 6 months of delivery and, in the other half, the antibodies became detectable by the end of the second pregnancy.

Source of anti-D for immunoprophylaxis

Anti-D is usually obtained from volunteer men and from women unable to bear children, preferably if they have already been immunized by transfusion or pregnancy. Those with low levels of anti-D are deliberately restimulated with D-positive red

cells. Plasma from these donors is harvested by apheresis and sent to a fractionation plant for processing. The possibility of using human monoclonal anti-D for prophylaxis might become a reality within the near future. Preliminary clinical trials look promising.

Detection of fetal red cells in the maternal circulation

Fetal red cells can be detected in a sample of maternal blood by the acid elution method of Kleihauer, which depends on the fact that fetal haemoglobin is more resistant to elution in an acid medium than adult haemoglobin. Thus, fetal haemoglobin is retained in the cell and the fetal red cell stains darkly with the counterstain, whereas adult haemoglobin elutes and the mother's red cells appear as ghosts. Fetal D-positive cells can be quantified in the maternal circulation by flow cytometry after fluorescent staining with anti-D, with as few as 0.05% of fetal cells being detected. This is the preferred method for the follow-up of large TPHs and also of the inadvertent transfusion of Rh-positive red cells to D-negative women. Rosetting techniques can be useful for the estimation of RhD-positive cells in an RhD-negative patient.

Fetal red cells can frequently be detected in the mother's circulation, particularly during the last trimester of pregnancy and after delivery. In about 85% of blood samples taken soon after delivery, the proportion of fetal cells to adult cells is less than 1 in 20 000 (equivalent to a TPH of less than 0.5 mL). In two to three samples per 1000 deliveries, the TPH will be of the order of 10 mL of whole blood (5 mL of red cells) or more. Such women, if delivering a D-positive infant, will not be protected by the standard UK anti-D Ig dose of 100 μg and additional protection should be given. All laboratories should standardize the conditions of the acid elution technique (or any other quantitative technique) in order to estimate the absolute amount of fetal red cells present in the maternal circulation.

Immunization by abortion, miscarriage and obstetric intervention

Abortion and miscarriage can induce the immunization of D-negative women; obviously the incidence is greater if the abortion is therapeutic and if it occurs in the second trimester rather than in the first. Amniocentesis, chorionic villus sampling, fetal blood sampling and other obstetric manoeuvres can also lead to immunization of D-negative women carrying a D-positive fetus.

Prediction of fetal Rh genotype by molecular methods

Knowledge of the molecular basis for D-negative phenotypes has made it possible to devise tests for predicting fetal D type from fetal DNA. This is valuable in determining whether the fetus of a woman with anti-D is at risk from HDN. Most methods involve

PCR tests that detect the presence or absence of *RHD*. For the PCR, it is important that primers are selected that distinguish between *RHD* and *RHCE*. Differences between the two genes in exon 7, the non-coding region of exon 10 and in intron 4 have usually been exploited for this purpose. It is also important to test for more than one region of *RHD*, so that hybrid genes responsible for partial D antigens do not give a false result, and to test for the *RHD*-pseudogene (*RHDψ*), so that this does not give rise to a false-positive result.

Until recently, the usual source of fetal DNA has been amniocytes, obtained by amniocentesis, with its inherent risk of fetal loss and feto-maternal haemorrhage. It is now possible to use sensitive PCR technology to determine fetal D type from the small quantities of free fetal DNA present in maternal plasma, as early as 12 weeks into the pregnancy. This non-invasive form of fetal D typing is now provided as a reference service in the UK and some other parts of Europe.

The MNS system

MNS was discovered by Landsteiner and his colleagues in 1927 and the MNS genes were the first blood group genes to be cloned, in 1986 and 1987. The MNS system now contains 43 antigens, but is relatively unimportant in clinical blood transfusion.

The antigens of the MNS system

M and N are inherited as codominant Mendelian traits, giving rise to three common genotypes *M/M*, *M/N* and *N/N*. The *Ss* locus, which is closely linked to *MN*, also consists of two codominant alleles, at least in Europeans and Asians, producing S or s antigens. In northern Europeans, haplotype frequencies are *MS*, 25%; *Ms*, 28%; *NS*, 8%; and *Ns*, 39%. The system also contains many variants. About 2% of black West Africans and 1.5% of African-Americans are S–S– and most of these lack the U antigen that is present when either S or s is expressed.

The MN antigens are carried on glycophorin A (GPA) (see Figure 14.1), which is encoded by the *GYPA* gene on chromosome 4. M and N differ by amino acids at positions 1 and 5 of the external N-terminus of GPA. There are about 1 million molecules of GPA per cell, yet their absence in the rare En(a–) phenotype does not affect red cell function or survival. The negative charge of the red cells is mainly due to the ionized COOH groups of sialic acid (neuraminic acid), which is mostly carried on the oligosaccharides of GPA and can be removed with neuraminidase. Hence, En(a–) cells have a reduced negative charge and behave serologically as if they have been neuraminidase treated. Glycophorin B (GPB; see Figure 14.1) carries the S and s determinants, which represent an amino acid substitution at position 29. GPB is encoded by *GYPB*, which is closely linked and homologous to *GYPA*. S–s–U– red cells lack GPB. The amino acid sequence at the N-terminus of GPB is identical to that of N-specific GPA and accounts for the weak reactivity of *M/M* cells with anti-N, provided they are S+ or s+. The numerous MNS variants mostly result from amino acid substitutions in GPA and GPB and from the formation of hybrid GPA–GPB molecules, formed by intergenic recombination between *GYPA* and *GYPB*. GPA and GPB are exploited as receptors by the malaria parasite *Plasmodium falciparum*.

The antibodies of the MNS system

Anti-M is uncommon and reacts with about 80% of random samples. It is naturally occurring, more common in infants than adults, but can be immune and can very rarely cause HDN.

Anti-N is also rare and reacts with about 70% of random samples. It is nearly always a cold-reactive IgM antibody. Because of the 'N' activity of GPB, at low temperatures anti-N reacts with, and can be completely absorbed by, *M/M* cells, except those of the M+N–S–s– phenotype. Useful anti-N lectin can be prepared from the seeds of *Vicia graminea*.

A cold-reacting N-like antibody (anti-Nf) has been described in certain patients undergoing renal dialysis, regardless of their MN group. Although it may cause confusion in cross-matching tests, anti-Nf is usually of little clinical importance, but has been reported to cause hyperacute renal graft rejection. Nf arises from the effects of minute amounts of formaldehyde (used to sterilize the dialyser coil) on the patient's red cells; these changed cells stimulate anti-Nf.

Anti-S, the rarer anti-s and anti-U are usually immune, IgG, and can cause HDN. They have also been implicated in HTRs. Anti-U only occurs in S–s– black people and reacts with all cells that have the S or s antigens and up to 50% of cells that are S–s–. Finding compatible blood for a patient with anti-U may prove difficult.

The Lutheran blood group system

Lutheran is a complex system comprising four pairs of allelic antigens: Lu^a and Lu^b, Au^a and Au^b, Lu6 and Lu9, Lu8 and Lu14. These represent single amino acid substitutions in the Lutheran glycoproteins. There are another 12 antigens of very high frequency. The incidence of Lu^a and Lu^b phenotypes in the UK population is as follows:

Lu(a+b–)   0.1%;
Lu(a+b+)   7.5%;
Lu(a–b+)   92.4%.

The rare Lu$_{null}$ phenotype, in which no Lutheran antigens are expressed, has three genetic backgrounds: (i) homozygosity for an inactive Lutheran gene; (ii) heterozygosity for an unlinked dominant suppressor gene, *In(Lu)*; and (iii) hemizygosity in males of a recessive X-linked suppressor gene, *XS2*. Only individuals with the recessive type completely lack the Lutheran glycoproteins and can make anti-Lu3.

Lutheran antibodies are uncommon and are not generally considered clinically significant, although anti-Lu^b may have caused mild delayed HTRs. Lu^a may be omitted from antibody screening cells.

The Lutheran glycoproteins bind the extracellular matrix glycoprotein laminin and might function as adhesion molecules.

The Kell blood group system

The Kell system consists of one triplet and four pairs of allelic antigens – K and k; Kp^a, Kp^b, and Kp^c; Js^a and Js^b; K11 and K17; K14 and K2 – all of which represent amino acid substitutions in the Kell glycoprotein, plus 11 high-frequency and three low-frequency antigens.

The incidence of the K/k phenotypes, the most important clinically, is as follows:

K+k−   0.2%;
K+k+   8.7%;
K−k+   91.1%.

K is rare in populations other than those of white people. Js^a is present in about 20% of black people, but is extremely rare in other ethnic groups. The very rare null phenotype of the Kell system, in which no Kell system antigens are expressed, is called K$_o$, and results from homozygosity for a variety of inactivating mutations in the *KEL* gene.

The Kell antigens are located on a glycoprotein of 93 kDa, which crosses the cell membrane once and has a large, glycosylated, C-terminal extracellular domain, maintained in a folded conformation by multiple disulphide bonds. Reduction of these bonds by 2-aminoethylisothiouronium bromide (AET) results in loss of expression of all Kell system antigens. The Kell glycoprotein has sequence and structural homology with a family of neutral endopeptidases that processes biologically important peptides. The Kell glycoprotein cleaves the biologically inactive peptide big endothelin-3 to produce endothelin-3, an active vasoconstrictor. Whether Kell performs this function *in vivo* is not known.

The Kell glycoprotein is linked by a single disulphide bond to the Kx protein, which is produced by an X-linked gene, *XK*. Absence of Kx protein, resulting from hemizygosity in males of a deletion of *XK* or *XK* inactivating mutations, gives rise to the McLeod phenotype, in which there is no expression of Kx antigens and weak expression of all Kell system antigens. This rare phenotype is also associated with McLeod syndrome (MLS), a neuroacanthocytosis that is usually characterized by late onset muscular, neurological and, occasionally, psychiatric disorders, and abnormally shaped red cells. In some cases, an X chromosome deletion is large enough to encompass *XK* and *CYBB*, a gene for a subunit of flavocytochrome b_{558}, which leads to MLS and chronic granulomatous disease (CGD). If boys with MLS and CGD are transfused, they are liable to make anti-Kx, which can cause severe HTRs and makes compatible blood very difficult to find. If possible, transfusion of these patients should be avoided.

Anti-K is an important antibody in white populations; it is nearly always immune, IgG and complement-binding. It has been the cause of severe HTRs and HDN. K antigen stimulates the formation of anti-K in about 10% of K-negative people who are given one unit of K-positive blood. This makes K the next most immunogenic antigen after D. About 0.1% of all cases of HDN are caused by anti-K; most of the mothers will have had previous blood transfusions. HDN caused by anti-K differs from Rh HDN in that anti-K appears to cause fetal anaemia by suppression or erythropoiesis, rather than immune destruction of mature fetal erythrocytes. Kell antigen is expressed by erythroid cells at a very early stage of erythropoiesis and anti-K probably facilitates immune destruction of early erythroid progenitors, before they become haemoglobinized. Anti-K is best detected by the IAT; anti-K does not always agglutinate red cells treated with enzymes, or suspended in low-ionic-strength solution.

Anti-k is a very rare antibody, which reacts with 99.8% of random blood samples. It is always immune and has been incriminated in some cases of mild HDN. Most other Kell system antibodies are rare and best detected by the IAT.

The Duffy blood group system

The allelic antigens Fy^a and Fy^b represent a single amino acid substitution in the extracellular N-terminal domain of the Duffy glycoprotein. Their incidence in the UK is as follows:

Fy(a+/−)   20%;
Fy(a+b+)   46%;
Fy(a−b+)   34%.

About 70% of African-Americans and close to 100% of West Africans are Fy(a−b−). They are homozygous for an *Fy^b* allele containing a mutation in a binding site for the erythroid-specific GATA-1 transcription factor, which means that Duffy glycoprotein is not expressed in red cells, although it is present in other tissues. The Duffy glycoprotein is the receptor essential for penetration of *P. vivax* merozoites into erythroid cells and the Fy(a−b−) phenotype confers resistance to *P. vivax* malaria. In West Africa, where other forms of malaria are common, *P. vivax* does not occur and it is tempting to speculate that the high incidence of Fy(a−b−) arose by natural selection when the parasite was previously prevalent. An identical GATA mutation is found in an *Fy^a* allele in Papua New Guinea, where *P. vivax* is endemic.

The Duffy glycoprotein (also called Duffy-Antigen Chemokine Receptor, DARC) is a red cell receptor for a variety of chemokines, including interleukin 8. It might function as a 'sink' or scavenger for the removal of unwanted chemokines.

Anti-Fy^a is not infrequent and is found in previously transfused patients who have usually already made other antibodies. It is IgG, often complement-fixing and can cause HTRs, but seldom HDN. It is best detected by IAT and does not react with red cells treated with the proteases papain and ficin. Anti-Fy^b is very rare and is always immune.

The Kidd blood group system

Kidd has two alleles, Jk^a and Jk^b, which represent a single amino acid change in the Kidd glycoprotein. Phenotype frequencies in the UK population are as follows:

Jk(a+b−)   25%;
Jk(a+b+)   50%;
Jk(a−b+)   25%.

A Kidd-null phenotype, Jk(a−b−), results from homozygosity for inactivating mutations in the Kidd gene, *SLC14A1*. It is very rare in most populations, but reaches an incidence of greater than 1% in Polynesians.

The Kidd glycoprotein is a urea transporter in red cells and in renal endothelial cells.

Anti-Jk^a is uncommon and anti-Jk^b is very rare, but they may both cause severe transfusion reactions and, to a lesser extent, HDN. Kidd antibodies have often been implicated in delayed HTRs; they are IgG and predominantly complement fixing, but may be difficult to detect because they tend to disappear and then reappear promptly in anamnestic responses. The antiglobulin test is the best method for detection; reactions will be enhanced if the cells have been protease-treated or if fresh serum is added as a source of complement. Patients who have made Kidd antibodies should always be given an antibody card.

The Diego blood group system

Diego is a large system of 21 antigens: two pairs of allelic antigens – Di^a and Di^b, Wr^a and Wr^b – plus 17 antigens of very low frequency. All represent single amino acid substitutions in band 3, the red cell anion exchanger. The original Diego antigen, Di^a, is very rare in white and black people, but relatively common in Mongoloid people, with frequencies varying between 1% in Japanese and 50% in some native South Americans. Anti-Di^a and -Di^b are immune and rare, but can cause HDN. Wr^a has a frequency of about 0.1%. Its high-frequency allelic antigen, Wr^b, is dependent on an interaction between glycophorin A and band 3 for its expression. Naturally occurring anti-Wr^a is present in approximately 1% of blood donors. Anti-Wr^a is often found in the serum of patients who have made other antibodies or who are suffering from autoimmune haemolytic anaemia. Very rarely, anti-Wr^a causes HDN.

The Dombrock blood group system

The allelic antigens Do^a and Do^b represent a single amino acid substitution on the Dombrock glycoprotein, a member of the ADP-ribosyltransferase family, which also expresses the high-incidence antigens Gy^a, Hy and Jo^a. Approximately 66% of northern Europeans are Do(a+). Gy(a−) red cells are also Do(a−b−) Hy$^-$ Jo(a−). Dombrock antibodies are extremely rare, immune and are best detected by IAT; they have been implicated in severe acute and delayed HTRs. Anti-Do^a and -Do^b reagents are rare and unreliable, so Dombrock typing is most easily achieved by molecular methods.

The Colton blood group system

Co^a and Co^b represent a single amino acid substitution in the water channel aquaporin-1. Colton phenotype frequencies in white people are:

Co(a+b−)   90.5%;
Co(a+b+)   9.0%;
Co(a−b+)   0.5%.

The extremely rare Colton-null phenotype, Co(a−b−), results from homozygosity for inactivating mutations in the Colton gene, *AQP1*.

Colton antibodies are very uncommon. Anti-Co^a has caused severe HDN, and has been implicated in acute and delayed HTRs.

Some other blood group systems

Yt^a and Yt^b of the Yt system represent a single amino acid change in red cell membrane acetylcholinesterase. Yt^a and Yt^b have frequencies of about 99.8% and 8% respectively. Anti-Yt^a and Yt^b are exceptional and most are of no clinical significance.

The Scianna system consists of five antigens: the allelic antigens Sc1 and Sc2 of high and low frequency respectively; the high-frequency antigens Sc3 and STAR; and the low-frequency antigen Radin (SC4). They are located on the adhesion protein ERMAP. Scianna antibodies are very rare and little is known of their clinical significance.

The Xg system comprises two antigens, Xg^a and CD99, encoded by separate, but homologous genes on the X chromosome; *CD99* is also expressed on the Y chromosome. The corresponding antibodies are rare and of no clinical significance.

The eight antigens of the Gerbich system – three of high frequency and five of low frequency – are located on glycophorins C and D, which are encoded by a single gene, *GYPC*. The 12 antigens of the Cromer system and eight antigens of the Knops system are carried on the complement regulatory glycoproteins decay accelerating factor (CD55) and complement receptor 1 (CD35) respectively. Antibodies of these three systems are not generally considered clinically significant. However, antibodies of the Knops system are relatively common and often obscure identification of other, clinically important antibodies, in the same serum. Once identified, Knops antibodies can be ignored from a clinical point of view.

Antigens with high or low frequency

There are many other antigens, of either very high or very low incidence, that have not been assigned to blood group systems. Anti-Vel, -Lan, -At^a, -AnWj and -MAM are examples of antibodies to high-frequency antigens (HFAs) that have caused HDN and/or HTRs. For those rare individuals who have formed antibodies to HFAs, the provision of compatible blood can be a problem; it is often necessary to approach the national or international panels of rare donors for compatible units.

Antibodies to low-frequency antigens (LFAs) are usually naturally occurring; they may occasionally give rise to unexpected incompatible cross-matches. Some antibodies to LFAs have caused HDN.

Polyagglutinable red cells

Erythrocyte polyagglutination is the agglutination of red cells irrespective of blood group by many sera from normal adults. Polyagglutinable red cells are not agglutinated by the patient's own serum. The abnormality is a property of the red cells, not of the sera, in contrast with panagglutination, which is the agglutination of most red cells by one serum.

There are two main categories of polyagglutination, acquired and inherited. The acquired forms can be subdivided into: (i) microbial, due either to the passive coating of red cells with bacteria or their products or to the action of microbial enzymes on red cell surface oligosaccharides (T, Tk, acquired B); and (ii) non-microbial, which is caused by somatic mutation (Tn). There are four types of inherited polyagglutination: Cad (a strong expression of Sd^a), congenital dyserythropoietic anaemia type II (CDAII or HEMPAS), NOR and Hyde Park. Lectins are required for the diagnosis of the different types of polyagglutination (Table 15.12).

T activation

T activation occurs transiently in some patients with an obvious microbial infection, especially *Vibrio cholerae*, *Clostridium perfringens*, *Diplococcus pneumoniae*, various streptococci and the influenza virus. These microbes produce sialidases, which remove sialic acid (*N*-acetylneuraminic acid, NANA) from the oligosaccharides of membrane sialoglycoproteins (Table 15.13) to expose the hidden T antigen (galactose linked to *N*-acetylgalactosamine), with an accompanying loss of negative surface charge. For T polyagglutination to occur, microbial sialidases must be present in sufficient quantity to neutralize the enzyme inhibitors normally present in plasma; the same is true for other forms of enzymic polyagglutination.

Most adult sera contain naturally occurring, cold-reacting, complement-fixing, IgM anti-T. Most cases of T activation are detected by the discrepancy in results of cell and serum ABO grouping. The correct ABO group can be obtained from tests at 37°C.

T polyagglutination may be associated with (i) haemolytic anaemia, (ii) haemolytic transfusion reactions (especially in children) caused by anti-T in transfused plasma, although this is still questionable, (iii) haemolytic uraemic syndrome and (iv) neonatal necrotizing enterocolitis.

Peanut lectin, *Arachis hypogaea*, is the most effective tool for identification of T -activated cells (Table 15.12).

Tk activation

Tk activation, like T activation, is transient and associated with infection. Endo-β-galactosidases produced by *Bacteroides fragilis*, various clostridia or *Candida albicans* remove β-galactose from ABH polysaccharide chains, exposing *N*-acetylglucosamine (Tables 15.7 and 15.13), with the consequent depression of ABH expression, without affecting the quantity of sialic acid on the red cell. Tk cells are specifically agglutinated by BSII lectin,

Table 15.12 Some characteristics of T, Tk, Tn and Cad polyagglutinable red cells.

	T	Tk	Tn	Cad
MN antigens	↓	Normal	↓	Normal
ABH antigens	Normal	↓	Normal	Normal
Most normal sera	+	+	+	+
Glycine soja lectin	+	−	+	+
Arachis hypogaea lectin	++	+	−	−
Bandeiraea simplicifolia lectin	−	+	−	−
Salvia sclarea lectin	−	−	+	−
Dolichos biflorus lectin (other than group A$_1$)	−	−	+	+
Polybrene* solution	−	+	+mf	+

*Polybrene is a positively charged polymer that agglutinates cells with a negative charge and fails to aggregate sialic acid-deficient cells.

↓, reduced reactivity of MN or ABH antigens; mf, mixed field.

Table 15.13 Structure of T, Tn and Tk antigens.

O-linked oligosaccharide of GPA and GPB	
NeuNAcα2→3Galβ1→3GalNAc–Ser/Thr	Normal
6	
↑	
2	
NeuNAc	
Galβ1→3GalNAc–Ser/Thr	T
GalNAc–Ser/Thr	Tn

A-, B- or H-active chains modified by endo-β-galactosidase	
GlcNAcβ1→3Galβ1→4GlcNAc–R	Tk

Gal = galactose; GalNAc = *N*-acetylgalactosamine; GlcNAc = *N*-acetylglucosamine; NeuNAc = *N*-acetylneuraminic acid (sialic acid); R = remainder of molecule; Ser/Thr = serine or threonine.

an extract from *Bandeiraea simplicifolia* (Table 15.12). These cells are also agglutinated by peanut lectin, probably due to the exposure of galactose, the next sugar in the chain.

Tn activation

Tn activation, unlike T and Tk, is a persistent abnormality caused by an abnormal clone of stem cells arising by somatic mutation. Tn is often associated with other haematological abnormalities, such as chronic haemolytic anaemia, leucopenia or thrombocytopenia, but may be present in healthy individuals. Somatic mutation leads to a deficiency of the galactosyltransferase that elongates the O-linked oligosaccharides on GPA, so that many of the O-glycans consist of only *N*-acetylgalactosamine, the immunodominant sugar of Tn (see Table 15.13). This loss results in a depression of M and N antigens, a loss of sialic acid and a negative charge similar to that found in T activation. Only some of the red cells are agglutinated by the anti-Tn present in all normal adult sera, giving a mixed field appearance in agglutination tests. Platelets also show two populations. *Salvia sclarea* lectin specifically agglutinates Tn-activated cells, and the exposed *N*-acetylgalactosamine molecules can be detected with *D. biflorus* lectin (but only in people who are not group A₁).

White cell and platelet antigens and antibodies

HLA and transfusion

The HLA system is covered in Chapter 23. Leucocyte reactive antibodies have in the past been reported, albeit transiently, in up to 96% of massively transfused patients. Complement-fixing lymphocytotoxic antibodies have been found in as many as 50% of patients receiving multiple transfusions of platelet concentrates over a 4-week period. This frequency is lower in immunosuppressed patients. In contrast, some patients never become HLA immunized, despite repeated transfusions, and are considered to be non-responders to HLA. Pregnancy can lead to HLA antibodies in approximately 15%, 25% and 35% of women after a first, second or third pregnancy respectively. Such antibodies are generally of class I specificity, with anti-HLA-B being approximately twice as prevalent as HLA-A antibodies.

HLA antibodies stimulated by pregnancy or transfusion are usually IgG, complement fixing; naturally occurring IgM antibodies produced without a known stimulus, usually HLA-B8 specific, can be found in about 1% of individuals. The clinical importance of HLA antibodies relates to their ability to mediate graft rejection. In pregnant women, IgG antibodies may cross the placenta but are not considered to be a cause of neonatal leucopenia or thrombocytopenia. HLA antibodies are the usual cause of immunological refractoriness to random donor platelet transfusions, but not all patients with HLA antibodies are refractory to platelet transfusions, and a small proportion of immunologically refractory patients have no detectable lymphocytotoxic antibodies. The management of patients who become immunologically refractory to platelet transfusions is described in Chapter 16.

Neutrophil-specific antigens and antibodies

Neutrophils carry not only class I HLA antigens, but also neutrophil-specific antigens, as shown in Table 15.14. The antibodies showing specificity to the following antigens are clinically important in: (i) alloimmune neonatal neutropenia (HNA-1a, -1b, -1c, -2a, -3a, -4a); (ii) febrile transfusion reactions (HNA-1a, -1b, -2a, and other unidentified antigens on FcRIIIb and CD18); (iii) transfusion-related acute lung injury, caused by the passive transfer of granulocyte-specific antibodies in donor plasma (HNA-1a, -1b, -2a, -3a, NB2, though less frequently than HLA); and (iv) autoimmune neutropenia, in adults or in infancy (ND and NE have only been defined by autoantibodies). The antigens of the HNA-1 system are expressed on neutrophil FcRIIIb.

In addition, neutrophils express polymorphic antigens that also occur on endothelial cells (EM antigens), monocytes (HMA antigens), monocytes plus lymphocytes (HNA-4, HNA-5), and granulocytes and lymphocytes (SL).

Working with granulocytes is cumbersome and typing, as well as antibody screening, should be left to specialized laboratories. The techniques used to detect neutrophil antigens and antibodies include EDTA-dependent granulocyte agglutination, immunofluorescence, cytotoxicity, opsonization, chemiluminescence, radioactive antiglobulin tests and the use of staphylococcal protein A. Of these, granulocyte agglutination and immunofluorescence antiglobulin techniques are the most widely

Table 15.14 Neutrophil antigens.

System	Antigen	Previous names	Frequency (%)*	Glycoprotein	Amino acid change
HNA-1	HNA-1a	NA1	61.2	FcγIIIb	Arg36, Asp65, Asp82, Val106
	HNA-1b	NA2, NC1	89.6		Ser36, Ser65, Asp82, Ile106
	HNA-1c	SH	< 0.01		Asp78
HNA-2	HNA-2a	NB1	90.8		
HNA-3	HNA-3a	5b			
HNA-4	HNA-4a	Mart[a]		CD11b	Arg61
HNA-5	HNA-5a	Ond[a]		CD11a	Arg766

*In white people.

used; each can detect a different range of antigen specificities and both techniques should be used in parallel when investigating samples for neutrophil antibodies. Both techniques will detect HLA antibodies, including non-complement fixing ones that are not detectable by the lymphocytotoxicity test (LCT).

The discrimination of granulocyte-specific antibodies from granulocyte-reactive antibodies such as anti-HLA, which also react with other leucocyte subsets, requires access to large panels of HLA-typed granulocytes and lymphocytes, the application of tests that detect non-complement-fixing lymphocyte-binding antibodies (e.g. immunofluorescence by flow cytometry) and monoclonal antibody capture assays, known as MAIGA (monoclonal antibody immobilization of granulocyte antigens).

Neutrophil antibodies can be found in as many as 3% of pregnant women, especially if their serum is tested against their partner's neutrophils. However, neonatal alloimmune neutropenia is very rare and, as expected, associated with the presence of potent IgG antibodies. Neutrophil autoantibodies are also usually IgG, although some cold-reacting IgM antibodies have also been reported; these may be cytotoxic. Soluble IgG-containing immune complexes, rather than granulocyte-binding (auto)antibodies, may cause the neutropenia associated with Felty's syndrome. Autoimmune neutropenia may also be caused by antibodies that prevent neutrophil precursor maturation, rather than by destroying mature neutrophils and some drug dependent antibodies may also act by binding to neutrophil precursors.

Platelet-specific antigens and antibodies

Platelets carry ABH, Lewis, li and P antigens, as well as HLA class I and several so-called platelet-specific antigens. The HLA class I antigens are predominantly HLA-A and HLA-B; HLA-C is only weakly expressed on platelets. In some individuals, HLA-A and HLA-B are barely, or not at all, detectable on the platelet surface. HLA antibodies are the single most important cause of immunological refractoriness to random donor platelet transfusions although platelet-specific antibodies occur in 3–9% of

cases, usually in association with HLA antibodies, and are also responsible for post-transfusion purpura (PTP) and neonatal alloimmune thrombocytopenia (NAIT) and, very occasionally, febrile transfusion reactions.

Over 20 antigens have been described as platelet specific, some of which are shown in Table 15.15. These include the antigens of the various HPA (human platelet antigen) systems, which are composed of a high-incidence 'a' allele (e.g. HPA-1a) and a low-incidence 'b' allele (HPA-1b).

Some of the HPA antigens are not truly platelet specific; the HPA-1 antigens are also found on endothelial cells, which might contribute to the severity of NAIT and PTP caused by anti-HPA-1a. The HPA-5 antigens have been described on activated T cells and probably also on endothelial cells, on the very late antigen-2 (VLA-2) membrane protein.

The genetic location of the HPA alleles is known for all of the HPA systems. All represent single nucleotide polymorphisms (SNPs) encoding amino acid substitutions at different positions on the platelet glycoproteins GPIIIa, GPIb, GPIIb and GPIa (Table 15.15); except HPA14w, which is a frameshift deletion. Typing for platelet antigens by serology is difficult: sera with appropriate specificity are rare, usually contaminated by HLA antibodies, and generally lack the adequate potency required for reliable typing. However, serology can now be replaced by PCR-based DNA typing methods.

Three alternative strategies for PCR typing have been widely used. In the first, restriction fragment length polymorphisms (RFLP), the relevant HPA genes are amplified with appropriate primers, and the alleles encoded subsequently discriminated with allele-specific restriction enzymes. The restriction enzymes are chosen for their ability to recognize the nucleotide sequence of one of the two alleles and to cleave the PCR-amplified DNA product of that particular allele. The length of the DNA fragments produced on cleavage by the enzymes are analysed by polyacrylamide gel electrophoresis, and the observed RFLP determines which of the two alleles was present. This approach is also known as PCR-ASRE (allele-specific restriction enzyme) typing.

Table 15.15 Platelet antigens.

System	Antigen	Previous names	Frequency (%)*	Glycoprotein	Amino acid change
HPA-1	HPA-1a	Zw^a, Pl^{A1}	97.6	GPIIIa	Leu33
	HPA-1b	Zw^b, Pl^{A2}	26.8		Pro33
HPA-2	HPA-2a	Ko^b	99.4	GPIb	Thr145
	HPA-2b	Ko^a, Sib^a	14.3		Met145
HPA-3	HPA-3a	Bak^a, Lek^a	87.7	GPIIb	Iso843
	HPA-3b	Bak^b	64.1		Ser843
HPA-4	HPA-4a	Yuk^b, Pen^a	> 99.9	GPIIIa	Arg143
	HPA-4b	Yuk^a, Pen^b	< 0.2†		Gln143
HPA-5	HPA-5a	Br^b, Zav^b	99.0	GPIa	Glu505
	HPA-5b	Br^a, Zav^a, Hc^a	20.0		Lys505
HPA-6w	HPA-6bw	Ca^a, Tu^a	< 0.01	GPIIIa	Arg489
					Gln489
HPA-7w	HPA-7bw	Mo	0.01	GPIIIa	Pro407
					Ala407
HPA-8w	HPA-8bw	Sr^a	< 0.01	GPIIIa	Arg636
					Cys636
HPA-9w	HPA-9bw	Max^a	< 0.01	GPIIb	Val837
					Met837
HPA-10w	HPA10bw	La^a	< 0.01	GPIIIa	Arg62
					Gln62
HPA-11w	HPA11bw	Gro^a	< 0.01	GPIIIa	Arg633
					His633
HPA-12w	HPA12bw	Iy^a	< 0.01	GPIb	Gly15
					Glu15
HPA-13w	HPA13bw	Sit^a	< 0.01	GPIa	Thr799
					Met799

*In white people.
†In Japan.

In PCR with sequence-specific oligonucleotides (SSO), the amplified DNA is blotted onto nylon membranes, then hybridized with SSO probes under conditions of sufficiently high stringency to allow only the SSO probes complementary to the amplified allele to bind. The bound probe can then be detected with immunoenzyme conjugates, which recognize haptenylated deoxyribonucleotides incorporated into the SSO probes, or by autoradiography if ^{32}P-labelled probes are used. In PCR SSP, allele sequence-specific primers are used to amplify individual alleles and the PCR product is visualized after electrophoresis through agarose and staining with ethidium bromide. All three PCR typing methods use DNA extracted from lymphocytes, as platelets, being anucleate, lack DNA. Alternatively, platelet mRNA can be converted to cDNA with reverse transcriptase before PCR amplification.

Serological techniques for platelet antibody detection in patients' sera include the platelet suspension immunofluores-

cence test (PSIFT, the 'gold standard' recommended for routine platelet serology), solid-phase technology and an antigen-capture ELISA technique known by the acronym MAIPA (monoclonal antibody-immobilization of platelet antigens). In the PSIFT, HPA-typed platelets are incubated with the patient's serum, washed, and any bound immunoglobulin detected with a fluorescent anti-Ig conjugate is visualized by ultraviolet microscopy or flow cytometry. In the solid-phase method, platelets are anchored onto the bottom of U-well microtitre plates by a polyclonal rabbit–anti-human platelet serum. Following incubation with the patient's serum, platelet-bound IgG is subsequently detected using anti-human IgG-coated indicator red cells.

In the MAIPA assay, donor platelets are incubated successively with the patient's serum and a mouse monoclonal antibody that recognizes a specific platelet membrane glycoprotein complex (e.g. anti-GPIIb-IIIa, anti-GPIa-IIa or anti-GPIb-IX), and then solubilized in a mild detergent such as Triton X-100. Immune complexes in the resulting supernatant are captured into the wells of an ELISA plate coated with goat–anti-mouse IgG. Any human antibody present in a captured monoclonal antibody–platelet glycoprotein trimolecular complex is detected with an anti-human Ig ELISA conjugate.

Other techniques that have been used for platelet serology, although much less frequently, include platelet agglutination, the platelet radioactive antiglobulin test, ELISA, ^{51}Cr release, monocyte chemiluminescence and complement fixation.

The platelet antibody specificity that most frequently causes PTP is anti-HPA-1a, found in 85% of cases; anti-HPA-1b has been reported in 5% and anti-HPA-3a in 7% of cases in Europe. Similarly, anti-HPA-1a is the most common cause of NAIT, having been reported in 80% of HPA-1a-negative mothers at the time of birth of an affected infant. Anti-HPA-5b has been found in 15% of NAIT cases, as have occasional examples of anti-HPA-1b and HPA-3a, in HPA-1a-positive mothers in Europe. Approximately 85% of babies affected by NAIT are born to HPA-1a-negative mothers, making anti-HPA-1a the major implicated antibody specificity.

Cross-matching for immunologically refractory patients

The major cause of immunological refractoriness to platelet transfusion is, by far, the presence of HLA-A and/or HLA-B antibodies in multitransfused patients. Quite often, such antibodies are found to react with the lymphocytes from the majority (and sometimes all) of the donors included in the panel. Platelet-specific antibodies may occur in 3–9% or less of refractory patients. Implicated specificities have included anti-HPA-1a and anti-HPA-1b, as well as anti-HPA-3a, anti-HPA-2b, HPA-15b, and in this setting platelet-specific antibodies are usually accompanied by HLA antibodies.

Management of immunological refractoriness can often be accomplished by transfusion of platelets obtained by apheresis from HLA-matched donors. Some degree of mismatching of donor–recipient phenotypes may be permissible. 'HLA-B-matched' platelets, which differ by one or more antigens (B1 to B4 matches) within a serologically cross-reactive group of HLA-A or -B antigens, can often provide satisfactory increments in platelet counts; for example, by transfusing platelets from an HLA-A1-A11-B8-B27 donor to an A1-A11-B8-B7 patient (B7 and B27 are cross-reactive). The best matched platelets are theoretically from 'A-matched' donors, who do not express any HLA-A or -B antigens that are not present on the recipient's lymphocytes. Donors with apparently 'homozygous' HLA phenotypes (e.g. A1-X-B8-X) can often provide 'A-matched' platelets for a variety of recipients (e.g. A1-A2-B8-B44) who have an HLA haplotype in common with the homozygous donor. All matched donor platelets must be gamma irradiated before transfusion to prevent potentially fatal graft-versus-host disease.

Because the provision of HLA-matched platelets is an extremely expensive service, it is strongly recommended that their use is properly justified by taking post-transfusion platelet counts 1 h or 24 h after transfusion. If HLA-matched, cross-match (LCT or solid phase) compatible platelets still do not provoke satisfactory increments and the presence of platelet-specific antibodies has been excluded, then it is recommended to revert to the transfusion of platelets from random donors. In immunological refractoriness to platelet transfusions, the provision of HLA-matched platelets may not be sufficient per se for obtaining satisfactory post-transfusion platelet increments; it could be that a previously unrecognized HLA specificity, detectable by cross-matching the donor's lymphocytes by LCT, might be present, or that platelet-specific antibodies might be involved. If a patient does not show good increments when transfused with HLA-matched platelets that gave negative LCT cross-matches, then cross-matching the donor's platelets by a method such as the solid-phase technique could prove valuable in selecting compatible donors.

Plasma protein antigens and antibodies

Many components of human plasma can be antigenic when whole blood or plasma is transfused. Problems associated with such antibodies represent one of the less well-investigated areas in blood transfusion. Urticarial reactions following the transfusion of blood or plasma components are not infrequent, although the culprit proteins are only rarely disclosed and are most likely to be ingested haptens present in donor plasma (e.g. chocolate, drugs). Quite often the antibodies causing the reactions are IgE. Antibodies to factor VIII are not known to cause transfusion reactions, although they will cause inhibition of the activity of transfused factor VIII. Antibodies to IgA can lead to serious anaphylactic reactions. Antibodies to IgG determinants may cause problems in blood grouping, but their role in transfusion reactions is debatable.

Gm antigens are polymorphic antigens on the heavy chains of IgG (γ-chains), present mainly on the Fc fragment, although a few are on the Fd fragment. There are many different Gm antigens and they are inherited in haplotypes. IgG myeloma proteins have shown that different Gm antigens are associated with different IgG subclasses (e.g. IgG1 can carry four different Gm determinants, whereas IgG3 can carry 13 and IgG4 none).

Typing for Gm antigens is carried out with test serum to inhibit the agglutination of red cells coated with selected IgG Rh antibodies, of known Gm status, by Gm-specific antibodies.

Gm antibodies are found in: (i) the sera of patients with rheumatoid arthritis; (ii) the sera of women who have been pregnant; (iii) children between the age of 6 months and 5 years who are Gm incompatible with their mothers' IgG; and (iv) some normal adults. Gm antibodies are of no significance in transfusion medicine.

Selected bibliography

General

Mollison PL, Engelfriet CP, Contreras M (1997) *Blood Transfusion in Clinical Medicine*, 10th edn. Blackwell Science, Oxford.

Red cell antigens

Avent ND (2002) Fetal genotyping. In: *Alloimmune Disorders of Pregnancy* (A Hadley, P Soothill, eds), pp. 121–39. Cambridge University Press, Cambridge.

Avent ND, Reid ME (2000) The Rh blood group system: a review. *Blood* 95: 375–87.

Cartron JP, Colin Y (2001) Structural and functional diversity of blood group antigens. *Transfusion Clinical Biology* 8: 163–99.

Chester MA, Olsson ML (2001) The ABO blood group gene: a locus of considerable genetic diversity. *Transfusion Medicine Reviews* 15: 177–200.

Danek A, Rubio JP, Rampoldi L *et al.* (2001) McLeod neuroacanthocytosis: genotype and phenotype. *Annals of Neurology* 50: 755–64.

Daniels G (2002) *Human Blood Groups*, 2nd edn. Blackwell Science, Oxford.

Daniels G, Poole J, de Silva M *et al.* (2002) The clinical significance of blood group antibodies. *Transfusion Medicine* 12: 287–95.

Economidou I, Hughes-Jones NC, Gardner B (1967) Quantitative measurements concerning A and B antigen sites. *Vox Sanguinis* 12: 321–8.

Hadley TJ, Peiper SC (1997) From malaria to chemokine receptor: the emerging physiologic role of the Duffy blood group antigen. *Blood* 89: 3077–91.

Henry S, Samuelsson B (2000) ABO polymorphisms and their putative biological relationships with disease. In: *Human Blood Cells. Consequences of Genetic Polymorphism and Variations* (M-J King, ed.), pp. 1–103. Imperial College Press, London.

Huang C-H, Blumenfeld OO (1995) MNS blood groups and major glycophorins. Molecular basis for allelic variation. In: *Blood Cell Biochemistry* (J-P Cartron, P Rouger, eds), vol. 6, pp. 153–88. Plenum, New York.

Issitt PD, Anstee DJ (1998) *Applied Blood Group Serology*, 4th edn. Montgomery Scientific Publications, Durham.

Lee S (1997) Molecular basis of Kell blood group phenotypes. *Vox Sanguinis* 73: 1–11.

Reid ME (2003) The Dombrock blood group system: a review. *Transfusion* 43: 107–14.

Rochna E, Hughes-Jones NC (1965) The use of purified ^{125}I-labelled anti-γ globulin in the determination of the number of D antigen sites on red cells of different phenotypes. *Vox Sanguinis* 10: 675–86.

Sneath IS, Sneath PHA (1955) Transformation of the Lewis groups of human red cells. *Nature* 176: 172.

Wagner FF, Flegel WA (2000) *RHD* gene deletion occurred in the *Rhesus box. Blood* 95: 3662–8.

Watkins WM (2001) The ABO blood group system: historical background. *Transfusion Medicine* 11: 243–65.

Yamamoto PI, Clausen H, White T *et al.* (1990) Molecular genetic basis of the histo-blood group ABO system. *Nature* 345: 229–33.

Yu L-C, Twu Y-C, Chou M-L *et al.* (2003) The molecular genetics of the human I locus and molecular background explaining the partial association of the adult I phenotype with congenital cataracts. *Blood* 101: 2081–8.

White cell and platelet antigens

Blanchette VS, Johnson J, Rand M (2000) The management of alloimmune neonatal thrombocytopenia. *Baillière's Clinical Haematology* 13: 365–90.

Hurd C, Cavanagh G, Ouwehand WH *et al.* (2002) Genotyping for platelet-specific antigens – techniques for the detection of single nucleotide polymorphisms. *Vox Sanguinis* 83: 1–12.

International Forum (2003) Detection of platelet-reactive antibodies in patients who are refractory to platelet transfusions, and the selection of compatible donors. *Vox Sanguinis* 84: 73–88.

Lucas GF, Metcalfe P (2000) Platelet and granulocyte polymorphisms. *Transfusion Medicine* 10: 157–74.

Metcalfe P, Watkins NA, Ouwehand WH *et al.* (2003) Nomenclature of human platelet antigens. *Vox Sanguinis* 85: 240–5.

Shastri KA, Logue GL (1993) Autoimmune neutropenia. *Blood* 81: 1984–95.

Webert KE, Blajchman MA (2003) Transfusion related acute lung injury. *Transfusion Medicine Reviews* 17: 252–62.

Protein antigens

Giblett E (1969) *Genetic Markers in Human Blood*. Blackwell Scientific, Oxford.

de Lange GG (1991) Allotypes and other epitopes of immunoglobulins. *Baillière's Clinical Haematology* 4: 903–26.

CHAPTER 16

Clinical blood transfusion

Marcela Contreras, Clare PF Taylor and John A Barbara

16

Introduction

This chapter describes pretransfusion testing of the recipient's blood, complications and adverse effects of blood transfusion, appropriate use of components and, finally, a description of the features of haemolytic disease of the newborn. The first section deals with aspects of blood donation and collection, and the preparation and storage of blood components.

The blood donor (Tables 16.1 and 16.2)

Blood donation shall in all circumstances be voluntary. Financial profit must never be a motive for the donor or for those collecting the donation.

These statements sum up the attitude of the World Health Organization and the International Society of Blood Transfusion towards the principle of blood donation. However, in a number of countries worldwide, whole blood donation and apheresis plasma donation are remunerated. There are data suggesting that the microbiological safety of donations from paid donors is inferior, and stringent post-donation testing and viral inactivation are required to enhance blood safety.

In general, blood donors should be healthy adults between the ages of 17–18 and 65–70 years. These age limits vary slightly worldwide, but a lower limit is set to take account of the high iron requirements of adolescence. An upper limit is necessary because with age there is an increase in medical conditions that might make blood donation more hazardous, and increase the

Table 16.1 Measures to protect the donor.

Age 17–70 years (60 at first donation)
Weight above 50 kg (7 st 12 lb)
Haemoglobin > 13 g/dL for men, 12 g/dL for women
Minimum donation interval of 12 weeks (16 weeks advised) and
    three donations per year maximum
Pregnant and lactating women excluded because of high iron
    requirements
Exclusion of those with:
    Known cardiovascular disease, including hypertension
    Significant respiratory disorders
    Epilepsy and other CNS disorders
    Gastrointestinal disorders with impaired absorption
    Insulin-dependent diabetes
    Chronic renal disease
    Ongoing medical investigation or clinical trials
Exclusion of any donor returning to occupations such as driving
    bus, plane or train, heavy machine or crane operator, mining,
    scaffolding, etc. because delayed faint would be hazardous

Table 16.2 Conditions in the donor that lead to deferral.

All potential donors provided with information, so those at risk of HIV through lifestyle will refrain from donation (sexual practices, piercing, tattooing)

Donors with history of hepatitis deferred until 12 months after recovery

Exclusion of all potential donors who have themselves received a blood transfusion (due to risk of third party vCJD transmission)

Exclusion of those who have received pituitary-derived hormones or cadaveric dura mater or corneal grafts, and those with family history of CJD

Exclusion of those whose travel history places them at risk of malaria, Chagas' disease (unless antibody test available) and SARS

Permanent exclusion of any donor who has had filariasis, bilharzia, yaws or Q fever

Exclusion for varying time periods following vaccinations

Exclusion after known exposure to infectious illnesses such as varicella

Exclusion of anyone with a malignant condition except fully excised BCC of skin

Exclusion of those with diseases of unknown origin, e.g. Crohn's disease

Donor deferral for most drugs based on the underlying illness, e.g. cardiovascular, diabetes, malignancy, anaemia

Exclusion of those taking teratogenic drugs or those that accumulate in the tissues

probability that coincidental accidents may be attributed to the act of giving blood. Pregnant and lactating women are not accepted as donors of allogeneic blood, again because of high iron requirements.

As donors should be fit, healthy individuals, no donations should be accepted from those who have ever suffered from cancer, diabetes, or heart or kidney disease. Those with severe allergic disorders should not give blood because recipients may develop temporary hypersensitivity reactions due to passively transfused antibodies.

Minor red cell abnormalities

Donors with minor red cell abnormalities, such as thalassaemia trait, sickle cell trait and hereditary spherocytosis, are perfectly acceptable, providing that the haemoglobin (Hb) screening test excludes anaemia. Red cells containing HbS have a limited survival under conditions of reduced oxygen tension and so should not be transfused to newborn infants and patients with hypoxia or sickle cell disease. Red cells with HbS obstruct leucodepletion filters and it is therefore advisable, in the UK, to defer such people from blood donation. Blood from donors with G6PD deficiency survives normally, unless the recipient is given oxidant drugs.

Volume of blood taken

Modem blood collection packs are designed to hold 450 ± 45 mL of blood, mixed with 63 mL of citrate–phosphate–dextrose–adenine (CPD-A) anticoagulant. The ratio of anticoagulant to blood must be maintained at the optimal level, and donations of less than 405 mL or more than 495 mL of blood should not be issued for clinical use. Healthy donors can generally withstand the loss of 450 mL of blood without any ill effect, but vasovagal reactions become more common in those who weigh less than 47.5–50.0 kg (105–110 lb), as the standard donation represents a greater proportion of their total blood volume. In some countries, such as China and Japan, 'underweight', otherwise healthy, donors may donate smaller volumes (250 mL) of blood into specially designed packs containing the appropriate volume of anticoagulant. In several countries, including the UK, double doses of red cells are collected by apheresis from suitable large donors; such units are very useful to decrease donor exposure in multitransfused patients such as those with β-thalassaemia major.

Haemoglobin estimation

A test to exclude anaemia is performed before donation. A convenient and widely used method depends upon the specific gravity of a drop of blood, obtained by means of a finger prick. An estimate of the Hb value can be made, depending upon whether the drop of blood sinks in a copper sulphate solution of known specific gravity. The standard for male donors is generally a solution of specific gravity 1.055, approximating to a Hb level of 13.0 g/dL. The equivalent for females is 1.053 (Hb of 12.0 g/dL), although lower limits have been introduced in some countries. The copper sulphate method tends to underestimate the Hb value and may lead to unnecessary rejection of donors. However, the specific gravity of whole blood does not depend solely upon the Hb content of red cells and a pathological rise in plasma protein level or total white cell count (e.g. myeloma, chronic myeloid leukaemia) may lead to an anaemic donor passing the Hb test. Many transfusion services use an additional method of Hb determination on donors who fail the copper sulphate test, or as an alternative screening test. A relatively inexpensive portable haemoglobinometer can reduce the number of unnecessary rejections by up to 30%.

Donation intervals

A donation of 450 mL of blood contains approximately 200 mg of iron, which is lost to the body. Studies have shown depletion of iron stores in those who give three or four blood donations per year, but overt iron deficiency anaemia is uncommon except in female donors of childbearing age. In general, donors are bled two or three times per year in the UK (minimum interval 16 weeks), but some donors are able to donate more frequently without any significant iron depletion. When it is standard practice to take donations at shorter intervals, appropriate monitoring and/or iron supplements are recommended. However, this is not a major problem in the UK, where the average annual donation rate is less than 1.5.

Hazards of blood donation

The most common hazard of blood donation is fainting, reported in between 2% and 5% of all donors, but being especially common in young people and in those donating for the first time, particularly if they are nervous or apprehensive. A sympathetic approach by blood collection staff, enforcement of an adequate rest period, and constant vigilance to detect warning signs of an impending vasovagal attack can help to avert this problem. Once a faint occurs, the standard treatment of rest in a horizontal position and elevation of the legs is usually sufficient. Delayed faints occurring after a donor has left the clinic are potentially hazardous and a contraindication to further donation. For this reason, those donors who are drivers, machine operators, scaffolders and so on should not return to work on the day of donation. Infection of the venepuncture site should be avoided by meticulous attention to skin cleansing and aseptic techniques. All blood collection packs are manufactured as integral sets, each needle is sterile, to be used only once. No pack should be reused (even on the same donor) if the initial venepuncture attempt fails. Bruising of the arm may occur, particularly when venous access has been difficult; firm pressure over the site for 2–3 min and an explanation to the donor are usually sufficient. In the very rare event of arterial puncture, elevation of the limb and firm pressure over the site for 10–15 min should be combined with prolonged rest if a whole donation has been taken, as the rate of blood donation under such circumstances is usually very rapid. Very occasionally, attempted venepuncture may result in trauma to the nerves in the arm, resulting in pain, paraesthesiae and numbness. Such symptoms generally resolve in a few days, but very rarely may take several months of recovery.

Hazards of allogeneic blood transfusion

A number of diseases have the potential to be transmitted by transfusion of blood or its components. Donor selection criteria and subsequent testing of all donations are designed to prevent such transmission (Table 16.3).

The viruses that pose the greatest potential risk for transmission by transfusion are those that have long incubation periods (often causing subclinical infection), and especially those that may be carried by asymptomatic individuals for many years, or even lifelong. Alternatively, some viruses that are transfusion tranmissible exhibit cell-associated latency. If the virus is latent in white blood cells, recrudescence of that virus stimulated by allogeneic transfusion can cause infection of the recipient.

More rarely, a few viruses causing acute infection can be transmitted in the short presymptomatic viraemic phase if this

Table 16.3 Measures to protect the recipient.

Donor selection
Donor deferral/exclusion
Microbiological testing of donations
Immunohaematological testing of donations
Stringent arm cleansing
Diversion of the first 20–30 mL of blood collected
Leucodepletion of cellular products
Post-collection viral inactivation steps, e.g. MB or SD treatment
Monitoring and testing for bacterial contamination
Pathogen inactivation, e.g. using psoralen technology
Safest possible sources of donors for plasma-based products

coincides with the time of blood donation. Such agents pose a risk only if recipients have not been previously infected and donors have become infected after visiting endemic countries.

Bacteria, especially skin contaminants and blood-borne parasites, are also potentially transmissible by blood transfusion.

The key transfusion transmissible agents are summarized in Table 16.4.

Hepatitis viruses

Donors with a history of hepatitis are deferred for 12 months.

When serum from an individual with hepatitis B virus is ultra-centrifuged and examined with the electron microscope, three types of particle may be seen. The large (42-nm diameter) Dane particle is the actual virus with its central nucleocapsid core, which has its own antigenic constituent HBc. The core contains partially double-stranded DNA and DNA polymerase, and is surrounded by a lipoprotein coat carrying the surface antigen (HBsAg). The other two types of particles are 20-nm rods and spheres and represent overproduction of surface antigen material. The HBe antigen is in soluble form and is present in the incubation period, during acute infection and during the first years of the carrier phase. HBeAg is a marker of high infectivity. Dane particles are very rare in the plasma of low-infectivity carriers.

All donations are tested for the presence of hepatitis B surface antigen (HBsAg) by sensitive enzyme-linked immunosorbent assays (ELISAs) that can detect at least 0.2 IU/mL of HBsAg.

Hepatitis C virus (HCV) is recognized as the cause of the majority of cases of what was previously known as non-A non-B (NANB) hepatitis. Although electron microscopic visualization of HCV has not been verified, its genome has been cloned and ELISAs have been developed in which cloned and/or synthetic peptides can react with antibody to HCV.

Individuals with a history of jaundice may be accepted as donors, provided that they have been shown to be negative for markers of HBV and HCV. Clinical jaundice may be due to causes other than hepatitis B and C, including non-viral causes; also the majority of donors who are positive for HBsAg have no such history, so there is no sense in rejecting all people who give

Table 16.4 Transfusion-transmissible agents.

Agents		Characteristics related to transfusion
Viruses		
Hepatotropic	HAV	Very rarely transfusion transmitted; no carrier state; faecal–oral transmission
	HBV	2- to 6-month incubation period; carrier state; readily transmissible by blood
	HCV	Majority of cases asymptomatic; carrier state; readily transmissible by blood
Retroviruses	HIV1 and HIV2	Carrier state and latent in WBCs; readily transmissible by blood
	HTLV-I and HTLV-II	Latent in WBCs
Herpesviruses	CMV	50% UK adults have been infected; latent in WBCs
	EBV	Most UK adults have been infected (therefore already exposed pretransfusion); latent in WBCs
Others	Parvovirus B19	Generally mild or asymptomatic, posing no transfusion risk except for non-immune aplastic anaemia patients and fetuses
		Approximately two-thirds of UK adults have been infected
		Seasonal variation (and epidemic years) in incidence rate
	West Nile virus	Recently exhibiting epidemic rates of transmission in summer months in North America
Bacteria		
Endogenous	*Treponema pallidum*	Inactivated by storage at 4°C
		No transfusion transmissions reported in the past 15 years
	Yersinia enterocolitica	Very occasional transmissions, usually contaminated red cells transfused late in the storage period
Exogenous	For example, *Staphylococcus epidermidis; micrococcus, sarcina*	Mainly skin commensals or contaminants
		Most common cause of platelet contamination
Parasites	Malaria	Only five verified transfusion cases reported in UK in 25 years (all *Plasmodium falciparum*)
	Chagas' disease	No transmission of *Trypanosoma cruzi* by transfusion has been reported in UK
Prions	Abnormal PrP	Possible transfusion risk from vCJD; two UK cases potentially transfusion transmitted

a history of clinical jaundice. In the UK, the incidence of HBsAg in first-time blood donors is approximately 1 in 2000 and in established donors (i.e. new infections) less than 1 in 100 000. Hepatitis B surface antigen-positive subjects are permanently excluded from donation, and should be under specialist follow-up, as they have an increased risk of developing chronic liver disease and hepatocellular carcinoma.

Although the transmission of hepatitis B by blood and blood components has been virtually eliminated, HBsAg testing will not exclude all donors capable of transmitting HBV, as the sensitivity of presently available techniques may allow as many as 10^4–10^6 HBV genome copies per millilitre of plasma to remain undetected. The introduction of screening for anti-HBc and/or HBV DNA would reduce the very low risk of transmission of HBV yet further, but is not justified in the UK because of the striking rarity of reports of post-transfusion hepatitis B in recent years.

In the USA, before screening for anti-HCV was introduced, about 10% of transfusions caused significant increases in transaminase activity in recipients. There were also occasional cases of symptomatic hepatitis. Acute HCV infection is usually mild, but a proportion of patients do develop chronic liver disease, with a risk of hepatocellular carcinoma. Confirmed rates of HCV positivity in the UK are 1 in 2000 for new donors and < 1 in 100 000 for repeat donors. Methods of heat inactivation and solvent–detergent treatment of factors VIII and IX prevent transmission of HCV. Haemophiliacs who have received effectively inactivated factor VIII have proved negative for anti-HCV, in contrast with those who received untreated concentrate.

Hepatitis A virus is rarely transmitted by transfusion. Any donor who has been in close contact with a case (e.g. household contact), or developed hepatitis A is deferred for 12 months.

Human immunodeficiency virus (HIV-I and HIV-2)

The classical descriptions and the vast majority of the literature on AIDS refer to HIV-1; a second retrovirus capable of causing AIDS, HIV-2, mainly occurs in West Africa.

Human immunodeficiency virus (HIV) can be transmitted both in cellular and plasma components. Most of the patients infected by the transfusion of blood components were transfused before the introduction of the screening of blood donations for HIV antibodies. The majority of recipients of blood products who were infected in the past were transfused before 1985 with unheated, non-pasteurized pooled plasma products, mainly factor VIII and factor IX. Thus, HIV infection became an important sequel to transfusion of factor VIII concentrates to haemophiliacs in the early 1980s, before the introduction of heat treatment and other viral inactivation methods. HIV is more heat labile than HBV, especially when in solution. Prolonged heat treatment and other viral inactivation methods of plasma products are effective means of protecting haemophiliacs from infection, although too late for those who were receiving regular factor VIII therapy in the late 1970s and early 1980s.

Albumin solutions are pasteurized, and carry no risk of HIV transmission. Similarly, i.m. immunoglobulin preparations are rendered safe from HIV infectivity by their manufacturing processes.

Blood and all fresh blood components (platelets, white cells, single donor plasma, fresh-frozen plasma and cryoprecipitate) are capable of transmitting HIV. Certain behaviour patterns place individuals at greater risk of HIV infection. Accordingly, male homosexuals and bisexuals, intravenous drug users and prostitutes are permanently deferred from blood donation. The sexual partners of such individuals and of haemophiliacs treated with blood products are also excluded. In addition, large areas of sub-Saharan Africa and South-East Asia have a high incidence of HIV seropositivity in the general population. Inhabitants of these areas and their partners are also considered to be at greater risk of HIV infection than heterosexual non-drug users in other areas of the world. Donor education and encouragement of those whose behaviour may have exposed them to HIV to exclude themselves from blood donation are highly cost-effective methods for the prevention of transmission of HIV infection by blood transfusion. Systems for donor deferral should continue to be in place, even in the presence of sensitive assays for the detection of infectious donors.

In most HIV-infected subjects, antibody develops within 3–4 weeks and it coexists with the virus thereafter. Hence, HIV seropositivity is an indicator of infectivity. The tests that lend themselves most readily to the rapid mass screening required in blood transfusion are all ELISA based. As many of the commercially available kits have some false-positive reactions, due mainly to cross-reactivity, confirmatory tests using alternative methodologies are carried out before a positive result is reported.

Routine screening, combined with the well-established donor education and self-deferral schemes, has reduced even further the already small risk of the transfusion of a contaminated donation. There have been only three documented cases of HIV transmission by transfusion in the UK since screening began. The small residual number of HIV transmissions through screened blood will arise through donations given in the 'window period' of infectivity, i.e. soon after the donor has been infected but before anti-HIV has become detectable (as in the three UK documented cases referred to), or through system errors. With current combined antigen–antibody screening techniques, the window period has been estimated to be less than 2 weeks on average. The prevalence of HIV antibodies in repeat UK blood donors is less than 1 in 100 000, and is 1 in 25 000 in new donors; there is no doubt that energetic donor education has contributed to this very low rate by excluding high-risk individuals. In England and Wales, it is estimated that the residual risk of HIV infection by transfusion at present, per donation, is approximately 1 in 8 million. Although small, the risk of HIV transmission by transfusion is greater in the USA (approximately 1 in 500 000–1 million donations) than in the UK. In order to reduce the length of the window period even more, i.e. to about 2 weeks, the USA and other countries (such as Thailand) introduced screening for HIV antigen at a considerable cost. In the USA, this has been replaced by nucleic acid testing (NAT) for HIV RNA, which reduces the window period to approximately 1 week. However, in areas of low HIV incidence, the number of extra donors detected by such screening will be extremely small. In the UK, combined antigen–antibody serological testing has proved extremely effective, although NAT for HIV has been introduced in some parts of the country.

Human T-cell leukaemia viruses (HTLV I and HLTV II)

Human T-cell leukaemia viruses (HTLV I and II) are related retroviruses. The importance of HTLV II is not clear; it appears to be associated with intravenous drug use in the Western world and has no known association with any clinical condition. However, HTLV I is endemic in the Caribbean, parts of Africa, and in Japan, where 3–6% of the population are seropositive. Infection with HTLV I is associated with at least two distinct clinical conditions; it can lead to adult T-cell leukaemia (ATLL), with an incubation period of approximately 20 years and, on rare occasions, to tropical spastic paraparesis (also known as HTLV I-associated myelopathy), which appears to have a shorter incubation period. Only about 1% of patients who are seropositive develop T-cell leukaemia. Both HTLV I and HTLV II are cell associated and not transmitted in plasma. In highly endemic areas, transmission of HTLV I by transfusion was relatively common before mandatory screening was introduced. Both tropical spastic paraparesis and ATLL have been associated with transfusion-transmitted HTLV I.

In areas of low prevalence of HTLV I and II infection, the cost benefit of mandatory screening of blood donations has been debatable. Routine serological screening is by ELISA, but confirmation of positive results can still cause difficulties because other retroviruses may cross-react. In certain cases, it may also be difficult to differentiate between HTLV I and HTLV II in the laboratory, despite the quite different clinical consequences of the two infections. The prevalence of anti-HTLV in previously untested UK blood donors is roughly 1 in 50 000 and screening became mandatory in 2002.

Cytomegalovirus

Although most cases of post-transfusion cytomegalovirus (CMV) infection are subclinical, the syndrome of post-transfusion infectious mononucleosis-like illness is well recognized, especially after the transfusion of large amounts of blood. The infection is characterized by fever, splenomegaly and atypical lymphoid cells in the peripheral blood, with a negative Paul Bunnell test. The usually benign course of CMV infection in recipients has meant that there has been no necessity to screen all donors for evidence of past infection. However, immunosuppressed individuals are at great risk from potentially fatal pneumonitis or disseminated cytomegalovirus infection, and these recipients require special measures to prevent CMV transmission.

The groups at particular risk are: premature babies weighing < 1500 g, bone marrow and other organ transplant recipients and pregnant women (the fetus is at risk). In such cases, if the patient (and the tissue donor) or the mother (in the case of neonates) lacks evidence of past CMV infection, then anti-CMV free blood and blood components should be provided. This may cause logistical problems, especially with platelet supplies, as the incidence of anti-CMV in the UK adult population is 50–60%. Although only a small number of antibody-positive donors may be capable of transmitting the infection, there is no test for infectivity. Thus, all antibody-positive donors should be considered as having the potential to transmit CMV. As CMV is cell associated, leucodepletion should provide similar levels of safety as serological testing, but this has not been proven prospectively in well-controlled clinical trials.

Syphilis

Each donation is tested by a serological test for syphilis. Although *Treponema pallidum* does not survive well at 4°C and red cell preparations are likely to be non-infective after 4 days' refrigeration, storage does not affect the positive serology. Passive transmission of the antibody to a recipient could cause diagnostic confusion. The organism is more likely to be transmitted in platelet concentrates, due to their room temperature storage and short shelf-life. Any donation from an individual giving a positive result is discarded, and subjects with positive tests are permanently debarred from donation, even after effective therapy. In the past, syphilis testing was believed valuable as a surrogate marker for lifestyles known to be associated with high risk of HIV infection. Sensitive HIV assays have reduced this usefulness.

Malaria

Malarial parasites remain viable in blood stored at 4°C, and are readily transmissible by blood transfusion. In some endemic areas, all recipients are treated with antimalarial drugs. In non-endemic areas, there is a real risk of failure to recognize post-transfusion malaria owing to the rarity of the infection. This fact, combined with increasing travel to tropical areas, necessitates the careful vetting of blood donors by direct questioning and, in some centres, by tests for malarial antibodies. Visitors who have recently travelled to a tropical area are treated similarly for 12 months after the visit, unless malaria antibody testing is available. Such testing has recently become available in the UK.

Other infections

There are no other protozoal or microbiological diseases (for which tests are available) that pose a significant problem in the context of blood transfusion in the UK. However, diseases such as Chagas' disease cause significant problems for the blood transfusion services in Latin America, and potential exposure of UK donors necessitates specific serological testing of those individuals to exclude the possibility of infection.

Bacteria

Although rare in absolute terms (approximately three cases are reported and confirmed per year in the UK), bacterial transmissions by transfusion constitute two-thirds of all microbial transmissions by this route and often prove fatal. The vast majority of such cases are due to contaminated platelet preparations that are more than 3 days old, because bacteria (mostly skin commensals) will proliferate easily at room temperature. This risk is now far greater than viral risks because of the introduction of interventions such as NAT for HCV. UK blood services are in the process of introducing enhanced methods of donor arm cleansing, 'diversion' of the first 20 mL of the donation to reduce the risk from skin contaminants and are considering routine bacterial screening of platelet preparations.

Prions

Variant Creutzfeldt–Jakob disease (vCJD), the human form of bovine spongiform encephalopathy (BSE), is considered a potential threat to blood safety. This risk is at present only applicable to the UK, where nearly 150 cases of vCJD had been reported at the beginning of 2004. Therefore, plasma for fractionation (and fresh-frozen plasma for infants and children not exposed to the risk of BSE in food) is obtained from the USA. Appropriate donor exclusions and the introduction of leucodepletion of all blood components are other precautionary interventions. It has been shown experimentally that BSE acquired in sheep, by eating contaminated beef, can be transmitted by blood transfusion to other sheep. As it is not known how many people could be infected with vCJD and because of the recent reports of two possible cases of vCJD transmission by blood transfusion, recipients of blood have now been excluded as blood donors in the UK. It has not been possible to detect abnormal prion in the blood of patients with vCJD; hence no screening tests are yet available for blood donations.

Laboratory tests on blood donations (Table 16.5)

Samples for laboratory testing are taken at the time of donation, to avoid later entry into the sterile blood pack. The routine tests are automated if large numbers of donor samples are tested daily.

Table 16.5 Microbial testing in England and North Wales.

HIV	ELISA (combined HIV_1 Ag plus anti-HIV_1, and anti-HIV_2)
HBV	HBsAg ELISA
HCV	Anti-HCV ELISA plus NAT on pools of 48 samples
HTLV	Anti-HTLV ELISA (on pools of 48 samples)
CMV	Anti-CMV for immunosuppressed recipients only.
Malaria	Antibody screening of potentially exposed donors
Chagas' disease	Antibody screening of potentially exposed donors
Bacteria	All donations are tested for antibody to syphilis; the option to test platelet preparations by culture methods is under review

All blood donors in the UK are tested at each donation for syphilis, HBsAg, anti-HIV 1 and 2 and antigen, anti-HCV, HCV RNA, and anti-HTLV. ABO and RhD grouping is determined routinely on each occasion. Typing for other Rh antigens (C, E, c and e) and K is now routinely performed on most, although not all blood donations, in the UK. Matching for such antigens is only performed in special cases such as alloimmunized patients and sickle cell disease patients. Ideally, girls and women of childbearing age should be matched for c and K, as anti-c and anti-K are, after anti-D, the major causes of severe HDN in the UK.

All donations are also screened for the presence of atypical red cell alloantibodies by testing against group O red cells that are selected to bear the most common blood group antigens. The incidence of clinically significant red cell alloantibodies in blood donors is very low (0.3%) compared with the incidence in potential recipients (1.5–3.0%). Donations with potent clinically significant alloantibodies are not issued to hospitals. Group O blood for emergency or 'flying squad' use, which may be given, in exceptional circumstances, to ungrouped recipients, should be given as red cells in additive solution (e.g. saline–adenine–glucose–mannitol, SAGM) to avoid problems that might be caused by high-titre anti-A,B in donor plasma. As soon as the patient's group is known, group-specific blood should be given. If group O platelets have to be given to non-O recipients, donors with high-titre anti-A,B should be excluded as the providers of the plasma used to suspend the platelets, or platelet-additive solutions can be used to replace most of the plasma.

Some donations are screened for CMV antibodies for patients in need of CMV-negative blood. Units from donors at risk are screened for malaria antibodies, Chagas' disease antibodies and for HbS (sickle trait).

Residual microbial risk of allogeneic blood transfusion

The residual risks of microbial transmission are now so low in the UK that prospective studies to determine them would need to be too large to be practical. Risk is therefore calculated from the length of the 'window period' (prior to laboratory delectability of the infection) and the rate of new infections for specific viruses. The calculated residual risks per donation in England and Wales for HIV, HBV and HCV are approximately 1 in 8 million, 1 in 1 million and 1 in 30 million respectively. These calculations are consistent with 'haemovigilence' reports in the UK Serious Hazards of Transfusion (SHOT) scheme. Indeed, acute microbial transmissions now constitute a mere 3% of all reported hazards, with 'incorrect blood component transfused' being the major reported risk. The low microbial risk is a result of a series of incremental safety interventions becoming ever more complex and costly.

In this context, pathogen inactivation–reduction is likely to prove very cost-*ineffective*, unless existing safety interventions can be reduced, or discontinued, or 'emerging' microbial risks are considered to pose a sufficient threat. In any case, if pathogen inactivation techniques such as photochemical inactivation are introduced, we need to ensure that the blood product is not affected in its immunogenicity or efficacy, and that the benefits of their introduction outweigh the risks.

Storage of blood

When blood is stored in a liquid state there is a progressive loss of viability of the red cells, and of red cell ATP, and depletion of 2,3-diphosphoglycerate (2,3-DPG). The purpose of modern anticoagulants that are used for the collection of blood is to reduce these changes to a minimum.

Anticoagulants and solutions for red cell preservation

The addition of 'rejuvenating' agents or purine nucleosides (adenosine, inosine) to standard anticoagulant solutions has been shown to improve significantly the viability of red cells (e.g. CPD-AI). Adenosine is effective in restoring the ATP content of stored red cells, whereas inosine restores the 2,3-DPG content. Adenosine is potentially toxic, although rapidly deaminated to inosine in the circulation. Inosine catabolism can raise serum uric acid levels. Hence, neither compound is used in routine practice, but adenine has been found to have a beneficial effect similar to that of adenosine without its side-effects.

Optimal additive solutions (e.g. saline-adenine-glucose-mannitol, SAGM)

Optimal additive plasma replacement solutions have been developed to improve viability of plasma-depleted red cells on storage, by maintaining both ATP and 2,3-DPG levels. SAGM (as well as ADSOL and Nutricel) medium provides good red cell storage conditions and is now the most usual preservative solution for red cells in the UK. A multiple 'top and bottom' blood collection pack is used (Figure 16.1). The blood donation is taken into the main pack, which contains standard CPD anticoagulant. After centrifugation, plasma and buffy coat are separated and transferred into empty satellite packs. The latter is pooled with three other buffy coats and the plasma from one of those donations. After a further gentle centrifugation, the platelet-rich plasma is expressed into a special platelet pack and the remainder of the buffy coat is discarded (Figure 16.2). Platelet concentrates are then suspended in CPD-plasma; they can be resuspended in 2:3 platelet additive solution and 1:3 plasma, especially for patients in whom exposure to plasma is contraindicated or when the potency of anti-A,B in group O platelets needs to be reduced for non-O recipients. As a separate procedure, the red cells left at the bottom of the pack are added to 100 mL of SAGM medium, contained in another satellite pack (i.e. in a closed system). The resulting red cells have flow characteristics equivalent to plasma-reduced blood and a storage life of 35–42 days (35 in the UK). Using this method, maximal amounts of plasma can be removed from blood donations for the manufacture of factor VIII and albumin, thus helping to meet the self-sufficiency targets for plasma products. At the same time, both platelets and an improved red cell product can be obtained. As stated above, in the UK, in order to decrease the possible risk of transmission of vCJD by transfusion, plasma for fractionation is imported from the USA.

Other anticoagulants and additive solutions

Heparin is now rarely used, and it can only be useful for blood that is to be transfused within 12 h of collection. This is because heparin is gradually broken down in storage and the blood then clots. Heparinized blood for neonatal cardiac surgery and exchange transfusion has been replaced by citrate–phosphate–dextrose–adenine (CPD-AI) blood, less than 3–5 days old, with no untoward effects. Some neonatologists use SAGM red cells for newborn infants, with success. For intrauterine transfusion, irradiated, white cell-depleted red cells are used.

CPD-AI solution has a final concentration of 9.25 mmol/L adenine and a slightly higher dextrose content than standard CPD. Red cell viability is well maintained for up to 5 weeks. Acid–citrate–dextrose (ACD) solution, which preserves red blood cells for only 21 days, is not used any more for red cells. However, ACD-A is the anticoagulant of choice for routine use in all apheresis platelet collections. CPD is used when collecting plasma donations by apheresis.

Storage changes of blood

Loss of red cell viability is the most important practical consideration. Progressive loss of viability varies according to the anticoagulant used. The time limit for storage of blood is set taking this into consideration. After transfusion of stored red cells, a proportion are removed from the circulation within the first 24 h. The remainder appear to survive normally. With increased length of storage, a greater proportion of red cells are

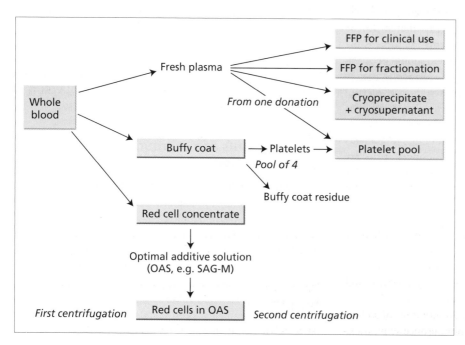

Figure 16.1 Diagrammatic representation of the preparation of components from whole blood by the 'top and bottom' or 'buffy coat' method. Items in boxes represent final components. FFP, fresh-frozen plasma.

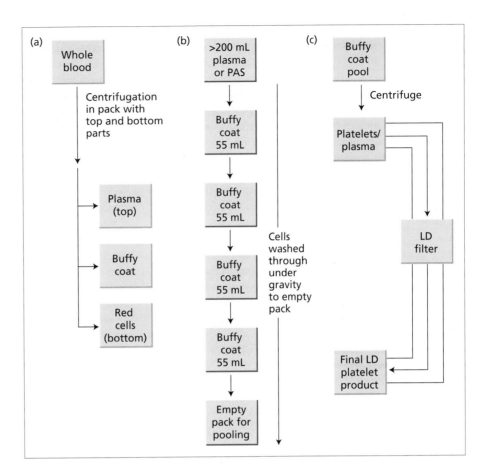

Figure 16.2 Preparation of leucodepleted pooled, buffy coat-derived platelet preparations. PAS, platelet additive solution; LD, leucodepletion.

removed within the first 24 h. The destruction at 24 h of more than 30% of the total number of cells transfused is considered unacceptable.

Depletion of ATP is progressive during storage of red cells, leading to changes in red cell shape (discs to spheres, loss of membrane lipid and increased rigidity). These changes can be partially reversed by incubation with purine nucleosides, and reduced by addition of adenine at the time of collection. ATP seems to be an important determinant of red cell viability, although not the only one.

Reduction in red cell 2,3-DPG during storage is less severe in CPD blood than in ACD: 2,3-DPG levels are normal in CPD and CPD-AI blood at 1 week. Reduced red cell 2,3-DPG levels increase the oxygen affinity of Hb, and the oxygen dissociation curve is shifted to the left, with less oxygen being given up to the tissues. The red cell 2,3-DPG level is restored to normal by approximately 24 h post transfusion. The clinical significance of the low 2,3-DPG level of stored red cells is only likely to be an important consideration in recipients with severe anaemia or coronary artery insufficiency. Even in massive transfusion of stored blood, depletion of red cell 2,3-DPG can probably be well tolerated if cardiac function is satisfactory.

Electrolyte changes are the result of equilibration of sodium and potassium levels across the cell membrane once active trans-port has been halted by the cooling of blood to 4°C. There is rapid restoration of electrolyte levels after transfusion.

The pH of blood decreases rapidly with storage, but most recipients can handle the acid load during transfusion without ill effect.

Frozen red cells

Red cells can be stored for a prolonged period without damage if glycerol is added before freezing. Thawed red cells must be washed free of glycerol before transfusion. This method of storage is expensive and time-consuming but is invaluable as a means of storing red cells with rare phenotypes. National banks for frozen rare cells have been established for this purpose. Freezing, thawing and washing is also an efficient way of removing plasma, platelets and leucocytes from red cells.

Blood components

Preparation and storage of other separate blood components (Figures 16.1 and 16.2)

After initial centrifugation, three components can be obtained from a whole blood donation: red cells, buffy coat and plasma (Figure 16.1). Fresh plasma is expressed from the top and red cells from the bottom of the pack, leaving the buffy coat in the original pack. The red cells are transferred to a pack containing an optimal additive solution (OAS) to preserve red cell function during storage. The plasma is then kept to resuspend the platelets, or frozen either for clinical use as fresh-frozen plasma (FFP) or it can be subjected to a fractionation process for the manufacture of IVIg, albumin, anti-D, specific antiviral immunoglobulins and coagulation factors. However, at present it is not permitted to use UK plasma for fractionation, owing to concerns over the possible transmission of vCJD by blood components.

The buffy coat layer contains most of the platelets, over 80% of the white cells and 5–10% of the red cells. This is pooled with three other buffy coats and > 200 mL of plasma from one of the donations, using a sterile connecting device (Figure 16.2). The pool undergoes a second gentle centrifugation step and the supernatant is used to produce a platelet preparation. The residue from the buffy coat pool, containing mainly white cells and some red cells, is then discarded.

The systems that enable the separation of buffy coats in a semiautomated manner are called blood separators, examples of which are Optipress and Compomat (Figure 16.2). Cellular components (red cells and platelets) and plasma may, at this stage, be individually filtered to leucodeplete to a level of $< 5 \times 10^6$ white cells per unit. The alternative is to use leucodepletion filters at the initial stage on whole blood, before separation of components. These two alternative methods are necessary because most whole blood filters also remove a significant number of platelets, making production of platelet concentrates from filtered whole blood impossible. In the UK, leucodepletion of all blood components has been mandatory since 1999.

Platelet preparations

Platelets do not survive well in stored blood. For all practical purposes, there are no viable platelets remaining in blood stored for 48 h at 4°C. Blood donations should be kept at room temperature after collection, and platelets separated as soon as possible. Although function is maintained when platelet preparations are stored at 4°C, post-transfusion survival is poor and any haemostatic effect is short lived. Storage at 20–22°C is therefore preferable. Platelets have a shelf-life of 5 days, in packs of plastics used for 'extended storage'. These allow the diffusion of oxygen into the pack, which, with constant gentle agitation, reduces the rate of fall of pH. The shelf-life of platelet preparations can be extended to 7 days, provided that systems are in place to monitor bacterial contamination.

Platelet pools provide an adequate adult dose of platelets and contain, on average 300×10^9 platelets, usually from four donations suspended in the plasma from one donation. White cell contamination should be reduced to a minimum in platelet concentrates, as this is the cause of non-haemolytic febrile transfusion reactions due mostly to the reaction of white cells with antibodies in the recipient and to cytokine release in storage. With leucodepletion, this is no longer a problem (Figure 16.2).

In the USA, platelets are prepared from individual donations by a method which leaves the platelet-rich plasma as a supernatant. Each platelet concentrate contains a minimum of 5.5×10^{10} platelets, suspended in 50 mL of plasma. An adult dose of platelets prepared in this way contains significantly more leucocytes than the platelet concentrates prepared by 'top and bottom' systems and which are considered to be leucocyte poor, even before leucodepletion.

The equivalent of two or even three adult doses of platelets (minimum 2.4×10^{11} each) may be obtained from one donor, with adequate platelet counts, by an apheresis procedure lasting approximately 90 min. At present, in the UK, approximately 40% of platelets are produced by this method, using Gambro, Baxter or Haemonetics cell separators. These preparations reduce donor exposure and are invaluable for the treatment of immunologically refractory thrombocytopenic patients requiring human leucocyte antigen (HLA)-matched platelets. However, they are expensive to produce and demanding on both staff and donors. A large HLA-typed donor panel is needed to provide HLA-compatible platelets. A proportion of apheresis platelet donors are also HPA typed.

Frozen platelets can be preserved in dimethyl sulphoxide (DMSO) or glycerol. The platelet recovery is significantly lower than with fresh preparations, but the post-transfusion survival is normal. Frozen platelets are very seldom used and are not available in the UK.

Granulocyte concentrates

Granulocytes are extremely labile; they must be separated from whole blood immediately after collection and transfused within hours of preparation. Granulocytes prepared from routine blood donations ('buffy coats') are heavily contaminated with red cells and platelets. Buffy coats from at least 10 donors are required to produce a therapeutic dose for an adult (at least 1×10^{10} granulocytes). Ten buffy coats also contain the equivalent of two units of red cells and 2.5 pools of platelets. Venesection of the recipient may therefore be required if daily buffy coats are indicated. Granulocyte concentrates prepared by apheresis are the only satisfactory means of achieving a therapeutic dose for an adult neutropenic patient. Sedimenting agents (gelatin, hydroxyethyl starch) must be added to the blood or given to the donor in order to obtain an adequate yield, unless the donor has chronic granulocytic leukaemia.

A directed donation from a suitable relative may sometimes be possible. Consent may then be obtained for the donors to have their counts boosted using steroids and granulocyte colony-stimulating factor (G-CSF), resulting in an excellent yield of granulocytes. In the UK, it is not permitted for non-directed volunteer donors to receive this medication. Average yields from unstimulated apheresis collections are 0.7×10^{10}; with the use of G-CSF and steroids, this can be increased to $5–10 \times 10^{10}$.

Fresh-frozen plasma

This plasma has been separated from whole blood (Figure 16.1) or obtained by apheresis, and frozen within 8 h, to a temperature that will maintain the activity of the labile factors V and VIII. FFP contains all coagulation factors and should be stored at –30°C or below for up to 24 months or even longer. When needed, the plasma is thawed rapidly at 37°C and then transfused without delay. A dose of 15 mL/kg is appropriate to correct abnormal coagulation in acquired coagulopathies when no concentrate is available. It may be used to reverse the effects of warfarin, and can be used to treat inherited coagulation factor deficiencies if the appropriate factor concentrates are not available.

Single units of FFP can be treated with methylene blue (MB) and exposed to visible light to inactivate pathogens that may be present in the plasma. If required, the MB can be removed before the plasma is rapidly frozen to –30°C. FFP can be pooled with around 1500 other units and treated with solvent–detergent (SD) in order to inactivate pathogens. Both these methods of viral inactivation reduce the levels of labile clotting factors in FFP. FFP or standard cryosupernatant are the products of choice for the treatment of thrombotic thrombocytopenic purpura (TTP) in the UK.

Cryoprecipitate

Cryoprecipitate is prepared from blood within 8 h of collection (Figure 16.1). Plasma is separated, frozen and allowed to thaw (classically at 4°C, overnight). After removal of the supernatant, the factor VIII:C, vW factor, fibrinogen, fibronectin and FXIII are left as a precipitate, which is then refrozen in approximately 15 mL of plasma, and stored at –30°C or below for up to 24 months. Each unit should contain a minimum of 70 IU of factor VIII:C and 140 mg of fibrinogen. Cryoprecipitate is now used mainly as a source of fibrinogen in cases of disseminated intravascular coagulation (DIC), hepatic failure and hypofibrinogenaemia. Where coagulation factor concentrate is not available, cryoprecipitate is effective in the management of von Willebrand's disease, but is not the product of choice. A standard adult dose of cryoprecipitate is 10 units, which are thawed at 37°C in about 10 min and should be used immediately.

Cryoprecipitate-poor plasma (cryosupernatant)

This term is used for the remaining plasma after the removal of cryoprecipitate. The main and specific indication for cryosupernatant is for plasma exchange in TTP. This is an immune-mediated condition in which there is an autoantibody directed against a vWF cleaving metalloproteinase. The resulting accumulation of high-molecular-weight (HMV) vWF multimers contributes to the pathophysiology of the condition with thrombosis in the microvasculature. Cryosupernatant supplies both more of the metalloproteinase, and lacks the HMW multimers, so it can be used to correct both abnormalities. It is stored frozen at –30°C or below for up to 24 months.

Table 16.6 Preoperative assessment.

Take a full history and examination, including previous surgical episodes and bleeding history

Arrange full blood count, group and antibody screen, routine chemistry, coagulation screen (if indicated) and tube for haematinics assessment (ferritin level for iron stores, vitamin B_{12} and folic acid), which can be put on hold pending full blood count (FBC) results

Consider autologous pre-deposit if patient is fit enough and greater than 50% likelihood of significant blood loss requiring transfusion or if rare atypical red cell antibodies are present

Consider using recombinant erythropoietin and/or intravenous iron sucrose, even with normal haemoglobin, at a dose of 600 IU/kg weekly for 4 weeks preoperatively

Prescribe iron and folic acid supplement if any suspicion of iron deficiency

Establish whether patient is taking regular aspirin, NSAIDS or warfarin and, whenever possible, make necessary arrangements to stop this drug 7 days preoperatively

The recipient (Table 16.6)

Preoperative assessment

Growing pressure on hospital beds and increasing use of day surgery means that a preoperative assessment should be performed before admission. This allows for efficient use of hospital resources and limits the number of cancelled operations. The key aims are to assess a patient's fitness to undergo surgery and anaesthesia, anticipate complications, arrange for supportive therapy to be available perioperatively and to liaise with the appropriate specialists regarding non-surgical management. This assessment needs to take place at a presurgical clinic at least 1 month before the planned date of surgery. After the clinic, it is imperative that the results are seen so that the necessary action can be taken for each patient.

Only a small proportion (1.0–1.5%) of potential recipients will have red cell alloantibodies other than anti-D; however, routine pretransfusion antibody screening will allow blood bank staff to identify those samples that need detailed investigation well in advance of the planned transfusion.

Laboratory tests

Pretransfusion group and screen

The ABO and RhD groups of all potential recipients should be determined before transfusion. No other blood groups are routinely tested or matched when selecting blood for transfusion. The need for blood is rarely so urgent that there is insufficient time to perform the ABO and RhD groups before transfusion, as rapid testing need take only 5–10 min. The patient's serum should also be screened for the presence of atypical red cell antibodies using a sensitive indirect antiglobulin technique, with two or three individual (not pooled) group O red cells selected to express, between them, all the common red cell antigens. If a positive result is obtained, further investigation using a red cell panel of 8–10 cells is required to identify the antibody.

For patients who have preformed antibodies, an antibody screen using a panel of cells that are negative for the pertinent antigen(s) should be used (i.e. panel of rr cells in the case of preformed anti-D). Only 1–2% of patients have clinically significant red cell alloantibodies. About 75% of these antibodies have Rh and/or K specificity. Therefore, patients with haematological diseases who are likely to need repeated transfusion over many years should ideally be phenotyped for the major red cells antigens; if this is not possible, at least RhD, C, c, E, e and K typing should be performed. Blood that is compatible with the patient's Rh and K type should be transfused, as this reduces the probability that they will produce antibodies. Ideally, girls and women of childbearing age should be transfused with K-negative red cells, but K typing is not necessary as only 9% will be positive.

Red cells for transfusion are selected to be of the same ABO and RhD group as the recipient. If clinically significant red cell alloantibodies are present in the recipient, units of blood lacking the relevant antigens are selected for compatibility testing, even if the maximum surgical blood ordering schedule (SBOS, see below) only requires 'group and screen' for that surgical procedure.

Compatibility testing (cross-match)

The donor red cells are routinely tested against the recipient serum or plasma in order to detect any potential incompatibilities, i.e. to identify any antibodies in the recipient that are reactive with antigens on the red cells of the selected donor. This test will provide a means of checking the ABO compatibility of donor and recipient. If the antibody screen is negative, then the cross-match should be as simple as possible, for example an immediate spin or indirect antiglobulin test at 37°C. This will detect ABO incompatibilities resulting from clerical or technical errors such as sample switching or erroneous group in the bag, or the presence of antibodies missed in the screening. The antiglobulin test can be performed in low-ionic-strength solution (LISS) in tubes or using gel (column) techniques (see Chapter 14) that decrease the incubation time and increase the sensitivity for the detection of some antibodies. Tests should be carried out at 37°C, not at room temperature, otherwise clinically insignificant cold antibodies will be detected, especially when LISS is used. This may cause confusion and inconvenience to the recipient (e.g. cancellation of planned surgery). Any clinically significant antibody will react at 37°C (see Chapter 14), and the techniques chosen should take this into account.

A group and screen policy used in combination with a maximum (or standard) surgical blood ordering schedule (MSBOS) can reduce the number of compatibility tests performed. Each hospital should agree its own MSBOS among the blood bank, surgeons and anaesthetists, through the Hospital Transfusion Committee (HTC). It is based on a retrospective comparison of the number of units of blood cross matched, and the number actually transfused for each elective surgical procedure. Procedures that are likely to require blood have a ratio of cross-matched:transfused blood below 2.5:1.0. All patients awaiting surgery have blood samples taken for grouping and antibody screening. As long as no atypical alloantibodies are detected, cross-matching is reserved for those in whom the need for blood is fairly certain. Operations for which blood is not usually required (such as hysterectomy and cholecystectomy) are not covered by cross-matched blood. If blood is unexpectedly needed, an abbreviated cross-match (using an immediate spin technique to ensure ABO compatibility) may be used safely, with minimal risk to the recipient. If atypical antibodies are detected, antigen-negative blood should be cross-matched before surgery if there is any minimal likelihood of blood being required.

Electronic cross-match

A number of hospitals with suitable blood bank computing systems now use a so-called 'electronic cross-match' or 'electronic issue'. A patient has group and screen performed on two separate occasions. If both screen results on the laboratory's computer system are negative, and if no blood has been transfused during this period, ABO and Rh compatible blood is issued directly via the computer with no further wet testing being performed. This makes it possible to reduce the number of operations for which blood is issued in advance even further, as the electronic cross-match is very quick. It also saves laboratory time, which can then be dedicated to more complex problems.

Antenatal testing

All women should have blood samples taken at antenatal booking for blood grouping and antibody screening. If no clinically significant antibody is detected, further samples should be tested at 28 weeks' gestation (see p. 271). Much of the emergency compatibility testing for possible Caesarean sections can be avoided by performing another antibody screen and group at admission, using either an abbreviated or electronic cross-match should blood be required.

Repeated transfusions

Patients who require repeat transfusion after an interval of more than 72 h must have a new sample sent before the next transfusion to detect any clinically significant antibody that may have been stimulated in an anamnestic response by the recent transfusion. Severe haemolytic transfusion reactions still occur due to failure to observe this simple rule; many could be avoided. In the case of an undetected haemolytic transfusion reaction, in addition to the antibody screen, a direct antiglobulin test (DAT) should be performed on the red cells of the new sample to detect any alloantibodies attached to donor red cells but not free in the serum.

Massive transfusion

If the total blood volume has been replaced within less than 24 h, compatibility testing becomes academic. In such patients, inter-donor incompatibility is a possible problem, but all donor sera should have been screened at the transfusion centre for the presence of potent atypical antibodies. When a pretransfusion alloantibody screen on the recipient has not detected any atypical antibodies and blood has been cross-matched without a problem then continued compatibility testing may be omitted. If a pretransfusion screen reveals the presence of an atypical antibody, the blood selected should be negative for the relevant antigen. Once transfusion has commenced, the antibody will be 'diluted out' and compatibility testing may no longer be reliable, unless the original serum sample is used for all testing. In practice, once 10 units have been transfused there is no need to continue to cross-match red cells for further transfusions, or to select antigen-negative red cells, if these are scarce.

Transfusion in autoimmune haemolytic anaemia

Ideally, patients with this condition should not be transfused. However, if transfusion is imperative, special serological techniques such as elution and absorption should be used to exclude the presence of alloantibodies, which may be masked by auto-antibodies. Blood should then be selected which is compatible with the alloantibody, if present, even though transfused red cells will be destroyed by the autoantibody at the same rate as the patient's own blood. Whenever possible, red cells should also be Rh- and K-compatible to reduce the possibility of further allo-immunization. Blood that does not express the antigen to which the autoantibody is directed against should be issued only when the autoantibody has restricted specificity and mimicks an alloantibody such as anti-e. However, if the patient is a female of childbearing age and is RhD-negative, with an autoantibody mimicking anti-e, then R_2R_2 (cDE/cDE) cells should not be given because of the high risk of RhD immunization.

Neonatal 'top-up' transfusion

Premature infants are amongst the most widely transfused patients, with 'top-up' transfusions being very frequent. Only the first pretransfusion sample needs to be tested, with no further sample testing until 4 months of age, as infants are not cap-able of making clinically significant antibodies in the first months of life. Ideally, the unit of red cells used for the first transfusion should be aliquoted into several (six to eight) satellite packs and used for the same infant until expiry, to decrease exposure to multiple donors. Measures should be in place in all neonatal units and their supporting laboratories to minimize the quantities of blood required for testing, by use of microsampling techniques and near-patient testing. Anaemia in this group is largely due to 'bleeding into the laboratory'. Erythropoietin has been extensively studied as an alternative to transfusion in the anaemia of prematurity but it does not consistently reduce the need for transfusion in this group.

Complications of blood transfusion

The frequency of the complications of blood transfusion will vary inversely with the care exercised in the preparation for, and especially in the supervision of the transfusion.

Although the majority of side-effects are mild, the overall incidence of complications is estimated at 2–5%. Immediate fatalities, although difficult to quantify accurately, are of the order of 1 in 100 000–500 000 patients transfused; 50% of these are caused by ABO incompatibilities, mainly due to failure to identify correctly the donor or recipient, at the time of sampling or at the time of transfusion. The wrong pack of blood, i.e. one intended for a different recipient, is reported to be given in 1 in 6000–30 000 transfusions. This is likely to be an underestimate due to underdetection and non-reporting of incidents. It follows that transfusions of blood and blood components should only be prescribed when there is a definite and appropriate clinical indication, when there are no feasible alternatives and when the benefits of transfusion are judged by the prescribing clinician to outweigh its short- and longer term risks.

The complications of blood transfusion can be conveniently divided into acute and delayed, immunological and non-immunological categories (Table 16.7).

Immunological complications

Sensitization to red cell antigens
As only the ABO and RhD antigens are routinely matched in blood transfusion; there is a constant possibility of sensitization to other red cell antigens. This is more likely in multitransfused patients. The consequences may be negligible but can lead to difficulty with compatibility testing, HDN and haemolytic transfusion reactions.

Haemolytic transfusion reactions
This is premature destruction of transfused red cells reacting with antibodies in the recipient. Red cell alloantibodies form in response to exposure, through previous transfusions or pregnancies, and are not naturally occurring. Such reactions may

Table 16.7 Hazards of transfusion

	Non-immune complications	Immune complications
Acute	Bacterial: acute sepsis or endotoxic shock	Febrile non-haemolytic transfusion reactions
	Hypothermia	Acute haemolytic transfusion reactions: intravascular (IgM), extravascular (IgG)
	Hypocalcaemia ($\downarrow Ca^{2+}$) in infants	Allergic reactions (urticarial)
	Air embolism rare	Anaphylactic reactions (anti-IgA)
		TRALI (transfusion-related acute lung injury)
Delayed (days to years after transfusion)	HIV	Delayed haemolytic transfusion reactions (due to anamnestic immune responses with red cell alloantibodies)
	Hepatitis C	Post-transfusion purpura (PTP)
	Hepatitis B	Transfusion-associated graft-versus-host disease (TA-GvHD)
	CMV	Immune modulation
	Others: parvovirus B19; hepatitis A; malaria; Chagas' disease; brucellosis; syphilis; vCJD?	

occur immediately after the transfusion, or may be delayed for anything up to 2–3 weeks.

Immediate haemolytic transfusion reactions

Immediate, intravascular destruction of recipient red cells should be avoidable. In practice, the main cause is error, when the incorrect blood component is transfused. The most severe reactions occur in major incompatibility, when a group O recipient with high-titre anti-A and/or anti-B, is transfused with group A, B or AB red cells. Less severe intravascular haemolysis occurs when group A red cells are transfused to a group B recipient, or vice versa, because group B and A subjects have less potent ABO antibodies than those of group O. More rarely, intravascular red cell destruction may occur when group O plasma is transfused, by mistake, to A, B or AB recipients. For this reason, group O blood should not routinely be used for non-O recipients; furthermore, this practice leads to unnecessary shortages of group O blood. If unavoidable, the group O blood must first be screened for the presence of high-titre haemolysins or be devoid of plasma.

In the UK, screening for high-titre ABO antibodies is routinely carried out at the blood centre and marked on the bag. ABO-compatible cryoprecipitate, FFP and platelet transfusions should be selected for all recipients, especially for children because of their smaller blood volume. Group A, B or AB plasma components are safe for group O recipients.

Occasionally, there is a laboratory error when antibodies in the recipient's plasma are not detected (or there is insufficient time to complete an antibody screen or compatibility test). In the UK haemovigilance system (SHOT), 30% of reported cases of incorrect blood components transfused were due to clerical or technical errors that originated in the hospital laboratory. The remainder of reports (70%) relate to clerical or administrative errors in the ward, collection of the blood from the blood bank, failure to confirm the identity of the patient when taking samples, mislabelling of the sample of blood or failure to perform proper checks before removing the units from the fridge or transfusing the blood. The serious consequences of such failures emphasize the need for set protocols for meticulous checks at all stages. If an identification mistake has been made, it is important to check, as a matter of urgency, that the units intended for the patient under study have not been misdirected to another recipient.

Intravascular red cell destruction is the most dangerous type of haemolytic transfusion reaction; it is associated with activation of the full complement cascade by IgM antibodies and is practically always due to ABO-incompatible blood transfusions (haemolytic anti-A,B, anti-A or anti-B present mainly in the recipient or, rarely, in the donor plasma). Most of these ABO incompatible transfusions are due to identification errors, and occur with an approximate frequency of 1 in 100 000 patients transfused. The mortality rate in such ABO-incompatible cases is 5–10%. In a further 10–15% of cases there is some morbidity.

The symptoms in the recipient are usually dramatic and severe; most are due to anaphylatoxins C3a and C5a that are liberated during complement activation (see Chapter 14), although the cytokines interleukin 1 (IL-I), IL-8 and tumour necrosis factor also play an important role. These molecules cause smooth muscle contraction, platelet aggregation, increased capillary permeability, and release of vasoactive amines and hydrolases from mast cells and granulocytes respectively. Typically, within less than 1 h of the start of the transfusion, when the reaction is symptomatic, the patient complains of heat or pain in the cannulated vein, throbbing in the head, flushing of the face, chest tightness, nausea and lumbar pain. These symptoms are

Table 16.8 Antibodies associated with haemolytic transfusion reactions.

Blood group system	Antibodies implicated in intravascular haemolysis	Antibodies implicated in extravascular haemolysis
ABO	A, B	
Hh	H (Bombay)	
Rh		All
Kell		K, k, Kp^a, Kp^b, Js^a, Js^b
Kidd		Jk^a, Jk^b, Jk^3
Duffy		Fy^a, Fy^b, Fy^3
MNS		M, S, s, U (some)
Lutheran		Lu^b (some)
Lewis	Le^a, Le^b, Le^{a+b}	
Cartwright		Yt^a (some)
Vel	Vel	Vel (some)
Colton		Co^a, Co^b
Dombrock		Do^a, Do^b

usually accompanied by tachycardia and hypotension. In severe cases, there is profound hypotension and collapse. Rigors and pyrexia usually follow. Intravascular destruction of red cells brings about liberation of thromboplastin-like substances that activate the coagulation cascade and lead to DIC. The bleeding diathesis and increased destruction of red cells (which may eventually involve the recipient's cells) further exacerbates the problem.

Intravascular destruction of red cells liberates Hb into the circulation. Once haptoglobins are saturated, Hb will also appear in the urine. If haemoglobinuria is very severe, haemosiderinuria may be seen. Renal complications consist of acute renal failure with oliguria and anuria, possibly the result of hypotension and/or the action of activated complement.

The initial symptoms may of course be modified or abolished in anaesthetized or heavily sedated patients, in whom evidence of DIC, hypotension or the presence of haemoglobinuria may be the first signs.

Haemoglobinaemia and haemoglobinuria may also be seen in severe extravascular haemolytic transfusion reactions (see below) and, occasionally, after the transfusion of lysed red cells. This may occur in the following circumstances: inappropriate warming and overheating of blood; exposure to extreme cold due to faulty storage conditions; lysis due to mechanical problems during administration; or due to the injection of 5% dextrose with the transfused red cells. Severe fulminant toxic symptoms leading to death, similar to those of intravascular haemolytic transfusion reactions, can be seen after the transfusion of bacterially infected blood, especially if it contains endotoxin-producing organisms (e.g. *Staphylococcus* and *Yersinia* species). Haemoglobinaemia and haemoglobinuria may also follow transfusion of blood to a patient with severe autoimmune haemolytic anaemia, due to an increase in the number of red cells in the circulation which will be subject to immune lysis.

Extravascular red cell destruction is mediated by IgG antibodies (Table 16.8). Mononuclear phagocytic cells have receptors for the Fc fragment of IgG1 and IgG3; the binding of IgG-coated cells to these receptors is inhibited by free IgG in plasma. There are no receptors for IgM on macrophages. Red cells sensitized with IgG1 and/or IgG3 antibodies, may or may not activate complement up to C3b only. If they do not, they are removed extravascularly (phagocytosis or cytotoxicity) by mononuclear phagocytic cells, predominantly in the red pulp of the spleen, where the plasma is largely excluded and the IgG on the red cells can compete with free IgG in the plasma. However, cells coated with IgG antibodies, which activate complement up to C3b, adhere to the C3b receptor on macrophages and monocytes. The presence of C3b on red cells greatly enhances the extravascular destruction of IgG-coated cells. This is because the binding to C3b receptors is not inhibited as there is no native C3b in plasma and consequently IgG-/C3b-coated cells are destroyed by phagocytosis or cytotoxicity, predominantly in the liver, where there are abundant macrophages (Kupffer cells) and a generous blood flow. As C3b is rapidly inactivated by the actions of factors H, I and proteases, a proportion of the cells re-enter the circulation coated with C3dg and are resistant to further lysis (Figure 16.3). Red cells coated with potent IgG antibodies, especially if they are C3b-binding, are destroyed mainly by cytotoxicity. Very rarely, red cell alloantibodies too weak to be detectable by routine pretransfusion testing may destroy donor red blood cells carrying the corresponding antigen.

The features of an immediate haemolytic transfusion reaction vary according to a number of factors: whether the red cells are destroyed within the circulation or in the reticuloendothelial (RE) system; the strength, class and subclass of antibody; the nature of the antigen; the number of incompatible red cells transfused; and the clinical state of the patient. When antibodies are present in the circulation in low titres and a large volume

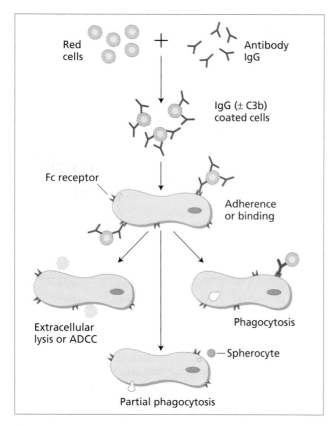

Figure 16.3 Mechanisms of extravascular destruction of red cells coated with IgG1 or IgG3 (± C3b). ADCC, antibody-dependent cell-mediated cytotoxicity.

of incompatible blood is given, all circulating antibody will bind to the incompatible red cells, coating them weakly without destroying them. There will then be no antibody detectable in the serum for a number of days until secondary antibody production is stimulated by the immune challenge. In the presence of an overloaded or poorly functioning RE system, large volumes of IgG-sensitized incompatible red cells can be present in the circulation with minimal or no premature removal, so the Hb level may be stable with little evidence of haemolysis. The DAT will be positive, but as there is no free antibody, elution techniques will be necessary for antibody identification.

Immediate extravascular destruction of red cells may be accompanied by hyperbilirubinaemia, occasionally haemoglobinaemia due to antibody-dependent cytotoxicity (in severe cases), fever and failure to achieve the expected rise in Hb level. The signs and symptoms are less severe and dramatic than in intravascular haemolysis and usually appear more than 1 h after the start of transfusion (Table 16.8). There may be no signs or symptoms at all. Renal failure is very rare, even when the antibody binds the earlier components of the complement cascade. The symptoms are attributed in a large degree to liberation of cytokines from mononuclear phagocytic cells after binding to

IgG-coated red cells and to liberation of C3a when complement is bound up to C3b. The mortality is extremely low, but, in an already sick patient, the added complication of destruction of transfused red cells may contribute to death.

The management of immediate haemolytic transfusion reactions should be to terminate the transfusion immediately the patient develops the appropriate signs or symptoms. The identity of the patient and the units transfused should be checked against the appropriate documentation. Blood samples must be taken for investigation as in Table 16.9.

The circulating blood volume should be restored and the blood pressure and urinary flow maintained using fluid challenges and furosemide (frusemide) infusion. Monitoring on a high-dependency unit may be required. The renal team should be involved early if urine output is poor (< 1 mL/kg/h) and haemofiltration may be necessary. Appropriate blood component therapy will be required if there is DIC.

All packs of transfused units should be returned to the blood bank. Pretransfusion samples should be tested in parallel. If no identification mistake is discovered immediately, a sample should be sent for bacteriological testing and all urine passed during the first 24 h should be measured and examined for Hb. Subsequent management depends upon awareness of the possible complications and prompt therapy if these occur. If the patient develops only a rise in temperature, unaccompanied by other symptoms, red cell incompatibility is unlikely and the transfusion should be slowed, under strict monitoring, but need not be stopped.

New technologies to prevent patient identification errors are under investigation in a number of countries. These generally involve bar-coded patient ID details on the patient's wristband and the use, both on the wards and in the laboratory, of a hand-held bar-code reader with all data collated by the transfusion computer system. These systems are likely to be developed in tandem with similar arrangements for pharmacy and drug prescriptions, as well as ordering of blood tests and other investigations for patients.

Delayed haemolytic transfusion reactions

Such reactions are neither predictable nor preventable. In the majority of cases, an individual has been previously sensitized to one (or more) red cell antigen(s) by previous transfusion or pregnancy. Antibody is not detectable in routine pretransfusion testing, but the transfusion of blood containing the antigens to which the recipient has been sensitized previously provokes a brisk anamnestic response that is characteristic of the secondary immune response. Within days, the antibody level rises and the transfused cells are removed from the circulation. The effects of the secondary immunization are usually seen about 5–10 days after the transfusion, when the recipient may already have left hospital.

The clinical features of this type of reaction are the triad of fever, hyperbilirubinaemia and anaemia. The degree of fall in

Table 16.9 Investigation of suspected acute haemolytic transfusion reaction.

Blood test	Rationale/findings
FBC	Baseline parameters, red cell agglutinates on film
Plasma/urinary Hb, haptoglobin, bilirubin	Evidence of intravascular or extravascular haemolysis
Blood group of patient and units transfused	Compare with retested pretransfusion sample, to detect ABO error. Unexpected ABO antibodies may arise from transfusion of incompatible plasma. Rechecking labels is often sufficient
DAT	Positive in majority. Compare with retested pretransfusion sample. May be negative if all incompatible cells destroyed
Compatibility testing	Repeat antibody screen and compatibility testing on pre- and post-transfusion samples. Elution of antibody from post-transfusion cells may aid antibody identification or confirm specificities in plasma in cases of non-ABO incompatibility
Urea, electrolytes and creatinine	Baseline renal function
Coagulation screen	Detection and monitoring of DIC
Blood cultures	In event of possible septic reaction caused by bacterial contamination of unit

Hb level will of course depend upon the number of incompatible units transfused.

The possibility of delayed haemolytic reactions underlines the importance of always taking fresh serum samples for antibody screening, direct antiglobulin test and compatibility testing if a transfusion has been given more than 72 h previously. Awareness of this complication may avoid unnecessary investigations to exclude infection when fever develops a few days after a transfusion. Most importantly, it will detect any alloantibody that will have been boosted by the transfusion, thus enabling the provision of compatible blood.

Reactions due to white cell and platelet antibodies

Febrile transfusion reactions
Febrile reactions are most frequently due to sensitization to white cell antigens and more rarely to platelet antigens. Together with urticaria, these are the most common type of immunological reaction to blood transfusion. Antibodies are directed usually against HLA antigens, or sometimes against granulocyte and platelet-specific antigens; they are stimulated by previous transfusions or pregnancies. Cytokines released from white cells during storage may also be pyrogenic. Characteristically, the onset of the reaction is delayed until 30–90 min after the start of the transfusion (depending upon the strength of antibody and the speed of transfusion). A rise in temperature may be the sole symptom, but the recipient may suffer chills, headache or rigors. There is no associated hypotension, lumbar pain or chest discomfort. These reactions are usually only troublesome rather than dangerous, except in very sick patients or in the presence of very potent lymphocytotoxic HLA antibodies.

The management of a simple, mild febrile transfusion reaction is to slow the rate of transfusion and treat the patient with an antipyretic such as paracetamol. Antihistamines are of no benefit. It is usually not necessary to discontinue the transfusion: more blood is probably wasted by premature termination of a unit due to a simple febrile reaction than for any other reason.

When a patient requiring repeated transfusions has a history of simple febrile reactions, the rate of transfusion should be kept slow and antipyretics should be prescribed prophylactically. If symptoms recur with repeated transfusions, buffy coat-poor red cells and platelets should be tried. If severe symptoms persist, tests for HLA antibodies (lymphocytotoxicity) should be carried out. If these are negative, platelet antibodies should be sought. Patients with troublesome symptoms in whom white cell antibodies have been demonstrated should be given white cell-depleted blood. Modern prestorage leucodepletion filters are highly efficient and can remove more than 98% of the white cells; the specification is that 99% of leucodepleted components should have $< 5 \times 10^6$ leucocytes. Red cells and platelets should be filtered as soon as possible after collection in the transfusion centre. In the UK, the incidence of febrile transfusion reactions has decreased significantly since the introduction of universal leucodepletion of blood components in 1999.

In countries where there is no universal leucodepletion policy, there is no need to administer white cell-depleted blood prophylactically, except in cases where prevention of sensitization to HLA and leucocyte/platelet antigens is essential (i.e. possible future consideration for bone marrow transplantation, especially in patients with aplastic anaemia).

Transfusion-related acute lung injury

Transfusion-related acute lung injury (TRALI) consists of pulmonary infiltrates on chest radiograph, accompanied by chills, fever, cough and dyspnoea with low oxygen saturation and low or normal central venous pressure. The clinical picture, depending on the severity, will be the same as acute lung injury (ALI) or acute respiratory distress syndrome (ARDS) due to other causes, and a differential diagnosis is essential. Symptoms develop very rapidly usually within 1–2 h, or up to 6 h after infusion of a plasma-containing component.

Management is essentially supportive, requiring high-dependency unit care, and careful attention to fluid balance. The reaction is due in most cases to passive transfer of leucoagglutinins (mostly anti-HLA class I or class II or granulocyte antibodies, i.e. anti-HNA) in donor plasma, leading to endothelial and epithelial injury, alveolar damage and inflammatory changes, mediated by cytokines and other inflammatory mediators. The donors are usually multiparous women; once identified as the source of a reaction, such donors should be removed from the panel, even although it is known that their plasma will not always lead to TRALI in recipients with the pertinent antigens. The incidence is unclear but may be in the region of 1 in 5000 transfusions. There appears to be a significant mortality rate from this condition.

Post-transfusion purpura

Post-transfusion purpura is a rare complication of blood transfusion, characterized by a sudden onset of severe thrombocytopenia 7–10 days after the transfusion of platelet-containing blood components, usually red cells. The patient always has a history of previous blood transfusions or pregnancies (thus it is far more common in women). The most frequent cause is the presence in the recipient of an antibody (anti-HPA-1a) against the platelet-specific antigen HPA-1a (PI^{A1}). It appears that the antigen–antibody reaction between the recipient's antibody and the donor platelets causes both transfused and autologous platelets to be prematurely destroyed, either by the formation of immune complexes (in a manner similar to the 'innocent bystander' mechanism) or by cross-reaction of the causative antibody with the patient's own platelets. The disease is self limiting but, in severe cases, or if bleeding occurs, prompt therapy with intravenous immunoglobulin or plasma exchange is indicated. Platelet transfusion is not recommended, as this may exacerbate the disease process.

Reactions due to plasma protein antibodies

Mild urticarial reactions without other symptoms are not uncommon during blood transfusion; they occur with an approximate incidence of 1% and are mediated by IgE antibodies, usually against plasma proteins or other allergens present in donor plasma. Mild urticarial reactions may be treated effectively with antihistamines, and do not always recur. There is no necessity to avoid transfusion of standard 'bank blood' unless symptoms are recurrent and severe. On the other hand, severe anaphylactic reactions accompanied by dyspnoea, wheezing, collapse and shock are rare and potentially fatal. Such reactions are associated with the presence of anti-IgA in an IgA-deficient recipient. These antibodies react with IgA in the transfused plasma and complement is activated, with the consequent liberation of anaphylatoxins C3a and C5a, leukotrienes and cytokines.

Milder reactions may be associated with anti-IgA of limited specificity. If an anaphylactic reaction occurs, the recipient should be treated promptly with adrenaline and tested for the presence of plasma protein antibodies. If anti-IgA is detected, plasma from IgA-deficient donors should be used in future, as well as well-washed red cells and platelets. Occasionally, washed cells may be indicated for patients with serious urticarial or severe hypersensitivity reactions due to non-IgA antibodies.

Non-immunological complications

Disease transmission

See p. 251.

Reactions due to bacterial pyrogens and bacteria

The presence of bacteria in transfused blood may lead either to febrile reactions in the recipient (due to pyrogens) or to the far more serious manifestations of septic or endotoxic shock. Bacterial-transmitted infections are considerably more frequent than serious acute manifestations of virus-transmitted infections in countries such as the UK (see p. 255).

Bacterial pyrogens are rarely the cause of reactions with present-day methods of manufacture and the sterilization of fluids and disposable equipment. Infection of stored blood is also extremely rare, but has a very high mortality in recipients. Skin contaminants are sometimes present in freshly donated blood but many (e.g. staphylococci) do not survive storage at 4°C. However, they will grow profusely in platelet concentrates stored at 22°C. A number of Gram-negative psychrophilic, endotoxin-producing contaminants found readily in dirt, soil and faeces (pseudomonads, coliforms) may very rarely enter a unit and grow readily under the storage conditions of blood (and even more rapidly at room temperature).

Healthy individuals who are bacteraemic at the time of donation may also act as a source of infection. The majority of such cases relate to transmission of *Yersinia enterocolitica*, which grows well in red cell components due to its dependence on citrate and iron.

Transfusion of heavily contaminated blood will usually lead to sudden, dramatic symptoms, with collapse, high fever, shock and DIC with haemorrhagic phenomena. These symptoms resemble, and may be more severe than, those of ABO incompatibility. Prompt recognition of the cause and administration of broad-spectrum intravenous antibiotics, in conjunction with the treatment of shock, are vital. The diagnosis should be confirmed by direct microscopic examination of the blood, and blood cultures from the recipient and the blood bag.

Prevention of this potentially disastrous complication of blood transfusion rests on stringent observation of procedures for aseptic techniques in blood collection and in the manufacture of anticoagulant solutions and packs. Packs should never be opened for sampling, and the unit should be transfused within 24 h if any open method of preparation has been used (for example, washed red cells, frozen–thawed blood). Blood should always be kept in accurately controlled refrigerators (with alarms), maintained strictly at 2–6°C, and a unit of blood should never be removed and taken to the ward or theatre until it is required. The practice of obtaining multiple units of blood for the same patient, and leaving unused units at room temperature (or in uncontrolled ward refrigerators) until needed must not be tolerated. Bacteria may cause haemolysis or clotting of blood and all units should be inspected for these before transfusion. Platelets should be inspected for discoloration, foaming and absence of swirling.

Circulatory overload

All patients, except those who are actively bleeding or fluid depleted, will experience a temporary rise in blood volume and venous pressure after the transfusion of blood and/or plasma. In young people with normal cardiovascular function, this will not cause any embarrassment, providing the total volume given and the transfusion rate are not excessive. In contrast, pregnant women, patients with severe anaemia, and the elderly with compromised cardiovascular function will not tolerate the increase in plasma volume, and acute pulmonary oedema may develop. In view of this possibility, concentrated red cells should be given to these patients more slowly over 4 h. Patients with severe chronic anaemia and cardiac failure may require partial exchange transfusion. In less severe cases, diuretics (oral or intravenous furosemide) should be given at the start of the transfusion and only one or two units of concentrated red cells should be transfused in any 24 h period. The patient should be observed carefully for early signs of cardiac failure (raised jugular venous pressure, crepitations at the lung bases, and symptoms of pulmonary oedema, cough and breathlessness). For this reason alone, transfusions should be given during the day, when staff are able to monitor the patient closely. Overnight transfusions should be avoided for the patient's safety and comfort. If circulatory overload occurs, transfusion should be discontinued, the patient propped upright and intravenous diuretics given. Emergency venesection for fluid overload should not be necessary if all precautions have been taken.

Thrombophlebitis

Thrombophlebitis is a complication of indwelling venous cannulae, and not specifically related to blood transfusion.

Air embolism

This is now practically unknown, as blood and blood components are administered from plastic bags.

Transfusion haemosiderosis

Haemosiderosis is a very real complication of repeated blood transfusions, and is being seen more commonly as long-term blood transfusion therapy improves the survival of patients suffering from some chronic anaemias. It is most commonly seen in thalassaemic individuals, who commence transfusions in early childhood. Each unit of blood has approximately 200 mg of iron, whereas the daily excretion rate is about 1 mg: the body has no way of excreting the excess. Unless a patient is actively bleeding, and therefore losing iron, iron accumulation is inevitable. Significant iron overload is generally present after approximately 50 units of blood have been transfused to an average-sized adult. It is routine practice to give thalassaemic patients the parenteral iron-chelating agent desferrioxamine or the oral iron chelator deferiprone (L1) when available, or a combination of both. This does not completely overcome the iron load administered with blood, but has substantially delayed the onset of problems due to haemosiderosis (see Chapters 3 and 6).

Transfusion of neocytes, or young red cells, looked promising as a means of decreasing the frequency of transfusions and of reducing the iron load. However, this practice is expensive and time-consuming and the trial results were not as favourable as expected. Patients who are transfusion dependent should receive blood which is less than 1 week old, which may help to increase the transfusion interval and therefore reduce the overall number of units required.

Complications of massive transfusion

Massive transfusion is usually defined as the replacement of the total blood volume within a 24-h period. Although a number of different problems may result from changes that occur in stored blood, it should not be forgotten that any patient who needs a massive blood transfusion is by definition already seriously ill. Too much attention may be paid to the theoretical problems caused by metabolic changes in stored blood, and not enough to the underlying clinical condition. The coagulopathy problems derived from massive transfusion are different in trauma from those in elective surgery.

Although the transfusion problems encountered in cardiac surgery were in the past similar to those of massive transfusion, the volume of blood transfused to such patients is now insufficient to merit the routine administration of fresh blood or FFP. When post-operative bleeding occurs, this is usually due to platelet dysfunction and/or reduced numbers. Platelet transfusion is then indicated.

Replacement of the total blood volume will inevitably lead to some dilution of platelets. Blood effectively has no functional platelets after 48-h storage and once 8–10 units of blood have been given to an adult, thrombocytopenia will usually be seen. The severity will vary from patient to patient; in most elective surgery patients, the thrombocytopenia will reach a critical level only after 20 units of blood have been transfused. Bleeding due to a slightly low platelet count is uncommon, so that the routine administration of platelets after a set number of units of blood is unnecessary. Regular monitoring of the platelet count in these situations is far more helpful; platelet administration may then be judged on the clinical condition and the platelet count. As a guide, platelet transfusion may be required if the platelet count falls below 80×10^9/L in the face of continued bleeding or surgical intervention. Red cell transfusion contributes to normal haemostasis by helping with the margination of platelets and responsiveness of activated platelets, so it is recommended to aim for Hb levels around 10 g/dL if possible.

Coagulation factors will also be diluted as stored blood is administered. Whole blood that has been stored for less than 14 days has adequate levels of most coagulation factors for haemostasis (whole blood is not available in the UK). Factors V and VIII are the most labile but, in conditions of patient 'stress', factor VIII is released from endothelial cells; deficiency of factor VIII sufficient to cause bleeding does not usually occur in these circumstances. If stored blood that is more than 14 days old is given, or if plasma-reduced blood or red cells in optimal additive solution have been used, replacement of coagulation factors may become necessary. Treatment should be monitored by coagulation studies and DIC screen; FFP and cryoprecipitate, as a source of fibrinogen, should be prescribed on the basis of results from the laboratory or near-patient testing. Disseminated intravascular coagulation associated with massive transfusion is most usually due to the underlying condition, such as trauma and/or prolonged shock, and not due to transfused blood per se.

Metabolic changes in stored blood include low pH, hypocalcaemia and hyperkalaemia. The reduced oxygen-carrying capacity of stored blood becomes significant only after 21 days' storage (for CPD-AI blood), and is due to low 2,3-DPG levels (see p. 256). Although excess citrate in transfused blood could cause toxicity theoretically, its metabolism in the liver is usually rapid. In practice, the only situations when citrate toxicity is a real problem is with extremely rapid transfusion (1 unit every 5 min), or in infants, especially if premature, having exchange transfusion with blood stored in citrate for longer than 5 days. Hypocalcaemia and hyperkalaemia are usually transient and rapidly corrected once the transfused blood is circulating. Acidosis is not usually significant, as citrate metabolism leads to an alkalosis. However, if a patient is severely shocked and undertransfused, acidosis may be a clinical problem. All these changes due to stored blood are exacerbated by hypothermia. Cardiac irregularities, in particular ventricular fibrillation, may result from transfusion of large quantities of cold blood. The optimal functioning of coagulation factors and of platelets is also temperature dependent and effectiveness is reduced by hypothermia. Thus, the use of a blood warmer and keeping the patient warm may be the most important measures to prevent the complications of massive transfusion. Unfortunately, this inevitably reduces the speed at which blood can be transfused, which may be a serious disadvantage when rapid transfusion is needed. When replacement therapy has failed, recombinant

activated factor VII (rFVIIa) has been reported as successful in treating the coagulopathy of massive transfusion. However, more evidence is needed.

The most important consideration in massive blood transfusion is to replace blood loss quickly and adequately with maintenance of normal tissue perfusion. Too little blood too late has far more serious consequences than massive blood transfusion itself.

Haemovigilance and SHOT

The interest in transfusion-transmitted infections has meant that transfusion medicine has developed significantly and great emphasis has been put on quality, audit and good manufacturing practice (GMP). However, there were no surveillance systems in place to assess the incidence and prevalence of transfusion risks. France instituted the first system of national haemovigilance in 1994. Haemovigilance is defined as 'the set of procedures of surveillance organized from the collection of blood and its components to the follow-up of its recipients, with the purpose of collecting and evaluating information on the undesirable and unexpected effects resulting from the use of blood products and of preventing their occurrence'.

SHOT (Serious Hazards of Transfusion), the UK haemovigilance system was introduced in 1996 (Figure 16.4). SHOT receives reports of major adverse events surrounding the transfusion of single or small pool blood components supplied by the UK National Blood Services (red cells, platelets, FFP, methylene blue-treated FFP and cryoprecipitate). It does not cover complications of fractionated plasma products except for some incidents related to anti-D Ig administration. It is a confidential and anonymized scheme of voluntary reporting, though the

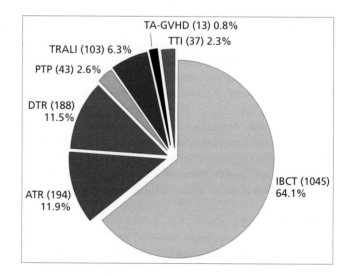

Figure 16.4 Cumulative data from 6 years of UK Haemovigilance (SHOT) reporting, 1996/97 to 2001/02. Completed questionnaires received, by transfusion incident, 1996/97–2001/02 ($n = 1630$).

European Directive will make reporting mandatory. Hospitals report events under the following categories:
- incorrect blood component transfused (IBCT), regardless of harm to recipients;
- acute transfusion reaction (ATR) within 24 h;
- delayed transfusion reaction (DTR) beyond 24 h;
- transfusion-associated graft-versus-host-disease (TA-GvHD);
- transfusion-related acute lung injury (TRALI);
- post-transfusion purpura (PTP);
- transfusion transmitted infection; (TTI) comprising
  - bacterial contamination;
  - post-transfusion viral infection;
  - other post-transfusion infection, e.g. malaria;
- 'Near miss' events (this has been introduced more recently).

Since 1996, the SHOT scheme has collected data on serious transfusion complications in the UK, from which to make firm recommendations for improvements in transfusion safety. The four UK Blood Services issue approximately 3.5 million blood components each year. Since 1996 there has been a year-on-year increase in the number of reports, with 405 eligible hospitals on the scheme. By the sixth year, participation was running at 93%. The increase in total reports is almost solely the result of an increase in 'incorrect blood component transfused' incidents.

Of 1630 fully analysed reports, the vast majority, i.e. 1045 (64.1%) were 'wrong blood' incidents. Of these, 193 were ABO-incompatible transfusions leading to 11 deaths and 41 cases of major morbidity, for example leading to intensive care unit admission; 92 were RhD incompatible, leading to possible RhD sensitization in females of childbearing potential.

Immune complications constituted 33.1% of reports, with 103 cases of possible TRALI, leading to 11 deaths that were definitely, or probably, related to transfusion, and a further 14 deaths possibly, making TRALI the second largest cause of transfusion-related mortality and morbidity after ABO incompatibility. A large proportion of cases reported as TRALI could not be confirmed in the laboratory.

TTI constituted less than 3% of reports. There were 36 confirmed TTIs of which the majority (22 cases) were of bacterial contamination (19 of platelets, three of red cells), resulting in six deaths.

The SHOT data demonstrate that in high-resource countries, microbiological, and especially virological, safety of the blood supply is advanced. Efforts should now be concentrated in preventing bacterial contamination and in other areas of transfusion medicine, such as the encouragement of appropriate use of blood, safe administration of blood components, accurate patient and sample identification, etc.

Appropriate use of blood and alternatives to allogeneic blood transfusion

In view of the inherent risks of blood transfusion and difficulties with donor recruitment due to escalating stringent donor selection criteria, blood components should only be transfused when the benefits outweigh the risks.

There are several reasons for aiming at reducing unnecessary allogeneic blood transfusion:
1 safety of the patient, by avoiding errors, as well as microbiological and immunological risks;
2 shortages of blood and increasing difficulties in the recruitment of blood donors;
3 cost containment;
4 high anxiety levels in patients that are disproportionate to the real residual risk of transfusion.

There are several alternatives to allogeneic blood transfusion, which can be classified as operational, biological and pharmacological, as listed below.

Operational alternatives

- Treatment of preoperative anaemia with haematinics, if appropriate, in a timely way at preassessment clinics.
- Autologous transfusion in all its forms. It seems that cell salvage is considerably more cost-effective than pre-deposit autologous transfusion. The value of preoperative haemodilution needs further assessment.
- Re-evaluation of transfusion triggers and algorithms for estimation of acceptable blood loss in surgery. Adherence to guidelines.
- Alternative fluid replacement (i.e. replace FFP with crystalloids or colloids when appropriate).
- Anaesthetic methods to reduce blood loss (e.g. hypotension).
- Enhancement of surgical haemostasis and new surgical technologies (e.g. water scalpels).
- Stopping aspirin, non-steroidal anti-inflammatory drugs (NSAIDS) and anticoagulants preoperatively.
- Post-operative haematinics.
- Near-patient testing in theatre.
- Miniaturizing blood sampling in intensive care units for premature babies and adults.
- Stem cell transplantation for transfusion-dependent patients (e.g. thalassaemia).

Biological alternatives

- Recombinant erythropoietin.
- Granulocyte colony-stimulating factor (G-CSF).
- Recombinant clotting factors.
- Recombinant activated factor (rVIIa).
- Fibrin glue in surgery.
- Probably in the future? Hb solutions and platelet substitutes.

Pharmacological alternatives

- Aprotinin in cardiac and liver surgery.
- Tranexamic acid infusion intra- or post-operatively.

- DDAVP® preoperatively in mild haemophiliacs.
- Intravenous iron, with or without recombinant erythropoietin (rEPO) preoperatively, especially in patients intolerant or unresponsive to oral iron.
- In the future? Oxygen carriers such as fluorocarbons.

Haemolytic disease of the newborn

Haemolytic disease of the newborn (HDN) is a condition in which the lifespan of the fetal/neonatal red cells is shortened due to maternal alloantibodies against red cell antigens inherited from the father. Maternal IgG can cross the placenta, thus IgG red cell alloantibodies can gain access to the fetus. If the fetal red cells contain the corresponding antigen then binding of antibody to red cells will occur. When the antibody is of clinical significance (e.g. anti-D, -c, -E, -K, -Jk^a), and of sufficient potency, the coated cells will be prematurely removed by the fetal mononuclear phagocytic system. The effects on the fetus/newborn infant may vary according to the characteristics of the maternal alloantibody.

The antibodies giving rise to HDN most commonly belong to the Rh or ABO blood group systems. The morbidity of Rh HDN is explained by the great immunogenicity of the D antigen; HDN due to anti-c is also important and its incidence comes second amongst the cases of severe HDN closely followed by the non-Rh antibody, anti-K. (The anaemia caused by anti-K is more properly called *alloimmune anaemia of the fetus and newborn* as it is due to direct inhibition of erythropoiesis by the antibody and haemolysis is not a feature.) Antibodies against antigens in almost all the blood group systems (e.g. Duffy, Kidd, etc.) and against the so-called 'public' and 'private' antigens, have also been responsible for HDN. However, IgM cannot cross the placenta and Lewis and P$_1$ antibodies, which occur frequently during pregnancy, are usually IgM and do not lead to HDN. Furthermore, the Lewis antigens are not fully developed at birth.

All women who have had previous pregnancies or blood transfusions may become immunized against 'foreign' red cell antigens. However, alloantibodies may be found in those with no such history, either because the antibodies are 'naturally occurring' or because a spontaneous abortion early in a previous pregnancy was unrecognized as such. Blood samples from all pregnant women must be tested early for the presence of atypical red cell antibodies (usually at 12–16 weeks, at the booking visit), and again at 28 weeks' gestation, even if no antibody was found at booking.

When anti-D, anti-c or anti-K are detected at booking, the strength of the antibody and the rate of rise (if any) in titre, or level in micrograms, during pregnancy must be carefully monitored by regular monthly blood sampling during the second trimester and fortnightly thereafter. If the level of any other clinically significant antibody is moderately high or high at 28 weeks, it should be monitored fortnightly until term. If the level

of anti-D is > 10 IU (2 µg) or anti-c > 20 IU, or if other antibodies have an IAT titre of 32 or greater, the fetus should be monitored by ultrasound/Doppler for evidence of anaemia and cardiac decompensation. At these levels, in the case of anti-D, -c or -K referral to a feto-maternal unit is advised. It should be noted that, in the case of potent anti-K, severe anaemia may occur relatively early during gestation.

Fetal and neonatal anaemia due to anti-D and anti-K tends to be more severe than that due to any other alloantibody. The next important in terms of severity is that due to anti-c. Anti-A,B is a common cause of HDN in group O mothers delivering group A or B infants (1 in 150 births), but the disease is usually mild; death *in utero* is unknown though exchange transfusion after birth may occasionally be required.

There are many significant differences between HDN due to ABO and Rh incompatibilities. The low incidence of infants requiring treatment for ABO HDN contrasts with the situation in Rh HDN. Furthermore, ABO HDN is found as frequently in the first pregnancy as in later pregnancies; subsequent infants may not be affected. In Rh HDN, a first pregnancy is usually unaffected (unless there has been prior immunization by abortion or transfusion), and subsequent Rh incompatible infants are affected to an equal degree or more severely. The majority of neonates affected with Rh HDN require some form of therapy.

Clinical features

In its least severe form, HDN manifests itself as mild haemolytic anaemia. The infant's red cells, coated with maternal IgG alloantibody, are removed prematurely from the circulation, causing slight jaundice (maximum on the second to third days of life) and mild anaemia during the second week of life. More severely affected infants show severe hyperbilirubinaemia in the neonatal period, a condition that was called *icterus gravis neonatorum*. Prompt treatment with exchange transfusion is necessary to prevent bilirubin impregnation of the basal ganglia and neurological damage, a condition known as *kernicterus*. This condition may be fatal, or lead to serious neurological deficit, with deafness, mental retardation, choreoathetosis and spasticity.

In the most severely affected cases, profound anaemia develops *in utero*, and intrauterine death may occur at any time from the eighteenth week of gestation. Affected fetuses are pale and oedematous, with marked ascites. The placenta is bulky, swollen and friable. This condition is known as *hydrops fetalis*, and had a high mortality rate until ultrasound-guided intravascular transfusions and improved intensive care facilities for very premature babies were introduced. The pathophysiology of hydrops is not fully understood, but extravascular haemolysis with fetal anaemia seems to play a major role by stimulating extramedullary erythropoiesis in the liver, with distortion of the hepatic circulation, leading to portal hypertension and impaired albumin production. Hypoalbuminaemia leads to ascites, oedema and pleural/pericardial effusions. In addition, the severe

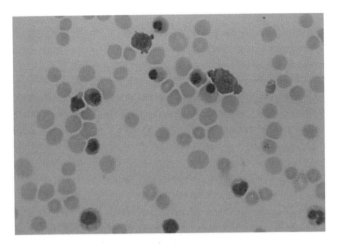

Figure 16.5 Blood film of a fetus affected by HDN, showing polychromasia and increased numbers of normoblasts.

anaemia leads to cardiac failure and tissue hypoxia, which damages the endothelium, leading to fluid extravasation into the extravascular space.

The blood film of a fetus affected by HDN shows polychromasia and increased numbers of nucleated red cells (Figure 16.5). In most cases (except a few due to ABO antibodies), the direct antiglobulin (DAT or Coombs') test on the infant's cells is positive owing to IgG coating.

Rh haemolytic disease of the newborn

Until the early 1970s (when Rh immunoprophylaxis was introduced), 0.5–0.75% of all births gave rise to infants affected by Rh HDN. Anti-D accounted for over 90% of all cases. Although anti-D HDN has decreased significantly as a cause, it remains the most important. Of all infants affected by Rh HDN, 10–20% died *in utero* or in the early neonatal period before effective therapy was possible. The disease due to anti-D is more severe than that due to most other alloantibodies (e.g. anti-c, -E) except for some cases of anti-K. Early detection of maternal alloantibodies, regular fetal monitoring and assessment of rises in antibody titres are prerequisites to a successful outcome.

Antenatal assessment of maternal blood

Rarely, anti-D may develop in a first pregnancy in a woman who has had no previous transfusions. However, it is not common for the antibody to reach high levels, and it is not usually detectable before 28 weeks; most of such cases become apparent after delivery. Conversely, in women who have had previous pregnancies or transfusions with Rh-positive red cells, anti-D may be detected early in pregnancy; regular monitoring of the level is necessary in order to plan the best type and timing of intervention. At present, the most objective means of quantifying anti-D levels routinely is with an automated analyser or,

rarely, by flow cytometry and not by manual titration. More important than the anti-D levels in determining the severity of HDN is the obstetric assessment of the fetus.

The ABO, Rh groups and antibody screen should be performed in all pregnant women at booking (usually around 16 weeks' gestation). All women should have the testing repeated once more at about 28 weeks to confirm the Rh group and to detect the presence of atypical antibodies. If clinically significant antibodies are detected, more frequent testing will be required (see below). If the mother is RhD-negative with no anti-D by 28 weeks, routine antenatal prophylaxis should be given (see below). Following delivery, all RhD-negative women who are unsensitized for RhD should be given prophylactic anti-RhD immunoglobulin if the infant is RhD positive (Figure 16.6).

The level of anti-D in the serum correlates approximately with the clinical severity of the HDN, but this is also affected by factors such as IgG subclass, rate of rise of antibody, past history and presence of maternal blocking antibodies. As a rough guide, levels below 4.0 IU/mL (0.8 µg/mL) require no action, whereas a level of > 4 and up to 10 IU/mL (2.0 µg/mL) indicates moderate risk; 10–20 IU/mL indicates high risk of HDN and levels greater than 20 IU/mL indicate a high risk of hydrops. Anti-D, -c and -K should be monitored monthly to 28 weeks and 2-weekly thereafter. Other red cell antibodies reacting by IAT should be re-tested at 28 weeks, titrated and the maternal serum should be tested for the presence of kell alloantibodies. If the anti-D level is > 10 IU, anti-c > 20 IU, or, for other antibodies the IAT titre is > 32, the fetus should be monitored by the fetal medicine specialist for evidence of anaemia. The strength and trend in titre of other maternal alloantibodies should be reported to the obstetrician, for fetal monitoring as appropriate.

Antenatal assessment of disease severity and treatment of haemolytic disease

The severity of the haemolytic process may be assessed by fetal medicine specialists by clinical and ultrasound monitoring, including Doppler flow velocity. The systolic velocity of the fetal middle cerebral artery is a reliable indicator of fetal anaemia (Figure 16.7). Measurement of the bile pigments in the amniotic fluid by spectrophotometry from week 28 onwards is less commonly used now in the UK. The absorbance of normal amniotic fluid over the range of wavelengths 400–600 nm forms a smooth curve when plotted on semi-logarithmic graph paper. When there is an excess of bilirubin, the curve shows a greatly increased absorbance, with a peak at about 450 nm. The increase in density at this wavelength over the normal absorbance is the measurement of severity.

If the non-invasive parameters of severity indicate a severely affected infant, the fetal medicine specialist can perform ultrasound-guided fetal blood sampling (FBS), from 18–20 weeks onwards. The fetal Hb deficit is measured (Figure 16.8) and, if necessary, an intravascular transfusion with fresh (< 5 days

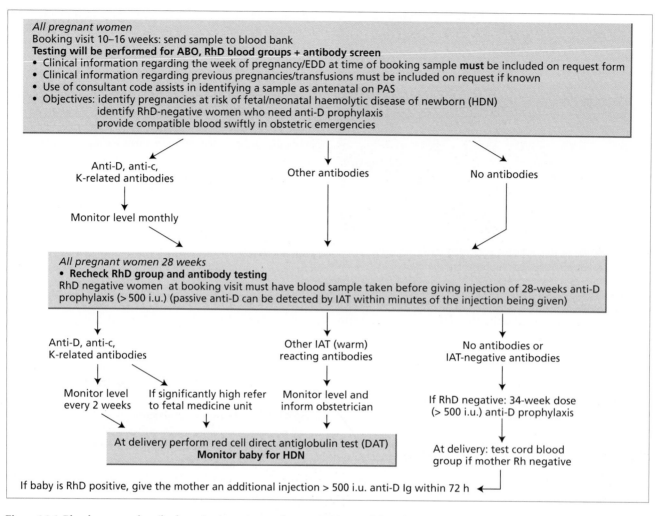

Figure 16.6 Blood group and antibody testing in pregnancy (source: *BCSH Guidelines for Blood Grouping and Antibody Testing During Pregnancy 1996*).

old) group O RhD-negative, CMV-negative, irradiated blood of the desired packed cell volume (PCV) can be administered. Such transfusions will be performed subsequently throughout pregnancy, with a frequency determined by the severity of the disease. Fetal blood sampling and amniocentesis carry a risk of immunizing a previously unsensitized RhD-negative woman carrying an RhD-positive fetus, due to leakage of fetal blood into the maternal circulation. Similarly, pre-existing low antibody levels may be 'boosted' by a new stimulus. Immunization to, or boosting of, other clinically significant red cell alloantibodies is not a rare occurrence. Although the risks of FBS are small in experienced hands, there are possible adverse effects on the fetus (e.g. bleeding through puncture of fetal vessels).

Intraperitoneal transfusion involves injection of antigen-negative donor red cells into the peritoneal cavity of the fetus (now rarely used). Blood with the same specification as used for intravascular transfusions, is used from 24 weeks of gestation. If ascites is already present, absorption of the red cells into the fetal circulation is slow and intravascular transfusion will continue to be the treatment of choice.

It is possible to determine the Rh genotype of the fetus from amniotic cells through DNA typing, thus avoiding further manipulations when the fetus is RhD negative. Fetal RhD genotyping is now possible by DNA extraction from maternal plasma from 16–18 weeks' gestation; this non-invasive technique is replacing amniocyte typing (see Chapter 15). If the partner is available, he too may be tested for the presence of the relevant antigen.

Premature delivery

Modern neonatal intensive care has dramatically increased survival rates of very premature infants born at 24–30 weeks' gestation. Nevertheless, morbidity is high and premature delivery is now, due to the success of intrauterine transfusions, rarely performed. It is sometimes considered at 36 weeks for

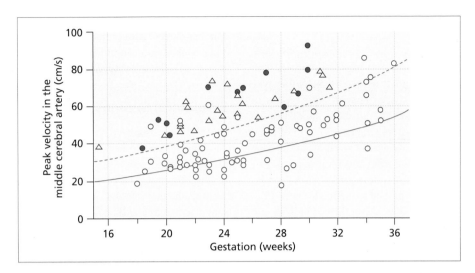

Figure 16.7 Middle cerebral artery Doppler. Peak velocity of systolic blood flow in the middle cerebral artery in 111 fetuses at risk for anaemia due to maternal red cell alloimmunization. Open circles indicate fetuses with either no anaemia or mild anaemia (≥ 0.65 multiples of the median Hb concentration). Triangles indicate fetuses with moderate or severe anaemia (< 0.65 multiples of the median Hb concentration). The solid circles indicate the fetuses with hydrops. The solid curve indicates the median peak systolic velocity in the middle cerebral artery and the dotted curve indicates 1.5 multiples of the median (courtesy of Professor Charles Rodeck).

Figure 16.8 Fetal Hb concentration of 48 hydropic (open circles) and 106 non-hydropic (closed circles) fetuses from red cell isoimmunized pregnancies at time of first blood sampling. Values are plotted on the reference range of fetal Hb for gestation. The individual 95% confidence intervals of the normal Hb for gestation define zone I and the individual 95% confidence intervals of the Hb for gestation of the hydropic fetuses define zone III. Zone II indicates moderate anaemia (courtesy of Professor Charles Rodeck).

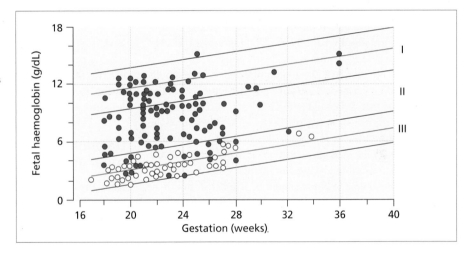

fetuses suffering from haemolytic disease due to antibodies other than anti-D, -c or -K. When the previous obstetric history is poor, the mother starts with a high level of anti-D and the partner is homozygous for D, or the fetus is known to be D positive, IVIg is given to carry the pregnancy to 20 weeks, when intrauterine transfusions can be started. In several countries, IVIg is the mainstay of therapy throughout pregnancy.

Assessment of severity in the newborn

Cord blood samples should be taken at delivery. The DAT may be positive, but is not a useful indication of severity or need for therapy. The best simple criterion of severity is the cord Hb level;

this is much more useful than a sample taken a few hours after birth, when rapid haemodynamic changes are occurring. The normal range of cord Hb levels is 13.6–19.6 g/dL. Most infants with levels in this range do not require therapy; more than 50% of affected babies have a level in the normal range. Where the cord Hb is below 12 g/dL, exchange transfusion will be necessary. It may also be indicated for a rising bilirubin level after birth, dependent upon the rate of rise and the maturity of the infant. Phototherapy may be given to reduce the rise in bilirubin levels but it is not a substitute for transfusion. Less severely affected infants may require small-volume transfusions of red cells at 2–3 weeks of age. In both of these instances, careful follow-up arrangements must be made as haemolysis may continue, causing further rises in bilirubin or need for additional top-up transfusion.

The infant's RhD group should be determined on the cord blood sample of all infants born to D-negative mothers with no preformed anti-D, to give anti-D Ig prophylaxis if they type as D-positive. A DAT is only performed on cord bloods of mothers who have made anti-D; the cord bloods of women given antenatal Rh prophylaxis should not have a DAT done as it may be positive due to the passive anti-D given. If intrauterine transfusions have been given, the ABO and Rh groups may be those of the donor, and the DAT may be negative. A DAT should be performed on the cord blood of all women who have IAT-reactive antibodies. If the DAT is positive, the cord Hb should be checked and the clinical state, Hb and bilirubin of the infant monitored for signs of HDN for 1 month.

Exchange transfusion

Exchange transfusion is effective therapy for HDN, removing from the infant's circulation sensitized red cells and plasma containing both maternal antibody and bilirubin. It also treats the anaemia.

An exchange transfusion of one blood volume will replace approximately 75% of the infant's red cells. It is usual to exchange relatively large volumes of blood (e.g. 160 mL/kg) slowly, via an umbilical vein catheter. The donor blood should be ABO compatible with mother and infant, and lack the antigen against which the maternal antibody is directed. A compatibility test should be performed against maternal serum. Blood in CPD-A1 of less than 5 days old with a PCV of 0.5–0.6 is suitable for exchange transfusions, regardless of the ABO group of the infant. If group O blood is used in all exchange transfusions, it should be devoid of high-titre ABO antibodies. CMV Ab-negative donations should be used for infants of less than 1200 g in weight. If possible, the blood should be irradiated, but there should be no delay to the exchange on account of this. Irradiated blood must be given to infants who have been transfused *in utero*, because they are at greater risk of TA-GvHD.

ABO haemolytic disease of the newborn

In 20% of births, the mother is ABO incompatible with her fetus. In A and B subjects, the anti-B and anti-A are predominantly IgM and do not enter the fetus. ABO HDN is usually restricted to group O mothers possessing IgG anti-A,B. In 15% of all pregnancies of white mothers, a group O mother carries a group A or B fetus, but the overall incidence of ABO HDN requiring treatment is extremely low. In absolute terms, however, exchange transfusion may be required in up to 1 in 3000 infants.

The lack of severity of ABO HDN can be accounted for by the widespread occurrence of A and B antigens, not only on red cells but also in plasma and on other cells, which will partially neutralize maternally derived ABO antibodies. Furthermore, the A and B antigens are not fully developed in the infant and the number of ABO sites is much smaller than in adults (see p. 227). Thus, only small amounts of the maternal antibody bind to infant red cells, and clinical sequelae are usually mild.

Serological findings

The mother is usually blood group O; IgG anti-A and anti-B can be demonstrated in her plasma after inactivating or inhibiting the IgM component with a reducing agent (2-mercaptoethanol or dithiothreitol, ZZAP). When infants are affected and require therapy, the maternal IgG anti-A or anti-B is almost always present in a titre greater than 64.

The infant will be group A or B and the DAT may be positive, only weakly positive or negative. In most cases, spontaneous agglutination will be observed if a drop of whole blood from the cord is rocked gently on a tile, especially if the cells are suspended in ABO-compatible plasma. Testing eluates from the red cells by IAT will reveal anti-A or anti-B specificity. Examination of the infant's blood film may show spontaneous agglutination of red cells, spherocytosis (not seen with Rh HDN), reticulocytosis, polychromasia and increased numbers of nucleated red cells.

Treatment

Severe anaemia is uncommon. Hyperbilirubinaemia is more often a problem which often subsides with phytotherapy, but may occasionally be serious enough to warrant exchange transfusion to prevent brain damage. Group O donor blood with low-titre anti-A,B should be used.

Haemolytic disease of the newborn due to other antibodies

After anti-D, the antibodies encountered most commonly as a cause of HDN are anti-c and anti-K (the former usually due to previous pregnancy and the latter usually due to previous maternal blood transfusions). The disease is generally less severe than that caused by anti-D, but may sometimes be serious enough to warrant early delivery and/or exchange transfusion, and occasionally requires treatment of the fetus. Anti-K of high titre may cause severe fetal anaemia. Assessment and treatment of the fetus and infant should be along the same lines as for anti-D. Blood that lacks the appropriate antigen should be given if intrauterine or exchange transfusion is required.

Although uncommon, practically all other red cell alloantibodies have been implicated in HDN requiring no therapy, small-volume transfusion or exchange transfusions.

Prevention of haemolytic disease of the newborn

The major success in HDN in the last 15 years is because of

the decrease in cases due to anti-D, so that other antibodies now account for a higher proportion of occurrences. This reduction has been achieved by the routine administration of 500 IU (100 µg) anti-RhD immunoglobulin to all RhD-negative mothers within 72 h of delivery of a RhD-positive infant. Extra doses of 50–75 IU (20–25 µg) per additional millilitre of red cells may be required for the small number of women (< 1%) who have a transplacental bleed greater than that covered by the standard dose (which covers 4 mL of packed cells). Anti-RhD immunoglobulin is also indicated after spontaneous or therapeutic abortion or threatened miscarriage and all procedures that might lead to a feto-maternal bleed (amniocentesis, external version, abdominal injury, chorionic villus sampling); the dose is 250 IU (50 µg) up to 20 weeks' gestation and 500 IU thereafter. It is critical that a Kleihauer acid elution test for detection and quantification of fetal red cells is performed on a maternal blood sample taken shortly after (within 1 h of) delivery and after each sensitizing event after 20 weeks. If the test shows > 4 mL of fetal cells, flow cytometry should be used to check the volume and give additional doses of anti-D as required. In several countries, and parts of the UK, the standard dose of anti-D Ig is 1250–1500 IU (250–300 µg).

Despite prophylaxis, new cases of sensitization to the D antigen still occur. Some may be due to an early unrecognized abortion and some to clerical and administrative errors (e.g. incorrect grouping of mother or child, or errors in the recording of groups). Failure of protection after delivery may result from omission of anti-D Ig (e.g. early discharge), an insufficient dose, or where primary immunization has already occurred during the pregnancy, now the most common cause of failure of conventional postnatal prophylaxis. Approximately 0.8–1.5% of Rh-negative women carrying a Rh-positive fetus become immunized during pregnancy.

To further reduce Rh immunization significantly, anti-RhD immunoglobulin should be given routinely during pregnancy to all RhD-negative women (usually 500 IU (100 µg) at 28 and 34 weeks, or a single dose of 1500 IU (300 µg) at 28 weeks). However, data from Canada suggest that a second dose of 300 µg may be needed for many women at 34 weeks, despite the larger dose at 28 weeks. The UK policy is to offer routine antenatal prophylaxis to all pregnant RhD-negative women, as it would significantly reduce the incidence of RhD sensitization in pregnant women. It is expected to offer D typing of the fetus from DNA extracted from maternal plasma before 28 weeks' gestation (see Chapter 15). This will avoid giving unnecessary routine antenatal Rh prophylaxis to women carrying RhD-negative fetuses.

The next most common causes of HDN requiring therapy are anti-c and anti-K. Any reduction in the cases due to anti-K could only be achieved by prevention of sensitization through transfusion of all women of childbearing potential with K-negative blood.

Selected bibliography

Barbara JAJ (2002) Transfusion transmitted infections. *Transfusion Alternatives in Transfusion Medicine* 4: 42–7.

Beauregard P, Blajchman MA (1994) Haemolytic and pseudo-haemolytic transfusion reactions: an overview of the haemolytic transfusion reactions and the clinical conditions that mimic them. *Transfusion Medicine Review* 7: 184–99.

Bowman IM (1990) Treatment options for the fetus with alloimmune haemolytic disease. *Transfusion Medicine Review* 4: 191–207.

British Committee for Standards in Haematology – Blood Transfusion Task Force (1988) Guidelines for transfusion for massive blood loss. *Clinical and Laboratory Haematology* 10: 265–73.

British Committee for Standards in Haematology – Blood Transfusion Task Force (1990) Guidelines on hospital blood bank documentation and procedures. *Clinical and Laboratory Haematology* 12: 209–20.

British Committee for Standards in Haematology – Blood Transfusion Task Force (1990) Guidelines for implementation of a maximum surgical blood order schedule. *Clinical and Laboratory Haematology* 12: 321–7.

British Committee for Standards in Haematology – Blood Transfusion Task Force (1990) Guidelines on hospital blood bank documentation and procedures. *Clinical and Laboratory Haematology* 12: 209–20.

British Committee for Standards in Haematology – Blood Transfusion Task Force (2004) Guidelines for the use of fresh frozen plasma, cryoprecipitate and cryosupernatant. *British Journal of Haematology* 126: 11–28.

British Committee for Standards in Haematology – Blood Transfusion Task Force (1996) Guidelines for pretransfusion compatibility procedures in blood transfusion laboratories. *Transfusion Medicine* 6: 273–83.

British Committee for Standards in Haematology – Blood Transfusion Task Force (1998) Guidelines for the clinical use of blood cell separators. *Clinical and Laboratory Haematology* 20: 265–78.

British Committee for Standards in Haematology – Blood Transfusion Task Force (1998) Guidelines on the clinical use of leucocyte-depleted blood components. *Transfusion Medicine* 8: 59–71.

British Committee for Standards in Haematology – Blood Transfusion Task Force (1999) Addendum for guidelines for blood grouping and red cell antibody testing during pregnancy. *Transfusion Medicine* 9: 99.

British Committee for Standards in Haematology – Blood Transfusion Task Force (1999) Guidelines for the estimation of feto-maternal haemorrhage. *Transfusion Medicine* 9: 87–92.

British Committee for Standards in Haematology – Blood Transfusion Task Force (1999) Guidelines of the administration of blood and blood components and the management of transfused patients. *Transfusion Medicine* 9: 227–38.

British Committee for Standards in Haematology – Blood Transfusion Task Force (2000) Guidelines for blood bank computing. *Transfusion Medicine* 10: 307–14.

British Committee for Standards in Haematology – Blood Transfusion Task Force (2001) Guidelines for the clinical use of red cell transfusions. *British Journal of Haematology* 113: 24–31.

British Committee for Standards in Haematology – Blood Transfusion Task Force (2003) Guidelines for the use of platelet transfusions. *British Journal of Haematology* 122: 10–23.

British Committee for Standards in Haematology – Blood Transfusion Task Force (2004) Transfusion guidelines on transfusion for neonates and older children. *British Journal of Haematology* 124: 433.

Brown P (2001) Creutzfeldt–Jakob disease; blood infectivity and screening tests. *Seminars in Haematology* 38: 2–6.

Contreras M (1998) Diagnosis and treatment of patients refractory to platelet transfusions. *Blood Reviews* 12: 215–21.

Engelfriet C, Reesink H (1999) Haemovigilance systems. *Vox Sanguinis* 77: 110–20.

Farese AM, Schiffer CA, MacVittie TJ (1997) The impact of thrombopoietin and related MpI-ligands on transfusion medicine. *Transfusion Medicine Reviews* 11: 243–55.

Hunter N, Foster J, Chong A et al. (2002) Transmission of prion diseases by blood transfusion. *Journal of General Virology* 83: 2897–905.

Lee D, Contreras M, Robson SC et al. (1999) Recommendations for the use of anti-D immunoglobulin for Rh prophylaxis. *Transfusion Medicine* 9: 93–7.

Linden JV, Kaplan HS (1994) Transfusion errors: causes and effects. *Transfusion Medicine Review* 7: 169–83.

Llewelyn CA, Hewitt PE, Knight RS et al. (2004) Possible transmission of variant Creutzfeldt-Jakob disease by blood transfusion. *Lancet* 363: 411–12.

McClelland DBL, Phillips P (1994) Errors in blood transfusion in Britain: survey of hospital haematology departments. *British Medical Journal* 308: 1205–6.

Mollison PL, Engelfriet CP, Contreras M (1997) *Blood Transfusion in Clinical Medicine*, 10th edn. Blackwell Scientific Publications, Oxford.

National Institute for Clinical Excellence (2003) Full guidance on the use of routine antenatal anti-D prophylaxis for RhD-negative women (www.nice.org.uk).

Norfok DR, Ancliffe PJ, Contreras M et al. (1998) Consensus Conference on Platelet Transfusion, Royal College of Physicians of Edinburgh 27–28 November, 1997. *British Journal of Haematology* 101: 609–17.

Petz L, Swisher SN (1989) *Clinical Practice of Blood Transfusion.* Churchill Livingstone, New York.

Poel van der CL, Seifried E, Schaasberg WP (2002) Paying for blood donations: still a risk? *Vox Sanguinis* 83: 285–93.

Sazama K (1990) Reports of 355 transfusion-associated deaths: 1976 through 1985. *Transfusion* 30: 583–90.

Simon TL, Marcus CS, Myhre BA et al. (1987) Effects of AS-3 nutrient additive solution on 42 and 49 days of storage of red cells. *Transfusion* 27: 178–82.

Stainsby D, Cohen H, Jones H et al. (2003) *Serious Hazards of Transfusion Annual Report 2001/02.* http://www.shotuk.org/SHOT%20Report%202001-02.pdf.

Stainsby D, Cohen H, Jones H et al. (2004) *Serious Hazards of Transfusion Annual Report 2003.* http://www.shotuk.org/SHOT%20Report%202003.pdf.

Strauss RG (1994) Neonatal transfusion. In: *Scientific Basis of Transfusion Medicine* (KC Anderson, PM Ness, eds), pp. 421–42. Saunders, Philadelphia.

Tannirandorn Y, Rodeck CH (1990) New approaches in the treatment of haemolytic disease of the fetus. In: *Bailliere's Clinical Haematology – Blood Transfusion: the impact of new technologies* (M Contreras, ed), pp. 289–320.

The TRAP Study Group (1997) Leucocyte reduction and UV-B irradiation of platelets to prevent allo-immunization and refractoriness to platelet transfusion. *New England Journal of Medicine* 337: 1861–9.

Turner M (2003) vCJD screening and its impilcations for transfusion-strategies for the future? *Blood Coagulation & Fibrinolysis* 14: 565–8.

UK Blood Transfusion Services (2002) *Guidelines for the Blood Transfusion Services in the United Kingdom*, 6th edn. The Stationery Office, London or http://www.transfusionguidelines.org.uk.

Williamson LM, Lowe S, Love EM et al. (1999) Serious hazards of transfusion initiative: analysis of the first two annual reports. *British Medical Journal* 319: 16–9.

World Health Organization (1992) *Guidelines for the Organization of Blood Transfusion Service* (WN Gibbs, AFH Britten, eds). WHO, Geneva.

CHAPTER 17

Phagocytes

Farhad Ravandi and Ronald Hoffman

Introduction

White blood cells have fundamental roles in defence against invading micro-organisms and the recognition and destruction of neoplastic cells as well as their role in acute inflammatory reactions. Furthermore, through their phagocytic function, white blood cells are influential in clearing senescent and apoptotic cells, hence allowing tissue repair and remodelling. Production of various cytokines by white blood cells influences the functions of other cells and affects processes such as cellular and humoral immunity, and allergic phenomena. The phagocytic actions of white blood cells can cause damage to the host tissue, leading to inflammation. This occurs either as a by-product of their microbial killing actions or as a direct attack on the host in autoimmune disorders.

Normal haemopoiesis, including generation of appropriate white blood cell number and constellation, is dependent upon intricately regulated signalling cascades that are mediated by cytokines and their receptors. Orderly function of these pathways leads to the generation of the normal constellation of haemopoietic cells, and their abnormal activation results in impaired apoptosis, uncontrolled proliferation and neoplastic transformation. Cytokines function in a redundant and pleiotropic manner; different cytokines can exert similar effects on the same cell type and any particular cytokine can have several differing biological functions. This complexity of function is a result of shared receptor subunits as well as overlapping downstream pathways, culminating in transcription of similar genes. Increased understanding of the role of cytokines and other growth factors in the control of normal haemopoiesis has led to better delineation of the pathogenetic events that affect the function and number of these cells.

In this chapter, we consider the normal production and function of white blood cells involved in phagocytosis and describe various disorders causing their altered number and activity.

Mechanisms of phagocyte function

Locomotion

Phagocytes are an important part of the innate host defence system, performing their function either as resident cells in tissues (e.g. macrophages) or as circulating defenders (e.g. neutrophils, eosinophils and monocytes). Phagocytosis of invading micro-organisms by both types of defender involves the synthesis of highly toxic derivatives of molecular oxygen by the respiratory burst NADPH oxidases and the delivery of stored antimicrobial proteases into the vacuoles containing microbes.

Circulating phagocytes such as neutrophils respond to spatial gradients of chemotaxin and move by alternating the extrusion and retraction of broad frontal lamellipodia that determine the direction of movement. As a result, the cell body elongates along the axis defined by the lamellar protrusion. As little as a 2% change in the concentration of the chemoattractant can be recognized by neutrophils. The signals generated by such gradients activate the cytoplasm of the cell for propulsive and retractive events. Movement of neutrophils is achieved by the contraction of an actin filamentous network in the cortical gel at the leading front. This dynamic network provides strength for the forming protrusions and serves as an anchor for adhesion molecules. ATP provides the energy for the movement of the cell.

Phagocytic cells possess a number of cell–cell adhesion receptors and ligands, which mediate their recruitment, migration and interaction with other immune cells (Table 17.1). These include members of the integrins, the immunoglobulin superfamily and the selectins. Migration of macrophages involves their adhesion to endothelial surfaces and their extravasation through to the extravascular space. This process is mediated by cytokine-regulated expression of intercellular adhesion molecules (ICAMs) on the surface of both phagocytes and endothelial cell. ICAMs share similar structure to the immunoglobulin (Ig)

Table 17.1 Phagocytic cell adhesion molecules.

Adhesion molecule	CD number	Cellular distribution	Ligand	Function
Integrin family				
Very late-acting antigens				
$\alpha_1\beta_1$ (VLA-1)	CD49a/29	Mo, EC	Collagen I, IV, laminin	Cell adherence to ECM
$\alpha_2\beta_1$ (VLA-2)	CD49b/29	Mo, EC, platelets	Collagen I, IV, laminin	
$\alpha_3\beta_1$ (VLA-3)	CD49c/29	Mo	Collagen I, laminin, fibronectin	Cell adherence to ECM
$\alpha_4\beta_1$ (VLA-4)	CD49d/29	Mo, eos, bas	Fibronectin, VCAM-1	Cell adherence to ECM and cell–cell adhesion matrix
$\alpha_5\beta_1$ (VLA-5)	CD49e/29	Mo, neut, EC	Fibronectin	Cell adherence to ECM
$\alpha_6\beta_1$ (VLA-6)	CD49f/29	Mo	Laminin	Cell adherence to ECM
Leucocyte integrins(LFA-1 family)				
$\alpha_D\beta_2$	–/18	Ma	?	
$\alpha_L\beta_2$ (LFA-1)	CD11a/18	Mo, Ma, granulocytes	ICAM-1, ICAM-2, ICAM-3	Cell–cell adhesion and cell–matrix adhesion
$\alpha_M\beta_2$ (CR3, Mac-1)	CD11b/18	Mo, Ma, granulocytes	ICAM-1, C3bi, fibronectin, factor X, microbial antigens	Endothelium adherence/extravasation
$\alpha_X\beta_2$ (p150,95)	CD11c/18	Mo, Ma, granulocytes	C3bi, fibronectin	Adhesion during inflammatory response
Cytoadhesins				
$\alpha_V\beta_3$ (vitronectin receptor)	CD51/61	Mo, EC	Vitronectin, fibronectin, collagen, thrombospondin, vWF	Cell adherence to ECM
$\alpha_R\beta_3$ (leucocyte response integrin)		Mo, granulocytes	Vitronectin, fibronectin, collagen, thrombospondin, vWF	Cell adherence to ECM
$\alpha_V\beta_5$	CD51/–	Mo	Vitronectin, fibronectin	Cell adherence to ECM
$\alpha_V\beta_7$	CD51/–	Ma	?	
Immunoglobulin superfamily				
ICAM-1	CD54	Mo, EC	$\alpha_L\beta_2$, $\alpha_M\beta_2$	Cell–cell adhesion
ICAM-2	CD102	Mo, EC	$\alpha_L\beta_2$	Cell–cell adhesion
ICAM-3	CD50	Mo, granulocytes	$\alpha_L\beta_2$	Cell–cell adhesion
VCAM-1	CD106	Ma, EC, dendritic cells	$\alpha_4\beta_1$	Recruitment
PECAM-1	CD31	Mo, EC, platelets	CD31, $\alpha_V\beta_3$	Transmigration
HCAM	CD44	Ubiquitous	Collagen I, IV, fibronectin	Extravasation
Selectin family				
L-selectin	CD62L	Mo, granulocytes	Carbohydrate determinants on EC	Migration, rolling on vessel wall
E-selectin	CD62E	Neutrophil, EC	Mo, neut, eos	Migration, rolling on vessel wall
P-selectin	CD62P	EC, platelets	Mo, neut, eos	Adhesion to activated platelets and EC

Bas, basophil; cd, cluster of differentiation; EC, endothelial cell; eos, eosinophil; ICAM, intercellular adhesion molecule; Mo, monocyte; Ma, macrophage; neut, neutrophil.

family and other Ig-like adhesion molecules such as VCAM-1, and serve as ligands for the β_2-integrins. The distribution and regulation of the three members of the ICAM family is different. ICAM-1 is expressed at a low level on endothelial cells; its expression is enhanced by the inflammatory cytokines such as interleukin 1 (IL-1), interferon-α (IFN-α) and IFN-γ. ICAM-2 is constitutively expressed on endothelial cells, with no response to the inflammatory cytokines. ICAM-3 is expressed by neu-

Table 17.2 Opsonic receptors mediating phagocytosis.

Receptor	Marker	Opsonic ligand	Binding affinity (Ka)	Cell type	Function
FcγRI	CD64	IgG1	High (50 nmol/L)	Monocytes, Macrophages, Neutrophils (after IFN-γ exposure)	Phagocytosis, Respiratory burst
FcγRII	CD32	IgG1 = IgG3≥ IgG4 = IgG2	Low (1 μM)	Neutrophils, monocytes, macrophages	Phagocytosis, Respiratory burst
FcγRIII		IgG1 = IgG3	Low (110 nmol/L)	Neutrophils, monocytes, macrophages	IIIB – Phagocytosis (requires CR1 or FcγRII)
IIIA	CD16a, 1 allotype NA1		Low (470 nmol/L)		
IIIB	CD16b, 2 allotypes NA1 and NA2				
FcαR	CD89 My43 IgM	IgA1, IgA2, secretory IgA1 and IgA2		Neutrophils, monocytes, macrophages, T- and B-cell subsets, NK cells, erythrocytes	Phagocytosis, Respiratory burst, Bacterial killing
CR1	CD35 4 alleles	C3b and C4b dimers	High (0.5 nmol/L)	All phagocytes, some T lymphocytes	Phagocytosis
CR3	CD11b/CD18 Mac1	C3bi	High (0.5 nmol/L)	All phagocytes, NK cells, γδ-T cells	Phagocytosis, Respiratory burst

CR, complement receptor; NK, natural killer.

trophils, monocytes and lymphocytes. Another member of the endothelial Ig superfamily, PECAM-1 (CD31), serves an important role in transmigration of neutrophils into mucosal or other body tissues.

The β₂-integrin family consists of three leucocyte restricted integrins, LFA-1 (CD11a/CD18), CR3 (MAC-1, CD11b/CD18) and p150/95 (CD11c/CD18). They share a common β-subunit, CD18, and three unique α-subunits, CD11a, CD11b, and CD11c. LFA-1 and ICAM-1 are both present on monocytes and mediate their attachment to endothelial cells and to lymphocytes bearing the corresponding receptor/ligand, thereby facilitating antigen presentation. Leucocyte adhesion deficiency (LAD) type I, described later in the chapter, is caused by the genetic deficiency of all three CD18 integrins. LAD-I neutrophils bind poorly to IL-1-stimulated endothelial cells and do not undergo transendothelial migration.

Selectins are expressed on all leucocytes (L-selectins) as well as post-capillary endothelial surfaces (E-selectins) and in platelet α-granules and endothelial cell Weibel–Palade bodies (P-selectins). Neutrophils, eosinophils, monocytes and macrophages constitutively express L-selectin. E- and P-selectins recognize oligosaccharide ligands on macrophages. Selectins

are implicated in the early interactions of phagocytes and endothelium. The interaction of E- and P-selectins on cytokine-activated endothelial cells, and L-selectins on macrophages with their appropriate ligands, targets phagocytic cells to the endothelium at sites of vascular injury and initiates the rolling movement of leucocytes along the vessel wall. The ligands for selectins have a similar structure containing carbohydrate groups typically as terminal structures of glycoproteins and glycolipids. A major selectin ligand, a sialylated and fucosylated tetrasaccharide related to the sialylated Lewis X blood group, is heavily expressed on quiescent neutrophils and monocytes.

Phagocyte receptors

Phagocytes express a number of surface receptors that are able to recognize microbial surfaces as well as altered tissue components and apoptotic bodies (Table 17.2). Furthermore, non-specific components of the innate immune response, such as the components of the complement cascade, can tag and thereby identify invading micro-organisms, thus allowing their opsonization via another family of receptors, leading to the uptake of complement-coated micro-organisms. This complement fixation can occur either via the classical pathway, which is activated by the prior binding of immune IgG or IgM to the organism or particle, or by antibody-independent activation of the alternative pathway. Similarly, other molecules such as matrix proteins (i.e. fibronectin and vitronectin) can act as opsonins allowing recognition and uptake by the phagocytic cells. Interestingly, in order to evade phagocytes, pathogenic bacteria such as *Streptococcus pneumoniae*, *Haemophilus influenzae* and *Neisseria meningitidis* have developed strategies such as production of polysaccharide capsules, which provide a shield against complement binding and activation, and recognition by scavenger receptors.

Two types of complement receptors, CR1 (CD35) and CR3 (CD11b/CD18) have been described. The CR1 receptor is a glycosylated protein with a molecular weight of 160–250 kDa and can be identified as CD35. CR1 is present on all phagocytes as well as some T lymphocytes. CR1 mediates phagocytosis of particles opsonized by C3b and regulates complement activation. CR3 is a member of the β_2-integrin family and is designated CD11b/CD18. It is composed of two polypeptide chains, an α-subunit of 185 kDa and a β-subunit of 95 kDa. CR3 is expressed on all phagocytes as well as natural killer cells and some $\gamma\delta$-T cells. Monocytes and macrophages express high levels of CR3; neutrophils have lower level expression that can increase rapidly through release from intracellular stores. CR3 can bind particles opsonized with C3bi as well as determinants on unopsonized microbes. The avidity of CR3 is enhanced by an amphipathic anion lipid called integrin-modulating factor (IMF-1) as well as by bacterial peptide fragments, C5a, LTB4, and cytokines such as tissue necrosis factor (TNF), granulocyte colony-stimulating factor (G-CSF) and granulocyte–macrophage colony-stimulating factor (GM-CSF). However, IFN-γ transiently decreases the binding capacity of both CR1 and CR3. Simultaneous cross-linking of two different receptor types also increases binding by CR3. For example, macrophages adhered to collagen ingest complement-coated particles less efficiently than macrophages adhered to fibronectin, which cross-links other integrin receptors. CR3 also plays a critical role in adherence dependent potentiation of the respiratory burst and secretory responses of neutrophils.

Phagocytes also express a number of receptors for the Fc portion of immunoglobulin molecules IgA, IgE, and IgG. They mediate opsonization of particles and micro-organisms enhancing their phagocytic uptake. The antigen binding site (Fab) of IgG binds to bacteria exposing the Fc binding site, which is in turn recognized by one of three classes of receptors, FcγRI, FcγRII or FcγRIII. FcγRIII is constitutively expressed in neutrophils with 100 000 to 300 000 copies per cell and is identified as CD16. Two isoforms, A and B, exist, which differ only with respect to their transmembrane and cytoplasmic domains. FcγRIIIB lacks both of these domains and is anchored by a glycosyl-phosphatidylinositol (GPI) protein and is therefore absent in patients with paroxysmal nocturnal haemoglobinuria. FcγRIIIB can trigger granule release but no associated respiratory burst.

However, FcγRIIIB and CR3, together with FcγRII, act synergistically to activate the respiratory burst. FcγRII (identified as CD32) is a constitutive low-affinity receptor with low expression (1000 to 4000 copies per cell) requiring dimeric IgG for binding. Cross-linking FcγRII stimulates oxygen radical production. FcγRI, identified as CD64, is not expressed on quiescent neutrophils but its expression is highly increased after exposure to IFNγ and a number of inflammatory mediators. It binds IgG1 and IgG2 with high affinity and promotes phagocytosis of bacteria opsonized by them. Polymeric IgA antibody can also function as an opsonin and is recognized by a specific IgA receptor (FcαR), which is widely distributed on the circulating haemopoietic cells but is more highly expressed in phagocytes found in secretions of the gut and the lung.

A number of miscellaneous receptors involved in phagocytosis have been described. The mannosyl/fucosyl receptors, otherwise known as the macrophage mannose receptors (MMR), are lectin-like molecules that bind mannose and fucose residues on the surfaces of yeasts, bacteria and parasites. These receptors are present only on the surface of macrophages and their expression is increased by IFN-γ. Their activation mediates endocytosis, phagocytosis and cytotoxicity by reactive oxygen intermediates. The receptors described to date are composed of eight and 10 contiguous C-type lectin domains. CD14 is the receptor for complexes of lipopolysaccharide (LPS)-binding protein with LPS, which coat Gram-negative bacteria and enhance phagocytosis. CD14 is constitutively expressed on monocytes and macrophages but its expression is modulated by cytokines. TNF, IL-1 and IL-6 increase its expression, whereas IFN-γ and IL-4 decrease it. CD14 expression can also be induced on neutrophils by various cytokines. CD14 is also a GPI-linked protein and is shed by monocytes.

Several receptors have also been implicated in the recognition and phagocytosis of apoptotic cells. Morphological changes in the apoptotic cells such as formation of characteristic membrane protuberances (blebs) lead to the exposure of phosphatidylserine (PS) and changes on surface sugars, which are recognized by phagocytic receptors. These include integrins of the $\alpha_v\beta_3$ or $\alpha_v\beta_5$ classes and the lipid scavenger receptors of both A and B classes. The membrane of apoptotic cells bind increased amounts of thrombospondin, a macrophage secretory product, that is recognized by both CD36 (thrombospondin receptor) and integrin $\alpha_v\beta_3$ (vitronectin receptor). Similarly, phagocytic lectin receptors bind carbohydrate determinants exposed on the surface of apoptotic cells. A specific receptor for PS, or PSR, has also been described, which acts alone or in association with CD36 to recognize the exposed PS. CD14 has also been reported to be involved in tethering of apoptotic lymphocytes via interaction with ICAMs.

Neutrophils also recognize the chemoattractant signals through receptors expressed on their cell surface. N-formyl-methionyl tripeptide receptors such as f-Met-Leu-Phe (FMLP) are similar to naturally occurring bacteria-derived factors. Each demonstrates time-dependent saturable binding kinetics and a high-affinity dissociation constant (K_D) for the specific chemoattractant. Approximately 50 000 FMLP receptors per cell with a K_D of 20 nmol/L have been demonstrated on human neutrophils. Thrombospondin also has chemotactic activity and binds neutrophils via specific receptors linked to Gi2 proteins, a subpopulation of which is also associated with the FMLP receptors. Neutrophils also have a specific receptor for the chemotactic cleavage product of C5a with a receptor expression of approximately 50 000–100 000 per cell and a binding affinity of 2 nmol/L.

Chemokines are a family of proinflammatory cytokines with potent chemotactic activity. They are small proteins (8–10 kDa), characterized by a pattern of conserved cysteine residues. CXC chemokines such as IL-8 are specific to neutrophils and are distinguished by having their first two cysteine residues separated by an amino acid. Whereas CC chemokines, including macrophage inflammatory protein-1α (MIP-1α) have the first two cysteine residues adjacent, are inactive for neutrophils, but attract monocytes, basophils, eosinophils and T-lymphocytes. Monocyte migration is also directed by monocyte chemotactic proteins (MCP). Eosinophil migration is directed by MIP-1α and RANTES (regulation on activation normal T-cell expressed and secreted protein) in addition to the CC chemokine, eotaxin. Phagocytic cells in general have a high expression of the receptors for these chemokines enabling them to recognize and respond to the appropriate chemoattractants.

Phagocytic signalling

The complex process of phagocytosis is regulated by events related to the activation of various receptors such as the FcγRs. Such receptor activation results in initiation of downstream signalling events through immunoreceptor tyrosine-based activation motifs (ITAMs). As a result of cross-linking of these receptors under appropriate conditions, downstream effector functions are activated, resulting in phagocytosis, stimulation of the respiratory burst, degranulation of bactericidal proteins and activation of transcription factors, in turn leading to enhanced expression of genes encoding cytokines and other inducible proteins.

Members of the Src family of tyrosine kinases (e.g. Lyn, Fgr and Hk) associate with FcγRs and are probably responsible for their tyrosine phosphorylation. The tyrosine-phosphorylated ITAMs then serve as binding sites for downstream kinases such as Syk, which propagate signals important for phagocytosis. Downmodulation of Syk in monocytes using antisense oligonucleotides results in decreased ability of these cells to ingest IgG-coated particles. Furthermore, macrophages that lack Syk demonstrate a profound reduction in FcγR-mediated tyrosine phosphorylation of p85 subunit of PI-3 kinase, SHIP, Shc and other important signalling proteins.

Phosphorylation and activation of members of the Rho/Rac family of GTPases as well as the ARF6 family are probably involved in cytoskeletal remodelling necessary to trigger phagocytosis. For example, inhibition of Rac1 or Cdc42 in murine macrophage models leads to impaired focal actin assembly beneath bound IgG-coated particles and blocks subsequent ingestion without affecting particle binding. Cdc42 and Rac1 appear to control different steps in the phagocytic process, namely pseudopod formation for the former and phagosome closure for the latter. The role of phospholipase C-γ (PLC-γ) and protein kinase C (PKC) isoforms in actin assembly, and the role of PI3 kinase (PI3K) pathways in membrane remodelling during phagocytosis are under investigation. Treatment of macrophages with PI3K inhibitors such as wortmannin and LY 294002 results in the failure of pseudopods to extend around particles.

Degranulation and secretion

Degranulation and secretion are processes whereby the contents of phagocytic storage granules are released into the phagocytic vacuoles (degranulation) or into the extracellular space (secretion). Degranulation and secretion can be triggered by invading micro-organisms, immune complexes, cytokines, chemotactic factors, and adhesion to tissue surfaces and activation of ICAMs. The processes of degranulation and secretion begin with the onset of phagocytosis. A number of morphological changes occur within the granules and they translocate and fuse their membranes with those of the phagocytic vacuoles formed by the invagination of the plasma membrane.

Cytoskeletal proteins are essential for this process facilitating granule transfer to plasma membrane or phagolysosomes. The exact cause of membrane fusion is unknown but the process is likely to involve the activation of several phospholipases leading to altered lipid composition of granule–phagosome or granule–plasma membrane contact points. Actin polymers act like a barrier between plasma membrane and granules, and in order for the membrane fusion to occur the granules have to go through the physical barrier of such cytoskeletal elements in the cell periphery. Furthermore, the repulsive negative charge on the surface of both membranes, related to the negatively charged phospholipids phosphatidylserine and phosphatidylethanolamine, is a further barrier that needs to be overcome. A number of soluble molecules capable of provoking the release of granule content into the extracellular space have been described. They include many chemotactic factors such as C5a, fMLP, PAF, LTB4, as well as phorbol myristate acetate (PMA) and several non-chemotactic interleukins, cytokines and growth factors such as TNF-α, IL-1, IL-6, IL-4, IL-6 and GM-CSF. Importantly, phagocytes are capable of rapidly replenishing cellular stores of proteins and forming new granules, thus allowing repeated degranulation and secretion.

Regulation of granule release is mediated by a number of factors such as calcium, guanine nucleotides and G-proteins, which regulate changes in the cytoskeleton, resulting in actin polymerization and clearing of the cytoskeleton along the plasma

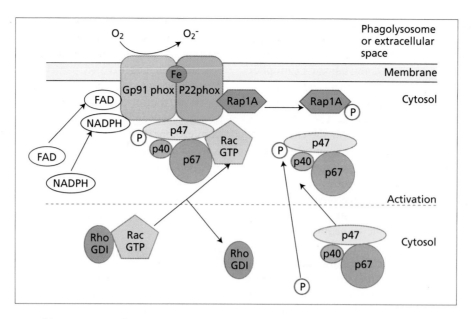

Figure 17.1 Components of the NADPH oxidase system. The components include a 47-kDa cytosolic protein (p47), a 67-kDa cytosolic protein (p67), a 40-kDa cytosolic protein (p40), cytosolic G-proteins (Rac1 and Pap1), and a membrane-bound cytochrome (*b*558). The cytochrome consists of haem containing p22-phox and gp91-phox. The gp91 subunit is a FAD-dependent flavoprotein shuttling electrons to molecular oxygen, forming O_2^-. The p47 component can be phosphorylated to various extents. In activated cells, the p40, p47 and p67 proteins translocate to membrane to form an activation complex with cytochrome *b*558. Similarly, the Rac1 and Rap1 proteins also translocate. The activated oxidase passes electrons from NADPH via FAD to oxygen, thereby generating superoxide.

membrane fusion site. These proteins include members of the annexin family, the calcium-binding protein calmodulin, protein kinase C and phospholipases.

Phagocytic killing – the respiratory burst

Activation of phagocytes is associated with a rapid and dramatic increase in oxygen consumption described as the respiratory burst. This process is non-mitochondrial and is mediated by the activation of a latent enzyme system referred to as NADPH oxidase, which transfers a single electron to molecular oxygen (O_2), forming the superoxide anion (O_2^-). The superoxide anion then dismutates to hydrogen peroxide (H_2O_2), a process occurring either spontaneously or through the catalytic function of superoxide dismutase. H_2O_2 then reacts with superoxide anion, forming the highly reactive hydroxyl radical (OH), which is highly microbicidal. This and other reactive oxidative products not only contribute to microbial killing but also activate metalloproteinases such as elastase and collagenase, leading to the surrounding tissue injury that often accompanies phagocyte activation.

The NADPH oxidase is a multicomponent enzyme, with several subunits located in various regions of the quiescent phagocytes (Figure 17.1). These subunits, called the phox (phagocyte oxidase) proteins, are identified by their molecular weight (e.g. p40

phox). In the quiescent neutrophil, p47 phox protein resides in the cytosol, along with p67 phox complexed with p40 phox. Activation of NADPH oxidase results from protein kinase C-mediated phosphorylation of p47 phox and the subsequent binding of the p47 phox phosphoprotein and the p67 phox–p40 phox complex to the membrane flavocytochrome b558 located primarily in the specific granules, gelatinase granules and secretary vesicles of neutrophils. The cytochrome *b*558 is the terminal component of the superoxide generating system allowing the efficient transfer of electrons from the cytoplasmic NADPH to the surface of phagolysosome or the extracellular surface, where oxygen is reduced to the superoxide anion. Other GTP-binding proteins such as Rap1A and Rac2, associate with the above molecules and regulate phagocyte activation and oxidase activity through their preferred substrate GTP (Figure 17.1).

Phagocytic killing – nitric oxide

Generation of reactive nitrogen intermediates through nitric oxide synthase (NOS) is another mechanism for phagocytic killing of microbes. Nitric oxide (NO) is the highly reactive free radical product of the oxidation of L-arginine in phagocytes during inflammation. Three distinct isoforms of NOS have been described in blood cells. Two are found in endothelial and neuronal cells and the third, the inducible NOS, is induced by cytokines, such as IFN-γ, in a number of cell types. Cofactors required for the activity of NOS include flavine adenine dinucleotide (FAD), flavine mononucleotide (FMN), NADPH and tetrahydrobiopterin. The calcium binding protein, calmodulin, is tightly bound to the macrophage NOS. The activity of NOS is also regulated by kinases and phosphatases and its production is influenced by other cytokines such as IL-4, IL-10, IL-8 and transforming growth factor β (TGF-β).

NO has an important role in the antimicrobial activity of both neutrophils and mononuclear phagocytes. In contrast to NADPH oxidase, which is active at the plasma and phagolysosome membrane, NOS is located in the cytoplasm and mediates defence against facultative intracellular pathogens, as well as other prokaryotic and eukaryotic pathogens. Its inhibitory effects are due to nitrosylation of proteins and interaction with transition metals at the active sites of enzymes. Furthermore, NO scavenges superoxide to form peroxynitrite ($OONO^-$), which can disrupt protein phosphorylation.

Phagocytic killing – antimicrobial proteins

Phagocytic cells such as neutrophils can kill micro-organisms using proteins present in various granules. The importance of such non-oxidative killing is evident in chronic granulomatous disease neutrophils that are still capable of killing many potent micro-organisms. Furthermore, this process is important for defence against organisms such as *Escherichia coli* and *Salmonella typhimurium*, which do not produce their own source of oxidants and are killed under anaerobic conditions. The contents of each phagocytic cell type are specific. Neutrophil antimicrobial proteins include defensins, serpocidins (including cathepsin G and azurocidin) and bacterial permeability-increasing protein (BPI). The antimicrobial proteins within neutrophils are summarized in Table 17.3.

These microbicidal proteins exert their killing effect through enzymatic means such as proteolysis or by non-catalytic mechanisms, and their combinations potentiate bactericidal activity. Cathepsin G is a serine protease that exerts its bactericidal action by binding to penicillin-binding proteins of bacteria and interfering with the synthesis of peptidoglycans. Azurocidin is another serine protease effective against a number of bacteria and fungi. Defensins constitute as much as 50% of neutrophil granule protein content and exert their cidal activity by inserting into hydrophobic channels, forming voltage-dependent ion channels in the lipid bilayer. BPI kills Gram-negative bacteria by binding to their LPS capsule and altering their bacterial

Table 17.3 Neutrophil microbicidal proteins.

Protein	Characteristics	Target organisms	Effects on target
Non-enzymatic proteins			
BPI	Highly cationic, neutralizes LPS, most potent cidal protein, not released from granule	Gram −ve bacteria	Binds lipid A region of LPS, increases bacterial membrane permeability, activates bacterial degradative enzymes
Defensins	Comprise 30% to 50% of azurophil granule protein	Gram +ve > −ve bacteria, fungi, viruses, mammalian cells	Increases membrane permeability
Lactoferrin	Cationic, stimulates hydroxyl radical formation	Gram +ve and −ve bacteria, fungi	Oxidative damage
Catalytic proteins and analogues			
Proteinase 3	Serine proteinase	*Escherichia coli, Streptococcus faecalis, Candida albicans*	Growth inhibition
Cathepsin G	Serine proteinase	Gram +ve and −ve bacteria, fungi	Inhibition of peptidoglycan synthesis
Azurocidin	Serine proteinase	Gram −ve bacteria	Non-catalytic mechanisms
Lysozyme	Cationic	Gram −ve bacteria, few Gram +ve bacteria	Potentiation of complement and H_2O_2 killing, cleavage of cell wall peptidoglycans
Elastase	No direct cidal activity		Co-active with lysozyme Potentiation of MPO–halide–H_2O_2 system

BPI, bacterial permeability inducing factor; LPS, lipopolysaccharide; MPO, myeloperoxidase.

membrane permeability to extracellular solutes. A mutant strain of *S. typhimurium*, which is resistant to BPI, has also been found to be resistant to neutrophil bactericidal activity under strict anaerobic conditions, demonstrating the importance of BPI in non-oxidative killing by neutrophils. Other neutrophil granule proteins include lactoferrin, which kills some Gram-negative bacteria by generating free radicals from iron bound to it, and lysozyme, which is involved in the digestion of killed bacteria in phagolysosomes of neutrophils. These antimicrobial proteins can also enhance the effects of other cidal mechanisms such as complement lysis and oxidative killing. Combinations of these proteins can also enhance their killing action, as seen with the combination of neutrophil lysozyme and elastase against Gram-negative bacteria. Some of the microbicidal proteins of the phagocytes have other effects at lower concentrations, such as stimulation of mast cell degranulation, release of proinflammatory molecules and monocytic chemotaxis, as well as regulation of phagocytosis and granulopoiesis.

Production, structure and dysfunction of phagocytes

White blood cells are produced from pluripotent stem cells located within the bone marrow. Development of white blood cells along different lineages is governed by external stimuli including cytokines, matrix proteins, and other cellular products within the marrow environment. The combination of specific cytokines and growth factors influence the maturation of white blood cell progeny along specific lineages. Although there is significant overlap between these growth factors, certain cytokines have been found to be associated with specific maturation pathways. Some of these cytokines are now manufactured commercially and are in clinical use to influence the speed of recovery of white blood cells following administration of chemotherapy.

Neutrophils (Figure 17.2a)

Development and function

Neutrophils are the predominant white blood cells involved in phagocytic killing of bacteria and certain fungi. They are also referred to as polymorphonuclear or segmented, owing to their characteristic lobulated nucleus (their nucleus is segmented into two to five lobes, connected by thin chromatin strands). They are at the end stage of maturation (Figures 17.3 and 17.4) and generally uniform in size (13 μm in diameter), with pink cytoplasm and fine azurophilic granules. The production of neutrophil leucocytes involves the action of a variety of growth factors including granulocyte colony-stimulating factor (G-CSF), granulocyte–macrophage-colony-stimulating factor (GM-CSF), IL-3, and macrophage colony-stimulating factor (M-CSF). Other factors such as IL-11, stem cell factor (SCF) and FLT-3 ligand enhance clonal neutrophil expansion *in vitro*. GM-CSF induces neutrophil, eosinophil and macrophage colony expansion *in vitro*, but there is no evidence that it induces neutrophil differentiation in the absence of G-CSF.

Neutrophils contain four types of granules that can be identified by marker enzymes or proteins (Table 17.4). The lysozyme-like azurophil granules, otherwise known as primary

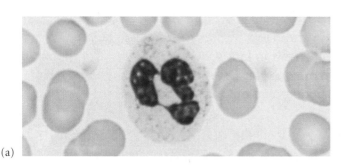

(a)

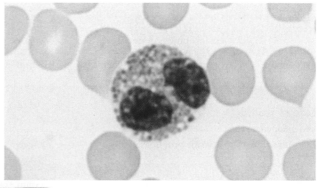

(b)

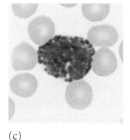

(c)

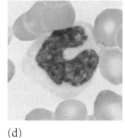

(d)

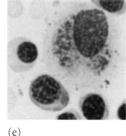

(e)

Figure 17.2 Morphology of phagocyte cell types.
(a) Neutrophil. (b) Eosinophil. (c) Basophil.
(d) Monocyte. (e) Macrophage.

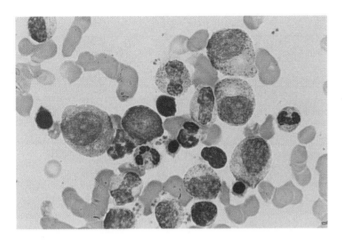

Figure 17.3 Stages of neutrophil maturation: shown are a myeloblast, a promyelocyte, several myelocytes and metamyelocytes, a band cell and a segmented neutrophil.

granules, present in the promyelocytes and all further stages of neutrophil differentiation and contain microbicidal proteins and acid hydrolases (such as myeloperoxidase, defensins, and lysozyme) involved in oxidative and non-oxidative killing of bacteria and fungi. These granules release their contents exclusively into phagocytic granules, with little discharge outside the cell except for release from disintegrating neutrophils. Specific or secondary granules are smaller than azurophil granules and contain other distinct hydrolases, as well as chemotactic,

opsonic, and adhesion protein receptors. They release their contents both into phagocytic vesicles and into the extracellular medium. Other granules, collectively known as tertiary granules, include secretory vesicles, which contain alkaline phosphatase, and gelatinase granules rich in gelatinase. Degranulation of neutrophils begins with the onset of phagocytosis and involves their translocation and fusion with phagocytic vacuoles created by invagination of the plasma membrane. Degranulation may also occur by reversed endocytosis as a result of the action of complement, aggregated immunoglobulin or certain cytokines. Although the release of granule contents is important for phagocytosis and bacterial killing, extracellular release can also lead to tissue injury and inflammation.

Neutrophils exist in one of three states: quiescent, activated or primed. They circulate in the blood in the quiescent state and react weakly to stimuli, thus limiting potential damage to vascular walls. Priming of neutrophils is a process that does not immediately stimulate an effector response but allows an exaggerated response upon later stimulation. Therefore, this is a mechanism whereby phagocytes are selectively activated upon recruitment to sites of infection and inflammation. Three main types of agonists are responsible for priming neutrophils, including chemotactic inflammatory mediators, serum immunoglobulin and complement opsonins, and inflammatory cytokines and growth factors. Upon neutrophil activation, a significant increase in oxygen consumption, termed respiratory burst, occurs leading to the production of reactive oxygen species responsible for microbial killing.

Figure 17.4 Neutrophil lifespan and stages of maturation. Of every 100 nucleated cells in the bone marrow, 2% are myeloblasts, 5% promyelocytes, 12% myelocytes, 22% metamyelocytes and bands and 20% mature neutrophils (i.e. about 60% developing neutrophils). The times indicated for the various compartments were obtained by isotopic labelling techniques. The ordinate shows the flux, and the abscissa the time, in each compartment. The stepwise increase in cell numbers through the dividing compartments represents serial divisions. Note that no mitoses occur after the myelocyte stage (reproduced with permisssion from Bainton DF, *Developmental Biology of Neutrophils and Eosinophils*, and Cronkite EP, Vincent PC, 1969, *Ser Haematology* 3: 3–43).

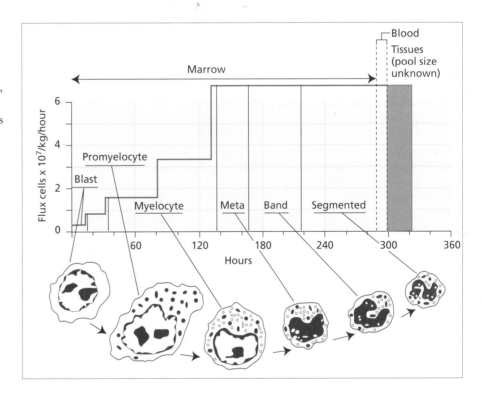

Table 17.4 Neutrophil granules and their contents.

Granule	Azurophilic (primary)	Specific (secondary)	Gelatinase (tertiary)	Secretory vesicles
Marker enzyme	Myeloperoxidase	Lactoferrin	Gelatinase	Alkaline phosphatase
Membrane	CD63, granulophysin, CD68, V-type H^+-ATPase	CD15, CD66, CD67, CD11b/CD18, Cytochrome b, fMLP-R, fibronectin-R, G-protein α-subunit, laminin-R, NB-1 antigen, 19-kDa protein, 155 kDa protein, Rap-1, Rap-2, SCAMP, thrombospondin-R, TNF-R, urokinase type plasminogen activator-R, VAMP-2, vitronectin	CD11b/CD18, cytochrome b, diacylglycerol-deacylating enzyme, fMLP-R, SCAMP, urokinase type plasminogen activator-R, VAMP-2, V-type H^+-ATPase	CD10, CD13, CD45, CD14, CD16, CD35 (CR1), CD11b/CD18, alkaline phosphatase, fMLP-R, SCAMP, urokinase type plasminogen activator-R, V-type H^+-ATPase, VAMP-2, C1q-receptor, decay activating factor
Matrix, microbicidal	Myeloperoxidase, nitric oxide (NO) synthase, lysozyme, BPI protein, defensins, serprocidins, elastase, cathepsins, proteinase 3, azurocidin (CAP 37)	Lactoferrin, lysozyme	Lysozyme	
Matrix, hydrolases	Acid β-glycerophosphatase, α-mannosidase, β-glucuronidase, β-glycerophosphatase, N-acetyl-β-glucosaminidase, sialidase	Gelatinase, collagenase, histaminase, heparanase, NGAL, sialidase	Gelatinase, acetyltransferase	
Matrix, other	Acid-mucopolysaccharide, heparin binding protein	β_2-microglobulin, urokinase-type plasminogen activator, vitamin-B_{12} binding protein	β_2-microglobulin,	Plasma proteins (including tetranectin)

Fmlp, f-Met-Leu-Phe; R, receptor; SCAMP, secretory carrier membrane protein; VAMP, vesicle associated membrane protein.

Neutrophils are the most numerous leucocytes comprising 65% of circulating phagocytes with a normal range in the peripheral blood of 1.5–7.7×10^9/L. The largest proportion of neutrophils is within the marrow (reserve pool), with circulating and tissue pools comprising smaller fractions (Figure 17.4). The circulating pool itself consists of a marginated pool of cells that are loosely adherent to the vascular endothelium and a freely circulating pool with the compartments in a constant state of dynamic equilibrium. Several factors including corticosteroids, exercise and infection can lead to an increase in the free circulating pool. Corticosteroids promote the release of neutrophils from the reserve pool into the circulation and prevent migration from the blood into the tissue pool. Endotoxin and some complement components (C5a) on the other hand, result in increased margination and reduction in the circulatory pool. The half-life of a circulating neutrophil is short (6–8 h) (Figure 17.4). In Figure 17.5, the variations in neutrophil morphology are shown. These include: (a) Barr body, a drumstick appendage to the neutrophils in females; (b) Pelger–Huët anomaly, with

bilobed nuclei; and (c) Alder–Reilly anomaly. Also shown are May–Hegglin (d), toxic granulation (e), hypersegmented neutrophils (f) and Chédiak–Hegasin (g).

The May–Hegglin anomaly is a rare autosomal dominant condition. The neutrophils contain basophilic inclusions of RNA, resembling Döhle bodies (Figure 17.5). Giant platelets with thrombocytopenia are common, leukopenia less so.

Disorders of neutrophil function and number

Neutrophilia

Leucocytosis or increased white blood cell count may be either due to a primary (congenital or acquired) marrow disorder or secondary to a disease process, a toxin or a drug (Table 17.5). Neutrophil counts are high in neonates and decrease to normal adult levels with ageing. Secondary leucocytosis not associated with leukaemia but with a very high white blood cell count ($> 50 \times 10^9$/L) is often referred to as leukaemoid reaction and can be associated with presence of Döhle bodies and toxic

Table 17.5 Causes of neutrophilia.

Primary	Hereditary
	Chronic idiopathic
	Familial myeloproliferative disease
	Leukaemoid reaction associated with congenital anomalies
	Leucocyte adhesion deficiency (LAD) types I and II
	Familial cold urticaria and leucocytosis
Secondary	Infection
	Stress
	Chronic inflammation
	Drugs (steroids, lithium, tetracycline)
	Non-haematological neoplasms
	Asplenia and hyposplenism
Neoplastic	Chronic myeloid leukaemia
	Other myeloproliferative disorders (myelofibrosis, PV, ET)

ET, essential thrombocythaemia; PV, polycythaemia vera.

granulation within the cytoplasm (Figure 17.5), as well as a 'left shift' (with presence in blood of myelocytes, metamyelocytes and band forms) and an elevated leucocyte alkaline phosphatase score (compared with a low score in chronic myeloid leukaemia, CML). In contrast with acute leukaemia, there is an orderly maturation and proliferation of all normal myeloid elements in the bone marrow. Leukaemoid reactions have been described in patients with osteomyelitis, empyema, septicaemia, tuberculosis, Hodgkin's disease, juvenile rheumatoid arthritis and dermatitis herpetiformis.

Leucocyte adhesion deficiency (LAD) is a congenital disorder, presenting with persistent leucocytosis, delayed separation of the umbilical cord, recurrent infections, impaired wound healing and defects of activation of neutrophils. The condition is caused by defects in adhesion of neutrophils to blood vessel walls. As a result, phagocytes do not migrate from the bloodstream to sites of infection. Two types of LAD have been described. In LAD-I, mutations of the gene encoding the β-subunit of the $β_2$-integrins (CD11b and CD18) have been detected. The molecular basis for the rare LAD-II is defective glycosylation of ligands on leucocytes recognized by selectin family of adhesion molecules. Clinical features in the two types are similar and, due to the defect in neutrophil migration, abscesses and other sites of infection are devoid of pus despite the striking neutrophilia. Treatment involves the use of prophylactic antibiotics and aggressive therapy of periodontal disease. Stem cell transplantation can be considered in patients with severe disease.

Hereditary neutrophilia has been described in a single family of four with leucocyte counts chronically in the range of

$20 \times 10^9/L$ to $70 \times 10^9/L$ as well as splenomegaly, widened diploë of the skull, and a high leucocyte alkaline phosphatase but without serious medical problems. Neutrophil function and adhesion to vessel walls in these patients are normal and the condition appears to have an autosomal dominant inheritance.

Chronic idiopathic neutrophilia is an association of a chronically elevated neutrophil count (in the range of $11 \times 10^9/L$ to $40 \times 10^9/L$) in healthy individuals without any associated clinical problems. In one series, several individuals were followed for up to 20 years without developing any disease.

Leukaemoid reactions have been described with congenital disorders such as amegakaryocytic thrombocytopenia, tetralogy of Fallot, dextrocardia with absent radii and in patients with Down's syndrome. The neutrophilia in Down's syndrome patients is transient but may be exaggerated in response to stress. A syndrome of growth retardation, hepatosplenomegaly and leucocytosis has been described as familial myeloproliferative disease with some affected individuals dying in early life and others remaining stable or even improving with time. These patients had low LAP scores and no detectable cytogenetic abnormality. Others have reported families with several generations of affected individuals with a variety of myeloproliferative disorders but without cytogenetic abnormalities.

Familial cold urticaria and leucocytosis is a syndrome of fever, urticaria, rash and muscle and skin tenderness on exposure to cold, which appears to be dominantly inherited. The onset of the disease is in infancy with urticaria, rash and leucocytosis generally occurring several hours after cold exposure. The skin rash is histologically characterized by intense infiltration by neutrophils.

Non-malignant causes of neutrophilia include acute infections with elevated counts in most bacterial infections. In cases of overwhelming infection, marrow depletion can occur, resulting in neutropenia rather than neutrophilia. Neutrophilia in chronic inflammatory processes is usually more modest in degree and can be accompanied by monocytosis. Modest elevation of neutrophil count is commonly seen in various forms of 'stress' such as exercise, adrenaline injection, myocardial infarction, post-operative period, post-ictal states and with emotional distress. This is probably due to the migration of neutrophils from the marginated pool to the circulatory pool. Mild neutrophilia has also been reported with unipolar depression. A number of drugs and drug reactions are commonly associated with increased neutrophil count. Steroids stimulate the release of neutrophils from the bone marrow and diminish their egress from the circulation resulting in chronic neutrophilia. This can be distinguished from neutrophilia due to infection by the distinct lack of band forms in the former. β-Agonists produce an acute neutrophilia by releasing neutrophils from the marginated pool. Other drugs known to produce neutrophil leucocytosis include lithium, which increases the production of CSF and potentiates its effects on myeloid colony formation, and tetracycline, which has been associated with counts as high as

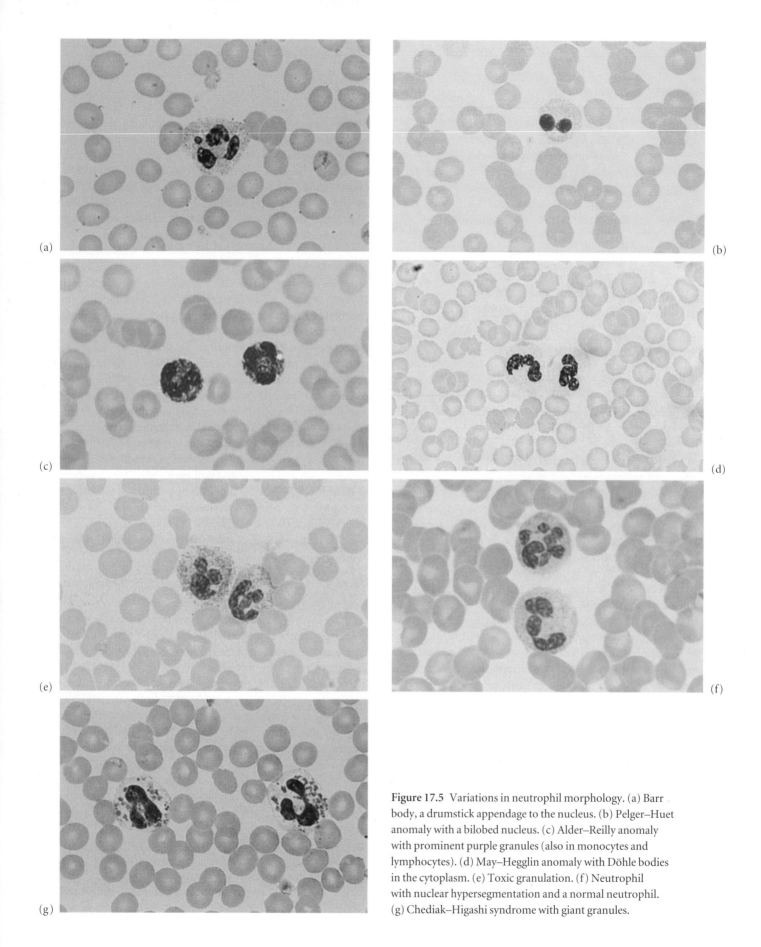

Figure 17.5 Variations in neutrophil morphology. (a) Barr body, a drumstick appendage to the nucleus. (b) Pelger–Huet anomaly with a bilobed nucleus. (c) Alder–Reilly anomaly with prominent purple granules (also in monocytes and lymphocytes). (d) May–Hegglin anomaly with Döhle bodies in the cytoplasm. (e) Toxic granulation. (f) Neutrophil with nuclear hypersegmentation and a normal neutrophil. (g) Chediak–Higashi syndrome with giant granules.

80×10^9/L. Growth factors such as G-CSF, GM-CSF and Neulasta (a pegylated form of G-CSF that prolongs its half-life in circulation) are commercially available and are used commonly to reduce the duration of neutropenia associated with chemotherapy and to mobilize stem cells for transplantation. Their use in healthy individuals for the latter purpose is associated with significant neutrophilia and a left shift.

Neutropenia

Neutropenia can be due to impaired production by the bone marrow, shift from the circulating pool to marginated pool, increased peripheral destruction, or a combination of these (Table 17.6). It has been defined as an absolute neutrophil count

Table 17.6 Causes of neutropenia.

Decreased production

Inherited	Reticular dysgenesis
	Dyskeratosis congenita
	Schwachman–Diamond–Oski syndrome
	Cyclic neutropenia
	Kostmann's syndrome
	Hyperimmunoglobulin-M syndrome
	Chronic idiopathic neutropenia
Acquired	Aplastic anaemia
	Bone marrow infiltration (leukaemia, lymphoma, tumours, tuberculosis, etc.)
	Severe infection
	Drug induced (cytotoxic chemotherapy, radiation, chloramphenicol, penicillins, cephalosporins, phenothiazine, phenylbutazone, gold, antithyroid drugs, quinidine, anticonvulsants, alcohol)
	Myelodysplastic syndrome
	Vitamin B_{12} or folate deficiency
	Pure white cell aplasia
	T-γ lymphocytosis and neutropenia
	Neutropenia associated with metabolic disorders

Increased peripheral destruction

Hypersplenism
Immune mediated
Drug induced
Associated with collagen vascular disease (Felty's syndrome, systemic lupus erythematosus)
Complement mediated (haemodialysis, cardiopulmonary bypass)

Altered distribution

Drugs
Stress

of more than two standard deviations below a normal mean value. There is a variation of neutrophil counts amongst different ethnic groups, with black people generally having slightly lower counts (lower limit of normal 1.2×10^9/L) compared with white people (lower limit of normal 1.5×10^9/L). The lower count in black population has been attributed to a relative decrease in the size of marrow storage pool. In patients whose neutropenia is related to decreased production, the propensity to develop infections is directly related to the degree and duration of neutropenia.

On the other hand, in patients whose neutropenia is to peripheral destruction or margination of neutrophils, there is no direct correlation between the degree of neutropenia and the propensity for infections. Conditions such as marrow failure states and neutropenia associated with chemotherapy can predispose patients to severe life-threatening infections, although this is more likely in patients with neutrophil counts below 0.5×10^9/L. Common organisms encountered in this setting are *Staphylococcus aureus*, *Pseudomonas aeruginosa*, *Escherichia coli* and *Klebsiella* species. On the other hand, patients with some congenital or immune forms of neutropenia can tolerate low counts for prolonged periods without any apparent increase in the incidence of infections.

Several well-defined inherited syndromes associated with neutropenia have been described. Moderate, asymptomatic neutropenia associated with specific ethnic groups such as American black people and Yemenite Jews has dominant inheritance. *Kostmann's syndrome or infantile agranulocytosis* is characterized by early onset of severe, recurrent infections, neutropenia and maturation arrest of myelopoiesis at the promyelocyte stage. Defects of granule production have been described in some patients. Both autosomal recessive and dominant inheritance, as well as sporadic cases, have been described. Recent studies have detected different inherited or spontaneous point mutations in the neutrophil elastase gene.

Other reported abnormalities include deficiency of antibacterial peptides, which correlates with the degree of periodontal disease. Development of additional genetic defects during the course of the disease, such as G-CSF receptor and *ras* gene mutations, and cytogenetic aberrations, indicates an underlying genetic instability. Progression to acute myeloid leukaemia (AML) and myelodysplastic syndrome (MDS) has been reported and may be associated with the mutations of G-CSF receptor gene. The majority of patients (over 90%) respond well to G-CSF, with a reduction in incidence of severe infections and use of intravenous antibiotics. It is plausible that G-CSF may accelerate the propensity for MDS/AML in the genetically altered stem and progenitor cells, especially in those with G-CSF receptor and *ras* mutations (82% and 50% of patients who transform, respectively). However, no association between the dose or duration of G-CSF therapy and malignant transformation has been identified and it is more likely that G-CSF may simply be an 'innocent bystander' that corrects neutropenia, prolongs patient survival and allows time for the malignant predisposition to declare itself. Haemopoietic stem cell transplantation should be considered particularly in those with a poor response to G-CSF.

Cyclic neutropenia is a rare, dominantly inherited disorder with variable expression, which is characterized by repetitive episodes of fever, pharyngitis, stomatitis and other bacterial infections attributable to recurrent severe neutropenia occurring every 15–35 days. The nadir neutrophil count, usually between zero and 200×10^9/L, lasts 3–7 days and is frequently associated with monocytosis. Cycling of red cell and platelet production is also observed in some cases. The bone marrow is characterized by transient arrest at the promyelocyte stage before each cycle. Both childhood and adult onset have been reported. Recent studies have shown that autosomal dominant and sporadic cases of this disease are due to a mutation in *ELA2*, the gene for neutrophil elastase (a chymotryptic serine protease of neutrophil and monocyte granules), located at chromosome 19p13.3. This enzyme is synthesized in neutrophil precursors early in the process of primary granule formation. A hypothesis at present suggests that the mutant neutrophil elastase functions aberrantly within the cells to accelerate apoptosis of the precursors, resulting in oscillatory production. The disorder is effectively treated with G-CSF, and no transformation to AML or MDS has been in these patients, with or without G-CSF therapy.

Schwachman–Diamond–Oski syndrome is an autosomal recessive disorder characterized by exocrine pancreas insufficiency, metaphyseal dysostosis and bone marrow dysfunction. Recurrent severe bacterial infections and susceptibility to leukaemia are the major causes of morbidity and mortality, although many affected individuals have relatively few problems with infections. Neutrophil count is commonly less than 500×10^9/L and many patients are also anaemic and thrombocytopenic. Bone marrow is usually hypoplastic and a number of neutrophil functional disorders such as chemotactic defects may be present. A variety of physical anomalies including short stature, strabismus, syndactyly, cleft palate and microcephaly may exist. The propensity to develop leukaemia and aplastic anaemia suggests that a stem cell defect may be present. Treatment involves the use of G-CSF in patients with recurrent infections, and the use of pancreatic enzyme supplements for the gastrointestinal insufficiency and steatorrhoea. Some anaemic patients respond to steroids.

Reticular dysgenesis is associated with neutropenia, lymphoid hypoplasia, and thymic hypoplasia with normal erythropoiesis and megakaryopoiesis. Patients have a hypoplastic marrow and low levels of IgM and IgG and die from overwhelming infections usually in early infancy. Dyskeratosis congenita is a rare disease characterized by abnormal skin pigmentation, nail dystrophy and mucosal leucoplakia. More than 80% of the affected individuals develop bone marrow failure, which is the major cause of death. The disorder is caused by defective telomere maintenance

in stem cells. The major X-linked form of the disease is due to mutations in the DKC1 gene located at Xq28 and coding for dyskarin, a nucleolar protein (see Chapter 12). Dyskerin is part of small nucleolar ribonucleoprotein particles involved in processing ribosomal RNA. It is also found in the telomerase complex, pointing to a possible link between these two processes. An autosomal dominant form is due to mutations in the RNA component of telomerase. Patients with this form of the disease are more severely affected in the later generations carrying the mutations, possibly due to the inheritance of shortened telomeres, and may be considered to have aplastic anaemia.

Neutropenia has been seen with immunological abnormalities such as hyper-IgM syndrome and X-linked agammaglobulinaemia. Hyper-IgM syndrome is an X-linked disorder characterized by lymphoid hyperplasia, low concentrations of IgG and IgA, but high concentration of IgM and severe neutropenia. A genetic defect in the T-cell CD40 ligand has been implicated as the cause of the disease. CD40 ligand is a 39-kDa protein expressed on the surface of activated CD4+ T cells, which delivers contact-dependent signals to CD40-expressing cells: B cells, monocytes, dendritic cells, epithelial cells, endothelial cells and fibroblasts. The loss of interaction between CD40 and its ligand results in an impairment of T-cell function, of B-cell differentiation and of monocyte function. Patients commonly die of overwhelming infections by the age of 5 years unless treated with intravenous immunoglobulin and long-term G-CSF.

Chronic benign neutropenia, chronic idiopathic neutropenia and autoimmune neutropenia are very similar in laboratory findings and differ only with regards to age of onset and association with other immune disorders. Chronic benign neutropenia commonly presents in older children or young adults. Patients are usually asymptomatic and have neutrophil counts in the range of $0.2–0.5 \times 10^9$/L. Bone marrow examination is commonly normocellular or occasionally moderately hypocellular. They usually have a peripheral monocytosis and often a benign course, although anecdotal cases progressing to acute leukaemia have been reported. Anti-neutrophil antibodies, detected in some patients, are not commonly present but antibodies to the stem cells or other precursors may be the inciting factor in these patients. As these patients generally have a benign course, treatment to increase neutrophil count should be reserved for those who have recurrent infections. Corticosteroids, splenectomy, cytotoxic agents and G-CSF have all been used successfully in this setting. Chronic benign neutropenia of infancy and childhood is probably a related disease, with the majority of patients presenting in the first year of life. There is no familial predisposition and anti-neutrophil antibodies are commonly detected. Furthermore, the neutropenia responds to immunosuppressive therapy, suggesting an immune mechanism. There is a compensatory increase in neutrophil precursors in the marrow. Some patients have a measurable defect of neutrophil mobility, otherwise described as 'lazy leucocyte syndrome'.

Infants of hypertensive mothers also commonly have

moderate to severe neutropenia lasting for several days. This is probably related to bone marrow suppression. Moderate to severe neutropenia can also occur in newborn infants as a result of transfer of maternal IgG anti-neutrophil antibodies in a manner similar to the rhesus haemolytic disease of the newborn. This isoimmune neutropenia develops antenatally and is due to maternal production of antibodies against antigens on fetal neutrophils.

Pure white cell aplasia is a rare condition associated with recurrent pyogenic infections and with thymoma in 70% of the affected patients. There is almost complete absence of myeloid precursors without any abnormality of erythroid or megakaryocytic precursors in the marrow. In the majority of patients, the marrow inhibitory activity is in the IgG and IgM fractions of serum but, in some, the inhibition is due to the lymphocytes. The immunoglobulin is directed against progenitor cells or myeloid precursors. The disorder has been associated with therapy with ibuprofen, certain natural remedies and chlorpropamide. If associated with thymoma, surgical removal of the thymus gland can partially correct the neutropenia. Other treatment options include corticosteroids, cyclosporin A, cyclophosphamide and intravenous immunoglobulin.

Humoral and cellular immune responses are responsible for the development of neutropenia in a number of settings. Autoimmune neutropenia due to circulating antibody can occur as an isolated condition or in association with other autoimmune disorders such as autoimmune thrombocytopenic purpura and autoimmune haemolytic anaemia. The antibodies may be directed at the mature neutrophils or morphologically identifiable myeloid precursors.

Inhibition of granulopoiesis by suppressor or cytotoxic T lymphocytes can occur in patients with collagen vascular disorders as well as in patients with T-γ lymphocytosis. Patients with T-γ lymphocytosis commonly present with recurrent infections at a median age of 55 years. There is a clonal proliferation of either CD3$^+$/CD56$^+$ T cells or CD3$^-$/CD56$^+$ natural killer (NK) cells. NK cells do not express CD5 and T-cell receptor (TCR) proteins, and their TCR locus is not rearranged, whereas CD3$^+$ large granular lymphocytes have rearranged TCR genes and are thought to represent *in vivo* activated cytotoxic T cells. The characteristic findings include peripheral blood lymphocytosis with most lymphocytes being large granular lymphocytes. Patients may also have lymphadenopathy and hepatosplenomegaly; the bone marrow is commonly normocellular with increased lymphocytes and arrested myelopoiesis at the myelocyte stage. The CD3$^+$ subset of the disease most commonly has an indolent course although most patients need treatment for recurrent episodes of life-threatening infections. G-CSF therapy is used in managing acute infections and methotrexate, prednisolone, cyclophosphamide or cyclosporin can be effective in improving neutrophil counts for sustained periods. In contrast, the CD3$^-$/CD56$^+$ NK-cell disorders are clinically aggressive, occurring in younger patients and presenting with fever, massive hepatosplenomegaly, jaundice and marrow infiltration with the abnormal clone. They typically have a rapidly progressive course unresponsive to combination chemotherapy.

Neutropenia is also associated with collagen vascular diseases such as systemic lupus erythematosus (SLE), and rheumatoid arthritis. IgG or IgM antibodies may be directed against mature neutrophils or their precursors. Recent advances have allowed better understanding regarding the mechanism of neutropenia and improved options for treatment. Target antigens for anti-neutrophil antibodies have been identified for both Felty's syndrome and for SLE. In Felty's syndrome, severe neutropenia is associated with rheumatoid arthritis, splenomegaly and leg ulcers. Therapy for neutropenia with methotrexate and cyclosporin A has been attempted with variable success. The efficacy of both GM-CSF and G-CSF in reversing neutropenia and decreasing the risk of infections in Felty's syndrome and SLE has been well documented. Of concern, however, have been flares of symptoms or development of leucocytoclastic vasculitis in some patients following the use of these cytokines. Recent results suggest that G-CSF should be administered at the lowest dose effective at elevating the neutrophil count above 1.0×10^9/L.

Drug-induced neutropenia is probably the commonest cause of isolated neutropenia. A thorough evaluation of the medication history of a patient with neutropenia is important for excluding drugs as the inciting factor. The mechanisms usually are by suppression of the bone marrow or immunological. The neutropenia commonly develops 1–2 weeks after initiation of the drug and resolves soon after discontinuation of the offending agent. Agents most commonly associated with this side-effect include antibiotics (such as penicillins, cephalosporins and chloramphenicol), anticonvulsants (e.g. carbamazepine and phenytoin), anti-inflammatory agents (e.g. gold, phenylbutazone), antithyroid drugs (e.g. carbimazole, methylthiouracil), hypoglycaemic agents (e.g. chlorpropamide), diuretics (e.g. hydrochlorothiazide, bumetanide) and phenothiazine. Cytotoxic agents used in cancer therapy are well known for this complication.

Other miscellaneous causes of neutropenia include viral infections (HIV, varicella, measles, rubella, infectious mononucleosis, influenza, hepatitis A and B, parvovirus and cytomegalovirus), overwhelming bacterial infections (by exhausting the neutrophil reserve pool), metabolic diseases (such as orotic aciduria, methylmalonic aciduria and glycogen storage disease type Ib), nutritional deficiency (deficiency of vitamin B$_{12}$, folate causing also hypersegmented nuclei – Figure 17.5 – or copper) and with hypersplenism.

Disorders of neutrophil function

A number of congenital and acquired conditions with abnormal neutrophil morphology (Figure 17.2a) and/or function have been recognized (Table 17.7). Some of these are associated with abnormal neutrophil numbers and were discussed earlier.

Table 17.7 Disorders of neutrophil morphology and/or function.

Functional defect	Congenital	Acquired
Minimal	Hereditary neutrophil hypersegmentation (AD) Pelger–Huet anomaly (AD) Alder–Reilly anomaly (AR) May–Hegglin anomaly (AD) Myeloperoxidase deficiency (AR)	Megaloblastic hypersegmentation Mucopolysaccharidoses
Adherence/migration	Leucocyte adhesion deficiency (AR) Neutrophil-specific granule deficiency (AR) Schwachman's syndrome (?AR) Hyper-IgE syndrome Job's syndrome (AR) Familial Mediterranean fever (AR)	Renal failure Diabetes Neonates Malnutrition Leukaemia
Phagocytic killing	Chronic granulomatous disease Papillon–Lefevre syndrome (AR)	Malnutrition Vitamin E deficiency Severe iron deficiency Neonates Diabetes Viral infections Sickle cell disease

AD, autosomal dominant; AR, autosomal recessive.

Chédiak–Higashi syndrome

Chédiak–Higashi syndrome is a rare autosomal recessive disorder characterized by oculocutaneous albinism, recurrent and severe bacterial infections, giant blue-grey granules in the cytoplasm of white blood cells (Figure 17.5f), a mild bleeding diathesis, progressive peripheral neuropathy and cranial nerve abnormalities. Morbidity results from patients succumbing to frequent bacterial infections or to an 'accelerated phase', a progressive lymphoproliferative syndrome. Patients eventually succumb to a profound pancytopenia. Neutrophils contain a highly inhomogeneous population of giant granules probably derived from coalescence of azurophil and secondary granules. The giant granules are seen more commonly in the bone marrow than peripheral blood, as many of the abnormal myeloid precursors are destroyed before release, leading to moderate neutropenia.

Neutrophils also have a deficiency of antimicrobial proteins as well as disordered degranulation and chemotaxis. Dysfunction of other elements of the immune system such as the cytotoxic T lymphocytes and natural killer cells contribute to the propensity for infection and the development of the accelerated phase of the disease. Mutations in the lysosomal trafficking regulator, or *CHS1/LYST* gene, located on chromosome 1q43, have been implicated as the cause of this disease. At present, treatment for the disorder is stem cell transplant, which alleviates the immune problems and the accelerated phase, but does not inhibit the development of neurological disorders that grow increasingly worse with age.

Chronic granulomatous disease

Chronic granulomatous disease (CGD) is an inherited disease characterized by severe and recurrent purulent bacterial and fungal infections, including pneumonia, lymphadenitis, hepatic abscesses and osteomyelitis. The majority of patients present in the first year of life with infections with catalase-positive organisms. Phagocytic cells of CGD patients are unable to produce superoxide anions, and their efficiency in bacterial killing is significantly impaired. In addition, a failure to switch off the inflammatory response leads to the formation of granules. All the subtypes of X-linked CGD are caused by mutations in the gene for the gp91-*phox* subunit of cytochrome *b* (CYBB) located at the XP21.1. There is a significant heterogeneity in the mutations in the gene, with most being family specific. This accounts for the clinical heterogeneity seen in the X-linked CGD. Other mutations in recessively inherited forms of the disease have also been described.

Diagnosis of CGD is suggested by failure of neutrophils to reduce nitroblue tetrazolium (NBT slide test). Diagnosis can be further established by directly measuring respiratory burst activity as oxygen consumption, O_2 production or H_2O_2 production. A severe deficiency of glucose-6-phosphate dehydrogenase (G6PD) in neutrophils, as seen in a rare X-linked disorder, can result in a greatly attenuated respiratory burst and a condition resembling CGD. Therapy involves prevention and early treatment of infections, aggressive parenteral antibiotic therapy for established infections, and use of prophylactic trimethoprim–

sulphamethoxazole. Recombinant human interferon-γ may augment the host defence and reduce the incidence of life-threatening infections by unknown mechanisms other than reversing the respiratory burst defect. Haemopoietic stem cell transplantation, if performed at the first signs of a severe course of the disease, is a valid therapeutic option for children with CGD having an HLA-identical donor.

Myeloperoxidase deficiency

Myeloperoxidase (MPO) deficiency is the most common inherited disorder of phagocytes and is inherited in an autosomal recessive manner. The gene encoding for MPO is located at 17q22–23 near the breakpoint of the translocation in acute promyelocytic leukaemia. Despite the key role of MPO in the microbicidal function of neutrophils, persons with MPO deficiency lack any clinical symptoms and therapy is not required except for incidences of fungal infections when aggressive antifungal therapy is indicated.

Neutrophil specific granule deficiency

Specific granule deficiency (SGD) is a rare congenital disorder characterized by recurrent bacterial and fungal infections of skin and lungs. The inheritance is autosomal recessive and, although the precise molecular defect has not been elucidated, recent data implicate functional loss of the myeloid transcription factor CCAAT/enhancer binding protein, C/EBP(epsilon), as important in the development of SGD. The neutrophils of these patients display atypical bilobed nuclei, lack expression of at least one primary and all secondary and tertiary granule proteins, and possess defects in chemotaxis, disaggregation, receptor upregulation and bactericidal activity. Similar neutrophil granule deficiencies have been described in some patients with leukaemia.

Papillon–Lefevre syndrome

This is a rare autosomal recessive disorder characterized by palmoplantar keratoderma and early-onset peridontitis. Pyogenic liver abscesses are an increasing recognized complication. Consanguinity is common and the disease is commonly manifested in the first 6 months of life, with early progressive loss of both primary and secondary dentition. A phagocytic defect in microbicidal activity and degradation of ingested material is thought to be present. This is attributed to loss of function mutations of the CTSC gene located on chromosome 11q14–q21, which encodes the protease, cathepsin G.

Eosinophils (Figure 17.2b)

Development and function

Eosinophils, which account for 5–10% of leucocytes (0.2×10^9/L) are similar to neutrophils morphologically except for the presence of a bilobed nucleus and numerous bright-orange cytoplasmic granules. There are three distinct granule popula-

tions including the round, uniformly electron-dense primary granules present mainly in the eosinophilic promyelocyte/myelocyte stages, secondary or specific granules, and the less well characterized small granules (Table 17.8).

Primary granules contain eosinophil peroxidase and Charcot–Leyden crystal protein. The eosinophil peroxidase is distinct from neutrophil myeloperoxidase and can mediate damage to micro-organisms and tissues and bronchoconstriction in asthma. Charcot–Leyden crystal protein is found in tissues and fluids in association with eosinophil inflammatory reactions and may have a role in respiratory disease.

The large specific granules contain the eosinophils' cytotoxic and proinflammatory proteins and account for more than 95% of granules in the mature eosinophils conferring the characteristic appearance of the cell. The eosinophil granules contain a number of enzymes similar to those in the neutrophil lysosomes, but lack lysozyme. Different cationic polypeptides are the major constituents of eosinophil granules and include the major basic protein (MBP), eosinophil cationic proteins (ECP) and eosinophil-derived neurotoxin (EDN). MBP is toxic to cells, including parasites and mammalian epithelial cells, and evokes release of mediators from basophils and mast cells. Eosinophils have a significant cytotoxic and proinflammatory function and play an important part in the pathogenesis of a number of allergic, parasitic and malignant disease processes.

Eosinophils are derived from bone marrow stem cell-derived, myeloid progenitors in response to a number of T-cell derived cytokines and growth factors including IL-3, GM-CSF and IL-5. Mast cells, macrophages, natural killer cells, endothelial cells and stromal cells also produce these cytokines. IL-5 is the most lineage-specific factor and plays an important role in regulation of terminal differentiation and post-mitotic activation of eosinophils. Therefore, IL-5 is a late-acting cytokine that is both necessary and sufficient for eosinophil development in vivo, a finding that has been confirmed by IL-5 transgenic and IL-5 knockout mice.

In normal individuals, eosinophils exist transiently in the circulation and localize specifically to certain tissues and organs exposed to the external environment. Eosinophils are recruited in response to early- and late-phase components of immediate hypersensitivity reactions as well as other immunologically mediated reactions. Their activation and recruitment involves the interaction of several adhesion pathways and chemotactic agents including the complement fragment C5a, platelet-activating factor (PAF), IL-3, IL-5, GM-CSF, IL-2, RANTES, eotaxins and the CD8+ T cell-derived lymphocyte chemoattractant factor (LCF).

The specificity and intensity of the microbicidal function of eosinophils differ from those of other leucocytes; their bactericidal activity is less efficient than that of neutrophils, but not because any deficiency of specific enzymes. In fact, eosinophil peroxidase is more bactericidal than myeloperoxidase. However, the major protective role of eosinophils in host defence is the

Table 17.8 Contents of eosinophil granules.

Granule	Protein content	Comment
Primary granule (Charcot–Leyden crystal protein-containing granule)	Charcot–Leyden crystal (CLC) protein	Weak lysophospholipase, carbohydrate binding properties
Specific granule (secondary granule)	Eosinophil peroxidase	
	Major basic protein (MBP)	Toxic to parasites
	Eosinophil cationic protein (ECP)	Ribonuclease, bactericidal, toxic to parasites
	Eosinophil derived neurotoxin (EDN)	Ribonuclease, toxic to parasites
	Eosinophil peroxidase (EPO)	Antibacterial
	Lysophospholipase	
	Acid phosphatase	
	Arylsulphatase B	
	Phospholipase A_2 (secretory)	Antibacterial
	Bactericidal permeability-increasing protein (BPI)	LPS binding, antibacterial
	NAMLAA	Antibacterial
	FAD	
	Catalase	
	Urokinase	
	CD63	Tetraspanin
	Proteoglycan	
	α_1-Antitrypsin	
Small-type granule	Arylsulphatase B	Lysosomal hydrolase
Secretory vesicle	Cytochrome $b558$	NADPH oxidase component
	CR3	β_2-Integrin

FAD, flavin adenine dinucleotide; NAMLAA, N-acetylmuramyl-L-alanine amidase.

destruction of metazoan parasites. Eosinophils readily degranulate in response to stimulation by antigens, cytokines and complexed or secretory IgA, IgE, and IgG. Proteins released from eosinophils result in histamine release from basophils and mast cells, and amplify the inflammatory response. They are also powerful toxins towards host cells, leading to tissue injury. A further role of eosinophils is in tissue repair and remodelling through the regulation of the deposition of extracellular matrix proteins.

Disorders of eosinophils

Eosinophilia

Eosinophilia is considered as an absolute eosinophil count of 0.5×10^9/L or more. Blood and tissue eosinophilia can be seen in a number of parasitic, neoplastic, collagen vascular and allergic diseases (Table 17.9). In these disorders, a variety of abnormal stimuli lead to the increased production and tissue localization of eosinophils. When no underlying cause can be identified, the hypereosinophilic syndrome (HES) may be present. Several reactive pulmonary and cutaneous eosinophilic syndromes (such as Churg–Strauss syndrome, Loeffler's syndrome and eosinophilic lymphofolliculosis or Kimura's disease) as well as

an eosinophilia–myalgia syndrome have also been described. Eosinophilia–myalgia syndrome is related to metabolites and contaminants in preparation of the drug L-tryptophan and presents with peripheral blood eosinophilia, fatigue and severe myalgia. It responds slowly to the cessation of L-tryptophan therapy in a number of the patients.

Hypereosinophilic syndrome is characterized by sustained eosinophilia of 30–70% of total leucocyte count ($> 1.5 \times 10^9$/L) for longer than 6 months, absence of other underlying causes of eosinophilia and evidence of organ dysfunction due to eosinophilic tissue infiltration. Presenting features include anorexia, weight loss, fever, sweating, thromboembolic episodes, heart failure, splenomegaly, and skin and central nervous system disease. Peripheral blood eosinophils have a variety of cellular abnormalities and bone marrow eosinophils are increased (30–60%), but myeloblasts are usually not. It has been difficult to assess the clonality of the hypereosinophilic syndrome, but some cases are clonally derived, as demonstrated by clonal karyotypic abnormalities and X-inactivation assays.

In most cases of idiopathic hypereosinophilic syndrome, however, the eosinophils are independent of growth factors, and the condition has features of a myeloproliferative syndrome. In some cases, a monoclonal population of activated T cells,

Table 17.9 Causes of eosinophilia.

Infections		
	Parasitic	Helminthic (filariasis, strongyloidosis, hydatid disease, onchocerciasis, etc.) Visceral larva migrans
	Non-parasitic	Coccidiomycosis Recovery from acute infections Cat scratch disease Cryptococcus
Allergic disease		Atopic diseases Drug hypersensitivity Bronchopulmonary aspergillosis
Pulmonary		Allergic bronchopulmonary aspergillosis Eosinophilic pneumonia Transient pulmonary infiltrates (Löffler's syndrome) Prolonged pulmonary infiltrates with eosinophilia Tropical pulmonary eosinophilia Allergic granulomatosis (Churg–Strauss syndrome)
Cutaneous		Eosinophilic lymphofolliculosis (Kimura's disease) Bullous pemphigoid Granulomatous dermatitis with eosinophilia (Well's disease) Eosinophilic fascitis (Shulman's syndrome) Atopic dermatitis Urticaria and angioedema
Connective tissue disorder		Vasculitis Serum sickness Eosinophilic fascitis
Immunological disorders		Wiskott–Aldrich syndrome Selective IgA deficiency Graft-versus-host disease
Neoplastic conditions		Eosinophilic leukaemia Lymphoma (Hodgkin's, T cell) Chronic myeloid leukaemia Acute myeloid leukaemia, M4Eo Some solid tumours
Miscellaneous		Eosinophilic myalgia syndrome Toxic oil syndrome Idiopathic hypereosinophilic syndrome

displaying abnormal combinations of surface markers, produces large amounts of IL-5, the presumed cause of the eosinophilia. IgE levels in serum can be very high, perhaps because of other cytokines released by the T cells. Treatment of the HES attempts to limit organ damage by controlling the eosinophil count and includes prednisolone, hydroxyurea, IFN-α and cytotoxic chemotherapy. In most cases, however, the disorder is fatal. Recently, it was reported that nine out of eleven patients treated with imatinib mesylate, a tyrosine kinase inhibitor specific to BCR-ABL, KIT and platelet-derived growth factor (PDGF) responded with a durable normalization of their peripheral blood and marrow eosinophil count. One of these patients had a complex chromosomal abnormality leading to the identification of a fusion gene, *FIP1L1–PDGFRα*, generated by an interstitial deletion on chromosome 4q12. The protein product of *FIP1L1–PDGFRα* has enhanced tyrosine kinase activity, may be pathogenic at least in some patients, transforms haemopoietic cells and is inhibited by imatinib.

Basophils and mast cells (Figure 17.2c)

Development and function

The functions of basophils and mast cells are similar but not identical. They express on their surface the receptor that binds with high affinity the Fc portion of IgE antibody (FcεIR) and they have large metachromatic (purple-black) granules rich in histamine, serotonin and leukotrienes. Basophils have a bilobed nucleus, in contrast to mast cells, which have a unilobed nucleus. More recent studies have demonstrated that despite their significant similarities, basophils and mast cells are terminally differentiated progeny of distinct bone marrow progenitors. Whereas basophils mature in the bone marrow and circulate in the blood, mast cells mature in the tissues. They both have significant roles in a number of allergic and inflammatory disorders as well as host defence mechanisms against parasites.

Mechanisms mediating the maturation of basophils and mast cells are different. Mast cells are derived from CD34+, c-Kit-positive progenitors and not monocytes or basophils. A complex array of cytokines, elaborated by T cells, macrophages and stromal cells, regulate the production of basophils and mast cells. The major growth and differentiation factor for basophils is IL-3, whereas the growth and development of mast cells requires the presence of stem cell factor (SCF).

Basophils are the least abundant leucocytes, accounting for less than 0.5% of bone marrow and peripheral blood leucocytes. Basophils arise from a common basophil–eosinophil progenitor cell, mature in the marrow over a period of 2–7 days and after release in the circulation last for up to 2 weeks. They are the key mediators of immediate hypersensitivity reactions such as asthma, urticaria and anaphylaxis. In addition, they have been implicated in delayed cutaneous hypersensitivity reaction. Basophils are stimulated by a number of mediators, such as IgE, IL-3, C5a, GM-CSF, insect venoms and morphine, to release the contents of their granules such as histamine.

The interaction between IgE and basophil/mast cell FcεIR and antigens bridging them results in basophil degranulation and initiation of their effects. The granules of basophils and mast cells contain sulphated glycosaminoglycans responsible for their intense staining as well as histamine, leukotriene D_4 (LTD_4), PAF, eosinophil chemotactic factor (ECF), and kallikrein responsible for type I immediate hypersensitivity reactions and chronic inflammation (Table 17.10). Histamine is derived from histidine by decarboxylation and is stored as a complex with heparin or chondroitin sulphate proteoglycans. The primary protease of mast cells, tryptase, is mainly released during the early phase of allergic response and is a marker of mast cell activation in chronic inflammatory diseases. Other neutral proteases such as carboxypeptidase B, chymase, and sulphatases are also released and degrade extracellular matrix proteins. Basophil and mast cell activation also leads to the elaboration of cytokines such as GM-CSF, TNF-α, IFN-γ, IL-3, IL-4 and IL-5, which serve to amplify the inflammatory response; TNF-α and GM-CSF recruit and prime neutrophils, IL-5 activates eosinophils and IL-4 enhances cell adhesion molecule expression on endothelial cells, recruits eosinophils into tissues and induces helper T cells to mediate IgE production by B cells.

Disorders of basophils and mast cells

High basophil numbers are commonly seen in patients with myeloproliferative disorders, in particular chronic myeloid leukaemia (CML). Basophil number can be strikingly elevated in patients with CML, accounting for over 20% of circulating leucocytes in the more advanced stages of the disease. They are a part of the neoplastic clone expressing the Philadelphia chromosome or the BCR–ABL fusion gene. In other myeloproliferative disorders such as myelofibrosis and polycythaemia vera, elevation of basophil numbers is usually more modest. Cases of AML with high levels of immature basophils have also been reported. Rarely, basophils may constitute over 80% of circulating leucocytes, a condition sometimes referred to as basophilic leukaemia. These patients may exhibit clinical features related to the release of histamine and other basophil granular contents, and their treatment can be difficult owing to the possibility of massive release of these mediators secondary to cellular lysis. Other causes of basophilia include ulcerative colitis, myxoedema, recovery from acute illness and drug allergies, although these conditions are usually associated only with modest elevations of circulatory basophils.

As discussed earlier, SCF or c-kit ligand is an important factor in mast cell development. Therefore, it is plausible that conditions leading to its excessive production and mutation of c-kit, leading to its constitutive activation, can cause mastocytosis. An increased number of tissue mast cells can be seen in a number of disorders, including atopy, parasitic diseases, Hodgkin's and other lymphoproliferative disorders, some neoplasms and rheumatoid arthritis.

Several conditions, ranging from isolated cutaneous mastocytomas to mast cell leukaemia, are associated with mast cell proliferation. Solitary mastocytomas generally regress spontaneously. The more common cutaneous mastocytosis or urticaria pigmentosa typically presents with multiple small round reddish-brown maculopapular lesions, which, when subjected to minimal trauma, lead to intense pruritus. In some patients, this disease progresses to the systemic variety, with involvement of bone marrow, spleen, liver and the gastrointestinal tract. Systemic mastocytosis can also occur without prior or concurrent cutaneous disease, and in association with haematological disorders, including leukaemias and lymphomas. Organ dysfunction may be secondary to the release of biochemical mediators by mast cells, such as peptic ulcer disease secondary to histamine release. Mast cell leukaemia, a rare condition, presents with circulating mast cells of abnormal morphology (accounting for up to 95% of circulating nucleated cells), peptic ulcer disease, constitutional symptoms, anaemia and

Table 17.10 Basophil and mast cell granules, and their contents.

Component	Function	Main physiological role	Other properties	Cell specificity
Protein				
Histamine	Binds to H_1, H_2, H_3 receptors	Hypersensitivity reactions and inflammation		Basophils, mast cells
Proteoglycan				
Heparin	Package of basic proteins into granules		Binds and stabilizes proteases	Connective tissue mast cells
Chondroitin sulphates	Package of basic proteins into granules		Binds and stabilizes proteases	Basophils
Enzymes				
Chymase	Inactivates bradykinin, activates angiotensin 1, activates precursor IL-1β	Affects microcirculation, modulates microcirculation, modulates skin, inflammation		Connective tissue mast cells
Tryptase	Cleaves C3 to C3a and C3b	Proinflammatory, stimulates neutrophil chemotaxis and adherence	Tetrameric when bound to heparin, monomer inactive, restricted substrate specificity, raised levels in mast cell disorders	Mast cells
	Activates metalloproteinase 3, inactivates fibrinogen Degrades calcitonin gene-related peptide	Regulates collagenase, attenuates fibrin deposition		
Cathepsin G-like protease				Connective tissue mast cell
Carboxypeptidase				Connective tissue mast cell
Other				
Charcot–Leyden crystal protein	Lysophospholipase	Phospholipid metabolism	Neutralizes pulmonary surfactant	Basophil
Major basic protein		Disrupts membranes		Basophil
Sulphatase				
Exoglycosidase				

hepatosplenomegaly. It should be distinguished from AML, which can develop in association with systemic mastocytosis.

Management of patients within all categories of mastocytosis includes careful counselling of patients and care providers, avoidance of factors triggering acute mediator release, treatment of acute and chronic mast cell mediator release, an attempt to treat organ infiltration by mast cells, and treatment of any associated haematological disorder. The agents and modalities commonly used in treating patients with mastocytosis include antihistamines, H_2-receptor blockers, adrenaline, steroids, cromolyn sodium, proton pump inhibitors, ultraviolet light with psoralen (PUVA), chemotherapy, radiation, IFN-α, cyclosporin, 2-chlorodeoxyadenosine and splenectomy. With increased availability of small-molecular-weight inhibitors of signal transduction, targeting of the constitutively active mutated c-kit has attracted more attention. Two classes of constitutive activating c-kit mutations have been reported. The more frequent occurs in the catalytic pocket coding region, with substitutions at codon 816, and the other in the intracellular juxtamembrane coding region. Therefore, kinase inhibitors that block mutated c-*kit* activity might be used as therapeutic agents in systemic mastocytosis. Imatinib mesylate inhibits both wild-type and juxtamembrane mutant c-Kit kinase activity, but has no effect on the activity of the D816V mutant, commonly seen in patients with mastocytosis. Therefore, imatinib mesylate does not appear to be an effective therapy for this disease. However, activity of imatinib has been reported in a subset of patients with associated eosinophilia, who express the *FIP1L1–PDGFRα* fusion gene.

Monocytes and macrophages (Figure 17.2d and e)

The mononuclear phagocyte system has been defined as a family of cells comprising bone marrow progenitors, blood monocytes and tissue macrophages. Monocytes develop from a pluripotent stem cell in the bone marrow, termed colony-forming unit – granulocyte, erythrocyte, monocyte, megakaryocyte (CFU-GEMM) and the more committed CFU-GM. This stem cell can commit to both the neutrophil and monocytic pathways. Cytokines and growth factors, such as monocyte colony-stimulating factor (M-CSF), GM-CSF and IL-3, allow the commitment along monocytic pathways. M-CSF, also known as colony-stimulating factor-1 (CSF-1), is the most important factor in the development of monocytes and macrophages, and is necessary but not sufficient for their activation.

Following their release into the circulation, monocytes rapidly partition between the marginating and circulating pools. The circulating monocytes have a highly convoluted surface and a lobulated nucleus. They can be further characterized by non-specific esterase and contain a single type of nucleus with staining characteristics of lysosomes. After migration into tissues, they become larger and acquire the characteristics of tissue macrophages. Monocytes contain lysosomal hydrolases and the intracellular enzymes elastase and cathepsin. After transformation into tissue macrophages they produce predominantly metalloproteases and metalloprotease inhibitors, lose expression of hydrolases, and express macrophage-specific genes and products such as inducible nitrous oxide synthase (NOS) and IFN-γ. Tissue macrophages are long-lived and self-sustaining cells.

Macrophage activation is the acquisition of competence to perform specific and complex functions as a result of exposure to a constellation of cytokines and other factors in their environment, rather than achievement of a universal activated state. Physiological factors from the host such as cytokines and growth factors as well as environmental factors from micro-organisms constitute this constellation and their combined effect is synergistic. Macrophage activating factor (MAF), identified as IFN-γ, as well as IL-2, IL-4, M-CSF and GM-CSF are either directly or indirectly, through IFN-γ, responsible for macrophage activation. They stimulate monocyte/macrophage proliferation, increase adhesive receptor expression and stimulate the production of proteolytic agents responsible for pathogen clearance.

Whereas production of IFN-γ by the T helper 1 cells (Th1) results in a cytocidal macrophage state, IL-4 and IL-13 produced by the Th2 population of T lymphocytes stimulate the antigen-presenting cell (APC) state. These cytokines then enhance macrophage stimulation of T cells by inducing class II MHC antigen and co-stimulatory molecule expression. Activated macrophages, in turn, produce cytokines that stimulate both types of helper T cells.

Several cytokines including IL-4, IL-10, IL-13 and TGF-β can inhibit different aspects of macrophage function. Furthermore, prostaglandin E$_2$, elaborated by macrophages as well as corticosteroids can suppress various actions of macrophages. These provide a feedback loop mechanism for the control of the immune response.

Disorders of monocyte/macrophages

Monocytosis and monocytopenia
Chronic inflammatory conditions, both infectious and immune in nature, are associated with monocytosis (Table 17.11). These

Table 17.11 Causes of monocytosis.

Inflammatory conditions
Infections
Tuberculosis
Bacterial endocarditis
Fever of unknown origin
Syphilis

Other
Systemic lupus erythematosus
Rheumatoid arthritis
Temporal arteritis
Polyarteritis
Ulcerative colitis
Sarcoidosis
Myositis

Malignant disorders
AML
Hodgkin's disease
Non-Hodgkin's lymphomas
Histiocytoses
Carcinomas
MDS

Miscellaneous
Cyclic neutropenia
Chronic idiopathic neutropenia
Kostmann's syndrome
Post splenectomy

include tuberculosis, bacterial endocarditis, syphilis, collagen vascular disease, sarcoidosis and ulcerative colitis. Monocytosis is also commonly seen in a number of haematological malignancies such as AML, Hodgkin's disease, non-Hodgkin's lymphomas, and histiocytosis. Decreased number of circulating monocytes has been reported with endotoxaemia, corticosteroid administration and hairy cell leukaemia.

Histiocytic disorders

As described above, bone marrow monocytes enter the circulation and transform into tissue-specific macrophages under the influence of the local environment thus becoming cells of the mononuclear phagocytic system (MPS). Dendritic cells also have their origin in the bone marrow and share common progenitors with macrophages. Progenitors of dendritic cells are released from the bone marrow and enter tissues in which they differentiate into functional, antigen-presenting dendritic cells. The ordinary tissue macrophages have IgG Fc receptors, whereas the tissue-based dendritic cells comprising the dendritic cell system (DCS), lack phagocytic capacity or Fc receptors, and are predominantly antigen-presenting cells. The dendritic Langerhans cells are found in virtually all tissues except the brain and are the major immunological cellular components of the skin and mucosa. Their racquet-shaped ultrastructural inclusions (Birbeck bodies) distinguish them from other tissue cells. They interact with and process antigen, then migrate to lymphoid organs, where, through interaction with T-cells, they generate cellular and humoral immune responses. This ability of dendritic cells to interact with T cells and other inflammatory cells contributes to the often varied clinical manifestations of the histiocytic disorders.

The histiocytic disorders comprise varied haematological disorders with cells of the MPS or the DCS involved in their pathogenesis. In general, disease associated with proliferation of histiocytes can be grouped into two different categories: inflammatory disorders and neoplastic (clonal) disorders (Table 17.12). In the more recent classifications by the World Health Organization Committee on Histiocytic/Reticulum Cell Proliferations, other disorders in which histiocytes are implicated such as storage diseases (Gaucher's and Niemann–Pick) have been excluded. Abnormal immune response mediated by cytokines has been proposed to be the inciting factor for the two more common disorders: Langerhans cell histiocytosis (LCH) and haemophagocytic lymphohistiocytosis (HLH). It is, however, unclear whether the histiocytes themselves or other immune cells are the defective cell population.

Langerhans cell histiocytosis

It has been recognized that the offending cells in the disorders previously referred to as 'histiocytosis X' (including eosinophilic granuloma, Letterer–Siwe disease and Hand–Sculler–Christian disease) have the characteristics of the epidermal Langerhans cells. These disorders, now collectively referred to as LCH, have

Table 17.12 Histiocytic disorders.

Disorders of varied biological behaviour
Related to dendritic cells
Langerhans cell histiocytosis
Juvenile xanthogranuloma and related disorders
Solitary dendritic cell histiocytoma

Related to macrophages
Haemophagocytic syndromes
  Primary – familial haemophagocytic histiocytosis
  Secondary – infectious, tumour associated, drug associated
    (e.g. phenytoin)
Rosai–Dorfman disease (sinus histiocytosis with massive
  lymphadenopathy)
Solitary macrophage histiocytoma

Clonal disorders
Related to monocytes
Leukaemia – FAB M4 and M5, acute myelomonocytic
  leukaemia, chronic myelomonocytic leukaemia,
  extramedullary monocytic tumours

Related to dendritic cells
Histiocytic sarcoma (malignant histocytosis) – localized or
  disseminated

Related to macrophages
Histiocytic sarcoma (malignant histiocytosis) – localized
  or disseminated

variable clinical features depending on the organs infiltrated by the responsible Langerhans and accompanying cells. The true prevalence of these disorders is seven cases per million. The majority of cases occur in children under 15 years of age, but they can occur at any age.

The aetiology of these disorders is far from clear, but a number of clues from their biology and epidemiology are emerging. Associations with malignancies and an inherited predisposition based on studies in identical twins have been suggested. No seasonal variations or geographic or racial clustering has been reported, disputing the possibility of an infectious aetiology. Flow cytometry and chromosomal analysis of cells from LCH infiltrates as well as methods to assess clonality based on X chromosome inactivation have suggested the possibility of a clonal nature, although no consistent chromosomal alterations have been reported so far.

However, it is now clear that LCH is characterized by a clonal proliferation of CD1a$^+$ cells. The Langerhans cells from the lesions of patients demonstrate several phenotypic changes that distinguish them from their normal counterparts. Differences in staining by the lectin, peanut agglutinin (PNA), expression of placental alkaline phosphatase (PLAP), expression of the interferon-γ receptor, and expression of co-stimulatory receptors such as CD86 and CD80 have been reported between LCH lesional cells and their normal counterparts. There is extensive expression of GM-CSF, IL-1, IL-3, IL-4, IL-8, TNF and LIF in the LCH lesions, suggestive of activation of T lymphocytes as well as recruitment of macrophages, eosinophils and granulocytes. The accumulation of IL-1 and prostaglandin E_2 may explain the association of these lesions with bone loss. It is of note that such increases in immunostimulatory and tissue-damaging cytokines are at local sites, usually without high systemic levels.

The diagnosis of LCH is based on a biopsy of the involved organs with the key diagnostic feature being the presence of pathological Langerhans cells, which can be identified by demonstration of either CD1a surface antigen, or the presence of Birbeck granules on electron microscopy (Figure 17.5). Mitoses are usually not present and when found have no prognostic significance. Early lesions are generally cellular and locally destructive with abundance of essentially normal Langerhans cells. As the lesions mature, there are fewer Langerhans cells with occasional necrosis.

The lesions of LCH occur in skin, bone, lymph nodes, liver, spleen, bone marrow, lungs, the central nervous system and the gastrointestinal tract. Clinical features are varied and depend on the organs involved. It may involve single organs or be multisystem, and assessment of organ function is important as it can have prognostic significance. Initial investigations should include a full blood count, assessment of renal and hepatic function, a skeletal survey and a technetium bone scan; these latter studies are complementary with the latter being more sensitive for early lesions. Other investigations include a chest radiograph, and possibly magnetic resonance imaging (MRI) of the brain to rule out central nervous system (CNS) involvement. Additional testing for diabetes insipidus and other organ involvement should be carried out as indicated.

Solitary or multifocal eosinophilic granuloma (SEG or MEG) is found mainly in older children and young adults and accounts for the majority of cases of LCH. Hand–Sculler–Christian disease occurs in younger children (2–5 years) and often presents with exophthalmos due to a tumour mass in the orbital cavity. Letterer–Siwe disease is the rarest and often most severe form of LCH, typically presenting with a scaly, seborrhoeic, eczematoid and, occasionally, purpuric or ulcerative rash in infants younger than 2 years. Bone involvement in LCH can lead to a tender swelling (as a result of infiltration of adjacent tissues) and inability to bear weight. On radiography, lesions appear as 'punched out' holes sometimes with sclerotic edges. Other clinical manifestations include rashes, which may be maculopapular, nodular or vesicular, ear discharge, lymphadenopathy, diabetes insipidus due to the involvement of hypothalamus and the pituitary, respiratory symptoms with radiographic changes such as micronodular infiltrates due to lung involvement, hepatomegaly with laboratory evidence of liver dysfunction, splenomegaly, CNS disease with ataxia, dysarthria, cranial nerve palsies and, rarely, gut involvement with diarrhoea, malabsorption and protein-losing enteropathy.

The prognosis of patients with LCH depends on age of onset, number of involved organs and degree of their dysfunction. In general, infants with multiorgan disease have the worst prognosis. There is also growing realization that multiple recurrences of the disease can occur indefinitely, and those patients with multisystem involvement can have long-term sequelae of their disease and/or its treatment. These include neurocognitive and psychosocial problems, neurological complications with a neurodegenerative pattern of CNS involvement, orthopaedic problems, hearing loss, and hypothalamic/pituitary axis deficiencies, leading to stunted growth and other endocrine problems.

Spontaneous resolution in a significant proportion of patients with LCH can occur and patients with a limited disease usually do not require systemic therapy. In contrast, patients with multifocal disease generally benefit from systemic therapy. Treatment options have included low-dose radiation for symptomatic single lesions, local injection of steroids, topical steroids, PUVA, non-steroidal anti-inflammatory drugs, high-dose systemic steroids, and systemic multi-agent chemotherapy regimens with agents such as prednisolone, vinblastine, vincristine, etoposide and 6-mercaptopurine. Other agents, that have been tested in patients with disease progression while on therapy include cyclosporin, antithymocyte globulin, 2-chlorodeoxyadenosine (2CDA), thalidomide, TNF inhibitors, anti-CD1a antibodies and haemopoietic stem cell transplantation.

Haemophagocytic lymphohistiocytosis

These disorders include primary (familial) and secondary (related to infections or malignancy) with the familial form affecting neonates and infants and occurring in 1–2 children per million white people per year. Males and females are equally affected and over two-thirds of cases occur in siblings. The familial form is an autosomal recessive disease without a well-defined genetic defect. Recently, several defects in genes important for immune functions have been reported in patients with familial HLH and include mutations in the genes for perforin, the γ-chain of IL-2 receptor and purine nucleoside phosphorylase.

It is hypothesized that the disease is caused by impaired lymphocyte-mediated cytotoxicity and defective triggering of apoptosis. Perforin, normally secreted by cytotoxic T cells and natural killer (NK) cells, can form cell death-inducing pores through which toxic granzymes may enter the target cell and trigger apoptosis. Mutations of the perforin gene have been reported in several patients with familial HLH and result in defective lymphocyte cytotoxic activity. The manifestations of the disease are thought to be mediated by such inflammatory cytokines as IFN-γ TNF-α, soluble IL-2 receptor, FAS ligand and GM-CSF. Such excess of proinflammatory cytokines results in tissue infiltration by lymphocytes and macrophages, leading to haemophagocytosis.

The secondary form of HLH is commonly precipitated by viral (particularly Epstein–Barr virus and other herpesviruses), bacterial, fungal and protozoan infections, often in an immunocompromised host. Other factors that have been associated with secondary HLH include malignancies (particularly lymphoproliferative disorders), autoimmune disorders, drugs (such as phenytoin) and Chédiak–Higashi disease. It is important to distinguish patients with the secondary form of the disease from individuals with familial HLH and a precipitant viral infection.

Clinical presentations of HLH commonly include fever, anorexia, malaise, irritability and vomiting. Hepatic and splenic enlargement, lymphadenopathy, pancytopenia, abnormal liver function, coagulopathy, and CNS signs and symptoms are also common. Other features include hypertriglyceridaemia, hypofibrinogenaemia, cerebrospinal fluid pleocytosis, and rashes. Marrow examination is often hyperplastic with increased numbers of haemophagocytic histiocytes. Histopathological features of lymph node or other involved tissue are often diagnostic, showing infiltration by lymphocytes and histiocytes and the characteristic prominent erythrophagocytosis and haemophagocytosis, which is essential for diagnosis. There are no specific diagnostic tests, but during the acute phase of the illness, the plasma concentrations of inflammatory cytokines IFN-γ, TNF-α, soluble IL-2 receptor and IL-6 are often markedly elevated.

Treatment of familial HLH has traditionally involved the use of corticosteroids, cyclosporin and etoposide. Although high initial responses are observed, disease recurrence within months is usual. Adequate control of CNS disease is important but the value of routine prophylaxis with intrathecal methotrexate is controversial. Patients are at high risk of opportunistic infections because of their underlying immune dysfunction and the effects of therapy. Age is an important prognostic factor with the higher likelihood of survival in children older than 2 years of age. Haemopoietic stem cell transplant from a matched sibling is the definitive treatment modality in patients with familial HLH.

Sinus histiocytosis with massive lymphadenopathy or Rosai–Dorfman syndrome is characterized as a benign, frequently chronic, painless lymphadenopathy involving the cervical nodes and less commonly other nodal areas. Other features may include fever, weight loss, extranodal disease in skin, soft tissues, orbits, upper respiratory mucosa, bone and other organs. Although the disease commonly occurs in the first two decades of life, all ages can be affected. Diagnostic evaluation of involved lymph nodes reveals infiltration by histiocytes and multinucleated giant cells associated with erythrophagocytosis. The proliferating histiocytes are morphologically distinguished from Langerhans cells of LCH by the absence of Birbeck granules on electron microscopy as well as their surface phenotype. Treatment is usually unnecessary and ineffective with the disease manifestations usually subsiding over several months to years.

Although monocytic leukaemias are included in the classification of histiocytic disorders, their discussion is beyond the scope of this chapter and will be dealt with elsewhere.

Suggested bibliography

Haemopoietic cell development
Metcalf D (1993) Hematopoietic regulators: redundancy or subtlety? *Blood* **82**: 3515–23.

Ogawa M (1993) Differentiation and proliferation of hematopoietic stem cells. *Blood* **81**: 2844–53.

Phagocytic cell function
Clutterbuck EJ, Sanderson CJ (1990) Regulation of human eosinophil precursor production by cytokines: a comparison of recombinant human interleukin-1 (rhIL-1), rhIL-3 rhIL-5 rhIL-6 and rh granulocyte–macrophage colony-stimulating factor. *Blood* **75**: 1774–9.

Dancey JT, Deubelbeiss KA, Harker LA *et al.* (1976) Neutrophil kinetics in man. *Journal of Clinical Investigation* **58**: 705–15.

Denburg JA (1992) Basophil and mast cell lineages *in vitro* and *in vivo*. *Blood* **79**: 846–60.

Gordon S (1995) The macrophage. *Bioessays* **17**: 977–86.

Malech HL, Gallin JI (1987) Current concepts: immunology. Neutrophils in human diseases. *New England Journal of Medicine* **317**: 687–94.

Mansour MK, Levitz SM (2002) Interactions of fungi with phagocytes. *Current Opinion in Microbiology* **5**: 359–65.

Prussin C, Metcalfe DD (2003) IgE, mast cells, basophils, and eosinophils. *Journal of Allergy and Clinical Immunology* **111**: S486–94.

Sanderson CJ (1992) Interleukin-5 eosinophils, and disease. *Blood* **79**: 3101–9.

Mechanisms of phagocyte function
Booth JW, Trimble WS, Grinstein S (2001) Membrane dynamics in phagocytosis. *Seminars in Immunology* **13**: 357–64.

Borregaard N, Cowland JB (1997) Granules of human neutrophilic polymorphonuclear leukocyte. *Blood* **89**: 3503–21.

Castellano F, Chavrier P, Caron E (2001) Actin dynamics during phagocytosis. *Seminars in Immunology* **13**: 347–55.

Cox D, Greenberg S (2001) Phagocytic signaling strategies: Fc(gamma)receptor-mediated phagocytosis as a model system. *Seminars in Immunology* **13**: 339–45.

Duffield JS (2003) The inflammatory macrophage: a story of Jekyll and Hyde. *Clinical Science (Lond)* **104**: 27–38.

Egesten A, Calafat J, Janssen H *et al.* (2001) Granules of human eosinophilic leucocytes and their mobilization. *Clinical and Experimental Allergy* **31**: 1173–88.

Fadok VA, Chimini G (2001) The phagocytosis of apoptotic cells. *Seminars in Immunology* **13**: 365–72.

Falcone FH, Haas H, Gibbs BF (2000) The human basophil: a new appreciation of its role in immune responses. *Blood* **96**: 4028–38.

Feger F, Varadaradjalou S, Gao Z *et al.* (2002) The role of mast cells in host defense and their subversion by bacterial pathogens. *Trends in Immunology* **23**: 151–8.

Garcia-Garcia E, Rosales C (2002) Signal transduction during Fc receptor-mediated phagocytosis. *Journal of Leukocyte Biology* **72**: 1092–108.

Sansonetti P (2001) Phagocytosis of bacterial pathogens: implications in the host response. *Seminars in Immunology* **13**: 381–90.

Watts C, Amigorena S (2001) Phagocytosis and antigen presentation. *Seminars in Immunology* **13**: 373–9.

Disorders of phagocyte function and number

Arceci RJ, Longley J, Emanuel PD (2002) Atypical cellular disorders. *Hematology (American Society of Hematology Education Program)* 297–314.

Bernini JC (1996) Diagnosis and management of chronic neutropenia during childhood. *Pediatric Clinics of North America* **43**: 773–92.

Cham B, Bonilla MA, Winkelstein J (2002) Neutropenia associated with primary immunodeficiency syndromes. *Seminars in Hematology* **39**: 107–12.

Etzioni A, Doerschuk CM, Harlan JM (1999) Of man and mouse: leucocyte and endothelial adhesion molecule deficiencies. *Blood* **94**: 3281–8.

Freedman MH, Alter BP (2002) Risk of myelodysplastic syndrome and acute myeloid leukemia in congenital neutropenias. *Seminars in Hematology* **39**: 128–33.

Fuleihan RL (1998) The X-linked hyperimmunoglobulin M syndrome. *Seminars in Hematology* **35**: 321–31.

Goldblatt D, Thrasher AJ (2000) Chronic granulomatous disease. *Clinical and Experimental Immunology* **122**: 1–9.

Henter JI (2002) Biology and treatment of familial hemophagocytic lymphohistiocytosis: importance of perforin in lymphocyte-mediated cytotoxicity and triggering of apoptosis. *Medical and Pediatric Oncology* **38**: 305–9.

Henter JI, Arico M, Elinder G *et al.* (1998) Familial hemophagocytic lymphohistiocytosis. Primary hemophagocytic lymphohistiocytosis. *Hematology Oncology Clinics of North America* **12**: 417–433.

Herring WB, Smith LG, Walker RI *et al.* (1974) Hereditary neutrophilia. *American Journal of Medicine* **56**: 729–34.

Heyworth PG, Curnutte JT, Rae J *et al.* (2001) Hematologically important mutations: X-linked chronic granulomatous disease (second update). *Blood Cells, Molecules and Diseases* **27**: 16–26.

Kyono W, Coates TD (2002) A practical approach to neutrophil disorders. *Pediatric Clinics of North America* **49**: 929–71, viii.

Lakshman R, Finn A (2001) Neutrophil disorders and their management. *Journal of Clinical Pathology* **54**: 7–19.

Lekstrom-Himes JA, Gallin JI (2000) Immunodeficiency diseases caused by defects in phagocytes. *New England Journal of Medicine* **343**: 1703–14.

Mason PJ (2003) Stem cells, telomerase and dyskeratosis congenita. *Bioessays* **25**: 126–33.

Putsep K, Carlsson G, Boman HG *et al.* (2002) Deficiency of antibacterial peptides in patients with morbus Kostmann: an observation study. *Lancet* **360**: 1144–9.

Roos D, Law SK (2001) Hematologically important mutations: leukocyte adhesion deficiency. *Blood Cells, Molecules and Diseases* **27**: 1000–4.

Rothenberg ME (1998) Eosinophilia. *New England Journal of Medicine* **338**: 1592–600.

Shastri KA, Logue GL (1993) Autoimmune neutropenia. *Blood* **81**: 1984–95.

Starkebaum G (2002) Chronic neutropenia associated with autoimmune disease. *Seminars in Hematology* **39**: 121–7.

Ward DM, Shiflett SL, Kaplan J (2002) Chediak–Higashi syndrome: a clinical and molecular view of a rare lysosomal storage disorder. *Current Molecular Medicine* **2**: 469–77.

Ward HN, Reinhard EH (1971) Chronic idiopathic leukocytosis. *Annals of Internal Medicine* **75**: 193–8.

Welte K, Dale D (1996) Pathophysiology and treatment of severe chronic neutropenia. *Annals of Hematology* **72**: 158–65.

Zeidler C, Welte K (2002) Kostmann syndrome and severe congenital neutropenia. *Seminars in Hematology* **39**: 82–8.

CHAPTER 18

Haemopoietic growth factors

18

Jenny L Byrne and Nigel H Russell

Haemopoiesis

Stable haemopoiesis is maintained by the activity of pluripotential stem cells, which are capable not only of differentiating to form all three haemopoietic cell lineages, but also of retaining the ability for self-renewal. These pluripotential stem cells give rise to more differentiated lineage-committed stem cells that in turn differentiate into mature blood cells.

Initially, measurements of the stem cell content of human bone marrow could only be inferred by the growth of erythroid, myeloid and megakaryocytic cell colonies (BFU-E, CFU-GM and CFU-Meg) in culture. It has been estimated that there are 1×10^6 pluripotential stem cells in human marrow, and assays for these primitive cells have been developed, such as the long-term culture-initiating cell (LT-CIC) assay. In 1984, the expression of a specific antigen (now designated the CD34 antigen) on the surface of a small percentage of immature marrow cells was identified. This CD34$^+$ fraction of cells does, in fact, contain a number of committed stem cells, but it is also capable of restoring haemopoiesis following myeloablative chemotherapy, indicating that it also contains the pluripotential cell fraction. Expression of the CD34 antigen appears to be stage specific and is lost upon further maturation. Studies have shown that cells expressing high levels of CD34 are the most primitive, and those with a CD34^{bright}, Thy-1$^+$, CD38$^-$, CD45RO$^+$ and rhodamine^{dull} profile are representative of true pluripotential stem cells and account for less than 10% of the CD34$^+$ cell fraction.

The role of haemopoietic growth factors in normal haemopoiesis

The survival, differentiation and proliferation of haemopoietic progenitor cells *in vivo* and *in vitro* are dependent on the presence of small, hormone-like polypeptide molecules referred to as haemopoietic growth factors or colony-stimulating factors (CSFs). A large number of these factors have now been cloned and their effects have been studied. Their effects are exerted upon cells following interaction with specific growth factor receptors situated on the cell surface, which in turn activate signal transduction pathways. Different CSFs act on bone marrow cells at different stages of maturation (Table 18.1). Some influence immature progenitors and increase the production of cells of several lineages [e.g. interleukin 3 (IL-3) and stem cell factor (SCF)], whereas others act on more committed progenitors and thus have a specific effect, leading to an increased production of cells of a particular subtype, e.g. Epo and granulocyte colony-stimulating factor (G-CSF). The evolutionary importance of these molecules is indicated by the significant homology that exists between the species for these growth factors and their receptors and the common use of certain receptor subunits and signalling pathways.

In addition, there is considerable overlap between the functions of different CSFs, for example IL-3, granulocyte–macrophage colony-stimulating factor (GM-CSF) and G-CSF all stimulate the production of mature neutrophils. This redundancy may arise because different CSFs act on cells at different stages of differentiation. Furthermore, the actions of CSFs may be subtly different in that some may promote survival of cells by inhibiting apoptosis, whereas others act to induce proliferation of these cells. There is also evidence that the actions of CSFs may be synergistic in their effects upon haemopoietic progenitors; for example, the addition of SCF and GM-CSF results in an increase in both the number of colonies formed and the number of cells in each colony.

Growth factor receptors

Haemopoietic growth factors act by binding to specific receptor molecules on the surface of haemopoietic progenitors. The

Table 18.1 Haemopoietic growth factors and their receptors.

Growth factor	Location of gene	Receptor	Cell source	Cells produced	Clinical use
IL-3	5q23–31	Low-affinity α-subunit (70 kDa) and β-subunit (120 kDa) common to IL-3/5 receptors	Fibroblasts, mast cells, T cells, NK cells, endothelial cells	Granulocytes, monocyte/macrophages, eosinophils, basophils, mast cells (erythrocytes if Epo also present)	Not in clinical use
GM-CSF	5q23–31	Low-affinity α-subunit (70 kDa) and β-subunit (120 kDa) common to IL-3/5 receptors	Fibroblasts, T cell macrophages, marrow stroma, endothelial cells	Granulocytes, monocyte/macrophages, eosinophils, megakaryocytes	Stem cell mobilization; post chemotherapy/bone marrow transplantation, use in graft rejection
G-CSF	17q21–22	Low-affinity monomer, high-affinity oligomer	Fibroblasts, marrow stroma, endothelial cells	Granulocytes	Stem cell mobilization, post-chemotherapy/bone marrow transplantation
SCF	12q22–24	145-kDa transmembrane protein	Fibroblasts, marrow stroma, endothelial cells	Granulocytes, monocyte/macrophages, erythrocytes, megakaryocytes	? Increase stem cell mobilization
Epo	7q21	166-amino-acid polypeptide	Kidney cells	Erythrocytes, megakaryocytes	Renal anaemia, MDS; anaemia secondary cancer
TPO	3q26–27	Product of c-mpl proto-oncogene	Liver and kidney cells	Megakaryocytes	Not in clinical use

molecular structure of a number of these growth factor receptors is now defined (Figure 18.1).

Some of the receptors have intrinsic tyrosine kinase domains that are activated upon ligand binding to the extracellular domain. Examples include the macrophage colony-stimulating factor (M-CSF) and SCF receptors.

The remaining CSF receptors all share a common Trp–Ser–X–Trp–Ser motif (where X can be any amino acid) near the transmembrane domain and are referred to as part of the cytokine receptor superfamily. Some of these receptors consist of a single chain, for example Epo and G-CSF receptors, whereas others are made up of two or more subunits, some of which are

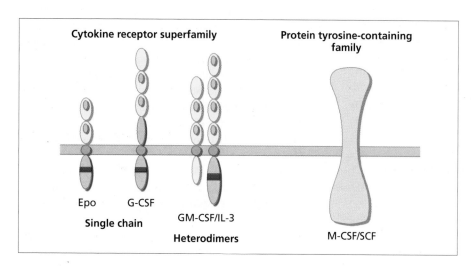

Figure 18.1 Cytokine receptor superfamily.

common to several receptors, for example the common sub-unit of GM-CSF and IL-3 receptors. Following ligand binding, homo- or heterodimerization occurs and leads to the activation of intrinsic or extrinsic tyrosine kinases, resulting in signal transduction.

Mutations of various CSF receptors have been described which may have clinical sequelae. For example, deletion at the C-terminal end of the cytoplasmic domain of the erythropoietin receptor leads to the development of familial erythrocytosis in humans. Mutations of the gene encoding the thrombopoietin receptor have been identified in all patients with congenital amegakaryocytic thrombocytopenia, a rare disorder characterized by severe hypomegakaryocytic thrombocytopenia in infancy, which develops into pancytopenia in later childhood. In the case of congenital neutropenia, for example Kostmann's syndrome, mutations of the G-CSF receptor appears to be acquired in patients and heralds transformation to myelodysplastic syndrome (MDS)/acute myeloid leukaemia (AML).

Signal transduction by growth factor receptors

Following growth factor binding to its receptor, a number of signal transduction pathways are activated. The first step in these signalling pathways involves the activation of a tyrosine kinase, either the intrinsic tyrosine kinase domain such as in M-CSF and SCF or an extrinsic tyrosine kinase molecule.

Jak/STAT signalling

Members of the family of Janus or Jak kinases are known to be associated with activated growth factor receptors. This association may either be constitutive, for example Epo receptor, or occur only after ligand binding, for example IL-3 receptor. Heterodimerization of the receptors allows these kinases to be brought into close proximity, resulting in cross-phosphorylation and activation of their kinase domains. Following activation, Jak kinases are able to phosphorylate another family of proteins known as the STAT proteins (signal *t*ransducers and *a*ctivators of *t*ranscription). Phosphorylated STAT proteins are then able to enter the nucleus and bind to DNA acting as transcription factors, and leading to a cellular response.

Ras-dependent signalling

Activated Jaks can also phosphorylate the protein Shc, which, in turn, associates with the adaptor protein Grb2. The latter associates with the nucleotide exchange factor Sos, which controls the GTPase activity of a small membrane-bound protein termed 'Ras'. Activated Ras in the GTP-bound state can then induce signalling via a number of phosphorylation cascades, including the MEK–MAP kinase pathway and the phosphatidylinositol

3-kinase (PI-3 kinase) pathway, which, in turn, lead to gene induction and a cellular response.

Recombinant growth factors

Following the discovery of haemopoietic growth factors and their effects on haemopoiesis, the genes encoding these proteins were identified. This has enabled recombinant human growth factors to be produced, and several of these have now become established for clinical use. Growth factors that have been synthesized and used in this way include G-CSF, GM-CSF, SCF, IL-3, erythropoietin and thrombopoietin. A large number of studies have been published reporting on the use of these growth factors in a number of different clinical settings. In view of the high costs of these agents it is important to carefully evaluate their use in terms of both clinical efficacy and cost–benefit ratio. In this regard, a number of groups have attempted to rationalize the use of haemopoietic growth factors by issuing clinical guidelines that recommend specific indications when they should be considered.

Erythropoietin

Physiology of erythropoietin secretion
(see also Chapter 2)

Erythropoietin (Epo) is an 18-kDa protein consisting of a 166-amino-acid polypeptide chain linked by two disulphide bonds. Following translation, it is heavily glycosylated, resulting in a final molecular weight of 30.4 kDa. The glycosylation is essential for its biological activity *in vivo* as removal of the sialic acid residues decreases its half-life significantly. It is encoded by a gene on the long arm of chromosome 7. In adult life, the gene is largely expressed by the peritubular fibroblast-like interstitial cells of the kidney and, to a lesser extent, by hepatocytes. In embryonic tissues, the liver is the major source of Epo production. Epo production is stimulated by hypoxia, which is detected by a DNA-binding complex termed hypoxia-inducible factor 1 (HIF1). HIF1, a transcription factor complex, is a key mediator of oxygen homeostasis and is regulated by a ubiquitin-mediated oxygen-dependent destruction of the α-subunit of the complex. It controls the expression of many genes that are regulated by hypoxia, including erythropoietin. Activation of HIF1 by hypoxia results in the rapid synthesis and release of Epo into the bloodstream, increasing levels by up to 1000-fold. Other factors may regulate Epo levels, including the red cell precursor mass (as high serum levels are found in aplastic anaemia).

Epo is a true hormone that circulates to the bone marrow and binds to Epo receptors on erythropoietic cells within the bone marrow. Epo plays no role in determining the lineage commitment of haemopoietic cells but, rather, binds to receptors on committed erythroid progenitor cells (BFUe and CFUe) and stimulates their growth, survival and differentiation. Erythroid progenitors, particularly CFUe, require continual exposure to Epo in order to survive, although their sensitivity to Epo varies widely, with only those progenitors requiring low Epo levels surviving and CFUe with high Epo requirements undergoing apoptosis during steady-state haemopoiesis when Epo levels are low. As Epo levels rise in response to tissue hypoxia, increasing numbers of erythroid progenitors are prevented from undergoing apoptosis, leading to an expansion of red cell production. An understanding of this is crucial to the appropriate use of Epo replacement therapy because when Epo levels are high nearly all available CFUe survive and, therefore, increased pharmacological doses of the drug cannnot lead to further expansion of erythropoiesis. Epo is not only a survival factor for erythroid progenitor cells but it also stimulates proliferation as well as RNA and protein synthesis in more differentiated erythroid cells.

The erythropoietin receptor is a member of the class 1 cytokine receptor family encoded by a gene on chromosome 19p13.3–p13.2. The binding of Epo to its receptor (Epo-R) induces receptor dimerization, which, in turn, induces phosphorylation of the pre-bound Jak2 kinase and hence phosphorylation of the Epo-R itself. The STAT5 protein is then able to bind to the phosphorylated Epo-R, leading to tyrosine phosphorylation of the STAT5 molecule. Phosphorylated STAT5 then disengages from the Epo-R, moving to the nucleus, where it activates Epo-inducible genes. Downstream events from this pathway lead to the upregulation of the anti-apoptotic protein bcl-xl, which promotes survival of erythroid progenitor cells.

Recombinant erythropoietin

Epo was the first haemopoietic growth factor to be cloned in 1985, and since then the use of recombinant erythropoietin (epoetin) has been shown to be effective in the management of the anaemia of chronic renal failure. At present, several different epoetin molecules are clinically available, including epoetin-α and epoetin-β, which vary in the number of sialic acid residues present and, more recently, darbepoetin-α. This is a modified, hyperglycosylated form of erythropoietin, which differs in five amino acids from the endogenous protein and has a threefold longer biological half-life than standard preparations and is suitable for weekly administration. More recently, other clinical uses of epoetin have emerged in the treatment of conditions in which defective endogenous Epo production can occur. These include the myelodysplasias, anaemia in patients with solid tumours and lymphoproliferative disorders, and anaemia associated with HIV infection, chronic disease and prematurity (Table 18.2).

The clinical uses of erythropoietin

The anaemia of renal failure
The use of recombinant Epo for the treatment of renal anaemia is a clearly established indication. Renal anaemia is an erythropoietin deficiency state and, although coexisting conditions, for example haematinic deficiency, blood loss or aluminium toxic-

Table 18.2 Clinical uses of erythropoietin.

Anaemia of chronic renal failure
Myelodysplastic syndrome
Anaemia associated with malignancy
Anaemia of chronic disease
AIDS
Anaemia of prematurity
Perisurgical uses

ity, can blunt the effectiveness of Epo therapy, nearly all patients with renal anaemia have a positive response, if adequate doses are given, resulting in an increase in haemoglobin (Hb) levels into the normal range. Most physicians accept a target Hb of 11 g as recommended by the European Best Practice guidelines. This can be achieved with an initial thrice-weekly loading schedule followed by a maintenance schedule of weekly subcutaneous therapy at a dose of 100 IU/kg. The use of epoetin and the correction of anaemia have been associated with an improved quality of life without evidence of a deterioration in renal function or dialysis efficiency. Furthermore, there is evidence for a reduction in mortality and morbidity in renal patients receiving optimal epoetin therapy.

For a decade, epoetin therapy has been considered safe. In 2002, however, a series of renal patients were reported who developed pure red cell aplasia due to the development of anti-erythropoietin antibodies. Serum from these patients was found to be inhibitory to erythroid colony formation in vitro. Almost all cases now reported have been associated with subcutaneous administration of epoetin-α, and in 2002 the prescribing information was changed to state that this preparation should no longer be given by this route in renal failure. Pure red cell aplasia (PRCA) due to epoetin therapy remains a rare event; however, it should be suspected in patients who have been on therapy for more than 3 months and who develop a sudden severe unexplained fall in their Hb, associated with reticulocytopenia, despite continuing epoetin treatment, and in whom no other cause of PRCA can be found. The diagnosis can be confirmed by the finding of low serum erythropoietin levels and the detection of anti-erythropoietin antibodies. Epoetin therapy should be withdrawn in favour of transfusions. Immunosuppression with cyclophosphamide has been reported to be of help in some patients, and correction of the anaemia has been reported following successful renal transplantation. Although this remains a rare complication, it has been recommended that monitoring of the reticulocyte count should now be a regular part of the monitoring of all patients receiving erythropoietin therapy.

Myelodysplasia
Anaemia is one of the commonest manifestation of myelodysplasia and repeat transfusions, which have been the major therapeutic

option for low-risk MDS such as RA and RARS, eventually lead to complications, particularly transfusional haemosiderosis. The anaemia particularly of low-grade MDS has been in part explained by increased apoptosis of haemopoietic cells in the bone marrow. Treatment of MDS patients with the cytokines G-CSF and Epo alone, or in combination, has been associated with reduced levels of imtramedullary apoptosis and enhanced haemopoiesis.

The efficacy of epoetin therapy has been explored both as a single agent and in combination with G-CSF. In one randomized double-blind placebo-controlled trial of 87 patients, 37% of the epoetin group responded with a 1–2 g rise in their Hb level compared with 11% of control subjects ($P = 0.007$). The subgroup of patients with RA had the highest response rate of 50%. Patients with low Epo levels of < 200 IU/L and who have low transfusion requirements have the highest response rate and guidelines produced by the British Committee for Standards in Haematology (BCSH) have suggested an 8-week trial of therapy in this subgroup. Most patients with MDS who are anaemic have appropriately high Epo levels, and it is unclear why a proportion have low levels. Dosage schedules of 10 000 IU three times per week have been recommended, although it has been suggested that a once-weekly dose of 40 000 IU may be as effective and may improve patient compliance.

A number of studies have combined G-CSF with epoetin in MDS patients with evidence of an enhanced effect. The synergy of these two cytokines is most pronounced in RARS, when responses are seen in approximately 50% of patients, whereas responses with epoetin alone are poor in this subgroup. A predictive model for response to epoetin has been developed based on steady-state erythropoietin levels (< 100, 100–500, > 500 IU/L) and monthly transfusion requirements (< 2 or > 2 units/month). The model provides a predictive score for Hb response of high (74% response rate), intermediate (23%) and poor (7%), with the group with the low epo levels and low transfusion requirements having the high response rate.

A practical recommendation is to start epoetin therapy alone in RA patients and in RARS patients, with a high predicted response as outlined above. The trigger for starting epoetin therapy is a Hb of 10 g or less, or patients who are becoming transfusion dependent. Most patients will require doses of greater than 30 000 IU per week and treatment can therefore be extremely expensive. G-CSF can be added to non-responders in a weekly schedule at a dose adjusted to keep the neutrophil count in the normal range. A trial of therapy should continue for 2–3 months and in responding patients gradual dose de-escalation can be attempted.

Unfortunately, although responses are well described in low-risk MDS, the patients who one might wish to benefit most from epoetin therapy, i.e. those with severe anaemia and transfusion dependency, appear the least likely to respond. Furthermore, the durability of response is not always clear from the published studies. The risk of epoetin-induced PRCA must also be considered, although this is likely to be difficult to diagnose in the setting of MDS and the risk of this complication occurring is unclear.

Use of erythropoietin in anaemia associated with malignant disease

Anaemia is common in patients both with solid tumours and haematological malignancy, as a consequence either of the disease or of its treatment. A number of individual studies have shown response rates between 28% and 80% for patients with cancer-related anaemia and a Hb of < 10 g/dL. At present, guidelines produced by the American Society of Clinical Oncology (ASCO) recommend treatment with epoetin for this group of patients. Patients with lymphoproliferative disease, particularly chronic lymphocytic leukaemia (CLL) and myeloma, often develop anaemia for which blood transfusion is required. Most anaemic patients with myeloma have been shown to have low Epo levels, and there is evidence that they greatly benefit from epoetin therapy. In 1996, Osterborg and colleagues found an improvement in Hb level and elimination of transfusion requirements in 60% of epoetin-treated patients compared with 24% in the control group. These results have been confirmed in other studies and have also shown not only an improvement in Hb and haematocrit levels, but also significant improvements in patient-assessed quality of life. At present, there are no reliable indicators of response to therapy, but with an appropriate dosage more than 80% of myeloma patients show a Hb increment of > 1 g/dL after 4 weeks of treatment.

It seems reasonable to recommend a 6-week trial of epoetin in patients with a Hb of < 10 g/dL and for symptomatic patients with a Hb of 10–12 g/dL, provided that other possible correctable causes of the anaemia have been excluded. A dose schedule of 10 000 IU three times per week with dose escalation for initially unresponsive patients is appropriate. Recently, a weekly schedule of epoetin-β given at a dose of 30 000 IU was found to be equivalent to 10 000 IU three times per week in patients with lymphoproliferative disease who had serum epo levels of < 100 IU/L, with > 70% of patients responding.

The use of epoetin as an alternative to blood transfusion in patients with cancer-related anaemia is low in the UK at present compared with the USA and some other European countries. However, its use in this setting is likely to increase and is consistent with the objective of avoiding unnecessary blood transfusion, as outlined in the NHS Circular on Better Blood Transfusion.

Other uses of erythropoietin

The anaemia associated with HIV infection is multifactorial and involves a direct effect of the virus on haemopoietic progenitor cells, as well as anaemia of chronic disease and peripheral destruction of red cells and the involvement of the bone marrow by lymphoma and by infection. Furthermore, the drugs used in the treatment of HIV or it complications, such as cytomegalovirus (CMV) infection, frequently cause marrow suppression. Several clinical trials have now demonstrated the benefit of epoetin therapy in some patients with HIV-associated anaemia. Improvements in Hb and a significant reduction in transfusion requirements have been seen in patients with an Epo level of < 500 IU/L, whether or not the patient is receiving anti-retroviral therapy.

Following allogeneic bone marrow transplantation (BMT), endogenous Epo production may be impaired, possibly related to the effect of cyclosporin. A number of studies have shown that epoetin can accelerate erythroid recovery and reduce transfusion requirements in the first few months post allogeneic transplant.

Epoetin has also been used perisurgically to enhance the collection of autologous blood pre-deposited before elective surgery and also to correct anaemia prior to surgery with the aim of reducing the requirement for donor blood. In a Canadian study, the use of Epo was found to reduce the need for transfusion in patients undergoing elective hip replacement surgery, whose initial Hb was < 13.5 g/dL, from 74% to 33%.

Granulocyte and granulocyte–macrophage colony-stimulating factors

Physiology of G-CSF and GM-CSF

G-CSF and GM-CSF are both glycosylated polypeptides in their natural form, which are the main regulators of granulocyte production. The gene for G-CSF is located on chromosome 17q, whereas that of GM-CSF is located on chromosome 5q. Both of these CSFs can be secreted by a variety of cell types, including monocytes/macrophages, T cells, endothelial cells and fibroblasts when appropriately stimulated *in vitro*. The levels of endogenous G-CSF can increase to detectable levels when there is a demand for increased granulocyte production such as in acute treatment-induced neutropenia, chronic neutropenic conditions and in acute infections in patients with or without underlying haematological disorders. G-CSF in peripheral blood is detected more often and in higher concentrations than GM-CSF, and there appear to be differences in their production and regulation. GM-CSF has more pleiotropic effects than G-CSF and stimulates the production of neutrophils, eosinophils and monocytes, although both have been primarily exploited for their effects on stimulating myelopoiesis. GM-CSF treatment results in the release of IL-1 and tumour necrosis factor from monocytes and hence its administration has been associated with fever.

Clinical uses of G-CSF and GM-CSF

Mobilization of peripheral blood stem cells

The use of CSFs for the mobilization of peripheral blood stem cells (PBSCs) from both patients and donors is recommended in both the BCSH guidelines and also the ASCO recommendations.

Mobilization of PBSC for autologous transplantation

It was first discovered in the 1960s that peripheral blood contains a small number of stem cells that can give rise to all three haemopoietic cell lineages. In the resting state, the number of these cells circulating in the peripheral blood is very low, whereas during haemopoietic recovery after myelosuppressive chemotherapy the number of circulating PBSC increases up to 100-fold. The administration of haemopoietic growth factors (G-CSF or GM-CSF) can also lead to a similar increase in the number of circulating PBSCs, and these can be readily collected by the use of continuous-flow cell separation and then used for autologous transplantation and to support high-dose therapy.

The combination of chemotherapy and subsequent administration of a growth factor (G-CSF or GM-CSF) appears to be synergistic and leads to a superior yield of PBSCs as enumerated by flow cytometric analysis of cells expressing the CD34 antigen. The minimum number of PBSCs required for complete and sustained haemopoiesis has been established at a level of 2×10^6 CD34$^+$ cells/kg, with optimal haemopoietic recovery occurring at doses of around 5×10^6/L. Various stem cell mobilization regimens have been employed, either using cyclophosphamide alone in doses ranging from 2 to 7 g/m^2 followed by G-CSF, or using combination chemotherapy regimens plus G-CSF, which may give superior yields and also have the advantage of efficacy against the underlying haemopoietic malignancy. Although high doses of cyclophosphamide may be more effective for PBSC mobilization, they are now less frequently used because of the higher toxicity that is associated with them (Figure 18.2).

The rationale behind obtaining PBSCs for autologous transplantation is that a number of studies have confirmed that restoration of haemopoiesis occurs more rapidly using PBSCs as the source of haemopoietic progenitors than when using autologous marrow. The use of PBSCs for autologous transplantation leads to a significant acceleration of neutrophil and platelet engraftment, and this may result in shorter hospitalization and reduced toxicity of the procedure. One of the early studies by Sheridan *et al.* (1992) showed a highly significant acceleration of platelet engraftment compared with historical bone marrow controls of 15 versus 39 days. Furthermore, this benefit of PBSC transplantation over bone marrow transplantation in terms of faster haemopoietic reconstitution has been confirmed in a randomized study of lymphoma patients. As a result of these findings, the use of PBSCs for autologous transplantation has become widespread and has virtually replaced autologous marrow in order to achieve rapid restoration of bone marrow function after high-dose therapy.

The efficacy of G-CSF and GM-CSF for autologous mobilization has been reported to be equal in terms of median progenitor cell yield and time to haematological recovery following transplantation. However, in view of the better toxicity profile of G-CSF, its use has generally been favoured for PBSC mobilization. Mobilization of sufficient PBSCs for autografting is not always successful, and factors associated with a failure to mobilize

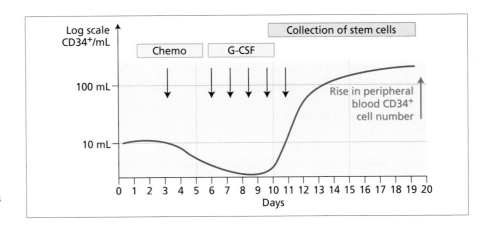

Figure 18.2 Mobilization of stem cells for autologous transplantation.

include heavy pretreatment with chemotherapy, especially alkylating agents, and also previous radiotherapy exposure. The use of additional growth factors for these patients, for example IL-3 and SCF, is being evaluated at present.

Mobilization of PBSCs for allogeneic transplantation
A number of randomized studies have also shown similar benefits of mobilized PBSCs compared with bone marrow for allogeneic transplantation. There are good data showing significant benefits for G-CSF-mobilized PBSC in terms of neutrophil and platelet recovery. One study has also reported a trend for improved survival and a significant increase in disease-free survival at 2 years for the PBSC recipients. Another has reported a shorter duration of hospitalization for those patients receiving G-CSF-mobilized PBSCs, resulting in a reduction in the total cost of the procedure.

One concern regarding the use of PBSCs for allogeneic transplantation was that there is a theoretical increased risk of graft-versus-host disease (GvHD) compared with the use of bone marrow, as unmodified PBSC grafts contain at least 1 log more T cells. However, this has not been apparent clinically, as a number of studies have not shown an increased risk of acute GvHD, although the incidence of chronic GvHD does appear to be raised.

The mobilization of PBSCs from normal donors has almost entirely been with G-CSF alone, which has an excellent safety record and low toxicity profile compared with GM-CSF, which tends to have more side-effects. In Europe, the usual schedule for G-CSF administration to normal donors has been 10 µg/kg per day given subcutaneously for four consecutive days. Higher doses of G-CSF have been used (12–16 µg/kg per day), which may result in a higher yield of progenitors, although this may result in greater toxicity. Using the standard dose of G-CSF of 10 µg/kg per day, the number of CD34+ cells in the peripheral blood peaks on days 5–6, reaching levels of between 20 and 140 µL before tailing off. The white cell count (WCC) usually peaks at between 30 and 65×10^9/L. There is no correlation between the WCC and the CD34+ cell count in the peripheral blood; however, a dose reduction of G-CSF is usually recommended if the WCC reaches levels of more than 70×10^9/L. With this regimen, leucapheresis is usually initiated on day 5 (i.e. the day following the fourth G-CSF injection), and the target of $> 4 \times 10^6$ CD34+ cells/kg recipient weight is usually achieved in one to two collections processing 2.5 times the blood volume (Figure 18.3). For the majority of donors, it is possible to collect PBSCs via the use of peripheral veins, although the use of long lines is occasionally necessary due to poor venous access.

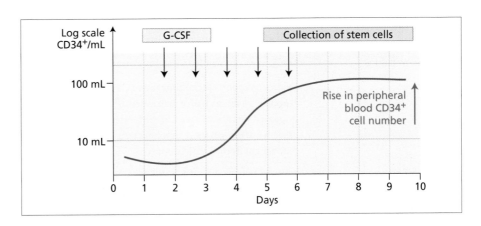

Figure 18.3 Mobilization of stem cells – sibling donors.

The advantages of PBSC donation for the donor include the avoidance of general anaesthesia, the less invasive procedure and the lack of hospitalization. Using this dose of G-CSF, the procedure is generally well tolerated but it is not a completely risk-free procedure. The commonest side-effects reported include bone pain (83%), headache (39%), fatigue (14%) and nausea (12%), which resolve rapidly with cessation of G-CSF therapy. More serious adverse effects have been reported in small numbers of patients (often using higher doses of G-CSF), including splenic rupture, severe pyogenic infection, exacerbation of ischaemic heart disease and precipitation of vaso-occlusive crisis in a patient with Hb SC disease. A number of relative contraindications of PBSC mobilization have been agreed, which include a history of autoimmune, inflammatory or thrombotic disease. There do not appear to be any long-term sequelae of a short course of G-CSF for PBSC mobilization. Studies investigating the long-term effects of PBSC donation have revealed no significant abnormalities in the blood counts of donors, their general health, the risk of development of leukaemia or other malignancy or any effect on fertility.

Use of colony-stimulating factors following haemopoietic progenitor cell transplantation

The use of CSFs to accelerate haemopoietic reconstitution after autologous and allogeneic progenitor cell transplantation is recommended both by the BCSH guidelines (Table 18.3) and the ASCO recommendations (2000 update) (Figure 18.4 and Table 18.4).

Colony-stimulating factors post autologous transplantation

High-dose myeloablative chemotherapy followed by autologous transplantation is a highly effective treatment for a number of haematological malignancies and has been widely used. Apart from the risk of disease relapse, the major complication of this approach is the possibility of procedure-related toxicity. This includes the risks of major haemorrhage, life-threatening infection, delayed or incomplete engraftment and organ damage from the ablative regimen, all of which may lead to prolonged hospitalization and increased procedural cost. Measures to reduce any of these potential problems will clearly be of benefit in terms of improved survival and also the cost–benefit of this treatment

Table 18.3 BCSH guidelines on the use of colony-stimulating factors in haematological malignancies.

Primary prophylaxis	Not routinely recommended unless the expected incidence of febrile neutropenia is greater than 40% (level IIa, grade B)
Secondary prophylaxis	Not routinely justified but indicated for tumours when delay/dose reduction would compromise overall survival (level III, grade B)
Adjunctive treatment	Not recommended for patients with uncomplicated febrile neutropenia (level Ib, grade A) but should be considered in patients with poor prognostic factors (level IV, grade C)
AML	Routine use of CSF is recommended after consolidation chemotherapy (level Ib, grade A); CSF is recommended following induction if it reduces hospital stay or antibiotic usage
ALL	G-CSF is indicated to reduce the severity of neutropenia following intensive phases of therapy (level Ib, grade A)
MDS	CSFs are indicated to reduce the severity of neutropenia in patients receiving intensive chemotherapy (level 1b, grade A). CSFs are also recommended on an intermittent basis for neutropenic patients with infection (level IV, grade C) but continuous prophylactic use is not justified
Aplastic anaemia	There is insufficient evidence to make any recommendations and so patients should be given CSFs on an individual therapeutic trial basis (level IV, grade C)
Bone marrow failure	G-CSF is recommended when improvement of the neutrophil count is appropriate (level III, grade B)
Lymphomas	Evidence supports the routine use of CSFs to reduce infection, chemotherapy delay and hospitalization especially when the risk of neutropenia sepsis exceeds 40% (level 1a, grade A); there is also evidence of improved survival with G-CSF supported dose intensification in elderly patients with HG NHL (level Ib, grade A); at present this cannot justify a change in policy for all lymphoma patients but elderly patients may benefit from G-CSF support
PBPC mobilization	CSFs are indicated for the mobilization of PBPCs
PBPC transplantation	CSFs are indicated to accelerate reconstitution after allogeneic and autologous transfusion

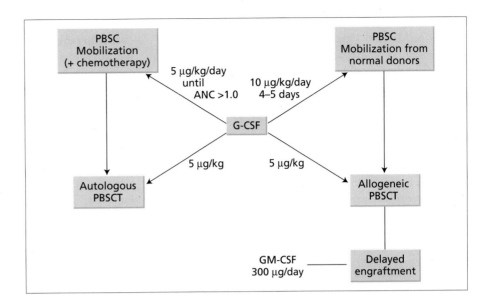

Figure 18.4 Role of haemopoietic growth factors in progenitor cell transplantation.

Table 18.4 Summary of ASCO recommendations (2000 update).

Primary prophylaxis	Routine use of CSFs not recommended; consider CSFs in high-risk patients, including the elderly
Secondary prophylaxis	Use of CSFs should be considered in patients with complicated febrile neutropenia
Chemotherapy	
AML	CSF treatment after induction therapy should be used if cost–benefits can be shown; CSFs for priming is not recommended outside the setting of clinical trials; CSFs are recommended after consolidation chemotherapy
ALL	G-CSF administration begun after completion of the first few days of chemotherapy of the initial induction or first post-remission course is recommended
MDS	Intermittent use of CSFs may be considered in patients with severe neutropenia and recurrent infection; prolonged or continuous treatment with CSFs is not recommended
AA	No specific recommendations
Lymphomas	No specific recommendations
PBSC mobilization	Use of CSFs is recommended for both patient and donor
	PBSC mobilization; higher CSF doses may be useful
Post HSC transplantation	Use of adjunctive CSFs is recommended post PBSC transplantation and after autologous and allogeneic BMT

approach. The administration of haemopoietic growth factors following autologous transplantation has therefore been introduced in an attempt to shorten the neutropenic period, decrease the frequency and severity of neutropenic septic episodes, and hence reduce the duration of hospitalization and thereby reduce the overall cost of the procedure. A number of randomized controlled trials have confirmed that the use of CSFs after autologous transplantation are beneficial in significantly shortening the duration of neutropenia and hospitalization. This did lead to a mean cost saving in at least one of the studies.

Both G-CSF and GM-CSF have been shown to be effective in hastening haemopoietic recovery following autologous transplantation. No large-scale prospective comparative studies have been performed addressing the relative efficacy of these two CSFs. In addition, the optimal timing, duration and dose of CSFs following autologous transplantation remains to be established.

The ASCO guidelines support the use of G-CSF at a dose of 5 µg/kg per day and 250 µg/m^2 per day for GM-CSF, and the commencement of CSFs up to 5 days after progenitor cell reinfusion. This dose should then be continued until the absolute neutrophil count (ANC) exceeds a minimum of 1×10^9/L. Further modifications to the dosage and scheduling of these growth factors may be possible to reduce costs without impairment of the beneficial clinical effects.

Colony-stimulating factors post allogeneic transplantation

The major complications of allogeneic transplantation are similar to those of autologous transplantation with the additional problems of GvHD and graft rejection. Therefore, as for autologous transplantation, the rationale for administration of growth factors following allogeneic transplantation is to accelerate myeloid recovery and reduce the incidence of infection, number of febrile days, antibiotic usage and duration of hospitalization. Available data from a number of studies have confirmed a clinical benefit in terms of neutrophil engraftment kinetics using either G- or GM-CSF following allogeneic transplantation from either sibling or unrelated donors. The degree of acceleration of neutrophil recovery, however, is also influenced by other factors, including the GvHD prophylaxis used and the source of haemopoietic progenitors infused, i.e. G-CSF-mobilized PBSCs versus bone marrow.

It is still not clear whether the enhanced haemopoietic reconstitution seen in patients receiving CSFs post transplant translates into improved transplant-related mortality rates and survival, although this has been suggested by some studies.

Initial concerns about the use of growth factors in the allogeneic setting leading to an increased risk of GvHD or to an increase in relapse rates for AML have proved to be unfounded despite the effects of growth factors on cytotoxic T cells and myeloid blast cells *in vitro*. As with autologous transplantation, the optimal cost-effective dose and schedule for the administration of CSFs following allogeneic transplantation remains to be established.

The problem of bone marrow graft failure or delayed haematological recovery (ANC $< 0.2 \times 10^9$/L by day +28) after transplantation is a problem mainly seen after allogeneic transplantation using unrelated donors, especially when a low cell dose has been infused. When this occurs, it usually results in prolonged hospitalization, increased treatment costs and a higher treatment-related mortality, mainly as a result of infective deaths. Few studies have examined the use of growth factors for the treatment of delayed engraftment, although there are some data to suggest that GM-CSF may be of benefit in this setting. The updated ASCO guidelines recommend a trial of CSFs for patients who experience delayed or inadequate neutrophil engraftment after PBSC transplantation, and suggest using a dose of GM-CSF 250 µg/m^2 per day for 14 days, followed by a 7-day break. This can be repeated for up to three courses if there is no effect with a dose escalation to 500 µg/m^2 per day for the third course.

Use of colony-stimulating factors to support standard chemotherapy

Neutropenia and neutropenic sepsis are the main dose-limiting complications of chemotherapy, with the risk of infection being directly related to the severity and duration of neutropenia. Although the mortality from neutropenic sepsis is low, such episodes require hospitalization and treatment with broad-spectrum antibiotics. They may also lead to the delay or dose reduction of subsequent courses of chemotherapy, which may have a deleterious effect on the response to treatment.

Primary prophylaxis

Although the addition of CSFs following chemotherapy has been shown to reduce the incidence of febrile neutropenia, this appears only to be cost effective for highly myelosuppressive dose-escalated regimens in which the incidence of febrile neutropenia reaches 40%. Routine use of CSFs for primary prophylaxis in patients receiving standard outpatient chemotherapy regimens is not recommended except in high-risk patient populations (e.g. the elderly, patients with AIDS-related non-Hodgkin's lymphoma, patients with pre-existing neutropenia or decreased immune function or patients with active infections).

Secondary prophylaxis

The use of CSFs in patients who have already experienced an episode of febrile neutropenia following a previous course of chemotherapy is justified in order to prevent further infection and also to maintain the delivery of full-dose chemotherapy on schedule.

Use of colony-stimulating factors for neutropenia

The routine use of haemopoietic growth factors in patients rendered neutropenic following standard chemotherapy but who remain afebrile cannot be justified. Although the duration of neutropenia may be reduced in patients treated with CSFs, this has not been shown to be of any clinical benefit as in general the neutropenia observed in such patients is profound but short. Even in the presence of neutropenic fever, there is only limited evidence that the addition of growth factors improves clinical outcome in terms of duration of hospitalization and antibiotic use despite a consistent reduction in the duration of neutropenia. Thus, current ASCO and BCSH guidelines recommend the use of CSFs only in febrile neutropenic patients who have adverse prognostic factors such as pneumonia, hypotension, multiorgan failure or invasive fungal infection or who are elderly.

Use of colony-stimulating factors in haematological disorders

A number of studies have investigated the role of haemopoietic CSFs in the treatment of patients with a number of haematological disorders in an effort to maintain chemotherapy dose intensity and to reduce the incidence of neutropenic sepsis.

Use of colony-stimulating factors in AML therapy

Randomized trials have shown that the administration of CSFs following acute myeloid leukaemia (AML) induction chemotherapy has consistently reduced the neutropenic period, with concurrent benefits in terms of hospitalization and antibiotic use. Some of these studies have also shown additional benefits in terms of clinical response rate, disease-free or overall survival, although this has not been consistently observed. Importantly, no adverse effects have been observed on the stimulation of leukaemic cell growth or drug resistance in any of these studies despite the fact that CSF receptors may be expressed on myeloid blasts. Elderly AML patients are most at risk from death from neutropenic sepsis, and recommendations at present are that this group should certainly be considered for CSF therapy. The use of CSFs for other AML patients can also be justified if it is considered that the reduction in hospitalization outweighs the cost of the CSF treatment. Comparative studies of G- and GM-CSF have not been performed, but available data seem to suggest that both CSFs are effective in this setting. Delaying the commencement of CSF 2–3 days following the completion of chemotherapy does not appear to reduce the efficacy and may be associated with some cost savings.

Similarly, the use of CSFs in a similar way following consolidation chemotherapy can also be justified as their use in this setting appears to result in a marked reduction in the duration of neutropenia and hospitalization.

The use of CSFs to 'prime' leukaemic blasts in an attempt to enhance their sensitivity to S-phase-specific cytotoxic agents has been investigated. The best-known AML chemotherapy regimen utilizing this approach is the 'FLAG' chemotherapy protocol, which combines fludarabine, cytosine arabinoside and G-CSF. In this case, G-CSF is given before and during the chemotherapy to sensitize the blast cells, and the fludarabine, being scheduled before the cytosine arabinoside, acts synergistically to increase the rate of accumulation of Ara-CTP in the blasts and lead to enhanced killing of these cells. No clear benefit in terms of response rates or survival has, however, been demonstrated using such an approach, and at present it is recommended that the use of CSFs in this setting should be restricted to clinical trials.

Myelodysplastic syndromes

Many patients with myelodysplasia suffer from chronic severe neutropenia, and among such patients the incidence of serious infections is high. Studies have demonstrated that administration of CSFs alone to such patients may be effective in improving neutrophil and also eosinophil counts and is well tolerated. Thus, the intermittent use of CSFs in patients with severe neutropenia and recurrent infection can be recommended. Indeed, the combination of CSFs together with erythropoietin may also be of benefit in MDS patients who are also anaemic owing to a synergistic effect on Hb. Furthermore, for patients with high-risk MDS who are receiving systemic chemotherapy, the administration of CSFs results in a shortening of neutropenia and reduction of the interval between induction and consolidation courses. The theoretical increased risk of transformation to overt AML has not been observed but, in view of this, prolonged or continuous use of CSFs cannot be recommended.

Acute lymphoblastic leukaemia

There is good evidence from randomized trials that G-CSF is effective in reducing the duration of neutropenia by up to 8 days in both adults and children receiving ALL induction chemotherapy. This was associated with a reduction in the number of infections and duration of hospitalization in some of the studies but had no effect on overall or disease-free survival. On the basis of these findings, it has been recommended that G-CSF is commenced after the first few days of induction or first post-remission course of chemotherapy.

Aplastic anaemia

There is limited evidence from clinical trials regarding the use of CSFs for patients with aplastic anaemia. There have been a number of sporadic reports of responses to G- and GM-CSF, especially in less severe cases. It also does not appear that the addition of prophylactic CSFs to immunosuppressive therapy reduces the number of infections developing in such patients. Therefore, it is suggested at present that the use of these agents for patients with aplastic anaemia should be restricted to clinical trials. The efficacy of a number of other haemopoietic growth factors is being evaluated at present, both alone and in combination with stem cell factor (SCF), erythropoietin, flt3-ligand and thrombopoietin. The data from these studies are awaited with interest.

Severe chronic neutropenia

Severe chronic neutropenia is defined as an absolute neutrophil count below 0.5×10^9/L lasting for months or even years. Causes include cyclic, idiopathic and congenital neutropenias, and G-CSF has been shown to be effective in all these categories, leading to durable responses in the neutrophil counts. In the case of inherited bone marrow failure syndromes such as Kostmann's syndrome, Schwachman–Diamond syndrome, Fanconi anaemia and dyskeratosis congenita, G-CSF may be effective in improving neutrophil counts in up to 90% of cases and may also reduce infections and improve survival; these infants previously suffered from severe pyogenic infections and had a median survival of less than 3 years. Adverse effects include mild splenomegaly, mild thrombocytopenia, osteoporosis and possibly malignant transformation.

The fact that some responders with congenital neutropenia have developed myelodysplastic syndromes or AML raises the possibility that G-CSF may play a role in the pathogenesis of these disorders in these patients. The issue is complicated because many of these disorders have a propensity for transformation into AML/MDS as part of their natural history. One registry study revealed a rate of AML/MDS of 12.5% after 8 years of treatment, with no significant relationships found between the age of onset of AML/MDS, patient gender, G-CSF dose or duration of G-CSF therapy. However, the cumulative acquisition of genetic aberrations was observed in the bone marrow cells from patients with Kostmann's syndrome who transformed, including *ras* mutations, the appearance of clonal cytogenetic abnormalities and the presence of G-CSF receptor mutations. It has been shown in murine models that G-CSF receptor defects may lead to the development of a hyperproliferative response to G-CSF, confer resistance to apoptosis and hence enhance cell survival.

It remains unclear whether G-CSF directly accelerates the propensity for transformation to AML/MDS in the genetically abnormal progenitor cells in these patients with inherited forms of bone marrow failure, especially those with G-CSF and *ras* mutations, or whether G-CSF simply prolongs patient survival and allows time for the malignant predisposition to declare itself. It is, however, noteworthy that G-CSF has also been shown to be effective in the management of patients with cyclic and idiopathic neutropenia, and in these patients there have been no cases of AML/MDS. Nevertheless, only careful follow-up of these patients will resolve this issue.

Hodgkin's disease and non-Hodgkin's lymphoma

Several studies have shown that the addition of G- or GM-CSF as primary prophylaxis in patients receiving chemotherapy for various lymphomas reduces the incidence of neutropenia, neutropenic sepsis, chemotherapy delays and duration of hospitalization. Furthermore, G-CSF has been used to permit a reduction in the interval between cycles of CHOP chemotherapy from 3-weekly to 2-weekly, which may translate into improved disease responses and survival. Overall, there is currently insufficient evidence to justify routine addition of CSFs for all patients with non-Hodgkin's lymphoma, but it may be considered in elderly patients.

Use of colony-stimulating factors in the paediatric population

Chemotherapy protocols for the treatment of paediatric malignancies are often considerably myelotoxic, and infants are particularly susceptible to neutropenic sepsis because of the immaturity of their immune systems. In addition, as many childhood cancers are potentially curable, there is a perceived higher cost–benefit ratio for the use of CSFs to support these chemotherapy regimens. As a result, there is generally a higher usage of CSFs for primary and secondary prophylaxis than in the adult population. The use of CSFs for patients with congenital neutropenias has already been discussed, and there are some data to support the use of CSFs in neonatal sepsis. Otherwise, the indications for the use of CSFs are similar to those for adults, and it appears to be that G-CSF is better tolerated than GM-CSF.

Use of GM-CSF as an adjunct to antifungal therapy

Invasive fungal infections have emerged as a cause of serious mortality and morbidity to immunocompromised patients. Host defences including appropriate cytokine responses and intact phagocyte function are necessary to combat opportunistic fungal infections such as candidiasis and aspergillosis. Bronchoalveolar macrophages, which are derived from peripheral blood monocytes, have a particularly important role in this regard, but this mechanism may be severely impaired in patients who are cytopenic following cytotoxic chemotherapy or who are treated with steroids (e.g. dexamethasone) that have a suppressive effect on macrophage function.

A number of CSFs have been investigated and studied *in vitro* for activity against fungal pathogens. The most promising results have been seen with GM-CSF, which has been shown to augment the antifungal activity of monocytes and macrophages. The main effects of GM-CSF on macrophages and monocytes are to enhance their phagocytic and metabolic functions, including increased synthesis and release of superoxide anions that are directly toxic to microbes, and to release other proinflammatory cytokines. This results in the inhibition and/or killing of *Candida albicans*, *Aspergillus hyphae*, *Cryptococcus*, *Pneumocystis*, *Leishmania* and *Mycobacteria* as well as other intracellular pathogens. GM-CSF has also been shown to block the ability of dexamethasone to suppress the activity of bronchoalveolar macrophages.

There have been several reports on the successful use of GM-CSF in conjunction with antimicrobial therapy in the management of patients with these opportunistic infections. This supports the clinical value of CSFs in this situation, although controlled trials are needed for full evaluation of their efficacy.

The role of G-CSF in the harvesting of granulocytes for transfusion

The development of bacterial and fungal infections continues to be a major complication for neutropenic patients. Despite the use of modern antibiotics and the use of haemopoietic growth factors to reduce the period of post-treatment neutropenia, infection remains a major cause of morbidity and mortality in these patients. The transfusion of normal granulocytes is a logical approach to the treatment of serious infections in neutropenic patients. Before the introduction of CSFs, initial studies of granulocyte transfusions in the 1960s using buffy coats were disappointing owing to difficulties in collecting adequate numbers of functional granulocytes from donors to raise the ANC in adult recipients by more than a few hundred cells per litre. This dose of cells is probably inadequate to treat an established infection.

More recently, it has been shown that the combined administration of dexamethasone and G-CSF to donors prior to leucapheresis can increase the yield of granulocytes collected up to 10×10^9/L in a single 2- to 3-h procedure using hydroxyethyl starch as a sedimenting agent. These cells appear to be functionally normal by both *in vitro* and *in vivo* measurements. This dose of cells can increase and maintain the blood neutrophil count at $0.5–1.0 \times 10^9$/L for up to 24 h after transfusion, and several reports have indicated a significant improvement in established infections. Adverse effects experienced by recipients are mainly febrile transfusion reactions, although there are theoretical concerns regarding pulmonary toxicity and HLA sensitization. G-CSF administration to donors is generally well tolerated. Further studies are required to determine the exact role for granulocyte transfusions in neutropenic patients with severe infection.

Exogenous production of colony-stimulating factors by tumours

Tumour-related leucocytosis is a paraneoplastic syndrome that has been reported occasionally in a number of different non-haematological malignancies, including lung carcinoma, mesothelioma, transitional cell carcinoma of the bladder, and renal and hepatocellular carcinomas among others. Autonomous production of haemopoietic CSFs such as G-CSF, GM-CSF and IL-6 by these tumours has recently been demonstrated. Although the mechanism for this aberrant expression of G-CSF m-RNA remains unclear, it appears that in the case of lung cancer this phenomenon is associated with a poor outcome.

Long-acting haemopoietic growth factors

Haemopoietic growth factors such as G-CSF and GM-CSF are highly effective at shortening the period of neutropenia following cytotoxic chemotherapy and hence reducing the incidence of infections. Although they are safe and effective, they have a short half-life, being rapidly cleared from the body predominantly through the kidneys. As a result, daily subcutaneous administration is required often for periods of 7–14 days. Attempts have therefore been made to modify these agents to increase their half-life and reduce the frequency of injections. The successful engineering of a sustained-duration G-CSF has now been achieved by the addition of a polyethylene glycol moiety to the G-CSF molecule (pegfilgrastim). This longer-acting cytokine binds to the same receptor and stimulates the proliferation and differentiation of neutrophils by the same mechanism as its shorter-acting counterpart. However, it is minimally cleared by the kidneys and has a much longer serum half-life. Furthermore, its clearance is neutrophil dependent and is therefore self-regulated. Initial clinical trials have shown that a single subcutaneous dose of the pegylated G-CSF per cycle of chemotherapy is sufficient and as effective as its shorter-acting derivative in reducing the neutropenic period. The safety profile and tolerability of pegylated G-CSF is also similar.

Thrombopoietin

Thrombopoietin (TPO) is an essential growth factor for stem cell maintenance and proliferation, although its major role is to enhance platelet production and function. It is the ligand for the receptor c-mpl, which is a member of the cytokine receptor superfamily and is expressed on megakaryocytes, platelets and also on pluripotential stem cells. TPO is mainly synthesized in the liver, and its levels are regulated by clearance through platelet binding. The effect of TPO in culture is to increase the number of CD34$^+$ stem cells, colony-forming units and long-term culture-initiating cells (LT-CIC) (repopulating cells). Indeed, TPO alone can be used to maintain bone marrow cells in culture for several months without loss of the primitive phenotype and with sustained high-level production of both megakaryocytic and non-megakaryocytic cells. Knockout mice lacking TPO or c-mpl expression are not only thrombocytopenic, but also have a serious deficiency in stem cell numbers.

Early hopes that TPO administration after myelotoxic treatment would lead to accelerated platelet recovery were borne out by animal studies. In non-human primates, a single dose of TPO given shortly after cytotoxic therapy was sufficient to alleviate thrombocytopenia and also appeared to potentiate the action of G- or GM-CSF by accelerating CD34$^+$ reconstitution. However, the dose and scheduling were important. Unfortunately, clinical trials with TPO in humans were less successful partly because of problems in scheduling the drug and also because of problems with platelet aggregation. Furthermore, the pharmaceutical development of a pegylated truncated thrombopoietin, termed *megakaryocyte growth and development factor* (MDGF), was halted because of the development of neutralizing antibodies in some patients who received the agent. These antibodies were able to cross-react with endogenous TPO, leading to profound thrombocytopenia. As a result, there are no growth factors with the ability to stimulate platelet production in use at present.

Stem cell factor

Stem cell factor (SCF) is an essential growth factor with both proliferative and anti-apoptotic functions and exerts its influence on both primitive and committed haemopoietic progenitors. It has been mainly used in conjunction with G-CSF due to the apparent synergy between these two CSFs. For example, this combination has been used in the laboratory to enhance the long-term expansion of human primitive haemopoietic cells and clinically to increase the yield of peripheral blood progenitor cells during mobilization. A randomized study comparing the efficacy of G-CSF alone and G-CSF combined with SCF in stem cell mobilization from heavily pretreated patients with non-Hodgkin's lymphoma and Hodgkin's disease showed that the combination led to a superior CD34$^+$ cell yield.

The SCF receptor, termed c-Kit, has an intrinsic tyrosine kinase domain and may be abnormally expressed in haemopoietic malignancies and other tumours (e.g. gastrointestinal stromal tumours, GIST). Recent advances have identified molecules that are able to target and inhibit specific tyrosine kinase inhibitors. This may represent an emerging modality for the treatment of AML, as activated endothelial cells have been shown to secrete haemopoietic growth factors such as SCF and GM-CSF, which may be necessary for leukaemic cell survival in a paracrine fashion. AML blasts themselves have been shown to express SCF (c-Kit) receptorsin approximately 50% of cases. These receptors may be responsible for AML blast proliferation and resistance to apoptosis as these cells may respond to growth stimuli provided by endothelial cells from the bone marrow microenvironment. Therefore, therapy directed at blocking SCF signalling might prove to be an effective therapy for the treatment of AML. Studies of different tyrosine kinase inhibitors in this regard are ongoing.

Interleukin 3

Interleukin 3 (IL-3) is a multipotential growth factor produced by activated T cells, monocytes/macrophages and stromal cells. It stimulates all haemopoietic lineages and induces proliferation, maturation and proliferation of pluripotential haemopoietic stem cells and also committed myeloid, erythroid and megakaryocytic cells. Human IL-3 was cloned in 1986 and recombinant IL-3 has been used in various clinical trials to speed haemopoietic recovery following cytotoxic chemotherapy. Initial phase I/II studies gave promising results with apparent faster regeneration, but this was not confirmed in phase III studies. Furthermore, the use of IL-3 alone in the treatment of patients with aplastic anaemia and myelodysplasia has been disappointing. The potential of IL-3 in conjunction with other growth factors to increase the yield of PBSCs for harvesting is being evaluated. Owing to the problems of toxicity and inflammatory side-effects induced by IL-3, it is no longer in clinical use. Instead, attention has switched to the development of synthetic chimeric growth factor receptor agonists that have greater *in vitro* biological activity and fewer side-effects.

Chimeric haemopoietic growth factors

The shared properties of haemopoietic growth factors and their receptors has enabled the construction of genetically engineered synthetic cytokines with higher affinities, increased biological activity and more favourable toxicity profiles. Synthokine (a high-affinity IL-3 analogue), myelopoietin (an IL-3 and G-CSF chimera) and promegapoietin (an IL-3 and thrombopoietin chimera) are all multilineage haemopoietic growth factors that are being evaluated in clinical trials. The advantage of these compounds is their potential ability to enhance platelet recovery in addition to their effect on neutrophil recovery.

Selected bibliography

ASCO (1994) American Society of Clinical Oncology recommendations for the use of hematopoietic colony-stimulating factors: evidence-based clinical practice guidelines. *Journal of Clinical Oncology* 12: 2471–508.

ASCO (1996) Update of recommendations for the use of hematopoietic colony-stimulating factors: evidence-based clinical practice guidelines. *Journal of Clinical Oncology* 14: 1957–60.

Basu S, Dunn A, Ward A (2002) G-CSF: function and modes of action (review). *International Journal of Molecular Medicine* 10: 3–10.

Bearpark A, Gordon M (1989) Adhesive properties distinguishing subpopulations of haemopoetic stem cells with different spleen colony forming and marrow repopulating capacities. *Bone Marrow Transplantation* 4: 625–8.

Bensinger W, Martin P, Storer B *et al.* (2001) Transplantation of bone marrow as compared with peripheral blood cells from HLA identical relatives in patients with haematologic cancers. *New England Journal of Medicine* 344: 175–81.

Blaise D, Kuentz M, Fortanier C *et al.* (2000) Randomised trial of bone marrow versus lenograstim-primed blood cell allogeneic transplantation in patients with early stage leukaemia: a report from the Societe Francaise de Greffe de Moelle. *Journal of Clinical Oncology* 18: 537–546.

Bowen D, Culligan D, Jowitt S *et al.* (2003) Guidelines for the diagnosis and therapy of adult myelodysplastic syndrome. *British Journal of Haematology* 120: 182–200.

Brenner M (ed.) (1994) *Cytokines and Growth Factors*. Baillière Tindall, London.

Broudy V (1997) Stem cell factor and haemopoiesis. *Blood* 90: 1345–64.

Byrne JL, Haynes AP, Russell NH (1996) Use of haemopoietic growth factors: commentary on the ASCO/ECOG guidelines. *Blood Reviews* 11: 16–27.

Casadevall N, Nataf J, Viron B *et al.* (2002) Pure red cell aplasia and anti-erythropoietin antibodies in patients treated with recombinant erythropoietin. *New England Journal of Medicine* 346: 1584–6.

Cazzola M, Mercuriali F, Brugnara C (1997) Uses of recombinant erythropoietin outside the setting of anaemia. *Blood* 89: 4248–67.

Freedman MH, Aler BP (2002) Malignant myeloid transformation in congenital forms of neutropenia. *Israeli Medical Association Journal* 4: 1011–14.

Haynes AP, Russell NH (1996) Clinical use of haemopoietic growth factors. In: *Recent Advances in Haematology* (A Hoffbrand, ed.). Churchill Livingstone, London.

Hellstrom-Lindberg H, Gulbrandsen N, Lindberg G *et al.* (2003) A validated decision model for treating the anaemia of myelodysplastic syndrome with erythropoietin and granulocyte colony-stimulating significant effects on quality of life. *British Journal of Haematology* 120: 1037–45.

Hochaus S, Wassmann B, Egerer G (1998) Recombinant human granulocyte and granulocyte-macrophage colony-stimulating factor (G-CSF and GM-CSF) administered following cytotoxic chemotherapy have a similar ability to mobilize peripheral blood stem cells. *Bone Marrow Transplantation* **22**: 625–30.

Holyoake T, Alcorn M (1994) CD34 positive haemopoietic cells: biology and clinical applications. *Blood Reviews* **8**: 113–24.

Hubel K, Dale D, Liles W (2002) Therapeutic use of cytokines to modulate phagocytic function in the treatment of infectious diseases: current status of granulocyte–macrophage colony-stimulating factor, macrophage colony-stimulating factor and interferon-gamma. *Journal of Infectious Diseases* **185**: 1490–501.

Ihle J, Kerr IM (1995) Jaks and Stats in signalling by the cytokine receptor superfamily. *Trends in Genetics* **11**: 69–74.

Kauchansky K (1995) Thrombopoietin: the primary regulator of platelet production. *Blood* **86**: 419–31.

Lee S, Radford J, Dobson L (1998) Recombinant human granulocyte colony stimulating factor (filgrastim) following high dose chemotherapy and peripheral blood progenitor cell rescue in high grade non-Hodgkin's lymphoma: clinical benefits at no extra cost. *British Journal of Cancer* **77**: 1294–9.

Ludwig H, Rai K, Blade J et al. (2002) Management of disease-related anaemia in patients with multiple myeloma or chronic lymphatic leukaemia: epoetin treatment recommendations. *The Haematology Journal* **3**: 121–30.

Mangi M, Newland AC (1999) Interleukin-3 in haematology and oncology; current state of knowledge and future directions. *Cytokines and Cellular Molecular Therapy* **5**: 87–95.

Maxwell PH, Pugh CW, Ratcliffe PJ (2001) The pVHL–hIF1 system. A key mediator of oxygen homeostasis. *Advances in Experimental Medical Biology* **502**: 365–76.

Nemuniatis J, Buckner CD, Singer JW et al. (1990) Use of recombinant GM-CSF in graft failure. *Blood* **76**: 245–53.

Nemunaitis J, Anasetti C, Storb R (1992) Phase II trial of recombinant human GM-CSF in patients undergoing allogeneic bone marrow transplantation from unrelated donors. *Blood* **79**: 2572–7.

Osterborg A, Brandberg Y, Molostova V et al. (2002) Randomised double blind placebo controlled trial of recombinant human erythropoietin in haematological malignancies. *Journal of Clinical Oncology* **20**: 2486–94.

Ozer H, Armitage J, Bennett C et al. (2000) Update of recommendations for the use of haematopoietic colony stimulating factors: evidence-based clinical practice guidelines. *Journal of Clinical Oncology* **18**: 3558–70.

Pagliuca A, Carrington PA, Pettengell R et al. (2003) Guidelines on the use of colony-stimulating factors in haematological malignancies. *British Journal of Haematology* **123**: 22–33.

Price T (2002) Granulocyte transfusion in the G-CSF era. *International Journal of Haematology* **76**: 77–80.

Rizzo JD, Lichtin A, Woolf S et al. (2002) Use of epoetin in patients with cancer: evidence based clinical practice guidelines of the American Society of Haematology. *Blood* **100**: 2303–20.

Russell NH, Gratwohl A, Schmitz N (1996) The place of blood stem cells in allogeneic transplantation. *British Journal of Haematology* **93**: 747–53.

Schmitz N, Linch DC, Dreger P et al. (1996) A randomized trial of filgrastim-mobilized peripheral blood progenitor cell transplantation versus autologous bone marrow transplantation in lymphoma patients. *Lancet* **347**: 3563–3567.

Sheridan WP, Begley CG, Juttner CA et al. (1992) Effect of peripheral-blood progenitor cells mobilized by filgrastim (G-CSF) on platelet recovery after high dose chemotherapy. *Lancet* **339**: 640–4.

Storek J, Gooley T, Siadek M et al. (1997) Allogeneic peripheral blood stem cell transplantation may be associated with a high risk of chronic graft versus host disease. *Blood* **90**: 4705–9.

Stroncek D, Clay M, Petzoldt M et al. (1996) Treatment of normal individuals with granulocyte colony-stimulating factor: donor experiences and the effects on peripheral blood CD34$^+$ cell counts and on the collection of peripheral blood stem cells. *Transfusion* **36**: 601–10.

CHAPTER 19

Lysosomal storage disorders

Atul B Mehta and Derralynn A Hughes

19

Introduction

Lysosomes

A vital feature of eukaryotic cells is the presence of internal membranes subdividing the interior of the cell and compartmentalizing cellular processes into organelles.

Lysosomes are membrane-bound intracellular organelles representing the major degradative compartment of mammalian cells. They are morphologically heterogeneous and are distinguished from other organelles by an operational definition that describes them as membrane-bound acidic organelles containing mature acid-dependent hydrolases and lysosome-associated membrane proteins (LAMPS) but lacking receptors for mannose 6-phosphate residues. Lysosomal hydrolases, active at acidic pH, catalyse the degradation of macromolecules imported from the cytoplasm by chaperones or derived from endocytosis, pinocytosis, phagocytosis or autophagocytosis. More than 50 different soluble hydrolases are responsible for the breakdown of lipids, proteins, nucleic acids, glycosaminoglycans and oligosaccharides.

The lysosomal membrane is also vital to protect the cytoplasmic components from the acid hydrolases. Protection against cell digestion is thought to be accomplished by LAMP proteins. These are transmembrane proteins with highly glycosylated intralysosomal domains, among the most densely N-glycosylated proteins so far reported. The lysosomal membrane is also involved in fusion with other organelles, in maintenance of an acidic intralysosomal pH and in the efflux of amino acids and mono- and oligosaccharides produced by the lysosomal hydrolases.

Soluble lysosomal enzymes are synthesized on the rough endoplasmic reticulum and acquire N-linked oligosaccharide side-chains in the Golgi apparatus. Here, asparagine-linked high-mannose residues are phosphorylated at position 6. This modification is specific for lysosomal enzymes and is essential for the routing of the enzymes to the lysosomal compartment via mannose 6-phosphate receptors (Figure 19.1). The receptor–lysosomal enzyme complex is translocated to a prelysosomal compartment where the complex is dissociated by the low pH. The mannose 6-phosphate receptor recycles back to the Golgi, whereas the enzyme accumulates in the lysosomes. The small proportion of newly synthesized enzyme that does not bind to the receptors is secreted into the interstitial fluid, where it may bind mannose 6-phosphate receptor located on the plasma membrane. This enzyme is then recovered by receptor-mediated endocytosis and transported to the lysosome. Trafficking signals for lysosomal membrane glycoproteins probably reside in the cytosolic tails of the proteins and differ from those of lysosomal enzymes. Knowledge of the sorting mechanism for lysosomal enzymes has been exploited in the development of enzyme replacement therapy of lysosomal storage disorders.

Pathophysiology of lysosomal storage disorders

In most lysosomal storage disorders, an inherited deficiency of a specific lysosomal enzyme results in the accumulation of undegraded substrates within the lysosome. In others, accumulation of storage product results from the deficiency or malfunction of activator proteins, transport proteins or enzymes responsible for the processing of other lysosomal macromolecules. The involvement of over 40 different genes has been characterized, with many exhibiting a large number of different mutations. The resulting diseases are grouped according to the major stored substance, for example mucopolysaccharidoses (MPS), sphingolipidoses and glycoproteinoses. Storage product within the lysosomes causes disruption of cellular organization and disturbance of normal function. Different lysosomal storage diseases have characteristic organ distribution patterns of the abnormal metabolites and therefore recognizable pathological manifestations. For example, in MPS III (Sanfilippo disease) there is accumulation of heparan sulphate, an essential component of the neuronal membrane. This results in mental retardation. In contrast, in MPS IV (Morquio disease) accumulation of keratan

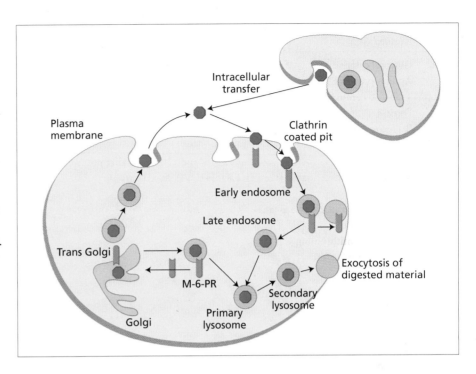

Figure 19.1 Routes of lysosomal enzyme cycling. Extracellular enzyme binds to the plasma membrane via mannose 6-phosphate receptors and is internalized by a clathrin-coated vesicle into an early endosome. As the early endosome acidifies to become a late endosome, the enzyme dissociates from the mannose 6-phosphate receptor, which recycles to the plasma membrane. The late endosome fuses with a primary lysosome derived from the Golgi apparatus to form a secondary lysosome, which may remain in the cell as a residual body or fuse with the plasma membrane in the process of exocytosis of digested products.

sulphate results in severe skeletal deformities. However, even within a discrete storage disorder there are often wide-ranging clinical manifestations. Individual mutations of the relevant enzymes give rise to variable levels of residual enzyme activity. This may result in different sites of storage and rates of accumulation producing clear genotype–phenotype correlations. More often, however, the genotype–phenotype relationship is unclear, with even siblings known to have the same mutation exhibiting disparate disease manifestations. This suggests that genetic or environmental factors other than residual enzyme level impacts upon the disease phenotype. Although knowledge of the genetics and biochemistry of the disorders has recently improved substantially, little is known of the pathological processes that actually result in end-organ damage. The enormous variability in symptom severity cannot be explained simply by differences in the overall burden of storage product but suggests a complex host reaction to abnormal cells. This may result in cytokine secretion, cellular proliferation, enhancement of other enzyme levels, and effects on metabolites and energy expenditure. In Gaucher's disease (GD), where storage cells are macrophages that play an essential role in host physiology and pathogenesis of inflammatory and immunological responses, a wide variety of enzymes, cytokines and coagulation factors are perturbed (Table 19.1). Interleukin 1 (IL-1), IL-6, IL-10 and tumour necrosis factor (TNF) have been implicated in GD pathogenesis. Elevated serum levels of IL-6, which is produced by macrophages, endothelial cells, fibroblasts and T cells, have been found to correlate with an index of severity in GD patients, and may be instrumental in the pathogenesis of B-cell dysregulation and

bone disease. IL-10, which in general inhibits the synthesis of other inflammatory cytokines, is also elevated and may represent an abnormal state of immune activation.

Prevalence

Few data are available on the frequency of lysosomal storage disorders. This is partly due to their rarity and the long observation period required to collect sufficient cases but also to incomplete ascertainment of cases. This is both because patients with minimal symptoms such as homozygotes for the Gaucher N370S mutation may not come to medical attention and also because of misdiagnosis of multisystem disorders such as Fabry disease. Studies in Europe, the USA and Australia suggest an overall birth prevalence of 1 in 5000–8000. In a study performed in the Netherlands, lipidoses were the most frequent as a group followed by mucopolysaccharidoses. Mucolipidoses and oligosaccharidoses were very rare. Metachromatic leucodystrophy, Krabbe's disease and Gaucher's disease were the most frequent individual disorders (Table 19.2).

Diagnosis

In the absence of an informative family history, diagnosis of lysosomal storage disorders requires a high degree of clinical suspicion. Levels of lysosomal enzymes may be measured in plasma or leucocytes using commercially available synthetic or naturally occurring labelled substrates. Storage product may be identified within biopsy specimens, plasma or urine. Once

	Elevated	Reduced
Plasma	Glucosyl ceramide	Total plasma cholesterol
	Apolipoprotein E	Low-density lipoprotein
	Transcobalamin II	High-density lipoprotein
	Ferritin	Apolipoprotein A-1
	β-Hexosaminidase	Apolipoprotein B
	α-Mannosidase	Factor XI
	β-Glucuronidase	Factor V and VIII (normalize post splenectomy)
	Angiotensin-converting enzyme	Factors II, VII, X, XII
	Lysozyme	
	Tartrate-resistant acid phosphatase	
	Chitotriosidase	
	Thrombin–antithrombin	
	Plasmin–antiplasmin	
	D-Dimer	
	Immunoglobulins	
	Paraprotein	
	IL-1	
	IL-6	
	IL-8	
	IL-10	
	TNF-α	
	M-CSF	
	Soluble CD14	
	CCL18/PARC	
Tissue	Glucosyl ceramide	
	β-Hexosaminidase	
	β-Glucuronidase	
	Galactocereobrosidase	
	Tartrate-resistant acid phosphatase	
	Non-specific esterase	
Hepatic	Alkaline phosphatase	
	Transaminases	

Table 19.1 Enzyme and cytokine disturbance in type 1 Gaucher's disease.

a candidate enzyme is identified analysis of the corresponding gene may identify a specific mutation and facilitate rapid screening of other family members. As effective treatment becomes available for a larger number of disorders it is increasingly important that patients should be diagnosed as early as possible as presymptomatic individuals may be candidates for early intervention.

Therapy

Effective treatment of lysosomal storage disorders self-evidently involves reduction of the stored compound and prevention of its reaccumulation. This has been achieved by replacement of the missing protein by stem cell transplantation and by infusion of the missing enzyme (enzyme replacement therapy, ERT). Many

patients with Gaucher's disease, metachromatic leucodystrophy, Krabbe's disease and mucopolysaccharidosis type I have undergone stem cell transplantation. Donation of stem cells has largely been from HLA-identical siblings but, as the highest level of enzyme activity will be supplied by donor cells from noncarriers, cord blood from unrelated donors has recently been used with good results.

Enzyme replacement therapy is now available or under investigation for several lysosomal storage disorders (Table 19.2). Recombinant human enzyme is produced in Chinese hamster ovary cells or human fibroblasts, chemically modified, purified and prepared for home infusion. ERT is effective in reducing the non-neuronopathic manifestations of a number of disorders, including Gaucher's type I and Fabry's disease. However, because enzyme does not cross the blood–brain barrier, it has not been

Table 19.2 Lysosomal storage disorders: biochemistry, prevalence and therapy.

Category	Disease	Alternative name	Enzyme deficiency	Stored material	Chromosome	Birth prevalence per 100 000	Therapy
Mucopolysaccharidosis	MPS I	Hurler Scheie, Hurler/Scheie	Iduronidase	Dermatan sulphate, Heparan sulphate	4p16.3	1.14	ERT, Phase 1–3, SCT
	MPS II	Hunter	Iduronate-2-sulphatase	Dermatan sulphate, Heparan sulphate	Xq27–28	0.74	ERT, Phase 1–3, SCT
	MPS III	Sanfilippo				(1.89)	SCT
		IIIA	Heparan-N-sulphatase	Heparan sulphate	17q25.3	0.88	
		IIIB	N-acetyl-glucosaminidase	Heparan sulphate	17q21.1	0.47	
		IIIC	Acetyl CoA glucosamine N-acetyl transferase	Heparan sulphate	Uncertain	0.07	
		IIID	N-acetyl-glucosamine-6-sulphatase	Heparan sulphate	12q14	0.09	
	MPS IV	Morquio				0.59	
		IVA	Galactose-6-sulphatase	Keratan sulphate	16q24	(0.22)	
		IVB	β-Galactosidase	Keratan sulphate	3p21–pter	(0.14)	
	MPS VI	Maroteaux–Lamy	Galactosamine-4-sulphatase	Dermatan sulphate	5q13–q14	0.43	ERT, Phase 1–2
	MPS VII	Sly	β-Glucuronidase	Dermatan sulphate, Heparan sulphate	7q21.1–q22	0.05	SCT, ERT, Preclinical
	MPS IX		Hyaluronidase	Hyaluronic acid	3p21.3		
Mucolipidoses	ML I	Sialidosis I	Neuraminidase	Sialic acid	10pter–q23	0.02	
	ML II	I Cell	UDP-N-acetyl glucosamine transferase	Many		(0.16)	SCT
	ML III	Pseudo-Hurler				(0.08)	
		IIIA	As ML II	Many			
		IIIC	Transferase-D-subunit	Many	16p		
	ML IV		Neuraminidase	Mucolipin	19p13.2–13.3		
Sphingolipidoses	GM1 gangliosidosis		β-Galactosidase	GM1-ganglioside, Keratan sulphate, Oligosaccharide, Glycolipids	3p21–3pter	0.5	SCT

Continued on next page

Table 19.2 (*cont'd*)

Category	Disease	Alternative name	Enzyme deficiency	Stored material	Chromosome	Birth prevalence per 100 000	Therapy
	GM2 gangliosidosis	Tay–Sachs	β-Hexosaminidase A	GM2-ganglioside Keratan sulphate Oligosaccharide Glycolipids	15q23–24	0.26	SCT
		Sandhoff	β-Hexosaminidase A and B	GM2-ganglioside Oligosaccharide	5q13		SCT
	GM2 gangliosidosis		GM2 activator	GM2-ganglioside Glycolipids	5q32–33		
	Globoid cell leucodystrophy	Krabbe	Galactocerebrosidase	Galactosyl-ceramides	14q31	0.71	SCT
	MLD		Arylsulphatase A	Sulphatides	22q13–3	1.09	SCT
	MLD		Saposin B activator	Sulphatides GM2-ganglioside Glycolipids	10q21		
	Fabry's disease		α-Galactosidase A	Globotriacylceramide	Xq22	0.85	SCT ERT Phase 1–4
	Gaucher's disease		Glucocerebrosidase	Glucosylceramide	1q21	1.75	ERT Phase 1–2 SCT
	Gaucher's disease		Saposin C activator	Glucosylceramide	10q21		
	Farber's disease		Ceramidase	Ceramide	8p22–21.2		SCT
	Niemann–Pick A and B		Sphingomyelinase	Sphingomyelin	22q13.1–13.2	0.4	ERT Preclinical
Oligosaccharidoses	α-Mannosidosis		α-Mannosidase	α-Mannosides	19p13.2–q12	0.09	SCT
	β-Mannosidosis		β-Mannosidase	β-Mannosides	4p	0.13	
	Fucosidosis		Fucosidase	Fucosides glycolipids	1p24	0.05	SCT
	Aspartylglucos-aminuria		Aspartylglucosaminidase	Aspartyl glucosamine	4q32–33	0.05	
	Schindler's disease		α-N-acetylgalactoseaminidase	N-acetylgalactosamineglycolipids	22q13.1–13.2		
Glycogen	Pompe's disease		α-Glucosidase	Glycogen	17q23	0.68	SCT ERT Phase 1–2

Category	Disease	Phenotype	Defect	Storage material	Gene locus	Frequency	Treatment
Lipid	Niemann–Pick C		Unknown	Cholesterol Sphingolipids	NPC1–18q NPC2–unknown	0.47	SCT SRT
	Wolman's disease and cholesterol ester storage disease		Acid lipase	Cholesterol ester	10q23.2–23.3	0.19	SCT ERT Preclinical
Monosaccharide amino acids and monomers	ISSD	Infantile sialic acid storage disease	Sialic acid transporter	Sialic acid glucuronic	6q14–q15	0.19	
	Salla disease		As ISSD	As ISSSD	As ISSD		
	Cystine		Cystine transporter	Cystine	17p13	0.52	
	Cobalamin F disease		Cobalamin transporter	Cobalamin	Unknown		
	Danon disease		Lamp-2	Cytoplasmic debris and glycogen	Xq24		
Peptides	Pycnodysostosis		Cathepsin k	Bone proteins	1q21		
S-acylated proteins ceroid lipofuscinosis	CLN	Batten's disease					
	CLN 1	Infantile	Palmitoyl protein thioesterase	Saposins	11p32		
	CLN 2	Late infantile	Pepstatin insensitive carboxypeptidase	Subunit C mitochondrial ATP synthase	11p15.5		
	CLN 3	Juvenile	Membrane protein	As CLN 2	16p21		
	CLN 4	Adult, kuf disease	Unknown	As CLN 2	Unknown		
	CLN 5	Late infantile, Finnish variant	Membrane protein	As CLN 2	13q22		
	CLN 6	Late infantile variant	Unknown	As CLN2	15q-q23		
	CLN 7	Late infantile variant	Unknown	Unknown	Unknown		
	CLN 8	Progressive epilepsy with mental retardation	Membrane protein	As CLN 2	8p23		
Multiple enzyme deficiencies	Multiple sulphatase deficiency		Multiple sulphatase enzymes	Sulphatides, glycolipids, glycosaminoglycans	Unknown	0.07	
	Galactosialidosis		Neuraminidase and β-galactosidase protective protein	Oligosaccharides, sialic acid	20q13.3	(0.04)	

demonstrated to prevent the onset and progression of neurological symptoms. Even attempts to administer missing enzymes into the spinal canal of patients with Tay–Sachs disease have failed, probably as a result of the limited access to the neuronal cells. Therefore, the effectiveness of ERT would appear to depend on the accessibility of the site of the pathology to exogenous enzyme and the ability of affected cells to internalize the enzyme.

Most recently, the strategy of decreasing the rate of synthesis of the stored component, so-called substrate reduction therapy (SRT), has been evaluated. The principle is to reduce the rate of substrate synthesis to approximately equal the rate of degradation using low-molecular-weight enzyme inhibitors. This may be especially effective in individuals with later onset forms of the diseases with detectable levels of residual enzyme activity. Furthermore, SRT may have therapeutic utility in crossing the blood–brain barrier. In addition, because low levels of enzyme may arise from misfolding or abnormal transport, the ability of pharmacological chaperones to rescue misfolded or unstable enzymes is under investigation at present. Low-molecular-weight analogues, receptor agonists and receptor antagonists diffuse into the cell and bind site-specifically to folding intermediates of the mutant protein and rescue it from degradation. Such enhancement of residual galactosidase A activity by galactose infusion has been used in the cardiac variant of Fabry's disease.

Finally, gene therapy is under investigation in animal models of lysosomal storage disorders and has been reported as an adjunct to ERT in Gaucher's disease.

Prognosis

The clinical course of infants diagnosed with a lysosomal storage disorder usually follows a predictable path of loss of learned skills and neurological deterioration until death results from infection and progressive organ damage. When onset is later, in adolescents and adults, the clinical course is more varied and the prognosis depends on the major organ systems affected.

Clinical manifestations

The key clinical features of the major lysosomal storage disorders are presented in Table 19.3. In view of recent advances in therapy, Gaucher's disease and Fabry's disease are presented in greater detail below.

Gaucher's disease

Gaucher's disease (GD) is due to deficiency of the enzyme glucocerebrosidase (GC), a lysosomal enzyme that hydrolyses glucosylceramide to glucose and ceramide (Figure 19.2). It is an autosomal recessive condition arising as a result of mutation within the GC gene. Affected individuals have a mutant enzyme with reduced activity, resulting in accumulation of the substrate (glucosylceramide) in lysosomes of reticuloendothelial (RE) cells. It is one of the commonest lysosomal storage disorders, with an estimated incidence of 1: 60–80 000 individuals.

Table 19.3 Lysosomal storage disorders: clinical features.

Category	Disease	Clinical features
Mucopolysaccharidoses	MPS I	Hurler's disease: developmental delay, ENT infections, coarse facial features, macrocephaly, thick skin, corneal clouding, hepatosplenomegaly, bony deformity including large skull, pelvic dysplasia, deformed vertebrae and shortened tubular bones (dysostosis multiplex)
		Scheie disease: mild skeletal abnormalities, stiff joints, corneal opacities, carpel tunnel syndrome, cardiac valvular abnormalities and respiratory infections
	MPS II	Like MPS I but without corneal clouding
	MPS III	Loss of acquired skills, aggression, hyperactivity, coarse hair, hirsutism, seizures, may become tetraspastic
	MPS IV	Disproportionate dwarfism, joint contractures, kyphoscoliosis, corneal clouding
	MPS VI	Like Hurler's disease but without neurological involvement
	MPS VII	Skeletal disease, hepatosplenomegaly, lethal hydrops, normal
Mucolipidoses	ML I	Early psychomotor retardation, hypotonia, truncal ataxia, upper motor neuron signs, corneal clouding
	ML II	Like Hurler's, mild corneal clouding and hepatosplenomegaly, prominent gum hypertrophy, severe dysostosis multiplex
	MLIII	Progressive arthropathy, bone lesions, low intelligence, cardiac valvular lesions, corneal clouding
	ML IV	Like ML 1

Table 19.3 (*cont'd*)

Category	Disease	Clinical features
Sphingolipidoses	GM1 gangliosidosis	Infantile: coarse features, seizures, progression to decerebrate rigidity and spastic quadriplegia by 2 years
		Juvenile: psychomotor and neurological degeneration over 2–10 years
		Adult: progressive cerebellar impairment, spasticity and intellectual impairment
	GM2 gangliosidosis	Tay–Sachs: motor weakness, psychomotor retardation, blindness, lapsing into vegetative state with decerebrate rigidity
		Sandhoff disease: like rapidly evolving Tay–Sachs disease
	Globoid cell leucodystrophy	Developmental delay and progressive neurological degeneration aged 3–9 months
	MLD	Flaccid paresis, lack of coordination and hyporeflexia, psychomotor retrogression, juvenile and adult forms have later onset, intellectual deterioration
	Fabry's disease	Left ventricular hypertrophy, renal impairment, angiokeratoma and acroparaesthesia
	Gaucher's disease	Type 1: hepatosplenomegaly, skeletal disease and pancytopenia
		Type 2: death from neurological complications by 2 years
		Type 3: slowly progressive neurodegenerative disorder
	Farber's disease	Hoarse cry, painful arthropathy, pulmonary infiltration, cherry-red spot, mental handicap, thickened heart valves
	Niemann–Pick	A: Hepatosplenomegaly, lymphadenopathy, neurological regression, epileptic seizures, macular cherry red spot
		B: Hepatosplenomegaly and pulmonary infiltration
		C: Psychomotor delay and regression
Oligosaccharidoses	α-Mannosidosis	Mild skeletal deformity, coarse facial features and moderate to marked mental retardation
	β-Mannosidosis	Hearing loss and swallowing difficulties
	Fucosidosis	Neurological degeneration, neurological impairment, seizures, angiokeratoma and mild skeletal dysplasia
	Aspartylglucosaminuria	Progressive psychomotor retardation, coarse facial features and mild skeletal dysplasia
	Schindler's disease	Progressive psychomotor retardation, blindness and seizures
Glycogen	Pompe's disease	Cardiomegaly, hepatosplenomegaly, muscular weakness and macroglossia
Lipid	Wolman's disease	Failure to thrive, malabsorption, adrenal gland enlargement and calcification, fatal by 1 year
	Cholesterol ester storage disease	Hypercholesterolaemia and premature atherosclerosis
Monosaccharide amino acids and monomers		
	ISSD	Visceral involvement, skeletal dysplasia, psychomotor retardation and early death
	Salla disease	Mental retardation, ataxia and near normal lifespan
	Cystinosis	Polyuria, thirst, failure to thrive, renal tubular acidosis, rickets, photophobia and hypothyroidism
	Cobalamin F disease	Stomatitis, glossitis, convulsions and developmental delay
	Danon disease	Cardiomyopathy, myopathy, variable mental retardation
Peptides	Pycnodysostosis	Short stature, osteosclerosis, short fingers, open fontanelle, hypodontia
Ceroid lipofuscinosis	CLN	Mental impairment, seizures, loss of vision and motor skills
Multiple enzyme deficiencies	Multiple sulphatase deficiency	Resemble a combination of MLD and Hurler's disease
	Galactosialidosis	Hypotonia, coarse features with facial oedema, retinal cherry-red spot

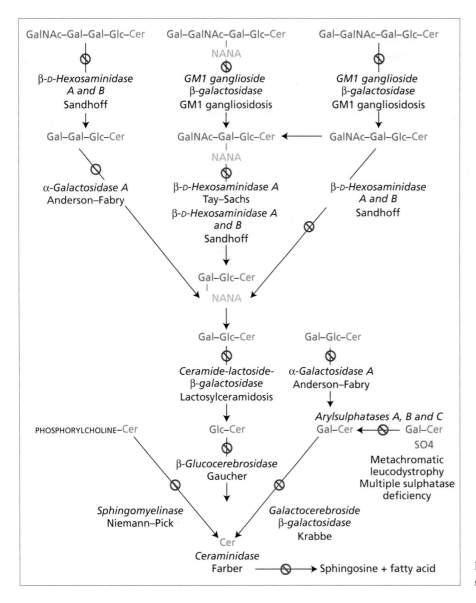

Figure 19.2 Biochemistry of lysosomal storage disorders.

Clinical features

Clinical manifestations are due to cellular and tissue damage consequent upon accumulation of abnormal RE cells in various tissues. Three main clinical phenotypes are observed (Table 19.4), determined in large part by the residual activity of the mutant enzyme. All three types are progressive disorders. The residual enzyme activity in type II is so low that abnormal cells accumulate in the central nervous system (CNS). This is the acute neuronopathic form of the disease, which presents with neurological complications in early infancy and usually leads to death before the age of 2 years. Type III GD is the subacute neuronopathic form that leads to a slowly progressive neurodegenerative disorder. Type I is the commonest form of GD and typically does not cause neurological disease. It is particularly common among

Table 19.4 Clinical manifestations of Gaucher's disease.

Manifestation	Type 1	Type 2	Type 3
Onset	1 year	< 1 year	2–20 years
Hepatosplenomegaly	++	+/–	+
Bone disease	++	–	+/–
Cardiac valve disease	–	–	+
CNS disease	–	+++	+/–
Oculomotor apraxia	–	+	+/–
Corneal opacities	–	+/–	+/–
Age at death	60–90 years	< 5 years	< 30 years

subjects of Ashkenazi Jewish origin; within this community, as many as 1 in 15–20 subjects are carriers, and approximately 1 in 800–1000 subjects are homozygous. Type I GD is a heterogeneous disorder that may present in childhood or in late adult life (> 60 years old). It is likely that many subjects are asymptomatic. Symptomatic individuals have hepatosplenomegaly, skeletal disease and bone marrow infiltration, leading to pancytopenia. Rarer manifestations of type I GD include renal involvement, pulmonary disease and skin involvement. Patients with type I GD have an increased incidence of malignancy generally and an increased incidence of haematological malignancies, especially B-lymphocyte disorders (myeloma, monoclonal gammopathy of undetermined significance) and myelodysplasia.

Laboratory features

Affected individuals have mutations within the GC gene; more than 300 different mutations have been described. The commonest mutation causing type I disease is a single basepair substitution in codon 370 (N370S), which accounts for approximately 70% of mutant alleles in affected Ashkenazi Jewish subjects. A basepair substitution in codon 444 (L444P) is the commonest mutation underlying neuronopathic GD. Diagnosis is confirmed by enzymatic assay of GC activity in leucocytes, fibroblasts and urine. However, enzymatic assay does not always identify heterozygote subjects and measured enzyme activity correlates poorly with clinical severity.

Splenic enlargement and marrow infiltration frequently lead to anaemia, leucopenia and thrombocytopenia.

Changes in serum immunoglobulins are frequent. Polyclonal hypergammaglobulinaemia is found in more than one-third of patients, and monoclonal gammopathy of undetermined significance (MGUS) is seen in up to 20%. Liver function tests are often abnormal, reflecting infiltration of the liver by Gaucher's cells leading to necrosis, fibrosis and, occasionally, even frank cirrhosis. There is an increased incidence of gallstones. The serum cholesterol level is typically lowered. GD is associated with a bleeding diathesis, attributable to abnormal platelet function and thrombocytopenia. Factor XI deficiency is commonly observed and is largely due to co-inheritance of other genetic abnormalities that are also common among Ashkenazi Jews.

The abnormal lipid-laden macrophages are readily detected on tissue biopsy (e.g. bone marrow aspirate, Figure 19.3), although biopsy is no longer considered necessary to make the diagnosis. The serum levels of ferritin, angiotensin-converting enzyme (ACE) and acid phosphatase are typically elevated. The enzyme chitotriosidase is derived from macrophages and is typically grossly elevated in untreated GD, and declines progressively with treatment. Levels may be as high as 30 000 units/L (normal range < 150 units/L); values below 1000 units/L generally indicate stable disease, and with prolonged (> 7 years) enzyme replacement therapy, values may even come down into the normal range (Figure 19.4). However, up to 6% of the population are deficient in this enzyme owing to a 24-basepair

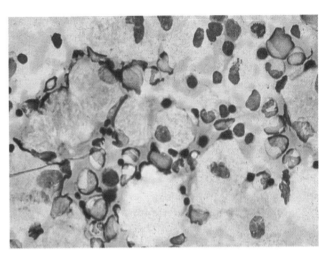

Figure 19.3 Gaucher's cells in the bone marrow.

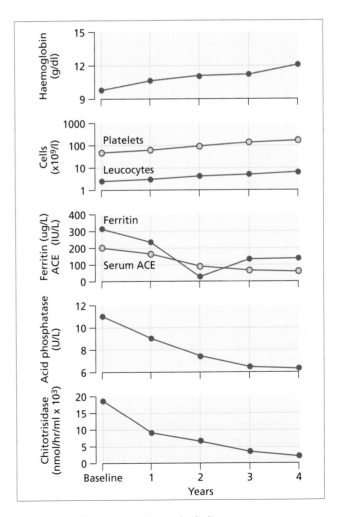

Figure 19.4 Clinical course in Gaucher's disease.

duplication in the chitotriosidase gene. These individuals cannot be monitored by measurement of plasma chitotriosidase activity. A new surrogate marker, pulmonary activation-regulated cytokine (Parc) (CCL18), is also elevated in plasma of patients with GD and may be useful for monitoring those patients with chitotriosidase deficiency. Parc is a member of the C-C chemokine family and its overexpression may be relevant to some of the pathophysiological features of GD such as abnormalities in neutrophil chemotaxis.

Treatment

All patients with GD should be evaluated by experienced physicians. Recombinant enzyme is made in Chinese hamster ovary (CHO) cells and additional mannose residues are added to the surface of the enzyme to facilitate uptake of the enzyme via the macrophage mannose receptor. This process allows treatment to be targeted to the RE system. GD is the first lysosomal storage disorder to be treated by enzyme replacement therapy (ERT), which has become the 'gold standard' of therapy for type I GD. Indications for ERT include significant pancytopenia (e.g. Hb < 10 g/dL, platelets < 100×10^9/L), skeletal disease and significant hepatosplenomegaly. High-dose ERT (> 100 units/kg every 2 weeks) is under evaluation at present for type II GD. The recombinant enzyme does not cross the blood–brain barrier and, although hepatosplenomegaly improves, ERT has little discernible impact on CNS disease.

However, ERT has recently (2003) been licensed for patients with type III GD, who typically have milder CNS abnormalities (e.g. ophthalmoplegia) in association with advanced systemic changes. ERT is administered by intravenous infusion (typically in the patient's home) every 1–2 weeks. The dose of therapy is titrated against the severity of clinical and laboratory changes. Type I patients with extensive bony disease and hepatosplenomegaly require 30+ units/kg every 2 weeks (60+ units/kg for type III), and these high doses should be continued for 2–3 years or more. Patients are monitored regularly with blood tests (the chitotriosidase assay is particularly helpful) and an annual skeletal MRI. Some patients with advanced type I and III disease may benefit from more frequent infusions (e.g. weekly) for the first year or more. The dose of ERT is gradually lowered as the disease burden declines. Patients with less advanced disease may require lower doses (e.g. 5–10 units/kg every 2 weeks), and some patients may only require monthly infusions. ERT is well tolerated and has been available for over 10 years. A small proportion of patients (< 10%) develop antibodies, but these are not usually neutralizing and do not affect treatment efficacy. Infusion reactions are rare and easily managed.

An oral form of therapy (Miglustat, Zavesca®) has recently been developed, and is licensed for mild to moderate type I disease. It is a form of SRT (see above). It is a small molecule that reduces the amount of substrate (glucosylceramide) being produced within lysosomes, such that patients with reduced residual enzyme activity will benefit. It is being evaluated at present in

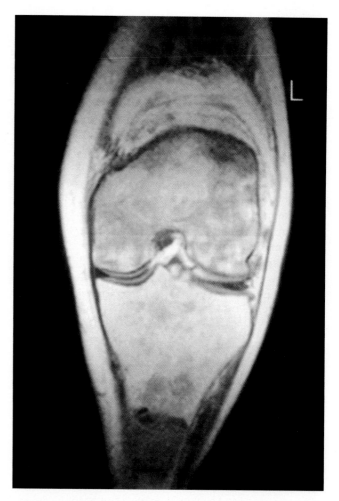

Figure 19.5 MRI scan showing skeletal changes in Gaucher's disease.

other lysosomal storage disorders (LSDs) (e.g. Tay–Sachs disease, Niemann–Pick type C) as its administration leads to reduction of a range of substrates in addition to glucosylceramide. SRT does cross the blood–brain barrier and is being evaluated in type III GD and in other LSDs affecting the CNS (e.g. Tay–Sachs).

Supportive therapy is frequently required. The skeletal disease in GD (Figure 19.5) is painful and patients may require analgesia. Prior to the use of ERT, patients frequently developed acute 'bone crisis' – episodic, severe pain, typically in the limbs and often precipitated by dehydration. Bisphosphonate therapy is under evaluation for its potential to reduce pain and rate of progression of skeletal disease. Blood component therapy may be required for pancytopenic patients. Splenectomy should be avoided if possible as splenectomized subjects are more likely to develop tissue infiltration in other organs (e.g. liver, lungs, skeleton). Allogeneic stem cell transplantation is a curative modality of therapy, and has a definite role in carefully selected children with neuronopathic GD.

Fabry's disease

Fabry's disease (or Anderson–Fabry disease) is an X-linked lysosomal storage disorder due to mutation within the gene for α-galactosidase A (αGal A) (Figure 19.2). The resulting inability to catabolize glycosphingolipids leads to progressive accumulation of the substrate globotriasylceramide (Gb_3) in a range of tissues. In contrast to GD, the lipid accumulation in Fabry's disease affects a range of cells (e.g. endothelial cells, epithelial cells, myocytes) within a broad range of tissues and organs, particularly the kidneys (leading to renal failure), heart (causing ventricular hypertrophy and conduction disturbances) and vasculature of the CNS. It is one of the commonest lysosomal storage disorders, with an incidence of approximately 1 in 100 000. It is panethnic.

Diagnosis

Diagnosis is by assay of αGalA activity in leucocytes and detection of molecular abnormalities within the αGalA gene. More than 200 different mutations have been described, and most lead to complete loss of enzyme activity. Tissue diagnosis is by renal, skin or cardiac biopsy.

Clinical features

Clinical features are legion. Although females are heterozygous, they are usually symptomatic and may be as severely affected as males. A skin rash (angiokeratoma) and pain in limbs (acroparaesthesia) are early symptoms (under 10 years old). In late childhood, reduced sweating, abdominal symptoms and lymphoedema are characteristic. Renal failure, cardiac failure, stroke, epilepsy and CNS/sensory organ involvement are later features. Life expectancy is 40–50 years for men and 50–65 years for most women.

Treatment

ERT for Fabry's disease has been available since 2001. Two formulations are available: a recombinant galactosidase that is translated in CHO cells and mannose terminated (agalsidase, Genzyme Corporation, MA, USA) and an enzyme of identical amino acid sequence that is translated in a human fibroblast cell line wherein post-translational modification is performed within the human cell itself (Transkarcytic Therapies, MA, USA). The infused enzyme in Fabry's disease must be taken up by lysosomes within cells in diverse organs and tissues; hence, targeting is of crucial importance. No direct comparative data on the two formulations are available, but in randomized placebo-controlled trials both preparations appear to be well tolerated and to have clinical efficacy. Intravenous infusions are administered every 2 weeks and have been shown to reduce substrate levels in plasma, urine and tissue biopsy. Beneficial clinical effects of ERT have been observed in renal and cardiac function, pain, hearing loss and gastrointestinal symptoms.

At present, protocols advise commencement of ERT in any Fabry sufferer – male or female – with pain, renal or cardiac disease, neurological abnormalities or significant vascular disease. It is clear that ERT will not reverse significant organ damage (e.g. renal failure) but may slow progression. In Fabry's disease, as in many other LSDs, the key to successful ERT may be prevention of substrate accumulation by early intervention in childhood.

Selected bibliography

Cox TM, Schofield JP (1997) Gaucher's disease: clinical features and natural history. *Baillière's Clinical Haematology* 10: 657–690.

Dell'Angelica IEC, Payne GS (2001) Intracellular cycling of lysosomal enzyme receptors: cytoplasm tails tales. *Cell* 106: 395–8.

Desnick RJ, Schuchmann EH (2002) Enzyme replacement and enhancement therapies: Lessons form lysosomal storage disorders. *Nature Reviews Genetics* 3: 954–66.

Fukuda MJ (1991) Lysosomal membrane glycoproteins: structure biosynthesis and trafficking. *Journal of Biological Chemistry* 266: 21327–30.

Mehta A (2002) New developments in the management of Anderson Fabry disease. *Quarterly Journal of Medicine* 95: 647–53.

Meikle PJ, Hopwood JJ, Clague AE *et al.* (1999) Prevalence of lysosomal storage disorders. *Journal of the American Medical Association* 281: 249–54.

Poorthuis B, Wevers RA, Kleijer WJ *et al.* (1999) The frequency of lysosomal storage diseases in the Netherlands. *Human Genetics* 105: 151–6.

Wraith JE (2001) Advances in the treatment of lysosomal storage disease. *Developmental Medicine and Child Neurology* 43: 639–46.

CHAPTER 20

Normal lymphocytes and non-neoplastic lymphocyte disorders

20

Mark T Drayson and Paul AH Moss

Introduction

The immune system has evolved in order to provide protection against infection. Its potential role in defence against malignant disease is also under investigation. The functions of the adaptive/specific immune system are mediated by lymphocytes, which circulate through a number of anatomical structures comprising *primary* and *secondary* lymphoid tissues.

The anatomy of the immune system

Lymphocytes are cells of the haemopoietic system and most derive ultimately from the haemopoietic stem cell in the bone marrow. The myeloid and lymphoid lineages diverge at an early time-point during differentiation, and this correlates with identification of a common myeloid progenitor (CMP) and common lymphoid progenitor cell (CLP). There are three classes of lymphocyte – B cells, T cells and NK cells – and these have different developmental pathways. T cells are generated in the thymus following the migration of prothymocytes from bone marrow to thymus followed by a complicated selection

process involving negative and positive selection of thymocyte precursors. Over 95% of thymocytes die in the thymus, but the minority population emerges from the thymus as single positive CD4$^+$ or CD8$^+$ T cells and enter the lymphoid system as naive precursors that can survive for many years.

Most B cells are generated from within the bone marrow, the 'B' in their name referring to an obscure avian structure called the bursa of Fabricius in which the B cells of birds develop. Naive mature B cells enter the lymphoid circulation but, if triggered by antigen in the periphery, a proportion of cells will return to the bone marrow as long-lived plasma cells that secrete immunoglobulin. Natural killer (NK) cells similarly appear to develop from within the environment of the bone marrow.

The bone marrow and thymus are therefore the sites of lymphocyte development and are known as the *primary* lymphoid organs. However, immune responses are initiated when lymphocytes encounter antigen and this occurs primarily in *secondary* lymphoid tissues such as lymph nodes and the spleen.

Lymphocytes circulate around the body tissues via the blood and lymphatic vasculature. Lymphatic vessels drain extravascular spaces and lymph nodes are collections of lymphoid tissue in lymphatic vessels, which are organized to optimize encounters between lymphocytes and antigen. Afferent lymph drains into the lymph nodes, bringing circulating lymphocytes and populations of antigen-loaded dendritic cells from regional tissue. Efferent lymph returns lymphocytes to the bloodstream, where naive cells continue this circulatory pattern in a continuing quest for antigenic encounter. Antigen-experienced lymphocytes migrate to a variety of tissues in order to mediate their effector functions. The pattern of homing is largely determined by the chemokine receptor profile on the lymphocyte.

Lymphocytes

B lymphocytes are the precursors of antibody-producing cells. Each B cell produces and expresses on its surface immunoglubulin (Ig) with a distinct specificity for antigen. The specificity of the Ig is determined by the way the Ig variable-region genes are rearranged during B lymphopoiesis. B cells that bind antigen through their surface Ig have to obtain accessory signals if they are to proliferate and differentiate into antibody-secreting cells. These can be provided by helper T cells, which recognize antigen that has been taken up and presented by the B cell.

T cells are functionally diverse. Their receptors for antigen – the T-cell receptor (TCR) – exist only as cell-surface molecules and are not secreted. T cells function by: (i) providing signals that help induce T cells and B cells to proliferate and differentiate; (ii) specifically deleting virally infected cells or foreign cells; and (iii) activating macrophages to enhance cellular cytotoxicity.

NK cells are able to kill cells that fail to express major histocompatibility complex (MHC) class I molecules on their surface. Many intracellular viral infections are able to downregulate surface MHC class I expression as a mechanism of immune evasion. Surface expression is also frequently reduced on malignant cells.

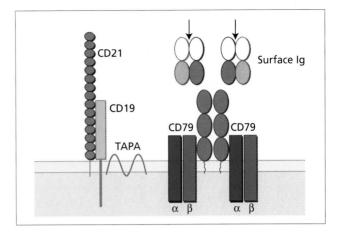

Figure 20.1 The structure of the antigen-specific receptor of B cells (BCR). Antibody (Ig) molecules on the surface of B cells provide their antigen-specific receptors. The green structures are the heavy (H) chains and the orange the light (L) chains. The antigen-combining – variable – regions are shown as open circles; the locations of the antigen-combining sites are indicated by arrows. The binding of antigen by B cells through their surface Ig can lead to antigen being internalized and can result, indirectly, in proliferation by the B cell and its differentiation to become an antibody-secreting cell or a memory cell. Signals delivered to the B cell when the surface Ig binds antigen are delivered through the α and β CD79 transmembrane signalling molecules and other surface Ig-associated molecules, including the complex of CD21 and CD19 with TAPA. CD21 binds the complement component C3d, which is derived from C3, and attaches to bacterial and other cell membranes; when CD21 and the surface immunoglobulin are cross-linked the stimulus for B-cell activation is considerably more than that delivered through the surface Ig alone. All B-cell surface Ig, such as plasma IgG and IgA, has two heavy and two light chains per molecule; IgA secreted from the body is a dimer and most IgM found in body fluids a pentamer of this basic four-chain structure.

The nature of the antigen-specific receptors on T and B cells

B-cell surface immunoglobulin

In the 1960s, Gell and Sell provided indirect evidence that the surface receptor for antigen on B cells was immunoglobulin, and this was confirmed in 1970 by a number of workers using fluorescent anti-Ig antibodies. In 1984, the TCR was identified by the use of subtraction libraries comparing cDNA expression between T and B cells. There are approximately 20 000 to 100 000 antigen-specific receptors on a lymphocyte and all the receptors on a single T cell or B cell are identical.

However, although the antigen receptors on a single cell have homogeneous antigen-recognition structures, they are different from the receptors on other B or T lymphocytes. During lymphoid development, a repertoire of billions of B and T cells is generated and all have slightly different antigen receptors on their surface. At the initiation of an immune response, only a few

of these cells are able to recognize the antigen and these are then expanded during their differentiation into effector cells. This is the basis of the *clonal selection* theory of immunology. The mechanisms that generate this great diversity of antigen receptors on lymphocytes are described in the next section. Figure 20.1 shows the structure of surface immunoglobulin on B cells.

T-cell receptors

T cells recognize peptides presented in association with MHC molecules. In humans, the MHC molecules are also known as human leucocyte antigens (HLAs) and there are two classes of MHC molecule. MHC class I molecules (Figure 20.2) are expressed by all nucleated cells except germ cells. They are not expressed by erythrocytes but are found on the surface of

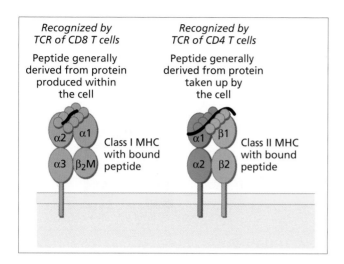

Figure 20.2 T cells recognize peptides held in MHC molecules. A class I MHC molecule is depicted on the left and a class II MHC molecule on the right. Some of the protein produced within each cell is broken down to peptides, which are presented on the cell surface in the peptide-binding groove of MHC molecules, usually class I (Figure 20.3). Extracellular molecules are taken up by antigen-presenting cells, broken down within the cell and presented on the cell surface in the peptide-binding groove of MHC molecules, usually class II (Figure 20.3). There are three isotypes of class II molecules, known as DP, DQ and DR, and three main class I isotypes, A, B and C. All of these are encoded within the MHC gene complex at 6p21.3. The genes encoding the peptide-binding grooves of each of these isotypes show extraordinary variability within the human population – 'allelic polymorphism' (Figure 20.5). The range of peptides that can be held by different MHC molecules varies. Consequently, this polymorphism is reflected in differences between individuals in the ability to recognize specific peptides. Any one TCR will only recognize a particular peptide within a particular groove structure. β_2-Microglobulin is a non-polymorphic Ig-like domain that is non-covalently associated with HLA class I MHC molecules; it stabilizes peptide binding and is essential for the expression of class I on the cell surface.

erythroblasts. The peptides seen by T cells in association with class I MHC molecules are, in most circumstances, derived from proteins produced from within the cell. This places MHC class I molecules in an excellent position to present peptides derived from viral proteins following intracellular viral infection (Figure 20.3). It is now clear that antigen-presenting cells are also able to take up proteins from outside the cell and process them such that peptides gain access to the MHC class I presentation. This process is called *cross-presentation* and may be particularly important in generating CD8$^+$ T cell responses to tumour-associated proteins.

MHC class I antigen presentation starts with the intracellular breakdown of proteins by a multimolecular proteolytic complex

known as a *proteasome*. These peptides are actively transported by TAP (transporter associated with antigen processing) proteins into the endoplasmic reticulum, where empty MHC class I molecules are being assembled. The nascent MHC molecules are able to 'fold' around the peptides, which make non-covalent interactions with the peptide-binding groove at the top of the molecule. This complex is then stabilized by the association of β_2-microglobulin before being transported to the cell surface. In this way, the cells are continuously advertising the peptide composition of the proteins that they are producing.

The selection of T cells during their development in the thymus involves the processes of *negative selection* and *positive selection*. T cells that have high affinity for self-peptides held in the groove of a self MHC molecule are deleted by apoptosis in a process known as *negative selection*. T cells with lower affinity for self peptide–MHC complexes are positively selected and survive to become peripheral T cells. T cells that recognize peptide presented by MHC class I molecules express a molecule CD8, which binds to the α3 domain of the MHC class I molecule (Figure 20.4). When any cell in the body presents immunogenic peptides, these may be recognized by a cytotoxic CD8 T lymphocyte that can then kill the target cell. This is most likely to occur as the result of virus infection when virus-encoded proteins are produced; it may also occur following the acquisition of a genetic mutation within a cell.

The other class of MHC molecule, MHC class II (Figure 20.2), is less widely expressed. The only cells that constitutively express large amounts of this class of MHC molecule are: (i) specialized antigen-presenting cells collectively known as dendritic cells; (ii) B lymphocytes; and (iii) thymic epithelial cells. Dendritic cells are derived from haemopoietic stem cells and codevelop with monocytes; they can be derived from blood mononuclear preparations by culture with granulocyte–macrophage colony-stimulating factor (GM-CSF) and interleukin 4 (IL-4). They migrate to many tissues, particularly epithelia, where they remain until activated by local tissue injury. On activation, they take up fluid and particles from their surrounding environment (Figure 20.3).

The pinocytotic activity in these cells can be induced by IL-1 and tumour necrosis factor (TNF) released at sites of injury. The pinocytotic vesicles fuse with an antigen-presenting endosomal compartment; proteolytic enzymes within this compartment are activated and proteins are broken down to peptides by the action of lysosomal enzymes. Class II molecules with peptide-binding grooves sealed by invariant chain (CD74) are inserted into the endosome wall. The invariant chain is digested and this allows peptides within the compartment to associate with MHC class II molecules. The MHC class II–peptide complex is then taken to the cell surface.

The scrutiny of antigen-presenting cells by T cells starts when dendritic cells have moved from peripheral tissues to the T cell-rich areas of adjacent secondary lymphoid organs. In that site they are known as interdigitating dendritic cells (IDCs),

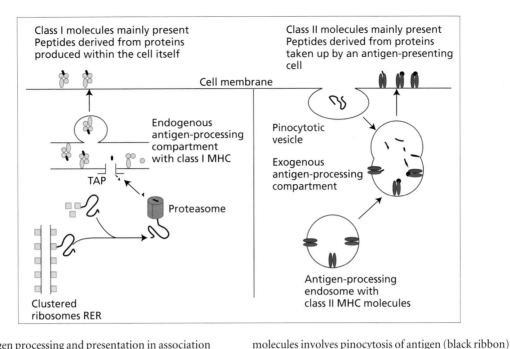

Figure 20.3 Antigen processing and presentation in association with MHC molecules. Left: Antigen presentation of proteins produced within cells is mainly the property of class I MHC molecules. A proportion of proteins (black ribbons) produced within a cell on ribosomes (yellow) are broken down to peptides (black fragments) within a cytoplasmic molecular complex known as a proteasome. The resulting peptides are actively transported by TAP proteins (blue) through the wall of specialized endoplasmic reticulum (ER) that has MHC class I molecules blue in its wall. The peptides and β_2-microglobulin associate with class I molecules and are then expressed on the cell surface (detailed in Figure 20.2). Right: Antigen presentation in association with class II MHC molecules involves pinocytosis of antigen (black ribbon) and fusion with an antigen-processing endosome, which has class II MHC molecules (magenta and blue) inserted in its wall. The antigen-presenting grooves of the class II MHC molecules are kept empty by the association with invariant chain (CD74). Fusion of the pinosome with the endosome heralds the activation of proteolytic enzymes; the invariant chain and the ingested proteins are broken down to peptides. The resulting peptides (black fragments) are assembled into the antigen-presenting groove of class II MHC molecules that are held in the endosomal wall. The HLA class II molecules with bound peptides are then carried to the cell surface (detailed in Figure 20.2).

which express increased amounts of MHC class II and constitutively express other molecules associated with T-cell activation such as CD40, CD80 (B7.1) and CD86 (B7.2). They also have markedly reduced capacity for pinocytosis. In the T zones of secondary lymphoid organs CD4+, and to a lesser extent CD8+, recirculating T cells are constantly migrating to the surface of IDCs, which they appear to scrutinize for the presence of an MHC–peptide complex to which they can bind with their T cell receptor. In this way, the T cells continually screen for the presence of peptides derived from both extra- and intracellular antigens (see section on immune responses).

The T-cell receptor (TCR) (Figure 20.4) has certain similarities to immunoglobulin in that it is made up of two non-identical polypeptide chains that have constant and variable regions. In addition, as described in the next section, the genes that encode for TCR and immunoglobulin are remarkably similar. The TCR has only one antigen binding site per molecule, as opposed to the two antigen binding sites of immunoglobulin.

There are two types of TCR. The most common is composed of a heterodimer of an α-chain and a β-chain. The minority population of $\gamma\delta$ TCRs is less well characterized, but they appear to recognize antigen in a different way from $\alpha\beta$ TCR. A number of different molecules are associated with the two TCR polypeptide chains in order to generate the TCR complex. This transmembrane signalling complex of molecules is collectively known as CD3 (detailed in Figure 20.4) and is linked to 'second messenger' signalling molecules, whose expression varies between different T-cell subsets and at different stages of T-cell differentiation. CD4 or CD8 molecules are closely associated with the CD3 complex and determine the class of MHC molecule to which the TCR can bind.

The polymorphism of major histocompatibility complex molecules

There is extensive polymorphism of the major histocompatibility complex (MHC) class I and class II molecules (Figure 20.5).

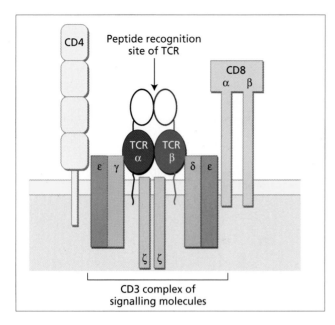

Figure 20.4 The αβ T-cell receptor complex. The αβ TCR is composed of two polypeptide chains, each with a variable (open ovoid) and constant (closed ovoid) domain. Peptide plus MHC is recognized by the combined variable regions. The TCR is surrounded by the CD3 complex of transmembrane signalling molecules. This is composed of four types of polypeptide chain, γ, δ, ε and ζ that are present as three pairs: ε with δ, ε with γ and a pair of ζ-chains or ζ plus η (a splice variant of ζ with a longer intracellular tail). Most monoclonal antibodies against CD3 are directed against antigenic determinants on CD3ε. Most peripheral T cells express CD4 or CD8 with their TCR. In the thymus, the TCR is first expressed on thymocytes that express both CD4 and CD8, allowing the possibility for selection on the basis of either class II or class I-recognizing properties (see section on T-cell development).

These were first recognized as targets for allograft rejection and the allelic forms of the MHC molecules differ in the fine structure of their MHC-binding grooves. This is reflected in differences in the range of peptides that different MHC alleles can present to T cells. Crossover during meiosis is relatively rare; consequently. the alleles on each chromosome 6 are usually inherited *en bloc* and are named the MHC haplotype of that chromosome. It follows that approximately one in four siblings share the same MHC haplotype on both chromosomes. For the purposes of stem cell transplantation, the patient and donor must usually be fully matched for HLA alleles and thus only 25% of siblings are appropriate for donation.

Highly inbred strains of mice have the same MHC haplotype on both chromosomes and accept grafts from each other. Analysis of the immune response of such mice indicates that some strains of mice are poor responders to certain antigens, whereas other strains produce high responses to the same antigen. Analysis of the response to different antigens does not necessarily show the same pattern for high and low responders. Cross-breeding experiments show that strains of mice responding well to a certain protein have an MHC allotype that is particularly good at presenting a peptide from the antigen to T cells. It is possible to rank the capability of particular alleles to present specific peptides to TCR.

Certain MHC alleles are associated with relative protection against specific infections. Conversely, some alleles, or combinations of alleles, are associated with a greater chance of developing autoimmunity. Many diseases, including diabetes mellitus, Graves' disease and ankylosing spondylitis, are distinctly more common in individuals with a particular MHC allele or MHC haplotype. It seems logical that in evolution most alleles have been retained because they have certain advantages without too many disadvantages. The advantages of an allele might relate to a particular infection that is prevalent in one part of the world, but almost unknown in another; for example, the HLA-B53 allele has a high prevalence in West Africa and is associated with relative protection from a potentially lethal form of malaria.

The generation of antigen-specific receptors on T and B lymphocytes

The genes that encode the antigen-combining or variable (V) part of the antigen-specific receptors of both B cells and T cells show marked similarities, which indicate that the gene complexes have evolved from a common precursor gene during the process of evolution. Both the immunoglobulin and TCR variable-region genes have to undergo a process of *gene rearrangement* from their germline configuration before they can encode an antigen recognition structure. This process is a key element in

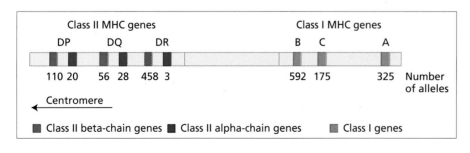

Figure 20.5 MHC polymorphism. This is a simplified diagram of the main genes that encode MHC class I and MHC class II molecules and their exceptional polymorphism.

Table 20.1 The variable region genes of human T- and B-cell antigen receptors.

Gene complex	Chromosomal location	Gene segments	
		Type	Approximate number
Ig heavy chain	14q32.3	V_H	51
		D_H	~27
		J_H	6
		C_H	10
Ig kappa light chain	2p12	V_κ	40
		J_κ	5
		C_κ	1
Ig lambda light chain	22q11	V_λ	~29
		J_λ	4
		C_λ	4
TCR alpha chain	14q11.2 (contains TCR δ locus)	V_α	~70
		J_α	61
		C_α	1
TCR delta chain	14q11.2 (between Vα and Jα of TCR α)	V_δ	~4
		D_δ	3
		J_δ	3
		C_δ	1
TCR beta chain	7q32.5	V_β	52
		D_β	2
		J_β	13
		C_β	2
TCR gamma chain	7p15	V_γ	12
		J_γ	5
		C_γ	2

C, constant regions; D, diversity segments; J, joining segments; V, variable sements.
Where the number of functional gene segments is uncertain, this is denoted by '~'. There are many non-functional gene segments (pseudogenes); these are disregarded in this table. Because TCR α- and δ-genes are encoded in the same gene complex on chromosome 14, successful rearrangement of the TCRα genes inevitably results in looping out of the δ-genes so that α- and δ-genes cannot be co-expressed.

the differentiation of lymphocytes from haemopoietic stem cells. The location and composition of the B- and T-cell receptor gene complexes and the details of their variable regions are given in Table 20.1. Although there are considerable differences in the organization of the gene complexes, the mechanism of variable-region gene rearrangement appears to be similar.

The genetic organization of the variable-region genes and the way in which they are rearranged can generate a huge diversity of antigen recognition structures for subsequent display on the surface of mature B and T lymphocytes. For T cells, this is the only way in which diversity of V region structure is achieved. In B cells, there is an additional mechanism that increases the variable-region gene repertoire. This is a *somatic hypermutation* mechanism that is activated during B-cell maturation in germinal centres and which introduces mutations into the rearranged immunoglobulin variable-region genes. It is discussed in detail in the section on antibody responses.

There are six pairs of genes that encode antigen-specific receptors – three for immunoglobulin (κ and λ light chains, and heavy chains) and three for TCRs (β, γ and a combined α and δ locus – see Table 20.1). Each has variable-region and constant-region gene segments and, before comparison of the individual members, the structure of the variable-region gene segments that encode immunoglobulin heavy chain and the way in which these are rearranged during B-cell development will be described to exemplify the common features.

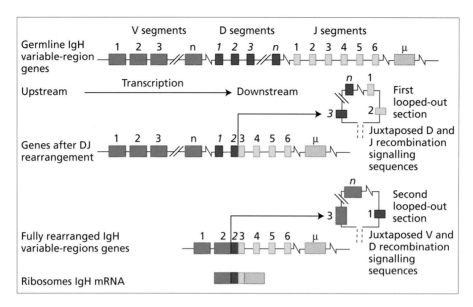

Figure 20.6 Immunoglobulin heavy-chain variable-region genes and their rearrangement. The germline structure of the variable-region gene complex is shown in the top line. The genes are present in this form in haemopoietic stem cells. The approximate number (*n*) of V_H, D_H and J_H segments are given in Table 20.1. The constant-region genes are downstream of the V region genes. The first of these, μ, encodes the IgM heavy chain constant-region domain. This is followed in sequence by δ, γ3, γ1, a non-functional pseudo-ε gene, α1, γ2, γ4, ε and α2. The boxes represent exons and lines introns. During rearrangement, first one of the J segments becomes aligned with one of the D segments and the intervening sequences are deleted; DJ rearrangement is always attempted on both chromosomes 14. The aligned DJ pair on one chromosome 14 then becomes linked to one of the V segments on that chromosome, and again intervening sequences are deleted. If this V

to DJ rearrangement is able to encode a variable region then there is no V to DJ rearrangement on the other chromosome; if it has been unsuccessful (e.g. the rearrangement is out of frame) the cell goes on to attempt to rearrange a V segment to the DJ on the other chromosome. The D to J and V to DJ alignment is made possible by the presence of recombinase signalling sequences that flank (i) the upstream end of each J segment and the downstream end of each D segment and (ii) the upstream end of each D segment and the downstream of each V segment. Additional diversity at the junctions between the rearranged V, D and J segments results in part from imprecise splicing and partially through the insertion of additional non-encoded (N) basepairs at the D to J and V to DJ junctions through the action of terminal deoxynucleotidyl transferase (tdt).

Rearrangement of immunoglobulin heavy chain variable-region genes

The heavy chain gene is located at 14q32.3 and the germline organization of the part of the gene that encodes for the variable region of IgH is shown at the top of Figure 20.6. The variable-region component of the immunoglobulin heavy chain gene is divided into three types of *gene segment*: V segments, D segments and J segments. A large number of individual V gene segments are encoded within the genome. The V gene segments are longer than J or D segments and encode much of the framework of the variable-region domain, together with the first and second hypervariable regions (known as the complementarity-determining regions – CDR1 and CDR2). The CDR1 and CDR2 regions encode two out of the three parts of the variable region that determine the antigenic specificity of the heavy-chain V region.

There are fewer D and J gene segments. The third hypervariable region (CDR3) is encoded at the site of joining of one of the

functional D segments with any one of the functional J segments and includes the downstream end of one of the V segments. Heavy-chain rearrangement involves two looping-out manoeuvres (Figure 20.6). In the first of these, one of the J segments becomes spliced to one of the D segments and the intervening sequences are deleted. Next, one of the two rearranged D–J pairs becomes linked to one of the V segments and again the intervening sequences are deleted. The association of segments appears to occur at random and the theoretical number of different variable region genes that might be generated in this way is the product of the number of functional V, D and J segments, i.e. ~8262. In practice, D to J and V to D–J joining is not exact and additional random nucleotides may be added at the point where the gene segments join. This results in very much greater diversity, which is seen only in CDR3 and which includes both the D to J and V to D–J junctions.

The diversity of CDR1 and CDR2 is therefore much less than that of CDR3. Junctional diversity in CDR3 is sufficiently

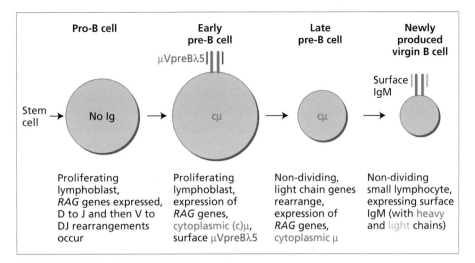

Figure 20.7 Outline of the main stages of B lymphopoiesis. The central process in B-cell formation is the rearrangement of Ig variable-region genes. For rearrangement of V-region genes to occur in either T or B cells, recombinase-activating genes (RAG) 1 and 2 have to be expressed. Absence of these genes totally blocks further differentiation towards B or T cells. After a successful heavy-chain VDJ has been made, a B cell must express the heavy chain with the surrogate light chain composed of V–pre-B and λ5 if further differentiation is to occur. Cells that fail to make either a productive heavy- or light-chain rearrangement destroy themselves by apoptosis.

great to allow the conclusion that B cells with the same CDR3 sequence are almost certainly derived from the same clone and this fact is used widely to identify the origin and relationship of malignant B cells. Further details about the process of rearrangement are given in the legend to Figure 20.6.

B lymphopoiesis

Sites of B lymphopoiesis

B-cell production starts in the fetal liver at the end of the first trimester of pregnancy and normally ceases at this site later in pregnancy. Subsequently, B cells are also produced in the bone marrow and production in this tissue continues throughout life such that approximately 2% of adult marrow mononuclear cells are B-cell progenitors. Some differences in the nature of

B-cell production occur during ontogeny; these are discussed at the end of this section.

Early signs of commitment of haemopoietic cells towards the B lineage

The events that occur as cells differentiate towards B cells are summarized in Figure 20.7. The associated phenotypic changes are set out in Table 20.2. The earliest signs associated with differentiation of haemopoietic cells towards the B lineage are the expression of CD19, CD24 and MHC class II molecules on the cell surface and CD22 inside the cell. These changes are followed by the expression of molecules such as recombinase-activating genes (RAG) 1 and 2, which are involved in immunoglobulin gene rearrangement. These genes act in both immunoglobulin and TCR gene rearrangement, and their absence totally blocks further differentiation towards B or T cells.

Table 20.2 Phenotypic changes during B-cell lymphopoiesis.

	Surface CD34	Cytoplasmic CD22 with surface CD19 and 24	Nuclear tdt	Surface CD10	Surface CD20	Cytoplasmic μ	Surface IgM
Pro-B cell	+	+	+	−	−	−	−
Early pre-B cell	+	+	+	+	−	−	−
Late pre-B cell	−	+	−	+	+	+	−
Virgin B cell	−	+	−	−	+	+	+

Almost always, heavy-chain rearrangement precedes light-chain gene arrangement. The first rearrangements to occur are in the joining of one of the J segments to one D segment, with the looping out of the intervening sequences (see previous section for details). The rearrangement or attempted rearrangement of D to J is completed on both chromosomes 14 before an attempt is made to rearrange the D–J to a V segment on one of the chromosomes. If this is successful, the rearranged V–D–J sequence will be transcribed together with the genes encoding the μ constant region. After translation of this transcript, the cell has cytoplasmic μ heavy chain and is known as a pre-B cell. During all the preceding stages of B lymphopoiesis cells showing differentiation towards B cells are known as pro-B cells.

When intact μ heavy chain is expressed, an essential further step has to take place if the B cell is to proceed to light-chain rearrangement. The μ chain is expressed on the cell surface at low level with a 'surrogate' light chain that is composed of two peptides, V–pre-B and λ5. If this surface expression does occur, the pre-B cell receives a signal for further differentiation to proceed, exits cell cycle and starts light-chain gene rearrangement. On the other hand, if the first attempt to rearrange V to D–J is not successful and no μ V–pre-B–λ5 complex is expressed at the surface, an attempt is made to rearrange a V segment to D–J on the other chromosome 14. If this also fails and the cell is still unable to express μ V–pre-B–λ5 at its surface, it will die by apoptosis. When the second heavy-chain rearrangement is successful, the cell proceeds, as above, towards light-chain gene rearrangement. The first expression of IgM on a B-cell surface marks the transition from pre-B cell to a newly produced virgin B cell.

Extensive analysis of variable-region genes in pre-B cells of mice has failed to identify cells with two functional VDJ rearrangements. One functional VDJ rearrangement can only be seen with a non-functional VDJ rearrangement or a D–J rearrangement. This *allelic exclusion* of antigen receptor genes means that only one functional antigen-binding protein is expressed on the surface of the cell.

The enzyme terminal deoxytransferase (TdT) is expressed during variable-region gene rearrangement and introduces non-encoded (N) sequences at the junctions of V to D–J and D to J. The enzyme is expressed both in pro-B cells in the marrow and in cortical thymocytes during TCR gene rearrangement. The expression of tdt is much greater in the bone marrow than in the fetal liver and, as a result, junctional diversity is less marked in the first B cells that are produced. These are mainly B1 cells, which are described later. The enzyme tdt is not expressed in late pre-B cells at the time of light-chain gene rearrangement and N sequences are not a feature of light chain V–J junctions. Normally, B cells will express only light chains encoded by one of their four light-chain gene complexes, i.e. they express either a κ-chain or a λ-chain. The ratio of κ-expressing B cells to λ-expressing B cells is closely regulated and in humans is close to 60:40. Major deviation from this ratio has been observed only in B-cell neoplasia, when there is massive expansion of a neoplastic clone of B cells. Disturbance of the κ/λ B cell ratio to > 10:1 or < 0.1:1 can therefore be taken as a reliable indicator of the presence of a neoplastic clone.

Intact heavy chains can be exported to the surface of a B cell only if they are complexed with light chain or surrogate light chain. This does not apply to free light chains, which are able to pass out of B cells and plasma cells. Physiological light chain production is always greater than that required to complex all the available heavy chain, and measurement of serum free light chain is now a useful tool in the management of paraproteinaemia. The heavy chains that are secreted in heavy chain disease get out of the cell only because they are truncated heavy chains.

There is a high death rate among B cell progenitors. In part, this reflects failure to pass essential landmarks during the process of immunoglobulin gene rearrangement. Sometimes this results from the generation of non-productive variable-region gene rearrangements. In other circumstances light chains may be produced that will not combine with the heavy chains available in a cell as not all light and heavy chains are compatible.

T-cell production and selection in the thymus

Although the earliest progenitors of T cells are produced in the bone marrow, the development and selection of most mature immunologically competent T cells occurs in the thymus. The thymus is an encapsulated gland that is organized into lobules by capsular septa. Within each lobule, there is a complex meshwork of epithelial and other cells that are responsible for regulating the development of prothymocytes into mature T cells. The subcapsular region of the thymus is divided into the more peripheral cortex and the deeper medulla. The lymphocytes of the cortex are more densely packed than those of the medulla, many in the outer cortex are in division and a high proportion of cells throughout the cortex are dying by apoptosis.

It has been estimated that 95% of all thymocytes die within the thymus either as a result of failure to rearrange their TCR genes in an expressible form or as a consequence of elimination during the T-cell selection process. During the development from prothymocytes to mature lymphocytes, T cells pass from the outer cortex, through the inner cortex and on through the medulla before emerging as immunocompetent T cells in the peripheral circulation. T cells whose TCR molecules fail to engage with MHC–peptide complexes within the thymus die by neglect, whereas those whose TCR can interact with these complexes are subject to *positive* and *negative selection (see below)*. The individual regions of the thymus play differential roles during the generation and selection of the T-cell repertoire.

The accessory cells of the outer and inner cortex are different. In the outer cortex, large epithelial cells called 'nurse cells' can be seen and there is massive proliferation of thymocytes in this part of the cortex, which is followed by TCR rearrangement. The epithelial cells of the deep cortex have branched dendritic processes rich in MHC class II molecules. These cells interconnect through cell junctions (desmosomes) that create a network through which cortical lymphocytes pass on their way to the medulla. There is now strong evidence that these thymic epithelial cells are critical in the positive selection of thymocytes, which have moderate affinity for MHC–peptide complexes. The boundary of the cortex and medulla is populated by macrophages (often called sentinel macrophages) that phagocytose cells undergoing apoptosis.

The medulla contains some epithelial cells and a number of bone marrow-derived IDCs that have broader processes than the cortical epithelial cells and express MHC class I and II antigens. It is here that the process of negative selection is mediated, in which T cells with high affinity for self MHC–peptide complexes are deleted. Structures known as 'Hassall's corpuscles', which are whorled aggregates of epithelial cells, can also be seen in the medulla. The function of these cells is obscure.

T-cell receptor gene rearrangements and phenotypic changes

Bone marrow-derived T-cell progenitors (prothymocytes) seed the subcapsular region of the thymic lobule (Figure 20.8). At this stage of ontogeny the cells have not started to rearrange their TCR genes, do not express the mature T-cell markers CD3, CD4 or CD8, and may not be irreversibly committed to the T-cell lineage. They may be identified by expression of CD7 and CD34. Interaction with the thymic stroma is accompanied by proliferation and expression of CD2, soon followed by cytoplasmic expression of CD3 genes. By this stage, the cell is committed to the T-cell lineage and TCR gene rearrangement is under way.

The configuration of the TCR and its genes is discussed in the section on antigen-specific receptors on T and B cells and is summarized in Figure 20.4 and Table 20.1. During early fetal development, the first cells to leave the thymus as mature T cells have successfully rearranged their γ and δ genes and express the γδ form of the TCR. Many γδ T cells do not express CD8 or CD4,

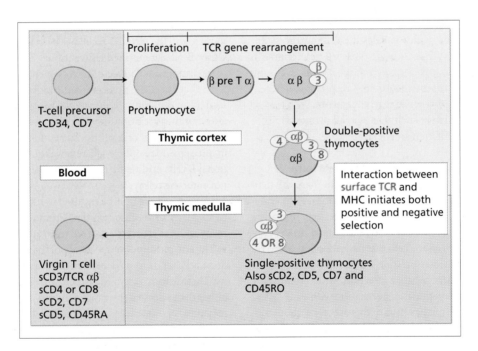

Figure 20.8 T-cell maturation in the thymus. Molecules within cells (red) or on a cell's surface (blue) are depicted without the prefix CD. T-cell progenitors enter the thymus from the marrow or other primary lymphoid site to become a prothymocyte. At this stage their TCR genes are in germline configuration. The proliferative potential and lack of commitment of prothymocytes is reflected in the ability of a single prothymocyte to populate an entire thymic lobe and generate a full T-cell repertoire. Prothymocytes proliferate in the outer cortex. Towards the end of the proliferative phase, TCR rearrangement starts: first β-chain genes are rearranged, then these are expressed with a surrogate α chain – pre-T α–. After this, α-chain genes rearrange. As with B cells, these rearrangements require *RAG1* and *RAG2* genes to be expressed, and junctional diversity is increased by the addition of N sequences using tdt. Selection occurs at the double-positive stage when the full TCR complex is expressed with CD3 and both CD4 and CD8. These cells are selected on their ability to recognize self peptide presented by a self MHC molecule at low avidity. Those cells recognizing peptide with class I go on to become single-positive CD8 expressors; those recognizing peptide with class II continue to express CD4 without CD8. Cells recognizing self peptide at high avidity and cells failing to recognize a self MHC molecule are deleted.

suggesting they may not be interacting with antigen in association with MHC class I or class II molecules. During fetal development of mice, sequential waves of γδ T cells populate different epithelial surfaces with different and restricted Vγ gene usage. This does not appear to be the case in humans, although considerably less is known about the ontogeny and function of γδ T cells in humans. Some γδ T cells develop in congenitally athymic animals and are probably thymus independent and may have different functions from those of thymus-processed cells. During later stages of human fetal development and throughout the rest of life, 85–98% of T cells that leave the thymus have undergone successful α and β-gene rearrangement and express the αβ TCR.

Rearrangement of the gene encoding the TCR β-chain occurs first with D to J rearrangements followed by V to D–J rearrangements. Successful rearrangement leads to low-level expression of the β-chain at the cell surface in a complex with CD3 and a surrogate α-chain analogous to λ5–V–pre-B in B-cell development. It is at this stage that the cell starts to express low levels of both CD4 and CD8; further β-chain gene rearrangement is halted and α-chain gene rearrangement starts (Figure 20.8). TCR α-chain gene rearrangement may involve sequential rearrangements of V–J pairs, which enables the cell to express different TCR α-chains until a successful TCR αβ heterodimer is generated. Unlike B cells, αβ T cells do not show allelic exclusion of TCR α-chains and approximately 30% of peripheral T cells have two functional TCR α-chain rearrangements. Both may be expressed at the cell surface such that a small proportion of T cells may express two different antigen receptors.

Selection of the TCR αβ T-cell receptor repertoire

CD8 and CD4 thymocytes are selected on the basis of their potential to recognize peptides held in association with either MHC class I or MHC class II molecules respectively. Immature αβ TCR thymocytes are subject to two selection processes – positive selection, which allows cells that have the potential to recognize foreign peptide in association with self-MHC to mature to functional T cells, and negative selection, which removes T cells that recognize self-peptides in association with a self-MHC molecule. As with B cells, exhaustion of this process without successful rearrangement results in cell death by apoptosis. Generation of a rearrangement that is positively selected by interaction with self-MHC is accompanied by cessation of further gene rearrangement, loss of RAG1, RAG2 and tdt expression and cessation of expression of the redundant CD4 or CD8 molecule. Although the selection forces that are imposed on αβ T cells are well defined, it is still unclear whether those γδ T cells that develop in the thymus undergo a similar selection process.

Overt and hidden self peptides

It is now clear that negative selection in the thymus does not cover all the peptides produced from proteins within the body. This applies particularly to intracellular proteins and to extracellular proteins in tissues that do not normally allow the egress of macromolecules, such as the anterior chamber of the eye. These proteins may therefore be immunogenic if administered systemically in an appropriate form.

Peripheral B cells

Two lineages of B cells are recognized. The B cells that are produced in haemopoietic tissues in red bone marrow throughout life are termed conventional B cells. The other lineage appears to originate during ontogeny in the fetal liver and this population is known as B1 B cells.

B1 B cells

Studies of B cell ontogeny in mice indicate that B cells produced in fetal liver differ from those subsequently produced in the bone marrow. These B cells produced in the liver persist in adults and are found particularly in the peritoneal cavity. The surface glycoprotein CD5 is associated with many of these cells in mice and the term B1 B cell has been suggested for these cells. Other B cells are termed conventional B cells. A number of features distinguish B1 B cells from conventional B cells:

1 B1 B cells are the predominant B cell type that is produced in fetal life and in humans during the first year after birth, whereas after this they are outnumbered by conventional B cells.
2 Unlike virgin B cells produced in adults, B1 B cells are capable of antigen-independent self-renewal in the periphery. Conventional B cells proliferate in response to antigen but otherwise do not enter the cell cycle.
3 B1 B cells can readily be restored to irradiated mice by transfer of fetal liver or B cells from the peritoneal cavity, but cannot be renewed from stem cells derived from adult bone marrow.
4 The antigen-binding specificity of the antibodies produced by these cells tends to have broad reactivity including autoreactivity. These features seem to result from selection at the B-cell level rather than selective rearrangements to particular V-region gene segments. N sequences at the D to J and V to DJ regions are not usually found. This reflects a lack of tdt expression in fetal liver.

The function of B1 cells and the background IgM antibody they produce is still far from clear. It has been suggested that they may produce play a regulatory role in immune responses and selection of the B cell repertoire and they certainly seem to have been conserved during the evolutionary divergence of rodents and primates.

Conventional B cells

The B cells produced in the marrow after the first year of life fall into this category. Three stages of conventional B cell differentiation can be identified:

Table 20.3 Differences between the three main types of human B cell found in adults.

	B-cell type		
	Marrow IgM⁺, IgD⁻	Recirculating	Marginal zone
Diameter		~8 μм	~10 μм
Chromatin	Condensed	Condensed	Open
Cytoplasm volume/basophilia	Scanty/little	Scanty/little	Moderate/moderate
Proliferating	No	No	No
Lifespan	About 3 days	4 or more weeks	3 or more weeks
Antigen-independent movement	Migrate from marrow to 2° lymphoid tissue	Migrate between the 2° lymphoid tissues	Remain in the marginal zones
Surface Ig	IgM	IgM and IgD	IgM or IgG or IgA
Memory or virgin	All virgin	Almost all virgin	Variable mixture of virgin and memory
Ig V-region mutations	None	Not present	Present in memory cells
Molecules expressed on the cell surface			
CD19, 20, 37, 40 and class II MHC	+ve	+ve	+ve
CD21, 39	−ve	+ve	+ve
CD5	−ve	some +ve	−ve
CD23	−ve	+ve	−ve
CD25	−ve	−ve	+ve
CD38	−ve	−ve	−ve
Capacity to respond to different classes of antigen			
Bacterial cell wall lipopolysaccharide	+	+	+
Bacterial capsular polysaccharide	−	−	+
Protein-based antigens	+	+	+

IgM⁺, IgD⁻ cells of the marrow are representative of newly produced virgin B cells.

1 newly produced virgin B cells;
2 recirculating B cells;
3 marginal zone B cells.

These three cell types do not represent different cell lineages, as recirculating cells are derived from newly produced virgin B cells and marginal zone cells mature from recirculating cells. Most newly produced virgin B cells die without becoming recirculating cells, and only some recirculating cells mature to become marginal zone cells. The three types of conventional B cell differ in phenotype (Table 20.3), which reflects marked differences in the signals that influence their survival and induce them to proliferate and differentiate. *Recirculation* is a process by which cells migrate continually between the follicles of secondary lymphoid tissues via blood and lymph. Most recirculating B cells are virgin cells, whereas the B cells of the marginal zones do not recirculate and are a mixture of virgin and memory cells. In some lymphoid organs that are regularly exposed to antigen, such as the palatine tonsils and Peyer's patches, most marginal zone cells are memory cells.

Newly produced virgin B cells

These cells are produced in the bone marrow in large numbers throughout life and represent the only way the recirculating pool can be replenished, as recirculating B cells do not proliferate unless they are activated by antigen. Antigen-driven proliferation of recirculating cells can generate memory cells, but most of these become marginal zone memory B cells.

If a newly produced virgin B cell encounters self antigen expressed on a cell surface, it may enter apoptosis within the marrow and in this way some, but by no means all, autoreactive B cells are eliminated. Soluble autoantigens binding to the antigen receptor of a newly produced virgin B cell may be taken up and processed, and the resulting peptides are presented on the cell surface in association with MHC molecules (Figure 20.3). These cells become programmed to seek cognate interaction with primed T cells, but die after 3 days without proliferating or secreting antibody if this interaction is not made. As most autoreactive T cells have been eliminated during thymic education, it follows that B-cell tolerance is heavily dependent on

T-cell tolerance. The consequences of a successful interaction between B cells that have taken up antigen and primed T cells are discussed later.

Recirculating B cells

These cells are small, non-dividing virgin B lymphocytes that are classically surface IgM$^+$ and IgD$^+$. They are in a constant state of migration between the follicles of secondary lymphoid organs. On their way to the follicles, they migrate through the T cell-rich zones that contain antigen-presenting cells and have an average lifespan of 4 or more weeks.

Marginal zone B cells

These cells were first identified as a major B-cell population in the spleen, where most of the cells are IgM$^+$, IgD$^-$. Some of these cells express surface IgG or IgA. Almost all of these cells in the tonsils and Peyer's patches have features of memory B cells as they have undergone immunoglobulin class switching and somatic hypermutation of their immunoglobulin variable-region genes.

Marginal zone cells respond to capsular polysaccharides

Marginal zone cells, like recirculating B cells, respond to T cell-dependent antigens and to bacterial cell wall lipopolysaccharides (thymus-independent type 1, TI-1, antigens). Unlike recirculating B cells, they will also respond to bacterial capsular polysaccharides. Capsular polysaccharides are thymus-independent type 2 (TI-2) antigens. These antigens do not evoke antibody responses until several months after birth, and levels of antibody produced in response to these antigens do not reach adult levels until 5 years of age. Antibodies to the capsular polysaccharides of *Streptococcus pneumoniae*, *Haemophilus influenzae* B and *Neisseria meningitidis* are important in eliminating these pathogens from the body. Infection with these encapsulated bacteria is a particular problem in patients with hypogammaglobulinaemia. They have been estimated to cause some 5 million deaths worldwide per year in infants under 5 years of age, mostly after the first 3–6 months of life, when antibody transferred from the mother has been lost.

It is quite unclear why immune responses against TI-2 antigens should be delayed for so long during ontogeny, whereas TD and TI-1 responses can occur before birth. It cannot simply be that antibodies against these antigens are harmful in early life, for they are present in the perinatal period as the result of maternal Ig transfer across the placenta. (See Figure 20.12 for responses to conjugate vaccines made up of capsular polysaccharide and an immunogenic protein.)

Peripheral T cells

The majority of peripheral T cells express αβ TCR. When these αβ T cells leave the thymus, most express either CD4 or CD8 on their surface and are restricted to the recognition of peptides in the context of MHC class II or class I molecules respectively. A minority of T cells express a γδ TCR.

CD4$^+$ and CD8$^+$ T cells and their functions

CD4$^+$ T cells can have one or more of a variety of functions:
1 the provision of signals, during immune responses, that induce proliferation or differentiation of T or B cells, generally known as *T-cell help*;
2 selection of B cells in germinal centres, which have undergone hypermutation in their Ig V-region genes;
3 activation of macrophages as is seen in delayed hypersensitivity reactions;
4 class II-restricted cytotoxic activity.

CD8$^+$ T cells include:
1 a large majority of HLA class I-restricted cytotoxic T cells;
2 a relatively small proportion of cells that can provide help; in this case, following activation by peptide presented with class I MHC molecules.

Although αβ T cells are selected to become CD4$^+$ or CD8$^+$ in the thymus, much of the functional diversity of these cells results from signals delivered when they are activated in the periphery. Virgin T cells have to undergo a process known as *priming*, which requires interaction with specialized antigen-presenting cells in the T zone of secondary lymphoid organs.

Cytotoxic T cells

Cytotoxic T cells kill target cells that present peptides they recognize in association with MHC molecules. The recognition and killing stages of T cell-mediated cytolysis require direct cell-to-cell contact, and only targets that are recognized through the TCR are killed. As with helper cells, cytotoxic T-cell precursors require antigen-specific priming before they acquire the ability to migrate into non-lymphoid tissues and kill cells that they recognize through their TCR.

There are two main killing mechanisms; in both of these, the target cell is induced to die by apoptosis without the effector cell being killed. The effector cells can go on to kill further targets. In one of the mechanisms, enzymes known as *granzymes* and pore-forming molecules termed *perforins* are transferred from the T cell to the target cell. Granzymes and perforins are present in granules that stain crimson and are easily seen against the featureless pale cytoplasm of cytotoxic T cells and NK cells in Jenner–Giemsa preparations. These features have given rise to the term large granular lymphocyte. This is misleading, for cytotoxic cells are generally no more than intermediate-sized lymphocytes (~10 μm in diameter). Similar granules are present in NK cells.

The second cytotoxic mechanism involves the expression of the Fas ligand (FasL) by the effector cell. The resulting engagement of Fas on the target cell induces the target to undergo apoptosis. Fas is a member of the TNF receptor family and FasL is an analogue of TNF-α and -β. Secreted TNF-β, sometimes termed lymphotoxin, will also induce some cells to enter apoptosis but is not targeted to a single cell, and in other situations it acts as a signal to induce differentiation or proliferation.

Expression of CD45R isoforms by T cells

The CD45 family of cell-surface glycoproteins is known collectively as *leucocyte common antigen*. Two of its isoforms, CD45RO and CD45RA, are expressed differentially on T cells. High relative expression of CD45RO appears to relate to whether the cells have been activated recently by antigen.

The lifespan of peripheral T cells

Once the peripheral T-cell pool is established, it can maintain itself without further input from the thymus. Even neonatal thymectomy in humans during cardiac surgery does not cause clinically noticeable immunodeficiency. This indicates that T-cell clones can be very long-lived and this certainly applies to CD45RA^{high} virgin T cells. Unlike the peripheral pool of recirculating B cells, which cannot replenish itself when depleted, small numbers of transferred recirculating T cells will proliferate to fill a depleted peripheral T-cell pool in a process known as *homeostatic proliferation*. Some experiments suggest that memory T-cell clones persist only if there is periodic restimulation by antigen, but other experiments indicate that in some instances this is not required.

Natural killer cells

NK cells are cytotoxic lymphocytes that lack expression of a T-cell receptor and whose primary function is to kill cells that have downregulated expression of MHC class I molecules. NK cells express a range of inhibitory and activating receptors and it is the balance of signals received through these molecules that determines whether or not the target cell will be killed.

The inhibitory signals include: (i) killer inhibitory receptors (KIRs) that bind to HLA-C or HLA-B alleles on the surface of the target cell and (ii) CD94–NKG2 heterodimers that bind to HLA-E. Activating receptors include: (i) activating forms of KIR molecules, whose ligands are uncertain at present; (ii) NKG2D, which binds to proteins such as MICA and ULBP expressed on cells under physiological stress; and (iii) the immunoglobulin receptor (FcR) CD16.

HLA class I expression is often downregulated on the surface of cells following viral infection and is also a common feature of malignant cells. This provides some protection from recognition by CD8$^+$ T cells but renders the cell susceptible to lysis by NK cells (Figure 20.9). Thus, CD8$^+$ T cells and NK cells can be viewed as having complementary recognition systems based on the level of HLA class I on the target cell. The ability of NK cells to recognize ligands such as MIC-A, which are expressed on the surface of damaged or stressed cells, demonstrates that NK cells may also have the ability to target cells at site of inflammation, irrespective of HLA class I expression level.

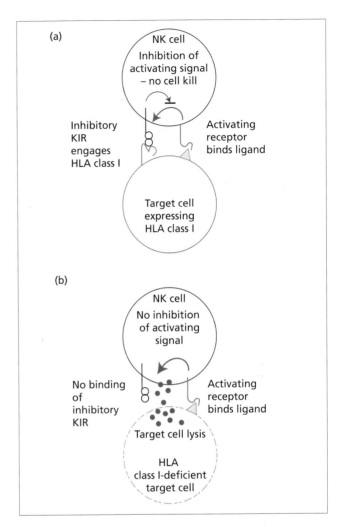

Figure 20.9 Mechanism by which NK cells kill target cells that fail to express HLA class I. NK cells express two classes of receptors which either activate (b) or inhibit (a) NK cell killing. The activatory receptors can bind to a range of ligands on the target cell whose expression is often constitutive. In contrast, the major forms of inhibitory receptor bind to HLA class I molecules. If HLA class I expression is downregulated on the target cell, no inhibitory signal is delivered to the NK cells and the target cell is killed.

The lytic mechanisms of NK cells seem to be the same as those used by cytotoxic T cells. NK cells proliferate in the presence of IL-2 and their activity can be augmented by exposure to interferon-γ. They characteristically express a range of receptors such as CD56 (NCAM) and CD57 but these are also expressed on a subset of T cells.

NKT cells

Natural killer T cells represent a small (< 1%) population of peripheral blood T cells and appear to be positioned somewhere between conventional T cells and NK cells in that they express a TCR but also a range of receptors typically associated with NK cells. Moreover, the TCR is invariant, with the same Vβ11Vα24 heterodimer being expressed on all cells. NKT cells recognize lipid antigens presented on the surface of CD1d molecules, CD1d being a protein with homology to MHC class I. It appears that NKT cells are activated very early in an immune response although their functional significance is uncertain.

Immune responses

The previous sections have indicated that antigen-driven T- and B-cell activation leading to antibody production or the generation of effector T cells requires a complex series of interactions between cells. In most primary immune responses this will occur only within secondary lymphoid tissue. The lymph nodes, mucosal lymphoid tissues and spleen contain the bulk of secondary lymphoid tissue. The outward appearance of the various secondary lymphoid tissues is markedly different, but their fine structure has many common features. In this section, the way in which immune responses occur in the different compartments of lymphoid tissues are considered.

There are two main sites of T-cell activation and T cell-dependent B-cell activation. These are the T zones and follicles. The general structure of a lymph node (Figure 20.10) is given first to provide a context for the detailed description that follows of the sites where immune responses occur and the molecular basis of T- and B-cell activation.

Lymph nodes have an afferent lymphatic supply that is fed by lymph draining the extravascular tissue spaces. This lymph

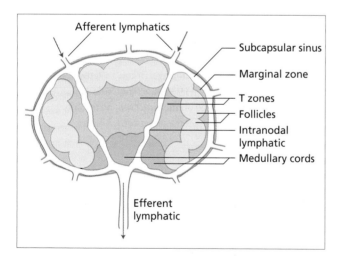

Figure 20.10 The main compartments of a lymph node. Note that the size of the marginal zone is variable; although it is often obvious in mesenteric lymph nodes, it may not be obvious in small nodes such as the popliteal nodes, particularly if these have not been sites of recent immune responses.

provides the main source of antigen for the node. Langerhans cells activated by local disturbance take up and process antigen, and then pass through afferent lymph into lymph nodes (Figure 20.11). The afferent lymph passes into the subcapsular sinus, which forms a lake of lymph that covers the cortical surface of the node. From the subcapsular sinus, lymph passes through intranodal lymph sinuses that surround and separate the cone-like segments that make up the solid tissue of the node. The intranodal lymphatics, as they pass the follicles and T zone, are difficult to see as they are crossed by fibrous cords. Attached to these and the walls of the tissue cones are macrophages and other poorly defined cells. Increased numbers of these cells in the intranodal lymph sinuses and similar cells in the subcapsular sinus are described by histopathologists as *sinus histiocytosis*. The intranodal lymph sinuses passing the medullary cords contain fewer fixed cells and are easier to identify. In the medulla, the intranodal lymph sinuses feed into the efferent lymphatic vessel that returns the lymph to the venous blood supply; in the case of the gut and lower half of the body, via the thoracic duct to the left subclavian vein.

The solid tissue of the node is made up of variable numbers of roughly cone-like segments (Figure 20.10). The base of each cone abuts onto the subcapsular lymph sinus in the cortex of the node and the apex is in the medulla. These cones fit together, but are separated by the intranodal lymphatic sinuses, to form the roughly kidney-shaped structure of lymph nodes. The cones have three main zones: the follicles in the cortex, the T zones and the medullary cords. The medullary cords form a convoluted apex to the cone. The contents and functions of each of these zones are described in detail in subsequent sections. The blood supply to the node enters and leaves the node through the medulla, and the specialized high endothelial venules through which recirculating B and T cells and newly produced virgin B cells enter the node are located in the T zones.

T zones – the primary sites of T- and B-cell recruitment into antibody responses

These zones are packed with migrating cells:
1 Interdigitating dendritic cells (IDCs) (Figure 20.11), permeate all parts of this zone. On their surface are processed peptides held in the antigen-presenting grooves of MHC molecules. IDCs enter the T zones of lymph nodes from the intranodal lymphatics. Those in mucosal lymphoid tissues probably come directly from local epithelia. IDCs in the spleen enter via the blood and include cells that have migrated from internal organs.
2 Virgin B and T cells and some memory cells enter the T zone by passing across specialized small blood vessels. In most T zones, these take the form of *high endothelial venules* that express a series of molecules that have ligands carried by recirculating and newly produced virgin B cells. Interaction between these pairs of molecules causes the lymphocytes to adhere to and

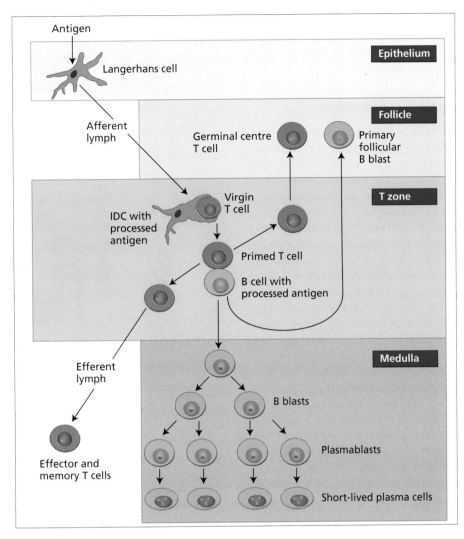

Figure 20.11 T-cell priming and T-cell-dependent B-cell activation in a lymph node. Local disturbance induces dendritic cells in the tissues to take up material from their surroundings. Ingested proteins are processed to peptides inside the cell (Figure 20.3). Dendritic cells that have taken up antigen migrate through afferent lymphatics to draining lymph nodes or through the blood to the spleen. By the time they reach a T zone, they have differentiated into interdigitating cells, which are specialized at presenting antigenic peptides, held in MHC molecules, to recirculating T cells. Virgin T cells migrating through the T zones move over the surface of the interdigitating cells and are activated if they meet antigen they recognize. As the result of this priming process, they move to the outer T zone and become targets for B cells that have taken up and processed antigen. The primed as opposed to virgin T cells are able to deliver co-stimulatory signals via CD40 and B7.1 and B7.2 to B cells that specifically engage their TCR. B cells activated in this way migrate to extrafollicular foci of B-cell proliferation – the medullary cords in lymph nodes – where they generate short-lived plasma cells. Other B cells migrate to follicles where they may form germinal centres. T cells, after a brief period of proliferation in the T zone, either leave the node as effector cells/recirculating memory T cells or migrate to follicles, where they proliferate further and participate in the selection of B cells that have mutated the Ig variable-region genes in germinal centres (Figure 20.14). The consequences of this cognate T cell–B cell interaction are described in more detail in the text.

cross the venules into the T zones. Migration of these cells to the T zone in the spleen occurs after adhesion to the marginal zone blood sinusoids.

3 Primed T cells locate towards the edges of the T zones. These cells are very efficient at interacting with B cells that have taken up and processed antigens. About one-half of the primed T cells have preformed CD40 ligand in granules in their cytoplasm. The presence of this preformed B-cell coactivation molecule is not characteristically found in recirculating memory T cells.

4 All B-cell types, including marginal zone memory B cells,

migrate to the outer T zones if they have taken up and processed antigen. Unlike recirculating B cells, they stay in the outer T zone until they make cognate interaction with a T cell, but those failing to make this encounter die within 3 days.

Responses to protein-based antigens in T zones

The series of stages leading to T-cell-dependent B-cell activation in the T zones is shown in Figure 20.11. T lymphocytes entering the T zone 'inspect' peptides held in MHC molecules of local IDCs and this interaction involves intimate contact between the two cells. If a T cell is able to recognize a peptide–MHC complex, it is activated through TCR signalling. Costimulation is provided by interaction between molecules such as CD80 and CD86 expressed on the IDCs and CD28, which is constitutively expressed by T cells. The effect of this interaction is to bring about changes in the T cell that are collectively called *T-cell priming*. These include the ability to express CD40 ligand and CTLA-4, a high-affinity ligand for CD80 and CD86. B cells cannot prime virgin T cells but are able to interact with primed T cells in the T zone (Figure 20.12).

Cytokines are produced by the T cell following this interaction and the nature of the cytokines produced in different situations is considered later. Short-term proliferation of the T and B cells is also induced, and most B cells migrate to local sites of antibody production. In the spleen this is the red pulp, and in lymph nodes the medullary cords. The lifespan of most of these plasma cells is 3 days. The extent of immunoglobulin class switching will depend on the conditions of dendritic cell activation and T-cell priming. In *primary* antibody responses, the plasma cells generated by B-cell activation in T zones do not have somatic mutations in their Ig V-region genes. On the other hand, in *secondary* responses, marginal-zone memory B cells that have somatic mutations in their V region genes can be induced to migrate to T zones on contact with antigen and give rise to short-lived plasma cells.

The other pathway of migration of T and B cells activated in T zones is to the follicles. Both antigen-specific B blasts and T blasts migrate to the follicles at an early stage in T-zone responses and give rise to *germinal centres*. This process is described in the section on follicular responses.

Responses to conjugate vaccines

Polysaccharides on bacterial cells are often poorly immunogenic but represent an important target for immune protection. One approach to overcoming this problem is to attach the polysaccharide to a carrier protein that elicits a strong T-cell immune response. The Hib conjugate vaccine provides an example of a large carbohydrate molecule that cannot elicit the help of thymus-processed T cells by itself. When conjugated to diphtheria toxoid, an aggregated glycoprotein, T-cell help can be obtained.

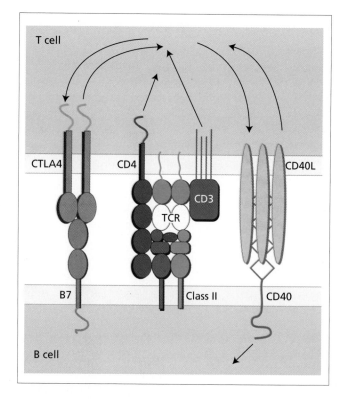

Figure 20.12 Surface molecules involved in T-dependent B-cell activation in T zones. B cells take up antigen that they bind specifically through their surface Ig. This is internalized, broken down to peptides and the peptides are presented on the B cell surface, held in the peptide-binding grooves of MHC class II molecules (Figure 20.3). Cross-linking of surface Ig by antigen induces the endocytosis of the antigen–antibody complex and signals upregulation of CD40 expression and *de novo* B7.1 and B7.2 expression. If this B cell interacts with a primed T cell that recognizes the peptide complex with class II MHC molecules, there will be costimulation through the molecule CD28, which is constitutively expressed by CD4 T cells, and this can result in further signalling through co-stimulatory molecules that are transiently expressed on the T cell surface; CD40 ligand exemplifies these transiently expressed signalling molecules. These interactions can lead to B- and T-cell proliferation and differentiation and may also induce cytokine secretion by the cells. Cytokine receptor expression by the B cell and the T cell is initiated or upregulated. The arrows indicate that TCR engagement induces CD40 ligand expression and that engagement of these molecules by their counterstructures on the B cell delivers further signals to the T cell. CD40 ligation induces Ig class switching in the B cell and migration as indicated in Figure 20.11.

After administration, the polysaccharide is bound by B cells with surface immunoglobulin that can recognize it and the conjugate molecule is internalized. The protein is broken down into peptides in the antigen-processing endosome and diphtheria toxin-derived peptides are presented on the cell surface. This

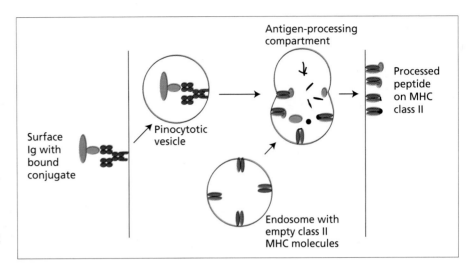

Figure 20.13 Processing of a conjugate vaccine between diphtheria toxoid (magenta) and the polyribosyl ribose phosphate of the capsule of *Haemophilus influenzae* B (green). A B cell with specificity for the capsular polysaccharide binds the conjugate vaccine with its surface Ig (black). The complex is endocytosed and the protein components are broken down to peptides (Figure 20.3). Peptides derived from the diphtheria toxoid are subsequently presented on the B-cell surface in association with class II MHC (blue and pink).

enables a Hib-specific B cell to obtain T-cell help from a diphtheria toxoid-specific T cell (Figure 20.13).

The follicles of secondary lymphoid tissues and germinal centres

These B-cell-rich areas are permeated by a dense network of follicular dendritic cells (FDCs). In follicles where no antigen-dependent activation is taking place, small recirculating B cells fill the spaces in the FDC network. In the first 3 weeks of T-dependent antibody responses, there is massive clonal expansion of B cells in follicles. This is associated with germinal centre formation. In the later stages of responses to protein antigens, small numbers of memory B blasts continue to proliferate in follicles for months or even a few years.

FDCs have the capacity to take up antigen in the form of antigen–antibody complexes and retain it for periods of many months. FDCs hold the antigen on their surface in a non-degraded form. In this respect they are completely different from Langerhans cells, IDCs and B cells, which process and present protein-based antigens to T cells. It seems likely that the antigen retained by these cells provides the drive for maintaining B-cell activation and indirectly T-cell activation during the months of the established phase of T-cell-dependent antibody responses.

Germinal centres – sites of antigen-driven clonal expansion of B cells that undergo mutation in their Ig V-region gene

Germinal centres are present in the first 3 weeks after immunization with protein-based antigens. Figure 20.11 indicates that some of the B blasts generated after cognate interaction with primed T cells migrate to follicles. Some of the antigen-specific T cells also migrate to the follicles. On arrival in the follicles, there is massive clonal expansion of the B cells such that the spaces in

the FDC network become filled with blasts. At this stage, changes occur in which the classical germinal centre structures of dark and light zones develop. The dark zone is formed by the blasts moving to the edge of the FDC network next to the T zone. These blasts, now termed centroblasts, activate the somatic hypermutation mechanism that acts on their rearranged immunoglobulin V-region genes. Centroblasts, like their precursors, have a cell cycle time of 7 h, but their numbers remain relatively constant. The hypermutation mechanism is specifically directed against the immunoglobulin V-region genes but is random in other respects.

The result is that the affinity of surface immunoglobulin for the original antigen may be either decreased or increased. Centroblasts continually give rise to centrocytes, non-dividing cells that migrate into the FDC network that forms the light zone of the germinal centre. Centrocytes either leave the light zone within 12 h or die *in situ*. They can leave the light zone only if they receive antigen-specific selection signals. The probable sequence of events occurring in fully developed germinal centres is shown in Figure 20.14.

Centrocytes pick up antigen from FDC. Their ability to do this will be determined by the affinity of their surface immunoglobulin for the antigen. In addition, they require signals from local T cells so they must process the antigen they have taken from FDCs and present the resulting peptides with class II MHC molecules to T cells. The T cells in the germinal centre are concentrated in the outer part of the light zone. They are antigen specific in that they were driven to enter the follicle after specific interaction with peptide on B cells in the T zone. This requirement for the B cells to receive T-cell help in the germinal centre protects against potential autoimmune responses, as those B cells that have developed reactivity against autoantigens are unlikely to receive selection signals from germinal centre T cells.

Centrocytes that survive selection within germinal centres leave the light zone as either plasmablasts or memory B cells. The plasmablasts migrate to distant sites of antibody production.

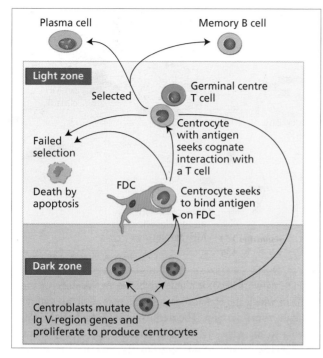

Figure 20.14 Selection of cells that have undergone Ig V-region gene hypermutation in germinal centres. The hypermutation mechanism is active in centroblasts, which are the rapidly dividing cells of the dark zone that give rise to centrocytes. Centrocytes die by apoptosis unless they (i) pick up and process antigen held on FDC and (ii) find a T cell in the germinal centre that recognizes the peptides from this antigen presented on centrocytes in association with self-class II. The T cell-dependent selection mechanism makes it unlikely that centrocytes with mutated Ig V-region genes that encode self-reactive antibody will be selected. Most B cells that are selected leave the germinal centre (i) to migrate to distant sites of antibody production, the gut or bone marrow, where they differentiate to become plasma cells and (ii) to differentiate into memory B cells. Some selected cells remain within the germinal centre and return to the dark zone as centroblasts.

Plasmablasts from follicles in the spleen or peripheral lymph nodes migrate to the bone marrow. Those activated in the gut or respiratory tract or the lymph nodes that drain these tissues migrate to the corresponding mucosal surfaces. In the bone marrow or the lamina propria of the gut, the plasmablasts differentiate into plasma cells. Unlike the plasma cells generated in T zones, most of these plasma cells have a lifespan of about 1 month.

Immunoglobulin class switching

Most, but not all, of the plasma cells and memory cells generated in follicles have undergone *switch recombination*. This is a pro-

cess by which the rearranged V-region genes become linked to heavy chain genes downstream from IgD. This process is similar to immunoglobulin variable gene rearrangement, with the DNA forming loops between complementary switch region genes that lie upstream of each set of heavy chain gene exons. The order of the heavy chain constant-region genes that encode the different heavy chain isotypes is located downstream from the variable-region genes: μ, δ, γ3, γ1, a non-functional pseudo-ε gene, α1, γ2, γ4, ε and α2. Thus, switching to γ2 involves looping out μ, δ, γ3, γ1, pseudo-ε and α1.

IgM and IgD are co-expressed on recirculating B cells. In this case, IgD is expressed without deletion of the μ-chain genes; this is achieved by differential splicing at the RNA level. The extent to which expression of other Ig isotypes can occur without μ and δ deletion is not clear, although this has been shown to occur in some neoplastic B-cell clones.

Class switching is triggered during interactions between T and B cells in the T zone of secondary lymphoid organs. It also occurs to a lesser extent during cognate interactions between centrocytes and T cells. The importance of interactions between CD40 and CD40 ligand to signalling class switching became apparent when X-linked hyper-IgM syndrome was mapped to mutation of the gene encoding CD40-ligand. Children affected by this mutation make antibody responses to protein antigens, but the antibody produced is all IgM and no germinal centres are formed. Interestingly, they do produce IgG in response to T-cell-independent antigens. Considerable evidence *in vitro* and some *in vivo* shows that cytokines can induce class switching. The best-characterized of these effects is the ability of IL-4 to induce switch recombination, first to γ1 and then ε. This will be discussed further in the section on T-helper subsets and cytokines.

Functional maturation of T cells during immune responses

T-cell priming

CD4 and CD8 cells can be primed in the T zones and undergo IL-2-dependent proliferation. This increases the number of antigen-specific T cells and alters the phenotype of the T cell. The level of adhesion molecules changes, as LFA-1 (CD11a, CD18 heterodimer), VLA molecules (heterodimers of CD29 and CD49) CD44 and CD2 are among those that may be upregulated. At the same time there is downregulation of some receptors such as CD62L (L-selectin), which is required for the entry of recirculating B and T cells from the blood to secondary lymphoid organs. The important effect of these changes is the expression of surface molecules that allow primed T cells to enter non-lymphoid tissues, particularly those that drain lymph into the lymphoid organs where their precursors were primed.

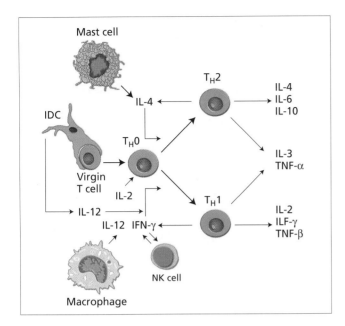

Figure 20.15 Maturation pathways of CD4$^+$ T helper cells. CD4$^+$ T cells that have been activated by antigen acquire the capacity to produce cytokines. The cytokines that they produce depends on the environment in which they are activated. Two main types of cytokine-producing T_H cell are recognized – T_H1 and T_H2 cells. The cytokines produced by T_H1 cells tend to promote further T_H1 cell formation and inhibit T_H2 cell formation, and IL-4 produced by T_H2 cells promotes further differentiation towards T_H2 cells. T_H1-promoting cytokines are also produced by activated macrophages, dendritic cells and NK cells, whereas mast cells produce IL-4.

Differentiation of primed T cells into effector cells

Most CD8$^+$ T cells differentiate into cytotoxic effector cells. Differentiation of primed CD4$^+$ cells is directed into one of two pathways (Figure 20.15). T_H1 cells produce cytokines that are associated with macrophage activation, granuloma formation and delayed hypersensitivity. These cytokines are principally IL-2, interferon-γ and TNF-β. In contrast, T_H2 cells produce cytokines associated with antibody production, particularly IL-4, IL-10 and, in some instances, IL-6, although the last of these is mainly produced by macrophages and osteoclasts. This bifurcation in the differentiation pathway for CD4$^+$ T cells is preceded by an uncommitted stage (T_H0).

The nature of antigen, its route of entry to the body, the cells that process and present the resulting peptides, and the genetic polymorphism of MHC molecules are some of the factors that may influence the way that CD4$^+$ T cells differentiate. CD4$^+$ T cells stimulated in the presence of IL-12, which is produced by macrophages, and dendritic cells are more likely to differentiate into T_H1 cells. Interferon-γ secreted by NK cells or T_H1 cells themselves has a similar effect, which is in part attributable to inhibition of differentiation towards T_H2 cells. In contrast, IL-4 produced either by NKT cells or T_H2 cells promotes production of T_H2 cells and inhibits T_H1 cell formation.

A feature of antigen-experienced T cells is that effector function can be evoked without co-stimulatory signals from a specialized antigen-presenting cell, such as those delivered via CD28 and CD40 ligand. This reflects an increased surface expression of the adhesion molecules LFA-1 and CD2 and a change in the isoform of CD45 from a high-molecular-weight form (CD45RA) to a low-molecular-weight form (CD45RO), which increases the efficiency of signal transduction through the TCR. Most T-effector cells have a short lifespan – probably 95% die by apoptosis within a few days without having encountered specific peptide on a target cell. Others survive to become memory T cells. Table 20.4 lists the main cytokines that have been reported to be produced by lymphocytes, together with actions attributed to these cytokines.

Inflammatory (T_H1) CD4 T cells

Macrophages work in concert with T_H1 cells to provide a major mechanism by which mycobacteria and other pathogens are destroyed. Inflammatory CD4$^+$ T cells enhance this activity through

Table 20.4 The cytokine and cytokine receptor families.

Cytokine family	Members of family	Type of receptor
β-Trefoil	IL-1α, IL-1β	Ig family
Haematopoietins	IL-2, IL-3, IL-4, IL-5, IL-6, IL-7, IL-9, IL-13, IL-15, GM-CSF	Class I cytokine receptor
	IL-10, interferons	Class II cytokine receptor
Tumour necrosis factor	TNF-α, TNF-β	Nerve growth factor receptor family
Cysteine knot	NGF	Nerve growth factor receptor family
	TGF-β	Serine threonine kinase
Chemokines	IL-8, MIP-1α, MIP-β, I-309, MCP1, MCP2, MCP3, γIP-10	Rhodopsin family

the action of cytokines following recognition of peptides presented by MHC class II molecules on macrophages.

Unlike cytotoxic T cells, effector functions activated in macrophages require hours or days to be accomplished.

Some T_H1 T cells have cytolytic potential and can kill infected macrophages by granzyme and perforin release or expression of Fas ligand. Recently, it has been shown that they can also kill by ADP release – this cytotoxic pathway has been found recently to result in the death of mycobacteria ingested by macrophages.

The balance between T_H1 and T_H2 cells

It is probably an unreasonable oversimplification to conclude that selective activation of inflammatory CD4 T cells (T_H1) leads to cell-mediated immunity, whereas selective activation of helper CD4 T cells (T_H2) leads to humoral immunity. In practice, there is unlikely to be a simple split between these two extremes, and intermediate effector cells probably exist. Tuberculoid leprosy exemplifies apparent dominance of a T_H1 response, and atopic disease seems to reflect an imbalance towards T_H2. Whether these extremes are due to the way the T cells were induced to differentiate or to a defect in the responsiveness of the T cells, or a combination of both of these, has to be determined. Nevertheless, manipulation of these cytokine networks provides a potential means of modifying established immune responses to avoid the complications associated with overactivity of either T_H1 or T_H2 cells.

Regulatory CD4+ T cells

Immunological tolerance is mediated by a number of mechanisms, including deletion of self-reactive B and T cells in the bone marrow and thymus respectively. In addition, it is now clear that a specialized population of T lymphocytes can actively suppress immune responses. These cells have been termed 'regulatory T cells' (Treg) and have a phenotype of CD4+ CD25+. Naturally occurring regulatory CD4+ T cells express high levels of CD25, the IL-2 receptor α-chain, and have been shown to suppress CD4 and CD8 T cells' responses to a range of stimuli, both *in vitro* and *in vivo*. In mice, CD4+ CD25+ regulatory T cells (Treg) are involved in maintenance of peripheral T-cell tolerance to self antigens and protection against autoimmunity. Human Treg appear to enrich within CD4+ CD25high T cells and constitute approximately 1–5% of peripheral blood CD4 lymphocytes. *In vitro*, Tregs are cytokine independent and require cell contact to mediate suppressive action. However, Tregs are able to induce other conventional CD4+ CD25− T cells to develop cytokine-dependent regulatory function, termed 'infectious tolerance', and this observation may in part explain the complex discrepancy between *in vitro* and *in vivo* observations regarding the role for cytokines in Treg function. The role of Treg in a range of human diseases is being explored at present.

Cytokines and their classification

Cytokines are soluble proteins produced by leucocytes and other cells that influence the behaviour of cells that carry cytokine receptors. Many are secreted, but others, such as TNF-α, are cell membrane proteins that are active when bound to the cell that produced them but also have activity as a soluble protein. The potency of cytokines *in vivo* has been exemplified clearly by the dramatic effects of recombinant granulocyte colony-stimulating factor (G-CSF) in inducing accelerated recovery of neutrophil counts after the administration of myelotoxic therapy and the effect of interferon-α in the management of haematological malignancies. It seems likely that many cytokines act only at very short range and some appear to be more potent as membrane-bound forms than as released proteins.

Analysis of the genes that encode cytokines and their receptors show that many of these are related. This is dramatically exemplified in the case of the common γ-chain that forms part of many of the class I cytokine receptors for the haematopoietin family of cytokines, including the receptors for IL-2, IL-4, IL-7, IL-9 and IL-15. Deficiency of this polypeptide is one of the causes of severe combined immunodeficiency (SCID). The families of cytokines are summarized in Table 20.4, and a fuller description of the known cytokines that act on cells of the immune system is given in Table 20.5.

Chemokines and their classification

Chemokines are a class of cytokines with chemoattractant properties and are all related in sequence. There are two groups, the CC chemokines, which have two adjacent cysteine residues in their sequence, and CXC chemokines, in which these two cysteine residues are separated by another amino acid. Chemokine receptors are integral membrane proteins linked to G-proteins and have seven membrane-spanning domains. They are classified according to the type of chemokine that they bind, i.e. CCR1–9 and CXCR1–5. Cells that express chemokine receptors are attracted towards an increasing concentration of chemokine molecules, and these interactions are critical to many functions of the innate and adaptive immune response (Table 20.5). Some chemokines are expressed in a constitutive fashion, whereas others are released in response to inflammation.

Interpretation of blood lymphocyte counts

Blood provides the most accessible view of the lymphoid system but it must be remembered that peripheral blood contains only around 2% of total body lymphocytes. The cells that are in the blood are in transit and many are recirculating T and B lymphocytes that will pass rapidly into secondary lymphoid organs in less than 30 min. Some memory T cells also recirculate, and

Table 20.5a The major chemokines within the CXC subgroup.

Chemokine	Production	Receptors	Cells that are attracted	Effects
Il-8	Monocytes Macrophages Fibroblasts	CXCR1 CXCR2	Neutrophils T cells	Inflammation Angiogenesis
β-TG	Platelets	CXCR2	Neutrophils	Inflammation
GROα,β,γ	Monocytes Endothelium	CXCR2	Neutrophils T cells Fibroblasts	Inflammation Angiogenesis
IP-10	Endothelium Monocytes T cell Fibroblasts	CXCR3	T cells NK cells Monocytes	Promotes T_H1 immunity Immunostimulation
SDF-1	Stromal cells	CXCR4	Stem cells Lymphocytes	Stem cell homing Haemopoiesis

Table 20.5b The major chemokines within the CC subgroup.

Chemokine	Production	Receptors	Cells that are attracted	Effects
MIP-1α	Monocytes T cells Fibroblasts	CCR1, 3, 5	Monocytes NK and T cells Dendritic cells	T_H1 immunity
MIP-1β	Monocytes Macrophages Neutrophils Endothelium	CCR1, 3, 5	Monocytes NK and T cells Dendritic cells	T_H immunity
MCP-1	Monocytes Macrophages Fibroblasts Keratinocytes	CCR2B	Monocytes NK and T cells Dendritic cells	T_H2 immunity
RANTES	T cells Endothelium Platelets	CCR1, 3, 5	Monocytes NK and T cells Dendritic cells	Inflammation T-cell activation
Eotaxin	Endothelium Monocytes Epithelium	CCR3	Eosinophils Monocytes T cells	Allergy

some memory B cells circulate in the blood without entering secondary lymphoid tissues unless activated by antigen. Effector T cells pass through the blood on their way to the tissues, and plasmablasts migrate via the blood to mucosae and bone marrow.

The numbers of different lymphocyte subsets that are normally found in the blood in different age groups is given in Table 20.6. These numbers are derived from studies in which whole blood was labelled by fluorescent dye/monoclonal antibody conjugates, followed by red cell lysis and flow cytometry. When this method is used to measure the proportion of lym-phocytes that belong to different subsets, much of the inter-laboratory variation in calculating absolute numbers of subsets can be attributed to the method of measuring the total WCC and the percentage of lymphocytes.

A wide range of results is to be expected between different individuals. The most consistent variation is seen in childhood, but from adolescence onwards age-related changes are small. Differences between the sexes are small and, excluding physio-logical lymphopenia, there is little difference between ethnic groups.

Table 20.5c The main cytokines that have been described as having activity on cells of the immune system.

Cytokine	Molecular family, M_r (kDa)	Cytokine produced by	Family and size of receptors	Receptors expressed by	Immunological actions
IL-1α	β-Trefoil (M_r 17.5 kDa)	Macrophage, epithelia	Ig superfamily; type I (CD121a, M_r 80 kDa) type I (CD121b, M_r 60–68 kDa)	Very broad, including T, B, and NK	Activates T, macrophage, is pyrogenic
IL-1β	β-Trefoil (M_r 17.3 kDa)	Macrophage, epithelia	As IL-1α	As IL-1α	Activates T, macrophage, is pyrogenic
IL-2 (TCGF)	Haematopoietin (M_r 15–20 kDa)	T_H0 and T_H1	CKR class I; α (CD25, M_r 55 kDa) +β (CD122, M_r 70–75 kDa) + γ_c (M_r 64 kDa)	Activated T, some B, NK, macrophage	Induces T growth and differentiation; also induces growth and differentiation of some B
IL-3 (multi-CSF)	Haematopoietin (M_r 14–30 kDa)	T, thymic epithelium	CKR class I; α (CD123, M_r 70 kDa) + β_c (KH97, M_r 120 kDa)	Haemopoietic, B, macrophage	Apart from effect on haemopoiesis, induces growth and differentiation of some B
IL-4	Haematopoietin (M_r 15–19 kDa)	T_H2, mast, marrow stroma	CKR class I; α (CD124, M_r 140 kDa) + γ_c	Activated B and some T, others	B growth, switch to IgG4 and IgE
IL-5	Haematopoietin (M_r 45 kDa)	T, mast, eosinophil	CKR class I; α (CD125, M_r 60 kDa) + β_c	Eosinophil and basophil	Eosinophil growth and differentiation; growth and differentiation of mouse but not human B
IL-6	Haematopoietin (M_r 26 kDa)	T, macrophage, some B, osteoclast, others	CKR class I; CD126 (gp80) + CD130 (gp130)	Activated B, plasma, T, macrophage, others	Inflammatory, cytokine induces acute phase reaction, plasmacytoma growth factor, influences T and B activity
IL-7	Haematopoietin (M_r 20–25 kDa)	Bone marrow and thymic stroma	CKR class I; CD127 (M_r 68 kDa) + γ_c	T and B progenitors, mature T	Pre-B and thymocyte growth, some action on mature T
IL-8	Chemokine, (M_r 7 kDa)	Lymphocyte, macrophage, granulocyte, endothelia, others	Rhodopsin family; CDw128 (M_r 40 kDa)	Neutrophil, basophil, some lymphocyte	Chemoattractant neutrophil basophil, inflammatory and angiogenic
IL-9	Haematopoietin (M_r 35 kDa)	T_H2	CKR class I; IL-9R (M_r 64 kDa) may associate with γ_c	T_H, macrophage	Growth T, erythroblast, mast and megakaryoblastic leukaemia lines
IL-10	Haematopoietin (M_r 35–40 kDa)	T_H0, T_H2, mφ	CKR class II; (M_r 90–110 kDa)	B, T	Suppresses macrophage activation by T_H1 and NK, with TGF-β induces B switch to IgA
IL-11	Haematopoietin? (M_r 23 kDa)	Fibroblasts	Unassigned; IL-11R (M_r 151 kDa)	Plasmacytoma, haemopoietic	Plasmacytoma, megakaryocyte and macrophage precursor growth factor

Cytokine	Structure (Mr)	Source	Receptor	Target	Actions
IL-12	Unassigned (Mr 35 + 40 kDa)	B, macrophage	CKR class I? IL-12R (Mr 180 kDa)	T, NK	Differentiation T_H0 to T_H1, promotes NK cytotoxic activity, induces IFN-γ secretion
IL-13	Haematopoietin (Mr 132 kDa)	T	CKR class I; (IL-13R may share components with IL-4R)	?	Growth and differentiation of B, like IL-4, suppresses production of IL-1-β, IL-6, TNF-α by activated macrophage
IL-14	Unassigned (Mr 60 kDa)	T, some B	Unassigned; IL-14R	B	B growth factor, inhibits Ig synthesis
IL-15	Probably haematopoietin (Mr 14 kDa)	Epithelial, macrophage	CKR class I; includes IL-2R-β and γc but not CD25	?	Actions like IL-2
GM-CSF	Haematopoietin (Mr 22 kDa)	T cells, macrophage	CKR class I; α (CDW116) + βc	GM series, Langerhans, others	GM precursor growth and differentiation, some plasmablasts
IFNγ	Haematopoietin (Mr 40–70 kDa)	T, NK	CKR class II; CDw119	Leucocyte, others	Macrophage and NK activation, expression MHC class I raised
IFNα	Haematopoietin, many isoforms (Mr 16–21 kDa)	Leucocytes	CKR class II; complex includes CD118	Most cells	Growth, differentiation of some B, expression MHC class I raised
NGF	Cysteine knot (Mr 26 kDa)	Nervous system, prostate	NGFR; (Mr 70–75 kDa)	Neurones, B, macrophage	Apart from role in nervous system, growth and differentiation B
TNFα	TNF family (Mr 52 kDa)	Activated mφ, NK, T, B, fibroblast	NGF family; type I CD120a, gp55; type II CD120b, gp75	Type I most cells, not resting T or red, type II haemopoietic	Induces apoptosis of some transformed cells synergizing with IFN-γ, inflammation, lymphocyte growth synergy with IL-6
TNFβ (lymphotoxin)	TNF family (soluble Mr 25 kDa)	Activated T and B	NGF family; as TNF-αRs		Induces apoptosis of some cells, inflammation, fibroblast growth factor
TGF-β	Cysteine knot, Mr 25 kDa × 2, there are three isoforms	Platelet, T, macrophage, others	Serine/threonine kinase; type I and II high and type III low affinity (Mr 53, 65 and 250–350 kDa) act in concert	Most	Inhibits cell growth, involved in wound repair and bone remodelling

This list is not comprehensive and some of the information about the function of these molecules is based upon studies *in vitro* that will not necessarily be found to be relevant to activity *in vivo*.

βc and γc, common receptors shared by more than one of the class I cytokine receptor family; CKR, cytokine; receptor family; CSF, colony-stimulating factor; 'growth', used to mean proliferation of cells; GM, granulocyte macrophage, IFN, interferon; Ig, immunoglobulin; IL, interleukin; kDa, kilodaltons; M_r, molecular ratio; NGF, nerve growth factor; R, receptor; TCGF, thymus cell growth factor; TGF, transforming growth factor; T_H, helper T cell; TNF, tumour necrosis factor. The word cell has been omitted, e.g. T for T cell.

Table 20.6 Normal ranges for lymphocyte subsets in the blood.

	Cell types	0–2 months		2–3 months		4–8 months		1–2 years		2–5 years		5–12 years		Adults	
Percentile		5	95	5	95	5	95	5	95	5	95	5	95	5	95
Total lymphocytes		3.2	8.5	2.9	8.8	3.6	8.8	2.2	8.3	2.4	5.8	1.8	5.8	1.0	3.4
CD3$^+$	All αβ and γδ T cells			2.1	6.5	2.3	6.5	1.5	5.4	1.6	4.2	0.9	2.6	0.60	2.5
CD4$^+$	Class II MHC-restricted αβ T cells	1.2	5.3	1.4	5.6	1.4	5.7	1.0	3.6	0.9	2.9	0.5	1.4	0.35	1.5
CD8$^+$	Class I MHC-restricted αβ T cells some γδ T cells and NK cells			0.7	2.5	0.7	2.5	0.6	2.2	0.6	1.9	0.4	1.2	0.23	1.1
CD4/CD8 ratio		1.1	4.5	1.1	4.4	1.1	4.2	1.0	3.0	0.9	2.7			0.66	3.5
CD3$^-$CD57$^+$ or CD56$^+$	NK cells					0.3	0.7			0.2	0.6			0.20	0.70
CD19$^+$ or sκ$^+$ or sλ$^+$	Total B cells					0.5	1.5			0.5	1.3			0.04	0.70

There is considerable variation in the normal ranges reported from different studies and this table is only intended to be illustrative.

Alteration of lymphocyte counts can result from the redistribution of lymphocytes, an absolute increase of lymphocyte numbers or a loss of lymphocytes. Redistribution of lymphocytes accounts for much of the marked differences in lymphocyte subset numbers found in serial measurements within a healthy individual. Some of these changes in lymphocyte numbers follow a diurnal pattern with peak levels at night and nadir in the morning; accordingly, time of sampling should be taken into account.

Increased numbers of effector cells in the blood usually reflects an active immune response. Analysis of the phenotype of these effector cells provides some information on the type of immune response, especially in differentiating between cytotoxic and inflammatory CD4$^+$ T cells. Particularly in viral infections, this response may be of sufficient magnitude to cause a lymphocytosis. Some non-malignant causes of lymphocytosis are given in Table 20.7.

Redistribution of lymphocytes is probably the cause of the lymphocytosis seen in *Bordetella pertussis* infection. Although lymphocytosis is uncommon in bacterial infections, in children over the age of 6 months the second and third weeks of infection with pertussis are usually associated with a lymphocytosis $> 10 \times 10^9$/L (in some cases $> 50 \times 10^9$/L). The lymphocytosis consists of small lymphocytes and is believed to be due to redistribution – a protein toxin from *B. pertussis* preventing migration across endothelium.

Acute infectious lymphocytosis is a benign disease, usually of children. In most cases there are no symptoms, but in some there is fever and in a small proportion gastrointestinal symptoms. Increase in the size of secondary lymphoid organs, anaemia and thrombocytopenia are rare. There is an increased number of small lymphocytes, persisting for 3–7 weeks, with an average peak level of $30–40 \times 10^9$/L. This is usually associated with an eosinophilia (average of 2×10^9/L), but the aetiology of the condition is unknown.

Table 20.7 Non-malignant causes of lymphocytosis.

Viral infections
Infectious lymphocytosis; infectious mononucleosis; cytomegalovirus infection; occasionally rubella, hepatitis, adenoviruses, varicella, HIV, human herpesvirus 6, mumps, chickenpox, dengue

Bacterial infections
Pertussis; occasionally healing tuberculosis, brucellosis, secondary and congenital syphilis, cat scratch fever, typhoid fever, diphtheria

Protozoal infections
Toxoplasmosis; occasionally malaria

Other conditions
Serum sickness; allergic drug reactions; splenectomy, dermatitis herpetiformis; metastatic melanoma; hyperthyroidism; congenital adrenal hyperplasia

Causes of primary lymphopenia have already been addressed in the section on primary immunodeficiency. Some lymphopenias predominantly reflect redistribution rather than a depletion of total body lymphocyte numbers. A dramatic short term lymphopenia is induced by corticosteroids. This causes the retention of lymphocytes in secondary lymphoid organs but these are released again after about 2 days and the blood lymphocyte counts return to near normal levels. Endogenous secretion of corticosteroids during acute illnesses may in part be responsible for the lymphopenias often seen in conditions such as heart failure or pneumonia. In many other conditions, lymphopenia reflects an increased rate of death of lymphocytes and/or a reduction in their rate of formation. Some of the causes of secondary lymphopenia are listed in Table 20.8. A normal absolute

Table 20.8 Causes of secondary lymphopenia.

Infections
Influenza; occasionally other viral infections, colorado tick fever, miliary tuberculosis, pneumonia, septicaemia, malaria, HIV

Loss of lymphocytes
Intestinal lymphangiectasia, Whipple's disease, severe right-sided heart failure, rarely inflammatory bowel disease, lymphatic fistula

Therapeutic procedures
Radiotherapy, anti-lymphocyte globulin, corticosteroids, cytotoxic drugs, purine analogues

Neoplastic conditions
Metastatic carcinoma, advanced Hodgkin's disease

Nutritional/metabolic
B_{12} or folate deficiency, zinc deficiency, uraemia

Other conditions
Systemic lupus erythematosus and other collagen vascular diseases, myasthenia gravis, aplastic anaemia, graft-versus-host disease, pancreatic necrosis, sarcoidosis, idiopathic

lymphocyte count can belie an underlying deficit of one or more lymphocyte subsets. This is often seen in HIV infection, when a severe deficit of CD4$^+$ T cells may be disguised by expansion of CD8$^+$ T cells.

Infectious mononucleosis

Infectious mononucleosis (IM) is caused by Epstein–Barr virus (EBV), which infects B lymphocytes. EBV enters B cells via CD21, a surface receptor for the C3d component of complement and, after the acute infection has been resolved, a lifelong subclinical infection is maintained, with a low frequency of infected B cells and detectable virus in the saliva – a main vehicle for contagion.

EBV infection of children usually results in immunity without developing typical clinical manifestations of IM. This immunity can be detected serologically and is associated with lifelong protection. Usually only after the age of 10 years is infection by EBV associated with the clinical manifestations of IM. In developing countries, the rate of seroconversion before the age of 10 years can be so high that clinically evident IM is rare. IM has its highest prevalence in young adults. It is uncommon after the age of 30 years and rare after the age of 40 years.

Clinical features of infectious mononucleosis

The symptoms of IM usually develop abruptly, with fatigue, malaise and feverishness after an incubation period of up to 7 weeks. These symptoms last for about 3 weeks. Sore throat occurs in over 80% of cases and is usually accompanied by anorexia and nausea. The sore throat develops in the first week and subsides in the second week, rarely generating severe symptoms or massive tonsillar/pharyngeal oedema. Sharply defined, red spots at the junction of the soft and hard palates are of diagnostic value. Positive throat swabs for β-haemolytic streptococci are frequently found. Bilateral, non-inflammatory cervical lymphadenopathy is almost invariable, and inguinal and axillary lymphadenopathy is usual. The spleen is palpable in more than one-half of cases, although only occasionally does it extend to the iliac crest. These secondary lymphoid organs increase in size in the first week and subside slowly after the second week. Slight hepatomegaly and jaundice occurs in about 10% of cases. Fever is present in most cases but of no characteristic type and may be transient. A few patients develop a fine macular rash, but rashes are more usually found as temporary reactions to penicillin and especially ampicillin.

Blood picture in infectious mononucleosis

In most patients, IM is associated with a leucocytosis; this peaks in the second and third weeks and usually persists for 1–2 months (the first week is occasionally associated with a leucopenia). In two-thirds of patients, the leucocytosis is from 10 to 20×10^9/L but in some cases may substantially exceed these levels. The leucocytosis is attributable to an absolute increase in numbers of both normal small lymphocytes and of activated T cells (atypical lymphocytes). Most of the activated cells are CD8$^+$ T cells but they also include CD4$^+$ T cells and CD3$^-$ NK cells. Most of these activated lymphocytes are cytotoxic for virus-infected cells and target viral peptides presented on MHC class I molecules. Although infection of B cells by EBV stimulates their proliferation, this appears to be controlled by the T-cell response such that the proportion of blood mononuclear cells that is EBV infected rarely exceeds 0.1%.

A peripheral neutrophilia may be seen early in the disease, but a neutropenia is equally common and eosinophilia is not unusual. Thrombocytopenia may occur and is occasionally severe. Anaemia is rare and then usually associated with anti-i antibodies. EBV infection may trigger a haemophagocytic syndrome in rare cases.

Serological changes in infectious mononucleosis

Three categories of antibody are produced as a result of EBV infection: (i) virus specific; (ii) heterophile; and (iii) autoimmune. The first virus-specific antibodies to appear are directed against the EBV capsid antigen (VCA). IgM anti-VCA antibodies probably develop during the incubation period and they peak in the second week of the illness followed by a rapid decline. IgG anti-VCA antibodies peak in the second to third weeks and persist for life. Most patients also have a transient response to EB early antigen (EA), which peaks in weeks 2–3. Antibodies to Epstein–Barr virus nuclear antigen (EBNA) do not develop until some weeks into the illness but are present lifelong in all patients by 6 months. Serological diagnosis of acute IM is most accurately made by the presence of IgM anti-VCA and anti-EA antibodies and the absence of anti-EBNA antibodies.

Paul and Bunnell demonstrated that patients with IM have serum agglutinins directed against sheep erythrocytes (heterophile antibodies) and that a serum titre in excess of 1:112 is highly suggestive of IM. Similar agglutinins are found in low titre in healthy individuals (directed against Forssman antigen) and in some leukaemias and lymphomas as well as serum sickness. However, in these conditions the heterophile antibody can be absorbed out on guinea pig red cells. Formalin-treated horse erythrocytes appear to be agglutinated exclusively by heterophile antibodies of IM, and this forms the basis of the *monospot test*. Heterophile antibodies provide the routine serological test for IM but are commonly negative, particularly in children and in patients over the age of 25 years. EBV-specific serodiagnostic tests should be applied in cases with a strong clinical suspicion but negative heterophile antibodies. Total serum immunoglobulin levels increase around 4 weeks following onset of symptoms, and raised levels may persist for many months. The greatest proportional increase is in IgM, but IgG may also be raised. The specificity of most of these Igs is unknown but a variety of autoantibodies may be found, including: cold-reactive anti-i antibodies; Donath–Landsteiner cold haemolysins; and, occasionally, antibodies against smooth muscle, thyroid, stomach, rheumatoid factors and antinuclear antibodies (ANAs).

Differential diagnosis and treatment of infectious mononucleosis

The diagnosis and course of IM are usually uncomplicated. Signs of significant respiratory, cardiovascular, intestinal, urinary or joint disease make consideration of other diseases mandatory; some of these other diseases are listed in Table 20.7. Perhaps the commonest problem is when the patient is heterophile antibody negative. In this situation, other viral infections, particularly cytomegalovirus (CMV), should be considered, with assay for CMV-specific IgM. Primary EBV infection is rare in older patients and there may not be conspicuous lymphadenopathy. Occasionally, the blood picture may raise the suspicion of a leukaemia, in which case immunophenotyping of the blood mononuclear cells may be appropriate. Persistent lymphadenopathy beyond a few weeks suggests the need for diagnostic biopsy, particularly if heterophile antibodies are negative, but also the possibility of a false-positive Monospot test should be considered. Virus-specific serology may be helpful in both these situations.

There is no specific therapy for IM. In patients with severe fever or lymphadenopathy, corticosteroids produce prompt lysis of fever and reduction of lymph node hyperplasia. Steroids may be indicated in management of associated haemolytic anaemia, thrombocytopenia, progressive neurological complications and incipient airway obstruction. Patients should be advised of the small risk of splenic rupture from minor abdominal trauma and contact sports should be avoided for several months.

X-linked lymphoproliferative syndrome (XLP; Duncan's syndrome) is a rare inherited X-linked condition in which there is a specific immunodeficiency against EBV. These individuals may die as a result of primary infection or the subsequent development of an EBV-driven B-cell lymphoma. Patients receiving immunosuppressive therapy for allografts and who are carriers of EBV can develop proliferations of B lymphocytes that carry the EBV genome. These cases of *post-transplant lymphoproliferative disease* are heterogeneous, and B-cell proliferations vary from a polyclonal diffuse B-cell hyperplasia to monoclonal B-cell lymphomas. There is evidence for a causal role by EBV in the development of Burkitt's lymphoma, in association with both HIV infection and in the form endemic in African children. In less than 20% of sporadic cases of Burkitt's lymphoma, EBV-associated DNA can be demonstrated in the lymphoma cells.

Selected bibliography

General reading

Janeway CA, Travers, P, Walport M *et al.* (2001) *Immunobiology: The Immune System in Health and Disease*, 5th edn. Current Biology, London.

Immunoglobulin genes and B lymphopoiesis

Melchers F, Haasner D, Grawunder U *et al.* (1994) The role of IgH and L chains and of surrogate H and L chains in the development of cells of the B lymphocyte lineage. *Annual Review of Immunology* 12: 209–25.

B1 B cells

Stall AM, Wells SM (1996) B-1 cells: origins and functions. *Seminars in Immunology* 8: 1–59.

T-cell receptor genes

Leiden JM (1993) Transcriptional regulation of T cell receptor genes. *Annual Review of Immunology* 11: 539–70.

The T-cell receptor complex

Cantrell D (1996) T cell antigen receptor signal transduction pathways. *Annual Review of Immunology* 14: 259–74.

Malissen B, Schmitt-Verhulst AM (1993) Transmembrane signalling through the T-cell-receptor–CD3 complex. *Current Opinion on Immunology* 5: 324–33.

T-cell development in the thymus

Anderson G, Moore NC, Owen JJT *et al.* (1996) Cellular interactions in thymocyte development. *Annual Review of Immunology* 14: 73–100.

Leucocyte molecules

Barclay, AN, Birkland, ML Brown *et al.* (1993) *The Leucocyte Antigen Facts Book.* Academic Press, London.

Mason D ed. (2001) *Leucocyte Typing VII.* Oxford University Press, Oxford.

Cytokines

Callard R, Gearing, A (1993) *The Cytokine Facts Book.* Academic Press, London.

Powrie F, Coffman RL (1993) Cytokine regulation of T cell function: potential for therapeutic intervention. *Immunology Today* **14:** 270–4.

Antibody responses

MacLennan ICM (1994) Germinal centres. *Annual Review of Immunology* **12:** 117–39.

Polysaccharide-based antigens (TI-2)

Mond JJ, Lees A, Snapper CM (1995) T cell-independent antigens type 2. *Annual Review of Immunology* **13:** 655–92.

Antigens based on bacterial cell wall lipopolysaccharides

Ulevitch RJ, Tobias PS (1995) Receptor-dependent mechanisms of cell stimulation by bacterial endotoxin. *Annual Review of Immunology* **13:** 437–57.

Effector T cells

Kägi D, Ledermann B, Bürki K *et al.* (1996) Molecular mechanisms of lymphocyte-mediated cytotoxicity and their role in immunological protection and pathogenesis *in vivo. Annual Review of Immunology* **14:** 207–32.

Immunodeficiency

Fischer A (1993) Primary T cell immunodeficiencies. *Current Opinion on Immunology* **5:** 569–78.

Hammarstrom L, Gillner M, Smith CI (1993) Molecular basis for human immunodeficiencies. *Current Opinion in Immunology* **5:** 579–84.

Clinical aspects of Immunology

Chappel H, Haeny M (1994) *Essentials of Clinical Immunology,* 4th edn. Blackwell Scientific Publications, Oxford.

The spleen

S Mitchell Lewis

21

The spleen has important diverse roles in homeostasis. Its normal functions are affected in a number of primary blood diseases as well as in other clinical disorders when its dysfunction may, in turn, give rise to haematological abnormalities. These haematological effects may be a minor phenomenon but in some cases they may come to dominate the clinical presentation. In such patients, especially those with a primary blood disorder, an assessment of spleen function is important in diagnosis, staging and clinical management. This is often useful for elucidating an abnormal blood picture.

Evolution of the spleen

The spleen is derived from a mesenchymal stem cell, which appears in the yolk sac of the embryo within 2 weeks of conception. The mesenchymal cell differentiates into reticulum cells, pluripotent stem cells and colony-forming units. Together with the liver, the spleen has a transient role in haemopoiesis from the third month, continuing until birth. From about 20 weeks, the bone marrow becomes a site of haemopoiesis, and this increases rapidly in the marrow during the last trimester of pregnancy, in both amount and extent of differentiation, while haemopoietic activity in the spleen disappears (Figure 21.1). There is no evidence of a specific inhibitor and the spleen remains a potential site for haemopoiesis, as the appropriate microenvironment is present, especially for the maintenance of erythropoiesis. The mechanisms for extramedullary haemopoiesis after birth are described below.

Structure and function

The normal spleen weighs about 150–250 g, but there is considerable variation between normal individuals and at various times in the same individual. At puberty, it weighs about 200–300 g, and after the age of 65 years its weight decreases to 100–150 g or less. In the adult, its length is 8–13 cm, its width is 4.5–7.0 cm, the surface area is 45–80 cm² and its volume less than 275 cm³. A spleen greater than 14 cm long is usually palpable (see later). It enlarges in a wide range of diseases, up to a massive 2 kg or more in weight in some blood disorders.

The spleen has a complicated structure and several different functions. Essentially, it consists of a connective tissue framework, vascular channels, lymphatic tissue, lymph drainage channels and cellular components of the haemopoietic and reticuloendothelial systems. There is white pulp, red pulp and an intermediate marginal zone, which lies at the periphery of the white pulp, blending into the red pulp.

The red pulp: splenic blood flow

The circulation within the spleen is illustrated in Figure 21.2. Blood is brought to the spleen via the splenic artery, and then, through its branches (the trabecular arteries), into the central arteries, which are sited in the white pulp. These central arteries run in the central axis of periarteriolar lymphatic sheaths; they give off many arterioles and capillaries, some of which terminate in the white pulp whilst others go on to enter the red pulp. In the red pulp there are sinuses, 20–40 μm in diameter, and connecting cords (Bilroth cords). The sinuses are lined by endothelial and adventitial cells with a basement membrane. The cords consist

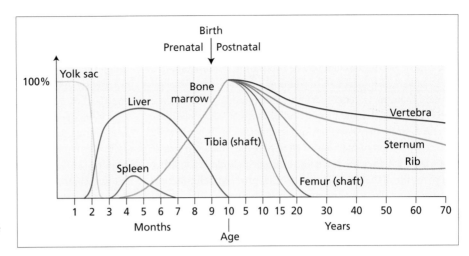

Figure 21.1 Site of erythropoietic tissue in fetus and throughout life.

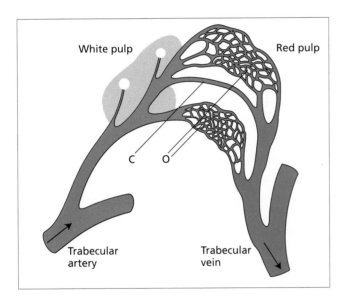

Figure 21.2 The circulation of the spleen. O, open system; C, closed system (see text).

of a fibroblast-like reticular meshwork containing numerous macrophages and erythrocytes. The cords and sinuses communicate by narrow inter-endothelial spaces in the sinus wall (open system).

A few arteries enter the sinuses directly and connect via the collecting vein to the trabecular vein (closed system).

There is thus both a rapid and a slow transit component in the splenic circulation. The rapid transit is of the order of 1–2 min; the slow mixing, which occurs notably when there is splenomegaly (see later), has a circulation time of 30–60 min or even longer. In normal subjects, the blood flows through the spleen as rapidly as through other organs, at a rate of about 5% of the blood volume per minute, so that each day the blood has repeated passages through the spleen. During the flow, by a process of

plasma skimming, the plasma and the leucocytes pass preferentially to the white pulp, while the red cells remain in the axial stream of the central artery. The passage of cells into the sinuses is controlled by their ability to squeeze through the interendothelial spaces, assisted by contraction of the reticular cells.

The red cells are normally flexible, whereas cells with abnormal membranes, or with inclusions that render them relatively inflexible, remain in the cords where they either become conditioned for later transit or are destroyed.

Phagocytosis and sequestration

Three mechanisms are involved in the action of the spleen: sequestration, phagocytosis and pooling. Sequestration is a reversible process whereby cells are temporarily trapped by adhesion to the reticular meshwork of the cords on their passage through the spleen. Phagocytosis is the irreversible uptake by macrophages of particulate matter, non-viable cells and viable cells which have been damaged by prolonged sequestration or by antibody coating. Pooling is the presence of an increased amount of blood in the spleen in continous exchange with the circulation.

The red cells are subject to a further hazard: as the blood passes through the spleen, the plasma flows freely, whereas the red cells which are trapped in the reticular meshwork have reduced velocity. This leads to a rise in the intrasplenic haematocrit with increased viscosity, resulting in slower flow.

In the presence of metabolically active macrophages, the densely packed red cells are deprived of oxygen and glucose. This stress increases membrane rigidity and reduces the natural deformability of the biconcave cell. This occurs especially as a result of excessive reaction to stress (e.g. because of an underlying abnormality of the red cell metabolic system, or because the cells are already spherical or antibody coated, or are fragmented or misshapen in other ways); they remain trapped in the cord space and there undergo phagocytosis.

Siderotic granules, Howell–Jolly (DNA) bodies, nuclear remnants and Heinz bodies are removed (culling or pitting) during temporary sequestration; after removal of the inclusions, the red cells return to the circulation. Sequestration of reticulocytes has been shown to occur in both humans and in experimental animals. In humans, reticulocytes may be retained in the splenic cords for a considerable proportion of their 2–3 days' maturation time, while they lose their intracellular inclusions, alter the lipid composition of their surface and become smaller in size. It is not clear whether the spleen has any special role at the other end of the life of the red cell in the normal process of elimination of senescent cells; it seems more likely that such cells are removed by the general reticuloendothelial system, including the spleen to some extent, and especially in the marrow.

Blood pooling

The normal red cell content of the spleen is 30–70 mL, or less than about 5% of the total red cell mass. When the spleen is enlarged, expansion of the vascular bed occurs. This results in a considerable pool with a high haematocrit and only a slow exchange of red cells with the general circulation. In myelofibrosis, hairy cell leukaemia and prolymphocytic leukaemia, as much as 40% of the red cell mass may be pooled in the spleen. This pooling will functionally exclude a relatively large volume of red cells from the main arteriovenous circulation, and thus be an important cause of anaemia. In such cases, it should be noted that the red cell mass, as measured by a radionuclide labelling technique, may give a misleadingly normal result, whereas the peripheral blood packed cell volume will give a more reliable measurement of the effectively circulating red cell mass. In splenomegaly due to cellular infiltration, the pool is less prominent. Conversely, in the congestive splenomegaly of portal hypertension, spleen size with an increased red cell pool is a dominant feature.

The normal spleen contains a reservoir of granulocytes, which is in dynamic equilibrium with the circulating granulocytes. It is 30–50% of the body's total marginating pool, with a mean transit time through the spleen of about 10 min. Splenic sequestration of granulocytes is thought to be responsible for the neutropenia that often occurs in patients with splenomegaly. Platelets have also been shown to have a significant reservoir in the spleen, and are rapidly interchangeable with the circulation. In normal subjects, 20–40% of the total platelet mass is pooled in the spleen and the platelets spend up to one-third of their lifespan there. The pool increases when the spleen is enlarged. This pooling and temporary sequestration must be distinguished from destruction of platelets in the spleen, which occurs in many cases of thrombocytopenia.

Plasma volume is controlled by a neurohumoral mechanism which affects distribution of water between intravascular and extracellular fluid compartments across the capillary wall. Under physiological conditions, the red cell volume is fairly constant, while the plasma volume undergoes continual transient variations that trigger off the necessary adjustments which ensure that the total blood volume remains constant. There is no evidence that the normal spleen is involved in this mechanism, but when the spleen is enlarged it does play a role; splenomegaly is frequently associated with an increased plasma volume, which may lead to a dilutional pseudo-anaemia. Possible mechanisms that have been suggested to explain expanded plasma volume in splenomegaly include the following:

1 The enlarged organ, acting as a large arteriovenous fistula, requires an expansion of blood volume to fill the additional intravascular space; in conditions where marrow erythropoietic activity is reduced, as in myelofibrosis, it may not be possible to maintain the normal red cell : plasma ratio and the additional volume is provided by plasma alone.

2 As splenomegaly increases, flow-induced portal hypertension may cause activation of the neurohumoral mechanism, augmented renal sympathetic nerve activity and secondary renal sodium retention with consequent fluid imbalance.

3 Protein alterations, especially increased globulin levels with reduced albumin, result in an alteration in colloid cellular osmotic pressure. This has been suggested as a factor in tropical splenomegaly and in cirrhosis.

In blood dyscrasias, the increase in plasma volume is directly proportional to the size of the spleen, less so in cirrhosis.

The white pulp: immunological function

The spleen is the largest single accumulation of lymphoid tissue in the body. It contains 25% of the T-lymphocyte pool and 10–15% of the B-lymphocyte pool. T cells are found predominantly in periarteriolar lymphatic sheaths, and B cells in germinal centres in the white pulp. These cells do not appear to arise in the spleen but to have migrated there from other sites of origin, such as the bone marrow and thymus. There is a constant flow of both T and B cells through the spleen; T cells are the more mobile cells and stay in the spleen for a few hours, while B cells settle in the follicles, where they release immunoglobulins. T-cell interaction with the corresponding B cells takes place mainly when they are juxtaposed in the periarteriolar sheath.

During the primary immune response CD8+ T cells act in association with macrophages to stimulate removal by phagocytosis of blood-borne bacteria as well as antigenic material such as damaged erythrocytes. Secondary stimulation with the antigen enhances antibody production, usually IgG. The antibody-coated cells come into contact with macrophages which have Fc receptors that enable immune-complex binding to occur.

The circulating immune complexes are then dealt with in two phases. Larger aggregates are removed by macrophage phagocytosis in the red pulp and marginal zone, while smaller aggregates are transported by B cells to the germinal centres. B cells produce immunoglobulins with antigen specificity and there is stimulation of immune response to soluble antigens as well as to particulate material. These are important mechanisms for protection against bacterial sepsis, especially from *Streptococcus pneumoniae*, *H. influenzae* type b and *Neisseria meningiditis*. The spleen also appears to acts as a defence against viral infections and intra-erythrocyte parasitic infections such as Plasmodium and Babesia.

The coated red cells lose pieces of their membrane, becoming more spherical and less flexible each time they traverse the endothelial pores and thus are trapped. Apart from the type of antibody, several other factors also influence the role of the spleen in immune red cell destruction (e.g. the number of macrophages present and the rate of splenic blood flow). Increased haemolysis results in an increased number of phagocytes accumulating in the splenic cords, with consequent increasing lysis in a spiralling system. Conversely, however, phagocytic action may be reduced, at least temporarily, as the damaged red cell load blockades the reticuloendothelial cells.

Coagulation factors

The spleen has a role in haemostasis and thrombosis. Experimental studies demonstrated increased factor VIII activity in haemophilic dogs after spleen transplantation, and reports of the successful treatment of haemophilia by splenic transplantation adds weight to the view that the spleen is an important organ for production and storage of factor VIII.

The spleen has not been identified as a site of production of other coagulation factors except, possibly, the lupus anticoagulant. It does, however, have a significant role in bleeding disorders, as its platelet pool is a source of platelet reserve so that patients with moderate thrombocytopenia are at risk of bleeding in the absence of normal splenic function. In immune thrombocytopenias, when the spleen is the focal organ of platelet destruction, splenectomy may induce remission but also removes the platelet pool as a reserve to protect the patient in the event of a recurrence of the thrombocytopenia.

Extramedullary haemopoiesis

Total haemopoiesis in the spleen has been described above. The potential for splenic haemopoiesis remains after birth and recurs in two circumstances:
1 compensatory erythroblastic hyperplasia when there is a haematological stress of severe anaemia, as in chronic haemolysis, megaloblastic anaemia and thalassaemia major;
2 in myelofibrosis, and occasionally in patients with secondary carcinomatosis and myeloid leukaemia, when there is myeloid metaplasia.

A number of theories have been postulated. Committed progenitor cells of all series have been demonstrated in the spleen, but it is not clear whether they arise from a pluripotential stem cell which is present in the spleen (as in the marrow), but normally dormant in the spleen, or whether they derive from the bone marrow, having escaped into the blood and become trapped in the splenic red pulp. In haematological stress, this may occur as a mechanical process when the marrow expands beyond its confines as a result of increased cellularity (as in severe anaemia). In myelofibrosis and myeloid metaplasia, the cause may be inadequate cell to cell interaction with the stroma, or injury to the endothelial cells of the bone marrow sinuses.

The activation of cytokines or other factors required for haemopoiesis may take place in the spleen in pathological conditions in which structural changes may produce a microenvironment more amenable to cell growth, or the cells themselves may alter their character as a result of dysplasia and develop a predilection to growth outside the marrow.

Splenomegaly and hypersplenism

Spleen size

An enlarged spleen is a frequent and important clinical sign. It is thus essential to have a reliable picture of the presence and extent of splenomegaly. The dimensions of the normal sized spleen are given on p. 358. In the adult, an enlarged spleen is usually palpable when its length exceeds 14 cm. However, the measurement of spleen size by means of a physical examination of the abdomen is unreliable, as minor enlargement is often undetected by palpation and even a grossly enlarged spleen may be missed in an obese person.

Conversely, a lax phrenic–colic ligament or loss of tone of abdominal wall may give rise to a wandering spleen, which will be palpable, as will one that is pushed downwards by a flattened diaphragm in obstructive airways disease.

Traditional radiographic imaging may also be misleading and difficult to interpret. However, in modern practice, reliable information is obtained by ultrasonic imaging, nuclear magnetic resonance imaging (MRI) and computerized tomography (CT) scan, all of which give an accurate representation of the anatomy of the spleen and its position in relation to adjacent organs (Figure 21.3). The major advantage of CT scanning is the excellent structural detail that it provides, but it gives no insight into splenic function, whereas the advantage of MRI is that it demonstrates comparatively fine detail of structure and is also capable of identifying function-related parameters that are sensitive to pathological changes.

Another method of scanning the spleen is by means of a scintillation camera following injection of radio isotope-labelled red cells after they have been manipulated by a procedure which ensures that they are removed from the circulation by the spleen. The most effective method is by exposing the red cells, which have been labelled with ^{51}Cr, ^{111}In or ^{99m}Tc, to a temperature of 49.5°C for precisely 20 min (Figure 21.3b). As this procedure is laborious and the images obtained are relatively crude, it has been largely overtaken by MRI and CT scanning; however, it has a major advantage in that it provides information on the functional size of the spleen. Functional asplenia or atrophy is

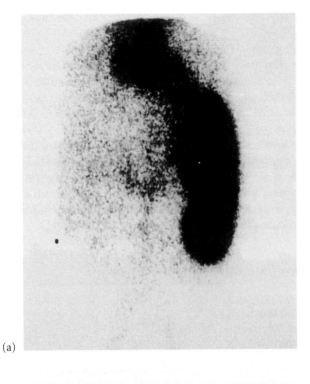

(a)

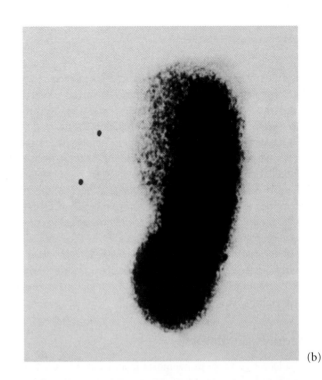

(b)

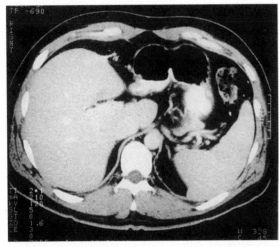

(c)

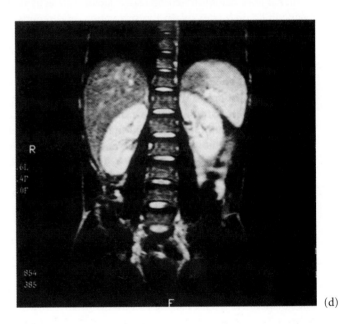

(d)

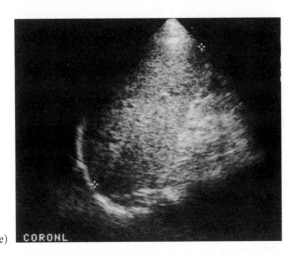

(e)

Figure 21.3 Imaging of the spleen by various methods. (a) Scan of spleen after administration of ^{111}In-labelled autologous red cells showing red cell pool in the spleen; the scan also shows blood flow in the heart. (b) Scan of the same patient as in (a) after administration of labelled heat-damaged red cells which have been taken up exclusively by the spleen. (c) Computerized tomography: transverse section showing liver (left) and spleen (right). (d) MRI: Coronal (longitudinal) section showing liver, spleen and kidneys. (e) Ultrasound scan of enlarged spleen.

well demonstrated by this procedure. It is also useful in diagnosing space-occupying lesions such as splenic cysts and tumour deposits, in determining whether an upper abdominal mass is of splenic origin, and in identifying abnormally positioned and accessory splenic tissue.

From the radionuclide image, the area (A) of the spleen can be obtained from the linear measurements. Several formulae have been proposed for estimating the volume of the spleen from these measurements. The following appears to be fairly reliable:

$$[\text{Spleen volume (mL)} = 9.9A - 540]$$

A method has been developed which combines tomographic imaging and conventional radionuclide scanning by means of single photon emission tomography (PET scan); this has potential value for detecting deep-seated functional lesions. It also provides an accurate three-dimensional measurement of spleen volume.

Causes of splenomegaly

Enlargement of the spleen may occur as a result of various pathological factors:

1 reactive increase of white pulp in inflammation and infection;
2 congestive expansion of the red pulp compartment;
3 increased blood pool;
4 increased macrophage function;
5 proliferative cellular infiltration;
6 extramedullary haemopoiesis;
7 storage disease;
8 cysts;
9 solid tumours.

Splenomegaly is thus a frequent and important clinical sign. The diseases in which it occurs are listed in Table 21.1.

The relative incidence of the cause of splenomegaly is subject to geographical variation. In Western countries, the leukaemias, malignant lymphomas, myeloproliferative disorders, haemolytic anaemias and portal hypertension account for most cases. Infective endocarditis is also relatively frequent. In tropical countries, however, the incidence of these haematological causes of splenomegaly is swamped by the great preponderance of splenic enlargement caused by the parasitic tropical infections: malaria, leishmaniasis and schistosomiasis. Malaria demonstrates how several pathogenetic mechanisms may be involved in splenomegaly. There are reactive lymphoid changes and the red pulp sinuses dilate with expanded microcyte phagocytic activity; this latter function removes intercellular parasites, leaving the red cells intact but with loss of membrane, thus causing the cells to sphere. These spherical cells are then sequestered by the mechanism described earlier, and the spleen increases further in size. Portal hypertension is an important cause of splenomegaly in most tropical countries but it is especially prevalent in north-eastern India and southern China. The 'tropical splenomegaly syndrome' is seen in large numbers of patients in New Guinea and Central Africa. Splenomegaly is also associated with haemoglobin C disease in West Africa, with haemoglobin E disease in the Far East and with thalassaemia syndromes, which have a wide distribution throughout the tropics. Because of the multiplicity of factors responsible for splenomegaly in such countries, more than one pathology may contribute to an increase in splenic size in a particular patient. The prevalence of malaria is thought to explain the anomaly of splenic enlargement in African adults with homozygous sickle cell disease. In haemoglobin S/C and haemoglobin S/β thalassaemia syndromes, the spleen remains enlarged in adults.

The role of the spleen in myeloproliferative disorders is described in Chapters 37 and 46 and in lymphoproliferative disorders in Chapters 38 and 45. In primary proliferative polycythaemia, the increase in spleen size is mainly due to vascularity, with expansion of the red pulp and an increased red cell pool. In myelofibrosis, the red cell pool is remarkably increased and the spleen size is further augmented by myeloid metaplasia and expansion of the reticular elements. In contrast, in chronic myeloid leukaemia and lymphoproliferative disorders the increase in size is attributed mainly to cellular infiltration, while vascularity and red cell pooling have only a minor influence.

Primary splenic tumours are rare; the usual primary tumours are melanoma and carcinoma of breast and lung. Metastatic carcinoma is also a rare event.

Hypersplenism

Hypersplenism is a clinical syndrome; it does not imply a specific causal mechanism. It has the following characteristic features:

1 enlargement of the spleen;
2 reduction in one or more of the cell lines in the peripheral blood;
3 normal or hyperplastic cellularity of the bone marrow, often with orderly maturation of earlier stages but paucity of more mature cells;
4 premature release of cells into peripheral blood, resulting in reticulocytosis and/or large immature platelets;
5 increased splenic red cell pool, decreased red cell survival and increased splenic pooling of platelets with shortening of their lifespan.

The diagnosis of hypersplenism is ultimately confirmed by the response to splenectomy, although an immediate remission may be followed in the longer term by partial relapse.

Most of the diseases listed in Table 21.1 can give rise to secondary hypersplenism. In these conditions, the haematological features of hypersplenism may be obscured or dominated by the primary disease, especially if it involves the marrow. Hypersplenism also occurs as a primary event, due to an unknown pathogenetic stimulus. It is sometimes termed primary splenic hyperplasia, splenic neutropenia or splenic anaemia, and it includes those cases of non-tropical primary splenomegaly in which there is no firm evidence for an underlying lymphoma.

Table 21.1 Causes of splenomegaly.

Haematological
Acute leukaemia
Chronic myeloid leukaemia*
Chronic lymphocytic leukaemia
Malignant lymphomas (some cases present as 'non-tropical primary splenomegaly')*
Chronic (primary) myelofibrosis*
Polycythaemia vera
Thrombocythaemia (some cases)
Hairy cell leukaemia*
Gaucher's disease*, Niemann–Pick disease, Langerhans cell histocytosis X*
Primary splenic hyperplasia
  'Non-tropical splenomegaly'
  Splenic anaemia/neutropenia
Thalassaemia
Sickle-cell disease, HbSC disease and other haemoglobinopathies
Haemolytic anaemias

Minor
Acute anaemia
Megaloblastic anaemia

Systemic
Acute infections: septicaemia, typhoid, infectious mononucleosis, cytomegalovirus
Subacute and chronic infections: tuberculosis, syphilis, brucellosis, subacute bacterial endocarditis, AIDS
Tropical parasitic infections (tropical splenomegaly*): malaria*, leishmaniasis*, schistosomiasis*, trypanosomiasis
Collagen diseases: systemic lupus erythematosus, rheumatoid arthritis (Felty)
Sarcoidosis
Amyloidosis
Cysts
Haemangiomas
Carcinoma (rare)
Congestive splenomegaly
  Portal hypertension
  Cirrhosis
  Splenic/portal/hepatic vein obstruction
  Congestive cardiac failure

*Common causes of splenomegaly.

Splenectomy

Surgical excision of the spleen has been a standard treatment for the diagnosis and management of a number of disorders associated with a hyperactive spleen and also when a normal spleen has an effect on an extrasplenic defect such as: an heredit-ary spherocytosis, when there are inflexible red cells that cannot readily traverse the red pulp cord; or in autoimmune acquired haemolytic anaemia, where removal of a major site for phagocy-tosis of antigen–antibody complex or damaged cells allows them to survive better in circulation.

Concern about the risks post splenectomy including sepsis in both children and adults has led to a search for alternative procedures for controlling hypersplenism while preserving some degree of splenic function. These include: (1) partial arterial embolization; (2) partial surgical amputation in selected patients in whom some splenic function may be preserved; (3) localized irradiation; and (4) immunosuppressive and cytotoxic drugs.

Apart from the removal of the spleen because of traumatic rupture or to facilitate surgery on contiguous organs, splenec-tomy is most commonly performed as a first choice in some hereditary haemolytic anaemias. In autoimmune haemolytic anaemias and thrombocytopenias, splenectomy or possibly splenic irradiation should be considered only after a course of immunosuppressive therapy; the results of spleen function studies (see later) may be helpful in supporting a clinical judge-ment. The role of splenectomy in myelofibrosis, lymphomas and other haematological conditions is discussed in the relevant chapters. When splenectomy is contemplated for any reason, the preoperative evaluation of the patient requires close coopera-tion between the surgeon and the haematologist; it is important to check liver function, to carry out ultrasound, CT, MRI or radionuclide scans, and to evaluate the hepatic and portal blood flow by means of Doppler ultrasound examination.

Complications of splenectomy

Immediate postoperative complications
These are bleeding, particularly when there is thrombocytopenia and subphrenic abscess. Haemorrhage usually comes from the peritoneal and diaphragmatic surfaces rather than from identi-fiable blood vessels. Frequently, no specific bleeding source is found at re-operation.

The incidence of subphrenic abscess is variable, and appears more likely to occur when adjacent organs are injured either by trauma or during surgery. Infection is also liable to occur following embolization.

Delayed complications
These include overwhelming post-splenectomy infection and a tendency to develop thrombocytosis with a risk of thromboem-bolic incidents.

Thrombocytosis

In the immediate postoperative period in uncomplicated splenectomy patients, the platelet count rises steeply to a max-imum of usually $600–1000 \times 10^9/L$, with a peak at 7–12 days. In a number of patients, the thrombocytosis persists indefinitely after splenectomy. This usually appears to be a consequence of continuing anaemia with a hyperplastic marrow; an inverse relationship exists between the severity of the anaemia and the height of the platelet counts. Although a reactive thrombocytosis is not usually associated with thromboembolic problems, the high platelet counts may have contributed to the serious and sometimes fatal episodes of pulmonary embolism that have occurred following splenectomy. Mesenteric infarction secondary to partial vein occlusion is more common in patients with myeloproliferative disorders who undergo splenectomy. Postoperative prophylaxis with heparin is usually needed. It is advisable to give antiplatelet therapy (e.g. aspirin 75 mg daily) as long as thrombocytosis is present.

Overwhelming postoperative infection

This may occur in adults as well as in children but it is in children, especially in the first few years of life, that splenectomy is more frequently associated with overwhelming bacterial infections. *Streptococcus pneumoniae* (pneumococcus) is the most common cause of infection but while *H. influenzae* type B, *Neisseria meningitidis* (mengococcus), *E. coli* and *Pseudomonas* are much less common, they are also associated with serious infection. Death is usually due to septicaemia or meningitis. The vulnerability of young children and their dependence on the spleen to deal with blood-borne infection can be explained by the general immaturity of their lymphoreticular systems. In the absence of the spleen, the defective reticuloendothelial clearance of an encapsulated rapidly growing organism such as pneumococcus may lead to a dangerous bloodstream concentration in too short a time for immunological defence to be mounted. Splenectomy should therefore be postponed until after the age of 5 if possible.

When splenectomy is being planned, the patient should be immunized against pneumococcal pneumonia, *H. influenzae* type B (HIB) and meningococcal infection. However, while pneumococcal vaccine contains antigens to a number of strains of *Streptococcus pneumoniae* it does not give complete protection because some strains are not covered and antibody response to the different antigens is variable. To obtain the maximum immune response, patients should, if possible, be immunized 2 to 3 months before splenectomy, and a booster dose should be given 5 years later. Most children will have received HIB vaccine but this should be checked; booster doses are not necessary for those who received the full course of three injections. Meningococcal vaccines are effective against types A and C but not against type B, the most prevalent in the West. The patient should also receive meningococcal C conjugate vaccine at a 6-month interval as this gives a higher and more lasting immunization against type C organism. Influenza vaccine is also recommended for asplenic or hyposplenic patients.

Postoperatively, lifelong prophylactic antibiotics should be advocated in all cases, but if this is not possible, antibiotics should be administered at least for the first 2 years after splenectomy, for all children up to 16 and when there is underlying impaired immune function. Oral penicillin 250 mg b.d. is usually recommended and patients who are allergic to penicillin should be offered erythromycin 250 mg b.d. When away from home, patients not allergic to penicillin should take a supply of amoxycillin to be used immediately if infective symptoms (pyrexia, malaise, shivering) develop; and penicillin-sensitive patients should increase their dose of erythromycin or change to a broader spectrum preparation. In all such cases, the patient should seek immediate medical help. When travelling to tropical areas, asplenic patients should be advised of the increased risk of severe Plasmodium infection and they must adhere scrupulously to antimalarial prophylaxis. *Neisseria meningitidis* and *H. influenzae* type B vaccines are also recommended for those travelling abroad. Education of patients or parents is perhaps the most important aspect of management, to ensure that they are alert to the possibility of infection, and know how to react. A card indicating that a splenectomy has been carried out should be carried.

Recurrence of symptoms

Accessory splenic tissue may be overlooked at operation; after splenectomy, it may enlarge and cause a recurrence of the symptoms for which the original operation was carried out. The haematological features of hyposplenism (see below) such as Howell–Jolly bodies and increased pitting, may be absent; CT and radionuclide scanning (Figure 21.4) will demonstrate the presence of a 'splenuncule' and identify its location for subsequent surgical removal should this be required.

Hyposplenism

Hyposplenism (excluding that induced by medical or surgical intervention) occurs in a wide range of conditions.

In some disorders such as sickle cell disease, gluten-induced enteropathy (coeliac syndrome) and dermatitis herpetiformis, hyposplenism occurs frequently; it is seen less frequently in Crohn's disease, ulcerative colitis and essential thrombocythaemia, and it occurs only occasionally in the other conditions listed in Table 21.2. Congenital absence of the spleen is rare and may be associated with organ transposition and with severe malformations of the heart and lungs.

After the age of 65–70 years, there is evidence of a decrease in splenic function. In old age, there is a rapid decrease in the weight of the spleen, together with increasing atherosclerotic vascular obstruction and fibrosis.

Patients with functional hyposplenism have impaired immunity to blood-borne bacterial and protozoal infections, and persistent thrombocytosis. Management is similar to that required post-splenectomy. It includes prophylactic antibiotics and vaccines (see above) and advice to the patients to seek

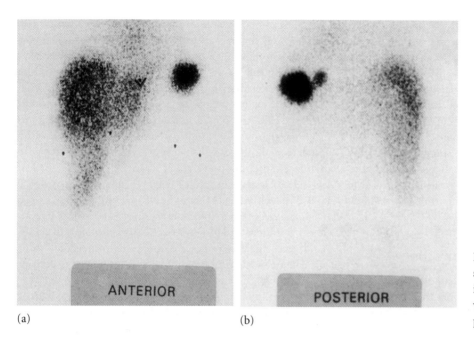

(a)   (b)

Figure 21.4 Demonstration of residual splenunculus by a scan of heat-damaged isotope-labelled red cells: (a) anterior view; (b) posterior view. Uptake is predominantly in the liver.

medical attention immediately in the event of illness or fever. Antiplatelet therapy is advisable when the platelet count is high.

Haematological effects of splenectomy or splenic atrophy

Characteristic blood changes occur following splenectomy. Similar changes are seen with atrophy of the spleen to less than 20% of normal size and when there is functional asplenia, with or without reduction in the size of the organ.

Red cell changes

The changes in red cell morphology include the presence of Howell–Jolly bodies and siderotic granules in some of the cells and target cell vacuoles due to pitting may be seen (see below). In a proportion of subjects, irregularly contracted or crenated, acanthocytic forms are also a feature (Figure 21.5). There is usually an increase in the number of reticulocytes in the circulation and occasionally isolated erythroblasts are seen. There is, however, no alteration in red cell survival.

As a rule, only some of the red cells leaving the marrow will contain siderotic granules and Howell–Jolly bodies. As the number of cells containing siderotic granules is related to the sideroblastic percentage in the bone marrow, the siderocyte count in the peripheral blood will be low in hyposplenism if there is no marrow pathology. In patients suffering from haemolytic anaemias, thalassaemia and sideroblastic anaemia, a major proportion of the circulating red cells may contain siderotic granules. The number of Howell–Jolly bodies is also variable and is most marked in conditions characterized by dyserythropoiesis.

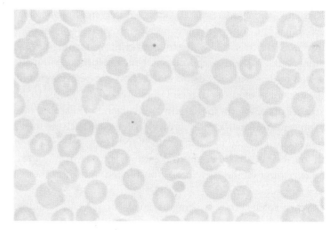

Figure 21.5 Blood film showing features of hyposplenism: Howell–Jolly bodies, target cells and contracted cells.

Other red cell inclusions may be prominent in the hyposplenic state: Heinz bodies are found following oxidative injury by drugs and in patients who have glucose-6-phosphate dehydrogenase deficiency or an unstable haemoglobin; precipitated α-chains are found in β-thalassaemia; and crystalline deposits of haemoglobin C in HbC disease.

Leucocyte changes

After splenectomy, there is a rise in the total leucocyte count. A neutrophil leucocytosis in the immediate postoperative period is, in the majority of subjects, later replaced by a significant and permanent increase in both lymphocytes and monocytes. After a few weeks, the neutrophil count returns to normal or near normal

Table 21.2 Causes of hyposplenism.

Congenital aplasia syndrome
Ageing
Haematological disorder
  Sickle cell disease
  Thrombocythaemia
  Myelofibrosis
  Malaria
  Lymphomas
Circulatory
  Splenic arterial/venous thrombosis
Autoimmune disease
  Systemic lupus erythematosus
  Rheumatoid arthritis
  Hyperthroidism
  Sarcoidosis
  Chronic graft-versus-host disease
  Combined immunodeficiency
Gastrointestinal (? immune basis)
  Gluten-induced enteropathy
  Dermatitis herpetiformis
  Crohn's disease
  Ulcerative colitis
  Tropical sprue
Infiltrations
  Lymphomas
  Sézary syndrome
  Myelomatosis
  Amyloidosis
  Secondary carcinomas, especially breast
  Cysts, e.g. hydatid
Nephrotic syndrome
Drugs
  Methyldopa
  Intravenous gammaglobulin
  Corticosteroids
Irradiation
Splenectomy and splenic embolization

levels. Minor increases in blood eosinophils and basophils have been noted after splenectomy but this is not a regular feature.

In response to infection, splenectomized subjects produce a much greater leucocytosis than persons with intact spleens. Often there is a marked left shift in the differential leucocyte count, with myelocytes and occasionally more primitive cells.

Platelet changes

As indicated above, the thrombocytosis post splenectomy is usually transitory and falls to normal or near normal values over the following 1–2 months. However, even if the platelet count has returned to normal values, occasional large and bizarre platelets can be seen in the blood films of many splenectomized subjects. Their presence suggests that these particular platelets are normally removed by the spleen.

Immunological effects

The spleen plays an important role in immunoglobin synthesis; a fall in the IgM fraction of the serum immunoglobulins is commonly found post splenectomy. IgG levels do not change while IgA and IgE increase. The removal of an organ with a unique ability to recognize and phagocytose circulating particulate antigens would be expected to have serious consequences. Despite these facts, splenectomy in adults without complicating disease is not usually associated with a substantially increased incidence of infection. It must be assumed, therefore, that an increase in activity of other lymphoreticular organs compensates for any defects in the immunological defence mechanisms that result from this operation.

Investigation of splenic function using radionuclides

The investigations described in this section are sometimes of clinical value; more frequently they have been undertaken to provide a better understanding of the pathophysiology of splenic function. Imaging techniques, especially when used in quantitative methods, allow a more extensive assessment of the various splenic mechanisms responsible for the production of anaemia. In hypersplenism, there may be thrombocytopenia and neutropenia as well as anaemia. There have been a number of studies of the role of the spleen using labelled platelets and white cells, as well as *in vivo* studies with red cells.

Apart from visualization of the spleen by ultrasound, MRI, CT scanning or radionuclide scanning, factors that may require elucidation are: the extent of splenic red cell and platelet destruction by the spleen; the degree of red cell pooling; the relative amounts of functioning and non-functioning tissue within the spleen; and the presence of extramedullary erythropoiesis. In cases of splenomegaly, it is possible to distinguish increased reticuloendothelial activity causing cell destruction from increased red cell content due to a large splenic pool, and from enlargement of the organ due to tumour infiltration. However, in practice, all three mechanisms may act at the same time.

Sites of red cell destruction

In vivo surface counting during survival studies with ^{51}Cr-labelled red cells provides a means for determining the sites of red cell destruction. The principle is that the destruction of red cells in an organ is manifested by an increase in radioactive counts over that organ relative to the count rate over other organs and in the blood. By this means, it is possible to identify the principal site of red cell sequestration and destruction, and to determine the relative activities of the spleen and liver in a haemolytic process. Four patterns of surface counting occur: (1) excess accumulation in the spleen alone; (2) excess accumulation in the liver alone; (3) no excess accumulation in either organ; and (4) excess accumulation in both organs. Some congenital haemolytic anaemias (hereditary spherocytosis and hereditary elliptocytosis) generally fall into group (1); auto-immune haemolytic anaemias into group (1) or (4); hereditary non-spherocytic haemolytic anaemia into group (3); and paroxysmal nocturnal haemoglobinuria and cases of intravascular haemolysis into group (3) or (4). In patients with haemolytic disease, the results taken in conjunction with the clinical details of the patients have some value in deciding whether splenectomy should be undertaken. A good response can be expected mainly in patients who show the first pattern. Although this test is no longer often used, from published reports and personal data, it appears to give a 90% positive prediction that there will be at least a partial response to splenectomy and a 70% prediction of a full response.

Measurement of splenic phagocytic and immunological function

Irreversible trapping of particulate matter is a function of the reticuloendothelial system. Colloid particles 1 μm in size or less will be taken up by the liver, larger particles by the spleen. There is a well-established relationship between splenic reticuloendothelial function and the rate at which heat-damaged red cells are removed from the circulation. The half-clearance time in normal subjects is about 8–16 min. Post splenectomy, the time is increased to 60–120 min or longer and significantly increased times also occur in conditions associated with splenic hypofunction (see Table 21.2).

In these conditions, a slow clearance rate may identify splenic hypofunction before the blood film shows Howell–Jolly bodies and other morphological features. This test also provides a reliable functional assessment of residual splenic tissue after splenectomy for immune thrombocytopenic purpura or autoimmune haemolytic anaemia, thus indicating the extent to which the splenuncle can be incriminated for the occurrence of relapse. Faster than normal clearance times have been observed in patients with haemolytic anaemia and in some patients with splenomegaly.

The curve of the clearance time is complex, as it comprises three overlapping components, namely, intrasplenic cell transit, sequestration and phagocytosis or irreversible extraction. These may be interpolated from the curve which shows blood flow, cell transit time and extraction ratio (Figure 21.6). There is also a rapid uptake of some of the labelled material by the liver. When the spleen is functioning normally, transit time is 5–10% per

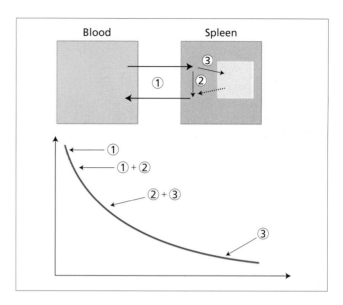

Figure 21.6 Curve of disappearance from circulation of heat-damaged red cells. The components of the curve reflect sequential transit pooling, sequestration and irreversible trapping of the cells. 1, blood flow; 2, cell transit time; 3, extraction rate.

minute, with extraction of 20–50% of the labelled cells. Using red cells coated with IgG (anti Rh(D)) antibody, splenic Fc-receptor phagocytic function can be measured.

Identification of platelet sequestration

When ^{51}Cr-labelled platelets are administered, combined measurements of radioactivity in the liver and spleen and in the blood show that normally about one-third of the platelets are promptly extracted from circulation by the spleen and are released later, with a subsequent monoexponential equilibration with the circulating platelets. A small fraction of the labelled platelets is taken up rapidly and irreversibly by the liver; this is assumed to be due to their being damaged by the labelling process. Splenomegaly is associated with a marked increase in splenic pooling; in contrast, in asplenia, nearly 100% of the labelled platelets are recovered in circulating blood. Surface counting and quantitative scanning have been used to identify the role of the spleen in thrombocytopenia. The clinical usefulness of such data in predicting the results of splenectomy in such patients is, however, debatable, as there is both sequestration and destruction of platelets in the spleen; sequestration is, as a rule, a temporary phase, which does not necessarily mean subsequent destruction, as with red cells.

Splenic red cell pool

A similar procedure to that for visualizing the spleen, but with undamaged, labelled red cells, provides a relatively simple method for measuring the splenic red cell volume. By quantitative imaging, the fraction of the administered radionuclide present in the spleen is measured 20–30 min after injection. Normally, the spleen contains 5% or less of the red cell volume (about 60 mL), and there is general correlation between splenic red cell volume and the physical size of the spleen. There is a proportionately greater pool in certain disorders; in these, the pool may be a major cause of splenomegaly. Discrepancies between the volume of the spleen and of the red cell pool suggest that the splenomegaly is due, at least in part, to cell or tumour infiltration. The extent of the splenic red cell pool should be taken into account when assessing the significance of anaemia; it also makes it possible to predict the degree to which anaemia will improve following splenectomy.

Plasma volume

Splenomegaly is often associated with an increased plasma volume and splenectomy is usually followed by a reduction in plasma volume. This means that in splenomegaly the blood count may give an exaggerated impression of anaemia, so that measurement of red cell and plasma volumes must be included in clarifying the cause of anaemia in conditions associated with splenomegaly.

Selected bibliography

Armas RR (1985) Clinical studies with spleen-specific radiolabelled agents. *Semin Nucl Med* **15**: 260–75.

Bowdler AJ ed. (2002) *The Complete Spleen: Structure, Function and Clinical Disorders*, 2nd edn. Humana Press, Totowa, NJ.

British Committee for Standards in Haematology (1996) Guidelines for the prevention and treatment of infection in patient's with an absent or dysfunctional spleen. *Br Med J* **312**: 430–4.

Buchanan GR, Holtkamp CA (1987) Pocked erythrocyte counts in patients with hereditary spherocytosis before and after splenectomy. *Am J Hematol* **25**: 253–7.

Caulier MT, Darloy F, Rose C et al. (1995) Splenic irradiation for chronic autoimmune thrombocytopenia purpura in patients with contraindications to splenectomy. *Br J Haematol* **91**: 208–11.

Corazzo R, Bullen AW, Hall R et al. (1981) Simple method of assessing splenic function in coeliac disease. *Clin Sci* **60**: 109–113.

Crane CG (1981) Tropical splenomegaly. Part 2: Oceania. *Clin Haematol* **10**: 976–82.

Davies JM, Barnes R, Mulligan D (2002) Update of guidelines for the prevention and treatment of infection in patients with an absent or dysfunctional spleen. British Committee for Standards in Haematology Working Party of the Haematology/Oncology Task Force. *Clin Med* **2**: 440–3.

Dokal IS, Deenmamode M, Lewis SM (1990) Detection and functional assessement of accessory splenic tissue (splenunculi) with radiolabelled heat damaged autologous erythrocytes. *Clin Lab Haematol* **12**: 287–93.

Fakunle YM (1981) Tropical splenomegaly. Part 1: Tropical Africa. *Clin Haematol* **10**: 963–75.

Ferrant A, Cauwe F, Michaux JL et al. (1982) Assessment of the sites of red cell destruction using quantitative measurements of splenic and hepatic red cell destruction. *Br J Haematol* **50**: 591–8.

Fishman D, Isenberg DA (1997) Splenic involvement in rheumatoid diseases. *Semin Arthritis Rheum* **27**: 141–155.

Giebink GS (2001) The prevention of pneumococcal disease in children. Review. *New Eng J Med* **345**: 1177–83.

Guidelines for the prevention and treatment of infection in patients with an absent or dysfunctional spleen. Working Party for the British Committee for Standards in Haematology. Clinical Haematology Task Force 1996. *Br Med J* **312**: 430–4.

Harrington WJ (Jr), Harrington TJ, Harrington WJ (Snr). (1990) Is splenectomy an outmoded procedure? *Adv Intern Med* **35**: 415–40.

Jonasson O, Spigos DC, Moyes MF (1985) Partial splenic embolisation: experience in 136 patients. *World J Surg* **9**: 461–7.

Liu DL, Xia S, Tang J et al. (1995) Allotransplantation of whole spleen in patients with hepatic malignant tumours or hemophilia A. *Arch Surgery* **130**: 33–9.

Messinezy M, Macdonald LM, Nunan TO et al. (1997) Spleen sizing by ultrasound in polycythaemia and thrombocythaemia: comparison with SPECT. *Br J Haematol* **98**: 103–7.

Musser G, Lazar G, Hocking W et al. (1984) Splenectomy for haematologic disease: the UCLA experience with 306 patients. *Ann Surg* **200**: 40–5.

Najean Y, Rain JD, Billotey C (1997) The site of destruction of autologous ^{111}In-labelled platelets and the efficiency of splenectomy in children and adults with idiopathic thrombocytopenic purpura: a study of 578 patients with 268 splenectomies. *Br J Haematol* **97**: 547–50.

Peters AM, Swirsky DM (1998) *Blood Disorders in Clinical Nuclear Medicine*, 3rd edn (MN Maisey, KE Britton, BD Collier, eds), pp. 525–39. Chapman & Hall, London.

Peters AM, Saverymutti SH, Danpure HJ et al. (1986) Radionuclides in haematology: cell labelling. *Methods Haematol* **14**: 70–109.

Peters AM, Saverymutti SH, Keshavarzian A et al. (1985) Splenic pooling of granulocytes. *Clin Sci* **68**: 283–9.

Pickering J, Campbell H (2000) An audit of the vaccinations and antibiotic prophylaxis practices amongst patients splenectomised in Lothian. *Health Bull* **58**: 390–5.

Pochedly C, Sills RH, Schwartz AD (1989) *Disorders of the Spleen: Pathophysiology and Management*. New York: Marcel Dekker.

Shadbolt C, Peters AM (2003) The spleen. In: *Nuclear Medicine in Radiological Diagnosis* (AM Peters, ed). Martin Dunitz, London.

Sty JR, Conway JJ (1985) The spleen: development and functional evaluation. *Semin Nucl Med* **15**: 276–98.

Tham KT, Teague MW, Howard CA et al. (1996) A simple splenic reticuloendothelial function test. *Am J Clin Pathol* **105**: 548–52.

Weiss L (1983) The red pulp of the spleen: structural basis of blood flow. *Clin Haematol* **12**: 375–93.

Zhang B, Lewis SM (1983) Splenic haematocrit and the splenic plasma pool. *Br J Haematol* **66**: 97–102.

Zhang B, Lewis SM (1987) Use of radionuclide scanning to estimate size of spleen *in vivo*. *J Clin Pathol* **40**: 508–11.

Zhang B, Lewis SM (1989) A study of the reliability of clinical palpation of the spleen. *Clin Lab Haematol* **11**: 7–10.

CHAPTER 22

Immunodeficiency diseases

A David B Webster

22

This chapter describes the clinical presentations and mechanisms of the immunodeficiency diseases, focusing on those disorders that affect lymphocytes and complement. Defects in neutrophils are dealt with in Chapter 17. Immunodeficiency is either primary or secondary to other diseases, transplantation and various drugs. Although the first description of a patient with primary immunodeficiency (PID) was half a century ago, it is only in the last decade that significant advances have been made in our understanding of the molecular mechanisms. Over 50 separate genetic defects in lymphocytes or monocytes/macrophages are now known, mostly very rare and presenting in infants and young children. However, the majority of patients with PID do not yet have a defined condition and are 'classified' as having 'common variable immunodeficiency – CVID'. This disorder, as well as many of the known single-gene defects causing PID, is associated with autoimmunity to blood cells and lymphoma, and affected patients are often referred to haematologists.

Primary immunodeficiency: introduction

Patients with PID can be broadly divided into three clinical groups: (i) those who present in infancy or early childhood with severe life-threatening infection (severe combined immunodeficiency, SCID); (ii) those presenting at any age with a defect predominantly affecting antibody production; and (iii) those with inherited complement deficiency. The first is a paediatric emergency, while those in the last group often remain undiagnosed for many years owing to the insidious onset of symptoms. In addition, there are rare inherited disorders affecting multisystems in which the immunodeficiency has a major influence on survival. There is a network of specialist centres in the UK for the diagnosis and management of PID, and most patients need referral. An

important role for general practitioners and specialists such as haematologists is to recognize the characteristic clinical features of PID, have facilities to screen for the most common disorders and to have a working collaboration with a local immunologist who can provide specialized diagnostic tests.

Severe combined immunodeficiency

The majority of patients with SCID present with severe persistent infection in infancy or early childhood. A typical scenario is failure to thrive during the first 2 years of life, episodes of protracted diarrhoea and persistent cough due to an opportunistic fungal respiratory infection (Figure 22.1). However, there are many exceptions to this 'classical' presentation, some patients having features that are not directly related to infection, such as skin rashes, severe autoimmune phenomena, lymphadenopathy and hepatosplenomegaly. The associated antibody deficiency leads to a susceptibility to bacterial infection, particularly with *Haemophilus influenzae*, pneumococci and enteric pathogens such as *Campylobacter jejuni*. The cellular immunodeficiency leads to chronic fungal infections that are often difficult to diagnose and treat, such as *Pneumocystis carinii*, *Aspergillus fumigatus* and *Candida albicans*; chronic viral infection is also common, particularly rotavirus enteritis and life-threatening varicella or cytomegalovirus infection. Chronic intestinal parasitic infections can occur, particularly in patients living in underdeveloped countries.

A few patients present later in childhood and, occasionally, as adults with a more insidious development of persistent opportunistic infection, the first manifestation in adults often being severe cutaneous warts caused by papillomaviruses. Such patients may remain undiagnosed for many years, with no easy explanation as to how they have survived through childhood

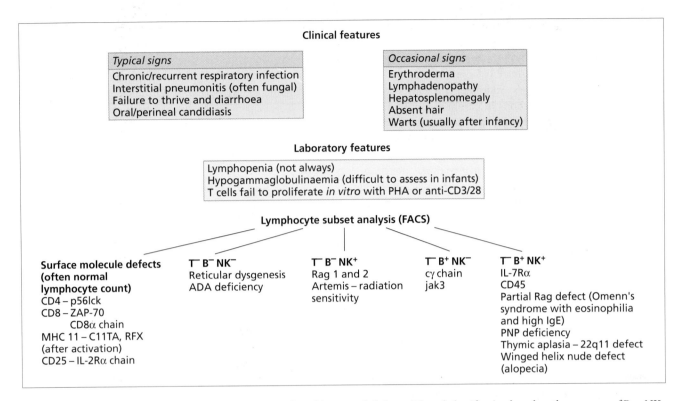

Figure 22.1 Clinical and laboratory features of severe combined immunodeficiency. The subclassification based on the presence of B or NK cells is used only as a guide to potential molecular defects.

without significant infection. Nevertheless, having presented as adults, the prognosis is poor and most die from opportunistic infection within 5 years.

Prevalence and initial diagnosis

Severe combined immunodeficiency is rare, estimated to occur in about 1 in 30 000–100 000 live births. Haematologists will usually play some part in the diagnosis as lymphopenia is a characteristic but not consistent feature. It is important that haematology laboratories provide normal age-related ranges for lymphocyte counts and that paediatricians appreciate that these are different to adult ranges. Most infants and young children with SCID are lymphopenic, so a full blood count is a valuable initial diagnostic aid. A family history suggesting autosomal or X-linked inheritance, such as early deaths from severe infection in family members, may support the diagnosis. Although it may be useful to identify deficiencies of lymphocyte subsets using fluorescence-activated cell sorter (FACS) analysis, most suspected cases should be urgently referred to a paediatric immunology centre with facilities to make a definitive molecular diagnosis and proceed to bone marrow transplantation (BMT). No time should be lost in trying to treat a current infection before referral to a specialist centre, as the earlier BMT is performed the better the outcome.

Subclassification of severe combined immunodeficiency

Infants and young children with SCID can be conveniently subclassified into those patients who lack both T and B lymphocytes (T⁻ B⁻ SCID) and those who retain B lymphocytes (T⁻ B⁺ SCID). Additional clues to the molecular diagnosis can be provided by the presence or absence of natural killer (NK) cells (Figure 22.1). This is only a guide to a molecular defect, and is less reliable in patients presenting later in life.

The most common molecular defects involve the recombinase-activating genes (*RAG1* and *RAG2*) and the genes coding for adenosine deaminase or the γ-chain shared by receptors for a number of cytokines involved in growth and development of lymphocytes. The clinical phenotype of *RAG* gene defects is particularly variable, ranging from a typical presentation with severe lymphopenia and infection when there is no *RAG* gene expression, to Omenn's syndrome, with lymphadenopathy, hepatosplenomegaly, autoimmune blood dyscrasias, severe skin rashes and eosinophilia when there is partial expression. The pattern of T-lymphocyte subset deficiency can be a useful guide to the molecular diagnosis. For example, a selective deficiency of CD8⁺ T cells suggests one of the rarer SCIDs caused by mutations in the genes coding for CD8α or ZAP-70. A few SCIDs can be diagnosed relatively easily; deficiency of adenosine deaminase and purine nucleoside phosphorylase can be diagnosed by measuring the enzymes in erythrocytes in a specialized laboratory; MHC class II deficiency can be diagnosed by the absence of these molecules on lymphocytes using FACS systems.

Thymic aplasia (DiGeorge's syndrome) is usually associated with hemizygous microdeletions in chromosome 22q11, and occasionally 10p, the underlying genetic mechanism not being understood. Although this is a relatively common cytogenetic abnormality, the consequences, which affect the embryonic development of the third and fourth pharyngeal pouch, are diverse and include cardiac defects, abnormal facies, thymic hypoplasia, cleft palate and hypocalcaemia due to parathyroid hypoplasia, the syndrome being referred to by the acronym 'CATCH 22'. Only a few of the affected infants and children have a significant immunodeficiency, and very few require either thymic transplantation or BMT. Circulating T-cell numbers often rise during childhood in those with severe lymphopenia in infancy, but about 50% of patients have lifelong minor defects in humoral immunity, often with low serum IgM levels.

Molecular diagnosis

A detailed family history is important because it may suggest an X-linked or autosomal recessive type of SCID, thus narrowing down the possibilities. The knowledge that a previous relative has suffered from a defined molecular defect clearly makes the diagnosis relatively straightforward, and if the mutation is known then the genotype can be confirmed within a few weeks in a specialized laboratory. Genetic counselling can be offered to the family and fetal diagnosis may be possible. However, most SCIDs are sporadic, and with facilities available at present it may take many months before the molecular defect is found. Routine rapid sequencing of potentially affected genes should soon be available in the UK, providing a specific diagnosis in most patients before long-term management decisions are taken.

Treatment

As for all patients with severe T-cell deficiency, patients should be immediately given prophylactic cotrimoxazole to prevent *Pneumocystis carinii* pneumonia, and immunoglobulin replacement therapy for the associated antibody deficiency. Some centres use antifungal prophylaxis while waiting for more definitive treatment. Blood transfusions should be irradiated to avoid graft-versus-host disease (GvHD) and all live vaccines are contraindicated.

Bone marrow or stem cell transplantation is the only curative option for most SCIDs. The various protocols used will not be discussed here, but the success rate for a complete HLA-matched sibling donor is more than 95%, with about 75% for a matched unrelated donor or haplo-identical sibling donor. In contrast to other indications for BMT, myeloablation is not required. There is usually split chimerism after transplanta-

tion, with the T cells being donor and the B cells being of recipient origin. Except for an identical related match, either a stem cell or whole marrow transplant followed by *in vivo* T-cell depletion is used to avoid GvHD. There is usually a period of some months before normal B-cell function is achieved, with about 20% of patients having persistent antibody deficiency requiring regular immunoglobulin replacement therapy. BMT is less successful in adolescents or adults because of thymic atrophy, and engraftment is less consistent in those retaining NK cells.

For those with ADA deficiency, enzyme replacement therapy with pegylated bovine ADA will often partially correct the immunodeficiency. However, this is usually inadequate, and there are additional problems with the production of antibodies to bovine ADA that neutralize the replaced enzyme. The most exciting curative development has been gene therapy, with complete restoration of immunity following transfection of the γc gene into the stem cells of infants with X-linked SCID. Unfortunately, the random nature of proviral integration into the host genome caused acute lymphoblastic leukaemia in two children associated with aberrant expression of LMO-2. This has led to a temporary cessation of gene therapy in the pioneering Paris centre, although other centres are continuing treatment with different vectors on selected patients, and are extending it to other types of SCID.

Combined immunodeficiency

A number of rare inherited defects significantly compromise both humoral and cellular immunity but do not usually lead to early death from severe infection (Table 22.1). These include defects in CD40 ligand (HIM-1), ataxia telangiectasia (AT) and other defects in DNA repair systems, and the Wiskott–Aldrich syndrome (WAS). A predisposition to cancer, particularly lymphoma, occurs in many of these syndromes. In WAS, the clinical features range from thrombocytopenia alone to a severe disease characterized by recurrent infection, severe eczema and B-cell lymphoma at an early age. Patients with ataxia telangiectasia usually die before the third decade from progressive ataxia and/or tumours, often compounded by recurrent infections due to an associated antibody deficiency. The mutated gene (ATM) is involved in cell cycle regulation and also appears to be a tumour suppressor, as it is frequently deleted in prolymphocytic and chronic lymphocytic leukaemia (CLL) cells. Another gene involved in DNA repair causes the Nijmegen breakage syndrome, affected patients also having progressive neurological disease and antibody deficiency, but having distinctive dysmorphic features.

Dysregulation of cytotoxic – and/or NK-cell function – can cause tissue damage during infection, often with bone marrow failure. For example, the dramatic expansion of CD8 cytotoxic T cells in X-linked lymphoproliferative syndrome (XLP) during Epstein–Barr virus (EBV) infection may cause acute liver failure,

Table 22.1 Combined immunodeficiency.

Designation	Genetic defect	Cellular abnormality	Specific features
Disorders of cytotoxic T cell/NK function causing acute organ damage after viral infections			
X-linked lymphoproliferative syndrome (XLP) (X)	SAP	Excessive CD8 T-cell expansion	Burkitt's-like lymphoma
Chediak–Higashi syndrome	Lyst	Deficient CTL and NK	Giant lysosomes in leucocytes
Griscelli syndrome	Myosin 5a or RAB27A		Encephalopathy in severe cases
Familial haemophagocytic syndrome	Perforin		
T-cell receptor defects			
Class 1 transporter defect	TAP 1 or 2	Absent Class 1 expression	Midline granulomas
CD3 receptor defects	CD 3γ or ε	CD3 signalling defect	
Disorders of DNA repair with chromosomal instability and sensitivity to X-radiation			
Ataxia–telangiectasia	ATM	Cell cycle checkpoint defect	Lymphomas, severe ataxia
Ataxia + immunodeficiency	Mre 11		Moderate ataxia
Nijmegen breakage syndrome	Nibrin	Cell cycle checkpoint DNA double-strand break–repair defect	Microcephaly
Ligase deficiency	Ligase 1 or 4		Growth retardation, lymphomas
Multisystem disorders			
Wiskott–Aldrich syndrome (X)	WASp	Defect in cytoskeletal integrity	Thrombocytopenia, small platelets lymphomas, vasculitis
Immune dysregulation polyendocrinopathy, enteropathy, X-linked syndrome (IPEX) (X)	FOXP3		Early onset diabetes, severe skin disease
Autoimmune polyendocrinopathy and ectodermal dysplasia	AIRE		Chronic mucocutaneous candidiasis
WHIM (waits, hypogammaglobinaemia infections, myelokathexis)	CXCR4	Chemokine receptor defect	Severe warts

These disorders are associated with variable patterns of immunoglobulin deficiencies and T cell abnormalities.
X, x-linked.

and the failure of a cytotoxic response to viruses in familial haemophagocytic lymphohistiocytosis and Chediak–Higashi syndrome can lead to uncontrolled viral replication and a massive acute phase response. The best explanation for the high incidence of midline granulomas in TAP (transporter associated with antigen processing) deficiency is that the failure to express MHC class 1 inhibitory molecules allows activated NK cells in the nasopharynx to damage adjacent tissues.

Secondary defects in cellular immunity

Chronic malnutrition is the most common cause of secondary T-cell deficiency worldwide, often exacerbated by AIDS in many underdeveloped countries in Africa. This explains the pandemic of tuberculosis at present in these countries and the very high mortality in children during epidemics of measles and other common viruses. Zinc, vitamin A and selenium have been em-

phasized as being important for normal immunity, with some evidence that maintaining adequate levels reduces mortality.

In developed countries, immunosuppressive and cytotoxic drugs used for autoimmune disease, malignancy and after transplantation are the main causes of T-cell defects, although only a minority of treated patients develop clinically significant immunodeficiency. An example is the increased EBV replication and development of EBV-triggered post-transplant lymphoproliferative disease (PTLD). Major trauma and surgery has a transient inhibitory effect on T-cell function and can rarely lead to fatal reactivation of cytomegalovirus.

Except in AIDS, and more recently in PTLD, clinicians usually make no attempt to regularly screen for T-cell defects in those taking immunosuppressive drugs or in malnourished elderly people. A simple circulating CD4+ T-lymphocyte count is probably a sufficient screening procedure, with counts of < 150/μL raising the alarm and prompting referral to an immunologist.

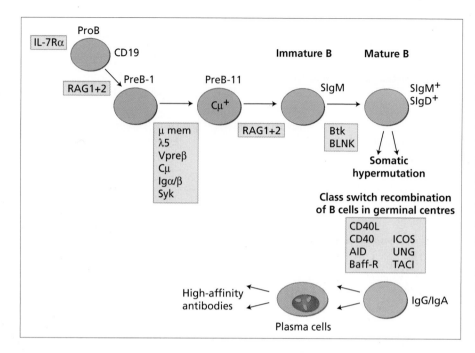

Figure 22.2 The stages in B-cell development. Genetic defects in molecules associated with arrest at various stages are shown in the coloured boxes. RAG, recombinase activating gene; μ mem, membrane-associated μ chain; Cμ, cytoplasmic μ expression; Btk, Bruton's tyrosine kinase; BLNK, B cell linker protein; ICOS, human *inducible co-st*imulator; AID, activation-induced cytidine deaminase; UNG, uracil–DNA glycosylase; BAFF-R, B-cell activation factor from the tumour necrosis factor family; TAC-I, transmembrane activator and calcium modulator and cyclophilin ligand interactor.

Primary antibody deficiency

This is the most common PID, affected patients having either a severe or partial failure to produce antibodies, usually with low levels of one or more of the main immunoglobulin classes. Most patients with severe primary antibody deficiency (PAD) present as adolescents or adults, although a carefully taken history will uncover a susceptibility to infection in about 20% during childhood. The most common of these disorders is a selective complete deficiency of immunoglobulin A (IgAD), this having a prevalence of about 1 in 700 white people. Most affected individuals are asymptomatic, and the defect may be recognized only during population surveys or during routine investigation of an unrelated problem. However, there is a raised incidence of IgAD in patients with various autoimmune disorders, particularly coeliac disease. Family studies show that IgAD is often genetically linked to a more severe antibody deficiency called *common variable immunodeficiency* (CVID). Furthermore, many patients with subtle defects in immunoglobulin production (i.e. IgG subclass defects, low serum IgA and/or deficiencies in producing IgG-specific antibodies), appear also to have a disorder genetically linked to CVID and IgAD.

A variety of rare single-gene defects cause severe antibody deficiency as a result of failure of development of B lymphocytes within the bone marrow. The best known is X-linked agammaglobulinaemia (XLA), caused by a defect in Bruton's tyrosine kinase (btk), an intracellular signalling molecule whose precise role in B-cell development is still unknown. Other rarer defects

involve surface ligands or intracellular signalling molecules involved in the differentiation of B cells (Figure 22.2). Recent work has identified a number of molecules critical for immunoglobulin class switching and somatic hypermutation, these processes being necessary for the generation of antibody diversity. The germline configuration of immunoglobulin genes on chromosome 14 consists of 'variable' V-region genes linked to the 'constant' region genes by a D–J segment. During the later stages of B-cell development in the bone marrow, functional immunoglobulin genes are assembled by recombination to produce a repertoire of IgM antibodies with low affinity. When these B cells encounter antigen, there is rapid proliferation to form the germinal centres in the secondary lymphoid apparatus, during which there is intense hypermutation in and around the rearranged V gene segments. Class-switch recombination occurs at this stage, a critical requirement being a signal within B cells stimulated via CD40-ligand expressed on the surface of activated T cells and CD40 on the B cell. Activation-induced cytidine deaminase (AID) is another molecule involved in class switching, its role being to deaminate doxycytidine to uracil, which then has to be excised and repaired for the immunoglobulin gene segment to be functional. Uracil–DNA glycosylase (UNG) is the most important molecule for this excision/repair step.

Genetic defects in any of these four molecules are very rare and characterized by a raised serum IgM, and usually very low IgG and IgA (hyper-IgM syndromes: HIM 1–4). However, each has some special features, for example defects in CD40 ligand cause susceptibility to opportunistic infection, particularly with cryptosporidia, and to unexplained sclerosing cholangitis and

Typical features	Occasional features
Chronic/recurrent bronchitis	Autoimmune disease, e.g. haemolytic anaemia,
Sinusitis/otitis media	neutropenia, thrombocytopenia, vitiligo
Pneumonia/septicaemia	Enteropathy
	Arthritis (usually mycoplasmal)
	Meningoencephalitis (usually enteroviral)
	Lymphoma

Diagnosis

Stage 1	Serum immunoglobins (+ serum immunoelectrophoresis)
	Baseline functional antibodies → if low, immunize and check response
	   e.g. to tetanus toxoid
	              pneumococcal polysaccharides
	IgG subclasses if total IgG <11 g/L

Stage 2	Consider secondary causes:
	1 Drugs – anti-inflammatory
	            anticonvulsant
	            immunosuppressive
	2 Increased loss –
	          nephrosis
	          enteropathy
	          lymphangiectasia
	3 Lymphoma

Stage 3	Lymphocyte subsets – absence of B cells suggests Btk, μ-chain defect, etc. Family history – XLP, X-HIM and XLA need to be excluded in males Exclude thymoma in those > 40 years (lateral chest radiograph) Most patients with B cells will be 'labelled' as having common variable immunodeficiency

Figure 22.3 Clinical features and diagnosis of antibody deficiency.

liver cancer at a young age; the AID and UNG defects cause lymphadenopathy with expanded germinal centres filled with IgM-committed B cells, a feature sometimes confused with follicular lymphoma. Only three patients with UNG defects have so far been described, but they may be prone to B-cell lymphoma as this is a frequent complication in the knockout mouse model.

Presenting features of antibody deficiency

Nearly all patients with severe PAD present with infection, although in a minority the hypogammaglobulinaemia is discovered during investigation of autoimmune or inflammatory bowel disease (Figure 22.3). There is usually a gradual escalation of bacterial infection in the respiratory tract, with recurrent bronchitis, persistent nasal catarrh and sinusitis, and otitis media in children. The organisms most commonly isolated are nontypeable *Haemophilus influenzae*, pneumococci and *Moraxella catarrhalis*.

A few patients present with an acute, life-threatening septicaemia, sometimes with meningitis caused by pneumococci, capsulated *H. influenzae* and occasionally meningococci. A minority are susceptible to chronic enteroviral infection, particularly with echoviruses, that cause an insidious meningoencephalitis and sometimes a dermatomyositic-like condition and/or myocarditis. Immunization with live attenuated vaccines is contraindicated, particularly with oral polio vaccine (OPV),

because some patients have subsequently developed paralytic poliomyelitis. About 10% of patients are prone to chronic mycoplasma infection, usually manifesting as arthritis or urethritis, but sometimes as deep abscesses in the lungs or elsewhere. As only a minority of patients are prone to enteroviral or mycoplasmal infection, it is likely that they lack additional protective factors for these specific organisms. In the bowel, campylobacter or giardia infection is common and often difficult to eradicate with standard therapy.

Individuals with IgAD are usually healthy and need take no special precautions with vaccines. However, they often make anti-IgA antibodies, which in a small minority are of sufficiently high titre and affinity to cause anaphylactic reactions during blood or blood product infusion. There is no consensus among immunologists on whether IgAD individuals should be routinely monitored for anti-IgA antibodies, mainly because there is very poor correlation between the level of these antibodies and severe reactions.

Common variable immunodeficiency

This is a diagnosis of exclusion, but typically patients present with infections after adolescence and have very low levels of serum IgG and IgM and unrecordable IgA. Some rare inherited single genes defects have recently been shown to cause the CVID phenotype [e.g. a defect in human *inducible co-st*imulator

(ICOS), X-linked lymphoproliferative syndrome (XLP), BAFF-R and TAC-I], but the majority appear to have a complex genetic disorder associated with increased production of inflammatory cytokines, particularly IFN-γ. This helps to explain the high incidence of inflammatory bowel disease and granulomatous infiltration of organs such as the spleen, liver and lungs, and the splenomegaly that often prompts a search for lymphoma. The incidence of stomach cancer and lymphoma is raised in CVID, the former probably due to *Helicobacter pylori* gastritis. There are some similarities between CVID and XLP, in that both are associated with a relative expansion in numbers of circulating CD8$^+$ T cells with restricted clonality, which in XLP are mainly committed to EBV peptides. Although XLP is a very rare disorder, the diagnosis should be excluded in male patients presenting with hypogammaglobulinaemia, particularly if they develop an EBV-related lymphoma. Hypogammaglobulinaemia associated with thymoma can mimic CVID at presentation but is classified separately because the prognosis is often poor due to a gradual deterioration of T-cell function.

There is evidence that at least 20% of CVID patients have an inherited dominant condition with a major susceptibility locus in the MHC region on chromosome 6, probably involving class II genes. However, the phenotype in affected family members varies from a mild subclinical selective deficiency of IgA (IgAD), to low IgG or IgG subclass deficiencies, with only the rare individual developing CVID with very low or absent serum levels of all immunoglobulin classes. Interestingly, IgAD is rare in Japanese people (1:80 000 of the population) but is relatively common in white people (1:700), with very few cases of CVID being reported in Japan. This geographical distribution suggests some selective advantage for the IgAD/CVID genotype, one possibility being that the associated upregulation of inflammatory cytokines has provided some protection during pandemics of infection with intracellular organisms such as mycobacteria.

Differential diagnosis of primary and secondary antibody deficiency

Figure 22.3 shows the procedures for investigating patients with suspected antibody deficiency. The family history may suggest an inherited defect. The pattern of the serum immunoglobulin deficiency can be helpful, with complete agammaglobulinaemia and absence of circulating B lymphocytes suggesting a B-cell maturation/differentiation defect. The presence of a normal or raised serum IgM, with very low IgG and IgA, suggests one of the HIM syndromes, whereas low IgG, unrecordable IgA and very low IgM suggests CVID. Some inherited 'single-gene' defects can be diagnosed easily by Western blot analysis of the relevant protein in lymphocytes and/or monocytes (e.g. XLA, XLP), but many patients remain undiagnosed because of the cost and the time it takes to search for mutations. The diagnosis of more subtle defects in antibody production relies on measuring specific antibodies before and after immunization. The problem here is

that there is very poor correlation between a specific failure to respond to various types of antigen (e.g. bacterial polysaccharides) and clinical symptoms and signs.

Secondary antibody deficiency must be excluded, being relatively common nowadays with many patients being treated with immunosuppressive and cytotoxic drugs. A variety of anti-inflammatory and anticonvulsant drugs have been associated with low serum immunoglobulins, and nearly 10% of patients treated for vasculitis with combinations of cyclophosphamide and steroids develop hypogammaglobulinaemia. The increasing use of combination therapy for malignancy and anti-B lymphocyte therapy for autoimmune disease is likely to be associated with an increase in the numbers of patients with secondary antibody deficiency. The mechanism for this complication is not known but is likely to be complex and involve polymorphisms in enzymes that metabolize specific classes of drugs. Other causes of secondary antibody deficiency such as increased loss from the kidney (nephrotic syndrome) can be easily eliminated, but protein loss from the bowel may be more difficult to confirm, particularly if the serum albumin is maintained (e.g. lymphangiectasia in the bowel due to tumours or venous congestion).

Hypogammaglobulinaemia is common in CLL, but usually the immunoglobulin levels are only moderately low and the clonal lymphocytosis confirms the diagnosis. Myeloma is often associated with profound depression of useful antibodies and, apart from the paraprotein, low immunoglobulin levels. Therefore, immunoelectrophoresis should be routine for all initial serum samples sent to the laboratory for immunoglobulin levels. Tests on urine for Bence Jones proteins may also be necessary to exclude atypical myeloma, particularly in patients presenting after 50 years of age. Some patients present with severe hypogammaglobulinaemia associated with malignant lymphoma, with uncertainty as to whether the patient has a primary antibody deficiency (e.g. CVID) with secondary lymphoma or a lymphoma with secondary immunodeficiency. Fortunately, such confusion does not alter management, and in most cases the sequence of events cannot be resolved.

Management of antibody deficiency

Most patients with suspected PID should be referred to a clinical immunologist with access to modern immunological tests. For severely affected patients, a combination of immunoglobulin replacement and periodic or prophylactic antibiotics (e.g. ciprofloxacin or a rotating regimen of amoxycillin, doxycycline and a quinolone) are required, but mild cases can often be managed with antibiotics alone. Most severely affected patients are given monthly intravenous immunoglobulin (400 mg/kg) or weekly subcutaneous infusions (100 mg/kg), the latter being recommended for infants and young children with difficult venous access. Morbidity and life expectancy depend on the type of immunodeficiency and the degree of organ damage at diagnosis; for example patients with XLA diagnosed early before there is lung damage will have an excellent prognosis if they are compliant with treatment. In contrast, CVID patients frequently develop chronic inflammation with granulomas in their lungs and livers, and a minority may have severe unexplained enteritis or autoimmune thrombocytopenia that can severely affect their quality of life. Other rarer PADs are associated with special complications, such as cholangitis and liver cancer in patients with CD40 ligand deficiency, and EBV-induced lymphoma in those with XLP. Protocols for management and follow-up therefore need to be tailored to the genetic defect.

In secondary antibody deficiency, prognosis depends on the primary disorder, but there is often recovery of antibody production if the offending drug is discontinued or the underlying disease remits. There is no consensus on the use of prophylactic immunoglobulin in CLL or myeloma, with many centres preferring to use prophylactic antibiotics for those prone to infection. Nevertheless, there are patients who benefit from prophylactic immunoglobulin therapy, particularly in the winter months.

Primary defects in innate immunity (IL-12/IFN-γ and NFκB pathways)

Experimental mouse models have clearly demonstrated the importance of IL-12 and IFN-γ and their corresponding receptors in protection against infection with intracellular pathogens, particularly mycobacteria. This work led to a search for defects in these proteins in rare cases of infants and young children presenting with chronic mycobacterial disease, including persistent local disseminated BCG infection following vaccination. Families have been reported with autosomal inherited defects involving the IFN-γ receptor, STAT-1, which is critical in the signalling pathway for this receptor, and in IL-12 and its receptor. Affected patients usually present with chronic atypical mycobacterial infection at an early age and are also prone to chronic *Salmonella* infection. A defect in NEMO (NFκB modulator) causes a rare X-linked severe immunodeficiency with ectodermal dysplasia. Defects in IRAK-4 (interleukin-1 receptor-associated kinase 4) have been found in patients prone to recurrent pneumococcal pneumonia.

Patients with IFN-γ receptor (R) defects either fail to express the R1 chain or partially express either the R1 or R2 chain. Partial expression allows signalling by high concentrations of IFN-γ, and affected patients may respond to IFN-γ therapy. The heterozygous dominant form of partial expression is the most common, the abnormal chains interfering with the signalling via Jak-1 and STAT-1 following binding of IFN-γ to the receptor complex (so-called 'dominant negative' effect). Patients with complete deficiency of the p40 chain shared by both IL-12 and IL-23, and of the IL-12β1 receptor can be helped by IFN-γ therapy, but the few patients described with STAT-1 deficiency do not respond.

Defects in complement components

Inherited defects in nearly all of the complement components have been reported since the first description of a patient with very low haemolytic complement activity in 1960. Complement is important for localizing infection with encapsulated bacteria during the first few hours and preventing blood-borne dissemination. This is achieved mainly by activation of the 'classical' pathway through immune complexes activating C1q, but also by direct activation of the 'alternative' pathway by microorganisms, sometimes amplified by plasma collectins such as mannose-binding lectin (MBL). The alternative pathway, triggered by the production of nascent C3b, acts as an amplification system for the classical pathway (Figure 22.4). The importance of inhibitors at various stages to prevent persistent activation and unwanted bystander damage to tissues is demonstrated by inherited deficiencies of C1 esterase inhibitor, which causes attacks of severe angioedema: another example is haemolytic anaemia caused by deficiency of decay accelerating factor (DAF). As defects in these 'control' systems are not associated with infection they will not be discussed here.

Most patients with inherited defects are homozygous for the mutated allele; these are very rare except for C2 deficiency, which affects about 1:10 000 white people. Defects in the early components of the classical pathway (C1, C2, C4) predispose to recurrent bacterial infection, but the main problem for affected patients is a susceptibility to immune complex disease such as systemic lupus erythematosus (SLE), glomerulonephritis and vasculitis. The rare patients with complete C3 deficiency suffer from severe bacterial infections from an early age, but are also prone to vasculitis and glomerulonephritis. Defects in the late components, which include the membrane attack complex, are associated with recurrent meningococcal and gonococcal infection, except for C9 deficiency, which is common in Japanese people and only occasionally predisposes to meningococcal meningitis. Recurrent meningococcal disease is a feature of complete deficiency of alternative pathway components (i.e. factors B, D, I, H and properdin); those with factor H deficiency have an additional susceptibility to vasculitic renal disease. The clinical significance of MBL deficiency is controversial, but there is good evidence that severe deficiency predisposes to sepsis in infants, possibly in those with inadequate antibody production. About 5% of white people have severe MBL deficiency, and there are many reports linking both complete and partial deficiency with a wide variety of infections.

Diagnosis and treatment of complement deficiencies

Functional assays of classical and alternative pathway haemolytic activity are available in most immunopathology laboratories as an initial screening test. Distinguishing primary from secondary

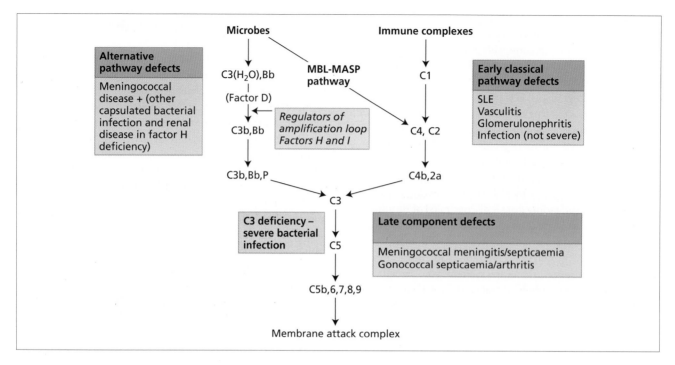

Figure 22.4 Diagram showing the sequential activation of the components of the classical and alternative complement pathways. Genetic defects in the various components are associated with the clinical complications shown in the adjacent coloured boxes.

hypocomplementaemia can sometimes be difficult during episodes of complement consumption, for example in active SLE, but the haemolytic activity rarely falls below 5% of normal, which is usual for primary defects. A specialized laboratory will measure individual components and search for the mutation, sometimes assisted by the type of inheritance (e.g. X-linked in properdin deficiency). Potentially affected family members should be screened. Regular replacement therapy for specific complement component deficiencies is not feasible but is theoretically possible on a temporary basis during an infection (compare with C1 inhibitor concentrate for hereditary angioedema). In practice, fresh-frozen plasma can be given, although it is not clear whether this adds any benefit to antibiotics that are clearly life-saving. Careful attention to maintaining protective levels of antibodies to pneumococci and meningococci by vaccination is sensible, and patients should be encouraged to take antibiotics as soon as they experience symptoms of infection; these prophylactic measures are best managed by an immunologist.

Selected bibliography

General

Bonilla FA, Geha RS (2003) Primary immunodeficiency diseases. *Journal of Allergy and Clinical Immunology* 111 (2 suppl.): S571–81.

Chapel H, Geha R, Rosen F (2003) Primary immunodeficiency diseases: an update. *Clinical and Experimental Immunology* 132: 9–15.

Ochs HD, Edvard Smith CI, Puck JM (eds) (1999) *Primary Immunodeficiency Diseases: A Molecular and Genetic Approach*. Oxford University Press, New York.

Diagnosis

Chapel H, Webster ADB (1999) Assessment of the Immune System. In: *Primary Immunodeficiency Diseases: A Molecular and Genetic Approach* (HD Ochs, CI Edvard Smith, JM Puck, eds), pp. 419–31. Oxford University Press, New York.

Folds JD, Schmitz Jl (2003) Clinical and laboratory assessment of immunity. *Journal of Allergy and Clinical Immunology* 111 (Suppl.): S701–11.

Gaspar R, Gillour KC (2001) Screening for genetic defects in primary immunodeficiencies. *CPD Bulletin for Immunology and Allergy* 2: 3–7.

B-lymphocyte defects

Conley MEJ, Rohrer L, Rapalus EC *et al.* (2000) Defects in early B-cell development: comparing the consequences of abnormalities in pre-BCR signaling in the human and the mouse. *Immunological Reviews* 178: 75–90.

Durandy A (2003) Mini-review. Activation-induced cytidine deaminase: a dual role in class-switch recombination and somatic hypermutation. *European Journal of Immunology* 33: 2069–73.

Rada C, Williams GT, Nilsen H *et al.* (2002) Immunoglobulin isotype switching is inhibited and somatic hypermutation perturbed in UNG-deficient mice. *Current Biology* 12: 1748–55.

Webster ADB (2001) Common variable immunodeficiency. In: *Humoral Immunodeficiences* (C Roifman, ed.). *Immunology and*

Allergy Clinics of North America 21: 1–22. WB Saunders, Philadelphia.

Treatment

Antoine C, Muller, S Cant A *et al.* (2003) Long-term survival and transplantation of haemopoietic stem cells for immunodeficiencies: report of the European experience 1968–99. *Lancet* 361: 553–60.

Hacein-Bey-Abina S, Fischer A, Cavazzana-Calvo M (2002) Gene therapy of X-linked severe combined immunodeficiency. *International Journal of Hematology* 76: 295–8.

Combined immunodeficiencies

Dupuis-Girod SJ, Medioni E, Haddad P *et al.* (2003) Autoimmunity in Wiskott-Aldrich syndrome: risk factors, clinical features, and outcome in a single-center cohort of 55 patients. *Pediatrics* 111: 622–7.

Notarangelo LD, Santagata S, Villa A (2001) Recombinase activating gene enzymes of lymphocytes. In: *Current Opinion in Haematology* (TP Stossel, ed.), pp. 41–6. Lippincott Williams & Wilkins, Boston.

IL-12 and IFN-γ

Dupuis S, Jouanguy E, Al Hajjar SE *et al.* (2003) Impaired response to interferon-alpha/beta and lethal viral disease in human STAT1 deficiency. *Nature Genetics* 33: 388–91.

Lammas DA, Casanova J-L, Kumararatne DS (2000) Clinical consequences of defects in the IL-12-dependent interferon-gamma (IFN-gamma) pathway. *Clinical and Experimental Immunology* 121: 417–25.

Complement

Barilla-LaBarca ML, Atkinson JP. (2003) Rheumatic syndromes associated with complement deficiency. *Current Opinion in Rheumatology* 15: 55–60.

Jack DL, Klein NJ, Turner MW (2001) Mannose-binding lectin: targeting the microbial world for complement attack and opsonophagocytosis. *Immunological Reviews* 180: 86–99.

Secondary immunodeficiency

Webster ADB (1997) Secondary immunodeficiency. In: *Encyclopaedia of Immunology* (IM Roitt, PJ Delves, eds). Saunders Scientific Publications, London.

CHAPTER 23

Haematology in HIV disease

Christine Costello

Acquired immunodeficiency syndrome

Viral structure

There are two subtypes of human immunodeficiency virus, HIV-1 and HIV-2. Infection with both viruses usually causes acquired immunodeficiency syndrome (AIDS), although those infected with HIV-2 tend to progress at a slower rate. HIV-1 and HIV-2 are retroviruses of the lentivirus subfamily and are sufficiently alike to be considered as one in terms of viral properties. Like all retroviruses, HIV replicates by forming a DNA provirus using the viral enzyme, reverse transcriptase. Retroviruses contain RNA in two subunits and have three genes central to their action: *gag* (group-specific antigen), coding for proteins within the viral particle; *pol*, coding for reverse transcriptase, which converts the RNA into DNA within the host cell; and *env*, which codes for envelope glycoproteins. In addition to these genes, the HIV genome contains several regulatory genes that modulate the rate of viral gene expression and the infectivity of the virus. The *tat* and *rev* genes act in positive feedback to enhance the processing and translation of RNA encoding the structural genes and proteins, whereas the *nef* gene appears to downregulate HIV replication.

It has been known for some years that different laboratory strains of HIV show considerable diversity of nucleotide sequence, which may result in antigenic variation, providing a means whereby the virus can escape humoral and cellular immune control. Using the polymerase chain reaction method for the amplification and subsequent analysis of viral genomes, it is now apparent that HIV genomes *in vivo* are even more diverse than those in laboratory strains.

Viral transmission

HIV transmission usually occurs by sexual contact, blood or blood products. It has been suggested that infected lymphocytes and macrophages are particularly effective at transmission but the infection of haemophiliacs given contaminated factor VIII demonstrates that extracellular viruses are potent.

Over one-half of patients in the UK with severe haemophilia have been infected with HIV, and of these two-thirds have died. No new cases of HIV infection from virally inactivated blood products have been detected since 1986. AIDS has been a new cause of death in thalassaemia major patients who have been regularly transfused. The risk is much lower in patients with sickle cell disease, as the frequency of transfusion is lower.

Latency

Although some cells are lysed directly by replicating HIV, the virus remains latent in others and so cannot be recognized by the immune system. Once a latently infected T cell is activated, however, viral replication begins and cell death follows.

Target cells

HIV produces its dominant effects on CD4$^+$ T cells, which are lysed or form syncytia with adjacent CD4$^+$ cells. CD4$^+$ antigen-presenting cells can harbour and release high titres of active virus. The CD4 antigen is the main receptor for HIV and CD4 antibodies and free CD4 antigens can block infection. However, CD4 alone is not sufficient for infection (e.g. mouse cells transfected with human CD4 will not necessarily become infected), and second receptors (CCR4 or CCR5) are required. CD4$^-$ cells, including brain cells and haemopoietic cells, may also be infected using such alternative receptors.

Clinical effects of human immunodeficiency virus

The outcome of HIV infection is divided into four stages (or groups) according to the Centers for Disease Control (CDC) (Table 23.1), and it is not yet clear what factors determine whether (or how rapidly) movement occurs from one stage to the other.

After the initial seroconversion, which is often associated with a febrile mononucleosis-like illness, patients who are HIV antibody-positive enter either group 2 (chronic asymptomatic infection) or group 3 (persistent generalized lymphadenopathy).

Persistent generalized lymphadenopathy, or extended lymphadenopathy syndrome, should be diagnosed only if enlarged lymph nodes in at least two extrainguinal sites have been present for 3 months. There is no evidence that progression into group 4 is different in these patients from those without node enlargement. Biopsy is not now routinely undertaken but may be necessary to exclude lymphoma or Kaposi's sarcoma in a node that suddenly enlarges or, occasionally, in pyrexia of unknown origin, to exclude infection with acid-fast bacilli.

Three histological patterns have been described in biopsies of lymph nodes from HIV antibody-positive patients. Type I is the most common pattern seen in persistent generalized lymphadenopathy in which there is follicular hyperplasia with or without paracortical hyperplasia. The germinal centres are greatly expanded and may show necrosis and haemorrhage (Figure 23.1a). There is a variable loss of surrounding mantle zone lymphocytes. Type II is also seen in persistent generalized lymphadenopathy but is less common and may herald the development of AIDS. There is diffuse lymphoid hyperplasia with loss of germinal centres. Type III pattern, seen in patients with established AIDS, is marked by the absence of lymphoid follicles and severe depletion of both T and B lymphocytes (Figure 23.1b).

Haematological changes

Infection with HIV is associated with a range of haematological abnormalities. The mechanisms for these changes are multiple: quantitative and qualitative marrow defects and immune cytopenias are a direct result of HIV infection, whereas the effects of opportunistic infections, lymphoma and a myriad of drugs against infection, malignancy or HIV itself play an important role. With such a varied assault on the haemopoietic system it is not surprising that peripheral blood and bone marrow abnormalities are common in HIV infection and increase in frequency with advancing disease.

Haemopoiesis

Cytopenia is common in HIV disease and is often associated with morphological abnormalities in peripheral blood and bone

marrow cells suggestive of myelodysplasia. It is likely that HIV directly affects marrow production either by direct infection of precursor cells or by infecting stromal or accessory cells, thereby inducing altered production of regulatory cytokines.

Studies of purified haemopoietic progenitors (CD34$^+$), as well as haemopoietic colonies obtained from semisolid culture, have yielded conflicting results with respect to the presence of HIV DNA, although HIV infection of monocytes/macrophages, promonocyte cell lines, megakaryocytes and eosinophils has been demonstrated as well as infection of bone marrow-derived fibroblast cell lines. Although susceptibility of marrow progenitor cells to infection by HIV *in vitro* has been demonstrated, the extent to which progenitor cell infection *in vivo* contributes to

Table 23.1 Stages of HIV infection according to the Centers for Disease Control (CDCI classification).

CDC 1	**Recently observed illness with seroconversion** (1)
CDC 2	**Well, no generalized lymphadenopathy** (2)
CDC 3	**Well, with generalized lymphadenopathy** (3)
CDC 4A	**Significant constitutional disease (ARC or AIDS)** Fever or night sweats for over 1 month (ARC) (4) Weight loss > 10% (ARC) (5) Diarrhoea for over 1 month, no cause (ARC)*(6) *Wasting syndrome (AIDS) weight loss and diarrhoea, or fever and weakness for over 1 month (7)
CDC 4B	**Neurological** *Dementia (disabling encephalopathy) (AIDS) (10) Myelopathy (11) Peripheral neuropathy (12)
CDC 4C1	**Infections in AIDS** *Diagnosed by definitive method* *Pneumocystis carinii* pneumonia (15) *Cerebral toxoplasmosis (16) *Cryptosporidiosis over 1 month (17) *Oesophageal *Candida* (18) *Bronchial *Candida* (19) *Cryptococcosis (20) *Mycobacterium avium* complex (MAC) (21) *CMV retinitis (22) *CMV oesophagitis (23) *CMV colitis (24) *CMV pneumonitis (25) *Other proven CMV (26) *Mucocutaneous HSV over 1 month (27) *Other HSV (28)

Table 23.1 (cont'd)

CDC 4C1	*Progressive multifocal leucoencephalopathy (PML 29)
	*Isosporiasis (30)
	*Histoplasmosis (31)
	*Coccidioidomycosis (32)
	*Extrapulmonary TB (33)
	*Pulmonary TB (46)
	*Recurrent salmonella septicaemia (34)
	*Recurrent bacterial chest infections (73)
	Diagnosed presumptively
	Pneumocystis carinii pneumonia (37)
	*Cerebral toxoplasmosis (38)
	Mycobacteriu–avium complex (MAC), only AFB+ (39)
	*Oesophageal *Candida* (40)
	PCP – recent symptoms, abnormal chest radiograph, $Pa_{O_2} < 9.3$ and no bacterial pathogen
CDC 4C2	Infections in ARC
	Oral hairy leucoplakia (43)
	Shingles, multidermatomal (44)
	Nocardis (45)
	Oral *Candida* (47)
CDC 4D	Neoplasms in AIDS
	Diagnosed by definitive method
	*Cerebral lymphoma (50)
	*Kaposi's sarcoma (51)
	*Non-Hodgkin's lymphoma (52)
	*Invasive cervical carcinoma (78)
	Diagnosed presumptively
	*Kaposi's sarcoma (55)
	*Cerebral lymphoma (66)
CDC 4E	**Possible HIV-associated disease (not AIDS)**
	Constitutional (not ARC or AIDS)
	Fatigue (59)
	Intermittent diarrhoea (60)
	Intermittent fevers/sweats (61)
	Weight loss < 10% (62)
	Infections
	Strongyloidosis (64)
	Leishmaniasis (65)
	Presumptive CMV disease (66)
	Aspergillosis (67)
	Microsporidiosis (68)
	Salmonella, septicaemia – one episode (69)
	Shigellosis (70)
	Campylobacter (71)
	Giardiasis (72)
	Amoebic dysentery (74)
	Other infections (75)

Table 23.1 (cont'd)

CDC 4E	*Neoplasms*
	Hodgkin's lymphoma (76)
	Invasive anal carcinoma (77)
	Other neoplasms (79)
	Skin
	Seborrhoeic dermatitis (82)
	Folliculitis (83)
	Dry skin (84)
	Frequent HSV (85)
	Psoriasis (86)
	HZV, shingles, one dermatome (87)
	Facial warts (88)
	Non-genital molluscum contagiosum (89)
	Other skin (90)
	Fungal toenail dystrophy (91)
	ZDV nail dyschromia (113)
	ENT
	Gingivitis (93)
	Aphthous ulcer (94)
	Angular stomatitis/cheilitis (95)
	Sinusitis, chronic (96)
	Otitis externa, chronic/recurrent (97)
	Haematological
	Thrombocytopenia, idiopathic = < 20 (100)
	Thrombocytopenia 21–150 (101)
	Anaemia, no cause except HIV (104)
	Haematological other (105)
	Neurological
	Aseptic meningitis (107)
	Guillain–Barré syndrome (108)
	Neurological other (109)
	Cardiovascular
	Cardiomyopathy (114)
	Cardiovascular other (115)
	Gastrointestinal
	Sclerosing cholangitis (116)
	Other GI (117)
	General other
	Arthralgia (102)
	HIV myopathy (103)
	Splenomegaly (111)
	ZDV myopathy (112)
	Primary gonadal failure (118)
	Endocrine other (119)
	General other (120)

*Denotes AIDS diagnosis. A CD4 count < 200 without an AIDS defining illness is considered as an AIDs diagnosis in the USA (but not in Europe).
Number in brackets is the diagnosis code.

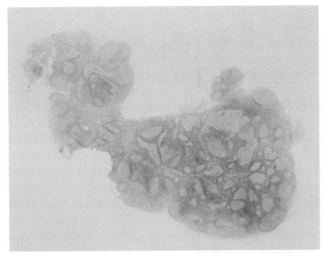

(a)

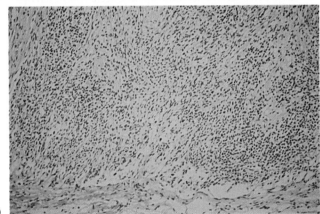

(b)

Figure 23.1 Lymph node biopsy in HIV disease. (a) Type I pattern, showing florid follicular hyperplasia with large irregular germinal centres; (b) type III pattern, showing marked depletion of T lymphocytes and lack of lymphoid follicles with germinal centres (courtesy of Professor K Henry).

abnormal haemopoiesis is uncertain, and it is likely that the effect of HIV on stromal or accessory cells is more important. Infection of marrow accessory cells, T lymphocytes, macrophages, fibroblasts and dendritic cells with HIV leads to overproduction of cytokines, such as tumour necrosis factor (TNF), interleukin 1 (IL-1) and interferons, which have inhibitory effects on marrow progenitor cells. *In vitro* infection of stromal cells leads to impaired colony growth. T-cell depletion of marrow enhances marrow colony production in HIV-infected patients and, when T-cell-depleted marrow is cocultured with increasing concentrations of circulating or marrow T cells, an inverse correlation of T cells with progenitor colony growth is observed. This inhibitory effect of T lymphocytes is not seen in patients who are not infected with HIV.

Cell cultures of bone marrow from patients with HIV infection show a normal response to recombinant growth factors but colony formation is suppressed when anti-HIV antibodies are added to the culture system. This effect is not seen in marrow cultures from seronegative donors, suggesting that anti-HIV antibodies exert a suppressant effect directly on HIV-infected progenitor cells or indirectly on HIV-infected marrow accessory cells.

Thrombocytopenia

Thrombocytopenia is common at all stages of HIV disease and may be the presenting feature. In many patients, an immune basis is strongly suggested by the presence of normal or increased numbers of megakaryocytes in the bone marrow, by the presence of platelet-associated IgG and complement in a high proportion of patients studied, and by the response to conventional treatment for immune thrombocytopenic purpura (ITP). However, thrombocytopenia in HIV disease may also result from marrow impairment, toxic drug effects or the effects of splenomegaly.

The specific mechanism of platelet autoimmunity remains unclear. Higher levels of platelet-bound IgG and complement are seen in HIV-related ITP than in classic ITP, and circulating immune complexes capable of binding normal platelets can be found in the serum. In contrast with classic ITP, the eluates of the platelet-associated immunoglobulins in HIV-associated ITP react against normal platelets in only a minority of patients. In HIV patients, unlike patients with classic ITP, platelet counts are not inversely related to platelet-bound IgG, although it is likely that the deposition of immune complexes leads to increased peripheral destruction of platelets by phagocytic cells. The nature of the immune complexes has been extensively studied. They lack HIV antigen and proviral DNA but contain anti-HIV gp120 and anti-antibodies directed against the anti-HIV antibodies. In some patients cross-reactivity of antibodies against HIV gp120/gp160 with platelet glycoprotein GPIIb/IIIa has been demonstrated.

Platelet kinetic measurements suggest that, in addition to peripheral platelet destruction, ineffective thrombopoiesis is a factor in producing thrombocytopenia in HIV-infected patients, and this may result from the deposition of immune complexes on megakaryocytes, invasion of megakaryocytes by HIV or thrombopoietic inhibitors induced by HIV. The commonly observed dysplastic changes in the megakaryocyte series suggest that dysplasia is an important cause of ineffective platelet production and may be the dominant factor in the thrombocytopenia of advanced HIV disease.

Thrombotic thrombocytopenic purpura has been described in HIV disease and responds to conventional treatment with plasma exchange. The pathophysiology is unclear, although it has been postulated that immune complex damage to platelets and endothelial cells is contributory.

Management of HIV-related ITP

Immune thrombocytopenia in HIV disease does not increase the risk of progression to AIDS so should not be viewed as an indicator of poor prognosis. The response to conventional treatment for ITP does not differ from classic ITP, although the approach to treatment is affected by the presence of HIV infection. Prednisolone is not satisfactory as a first-line treatment because of the risk of potentiating or reactivating infections. If other treatments fail, then prednisolone therapy should be covered with prophylactic antimicrobials against *Pneumocystis carinii* and mycobacteria, at least in patients with significantly reduced CD4 counts. Intravenous immunoglobulin is effective in HIV-related ITP and should probably be the first-line treatment, although the effect is usually only transient. Many patients, however, do not need active treatment and a conservative approach is justified, with intervention only if bleeding occurs, if an invasive procedure is planned, or if the platelet count is judged to be perilously low. Platelet transfusion may permit an adequate, if short-lived, increment sufficient to allow an investigative procedure such as endoscopic biopsy or lumbar puncture.

Splenectomy improves the platelet count in the majority of patients, but may not be justified in a person with advanced HIV disease. It does, however, have a role to play in the management of severe and troublesome ITP in the earlier stages of HIV disease, and there is no evidence that splenectomy contributes to the development of AIDS.

Some patients with HIV-associated thrombocytopenia respond to antiretroviral therapy. This effect was first described using zidovudine, but other agents may have a similar effect. It is likely that antiretroviral treatment exerts its effect by permitting more effective platelet production rather than by decreasing peripheral platelet destruction, thereby emphasizing the two mechanisms involved in HIV-associated thrombocytopenia.

Intravenous anti-D immunoglobulin is effective in a high proportion of RhD-positive patients with ITP and is generally well tolerated, with significant immune haemolysis being uncommon. The mode of action is likely to be Fc receptor blockade by anti-D-coated red blood cells. Patients who have been splenectomized have a much lesser chance of response as the spleen is the primary site of removal of antibody-coated cells.

Other treatment options in HIV-related ITP include danazol, vincristine, interferon-α and extracorporeal immunoabsorption; all have limited success.

Neutropenia

Neutropenia increases in incidence as HIV disease progresses, although it may be present in asymptomatic individuals. Impaired haemopoiesis, as discussed above, is the major factor, although in some patients immune neutrophil destruction may contribute. Antineutrophil antibodies have been detected in some HIV antibody-positive patients by using a granulocyte immunofluorescence technique, but there is poor correlation with the neutrophil count.

In general, neutropenia is well tolerated in HIV-positive individuals, although the risk of infection increases once the neutrophils fall to below 0.5×10^9/L, especially if a central venous catheter is *in situ*.

The responsiveness of HIV patient bone marrow culture to recombinant growth factors *in vitro* has led to the clinical use of recombinant granulocyte–macrophage colony-stimulating factor (GM-CSF) and granulocyte colony-stimulating factor (G-CSF) to reverse neutropenia. Following the administration of recombinant GM-CSF, a rapid dose-dependent increase in neutrophils, bands, eosinophils and monocytes is observed, although there is no increase in haemoglobin or platelets. The effect is reversed when GM-CSF is discontinued. G-CSF is the treatment of choice as it is better tolerated, and reports suggest that doses as low as 100–200 µg are capable of significantly elevating the neutrophil count, although conventional doses are more frequently used. Therapy with marrow-suppressant drugs such as ganciclovir or chemotherapeutic agents may thereby be continued.

There are no convincing studies to suggest that GM-CSF or G-CSF increase HIV-p24 antigenaemia.

Anaemia

The degree of anaemia increases with progression of HIV disease irrespective of other factors, including drug therapy (especially zidovudine), reticuloendothelial iron block, intercurrent infections, especially with atypical mycobacteria, marrow infiltration with lymphoma and haemophagocytic syndrome. It is unlikely that autoimmune haemolysis contributes, although a positive direct antiglobulin reaction is seen in 6–43% of HIV antibody-positive patients and may result from IgG or complement on the surface of the red cells. Although specific antibodies directed against a phospholipid antigen on the red cell could account for the positive antiglobulin test, in many patients this results from non-specific deposition of circulating immune complexes.

Reduced vitamin B_{12} levels have been reported in 10–35% of patients infected with HIV and, although many of these patients have gastrointestinal symptoms or late-stage HIV disease, reduced levels are also described in early, asymptomatic disease. The serum transcobalamin II cobalamin-binding capacity is significantly raised in asymptomatic patients with HIV infection, regardless of the vitamin B_{12} level; this suggests a stage of negative cobalamin balance.

The most likely mechanism underlying the reduced serum cobalamin in HIV disease is malabsorption. Malabsorption of cobalamin assessed by a Schilling test has been demonstrated in some patients with AIDS, and colonic and duodenal biopsies show chronic inflammation within the lamina propria. *In situ* hybridization of the specimens shows HIV to be present within mononuclear cells. Partial villous atrophy in the absence of enteropathogens has been shown in patients at all stages of disease, and HIV antigen p24 is present within the intestinal mucosa of patients presenting with gastrointestinal complaints. There is also some evidence that damage occurs to the gastric mucosa in patients with HIV disease, resulting in a reduced ability to secrete acid and enzymes, which may cause difficulty in releasing cobalamin from protein-binding in food. This might explain the observation that in some HIV patients with reduced cobalamin levels, the Schilling test, in which cobalamin unattached to food is presented to the intestine, is normal.

Cobalamin levels tend to fall along with CD4 cell counts in those patients progressing to AIDS and thus falling serum cobalamin levels are a predictor of disease progression.

Anaemia in HIV disease is not usually due to or compounded by vitamin B_{12} deficiency and would not be expected to improve with vitamin B_{12} therapy.

The major cause of anaemia in HIV disease is impaired erythropoiesis secondary to marrow dysfunction and impaired response to erythropoietin. The anaemia has the characteristics of the anaemia of chronic disease, usually being normochromic, normocytic with a low or normal reticulocyte count. As with other cytopenias, inhibitor cytokines play a central role. In addition, there is an inappropriately low serum level of erythropoietin for the degree of anaemia. Treatment with recombinant erythropoietin may be helpful in patients with an endogenous erythropoietin level of < 500 IU/L. For most patients with severe anaemia, however, management is with red cell transfusions when clinically indicated. An occasional patient develops chronic red cell aplasia following parvovirus infection and may be helped by infusions of intravenous immunoglobulin.

Drugs may cause or exacerbate anaemia, the main culprits being zidovudine, ganciclovir and chemotherapeutic agents, all of which lead to marrow suppression; primaquine and dapsone may provoke oxidative haemolysis in patients with glucose-6-phosphate-dehydrogenase deficiency and even, in high dose, in patients with normal enzyme levels.

Bone marrow changes

Myelodysplasia

Abnormalities in the bone marrow are very common at all stages of HIV disease (Table 23.2), increasing in frequency as the disease progresses. The most common abnormal finding is of dysplasia affecting one or more of the cell lines. In general, the more advanced the disease, the more marked the dysplasia, and, although erythroid dysplasia is the most common finding, being recognized in over 50% of HIV-infected patients, abnormal granulocytic and megakaryocytic development is encountered in approximately one-third of patients.

Dyserythropoiesis may be manifest by florid megaloblastic change. This is unrelated to serum cobalamin and folate levels, or to drug therapy with zidovudine or folate antagonists, although these drugs may accentuate it. Erythroblasts are often bi- or multinucleated, with an irregular nuclear outline and basophilic stippling (Figure 23.2). Abnormal sideroblasts including ringed forms may be present. The frequently observed reticuloendothelial iron block is likely to be secondary to concurrent infection or chronic disease. Erythropoiesis appears disorganized on trephine biopsy with poorly formed erythroid islands.

Dysplastic features in megakaryocytes are common, occurring in over one-third of marrows and including nuclear hypolobulation and micromegakaryocytes (Figure 23.3). On trephine biopsy, megakaryocyte hyperplasia and clustering may be very pronounced. Increased numbers of naked megakaryocytic nuclei are a consistent feature.

Granulocytic dysplasia may be apparent at all stages of maturation, with giant metamyelocytes, nuclear abnormalities including detached nuclear fragments and Pelger cells reflecting

Table 23.2 Features of bone marrow in HIV disease.

Dysplasia	70% of marrows show some dysplastic features
	Erythroid dysplasia 60%
	Granulocytic dysplasia 30%
	Megakaryocytic dysplasia 40%
Cellularity	Increased in over 50%
	Hypocellular 15%
Fibrosis	Seen in 20–50% of trephines and may make aspiration difficult
Reticuloendothelial iron block	Common manifestation of chronic disease
Histiocytes	Increased and may show haemophagocytosis
Plasma cells	Increased and may be atypical
Opportunistic infections	Culture or examination of slides may show acid-fast bacilli (AFB), leishmania, histoplasma, pneumocystis, cryptococcus
Granulomas	Seen in infection with AFB and cryptococcus
Lymphoid aggregates	Reactive nodules
AIDS-related lymphoma (ARL)	20% of patients with ARL have bone marrow involvement

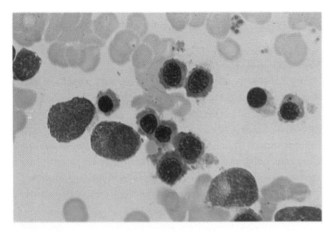

Figure 23.2 Erythroid dysplasia in HIV disease.

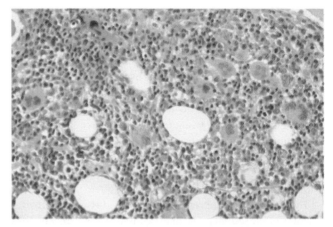

Figure 23.4 Bone marrow trephine biopsy in HIV disease, showing hypercellularity and increased numbers of dysplastic megakaryocytes.

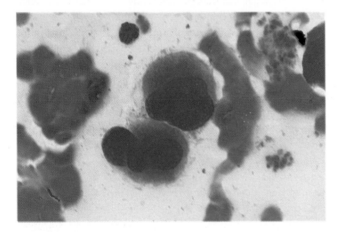

Figure 23.3 Dysplastic megakaryocytes in HIV disease.

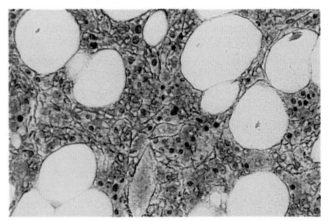

Figure 23.5 Bone marrow trephine biopsy in HIV disease, showing increased fibrosis.

dysfunctional nuclear maturation. On trephine biopsy, the atypical localization of immature precursors, a feature that has been highlighted in primary myelodysplastic syndrome, is sometimes observed in HIV marrows. Apoptosis is increased. In non-HIV patients, granulocytic dysplasia may precede acute leukaemia. Although several HIV antibody-positive patients with acute myeloid leukaemia have been described, the role of myelodysplasia in the evolution of acute leukaemia in HIV disease is uncertain. Its rarity and the failure to detect chromosomal abnormalities in patients with marked dysplastic changes suggest that myelodysplasia in the setting of HIV disease is not generally a pre-leukaemic state, thus differing from the classic myelodysplastic syndrome. The term 'HIV-related myelodysplasia' has been coined to describe the changes in HIV disease.

Ultrastructure studies of bone marrow cells from patients infected with HIV have shown abnormalities in erythroid cells, marrow granulocytes, plasma cells and stromal cells, which were attributed to a direct effect of HIV infection. No definite viral particles were detected at electron microscopy level, although the presence of incomplete virus particles was not excluded. The abnormalities in stromal cells lend credence to the hypo-

thesis that disturbances in the microenvironmental regulation of haemopoiesis may contribute to cytopenias.

Cellularity

Marrow from HIV-infected patients is sometimes difficult to aspirate and the trails are of decreased cellularity. The true marrow cellularity is better appreciated on trephine biopsy, which is hypercellular in a majority of patients (Figure 23.4). The difficulty in aspiration may in part be due to the increased reticulin fibrosis seen especially in hypercellular marrows (Figure 23.5). Hypercellularity of the marrow in the face of peripheral cytopenia is a very common finding in HIV disease and is likely to reflect myeloid dysplasia and ineffective haemopoiesis. Indeed, there is a correlation between observed marrow dysplastic changes and the peripheral blood findings of anaemia and leucopenia.

Red cell hypoplasia has been described in patients with HIV disease and may be associated with infection with B19 parvovirus and disseminated *Mycobacterium avium intracellulare*. Severe erythroid hypoplasia has also been described in patients receiving therapy with zidovudine.

Gelatinous transformation (serous fat atrophy) is common in marrow from HIV patients and has been described previously in patients with severe malnutrition and weight loss.

Histiocytes

Increased numbers of histiocytes are often seen in the bone marrow and in many patients haemophagocytosis is striking. Reactive haemophagocytosis has been described in patients suffering from a wide variety of viral, bacterial, fungal and parasitic infections and is more common in immunosuppressed patients. In many of the patients with HIV infection who show increased numbers of marrow histiocytes, there is no obvious infective cause and it is likely that HIV itself is the trigger to histiocyte proliferation and phagocytosis, probably by initiation of cytokine production, resulting in macrophage stimulation. It is likely that as a result of HIV infection the marrow produces a histiocytic reaction, which varies from increased numbers of histiocytes to a full-blown haemophagocytic syndrome with severe pancytopenia.

Plasma cells

Plasma cells are often strikingly increased in the marrow of HIV-infected patients. They may represent a physiological response to antigenic stimulation by viruses or other infective agents, or may be secondary to dysregulated B-cell proliferation due to HIV. The marrow plasmacytosis is not confined to those patients with advanced HIV disease in whom opportunistic infections could be implicated, but is seen also in patients at an early stage who have no concurrent infections. The plasma cells are often morphologically abnormal and may appear in clusters. A polyclonal increase in gammaglobulins occurs in most HIV patients. Paraproteinaemia occurs in approximately 9% of homosexual HIV antibody-positive men without AIDS. This is much higher than the incidence of paraproteins in healthy people of similar age and may result either from changes in T-cell regulation or from the activation of B lymphocytes directly infected by HIV. The prognostic significance of paraproteinaemia in HIV antibody-positive patients is unknown. It does not appear to be more common in patients developing non-Hodgkin's lymphoma (NHL), although this also occurs in the setting of clonal B-cell activation. Some of the paraproteins have activity against HIV *gag* and *pol* gene products and may represent a vigorous immune response to HIV infection.

Multiple myeloma has been described in a few patients with HIV disease and occurs at a much younger age than in the general population.

Lymphoid aggregates

Lymphoid aggregates are identified in one-third of trephine biopsies and are likely to be benign manifestations of infection with HIV rather than a response to opportunistic infections or a herald of malignant lymphoma.

Opportunistic infections

Bone marrow examination and culture have a contribution to make to the diagnosis of opportunistic infections. Trephine biopsy may yield histochemical evidence of acid-fast bacilli or fungal organisms (Figure 23.6). Acid-fast bacilli (both *Mycobacterium tuberculosis* and atypical mycobacteria) may be cultured from the bone marrow of patients with disseminated infection. The bone marrow may be the only site of culture, despite culturing of blood, induced sputum and bronchoalveolar lavage.

Disseminated infection with *Leishmania donovani-infantum* and *Histoplasma capsulatum* may be diagnosed on the basis of marrow examination (Figures 23.7, 23.8 and 23.9). Clinically, these infections may be atypical in immunosuppressed patients and serological tests are not always helpful. Marrow aspirate and trephine biopsy material, as well as marrow culture, are useful in the monitoring of response to treatment.

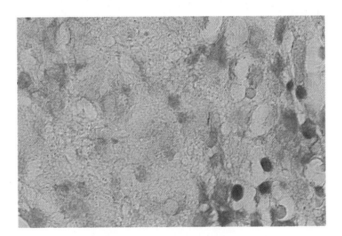

Figure 23.6 Acid-fast bacilli in trephine biopsy in HIV disease.

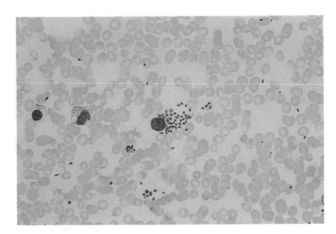

Figure 23.7 Leishman–Donovan bodies in macrophage in bone marrow of patient with AIDS.

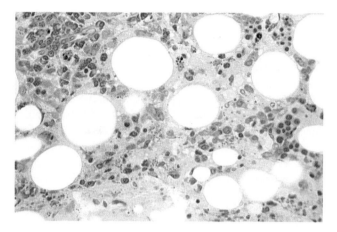

Figure 23.8 Leishman–Donovan bodies in trephine biopsy of patient with AIDS.

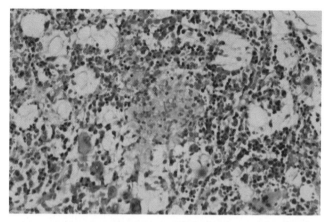

Figure 23.10 Bone marrow trephine biopsy from a patient with AIDS, showing well-defined granuloma.

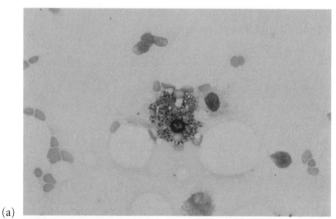

(a)

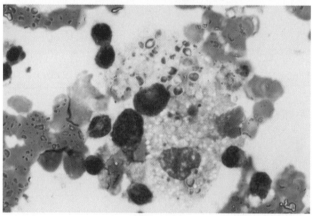

(b)

Figure 23.9 (a and b) *Histoplasma capsulatum* in macrophage in bone marrow of patient with AIDS.

tion that the major risk factor for infection with *Mycobacterium avium–intracellulare* is the level of immune dysfunction.

Granulomas (Figure 23.10) may be seen in marrows of patients secondarily infected with mycobacteria and have also been described in cryptococcal infection. Well-formed granulomas are not often associated with atypical mycobacteria and, when associated with *M. tuberculosis*, caseation is usually conspicuously absent.

Clinical value of bone marrow examination

Examination of the bone marrow is useful in the diagnosis and staging of AIDS-related lymphoma, marrow infiltration being seen in approximately one-fifth of patients; in some patients the marrow represents the initial evidence of lymphoma. Kaposi's sarcoma is extremely rare in the bone marrow.

Culture of marrow aspiration and careful examination of slides from aspirate and trephine biopsy are of value in the diagnosis of opportunistic infections and in the monitoring of treatment.

Immune thrombocytopenia can be suspected on the evidence of plentiful megakaryocytes in the marrow, along with peripheral thrombocytopenia. The value of marrow examination in elucidating the cause of anaemia and leucopenia is less obvious but has occasionally yielded an unexpected diagnosis of disseminated leishmaniasis or histoplasmosis in patients with pancytopenia.

The clinical value of bone marrow examination is in:
1 microbiological culture in patients with fever of unknown cause;
2 exclusion or staging of lymphoma;
3 diagnosis of immune thrombocytopenic purpura;
4 elucidation of cytopenias (value less clear).

Lupus anticoagulant

The lupus anticoagulant has been described in patients infected with HIV. This circulating anticoagulant is an IgG or IgM

Cryptococci and *P. carinii* have been demonstrated in marrow aspirates and trephine biopsies in patients infected with HIV. Patients in whom opportunistic organisms are present in the bone marrow are profoundly immunosuppressed, as manifest by very low CD4 cell counts. This is in keeping with the observa-

immunoglobulin, which inhibits *in vitro* activity of the prothrombin activator complex, thus prolonging the partial thromboplastin time and, to a lesser extent, the prothrombin time.

Thrombotic events in patients with AIDS are rare when compared with patients with the lupus anticoagulant in other settings, where thromboembolic phenomena are common. Patients with a prolonged partial thromboplastin time secondary to a lupus anticoagulant do not appear to be at increased risk of bleeding.

The pathophysiological basis for the development of the lupus anticoagulant in HIV disease is not understood, but an association with active opportunistic infection, especially with *P. carinii* has been suggested.

Anticardiolipin antibodies have also been described in HIV disease but do not correlate with the presence of a lupus anticoagulant.

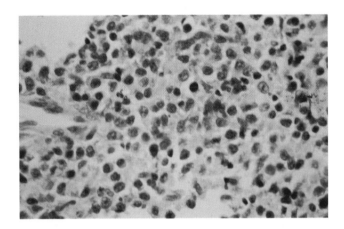

Figure 23.11 Diffuse large-cell lymphoma (courtesy of Professor K Henry).

AIDS-related lymphoma

It has long been recognized that patients with both inherited and acquired abnormalities of cellular immunity have an increased incidence of non-Hodgkin's lymphoma. The incidence of lymphoproliferative disorders in patients with primary immunodeficiency diseases, such as ataxia telangiectasia or the Wiscott–Aldrich syndrome, is approximately 100 times greater than expected; NHL in allograft recipients has an incidence 60 times that of the general population. In a similar way to these patients, individuals infected with HIV have defective cellular immunity and are thus at risk of developing B-cell malignancy, which is recognized as an AIDS-defining diagnosis. Both systemic and cerebral NHL occur in this population with the relative risk being approximately 100-fold higher than that expected in the general population.

The introduction of combination highly active anti-retroviral treatment (HAART) in the late 1990s has led to a reduction in AIDS-defining illnesses, including NHL. Adjusted incidence rates show a decline in incidence of AIDS-related lymphoma (ARL) from 1992 to 1996, and from 1997 to 1999, with a relative risk ratio of 0.58. This decline is most marked for cerebral lymphoma but is also significant for systemic disease. There remains, however, a significant risk among patients on HAART, and a higher risk in those who do not have access to HAART, either because of economic restrictions or because they are unaware of their HIV status. Overall, it is estimated that approximately 10% of HIV-infected individuals will develop NHL.

Histopathology

Over 90% of systemic ARL are high-grade B-cell tumours and within the WHO/REAL classification approximately two-thirds are diffuse large cell lymphomas (20% of which are confined to the central nervous system), whereas one-third are Burkitt's

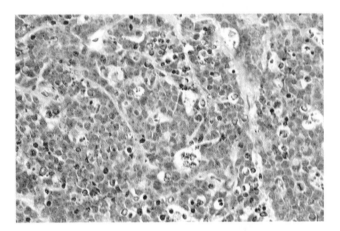

Figure 23.12 Burkitt's lymphoma: small non-cleaved lymphoma with scattered macrophages giving characteristic 'starry-sky' appearance (courtesy of Professor K Henry).

lymphoma (Figures 23.11 and 23.12). The incidence of T-cell lymphoma is also increased but only five- to tenfold. In addition, two uncommon lymphoproliferative disorders that are associated with human herpesvirus 8 are seen in this population: primary effusion lymphoma (PEL) or body-cavity lymphoma and multicentric Castleman's disease. Histologically, PEL is a CD30[-](Ki-1)-positive anaplastic large cell lymphoma.

Occasionally, low-grade B-cell lymphomas are reported in HIV patients but there is no epidemiological evidence that these cases have increased in parallel with the AIDS epidemic and no evidence that these patients respond differently to treatment when compared with non-HIV-infected individuals. A few patients with B-cell acute lymphoblastic leukaemia (FAB L3) in HIV disease have been described, and it is likely that these cases represent peripheral blood involvement with Burkitt's lymphoma.

Aetiology

In all groups of immunosuppressed patients it seems that malignant lymphoma arises in the setting of polyclonal B-cell proliferation secondary to impaired T-cell surveillance. Reactivation of latent Epstein–Barr virus (EBV) infection is likely to play a significant role in this proliferation. Following primary infection with EBV, some B cells appear to switch to a latency 1 pattern expressing only EBNA-1, a nuclear antigen, and these cells may escape destruction by cytotoxic T lymphocytes and persist, thus permitting reactivation of EBV, long-term stimulation and proliferation of B lymphocytes resulting in the development of NHL.

Some B-cell lymphomas from patients with ataxia telangiectasia have been shown to contain the EBV genome and several studies have documented its presence in the vast majority of B-cell lymphomas from allograft recipients. The EBV genome is a uniform finding in endemic African Burkitt's lymphoma, although it is uncommon in the sporadic type. The precise role of EBV in the development of ARL is controversial; EBV genomic sequences or EBV proteins have been demonstrated in fewer than one-half of HIV-associated Burkitt's lymphoma, although they have been shown in the majority of systemic and primary cerebral lymphomas.

HIV itself is unlikely to be directly involved in the malignant transformation of B-lymphocytes. No HIV sequences have been detected in B-lymphoma tissues and they are not detected in the reactive B-cell hyperplasia commonly seen before the evolution of lymphoma. HIV may, however, indirectly encourage the development of lymphoma by initiating the release of cytokines such as IL-1, IL-6, IL-10, TNF and B-cell growth factors, which stimulate B-cell proliferation.

The continuous stimulus to B lymphocytes may permit mutations in critical oncogenes or tumour-suppressor genes, eventually resulting in malignant transformation. The development of multiple clonal rearrangements of immunoglobulin genes within the reactive lymphadenopathy lesions of HIV-infected patients may represent precursors to the development of lymphoma.

Specific chromosomal translocations have been described in endemic, sporadic and HIV-related Burkitt's lymphoma in which t(8;14), t(8;22) or t(8;2) are commonly found. These translocations permit deregulation of the c-*myc* oncogene, which might encourage malignant transformation.

Some data suggest that the HIV diffuse large cell lymphomas are primarily driven by rearrangements of the oncogene *bcl* 6. In addition, mutations in the *p53* cancer-suppressing gene have been found in about 40% of cases of ARL, mostly Burkitt's.

In summary, it is likely that lymphoma in HIV disease arises from the chronic stimulation of B lymphocytes by EBV or cytokines that are produced as a result of HIV infection. In the setting of defective cellular immunity, this stimulation of B lymphocytes may lead to mutation in critical oncogenes or tumour-suppressor genes, permitting c-*myc* activation, clonal selection and the development of malignant lymphoma.

Clinical picture

In more than one-half of the patients with ARL, this is the presenting feature of AIDS. Data from the CDC relating to patients in whom lymphoma was the AIDS-defining diagnosis suggest that Burkitt's lymphoma is seen at a younger age than diffuse large cell lymphoma, the incidence of which increases with age. Primary cerebral lymphomas occur equally in all age groups and are of the immunoblastic type.

The majority (up to 98%) of patients with systemic ARL present with extensive disease and systemic (B) symptoms. Extranodal lymphoma is very common, occurring in the majority of patients at presentation: frequently, the disease is exclusively extranodal. The most common extranodal sites of lymphoma in HIV patients are gastrointestinal tract, liver, meninges (up to 20%), lung, bone marrow (approximately 20%) and oropharynx. Lymphoma in unusual sites such as the heart, adrenals, kidneys, skin, testes, mouth, muscle, soft tissue, anus and rectum occur more frequently in HIV-infected patients.

Primary cerebral lymphoma can be difficult to distinguish from cerebral toxoplasmosis and magnetic resonance imaging (MRI) may be more sensitive than computerized tomography (CT) in making the distinction, although only brain biopsy can make a definitive diagnosis. In practice, however, a trial of anti-toxoplasma therapy is fully justified, with brain biopsy being only rarely indicated. The presence of EBV, detected by polymerase chain reaction in cerebrospinal fluid, may give a clue to the diagnosis without recourse to biopsy in many patients with HIV-associated primary cerebral lymphoma.

Management

Patients with HIV disease are already at risk of opportunistic infections as a result of HIV-related immune suppression; chemotherapy would be expected to increase this risk. Furthermore, the bone marrow in AIDS patients is frequently impaired and likely to be seriously compromised as a result of marrow-toxic chemotherapeutic agents. The immunosuppressive effects of chemotherapy may precipitate acceleration of the HIV disease itself. Management therefore poses considerable problems with this group of patients.

However, the advent of HAART, improved prophylaxis against opportunistic infections and intrathecal prophylaxis support a more aggressive approach to treatment for systemic ARL, with better outcomes being reported. Many units now use standard-dose chemotherapy and are reporting response rates and overall survival that approach those in the immunocompetent. The prognosis for primary cerebral lymphoma remains very poor such that palliative treatment is usually the only option.

Table 23.3 Features of AIDS-related non-Hodgkin's lymphoma.

Histopathology (%)	Diffuse large cell (DLC)	65 (including primary cerebral lymphoma)
	Small cell non-cleaved (Burkitt's)	33
	Primary effusion lymphoma	2
EBV implicated (%)	Burkitt's	< 50
	Systemic DLC	80
	Primary cerebral lymphoma	100
	Primary effusion lymphoma	100
Prognosis features for AIDS-related NHL*		
Major adverse prognostic factors	Prior AIDS diagnosis	
	CD4 count < 100/μL	
	ECOG performance status > 2	
	Primary cerebral origin	
Minor adverse prognostic factors	Bone marrow involvement	
	Extranodal disease	
	Raised serum LDH	
	Age > 35 years	

*Good prognosis defined by less than two major adverse prognostic factors; poor prognosis is defined by more than one major adverse prognostic factor.

In centres without access to HAART, a prognosis-stratified approach to the management of ARL may be taken. Patients falling into the poor prognosis group (Table 23.3) may be treated with palliative intent using a combination of prednisolone, vincristine and bleomycin, with radiotherapy for localized symptomatic lesions. The life expectancy for these patients is 3–6 months. Patients with a better prognosis may be treated with combination chemotherapy such as CHOP (cyclophosphamide, doxorubicin, vincristine and prednisolone) or mBACOD (methotrexate, bleomycin, doxorubicin, cyclophosphamide, vincristine and dexamethasone), perhaps with the support of granulocyte colony-stimulating factor. Complete remission rates are approximately 60%. The role of rituximab (a monoclonal antibody directed against CD20) in ARL is under investigation.

Following chemotherapy, 40% of the patients with good prognostic features will remain in remission until another AIDS-related illness such as opportunist infection occurs. Recent studies show higher median survivals with little change in response rate for ARL, suggesting that the improved duration of survival is related to reduced deaths from opportunistic infections in the HAART era among patients who have durable remissions of their ARL.

The concomitant use of antiretroviral agents with chemotherapy is generally accepted practice with the possible exceptions of zidovudine, which significantly adds to the myelosuppression of combination chemotherapy, and didanosine, which may worsen the peripheral neuropathy caused by vincristine. Little is known about the pharmokinetic interaction of protease inhibitors and non-nucleoside reverse transcriptase inhibitors with chemotherapy.

It is routine practice to instigate prophylaxis against pneumocystis, M. avium intracellulare and toxoplasmosis in individuals receiving chemotherapy for ARL.

As there is a high rate of meningeal involvement in systemic ARL, intrathecal chemotherapy should be given to patients with meningeal disease or at high risk of cranial disease by virtue of Burkitt's histology or extensive paranasal sinus and base of skull disease. Most centres also recommend prophylactic chemotherapy for patients with bone marrow involvement.

A recent development in ARL chemotherapy has been the introduction of infusional therapy with CDE (cyclophosphamide, daunorubicin and etoposide) or EPOCH (etoposide, prednisolone, vincristine, cyclophosphamide and daunorubicin). In a recent study by Little and co-workers, a dose-adjusted EPOCH regimen with suspension of HAART achieved a complete remission in 74% of patients and at 53 months median follow-up, disease-free and overall survival were 92% and 60% respectively. A multicentre trial is under way to confirm these results.

The dose-adjusted strategy was developed to reduce haematological toxicity while maintaining maximum drug doses. In vitro studies have shown that tumour cells are relatively less resistant to prolonged low-concentration exposure compared with brief high concentration exposure. In addition, infusional therapy is more effective against highly proliferative tumours such as ARL.

The question is raised as to whether treatment with HAART alters the biology of the tumour, making it less resistant to chemotherapy. Low BCL-2 and high CD10 expression are observed, both implying a germinal centre origin, a feature associated with good-prognosis disease. The high expression of p53 indicates a highly proliferative tumour, but in HAART-treated patients this is not associated with a poor outcome.

In Little's study, discontinuing HAART during chemotherapy led to increases in viral load, which fell below baseline within 3 months of resuming treatment, and decreases in CD4 cells, which recovered within 4 months of reintroducing HAART. This suggests that withholding antiretroviral treatment does not significantly worsen the AIDS prognosis while avoiding the potentially adverse effects on lymphoma treatment.

Hodgkin's disease

The incidence of Hodgkin's disease is increased up to eightfold in HIV-infected individuals and is strongly associated with EBV. Most patients present with advanced disease and extranodal involvement with poor prognosis subtypes – mixed cellularity or lymphocyte depleted. The outcome of therapy is poor with opportunist infections and poor marrow reserve, making treatment difficult.

Drugs used in HIV disease

Inevitably, in a disease that results in opportunistic infections and opportunistic malignancies, multiple drug therapy is common, especially in patients with advanced disease. These are the very patients who commonly have compromised bone marrow function, and thus it is not surprising that marrow-toxic antiretroviral, antimicrobial and antimitotic drugs may have profound effects on their blood picture.

The introduction of HAART has transformed the prognosis in HIV infection with dramatic reductions in opportunistic infections and mortality. Long-term survival now seems possible, although deaths from HIV-associated liver disease and lymphoma are increasing as patients survive longer. At present, guidelines recommend initiating treatment when the CD4 count falls below 350 cells/μL or when the viral load (plasma HIV RNA) is in excess of 30 000 copies/mL in asymptomatic individuals. Patients who present with clinical manifestations of HIV should also receive treatment.

Antiretroviral agents

Antiretroviral drugs fall into three groups:
1 Nucleoside analogues, such as zidovudine, are phosphorylated within cells to their active triphosphate metabolites, which are incorporated into nucleic acids. They prevent the formation of double-stranded DNA from viral RNA by reverse transcriptase. Nucleotide analogues, for example tenofovir, have recently become available and work by a similar mechanism.

2 Non-nucleoside reverse transcriptase inhibitors prevent the same process; they are not incorporated into nucleic acids but bind directly to reverse transcriptase.
3 Protease inhibitors inhibit the viral protease that is responsible for cleaving precursor proteins, thereby preventing formation of fully formed infectious viral particles.

HAART usually comprises three or more drugs in combination. The usual starting combination is two nucleoside analogues, together with either a protease inhibitor or a non-nucleoside reverse transcriptase inhibitor. Treatment failure as determined by viral load, CD4 cell count or clinical progression requires a new regimen, with substitution or addition of at least two new agents. Newer agents including attachment inhibitors, fusion inhibitors, coreceptor antagonists and integrase inhibitors are undergoing clinical trials at present.

Prophylaxis against opportunistic infections

The timing of institution of primary prophylaxis differs according to the infective agent. In the prevention of *P. carinii* infection, a CD4 cell count of less than 200 cells/μL indicates a requirement for prophylactic treatment, for *Toxoplasma gondii*, less than 100 cells/μL, and for *M. avium*, less than 50 cells/μL.

Haematological toxicity of drugs used in HIV disease

Antiretroviral agents

Haematologically the most toxic antiretroviral agent is the nucleoside analogue, zidovudine. This was the first drug shown to be inhibitory to HIV and was initially used in larger doses than employed at present. Anaemia was the most common haematological toxic effect and repeated blood transfusions were frequently necessary, especially in patients with advanced disease. Marrow hypoplasia was often severe. New combination treatments with antiretroviral agents now permit smaller doses of zidovudine to be used with consequent reduced toxicity. Other nucleoside analogues such as didanosine (ddI), zalcitabine (ddC) and lamuvidine (3TC) have a low incidence of marrow toxicity. Protease inhibitors such as saquinavir, ritonavir and indinavir do not appear to suppress haemopoiesis.

Antimicrobial agents

Cotrimoxazole
Cotrimoxazole is effective both in the treatment and prevention of *P. carinii* pneumonia (PCP). A high proportion of HIV-infected patients, however, experience adverse effects from this drug combination, thus limiting its use. The most common problem is nausea, although this is less troublesome with intravenous administration. Skin reactions are commoner in the

HIV-infected population and the Stevens–Johnson syndrome is a potentially life-threatening complication. The dose of cotrimoxazole used in the treatment of PCP is high, and bone marrow toxicity is common due to the effects on folic acid metabolism and possibly to the suppression of DNA synthesis of marrow cells. Treatment with folic acid or folinic acid does not reduce the severity of marrow suppression and its attendant pancytopenia.

Pentamidine

Pentamidine isethionate is very effective against *P. carinii* but has major toxic side-effects of hypotension, hypoglycaemia, renal damage and bone marrow suppression, although the latter is less frequent than with cotrimoxazole. Nebulized pentamidine is less toxic and can be used in the treatment of mild or moderate PCP or in prophylaxis.

Dapsone

Dapsone is used as an agent for PCP prophylaxis and in combination with trimethoprim for the treatment of PCP but can cause haemolytic anaemia at high dosage and special care must be taken to exclude glucose-6-phosphate dehydrogenase deficiency in susceptible individuals.

Fansidar

This combination of sulphadoxine and pyrimethamine has been shown to be an effective prophylactic combination against PCP and may also provide effective prophylaxis against toxoplasmosis. In a twice-weekly regimen, haematological side-effects are uncommon, but long-term administration may lead to cytopenias, especially if other folate inhibitors such as cotrimoxazole are also administered. Fansidar is rarely used now because of severe skin rashes.

Ganciclovir

Ganciclovir (dihydrophosphoguanine) is a derivative of acyclovir and is effective when given intravenously in serious cytomegalovirus (CMV) infection, including CMV retinitis. It produces severe bone marrow suppression, especially neutropenia, in a high percentage of patients and this is probably worsened by concurrent administration of zidovudine. Valganciclovir, an oral prodrug of ganciclovir, has recently been shown to be as effective for induction treatment of CMV retinitis as ganciclovir, and has a similar degree of haematological toxicity. Oral ganciclovir is less marrow toxic than the intravenous preparation but is ineffective as treatment of CMV though may be useful for prophylaxis.

Antimitotic agents

Kaposi's sarcoma

The vinca alkaloids vinblastine and vincristine are both effective agents against Kaposi's sarcoma. Vinblastine is more toxic to the bone marrow than vincristine, especially when used in combination with doxorubicin. Bleomycin, also effective in Kaposi's sarcoma, does not usually lead to marrow suppression, whereas etoposide, another very effective agent, can lead to severe neutropenia. The suppressive effects of antimitotic agents are more pronounced in advanced HIV disease when the marrow is already compromised by the effects of HIV and, possibly, by concurrently administered antimicrobial or antiretroviral agents.

AIDS-related lymphoma

The problems of chemotherapy in NHL associated with HIV infection have been discussed earlier. As in Kaposi's sarcoma, the more powerful combinations of chemotherapeutic agents are significantly immunosuppressive and run the risk of precipitating opportunistic infections at the same time as provoking serious bone marrow suppression.

Hepatitis C in HIV disease

Hepatitis C virus (HCV) is especially common among haemophiliacs and intravenous drugs users, most of whom carry both viruses. As deaths from HIV disease are declining as a result of HAART, liver disease has become an increasing cause of morbidity and mortality. The immunodeficiency associated with HIV infection accelerates the course of HCV infection and the hepatotoxicity of anti-HIV drugs poses particular problems.

HIV antibody-positive patients who fulfil standard criteria for chronic hepatitis C (persistent elevated aminotransaminase levels, detectable serum HCV-RNA and necroinflammatory activity with portal or bridging fibrosis in the liver biopsy) respond less well to combination treatment with interferon-α and ribavirin than HIV antibody-negative patients, although this is linked to the degree of immunosuppression. Slow-release interferon-α, covalently bound to polyethylene glycol (pegylated form) can provide continuous exposure to interferon-α with a single weekly injection. Ribavirin can cause haemolytic anaemia, although this is not usually severe. Care should be taken when it is prescribed along with other nucleoside analogues (especially zidovudine) that cause bone marrow suppression and ddI, which causes severe mitochondrial toxicity.

Selected bibliography

Bain BJ (1997) The haematological features of HIV infection. *British Journal of Haematology* 99: 1–8.

Bain BJ (1998) Lymphomas and reactive lymphoid lesions in HIV infection. *Blood Reviews* 12: 154–62.

Bower M (2002) The management of lymphoma in the immunosuppressed patient. *Best Practice and Research in Clinical Haematology* 15: 517–32.

Caldena V, Chermann JC (1992) The effects of HIV on hematopoiesis. *European Journal of Haematology* 48: 181–6.

Centres for Disease Control and Prevention (CDC) (1992) Revised classification system for HIV infection and expanded surveillance care definition for AIDS among adolescents and adults. Centres for Disease Control and Prevention (CDC), Atlanta, GA, 1992. *Morbidity and Mortality Weekly Report* **41**: 1–19.

Cohen AJ, Philips TM, Kessler CM (1986) Circulating coagulation inhibitors in the acquired immunodeficiency syndrome. *Annals of Internal Medicine* **104**: 175–80.

Coyte TE (1997) Haematological complications of human immunodeficiency virus infection and the acquired immunodeficiency syndrome. *Medical Clinics of North America* **81**: 449–70.

Doweiko JP (1993) Management of the hematologic manifestations of HIV disease. *Blood Reviews* **7**: 121–6.

Harriman GR, Smith PD, Horne MK *et al.* (1989) Vitamin B12 malabsorption in patients with acquired immunodeficiency syndrome. *Archives of Internal Medicine* **149**: 2039–41.

Henry DH, Beall GN, Benson CA *et al.* (1992) Recombinant human erythropoietin in the treatment of anaemia associated with human immunodeficiency virus (HIV) infection and zidovudine therapy. Overview of four clinical trials. *Annals of Internal Medicine* **117**: 739–48.

Henry K, Costello C (1994) HIV-associated bone marrow changes. *Current Diagnostic Pathology* **1**: 131–41.

Holland HK, Spivak JL (1990) The haematological manifestations of acquired immune deficiency syndrome. *Baillières Clinical Haematology* **3**: 103–14.

Kaczmarski RS, Mufti GJ (1993) The pathophysiology and management of HIV-associated haematological abnormalities. *Haematologia* **25**: 1–17.

Karcher DS, Frost AR (1991) The bone marrow in human immunodeficiency virus (HIV)-related disease. *American Journal of Clinical Pathology* **95**: 63–71.

Karpatkin S (1990) HIV-related thrombocytopenia. *Baillière's Clinical Haematology* **3**: 115–38.

Levine AM (2000) Acquired immunodeficiency syndrome-related lymphoma: clinical aspects. *Seminars in Oncology* **27**: 442–53.

Levine AM (2001) Anaemia in HIV Infection. *Journal of the International Association of Physicians in AIDS Care* Winter (Suppl.): 61–72.

Little RF, Pittaluga S, Grant N *et al.* (2003) Highly effective treatment of acquired immunodeficiency syndrome-related lymphoma with dose-adjusted EPOCH: impact of antiretroviral therapy suspension and tumour biology. *Blood* **101**: 4653–9.

Miles SA (1992) Hematopoietic growth factors as adjuncts to antiretroviral therapy. *AIDS Research on Human Retroviruses* **8**: 1073–80.

Moses A, Nelson J, Bagby GC Jr (1998) The influence of human immunodeficiency virus-I on hematopoiesis. *Blood* **91**: 1479–95.

Panel of Clinical Practices for Treatment of HIV Infection (1999) Guidelines for the use of antiretroviral agents in HIV-infected adults and adolescents, 5 May 1999, online. Available: http://www.hivatis.org (16 December 1999).

Rodriguez-Rosado R, Garcia-Samaniego J, Soriano V (1999) Hepatitis C, an emerging problem in HIV-infected patients. *AIDS Review* **1**: 22–8.

Scaradovou A (2002) HIV-related thrombocytopenia. *Blood Reviews* **16**: 73–6.

Wickramasinghe SN, Beatty C, Sheils S *et al.* (1992) Ultrastructure of the bone marrow in HIV infection: evidence of dyshaemopoiesis and stromal cell damage. *Clinical and Laboratory Haematology* **14**: 213–29.

CHAPTER 24

Histocompatibility

24

Ann-Margaret Little, Steven GE Marsh and J Alejandro Madrigal

The major histocompatibility complex and human leucocyte antigens

In the 1950s, three independent scientists, Jean Dausset, Rose Payne and Jon van Rood, described the presence of alloantibodies in the sera of individuals exposed to genetically non-identical tissues such as the fetus in pregnancy and/or blood cells after transfusion. These alloantibodies were subsequently shown to react against protein antigens, encoded by a genetic region called the major histocompatibility complex (MHC). The MHC had also independently been identified in animal models of skin transplantation and tumour immunology, when genetically different strains of mice were shown to reject transplants from one another. Genetically identical mice could accept such transplants without rejection.

These observations led to theories of self–non-self discrimination, and the elucidation of the genetics of the MHC genes encoding the protein 'histocompatibility' (or transplantation) antigens. Analysis of the structure and function of histocompatibility antigens has led to the establishment of routine transplant protocols for both solid organ and haemopoietic stem cells between genetically disparate individuals.

The MHC in humans is located on the short arm of chromosome 6 (6p21.3). This region of the genome has been studied extensively and fully sequenced as part of the human genome project (www.sanger.ac.uk/HGP/Chr6/). The MHC is an extremely gene-dense region of the genome and it can be divided into 'three' subregions, based on the type of genes found.

The genes encoding histocompatibility antigens are located within the MHC class I and II regions (Figure 24.1). These genes are called HLA genes (defined as human leucocyte antigens – although originally called human locus-A). HLA genes found in the class I region differ in structure from those found in the class

II region and, as a result, the encoded proteins also differ. HLA class I genes encode a polypeptide of ~340 amino acids. This polypeptide is found as a cell-surface transmembrane glycoprotein and is associated with the soluble protein β_2-microglobulin (β_2m) encoded by a gene on chromosome 15.

There are three classical class I genes: HLA-A, HLA-B and HLA-C. Their encoded proteins are expressed on virtually all nucleated cells within the body and also on platelets. The expression of HLA class I proteins varies for different types of tissues. For example, expression is high on lymphocytes but low on hepatocytes and tissues constituting the nervous system. In addition, there are class I genes encoding non-classical class I molecules called HLA-E, HLA-F and HLA-G. The tissue distribution of these molecules is more restricted than that of HLA-A, B and C, and this is a reflection of their differing function. These molecules are not considered as transplantation antigens.

HLA class II molecules are overall similar in structure to HLA class I molecules. They are also composed of two polypeptide chains (α and β); however, both are encoded by MHC genes. HLA class II molecules, unlike class I, have a restricted tissue distribution. They are expressed on haemopoietic cells such as B cells, dendritic cells, macrophages and also activated (but not resting) T cells. There are three classical class II molecules: HLA-DR, HLA-DQ and HLA-DP. In addition, there are other non-classical class II molecules encoded by the HLA-DM and HLA-DO genes. These non-classical class II molecules are not transplantation antigens, but do contribute to the antigen-presenting function of class II molecules.

The class III region of the MHC does not contain any HLA genes. This region contains genes encoding proteins with various different functions, including proteins involved in the immune response such as TNFα and -β and complement components C2, C4 and Bf.

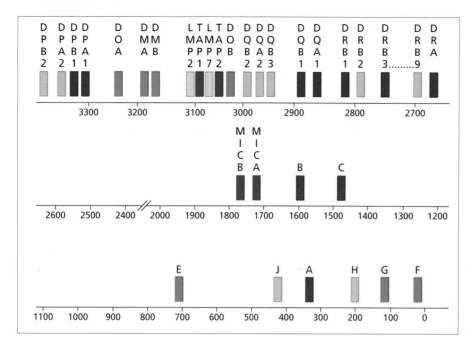

Figure 24.1 The major histocompatibility complex. Approximate location of HLA-A, -B, -C, -DRA, -DRB, -DQA, -DQB, -DPA and -OPB genes are indicated. Other related genes are also present.

Structure of HLA proteins

The X-ray crystallographic structure of the extracellular domains of several HLA class I and II proteins has been obtained. The structures are divided into four domains, as illustrated in Figure 24.2. The two most membrane-distal domains, α_1 and α_2 for HLA class I and α_1 and β_1 for HLA class II, form a β-pleated sheet, surrounded on both sides by two α-helices. In both class I and II structures, a short peptide was found bound in the cleft formed. Thus, both class I and class II proteins can be considered as trimolecular proteins consisting of three subunits: HLA heavy chain, β_2-microglobulin and peptide form class I molecules, and HLA α- and β-chains and peptide form class II molecules.

Antigen processing and presentation

Peptide binding to HLA class I and II proteins plays an important role in the function of these molecules. The way in which peptides are derived and the binding procedure differs for the two classes of molecules, and this is reflected in the different function of these molecules.

HLA class I molecules are assembled within the endoplasmic reticulum (ER). The heavy chain is directed to the ER via a leader peptide sequence. Within the lumen of the ER, the extracellular domains of the heavy chain associate with β_2-microglobulin. This association is mediated by ER-resident chaperones including calnexin and calreticulum.

Association with peptide also occurs within the ER. Peptides are derived from the cytoplasmic degradation of molecules that takes place in the proteasome, a multicatalytic protein complex. Peptides produced by the proteasome are actively transported into the ER via a transmembrane peptide pump called TAP (transporter associated with antigen processing). Association between HLA class I heavy chain–β_2-microglobulin complex and peptide is catalysed by another ER resident chaperone called tapasin.

Once the class I trimolecular complex is formed, the molecule can leave the ER and complete its journey to the cell surface via the Golgi apparatus.

The journey of a class II molecule differs from that of a class I

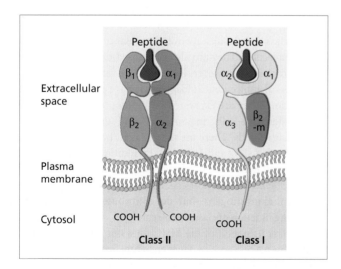

Figure 24.2 HLA class I and II molecules showing protein domains and bound peptide.

molecule. Both α- and β-chains are directed to the ER, where a complex of three αβ chains and three invariant chains is formed. The invariant chain (Ii) is also a transmembrane protein. Association of HLA class II molecules with Ii effectively blocks the peptide binding site on the class II molecule, thus preventing association of ER-resident peptides. Invariant chain cytoplasmic tail sequences direct the class II molecule through the Golgi apparatus, but, unlike class I molecules, the class II molecules make a detour to endosomal vesicles before arriving at the cell surface. The non-classical HLA-DM and HLA-DO molecules are located within endosomal vesicles, and it is here that the Ii chain is cleaved, leaving a peptide, called CLIP, to block the class II peptide binding cleft. Specific peptide binding is catalysed by HLA-DM, and may also be aided by HLA-DO. The peptides that bind to class II molecules are derived either from internalization of cell surface or from extracellular proteins. Thus, the antigen presentation pathway for HLA class II molecules differs from that of HLA class I molecules by directing the class II molecules to a location where they can bind peptides that differ from those presented by class I molecules.

HLA function

Once presented at the cell surface, HLA molecules are subjected to surveillance by circulating T cells and natural killer (NK) cells. Both of these cell types possess receptors that can recognize and interact with HLA molecules. Typically, T cells expressing the CD4 molecule recognize HLA class II molecules, and T cells expressing CD8 recognize HLA class I molecules. The specificity of interaction is determined during development of T cells within the thymus, such that circulating T cells should not interact with HLA molecules presenting peptides derived from normally expressed self proteins. However, the presentation of non-self peptides, for example peptides derived from viral or bacterial proteins, or aberrant expression of tumour antigens, can initiate activatory signals mediated by the T-cell receptor, resulting in the generation of an immune response against infected cells.

The interactions between HLA molecules and NK cell receptors play an important role in the function of NK cells. NK cells primarily function in innate immune responses. These cells express a range of receptors that can elicit either activatory or inhibitory signals. It is the balance between the two opposing signals that determines the action of an NK cell. Typically, interaction between HLA molecule and corresponding NK receptor resulting in a negative signal will outweigh any activatory signals; thus, the NK cell will not attack the cell expressing the HLA molecule. However, if a cell has lost expression of HLA molecules such as after malignancy or virus-induced downregulation, then the absence of the inhibitory signal will result in the activatory signal being dominant and allow NK cell-mediated attack on the target cell.

HLA nomenclature

The naming of HLA specificities falls under the remit of the WHO Nomenclature Committee for Factors of the HLA System. The Committee names HLA genes, alleles and serologically defined antigenic specificities. The names of the antigens, which were originally defined using either serological or cellular techniques, are a combination of letters that indicate the gene encoding the antigen and numbers assigned in chronological order of their description. An example of an individual's HLA type determined by cellular and serological methods is A1, A2; B7, B13; Cw6, Cw7; Dw1, Dw13; DR1, DR4; DR53; DQ5, DQ8; DPw1, DPw4.

The numbering of antigens encoded by HLA-A and -B genes is in a single series for historical reasons, as these antigens were originally believed to represent the products of a single gene. The use of a lower case 'w' between the gene name and antigen number to indicate a provisional specificity has been used, although in most cases these have been removed. The exceptions are Bw4 and Bw6, which represent public epitopes rather than distinct antigens, HLA-C antigens (e.g. Cw1), to distinguish them from complement factors, and the HLA-D and HLA-DP antigens defined by cellular techniques.

Many HLA antigens have been characterized by serological methods into two or more subtypes, which are called 'splits', with the parent antigen called 'broad'. Thus, both A23 and A24 are splits of the broad antigen A9. It is convention to indicate the broad antigen specificity in parentheses following the designation of the split, for example A23(9) or A24(9). A full listing of all the serologically and cellularly defined HLA antigens is given in Table 24.1.

Since 1987, the WHO Nomenclature Committee for Factors of the HLA System has assigned official names to HLA allele sequences. It was recognized that a single antigenic specificity, such as HLA-A2, defined by serology could be subdivided still further by DNA sequencing. Each allele is given a numerical designation that may be up to eight digits in length. The gene name is followed by an asterisk (*) and then the numerical designation; the first two digits indicate the allele group, which often corresponds to the broad serological antigen encoded by the allele. The third and fourth digits are used to list subtypes, numbers assigned in the order in which the DNA sequences have been determined. Alleles whose numbers differ in the first four digits must differ in one or more nucleotide substitutions that change the amino acid sequence of the encoded protein. The fifth and six digits are used to name alleles that differ only by synonymous nucleotide substitutions (also called silent or noncoding). The seventh and eighth digits are used to name alleles that differ in either intron, or 3′- or 5′-regions of the gene. Lastly, an allele may have a suffix indicating an aberrant expression; for example an N indicates that it is a null allele with no protein being expressed, an L indicates low cell-surface expression, and an S indicates that the molecule is expressed only in a soluble form.

Table 24.1 Complete listing of recognized serological and cellular HLA specificities.

A	B		C	D	DR	DQ	DP
A1	B5	B70	Cw1	Dw1	DR1	DQ1	DPw1
A2	B7	B71(70)	Cw2	Dw2	DR103	DQ2	DPw2
A203	B703	B72(70)	Cw3	Dw3	DR2	DQ3	DPw3
A210	B8	B73	Cw4	Dw4	DR3	DQ4	DPw4
A3	B12	B75(15)	Cw5	Dw5	DR4	DQ5(1)	DPw5
A9	B13	B76(15)	Cw6	Dw6	DR5	DQ6(1)	DPw6
A10	B14	B77(15)	Cw7	Dw7	DR6	DQ7(3)	
A11	B15	B78	Cw8	Dw8	DR7	DQ8(3)	
A19	B16	B81	Cw9(w3)	Dw9	DR8	DQ9(3)	
A23(9)	B17	Bw4	Cw10(w3)	Dw10	DR9		
A24(9)	B18	Bw6	Dw11(w7)	DR10			
A2403	B21		Dw12	DR11(5)			
A25(10)	B22		Dw13	DR12(5)			
A26(10)	B27		Dw14	DR13(6)			
A28	B2708		Dw15	DR14(6)			
A29(19)	B35		Dw16	DR1403			
A30(19)	B37		Dw17(w7)	DR1404			
A31(19)	B38(16)		Dw18(w6)	DR15(2)			
A32(19)	B39(16)		Dw19(w6)	DR16(2)			
A33(19)	B3901		Dw20	DR17(3)			
A34(10)	B3902		Dw21	DR18(3)			
A36	B40		Dw22				
A43	B4005		Dw23	DR51			
A66(10)	B41						
A68(28)	B42		Dw24	DR52			
A69(28)	B44(12)		Dw25				
A74(19)	B45(12)		Dw26	DR53			
A80	B46						
	B47						
	B48						
	B49(21)						
	B50(21)						
	B51(5)						
	B5102						
	B5103						
	B52(5)						
	B53						
	B54(22)						
	B55(22)						
	B56(22)						
	B57(17)						
	B58(17)						
	B59						
	B60(40)						
	B61(40)						
	B62(15)						
	B63(15)						
	B64(14)						
	B65(14)						
	B67						

Broad specificities are indicated in parentheses.

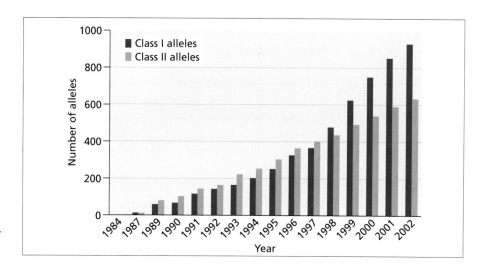

Figure 24.3 The increase in number of HLA alleles identified by year.

For example, the A*24020101 and A*24020102L alleles differ only by a single nucleotide that lies within an intron at a splice site. A*24020101 is expressed at normal levels on the cell surface; however, A*24020102L is expressed at very low levels on the cell surface due to the splice mutation.

Many new HLA alleles are reported each year (Figure 24.3). Details of the most recent advances in HLA nomenclature can be found in the latest WHO Nomenclature Committee for Factors of the HLA System Report or by accessing the IMGT/HLA Sequence Database, the official database of the Nomenclature Committee (www.ebi.ac.uk/imgt/hla).

HLA polymorphism

The outstanding feature of HLA genes and the proteins encoded by the genes is the extensive polymorphism exhibited. At each of the genes, there are multiple possible variants (Tables 24.2 and 24.3). These variants are called alleles. The nucleotide sequence differences between HLA alleles at a given locus can be translated into the protein sequence and analyses of the polymorphism has demonstrated that most variation exists within the peptide-binding domains. Experimental data support this by showing that different HLA proteins can bind peptides with different sequences. Thus, one of the functions of HLA polymorphism is to allow the presentation of different peptides to the immune system. As there are six antigen-presenting 'classical' HLA molecules (HLA-A, -B, -C, -DR, -DQ, -DP), and most individuals are heterozygous for these loci; one can see that potentially each individual has 12 different HLA molecules, each of which can bind thousands of different peptides. The existence of a polymorphic polygenic antigen-presenting system gives each individual the capacity to elicit immune responses against a wide variety of protein antigens.

HLA polymorphism also varies within different populations.

Table 24.2 Number of HLA alleles and serologically defined antigens, by June 2003.

HLA gene	No. of alleles	No. of antigens
A	282	24
B	540	49
C	136	9
DRA	2	–
DRB1	342	20
DRB3	39	1
DRB4	12	1
DRB5	17	1
DQA1	20	–
DQB1	55	7
DPA1	20	–
DPB1	106	–

Variation in climate, geography and infectious agents are all factors that are considered to have influenced the evolution of HLA polymorphism, therefore it is not surprising to find that different ethnic groups display different HLA types.

Thus, HLA polymorphism functions as an advantage both at the level of an individual and population. The extreme diversity found makes it extremely likely that that someone somewhere should possess an HLA molecule that can be effective in generating an immune response against any infectious agent.

HLA associations with disease

As both HLA class I and class II molecules control the positive and negative selection of T-cell receptors in the thymus, it is not surprising to find many associations between HLA loci and

Table 24.3 Complete listing of defined HLA alleles and serological specificities, by June 2003.

HLA-A alleles	HLA-A antigen specificity	HLA-B alleles	HLA-B antigen specificity	HLA-C alleles	HLA-C antigen specificity	HLA-DR alleles	HLA-DR antigen specificity	HLA-DQ alleles	HLA-DQ antigen specificity	HLA-DP alleles	HLA-DP antigen specificity
A*010101	A1	B*070201	B7	Cw*0102	Cw1	DRA*0101	–	DQA1*010101	–	DPA1*010301	–
A*010102	–	B*070202	B7	Cw*0103	Cw1	DRA*010201	–	DQA1*010102	–	DPA1*010302	–
A*0102	A1	B*070203	B7	Cw*0104	–	DRA*010202	–	DQA1*010201	–	DPA1*0104	–
A*0103	A1	B*0703	B703	Cw*0105	–			DQA1*010202	–	DPA1*0105	–
A*0104N	Null	B*0704	B7	Cw*0106	–	DRB1*010101	DR1	DQA1*0103	–	DPA1*0106	–
A*0106	–	B*0705	B7	Cw*0107	–	DRB1*010102	–	DQA1*010401	–	DPA1*0107	–
A*0107	A1	B*0706	B7	Cw*020201	Cw2	DRB1*010201	DR1	DQA1*010402	–	DPA1*0108	–
A*0108	A1	B*0707	B7	Cw*020202	Cw2	DRB1*010202	DR1	DQA1*0105	–	DPA1*020101	–
A*0109	–	B*0708	–	Cw*020203	Cw2	DRB1*0103	DR103	DQA1*0106	–	DPA1*020102	–
A*020101	A2	B*0709	B7	Cw*020204	Cw2	DRB1*0104	DR1	DQA1*0201	–	DPA1*020103	–
A*020102	A2	B*0710	–	Cw*020205	–	DRB1*0105	–	DQA1*030101	–	DPA1*020104	–
A*020103	A2	B*0711	B7	Cw*0203	–	DRB1*0106	–	DQA1*0302	–	DPA1*020105	–
A*020104	A2	B*0712	B7	Cw*0204	–	DRB1*0107	–	DQA1*0303	–	DPA1*020106	–
A*020105	A2	B*0713	–	Cw*0205	–	DRB1*0108	–	DQA1*0401	–	DPA1*020201	–
A*020106	–	B*0714	–	Cw*030201	Cw10(w3)	DRB1*030101	DR17(3)	DQA1*050101	–	DPA1*020202	–
A*0202	A203	B*0715	B7	Cw*030202	Cw10(w3)	DRB1*030102	DR17(3)	DQA1*050102	–	DPA1*020203	–
A*0203	A203	B*0716	–	Cw*030301	Cw9(w3)	DRB1*030201	DR18(3)	DQA1*0502	–	DPA1*0203	–
A*0204	A2	B*0717	B7	Cw*030302	Cw9(w3)	DRB1*030202	DR18(3)	DQA1*0503	–	DPA1*0301	–
A*0205	A2	B*0718	–	Cw*030303	Cw9(w3)	DRB1*0303	DR18(3)	DQA1*0504	–	DPA1*0302	–
A*0206	A2	B*0719	–	Cw*030401	Cw10(w3)	DRB1*0304	DR17(3)	DQA1*0505	–	DPA1*0401	–
A*0207	A2	B*0720	–	Cw*030402	Cw10(w3)	DRB1*030501	DR17(3)	DQA1*060101	–		
A*0208	A2	B*0721	–	Cw*0305	–	DRB1*030502		DQA1*060102	–		
A*0209	A2	B*0722	–	Cw*0306	–	DRB1*0306	DR3	DQB1*0201	DQ2	DPB1*010101	DPw1
A*0210	A210	B*0723	–	Cw*0307	Cw3	DRB1*0307	DR3	DQB1*0202	DQ2	DPB1*010102	DPw1
A*0211	A2	B*0724	B7	Cw*0308	–	DRB1*0308	–	DQB1*0203	DQ2	DPB1*020102	DPw2
A*0212	A2	B*0725	–	Cw*0309	Cw3	DRB1*0309	–	DQB1*030101	DQ7(3)	DPB1*020103	DPw2
A*0213	A2	B*0726	B7	Cw*0310	Cw3	DRB1*0310	DR17(3)	DQB1*030102	DQ7(3)	DPB1*020104	DPw2
A*0214	A2	B*0727	–	Cw*0311	–	DRB1*0311	DR17(3)	DQB1*0302	DQ8(3)	DPB1*020105	DPw2
A*0215N	Null	B*0728	–	Cw*0312	–	DRB1*0312	DR3	DQB1*03032	DQ9(3)	DPB1*020106	DPw2
A*0216	A2	B*0729	–	Cw*0313	–	DRB1*0313	–	DQB1*03033	DQ9(3)	DPB1*0202	DPw2
A*021701	A2	B*0730	–	Cw*0314	–	DRB1*0314	DR3	DQB1*0304	DQ7(3)	DPB1*030101	DPw3
A*021702	A2	B*0731	–	Cw*0315	–	DRB1*0315	–	DQB1*030501	DQ8(3)	DPB1*030102	DPw3
A*0218	A2	B*0801	B8	Cw*04010101	Cw4	DRB1*0316	–	DQB1*030502	–	DPB1*0401	DPw4
A*0219	–	B*0802	B8	Cw*04010102	–	DRB1*0317	–			DPB1*0402	DPw4
A*022001	A2	B*0803	B8	Cw*040102	Cw4	DRB1*0318	–	DQB1*0306	DQ3	DPB1*0501	DPw5
A*022002	A2	B*0804	–	Cw*0403	–	DRB1*0319	–	DQB1*0307	–	DPB1*0601	DPw6

A*		B*		Cw*		DRB1*		DQB1*		DPB1*	
A*0221	A2	B*0805	–	Cw*0404	–	DRB1*0320	–	DQB1*0308	–	DPB1*0801	–
A*0222	A2	B*0806	B8	Cw*0405	–	DRB1*0321	–	DQB1*0309	–	DPB1*0901	–
A*0224	A2	B*0807	B8	Cw*0406	–	DRB1*0322	–	DQB1*0310	DQ8(3)	DPB1*1001	–
A*0225	A2	B*0808N	Null	Cw*0407	Null	DRB1*0323	DR4	DQB1*0311	–	DPB1*110101	–
A*0226	–	B*0809	B8	Cw*0408	Null	DRB1*040101	DR4	DQB1*0312	–	DPB1*110102	–
A*0227	–	B*0810	B8	Cw*0409N	Cw4	DRB1*040102	DR4	DQB1*0313	–	DPB1*1301	–
A*0228	–	B*0811	–	Cw*0410	Cw5	DRB1*0402	DR4	DQB1*0401	DQ4	DPB1*1401	–
A*0229	A2	B*0812	–	Cw*0501	Cw5	DRB1*040301	DR4	DQB1*0402	DQ4	DPB1*1501	–
A*0230	–	B*0813	–	Cw*0502	Cw5	DRB1*040302	DR4	DQB1*050101	DQ5(1)	DPB1*1601	–
A*0231	A2	B*0814	–	Cw*0503	–	DRB1*0404	DR4	DQB1*050102	DQ5(1)	DPB1*1701	–
A*0232N	Null	B*0815	–	Cw*0504	–	DRB1*040501	DR4	DQB1*050201	DQ5(1)	DPB1*1801	–
A*0233	–	B*0816	–	Cw*0505	–	DRB1*040502	DR4	DQB1*050202	–	DPB1*1901	–
A*0234	A2	B*1301	B13	Cw*0602	Cw6	DRB1*040503	DR4	DQB1*050301	DQ5(1)	DPB1*200101	–
A*0235	–	B*1302	B13	Cw*0603	–	DRB1*040504	–	DQB1*050302	DQ5(1)	DPB1*200102	–
A*0236	–	B*1303	–	Cw*0604	–	DRB1*0406	DR4	DQB1*0504	DQ5(1)	DPB1*2101	–
A*0237	–	B*1304	–	Cw*0605	Cw6	DRB1*040701	DR4	DQB1*060101	DQ6(1)	DPB1*2201	–
A*0238	–	B*1306	–	Cw*0606	–	DRB1*040702	DR4	DQB1*060102	DQ6(1)	DPB1*2301	–
A*0239	–	B*1307N	Null	Cw*0607	–	DRB1*0408	DR4	DQB1*060103	DQ6(1)	DPB1*2401	–
A*0240	–	B*1308	–	Cw*070101	Cw7	DRB1*0409	DR4	DQB1*0602	DQ6(1)	DPB1*2501	–
A*0241	A2	B*1309	–	Cw*070102	Cw7	DRB1*0410	DR4	DQB1*0603	DQ6(1)	DPB1*260101	–
A*0242	A2	B*1310	–	Cw*07020101	Cw7	DRB1*0411	DR4	DQB1*060401	DQ6(1)	DPB1*260102	–
A*0243N	Null	B*1401	B64(14)	Cw*07020102	Cw7	DRB1*0412	–	DQB1*060402	DQ6(1)	DPB1*2701	–
A*0244	–	B*1402	B65(14)	Cw*0703	–	DRB1*0413	DR4	DQB1*060501	DQ6(1)	DPB1*2801	–
A*0245	–	B*1403	B14	Cw*070401	Cw7	DRB1*0414	DR4	DQB1*060502	DQ6(1)	DPB1*2901	–
A*0246	A2	B*1404	–	Cw*070402	Cw7	DRB1*0415	DR4	DQB1*0606	–	DPB1*3001	–
A*0247	–	B*1405	–	Cw*0705	–	DRB1*0416	DR4	DQB1*0607	–	DPB1*3101	–
A*0248	–	B*140601	B14	Cw*0706	Cw7	DRB1*0417	DR4	DQB1*0608	DQ6(1)	DPB1*3201	–
A*0249	–	B*140602	B14	Cw*0707	–	DRB1*0418	–	DQB1*0609	DQ6(1)	DPB1*3301	–
A*0250	A2	B*15010101	B62(15)	Cw*0708	–	DRB1*0419	DR4	DQB1*0610	–	DPB1*3401	–
A*0251	–	B*15010102N	Null	Cw*0709	–	DRB1*0420	DR4	DQB1*061101	DQ1	DPB1*3501	–
A*0252	–	B*150102	B62(15)	Cw*0710	–	DRB1*0421	DR4	DQB1*061102	DQ1	DPB1*3601	–
A*0253N	Null	B*150103	B62(15)	Cw*0711	–	DRB1*0422	DR4	DQB1*0612	DQ1	DPB1*3701	–
A*0254	–	B*150104	B62(15)	Cw*0712	–	DRB1*0423	DR4	DQB1*0613	–	DPB1*3801	–
A*0255	–	B*1502	B75(15)	Cw*0713	–	DRB1*0424	DR4	DQB1*0614	DQ6(1)	DPB1*3901	–
A*0256	–	B*1503	B72(70)	Cw*0714	Cw7	DRB1*0425	DR4	DQB1*0615	–	DPB1*4001	–
A*0257	–	B*1504	B62(15)	Cw*0715	–	DRB1*0426	DR4	DQB1*0616	–	DPB1*4101	–
A*0258	–	B*1505	B62(15)	Cw*0716	–	DRB1*0427	–	DQB1*0617	–	DPB1*4401	–
A*030101	A3	B*1506	B62(15)	Cw*080101	Cw8	DRB1*0428	DR4	DQB1*0618	–	DPB1*4501	–
A*030102	A3	B*1507	B62(15)	Cw*080102	Cw8	DRB1*0429	DR4	DQB1*0619	–	DPB1*4601	–
A*030103	A3	B*1508	B75(15)	Cw*0802	Cw8	DRB1*0430	–	DQB1*0620	–	DPB1*4701	–
A*0302	A3	B*1509	B70	Cw*0803	Cw8	DRB1*0431	DR4			DPB1*4801	–

Continued on next page

Table 24.3 (cont'd)

HLA-A alleles	HLA-A antigen specificity	HLA-B alleles	HLA-B antigen specificity	HLA-C alleles	HLA-C antigen specificity	HLA-DR alleles	HLA-DR antigen specificity	HLA-DQ alleles	HLA-DQ antigen specificity	HLA-DP alleles	HLA-DP antigen specificity
A*0303N	Null	B*1510	B71(70)	Cw*0804	Cw8	DRB1*0432	DR4			DPB1*4901	—
A*0304	A3	B*151101	B75(15)	Cw*0805	—	DRB1*0433	—			DPB1*5001	—
A*0305	A3	B*151102	B75(15)	Cw*0806	—	DRB1*0434				DPB1*5101	—
A*0306	—	B*1512	B76(15)	Cw*0807	—	DRB1*0435				DPB1*5201	—
A*0307	—	B*1513	B77(15)	Cw*0808	—	DRB1*0436				DPB1*5301	—
A*0308	—	B*1514	B76(15)	Cw*0809	—	DRB1*0437				DPB1*5401	—
A*0309	—	B*1515	B62(15)	Cw*120201	—	DRB1*0438				DPB1*5501	—
A*110101	A11	B*1516	B63(15)	Cw*120202	—	DRB1*0439				DPB1*5601	—
A*110102	A11	B*15170101	B63(15)	Cw*120203	—	DRB1*0440				DPB1*5701	—
A*1102	A11	B*15170102	B63(15)	Cw*120301	—	DRB1*0441				DPB1*5801	—
A*1103	A11	B*1518	B71(70)	Cw*120302	—	DRB1*0442	DR4			DPB1*5901	—
A*1104	A11	B*1519	B76(15)	Cw*120401	—	DRB1*0443	—			DPB1*6001	—
A*1105	A11	B*1520	B62(15)	Cw*120402	—	DRB1*0444	—			DPB1*6101N	Null
A*1106	—	B*1521	B75(15)	Cw*1205	—	DRB1*070101	DR7			DPB1*6201	—
A*1107	A11	B*1523	—	Cw*1206	—	DRB1*070102	DR7			DPB1*6301	—
A*1108	—	B*1524	B62(15)	Cw*1207	—	DRB1*0703	DR7			DPB1*6401N	Null
A*1109	—	B*1525	B62(15)	Cw*1208	—	DRB1*0704	DR7			DPB1*6501	—
A*1110	A11	B*1526N	Null	Cw*140201	—	DRB1*0705	—			DPB1*6601	—
A*1111	—	B*1527	B62(15)	Cw*140202	—	DRB1*0706	—			DPB1*6701	—
A*1112	A11	B*1528	B62(15)	Cw*1403	—	DRB1*080101	DR8			DPB1*6801	—
A*1113	A11	B*1529	B15	Cw*1404	—	DRB1*080102	—			DPB1*6901	—
A*2301	A23(9)	B*1530	B62(15)	Cw*1405	—	DRB1*080201	DR8			DPB1*7001	—
A*2302	—	B*1531	B75(15)	Cw*150201	—	DRB1*080202	DR8			DPB1*7101	—
A*2303	—	B*1532	B62(15)	Cw*150202	—	DRB1*080203	DR8			DPB1*7201	—
A*2304	—	B*1533	B15	Cw*1503	—	DRB1*080302	DR8			DPB1*7301	—
A*2305	—	B*1534	B15	Cw*1504	—	DRB1*080401	DR8			DPB1*7401	—
A*2306	—	B*1535	B62(15)	Cw*150501	—	DRB1*080402	DR8			DPB1*7501	—
A*2307N	Null	B*1536	—	Cw*150502	—	DRB1*080403	DR8			DPB1*7601	—
A*2308N	Null	B*1537	B70c	Cw*1506	—	DRB1*080404	DR8			DPB1*7701	—
A*2309	—	B*1538	—	Cw*1507	—	DRB1*0805	DR8			DPB1*7801	—
A*24020101	A24(9)	B*1539	B62(15)	Cw*1508	—	DRB1*0806	DR8			DPB1*7901	—
A*24020102L	Low A24	B*1540	—	Cw*1509	—	DRB1*0807	DR8			DPB1*8001	—
A*240202	A24(9)	B*1542	—	Cw*1510	—	DRB1*0808	—			DPB1*8101	—
A*240203	A24(9)	B*1543	—	Cw*1511	—	DRB1*0809	DR8			DPB1*8201	—
A*240301	A2403	B*1544	—	Cw*1601	—	DRB1*0810	DR8			DPB1*8301	—
A*240302	A2403	B*1545	B62(15)	Cw*1602	—	DRB1*0811	DR8			DPB1*8401	—

A*		B*		Cw*		DRB1*		DPB1*	
A*2404	A24(9)	B*1546	B72(70)	Cw*160401	—	DRB1*0812	DR8	DPB1*8501	—
A*2405	A24(9)	B*1547	—	Cw*1701	—	DRB1*0813	—	DPB1*8601	—
A*2406	A24(9)	B*1548	B62(15)	Cw*1702	—	DRB1*0814	DR8	DPB1*8701	—
A*2407	A24(9)	B*1549	—	Cw*1703	—	DRB1*0815	—	DPB1*8801	—
A*2408	A24(9)	B*1550	B70	Cw*1801	—	DRB1*0816	DR8	DPB1*8901	—
A*2409N	Null	B*1551	—	Cw*1802	—	DRB1*0817	DR8	DPB1*9001	—
A*2410	A2403	B*1552	—			DRB1*0818	—	DPB1*9101	—
A*2411N	Null	B*1553	—			DRB1*0819	—	DPB1*9201	—
A*2413	A24(9)	B*1554	—			DRB1*0820	—		
A*2414	A24(9)	B*1555	B15			DRB1*0821	—		
A*2415	—	B*1556	—			DRB1*0822	—		
A*2417	—	B*1557	—			DRB1*0823	—		
A*2418	—	B*1558	B15			DRB1*0824	—		
A*2419	—	B*1560	—			DRB1*090102	DR9		
A*2420	—	B*1561	—			DRB1*0902	—		
A*2421	—	B*1562	—			DRB1*100101	DR10		
A*2422	A9	B*1563	—			DRB1*100102	DR10		
A*2423	A24(9)	B*1564	—			DRB1*110101	DR11(5)		
A*2424	—	B*1565	—			DRB1*110102	DR11(5)		
A*2425	—	B*1566	—			DRB1*110103	DR11(5)		
A*2426	—	B*1567	—			DRB1*110104	DR11(5)		
A*2427	—	B*1568	—			DRB1*1102	DR11(5)		
A*2428	—	B*1569	—			DRB1*1103	DR11(5)		
A*2429	—	B*1570	B62(15)			DRB1*110401	DR11(5)		
A*2430	—	B*1571	B62(15)			DRB1*110402	DR11(5)		
A*2431	—	B*1572	—			DRB1*1105	DR11(5)		
A*2432	—	B*1573	B62(15)			DRB1*1106	DR11(5)		
A*2433	A2403	B*180101	B18			DRB1*1107	DR11(5)		
A*2434	—	B*180102	B18			DRB1*110801	DR11(5)		
A*2435	Null	B*1802	B18			DRB1*110802	DR11(5)		
A*2436N	Null	B*1803	B18			DRB1*1109	DR11(5)		
A*2501	A25(10)	B*1804	—			DRB1*1110	DR11(5)		
A*2502	A10	B*1805	B18			DRB1*1111	DR11(5)		
A*2503	—	B*1806	B18			DRB1*111201	—		
A*2504	—	B*1807	—			DRB1*111202	DR11(5)		
A*2601	A26(10)	B*1808	—			DRB1*1113	DR11(5)		
A*2602	A26(10)	B*1809	B18			DRB1*1114	DR11(5)		
A*2603	A26(10)	B*1810	—			DRB1*1115	—		
A*2604	A26(10)	B*1811	—			DRB1*1116	DR11(5)		
A*2605	A26(10)	B*1812	—			DRB1*1117	—		
A*2606	A26(10)	B*1813	—			DRB1*1118	—		

Continued on next page

Table 24.3 (cont'd)

HLA-A alleles	HLA-A antigen specificity	HLA-B alleles	HLA-B antigen specificity	HLA-C alleles	HLA-C antigen specificity	HLA-DR alleles	HLA-DR antigen specificity	HLA-DQ alleles	HLA-DQ antigen specificity	HLA-DP alleles	HLA-DP antigen specificity
A*2607	A26(10)	B*1814	–			DRB1*1119	DR11(5)				
A*2608	A26(10)	B*1815	–			DRB1*1120	DR11(5)				
A*2609	A26(10)	B*1817N	–			DRB1*1121	DR11(5)				
A*2610	A10	B*1818	–			DRB1*1122	–				
A*2611N	Null	B*2701	B27			DRB1*1123	DR11(5)				
A*2612	–	B*2702	B27			DRB1*1124	–				
A*2613	–	B*2703	B27			DRB1*1125	DR11(5)				
A*2614	–	B*2704	B27			DRB1*1126	DR11(5)				
A*2615	–	B*270502	B27			DRB1*112701	DR11(5)				
A*2616	–	B*270503	B27			DRB1*112702	DR11(5)				
A*2617	–	B*270504	B27			DRB1*1128	–				
A*2618	–	B*270505	B27			DRB1*1129	DR11(5)				
A*29010101	A29(19)	B*2706	B27			DRB1*1130	–				
A*29010102N	Null	B*2707	B27			DRB1*1131	–				
A*2902	A29(19)	B*2708	B2708			DRB1*1132	–				
A*2903	–	B*2709	B27			DRB1*1133	–				
A*2904	–	B*2710	B27			DRB1*1134	–				
A*2905	–	B*2711	B27			DRB1*1135	–				
A*2906	–	B*2712	–			DRB1*1136	–				
A*3001	A30(19)	B*2713	B27			DRB1*1137	–				
A*3002	A30(19)	B*2714	–			DRB1*1138	–				
A*3003	A30(19)	B*2715	–			DRB1*1139	–				
A*3004	A30(19)	B*2716	–			DRB1*1140	–				
A*3006	–	B*2717	B27			DRB1*1141	–				
A*3007	–	B*2718	–			DRB1*1142	–				
A*3008	–	B*2719	B27			DRB1*1143	–				
A*3009	–	B*2720	B27			DRB1*120101	DR12(5)				
A*3010	–	B*2721	–			DRB1*120102	DR12(5)				
A*3011	A30(19)	B*2723	–			DRB1*120201	DR12(5)				
A*3012	–	B*2724	–			DRB1*120202	DR12(5)				
A*310102	A31(19)	B*2725	–			DRB1*120302	DR12(5)				
A*3102	–	B*350101	B35			DRB1*1204	DR5				
A*3103	–	B*350102	B35			DRB1*1205	DR12(5)				
A*3104	A31(19)	B*3502	B35			DRB1*1206	DR12(5)				
A*3105	A31(19)	B*3503	B35			DRB1*1207	–				
A*3106	–	B*3504	B35			DRB1*1208	–				

A		B		DRB1	
A*3107	—	B*3505	B35	DRB1*130101	DR13(6)
A*3108	—	B*3506	B35	DRB1*130102	DR13(6)
A*3201	A32(19)	B*3507	B35	DRB1*130201	DR13(6)
A*3202	A32(19)	B*3508	B35	DRB1*130202	DR13(6)
A*3203	—	B*350901	B35	DRB1*130301	DR13(6)
A*3204	—	B*350902	B35	DRB1*130302	DR13(6)
A*3205	—	B*3510	B35	DRB1*1304	DR13(6)
A*3206	—	B*3511	B35	DRB1*1305	DR13(6)
A*3207	—	B*3512	B35	DRB1*1306	DR13(6)
A*3301	A33(19)	B*3513	B35	DRB1*130701	DR13(6)
A*3303	A33(19)	B*3514	B35	DRB1*130702	DR13(6)
A*3304	—	B*3515	B35	DRB1*1308	DR13(6)
A*3305	A33(19)	B*3516	B35	DRB1*1309	—
A*3306	—	B*3517	B35	DRB1*1310	DR13(6)
A*3401	A34(10)	B*3518	B35	DRB1*1311	DR13(6)
A*3402	A34(10)	B*3519	B35	DRB1*1312	DR13(6)
A*3403	—	B*3520	B35	DRB1*1313	DR13(6)
A*3404	—	B*3521	—	DRB1*131401	DR13(6)
A*3601	A36	B*3522	—	DRB1*131402	DR13(6)
A*3602	—	B*3523	—	DRB1*1315	—
A*3603	A36	B*3524	—	DRB1*1316	DR13(6)
A*4301	A43	B*3525	—	DRB1*1317	DR13(6)
A*6601	A66(10)	B*3526	B35	DRB1*1318	DR13(6)
A*6602	A66(10)	B*3527	B35	DRB1*1319	DR13(6)
A*6603	A10	B*3528	—	DRB1*1320	DR13(6)
A*6604	—	B*3529	B35	DRB1*1321	—
A*680101	A68(28)	B*3530	B35	DRB1*1322	DR13(6)
A*680102	A68(28)	B*3531	—	DRB1*1323	—
A*6802	A68(28)	B*3532	B35	DRB1*1324	—
A*680301	A28	B*3533	—	DRB1*1325	—
A*680302	A28	B*3534	—	DRB1*1326	—
A*6804	A68(28)	B*3535	B35	DRB1*1327	DR13(6)
A*6805	A68(28)	B*3536	—	DRB1*1328	—
A*6806	—	B*3537	—	DRB1*1329	DR6
A*6807	—	B*3538	—	DRB1*1330	—
A*6808	A68(28)	B*3539	—	DRB1*1331	—
A*6809	—	B*3540N	—	DRB1*1332	—
A*6810	—	B*3541	B35	DRB1*1333	—
A*6811N	Null	B*3542	B35	DRB1*1334	—
A*6812	A28	B*3543	B35	DRB1*1335	—
A*6813	—	B*3544	B35	DRB1*1336	DR13(6)

Continued on next page

Table 24.3 (cont'd)

HLA-A alleles	HLA-A antigen specificity	HLA-B alleles	HLA-B antigen specificity	HLA-C alleles	HLA-C antigen specificity	HLA-DR alleles	HLA-DR antigen specificity	HLA-DQ alleles	HLA-DQ antigen specificity	HLA-DP alleles	HLA-DP antigen specificity
A*6814	–	B*3701	B37			DRB1*1337	–				
A*6815	–	B*3702	–			DRB1*1338	–				
A*6816	A68(28)	B*3703N	Null			DRB1*1339	–				
A*6817	–	B*3704	–			DRB1*1340	–				
A*6818N	Null	B*3705	Null			DRB1*1341	–				
A*6819	–	B*3801	B38(16)			DRB1*1342	DR13(6)				
A*6820	–	B*380201	B38(16)			DRB1*1343	–				
A*6821	–	B*380202	B38(16)			DRB1*1344	–				
A*6822	–	B*3803	B16			DRB1*1345	–				
A*6901	A69(28)	B*3804	–			DRB1*1346	–				
A*7401	A74(19)	B*3805	B38(16)			DRB1*1347	–				
A*7402	A74(19)	B*3806	–			DRB1*1348	–				
A*7403	A74(19)	B*3807	–			DRB1*1349	–				
A*7404	–	B*3808	–			DRB1*1350	–				
A*7405	A74(19)	B*390101	B3901			DRB1*1351	–				
A*7406	A74(19)	B*390103	B3901			DRB1*1352	–				
A*7407	–	B*390104	B3901			DRB1*140101	DR14(6)				
A*7408	–	B*390201	B3902			DRB1*140102	DR14(6)				
A*8001	A80	B*390202	B3902			DRB1*1402	DR14(6)				
		B*3903	B39(16)			DRB1*1403	DR1403				
		B*3904	B39(16)			DRB1*1404	DR1404				
		B*3905	B16			DRB1*1405	DR14(6)				
		B*390601	B39(16)			DRB1*1406	DR14(6)				
		B*390602	B39(16)			DRB1*140701	DR14(6)				
		B*3907	B39(16)			DRB1*140702	DR14(6)				
		B*3908	B39(16)			DRB1*1408	DR14(6)				
		B*3909	B39(16)			DRB1*1409	–				
		B*3910	B39(16)			DRB1*1410	DR14(6)				
		B*3911	B39(16)			DRB1*1411	DR14(6)				
		B*3912	B39(16)			DRB1*1412	DR14(6)				
		B*3913	B39(16)			DRB1*1413	DR14(6)				
		B*3914	–			DRB1*1414	DR14(6)				
		B*3915	–			DRB1*1415	DR8				
		B*3916	–			DRB1*1416	DR6				
		B*3917	–			DRB1*1417	DR6				
		B*3918	–			DRB1*1418	DR6				

Allele	Serotype	Allele	Serotype
B*3919	—	DRB1*1419	DR14(6)
B*3920	—	DRB1*1420	DR14(6)
B*3922	—	DRB1*1421	DR14(6)
B*3923	B39(16)	DRB1*1422	DR14(6)
B*3924	B39(16)	DRB1*1423	—
B*3925N	—	DRB1*1424	—
B*3926	—	DRB1*1425	—
B*400101	B60(40)	DRB1*1426	DR14(6)
B*400102	B60(40)	DRB1*1427	DR14(6)
B*400103	B60(40)	DRB1*1428	—
B*4002	B61(40)	DRB1*1429	DR14(6)
B*4003	B61(40)	DRB1*1430	—
B*4004	B61(40)	DRB1*1431	—
B*4005	B4005	DRB1*1432	—
B*40060101	B61(40)	DRB1*1433	—
B*40060102	B61(40)	DRB1*1434	—
B*4007	B60(40)	DRB1*1435	—
B*4008	—	DRB1*1436	—
B*4009	B61(40)	DRB1*1437	—
B*4010	B60(40)	DRB1*1438	—
B*4011	B40	DRB1*1439	—
B*4012	—	DRB1*1440	—
B*4013	—	DRB1*1441	—
B*4014	—	DRB1*1442	—
B*4015	—	DRB1*1443	—
B*4016	B61(40)	DRB1*150101	DR15(2)
B*4018	—	DRB1*150102	DR15(2)
B*4019	—	DRB1*150103	—
B*4020	—	DRB1*150104	—
B*4021	Null	DRB1*150201	DR15(2)
B*4022N	—	DRB1*150202	DR15(2)
B*4023	—	DRB1*150203	DR15(2)
B*4024	—	DRB1*1503	DR15(2)
B*4025	B21	DRB1*1504	DR15(2)
B*4026	B61(40)	DRB1*1505	DR15(2)
B*4027	—	DRB1*1506	DR15(2)
B*4028	—	DRB1*1507	DR15(2)
B*4029	B61(40)	DRB1*1508	DR2
B*4030	—	DRB1*1509	—
B*4031	B60(40)	DRB1*1510	—
B*4032	—	DRB1*1511	—

Continued on next page

Table 24.3 (cont'd)

HLA-A alleles	HLA-A antigen specificity	HLA-B alleles	HLA-B antigen specificity	HLA-C alleles	HLA-C antigen specificity	HLA-DR alleles	HLA-DR antigen specificity	HLA-DQ alleles	HLA-DQ antigen specificity	HLA-DP alleles	HLA-DP antigen specificity
		B*4033	–			DRB1*1512	–				
		B*4034	B60(40)			DRB1*1513	–				
		B*4035	–			DRB1*160101	DR16(2)				
		B*4036	–			DRB1*160102	DR16(2)				
		B*4037	–			DRB1*160201	DR16(2)				
		B*4038	–			DRB1*160202	DR16(2)				
		B*4039	–			DRB1*1603	DR2				
		B*4040	–			DRB1*1604	DR16(2)				
		B*4042	–			DRB1*1605	DR16(2)				
		B*4043	–			DRB1*1607	–				
		B*4044	–			DRB1*1608	–				
		B*4101	B41								
		B*4102	B41			DRB2*0101	–				
		B*4103	B41								
		B*4104	–			DRB3*010101	DR52				
		B*4105	–			DRB3*01010201	DR52				
		B*4106	–			DRB3*01010202	DR52				
		B*4201	B42			DRB3*010103	DR52				
		B*4202	B42			DRB3*010104	DR52				
		B*4204	–			DRB3*0102	DR52				
		B*44020101	B44(12)			DRB3*0103	–				
		B*44020102S	–			DRB3*0104	–				
		B*440202	B44(12)			DRB3*0105	–				
		B*440203	B44(12)			DRB3*0106	DR52				
		B*440301	B44(12)			DRB3*0107	DR52				
		B*440302	B44(12)			DRB3*0108	–				
		B*4404	B44(12)			DRB3*0109	–				
		B*4405	B44(12)			DRB3*0110	–				
		B*4406	B44(12)			DRB3*0201	DR52				
		B*4407	B44(12)			DRB3*020201	DR52				
		B*4408	B44(12)			DRB3*020202	DR52				
		B*4409	B12			DRB3*020203	DR52				
		B*4410	B44(12)			DRB3*020204	DR52				
		B*4411	–			DRB3*0203	DR52				
		B*4412	B44(12)			DRB3*0204	–				
		B*4413	B44(12)			DRB3*0205	–				

Allele	Serology
B*4414	B12
B*4415	B12
B*4416	B47
B*4417	B44(12)
B*4418	–
B*4419N	Null
B*4420	–
B*4421	–
B*4422	–
B*4423N	Null
B*4424	–
B*4425	–
B*4426	–
B*4427	B44(12)
B*4428	–
B*4429	–
B*4430	–
B*4431	B44(12)
B*4432	–
B*4501	B45(12)
B*4502	–
B*4503	–
B*4504	–
B*4505	–
B*4506	–
B*4601	B46
B*4602	B46
B*47010101	B47
B*47010102	B47
B*4702	B47
B*4703	–
B*4704	–
B*4801	B48
B*4802	B48
B*4803	B48c
B*4804	B48
B*4805	B48
B*4806	–
B*4807	B48
B*4901	B49(21)
B*4902	B49(21)

Allele	Serology
DRB3*0206	–
DRB3*0207	DR52
DRB3*0208	DR52
DRB3*0209	DR52
DRB3*0210	DR52
DRB3*0211	DR52
DRB3*0212	–
DRB3*0213	–
DRB3*0214	–
DRB3*0215	–
DRB3*0216	–
DRB3*0217	–
DRB3*030101	DR52
DRB3*030102	DR52
DRB3*0302	DR52
DRB3*0303	–
DRB4*01010101	DR53
DRB4*0102	DR53
DRB4*01030101	DR53
DRB4*01030102N	Null
DRB4*010302	DR53
DRB4*010303	DR53
DRB4*010304	–
DRB4*0104	–
DRB4*0105	DR53
DRB4*0106	–
DRB4*0201N	Null
DRB4*0301N	Null
DRB5*010101	DR51
DRB5*010102	DR51
DRB5*0102	DR51
DRB5*0103	–
DRB5*0104	–
DRB5*0105	–
DRB5*0106	–
DRB5*0107	DR51
DRB5*0108N	Null
DRB5*0109	–
DRB5*0110N	Null
DRB5*0202	DR51

Continued on next page

Table 24.3 (cont'd)

HLA-A alleles	HLA-A antigen specificity	HLA-B alleles	HLA-B antigen specificity	HLA-C alleles	HLA-C antigen specificity	HLA-DR alleles	HLA-DR antigen specificity	HLA-DQ alleles	HLA-DQ antigen specificity	HLA-DP alleles	HLA-DP antigen specificity
		B*4903	–			DRB5*0203	–				
		B*5001	B50(21)			DRB5*0204	–				
		B*5002	B45(12)			DRB5*0205	–				
		B*5004	B50(21)								
		B*510101	B51(5)			DRB6*0101	–				
		B*510102	B51(5)			DRB6*0201	–				
		B*510103	B51(5)			DRB6*0202	–				
		B*510104	B51(5)								
		B*510105	B51(5)			DRB7*010101	–				
		B*510201	B5102			DRB7*010102	–				
		B*510202	B5102								
		B*5103	B5103			DRB8*0101	–				
		B*5104	B51(5)								
		B*5105	B51(5)			DRB9*0101	–				
		B*5106	B51(5)								
		B*5107	B51(5)								
		B*5108	B51(5)								
		B*5109	B51(5)								
		B*5110	–								
		B*5111N	Null								
		B*5112	–								
		B*511301	–								
		B*511302	–								
		B*5114	–								
		B*5115	–								
		B*5116	B52(5)								
		B*5117	B51(5)								
		B*5118	B51(5)								
		B*5119	–								
		B*5120	–								
		B*5121	–								
		B*5122	–								
		B*5123	–								
		B*5124	B51(5)								
		B*5126	–								
		B*5127N	–								

B*5128	B51(5)
B*5129	B51(5)
B*520101	B52(5)
B*520102	B52(5)
B*520103	B52(5)
B*5202	—
B*5203	—
B*5204	B52(5)
B*5301	B53
B*5302	—
B*5303	—
B*5304	—
B*5305	—
B*5306	—
B*5307	B53
B*5308	—
B*5309	—
B*5401	B54(22)
B*5402	B54(22)
B*5501	B55(22)
B*5502	B55(22)
B*5503	B55(22)
B*5504	B55(22)
B*5505	B22
B*5507	B54(22)
B*5508	B56(22)
B*5509	—
B*5510	B55(22)
B*5511	—
B*5512	—
B*5601	B56(22)
B*5602	B56(22)
B*5603	B22
B*5604	B56(22)
B*5605	B56(22)
B*5606	—
B*5607	B56(22)
B*5608	—
B*570101	B57(17)
B*570102	B57(17)
B*5702	B57(17)

Continued on next page

Table 24.3 (cont'd)

HLA-A alleles	HLA-A antigen specificity	HLA-B alleles	HLA-B antigen specificity	HLA-C alleles	HLA-C antigen specificity	HLA-DR alleles	HLA-DR antigen specificity	HLA-DQ alleles	HLA-DQ antigen specificity	HLA-DP alleles	HLA-DP antigen specificity
		B*570301	B57(17)								
		B*570302	B57(17)								
		B*5704	B57(17)								
		B*5705	–								
		B*5706	–								
		B*5707	–								
		B*5708	B57(17)								
		B*5709	–								
		B*5801	B58(17)								
		B*5802	B58(17)								
		B*5804	–								
		B*5805	–								
		B*5806									
		B*5901	B59								
		B*670101	B67								
		B*670102	B67								
		B*6702	–								
		B*7301	B73								
		B*7801	B78								
		B*780201	B78								
		B*780202	B78								
		B*7803	–								
		B*7804	–								
		B*7805	–								
		B*8101	B81								
		B*8201	–								
		B*8202	–								
		B*8301	–								

immune system disorders such as autoimmune disease. The first strong association described is that of HLA-B27 with ankylosing spondylitis and related spondylarthropathies, where over 95% of affected individuals possess an HLA-B*27 allele. Despite tremendous effort to discover the immunological basis for the association between B27 and AS, the answer is still unknown. HLA type has also been associated with susceptibility to and protection from infectious diseases. Individuals possessing HLA-B*5301, an allele prevalent within African populations, are more likely to be resistant to severe malaria. This association is supported by experiments showing the B53 allotype can present a peptide derived from the malaria parasite.

HLA class II molecules are restricted in their tissue distribution. However appropriate stimulation can induce the expression of class II molecules on tissue where they are not normally expressed. This aberrant HLA class II expression may contribute to an autoimmune reaction by providing HLA/peptide complexes not encountered during T-cell receptor education in the thymus. Amongst the many associations between HLA class II molecules and autoimmune and/or inflammatory disease is rheumatoid arthritis and HLA-DR4. This association has been linked to the presence of an epitope contributed by residues 67, 70, 71 and 74 of the β-chain that contributes to a pocket (P4) in the peptide-binding site, thus supporting the role of peptide binding in the disease.

For other associations between HLA and disease, the answer has been found. Haemochromatosis has been associated with haplotypes possessing HLA-A*03. Genetic mapping has identified the gene, *HFE*, responsible for this association. Thus associations between HLA and disease may not be directly related to the HLA allotype but may be due to the presence of other genes that are closely linked or are hitch-hiking within particular HLA haplotypes.

More recently, associations between HLA type and hypersensitivity to drugs have been reported. A high number of patients receiving abacavir, an inhibitor of HIV-1 reverse-transcriptase, who subsequently demonstrated life-threatening hypersensitivity have been found to possess haplotypes containing HLA-B*5701 and HLA-DRB1*0701. The mechanism for such association is currently not known.

HLA matching in transplantation

The benefits of HLA polymorphism in allowing the generation of immune responses against a wide range of antigens is completely negated when transplantation of organs and cells between genetically disparate individuals is considered.

Typically, an individual will possess T cells capable of reacting against a foreign antigen at a frequency of 1 in 10^4–10^5. However, if cells from two HLA disparate individuals are mixed, the frequency of responding cells can be as high as 1–10%. These responding cells are called alloreactive cells.

Alloreactions are responsible for the inability to transplant organs and cells between genetically different individuals. To overcome alloreactivity, it is necessary to define the HLA type of donor and recipient, and to select an HLA-matched donor wherever possible. In solid organ transplantation, HLA matching is encouraged for kidney transplants, where outcome data support a beneficial role of HLA matching. However, immunosuppressive therapy is extremely effective in renal transplantation, and this allows for imperfect matching to be performed, yet it is critical to avoid transplantation of mismatched donor kidneys possessing HLA types against which the patient may have raised alloantibodies as a result of a previous mismatched transplant, pregnancy or blood products. The presence of such alloantibodies can lead to hyperacute rejection. HLA matching for other solid organs such as liver and heart and lung is not usually performed. The liver appears to be an immunoprivileged site that tolerates HLA mismatches, whereas heart and lung transplants are usually performed on patients for whom no other chance of life is possible thereby not allowing for selection of HLA-matched donors. Alloreactions mediated following solid organ transplants are usually only directed at the transplanted organ.

Patients receiving blood products, for example random pooled platelets, can produce antibodies against the HLA molecules present on the transfused platelets. The presence of anti-HLA antibodies can lead to platelet refractoriness, and for these patients it is advised to seek HLA-matched platelet donors.

Alloreactions occurring after haemopoietic stem cell transplantation can result in the failure of the graft to engraft or graft-versus-host disease (GvHD), in which donor cells mediate attack on various tissues within the host's body. The risks of graft rejection and GvHD are reduced significantly if the donor cells are histocompatible with those of the patient. The perfect donor is an identical twin. However, this will only be the case for very few patients. The chances of finding an HLA-matched sibling as a potential donor for a patient is theoretically 1 in 4 (25%). Therefore, again, the majority of patients will not be able to find a suitable donor within their family.

Another source of HLA-matched donors are the various volunteer donor registries that exist throughout the world. The first volunteer donor register, The Anthony Nolan Trust, was established in London in 1974 at a time when unrelated donor transplants were viewed as experimental. Since this time, the success of unrelated donor transplants has increased and the use of unrelated volunteer donors is acceptable practice. There are now over 50 volunteer donor registers throughout the world. In addition, the successful use of cord blood derived stem cells for transplantation has driven the establishment of cord blood banks in many countries. In total there are 8.5 million potential donors/cord blood units registered worldwide. Details on both volunteer donor and cord blood registries can be found on www.bmdw.org.

Histocompatibility testing procedures

Detection of HLA polymorphisms can be performed by either targeting the DNA sequence of the HLA gene or by analysis of the encoded protein directly.

Serology

Serology describes the use of antibodies to detect epitopes on target antigens. HLA polymorphism results in the presence of different antigenic epitopes on the protein molecule. Antibodies used to define these antigenic epitopes can be found in multiparous women, and can also be created using monoclonal antibody technology. The latter has the advantage of being available in unlimited supply. Serology involves the incubation of peripheral blood mononuclear cells (PBMCs) or separated B cells for class II typing, with serum containing antibodies of known anti-HLA specificity. If the PBMCs express the appropriate HLA molecules then binding between the antibodies in the serum and the PBMCs will occur. This binding will result in lysis of the PBMCs after the addition of complement components. The cells can be stained in order to detect which cells are alive (no reaction) and which cells are dead (positive reaction). The pattern of positive and negative reactions is then interpreted to give an HLA type.

In order to obtain a full tissue type, panels of antisera have to be screened to cover the range of recognized HLA specificities. Despite the number of serological reagents that have been analysed, there are many HLA class I and II polymorphisms that remain undetected by serology (Table 24.2). Many of these polymorphisms are not present on the surface of the HLA molecules, but are found within the peptide binding site, and could alter the peptide binding specificity of the HLA molecule and hence the antigen presentation function of the molecule.

DNA methods

The introduction of polymerase chain reaction (PCR) methodologies for analysis of DNA has led to the establishment of rigorous DNA-based methodologies that can be applied for genetic diagnostics. DNA-based methods are now used routinely for histocompatibility typing.

The most frequent HLA class I antigen in populations of caucasoid Europeans, and the first HLA antigen to be defined, HLA-A2, encompasses three serological variants. Sequencing analyses have shown that at least 70 alleles encode the HLA-A2 specificity. Of these 70 alleles, 59 differ by substitutions that are predicted to influence the antigen-presentation function of the HLA-A2 molecule, and four alleles (A*0215N, A*0232N, A*0243N and A*0253N) contain mutations that prevent expression of the HLA-A2 antigen.

For HLA class I molecules, the polymorphism is mostly localized within the α1 and α2 domains, which are encoded by exons

2 and 3, respectively, of the class I gene. For HLA class II, the α1 domain of the β-chain, encoded by exon 2, is most polymorphic for DRB1, whereas for DQ and DP, the polymorphism extends to both the α1 and β1 domains. Thus, DNA methods for HLA class I typing focus predominantly on exons 2 and 3, whereas for HLA class II, exon 2 is targeted.

Sequence-specific oligonucleotide and sequence-specific primer methods

The most widely used DNA-based methods for HLA typing are PCR sequence-specific primers (PCR–SSP) and PCR sequence-specific oligonucleotide probing (PCR–SSOP). Both methods use DNA primers (sequence-specific primers, SSPs) or probes (sequence-specific oligonucleotides, SSOs) that react with polymorphic sequence motifs present within the nucleotide sequence of HLA alleles. The presence of a positive reaction indicates that the polymorphism defined by the primer or probe is present in the DNA sample, whereas a negative reaction defines the absence of that particular sequence polymorphism. For PCR-SSO typing, the target DNA molecule is amplified by locus (e.g. all HLA-A alleles are amplified in one PCR) or group-specific PCR. The PCR product (amplicon) is immobilized directly onto a nylon or nitrocellulose membrane, such that multiple amplicons from different individuals can occupy each membrane.

Most procedures utilize a 96-well plate format or multiples thereof; thus, this approach is ideal for the laboratory with a large-scale throughput such as screening of potential donors for bone marrow donor registries. Each membrane is subsequently incubated with a labelled (e.g. digoxigenin) oligonucleotide probe. If the amplicon contains the DNA sequence that is complementary to the probe sequence then the probe will anneal to the amplicon and remain bound to the membrane. Probes that do not bind will be lost after washing of the membrane. Bound probes are identified by a chemiluminescent secondary reaction using, for example, an alkaline phosphatase-labelled anti-digoxigenin antibody. After identification of the positive reactions, the HLA type can be assigned usually with the help of computer software.

Alternatively, in the reverse dot-blot assay, the probes are pre-immobilized onto a membrane support and a single amplicon (from one individual) is incubated with the membrane.

PCR–SSP typing utilizes multiple PCR primer pairs, all used independently on the same sample of DNA (Figure 24.4). The primer pairs are designed such that the 3′ end defines the specificity of the primer with the target sequence. To obtain a full HLA type requires numerous primer pairs that have been designed to operate under identical PCR amplification conditions. If the target sequence for a primer pair is present in the sample DNA, a PCR product will be produced, whereas if the target sequence is not present, there will be no PCR product. The presence and absence of PCR products can be visualized after agarose gel electrophoresis.

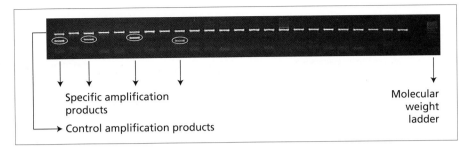

Figure 24.4 Example of PCR–SSP test. An ethidium bromide-stained agarose gel containing electrophoresed PCR products. In this example, 24 PCR primer mixes have been utilized to determine HLA-DRB1*11 subtype. Each lane on the gel contains the product from amplification of a non-polymorphic region of the genome. The presence of this product indicates successful amplification. A second band is observed in lanes 1, 3, 6 and 9, where specific amplification of a polymorphic region from an HLA gene is achieved. If no second band is present then the individual being tested does not possess the complementary HLA polymorphism. The pattern of positive and negative reactions (presence and absence of second bands) is interpreted to give the HLA type (courtesy of Franco Tavarozzi, the Anthony Nolan Trust).

The resolution of the typing results obtained by SSO and SSP methods can vary depending on the number of probes or primer mixes utilized, with an increasing number required for higher resolution.

Regardless of the number of typing reagents used with SSP and SSO methods, the end result is the presence or absence of a reaction between a probe or primer of a known sequence, with the target HLA sequence. Thus, the data generated can be directly related to the DNA sequence of the HLA alleles possessed by an individual.

Direct sequencing

The generation of a database of known nucleotide sequences of HLA alleles has had a tremendous impact on the transfer of methodologies from serology to DNA-based techniques. Improvements with automated instrumentation for DNA sequencing has also made this methodology an affordable alternative technique for HLA typing. The sequencing techniques utilized for HLA typing involve PCR amplification and direct sequencing of the PCR product. The strategies developed have focused on the amplification of DNA fragments containing the polymorphic exons, which, for the majority of class I alleles, extends to a fragment containing exons 2 and 3 (and exon 4 for increased resolution) and usually exon 2 is targeted for class II analysis. HLA-DQB1 benefits from analysis of both exon 2 and exon 3. As most loci are heterozygous, assignment of HLA type is dependent on the use of software that is capable of assigning heterozygous positions. In addition, an up-to-date database of all known HLA sequences is required (Figure 24.5).

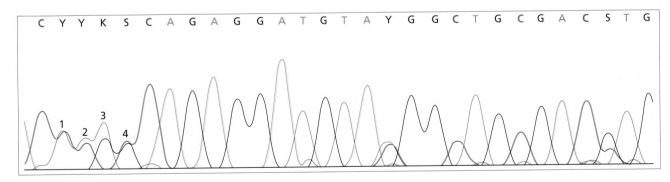

Figure 24.5 Electropherogram of sequencing results from analysis of a heterozygous locus. The sequence is read from left to right. For this short stretch of nucleotides, many different results are possible. Heterozygous positions are given appropriate IUB codes. First heterozygous position (marked 1): CC or CT, continuing to second heterozygous position (marked 2): CCC or CCT or CTC or CTT, continuing to third heterozygous position (marked 3): CCCG or CCCT or CCTG or CCTT or CTCT or CTCG or CTTT or CTTG, continuing to fourth heterozygous position (marked 4): CCCGG or CCCGC or CCCTG or CCCTC or CCTGG or CCTGC or CCTTG or CCTTC or CTCTG or CTCTC or CTCGG or CTCGC or CTTTG or CTTTC or CTTGG or CTTGC, etc. (courtesy of Steven T Cox, the Anthony Nolan Trust).

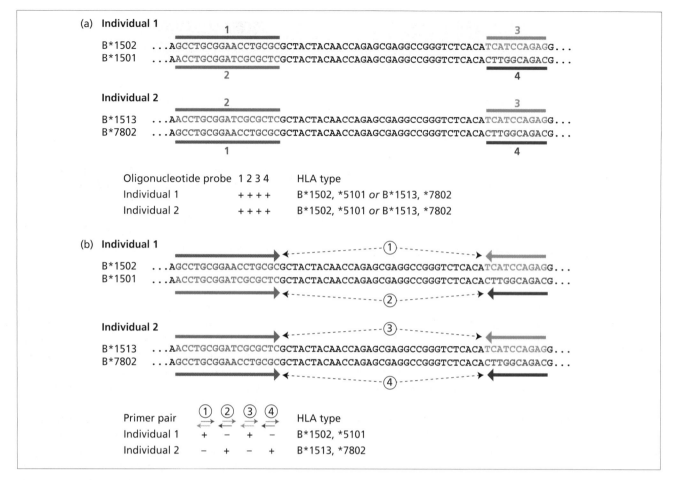

Figure 24.6 Example of SSO ambiguities. (a) The use of oligonucleotide probes to detect complementary DNA sequences. As HLA alleles share sequence motifs, two different heterozygous loci in two individuals can give the same pattern of reactivity with oligonucleotide probes. (b) The use of PCR primer pairs allows linkage of cis motifs (on same haplotype) and resolves the ambiguity.

The advantages of DNA based methods over serology are numerous and include the ease with which typing reagents (primers, probes) can be synthesized and the interpretation of the data as directly relating to nucleotide sequence, whereas the data obtained utilizing polyclonal antisera requires an extensive knowledge of cross-reactivities of sera with different HLA antigens. In addition, the storage of material is simplified for DNA typing, as live cells are not required.

Ambiguities

SSO and direct sequencing methods can generate ambiguous results as both alleles in a heterozygous combination are analysed together. Therefore, it can be difficult to determine whether a sequence motif is in the cis or trans orientation as compared with a different motif (Figure 24.6). This problem can be overcome by performing allele-specific amplification on samples with ambiguities prior to analysis by SSO or sequencing. Fewer ambiguities are obtained using PCR–SSP.

Conformational methods

An alternative approach for the definition of HLA polymorphism is to directly analyse differences in DNA conformation as detected by their differential mobilities in polyacrylamide gel electrophoresis (PAGE). Conformational methods offer the advantage of utilizing a minimum number of reagents. Both single- and double-stranded DNA molecules can be analysed by conformational methods. The limitations of single-strand conformation polymorphism (SSCP) is that only DNA fragments of 200–400 nucleotides in length can be analysed. With heteroduplex analysis, longer DNA fragments can be analysed. The major limitations of both SSCP and heteroduplex analysis are in the complexity of the banding patterns that are visualized by

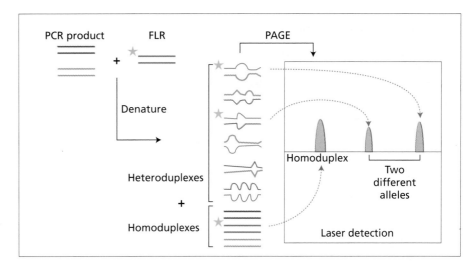

Figure 24.7 Reference strand-mediated conformational analysis (RSCA) methodology (see text for details).

conventional polyacrylamide electrophoresis. The lane-to-lane and gel-to-gel variations inhibit such approaches for direct HLA typing, and these methods have been most widely utilized for subtyping of HLA types and for donor–patient matching analyses.

Improvements with conformational methods for direct HLA typing have been aided by the use of sensitive detection systems and automated analysis software. Reference strand-mediated conformational analysis (RSCA) is a method that can be used to achieve high-resolution results without the ambiguities seen by direct sequencing.

RSCA begins with PCR to produce DNA from the locus of interest, for example HLA-A. The PCR product is hybridized with a locus-specific fluorescent labelled reference (FLR) DNA fragment. Heating the DNA mixture causes the double-stranded DNA molecules to separate. Subsequent cooling allows reformation of the original DNA molecules (homoduplexes) and, in addition, heteroduplexes can form (Figure 24.7). The resulting mixture of heteroduplexes and homoduplexes is separated by non-denaturing PAGE in an automated DNA sequencer. Only those duplexes containing a fluorescent duplex will be detected. The mobility of each fluorescent duplex is measured and comparisons are made with control duplexes analysed in the same gel, and control markers within each lane, allowing the assignment of a value indicative of HLA type. For a heterozygous locus, one homoduplex and two heteroduplex signals are detected. RSCA has been applied for the typing of class I and class II loci, and has also been used as a quick and effective method for assessing histocompatibility for HLA loci between donor and patients.

Cellular assays

Cellular methods for assessing potential alloreactivity between patient and donor can also be utilized for the selection of

the most appropriate haemopoietic stem cell (HSC) donor. The mixed lymphocyte culture (MLC) assay has been used since the 1960s. MLC measures the reactivity of donor T cells against alloantigens expressed by patient cells, i.e. graft-versus-host direction. By mixing both donor and patient cells together, any allo-reactions that occur will cause the responding donor cells to proliferate and incorporate [^{3}H]thymidine, which can be measured. The patient cells are prevented from proliferating by being gamma irradiated prior to the mixing of cells. However, since the introduction of DNA-based methods for HLA class II typing, the MLC reaction is infrequently utilized. Indeed, studies have indicated that positive MLC reactions in the absence of detectable HLA class II mismatches are not indicators of the development of GvHD post BMT.

More sensitive cellular assays have been developed to measure HLA disparity. The cytotoxic T-lymphocyte precursor (CTLp) assay uses limiting dilution analysis (LDA) to measure the frequency of donor CTL responding to predominantly HLA class I mismatches on patient cells. High frequencies of CTLp have been shown to be strongly associated with HLA class I mismatches, which may have escaped detection by the conventional low to medium level of resolution typings, which, until recently, were widely used for class I matching. Similarly, the helper T-lymphocyte precursor (HTLp) assay measures the HTL response of the donor to HLA class II mismatches, with HLA-DR mismatches associated with high HTLp frequencies with no apparent contribution from HLA class I mismatches. Both CTLp and HTLp assays can be combined in a single LDA, thus minimizing the use of often valuable material.

The drawback of cellular assays is that they take up to 2 weeks to perform, and they require viable cells from both donor and patient. With more widespread use of high-resolution HLA typing techniques, the number of laboratories performing cellular assays has decreased significantly.

Other genetic polymorphisms

HLA polymorphisms clearly play an important role in determining the outcome of a HSC transplant. There are also other genetic polymorphisms that have been demonstrated to influence outcome. Minor histocompatibility antigens (mHA) are also alloantigens that are capable of initiating an immune response when their genes are mismatched for patient and donors, despite the presence of HLA matching. Minor histocompatiblity antigens are peptides derived from normal self-proteins that possess polymorphisms. A donor and patient may share HLA type, but differ in the polymorphism found in the mHA gene. Several human mHA have been defined, for example HA1, HA2, HA3, etc. The genes encoding several of these mHA have been described, and this has allowed the development of typing procedures for these genes using techniques such as PCR–SSP.

There is therefore a choice in techniques that may be utilized for optimum donor selection for patients requiring a HSC transplant. Each methodology has its advantages and disadvantages. It is now accepted practice that DNA-based typing should be performed on all related and unrelated donors and patients. Serology and cellular assays may be used to complement the outcome of the DNA typings. A major challenge for the future of histocompatibility typing for HSC transplantation will be to acquire a greater understanding of what types of mismatches are acceptable in that they do not result in adverse alloreactions, and also to know which mismatches are detrimental. It is likely that more sensitive and reproducible cellular assays may play a role in determining these mismatches. The use of ELISPOT (enzyme-linked immunospot) assay and real-time PCR methods for detecting low numbers of cytokine-producing cells may become additional tools for the histocompatibility laboratory in the future.

Selected bibliography

History

Klein J (1986) *Natural History of the Major Histocompatibility Complex.* John Wiley, New York.

HLA molecular structure

Bjorkman PJ, Saper MA, Samraoui B *et al.* (*1987*) Structure of the human class I histocompatibility antigen, HLA-A2. *Nature* 329: 506–12.

Brown JH, Jardetzky TS, Gorga JC *et al.* (1993) Three-dimensional structure of the human class II histocompatibility antigen HLA-DR1. *Nature* 364: 33–9.

Antigen processing and presentation

Antoniou AN, Powis SJ, Elliott T (2003) Assembly and export of MHC class I peptide ligands. *Current Opinion in Immunology* 15: 75–81.

Robinson JH, Delvig AA (2002) Diversity in MHC class II antigen presentation. *Immunology* 105: 252–62.

HLA function

Bankovich AJ, Garcia KC (2003) Not just any T cell receptor will do. *Immunity* 18: 7–11.

Davis SJ, Ikemizu S, Evans EJ *et al.* (2003) The nature of molecular recognition by T cells. *Nature Immunology* 4: 217–24.

Trowsdale J (2001) Genetic and functional relationships between MHC and NK receptor genes. *Immunity* 15: 363–74.

Vilches C, Parham P (2002) KIR: Diverse, rapidly evolving receptors of innate and adaptive immunity. *Annual Review of Immunology* 20: 217–51.

HLA nomenclature

Marsh SGE, Parham P, Barber LD (2000) *The HLA Facts Book.* Academic Press, London.

Marsh SGE, Albert ED, Bodmer WF *et al.* (2002) Nomenclature for factors of the HLA system. *Tissue Antigens* 60: 407–64.

HLA polymorphism

Little A-M, Parham P (1999) Polymorphism and evolution of HLA molecules. *Reviews in Immunogenetics* 1: 105–23.

HLA matching in transplantation

Madrigal JA, Scott I, Arguello JR *et al.* (1997) Factors influencing the outcome of bone marrow transplants using unrelated donors. *Immunological Reviews* 157: 153–66.

Petersdorf EW, Anasetti C, Martin PJ *et al.* (2003) Tissue typing in support of unrelated hematopoietic cell transplantation. *Tissue Antigens* 61: 1–11.

Tiercy J-M, Villard J, Roosnek E (2002) Selection of unrelated bone marrow donors by serology, molecular typing and cellular assays. *Transplant Immunology* 10: 215–21.

Histocompatibility testing procedures

Bidwell JL, Navarrete C (2000) *Histocompatibility Testing.* Imperial College Press, London.

Powis SH, Vaughan RW (2003) *MHC Protocols.* Humana Press, New Jersey.

Minor histocompatibility antigens

Flalkenburg JHF, Marijt WAF, Heemskerk MHM *et al.* (2002) Minor histocompatibility antigens as targets of graft-versus-leukemia reactions. *Current Opinion in Haematology* 9: 497–502.

Mutis T, Blokland E, Kester M *et al.* (2002) Generation of minor histocompatibility antigen HA-1-specific cytotoxic T cells restricted by nonself HLA molecules: a potential strategy to treat relapsed leukaemia after HLA mismatched stem cell transplantation. *Blood* 100: 547–52.

Simpson E, Scott D, James E *et al.* (2002) Minor H antigens: genes and peptides. *Transplant Immunology* 10: 115–23.

CHAPTER 25

Stem cell transplantation

Charles Craddock and Ronjon Chakraverty

25

Introduction

The demonstration in the 1950s that infused bone marrow cells possess the ability to reconstitute the haemopoietic system of lethally irradiated recipients formed the basis for the development of stem cell transplantation (SCT) as a treatment for leukaemia and bone marrow failure. After decades of refinement, transplantation of allogeneic and autologous haemopoietic stem cells has become an increasingly safe and effective procedure and now plays a major role in the management of malignant and non-malignant haematological disorders. It was initially postulated that the curative potential of SCT simply reflected the ability to deliver myeloablative chemo/radiotherapy without the risk of permanent marrow aplasia. Although this is undoubtedly the case in recipients of autologous transplants, there is now conclusive evidence of an additional immunologically mediated graft-versus-leukaemia (GvL) effect after transplantation of allogeneic stem cells. This has permitted the introduction of non-myeloablative transplant regimens and, together with increased donor availability, has markedly increased the number of patients eligible for allogeneic transplantation. Taken together, these developments have resulted in a dramatic expansion in the numbers of stem cell transplants performed over this period in Europe and worldwide (Figure 25.1 and Table 25.1).

Immunological basis of stem cell transplantation

The major complications of allogeneic SCT are caused by the immunological responses triggered by the infusion of donor haemopoietic progenitors and lymphocytes into an immunosuppressed host. These can either take the form of a host-versus-graft (HvG) or a donor-derived graft-versus-host (GvH) response. Clinically, the HvG response can result in graft rejection, whereas a GvH response may manifest itself either as graft-versus-host disease (GvHD) or as a GvL reaction. It is now possible to blunt the HvG reaction by optimizing the immunosuppressive properties of the conditioning regimen and, consequently, graft rejection is rare in most clinical settings. In contrast, GvHD and disease relapse are still major complications of allogeneic transplantation and novel approaches that manipulate the GvH response to therapeutic advantage are needed. By contrast, autologous SCT, in which the patient serves as his/her own stem cell donor, is an immunologically unremarkable event.

Antigens and cellular effectors

The antigens against which HvG and GvH responses are directed include the products of highly polymorphic genes lying within the major human leucocyte antigen (HLA) complex and minor histocompatibility antigens (minor H antigens) encoded by genes lying outside the HLA system. These antigens and the methods employed to identify them have been reviewed in Chapter 20. In very general terms, the degree of difference or 'incompatibility' between the donor and recipient will define the risk of graft rejection and/or GvHD. Thus, in situations where the donor is genetically identical to the recipient (syngeneic transplantation), graft rejection or significant GvHD are not observed.

If the donor and recipient are mismatched for either class I or II HLA antigens, immune responses may be generated against

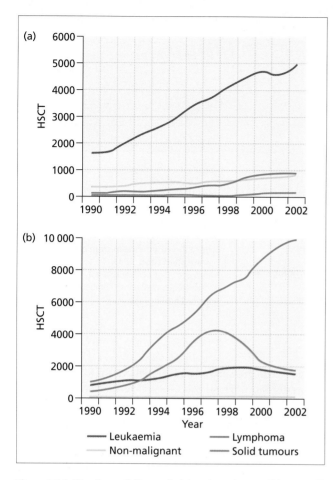

Figure 25.1 Numbers of allogeneic (a) and autologous (b) stem cell transplants performed within Europe 1900–2002 (EBMT data courtesy of Professor A Gratwohl).

Legend:
- Leukaemia
- Lymphoma
- Non-malignant
- Solid tumours

HLA antigens or minor H antigens. Single class I or class II mismatches are in general well tolerated, but greater degrees of mismatch are associated with increased rates of graft rejection or GvHD. At present it is not known whether it will be possible to define 'permissive' mismatches that have no impact on clinical outcome, although such information would clearly be of value in guiding the choice of unrelated donors.

If both recipient and donor are HLA identical, immune reactivity is limited to minor H antigens. These are polymorphic antigens, which include proteins such as HA-1, HA-2 and HA-8. In addition, the protein H-Y is coded for by a gene on the Y chromosome and is therefore only expressed on male cells. Female donors, specifically multiparous individuals, may have been primed against such antigens and, as a consequence, have circulating T-cells that can recognize host cells expressing these proteins. This is likely to underlie the increased risk of GvHD in male recipients of female grafts. The tissue specificity of minor H antigen expression influences the clinical presentation of the GvH response and it is of interest that minor H antigens such

as HA-1 and HA-2 are expressed exclusively on haemopoietic cells.

The most important cells with the capacity to recognize these antigenic differences and mount an injurious immune response are CD4$^+$ and CD8$^+$ T cells. A central role for donor-derived T cells in both GvHD and GvL is demonstrated by the observation that, although depletion of T cells from the donor stem cell inoculum reduces the risk of GvHD, this comes at the price of an increased risk of disease relapse. In the setting of class I HLA disparity, natural killer (NK) cells may also be important cellular effectors. NK cells express receptors termed killer immunoglobulin-like receptors (KIRs), which can interact with HLA class I molecules. KIR activation produced by interaction with a cognate class I ligand may inhibit NK alloreactivity. Conversely, NK-mediated lysis will be triggered if the appropriate inhibitory KIR ligand is not presented on the target cell. Consequently, NK-mediated killing of host targets is determined by their expression of HLA class I ligands.

Graft-versus-host disease

GvHD is a complex immunological disorder in which donor T cells with specificity for recipient antigens not expressed in the donor initiate tissue damage. The recipient, as a result of immunosuppression or immunodeficiency, is incapable of rejecting the T cells mediating the alloreactive response. Conditioning induced tissue injury leads to the release of proinflammatory cytokines and altered chemokine or adhesion molecule expression. These changes impact upon the developing GvH response, leading to cytokine dysregulation and enhanced trafficking of cellular effectors to GvHD target organs. Induction of GvHD (Figure 25.2) requires the interaction of donor T cells with host antigen-presenting cells (APCs), most probably dendritic cells within secondary lymphoid organs, such as lymph nodes and gut-associated lymphoid tissue.

Host APCs are activated by proinflammatory cytokines, such as TNF-α or IL-1β, which are released following tissue damage induced by the conditioning regimen. APCs upregulate the surface expression of co-stimulatory molecules and HLA molecules loaded with peptides derived from host antigens and, in addition, secrete inflammatory chemokines (e.g. MIP-1α). Donor CD4$^+$ and CD8$^+$ T cells with anti-host specificity interact with host APC, become activated, expand and develop effector functions that lead to the secretion of activating cytokines (e.g. TNF-α, interferon-γ) or the induction of perforin or Fas ligand pathways required for cellular cytotoxicity. Altered expression of homing molecules (e.g. the integrin α4β7) permits trafficking of alloreactive T cells from secondary lymphoid tissue to damaged non-lymphoid tissues (especially skin, gut and liver).

T cells aid recruitment of other cellular effectors such as neutrophils, eosinophils, macrophages and NK cells, which together cause the epithelial injury characterizing the clinical manifestations of GvHD. Importantly, GvHD at its initiation is

Table 25.1 Current indications for SCT.

	Autologous SCT	Allogeneic SCT	
		Sibling transplantation	VUD transplantation
AML first CR			
Good-risk cytogenetics	NR	NR	NR
Standard-risk cytogenetics	R	R	NR
Poor-risk cytogenetics	R	R	R
AML second CR	R	R	R
ALL first CR (normal cytogenetics)	D	R	NR
ALL first CR (t9:22)	R	R	R
ALL second CR	R	R	R
CML first CP	NR	R	R (after trial of imatinib)
MDS	NR	R	R
Myeloma	R	R	D
Hodgkin's disease first CR	NR	NR	NR
Hodgkin's disease relapsed	R	R	D
NHL DLBCL first CR	D	R	D
NHL DLBCL relapse	R	R	D
NHL follicular	D	R	D
Aplastic anaemia	NR	R	D
Haemoglobinopathies	NR	R	D

R, recommended; D, developmental; NR, not recommended.

an antigen-specific adaptive immune response but, as the immune response develops, it becomes less specific so that cells lacking the relevant antigens are targeted in the ensuing response. It follows that efforts designed to prevent or treat GvHD are likely to be more successful prior to or at the point of induction of the alloreactive response.

Graft-versus-leukaemia effect

The importance of an immunologically mediated GvL effect in contributing to the curative effect of allogeneic SCT is supported by the observations that T-cell depletion (TCD) increases the risk of relapse and that patients who develop GvHD have a lower risk of disease relapse. Conclusive evidence was provided by the demonstration that infusion of donor lymphocytes can produce durable remissions in patients who have relapsed after allogeneic SCT. It has subsequently been shown that donor lymphocyte infusion (DLI) is a remarkably effective salvage therapy in chronic myeloid leukaemia (CML), with > 80% of patients achieving a sustained molecular remission. Durable responses can also be achieved in patients with acute leukaemia, myeloma and lymphoma albeit at a much lower rate.

As would be predicted, DLI can be complicated by the development of GvHD although the risk of this life-threatening complication is reduced if donor lymphocytes are infused using an escalating dose schedule rather than in a single 'bulk' infusion.

Experimental data suggest that CD8+ T cells are the major effectors of GvL, although there is increasing evidence that other cells, including CD4+ and NK cells, play a role. The identity of the antigens recognized in a GvL reaction remains an area of conjecture. Candidates include ubiquitous or haemopoietic specific minor H antigens (e.g. HY and HA-1 respectively), leukaemia-specific antigens such as product of the BCR–ABL fusion gene or proteins that are overexpressed on leukaemic cells such as proteinase 3 or WT1.

Immune reconstitution

Allogeneic SCT is followed by a prolonged period of cellular and humoral immunodeficiency while donor-derived immune reconstitution occurs. This is exacerbated by T-cell depletion of the graft, coexisting GvHD or prolonged immunosuppressive therapy. Thymic function is reduced in adults and may be further compromised by the effects of chemoradiotherapy and chronic GvHD. As a consequence, the number of naive donor T cells generated from CD34+ progenitors within the thymus in the first months after transplantation is low. The T-cell repertoire as a consequence is limited and mostly dependent upon expansion of donor memory T cells.

Significant HLA mismatching between donor and recipient may also lead to 'holes' within the T-cell repertoire due to a failure of thymocytes or mature T cells to interact with peptides

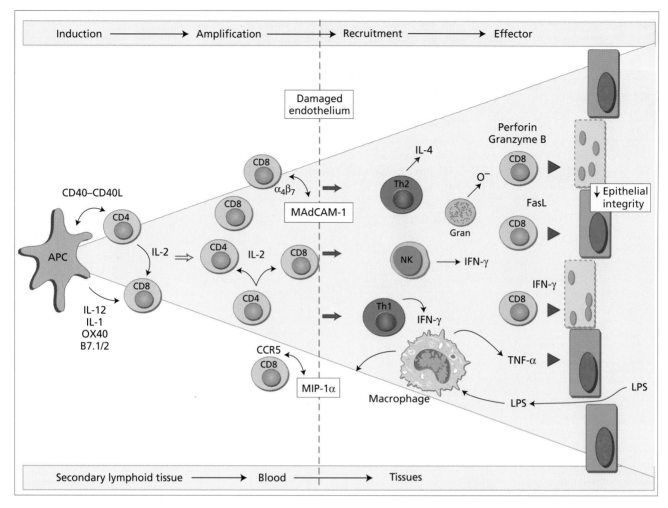

Figure 25.2 Pathophysiology of GvHD. APC, antigen-presenting cell; CD40L, CD40 ligand; FasL, Fas ligand; LPS, lipopolysaccharide; MAdCAM-1, mucosal addressin cell adhesion molecule-1; MIP-1α, macrophage inflammatory protein-1α.

presented in the context of 'foreign' host HLA molecules. Quantitative B-cell deficiency is present in virtually all patients in the first months post transplant, and may persist for a number of years as a consequence of reductions in the number of marrow B-cell precursors. This defect in B-cell production is often multifactorial; causes including damage to the bone marrow stroma, the deleterious effect of inflammatory cytokines and the lympholytic effects of glucocorticoid therapy.

Stem cell engraftment

Biology of stem cell engraftment

Restoration of haemopoiesis after myeloablative therapy is dependent on the transplantation of long-term reconstituting cells (LTRCs). These cells are defined by their capacity for self-renewal as well as their ability to differentiate into all

haemopoietic lineages. Their proliferative capacity is such that transplantation of as few as 100 LTRC can restore haemopoiesis in a lethally irradiated mouse. The cell-surface glycoprotein CD34 is widely used at present as a stem cell marker in clinical transplantation, and is expressed on both committed haemopoietic progenitors as well as LTRCs.

Durable engraftment of allogeneic stem cells is augmented by graft-facilitating donor CD8+ T cells, which usually overcome any residual HvG response generated by host T cells that have survived the conditioning regimen. Thus, the major factors determining engraftment are the intensity of host immunosuppression delivered by the conditioning regimen, the numbers of donor T cells in the stem cell inoculum and the degree of genetic disparity between donor and host.

It was previously assumed that engraftment of allogeneic cells was dependent upon the creation of 'space' within the bone marrow cavity. However, the demonstration that durable engraftment can be achieved using a non-myeloablative dose

Table 25.2 Comparison of cellular composition of typical bone marrow harvest compared with G-CSF-mobilized PBSC (after two aphereses).

	CD34 cells (×10⁶)	CD 34 cells (×10⁶/kg)	CD3 cells (×10⁶)	CD3 cells (×10⁶/kg)
Peripheral blood	240	7.4	11 519	281
Bone marrow	151	4.2	1745	71

Data courtesy of Dr D McDonald.

of total body irradiation (TBI) (200 cGy) has challenged this concept and emphasized the critical importance of pretransplant immunosuppression in securing donor engraftment. The other major determinant of engraftment is the number of stem cells transplanted (see below). The use of granulocyte colony-stimulating factor (G-CSF)-mobilized peripheral blood stem cells (PBSCs) makes it possible to transplant significantly higher stem cell doses than is possible if harvested bone marrow is used. Consequently, PBSCs now play a critical role in optimizing engraftment in settings when T-cell depletion or HLA disparity are present.

Incorporating these principles into clinical practice has markedly reduced the risk of graft failure such that it occurs in less than 1% of patients undergoing an HLA-identical sibling allograft, and less than 5% of those transplanted from an unrelated donor providing a myeloablative conditioning regimen is used. In autologous SCT, when a HvG reaction is absent, graft failure is very rare providing that an adequate stem cell dose is used.

Stem cell dose and source

In allogeneic transplants the size of the transplanted stem cell inoculum plays an important role in determining outcome in recipients of both matched sibling and volunteer unrelated donor (VUD) transplants. This effect is predominantly mediated through a reduction in transplant-related mortality (TRM), consequent upon accelerated immune reconstitution in recipients of a higher stem cell dose; 2×10^6 CD34 cells/kg (2×10^8 mononuclear cells/kg if bone marrow is being used) is considered the lowest acceptable stem cell dose but, as outcome is improved with higher doses, most centres aim for a dose in the region of 4×10^6 CD34 cells/kg. Reports of an increased incidence of chronic GvHD if more than 8×10^6 CD34 cells/kg are transplanted suggest that $4-8 \times 10^6$ CD34 cells/kg should be regarded as the desirable stem cell dose.

There remains considerable debate concerning the optimal source of stem cells in allogeneic transplants. The use of PBSCs is associated with earlier neutrophil and platelet engraftment and, in patients with advanced leukaemia, this may translate into a lower TRM. However, transplantation of PBSCs results in an increased incidence of chronic GvHD, reflecting the five- to tenfold greater dose of T cells transplanted if mobilized cells are used in preference to bone marrow-harvested cells (Table 25.2).

Thus, the use of PBSCs has become commonplace in patients being allografted for advanced leukaemia, when TRM is a major cause of treatment failure, but bone marrow is still preferred in diseases such as aplastic anaemia, when chronic GvHD is an important cause of treatment failure. The increasing use of PBSCs has obvious implications for allogeneic stem cell donors. G-CSF in the doses used for stem cell mobilization (10–15 μg/kg × 4–6 days) is in general well tolerated (Chapter 18). However, the attendant side-effects in the form of myalgia, bone pain, headache coupled with a 2–5% chance a bone marrow harvest being required because of failure to mobilize sufficient progenitors makes careful counselling an essential part of the donor work-up.

In the past decade, umbilical cord blood (CB) cells, harvested at the time of delivery, have been used as a source of allogeneic stem cells. CB is rich in LTRCs and haemopoietic progenitors, and durable engraftment can be reliably obtained in infants and children. Moreover, the incidence of severe acute GvHD is significantly lower with mismatched CB than would be expected using a comparable unrelated donor. It is theoretically possible that the lower numbers and naive phenotype of T cells contained in CB collections will be associated with a reduced GvL effect but no increase in relapse risk has yet been reported in CB transplants.

Given the difficulties which can be experienced in obtaining stem cell collections from unrelated donors, the relative ease of access to CB banks has resulted in this becoming an increasingly important stem cell source in paediatric transplantation. However, in older patients delayed engraftment is commonly observed because of the lower cell doses (per kilogram of body weight) transplanted and this has limited their use in adults. Therefore, approaches that improve engraftment, such as *ex vivo* expansion of haemopoietic progenitors or the use of more than one donation, will be needed before CB is widely used in adult transplantation.

In patients undergoing autologous transplantation PBSC are now almost universally used in preference to bone marrow harvests. The accepted minimum number of PBSC required for engraftment after autologous SCT is 2×10^6 CD34⁺ cells/kg. Although increasing the stem cell dose hastens neutrophil and platelet engraftment, there is little evidence that transplantation of more than 5×10^6 CD34⁺/kg is beneficial and there remain concerns that higher stem cell doses may be associated with an increased risk of tumour contamination.

Stem cell manipulation

Characterization of the stem cell phenotype has permitted the development of strategies by which PBSC grafts can be manipulated *ex vivo*. By using CD34-specific antibodies conjugated with magnetic beads, highly efficient enrichment of CD34$^+$ cells can be achieved. This technology also allows, as a consequence of passive depletion of CD34$^-$ cells, efficient depletion of either contaminating malignant cells in autologous grafts or donor T cells in allogeneic stem cell harvests. The former is of potential importance, although so far unproven, in reducing relapse rates in recipients of autologous transplants, whereas the latter is an effective form of GvHD prophylaxis in allogeneic transplant recipients.

Conditioning regimens: basic principles

The combination of drugs and radiotherapy that is administered before stem cell infusion is termed the conditioning or preparative regimen. In the setting of allogeneic SCT, the conditioning regimen serves two purposes: host immunosuppression to prevent graft rejection and myeloablation in order to achieve tumour eradication. Considerable experience has been gained over the past three decades in the design and delivery of myeloablative conditioning regimens. However, they are still associated with significant toxicity, which precludes their use in patients older than 50–55 years old (45–50 years for recipients of VUD transplants).

The recent demonstration that durable donor engraftment can be reliably achieved using a non-myeloablative preparative regimen, coupled with increased awareness of the potency of the GvL reaction, has led to the development of a range of reduced-intensity conditioning (RIC) regimens. These protocols are associated with a markedly reduced TRM than that which would be observed using a myeloablative regimen. As a result, allogeneic transplantation can now be safely performed in many patients in whom it would previously have been contra-indicated on the grounds of age or comorbidity (Chapter 26). Experience with RIC regimens is limited, however, and longer follow-up is needed before their ability to produce long-term disease-free survival can be accurately assessed.

In autologous SCT when there is no alloreactive response, myeloablative conditioning regimens are better tolerated, allowing autografting to be safely performed in patients up to the age of 70.

Myeloablative conditioning regimens in allogeneic stem cell transplantation

The two commonest myeloablative conditioning regimens used in allogeneic SCT utilize combinations of cyclophosphamide (Cy) and either TBI or busulphan (Bu).

Cyclophosphamide/total body irradiation (Cy/TBI)

Cyclophosphamide is an alkylating agent which, when administered in the doses routinely used in myeloablative conditioning regimens (120–200 mg/kg), has both immunosuppressive and anti-leukaemic properties. It is a prodrug that must be metabolized by the P450 system in the liver to produce metabolically active derivatives, principally phosphoramide mustard, which exert their cytotoxic activity through the production of interstrand DNA links. The two major complications of cyclophosphamide at the doses employed in allogeneic transplantation are haemorrhagic cystitis and cardiac toxicity. The former results from the toxic effects of a cyclophosphamide metabolite, acrolein, upon the uroepithelium and can be reduced by the use of the thiol sodium 2-mercaptoethanesulphonate (Mesna); the latter is very rare at doses of cyclophosphamide below 150 mg/kg.

TBI also has immunosuppressive and anti-leukaemic properties when administered in myeloablative doses (typically 12–14 Gy). The degree of immunosuppression produced by TBI-containing regimens is related to the total dose of irradiation delivered. The use of higher TBI doses is therefore an effective method of optimizing engraftment in settings such as TCD or unrelated donor transplantation when the risk of graft failure might otherwise be increased. Haematological malignancies are highly radiosensitive and the risk of disease relapse can be reduced if a higher dose of TBI is used. Early complications associated with the use of TBI include nausea, vomiting, diarrhoea and parotitis, which can usually be managed symptomatically. More seriously, TBI increases the risk of both pneumonitis and venoocclusive disease (VOD) of the liver. Long-term complications include cataract formation, hypothyroidism, infertility and, in children, growth retardation. Radiobiological principles predict that the toxicity of TBI can be reduced by either decreasing the overall dose of radiation administered or, as is now common, by giving it in a fractionated form over a number of days (e.g 14.4 Gy divided into eight fractions over 4 days).

Busulphan/cyclophosphamide (Bu/Cy)

Bu/Cy is a myeloablative preparative regimen which has the advantage of not requiring the presence of irradiation facilities on site. Busulphan is an oral alkylating agent with potent activity against leukaemic progenitors and is widely used in both allogeneic and autologous transplantation. Major complications associated with the use of high-dose busulphan (14–16 mg/kg) are VOD, infertility and pulmonary and CNS toxicity. There is considerable interpatient variability in busulphan pharmacokinetics, which is of clinical importance given the increased risk of VOD in patients who develop high plasma busulphan levels. Measurement of busulphan levels during the course of its administration allows appropriate dose adjustment and safer use of this agent. Seizures, a complication associated with the administration of high dose of busulphan, can be prevented by the use of prophylactic phenytoin or diazepam.

In non-malignant disorders such as aplastic anaemia, cyclophosphamide alone can be used as a conditioning regimen and is sufficiently immunosuppressive to permit engraftment of allogeneic stem cells, provided that an adequate stem cell inoculum is transplanted.

Comparisons of myeloablative conditioning regimens

The two central questions in the design of myeloablative conditioning regimens are: 'is there any survival benefit to be gained from intensifying the conditioning regimen?' and, secondly, 'are Cy/TBI and Bu/Cy equally effective preparative regimens'? In patients receiving a Cy/TBI allograft, prospective studies have failed to demonstrate any improvement in survival if an increased dose of TBI is used. Although the use of a higher TBI dose reduces the risk of leukaemic relapse, this benefit is offset by a concomitant increase in TRM. Similarly, there is no evidence that addition of busulphan to a Cy/TBI regimen has any impact on disease-free survival.

The decision whether to use Cy/TBI or Bu/Cy as a conditioning regimen has been examined in a number of randomized studies. Although both regimens appear equally effective for patients undergoing a sibling allograft for CML in first chronic phase, there appears to be some benefit attached to the use of a TBI-based regimen in patients with advanced leukaemia. The optimal conditioning regimen in patients who are being transplanted using an unrelated donor has not been determined. The greater degree of HLA disparity results in a higher risk of graft failure than that observed using an HLA-identical sibling and many groups therefore elect to use a TBI-based regimen. It should be noted, however, that equivalent results have been reported by a number of groups using a Bu/Cy regimen.

Strategies for graft-versus-host disease prophylaxis

The commonest method of GvHD prophylaxis utilizes post-transplant immunosuppression in the form of intravenous cyclosporin (2.5–5 mg/kg per day) and methotrexate (e.g. four doses of 10 mg/m^2 administered on days 2, 4, 8 and 12 post transplant). Cyclosporin and other related agents, such as tacrolimus, decrease T-cell activation by inhibiting the calcineurin-dependent secretion of IL-2. Increasing the intensity of immunosuppression reduces the risk of GvHD but is also associated with a higher rate of disease relapse consequent upon a decreased GvL effect.

Depletion of T cells from the donor stem cell inoculum is also an effective form of GvHD prophylaxis. TCD can be achieved *ex vivo* by manipulating the stem cell inoculum or *in vivo* by administration of T cell-depleting antibodies such as anti-thymocyte globulin (ATG) or alemtuzumab (a humanized monoclonal antibody which recognizes CD52). Although a highly effective method of GvHD prophylaxis, TCD is associated with an increased risk of relapse and graft failure, and delays immune reconstitution increasing the risk of post-transplant infections such as CMV. It is therefore difficult to show any overall benefit of TCD on patient survival. Alternative approaches that allow the selective depletion of T cell subsets (CD4$^+$ or CD8$^+$) are being explored and are of interest in terms of defining approaches that may permit dissociation of GvHD and GvL.

Clearly, the form of GvHD prophylaxis used for any particular patient should be selected with their individual risk of both GvHD and relapse in mind. Thus, it may be desirable to avoid the use of TCD in patients with advanced leukaemia in whom the risk of relapse is high. In contrast, patients with a low risk of disease recurrence may benefit from more intensive GvHD prophylaxis. It should also be remembered that patients receiving a TCD graft require a more intensely immunosuppressive conditioning regimen in order to overcome the increased risk of graft rejection.

Conditioning regimens in autologous stem cell transplantation

Conditioning regimens in autologous SCT are designed with dose intensification in mind, and are limited mainly by considerations of extramedullary toxicity. High-dose melphalan (200 mg/m^2) is the standard conditioning regimen in myeloma autografts. BEAM (BCNU 300 mg/m^2, etoposide 800 mg/m^2, cytosine arabinoside 1600 mg/m^2 and melphalan 140 mg/m^2) is widely used in patients with lymphoma. Both Bu/Cy and Cy/TBI are effective preparative regimens for patients with acute leukaemia. A number of other drug combinations incorporating melphalan, busulphan and thiotepa are used in solid tumours. The major extramedullary toxicities of these regimens (in addition to those described already for Cy/TBI and Bu/Cy) are mucositis and gastrointestinal toxicity. Disappointingly, there are little prospective randomized data on which to base the choice of conditioning regimens in autologous SCT. In myeloma, a randomized comparison between a TBI-containing regimen and high-dose melphalan alone demonstrated no benefit associated with the use of TBI. There are, however, no large randomized studies of preparative regimens in lymphoma.

Management of patients undergoing stem cell transplantation

The use of PBSCs coupled with improved supportive care has decreased the mortality of autologous transplantation to 1–3% in most centres. The morbidity and mortality of allogeneic SCT has also continued to fall over the last two decades, largely thanks to more accurate tissue typing and advances in the detection and management of infectious complications. Nonetheless, organ toxicity, GvHD and infections consequent upon delayed immune reconstitution mean that this procedure remains associated with a TRM in excess of 10%, even in the most favourable of circumstances. There also remain significant long-term complications after allografting, which can significantly compromise a patient's quality of life.

Practicalities of stem cell infusion and supportive care

Stem cell products are infused in the same way as other blood products, except that on-line blood filters should not be used. They must not be irradiated. Cryopreserved products are usually defrosted in a water bath at the bedside and then infused without delay. The most common side-effect of the DMSO cryopreservative is nausea but, as it is excreted by the lungs, a garlic-like odour is also observed for 2–3 days after stem cell infusion. Damage to red blood cells releases free haemoglobin, which can precipitate acute renal failure, and thus patients should be adequately hydrated and their urine output monitored closely. The supportive care of patients with neutropenia is discussed extensively in Chapter 36 and will not be repeated here.

Appropriate and timely use of blood products is required during the period of myelosuppression post transplant. All cellular blood products should be irradiated using 25 Gy prior to administration in order to prevent transfusion-related GvHD. This should be commenced 6 weeks prior to transplant and is continued for 6 months after an autograft or indefinitely for allogeneic transplants. In patients undergoing allogeneic SCT, where there is a major ABO incompatibility between donor and recipient (for example, a group O recipient receiving group A bone marrow), the graft must be depleted of red cells prior to administration unless PBSCs are being transplanted, in which case red blood cells are effectively depleted during leucapheresis. The subsequent choice of blood group for platelets or red cells depends upon the precise nature of the ABO incompatibility, the time from SCT and the results of blood grouping. Delayed erythroid engraftment or haemolysis, caused by continuing synthesis of isohaemagglutinins by host lymphocytes, may occur several weeks after stem cell infusion and is associated with the presence of a positive direct antiglobulin test and anti-donor red cell antibodies in serum or red cell eluates.

Complications of allogeneic stem cell transplantation

Early complications (day 0–90)

Graft failure

Primary graft failure is defined as the failure to achieve a neutrophil count $> 0.5 \times 10^9$/L within 28 days of stem cell infusion, and most commonly occurs as a consequence of graft rejection. It is rare except in the setting of TCD or where there is marked donor–host HLA disparity, such as that seen using a

mismatched unrelated or family donor. Investigations in patients with suspected graft failure should include a bone marrow aspirate and trephine (which should be urgently processed) and chimerism studies. Patients with evidence of donor chimerism, whose bone marrow examination demonstrates engrafting myeloid and erythroid progenitors, may benefit from G-CSF support. However, patients with no evidence of engraftment or absence of donor chimerism are candidates for urgent intervention in the form of a second transplant from the same donor or an infusion of cryopreserved autologous stem cells.

The mortality of primary graft failure is in excess of 50%, and it is therefore important to consider performing an autologous harvest in patients, such as unrelated donor recipients, where there is a significant risk of graft failure. Secondary graft failure occurring after initial evidence of engraftment occurs in up to 5% of mismatched or unrelated donor transplants but is extremely rare after a sibling allograft. The aetiology of secondary graft failure is often complex, but causes that need to be considered include late graft rejection, drugs (cotrimoxazole and ganciclovir), viral infection (CMV and parvovirus), disease relapse and, rarely, hypersplenism.

Acute graft-versus-host disease

Acute GvHD occurs at or near the time of engraftment in 40–70% of patients undergoing allogeneic SCT and is characterized by the presence of rash, diarrhoea or abnormal liver function tests. Risk factors for the development of acute GvHD include increased recipient age, HLA mismatch and the use of a female donor. Children and recipients of cord blood transplants have a lower risk of acute GvHD.

Skin GvHD typically presents as a maculopapular rash involving the face, neck, palms and soles, but may extend to involve the whole body (Figure 25.3). In the worst cases, it progresses to erythroderma, with bullae formation and painful blistering. Histology shows apoptosis at the base of dermal crypts, dyskeratosis, and evidence of lymphocytes in a perivascular distribution or adjacent to dyskeratotic keratinocytes. Gastrointestinal involvement presents with nausea, vomiting, secretory diarrhoea and/or abdominal pain. In patients with more severe gastrointestinal GvHD, abdominal pain and distension in association with voluminous, occasionally bloody, diarrhoea may occur. Gastric, antral and rectal biopsies have a high diagnostic yield with diagnostic features including the presence of apoptotic cells in the base of crypts and a lymphocytic infiltrate. A well-defined manifestation of upper gut GvHD is the development of anorexia and nausea – both of which usually resolve rapidly if treated with low-dose methylprednisolone (1 mg/kg). A rising bilirubin and raised alkaline phosphatase are the initial features of liver GvHD, which typically develops later than skin or gut GvHD. Liver histology is diagnostic and demonstrates a portal tract lymphocytic infiltration, pericholangitis and bile duct loss.

Accurate and early diagnosis of acute GvHD is essential for effective management of this potentially life-threatening distion of cyclosporin levels may be sufficient to control symptoms. Approximately 70% of patients will improve significantly with oral or intravenous corticosteroid therapy, but a number will either fail to respond or relapse when immunosuppression is tapered. Individuals with steroid refractory acute GvHD have a poor prognosis and require second-line therapy using equine or rabbit anti-thymocyte globulin (ATG). Although a proportion of patients will respond to second-line therapy, steroid refractory acute GvHD remains associated with a non-relapse mortality in excess of 80%. Prophylactic administration of antimicrobial and antifungal agents is essential in all patients receiving high-dose steroids for treatment of GvHD.

Infectious complications

The organisms responsible for infectious complications after allogeneic SCT depend primarily on the time from stem cell infusion (Figure 25.4). Active steps should be taken to prevent the risk of infection and patients should be cared for in single rooms, preferably with laminar air flow or high-efficiency particulate air filtration. A number of effective prophylactic strategies have been developed in allograft patients. Evidence supports the use of triazole antifungals, for example fluconazole (100–400 mg daily), as an effective means of reducing *Candida* infection. Aciclovir (200–400 mg q.d.s.) is administered to prevent herpes simplex virus (HSV) reactivation. Quinolone antibiotics (e.g. ciprofloxacin 500 mg b.d.) are used by some units to reduce the risk of severe Gram-negative infections, although the evidence supporting this measure is inconclusive and practice should be guided by advice from local microbiologists concerning the prevalence and sensitivity of drug-resistant organisms. Patients should receive cotrimoxazole (480 mg b.d. three times per week) upon recovery from aplasia (neutrophils $> 1.0 \times 10^9/L$) to prevent *Pneumocystis carinii* infection. If allergic to cotrimoxazole, nebulized pentamidine (300 mg monthly) can be substituted.

Allogeneic recipients, particularly recipients of TBI-containing regimens, continue to be at long-term risk from infections by encapsulated bacteria such as *Streptococcus pneumoniae* and *Haemophilus influenzae* and require lifelong penicillin prophylaxis (250 mg b.d.) or erythromycin (250 mg b.d.) if allergic to penicillin. Antibody titres to diseases for which childhood vaccination is performed decline after SCT. Revaccination is therefore recommended, particularly in allograft recipients, and most centres commence such a programme 12 months post transplant.

Cytomegalovirus infection and disease

Human cytomegalovirus (CMV) is a ubiquitous herpesvirus that infects up to 60% of healthy adults. CMV reactivation occurs commonly after allogeneic SCT, giving rise either to an asymptomatic infection or, less commonly, to end-organ damage (CMV disease) and death. Patients at the highest risk of CMV reactivation are seropositive recipients, especially those who

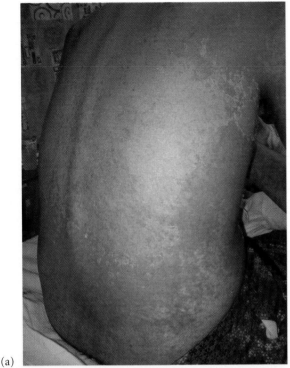

(a)

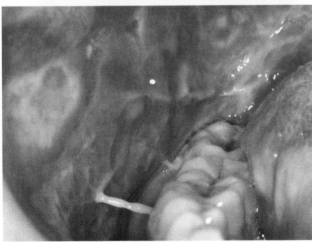

(b)

Figure 25.3 Acute skin GvHD: (a) acute cutaneous GvHD; (b) chronic oral GvHD.

order. When possible, diagnostic biopsies should be taken both to confirm the presence of GvHD and to assist in the exclusion of other aetiologies. It is also important to stage GvHD accurately and the criteria devised by Glucksberg are widely used (Table 25.3). This staging system is a reliable indicator of prognosis and guides the intensity of treatment required. Grade 2–4 acute GvHD should be treated with high-dose methylprednisolone (typically 2 mg/kg daily) which is tapered according to response. In the setting of limited skin GvHD and upper gut GvHD topical or oral steroids (1 mg/kg) coupled with optimiza-

(a)

Table 25.3 Glucksberg staging of acute GvHD: (a) clinical staging of acute GvHD; (b) clinical grading of acute GvHD.

Stage	Skin	Liver bilirubin	Gut
+	Maculopapular rash < 25% body surface	34–51 µmol/L	Diarrhoea, 500–1000 mL/day or persistent nausea
++	Maculopapular rash 25–50% body surface	51–102 µmol/L	Diarrhoea, 1000–1500 mL/day
+++	Generalized erythroderma	102–255 µmol/L	Diarrhoea > 1500 mL/day
++++	Desquamation and bullae	> 255 µmol/L	Pain with, without ileus

(b)

Overall grade	Skin	Liver	Gut	Functional impairment
0 (none)	0	0	0	0
I (mild)	+ to ++	0	0	0
II (moderate)	+ to +++	+	+	+
III (severe)	++ to +++	++ to +++	++ to +++	++
IV (life-threatening)	+ to ++++	++ to ++++	++ to ++++	+++

Reproduced with permission from Blume KG, Forman SJ, Appelbaum FR, eds (2004) *Thomas' Hemopoietic Stem Cell Transplantation*, 3rd edn. Blackwell Science, Oxford.

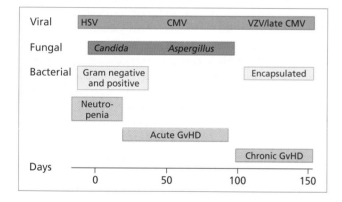

Figure 25.4 Infectious complications occurring after allogeneic SCT.

receive TCD or unrelated donor grafts and patients who develop GvHD, requiring steroid therapy. Primary infection of seronegative patients may occur as a result of the infusion of stem cell or blood products from a CMV-positive donor but is rare. Nonetheless, all seronegative transplant recipients should receive CMV-negative or leucodepleted blood products to limit the possibility of primary infection.

CMV reactivation occurs in 40–80% of at-risk patients and, until recently, a substantial number of such patients progressed to develop CMV disease. As a result, CMV was the commonest cause of infectious death after allogeneic transplantation. It is now possible to detect low levels of CMV infection post transplant, using either polymerase chain reaction (PCR)-based detection of CMV nucleic acids or detection of pp65 antigen in peripheral blood leucocytes (CMV antigenaemia). The introduction of these sensitive diagnostic techniques, coupled with the development of effective antiviral drugs, has markedly reduced the incidence of CMV disease. Nonetheless, CMV remains a significant cause of mortality in recipients of unrelated donor and T cell-depleted transplants. The most common manifestation of CMV disease is pneumonitis, which presents as progressive dyspnoea and hypoxia 30–80 days post transplant. CMV related gastrointestinal ulceration, hepatitis and retinitis are seen only rarely after SCT.

Prevention of CMV disease in at-risk patients (all CMV seropositive patients and any patient with a seropositive donor) has relied on the use of ganciclovir (5–10 mg/kg), a nucleoside analogue that inhibits viral thymidine kinase. The major side-effect of ganciclovir is myelosuppression, which is especially problematic after SCT. Two strategies have been devised to reduce the risk of CMV disease and death in allograft recipients. The first is based on pre-emptive treatment of patients who develop evidence of CMV infection. Ganciclovir therapy is continued until patients have a sustained period without evidence of CMV viraemia. Using this 'pre-emptive approach', ganciclovir use is restricted to patients who reactivate CMV and, consequently, a proportion of patients will not require ganciclovir therapy, thereby avoiding its attendant toxicities. Randomized studies have confirmed that this approach reduces the risk of CMV disease and death after sibling allogeneic transplantation.

Alternatively all at-risk patients can receive ganciclovir prophylactically from the time of engraftment until a defined time post transplant (usually 90 days), regardless of whether there is evidence of CMV infection. Although this approach is effective in reducing the incidence of both CMV infection and disease post transplant, it increases patient exposure to ganciclovir and is associated with a greater risk of neutropenia and bacterial and fungal infection. For this reason, a pre-emptive approach to prevention of CMV disease is generally preferred. The effective treatment of CMV infection delays the development of an immune response to CMV and as a result late (beyond 100 days post transplant) CMV reactivation and disease is increasingly observed.

Two other agents are valuable in the management of CMV infection and disease. Foscarnet, a DNA polymerase inhibitor, has less myelotoxicity than ganciclovir and is effective as part of a pre-emptive approach, although it is associated with significant nephrotoxicity. Cidofovir is also an effective agent that has the ability to salvage patients with ganciclovir-refractory CMV disease (particularly pneumonitis), although it is nephrotoxic and not recommended in patients with significant renal impairment. High-titre CMV immunoglobulin may also be of value in the treatment of CMV pneumonitis.

Other members of the herpesvirus family have the potential to cause significant morbidity after allogeneic SCT. The incidence of HSV, which used to be very common in the first 30 days after SCT, has been sharply reduced by the use of prophylactic aciclovir. Reactivation of varicella zoster virus (VZV) occurs in up to 50% of at-risk patients after allogeneic SCT, and typically presents as shingles with severe pain and a dermatomal vesicular eruption. Less commonly, VZV reactivation presents with atypical pain (headache or undiagnosed abdominal pain) in the absence of a rash. Prompt treatment of VZV infections with high-dose intravenous aciclovir is indicated after allogeneic SCT, both to prevent dissemination but also to reduce the severity of post-herpetic neuralgia. HHV-8 is also increasingly being reported in association with a syndrome variously associated with delayed engraftment, encephalitis and hepatitis.

Fungal infections

Fungal infections remain a major complication of SCT, reflecting the absence of accurate diagnostic tests and the inadequacy of therapies available at present. A high index of clinical suspicion is therefore required in transplant patients, particularly allografts, and most units administer systemic antifungal therapy early in the course of the management of neutropenic fever. Risk factors for the development of fungal infection include prolonged neutropenia after SCT, the use of high-dose corticosteroids for treatment of GvHD and a history of prior fungal infection.

Effective strategies exist for the prophylaxis and treatment of infection with yeasts (Candida spp.) but are lacking for moulds such as Aspergillus spp. Candida infections typical manifest as oral thrush and, less commonly, as oesophageal candidiasis. Hepatosplenic candidiasis is seen occasionally, presenting with high spiking fevers at the time of engraftment in association with abnormal liver function tests. Ultrasound or computerized tomography (CT) imaging of the liver and spleen will confirm the diagnosis. Prophylactic use of fluconazole (100 mg daily) has proved effective in reducing the incidence of both superficial and invasive candidiasis. Patients who develop either hepatosplenic candidiasis or candidaemia should be treated with systemic antifungals, usually amphotericin B and any indwelling catheter must be removed.

Clinical features of Aspergillus infection develop before or shortly after engraftment usually manifesting as an antibiotic-resistant fever in association with a markedly elevated CRP. End-organ infection, most commonly invasive pulmonary aspergillosis (IPA) or, rarely, cerebral or hepatosplenic aspergillosis, can develop rapidly over a period of days. Accurate diagnosis of Aspergillus infections remains problematic as spores are only rarely cultured from lavage fluid or infected tissues, and the sensitivity and specificity of other diagnostic techniques are low. Contradictory results have been obtained using galactomannan detection assays and the initially encouraging results with PCR technology have not been confirmed by all groups. In practice, many units base management decisions on the results of a chest CT, which should be obtained in all patients with a neutropenic fever that has persisted for more than 72 h. Although the characteristic radiographic features of peripheral nodular shadows, with or without evidence of cavitation or a 'halo' sign, may take weeks to develop, the presence of any significant pulmonary infiltrate substantially increases the likelihood of Aspergillus infection and is an indication for the commencement of high-dose amphotericin therapy. Conversely, the likelihood of developing IPA in a patient with a normal chest CT is low.

Many patients fail to tolerate treatment with conventional amphotericin because of infusion reactions or nephrotoxicity. Liposomal preparations (Abelcet®, Ambisone®), although significantly more expensive, are much better tolerated and also allow dose escalation in patients in whom there is a high degree of clinical suspicion of fungal infection. Newer drugs such as voriconazole and caspofungin, used alone or in combination with liposomal preparations of amphotericin, are likely to improve therapeutic options in this population of patients, but their precise role remains to be established.

Organ toxicity

Gastrointestinal toxicity

Mucositis is universally observed in patients transplanted using a myeloablative conditioning regimen. It typically develops in the first few days after stem cell infusion and peaks approximately 8 days post transplant. The severity of mucositis is closely correlated with both the intensity of the conditioning regimen and the use of methotrexate as GvHD prophylaxis. Patients with severe mucositis should receive adequate (often opiate) analgesia and be monitored for evidence of airway obstruction.

Table 25.4 Causes of abnormal liver function tests after allogeneic SCT.

Precipitant	Clinical presentation
Veno-occlusive disease	Hyperbilirubinaemia associated with weight gain, ascites and painful hepatomegaly
Drugs	Cyclosporin (hyperbilirubinaemia), fluconazole (raised AST)
Haemolysis	Fall in Hb associated with unconjugated hyperbilirubinaemia and positive Coombs' test
Biliary obstruction	Dilated biliary tree associated with gall bladder 'sludge' or cholelithiasis
Infection	Viral hepatitis, fungal infection (disseminated aspergillosis or candidiasis), cholangitis lenta

Allogeneic SCT recipients may require parenteral nutritional support during this period. In patients who develop symptoms of severe oesophagitis, the possibility of superadded infection with *C. albicans* or HSV must be considered, the latter typically being associated with intractable vomiting. Nausea, vomiting and anorexia are common complications associated with cytoreductive therapy. Given the range of underlying conditions that may be associated with these symptoms, upper gastrointestinal endoscopy is strongly recommended in patients, providing that their mucositis has resolved sufficiently to allow the procedure to be performed safely.

Diarrhoea and/or abdominal pain are common manifestations of conditioning toxicity. Alternative causes of diarrhoea in the first few weeks post transplant include enteritis due to *Clostridium difficile*, rotavirus or CMV, acute GvHD and pancreatitis. VZV reactivation can occasionally present with severe abdominal pain, usually in association with markedly deranged liver function tests.

Liver toxicity

Abnormal liver function tests are commonly observed after allogeneic SCT, and causes include VOD, drugs, infectious-related complications, cholelithiasis and acute GvHD (Table 25.4). VOD is a clinical syndrome characterized by a triad of hyperbilirubinaemia (> 34 μmol/L), weight gain (> 5% baseline) and painful hepatomegaly. It is associated with evidence of damage to sinusoidal endothelial cells and hepatocytes, and subsequent damage to the central veins in zone 3 of the hepatic acinus. In severe cases, hepatic venular occlusion and widespread zonal disruption may lead to portal hypertension, hepatorenal syndrome, multiorgan failure and death. Risk factors for the development of VOD include the use of conditioning regimens containing busulphan or higher doses of TBI, pretransplant abnormalities of liver function tests, previous abdominal irradiation and recent exposure to the anti-CD33 antibody gemtuzumab ozogamicin (Mylotarg).

A diagnosis of VOD is most commonly made on clinical criteria. Doppler studies demonstrating evidence of reversal of portal flow support the diagnosis. Definitive diagnosis requires transjugular venous liver biopsy. which has a significant morbidity in the early post-transplant period and is therefore often avoided. It is important to exclude other causes of hyperbilirubi-

naemia, particularly cyclosporin toxicity, haemolysis (typically consequent upon donor, recipient ABO mismatch) and the hepatitis of sepsis (cholangitis lenta). Management is supportive, consisting of careful fluid balance, the judicious use of diuretics and, where necessary, haemofiltration. There is now convincing evidence that defibrotide can effectively treat up to 40% of patients with severe VOD.

Renal toxicity

Impairment of renal function is frequently observed after allogeneic SCT unless careful attention is paid to fluid balance and the nephrotoxic potential of drugs commonly used during SCT, especially cyclosporin, amphotericin B, aminoglycosides and loop diuretics. Cyclosporin-related renal toxicity is usually easily reversible by temporary omission and dose reduction. Occasionally, cyclosporin toxicity manifests itself as a microangiopathic haemolytic anaemia with features of thrombotic thrombocytopenic purpura/haemolytic uraemic syndrome. Withdrawal of the drug is mandatory and plasmapheresis may be required.

Pulmonary infections and non-infectious complications

A variety of non-infectious pulmonary complications can occur after allogeneic SCT. Pulmonary oedema is common in the first few weeks after transplant, consequent either upon increased capillary hydrostatic pressure caused by fluid overload or upon increased capillary permeability due to irradiation or sepsis. Idiopathic pneumonia syndrome, defined as diffuse lung injury occurring after SCT for which no infectious or non-infectious aetiology can be identified, typically occurs 30–50 days post transplant. The classic presentation includes dyspnoea, nonproductive cough, hypoxaemia and non-lobar infiltrates on chest radiograph, which can progress rapidly to acute respiratory distress syndrome. Treatment is supportive but frequently unsatisfactory, and steroids have little effect upon outcome. Diffuse alveolar haemorrhage is seen predominantly in patients undergoing autologous SCT, but can also be seen in allogeneic recipients. This complication usually occurs within the first 2–3 weeks of transplantation and presents with dyspnoea, haemoptysis and hypoxaemia. Radiographic changes include interstitial or alveolar shadowing. Definitive diagnosis requires bronchoscopy, which shows fresh blood on repeated lavage. Recognition of this disorder is essential as early intervention with high-dose steroids may significantly improve survival.

A range of pulmonary infections occur after allogeneic SCT. In the first month, post-transplant bacterial and fungal pneumonias are common. Viral infections such as CMV, respiratory syncitial virus (RSV) and parainfluenza are important causes of pneumonitis and typically occur in the first 90 days post transplant. PCP infection and toxoplasmosis infection are still seen occasionally in the first few months post transplant in patients who do not receive or are not compliant with cotrimoxazole prophylaxis.

Intensive care support

The outcome of patients admitted to the intensive care unit after allogeneic SCT is very poor, and consultation with intensivists at an early stage in their care is essential. Interventions such as non-invasive ventilatory support, if used early, may reduce the requirement for mechanical ventilation. Patients with isolated respiratory failure requiring mechanical ventilation have a mortality in the range 80–95%, although a significant proportion of those who can be weaned from the ventilator may become long-term survivors. The development of combined hepatic and renal dysfunction in patients who are ventilated is associated with an extremely gloomy prognosis. It is therefore important that the complex decisions regarding the appropriateness or otherwise of intensive support in SCT patients are based on a realistic assessment of the probability of long-term survival.

Late complications of allogeneic stem cell transplantation

As the results of allogeneic SCT have improved, its long-term complications have come to be better recognized and represent an increasingly important cause of morbidity in patients who might otherwise be considered to be cured of their underlying disease.

Chronic graft-versus-host disease

Chronic GvHD refers to a complex syndrome occurring more than 100 days after allogeneic SCT and is its commonest long-term complication. Registry data show an incidence of chronic GvHD of approximately 33% in patients undergoing transplantation from HLA-identical siblings, rising to 66% in patients receiving grafts from unrelated donors. Risk factors for the development of chronic GvHD include increased recipient age, the use of PBSC or an unrelated or HLA-mismatched donor as a stem cell source, and the presence of prior acute GvHD. Chronic GvHD may develop directly from acute GvHD (progressive), after the resolution of an episode of acute GvHD, or de novo in patients with no history of chronic GvHD. The clinical manifestations are summarized in Figure 25.5 and are characterized by features of both immunodeficiency and 'autoimmunity'. At present, chronic GvHD is classified as limited or extensive (Table 25.5), although the utility of this staging system is under

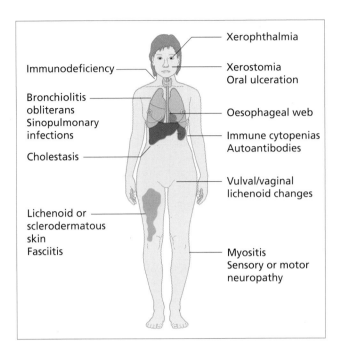

Figure 25.5 Clinical manifestations of chronic GvHD.

review. Patients with progressive-type onset, extensive skin involvement, a platelet count $< 100 \times 10^9$/L and a poor performance status have a particularly poor prognosis. Current treatment is unsatisfactory and involves immunosuppression with cyclosporin or prednisolone, which are continued for approximately 6 months prior to a gradual reduction in responding patients. Second-line therapies include tacrolimus, mycophenolate mofetil, thalidomide and extracorporeal photopheresis.

Secondary malignancies

The incidence of solid tumours in recipients of allogeneic SCT is increased compared with control populations and includes a higher rate of skin or buccal cavity squamous cell carcinoma and melanoma. In the largest study to date, the cumulative incidence of all solid tumours was 2.2% at 10 years and 6.7% at 15 years, although the latter figure may represent an overestimate. Risk factors for the development of secondary malignancies include the use of TBI in the conditioning regimen and the presence of chronic GvHD. Post-transplant lymphoproliferative disorder (PTLD) includes a spectrum of Epstein–Barr virus (EBV)-driven B-cell hyperproliferative states that range from polyclonal benign proliferations to life-threatening neoplastic disease. Most cases of PTLD involve EBV-seropositive donors and present with lymphadenopathy and fever. In contrast to the PTLDs that develop following solid organ transplants, the majority of cases after SCT are of donor origin and arise as a result of inadequate T-cell control of proliferation of EBV-infected B-cells. Risk factors for the development of PTLD include T-cell depletion, HLA disparity and ATG therapy. Treatment involves cessation

---

Limited chronic GvHD

Either or both

Localized skin involvement

Hepatic dysfunction as a result of chronic GvHD

Extensive chronic GvHD

Either

Generalized skin involvement

Or

Localized skin involvement and/or hepatic dysfunction as a result of chronic GvHD

Plus

Liver histology showing chronic aggressive hepatitis bridging necrosis or cirrhosis

Or

Involvement of eye (Schirmer test with < 5-mm wetting)

Or

Involvement of minor salivary glands or oral mucosa demonstrated on labial biopsy

Or

Involvement of any other target organ

Table 25.5 Classification of chronic GvHD.

Reproduced with permission from Blume KG, Forman SJ, Appelbaum FR, eds (2004) *Thomas' Hemopoietic Stem Cell Transplantation*, 3rd edn. Blackwell Science, Oxford.

of immunosuppressive therapy, donor lymphocyte infusion or anti-CD20 monoclonal antibody (Rituximab®).

Growth, puberty and fertility

Retarded growth is seen predominantly in children who have received irradiation, particularly cranial irradiation. Growth retardation is multifactorial and, although growth hormone levels may be diminished as a consequence of hypothalamic or pituitary irradiation, this does not entirely account for the observed reduction in height. Gonadal failure (both testicular and ovarian) is a common consequence of myeloablative conditioning regimens, particularly those which contain TBI or busulphan. Although prepubertal girls receiving cyclophosphamide alone (as for transplantation in severe aplastic anaemia) are likely to experience a normal puberty, most receiving other preparative regimens will fail to regain normal ovarian function and will require sex hormone replacement therapy for the induction of puberty. Thereafter, sex hormone replacement is indicated to maintain the menstrual cycle and normal bone turnover/mineralization, but the optimal duration of therapy and the potential long-term risks of hormone replacement therapy in this setting is unknown. Although ~10% of women who receive TBI-containing regimens may have some recovery of gonadal function, the overall incidence of pregnancy is very low. In males, cryopreservation of sperm should be performed at diagnosis.

Complications of autologous stem cell transplantation

The major toxicities of autologous SCT relate to immediate or delayed organ failure caused by the conditioning regimen (Table 25.6) or complications consequent upon neutropenia or thrombocytopenia. Late complications are rare but include

Organ	Complications
Lung	Diffuse alveolar haemorrhage; interstitial pneumonitis especially in recipients of bleomycin or TBI-containing regimens
Gastrointestinal	Mucositis, nausea, diarrhoea
Hepatic	Asymptomatic elevations of bilirubin or AST; veno-occlusive disease (especially in recipients of Bu-containing regimens)
Renal	Prerenal acute renal failure; renal toxicity, nephrotoxic antibiotics interstitial nephritis
Cardiac	Arrhythmias; cardiac failure (cyclophosphamide)

Table 25.6 Immediate complications of autologous stem cell transplantation.

pulmonary fibrosis in patients who have received busulphan and BCNU, and gonadal failure particularly in recipients of TBI- or busulphan-containing regimens. Female but not male recipients of BEAM chemotherapy may recover some gonadal function. The development of myelodysplasia and acute myeloid leukaemia (AML) is a well-recognized late complication. It appears that prior chemotherapy is the most important factor in the development of t-MDS or t-AML, as the leukaemia-associated cytogenetic abnormality can frequently be detected in the infused stem cell inoculum.

Management of relapse

Disease relapse after allogeneic SCT indicates resistance of cells within the malignant clone to the conditioning regimen, coupled with an ability to evade tumour surveillance by the donor immune system. Possible mechanisms for tumour evasion include downregulation of HLA class I or II expression, absence of co-stimulatory molecules or location of residual cells in privileged sites such as the central nervous system or testes. Relapse after autologous SCT is caused either by failure of the conditioning regimen to eradicate malignant haemopoiesis or infusion of contaminating tumour at the time of transplantation.

The management of relapse after allogeneic SCT has been transformed by the use of donor lymphocytes. DLI is remarkably effective in patients who have relapsed after allografting for CML, and up to 80% of patients treated in cytogenetic relapse will achieve a durable molecular remission. Responses to DLI are less commonly observed in patients who have relapsed after an allograft for acute leukaemia (AML or acute lymphoblastic leukaemia, ALL), myeloma or lymphoma, although durable responses can occur particularly if donor lymphocytes are administered after cytoreductive therapy. The major complications of DLI are myelosuppression and GvHD. Myelosuppression is most commonly observed in patients with overt haematological relapse and may require treatment with G-CSF and, occasionally, transfusion of donor PBSC. In early studies, DLI was administered as a single 'bulk' infusion and associated with a significant risk of severe GvHD. However, the recognition that the use of an escalating schedule of administration substantially reduces the risk of severe GvHD without compromising its efficacy has markedly reduced the toxicity of DLI.

Patients who relapse after autologous SCT may respond to further conventional chemotherapy, although this will only rarely result in long-term disease-free survival. In a small group of patients, allogeneic SCT may be indicated, although this will be associated with an increased TRM. Patients with myeloma in whom the duration of response to the first transplant was greater than 2 years may benefit from a second autograft.

Donor choice

An HLA-identical sibling donor is identifiable in only one-third of patients eligible for allogeneic SCT. Thanks to the rapid expansion of unrelated donor registries, approximately 8 million volunteer unrelated donors (VUDs) are now registered worldwide. As a result, it is possible to identify a suitable unrelated donor in up to 60% of Caucasians, although this figure is lower in other ethnic groups. Initial results with unrelated donor transplantation were characterized by a high TRM and an increased incidence of severe GvHD. In the last decade, there has been a marked improvement in outcome of unrelated donor SCT. Instrumental in this improvement in outcome has been the development of more accurate tissue typing techniques. In patients undergoing unrelated donor SCT, the availability of molecular typing at class I and II loci of the HLA complex has transformed the process of donor selection, since it is now clear that the presence of multiple disparities at class I or class II loci is associated with a worse transplant outcome. As yet, we lack sufficient information to allow us to identify whether specific allelic mismatches are of particular clinical significance.

Recent improvements in outcome using haploidentical donors make this an increasingly attractive alternative to unrelated donor transplantation. Until recently, haploidentical transplants have been associated with unacceptable rates of graft failure and GvHD. However, the ability to maximize the stem cell dose, using GCSF-mobilized progenitors, coupled with the development of efficient methods of TCD, has significantly improved outcome particularly in children.

Predicting outcome after allogeneic SCT is an imprecise science but analysis of registry data has allowed the identification of a number of risk factors that have been used to construct a robust prognostic score for patients allografted for CML (Table 25.7). The general principles encapsulated in this approach are also applicable to other diseases such as acute leukaemia where similar factors have been shown to affect outcome. In unrelated donor transplants patient CMV status also has a significant impact on outcome, with a marked increase in TRM in CMV-positive patients.

Table 25.7 Predictors of transplant outcome in patients undergoing allogeneic SCT for CML (Gratwohl et al., 1998).

Patient age

Donor match (sibling versus unrelated donor)

Donor sex (female–male associated with worse outcome)

Disease stage

Time from diagnosis to transplant (applies for patients with CML first CP)

Patient CMV serostatus (if undergoing VUD transplant)

Future developments in stem cell transplantation

Autologous stem cell transplantation

The commonest cause of failure after autografting is disease recurrence. Attempts to decrease disease relapse revolve around reducing the risk of contamination of the stem cell inoculum or the use of more effective conditioning regimens. By incubating stem cell harvests with a retrovirus, it is possible to 'tag' infused cells and demonstrate that cells within the transplanted stem cell inoculum do indeed contribute to disease relapse. However, attempts to decrease the risk of relapse using purging techniques have yielded disappointing results. Thus, although it is possible achieve up to a four-log reduction in the number of contaminating plasma cells, randomized studies have shown this does not reduce the relapse rate in patients autografted for myeloma.

The inability of conditioning regimens to eradicate malignant haemopoiesis at present is underlined by the observation that relapse rates remain high in CML and myeloma, even if syngeneic donors are used. Most of the drugs contained in preparative regimens are already administered at close to the limit of extramedullary toxicity and therefore there is little room for further dose escalation. Reducing the risk of relapse will depend either on altering the mode of delivery of agents used at present or the development of new therapies. The scope for optimizing drug delivery is demonstrated by the recent development of an intravenous preparation of busulphan, which results in a more predictable pharmacokinetic profile. Preliminary studies suggest that this approach may decrease the risk of VOD. Haematological malignancies are radiosensitive and there is interest in the possibility of increasing the effective dose of irradiation delivered to the marrow without increasing organ toxicity using radiolabelled immunoconjugates. Early-phase clinical studies using β-emitters (e.g. ^{131}I or ^{90}Y) conjugated to myeloid-specific antigens, such as CD45 or CD66, demonstrate that such an approach is feasible, and phase II studies in myeloma and lymphoma are ongoing.

Allogeneic stem cell transplantation

Major factors limiting the successful application of allogeneic SCT include regimen-related toxicity, GvHD, infectious complications and disease relapse. The use of RIC regimens to reduce the toxicity of allografting is discussed elsewhere. TCD remains the most highly effective method of GvHD prophylaxis, particularly when unrelated donors are used. A major limitation in the effective use of TCD is the increased rate of infectious complications associated with this manoeuvre. The possibility of accelerating immune reconstitution after allogeneic SCT by transfer of antigen-specific cytotoxic T lymphocytes to viruses such as CMV and EBV is being explored at present. Such cells can be generated either by culturing donor lymphocytes with candidate antigens or by direct selection from donor blood using HLA tetramers. Alternatively, infusion of donor lymphocytes from which alloreactive T cells have been depleted may hasten immune reconstitution without incurring a risk of GvHD. In one approach, alloreactive T cells are depleted from the stem cell inoculum by incubating them *ex vivo* with recipient APCs. Activated T cells, defined by the expression of CD25, are then removed using magnetic selection techniques or an immunotoxin. Alternatively, blockade of APC-mediated costimulation (for example, using CTLA-4–Ig or antibodies to B7) may induce anergy or deletion of alloreactive T cells. Co-infusion of naturally occurring or *ex vivo* expanded CD4+ CD25+ regulatory T cells may also inhibit conventional T cells from inducing GvHD. These strategies are all under intense investigation at the present time.

Reducing the risk of relapse after allogeneic SCT can be achieved either by increasing the intensity of the conditioning regimen or by optimizing the GvL effect. Incorporating radioimmunotherapy into the preparative regimen shows promise in the setting of allogeneic SCT and may prove of value in patients with advanced leukaemia, in whom relapse is the most important cause of treatment failure. Alternatively, patients judged to be at a high risk of relapse may benefit from prophylactic DLI, administered with the aim of boosting a GvL response. Such an approach is limited by the fact that administration of donor lymphocytes within the first 12 months of SCT is associated with a high rate of GvHD, particularly if an unrelated donor has been used. Consequently, there is great attraction in the use of donor lymphocytes that recognize residual host leukaemia. Early clinical studies examining the use of lymphocytes generated against minor H antigens or leukaemia-specific antigens such as WT1 and proteinase 3 are recruiting at present. If successful, such an approach, coupled with a TCD transplant, may offer the possibility of disassociating GvHD from GvL.

Selected bibliography

Appelbaum FR (2000) Is there a best conditioning regimen for acute myeloid leukemia? *Leukemia* 14: 497–501.

Aversa F, Tabilio A, Cunningham I *et al.* (1998) Treatment of high-risk acute leukaemia with T-cell-depleted stem cells from related donors with one fully mismatched HLA haplotype. *New England Journal of Medicine* 339: 1186–93.

Bacher-Lustig E, Rachamin N, Li H *et al.* (1995) Megadose of T cell-depleted bone marrow overcomes MHC barriers in sublethally irradiated mice. *Nature Medicine* 1: 1268–73.

Brenner MK, Rill DR, Moen RC *et al.* (1993) Gene-marking to trace origin of relapse after autologous bone-marrow transplantation. *Lancet* 342: 1134–7.

Clift R, Buckner CD, Appelbaum FR *et al.* (1990) Allogeneic marrow transplantation in patients with acute myeloid leukameia in first remission: a randomized trial of two irradiation regimens. *Blood* 76: 1867–71.

Crawford S, Petersen FB (1992) Long-term survival from respiratory failure after marrow transplantation for haematolgical malignancy. *American Review of Respiratory Disease* **145**: 510–14.

Ferry C, Socie G (2003) Busulfan-cyclophosphamide versus total body irradiation plus cyclophosphamide as preparative regimen before allogeneic hematopoietic stem cell transplantation for acute myeloid leukemia. *Experimental Hematology* **31**: 1182–6.

Gratwohl A, Hermans J, Goldman J *et al.* (1998) Risk assessment for patients with chronic myeloid leukaemia before allogeneic bone marrow transplantation. *Lancet* **352**: 1087–92.

Hansen J, Gooley T, Martin P *et al.* (1998) Bone marrow transplants from unrelated donors for patients with chronic myeloid leukemia. *New England Journal of Medicine* **338**: 962–8.

Ho VT, Soifer RJ (2000) The history and future of T-cell depletion as graft-versus-host disease prophylaxis for allogeneic hematopoietic stem cell transplantation. *Blood* **98**: 3192–204.

Kolb H, Schattenberg A, Goldman J *et al.* (1995) Graft-versus-leukemia effect of donor lymphocyte transfusions in marrow grafted patients. European Group for Blood and Marrow Transplantation Working Party Chronic Leukemia. *Blood* **86**: 2041–50.

Laughlin MJ, Eapen M, Rubinstein P *et al.* (2004) Outcome after transplantation of cord blood or bone marrow from unrelated donors in adults with leukaemia. *New England Journal of Medicine* **351**: 2265–75.

Mackinnon S, Papadopoulos E, Carabasi M *et al.* (1995) Adoptive immunotherapy evaluating escalating doses of donor leucocytes for relapse of chronic myeloid leukemia after bone marrow transplantation: separation of graft-versus-leukemia effect from graft-versus-host disease. *Blood* **86**: 1261–8.

McSweeney PA, Niederwieser D, Shizuru JA *et al.* (2001) Hematopoietic cell transplantation in older paients with hematologic malignacies: replacing high-dose cytotoxic therapy with graft-versus-tumor effects. *Blood* **97**: 3390–400.

Moss PA, Cobbold M, Craddock C (2003) The cellular immunotherapy of viral infections. *Transfusion Medicine* **13**: 405–15.

Petersdorf EW, Mickelson EM, Anasetti C *et al.* (1999) Effect of HLA mismatches on the outcome of hematopoietic transplants. *Current Opinion in Immunology* **11**: 521–6.

Rocha V, Labopin M, Sanz G *et al.* (2004) Transplants of umbilical-cord blood or bone marrow from unrelated donors in adults with leukaemia. *New England Journal of Medicine* **351**: 2276–85.

Schmitz N, Linch DC, Dreger P *et al.* (1996) Randomised trial of filgrastim-mobilized peripheral blood progenitor cell transplantation versus autologous bone-marrow transplantation in lymphoma patients. *Lancet* **347**: 353–7.

Sierra J, Storer B, Hansen J *et al.* (1997) transplantation of marrow cells from unrelated donors for treatment of high-risk acute leukemia: the effect of leukemic burden, donor HLA matching and marrow cell dose. *Blood* **89**: 4226–35.

Slavin S, NaglerA, Naparstek E *et al.* (1998) Nonmyeloablative stem cell transplantation and cell therapy as an alternative to conventional bone marrow transplantation with lethal cytoreduction for the treatment of malignant and nonmalignant hematologic diseases. *Blood* **91**: 756–63.

Socie G, Tone JV, Wingard JR *et al.* (1999) Long-term survival and late deaths after allogeneic marrow transplantation. Late Effects Working Committee of the International Bone Marrow Transplant Registry. *New England Journal of Medicine* **341**: 14.

Socie G, Salooja N, Cohen A *et al.* (2003) Nonmalignant late effects after allogeneic stem cell transplantation. *Blood* **101**: 3373–85.

Vogelsang GB (2001) How I treat chronic graft-versus-host disease. *Blood* **97**: 1191–201.

Yu C, Storb R, Mathey B *et al.* (1995) DLA-identical bone marrow grafts after low-dose total body irradiation: effects of high dose corticosteroids and cyclosporin on engraftment. *Blood* **86**: 4376–81.

CHAPTER 26

Non-myeloablative transplantation

Kirsty J Thomson, Michael Potter and Stephen Mackinnon

Introduction

Conventional allogeneic transplantation

In patients with haematological malignancy, bone marrow transplantation from an allogeneic donor has become a well-established mode of treatment for selected patient groups.

The rationale behind this therapeutic procedure is that conditioning treatment is administered in doses designed to ablate the host haemopoietic tissue and, with it, the remnants of the malignancy. The incoming donor graft is then introduced, in the face of minimal resistance from the depleted endogenous immune system, to repopulate the empty marrow and rescue the patient from death due to aplasia. This then largely mimics the technique of high-dose therapy with autologous stem cell rescue (autograft), with the additional benefit of guaranteed tumour-free replacement stem cells.

The disadvantages of this allografting technique, however, relate both to the formidable toxicity of the radio- and chemotherapy used in the conditioning regimens and to the morbidity and mortality ascribable to graft-versus-host disease (GvHD) – the immunological consequence of engrafting an allogeneic immune system – and its treatment.

These effects can be marked in certain groups, for example in older patients, such that allogeneic transplants have conventionally been utilized only in those under the age of 50–55 years, in the absence of concomitant medical problems. As most haematological malignancies peak in presentation after the age of 50, the majority of affected patients have not been considered for allogeneic transplantation. In addition, the procedure-related mortality for certain patient cohorts (e.g. those with Hodgkin's lymphoma, multiple myeloma) when treated with conventional allografts has historically been particularly high – whether because of the pattern of prior treatments, disease-related end organ damage, or other host/disease factors – and clinicians

have therefore tended not to offer this line of therapy in such situations.

There is, however, considerable evidence supporting the existence of a graft-versus-malignancy (GvM) effect, whereby an immune response, mediated by T lymphocytes from the incoming allograft, is directed at the host-derived residual tumour cells. Evidence in support of this concept first emerged over 20 years ago, with the observation of an association between the occurrence of graft-versus-host disease and a reduction in relapse rates, and has been further supported by the finding of similarly reduced relapse rates when allogeneic donors are compared with syngeneic donors, and when T cells are not depleted from the incoming graft. Most recently, there has also been the observation that durable disease responses can be obtained, in patients in whom relapse has occurred post allograft, by the direct infusion of additional donor lymphocytes. The disease in which this has been most comprehensively demonstrated is chronic myeloid leukaemia. Not only has the donor lymphocyte infusion (DLI) responsiveness of this disease been shown, it has also been noted that the graft-versus-leukaemia (GvL) effect can be separated from the GvHD effect by incremental increase in CD3 doses, administered at increasing times from transplant. This concept that a therapeutic window exists in which an optimal T-cell dose infused at an appropriate time following allograft will result in an isolated anti-tumour effect has been of particular interest to those attempting to manipulate the donor allogeneic effect in the context of reduced-intensity conditioning.

Reduced-intensity conditioning

Principles

As a potential solution to the problems of excessive regimen-related toxicity, the reduced-intensity or non-myeloablative allograft, was introduced in the mid-1990s.

Table 26.1 Advantages/disadvantages of reduced-intensity conditioning relative to conventional myeloablative regimens.

Advantages	Disadvantages

Transplants available in
  Older patients
  Those with comorbid conditions
  Patients with prior autograft
  In non-malignant conditions in which
    feasibility relies on minimal TRM
	Curative potential of myeloablation is lost
	Reliance on GvL effect risks continuing
	  morbidity/mortality from associated GvHD

Some regimens allow outpatient transplantation.

Here, the conditioning regimens are designed principally to immunosuppress the host sufficiently to allow donor engraftment, cure of disease being delivered subsequently by the allogeneic GvL effect. Although the regimens contain varying degrees of anti-tumour activity in order to control the malignancy until the incoming lymphoid compartment is sufficiently reconstituted to exert such a GvL effect, the aim of the conditioning therapy is no longer principally to eradicate disease, and thus toxicity is significantly reduced. In this way, the benefits of allogeneic transplantation can potentially be extended to patients who would generally not be considered candidates for conventional myeloablative transplant regimens (Table 26.1). Although all the regimens devised are broadly grouped together as 'reduced-intensity' or 'mini-' transplants, there is significant disparity in the relative degree of immunosuppression and myelosuppression involved (Figure 26.1). With minimally myelosuppressive or truly non-myeloablative regimens, patients can be conditioned such that donor neutrophil engraftment occurs in the absence of recipient granulocyte aplasia, and this preservation of circulating granulocyte numbers thus reduces the risks of serious bacterial sepsis, so the treatment can even be delivered in an outpatient setting. Conversely, the more myelosuppressive or 'reduced-intensity' regimens cause observable aplasia and carry greater toxicity but have the advantage of greater debulking of residual disease, which may be of importance in those malignancies which are aggressive and propagate rapidly.

To facilitate durable engraftment, the host has to be adequately immunosuppressed in order that the incoming stem cells are not rejected. This is often achieved by using the purine analogue, fludarabine, in combination with either low-dose total body irradiation (TBI) or alkylating drugs such as cyclophosphamide, melphalan or busulphan. Some regimens incorporate, in addition, anti-T-cell serotherapy with either alemtuzumab or anti-thymocyte globulin (ATG) to reduce the incidence of GvHD, although this must be balanced against the need for T cells to facilitate engraftment, contain viral infection and mediate subsequent GvL effects.

Finally, it is important to note that the kinetics of engraftment are significantly altered in non-myeloablative transplantation, although, once again, this is regimen dependent. Given that non-reversible myeloablation is not the aim, host haemopoiesis remains potentially functional, although suppressed, to varying degrees depending on the conditioning approach. This gives rise to a situation of mixed chimerism, whereby assays can detect cells of both recipient and donor origin in peripheral blood. In general, the more intensive regimens – those rendering the host temporarily aplastic – tend to lead to rapid full donor reconstitution, although mixed chimerism can re-emerge subsequently, whereas the minimally myelosuppressive regimens tend to result in a state of initial mixed chimerism. In this situation, a graft-versus-host haemopoiesis effect is required to gradually convert to full donor haemopoiesis. Once again, depending on the underlying condition being treated, rapidly eradicating host haemopoiesis and thus potentially residual malignancy may be a priority. The techniques available for detecting chimerism are usually either cytogenetic, e.g. fluorescence *in situ* hybridization (FISH) to detect sex chromosomes where there is a donor/recipient gender mismatch, or molecular, commonly a polymerase chain reaction (PCR)-based method utilizing microsatellite disparities.

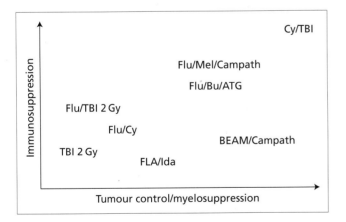

Figure 26.1 Comparing the relative myelosuppressive and immunosuppressive properties of various reduced-intensity conditioning regimens. Abbreviations: TBI, total body irradiation; flu, fludarabine; cy, cyclophosphamide; FLA/Ida, fludarabine, cytarabine, idarubicin; mel, melphalan; bu, busulphan; ATG, anti-thymocyte globulin; BEAM, carmustine, cytarabine, etoposide, melphalan.

Regimens

Initial reports from Giralt *et al.* (1997) demonstrated that conditioning with fludarabine, idarubicin and cytarabine in 15 patients with acute myeloid leukaemia (AML)/myelodysplastic syndrome (MDS) could result in successful engraftment and complete remission, in some cases of reasonable duration (Table 26.2). This regimen, however, proved insufficiently immunosuppressive to support consistent engraftment in chronic myeloid leukaemia (CML). The same group went on to demonstrate successful engraftment and encouragingly long-lived disease responses in a cohort of 86 patients with haematological malignancies using a purine analogue and melphalan combination, albeit with 34% of patients developing grade II–IV acute GvHD, and with a transplant-related mortality (TRM) at 2 years of 45%. This study also examined the use of a cladribine/melphalan combination, which proved unacceptably toxic.

Other centres were experimenting with radiotherapy-containing regimens, in the expectation that minimizing myelo-suppression while providing sufficient immunosuppression to facilitate engraftment would lessen treatment toxicity and even allow transplantation to occur in the outpatient setting. The regimens implemented built on pre-existing data from canine models using MHC-identical littermates which had demonstrated the threshold doses required, first, for causing lethal aplasia and, second, for allowing donor stem cell engraftment. Subsequently it was shown that similar engraftment could also be achieved with incremental reductions in TBI doses if immunosuppressive drugs were additionally administered, the TBI required varying with the drugs chosen.

These findings were then translated into a clinical model of low-dose TBI-based conditioning in HLA-matched related transplants for patients with haematological malignancies, with the majority of transplants being performed in the outpatient setting. The conditioning consisted of a single fraction of 2 Gy TBI given on the day of stem cell return, with immunosuppression thereafter by cyclosporin A (CyA) and mycophenolate mofetil (MMF). Although initial engraftment occurred in all patients, with most avoiding severe cytopenia, 20% of the first 45 rejected following discontinuation of their immunosuppression. The protocol was adjusted to include fludarabine in the conditioning, and rejection was seen thereafter in only 3%. Acute GvHD grade II–IV occurred in 46%, and, of the total 192 patients, 59% were alive at a median follow-up of 289 days. Transplant-related mortality was 22% and the remaining 18% died of their underlying disease, with 2-year overall survival and progression-free survival estimates of 50% and 40% respectively.

Given these results, this regimen was then used in a study of 77 HLA-matched unrelated donor allografts. Sustained engraftment was seen in 78% of patients, with rejection more common in those patients whose stem cell source was bone marrow (7/17; 41% rejected) rather than peripheral blood (10/60; 17%). Data are also available for a cohort of 52 patients with both matched and mismatched unrelated donors; with a median follow-up of 19 months, overall survival and progression-free survival figures were 35% and 25% respectively. Further studies are ongoing with peripheral blood stem cells (PBSC) only as stem cell source, and with modifications to post-transplant immunosuppression in an attempt to reduce late rejection events.

Each of the above regimens involves reinfusing an unmanipulated T-replete graft. As discussed in the previous section, although there are reasons for preferring this approach, it does confer significant risks of acute and chronic GvHD, with the attendant morbidity and mortality. The alternative involves a degree of T-cell depletion of the incoming stem cells, and, in the non-myeloablative setting, this has tended to be done by the use of anti-lymphocyte antibodies *in vivo*. These antibodies are given as part of the conditioning and thus fulfil a dual role, immunosuppressing both host and, as a result of their persistence *in vivo*, incoming donor T cells. The antibodies most commonly used are (ATG) or alemtuzumab (Campath-1H), the former being a mixed product with wide-ranging specificities including T lymphocytes, and the latter an anti-CD52 monoclonal antibody, which targets a variety of cell-types, including T cells, B cells and monocytes.

Slavin *et al.* reported the use of ATG, busulphan and fludarabine, first in 26 patients with either haematological malignancies or genetic disease and subsequently in a further 23 patients, all of whom had lymphoma. This regimen has incorporated subsequent donor lymphocyte infusions (DLIs) to compensate for the T depleting effect of *in vivo* ATG, and disease-free survival was 81% at median follow-up 240 days for the former group and 43% at 675 days for the latter group. Subsequent results have been particularly encouraging for patients with chronic myeloid leukaemia.

Finally, several groups have used regimens containing alemtuzumab (Campath-1H) or, less commonly, Campath-1G. While the most prevalent approach is to combine alemtuzumab with fludarabine and an alkylating agent, many other combinations are under investigation, and the optimal antibody and chemotherapy schedule remains to be established. Kottaridis *et al.* reported a series of 44 patients with haematological malignancies conditioned with alemtuzumab, fludarabine and melphalan, and observed sustained engraftment in 42 of the 43 evaluable patients. Only two patients developed grade II GvHD, with no grade III–IV, and, at a median follow-up of 9 months, progression-free survival was 75%. Other approaches include the use of alemtuzumab, fludarabine and busulphan in MDS in a series of 23 patients, which resulted in 2-year actuarial disease-free survival of 39%, and the use of Campath-1G with BEAM (carmustine, etoposide, cytarabine, melphalan) chemotherapy in lymphoid malignancies, following which 57% of 30 patients studied were disease-free at a median follow-up of 1.3 years.

One of the most striking features of the alemtuzumab-containing regimens is the reduction in GvHD rates. As mentioned above, grade II–IV GvHD has been reported to affect < 5% of

Table 26.2 Reduced-intensity conditioning regimens.

Reference	Disease	No. of patients	Donor	Conditioning regimen	GvHD	Outcome
Giralt et al. (1997)	AML/MDS	15	Related	Flu/Ida/Ara-C 2-CDA/Ara-C	Acute (grade II–IV) 20%	Median follow-up 100 days CR in 8, OS 6
Giralt et al. (2001)	HM	86	Related/unrelated	Flu/mel 2-CDA/mel	Acute (grade II–IV) 34% Chronic 21%	Two-year TRM 45% DFS 23%
McSweeney et al. (2001)	HM	45	Related	200 cGy TBI	Acute (grade II–IV) 47% Chronic > 60%	Median follow-up 417 days OS 67%, NRM 7%, RM 27%
Niederwieser et al. (2003)	HM	52	Unrelated	200 cGy TBI/flu	Acute (grade II–IV) 63% Chronic 30%	Median follow-up 19 months OS 35%, DFS 25% NRM 38%, RM 27%
Slavin et al. (1998)	HM/GD	26	Related	Flu/bu/ATG	Acute (grade II–IV) 38% Chronic 35%	Median follow-up 8 months OS 85%, DFS 81%
Nagler et al. (2000)	LM	23	Related	Flu/bu/ATG	Acute (grade II–IV) 35% Chronic 18%	Median follow-up 675 days DFS 43%
Kottaridis et al. (2000)	HM	44	Related	Flu/mel/alem	Acute (grade II) 4%	Median follow-up 9 months PFS 75%
Lush et al. (2001)	LM	30	Related/unrelated	BEAM/Campath-1G	Acute (grade I–II) 23%	Median follow-up 1.3 years DFS 57%

Abbreviations: AML/MDS, acute myeloid leukaemia/myelodysplastic syndrome; flu, fludarabine; ida, idarubicin; CR, complete remission; OS, overall survival; 2-CDA, 2-chlorodeoxyadenosine; mel, melphalan; TRM, transplant-related mortality; DFS, disease-free survival; HM, haematological malignancy; TBI, total body irradiation; NRM, non-relapse mortality; RM, relapse mortality; GD, genetic disorders; ATG, anti-thymocyte globulin; alem, alemtuzumab; BEAM, carmustine, Ara-C, etoposide, melphalan; PFS, progression-free survival.

patients receiving matched related allografts, and even in the unrelated setting a series of 47 patients, 20 of whom were mismatched for HLA class I and/or class II alleles, yielded grade II–IV GvHD in 21%, with grade III–IV in only 6%. This compares extremely favourably to those regimens that lack T-cell depletion, with the use of an unrelated donor in the fludarabine and melphalan study described earlier leading to a 25% mortality from acute GvHD.

Infections

A major cause of morbidity and mortality in allogeneic transplantation is infection. There has been some speculation that the use of reduced-intensity conditioning may alter the incidence and characteristics of such infection, for example by using regimens in which mucositis is reduced and by avoiding the lung injury associated with high-dose radiotherapy. Predictably, the profile of infection varies according to the conditioning regimen employed, with those minimally myelosuppressive regimens causing little or no neutropenia (e.g. fludarabine and low-dose TBI) resulting in less risk of early bacterial and fungal infection. Regarding the risk of opportunistic infection, particularly post-engraftment viral infection, this varies with the degree of immunosuppression inherent in the protocol. For example, lymphoid reconstitution is delayed in patients conditioned with regimens including T-cell-depleting antibodies such as alemtuzumab, with its *in vivo* T-depleting effect on the incoming allograft. This results in a high rate of cytomegalovirus (CMV) reactivation, although, with appropriate surveillance and prompt treatment, no excess of disease. This rate of reactivation, however, is not significantly different from similar T-depleted myeloablative regimens, and perhaps the only difference that is suggested between myeloablative and non-myeloablative regimens in the context of viral infection is a reduction in mortality following early respiratory virus infections in the latter group, presumably as they lack the pulmonary toxicity of myeloablative doses of TBI.

Finally, as would be expected, those protocols which contain no T-cell depletion result in significantly higher rates of acute and chronic GvHD, with the concomitant excess of infection that this entails.

In summary, therefore, the risks of infection appear to relate to the degree and length of neutropenia, degree of T depletion and incidence of GvHD – which vary considerably between reduced-intensity protocols – and are similar to those seen in myeloablative protocols, if matched for these risk factors. The possible exception to this seems to be a reduced mortality from respiratory infection in the absence of ablative doses of TBI.

Graft rejection/source of stem cells

Both bone marrow and granulocyte colony-stimulating factor (G-CSF) mobilized PBSCs have been used extensively in reduced-

intensity conditioning transplants. The experience with myeloablative regimens would suggest that the use of PBSCs results in more rapid engraftment and in higher rates of chronic GvHD.

There are few specific data in the reduced-intensity setting that address rates of GvHD/engraftment with differing stem cell source, although the Seattle group – using a minimally myelosuppressive regimen – did describe significantly increased rejection when the source of stem cells used was bone marrow rather than PBSCs. Further studies with this protocol therefore have been carried out with only PBSCs as the stem cell source. In addition, the earliest regimen used by this group contained low-dose TBI only, and gave rejection rates of 20%, a figure reduced to 3% by the addition of fludarabine to provide further host immunosuppression.

The more intensive regimens have been associated with significantly less graft rejection, irrespective of stem cell source, with one alemtuzumab-based regimen resulting in rejection in < 3% using PBSCs from sibling donors and 6% using bone marrow from unrelated donors.

Donor type/graft-versus-host disease

Regarding donor type, the early experience with reduced-intensity conditioning using sibling donors has been successfully extended to unrelated donors, either HLA-matched or 1–2 allele mismatched. As expected, the rates of GvHD increase with the use of unrelated, and particularly mismatched, donors, with substantially greater rates of GvHD when the regimens are T-cell replete. For example, the low-dose TBI-based regimens give acute (grade II–IV) GvHD rates of ~45% and ~60% in the sibling and unrelated setting respectively, whereas a T-deplete alemtuzumab-based regimen gives acute (grade II–IV) GvHD rates of 5% and ~20% in the sibling and unrelated settings. Chronic GvHD rates follow a similar pattern.

It had been proposed that the absence of the inflammatory response induced by myeloablative doses of TBI or chemotherapy would lead to generally less acute GvHD in reduced-intensity transplants when compared with the myeloablative setting, but this has not been confirmed.

It would be fair to conclude that there do not appear to be any particular characteristics of GvHD incidence intrinsic to reduced-intensity conditioning, rather that there are substantial differences seen depending on the degree of T-cell depletion in the non-myeloablative regimen used, and that these incidences are similar to those seen in myeloablative transplantation.

Disease-specific outcomes

Multiple myeloma

For the vast majority of patients, multiple myeloma is currently an incurable disease.

Standard treatment involves initial cytoreductive chemotherapy preceding high-dose therapy, with autologous PBSC rescue. While this strategy can result in several years of progression-free survival, there is a continual decline in disease-free survival (DFS), and relapse is generally considered inevitable.

The only prospect for long-term DFS has been allogeneic transplantation with conventional ablative conditioning. However, only a small number of patients are eligible for this treatment for reasons of age/comorbidity/donor availability, and the combination of TRM and disease relapse remains formidable, even in those deemed suitable. Although the historical reported TRM rates are now improving, with advances in supportive care, such non-relapse mortality remains usually in excess of 30%, even in highly selected younger patients with HLA-matched sibling donors. There is, however, evidence for a GvM effect, with demonstration of responses following donor lymphocyte infusion for relapse following conventional allograft, in the order of 40–60%.

The combination, therefore, of allogeneic transplantation as the only demonstrably curative treatment, evidence for a GvM effect, and a high attrition rate from transplant-related causes when conventional conditioning is used, makes this disease an attractive candidate for reduced-intensity conditioning regimens (Table 26.3).

Peggs et al. reported a series of 20 patients (12 HLA-matched related donors, eight unrelated donors) conditioned with alemtuzumab, fludarabine and melphalan. As expected in this setting of T-cell depletion, GvHD rates were encouragingly low, with only 3/20 patients developing grade II acute GvHD and none developing grade III or IV. Unfortunately, the disease responses post transplant presumably also reflect the degree of donor T-cell depletion, with only two patients in complete remission (CR) at 6 months, four in partial remission (PR) and two with minimal response. Donor lymphocytes in escalating doses were given to 14 patients, with seven demonstrating further disease responses – mostly but not exclusively those who also developed GvHD – but these responses were once again not durable, with a 2-year progression-free survival of only 30%.

This and other early experience in myeloma would suggest that debulking of disease to a minimum prior to the allograft, and certainly to a stable plateau, may be necessary to minimize the chance of early progression post transplant, and several groups have addressed this question, with protocols including high-dose chemotherapy with autologous stem cell rescue prior to the allogeneic procedure.

Maloney et al. reported a series of 54 patients treated with induction chemotherapy followed by high-dose melphalan and autologous stem cell rescue. At a median of 62 days later, patients were then conditioned with 2 Gy TBI and stem cells from HLA-matched related donors were returned, with CyA and MMF given as additional immunosuppression. Overall survival at a median follow-up of 552 days was 78%, with a TRM of 17% and extensive chronic GvHD in 46%. Of the 48 patients not in CR at study entry, 25 (52%) subsequently achieved CR and, of those patients (plus the six who entered the study in CR), only three have relapsed. Outcome, in terms of both TRM and disease response, was better in those transplanted with chemoresponsive disease, and the overall progression-free survival at 2 years was estimated at 55%.

A similar tandem approach has been reported by Kroger et al. in 17 patients (nine with HLA-matched related donors) with non-progressive myeloma, who received a melphalan autograft as above, and then were conditioned with fludarabine, melphalan and ATG, prior to stem cell infusion. Complete remission occurred in 72% post procedure, exclusively in those with proven chemosensitive disease, and the estimated progression-free survival at 2 years was 56%.

The follow-up in these studies is currently relatively short, and a true assessment of efficacy is not yet possible, but the early experience suggests that cytoreduction with an autograft may be obligatory if allogeneic transplantation with reduced-intensity conditioning is to be successful in this disease. In addition, the responses in these studies have usually been associated with the presence of GvHD, and there is currently little evidence for a GvM effect occurring in the absence of such GvHD.

Non-Hodgkin's lymphoma

Low-grade non-Hodgkin's lymphoma

This group of conditions, although indolent and frequently consistent with lengthy survival from the time of diagnosis, remain incurable with conventional chemotherapy. High-dose chemotherapy has been used in association with autologous stem cell rescue, and can generate prolonged DFS, but there is a continuing risk of relapse, and a plateau is not apparent on DFS curves.

Where allogeneic transplantation has been employed, the familiar pattern of reduced relapse risk offset by a significant risk of procedure-related mortality has proved prohibitive in the majority of patients. Treatment toxicity is particularly pronounced in the presence of a preceding autograft, and increases with increasing age, rendering the majority of patients with low-grade non-Hodgkin's lymphoma (NHL) ineligible, given the predominance of older patients in the affected cohort.

This has therefore been a particularly attractive setting for transplantation with reduced-intensity conditioning, and several groups have reported series of patients treated in this way, many of whom have relapsed following previous autograft procedures, and some of whom have chemorefractory disease (Table 26.3).

Encouraging results have been reported in a cohort of 20 patients conditioned with cyclophosphamide and fludarabine, nine of whom also received rituximab. Although numbers are relatively small, and 12 of the patients were in complete remission already at the time of transplant, all patients achieved a durable complete remission post procedure, with no disease relapses at a median follow-up of 21 months. In addition, of the six patients who were tested for minimal residual disease by

Table 26.3 Disease-specific outcome according to regimen.

Reference	No. of patients	Conditioning	GvHD	Outcome
Myeloma				
Peggs *et al.* (2003)	20	Flu/mel/alem	Acute (grade II) 15%	Two-year OS 71%; cPFS 30%, NRM 15%
Maloney *et al.* (2003)	54	(mel autograft 1st) 200 cGy TBI	Acute (grade II–IV) 38% Chronic 46%	Median follow-up 552 days OS 78% PFS at 2 years 55%
Kroger *et al.* (2002)	17	(mel autograft 1st) Flu/mel/ATG	Acute (grade II–III) 38% Chronic 40%	PFS at 2 years 56%
Low-grade NHL				
Khouri *et al.* (2001)	20	Cy/flu/ritux	Acute (grade II–IV) 20% Chronic 64%	DFS at 2 years 84%
Morris *et al.* (2002)	46 (94 all diagnoses)	Flu/mel/alem	Acute (grade II–IV) 13% Chronic 5%	TRM at 3 years 10% PFS at 4 years 65%
Fibich *et al.* (2002)	13	Flu/bu/ATG	Acute (grade II–III) 54% Chronic 31%	Median follow-up 652 days OS 93%, DFS 77%
Faulkner *et al.* (2004)	51 (65 all diagnoses)	BEAM/Campath-1G or BEAM/alem	Acute (grade I–II) 17%	EFS at 2 years 69%
High-grade NHL				
Morris *et al.* (2002)	48	Flu/mel/alem	As above	OS at 3 years 35% PFS at 3 years 29% TRM at 3 years 37%
Faulkner *et al.* (2004)	14	BEAM/Campath-1G or BEAM/alem	As above	EFS at 2 years 17% RR at 2 years 68%
Corradini *et al.* (2002)	10 (45 all diagnoses)	Flu/cy/thiotepa	Acute (grade II–IV) 47%	Median follow-up 385 days 70% CR
Spitzer *et al.* (2003)	20	Cy/ATG or anti-CD2/TI	Acute (grade II–IV) 45%	Follow-up 13–52 months DFS 25%

Abbreviations: flu, fludarabine; CR, complete remission; OS, overall survival; mel, melphalan; TRM, transplant-related mortality; DFS, disease-free survival; TBI, total body irradiation; NRM, non-relapse mortality; RR, relapse rate; ATG, anti-thymocyte globulin; alem, alemtuzumab; BEAM, carmustine, Ara-C, etoposide, melphalan; PFS, progression-free survival; cPFS, current progression-free survival; NRM, non-relapse mortality; ritux, rituximab; cy, cyclophosphamide; EFS, event-free survival; CR, complete remission; TI, thymic irradiation; bu, busulphan.

PCR for the *Bcl-2* gene rearrangement before transplant, all subsequently achieved molecular remission. This gave a 2-year actuarial DFS of 84%, although with a cumulative incidence of chronic GvHD of 64%.

The use of T-depleting regimens has also been reported. Morris *et al.* conditioned 46 patients with low-grade NHL [31 follicular NHL, 12 chronic lymphocytic leukaemia (CLL)] with alemtuzumab, melphalan and fludarabine. Most were in partial remission at the time of the transplant, and 25% had had prior autograft procedures. The TRM at 3 years was 10%, with 4-year actuarial overall survival of 69% and progression-free survival of 65%. Eleven patients received DLI for residual disease or disease progression, of whom six responded. Thus, this regimen can be given to relatively heavily pretreated patients with an extremely low incidence of GvHD and a respectable procedure-related mortality. Although the infused graft is T depleted by the alemtuzumab *in vivo*, the conditioning regimen has cytoreductive capacity which appears, so far, to protect from the potential relapse risk conferred by the loss of alloreactive T cells in the initial post-transplant period.

Another T-depleting regimen (fludarabine, busulphan and ATG) was described in 13 patients with CLL, of whom 12 were alive at a median follow-up of 652 days, and 10 of whom were disease-free, as assayed by flow cytometry for minimal residual disease in bone marrow.

The combination of alemtuzumab with BEAM has also been employed with low TRM in patients with lymphoma. Faulkner et al. reported a cohort of 51 patients with low-grade lymphoproliferative disease (including five with Hodgkin's lymphoma), conditioned with BEAM-Campath, whose actuarial event-free survival (EFS) at 2 years was 69%, with a relapse rate of 10%. Rituximab has also been added to this schedule to maximize cytoreduction, and preliminary results have been encouraging, with three out of five patients alive in molecular remission at a median follow-up of 521 days.

In addition, data on 77 patients with CLL collated by the Chronic Leukaemia Working Party of the European Bone Marrow Transplant group, albeit with heterogeneous conditioning regimens, showed a 1-year TRM of 18% and event-free and overall survival at 2 years of 56% and 72% respectively.

Therefore, it can be seen that this approach shows promise in the management of the low-grade lymphomas. There is some evidence supporting the presence of a GvL effect, the regimens have relatively low procedure-related mortality, and, although disease control pre-transplant is important, the indolent nature of the disease makes the risk of relapse in the period immediately post engraftment, before the generation of an effective anti-tumour allogeneic, less of an issue than in some of the other haematological malignancies discussed. The very indolence of the disease, however, means that it is still too early to comment on the efficacy of any of these regimens in effecting cure, and data emerging as these cohorts mature will be critical.

High-grade non-Hodgkin's lymphoma

Overall, high-grade NHL is curable in approximately 40–50% of affected individuals, a proportion of whom have relapsed and been salvaged by second-line treatment followed by autograft as consolidation. Almost inevitably, therefore, those patients who have up until now been considered for allogeneic transplantation with conventional conditioning have failed a previous autograft and been in, at best, a third complete remission. Transplant-related mortality in this situation has been reported from around 30% to in excess of 50%.

Several groups have therefore explored the use of reduced-intensity conditioning regimens (Table 26.3).

Morris et al., in the cohort described above, also reported 47 patients with high/intermediate-grade NHL. Most were again in partial remission at the time of transplant, and 70% had had a prior autograft. The TRM at 3 years was 37%, with actuarial overall survival and progression-free survival at 4 years of 35% and 29% respectively. Seven patients received DLI, of whom three responded.

The BEAM–Campath regimen has also been used in high/ intermediate-grade NHL, with a less encouraging event-free survival than in low-grade disease (17% at 2 years), and a correspondingly high relapse rate (68% at 2 years). Responses to DLI given for disease progression were poor, and this group now plan to reduce post-transplant immunosuppression in an attempt to combat early relapse.

Corradini et al. described 10 patients with high-grade NHL who received conditioning with thiotepa, fludarabine and cyclophosphamide before reinfusion of a T-replete graft. Non-relapse mortality was relatively low and, at the time of reporting, seven of the patients were alive in complete remission.

In addition, Spitzer et al. reported a series of 20 patients with diffuse large B-cell lymphoma, 17 of whom had chemorefractory disease, who were conditioned with cyclophosphamide, ATG or anti-CD2 antibody and thymic irradiation. Eight patients had a disease response, and, of these, five were alive and progression free at 13–52 months' follow-up (25%). Four of these five patients had chronic GvHD.

There have been many other reports of the use of different conditioning regimens on small numbers of patients with high-grade disease. In general, the data on high-grade disease are less encouraging than on low-grade disease, with usually higher procedure-related mortality and poorer disease response rates, although progression-free survival with 1–2 year follow-up is certainly being seen in a proportion of these otherwise incurable patients.

The generally inferior disease responses seen may partly reflect the more rapid tempo of disease growth when compared with low-grade disease, meaning that the risk of early relapse or progression is relatively higher during the period post transplant prior to the development of a significant allogeneic effect. Furthermore, donor lymphocyte infusions may be unable to exert a sufficiently robust GvL effect within the timescale needed, if administered in the presence of relapsing disease.

In an attempt to maximize disease reduction prior to allogeneic transplantation, and therefore minimize the risk of progression/ relapse prior to the establishment of an allogeneic GvL effect, cytoreduction with high-dose chemotherapy plus autologous stem cell rescue prior to allogeneic transplantation is also being explored.

Hodgkin's lymphoma

In Hodgkin's lymphoma, significant numbers of patients who relapse following standard first-line therapy can be salvaged by reinduction treatment and then consolidation with autologous stem cell rescue. There is, however, a cohort that subsequently relapses, and in whom allogeneic transplantation with conventional conditioning has proved effective in reducing relapse rates but at a prohibitive cost in terms of procedure-related mortality, resulting in no increase in overall survival.

Once again, reduced-intensity conditioning has been attempted in this cohort with reasonable early results (Table 26.4). Using an alemtuzumab-containing regimen, Peggs *et al.* describe results in 41 patients. Transplant-related mortality was 9%, and 16 patients received donor lymphocyte infusions for residual/ progressive disease post-transplant. Of those, nine had demonstrable responses, giving a current progression-free survival at 4 years of 42%, and demonstrating the existence of a therapeutically beneficial GvL effect.

The strategy described previously using preceding high-dose chemotherapy with autologous stem cell rescue has also been used in patients with high-risk Hodgkin's lymphoma. Carella *et al.* described 17 patients treated with a BEAM autograft, followed by fludarabine/cyclophosphamide conditioning and stem cell return from HLA-matched sibling donors. Responses were seen in 11 patients (CR in nine), and 11 were alive (six in ongoing CR) at a median follow-up of 566 days. Of note, the best disease responses were seen in those patients who achieved full donor status and in whom GvHD developed, again suggesting the presence of an allogeneic graft-versus-lymphoma effect.

Chronic myeloid leukaemia

As CML is the disease in which response to allogeneic donor lymphocyte infusion was first and most comprehensively demonstrated, it is an obvious candidate for the reduced-intensity conditioning approach (Table 26.4).

Or *et al.* described 24 patients transplanted in first chronic phase, using fludarabine, busulphan and ATG. The incidence of significant acute GvHD was 54%, and, at a median follow-up of 42 months, 21 of the 24 patients remained well, and in complete molecular remission, giving an actuarial 5-year DFS of 85%.

Elsewhere, use of a similar regimen, involving fludarabine plus busulphan as conditioning, was described in 44 patients

Table 26.4 Disease-specific outcome according to regimen.

Reference	No. of patients	Conditioning	GvHD	Outcome
Hodgkin's lymphoma				
Carella *et al.* (2001)	17	(BEAM autograft first) Flu/cy	Acute (grade II–IV) 24%	Median follow-up 566 days OS 65%, DFS 35%
Peggs *et al.* (2003)	41	Flu/mel/alem	Acute (grade II–IV) 12%	OS at 4 years 63% cPFS at 4 years 42%
Chronic myeloid leukaemia				
Or *et al.* (2003)	24	Flu/bu/ATG	Acute (grade II–IV) 54%	DFS at 5 years 85%
Bornhauser *et al.* (2001)	44	Flu/bu +/–ATG	Acute (grade II–IV) 43%	TRM 34% DFS at 2 years 50% (first CP)
AML/MDS				
Giralt *et al.* (1997)	15	Flu/ida/Ara-C 2-CDA/Ara-C	Acute (grade II–IV) 20%	Median follow-up 100 days CR in 8, OS 6
Parker *et al.* (2002)	23	Flu/bu/alem	Acute (grade II–IV) 17% Chronic 15%	OS at 2 years 48% DFS at 2 years 39%
Kroger *et al.* (2003)	37	Flu/bu/ATG	Acute (grade II–IV) 37% Chronic 48%	DFS at 3 years 38%
Feinstein *et al.* (2003)	18	200c Gy ± flu	Acute (grade II–IV) 45% Chronic 40%	OS at 1 year 54% PFS at 1 year 42% NRM at 1 year 17%
Sayer *et al.* (2003)	113	Flu/bu or TBI	–	Median follow-up 12 months RM 26%, NRM 26%

Abbreviations: flu, fludarabine; ida, idarubicin; bu, busulphan; cy, cyclophosphamide; CR, complete remission; OS, overall survival; 2-CDA, 2-chlorodeoxyadenosine; TRM, transplant-related mortality; DFS, disease-free survival; TBI, total body irradiation; NRM, non-relapse mortality; RM, relapse mortality; ATG, anti-thymocyte globulin; alem, alemtuzumab; BEAM, carmustine, Ara-C, etoposide, melphalan; PFS, progression-free survival; cPFS, current progression-free survival; CP, chronic phase.

with CML, with 34 patients also undergoing T-cell depletion via ATG. Again, acute GvHD occurred in a significant proportion, and at a median follow-up of 562 days TRM was substantial, at 34%, with 50% of the patients transplanted in chronic phase alive and disease free at 2 years. This form of transplantation is therefore a viable option in patients with CML in first chronic phase, with ample capacity for inducing disease responses by the administration of donor lymphocytes.

Acute myeloid leukaemia/myelodysplastic syndrome

Giralt *et al.* first demonstrated the feasibility of the non-myeloablative approach in a group of 15 patients with refractory or relapsed AML/MDS who were conditioned with either fludarabine/cytarabine/idarubicin or cladribine/cytarabine prior to infusion of stem cells from sibling donors (Table 26.4). Toxicity was acceptably low, and eight patients achieved remission post transplant, although responses were short-lived, as expected, in this high-risk group, and relapse occurred in all but two by a median follow-up of 100 days. The same group reported on the use of fludarabine and melphalan in these patients, and found that the additional cytoreduction conferred by this regimen resulted in improved DFS.

Following this, Parker *et al.* evaluated a fludarabine, busulphan and alemtuzumab-containing regimen in 23 patients with MDS. Early TRM was 9%, with a 2-year actuarial overall survival of 48% and DFS of 39%. Thus, transplantation with reduced-intensity conditioning was deemed a feasible approach for those patients considered inappropriate for conventional conditioning because of age or comorbidity, yielding similar results to those found in patients fit for the fully conditioned regimen. Of note, those individuals who fared best were those with good- or intermediate-risk cytogenetics and a low or intermediate International Prognostic Scoring (IPS) system score.

In those with high-risk MDS, Kroger *et al.* reported on 12 patients conditioned with fludarabine, busulphan and ATG. The results were consistent with the above observation regarding outcome-related to overall risk status, with a 2-year actuarial DFS of 12%, treatment toxicity and disease relapse both contributing to the generally poor outcome.

Furthermore, the same group subsequently published a study of 37 patients with MDS or secondary AML, in half of whom the donor was related, who were ineligible for conventionally conditioned transplants. The group received fludarabine, busulphan and ATG as reduced-intensity conditioning. The overall TRM was 27%, with significantly higher mortality in those with poor-risk cytogenetics (75% vs. 29%) or with an HLA-matched unrelated donor (45% vs. 12%). Thirty-two per cent of patients relapsed, and actuarial DFS at 3 years was 38%, with a median follow-up of 20 months. One further observation was that the development of chronic GvHD conferred a relative protection from disease relapse (15% vs. 70%).

Eighteen patients with AML (*de novo* 13, secondary 5) in first CR who had a sibling donor but were ineligible for conventional conditioning were reported by Feinstein *et al.* in 2003. Reduced-intensity conditioning was performed with fludarabine and 2 Gy TBI (8) or 2 Gy TBI alone (10). With a median follow-up of 766 days, 10 of the 18 patients (56%) had died, seven of whom had suffered a relapse. Of the eight survivors, seven were in continuing CR.

Finally, Sayer *et al.* reported on 113 patients with acute myeloid leukaemia ineligible for conventional transplants who were receiving reduced-intensity conditioning, consisting of fludarabine and busulphan or TBI. Apart from once again demonstrating the feasibility of such conditioning in these patients, this study identified certain poor prognostic factors. These included low Karnofsky performance scores and the presence of unrelated donors, but the most striking association was that between the level of residual disease at the time of transplant and subsequent outcome. With a median follow-up of 12 months, the probability of EFS was 49% for patients in morphological remission on bone marrow examination, 24% in patients with 5–20% blasts, and 14% in patients in whom > 20% blasts remained.

Thus, reduced-intensity conditioning shows some promise in those patients with AML/MDS ineligible for transplantation using conventional regimens, although follow-up is generally relatively short. Furthermore, outcome is significantly affected by the presence of poor-risk features such as high-risk cytogenetic changes, chemorefractory disease, unrelated donors and low IPS and Karnofsky performance scores. These factors should be considered when selecting patients for such procedures. In addition, there seems to be, in common with other malignancies, a beneficial effect conferred by the presence of chronic GvHD on the risk of disease recurrence.

In conclusion, although allogeneic transplantation with conventional conditioning should still be considered the procedure of choice in AML/MDS, if patients are ineligible for such treatment, reduced-intensity conditioning is a viable alternative.

Non-haematological malignancy

Reduced-intensity conditioning also has potential application in the treatment of solid tumours, where an allogeneic GvM effect may also be inducible (Table 26.5). Renal cell carcinoma is an attractive candidate for such immunotherapy, as some patients respond to immunomodulatory cytokines, and spontaneous regression of metastatic disease is occasionally seen. Childs *et al.* reported on 19 patients with refractory metastatic renal cell carcinoma conditioned with cyclophosphamide and fludarabine, a regimen with no anti-tumour effect. Disease responses with reduction in metastatic lesions were seen in 10 (53%) of the cohort, with three complete responses. All three remain in CR at a median follow-up of 402 days, and only two of the patients with PR have progressed within that time.

Table 26.5 Disease-specific outcome according to regimen.

Reference	No. of patients	Conditioning	GvHD	Outcome
Non-haematological malignancy				
Childs *et al.* (2003)	19	Flu/cy	Acute (grade II–IV) 53%	Median follow-up 402 days OS 43%, DFS 16%
Ueno *et al.* (2003)	23	Flu/mel	Acute (grade II–IV) 39% Chronic 43%	Follow-up 19–1119 days NRM 22% Disease response 45%
Inherited defects				
Horwitz *et al.* (2001)	10	Flu/cy/ATG	Acute (grade II–IV) 30%	Median follow-up 17 months Engraftment, reduced infection in 8/10 patients
Amrolia *et al.* (2000)	8	Flu/mel/ATG	No acute (grade II–IV)	Median follow-up 12 months Good immune function in 75%

Abbreviations: flu, fludarabine; cy, cyclopsosphamide; OS, overall survival; mel, melphalan; DFS, disease-free survival; NRM, non-relapse mortality; ATG, anti-thymocyte globulin.

The median time to disease response was 4 months, and evidence for a GvM effect was the occurrence of responses only following withdrawal of immunosuppression and conversion to full donor status, in addition to the association between GvHD and disease regression.

Given the observation that conversion from mixed chimerism seemed a necessary precondition for response, other groups have experimented with regimens yielding rapid full donor status, for example a fludarabine/melphalan combination, where only donor haemopoiesis was detected by 30 days post transplant, and responses were subsequently shown in 8 out of 15 (57%) of patients with metastatic renal cell carcinoma.

There has also been considerable interest in reduced-intensity conditioning in transplantation for treating breast cancer, following the earlier observations that an allogeneic effect occurred in some patients with regression of liver deposits following conventional myeloablative conditioning. The same fludarabine/melphalan regimen mentioned above was also administered to eight patients with refractory metastatic breast cancer, with three of the eight (37%) showing responses, two of which were complete. Once again, responses were associated with the withdrawal of immunosuppression or the development of significant GvHD.

Other solid tumours are also being studied, including colon carcinoma, hepatocellular carcinoma, and sarcomas of varying origin, and this is clearly an area with considerable potential but where definitive benefit remains to be demonstrated.

Inherited defects

A further group of disorders in which non-myeloablative transplantation has potential utility is in treating congenital defects of the lymphohaemopoietic system (Table 26.5). In this situation, the aim is to produce a state of mixed chimerism sufficient to provide a source of the defective gene product. There is usually no requirement for the incoming graft to completely supplant recipient haemopoiesis, as adequate function can be restored with only partial reconstitution of the defective cell population, and in addition there is no requirement for a graft-versus-host effect other than the relatively minor degree of graft-versus-lymphohaemopoietic effect necessary to ensure stable engraftment. While conventional conditioning has been used in these conditions, the procedure-related mortality and morbidity has proven prohibitive in many instances, which is not surprising given that the majority of these conditions are compatible with relatively lengthy lifespans when compared with the malignancies that constitute most candidate diseases for allogeneic transplantation.

Allogeneic transplantation has been shown to be curative in sickle cell disease, and there are anecdotal case reports of success using reduced-intensity conditioning regimens in this disease. In addition, transplantation with conventional conditioning has been demonstrated to be an effective intervention in other haemoglobinopathies, such as the thalassaemias, although toxicity becomes limiting where significant pretransplant end-organ damage is present, thus making this another attractive patient group for the reduced-intensity approach.

Regarding enzyme defects, a series of 10 patients with chronic granulomatous disease conditioned with cyclophosphamide, fludarabine and ATG has been reported, with 33–100% of neutrophils being of donor origin in eight of the recipients (graft rejection occurred in two) at a median follow-up of 17 months. A concomitant clinical response was seen, with only four episodes of significant bacterial infection in those eight patients post engraftment.

Amrolia et al. reported a series of eight patients with congenital immunodeficiencies (two CD40L deficiency, one X-linked lymphoproliferative disorder, one adenine deaminase deficiency, four unclassified severe or combined immunodeficiencies) who underwent conditioning with fludarabine, melphalan and ATG. One patient died of relapsed disease, while six of the remaining seven were evaluable at median follow-up of 1 year, and all showed improvement in phytohaemagglutinin stimulation indices. In addition, the patients with CD40L deficiency both show increased expression of the affected receptor, and the patient with adenine deaminase deficiency has increased levels of the appropriate metabolites.

Other conditions

First, it is important to mention aplastic anaemia, the condition in which, arguably, reduced-intensity conditioning became first established. Conditioning for HLA-matched sibling allografts with cyclophosphamide alone was introduced in 1969. Graft rejection was high, however, and ATG was added to the regimen in the late 1970s. Although various regimens have been employed since then, the use of a non-myeloablative approach has remained both popular and successful in transplantation for this condition.

Reduced-intensity conditioning has also been studied in patients with acute lymphoblastic leukaemia. Results so far have been modest, with high procedure-related mortality and little chance of effective salvage unless the patient is in a stable complete remission.

Treatment of myelofibrosis has also been attempted via non-myeloablative conditioning, with encouraging results, although numbers are small and follow-up preliminary.

There exist anecdotal reports of resolution of pre-existing autoimmune diseases such as psoriasis and ulcerative colitis in individuals who have undergone conventional allografts because of other pathology. There has also therefore been some interest in the use of reduced-intensity conditioning in autoimmune conditions such as systemic lupus erythematosus (SLE), although it must be remembered that chronic GvHD can manifest with syndromes resembling autoimmune diseases, and that complete removal of recipient lymphopoeisis may well be necessary to induce complete remission.

In addition, animal modelling has demonstrated that donor-specific tolerance to a solid organ allograft can be induced by preceding or concomitant stem cell transplantation. This is demonstrated in a report documenting the successful acceptance of a donor kidney in two patients with myeloma and end-stage renal failure who underwent combined bone marrow and renal transplantation following reduced-intensity conditioning. Post-transplant immunosuppression was tapered rapidly, and despite donor chimerism being lost by 100 days post procedure, a state of lasting tolerance to the solid-organ allograft was established.

Conclusion

It can therefore be seen that allogeneic transplantation with reduced-intensity conditioning can be successfully performed in individuals with a wide variety of different diseases. Procedure-related toxicity has proven significantly less of a problem than in conventional conditioning, and has provided a means of delivering potentially curative treatment in many situations where this has previously not been possible. Longer follow-up and greater numbers are clearly required to delineate the exact potential for cure in the various different diseases, but encouraging results have been published thus far.

The major challenges for this field remain the identification of the optimal conditioning regimen for particular disease groups and, crucially, the manipulation of the allogeneic effect so as to promote GvM while avoiding undesirable GvHD. While GvM responses are often seen following the development of GvHD, some disease responses have been observed in the absence of GvHD, and attempts are being made to target, for example, overexpressed/abnormal tissue antigens or haemopoietic minor histocompatability antigens which may be relevant for such anti-tumour activity. If, for example, appropriate T-cell clones can be generated and expanded ex vivo, or generated in vivo by vaccination of donors, transplantation with non-myeloablative conditioning could provide an ideal platform for subsequent adoptive cellular therapy.

Selected bibliography

Amrolia P, Gaspar HB, Hassan A et al. (2000) Nonmyeloablative stem cell transplantation for congenital immunodeficiencies. Blood 96: 1239–46.

Bornhauser M, Kiehl M, Siegert W et al. (2001) Dose-reduced conditioning for allografting in 44 patients with chronic myeloid leukaemia: a retrospective analysis. British Journal of Haematology 115: 119–24.

Carella AM, Beltrami G, Carella M et al. (2001) Immunosuppressive non-myeloablative allografting as salvage therapy in advanced Hodgkin's disease. Haematologica 86: 1121–3.

Chakraverty R, Peggs K, Chopra R et al. (2002) Limiting transplantation-related mortality following unrelated donor stem cell transplantation by using a nonmyeloablative conditioning regimen. Blood 99: 1071–8.

Childs R, Chernof A, Contentin N et al. (2000) Regression of metastatic renal-cell carcinoma after nonmyeloablative allogeneic peripheral-blood stem-cell transplantation. New England Journal of Medicine 343: 750–8.

Corradini P, Tarella C, Olivieri A et al. (2002) Reduced-intensity conditioning followed by allografting of hematopoietic cells can produce clinical and molecular remissions in patients with poor-risk hematologic malignancies. Blood 99: 75–82.

Faulkner RD, Craddock C, Byrne JL et al. (2004) BEAM-Campath reduced intensity allogeneic stem cell transplantation for lymphoproliferative diseases: GvHD, toxicity and survival in 65 patients. *Blood* **103**: 428–34.

Feinstein LC, Sandmaier BM, Hegenbart U *et al.* (2003) Non-myeloablative allografting from human leucocyte antigen-identical sibling donors for treatment of acute myeloid leukaemia in first complete remission. *British Journal of Haematology* **120**: 281–8.

Fibich C, Stewart D, Luiders J *et al.* (2002) Allogeneic stem cell transplantation for chronic lymphatic leukemia (CLL) with ATG-containing conditioning: Evidence for improved survival and preservation of graft versus leukemia effect. *Blood* **100**: 798a.

Giralt S, Estey E, Albitar M *et al.* (1997) Engraftment of allogeneic hematopoietic progenitor cells with purine analog-containing chemotherapy: harnessing graft-versus-leukemia without myeloablative therapy. *Blood* **89**: 4531–6.

Giralt S, Thall PF, Khouri I *et al.* (2001) Melphalan and purine analog-containing preparative regimens: reduced-intensity conditioning for patients with hematologic malignancies undergoing allogeneic progenitor cell transplantation. *Blood* **97**: 631–7.

Haddad N, Rowe JM (2004) Current indications for reduced-intensity allogeneic stem cell transplantation. *Clinical Haematology* **17**: 377–86.

Ho AY, Devereux S, Mufti GJ, Pagliuca A (2003) Reduced-intensity rituximab-BEAM-Campath allogeneic haematopoietic stem cell transplantation for follicular lymphoma is feasible and induces durable molecular remissions. *Bone Marrow Transplantation* **31**: 551–7.

Horwitz ME, Barrett AJ, Brown MR *et al.* (2001) Treatment of chronic granulomatous disease with nonmyeloablative conditioning and a T-cell-depleted hematopoietic allograft. *New England Journal of Medicine* **344**: 881–8.

Khouri IF, Saliba RM, Giralt SA *et al.* (2001) Nonablative allogeneic hematopoietic transplantation as adoptive immunotherapy for indolent lymphoma: low incidence of toxicity, acute graft-versus-host disease, and treatment-related mortality. *Blood* **98**: 3595–9.

Kottaridis PD, Milligan DW, Chopra R *et al.* (2000) *In vivo* Campath-1H prevents graft-versus-host disease following non-myeloablative stem cell transplantation. *Blood* **96**: 2419–25.

Krishnamurti L, Blazar BR and Wagner JE (2001) Bone marrow transplantation without myeloablation for sickle cell disease. *New England Journal of Medicine* **344**: 68.

Kroger N, Bornhauser M, Ehninger G *et al.* (2003) Allogeneic stem cell transplantation after a fludarabine/busulfan-based reduced-intensity conditioning in patients with myelodysplastic syndrome or secondary acute myeloid leukemia. *Annals of Hematology* **82**: 336–342.

Kroger N, Schwerdtfeger R, Kiehl M *et al.* (2002) Autologous stem cell transplantation followed by a dose-reduced allograft induces high complete remission rate in multiple myeloma. *Blood* **100**: 755–60.

Lokhorst HM, Schattenberg A, Cornelissen JJ *et al.* (2000) Donor lymphocyte infusions for relapsed multiple myeloma after allogeneic stem-cell transplantation: predictive factors for response and long-term outcome. *Journal of Clinical Oncology* **18**: 3031–3037.

Lush RJ, Haynes AP, Byrne J *et al.* (2001) Allogeneic stem-cell transplantation for lymphoproliferative disorders using BEAM-Campath (+/– fludarabine) conditioning combined with post-transplant donor-lymphocyte infusion. *Cytotherapy* **3**: 203–10.

Maloney DG, Molina AJ, Sahebi F *et al.* (2003) Allografting with non-myeloablative conditioning following cytoreductive autografts for the treatment of patients with multiple myeloma. *Blood* **102**: 3447–54.

McSweeney PA, Niederwieser D, Shiruzu JA *et al.* (2001) Hematopoietic cell transplantation in older patients with hematologic malignancies: replacing high-dose cytotoxic therapy with graft-versus-tumor effects. *Blood* **97**: 3390–400.

Morris E, Thomson K, Craddock C *et al.* (2002) Long term follow-up of an alemtuzumab (Campath-1H) containing reduced intensity allogeneic transplant regimen for non-Hodgkin's lymphoma (NHL). *Blood* **100** (11): 139a.

Nagler A, Slavin S, Varadi G *et al.* (2000) Allogeneic peripheral blood stem cell transplantation using a fludarabine-based low intensity conditioning regimen for malignant lymphoma. *Bone Marrow Transplantation* **25**: 1021–8.

Or R, Shapira MY, Resnick I *et al.* (2003) Nonmyeloablative allogeneic stem cell transplantation for the treatment of chronic myeloid leukemia in first chronic phase. *Blood* **101**: 441–5.

Parker JE, Shafi T, Pagliuca A *et al.* (2002) Allogeneic stem cell transplantation in the myelodysplastic syndromes: interim results of outcome following reduced-intensity conditioning compared with standard preparative regimens. *British Journal of Haematology* **119**: 144–54.

Peggs KS, Mackinnon S, Williams CD *et al.* (2003) Reduced-intensity transplantation with *in vivo* T-cell depletion and adjuvant dose-escalating donor lymphocyte infusions for chemotherapy-sensitive myeloma: limited efficacy of graft-versus-tumor activity. *Biology of Blood Marrow Transplantation* **9**: 257–65.

Peggs KS, Thomson K, Chopra R *et al.* (2003) Long term results of reduced intensity transplantation in multiply relapsed and refractory Hodgkin's lymphoma: evidence of a therapeutically relevant graft-versus-lymphoma effect. *Blood* **102**: 694a.

Sayer HG, Kroger M, Beyer J *et al.* (2003) Reduced intensity conditioning for allogeneic hematopoietic stem cell transplantation in patients with acute myeloid leukemia: disease status by marrow blasts is the strongest prognostic factor. *Bone Marrow Transplantation* **31**: 1089–95.

Slavin S, Nagler A, Naparstek E *et al.* (1998) Nonmyeloablative stem cell transplantation and cell therapy as an alternative to conventional bone marrow transplantation with lethal cytoreduction for the treatment of malignant and nonmalignant hematologic diseases. *Blood* **91**: 756–63.

Spitzer TR, McAfee SL, Bimalangshu RD *et al.* (2001) Durable progression-free survival (PFS) following non-myeloablative bone marrow transplantation (BMT) for chemorefractory diffuse large B cell lymphoma (B-LCL). *Blood* **98**: 2813a.

Storb R, Weiden PL, Sullivan KM *et al.* (1987) Second marrow transplants in patients with aplastic anemia rejecting the first graft: use of a conditioning regimen including cyclophosphamide and antithymocyte globulin. *Blood* **70**: 116–21.

Ueno NT, Cheng YC, Rondon G *et al.* (2003) Rapid induction of complete donor chimerism by the use of a reduced-intensity conditioning regimen composed of fludarabine and melphalan in allogeneic stem-cell transplantation for metastatic solid tumors. *Blood* **102**: 3829–36.

CHAPTER 27

Gene therapy of haemopoietic disorders

27

Raphaël F Rousseau and Malcolm K Brenner

Introduction

Somatic cell gene transfer may be used to correct a deficit in a cell, to enhance or inhibit its pre-existing function, or to provide the cell with an entirely new capacity. This broad range of actions means that gene transfer may in principle contribute to the therapy of almost every disease in haematology. For principle to be turned into practice, however, investigators will need to overcome a formidable array of regulatory and technical barriers. The delay in the introduction of successful gene therapeutics that followed the initial hyperbole has led many to conclude that the entire field is devoid of clinical relevance. While this nihilistic viewpoint may yet be proven correct, it is more likely that the power of gene transfer will allow it to make essential contributions to otherwise intractable haematological problems. It is the purpose of this chapter to describe potential applications, current problems and future solutions.

For gene transfer to be of benefit, a number of criteria need to be met. First, the transferred gene's function should be understood. If, for example, a gene is active only during fetal development, there may be little purpose in attempting gene therapy for an adult. Similarly, genetic disorders in which the abnormal gene produces a transdominant effect (for example sickle cell anaemia) cannot be corrected simply by transferring a normal gene. Second, it will be necessary to have vectors that transfer the genes efficiently, safely and (ideally) in a targeted fashion, so that the correct cells are transduced. Moreover, for many applications the products of the transgenes need to be regulated, in terms of the quantity and timing of the material produced. While many gene transfer techniques are available, none meets these needs in full, and many fall far short of the desired goals. Hence,

the practice of gene therapy has to a large extent consisted in a careful selection of disease entities and treatment strategies that can exploit the limited strengths of current vectors, while avoiding their very substantial weaknesses. Undoubtedly, as our capacity to prepare safe, efficient, targeted and regulatable gene transfer vectors improves, the range of disorders that will be amenable to such treatment will grow. But, for the moment, ambition must be tempered by ability. Fortunately, for haematological diseases in general, and for malignant haematological diseases in particular, even current vectors provide us with opportunities to explore worthwhile clinical applications.

Gene transfer vectors for haemopoietic cells

A prerequisite for gene therapy for haematological diseases is successful transduction of target cells, which may include a malignant cell population, haemopoietic stem cells (HSCs), cells of the immune system or (for haemophilia) the cells of other organ systems (Table 27.1). The aim of transducing malignant cells is to reduce tumorigenicity or enhance immunogenicity, while the aim of transducing normal cells is to correct functional defects, or (in malignant disease) to permit cytotoxic drug dose escalation and to improve the outcome of stem cell transplant procedures. The major constraints for gene transfer strategies are the efficiency of gene delivery to target cells and the safety of the vectors used, in terms of immediate toxicity and the induction of mutational events following transgene integration; the importance of each is dependent on the vector system used.

Table 27.1 Advantages and disadvantages of vector systems.

Vector	Advantages	Disadvantages	Current uses
Retrovirus	Stable integration into dividing cells Minimal immunogenicity Stable packaging system	Low titre Only integrates in dividing cells Limited insert size Risk of silencing Risk of insertional mutagenesis	Marker studies Gene therapy approaches using haemopoietic stem cells or T cells Transduction of tumour cells
Adeno-associated virus (AAV)	Integrates into dividing cells Infects wide range cell types	No stable packaging cell line Very limited insert size	Gene therapy approaches using haemopoietic stem cells
Lentivirus	Integrates into dividing cells Integrates into non-dividing cells	No stable packaging system Complex safety issues	No approved trials as yet
Adenovirus	Infects wide range cell types Infects non-dividing cells High titres High level of expression Accepts 12- to 15-kb DNA inserts	Highly immunogenic Non-integrating	Direct *in vivo* applications Transduction of tumour cells
Herpesvirus	High titres Transduces some target cells at high efficiency Accepts large DNA inserts	No packaging cell lines Non-integrating Difficult to scale up for human use May be cytotoxic to target cell	Transduction of tumour cells Neurological disorders
Liposomes and other physical methods using naked DNA	Easy to prepare in quantity Virtually unlimited size	Very inefficient entry into target cell Non integrating	Topical applications Transduction of tumour cells

Retroviruses

Murine retroviruses, particularly the Moloney murine leukaemia virus (MoMuLV), have been used extensively as gene delivery systems, especially in gene marking studies. They are single-stranded RNA viruses that are transcribed by reverse transcriptase into double-stranded DNA that can integrate into host DNA. In a clinical vector, the packaging signal and long terminal repeats (LTRs) are retained, while the structural and replicative genes (*gag*, *pol* and *env*) of a murine retrovirus are replaced by one or more genes of interest, driven either by the retroviral promoter in the 5'-LTR or by an internal promoter, leaving room for up to 5 kb of transgene. The retroviral constructs are made in cell lines in which the missing retrovirus genes are present in *trans* and thus reproduce and package a vector that is not replication competent. After production of viral particles and infection of target cells, the vector is uncoated in the cytosol and the RNA is transcribed via reverse transcriptase into DNA, which integrates into the host genome. Thus, the transferred gene not only survives for the entire lifespan of the transduced cell, but is also present in that cell's progeny.

The host range of MoMuLV viruses is determined by the gp70 envelope protein, which interacts with their cellular receptors, and the genetic information they convey is integrated into the host cell DNA. Hence, these vectors are ideal for transferring genes into rapidly dividing cell populations, such as haemopoietic stem cells or lymphocytes. However, retroviral vectors have several disadvantages. Because expression of the transferred gene requires viral integration of the genome, and hence a population of dividing cells, the efficiency of transfer to many types of cell may be low. It is possible to increase efficiency by bringing vector particle and target cell into close physical apposition, for example by performing transduction on substances such as fibronectin, but, even then, overall levels of transfer leave much to be desired. *In vivo* gene transfer in many clinical studies has been disappointingly low, perhaps because the cytokines used to induce target cells into cycle also commit them to differentiation. Further, because the integration events themselves occur largely at random in the host cell DNA, regulatory genes could conceivably be damaged, contributing to oncogenesis. This hypothetical concern became reality with the development of T-cell leukaemias in two children with X-linked common gamma-chain severe combined immunodeficiency who were treated by retrovirus-mediated gene transfer of the absent cytokine receptor gene. Both had proviral integration sites proximate to the *LMO-2* gene, which is critical for T-cell growth and has been implicated in other spontaneous leukaemic transformations. Finally, retroviral vectors are not well suited for use *in vivo*, since they are generally unstable in primate complement, and as yet they cannot be targeted to specific cell types.

The development of pseudotyped particles, in which a retroviral vector genome is incorporated into an envelope derived all or in part from a different virus, may improve the *in vivo* stability of retroviral vectors and alter their target cell range.

Adenoviruses

In approaches in which short-term gene transfer may be adequate (for example the generation of anti-tumour vaccines), adenoviral vectors are an alternative delivery system. First-generation adenoviral vectors are *E1* (early protein) deletion mutants and therefore are not replication competent. These vectors infect a wide range of cell types and, unlike retroviruses, can transfer cDNA sized up to 10 kb even into non-dividing cells. The vectors are reasonably stable *in vivo* and can be used to infect cells *in situ*. Examples include gene transfer into respiratory epithelium (the *CFTR* gene in cystic fibrosis) or liver (genes encoding factor VIII and factor IX in haemophilia A or B). However, adenoviral vectors are generally non-integrating, so that the gene products are expressed from episomal DNA. The episome is often lost after cell division and can be inactivated or lost even in a non-dividing cell. Thus, adenoviral vectors are unsuited for any application that requires long-term expression in a rapidly turning over cell population. A more important limitation is that most adenoviral vectors are immunogenic. Immune responses are generated against the vector proteins themselves (often preventing read-ministration of the vector), as well as against low levels of adenoviral proteins, expressed even when cells are transduced by defective viruses. Moreover, concurrent expression of adenoviral genes appears to increase the probability of developing an immune response to the transgene product. Even before these adaptive immune responses are generated by adenoviruses, vector entry into many cell types triggers an innate immune response, with the release of cytokines, such as interleukins 6 and 8 and the development of a potentially highly destructive local inflammatory response. Finally, adenoviral damage to vascular endothelium and to other organ systems may cause a potentially lethal disseminated intravascular coagulopathy, or a more chronic hepatocyte hypertrophy and hepatic fibrosis. Since deletion of the E1 region alone does not prevent these toxicities, subsequent generations of adenovectors have been prepared that lack more than one set of adenoviral genes. Although showing less immunogenicity and toxicity and more durable transgene expression in some studies, such modified vectors produced little or no benefit in others, at least in part because of the persistent induction of innate immunity. Indeed, administration of an *E1/E4*-deleted vector has been linked to the death of a patient with ornithine transcarbamylase deficiency after adenoviral gene transfer via the hepatic artery.

The ultimate attenuated adenovector is the helper-dependent or 'gutless' vector, in which virtually all of the adenoviral genes have been removed and replaced with the gene of interest and its promoter, together with irrelevant DNA to allow packaging in the viral envelope. In this system, one virus (helper) contains all viral replication genes and the other contains only the therapeutic gene sequence, the viral inverted terminal repeats (ITRs) and the packaging recognition signal. Helper-dependent vectors have shown a much higher therapeutic index than conventional adenovectors in several different models. Importantly, they also seem to be much less immunogenic, so that transduced post-mitotic cells (muscle or liver, for example) may secrete vector-derived proteins over many months, a prime consideration in the treatment of many deficiency disorders. However, the manufacture of these viruses is currently difficult to scale up and there is a continued problem with contaminating helper virus, although the amounts may be less than 0.1%.

Adeno-associated viruses

Adeno-associated viruses (AAVs) are human parvoviruses that normally depend on a helper virus (adeno- or herpesvirus) for productive infection. Structurally, AAV is a DNA parvovirus, containing two palindromic-inverted terminal repeats (ITR). When linked with two gene products from the *rep* gene region, these repeats favour site-specific integration of chromosome 19 by the AAV. Thus, AAVs, like retroviruses, should persist for the entire life of the host cell and its progeny. Because genomic integration by AAVs is relatively site specific, the risk of oncogenesis is theoretically low. Moreover, AAVs may integrate the genomes of non-dividing cells and become permanently expressed even in resting or post-mitotic cells. Vectors based on AAVs have been developed as gene transfer vehicles able to transduce a wide variety of cells including non-dividing cells. There is no known disease associated with AAVs and, since the AAV vector genome lacks viral coding sequences, the vector itself has not previously been associated with toxicity or inflammatory responses, although data from a study in haemophilia, described below, have led to questioning of this dogma. AAVs may certainly generate neutralizing antibodies that may limit repeat administration although the availability of additional AAV vector serotypes may overcome this problem and allow additional cell types to be targeted. The major limitations of the AAV vectors are the small size (ca. 3.5 kb) of insert and the labour-intensive large-scale production required for clinical trials, caused in part by difficulty in developing high-titre producer cell lines free of contaminating helper adenoviruses.

Herpes viruses

Vectors derived from herpes simplex viruses (HSVs) can be used to transduce neuronal cells in a variety of preclinical models, and in some rodent tumour cell lines. Herpes-based vectors have a number of potential advantages over alternative systems in terms of their titre, the size of the gene insert, and their safety. Herpes-based vectors lack essential genes for toxicity and/or infectivity (such as glycoprotein H or gH), but can be grown to high titre in a complementing cell line. In non-complementing cell lines that are permissive for herpesvirus growth, these vectors are restricted to a single cycle of replication, leading to the release of non-infectious virus. Improvements of this vector platform include the development of amplicons, in which plasmids are packaged as large tandemly repeated DNA in place of the wild-type HSV genome. Amplicons retain the outstanding transducing abilities of the original vector while reducing the risk of immunization and increasing the probability of generating stable transfectants of normal and malignant haemopoietic cells. Further enhancements include combination with other vectors and the generation of hybrid vectors with stable integrating capabilities into the genome of the host cell. These vectors have yet to be used for gene therapy of haemopoietic disease.

Human immunodeficiency viruses and other lentiviral vectors

Human immunodeficiency virus (HIV) vectors efficiently transduce primitive haemopoietic progenitors and primary acute leukaemia cells. HIV also infects and integrates into non-dividing and post-mitotic cells using as yet unidentified viral components. Technical problems remain before lentiviruses can readily be used for clinical application. For example, the toxicity of some HIV proteins has made generation of stable packaging cells difficult. In addition, there are safety concerns with these vectors – in particular the use of HIV-derived vector systems raises the possibility that wild-type or mutant infectious HIV may be generated during vector production. Efforts to increase safety include the development of third-generation, self-inactivating (SIN) lentiviral vectors in which the parental HIV-1 enhancer and promoter sequences from the lentivirus 3′-LTR have been deleted. When the SIN vector infects the target cells, they are incapable of transcribing vector-length RNA, and are thus incapable of further replication, reducing the likelihood of generating replication-competent retroviruses. SIN vectors should be regarded as the lentiviral vectors of choice for clinical trials and exploration of their value – initially in the treatment of AIDS – has begun.

Liposomes and other physical gene transfer methods

Clinical experience with the available physical methods of gene transfer has primarily involved cationic liposome–DNA complexes which fuse with the cell membrane and enter the endosomal uptake pathway. DNA released from these endosomes may then pass through the nuclear membrane and be expressed. The main advantage of liposomes is that they are non-toxic and can be given repeatedly. In some cell types, high levels of gene transfer have been obtained by this method. Liposomes are rather unstable *in vivo*, but liposomal transfer by local injection of human melanoma cells *in situ* has resulted in the expression of a new gene (HLA-B7). However, the DNA transferred by liposomes does not integrate the genome and, despite the incorporation of a variety of ligands into the liposome–DNA complex, the ability to target these vectors is still quite limited.

Successful gene transfer *in vivo* has also been reported with use of a bio-ballistic ('gene gun') technique in which DNA coated onto colloidal gold particles is driven at high velocity by gas pressure into the cell. It is not yet clear whether this approach can be used to transduce normal or malignant haemopoietic progenitor cells with sufficient efficiency to allow therapeutic application in humans. Localized electroporation of plasmid DNA using microelectrodes has also proved to be highly effective for *ex vivo* and *in vivo* transduction of cells from muscle and skin and may be followed by significant transgene expression.

Hybrid vectors

None of the vectors currently available is suitable for every potential application of gene transfer in haematological disease, and none is free of significant limitations and adverse effects. Ultimately, therefore, entirely new synthetic or semisynthetic vectors will have to be developed. Possibilities include the generation of hybrid viral vectors, which may combine, for example, the *in vivo* stability of adenoviruses and the integrating capacity of retroviruses. Alternatively, fully synthetic vectors will be developed by combining components from multiple different viruses, allowing safe, efficient and specific gene transfer and regulation. In the meantime, gene therapy protocols for haematological disease will require investigators to circumvent the limitations of current vectors and choose their agents on the basis of the most important feature required. For example, a requirement for long-term gene expression by the progeny of haemopoietic stem cells dictates an integrating vector such as a retrovirus, whereas a protocol specifying transient expression of differentiated malignant cells and their transduction *in vivo* would favour adenoviral vectors.

Targeting

To target viral vectors to specific cells or organ systems, it is usually necessary not only to add a targeting ligand to provide the new specificity, but also to disrupt pre-existing ligands ('detargeting') so that the new specificity replaces, rather than adds to, the old. Moreover, the new ligands should allow the virus to enter the cells by membrane fusion or active transport, through the same intracellular pathway as the native vector. For adenoviruses in particular, retargeting may also be an important means of limiting virus-induced toxicity to vulnerable organs. Type 5 adenoviruses, from which most human adenovectors have been derived, bind to at least two molecules on their target cells – the Coxsackie adenovirus receptor (CAR) and cell-surface integrins (usually $\alpha v\beta_3$ or $\alpha v\beta_5$). Domains on the adenoviral knob protein mediate binding. Since the sequence and crystal structure of this protein is known, one can identify new ligand sequences and incorporate them into positions that disrupt pre-existing patterns of binding and establish new ones. The complexity of the process has hampered efforts to effectively retarget viral vectors. Retargeting may be much simpler with liposomal vectors, whose intrinsic targeting capabilities are limited, so that simple addition of a ligand could secure the desired effect. Despite the appeal of these retargeting strategies, the only *in vivo* success reported to date has been infection of liver cells through directed binding to the asialoglycoprotein receptor.

Regulation of transgene expression

Most effective gene therapies will require regulation of the transgene. Two approaches are available. The first relies on endogenous regulatory elements, by replacing the defective sequence with an inserted wild-type sequence – the process of homologous recombination. Several approaches have been suggested by which this may be accomplished, but as yet none have had a high enough efficiency for clinical use. Nonetheless, in animal models of several diseases (Crigler–Najar disease or UDP-glucoronysyl transferase deficiency, α_1-antitrypsin deficiency and the factor IX deficiency of haemophilia B) these approaches have produced promising results.

For most disorders, regulatory elements may need to be introduced with the transgene. Several regulatory structures are being developed with the intention of using small molecules to control transgene expression. The three systems closest to clinical use are regulated by rapamycin or tetracycline and their analogues, or by the anti-progestin agent mifepristone (RU486). By modifying a given DNA-binding domain, it is possible to alter the target sequence that is bound, allowing a repressor and an inducer to be present in the same cell. Similarly, by modifying the receptor for the small molecule regulator it is possible to use two different oral agents, one to upregulate and one to downregulate production. This provides a lower background than an inducible system alone, and a higher level of maximum expression than a repressor alone. Alternatively, the system could be used to turn on two separate genes. None of these systems has yet entered clinical study.

Applications of gene transfer (Table 27.2)

Haemoglobinopathies

Sickle cell disease and thalassaemia have both attracted considerable interest as disease targets for gene transfer approaches, as the available treatments are unsatisfactory and the molecular basis of the diseases is well characterized. To date, most emphasis has fallen on thalassaemia, which also has the distinction of being the earliest disease for which gene therapy was attempted.

Table 27.2 Examples of early clinical trials for the treatment of malignant haemopoietic disorders approved by the Recombinant Advisory Committee of the National Institutes of Health (USA).

Target cell	Approach	Institution	Investigators
Leukaemia cells	Transduce with CD40L	Baylor College of Medicine UCSD	M Brenner, R Krance, H Heslop Thomas Kipps
Donor T cells after allogeneic BMT	Mark EBV-specific CTLs to prevent EBV lymphoma after transplant	St Jude Children's Research Hospital, Baylor College of Medicine	H Heslop, M Brenner, C Rooney
	Transduce donor T cell used to treat relapse with Tk	Human Gene Therapy Research Institute, Northwestern University	C Link, R Burt, A Traynor
	Transduce donor T cell used to treat relapse with Tk	Fred Hutchinson Cancer Research Institute	M Flowers, S Riddell
	Transduce donor T cell used to treat relapse with Tk	University of Washington, City of Hope National Medical Center, University of South Carolina, MD Anderson Cancer Center, Indiana University, University of Alabama	W Bensinger, P Parker, J Henslee Downey, S Abhyanker, S Giralt, K Cornetta, M Carabasi
	Transduce donor minor antigen specific clones used to treat relapse with Tk	Fred Hutchinson Cancer Research Institute	E Warren
Marrow mononuclear cells in autologous transplantation	Mark marrow to ascertain source of relapse	St Jude Children's Research Hospital	M Brenner, J Mirro, C Hurwitz, V Santana, J Ihle
	Mark marrow to compare purging regimens	St Jude Children's Research Hospital	M Brenner, R Krance, H Heslop, V Santana, J Ihle

Tk, thymidine kinase; CTLs,: cytotoxic T lymphocytes; BMT, bone marrow transplantation; EBV, Epstein–Barr virus.

The ensuing furore about the unethical conduct of this first study in Israel and Italy in the 1970s was a major contributor to the establishment of the regulatory environment, which now encumbers the field. Since that time, the feasibility of effective gene therapy for thalassaemia has greatly increased based on an improved understanding of the normal regulation of the β-globin gene and the increased efficiency of vector systems. Initial studies showed that murine retroviral vectors expressing the β-globin genes could transduce murine and human haemopoietic stem cells, but levels of expression were low. As described in Chapters 2 and 6, it then became apparent that regulation of the β-globin locus depended on a 25-kb sequence termed the locus control region (LCR), which was located ~60 kb upstream of the adult β-globin gene. Retroviral vectors composed of functional fragments of the LCR fragments and globin gene sequences were generated but were found to rearrange on integration in target cells, apparently as a result of cryptic splice sites that resulted in internal deletions in the LCR/globin minigene. This problem, coupled with a low efficiency of gene transfer into human stem cells by murine retroviral vectors, led many to abandon the approach altogether. More recently, however, it has been shown that lentiviral vectors, which can package much longer sequences than murine retroviruses, could contain larger fragments of the LCR together with the globin locus. These vectors could integrate unrearranged LCR/globin genes at high efficiency in human stem cells. Pseudotyping these vectors allowed them to transduce murine stem cells and their use in β^0-thalassaemic heterozygote and then homozygous mice resulted in long-term clinical improvement, including increased haemoglobin and haematocrit and a drop in the reticulocyte count.

Similar success with this vector system has been reported in sickle cell mice that received stem cells transduced to express an anti-sickling β-globin variant. Up to 48% of total haemoglobin originated from the transgene. If preclinical data continue to support this lentiviral approach, efforts will undoubtedly be made to bring it into the clinical setting. For thalassaemic and sickle cell disease patients, however, adequate engraftment of gene-modified cells will almost certainly require drug- or radiation-mediated ablation of uncorrected marrow progenitor cells. Such treatment will invariably have a finite risk of severe morbidity and mortality, so that the increase in safety of gene therapy over allogeneic transplantation may not be as striking as had been hoped: the cure rate in otherwise healthy thalassaemic patients transplanted from MHC-identical siblings is already more than 90%.

Haemophilia

Haemophilia is an attractive target for gene therapy, since production of even modest quantities of factor VIII or factor IX may be sufficient to improve levels in the blood and hence disease phenotype. For a similar reason, direct measurement of transgenic factor levels in the blood is an excellent marker of the success of the treatment and allows rapid analysis of outcome.

The availability of both small and large animal models of the disease has facilitated preclinical investigation and ensured that this disorder has been one of the most popular non-malignant disorders for a gene therapy approach. Because the factor VIII gene is large, most clinical studies of haemophilia A have focused on B-domain deleted mutants of the gene. For haemophilia B, the much smaller factor IX gene fits comfortably into most vector systems.

Of note, the target cell for gene therapy of haemophilia has not so far been of haemopoietic origin. Instead, fibroblasts, hepatocytes and muscle cells have all been genetically modified for treatment of the disease, using a range of vector systems including plasmids, retroviruses, AAVs and adenoviruses.

Clinical trials

Plasmid

The first clinical trial used a plasmid carrying a selectable marker and a B domain-deleted factor VIII cDNA, and introduced it by electroporation into patients' cultured skin fibroblasts. After *ex vivo* selection and expansion, cells were implanted into the patients' omenta. The first patients had a reduced frequency of spontaneous bleeds and of factor infusions. However, although factor VIII activity was above baseline in three out of six patients, it rarely reached the target level of > 2% required for major clinical benefit. After several months, the benefits and the factor VIII disappeared, presumably due to death or destruction of the transduced cells. It is not clear if this highly labour-intensive approach will ever be suited to widespread exploitation.

Adeno-associated viral vectors

Two widely reported subsequent clinical studies for haemophilia used adeno-associated viral vectors and targeted either skeletal muscle or liver. As described in the 'Vector systems' section above, AAV vectors have a limited size capacity for transgenes and have so far only been used clinically to treat factor IX deficiency. It is of note, however, that preclinical studies suggest that factor VIII can be delivered by AAV vectors in portions by using two vectors that subsequently concatemerize as DNA in the nucleus, or that encode separate protein subunits that assemble in the cell or even by using a dwarf promoter in a single vector. The first trial of AAV-mediated factor IX gene transfer used intramuscular injections and was based on successful preclinical studies in mice and haemophilic dogs. AAV–factor IX was administered at intramuscular sites in the legs and arms in a dose escalation design, although the highest doses administered [2×10^{12} virus particles (vp)/kg] were well below those required for efficacy in animal studies. Production of factor IX was hampered by the low efficiency of the required post-translational modifications in skeletal muscle, and by the propensity for inhibitory antibody formation as the dose per site was raised, which meant that dose escalation required injection of progressively larger numbers of intramuscular sites. Muscle biopsies showed gene transfer and expression of factor IX in 8/8 subjects. Unfortunately, circulating levels remained < 1%.

Infusion of AAVs into the portal vein results in high-level expression of factor IX in mice and in haemophilic dogs. Compared with muscle as a target tissue, there is more than a log difference in the amount of factor IX produced for a given dose of virus, probably because hepatocytes more efficiently secrete factor IX into the circulation. The clinical study encountered problems early on when vector sequences were detected in semen from treated subjects, raising the spectre of germline transmission. After it was shown that vector sequences were cleared from the semen over time, the study restarted. High and collaborators report that the third dose (5×10^{12} vp/kg) resulted in circulating levels of factor IX around 10% for 4–5 weeks after infusion, but this was followed by a gradual reduction in levels to the pretreatment baseline (< 1%). Accompanying the fall was a transaminitis, indicating hepatocyte damage, perhaps by an immune response. The study has now been halted.

Adenoviral vectors

Adenovectors transduce hepatocytes at high efficiency, are roomy and express large quantities of transgene product. Unlike AAVs, they are easy to make in large quantities. All these features make them attractive for haemophilia gene therapy. However, they are also hepatotoxic, immunogenic and generally produce short-term expression, which in general has deterred investigators from using them to treat genetic disorders. The development of helper dependent 'empty' adenoviral vectors with lower hepatotoxicity and prolonged expression (in some models) inspired efforts to use them to treat factor VIII deficiency in humans, particularly since experiments in non-human primates had yielded circulating levels of 3–8% of normal. Sadly, if predictably, a phase I dose escalation study of a helper-dependent adenoviral vector for haemophilia A failed at the lowest (subtherapeutic) dose level, when the first subject experienced transient thrombocytopenia and transaminitis, probably as a result of toxicity from adenovector capsid proteins. Since these were the same problems experienced by patients prior to the first fatality from adenoviral vector treatment, there was little tolerance for these types of adverse events in patients with a genetic disorder, and the study was abandoned. Additional preclinical studies will be required to determine whether helper-dependent adenoviral vectors will ever be of value in the treatment of genetic disease, or whether this vector system will essentially be confined to applications in malignant disease, in which adverse events are a more accepted aspect of treatment.

Retroviral vectors

A phase I study conducted in 13 patients with haemophilia A used a retroviral vector derived from the classical Moloney murine leukaemia virus rendered replication deficient and carrying a B domain-deleted gene encoding for human factor VIII. While this vector has been extensively used in gene therapy clinical trials using *ex vivo* gene transfer, the originality of this study resides in the choice of an intravenous route of administration. Safety monitoring indicated that this route of administration was safe and well tolerated. Tests performed at regular intervals demonstrated the absence of replication-competent retroviruses (even though one patient's semen tested positive by PCR). There was no exacerbation of pre-existing viral diseases, such as HIV or HCV. No factor VIII inhibitors were detectable after retrovirus administration but non-neutralizing antibodies to murine leukaemia virus developed in all subjects. PCR for retroviral sequences tested positive in 90% of the peripheral blood mononuclear cell (PBMC) samples after 29 weeks. At 1 year, 75% of the PBMC samples remained positive by PCR, even in subjects who had received the lowest retrovirus dose. Unfortunately, factor VIII activity unrelated to exogenous treatment remained low (1.1–19%) and transient, with nine subjects having factor VIII higher than 1% on at least two occasions 5 or more days after infusion of exogenous factor VIII. Of note, pharmacokinetic parameters of exogenously administered factor VIII showed an increased half-life and area under the curve compared with prestudy values. Bleeding frequency may have been lowered in five patients. As for many approaches using retroviral constructs, the long-lasting detection of retroviral sequences by PCR is counterbalanced with the loss of transgene expression, a finding as yet not fully elucidated. Alas, the recent insertional mutagenesis event observed in the French study conducted in patients with X-SCID does not incite optimism in getting approval for gene transfer approaches using retroviral vectors.

Therefore, for the moment, gene therapy of haemophilia is promising but will likely only become a clinical reality when safer and more efficient and longer lasting gene delivery systems can be developed.

Treatment of haemopoietic malignancies

Several approaches may use gene transfer as part of the clinical arsenal against haemopoietic malignancies:
- *modification of tumour cells*, by repairing genetic defects thought to be responsible for the malignant proliferation, for example by restoring genes controlling cellular division or that induce programmed cell death (apoptosis);
- *sensitization of normal tissues or malignant cells in order to modify their therapeutic index*, by introducing into the malignant cells genes encoding for an enzyme that can transform a non-toxic prodrug into an active drug; or by introducing into normal tissues genes that can protect them against the effects of anti-tumour toxic drugs;
- *modulation of tumour invasiveness*, by delivering genes that can inhibit the growth of new blood vessels in order to impede nutrient supply to the tumour cells (inhibition of neoangiogenesis);
- *enhancement of the anti-tumour immune response*, either by inducing the recognition of tumour cells by the host's immune system, or by enhancing the cytotoxic function of immune effectors;

• *gene marking*: even though gene marking is not *per se* a therapeutic intervention, this approach has helped investigators understand the behaviour and outcome of transduced cells once administered back to the patient.

Tumour correction

Many of the molecular aberrations leading to cancer alter key regulatory, survival and differentiation steps in the cell cycle; others lead to the production of abnormal fusion products, with subsequent gain or loss of critical functions of the cellular cycle.

In theory, gene therapy could be used to replace an inactive gene with an active one, or to neutralize an abnormal function gained by a mutated gene. While the introduction of genetic material into haemopoietic cells, either to correct or to block a defect involved in malignant transformation, is appealing, it is also technically extremely challenging. Not only is highly efficient transduction of target cells required, but also many of the mutations leading to cancer are effectively dominant, and simple introduction of a wild-type gene would not be of benefit. Under these circumstances, the abnormal gene product must be silenced. Several strategies for silencing are being evaluated, including antisense molecules that are oligonucleotides specifically designed to interfere with DNA or mRNA and prevent transcription or translation, and ribozymes that are RNA molecules that specifically cleave mRNA and intrabodies obtained by modifying genes encoding antibodies so that the antigen-binding domain is expressed intracellularly. More recently, RNA interference, for example with siRNA (small interfering RNA), has proven to be an extremely potent means of diminishing gene expression. All these approaches, however, still suffer from the key limitation of poor delivery to the tumour cell, a particular concern for haematological malignancy, in which broad, multiorgan distribution is essential.

These challenges notwithstanding, several clinical and many preclinical studies have attempted to correct the function of haematological malignancies. Synthetic oligonucleotides complementary to the junction transcripts of *BCL–ABL* fusion gene have been shown to block *in vitro* proliferation of Philadelphia-positive leukaemia cells without impairing the growth capabilities of normal bone marrow progenitors. Antisense-treated mice with severe combined immunodeficiency (SCID) injected with Philadelphia-positive leukaemia cells confirmed the capability of *BCR-ABL* antisense oligonucleotides to temporarily suppress the progression of the disease and to significantly enhance survival of the treated animals. A DNA–RNA hybrid ribozyme designed to cleave *BCR–ABL* mRNA was incorporated into a liposome vector and transfected into EM-2 cells, a cell line derived from a patient with blast crisis of chronic meyeloid leukaemia (CML). The ribozyme decreased levels of detectable *BCR–ABL* mRNA in these cells, inhibited expression of the *BCR–ABL* gene product, p210BCR–ABL, and inhibited cell growth.

Ribozymes against the multidrug resistance gene *MDR1* RNA have been shown to overcome retinoic acid (RA) resistance in acute promyelocytic leukaemia cells. Expression of *MDR1* transcripts was decreased in HL60 cells expressing the *MDR1* RNA ribozyme, allowing RA to inhibit cellular proliferation and induce differentiation of HL-60 cells in a dose-dependent manner, suggesting reversal of drug resistance in HL-60 cells by the *MDR1* ribozyme. Other antisense oligonucleotides are targeted to transcriptional products from proto-oncogenes (such as *myb* and *myc*) known to induce proliferation and/or downregulation of differentiation of normal haemopoietic progenitors. Several clinical studies have been reported using antisense oligonucleotides targeting the c-*myb* or the *p53* genes, either as marrow-purging agents for chronic- or accelerated phase CML patients or intravenously in patients with refractory acute myeloid leukaemia (AML) or CML in blast crisis. There have been no toxicities but no significant clinical responses. More encouragingly, an antisense *Bcl-2* oligonucleotide has also been administered in patients with refractory non-Hodgkin's lymphoma, with objective clinical and biological responses.

The above results emphasize that effective exploitation of a tumour correction strategy using gene transfer will require significant improvements in vector efficiency and targeting. Until these come to pass, the tumour correction strategy will probably be dominated by the development of novel rationally targeted small molecules.

Sensitization of normal tissues or tumour cells

Prodrug-metabolizing enzyme (PDME)

Introduction of a gene encoding an enzyme that metabolizes an otherwise inert molecule into a cytotoxic agent has frequently been used in anti-tumour gene therapy. Although the herpes simplex thymidine kinase–ganciclovir system has been the most widely used, in fact more than 20 such PDME systems are currently in various stages of development and/or clinical trials. For all of these, the concept is that the gene encoding the prodrug-metabolizing enzyme is expressed in the cancer cell, and metabolizes a small molecule to an active moiety, which then kills the tumour cell directly. The molecule may also diffuse either through intercellular gap junctions or in the extracellular space and destroy adjacent tumour cells. In this way, transduction of even a small proportion of tumour cells can produce a large 'bystander' effect on adjacent tumour tissue. This in turn, compensates for the low efficiency of transduction achieved by currently available vectors and may help to destroy a large tumour burden.

Initially, brain tumours were the target for this approach. A number of paediatric and adult clinical studies have been performed using retroviral and subsequently adenoviral vectors encoding herpes simplex thymidine kinase (HSV-Tk) or cytosine deaminase, which converts fluorocytosine to fluorourosil.

In haemopoietic malignancies that lack gap junctions and are widely distributed, the lack of any potential bystander effect has essentially precluded direct cytotoxicity mediated by PDME *in vivo*. Instead, PDME has been used as a means of controlling T-cell immunotherapies. For example, graft-versus-host disease (GvHD) may occur when donor T cells are given to patients after allogeneic stem cell transplantation in an effort to treat relapse of leukaemia or lymphoma (graft versus tumour effect) or post-transplant infections. Several groups have infused donor T cells transduced with the HSV-Tk gene and reported successful abrogation of unwanted GvHD by treating the patients with ganciclovir. More recently efforts have been made to induce expression of the death signal Fas in donor T cells. An inducible construct is used in which Fas expression occurs only in the presence of a small molecule (chemical inducer of dimerization) that dimerizes two individually inactive components of a Fas transcriptional regulator, leading to expression of the Fas receptor and cell death on exposure to the ligand.

If T-cell immunotherapy for haematological malignancy becomes more widespread and more effective, these suicide mechanisms will become extremely important in ensuring that the regimens are acceptably safe.

Transfer of drug resistance genes to haemopoietic stem cells (HSC)

The transfer of drug resistance genes to haemopoietic cells has been used to protect these cells from the myelosuppression associated with chemotherapy and as a strategy for the *in vivo* selection and amplification of genetically modified cells. Several drug resistance genes have been evaluated in preclinical studies, including *MDR*, dihydrofolate reductase, nitrobenzylmercaptopurine riboside and methylguanine DNA methyltransferase. Of these, the human multidrug resistance 1 (*MDR1*) gene has been evaluated in clinical trials. The *MDR1* product, P-glycoprotein, functions as a drug efflux pump and confers resistance to many chemotherapeutic agents, thereby allowing 'dose-intensive' therapy with little marrow suppression. Early clinical studies showed minimal transfer, little expression and no protection, but with new-generation retroviral vectors and the use of stromal support elements, transduction efficiency of the HSC has improved. While it has been possible to show modest *in vivo* selection of gene modified cells after chemotherapy, as yet no convincing protection of human stem cells *in vivo* has been observed. Concerns about this approach include the risk of transferring drug resistance genes to neoplastic cells in the HSC graft, thus promoting a drug-resistant relapse, and the possibility of inducing myeloproliferation.

Modification of the tumour environment with anti-angiogenesis gene therapy

Because angiogenesis is a prerequisite for the development of metastatic disease for solid tumours, and probably for leukaemias and lymphomas as well, inhibition of new blood vessel formation may impede the spread of disease. A number of different large and small molecule inhibitors are currently under study, and some of these are suitable for a gene therapy approach. For example, endostatin, a 20-kDa fragment of collagen XVIII, can efficiently block angiogenesis, but the recombinant protein is difficult and expensive to produce and is somewhat unstable. Delivery of endostatin in murine tumour models by several different vector systems has been able to overcome this limitation. Similarly, angiostatin, a fragment of plasminogen, also functions as a large-molecule inhibitor of vessel growth and impedes metastatic tumours. This too can be transferred (for example by adeno-associated virus vector) to produce benefit in animal models of malignant brain tumours.

Much remains to be learned about the most appropriate route and cell of delivery of angiogenesis inhibition, but, as with any protein-based therapeutic, gene transfer should allow a continuous delivery of the drug rather than the peak and trough concentrations that result from most forms of injection, and may thereby produce a more sustained and effective response.

Gene modification of the immune response

Immunotherapy represents one of the most appealing of new anti-tumour approaches for haematological malignancy. Identification of antigens expressed on tumour cells and the improvements made in gene transfer techniques, together with a better understanding of the molecular and cellular mechanisms involved in the immune response against cancer, have given investigators tools to manipulate the immune system to induce an efficient immune response in the tumour-bearing host.

Tumour cell-based vaccines against haematological malignancies

Autologous tumour cells isolated from the patient's own tumour and treated (for example by irradiation) so that they no longer grow *in vivo* have long been tried as tumour vaccines, with limited success. Interest was greatly revived, however, when it was shown that genetic modification of tumour cells could increase their immunogenicity and induce an effective response not only against the gene-modified tumour, but also against unmodified tumour cells elsewhere in the individual. Tumour cells may be transduced with cytokine or co-stimulatory molecule genes, or with foreign major histocompatibility complex (MHC) molecules.

For applications in haemopoietic malignancies, particularly leukaemia and myeloma, transduced autologous cell lines are often difficult to prepare because the cells are either difficult to obtain from the patient or do not grow or survive *ex vivo*. Where autologous tumour cells cannot be obtained, a standardized immunogenic allogeneic tumour cell is a possible alternative. One potential drawback of the allogeneic approach is that the tumour antigens present in the host may be absent in the tumour line. The use of polyvalent tumour cell preparations may overcome this limitation. Another problem is that shared antigens may not be expressed in the context of the patient's own MHC, making them unrecognizable by the host immune system. This problem may be overcome if the tumour cell antigens are taken up, processed and presented by host professional antigen-presenting cells (APCs). Finally, the immune response to the allogeneic MHC molecules will likely be more potent than to the weaker tumour antigens, and the gene-modified tumour cells may be lysed before tumour-reactive T cells are recruited. However, the highly immunogenic foreign MHC molecules might also act as an immune adjuvant and thereby enhance the anti-tumour immune response.

Clinical experience with gene-modified tumour cells

Among the many immunomodulatory gene products tested to date, vaccination with irradiated cells engineered to secrete GM-CSF (granulocyte–macrophage colony-stimulating factor) has been shown to induce the most potent, specific and long-lasting immunity in several murine tumour models. In patients with melanoma and renal cell carcinoma, local and systemic immune delayed-type hypersensitivity and transient tumour regressions were induced by GM-CSF-expressing autologous tumour cells. IL-2 and IL-12 have also emerged as potent immunomodulatory molecules in several murine and human tumours. In patients with several types of tumour including melanoma, renal cell carcinoma, glioblastoma, colon carcinoma and neuroblastoma, phase I trials of IL-2-gene transduced tumour cells showed no toxic effect of IL-2 production *in vivo*. Furthermore, preliminary results in these studies showed a positive effect of IL-2 on the specific immune response.

In haematological malignancy, considerable recent interest has focused on the CD40/CD40L system. CD40, a cell-surface receptor of the tumour necrosis factor (TNF) receptor family, was identified as a molecule expressed during all stages of B-cell development and differentiation. The ligand for CD40 (CD40L or CD154) is mainly expressed on activated CD4+ T cells and on professional APCs. The interactions between B-cell CD40 and T-cell CD40L play an important role in T-cell-dependent activation of B cells and in the processing of antigen by B cells. Moreover, CD40 ligation induces B7 expression by leukaemic B cells and enhances the ability of B cells to act as APCs. Preclinical experiments in mice with CD40-positive B-cell leukaemia have shown tumour reduction and a significant benefit in survival when animals received a vaccine consisting of tumour cells admixed with syngeneic fibroblasts engineered to secrete CD40L and IL-2. This approach is currently being tested in a phase I trial in patients with acute lymphoblastic and myeloid leukaemia and is producing high levels of immunity. Recent administration of human B-chronic lymphocytic leukaemia cells expressing murine CD40L has provided evidence that this approach may also enhance anti-tumour immunity *ex vivo* and *in vivo*, with evidence also of tumour responses. Other immunomodulatory molecules, such as IL-2, IL-4, IL-12, TNF-α, GM-CSF and B7.1

(CD80), have similarly induced anti-leukaemia activity in several preclinical vaccine models.

Gene modified dendritic cells

'Professional' APCs such as dendritic cells (DCs) may be modified to express candidate tumour antigens by gene transfer using viral or non-viral vectors. The advantage of these cells over whole tumour cell vaccines is their expression of high levels of co-stimulatory molecules that may enable them to recruit T-cell responses even to weak tumour-associated antigens. Most clinical studies have used peptide-, protein- or mRNA-derived antigens or tumour cell lysates and apoptotic bodies to load the DC with tumour-associated epitopes. However, gene transfer can also be used to directly transfer a validated tumour-associated gene intended to be the target for an immune response. For example, DCs can be transduced to express the Epstein–Barr virus (EBV) latency gene *LMP-2*, and generate cytotoxic T cells that are highly specific for this weak tumour-associated antigen, present on the malignant cells of EBV-positive Hodgkin's disease and nasopharyngeal carcinoma.

These *LMP-2*-specific T cells are being evaluated in a series of clinical studies described in the following section.

Cancer therapy with gene-modified T cells

Several studies have suggested the feasibility and apparent clinical efficacy of adoptive transfer of cytotoxic T lymphocytes (CTLs) directed at viral or tumour antigens. Gene transfer offers the potential for improving these approaches. The earliest modifications simply used genetic markers (e.g. *neo*) transferred by retroviral vectors, enabling investigators to determine the survival and homing of virus-specific T cells infused in patients with EBV-associated post-transplant lymphoproliferative disorder (PTLD), or Hodgkin's disease or nasopharyngeal carcinoma, and to discover if they mediated any adverse effects.

More recently, the approach has been used to protect T cells against tumour-induced downregulation. While clinical studies using infusions of CTL against EBV-related malignancies have been promising, with some complete tumour responses, most patients with aggressive relapsed EBV-positive Hodgkin's disease ultimately progress. This may in part be due to the lack of specificity of the EBV-specific CTLs for the subdominant LMP1 and LMP2 antigens that are present on the Hodgkin's tumour cells and may be overcome using gene-modified dendritic cells as described above. In addition, however, many haematological malignancies, including EBV-positive Hodgkin's disease, secrete immunosuppressive cytokines and chemokines that affect CTL function and APC activity.

Gene transfer can be used to overcome both types of problems. In Hodgkin's disease, for example, dendritic cells transduced with adenoviral vectors encoding either LMP2 or a mutated LMP1 will generate CTL with high cytolytic activity *in vitro* to LMP2- or LMP1-positive cancer cells. These effectors can then be made resistant to the immunosuppressive cytokines secreted

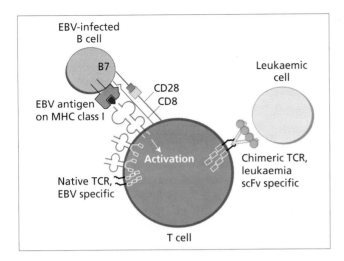

Figure 27.1 EBV-specific T cell redirected towards leukaemia-specific antigens by means of a chimeric TCR leukaemia scFv-specific.

by the Hodgkin Reed–Sternberg cell. The cytokine which has the most devastating effects on CTL proliferation and function is transforming growth factor beta (TGF-β). This cytokine is secreted by many haematological malignancies and allows the leukaemia/lymphoma to escape the immune response. Effector cells can be transduced with a retrovirus vector expressing a dominant-negative TGF-β type II receptor (DNR), which prevents formation of the functional tetrameric receptor. Cytotoxicity, proliferation and cytokine release assays showed that exogenous TGF-β has minimal inhibitory effects on DNR-transduced CTLs. This combination of tumour-specific and tumour-resistant CTLs may prove highly effective for therapy.

Chimeric receptor-expressing cytotoxic T cells for tumour therapy

One can generate chimeric T/B cell receptors by joining the heavy- and light-chain variable regions of a monoclonal antibody to form a single-chain Fv (scFv) and coupling this in turn to the T-cell receptor (TCR) ζ-chain (Figure 27.1) or Fc-γ immune receptor domain. When these chimeric receptor genes are introduced into T cells, antigen stimulation of the extracellular component of the chimeric receptor results in tyrosine phosphorylation of immune receptor activation motifs present in the cytoplasmic domain, initiating T-cell signalling to the nucleus.

Primary T cells genetically modified to express chimeric receptors derived from antibodies and specific for tumour or viral antigens have considerable therapeutic potential. Chimeric T-cell receptors allow the recognition specificity of T lymphocytes to extend beyond classical T-cell epitopes and can therefore be applied to every malignancy that expresses a tumour-associated antigen for which a monoclonal antibody (MAb) exists. Unlike conventional T-cell receptors, these chimeric receptors will be

active even if the tumour cells are MHC class I negative. Chimeric receptor transduced T cells have numerous advantages over immunotherapies based on monoclonal antibodies or T lymphocytes alone. As there is no need to select and expand tumour-specific antigens from scanty precursors, large populations of antigen-redirected T lymphocytes can be obtained in a matter of weeks. Moreover, chimeric T-cell receptors are MHC unrestricted, so that tumour escape by downregulation of MHC class I molecules and defects in antigen processing are bypassed. As both CD4+ and CD8+ T cells can express the same chimeric receptor, the full network of T-cell function is directed against tumour cells. The presence of chimeric TCR-mediated effector function may be more likely to produce tumour cell lysis than humoral immune responses alone.

The perforin/granzyme killing mechanism may be effective against cells that are relatively resistant to antibody and complement, while cytokine secretion upon T-cell activation by tumour antigen recruits additional components of the immune system, amplifying the anti-tumour immune response. Furthermore, unlike intact antibodies, T cells can migrate through microvascular walls, extravasate and penetrate the core of solid tumours to exert their cytolytic activity. Finally, a single T lymphocyte can sequentially kill a multiplicity of target cells.

Adoptively transferred chimeric receptor-transduced cells have been protective in murine tumour models and many investigators have succeeded in expanding human peripheral blood T cells expressing similar receptors. Among these have been cells targeted to the pan-B-cell markers CD19 and CD20. In the presence of CD80 and interleukin 15 (IL-15), these chimeric peripheral T cells can persist in tumour-bearing SCID Beige mice and eradicate disseminated intramedullary B-cell tumours. Similarly, CD20 chimeric receptor-transduced T cells from patients with chronic lymphocytic leukaemia (CLL) effectively lyse autologous tumour cells. While CD19 and CD20 are expressed on normal B cells which would then also become the targets of chimeric receptor-expressing T cells, this cross-reactivity would not be considered an absolute contraindication to their use in patients with advanced B-cell malignancies. Other targets for the treatment of haemopoietic malignancies include anti-CD33-specific chimeric constructs.

Though promising *in vitro* and in mice, in humans *in vivo*, chimeric receptor-expressing T cells have so far proved clinically disappointing, as they are short-lived or rapidly inactivated in the circulation. Clearance of modified T-effector cells by immune effector mechanisms may be delayed by humanization of currently available hybridoma antibodies or by the generation of fully human single-chain antibodies by phage display technology. But optimally sustained function may require chimeric receptor molecules that are coupled to the enhanced intracellular signalling mechanisms associated with co-stimulator molecules, such as CD28, or that are transferred into virus-specific T cells with established *in vivo* activity. Clinical trials adopting these approaches are imminent.

Conclusion

We have far to go before gene transfer will have any measurable impact on haematological diseases. But as we continue to make incremental advances in the application of this complex but potent methodology, we can expect to see gene therapies increasingly supplement, and perhaps ultimately supplant, many conventional therapies in haematology.

Selected bibliography

Viral and non-viral vectors for gene therapy

Buchschacher GL Jr, Wong-Staal F (2000) Development of lentiviral vectors for gene therapy for human diseases. *Blood* **95**: 2499–504.

Burton EA, Bai Q, Goins WF, Glorioso JC (2002) Replication-defective genomic herpes simplex vectors: design and production. *Current Opinion in Biotechnology* **13**: 424–8.

Chen SY, Bagley J, Marasco WA (1994) Intracellular antibodies as a new class of therapeutic molecules for gene therapy. *Human Gene Therapy* **5**: 595–601.

Hitt MM, Graham FL (2000) Adenovirus vectors for human gene therapy. *Advances in Virus Research* **55**: 479–505.

Kay MA, Glorioso JC, Naldini L (2001) Viral vectors for gene therapy: the art of turning infectious agents into vehicles of therapeutics. *Nature Medicine* **7**: 33–40.

Persidis A (1998) Ribozyme therapeutics. *Nature Biotechnology* **15**: 921–2.

Rossi FM, Blau HM (1997) Recent advances in inducible gene expression systems. *Current Opinion in Biotechnology* **9**: 451–6.

Russell DW, Kay MA (1999) Adeno-associated virus vectors and hematology. *Blood* **94**: 864–74.

Salmon P, Kindler V, Ducrey O *et al.* (2000) High-level transgene expression in human hematopoietic progenitors and differentiated blood lineages after transduction with improved lentiviral vectors. *Blood* **96**: 3392–8.

Sutton RE, Wu HT, Rigg R *et al.* (1998) Human immunodeficiency virus type 1 vectors efficiently transduce human hematopoietic stem cells. *Journal of Virology* **72**: 5781–8.

Templeton NS (2001) Developments in liposomal gene delivery systems. *Expert Opinion on Biological Therapy* **1**: 567–70.

Wang H, Prasad G, Buolamwin JK, Zhang R (2001) Antisense anti-cancer oligonucleotide therapeutics. *Current Cancer Drug Targets* **1**: 177–96.

Wickham TJ (2000) Targeting adenovirus. *Gene Therapy* **7**: 110–14.

Gene therapies for the treatment of haemophilias and sickle-cell disease

Kay MA, Manno CS, Ragni MV *et al.* (2000) Evidence for gene transfer and expression of factor IX in haemophilia B patients treated with an AAV vector. *Nature Genetics* **24**: 257–261.

Kren BT, Bandyopadhyay P, Steer CJ (1998) *In vivo* site-directed mutagenesis of the factor IX gene by chimeric RNA/DNA oligonucleotides. *Nature Medicine* **4**: 285–90.

Pawliuk R, Westerman KA, Fabry ME *et al.* (2001) Correction of sickle cell disease in transgenic mouse models by gene therapy. *Science* **294**: 2368–71.

Powell JS, Ragni MV, White GC 2nd *et al.* (2003) Phase 1 trial of FVIII gene transfer for severe hemophilia A using a retroviral construct administered by peripheral intravenous infusion. *Blood* **102**: 2038–45.

Rivella S, May C, Chadburn A *et al.* (2003) A novel murine model of Cooley anemia and its rescue by lentiviral-mediated human beta-globin gene transfer. *Blood* **101**: 2932–9.

Roth DA, Tawa NE Jr, O'Brien JM *et al.* (2001) Nonviral transfer of the gene encoding coagulation factor VIII in patients with severe hemophilia A. *New England Journal of Medicine* **344**: 1735–42.

Scallan CD, Lillicrap D, Jiang H, Qian X *et al.* (2003) Sustained phenotypic correction of canine hemophilia A using an adeno-associated viral vector. *Blood* **102**: 2031–7.

Snyder RO, Miao C, Meuse L *et al.* (1999) Correction of hemophilia B in canine and murine models using recombinant adeno-associated viral vectors. *Nature Medicine* **5**: 64–70.

Targeting oncogenes in malignant haemopoietic disorders

Bayever E, Iversen PL, Bishop MR *et al.* (1993) Systemic administration of a phosphorothioate oligonucleotide with a sequence complementary to p53 for acute myelogenous leukemia and myelodysplastic syndrome: initial results of a phase I trial. *Antisense Research and Development* **3**: 383–90.

Bishop MR, Jackson JD, Tarantolo SR *et al.* (1997) *Ex vivo* treatment of bone marrow with phosphorothioate oligonucleotide OL(1)p53 for autologous transplantation in acute myelogenous leukemia and myelodysplastic syndrome. *Journal of Hematotherapy* **6**: 441–6.

Calabretta B, Sims RB, Valtieri M *et al.* (1991) Normal and leukemic hematopoietic cells manifest differential sensitivity to inhibitory effects of c-myb antisense oligodeoxynucleotides: an *in vitro* study relevant to bone marrow purging. *Proceedings of the National Academy of Sciences of the United States of America* **88**: 2351–5.

Snyder DS, Wu Y, Wang JL *et al.* (1993) Ribozyme-mediated inhibition of bcr-abl gene expression in a Philadelphia chromosome-positive cell line. *Blood* **82**: 600–5.

Waters JS, Webb A, Cunningham D *et al.* (2000) Phase I clinical and pharmacokinetic study of Bcl-2 antisense oligonucleotide therapy in patients with non-Hodgkin's lymphoma. *Journal of Clinical Oncology* **18**: 1812–23.

Webb A, Cunningham D, Cotter F *et al.* (1997) BCL-2 antisense therapy in patients with non-Hodgkin lymphoma. *Lancet* **349**: 1137–41.

Suicide gene therapy in malignant haemopoietic malignancies

Sorrentino BP, Brandt SJ, Bodine D *et al.* (1992) Selection of drug-resistant bone marrow cells *in vivo* after retroviral transfer of human MDR1. *Science* **257**: 99–103.

Thomis DC, Marktel S, Bonini C *et al.* (2001) A Fas-based suicide switch in human T cells for the treatment of graft-versus-host disease. *Blood* **97**: 1249–57.

Tiberghien P, Cahn JY, Brion A *et al.* (1997) Use of donor T-lymphocytes expressing herpes-simplex thymidine kinase in allogeneic bone marrow transplantation: a phase I–II study. *Human Gene Therapy* 8: 615–24.

Verzeletti S, Bonini C, Marktel S *et al.* (1998) Herpes simplex virus thymidine kinase gene transfer for controlled graft-versus-host disease and graft-versus-leukemia: clinical follow-up and improved new vectors. *Human Gene Therapy* 9: 2243–51.

Vaccines against malignant haemopoietic malignancies

Cardoso AA, Schultze JL, Boussiotis VA, Freeman GJ *et al.* (1996) Pre-B acute lymphoblastic leukemia cells may induce T-cell anergy to alloantigen. *Blood* 88: 41–8.

Cardoso AA, Seamon MJ, Afonso HM, Ghia P *et al.* (1997) *Ex vivo* generation of human anti-pre-B leukemia-specific autologous cytolytic T cells. *Blood* 90: 549–61.

Dilloo D, Brown M, Roskrow M, Zhong W *et al.* (1997) CD40 ligand induces an anti-leukemia immune response *in vivo*. *Blood* 90: 1927–33.

Kato K, Cantwell MJ, Sharma S, Kipps TJ (1998) Gene transfer of CD40-ligand induces autologous immune recognition of chronic lymphocytic leukemia B cells. *Journal of Clinical Investigation* 101: 1133–41.

Ranheim E, Kipps T (1993) Activated T cells induce expression of B7/BB1 on normal or leukemic B cells through a CD40-dependant signal. *Journal of Experimental Medicine* 177: 925–35.

Rousseau RF, Bollard CM, Heslop HE (2001) Gene therapy for paediatric leukaemia. *Expert Opinion in Biological Therapy* 1: 663–74.

Rousseau RF, Hirschmann-Jax C, Takahashi S, Brenner MK (2001) Cancer vaccines. *Hematology Oncology Clinics of North America* 15: 741–73.

Vereecque R, Buffenoir G, Preudhomme C *et al.* (2000) Gene transfer of GM-CSF, CD80 and CD154 cDNA enhances survival in a murine model of acute leukemia with persistence of a minimal residual disease. *Gene Therapy* 7: 1312–16.

Wierda W, Cantwell M, Woods S *et al.* (2000) CD40-ligand (CD154) gene therapy for chronic lymphocytic leukemia. *Blood* 96: 2917–24.

Adoptive immune therapies against malignant haemopoietic malignancies

Bollard CM, Rossig C, Calonge MJ *et al.* (2002) Adapting a transforming growth factor beta-related tumor protection strategy to enhance antitumor immunity. *Blood* 99: 3179–87.

Brentjens RJ, Latouche JB, Santos E *et al.* (2003) Eradication of systemic B-cell tumors by genetically targeted human T lymphocytes co-stimulated by CD80 and interleukin-15. *Nature Medicine* 9: 279–86.

Falkenburg JHF, Willemze R (2004) Minor histocompatibility antigens as targets of cellular immunotherapy in leukaemia. *Clinical Haematology* 17: 415–25.

Finney HM, Lawson AD, Bebbington CR, Weir AN (1998) Chimeric receptors providing both primary and co-stimulatory signaling in T cells from a single gene product. *Journal of Immunology* 161: 2791–7.

Gottschalk S, Edwards OL, Sili U *et al.* (2003) Generating CTLs against the subdominant Epstein–Barr virus LMP1 antigen for the adoptive immunotherapy of EBV-associated malignancies. *Blood* 101: 1905–12.

Heslop H, Ng C, Li C (1996) Long-term restoration of immunity against Epstein–Barr virus infection by adoptive transfer of gene-modified virus-specific T lymphocytes. *Nature Medicine* 2: 551–5.

Heslop HE, Savoldo B, Rooney CM (2004) Cellular therapy of Epstein–Barr-virus-associated post-transplant lymphoproliferative disease. *Clinical Haematology* 17: 401–13.

Kolb H-J, Rank A, Chen X *et al.* (2004) In-vivo generation of leukaemia-derived dendritic cells. *Clinical Haematology* 17: 439–51.

Pule M, Bollard CM, Heslop HE (2002) Genetically engineered T-cells for adoptive immunotherapy. *Current Opinion in Molecular Therapies* 4: 467–75.

Rooney CM, Smith CA, Ng C *et al.* (1995) Use of gene-modified virus-specific T lymphocytes to control Epstein–Barr virus-related lymphoproliferation. *Lancet* 345: 9–13.

CHAPTER 28

The molecular basis of leukaemia and lymphoma

28

Peter J Campbell, Anthony J Bench and Anthony R Green

Introduction

The average human produces many billions of red cells and neutrophils each day. This process is exquisitely responsive to physiological stresses such as infection and blood loss, and is able to increase output by up to 10-fold at such times. The haemopoietic system maintains such a prodigious yet appropriately balanced output through tight control of stem cell proliferation, lineage commitment and differentiation. It is corruption of these processes that results in haematological malignancy.

Studies of leukaemia and lymphoma have led the way in providing paradigms of general relevance to cancer biology. Present models posit a 'multiple-hit' process in which critical cellular pathways are corrupted by accumulating genetic damage, resulting in an autonomous, proliferating stem cell clone. The phenotype of the malignancy is determined by the particular pathways that are corrupted, often in a quite stereotypic fashion. Thus, specific tumour types are associated with particular genetic alterations that are not seen in other haematological malignancies.

This chapter will review what we understand of the molecular pathogenesis of leukaemia and lymphoma. The first section describes several basic principles germane to the pathogenesis of haematological malignancies, including aspects of clonality and clonal evolution, the concept of the 'leukaemic stem cell' and genotype–phenotype correlations. The second section covers the nature of acquired gene alterations associated with haematological malignancies, including chromosomal rearrangements, point mutations and epigenetic effects. In the third section, we illustrate the consequences of such alterations. It is beyond the scope of the chapter to provide an exhaustive list of causative mutations and pathways in all haematological malignancies: instead we illustrate the underlying principles by describing five

specific examples of malignancies with corruption of distinct cellular processes: tyrosine kinase signalling (the myeloproliferative disorders); intracellular signal transduction (juvenile myelomonocytic leukaemia); regulation of gene transcription (acute myeloid leukaemia); cell cycle control (mantle cell lymphoma); and apoptosis (follicular lymphoma).

Basic concepts of haematological neoplasia

Clonality

Studies of haematological malignancies have led the way in establishing the clonal origins of tumours. This is mainly because normal and malignant haemopoietic cells are readily accessible, can be grown in culture and have been well-characterized at a molecular level. Three main lines of evidence suggest that haematological tumours each arise from a single ancestral cell and thus are 'clonal'.

First, in almost all lymphoproliferative disorders and a minority of acute myeloid leukaemias, the tumour population carries a unique rearrangement of either an immunoglobulin (*IGH*) or TcR gene, the exceptions being very primitive acute lymphoblastic leukaemia (ALL) and lymphoma. In contrast, non-malignant disorders causing proliferation of lymphocytes are characterized by a polyclonal pattern of antigen receptor rearrangement. This is persuasive evidence for a clonal origin of lymphoid malignancies and suggests that a key transformation event occurred at or after gene rearrangement.

Second, evidence for clonality also derives from studies of X-chromosome inactivation patterns from female patients

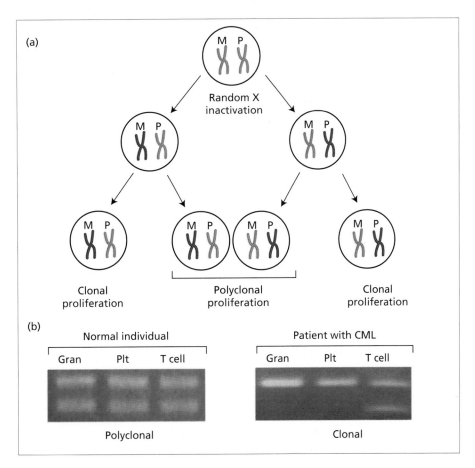

Figure 28.1 X-chromosome inactivation patterns. (a) X-inactivation patterns in clonal and polyclonal proliferations. Early in female embryogenesis, each cell randomly inactivates either the maternal or paternal X chromosome. The pattern of X inactivation is faithfully passed on to all progeny cells and, as a result, women are mosaic with respect to X inactivation. As a clonal proliferation arises from a single cell, all of the proliferating cells will carry the same inactive X chromosome. By contrast, a polyclonal proliferation will be mixed, with some cells carrying an inactive maternal X chromosome, and others carrying an inactive paternal X chromosome. (b) Reverse transcription polymerase chain reaction (RT-PCR) analysis of X-chromosome inactivation patterns. Transcripts from the polymorphic X-linked *IDS* gene were amplified by RT-PCR from granulocytes (gran), T cells and platelets (plt) obtained from a patient with CML, and a normal individual. Note that two products (representing the maternally and paternally derived X chromosomes) are obtained in cells from the normal individual and in T cells from the patient. By contrast, only one allele is active in granulocytes and platelets from the patient.

(Figure 28.1). The process of X-chromosome inactivation is random and occurs early in fetal development. In women, a polyclonal proliferation therefore contains a mixture of cells, some of which carry an active maternal X chromosome, whereas others contain an active paternal X chromosome. By contrast, a clonal proliferation contains cells that carry either an active maternal or an active paternal X chromosome. Unfortunately, the diagnostic utility of such studies is limited by the fact that many normal women develop, as they age, a skewed pattern of X inactivation in their blood cells.

Third, acquired cytogenetic or molecular changes that arise during the development of a malignancy can also be used as clonal markers. For example, in chronic myeloid leukaemia (CML) the Philadelphia (Ph) translocation can be found in multiple different blood cell types, including neutrophils, monocytes, basophils and B cells, suggesting that the disease arises in a multipotent stem cell.

If it is accepted that lymphoma and leukaemia are clonal disorders, in which the vast number of autonomous malignant cells that are present at diagnosis all derive from a single cell, several questions are immediately prompted. How does this single cell acquire sufficient genetic damage to become so disordered? What is the nature of the ancestral cell? Is the phenotype of the malignancy determined by the genetic changes, by the characteristics of the ancestral cell in which they occurred or by both? These questions will be addressed in turn.

Figure 28.1 X-chromosome inactivation patterns. (a) X-inactivation patterns in clonal and polyclonal proliferations. Early in female embryogenesis, each cell randomly inactivates either the maternal or paternal X chromosome. The pattern of X inactivation is faithfully passed on to all progeny cells and, as a result, women are mosaic with respect to X inactivation. As a clonal proliferation arises from a single cell, all of the proliferating cells will carry the same inactive X chromosome. By contrast, a polyclonal proliferation will be mixed, with some cells carrying an inactive maternal X chromosome, and others carrying an inactive paternal X chromosome. (b) Reverse transcription polymerase chain reaction (RT-PCR) analysis of X-chromosome inactivation patterns. Transcripts from the polymorphic X-linked *IDS* gene were amplified by RT-PCR from granulocytes (gran), T cells and platelets (plt) obtained from a patient with CML, and a normal individual. Note that two products (representing the maternally and paternally derived X chromosomes) are obtained in cells from the normal individual and in T cells from the patient. By contrast, only one allele is active in granulocytes and platelets from the patient.

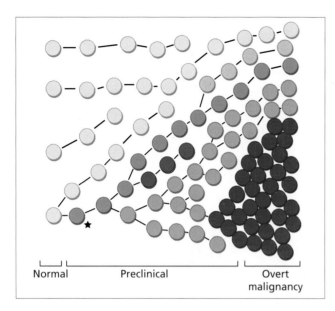

Normal   Preclinical   Overt malignancy

Figure 28.2 Clonal evolution of malignancy. The process starts in a single green cell (*) that acquires a mutation providing a slight selective advantage. Subsequently, the progeny of this cell acquire further mutations (blue, pink and red). Some mutations may be deleterious, and the corresponding clone dies out (blue). With time, a clone can acquire further mutations, leading to increasingly aggressive behaviour. Note that the overt malignancy is heterogeneous and contains a dominant subclone (red) as well as other less prevalent subclones (green and pink), which carry overlapping but distinct sets of mutations.

Clonal evolution

Most malignancies are thought to be the result of several mutations, acquired sequentially and randomly, rather than one single catastrophic mutation (Figure 28.2). Conceptually similar to the Darwinian natural selection, malignancy starts with a change in the genetic material of an ancestral cell that provides a slight selective advantage. Descendants of that abnormal cell subsequently acquire additional mutations, further increasing the selective advantage, and so the abnormal population expands until it eventually results in clinically overt disease. As the mutations are random events, some of them will be deleterious and may result in extinction of the corresponding subclone. Many different subclones, all deriving from the same original ancestral cell, will exist within the tumour population, and subtle differences in, for example, proliferative capacity or drug resistance may be evident. The several mutations that occur in a given tumour often occur in genes involved in interlinked or cooperating pathways, a theme developed in more detail later in this chapter.

Several lines of evidence demonstrate that more than one mutation is necessary for full malignancy. In both cell culture assays and murine models used to assess translocations found in leukaemia, the fusion gene alone is usually insufficient to induce a leukaemic phenotype. In mouse studies, transplantation of haemopoietic stem cells transformed by a fusion gene often result in leukaemia only after a long latency, suggesting that further events are required for neoplasia. Consistent with this concept, the latency can be shortened by the administration of mutagenic agents such as nitrosourea.

In humans, there is also evidence that a single mutation is not sufficient for the full malignant phenotype. First, individuals who inherit a mutated *RUNX1* gene in all their cells develop a clonal leukaemia (i.e. from only one of their cells) in later life, suggesting that additional events are needed to cooperate with the *RUNX1* mutation. Second, translocations associated with childhood leukaemia can be detected at birth, several years before the leukaemia develops. In children who develop acute leukaemia associated with the t(12;21) and t(8;21) translocations, testing of DNA extracted from the Guthrie blood spot taken just after birth has demonstrated that cells carrying the same translocation were present in the first few days of life. Third, it has been observed that normal individuals may harbour very low levels of fusion transcripts that are normally associated with leukaemia, such as the BCR–ABL transcript of CML or PML–RARα of acute promyelocytic leukaemia. These results suggest that cells carrying these translocations need further events to transform them or that the mutation occurred in a cell incapable of sustaining a long-term self-renewing malignancy.

The model of clonal evolution also proposes that a population of malignant cells contains subclones that have acquired distinct secondary changes, and which may therefore exhibit different biological characteristics. Drug resistance serves as a paradigm for this observation. In studies of CML patients who initially respond to the tyrosine kinase inhibitor imatinib, but subsequently become resistant, the resistance is often mediated by point mutations that affect the imatinib binding site of the BCR–ABL fusion protein. These mutations can be found in samples taken before the patients started imatinib thus demonstrating that the drug provided a selective advantage to a pre-existing subclone of leukaemic cells. Similarly, patients who relapse after intensive chemotherapy for acute leukaemia will sometimes be found to harbour an apparently new cytogenetic or molecular abnormality that in retrospect was present as a low level subclone in samples from the original presentation.

The 'malignant stem cell'

Myeloid malignancies

A central feature of haematological and other malignancies is a capacity for malignant cells to self-renew. Self-renewal is also a feature of normal stem cells, and this has resulted in the suggestion that tumours result from transformation of a stem cell, a concept that would also explain how the original transformed cell and its progeny survive long enough to allow the acquisition

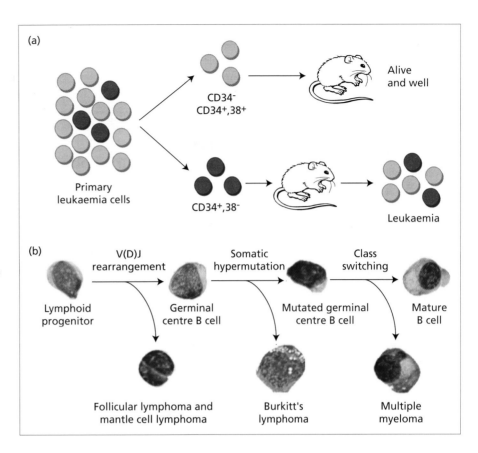

Figure 28.3 The cell of origin for haematological malignancies. (a) AML arises in a haemopoietic stem cell. Primary human AML samples contain a small number of leukaemia stem cells (red) with surface markers similar to normal haemopoietic stem cells (i.e. CD34$^+$, CD38$^-$). Transplantation of leukaemic stem cells but not the majority of leukaemia cells (orange) recapitulates the leukaemia in immunodeficient mice. (b) B-cell lymphomas may arise in committed B-cell progenitors. Normal maturation of B cells involves rearrangement and class switching of immunoglobulin genes. Mistakes occurring during these recombination events can result in leukaemogenic chromosome translocations. Analyses of sequences adjacent to the translocation breakpoints suggest that translocations occur at different stages of differentiation in distinct B-cell lymphomas.

of secondary mutations. An alternative hypothesis is that the original mutation does occur in a more mature cell, normally destined to differentiate and die, but the initiating event is sufficient to confer the ability to self-renew. It may well be that these different models operate in distinct types of malignancy.

Studies of myeloid malignancies have provided the first experimental evidence to support the existence of tumour stem cells. In patients with CML, cells representing multiple different haemopoietic lineages carry the *BCR–ABL* fusion gene and its protein product. Moreover, the fact that CML blast crisis can be either myeloid or lymphoid suggests that the original transformed cell had both myeloid and lymphoid potential (see also Chapter 37).

In AML, a leukaemic stem cell has been identified following transplantation of primary human AML cells into immunodeficient mice (Figure 28.3a). Leukaemic stem cells are relatively rare (most of the cells in a given leukaemia represent partially differentiated progeny), have the same surface markers as normal haemopoietic stem cells and are the only cells from the primary leukaemia capable of generating leukaemia in recipient mice.

These properties of leukaemic stem cells have significant implications for the treatment of malignant haematological disorders. A curative strategy must eliminate all malignant cells with the ability to self-renew and hence the capacity to regener-

ate the malignancy. Moreover, a fraction of leukaemic stem cells, like their normal counterparts, are metabolically inactive and in G_0, and so many conventional cell cycle-specific cytotoxics will be ineffective.

Lymphoid malignancies

In contrast to the myeloid malignancies, most lymphoid malignancies do not appear to result from transformation of a haemopoietic stem cell. Instead, lymphoid tumours arise from cells already committed to lymphoid differentiation, perhaps reflecting in part the fact that lymphocytes retain the potential for self-renewal and proliferation following exposure to antigen. Translocations associated with lymphoid tumours frequently reflect mistakes that occur during the normal process of antigen receptor rearrangement. During normal B-cell development, the *IGH* locus sequentially undergoes V(D)J rearrangement, somatic hypermutation and class switching. In B-cell malignancies, the timing of an associated translocation can therefore be inferred from analysis of the immunoglobulin locus sequence adjacent to the breakpoint (Figure 28.3b).

The cell of origin for mantle cell lymphomas and follicular lymphomas may well be pregerminal and germinal centre B cells undergoing immunoglobulin gene rearrangement. The breakpoints of the t(11;14) and the t(14;18) translocations tend to occur between the D and J segments of the *IGH* locus, suggesting that they arise from mistakes of DJ recombination. In Burkitt's lymphoma, the c-*MYC* gene is frequently juxtaposed with a fully V(D)J rearranged and hypermutated *IGH* variable region in the t(8;14) translocation. Breakpoints are found clustered in the VJ sequences that are particular targets for somatic hypermutation, suggesting that the double-stranded DNA breaks effected during hypermutation may cause the translocations. Class switch recombination appears to be responsible for many of the translocations that occur in multiple myeloma, because the breakpoints are found in immunoglobulin heavy-chain switch regions.

These observations provide evidence that the translocations associated with different B-cell malignancies occur at distinct times within B-cell ontogeny. However, two caveats should be emphasized. First, *IGH* translocations may not represent initiating events. It remains formally possible that an unknown earlier lesion precedes the translocation and occurs in a more primitive cell. Second, transformed cells undergo partial differentiation even after acquiring an *IGH* translocation. For example, follicular lymphoma cells have both the histological appearances and gene expression signatures of germinal centre cells. For this continued differentiation to occur, the pregerminal centre cell with the t(14;18) translocation must have been able to participate in an antigen-driven germinal centre response. Consistent with this idea, there is evidence for on-going somatic hypermutation within the tumour clone.

Phenotype–genotype correlations

One of the most striking properties of leukaemias and lymphomas is the close relationship between certain cytogenetic or molecular abnormalities and unique morphological and clinical features. For example, the cells of Burkitt's lymphoma are characterized by a very distinctive morphological appearance and are almost universally associated with translocations involving the *MYC* gene. Similar strong associations occur between acute myelomonocytic leukaemia with abnormal eosinophil precursors (M4Eo AML) and the inv(16) abnormality, acute promyelocytic leukaemia and the *PML–RARα* fusion gene, and mantle cell lymphoma and the t(11;14) translocation.

There are two potential explanations for such associations. The nature of the chromosome rearrangement may determine the phenotype of the resultant leukaemia. Alternatively, a specific chromosome rearrangement may only occur in, or provide a selective advantage for, progenitor cells committed to a particular lineage. Both models may well be correct. For example, different subtypes of AML associated with distinct translocations, and which appear very different morphologically, contain leukaemic stem cells that appear identical in their pattern of cell surface markers. Thus, it seems that in AML it is the acquired genetic alterations that determine distinct phenotypes, and not the characteristics of the target cell. By contrast, several translocations involving the *IGH* or *TCR* loci are thought to be restricted to lymphoid tumours because sequences adjacent to the oncogenes mimic sequences involved in *IGH* rearrangement. The translocations may therefore only occur in cells at particular stages of lymphoid differentiation.

Nature of acquired genetic abnormalities

Translocations

The best-understood genetic abnormalities in haematological malignancies are chromosomal translocations. Balanced translocations involve a reciprocal exchange of genetic material between two chromosomes and may result in aberrant function of genes adjacent to the breakpoint (see also Chapter 30). Two common mechanisms have been described (Figure 28.4).

First, a fusion gene may be generated and encode a fusion protein with oncogenic properties. This mechanism is seen in many of the translocations associated with myeloid malignancies and some associated with ALL. Fusion proteins contain a combination of functional modules donated by the two partner proteins. As a consequence, the fusion protein is endowed with novel functions. For example, in fusion proteins that involve a tyrosine kinase, the partner protein invariably contributes a dimerization domain that allows the fusion protein to form oligomers spontaneously, thus resulting in constitutive activation of the kinase.

A fusion gene can also result from an interstitial deletion (such as deletion of chromosome 4 giving rise to the *FIP1L1–PDGFRA* fusion gene in chronic eosinophilic leukaemia) or inversion of

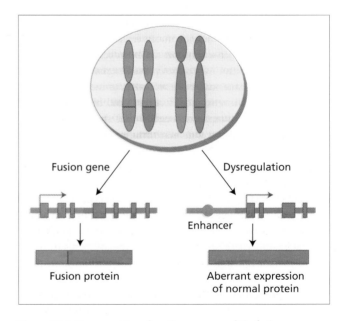

Figure 28.4 Recurrent translocations may result in fusion gene formation or transcriptional dysregulation of an intact target gene.

part of a chromosome (such as inversion 16 in the M4Eo subtype of AML).

The second category of translocations results in a structurally intact gene being placed next to regulatory elements from a gene on the partner chromosome. This scenario is frequently observed in lymphoid malignancies in which the normal process of antigen receptor rearrangement goes awry and results in translocations involving immunoglobulin or *TCR* loci. For example, in some B-cell tumours, genes such as *MYC* and *BCL2* are aberrantly expressed in B-cell precursors because they have been placed under the control of enhancers from one of the immunoglobulin loci. Similarly, in some cases of T-cell ALL, the *SCL* and *HOX11* genes are ectopically expressed in T-cell precursors when they relocate next to enhancers from the *TCR* loci. In addition, transcriptional dysregulation can occur as a consequence of deletions, such as chromosome 1 deletions resulting in dysregulation of the *SCL* gene (also known as *TAL1*) in T-ALL.

All balanced translocations give rise to two abnormal chromosomal products, one of which is usually implicated as the pathogenetic culprit. However, it is increasingly recognized that the other chromosomal product may also influence tumorigenesis. For example, in CML associated with the t(9;22) translocation, it is clear that the Philadelphia (derivative 22) chromosome carries the *BCR–ABL* fusion gene, which is central to the development of this leukaemia. However, in a subset of patients, the derivative 9 chromosome also carries a deletion that spans the translocation breakpoint. These deletions are thought to arise at the time of the Ph translocation and are associated with a particularly poor prognosis, perhaps reflecting the loss of one or more tumour-suppressor genes.

Similarly, in acute promyelocytic leukaemia, the t(15;17) translocation results in production of a *PML–RARα* fusion transcript from the derivative 15 chromosome, and considerable evidence supports a pivotal role for this transcript in the genesis of this form of leukaemia. However, in 70–80% of patients, the derivative 17 chromosome also expresses an *RAR–PMLα* transcript, which encodes a fusion protein that has functional domains capable of binding the p53 protein, and which influences the development of leukaemia in a mouse model.

What causes translocations to occur in the first instance? In the case of lymphoid tumours, chromosomal rearrangements and mutation are a feature of normal lymphocyte development. Rearrangements of immunoglobulin genes and the *TCR* genes require a series of double-stranded DNA breaks, with loss of intervening sequence and religation, and oncogenic translocations are likely to represent rare mistakes that arise during this process. There may be several reasons why certain genes are preferentially involved in these translocations. First, motifs similar to those recognized by the immunoglobulin or *TCR* recombinase have been found adjacent to the *BCL2* and *SCL* genes, which are involved respectively in the t(14;18) translocation of follicular lymphoma and the t(1;14) associated with T-ALL. Second, it is probable that dysregulation of only certain genes will confer a selective advantage on B- or T-cell progenitors. Third, physical proximity may play a role, as partner genes of *IGH* translocations are more likely to collocalize with the *IGH* locus in the same spatial zone of the interphase nucleus.

For myeloid cells, the mechanism of translocation is poorly understood. Central to most models is a double-stranded break in genomic DNA. These breaks occur spontaneously, but can be increased in frequency by exposing marrow cells to ionizing radiation or other DNA-damaging agents, known risk factors for leukaemia. Normal repair mechanisms, such as homologous recombination or non-homologous end joining, then attempt to join the broken ends of DNA. However, these mechanisms are not infallible, and it is conceivable that they could misrepair two simultaneous breaks on different chromosomes to generate a translocation. Germline mutations in DNA repair genes (such as the ataxia telangiectasia gene) certainly increase the frequency of chromosome rearrangements and the incidence of many cancers, including leukaemias. It may also be relevant that Alu repeat sequences appear to cluster at or near translocation breakpoints in CML and other malignancies, as it has been suggested that the Alu core sequence acts as a binding site for proteins mediating homologous recombination and DNA repair.

Consensus sites for topoisomerase II binding may play a role in some translocations, particularly those involving the *MLL* locus. Topoisomerase inhibitors, such as etoposide and anthracyclines, are well-recognized causes of therapy-related leukaemia, often associated with translocations involving the *MLL* gene on chromosome 11q23. Topoisomerase II creates double-stranded breaks during execution of its function of relaxing overwound DNA, and it appears that topoisomerase II inhibitors may stabilize complexes that are formed between the enzyme and free DNA ends, thus increasing the likelihood that those ends might participate in a translocation.

Deletions and aneuploidy

Chromosome deletions and disorders of chromosome number (aneuploidy) are among the most frequent karyotypic abnormalities seen in haematological malignancies, and result in an increase or decrease in the copy number of many genes. Increases in chromosome number are seen frequently in haematological malignancy. Hyperdiploidy is the most frequent cytogenetic abnormality of childhood ALL, and any chromosome can be duplicated. Trisomy 8 is the most common numeric abnormality of clonal myeloid disorders and can be seen in AML, myelodysplasia and myeloproliferative disorders. Presumably, quantitative chromosomal changes of this sort give rise to altered expression levels of oncogenes or tumour-suppressor genes that contribute to tumorigenesis. However, within an individual tumour that exhibits a complex karyotype, many of the changes may not be directly pathogenic in themselves, but merely serve as markers of genomic instability (see also Chapters 30 and 33).

Chromosomal deletions are large, frequently spanning several megabases and encompassing numerous genes. Identifying the key molecular consequences of a deletion is therefore a difficult task. Studies of retinoblastoma demonstrated that deletions may act to remove the remaining normal copy of a tumour-suppressor gene (*RB*), the other allele of which has been inactivated by mutation. This model seems to apply to mantle cell lymphoma, in which 11q deletions remove one copy of the *ATM* gene in up to 50% of cases. Careful screening of the remaining allele in tumour samples of patients with an 11q deletion revealed inactivating mutations in virtually all cases, suggesting the importance of inactivating both copies of the *ATM* gene in this disease.

However, this 'two-hit' model may well not hold for many of the deletions associated with haematological malignancies. Several deletions have been studied in considerable detail, including the 5q and 20q deletions associated with myeloid malignancies. The usual strategy has been to define a common deleted region that is lost in all cases and then to search for mutations in the remaining allele of genes within the common deleted region. This approach has so far failed to identify target genes, and it is likely that the pathogenetic mechanisms are more complex than originally envisaged for at least two reasons. First, loss of one copy of a gene can be sufficient to affect cellular behaviour – a situation termed haploinsufficiency. As the remaining allele of such genes would be structurally intact and unmutated, their identification presents considerable challenges. Second, it may be necessary for a deletion to remove more than one critical target gene in order to exert a tumorigenic effect. Indeed, different combinations of critical genes may be removed by deletions of varying sizes that affect a given region.

Small-scale mutations

Most of our understanding of the molecular pathogenesis of haematological malignancies has come from studies of chromosomal abnormalities, particularly because chromosome translocations identify the site of key target genes. However, smaller mutations, undetectable at the cytogenetic level, also play a critical role in promoting malignancy. There are many ways in which small-scale mutations can enhance or disrupt protein function, ranging from amino acid substitution, through internal tandem duplication to premature protein truncation. The discovery of these mutations requires careful screening of candidate genes in patient samples, and it is likely that many examples are yet to be identified.

Several activating mutations have been identified. For example, the importance of stem cell factor (SCF) and its receptor, KIT, for the normal growth and survival of mast cells led to a search for mutations in these genes in systemic mastocytosis. It is now clear that up to 40% of cases, particularly those with bone marrow involvement, have an activating point mutation in the *KIT* gene, most frequently Asp816Val. This mutation substitutes

a hydrophobic residue into the activation loop of the kinase domain of c-KIT, probably increasing the ease with which it switches to an active configuration and stabilizing it in this conformation. FLT3, another receptor tyrosine kinase, is activated by internal tandem duplications, which are seen in 20% of cases of AML. Although the amount of DNA duplicated varies, it is always transcribed in frame and leads to constitutively active tyrosine kinase activity, conferring a growth advantage on the cells and a poor prognosis for the patient. In a further 7% of AMLs, constitutive activation of FLT3 occurs through a single amino acid substitution of a hydrophobic residue for Asp835, analogous to the *c-KIT* mutations in systemic mastocytosis.

One of the most common family of genes to be mutated in tumours of all cell types is the RAS family. Up to 20% of all cancers have mutations in a RAS family member, most commonly KRAS and NRAS. The RAS family members are critical components of multiple signal transduction networks, especially those that transmit extracellular growth signals to the nucleus. The mutations found in cancers all compromise the GTPase activity of the RAS protein, promoting accumulation of the active GTP-bound isoform, thus leading to a permanent 'switched on' state.

Inactivating point mutations are commonly seen also. Screening of patients with lymphomas suggests that important cell cycle regulators such as the p53 and retinoblastoma genes are frequently mutated and non-functional. These are often secondary events, occurring during clinical evolution, and their presence usually correlates with poor prognosis, transformation to higher grade disease and/or drug resistance. Such tumour-suppressor genes generally require both alleles to be mutated or deleted to promote tumorigenesis. However, heterozygous inactivating point mutations of the gene encoding the transcription factor C/EBPα are found in 20% of cases of M2 AML. Within the haemopoietic system, this gene is expressed exclusively in and is critical to the differentiation of myelomonocytic cells. The mutation leads to premature truncation of the full-length protein, but leaves intact the translation of a smaller protein initiated downstream of the mutation. The smaller protein then acts in a 'dominant negative' manner to block the function of the wild-type protein translated from the intact allele, leading to a differentiation block in myelomonocytic cells. Hence, although heterozygous, mutations of this sort can be functionally equivalent to homozygous loss-of-function mutations.

Epigenetic effects

There is a mounting body of evidence that, in addition to genetic changes, tumorigenesis also involves epigenetic alterations that affect gene function without altering the nucleotide sequence. In a normal cell, epigenetic mechanisms control several important functions, including transcription, DNA replication, imprinting and X-inactivation.

DNA methylation is generally associated with transcriptional silencing of the neighbouring gene. Disordered patterns of DNA methylation have been found in a wide variety of haematological malignancies. There is global genomic hypomethylation evident in CLL lymphocytes and AML blasts compared with normal haemopoietic cells. In addition, certain candidate genes implicated in neoplasia can be either hyper- or hypomethylated compared with normal cells. DNA hypomethylation has been identified at a number of loci implicated in haematological malignancies, including *BCL2* (in CLL), *TNF-β* (in CML and AML), *H-RAS* (in CLL) and *FMS* (in AML). Given that hypomethylation generally promotes transcriptional activity, it is certainly plausible that such epigenetic changes could cause overexpression of these oncogenes. Conversely, DNA hypermethylation of several tumour-suppressor genes, such as *p16(INK4A)*, E-cadherin and *HIC1*, has also been described in CLL and AML.

Histone modification has also emerged as a key epigenetic mechanism that regulates transcription, and disorders of histone acetylation are well described in leukaemia. Histone acetylation is controlled by two opposing families of enzymes, histone acetyltransferases, which promote a relaxation of chromatin structure, and histone deacetylases (HDACs), which generate a closed chromatin configuration together with transcriptional repression. Several transcription factor fusion proteins are thought to act by recruiting HDACs and other repressor molecules that silence target genes that are important for normal differentiation, thus resulting in maturation arrest.

It is clear that epigenetic modifications are widespread in haematological malignancies. Most are thought unlikely to represent initiating lesions, but probably reflect downstream consequences of the primary genetic changes. Nonetheless, if various different initiating events act through a shared epigenetic mechanism, the latter may represent a fertile source of targets for novel therapies with broad applicability. This concept underlies the interest at present in developing therapeutic inhibitors of HDACs and DNA methyltransferases.

Consequences of acquired genetic abnormalities

This section illustrates the mechanisms by which acquired genetic changes may result in malignant transformation. Five specific examples have been chosen to illustrate how distinct cellular processes may be corrupted: tyrosine kinase signalling (the myeloproliferative disorders); intracellular signal transduction (juvenile myelomonocytic leukaemia); regulation of gene transcription (AML); cell cycle control (mantle cell lymphoma); and apoptosis (follicular lymphoma).

Tyrosine kinases and myeloproliferative disorders

Tyrosine kinases are critical for the response of haemopoietic progenitor cells to external growth stimuli. The binding of a ligand to the extracellular surface of a receptor tyrosine kinase (RTK) promotes receptor dimerization, which, in turn, stimulates autophosphorylation of specific tyrosine residues within the intracellular aspect of the protein. The dimerization and increased kinase activity result in recruitment of effector molecules

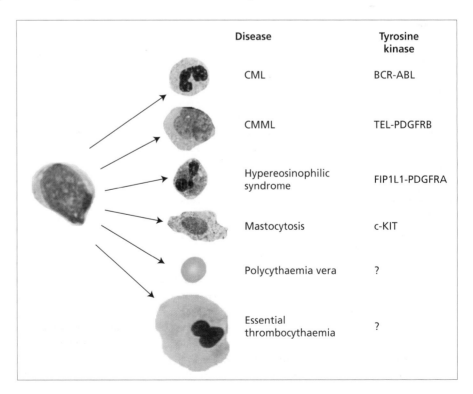

Figure 28.5 Tyrosine kinase genes are frequent targets for mutation or rearrangement in a number of myeloproliferative disorders. However, the molecular mechanisms underlying polycythaemia vera, essential thrombocythaemia and myelofibrosis remain obscure.

Disease	Tyrosine kinase
CML	BCR-ABL
CMML	TEL-PDGFRB
Hypereosinophilic syndrome	FIP1L1-PDGFRA
Mastocytosis	c-KIT
Polycythaemia vera	?
Essential thrombocythaemia	?

and activation of the downstream signalling pathway. Cytoplasmic tyrosine kinases are also thought to be activated by phosphorylation and dimerization.

Myeloproliferative disorders are associated with activation of several tyrosine kinases (Figure 28.5). In some of these diseases, activation of the tyrosine kinase stems from formation of a fusion protein, which undergoes spontaneous dimerization (Figure 28.6a). However, kinase activity can also be increased by more subtle mutations (e.g. c-KIT in mastocytosis). As a consequence of these changes, the corresponding signalling pathway is activated and this provides the transformed cell with a proliferative or survival advantage.

In CML, the *BCR* gene becomes fused in frame with the *ABL* tyrosine kinase gene as a consequence of the Ph translocation (Figure 28.6b). This usually results in the formation of a fusion protein with molecular weight of 210 kDa (hence p210$^{BCR-ABL}$). The fusion protein affects multiple different cellular processes, including intracellular signalling, apoptosis, transcriptional regulation and cellular adhesion. Transgenic mouse models have demonstrated that BCR–ABL is capable of inducing dramatic expansion of myeloid precursors *in vivo*, and can produce a phenotype that resembles the human form of the disease.

Several critical domains in the fusion protein have been mapped, and have provided important insights into its biological activity (Figure 28.6b). The coiled-coil domain in the first exon of *BCR* provides a dimerization motif that results in spontaneous dimerization and constitutive kinase activity. Other domains implicated in oncogenicity are the SH2 domain and the C-terminal actin-binding domain, both in the ABL portion; these domains appear to be important for interaction with regulatory molecules and subcellular localization of the fusion protein.

Numerous downstream pathways are affected by the presence of the BCR–ABL protein, including the RAS, PI3K, STAT and MAP kinase signalling cascades. The breadth of the pathways perturbed explains the protean effects of the fusion protein. For example, activation of the RAS pathway is thought to contribute to the increased cell division and proliferation seen in CML cells; altered interaction with the actin cytoskeleton and adhesion complexes may underlie the diminished adhesion to inhibitory bone marrow stromal cells; and STAT5-dependent upregulation of BCLXL is implicated in the reduced apoptosis of CML progenitors.

As shown in Figure 28.6b, a smaller protein, p190$^{BCR-ABL}$, is found in Ph-positive ALL, in which the breakpoint occurs in an earlier intron of the *BCR* gene than that usually seen in CML. The p190$^{BCR-ABL}$ has a higher level of constitutive tyrosine kinase activity than the p210$^{BCR-ABL}$ protein, and it is thought that this may contribute to the more aggressive behaviour of the ALL. A p230$^{BCR-ABL}$ isoform is also found rarely patients with CML. In some cases, it is associated with a morphological picture resembling chronic neutrophilic leukaemia and less frequent

transformation to blast crisis. These variants illustrate how even seemingly small structural differences in a fusion protein can cause substantial differences in disease phenotype.

PDGFRβ is a fusion partner for several translocations seen in a clinical syndrome of atypical (BCR–ABL negative) CML or myelomonocytic leukaemia with eosinophilia. Patients often exhibit a degree of myelofibrosis, with splenomegaly being found in about one-half of the reported cases, and there is a striking male preponderance. The first of these translocations to be described was the t(5;12), which results in a TEL–PDGFRβ fusion protein, but a number of other fusion partners have been identified, all of which contribute a dimerization domain (Figure 28.6c). In the TEL–PDGFR-β fusion, the first 154 amino acids of the TEL transcription factor are fused in frame with the carboxy-terminus of PDGFR-β. The TEL portion contains the helix–loop–helix protein interaction domain, which permits spontaneous dimerization of the fusion protein, even in the absence of ligand binding, and there is evidence that the fusion protein has constitutive tyrosine kinase activity. Downstream signalling in cells expressing the *TEL–PDGFRβ* fusion gene is also qualitatively abnormal. The TEL–PDGFR-β protein phosphorylates and activates STAT1 and STAT5 proteins, pathways that wild-type PDGFR-β does not use.

RAS family signalling and juvenile myelomonocytic leukaemia

Juvenile myelomonocytic leukaemia (JMML) is a rare disorder of childhood characterized by a marked expansion of both myeloid and monocytic lineages, with varying degrees of dysplasia and exquisite sensitivity to granulocyte–macrophage colony-stimulating factor (GM-CSF) in colony assays. These features reflect the fact that components of the GM-CSF receptor signalling pathway are frequently mutated in JMML (Figure 28.7).

Mutations in the N-*RAS* gene are seen in many haematological malignancies, including AML, myelodysplastic syndrome (MDS) and chronic myelomonocytic leukaemia (CMML), especially in the subtypes of these diseases, which have a monocytic component. Analyses of samples from patients with JMML have shown point mutations in N-*RAS* in about 40% of cases. The point mutations cause single amino acid substitutions, which result in constitutively active forms of the protein and thus dramatically enhance signalling from the GM-CSF receptor.

The neurofibromin (*NF1*) gene is also a target for mutations in JMML, but in this case the result is loss of NF1 activity. The incidence of JMML is increased in neurofibromatosis type 1, an autosomal dominant disorder caused by inactivating mutations in the *NF1* gene. This gene encodes a protein that directly interacts with and inhibits the activity of RAS proteins. Patients who have both neurofibromatosis type 1 and JMML have a high frequency (60%) of inactivating mutations of the second *NF1* allele in the leukaemic cells. Furthermore, inactivating *NF1* mutations are found in sporadic cases of JMML without the

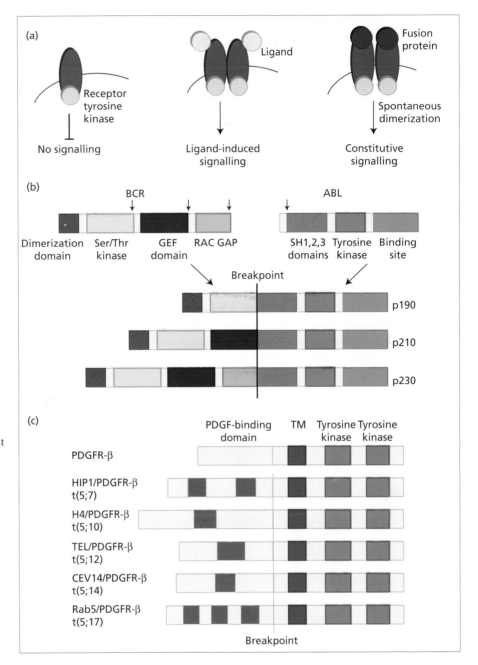

Figure 28.6 Tyrosine kinase fusion proteins are constitutively active as a consequence of spontaneous dimerization. (a) Diagram indicating how tyrosine–kinase fusion proteins mimic ligand-induced activation. (b) CML is caused by fusion of the *BCR* gene on chromosome 22 to the *ABL* gene on chromosome 9. The tyrosine kinase domain of the *ABL* gene (green) is retained in all the different fusion transcripts, and becomes constitutively activated in the fusion protein. Different breakpoints within the *BCR* gene (arrows) lead to different-sized fusion proteins, which have different phenotypic effects, but all of which retain the dimerization motif (red). (c) Five different fusion partners for *PDGFRβ* have been identified in translocations causing a myeloproliferative syndrome. The *PDGFRβ* gene contributes a tyrosine kinase domain (green), whereas all the fusion partners contribute a dimerization motif (red).

clinical syndrome of neurofibromatosis. It appears, therefore, that *NF1* acts as a tumour-suppressor gene, and that inactivation of both alleles allows unchecked signalling through the RAS pathway.

A similar story has been discovered for a gene, *PTPN11*, which encodes a tyrosine phosphatase, SHP2. Germline mutation of this gene can cause a developmental disorder, Noonan's syndrome, which is associated with an increased incidence of JMML. Up to 34% of non-syndromic patients with JMML have somatic mutations of *PTPN11* in the leukaemic cells. The muta-

tions all cause amino acid substitutions clustering in the N-terminal SH2 domain of the protein, which are thought to result in enhanced phosphatase activity. Like RAS, SHP2 signals through the MAP kinase pathway, and cell lines expressing the mutant proteins show a growth advantage over untransformed cell lines.

Thus within the GM-CSF receptor signalling pathway, activation of a positive component (such as RAS) has the same pathological consequences as inactivation of an inhibitory component (NF1). Moreover, the mutations in N-*RAS*, *NF1*

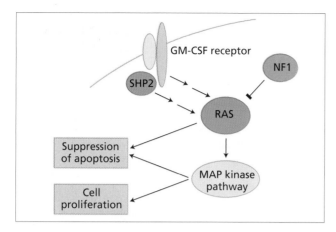

Figure 28.7 Distinct components of the GM-CSF signalling pathway may be mutated in JMML. Acquired activating mutations (green) are frequently found in the *RAS* gene and in the SHP2 phosphatase encoded by the *PTPN11* gene, leading to increased activity of the MAP kinase pathway. Inactivating mutations (red) of the inhibitory *NF1* gene are also associated with JMML. The three types of mutation are mutually exclusive, suggesting that each alone is sufficient to dysregulate GM-CSF receptor signalling.

and *PTPN11* are mutually exclusive. In other words, individual patients carry mutations in only one of these genes, suggesting that mutation of just one component is sufficient to activate the signalling pathway.

The core binding factor complex and acute myeloid leukaemia

Genes encoding transcription factors are common targets for rearrangements or mutation in acute leukaemia. Many of these translocations have been found to play important roles in regulating the behaviour of normal haemopoietic stem or progenitor cells, implying that perturbation of normal transcription programmes can be particularly leukaemogenic. Individual transcription factors usually function as part of a multiprotein complex, and it has become clear that different components of a given complex may be involved in distinct forms of acute leukaemia.

These principles are exemplified by the core binding factor (CBF) complex, made up of RUNX1 (also known as AML1 and CBF-α) and CBF. The normal CBF dimer recognizes and binds specific DNA sequences through the RUNX1 subunit and regulates many genes important for the differentiation of haemopoietic cells, such as interleukin 3 (IL-3), GM-CSF and the enhancer for immunoglobulin heavy chain (Figure 28.8a). Adjacent binding sequences in the DNA are important for other transcription factors, and it seems that the CBF dimer acts as a transcriptional organizer by recruiting other transcription factors into a large multimeric complex that regulates expression of target genes. Mice lacking RUNX1 fail to develop definitive haemopoiesis, confirming the vital importance of the CBF dimer for normal haemopoietic differentiation.

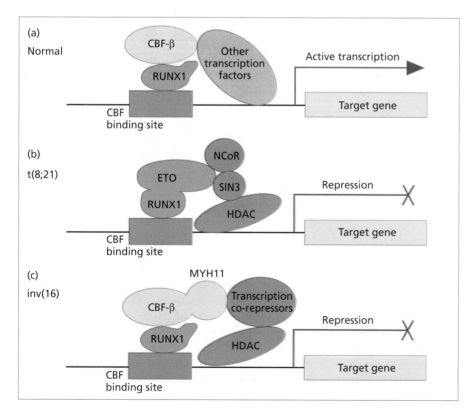

Figure 28.8 The genes encoding components of the CBF transcription factor complex are frequent targets in AML. (a) RUNX1 binds a specific DNA sequence motif, and recruits CBF-β to form a heterodimeric complex. This then acts as a transcriptional organizer, attracting other specific transcription factors and promoting target gene transcription. (b) The t(8;21) translocation results in fusion of RUNX1 to the ETO protein, which recruits a series of transcriptional repressors, including histone deacetylases, leading to target gene inactivation. (c) In cells carrying the inv(16) rearrangement, the CBF-β–MYH11 fusion protein binds to RUNX1 and then recruits transcriptional repressors.

The genes for the two CBF subunits represent the most commonly involved genes in acute leukaemia translocations, with the t(12;21) (*TEL–RUNX1*) found in 25% of childhood ALL, the t(8;21) (*RUNX1–ETO*) in 15% of AML (Figure 28.8b) and the inv(16) (*SMMHC–CBFβ*) found in 10% of AML (Figure 28.8c). How do the translocations involving *RUNX1* and *CBFβ* mediate their leukaemogenic effects? Dominant negative inhibition appears to be central to the process. *In vitro* experiments confirm that binding of wild-type *RUNX1* to gene enhancers is inhibited in the presence of *RUNX1–ETO*. Moreover, mice carrying the *RUNX1–ETO* fusion gene together with a wild-type *RUNX1* allele have exactly the same embryonic lethality phenotype as mice completely lacking *RUNX1*.

The mechanisms by which the fusion genes exert their dominant inhibitory effects are beginning to be understood. The fusion partners of the *CBF* genes appear to recruit nuclear co-repressor complexes, leading to transcriptional inhibition of target genes. In fact, in the *RUNX1–ETO* translocation, the *ETO* moiety recruits a complex comprising three proteins, N-CoR, SIN3 and a histone deacetylase, resulting in histone deacetylation, a change in chromatin structure and target gene repression (Figure 28.8b). Similarly, the CBF-β–MYH11 fusion protein of inv(16) complexes with the normal RUNX1 subunit through the CBFβ moiety, and recruits several transcription repressors via the MYH11 component (Figure 28.8c). The end result is similar for both situations – transcriptional silencing of genes required for normal differentiation and a consequent maturation arrest.

However, rearrangement of an individual transcription factor gene is not sufficient to give rise to acute leukaemia, an observation consistent with the multistep theory of tumorigenesis discussed above. Instead, there is mounting evidence for a model in which development of AML requires both a block to differentiation, frequently provided by subversion of a transcription factor gene, together with a proliferative signal, frequently provided by an altered tyrosine kinase. Consistent with this idea, the FLT3 receptor tyrosine kinase is activated in 25% of AML, and has been shown to cooperate with PML–RAR in a mouse model of acute promyelocytic leukaemia.

Cell cycle control, apoptosis and lymphoma

There is an intimate relationship between the cell cycle and apoptosis. Each phase of the cell cycle is tightly controlled by specific molecular 'checkpoints', which monitor for DNA damage and mitotic spindle formation before permitting cell cycle progression. If a checkpoint recognizes damage to the DNA or mitotic apparatus, this triggers programmed cell death (apoptosis). The enzymes involved in cell cycle control and apoptosis are among the commonest targets of mutation in all cancers, including haematological malignancies.

Figure 28.9a summarizes some of the ways in which cell cycle control may be corrupted in mantle cell lymphoma (MCL). The characteristic chromosomal abnormality associated with this disease is a t(11;14) translocation, leading to juxtaposition of cyclin D1 gene (also known as *BCL1*) with an *IGHJ* segment. Cyclin D1 functions late in G_1 phase, immediately before entry to S-phase, and binds and activates two kinases, CDK4 and CDK6. The cyclin–CDK complex then phosphorylates and inactivates the retinoblastoma (Rb) protein, which is then unable to repress transcription of genes important for the transition to S-phase. Experimental evidence confirms that forced overexpression of cyclin D1 similar to that seen in mantle cell lymphoma leads to a shortened G_1 phase, but overexpression in itself is not sufficient to induce lymphoma in transgenic mice.

Cooperating mutations and epigenetic changes have been found in other genes in the cyclin D1–CDK4-Rb pathway in patients with mantle cell lymphoma. In one study, deletions of *p16(INK4A)*, which codes for an inhibitor of the cyclin D1–CDK4 complex, were seen in 40% of mantle cell lymphomas, and deletions of Rb were present in a further 40% of cases. These additional mutations in genes of the cyclin D1 pathway correlated with markers of active cell proliferation and more aggressive clinical behaviour. Furthermore, epigenetic modifications have been found, such as hypermethylation of *p16(INK4A)*, which may also reflect gene inactivation. This pattern of several co-existing and synergistic mutations in the same pathway contrasts with the situation in JMML, in which mutations in different components of the RAS–MAP kinase pathway tend to be mutually exclusive.

Up to one-half of all mantle cell lymphomas also exhibit deletions of 11q and the deleted region includes the locus of the *ATM* gene. The *ATM* gene is essential for checkpoint controls at the G_2–M transition in particular, and is activated by double-stranded breaks in DNA (Figure 28.9b). The remaining *ATM* allele in patients with 11q deletions is almost invariably affected by inactivating mutations, resulting in aberrant splicing, truncation or abnormal structure of the protein. Similarly, in the absence of 11q deletions, biallelic point mutations in *ATM* have been found in mantle cell lymphoma, and patients with a germline mutation in the *ATM* gene (heterozygote carriers for ataxia telangiectasia) have a marked increase in incidence of malignant lymphomas. Taken together, these observations support the hypothesis that *ATM* functions as a tumour-suppressor gene in mantle cell lymphoma.

Follicular lymphoma is characterized by overexpression of the anti-apoptotic protein BCL2 (Figure 28.9b), as a result of a translocation t(14;18) in which the *BCL2* gene is placed under control of an *IGH* enhancer. Increased levels of BCL2 protect the lymphoma cells from a range of apoptotic signals, suggesting a model whereby cells do not have a proliferative advantage as such, but accumulate through lack of cell death. BCL2 overexpression will also reduce the ability of chemotherapeutic agents to induce apoptosis, and this may explain why it is notoriously difficult to cure patients with follicular lymphoma. Transgenic mice in which *BCL2* is placed under control of an *IGH* enhancer

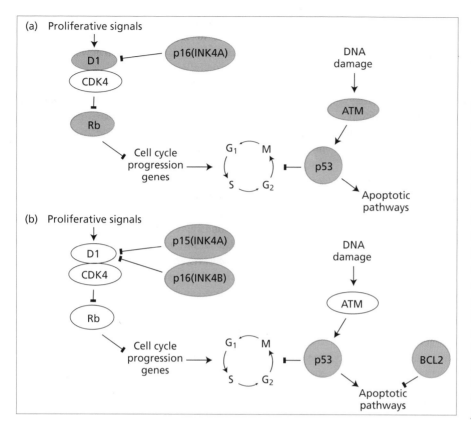

Figure 28.9 Pathways controlling the cell cycle and apoptosis are corrupted in mantle cell and follicular lymphomas. (a) In mantle cell lymphoma, cyclin D1 is frequently upregulated (green) by the t(11;14) translocation, leading to enhanced progression through the G₁–S transition. Inactivating mutations (red) in the inhibitory proteins p16(INK4A), Rb, p53 and ATM may cooperate to exaggerate this effect and dysregulate other cell cycle checkpoints and apoptotic pathways. (b) Follicular lymphoma is characterized by overexpression of the anti-apoptotic factor BCL2. Transformation to high-grade lymphoma is associated with inactivating mutations or deletions affecting *p53*, *p15(INK4B)* and *p16(INK4A)*.

show an accumulation of mature B cells, propensity to autoimmune diseases and follicular hyperplasia. Malignant lymphomas only develop in the mice after a long latency, and tend to be associated with disruption of other key genes, such as the cell cycle regulator *MYC*.

In human disease, follicular lymphoma may terminate in an aggressive, chemotherapy-resistant large cell transformation. Numerous second hits have been associated with this transformation, and these mutations preferentially involve cell cycle regulators such as those involved in mantle cell and other lymphomas. In particular, deletions involving *p15(INK4B)* and *p16(INK4A)* are found in 70% and *p53* mutations in up to 30% of transformed follicular lymphomas. Presumably these additional mutations confer a proliferation advantage on the cells, resulting in the more aggressive growth.

Summary

The cellular and molecular basis for many haematological malignancies is beginning to be understood, and these studies have already established numerous fundamental principles of broad relevance to cancer biology. This understanding of molecular pathogenesis is transforming the modern practice of clinical haematology. The diagnosis and classification of lymphomas

and leukaemias has been revolutionized by the discovery of causative cytogenetic and molecular abnormalities that allow more accurate definition of clinical subtypes with distinct prognosis and treatment response rates. Moreover, drugs such as imatinib for CML and ATRA for acute promyelocytic leukaemia are the first examples of molecularly targeted therapies, and are likely to herald a new era in the treatment of haematological and other malignancies.

Selected bibliography

Basic concepts

Dick JE (1996) Human stem cell assays in immune-deficient mice. *Current Opinion in Hematology* **3**: 405–9.

Greaves MF, Wiemels J (2003) Origins of chromosome translocations in childhood leukaemia. *Nature Reviews Cancer* **3**: 639–49.

Jordan CT (2002) Unique molecular and cellular features of acute myelogenous leukemia stem cells. *Leukemia* **16**: 559–62.

Kuppers R, Klein U, Hansmann ML *et al.* (1999) Cellular origin of human B-cell lymphomas. *New England Journal of Medicine* **341**: 1520–9.

Shaffer AL, Rosenwald A, Staudt LM (2002) Lymphoid malignancies: the dark side of B-cell differentiation. *Nature Reviews Immunology* **2**: 920–32.

Nature of acquired genetic alterations

Gilliland DG, Griffin JD (2002) The roles of FLT3 in hematopoiesis and leukemia. *Blood* **100**: 1532–42.

Herman JG, Baylin SB (2003) Gene silencing in cancer in association with promoter hypermethylation. *New England Journal of Medicine* **349**: 2042–54.

Willis TG, Dyer MJ (2000) The role of immunoglobulin translocations in the pathogenesis of B-cell malignancies. *Blood* **96**: 808–22.

Consequences of acquired genetic abnormalities

Boultwood J (2001) Ataxia telangiectasia gene mutations in leukaemia and lymphoma. *Journal of Clinical Pathology* **54**: 512–16.

Goldman JM, Melo JV (2003) Chronic myeloid leukemia: advances in biology and new approaches to treatment. *New England Journal of Medicine* **349**: 1451–64.

Gupta R, Knight CL, Bain BJ (2002) Receptor tyrosine kinase mutations in myeloid neoplasms. *British Journal of Haematology* **117**: 489–508.

Sanchez-Beato M, Sanchez-Aguilera A, Piris MA (2003) Cell cycle deregulation in B-cell lymphomas. *Blood* **101**: 1220–35.

Speck NA, Gilliland DG (2002) Core-binding factors in haematopoiesis and leukaemia. *Nature Reviews Cancer* **2**: 502–13.

Tartaglia M, Niemeyer CM, Fragale A *et al.* (2003) Somatic mutations in PTPN11 in juvenile myelomonocytic leukemia, myelodysplastic syndromes and acute myeloid leukemia. *Nature Genetics* **34**: 148–50.

CHAPTER 29

Diagnosis and classification of acute leukaemia

Barbara J Bain

Introduction

The diagnosis of acute leukaemia usually follows the presentation of a patient with clinical features suggestive of this disease, with relevant laboratory evaluation therefore being performed. Less often, the diagnosis is an incidental one when a blood count is requested because of an unrelated condition. In some patients, an unequivocal diagnosis of acute leukaemia can be made from a blood count and blood film but in other patients bone marrow aspiration is required for diagnosis. When a bone marrow aspirate is not essential for diagnosis, it is nevertheless necessary for further classification and to provide optimal material for cytogenetic analysis. In a small minority of patients, in whom a hypocellular or fibrotic bone marrow leads to a poor aspirate being obtained, only a trephine biopsy permits a definitive diagnosis of acute leukaemia. In other patients, this procedure is not essential. Immunophenotyping is a necessary part of the initial evaluation unless the leukaemia is obviously myeloid. With the increasing use of immunophenotyping, cytochemical stains are now less used, but they continue to have a role in the confirmation of a diagnosis of acute myeloid leukaemia; they have no role in the diagnosis of acute lymphoblastic leukaemia unless immunophenotypic analysis is not available. Cytogenetic analysis should be performed in all patients with acute leukaemia, since knowledge of the karyotype is essential for determining the prognosis and for choice of optimal treatment. Molecular genetic analysis is not yet a routine part of diagnosis but is likely to become so. The place of different modes of investigation in the diagnosis and classification of acute leukaemia is summarized in Table 29.1.

Table 29.1 The role of different laboratory procedures in the diagnosis and classification of acute leukaemia.

Investigation	Role
Full blood count and blood film	Essential in all patients
Bone marrow aspirate	Essential in all patients
Bone marrow trephine biopsy	Selective, necessary in patients with a hypocellular or fibrotic marrow
Cytochemical stains	Selective, useful if a leukaemia is not obviously myeloid
Immunophenotyping	Indicated in all patients in whom the leukaemia is not obviously myeloid; can provide means of monitoring for minimal residual disease
Cytogenetic analysis	Essential in all patients, best performed on a bone marrow aspirate
Molecular genetic analysis including fluorescence *in situ* hybridization (FISH)	Selective; is likely to become more important if monitoring for minimal residual disease is found to be necessary for optimizing treatment
Storage of bone marrow films wrapped in aluminium foil at −20°C	Useful if cytochemistry or molecular genetic analysis is retrospectively found to be necessary
Storage of DNA	Appropriate in a research setting

Table 29.2 A summary of the FAB classification of acute leukaemia.

Categories of AML	Categories of ALL
M0, AML with minimal evidence of myeloid differentiation	L1, ALL with fairly small uniform lymphoblasts
M1, AML without differentiation	L2, ALL with more pleomorphic lymphoblasts
M2, AML with differentiation	L3, ALL with basophilic vacuolated lymphoblasts*
M3 and M3 variant, acute promyelocytic leukaemia and its hypogranular/microgranular variant	
M4, acute myelomonocytic leukaemia	
M5, acute monoblastic (M5a) or monocytic (M5b) leukaemia	
M6, acute leukaemia with at least 50% erythroblasts in the bone marrow	
M7, acute megakaryoblastic leukaemia	

*In the WHO classification, cases with L3 morphology, with a mature B-cell immunophenotype and with Burkitt's lymphoma-related translocations would not be categorized as ALL.

It is insufficient to merely make a diagnosis of acute leukaemia, or even of acute myeloid leukaemia (AML) or acute lymphoblastic leukaemia (ALL). Further classification is essential in order to determine the prognosis and select the most appropriate treatment. Further classification is also essential in order to advance our knowledge, for the ultimate benefit of patients as well as for the advancement of scientific knowledge of both normal and abnormal haemopoiesis.

When facilities are limited, acute leukaemia can be classified on the basis of cytology and cytochemistry, as initially proposed by the French–American–British (FAB) group. This will mean that some cases of AML with minimal evidence of myeloid differentiation could be misclassified as ALL, but the diagnosis will be correct in the great majority of cases. If cytology and cytochemistry are supplemented by selective immunophenotyping in all cases that are not obviously myeloid, the diagnosis will be further refined. Cases of acute megakaryoblastic leukaemia and of acute myeloid leukaemia without cytological or cytochemical evidence of differentiation will be recognized and a positive, rather than default, diagnosis of ALL will be made. Cases of acute biphenotypic leukaemia will remain unrecognized without more extensive use of immunophenotyping. This approach leads to assignment to eight FAB categories of AML and three FAB categories of ALL, as summarized in Table 29.2 (Figures 29.1–29.23). It is also possible to classify acute leukaemia purely on the basis of the immunophenotype, as proposed by the European Group for the Immunological Characterization of Leukaemias (EGIL). This approach is not recommended as it ignores important

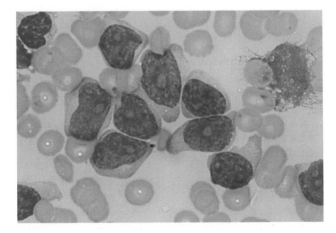

Figure 29.1 Acute myeloid leukaemia, FAB M0 type. Blast cells with no evident features of differentiation and with negative reactions for Sudan black B and myeloperoxidase. On immunophenotypic analysis, all B and T markers were negative but there was expression of CD13 and CD33. Without immunophenotyping such cases cannot be distinguished from L2 acute lymphoblastic leukaemia. Bone marrow film, MGG.

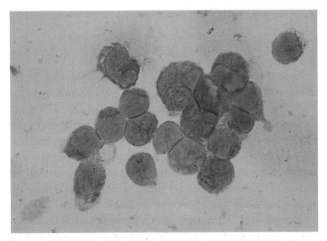

Figure 29.2 Acute myeloid leukaemia, FAB M0 type. Blast cells express CD13. Cytospin preparation, alkaline phosphatase–anti-alkaline phosphatase (APAAP) technique.

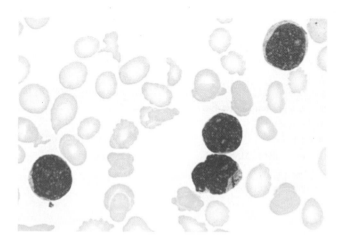

Figure 29.3 Acute myeloid leukaemia, FAB M1 type. Blast cells are small to medium in size with a high nucleocytoplasmic ratio and one of them contains an Auer rod. Sudan black B and peroxidase reactions were positive. Peripheral blood film, MGG.

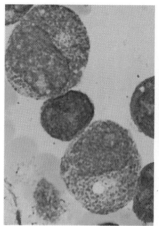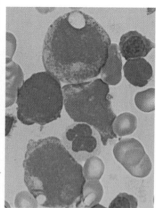

Figure 29.5 Acute myeloid leukaemia, FAB M2 type. There is differentiation to promyelocytes and in one of the two patients there is one neutrophil and a blast cell containing an Auer rod. Bone marrow, MGG.

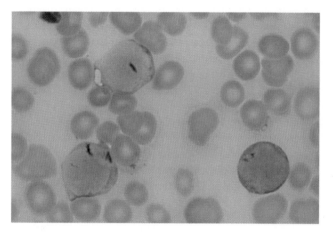

Figure 29.4 Acute myeloid leukaemia, FAB M1 type. Blast cells containing Auer rods. Peripheral blood film, myeloperoxidase reaction.

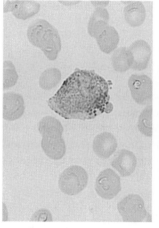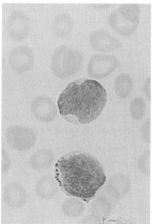

Figure 29.6 Acute myeloid leukaemia, FAB M2 type. In this patient there is basophil differentiation and characteristic granules are seen in the blast cells. Peripheral blood film, MGG.

information and leads to patients with the same type of disease being assigned to different categories. For example, patients with FAB M2 AML associated with t(8;21)(q22;q22) could be assigned to the EGIL category of 'AML of myelomonocytic lineage' or if, as not infrequently occurs, there were aberrant expression of CD19, to the EGIL category of 'AML with lymphoid antigen expression'. The optimal approach to the classification of acute leukaemia is one that seeks to identify real biological entities, using all the information available. Approaches based on morphology, immunophenotyping and cytogenetic analysis (MIC classification), or with the addition of molecular genetic analysis (MIC-M classification) have been proposed and this approach has been adopted in part by the World Health Organization (WHO) classification.

The roles of specific techniques in diagnosis and classification

Morphology and cytochemistry

A blood film, bone marrow aspirate film and manual differential counts of blood and bone marrow films should be performed in all patients. The WHO expert group advises a 200-cell differential count on a peripheral blood film and a 500-cell differential count on a bone marrow film. Performing a 500-cell differential count on the bone marrow is particularly important if the percentage of blasts cells is at a level that is critical for diagnosis (around 20%) since the precision of the count is otherwise poor. The erythroid, granulocytic/monocytic and megakaryocyte

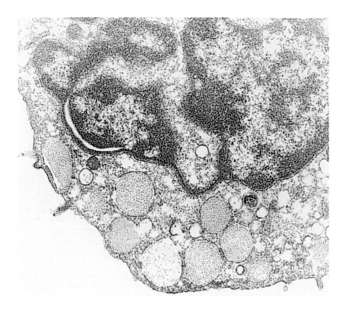

Figure 29.7 Acute myeloid leukaemia, FAB M2, same patient as in Figure 29.6 demonstrating that the cytoplasmic granules show the characteristic stippled pattern of basophil granules. Ultrastructural examination, lead and uranyl acetate stain.

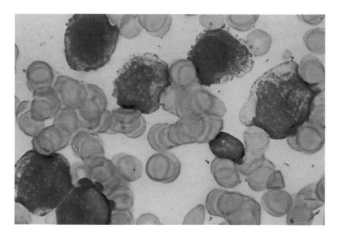

Figure 29.8 Acute hypergranular promyelocytic leukaemia, FAB M3 category of acute myeloid leukaemia. Blast cells are in a minority, the dominant cell being a hypergranular promyelocytes, some with bundles of Auer rods. Bone marrow film, MGG.

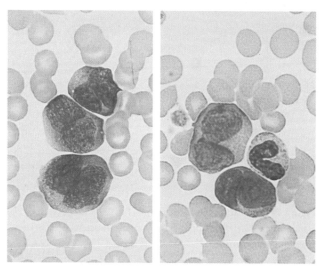

Figure 29.9 Acute hypogranular or microgranular promyelocytic leukaemia, FAB M3 variant category of acute myeloid leukaemia. The leukaemic cells are either blast cells or highly abnormal promyelocytes with a characteristic lobed nucleus in which a broad isthmus joins two distinct lobes. The abnormal promyelocytes, particularly those in the circulating blood, show few if any granules on light microscopy. Bone marrow film, MGG.

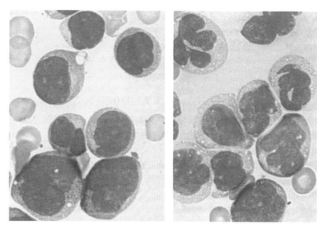

Figure 29.10 Acute myeloid leukaemia, FAB M4 category. There are some blasts showing granulocytic differentiation and others showing monocytic differentiation. Granulocytic differentiation is more obvious in the bone marrow (left) and monocytic in the peripheral blood (right). In this case the granulocytic differentiation is neutrophilic but sometimes it is eosinophilic (Figure 29.12) or, rarely, basophilic. Bone marrow and peripheral blood films, MGG.

lineages should be assessed for dysplastic features and the presence of Auer rods should be noted. The eosinophil count should be noted, as should the presence of eosinophil precursors with atypical large pro-eosinophilic granules with basophilic staining characteristics [suggestive of a the presence of inv(16)(p13q22) or t(16;16)(p13;q22)] (Figure 29.12). The features of hypergranular promyelocytes (cytoplasm packed with brightly staining granules, bundles of Auer rods, giant granules) should be sought (Figure 29.8) and, equally importantly, the characteristic cytological features of hypogranular or microgranular promye-

locytes (bilobed nuclei with a broad isthmus joining the two lobes and sometimes fine dust-like granules) (Figure 29.9) should be identified.

If cytochemistry is to be performed, the most useful reactions are (i) a myeloperoxidase reaction or Sudan black B or

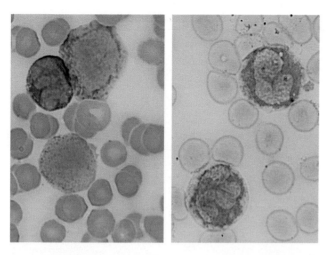

Figure 29.11 Acute myeloid leukaemia, FAB M4 category. Both Sudan black B (left) and alpha naphthyl acetate esterase (right) reactions are positive.

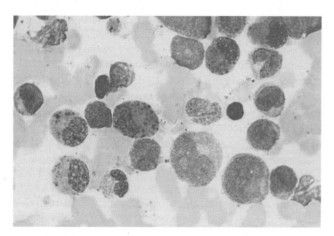

Figure 29.12 Acute myeloid leukaemia, FAB M4 category, with eosinophilic differentiation. This category of AML is often referred to as M4Eo AML, although this is not a FAB category. There are mature eosinophils and eosinophil precursors. The latter have large pro-eosinophilic granules, which have basophilic staining characteristics. Bone marrow film, MGG.

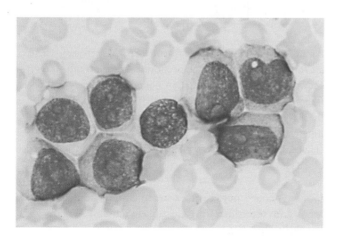

Figure 29.13 Acute myeloid leukaemia, FAB M5a category. The blasts are large with abundant cytoplasm. They show little signs of differentiation, but one cell has an indented nucleus. Nucleoli are large and prominent. Sometimes there are fine azurophilic granules. Bone marrow film, MGG.

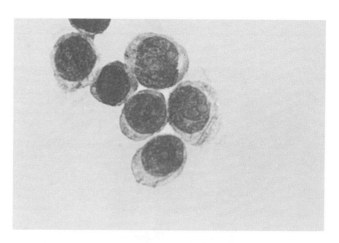

Figure 29.14 Acute myeloid leukaemia, FAB M5a category. The monoblasts in this patient show no nuclear lobulation. One cell contains a ribosomal–lamellar complex, the nature of which was confirmed on ultrastructural examination. Cytospin preparation, MGG.

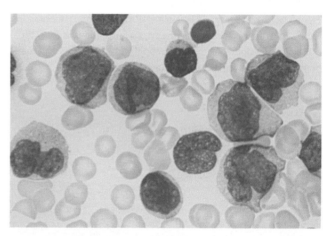

Figure 29.15 Acute myeloid leukaemia, FAB M5b category. Monocytic differentiation is apparent. Bone marrow film, MGG.

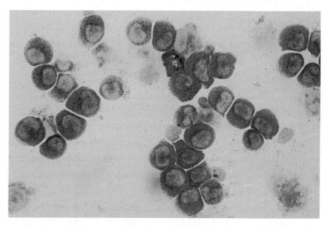

Figure 29.16 Acute myeloid leukaemia, FAB M5a category. Strong non-specific esterase activity. Cytospin preparation, alpha-naphthyl-acetate esterase reaction.

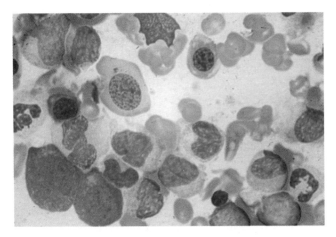

Figure 29.17 Acute myeloid leukaemia, FAB M6 showing erythropoiesis that is dysplastic and grossly megaloblastic; there is an excess of proerythroblasts but also of immature granulocytes, including blast cells. Bone marrow film, MGG.

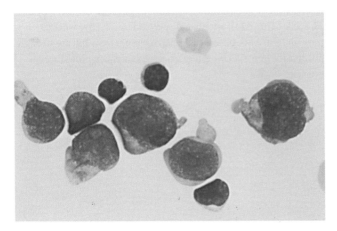

Figure 29.18 AML with an immature erythroid phenotype. The 'blast cells' do not show any cytological features of differentiation but were shown by reactivity with anti-glycophorin A antibodies to be primitive erythroid cells. This type of AML was not included in the FAB classification but could be designated 'M6 variant'. Cytospin preparation, MGG.

(ii) an alpha-naphthyl acetate esterase reaction (either alone or in combination with naphthol AS-D chloroacetate esterase, to facilitate the recognition of FAB M4 AML). A periodic acid–Schiff (PAS) stain can contribute to the recognition of FAB M3 and M3 variant AML because of the blush-like positivity that fills the cytoplasm and it can also highlight the presence of dysplastic erythroblasts and megakaryocytes. In ALL, particularly B-lineage ALL, a characteristic pattern of 'block positivity' is often seen (Figure 29.24); however, a PAS stain is no longer indicated in suspected ALL, unless there is no access to immunophenotyping. Similarly, an acid phosphatase stain for the recognition of Golgi zone staining in T-lineage ALL (Figure 29.25) is redundant if immunophenotyping is available.

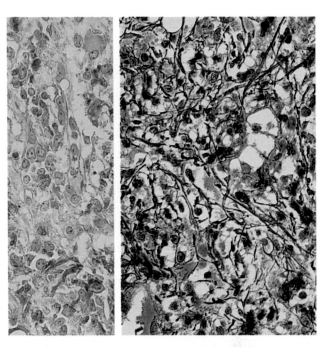

Figure 29.19 Acute myeloid leukaemia, FAB M7 category. Bone marrow trephine biopsy shows blast cells (left) and increased reticulin deposition (right).

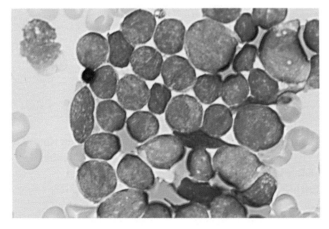

Figure 29.20 Childhood acute lymphoblastic leukaemia, FAB L1 type. The blast cells have a high nucleocytoplasmic ratio, lack visible nucleoli and are relatively small. This patient's leukaemic cells were of B-lineage and expressed CD10. Bone marrow film, MGG.

Immunophenotyping

Immunophenotyping is now usually performed largely by flow cytometry using anticoagulated whole blood or bone marrow samples in which red cells have been selectively lysed. Antibodies that are directly labelled with fluorochromes are generally used since this permits two-colour or three-colour analysis, by which

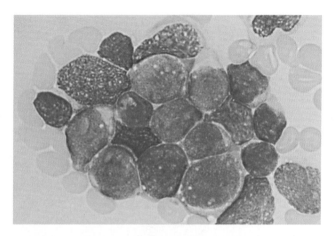

Figure 29.21 Childhood acute lymphoblastic leukaemia, FAB L2 type. The blast cells are mainly large and have one or two prominent nucleoli, which range in size from small to large. Bone marrow film, MGG.

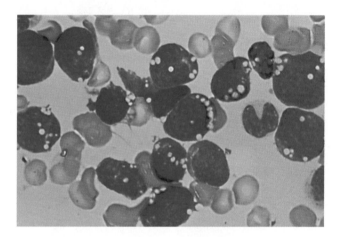

Figure 29.22 'Acute lymphoblastic leukaemia' of Burkitt type, FAB L3 type. The blast cells have prominent cytoplasmic basophilia and are heavily vacuolated. The immunophenotype was that of a mature B cell with expression of surface membrane immunoglobulin and the case would therefore be classified as non-Hodgkin's lymphoma rather than ALL in the WHO classification. Bone marrow film, MGG.

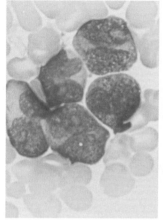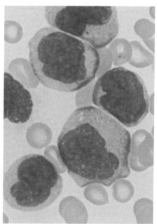

Figure 29.23 Acute hypogranular promyelocytic leukaemia, FAB M3 variant category of acute myeloid leukaemia (left) contrasted with acute monocytic leukaemia, FAB M5b type (right). The cells of monocyte lineage have more abundant cytoplasm and the nucleus is often kidney shaped rather than there being two distinct lobes. The cells of M3 AML are strongly peroxidase-positive whereas those of M5b AML have weaker peroxidase activity but are strongly positive for non-specific esterases, such as alpha naphthyl acetate esterase.

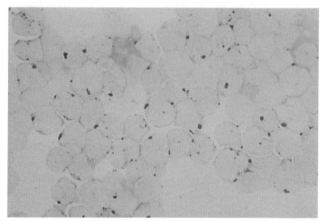

Figure 29.24 Acute lymphoblastic leukaemia, periodic acid–Schiff (PAS) stain showing a single block of PAS-positive material in each blast cell; this is therefore referred to as 'block positivity'. Cytospin preparation of cerebrospinal fluid, PAS stain.

co-expression of antigens can be evaluated. Forward light scatter (proportional to cell size) and sideways light scatter (determined by cell structure, including granularity) can be analysed and related to antigen expression. Techniques for detection of cytoplasmic and nuclear antigen expression are essential, the former for detecting the earliest expression of lineage-related antigens, such as CD3, CD13 and CD22 and for the detection of cytoplasmic antigens (myeloperoxidase) or cytoplasmic epitopes (CD79a), and the latter for detection of the nuclear expression of terminal deoxynucleotidyl transferase (TdT). Although expression of a specific antigen is often reported as a percent-

age, with an arbitrary cut-off point (such as 20%) for a marker to be considered positive, visual analysis of clusters is also important. For example, making a distinction between leukaemic B-lineage lymphoblasts and normal immature B-lineage cells (haematogones) is facilitated by observing (i) the stronger expression of TdT and the weaker expression of CD10 and CD19 by haematogones; (ii) the heterogeneous expression of different antigens in comparison with the more homogeneous expression by leukaemic lymphoblasts; and (iii) lack of aberrant myeloid

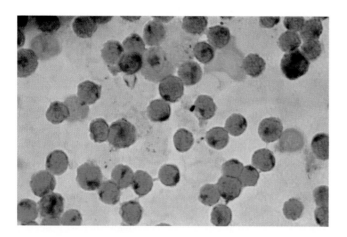

Figure 29.25 T-lineage acute lymphoblastic leukaemia showing acid phosphatase activity restricted to the Golgi zone. Cytospin preparation, acid phosphatase reaction.

antigen expression, which is seen in some leukaemic lymphoblasts, and in appropriate synchronous expression of lymphoid antigens in comparison with the asynchronous expression that can occur in leukaemia. Some of these subtle differences are obscured if only the percentage of positive cells is considered.

Analysis may be performed on 'gated' cells, with gating, for example, on cells characterized by CD45 expression and sideways light scatter. However, it is important that all data are initially collected ungated so that no information is lost; if subsequent analysis employs gating, the final report must make clear what gating procedure was followed and what percentage of cells fell within the gate. It should be noted that some monoblasts and the hypergranular promyelocytes of M3 AML often do not fall within the 'blast window' and that some B-lineage lymphoblasts do not express CD45, so gating must be done with care.

Various panels of antibodies have been proposed for the diagnosis and further classification of acute leukaemia, for example by the USA–Canadian Consensus Group and by the British Committee for Standards in Haematology (BCSH) (Table 29.3). In addition, the WHO expert group has modified the EGIL proposals for diagnosis of acute biphenotypic leukaemia (Table 29.4) and, if immunophenotyping is done for this purpose, then it is recommended that all these antibodies are included so that classification is uniform between different countries and centres. If there is a possibility of a monoclonal antibody being used in therapy (e.g. Myelotarg, anti-CD33, in AML) then it should be included in the diagnostic panel.

Table 29.3 Panels of monoclonal (or polyclonal) antibodies recommended by the British Committee for Standards in Haematology (BCSH) and by the US–Canadian Consensus Group for the Diagnosis and Classification of Acute Leukaemia.

		BCSH	Consensus group
Primary panel	B lymphoid	CD19, cCD22, cCD79a, CD10	CD10, CD19, anti-kappa, anti-lambda
	T lymphoid	cCD3, CD2	CD2, CD5, CD7
	Myeloid	CD13, CD117, anti-cMPO	CD13, CD14, CD33
	Not lineage specific	Nuclear TdT	CD34, HLA-DR
Secondary panel	B lymphoid	μ, SmIg (anti-kappa and anti-lambda), CD138	CD20, Sm/cCD22
	T lymphoid	CD7	CD1a, Sm/cCD3, CD4, CD8
	Myeloid	CD33, CD41, CD42, CD61, anti-glycophorin A	CD15, CD16, CD41, CD42b, CD61, CD64, CD71, CD117, anti-cMPO, anti-glycophorin A
	Not lineage specific	CD45	CD38, nuclear TdT
	Non-haemopoietic	MAb for the detection of small round cell tumours of childhood	
Optional	B lymphoid	CD15 (a myeloid marker often expressed on *MLL*-rearranged B lymphoblasts) and 7.1/NG2 (also for *MLL*-rearranged ALL)	
	T lymphoid	Anti-TCRαβ, anti-TCRγδ	
	Myeloid	Anti-lysozyme, CD14, CD36, anti-PML (MAb PLl-M3), HLA-DR (for negativity in M3 AML)	

c, cytoplasmic; CD, cluster of differentiation; MAb, monoclonal antibody; MPO, myeloperoxidase; Sm, surface membrane; TCR, T-cell receptor; TdT, terminal deoxynucleotidyl transferase.

Table 29.4 WHO criteria for the diagnosis of biphenotypic leukaemia.

Score*	B lineage	T lineage	Myeloid
2	cCD79a, cIgM cCD22	CD3 (c or Sm anti-TCR (αβ or γδ)	MPO
1	CD19 CD10 CD20	CD2 CD5 CD8 CD10	CD117 CD13 CD33 CD65
0.5	TdT CD24	TdT CD7 CD1a	CD14 CD15 CD64

*If > 2 points is scored for both myeloid and one of the lymphoid lineages the case is classified as biphenotypic; in the original EGIL recommendations CD117 scored 0.5 rather than 1.
c, cytoplasmic; CD, cluster of differentiation; Ig, immunoglobulin; MPO, myeloperoxidase; Sm, surface membrane; TCR, T-cell receptor; TdT, terminal deoxynucleotidyl transferase.

A secondary role for immunophenotyping is that of defining a leukaemia-related phenotype in an individual patient that can subsequently be used for monitoring minimal residual disease (MRD) (Figure 29.26). For this purpose, an extended antibody panel permits the defining of a leukaemia-associated immunophenotype in a larger proportion of patients. Table 29.5 shows the types of leukaemia-related phenotype that can be used for MRD monitoring.

The use of immunophenotyping to indicate prognosis or as a surrogate marker for a cytogenetic/molecular genetic subset of acute leukaemia is not generally of any great importance. An exception to this may be the rapid recognition of an immunophenotype typical of M3 AML (Figure 29.27) but, even in this instance, if molecular techniques are available they are generally preferred.

Cytogenetic analysis

Cytogenetic analysis will be discussed in detail in Chapter 30, but its role in the classification of acute leukaemia will be dealt with in this chapter. When resources permit, it should be carried out in all patients for the following reasons: (i) patients with AML can be assigned to three broad prognostic groups and their

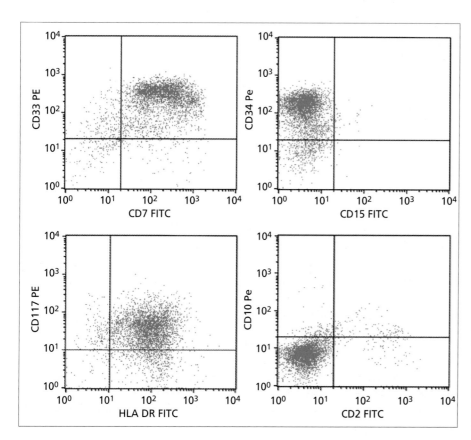

Figure 29.26 Scatterplot of flow cytometry immunophenotyping in acute myeloid leukaemia; there is expression of CD7, CD33, CD34, CD117 and HLA-DR. The co-expression of myeloid markers and CD7 could be used in this patient for the identification of minimal residual disease (with thanks to Mr Ricardo Morilla).

Table 29.5 Leukaemia-associated immunophenotypes that can be identified at diagnosis of acute leukaemia and can subsequently be used to monitor minimal residual disease.

Type of abnormality	Example
Aberrant expression of an antigen more appropriate to another lineage	Lymphoid-associated antigens, such as CD2, CD4, CD5, CD7, CD19 or CD20, on myeloid cells Myeloid-associated antigens, such as CD13, CD15, CD33, CD65 or CD66c, on lymphoid cells Natural killer or T-lineage-associated antigens, such as CD56, expressed on B lymphoblasts
Asynchronous expression of antigens or failure to express expected antigens synchronously	Co-expression of terminal deoxynucleotidyl transferase, CD10 and strong CD34 with cytoplasmic μ chain or strong CD19, CD20, CD21 or CD22 Co-expression of CD34 or terminal deoxynucleotidyl transferase with CD11b, CD14, CD15, strong CD33 or CD65 Failure to express CD13 and CD33 synchronously
Abnormally weak or abnormally strong antigen expression	Increased expression of CD10 Increased expression of CD33
Expression of antigens that are not usually expressed in the tissue being examined	Presence in the bone marrow of cells (i) expressing CD1a or (ii) expressing both cytoplasmic CD3 and either terminal deoxynucleotidyl transferase or CD34 or (iii) co-expressing CD4 and CD8

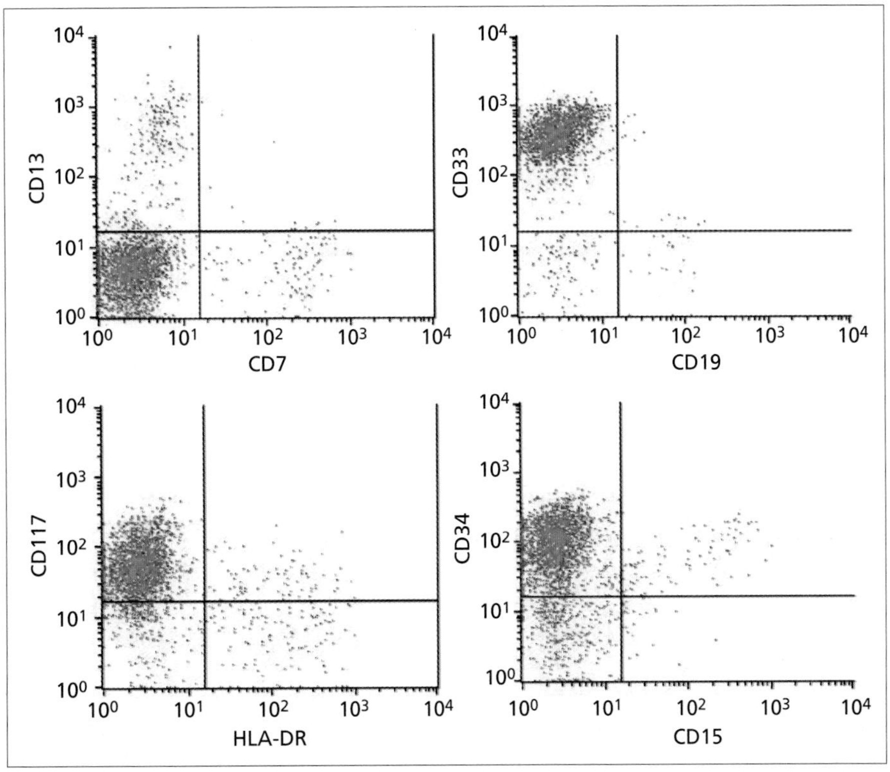

Figure 29.27 Scatterplot of flow cytometry immunophenotyping in acute promyelocytic leukaemia (FAB category M3); there is expression of CD33, CD34 and CD117 but CD13 and HLA-DR are not expressed. CD33 is more consistently expressed than CD13 in M3 AML and lack of expression of HLA-DR is characteristic (with thanks to Mr Ricardo Morilla).

treatment can be modified accordingly; (ii) specific categories of AML requiring very specific therapeutic strategies can be identified (particularly M3 and M3 variant); and (iii) it facilitates the recognition of therapy-related acute leukaemia and the distinction between alkylating agent-related and topoisomerase-II-interactive drug-related leukaemia. Cytogenetic analysis is essential if the WHO classification of AML is to be used.

Table 29.6 The role of detection of molecular genetic abnormalities in acute leukaemia.

Abnormality detected	Relevance of detection
PML–RARA fusion in AML	Use of all-*trans*-retinoic acid and possibly arsenic trioxide; good prognosis so overtreatment should be avoided
AML1–ETO fusion in AML	Good prognosis, overtreatment should be avoided
CBFB–MYH11 in AML	Good prognosis, overtreatment should be avoided
High hyperdiploidy in ALL	Good prognosis, overtreatment should be avoided
ETV6–AML1 fusion in ALL	Relatively good prognosis, overtreatment should be avoided; particularly sensitive to asparaginase
BCR–ABL fusion in AML, ALL or acute biphenotypic leukaemia	Poor prognosis in AML and ALL, intensive treatment may be justified and the therapeutic use of tyrosine kinase inhibitors could be considered
MLL–AF4 fusion in infant acute leukaemia	Poor prognosis, intensive treatment with drugs directed at both lymphoblasts and myeloblasts is justified
FLT-3 internal tandem duplication in AML	Use of tyrosine kinase inhibitors may prove relevant
Any abnormal fusion gene, a rearranged immunoglobulin or T-cell receptor gene or *WT1* overexpression	Potential for monitoring of minimal residual disease

Molecular genetic analysis

Molecular genetic analysis has been discussed in Chapter 28, but its role in the classification of acute leukaemia will be dealt with in this chapter. It has the following advantages over conventional cytogenetic analysis: (i) it can yield results when cytogenetic analysis has failed or when only normal metaphases are seen; (ii) it can confirm the presence of a specific fusion gene in patients with a variant rather than a classical translocation; (iii) it will detect some relevant abnormalities that cannot usually be detected by cytogenetic analysis, e.g. *ETV6–AML1* (*TEL–AML1*) fusion in B-lineage ALL associated with a usually cryptic t(12;21)(p12;q22) translocation; (iv) it will detect other molecular abnormalities that do not have any cytogenetic correlate because they are always submicroscopic events, e.g. *GATA1* mutation in transient abnormal myelopoiesis or acute megakaryocytic leukaemia in Down's syndrome, or internal tandem duplication of *FLT-3*, seen in multiple morphological subtypes of AML; and (v) it can give rapid results so that clinical decisions can be based on the analysis. However, it should be noted that molecular genetic analysis will only permit the detection of abnormalities that are specifically sought whereas in conventional cytogenetic analysis all chromosomes are assessed. At present, molecular genetic analysis is applied selectively, to supplement cytogenetic analysis in the recognition of specific categories of good-prognosis and poor-prognosis AML and ALL. The most useful techniques include fluorescence *in situ* hybridization (FISH) (both for the detection of specific fusion genes and for the detection of high hyperdiploidy), the reverse transcriptase polymerase chain reaction (RT-PCR) and immunofluorescence to demonstrate the abnormal microparticulate distribution of PML protein in M3 and M3 variant AML. The last technique is important since it can be done more speedily than conventional cytogen-

etic analysis and can thus permit the early application of optimal specific treatment. This and other molecular abnormalities that are often sought in acute leukaemia are shown in Table 29.6.

A potential future use for molecular genetic analysis is the monitoring of minimal residual disease, if this is shown to give clinically useful information. Suitable techniques include the monitoring of the transcript of a fusion gene or the identification of a patient-specific T-cell receptor (TCR) or immunoglobulin gene rearrangement. A further potential use for molecular genetics is for the identification of abnormal gene expression, e.g. *FLT-3* expression, that may indicate that leukaemic cells will be susceptible to tyrosine kinase inhibitors or other specific drugs.

The classification of acute leukaemia

The WHO criteria for the diagnosis and classification of acute myeloid leukaemia

The WHO criteria for the diagnosis of AML are shown in Table 29.7. The most important differences from the FAB criteria are (i) the lowering of the threshold for the percentage of blast cells to 20% in the blood or bone marrow; and (ii) the recognition of cases of acute leukaemia with an even lower blast count if specific acute leukaemia-associated cytogenetic or molecular genetic abnormalities are present.

The WHO classification of AML is hierarchical. Therapy-related cases are first recognized and assigned to subcategories related to alkylating agents/radiotherapy, topoisomerase II-interactive drugs or 'other'. Cases associated with certain specified cytogenetic or molecular genetic rearrangements (those shown in Table 29.7) are then assigned to a category of 'AML

Table 29.7 WHO criteria for the diagnosis of acute myeloid leukaemia.

Blast cells are 20% or more in either peripheral blood or bone marrow

Presence of
    t(8;21)(q22;q22) or *AML1–ETO* fusion gene
    inv(16)(p13q22) or t(16;16)(p13;q22) or *CBFB–MYH11* fusion gene
    t(15;17)(q22;q12) and variants or *PML–RARA* fusion gene or variants
    Translocation with an 11q23 breakpoint and *MLL* gene rearrangement

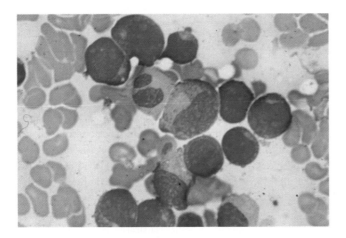

Figure 29.28 Acute myeloid leukaemia associated with t(8;21)(q22;q22) showing FAB M2 morphology with dysplastic maturing granulocytes. The basophilic cytoplasm of the blast cells and the prominent Golgi zone is characteristic of this type of acute leukaemia. This translocation leads to formation of an *AML1(RUNX1)–ETO* fusion gene. These cases are assigned to the WHO category of AML with recurrent cytogenetic abnormality. Bone marrow film, MGG.

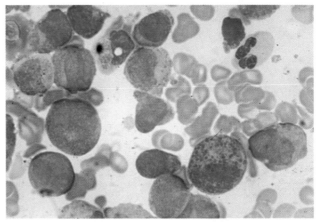

Figure 29.29 Acute myeloid leukaemia associated with inv(16)(p13q22) showing FAB M4 morphology plus abnormal eosinophil maturation, often referred to as M4Eo. There is an eosinophil myelocyte with prominent pro-eosinophilic granules, which have basophilic staining characteristics. This chromosomal inversion leads to formation of a *CBFB–MYH11* fusion gene. These cases are assigned to the WHO category of AML with recurrent cytogenetic abnormality. Bone marrow film, MGG.

with recurrent genetic abnormalities' (Figures 29.28–29.34). Remaining cases are next assessed for bilineage or trilineage dysplasia, and if this is found they are assigned to the category of 'AML with multilineage dysplasia'. The criteria for significant dysplasia are that at least 50% of cells of at least two lineages must be dysplastic. Cases with multilineage dysplasia are further categorized as (i) with an antecedent myelodysplastic syndrome or myelodysplastic/myeloproliferative disorder and (ii) without any such antecedent disease. After cases have been assigned to the category of 'AML with multilineage dysplasia' any remaining cases, including those with other recurrent cytogenetic or molecular genetic abnormalities, are assigned to 'AML, not otherwise specified' and are subcategorized on morphological grounds in a manner similar to that used in the FAB classification but with three extra categories. These extra categories are: (i) acute basophilic leukaemia (Figure 29.35); (ii) acute panmyelosis with myelofibrosis; (iii) myeloid sarcoma. An algorithm showing how the WHO classification is applied is shown in Figure 29.36.

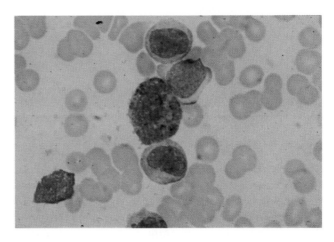

Figure 29.30 Acute myeloid leukaemia associated with t(16;16) (p13;q22). There are three blast cells and one eosinophil myelocyte with prominent pro-eosinophilic granules; the same fusion gene is found as in patients with inv(16)(p13q22), and the same cytological features. These cases are assigned to the WHO category of AML with recurrent cytogenetic abnormality. Bone marrow film, MGG.

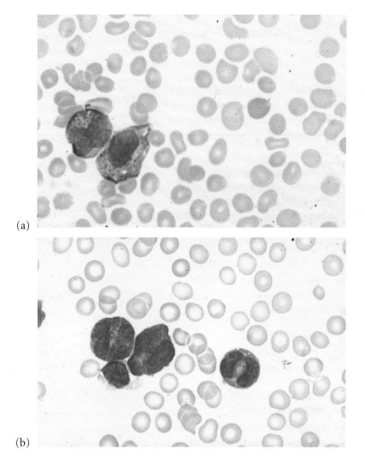

(a)

(b)

Figure 29.31 Peripheral blood films from two patients with acute promyelocytic leukaemia associated with t(15;17)(q22;q21): (a) acute hypergranular promyelocytic leukaemia showing two hypergranular promyelocytes; (b) acute hypogranular promyelocytic leukaemia showing characteristic bilobed nuclei. This translocation leads to formation of a *PML–RARA* fusion gene. These cases are assigned to the WHO category of AML with recurrent cytogenetic abnormality. MGG.

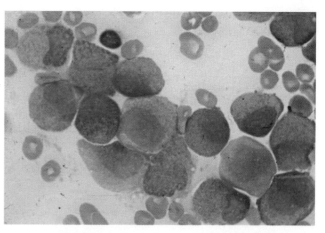

Figure 29.32 Acute myeloid leukaemia associated with t(11;17)(q23;q21); cytological features are closer to FAB M2 category although two hypergranular promyelocytes are apparent. M3-like or M2/M3 are convenient morphological designations for this type of AML. These cases are assigned to the WHO category of AML with recurrent cytogenetic abnormality but it should be noted that this type of leukaemia, which is associated with formation of a *PLZF–RARA* fusion gene, differs in several respects from acute promyelocytic leukaemia (whether classical or hypogranular) associated with t(15;17)(q22;q21) and a *PML-RARA* fusion gene. Bone marrow film, MGG.

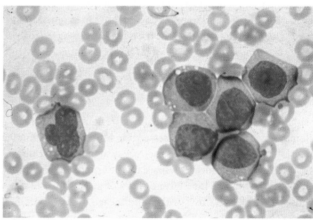

Figure 29.33 Acute myeloid leukaemia associated with t(9;11)(p21–22;q23) showing FAB M5a morphological features. This translocation leads to formation of a *MLL–AF9* fusion gene. These cases are assigned to the WHO category of AML with recurrent cytogenetic abnormality. Peripheral blood, MGG.

Other integrated approaches to the classification of AML

The WHO classification specifies four cytogenetic/molecular genetic categories but does not include other less common but nevertheless clearly defined categories. Of the four categories included, two are discrete entities with an overall good prognosis. These are, first, cases with an *AML1–ETO* fusion gene, whether or not t(8;21)(q22;q22) is present or detected, and, second, cases with a *CPFB–MYH11* fusion gene, whether or not inv(16) (p13q22) or t(16;16)(p13;q22) is present or detected. The WHO classification includes 'acute promyelocytic leukaemia, AML with t(15;17)(q22;q12) (*PML–RARA*) and variants'. This approach tends to blur the very real differences between acute promyelocytic leukaemia (either classical or variant) with a *PML–RARA* fusion gene and other cases with variant translocations involving *RARA* but not *PML*. Since AML with t(11;17) (q23;q21) and a *PLZF–RARA* fusion gene (Figure 29.32) responds neither to all-*trans*-retinoic acid (ATRA) nor to arsenic trioxide,

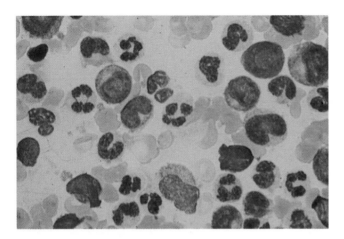

Figure 29.34 Acute myeloid leukaemia associated with t(11;19)(q23;p13.1) showing FAB M2 morphological features. This translocation leads to formation of a *MLL–ELL* fusion gene. These cases are assigned to the WHO category of AML with recurrent cytogenetic abnormality. Bone marrow film, MGG.

it seems important that it is *not* regarded as the same disease as acute promyelocytic leukaemia with a *PML–RARA* fusion gene. Defining optimal therapy for these and other even less common leukaemias with *RARA* rearrangement necessitates each of them being recognized as a discrete entity. The WHO classification also groups together all cases with an 11q23 breakpoint and rearrangement of the *MLL* gene, despite the very clear differences between different subtypes of leukaemia with *MLL* rearrangement. The European 11q23 Workshop (see Bain 2001) found that different *MLL* fusion genes were associated with different age ranges, different proportions of AML and ALL, different proportions of M4, M5a and M5b AML and different proportions of *de novo* and therapy-related cases. Although this does not yet have any therapeutic implications, these are clearly all different diseases and they would probably be better not aggregated into a single category.

In addition to the cytogenetic/molecular genetic entities recognized by the WHO classification there are other similar subtypes of AML with characteristic disease features which could be recognized. Some of these are summarized in Table 29.8 (Figures 29.37 and 29.38). The existence of categories of AML with a specific molecular genetic abnormality but without any specific associated cytogenetic abnormality should also be acknowledged. Important among these is AML, often FAB type M1, associated with mutation of the *CEBPA* gene; this is found in as many as 10% of cases of AML and appears to be associated with a good prognosis, particularly if there is no coexisting *FLT-3* abnormality. Recognition of this category of AML could be important in order to avoid overtreatment of good-prognosis patients.

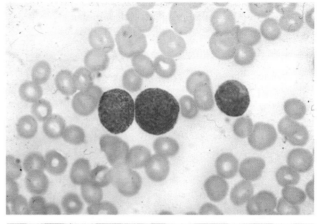

(a)

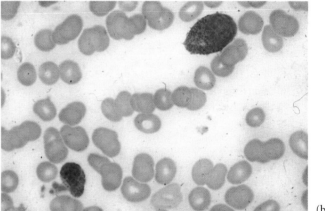

(b)

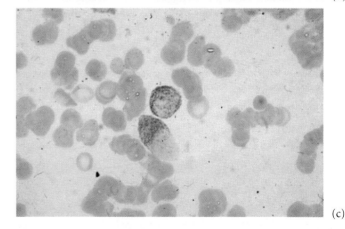

(c)

Figure 29.35 Peripheral blood film in acute basophilic leukaemia stained by MGG, showing large purple granules (a and b), and stained with toluidine blue stain showing metachromatic staining (c).

The WHO classification of acute lymphoblastic leukaemia

The most important alterations to the FAB classification made by the WHO group is that there is a clear separation of precursor-B and precursor-T lymphoblastic leukaemia/lymphoma

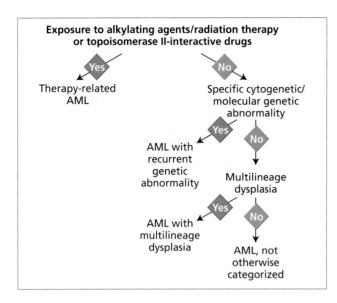

Figure 29.36 Flow chart showing how the WHO hierarchical classification is applied.

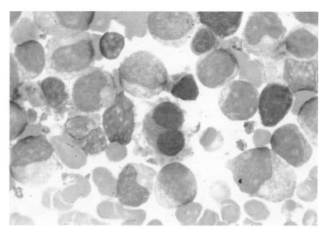

Figure 29.37 Acute myeloid leukaemia associated with inv(3)(q21q26) showing a binucleate micromegakaryocyte. Bone marrow film, MGG.

from cases with the immunophenotype of a mature lymphoid cell, whereas cases with a leukaemic presentation and those with a lymphomatous presentation are grouped together. The practical implication is that most cases categorized in the FAB classification as L3 ALL are reassigned to the category of Burkitt's lymphoma since they express surface membrane immunoglo-

bulin, do not usually express TdT, and have the same translocations that are found in Burkitt's lymphoma with a lymphomatous presentation. This reassignment is of some clinical relevance since it has been recognized for some time that these patients do much better with alternative intensive chemotherapeutic regimens rather than with chemotherapy that would be appropriate for ALL. There remain a small number of cases of L3 ALL that have a precursor-B cell immunophenotype, e.g. cases with

Table 29.8 Cytogenetic/molecular genetic entities not included in the WHO classification of AML.

Cytogenetic abnormality	Molecular genetic abnormality	Disease characteristics
t(9;22)(q34;q11)	BCR–ABL fusion gene	Mainly *de novo* but may follow topoisomerase II-interactive drugs, most often FAB M0 or M1, poor prognosis
t(6;9)(p23;q34.3)	DEK–CAN fusion gene (also known as DEK–NUP214)	Therapy related (either alkylating agent or topoisomerase II-interactive drugs) or *de novo*, most often FAB M2, may have Auer rods, dysplastic features and basophilic differentiation, poor prognosis
inv(3)(q21q26) or t(3;3)(q21;q26)	Dysregulation of EVI1	Therapy related or *de novo*, association with diabetes insipidus, multiple FAB categories, megakaryocyte numbers preserved, trilineage dysplasia with prominent megakaryocyte dysplasia, poor prognosis
t(8;16)(p11;p13)	MOZ–CBP fusion gene	Mainly *de novo* but may follow topoisomerase-II-interactive drugs, often FAB M5 with phagocytic blast cells and abnormal coagulation, poor prognosis
t(1;22)(p13;q13)	RBM15–MKL1 fusion gene (also known as OTT–MAL)	Acute megakaryoblastic leukaemia in infants, may originate in intrauterine life, often low percentage of bone marrow blast cells, intermediate prognosis
t(16;21)(p11;q22)	FUS–ERG fusion gene (also known as TLS–ERG)	Mainly FAB M1 and M2 AML, poor prognosis

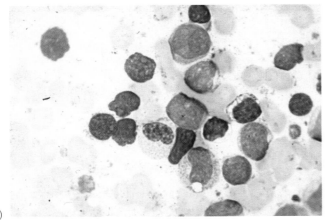

(a)

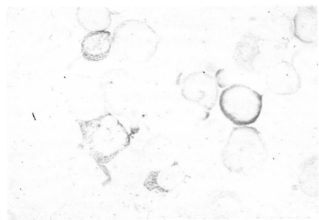

(b)

Figure 29.38 Acute myeloid leukaemia associated with t(6;9)(q23;q34); (a) MGG stained bone marrow film showing FAB M2 morphological features; there are two degranulated basophil precursors, one of which has some residual basophilic granules; (b) toluidine blue-stained bone marrow film, illustrating that many of the blast cells are also of basophil lineage.

t(1;19)(q23;p13), which should continue to be categorized as ALL.

Conclusion

The diagnosis and further classification of acute leukaemia requires a full assessment of the medical history, family history and physical findings, and careful assessment of cytological features in blood and bone marrow. The use of cytochemistry is selective. Application of immunophenotyping can be selective but is tending to become universal when facilities are readily available. Ideally, cytogenetic analysis should be universally applied, with molecular analysis being used selectively. Careful and detailed evaluation is important for the care of individual patients and for the advancement of knowledge.

Acknowledgement

Many of the illustrations in this chapter are taken from the equivalent chapter written by Professor Daniel Catovsky in the previous edition of this book.

Selected bibliography

Bain BJ (1998) The classification of acute leukaemia: the necessity for incorporating cytogenetic and molecular genetic information. *Journal of Clinical Pathology* **51**: 420–3.

Bain BJ (2001) *Leukaemia Diagnosis*, 3rd edn. Blackwell Publishing, Oxford, pp. 97–101.

Bain BJ, Barnett D, Linch D, Matutes E, Reilly JT (2002) Revised guideline on immunophenotyping in acute leukaemias and chronic lymphoproliferative disorders. *Clinical and Laboratory Haematology* **24**: 1–13.

Bene MC, Castoldi G, Knapp W *et al.* (EGIL) (1995) Proposals for the immunological classification of acute leukemias. *Leukemia* **9**: 1783–6.

Bennett JM, Catovsk, D, Daniel MT *et al.* (1976) Proposals for the classification of the acute leukaemias (FAB cooperative group). *British Journal of Haematology* **33**: 451–8.

Bennett JM, Catovsky D, Daniel MT *et al.* (1985) Criteria for the diagnosis of acute leukemia of megakaryocytic lineage (M7): a report of the French–American–British cooperative group. *Annals of Internal Medicine* **103**: 460–2.

Bennett JM, Catovsky D, Daniel MT *et al.* (1991) Proposal for the recognition of minimally differentiated acute myeloid leukaemia (AML M0). *British Journal of Haematology* **78**: 325–9.

Brunning RD, Matutes E, Harris NL *et al.* (2001) Acute myeloid leukaemia: introduction. In: *World Health Organization Classification of Tumours: Pathology and Genetics of Tumours of Haematopoietic and Lymphoid Tissue* (ES Jaffe, NL Harris, H Stein, JW Vardiman, eds), pp. 77–80. IARC Press, Lyon.

Brunning RD, Matutes E, Borowitz M *et al.* (2001) Acute leukaemias of ambiguous lineage. In: *World Health Organization Classification of Tumours: Pathology and Genetics of Tumours of Haematopoietic and Lymphoid Tissues* (ES Jaffe, NL Harris, H Stein, JW Vardiman, eds), pp. 106–7. IARC Press, Lyon.

First MIC Cooperative Study Group (1986) Morphologic, immunologic, and cytogenetic (MIC) working classification of acute lymphoblastic leukaemias. *Cancer Genetics and Cytogenetics* **23**: 189–97.

Second MIC Cooperative Study Group (1988) Morphologic, immunologic and cytogenetic (MIC) working classification of the acute myeloid leukaemias. *British Journal of Haematology* **68**: 487–94.

Preudhomme C, Sagot C, Boissel N *et al.* (2002) Favourable prognostic significance of CEBPA mutations with *de novo* acute myeloid leukemia: a study from the acute Leukemia French Association (ALFA). *Blood* **100**: 2717–23.

Stewart CC, Behm FG, Carey JL *et al.* (1997) US–Canadian consensus recommendations on the immunophenotypic analysis of hematologic neoplasia by flow cytometry: selection of antibody combinations. *Cytometry* **30**: 231–5.

Cytogenetics of leukaemia and lymphoma

Christine J Harrison

Introduction

Cytogenetics has contributed significantly to the understanding of the genetics of leukaemia and lymphoma over the last 40 years. Chromosomal rearrangements result in the movement of a gene to a new chromosomal location, thus bringing it under the influence of another gene, which may control its expression. This occurs in one of two ways: (i) deregulation of expression, causing abnormal expression of a gene; or (ii) by the generation of a new fusion gene product with aberrant activity. These observations have confirmed the importance of cytogenetic rearrangements in leukaemogenesis and recognized the concept of malignancy as an acquired genetic disorder. The purpose of a cytogenetic investigation in a haematological disorder is to determine whether the karyotype (chromosomal make-up) of the affected cells is abnormal (i.e. different from the constitutional karyotype). Chromosomal findings are important for the classification and diagnosis of the disorder. In acute leukaemia, the karyotype is an independent prognostic factor, now with an impact on therapy. Cytogenetic investigation during the course of an indolent leukaemia may be used to predict transformation to a more aggressive phase. The outcome of bone marrow transplantation can be determined by cytogenetics if the donor and recipient are of opposite sex or if a chromosomal abnormality was found at diagnosis. Successful engraftment can then be distinguished from regeneration of host cells and impending relapse. In this chapter, cytogenetic nomenclature and techniques for studying chromosomes in haematological malignancies are presented first. Then follows a description of the main cytogenetic abnormalities under the headings of the different haematological disorders with which they are associated. Where known, the genes involved will be named, together with a description of the genetic consequences of the chromosomal rearrangement. The diagnostic and prognostic importance of the abnormalities will be discussed.

Techniques

Chromosome preparation: band staining

In the haematological disorders, bone marrow and peripheral blood, or cells from lymph node biopsies of lymphomas, are investigated for the presence of dividing malignant cells. Chromosomes are visible only in the condensed form that they adopt in metaphase of cell division (mitosis). They are arrested in metaphase by the spindle poison colcemid and are stained by so-called banding techniques, the standard one being trypsin–Giemsa (or G) banding. This produces a specific banding pattern, clearly visible with bright-field microscopy, in which darkly staining regions of chromatin alternate with lighter staining regions. The banding pattern of each chromosome pair is unique, allowing positive identification of every chromosome (Figure 30.1). At mid-metaphase, a total of 240–330 bands can be seen over the whole karyotype. This increases to 850 or more in prometaphase. Chromosomal analysis has led to the description of many cytogenetic changes acquired in haematological malignancies. It also provides important information on the heterogeneity of cell populations and can detect several abnormalities simultaneously in a single cell. However, it is limited to cells which are mitotically active and must be representative of the malignant clone.

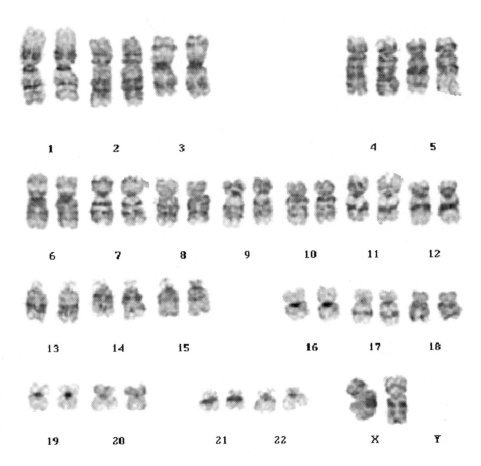

Figure 30.1 Karyogram of a G-banded metaphase from a normal female, 46,XX. Note the 22 pairs of autosomes, 1–22, and the two X chromosomes.

Molecular techniques

Chromosomal abnormalities that cannot be resolved by G banding may be discovered by molecular cytogenetic techniques, otherwise known as FISH (fluorescence *in situ* hybridization). The increasing number of FISH techniques have become an integral part of cytogenetic analysis and must be regarded as complementary, not replacement, tools. FISH analysis requires some pre-knowledge of the abnormality in order to select the appropriate probes, now available to an infinite number of genes and DNA sequences as a result of the Human Genome Mapping Project. Probes are available to each chromosome pair, known as chromosome paints, which can confirm suspected rearrangements and facilitate the analysis of complex chromosomal rearrangements. One of the most appealing aspects of FISH has become the ability to detect a number of targets in several colours at the same time in the same cell. Ultimately, 24-colour FISH (multiplex-FISH or SKY, differing only in the imaging system used to discriminate the fluorochromes) extends the painting technique for the simultaneous analysis of all chromosomes (Figure 30.2). Multiple-colour chromosome band-specific probes now exist (Figure 30.3).

Centromeric, subtelomeric or locus-specific probes can be used to detect aneuploidy, loss or amplification at a particular locus, or subtle/cryptic translocations. The advantage of FISH over cytogenetics is that it can be used to investigate chromosomes and genes in the non-dividing interphase cells as well as metaphases. For interphase FISH assays, it is possible to score large numbers of cells, which is helpful in cases where the mitotic cells are not representative of the malignant clone. Dual-colour translocation probes are now in routine use for interphase FISH detection of important translocations. They consist of probes specific for each of the genes disrupted in the translocation, labelled with different fluorochromes, usually red and green. Single fusion (S-FISH) dual-colour probe sets contain sequences for part of the genes involved in a translocation, and give one red, one green and one red/green (yellow) signal in cells carrying the translocation (Figure 30.4). One limitation of S-FISH for the detection of a fusion gene is the false-positive rate (the frequency with which the signals randomly collocalize in normal cells). Two improvements have increased the sensitivity of FISH and significantly reduced the false-positive rate. One has been the introduction of a third probe labelled with an alternative fluorochrome, giving an extra signal in a third colour, and another the use of two probes which span the breakpoints of both genes, giving a dual fusion in the positive cells. Since the chance occurrence of this signal pattern is virtually zero, this is the most sensitive approach to use.

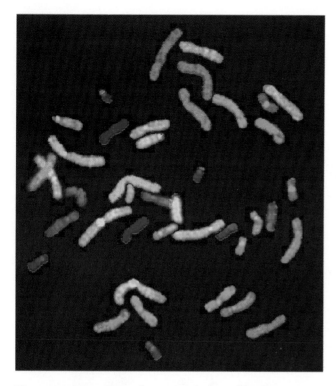

Figure 30.2 Normal metaphase painted in 24 colours by multiplex-FISH. Each chromosome pair is seen as a different colour, discriminated by sophisticated computer software.

In addition to FISH, other molecular techniques can be exploited to look for genetic abnormalities in malignant tissue. DNA can be investigated by Southern blotting to discover the presence of a deletion or a translocation in which a particular gene is deleted or disrupted in the creation of an aberrant fusion product. The polymerase chain reaction (PCR) with appropriate primers has now superseded Southern analysis for the detection

of fusion transcripts arising from translocations. PCR may be performed on genomic DNA when the breakpoints are tightly clustered, or on RNA transcripts using reverse transcriptase PCR (RT-PCR) when breakpoints are more variable. Gene expression may be quantified using real-time PCR. This technique can be used to track the abnormal clone throughout the course of the disease and thus will quantitatively detect minimal residual disease in patients who have achieved complete remission. There is currently intense interest in the use of DNA microarrays to determine global gene expression patterns, which may be of both diagnostic and prognostic value.

Terminology

Normal human somatic cells contain a diploid set of 46 chromosomes in 23 pairs: 22 pairs of autosomes, numbered 1–22, and a pair of sex chromosomes, XX (female) and XY (male), as shown in the karyogram (Figure 30.1). Each chromosome has a long (q) and a short (p) arm, separated by a primary constriction, the centromere. The chromosome arms are divided into regions and subregions based on the bands, and are numbered from the centromere outwards towards the ends (telomeres). This enables abnormalities to be described in terms of the affected region of the chromosome. Thus, 11q23.2 refers to the long arm of chromosome 11, region 2, subregion 3, subsubregion 2 (Figure 30.5).

Chromosomal abnormalities may be random or clonal. For the purposes of chromosomal classification, only clonal abnormalities are considered. These may be numerical or structural. Numerical changes result in gain or loss of one or more chromosomes. Gain of any single individual chromosome results in trisomy for that chromosome (indicated by the prefix +). The loss of a chromosome results in monosomy for that chromosome (indicated by the prefix −). Cells with numerical changes

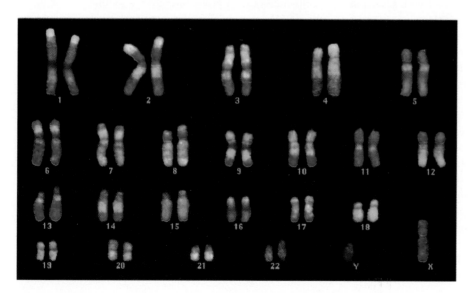

Figure 30.3 Karyogram of a normal male painted in seven colours in such a way as to produce coloured bands along the chromosome arms (Rx-FISH) allowing identification of the individual chromosome pairs.

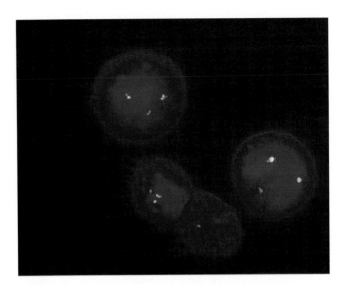

Figure 30.4 Four interphase nuclei showing individual signals specific for the ABL (red) and BCR (green) genes on the normal chromosomes 9 and 22 respectively and the BCR/ABL fusion (red/green collocalized signals appearing yellow) indicating the presence of the Philadelphia chromosome.

show a change of ploidy from the normal diploid complement and are classified by the number of chromosomes as less than (hypo) or greater than (hyper) the nearest ploidy number as follows: near-haploid, 23–29 chromosomes; low hypodiploid, 30–39 chromosomes; high hypodiploid, 40–45 chromosomes; diploid, normal 46 chromosomes; pseudo-diploid, 46 chromosomes with an abnormal chromosome complement; low hyperdiploid, 47–50 chromosomes; high hyperdiploid, 51–65 chromosomes; hypo- or hypertriploid, 69 ±, range 66–80 chromosomes; near-tetraploid, 92 ±, range 81–103 chromosomes.

Structural abnormalities result from chromosomal breakage. They include deletions (del) when part of a chromosome arm is missing [e.g. del(11)(q23) is loss of chromosomal material distal to the breakpoint 11q23] or translocations (t) when chromosomal material is exchanged with another chromosome [e.g. t(4;11)(q21;q23) indicates that material distal to the breakpoint on chromosome 4 at 4q21 is exchanged with material distal to the 11q23 breakpoint]. Translocations may be balanced, which assumes a reciprocal exchange with no loss of chromosomal material, or unbalanced, in which one of the derived chromosomes (der) is missing. A reciprocal translocation may be simple, involving two chromosomes, or complex, between three or more chromosomes. Inversion (inv) describes the inversion of the segment of a chromosome lying between two bands. The description of the chromosomal make-up of the cell is called the karyotype and is written strictly according to an International System for Human Cytogenetic Nomenclature. By convention, this lists the number of chromosomes in the cell,

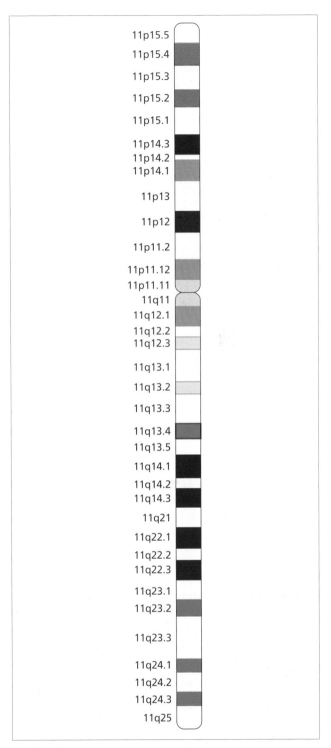

Figure 30.5 Schematic representation (ideogram) of the G-banding pattern of chromosome 11.

followed by the sex chromosomes, followed by a description of the abnormal chromosomes in numerical order. The number of cells with that karyotype then follows in square brackets. Thus, 50,XY,−7,+8,t(9;22)(q34;q11),+13,+19,+der(22)t(9;22) (q34;q11)[18]/46,XY[2] describes a bimodal cell population in which 18 cells belong to an abnormal clone and two are chromosomally normal. Each cell in the abnormal clone has 50 chromosomes with loss of chromosome 7, gains of chromosomes 8, 13 and 19, a balanced translocation between chromosomes 9 and 22 with breaks at 9q34 and 22q11 and an additional copy of the derived chromosome 22 from this translocation.

Cytogenetic and molecular genetic events

Oncogene activation by chromosomal translocation

Many human oncogenes are located at breakpoints consistently found in chromosomal changes in leukaemia and lymphoma. The gene situated at the other breakpoint of a translocation is likely to be a gene of functional importance. As a result of the translocation, genes that are normally separated are brought together. In this new location, they will be subject to control by their new rather than their normal neighbouring genes, leading to deregulation and abnormal expression. Alternatively, a new fusion gene with aberrant activity will be generated.

Recessive genes, translocations and leukaemogenesis

Leukaemias associated with total or partial chromosome loss suggest that malignancy can result from the unmasking of a recessive malignant gene by the loss of its normal allele. It has been generally assumed that deletions mark the site of tumour-suppressor genes, which behave according to Knudson's two-hit hypothesis of tumour-suppressor gene inactivation. In this model, one allele of the gene could be inactivated by a micro-deletion or point mutation or transcriptionally silenced by methylation of the promoter, with the second allele subsequently deleted. A haploinsufficiency model of tumour-suppressor gene inactivation is also possible, in which inactivation of one copy of a target gene, for example by deletion, could be sufficient to contribute to the pathogenesis of a haematological malignancy. Partial or total trisomies would also be expected to perturb gene dosage. An increase in the number of copies of a given proto-oncogene per cell might result in malignant transformation. At present, this is largely speculative, but amplification of proto-oncogenes has been demonstrated in association with homogeneously staining regions (HSRs) and double minutes (DMs). Amplification of the genes *MLL* and *AML1* has been reported in acute myeloid leukaemia (AML) and acute lymphoblastic leukaemia (ALL) respectively. In AML, amplification of c-*MYC* has been described in association with the increased expression of this oncogene.

The main chromosomal abnormalities found in chronic myeloid leukaemia (CML), AML, T- and B- lineage ALL, mature B-cell leukaemias, lymphomas and plasma cell dyscrasias will be discussed, together with their molecular, biological and clinical importance, in the following sections.

Chronic myeloid leukaemia (see also Chapter 37)

The most consistent chromosomal abnormality associated with a haematological malignancy is the Philadelphia chromosome (Ph), described in 1960 as the first cytogenetic abnormality to be associated with human malignancy. The Ph is the derived chromosome 22 from the translocation t(9;22)(q34;q11) (Figure 30.6). In CML, this translocation is found in 92% of patients. Of these patients, approximately 5% have a variant translocation, with the reciprocal chromosome apparently being other than chromosome 9, and 4% have a complex translocation, clearly involving chromosomes 9 and 22 with one or more additional chromosomes. The t(9;22) joins 3′ sequences of the *ABL* gene at 9q34 to the 5′ sequences of the *BCR* gene at 22q11, giving rise to the *BCR–ABL* fusion gene. Breakpoints within *BCR* occur within a 5.8-kb region, termed the major breakpoint cluster region (M-BCR), either between exons 13 and 14 (b2a2) or between exons 14 and 15 (b3a2) This transcribes an aberrant 8.5-kb mRNA, encoding a chimeric p210 protein with enhanced tyrosine kinase activity. Up to 8% of CML patients are Ph negative, without apparent rearrangement of chromosomes 9 or 22, in which the BCR–ABL fusion transcript is detectable by molecular analysis. In some cases, the *BCR–ABL* fusion is present on a cytogenetically normal chromosome 22 as a result of a cryptic insertion of *ABL* into *BCR*. In others, *BCR* is inserted into *ABL* on chromosome 9 (Figure 30.7). Several molecular methods have been utilized to detect the *BCR–ABL* rearrangement. FISH detects the juxtaposition or disruption of *BCR* and *ABL* genes in

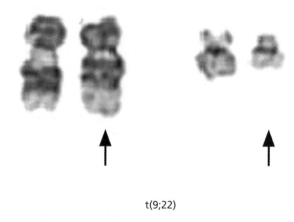

t(9;22)

Figure 30.6 Partial karyogram of chromosomes 9 and 22 from a patient with CML, showing t(9;22). The normal chromosome of each pair is on the left and the abnormal (translocated) chromosomes are on the right (arrowed).

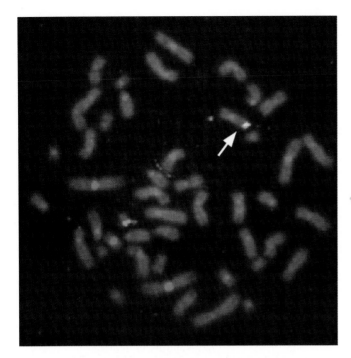 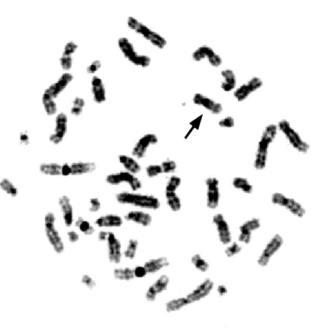

Figure 30.7 The same metaphase from a patient with CML examined by FISH (left) and G banded chromosomal analysis (right). Although the chromosomes 9 and 22 are apparently normal by G-banding, the BCR–ABL fusion is formed by the cryptic insertion of BCR into ABL on chromosome 9 (red/green–yellow signal) (arrowed). ABL (red) and BCR (green) signals are also visible on the normal chromosomes 9 and 22 respectively.

metaphase and interphase cells (Figure 30.4); Southern blotting determines whether the *BCR* gene is rearranged from analysis of genomic DNA; RT-PCR determines the presence of BCR–ABL mRNA; and Western blotting analyses cell lysates to determine the presence of BCR–ABL protein. These approaches are particularly useful in patients whose karyotype is normal or ambiguous.

As BCR–ABL is consistently transcribed, whereas ABL–BCR is not, the BCR–ABL transcript was identified to play the aetiological role in the development of CML. It is now known from RT-PCR and FISH studies that extensive deletions of *ABL*- and *BCR*-derived sequences are seen around the translocation breakpoint on the derivative chromosome 9 in up to 30% of patients at diagnosis, which may account for the lack of expression of the reciprocal transcript. Such deletions have been associated with a poorer outcome. Since patients with complex/ variant translocations have a higher incidence of deletion, it may be the deletion itself rather than the type of translocation that is linked to the poorer prognosis in these patients.

The progression of CML from chronic phase to blastic transformation is accompanied by additional abnormalities in 80% patients. These changes include duplication of the Ph, isochromosome 17 [i(17)(q10)], +8 and +19, either as a single change or in any combination. In the chronic phase, 5–10% of Ph-positive patients have additional chromosomal changes. The significance of additional changes at diagnosis of CML is not clear and may be an indication of genetic instability rather than a sign of early progression. However, any additional change detected after diagnosis during serial chromosomal analyses is generally predictive of impending transformation.

Patients have been successfully treated with interferon-α, with approximately 80% achieving a haematological response measured by a reduction in the number of Ph-positive cells in the bone marrow. The demonstration that BCR–ABL encodes a receptor tyrosine kinase led to the discovery of new therapeutic strategies in which an inhibitor of the tyrosine kinase domain of the BCR–ABL chimeric protein, imatinib mesylate (STI571 or Gleevec/Glivec), was found to be effective in treatment. The cytogenetic response with this drug is highly successful, although the results from long-term follow-up are not yet available.

Acute myeloid leukaemia (see also Chapter 31)

The majority of cases of AML (70%) are characterized by one of a variety of chromosomal abnormalities, many of which have now been molecularly characterized. These abnormalities correlate closely with morphological and clinical features and are a key determinant in outcome. They identify distinct biological subsets of disease, to which therapeutic approaches can be

Table 30.1 Significant chromosomal abnormalities in AML.

Chromosomal rearrangement	Genes	Genes	FAB type	Other clinical features	Prognosis
t(1;22)(p13;q13)	OTT	MAL	M7	Infants	
inv(3)q21q26)	EVI1			Trilineage dysplasia, dysmegakaryopoiesis	Poor
t(3;21)(q26;q22)	EVI1/MDS1/EAP	AML1		Therapy related	
+4			M2, M4	MDS	
−5				Therapy related	Poor
t(5;11)(q35;p15)	NSD1	NUP98	M2, M4	Infants	
t(6;9)(q23;q34)	DEK	CAN	M2	Basophilia	
−7				Therapy related	Poor
t(7;12)(q36;p13)	HLXB9	ETV6		Infants	
+8			M1, M4, M5		
t(8;16)(p11;p13)	MOZ	CBP	M4, M5	Erythrophagocytosis	
t(8;21)(q22;q22)	ETO	AML1	M2	Chloromas, Auer rods	Good
+9			M6		
t(9;11)(p21;q23)	AF9	MLL	M5 (M4)		
t(9;22)(q34;q11)	ABL	BCR-M or m	M0/1, M2		
+11			M0, M1		
t(11;17)(q23;q21)	PLZF	RARα	M3	ATRA and arsenic resistant	
+13			M0, M1		
t(15;17)(q22;q21)	PML	RARα	M3	ATRA sensitive	Good
inv(16)(p13q22)	MYH11	CBFβ	M4	Abnormal eosinophils	Good
del(20q)			M6		
+21			M4		
+22			M4Eo		

specifically tailored. This is particularly relevant to patients with good-risk cytogenetic features. The French–American–British (FAB) classification of AML consists of eight main groups (M0–M7) with two subtypes M3V (variant) and M4Eo (with increased or abnormal eosinophils). Those chromosomal abnormalities most commonly associated with AML, where known, the genes involved, their FAB types and associated clinical features are given in Table 30.1.

Good-risk cytogenetic groups

t(8;21)(q22;q22)

This translocation (Figure 30.8a) occurs predominantly in FAB type M2 (acute myeloid leukaemia with granulocytic maturation at or beyond promyelocyte stage) and a number of cases of M4 (myelomonocytic leukaemia). It fuses the core binding factor alpha gene (CBFα, AML1 or RUN1) on chromosome 21 with ETO on chromosome 8 to produce a novel chimeric gene, which is frequently accompanied by the loss of a sex chromosome (−Y in males and −X in females). In up to 8% of cases, the translocation is cryptic, requiring alternative molecular detection methods as described above. The translocation is found in all

age groups, but is most common under the age of 40 years. It is associated with a good outcome and, in current treatment trials, is considered as good risk and treated accordingly.

inv(16)(p13q22), t(16;16)(p13;q22)

These abnormalities of chromosome 16 are found in AML M4 and are notable for their association with abnormal eosinophilia (M4Eo) and a good prognosis. The inv(16)(p13q22) (Figure 30.8b) involves an in-frame fusion of the smooth muscle myosin heavy-chain gene, MYH11, normally on 16p13 and another core binding factor gene, CBFβ, normally on 16q22. This subtle chromosomal change has frequently been overlooked by cytogenetic analysis of poor-quality preparations, therefore FISH and RT-PCR have become routine detection methods.

t(15;17)(q22;q21)

The translocation t(15;17)(q22;q21) (Figure 30.8c) is specific for AML M3 and M3v (acute promyelocytic leukaemia) and is most often found in patients < 35 years old. It results in the rearrangement of the retinoic acid receptor alpha (RARα) gene, located at 17q21, which is fused to the PML gene on chromosome 15, a gene which is transcribed in normal haemopoietic cells. Thus,

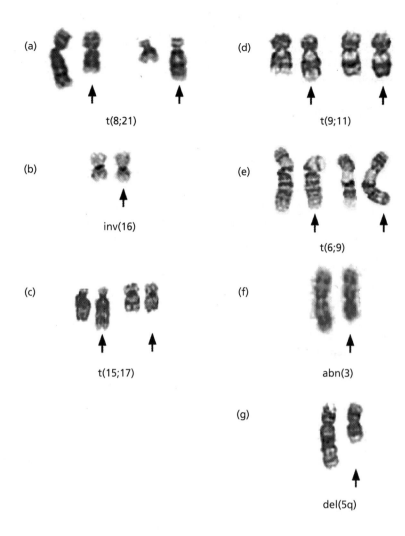

(a)

t(8;21)

(b)

inv(16)

(c)

t(15;17)

(d)

t(9;11)

(e)

t(6;9)

(f)

abn(3)

(g)

del(5q)

Figure 30.8 Partial karyograms from marrow cells of patients with acute myeloid leukaemia, each showing a chromosomal rearrangement. The normal chromosomes are on the left and the abnormal ones are on the right (arrowed).

the chimeric gene appears to play a role in the differentiation block that occurs in AML M3. The prognosis in these patients is good and of particular interest is their response to treatment with all-*trans*-retinoic acid (ATRA). This acts by converting the PML–RAR-α fusion protein from a transcriptional repressor to a transcriptional activator, thus inducing terminal differentiation of the leukaemic clone. This has conferred significant improvements in survival in combination with standard therapy. ATRA has now been adopted as a component of first-line therapy for this disease, highlighting the importance of accurate identification of this chromosomal abnormality. FISH and RT-PCR have become important tools in the detection of *PML–RARα*, as described for *BCR–ABL*. In AML M3, patients have been identified with atypical karyotypic features. These include the rare alternative translocation t(11;17)(q23;q21), whereby *RARα* is fused to the *PLZF* gene. The identification of these variants is important as, unlike the classic t(15;17) cases, they are resistant to ATRA.

Among these three groups of patients with favourable primary cytogenetic abnormalities t(8;21), inv(16) and t(15;17), the significance of additional chromosomal abnormalities has been a subject of some controversy; however, the majority of studies suggest that they do not have a major impact on prognosis.

Other chromosomal abnormalities

Abnormalities of 11q23 (see also Chapter 33)

Chromosomal rearrangements of 11q23 involving the *MLL* gene have been described most frequently in infants presenting at < 1 year of age. Numerous partner genes have been identified, but in AML, particularly M5 (monocytic leukaemia), the translocation t(9;11)(p21;q23), involving *AF9*, is the most common (Figure 30.8d). Although this translocation provides the best outcome compared to other *MLL* translocations in AML, survival is relatively short.

t(6;9)(p23;q34)

Bone marrow basophilia has been reported in a number of patients with the translocation, t(6;9)(p23;q34) (Figure 30.8e). Patients are often < 30 years of age and outcome is generally poor. The breakpoint at 9q34 is different from the Ph and interrupts a gene known as *CAN*. As a result of the translocation, *CAN* fuses with the gene *DEK* on 6p23 and encodes a DEK/CAN protein.

inv(3)(q21q26), t(3;3)(q21;q26)

Abnormalities involving chromosome bands 3q21 and 3q26 are found in all FAB types and are associated with an extremely poor prognosis (Figure 30.8f). Trilineage myelodysplasia, abnormalities of the megakaryocyte series and abnormal thrombopoiesis are common in this patient group. Three genes have been mapped to 3q26; *EVI1*, *EAP* and *MDS1/EVI1*. Aberrant expression of *EVI1* has been demonstrated in patients with 3q26 abnormalities.

Other chromosomal abnormalities specific to childhood AML include t(1;22)(p13;q13). This translocation occurs in less than 1% of childhood cases of AML and yet has been found in almost 100% of infants with M7 (megakaryoblastic leukaemia), usually as the sole cytogenetic change. This translocation fuses the *MAL* and *OTT* genes on chromosomes 22 and 1 respectively. The resulting OTT–MAL fusion protein regulates *HOX* gene expression. The cryptic translocation t(5;11)(q35;p15.5) is associated with a deletion of the long arm of chromosome 5. It involves *NUP98* at 11p15 with *NSD1*. The rare but recurrent translocation t(7;12)(q36;p13) is restricted to infants with AML, is cryptic and involves *ETV6* (*TEL*) at 12p13 and *HLXB9* at 7q36.

There are a number of chromosomal changes which occur in all FAB types. These include deletions of chromosome 5 [del(5q)] (Figure 30.8g), in which a variable portion of the long arm is missing. The proximal breakpoints vary but the distal breakpoint usually involves 5q31–q33, including the commonly deleted segment, which has been mapped to 5q31 in AML and MDS, the proposed site of a tumour-suppressor gene. The location of myeloid growth factor genes on 5q and the acquired hemizygosity of these genes in clones with monosomy 5 or del(5q) are subject to numerous investigations into the mechanisms of leukaemogenesis associated with this chromosomal change. Nevertheless, the relationship between these genetic events and neoplastic change remains elusive.

Monosomy 7 or del(7q) also frequently occur. Although the extent of the deletion of 7q is variable, two commonly deleted regions have been mapped by molecular methods to 7q22 and 7q32–q33.

Acquired hemizygosity of 17p in clones with i(17)(q10) or del(17p) has been shown to be associated with mutations of the *p53* gene, a tumour-suppressor gene, located on 17p. The oncogeneic potential of the mutated form of this gene suggests that these chromosomal abnormalities are of prime importance for malignant transformation.

Trisomy 8 is a common abnormality in AML. It often accompanies other chromosomal changes as a secondary abnormality. Thus, it has been difficult to evaluate this change in terms of risk.

The detection of trisomy 8 is amenable to FISH-based techniques using centromeric probes and chromosome painting, particularly when metaphases are of poor quality. Interphase-FISH using centromeric probes has demonstrated that trisomy 8 may be present in a greater proportion of patients than originally thought.

Abnormalities of chromosomes 5 and 7 (monosomy or partial long-arm deletion) and abnormalities of 3q, particularly in association with a complex karyotype (usually described as four or more structural and/or numerical changes in the same clone), predict an adverse prognosis. They are found most frequently in adults over the age of 55 years and are invariably associated with a particularly poor treatment response.

Secondary leukaemia

Chromosomal abnormalities have been described in up to 90% of cases of AML following cytotoxic treatment and arising as a secondary malignancy (s-AML). A similar incidence of abnormalities is found in patients with AML who have been exposed to environmental genotoxic agents. The chromosomes most frequently involved are 5 and 7. The clones tend to have highly complex karyotypes and these patients have a poor response to treatment. A t(3;21)(q26;q22) has been described in a number of s-AML cases, which fuses *MDS1–EVI1* with *AML1*. Other abnormalities involving the *AML1* gene and rearrangements of 11q23, including the translocation t(4;11)(q21;q23), are found in s-AML following treatment with topoisomerase II inhibitors, such as epipodophyllotoxins. Cytogenetic analysis was important in establishing the existence of leukaemia induced by these drugs and distinguishing them from cases induced by other alkylating agents.

Myelodysplastic syndromes
(see also Chapter 40)

The myelodysplastic syndromes (MDS) are a collection of five clinicopathological entities occurring most frequently in the elderly, with a wide spectrum of clinical behaviour and survival outcome. Between 40% and 70% of patients with primary MDS have chromosomal abnormalities. In secondary (therapy related) MDS, the incidence is much higher. The detection of a clonal cytogenetic change is useful in difficult cases to establish the definitive diagnosis of MDS. Cytogenetic findings are an independent prognostic variable and have been instrumental in predicting the likelihood of progression from MDS to AML. In classification systems, such as that of the World Health Organization, cytogenetics is now mandatory to the prognostic scoring of a newly diagnosed patient. Many of the karyotypic changes are similar to those found in AML and the myeloproliferative disorders. In general, they are unbalanced, with chromosome loss, deletion and unbalanced translocations. The most common single abnormalities are del(5q), monosomy 7, trisomy 8 and del(20q). However, multiple chromosomal changes are common. A complex karyotype, which may include the abnormalities listed above, carries a higher incidence of progression to acute leukaemia and signifies a particularly grave prognosis. An abrupt change from a simple to highly complex karyotype heralds leukaemic transformation in patients who previously had a stable clinical course over many years, thereby advocating serial monitoring of patients with stable disease.

The 5q minus syndrome

Deletion of a portion of the long arm of chromosome 5 is found in a wide spectrum of haematological disorders, including AML, secondary leukaemia and myeloproliferative disorders. However, the term '5q minus syndrome' refers specifically to a condition first described by Van den Berghe and colleagues in 1974 in which a clone with del(5q) is the sole chromosomal abnormality. A commonly deleted segment of 5q has been identified at 5q33, which is different from that defined for AML and MDS and is likely to harbour a different tumour-suppressor gene. Most affected patients are elderly females with severe refractory anaemia, without an excess of blasts, with no underlying haematological disorder and no significant history of exposure to drugs or toxins. Generally they have a favourable outcome and relatively long survival, with only ~10% of patients progressing to AML. Additional abnormalities which may be present and influence survival adversely include del(7q), −7, +8, +11, −17 and +21.

Myeloproliferative disorders
(see also Chapter 46)

The myeloproliferative disorders (MPDs) are a group of disorders defined by proliferation of one or more lineages of the myeloiderythroid series. This includes polycythaemia rubra vera, idiopathic myelofibrosis, undifferentiated MPD and essential thrombocythaemia (ET). Chromosomal abnormalities are seen in 30–40% of patients, although rarely in ET. There is no pathognomonic chromosomal abnormality associated with these disorders, but cytogenetic investigation is important to rule out Ph-positive CML. Some consistent chromosomal abnormalities have been described, including del(20)(q11), +8, +9, del(13)(q13–q31) and partial trisomy 1q, which seem to be associated with a poor prognosis. Frequently, the detection of a chromosomal abnormality in these cases is the only way to distinguish a malignant clone from a non-malignant hyperplasia.

Translocations in atypical MPD involving the chromosome band 8p11, most frequently t(8;13)(p11;12) and t(8;9)(p11;q34), define a rare group of patients described as 8p11 myeloproliferative syndrome. These translocations disrupt the fibroblast growth factor receptor-1 gene (*FGFR1*), a receptor protein tyrosine kinase that maps to 8p11. Patients with rearrangements of *FGFR1* have distinctive clinical features, notably prominent eosinophilia. In a similar manner, translocations involving 5q33 disrupts the platelet-derived growth factor beta receptor (PDGF-β), another receptor tyrosine kinase which maps to 5q33. The first such translocation to be reported was t(5;12)(q33;p13), in which *PDGFβ* fuses with the *ETV6* gene at 12p13. In these translocations, it seems that deregulation of *PDGFβ* as *FGFR1* leads to a consistent clinical phenotype that might be better classified as a distinct subtype of chronic MPD. In a similar manner to that described for CML, these patients respond to treatment with imatinib mesylate.

Acute lymphoblastic leukaemia
(see also Chapters 32 and 33)

Clonal chromosomal abnormalities are found in up to 80% of patients with ALL. They are closely related to the biology of the disease and indicate the genes involved in leukaemogenesis. Cytogenetic classification is based on the number of chromosomes and structural changes, which are important in both childhood and adult ALL to distinguish good- from high-risk patients. Significant chromosomal abnormalities and the genes involved are listed in Table 30.2. Cytogenetic studies in ALL are particularly difficult owing to the frequent low mitotic index of the abnormal blasts and the notoriously poor chromosome morphology. This can be largely overcome by using FISH or RT-PCR to screen for the significant chromosomal abnormalities.

B-precursor ALL

t(9;22)(q34;q11)
Of significance is the Ph chromosome, which is associated with a particularly poor outcome in ALL. This abnormality occurs more frequently in adults (in whom it accounts for up to 20% cases, increasing exponentially with age) than in children (among whom it is found in 2–3% cases). The Ph translocation, t(9;22)(q34;q11), in ALL is cytogenetically indistinguishable from that found in CML (Figure 30.6). In the majority of cases of ALL, the breakpoint in *BCR* occurs between exons 1 and 2 (e1 and e2) in the minor breakpoint cluster region (*m-BCR*) and exons 1 and 2 of *ABL* (e1a2). This generates a 7-kb mRNA giving rise to a p190 protein product. In some cases, the breakpoint is in M-BCR, resulting in the production of the p210 protein product as found in CML. Both result in raised tyrosine kinase activity, which induces the increased growth of the clone. As described for CML, FISH provides an accurate method of detection of this abnormality in poor-quality metaphases. The use of RT-PCR for the detection of mRNA in Ph-positive cases can be used to monitor the clone in remission with much greater sensitivity than that achieved by cytogenetic analysis. The two

Table 30.2 Significant chromosomal abnormalities in ALL.

Immunophenotype	Chromosomal rearrangement	Genes	Genes	Associated features	Prognosis
c-/pre-B ALL	HeH				Good
	near-haploidy				Very poor
	t(1;19)(q23;p13)	PBX1	E2A		Medium
	t(4;11)(q21;q23)	AF4	MLL	High WBC, infants	Very poor
	t(9;22)(q34;q11)	ABL	BCR-M or m	Higher incidence in adults	Very poor
	t(12;21)(p13;q22)	ETV6	AML1	Children	Good
	t(17;19)(q22;p13)	HLF	E2A	Variant t(1;19)	
T ALL	t(1;14)(p32;q11)	TAL1	TCRδ		
	t(5;14)(q35;q32)		HOX11L2		
	t(7;9)(q35;q32)	TCRβ	TAL2		
	t(7;9)(q35;q34)	TCRβ	TAN1		
	t(7;11)(q35;p13)	TCRβ	RBTN2		
	t(7;14)(p15;q11)	TCRγ	TCRδ		
	t(8;14)(q24;q11)	c-MYC	TCRα		
	del(9p)	p16			Poor
	t(10;14)(q24;q11)	HOX11	TCRα		
	t(11;14)(p13;q11)	RBTN2	TCRδ		
	t(11;14)(p15;q11)	RBTN1	TCRδ		
	inv(14)(q11;q32)	TCRα	IgH		
Mature B ALL	t(2;8)(p12;q24)	Igκ	c-MYC	L3	
	t(8;14)(q24;q32)	c-MYC	IgH	L3	
	t(8;22)(q24;q11)	c-MYC	Igλ	L3	

molecular variants of Ph-positive ALL do not apparently correlate with either different clinical features or with prognosis.

t(1;19)(q23;p13)

The translocation t(1;19)(q23;p13) fuses the *E2A* gene at 19p13 with the *PBX1* gene at 1q23 to form the *E2A/PBX1* fusion gene. The translocation is strongly associated with a pre-B immunophenotype and it occurs in two forms, a balanced translocation, t(1;19), and an unbalanced form, der(19)t(1;19) (in which the reciprocal product, der(1)t(1;19), is lost and the normal chromosome 1 is duplicated) (Figure 30.9a). Clinically, patients with the two forms appear identical, but the unbalanced form is associated with a significantly better prognosis than the balanced form. FISH probes directed to *E2A* reliably detect balanced and unbalanced forms of t(1;19) and the other rare abnormalities involving *E2A*.

t(17;19)(q21;p13)

The translocation t(17;19)(q21;p13) is a variant of t(1;19) resulting in the fusion of *E2A* with the hepatic leukaemia factor (*HLF*) gene on chromosome 17. Although limited numbers of patients have been reported, the prognosis is poor.

MLL rearrangements

The translocation t(4;11)(q21;q23) (Figure 30.9b) is the most frequently occurring *MLL* rearrangement in ALL, in which *MLL* fuses with AF4 located to chromosome band 4q21. This translocation identifies a particularly well-defined subgroup with a number of associated high-risk features, including white blood cell count > 50 × 10^9/L (frequently > 100 × 10^9/L) and a pre-B immunophenotype with some expression of myeloid features. It is most common in infants with ALL and in adults it is found more frequently in patients over the age of 40 years. The translocation occurs rarely between the ages of 2 and 10 years. A poor prognosis is associated with infants and adults. *MLL* is involved in a large number of translocations with a range of partner genes, many of which have been molecularly identified. A dual-colour FISH probe is available which reliably detects all *MLL* rearrangements. The identification of the subtle translocation t(11;19)(q23;p13) is shown in Figure 30.10.

t(12;21)(p13;q22)

This translocation occurs in up to 25% of children and 3% of adults with B-lineage ALL. In spite of this high incidence, it was discovered much later than the other ALL associated abnormal-

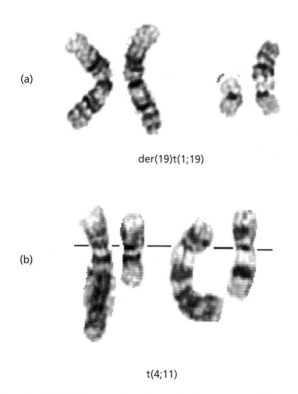

(a)

der(19)t(1;19)

(b)

t(4;11)

Figure 30.9 Partial karyograms of translocations seen in ALL, der(19)t(1;19) (a) and t(4;11) (b). Abnormal chromosomes 19 and 4 are on the right and abnormal 11 is on the left. Note that the two copies of chromosome 1 accompanying t(1;19) are normal.

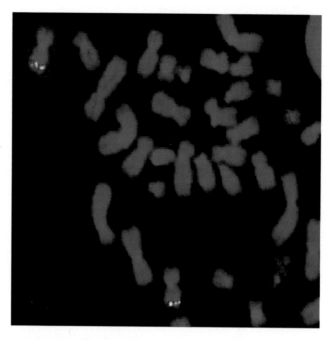

Figure 30.10 Metaphase from a patient with ALL showing the t(11;19) by FISH The probe set comprises two probes, 5′ and 3′ of *MLL* bcr, labelled with red (5′ distal) and green (3′ proximal). The red/green–yellow fusion signal is seen on the normal chromosome 11. As a result of the translocation the two probes become separated, the 5′ probe remains on the abnormal chromosome 11 (green signal) and the 3′ probe is relocated to chromosome 19 (red signal).

ities. The reason was that it is invisible by G-banded chromosomal analysis and was brought to light by chance chromosome painting in 1994. The translocation results in the fusion of the *ETV6* gene on chromosome 12 with *AML1* on chromosome 21. The *ETV6–AML1* fusion can be reliably detected by dual-colour FISH using specific probes (Figure 30.11) and by RT-PCR. Initial reports associated this translocation with a good prognosis. This has been reviewed as a number of patients have been shown to experience a late relapse. Deletions of the homologous *ETV6* allele have been reported in the majority of cases, which is believed to be a significant initiating event in the development of leukaemia in patients with t(12;21).

Ploidy

Ploidy classification embraces a heterogeneous group of numerical chromosomal changes, with an important role in prognosis. In particular, the high hyperdiploid group (which includes patients with 51–65 chromosomes) has been consistently shown to have the best outcome compared with any other chromosomal group in ALL. Chromosomal gains are non-random, with chromosomes 4, 6, 10, 14, 18, 17, 21 and X most frequently gained (Figure 30.12). The good prognosis has been linked to the gains of chromosomes 4, 10, 17 and 18. Interphase FISH using chromosome-specific centromere probes can be success-

fully used to look for high hyperdiploid clones in bone marrow samples which fail to achieve a cytogenetic result (Figure 30.13). Structural chromosomal changes accompany chromosomal gain in more than 50% of high hyperdiploid cases. It appears that structural change does not compromise the excellent prognosis of this group. It is of particular interest that high hyperdiploidy is the most frequent abnormal finding in children and a rare finding in adults. It is important to exclude the presence of one of the poor-risk translocations in a high hyperdiploid clone before designating the patient as good risk. In contrast to high hyperdiploidy, near-haploidy (23–29 chromosomes) and low hypodiploidy (30–39 chromosomes), both rare findings in ALL, are associated with an extremely poor prognosis. The chromosomes gained to the haploid chromosome set reflect the same additional chromosomes as seen in the high hyperdiploid patients. These abnormal clones often have an accompanying cell population with an exact doubling of their chromosome number. Although this resembles a classic good-risk high hyperdiploid karyotype, it confers no change to the dismal prognosis of these patients. Near-triploidy and near-tetraploidy are rare in childhood ALL, but in adults they account for approximately 5% of patients, in whom they are associated with a poor outcome.

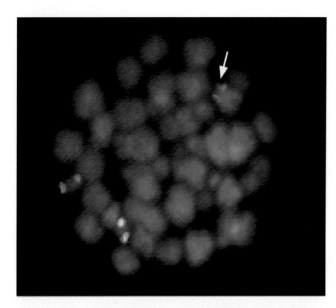

Figure 30.11 Metaphase from an ALL patient with t(12;21) showing the *ETV6–AML1* fusion on the abnormal chromosome 21 (red/green-yellow fusion signal). A small red signal from part of AML1 identifies the abnormal chromosome 12 (right hand red signal; arrowed), while the other red signal (left hand) indicates the normal chromosome 21. There is no complementary green signal seen on the homologous chromosome 12 indicating that an *ETV6* deletion accompanies the translocation in this patient.

Mature B-cell ALL

More than 80% of mature B-cell ALL (ALL L3) have one or other of three translocations consistently found in Burkitt's lymphoma: t(8;14)(q24;q32) (approximately 80%), t(2;8)(p12;q24) (6%) or t(8;22)(q24;q11) (14%) (Figure 30.14a–c). Chromosomes 14, 2 and 22 code for the immunoglobulin heavy-chain (*IgH*), and light-chain kappa (*Igκ*) and lambda (*Igλ*) genes respectively. The oncogene c-*MYC* is located at chromosome band 8q24. As a result of each translocation, the coding regions for c-*MYC* are brought into close proximity with one of the *Ig* genes. The recombination of *Ig* genes with c-*MYC* upregulates c-MYC expression, resulting in uncontrolled expansion of a malignant B-cell clone.

Although the translocation appears identical in African Burkitt's lymphoma (which occurs endemically in equatorial Africa and is associated with the presence of the Epstein–Barr virus (EBV) in more than 90% cases) and in sporadic cases (found in Europe and North America, in the absence of viral infection), a difference is seen at the molecular level. In sporadic cases, breakpoints occur either within or 5′ of c-*MYC* and in the switch region of *IgH*, c-*MYC* is structurally altered as a result of this translocation. Most endemic African Burkitt's lymphomas involve the *IgH* J_H region, c-*MYC* is not rearranged and break-

points are scattered widely over a 300-kb region upstream of the gene.

T-lineage ALL

The overall incidence of cases T-ALL classified by immunophenotyping is approximately 10% in childhood and 18% in adult ALL. The main chromosomal changes are shown in Table 30.2. The chromosomal abnormality detection rate by cytogenetic analysis is extremely low. It has been reported that ~20% of cases have translocations mapping to the chromosomal regions encoding one of the four T-cell receptor (*TCR*) genes, alpha/delta (*TCRα/δ*), beta (*TCRβ*) and gamma (*TCRγ*) at 14q11, 7q32 or 7p15 respectively. These translocations juxtapose a *TCR* promoter/enhancer element to one of many transcription factors located at or near the breakpoints of the partner chromosomes. Molecular studies have indicated that the incidence of these rearrangements is much higher than reported by cytogenetics alone. Similarly, molecular techniques have demonstrated hemi- and homozygous loss of genes located at 9p21-p22 in up to 80% of childhood cases of T-ALL, many without cytogenetic evidence of deletion of 9p. The genes of interest are two related tumour-suppressor genes, *MTS1* and *MTS2* otherwise known as *p16(INK4a)* and *p15(INK4b)*. These genes encode proteins that act as inhibitors of cyclin D-dependent serine-threonine kinases, which are necessary for the transition from G1 to S phase of the cell cycle. Further, it has been demonstrated that deletions of *TAL1* and the cryptic translocation t(5;14)(q35;q32), involving transcriptional activation of *HOX11L2*, occur in 45% of T-ALL. Also found, but not exclusive to T-ALL, are abnormalities of the long arm of chromosome 6 (6q), in approximately 12% patients.

Chronic lymphoproliferative disorders
(see also Chapter 38)

These disorders are characterized by the malignant proliferation of mature lymphocytic cells in the bone marrow and peripheral blood. Chronic lymphocytic leukaemia (CLL) and prolymphocytic leukaemia (PLL) are predominantly B-cell disorders. T-cell disorders account for only 5% of cases. Both mature B and T cells are particularly inert in culture and have to be stimulated into mitosis for cytogenetic analysis with mitogens, which even then may fail to stimulate the abnormal cells. Thus, it has been difficult to estimate the frequency of chromosomal abnormalities. The use of FISH, directed to the common changes, has increased the abnormality detection rate to approximately 80%. The major cytogenetic changes are listed in Table 30.3. In B-cell CLL these include trisomy 12, del(13q), del(11)(q22–q23), which includes the *ATM* gene (mutated or deleted in ataxia telangiectasia), and deletions or translocations of 17p13, usually resulting in loss of the p53 gene. In contrast to other low-grade B cell disorders, abnormalities

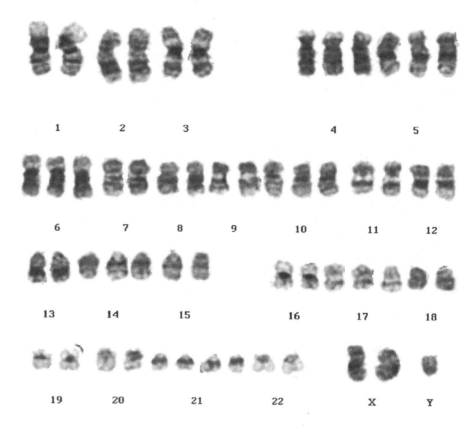

Figure 30.12 Karyogram of a hyperdiploid cell (55 chromosomes) from a male patient with ALL. Note the three copies of chromosomes 4, 6, 10, 14 and 17, the four copies of chromosome 21 and the additional X chromosome. This karyotype is associated with good prognosis in children.

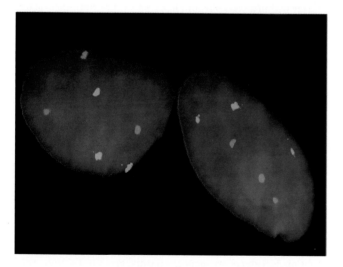

Figure 30.13 Two interphase nuclei from the bone marrow of an ALL patient with hyperdiploidy. The application of specific centromere probes has shown additional copies of chromosomes 10 and 17 indicated by the three red and green signals respectively.

Table 30.3 Significant chromosomal abnormalities in CLL.

Chromosomal abnormality	Genes	Genes	Incidence (%)
t(2;14)(p13;q32)	Bcl-11A	IgH	< 1
del(6q)			6
del(11q)			18
trisomy 12			16
del(13q)	RB1		55
t(14;18)(q32;q22)	IgH	Bcl-2	< 1
del(17p)	p53		7
t(14;19)(q32;q13)	IgH	Bcl-3	< 1

affecting the *IgH* locus at 14q32 are rare in B CLL. The translocation t(14;19)(q32;q13) has been reported in a number of cases. In view of the association with small lymphocytic lymphoma this is listed in the malignant lymphoma section. T-cell cases

(large granular lymphocytic leukaemia) may rarely have an inversion of chromosome 14, inv(14)(q11q32), and/or translocations involving 14q11, often accompanied by trisomy 7 and del(6q). Specifically in T-PLL, deletions or mutations of the *ATM* gene occur in association with abnormalities of 14q11.

Recent studies have shown that the mutational status of the *IgH* variable region (V_H) is an important prognostic factor in CLL. By comparison, trisomy 12 and del(13q) do not have independent prognostic significance. Abnormalities of 11q and 17p usually occur in patients with non mutated V_H genes and are associated with a shorter median treatment free interval and

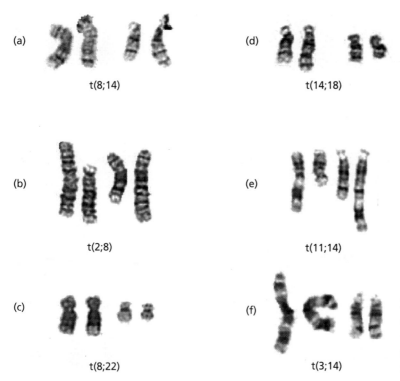

(a) t(8;14)

(b) t(2;8)

(c) t(8;22)

(d) t(14;18)

(e) t(11;14)

(f) t(3;14)

Figure 30.14 Partial karyograms from marrow cells of patients with Burkitt's lymphoma/mature B ALL (a–c) and NHL (d–f). The abnormal chromosomes are on the right. Note that the breakpoints involve the immunoglobulin genes in these karyotypes.

overall survival compared to patients with non mutated V_H genes who lack these genomic deletions.

Malignant lymphomas

Non-Hodgkin's lymphomas

Chromosomal analysis of lymph nodes in the non-Hodgkin's lymphomas (NHL) reveals 80–90% with karyotypic abnormalities. In patients with bone marrow involvement, the abnormal clone can frequently be found in bone marrow and peripheral blood cells. The prognosis of individual patients is highly dependent on clinical parameters including age, performance status and tumour burden. However, certain chromosomal abnormalities, while not disease specific, can provide additional prognostic information.

Burkitt's lymphoma

The cytogenetics of Burkitt's lymphoma are described above with mature B-cell ALL.

Non-Hodgkin's, non-Burkitt's lymphomas

The most consistent cytogenetic abnormalities in NHL are listed in Table 30.4. Follicular lymphoma, the most common B-cell malignancy, is associated with the translocation t(14;18)(q32;q21), which is found in ~90% cases (Figure 30.14d). The breakpoint on chromosome 14 occurs in the *IgH* locus within or directly

adjacent to a J_H segment. The breakpoints on chromosome 18 cluster within a 5.4-kb region flanking a transcriptionally active locus termed *Bcl-2*, also named *CCND2*, a putative oncogene which inhibits apoptosis (programmed cell death). The t(14;18) causes dysregulation and increased expression of *Bcl-2*, both by transcriptional activation and by abnormal post-transcriptional regulation of Bcl-2 mRNA, inhibiting apoptosis. Transformation of follicular lymphoma into a high-grade lymphoma is often accompanied by karyotypic evolution.

Mantle cell lymphoma is typically characterized by the proliferation of small lymphocyes with irregular nuclei, derived from the normal follicular mantle zone. The translocation t(11;14)(q13;q32) is the characteristic chromosomal abnormality seen in approximately 70% of cases (Figure 30.14e), sometimes in association with other abnormalities. The breakpoint on chromosome 14 is found within the J_H segment of the *IgH* gene, the breakpoints on chromosome 11 are clustered to within eight nucleotides of an oncogene termed *Bcl-1*, or *CCND1*, a cell cycle control element. The gene product, cyclin D1, is overexpressed. Dual fusion, dual-colour FISH with *IgH* and *Bcl-1* probes, has become the most sensitive method for detection of this translocation.

Small lymphocytic lymphoma or atypical CLL is associated with a t(14;19)(q32;q13). This involves the fusion of *IgH* with *Bcl-3*, a transcription factor normally located at 19q13.

Diffuse large-cell B-cell lymphomas (DLCL) are the most heterogeneous of lymphoma subtypes and can develop at different stages of B cell maturation. Up to 90% have clonal

Table 30.4 Significant chromosomal changes in NHL.

Chromosomal abnormality	Genes	Genes	Incidence (%)	Type
t(2;8)(p12;q24)	Igκ	c-MYC	100	Burkitt's
t(8;14)(q24;q32)	c-MYC	IgH	100	Burkitt's
t(8;22)(q24;q11)	c-MYC	Igλ	100	Burkitt's
t(2;3)(p12;q27)	Igκ	Bcl-6	10	DLCL
t(3;14)(q27;q32)	Bcl-6	IgH	10	DLCL
t(3;22)(q27;q11)	Bcl-6	Igλ	10	DLCL
t(2;5)(p23;q35)	ALK	NPM	72	Anaplastic large cell
7q			~40	SMZL, SLVL
t(9;14)(p13;q32)	PAX5	IgH		Lymphoplasmacytoid
t(11;14)(q13;q32)	Bcl-1	IgH	> 95	Mantle cell
t(11;18)(q21;q21)	AP12	MLT	30	Low-grade MALT
t(14;18)(q32;q21)	IgH	Bcl-2	> 90	Follicular
t(14;19)(q32;q13)	IgH	Bcl-3	> 1	

chromosomal abnormalities, of which ~50% are translocations involving *IgH*, whose most common partners are *Bcl-2* (20%), *c-MYC* (10%) and *Bcl-6* at 3q27 (7%) (Figure 30.14f). In contrast to *Bcl-2* and *c-MYC* rearrangements, which invariably involve the *Ig* loci, *Bcl-6* is frequently juxtaposed to non-*Ig* genes as a result of translocations with a variety of different partner chromosomes, occurring in up to 40% of DLCL. *Bcl-6* codes for a novel zinc finger protein sharing homologies with several known transcription factors. A further 5% of DLCL *Ig* translocations involve either the *Bcl-8* gene at 15q11, the *NFKB2* gene at 10q24 or a series of clustered genes at 1q21 which include *MUC1*. Chromosomal gains in DLCL include trisomies of chromosomes 3, 7, 11, 12 and 18. Chromosomal segments shown to be commonly amplified include the genes *Bcl-2, c-MYC, REL* (2p) *GLI, CDK4* and *MDM2* (12q), while commonly deleted regions include 1p, 1q, 3p, 3q, 6q and 7q. Although the presence of *Bcl-2* gene translocations has no prognostic significance, overexpression of Bcl-2 protein, which may occur in the absence of *Bcl-2* rearrangements, correlates with both short disease free and overall survival. Similarly, p53 mutations, overexpression of p27 and cyclin D3 with concurrent disruption of *p16(INK4a)*, p14 and *ARF* genes on 9p, correlate with aggressive disease and short survival.

Lymphoplasmacytoid lymphoma is associated with the t(9;14)(p13;q32), which juxtaposes the *PAX5* gene on chromosome 9 to the *IgH* gene, resulting in *PAX5* overexpression.

Anaplastic large-cell lymphoma is a specific morphological entity of T or null cell immunophenotype, with expression of CD30 and epithelial membrane antigen, occurring more frequently in childhood lymphoma. The translocation t(2;5)(p23;q35) is specific for this lymphoma type, and results in the fusion of the nucleophosmin (*NPM*) gene at 5q35 to the anaplastic lymphoma kinase gene (*ALK*) at 2p23, producing the NPM–ALK fusion protein. Rare variants have been described which involve *ALK* but not *NPM*.

Plasma cell dyscrasias (see also Chapter 41)

Multiple myeloma is a relatively common haematological malignancy in which the outlook for patients is poor. Detailed cytogenetic investigations of myeloma have increased in importance following the demonstration that they have prognostic significance. Chromosomal analysis is difficult owing to the small numbers and the low mitotic index of plasma cells in the bone marrow of these patients. With careful attention to culture times and conditions, successful cytogenetic results have been achieved, revealing highly complex karyotypes from which recurring chromosomal abnormalities have emerged. These include specific numerical changes giving rise to characteristic patterns of hyperdiploidy, with gains of chromosomes 3, 5, 7, 9, 11, 15, 18, 19 and 21, the loss of chromosome 13 and hypodiploidy. Hyperdiploidy is often accompanied by abnormalities of chromosome 1, specifically the unbalanced translocation, der(1;16)(q10;p10). The application of FISH techniques has substantially improved the interpretation of complex karyotypes and has shown that cytogenetic analysis alone underestimates the incidence of chromosomal abnormalities in myeloma.

The most significant structural chromosomal changes in myeloma, as shown in Table 30.5, are rearrangements involving the switch regions of the *IgH* gene with other partners at a high incidence of 75%. Four of these appear to be significant primary rearrangements. These are *CCND1* (*Bcl-1*) in the translocation t(11;14)(q13;q32); two genes *FGFR3* and *MMSET*, which are simultaneously involved in t(4;14)(p16;q32); to a lesser extent *c-MYC* in t(8;14)(q24;q32), *IRF4* in t(6;14)(p25;q32) and *MAF* in the t(14;16)(q32;q23).

Monosomy 13 and deletions of the long arm, specifically involving the chromosomal band 13q14, also frequently occur in myeloma. They are associated with a poor prognosis, particularly in association with raised serum β_2-microglobulin levels,

Table 30.5 Significant chromosomal abnormalities in myeloma.

Chromosomal abnormality	Genes	Genes	Incidence (%)
t(4;14)(p16;q32)	FGFR3/MMSET	IgH	15
t(6;14)(p25;q32)	IRF4	IgH	15
t(8;14)(q24;q32)	c-MYC	IgH	5
t(11;14)(q13;q32)	CCND1	IgH	16
t(14;16)(q32;q23)	IgH	MAF	5
del(13q)			40–80

and the progression of monoclonal gammopathy of undetermined significance (MGUS) to myeloma. As a result of these significant findings, interphase FISH has now become the method of choice for the detection of *IgH* rearrangements and deletions involving 13q14. The same chromosomal changes have been identified from cytogenetic and FISH analysis of MGUS, plasma-cell leukaemia and systemic monoclonal immunoglobulin light chain amyloidosis.

Summary

Cytogenetic analysis of the malignant cells of patients with haematological malignancies has contributed to advances in diagnosis, prognosis and patient management. The results have impinged on treatment, leading to an improved outlook for a significant number of patients. The development of molecular cytogenetic techniques has overcome some of the limitations of G-banded cytogenetic analysis and has offered opportunities to uncover abnormalities not identified by conventional methods. Chromosomal and genetic probes have added a new dimension to chromosome analysis, enabling the detection of subtle chromosomal changes in DNA and RNA from malignant tissues and extending chromosome analysis to interphase cells. These advances have led to a considerable expansion in the scientific knowledge of haematological malignancies. From the discovery of many leukaemia-specific cytogenetic changes, subsequent sequencing and cloning of the genes involved has uncovered a variety of biochemical pathways involved in leukaemogenesis, to which specific therapy is beginning to be targeted. Continued interaction of cytogenetics and molecular biology promises to lead to the detection of many more leukaemia-specific genes and continue the contribution to a better understanding of leukaemogenesis.

Selected bibliography

Bergsagel PL, Kuehl WM (2001) Chromosome translocations in multiple myeloma. *Oncogene* **20**: 5611–22.

Grimwade D (2001) The clinical significance of cytogenetic abnormalities in acute myeloid leukaemia. *Best Practice and Research in Clinical Haematology* **14**: 497–529.

Harrison CJ, Foroni L (2002) Cytogenetics and molecular genetics of acute lymphoblastic leukemia. *Review of Clinical and Experimental Hematology* **6**: 91–113.

Heim S, Mitelman F (1995) *Cancer Cytogenetics*, 2nd edn. Wiley-Liss, New York.

ISCN (1995) *An International System for Human Cytogenetic Nomenclature*, pp. 1–114. Karger, Basle.

Oscier DG, Gardiner AC (2001) Lymphoid neoplasms. *Best Practice and Research in Clinical Haematology* **14**: 609–30.

Rabbitts TH (1994) Chromosomal translocations in human cancer. *Nature* **372**: 143–9.

Secker-Walker LM (1997) *Chromosomes and Genes in Acute Lymphoblastic Leukaemia*. Chapman & Hall, New York.

CHAPTER 31

Acute myeloid leukaemia

Alan K Burnett

Epidemiology of disease

Acute myeloid leukaemia (AML) has an incidence of 2–3 per 100 000 per annum in children, rising to 15 per 100 000 in older adults. It can occur at all ages but has its peak incidence in the seventh decade (Figure 31.1). The incidence does not appear to be increasing beyond that expected in an ageing population. The fact that most cases occur in older patients has important implications for treatment strategies, in that biological variation associated with chemoresistance and comorbidity, which limits treatment options, increases with age.

Pathophysiology

The more carefully AML is studied, the clearer it becomes that there is considerable heterogeneity between cases with respect to morphology, immunological phenotype, associated cytogenetic and molecular abnormalities and, more recently, patterns of gene expression. This is reflected in the substantially different responses to treatment. Some entities are becoming so distinct that they are regarded as different diseases with specific approaches to treatment.

Acute myeloid leukaemia is a malignant clonal disorder of immature cells in the haemopoietic hierarchical system. Leukaemic transformation is assumed to occur in many cases at, or near, the level of the haemopoietic stem cell before it has embarked on any lineage commitment. Some cases may originate at a slightly later stage in cells that are committed to lineage differentiation. These cells have abnormal function characterized by a failure to progress through the expected differentiation programme and/or to die by the process of apoptosis. Associated with this may be the retention of the stem cell characteristic of self-renewal. This leads to the accumulation of a clone of cells, which dominates bone marrow activity and leads to marrow failure. The potential for arrest of haemopoiesis at different time points partially

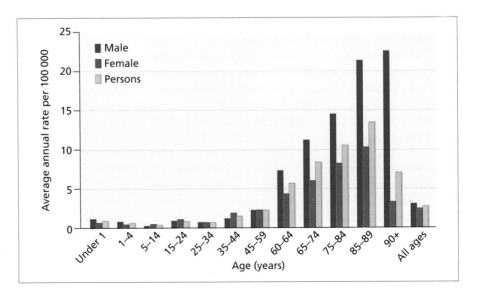

Figure 31.1 Age distribution of AML in the population of Wales: a population study.

explains why there can be such a variation in the leukaemic or 'blast' population characterizing the individual case. Adenopathy or organomegaly can occur but are not usual features. Extramedullary disease can occur, including cerebrospinal infiltration, but this is not usual, unlike in lymphoblastic leukaemias. Similarly, most patients present with low peripheral blood counts. While in the majority of cases no direct cause is found, there is an association with irradiation, smoking, some rare congenital abnormalities and chemical exposure. Perhaps the most frequently identified cause is progression from other myeloproliferative disorders, e.g. myelodysplasia, or as a consequence of prior chemotherapy for another malignancy.

Non-random chromosome abnormalities are found in the majority of cases. These may be structural (gain or loss of material) or reciprocal balanced translocations. The significance of these changes is developing at a steady pace and will be discussed below as far as the clinical implications are concerned.

Several molecular changes have also been discovered, either by association with the known cytogenetic abnormalities or somewhat by chance (Table 31.1). There is a variable level of proof at this stage as to whether the recognized molecular abnormalities are sufficient in themselves to cause leukaemia. The most common molecular mutation associated with AML has been found in the FLT receptor.

FMS-like tyrosine-3 (FLT-3) is a member of the platelet-derived growth factor receptor (PDGF-R) subfamily or receptor kinases and is most similar to FMS, KIT and the PDGF receptors. The receptor is expressed in haemopoietic cells restricted to the CD34-positive fraction and a CD34-negative subfraction of dendritic cell precursors. It is also expressed on neural tissues. Normal FLT-3 receptor is expressed on AML blasts in most cases and can be overexpressed or asynchronously expressed in that it can be expressed not strictly in association with CD34 expression. Most mutations are present in the juxtamembrane domain of the receptor and comprise internal tandem repeats of variable size that are always in frame and therefore expressed. Such mutations are found in approximately 25% of AML cases. Additional point mutations have been found on the activation loop of the interrupted kinase domain, usually at aspartate-835. The consequence of these mutations are activation of the receptor by phosphorylation, which promotes proliferation and resistance to apoptosis. Not only is the mutation the commonest mutation in AML, but a large clinical experience confirms that it is strongly predictive of relapse. Mutations are associated with high white cell counts and blast percentage at diagnosis. They are not uniformly distributed across the FAB or cytogenetic subgroups, being rare in FAB M0, M6 and M7 and most common in M3. The incidence is highest in patients with t(15;17), trisomy 8 and normal karyotype and uncommon in other favourable groups and in virtually all poor-risk cytogenetic groups.

There is an increasing belief that most tumours are a result of multiple 'hits' or molecular changes and that a single change may be insufficient to cause the full leukaemic phenotype. In AML, the phenotype is a consequence of both a proliferative lesion and a failure of differentiation, and it seems probable that molecular abnormalities which affect both functions are required. This understanding is already leading to the concept of therapeutic agents which inhibit the molecular consequences of these abnormalities.

Disease classification

The disease is confirmed by an excess of primitive 'blast' cells in the bone marrow, originally in the FAB classification required to be at least 30%. The French–American–British (FAB) morphological classification has been useful in developing a common vocabulary, but has little predictive value with the widespread use of genetic markers. The new system now recognizes 11 subtypes (see Chapter 29). Quality cytochemistry can provide valuable additional diagnostic information. Further precision can be added by immunophenotyping. Although widely used, in many cases where high-quality morphology and cytochemistry is available it is not strictly required to confirm the diagnosis as AML. As will be discussed later, the leukaemic blasts may demonstrate an 'aberrant' immunophenotype which can have potential use in monitoring response to treatment.

Cytogenetics (see also Chapter 30)

The recognition of non-random chromosome abnormalities associated with the various types of AML has had a major impact on the understanding of disease and has opened the way to unravel the molecular genetic defects and aids in the appropriate choice of treatment. A typical range of the more common abnormalities is shown in Figure 31.2. Some of the consequential molecular changes have been carefully investigated and, in the case of some of the reciprocal translocations, the molecular breakpoints have been cloned. Some of these are illustrated in Table 31.1.

The morphological, cytogenetic, immunological and molecular abnormalities are frequently associated as illustrated in Table 31.2. This, together with clinical response data, has led to a recognition that a predominantly morphological classification is no longer adequate to define some subsets which are better recognized as distinct clinically relevant entities based on cytogenetics. This has resulted in a new classification devised on behalf of the World Health Organization (WHO) (Chapter 29). Another key change in the revision is that the lower threshold blast percentage in the bone marrow is now set at 20%. From a therapeutic point of view, this transfers the proportion of patients with myelodysplastic syndrome [subgroup – refractory anaemia with excess blasts in transformation (RAEBt)] to acute leukaemia. It is still to be convincingly shown that these patients will benefit from a 'leukaemia approach' to their management.

Table 31.1 Examples of genes involved in cytogenetic abnormalities found in AML (adapted from Caligiuri *et al.* 1997).

Cytogenetic abnormality	Genes involved (gene activation)	Protein	FAB type
inv(3)(q21;q26)	*Ribophorin 1* (3q21)	RER transmembrane glycoprotein	MDS, M0, M1, M2, M4,
	EVI1 (3q26)	Multiple zinc fingers	M5, M6, M7
t(3;3)(q21;q26)	*Ribophorin 1* (3q21)	RER transmembrane glycoprotein	MDS, M1, M2, M4, M6
	EVI1 (3q26)	Multiple zinc fingers	
t(1;11)(p32;q23)	*AF1p* (1p32)	Murine eps 15 homologue	M0, M5
	ALL1 (11q23)	*Drosophilia* trithorax homologue	
t(1;11)(q21;q23)	*AF1q* (1q21)	No homology to any known protein	M4
	ALL1 (11q23)	*Drosophilia* trithorax homologue	
t(3;21)(q26;q22)	*EVI1* (3q26)	Multiple zinc fingers	MDS
	AML1 (21q22)	CBF-α *Drosophilia* runt homologue	
t(3;21)(q26;q22)	*EAP* (3q26)	Ribosomal protein L22	MDS
	AML1 (21q22)	*Drosophila* runt homologue	
t(6;9)(p23;q34)	*DEK* (6p23)	Nuclear protein	MDS, M1, M2, M4
	CAN (9q34)	Nucleoporin	
t(6;11)(q27;q23)	*AF6* (6q27)	GLGF motif	M4, M5
	ALL1 (11q23)	*Drosophilia* trithorax homologue	
t(7;11)(p15;p15)	*HOXA9* (7p15)	Class I homeobox	MDS, M2, M4
	NUP98 (11p15)	Nucleoporin	
t(8;21)(q22;q22)	*ETO* (8q22)	Zinc finger	MDS, M2
	AML1 (21q22)	CBF-α *Drosophilia* runt homologue	
t(9;11)(p22;q23)	*AF9* (9p22)	Nuclear protein, ENL homology	M4, M5
	ALL1 (11q23)	*Drosophilia* trithorax homologue	
t(10;11)(p12;q23)	*AF10* (p12)	Leucine zipper; zinc finger	
	ALL1 (11q23)	*Drosophila* trithorax homologue	M4, M5
+11	*ALL1* (11q23)	*Drosophila* trithorax homologue	M1, M2
t(11;17)(q23;q21)	*ALL1* (11q23)	*Drosophila* trithorax homologue	
	AF17 (17q21)	Leucine zipper; zinc finger	M5
t(11;19)(q23;p13.1)	*ALL1* (11q23)	*Drosophila* trithorax homologue	
	ELL (19p13.1)	Transcription enhancer	M4, M5
t(11;19)(q23;p13.3)	*ALL1* (11q23)	*Drosophila* trithorax homologue	
	ENL (19p13.3)	Transcription factor	M4, M5
t(12;22)(p13;q11)	*TEL* (12p13)	ETS-related transcription factor	
	MN1 (22q11)	Nuclear protein	MDS, M1, M4, M7
t(15;17)(q22;q11–12)	*PML* (15q21)	Zinc finger	
	RARα (17q21)	Retinoic acid receptor-α	M3
inv(16)(p13;q22)	*MYH11* (16p13)	Smooth muscle myosin heavy chain	
	CBFβ (16q22)	Heterodimerizes with AML1	M4Eo
t(16;16)(p13;q22)	*MYH11* (16p13)	Smooth muscle myosin heavy chain	
	CBFβ (16q22)	Heterodimerizes with AML1	M4Eo
t(16;21)(p11;q22)	*FUS* (16p11)	RNA-binding protein	
	ERG (21q22)	ETS-related transcription factor	M1, M2, M4, M5

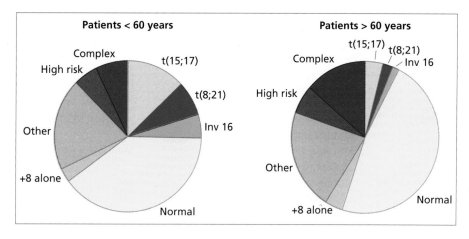

Figure 31.2 Distribution of common cytogenetic abnormalities in patients aged less than or more than 60. Data derived from UK Medical Research Council Database after Grimwade *et al.* (1998, 2001).

Table 31.2 The association of morphology (FAB group) with cytogenetics, and immunophenotype in AML.

MIC group	FAB	Immunological markers						Karyotype
		CD7	CD19	CD13	CD33	GPA	CD41	
M2/t(8;21)	M2	–	–	+	+	–	–	t(8;21)(q22;q22)
M3/t(15;17)	M3, M3v	–	–	+	+	–	–	t(15;17)(q22;q12)
M5a/del(11q23)	M5a (M5b, M4)	–	–	+	+	–	–	t/del(11)(q23)
M4Eo/inv(16)	M4Eo	–	–	+	+	–	–	del/inv(16)(q23)
M1/t(9;22)	M1 (M2)	–	–	+	+	–	–	t(9;22)(q34;q11)
M2/t(6;9)	M2 or M4 with basophilia	–	–	+	+	–	–	t(6;9)(p21–22;q34)
M1/inv(3)	M1 (M2, M4, M7) with thrombocytosis	–	–	+	+	–	–	inv(3)(q21;q26)
M5b/t(8;16)	M5b with phagocytosis	–	–	+	+	–	–	t(8;16)(p11;p13)
M2Baso/t(12p)	M2 with basophilia	–	–	+	+	–	–	t/del(12)(p11–13)
M4/+4	M4 (M2)	–	–	+	+			+4

*+, Positive; –, negative; no symbol, not specified by MIC Workshop.
Abbreviations: FAB, French–American–British Classification; TdT, terminal deoxynucleotidyl transferase; GPA, glycophorin A.

Treatment

Aspirations for treatment

Given the age distribution of patients who will present with the disease, it must first be decided what the goals of treatment are in an individual patient. In young people, there is little doubt that there is the prospect of significant benefit to be gained from an intensive approach. With increasing age, which is often associated with comorbidity and less responsive disease, the balance of benefit changes to a more palliative approach. Much of what is known about the prospects of successful treatment is derived from large clinical trials. In young patients, these results are usually representative of what can be expected for any age-matched patients. However, only a selected minority of older patients (aged > 60 years) will enter trials, so trial-derived information may be less transferable to the whole population in this age group. A substantial majority of older patients are not considered fit for the usual intensive approach and the priority for such patients is palliative care, optimization of quality of life and minimal hospitalization. Examination of survival in population studies illustrates the dominant effect of age (Figure 31.3).

Treatment strategy

The initial clinical priority is to apply chemotherapy to improve marrow function by inducing complete remission (CR). Conceptually, this means an approximate two log reduction in tumour burden. This becomes compatible with a bone marrow which appears normal morphologically and is functionally able to produce normal numbers of circulating cells. The traditional

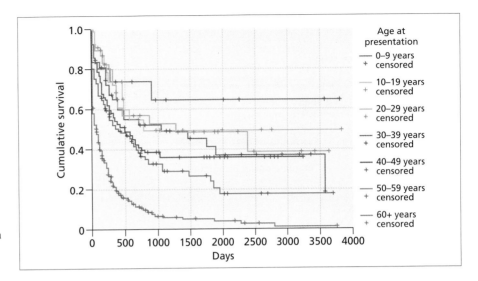

Figure 31.3 Survival of AML in relation to patient age. Data from a Welsh population database.

consensus definition of CR is based on these premises, i.e. < 5% blast cells in a cellular marrow durable for at least 28 days with a peripheral neutrophil count of $1.5 \times 10^9/L$ and platelet count of $> 100 \times 10^9/L$, and absence of extramedullary disease. In some cases, these criteria may be met but the morphology is dysplastic. It is not clear whether this is associated with a greater risk of relapse. Similarly, some patients meet the marrow criteria but do not achieve full peripheral regeneration. In some circumstances, these features may represent a pre-existing dysplastic state; in others it may represent the effects of overtreatment of that particular individual. In the former case, this may have adverse connotations while in the latter it represents optimum treatment. As more sophisticated molecular techniques have become available, it is clear that it is still possible to detect residual disease when all morphological and functional criteria are met. Such techniques (RT-PCR) are capable of detection at a level of 1 in 10^4 or 1 in 10^5 residual cells, but such markers are available for only a minority of cases in which the molecular lesion has been characterized (see also Chapter 34). When it is possible (i.e. in an individual who is heterogeneous for an X-linked marker) to use molecular markers of clonality, it has been noted that in some cases marrow remissions are clonal when they would be expected to represent both alleles of the clonal marker. Sometimes the molecular signature is that of the same clone as the leukaemic cells, suggesting that what the remission represents is a precursor or differentiated state of the malignant clone. It has also been noted that clonal remissions may be derived from the uninvolved allele.

Clinical experience has demonstrated that further intensive post-remission treatment is required to 'consolidate' CR. This is delivered at the same intensity as induction, to achieve further cytoreduction. Under these circumstances, it is possible to achieve disease levels that are beyond the level of molecular detection. It is not clear how many intensive consolidation courses are required, but two or three are generally used in younger patients, and a stem cell transplant may be included. Where intensive induction and consolidation can be given, e.g. in younger patients, maintenance chemotherapy is not required. A pictorial description of treatment is shown in Figure 31.4.

Treatment details

Induction of remission

The backbone of treatment for 30 years has been the combination of daunorubicin and cytosine arabinoside (Ara-C). Usually daunorubicin is given for 3 days in a dose of 45–50 mg/m². Ara-C is given for 7–10 days as a continuous infusion or by bolus doses of 100–200 mg/m²/day. Many clinical trials have been conducted which have tested variations of this standard of care. Alternatives to daunorubicin (adriamycin, mitoxantrone, idarubicin, aclarubicin) or different doses have not yet been shown to be superior overall, although current studies are exploring higher anthracycline doses. Idarubicin may achieve a better quality of remission, as reflected in a reduced relapse risk in younger patients, but it is more myelosuppressive and limits the intensity of consolidation treatment. In general, on a dose-equivalent basis, daunorubicin remains the anthracycline of choice. Higher doses (3 g/m²) of Ara-C in induction have been tested in recent years, with mixed results and no convincing evidence of overall benefit. Intermediate doses (400 mg/m²/day versus 200 mg/m²/day) have recently been tested in younger patients without demonstrating a difference.

Comparison of induction treatment is not simply measured by the rate of remission. By achieving a greater degree of cytoreduction, without necessarily getting more patients into CR, one treatment may be superior because it results in less subsequent relapses (Figure 31.4). The beneficial effect of the addition of a third drug to the induction combination has some evidence to support it. This will usually be etoposide or thioguanine. A large comparative study did not show any difference between these

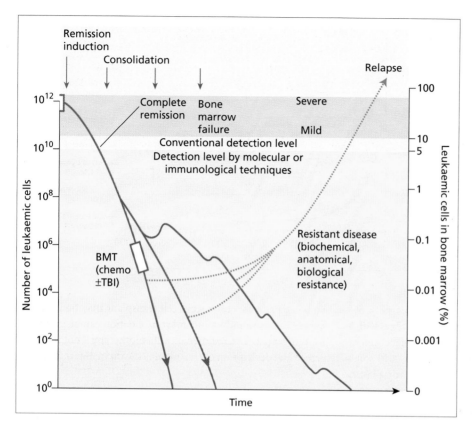

Figure 31.4 Diagnostic presentation of treatment strategy.

two drugs when used at the third drug in combination with daunorubicin and Ara-C. The majority of patients who are going to enter remission will do so after one course of treatment. If an incomplete response is obtained then a second course of the same combination is indicated. A further group will enter remission, but these patients have thus shown themselves to have less sensitive disease, and this is reflected in a modestly increased risk of relapse later. If patients fail to achieve a substantial reduction in marrow blasts in the first course or fail to enter complete remission with a second course, they should be considered refractory to the drugs used up to that point and transferred to an alternative treatment schedule.

Supportive care (see also Chapter 36)
It is unusual for induction chemotherapy not to clear most of the leukaemic blasts; however, this is at a cost of 3–4 weeks of severe pancytopenia. Several components of supportive care have to be in place during this period. Careful monitoring of biochemical parameters of renal and hepatic function and coagulation is required. Central venous access is now considered essential, together with high-quality and readily available blood product support.

A priority is the prevention and management of infection. Most patients will receive prophylactic oral antibiotics and antifungals to minimize the risk of infection during the neutropenic period, although the routine use of the latter can still be debated. Since hospital-acquired infections are becoming an increasing problem, it can be safer for the patient to be at home provided that close monitoring can be undertaken in the day hospital and that rapid readmission to specialist care is available.

In spite of prophylactic measures, most patients will become febrile during neutropenia. This must be considered as an indication of a serious, and potentially fatal, infection. The common pathogens are staphylococcal, caused by the use of central catheters, and, increasingly, fungal infections – *Candida* and *Aspergillus*, which are related to the duration of severe neutropenia which results from the more intensive chemotherapy now used. Particular patterns of infection will be determined within individual institutions, which will dictate the particular approach to empirical antimicrobial intervention. Fungal infections are a particular problem, not only related to more intensive treatment, but because of continuous building works which are a usual feature of hospital environments. Guidance on intervention should not only be literature evidence based but should incorporate local microbiological issues, as exemplified in Figure 31.5. Nursing expertise is an essential component. It seems probable that improvements in remission rates in recent years can largely be attributed to better supportive care and nursing skills which have enabled more intensive treatment to be given safely.

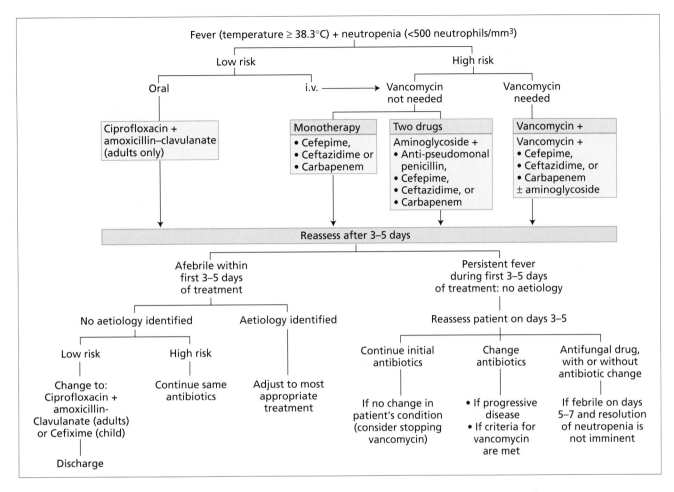

Figure 31.5 Management of febrile neutropenia (adapted from Hughes *et al.* 2002).

Recombinant growth factors (G-CSF or GM-CSF) have a potential use in two respects. If they can curtail the duration of neutropenia there will be less risk of death during the aplastic phase following induction chemotherapy. This may increase the rate of remission. Second, as many leukaemia cells exhibit receptors for these growth factors, it may be possible to pretreat the patient with growth factor to bring the leukaemic cells into the cell cycle and thereby make them more susceptible to chemotherapy. Extensive studies using G-CSF or GM-CSF to curtail neutropenia have been carried out. Some general conclusions can be made. The duration of neutropenia can be reduced by a few days, but it is less easy to demonstrate a reduction in episodes of febrile neutropenia. There is generally no improvement in remission rate. Growth factor use has not increased leukaemic growth or involved relapse.

The reasons for incorporating growth factors or not into routine practice are primarily economic. Their use may enable patients to leave hospital earlier. If the local policy is to hospitalize patients during neutropenia, this may save resources. Fewer studies have been carried out to see whether growth factor

'priming' of the leukaemic population would be advantageous. They have generally been unsuccessful but a recent positive study may rekindle interest in this approach.

Results of induction treatment

With this approach to treatment, 50–85% of patients will achieve remission. Of those who do, about 70% will require one course. A number of factors influence the prospects of achieving remission. Age is a dominant and independent risk factor and a continuous variable. Eighty per cent of patients < 60 years will achieve CR, but this prospect diminishes with age (Table 31.3). Clinical performance score at diagnosis is also highly predictive. In younger patients, fewer patients tend to present with poorer performance scores so this prognostic factor does not move the overall remission rate to any great extent. A larger proportion of older patients will have a poorer risk score and therefore the score has more predictive impact. The distribution of cytogenetic subtypes is related to age, with more responsive subtypes more frequently seen in younger patients and less responsive patients, aggregating in older patients. Tumour burden at

Age	< 35	35–55	55–60	61–65	66–70	71–75	75+
Complete remission (%)	88	82	77	62	63	48	59

Table 31.3 Relationship of complete remission rate to patient age. Patients were all given intensive chemotherapy (data derived from the UK Medical Research Council AML Trial database).

diagnosis, as represented by white blood count, serum albumin or lactate dehydrogenase (LDH) levels, will adversely impact on response to induction treatment. It is now possible to measure a number of proteins in the leukaemic blasts which are involved in drug efflux. These 'resistance' proteins, for example P-gp, tend to be more frequent in older patients, and to correlate with a lower remission rate. If patients have had an antecedent haematological disorder, e.g. myelodysplasia, the remission rate will be about 20% lower than in age-matched groups. About 10–25% of patients embarking on intensive induction chemotherapy will die during the aplastic phase from non-leukaemic causes, which is essentially a failure of supportive care. Induction deaths tend to be associated with the adverse features already mentioned.

Consolidation treatment

Having achieved remission, the priority is to prevent relapse. Optimization of induction treatment is still required as it will influence the quality of remission and thereby the subsequent rate of relapse. Three options are available for younger patients once remission has been achieved – further chemotherapy at induction level of intensity; chemotherapy with autologous stem cell transplantation; or allogeneic stem cell transplant with or without prior chemotherapy. Chemotherapy will usually involve a further two or three chemotherapy courses. At this point in the treatment, there is a theoretical logic in using different drugs to minimize the risk of selecting chemoresistant leukaemic clones. Combinations, using Ara-C at increased dosage, amsacrine, etoposide and alternative anthracyclines, are often used (Figure 31.6). Few studies have made direct comparisons between specific combinations, but rather they try to work out how many consolidation courses are needed. Two or three courses that are intensive enough to induce 3–4 weeks' neutropenia appears to be achievable but is reaching the limit of tolerability and compliance. High-dose Ara-C (3 g/m^2 on alternate days over 5 days) has been shown to be superior to lower doses (400 mg/m^2 or 100 mg/m^2), but no studies have so far studied intermediate Ara-C doses, which may be just as effective with less toxicity. It has been suggested that high-dose Ara-C is more effective in the most responsive subtypes of disease i.e. those with lower risk disease, based on cytogenetic prognostic markers. Overall, 50–55% of younger patients who enter remission will relapse – usually within the first 2 years. In older patients, the risk is much higher, at 80%.

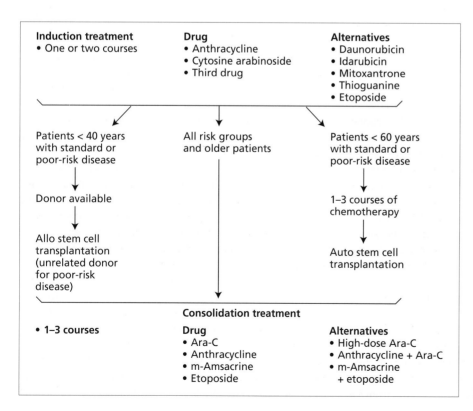

Figure 31.6 Treatment options in AML.

Allogeneic stem cell transplantation

There is little doubt that the most effective way to prevent leukaemic relapse in younger patients is allogeneic transplantation from an HLA-compatible sibling donor. Most of the extensive data available are derived from patients in whom the graft was of bone marrow. In these circumstances, the relapse risk will be reduced from 45% to about 20%. As there are non-leukaemic causes of death, the overall expectation of cure for recipients of allo-BMT is around 60%. Some of these survivors will have morbidities that survivors of chemotherapy will avoid, and this needs to be taken into account when advising patients. As the risk of transplant complications, graft-versus-host disease (GvHD) and infections, in particular, increases with age, this approach is normally limited to patients under 45 years, although the precise age cut-off remains controversial and will be a matter of the relative risk of the transplant, and of disease recurrence.

Some transplant-related factors may predict for a more favourable outcome, such as a male donor, a cytomegalovirus (CMV)-negative donor when the host is CMV negative and a higher cell count in the graft, and so influence the decision to undergo the treatment. The extent to which the high-dose preparative regimen that is necessary to ensure engraftment or the immunological reactivity of the donor marrow via donor T cells eliminates residual leukaemia has been debated extensively. At least some contribution from the immunological effect of 'graft-versus-leukaemia' is assumed. Experience with donors who are mismatched at more than one HLA locus has not been encouraging, but using fully matched unrelated donors has become more reliable, particularly with the development of molecular methods of tissue typing. In expert hands, in carefully selected young patients, this approach may be equivalent to having a sibling donor.

Once remission has been achieved there is probably no definite requirement to administer more than one course of consolidation chemotherapy before the allograft. But this usually happens because of the time required to identify a donor and make the necessary arrangements for the transplant. It does not appear that variations in transplantation protocols have a major effect on overall survival, e.g. choice of myeloablative schedule, GvHD prophylaxis or whether bone marrow or peripheral blood is the source of stem cells.

Because the applicability of transplant is limited, by treatment-related complications, to younger patients, and yet has a very powerful anti-leukaemic effect, there is recent interest as to whether a non-ablative allogeneic transplant will have a role for older patients. This approach does not require the traditional intensive treatment to ablate the host marrow but provides enough immunosuppression to enable the donor stem cells to engraft. Over a period of weeks, the host haemopoiesis becomes donor, i.e. changes from host to mixed to donor chimerism. Other clinical indications have demonstrated that full chimeric engraftment in older patients can be achieved with treatment modalities that are not ablative to the bone marrow. The hope is that this provides sufficient graft-versus-leukaemia (GvL) effect. In AML, in a conventional allogeneic transplant, it is not clear how important the GvL effect is, so it remains to be seen whether non-ablative transplants have a role in consolidation of AML in older patients.

Autologous stem cell transplantation

(see also Chapter 25)

For younger patients who lack donors, harvesting stem cells from the bone marrow or peripheral blood during remission and using them after a period of cryopreservation for haematological rescue after myeloablative chemo-radiotherapy has been widely used. This approach has also been shown to be a more effective way of preserving remission compared with chemotherapy. The treatment-related mortality is lower (5–10%) than with allogeneic transplant, but it lacks a GvL mechanism so the relapse risk is higher (around 35–40%). This results in an overall survival of 50–55% of those who receive this approach. Because the complications are not particularly age related, patients up to their mid-50s can safely undergo this procedure, but the results of autologous transplant in older patients (over 60 years) is not encouraging.

Patients who receive the autograft early in remission (e.g. within 3 months) do less well than those treated at 3–6 months because of a higher relapse rate. This may reflect patient selection, but it has also been interpreted to mean that, for an autograft to be successful, consolidation chemotherapy beforehand has an important role in cytoreduction of leukaemia cells before the marrow is harvested, so-called 'in vivo' purging of disease. Initially there was concern that returning stem cells to patients would be illogical unless efforts were made to eliminate contaminating leukaemia cells first – so called 'ex-vivo' purging. Various chemical, cellular and immunologically based techniques were used without clear evidence of benefit. Most clinical experience was gained using 'unpurged' bone marrow supporting myeloablative chemoradiotherapy, which was usually cyclophosphamide with total body irradiation or busulphan with cyclophosphamide.

One of the problems with the use of autologous bone marrow has been delayed peripheral blood count recovery, particularly of platelets. This seems to be a feature of AML and is less obvious in other disease indications. Recent attention has turned to using peripheral blood or combining peripheral blood and marrow stem cells to ameliorate this problem. This has improved haemopoietic recovery but may be associated with an increased risk of relapse, thus giving no overall survival advantage.

Comparison of consolidation options

For patients under 55 or 60 years, all three treatment options are available, so the dilemma is which treatment approach to take. About 45% of patients entering remission will survive with chemotherapy alone. Of those who receive an allogeneic or autologous stem cell transplant, 55–60% and 50%, respectively, will survive. Patients who receive a transplant are not equivalent to patients receiving chemotherapy alone. They have survived long enough to receive the transplant, whereas those who could not have the transplant may not have done so because they relapsed. Some studies demonstrate that 40% of patients with a donor do not receive an allograft.

Another less frequently considered option is to delay the transplant until there is disease recurrence. Primary treatment of relapse with transplantation is associated with a high rate of failure, so it is necessary to establish a second remission first. It is possible, however, to salvage overall about 15% of patients who relapse from chemotherapy. Based on risk factors, it is possible to define those patients who, if they relapse, are likely to enter a second remission. In this subgroup the transplant can therefore be delayed because, if first-line treatment does fail, a second CR can be reliably obtained and a transplant delivered. If there is a low chance of second remission, there is a stronger case for transplant as part of first-line treatment.

Several prospective randomized trials have compared chemotherapy with autologous transplantation and allograft with chemotherapy. In the latter case, these comparisons are not truly randomized comparisons but rather comparing patients who are found to have donors – and assumed to be intended to receive an allograft – with those for whom no donor is found. This 'donor versus no-donor' comparison is a substitute for the randomization. Although the conclusions are not universal, and in spite of the superior ability of autograft to reduce the risk of relapse, there have been no differences in survival between these approaches. When those with donors are then compared overall there is only a modest survival benefit in favour of allotransplant. When the cytogenetic risk of relapse is taken into account, as will be discussed below, it would appear that transplantation is not required for good-risk patients, and in the absence of an emerging improvement for poor-risk patients allogeneic transplant including from unrelated donors is the chosen approach. There is a prospect that chemotherapy may continue to improve so the question of whether allograft will continue to be the best option for standard-risk patients remains open.

Factors influencing the risk of relapse

As treatment of disease in younger patients has improved, so the heterogeneity of disease has also become apparent with respect to differences in relapse risk. On multivariate analysis a number of factors have emerged that can predict the risk of relapse irrespective of treatment schedules used, including stem cell transplantation.

Cytogenetics (see also Chapter 30)

Patients with t(8;21) and inv(16) have a high remission rate, a lower risk of relapse and a higher rate of second remission, and have a 5-year survival of 65–75%. These patients tend to have

lower expression of the 'resistance proteins' and a low frequency of FLT-3 receptor mutations (to be described below). Acute promyelocytic leukaemia (APL) is now regarded as a separate entity which is uniquely responsive to retinoic acid. In most cases, the disease is characterized by t(15;17), which predicts sensitivity for a differentiation and apoptotic response to retinoic acid. These abnormalities are frequently associated with additional abnormalities such as –X or Y or 9q– in the case of t(8;21), and trisomy 8 in the case of t(15;17). These additional changes do not adversely affect the favourable prognosis. Similarly, the FLT-3 mutation is expressed in about 35% of APL cases but does not affect prognosis in this group of patients. Together, these good-risk patients make up about 25% of patients under 60 years (Figure 31.2), with a tendency to accumulate in the younger age groups. When good-risk patients occur in the older group, they continue to represent a more favourable group, with a survival of 35% compared with an overall survival of 15–20% in that age group in those treated with intensive chemotherapy.

About 15% of younger patients have cytogenetic abnormalities which are associated with a lower remission rate and a relapse risk on conventional chemotherapy of 85%. These can be identified as –5, del(5q), –7, abnormal 3q, t(9;22), and complex (more than three unrelated changes). Such patients need to be identified early because, even if a remission is achieved, it will be short-lived. Currently, transplantation represents the only viable treatment, but even that is associated with a high relapse risk.

Patients who do not fall into the categories described are regarded as standard risk. They have a 5-year survival of 40–45% (Figure 31.7). The impact of this risk stratification is apparent irrespective of chemotherapy used or whether patients receive an allograft or autograft. There are some minor discrepancies between published series, e.g. trisomy 8 and 11q23 are regarded as poor risk in some series. In larger series, it emerges that 11q23 cases with a t(10;11) rearrangement are poor risk (17% survival), whereas other series show in excess of 50% survival in younger patients.

In older patients, the overall survival of chemotherapy is around 15–20% at 5 years; it is therefore less easy to delineate cytogenetic risk subgroups. Adverse groups are more frequent, and favourable subgroups are less common. This in part accounts for the poorer prognosis of AML in older patients. It is still possible to derive a hierarchical risk stratification in the older patients based on similar criteria already described for younger patients. Some extremely poor subgroups can be identified (Figure 31.7b).

Age

Increasing age from children to the elderly who are given intensive chemotherapy is associated not only with a poorer chance of achieving remission but also with an increasing risk of relapse, even allowing for obvious differences in comorbidities and distribution of cytogenetic risk groups. Leukaemias in the elderly

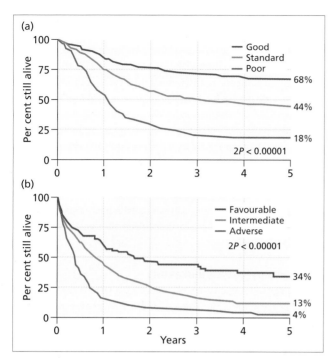

Figure 31.7 The impact of cytogenetic risk groups on treatment outcome. (a) The survival of patients aged < 60 years with good-risk abnormalities, t(8;21); inv (16); t(15;17), with or without other abnormalities. Poor risk is associated with changes involving chromosome 5 or 7, del 3q or complex abnormalities (more than three abnormalities). The standard-risk group comprises patients who do not have the abnormalities included in the good- or poor-risk categories. (b) The outcome for patients > 60 years old with these abnormalities who were treated with intensive chemotherapy. The relative proportion of those abnormalities in each age group is shown in Figure 31.2.

more frequently express the drug transport proteins associated with chemoresistance, as will be discussed below.

Response to induction chemotherapy

Patients who enter remission with the first course will have a lower relapse risk than those who require a further course. This has been recognized in various ways. For example, the presence of residual blasts in the bone marrow on day 14 can be used as a reason to give additional treatment. The blast percentage in the bone marrow assessed on recovery from the first treatment course has been shown to be highly predictive, i.e. patients who have more than 20% blasts, even though remission is subsequently achieved, will have a high relapse risk. Both cytogenetics and age are related to this response. When the morphological appearances are related to cytogenetic risk group, it is clear that, for good-risk patients, failure to clear the marrow with the first course is not an adverse feature, whereas in poor-risk patients even those who clear blasts in the first course will have a poor

Table 31.4 Relationship between blast status and cytogenetic group after course 1.

Cytogenetic group	CR (%)	PR (%)	RD (%)
Favourable	77	68	76
Standard	49	41	16
Poor	26	24	4

CR, complete remission; PR, partial remission; RD, resistant disease.

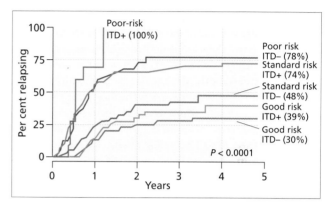

Figure 31.8 The impact of the presence of a *FLT-3* mutation on relapse risk in each of the risk groups as shown in Figure 31.7a. The presence of a mutation in good-risk patients is predominantly in the t(15;17) group but does not significantly change the relapse risk in good-risk patients.

prognosis. In standard cytogenetic risk patients, it is those who fail to clear the marrow that have an adverse risk. From such data, a risk definition incorporating cytogenetics and marrow response can be obtained which identifies the standard cytogenetic risk group that fails to clear the marrow in the poor-risk group (Table 31.4). This can be further related to age (Table 31.3), which suggests that the impact of older age is clearest in the standard risk patients who clear marrow blasts.

FLT-3 mutations

Not only has this mutation emerged as the most frequent in AML but several large series conclude that it is also a major prognostic factor, particularly for predicting relapse. It provides additional refinement to cytogenetic predictive groups (Figure 31.8). At the moment, there are insufficient data to suggest that patients with a mutation will benefit from a transplant.

Performance score

In older patients, standard assessments of performance vary considerably. These scores are highly predictive for induction treatment success, and also will inevitably relate to which patients are considered candidates for an intensive approach to treatment.

White blood count

High tumour load is an adverse feature for both induction and relapse risk. The threshold for risk is not definitive. A count of 50×10^9/L is often quoted. In subgroups a prognostic influence is apparent at much lower counts, e.g. in APL a white count at diagnosis of greater than 10×10^9/L is usually agreed as predictive of a higher relapse risk. The impact of a high white count is less than that of cytogenetics but may have isolated value when cytogenetics is not available.

Resistance proteins

One of the important biological differences between disease in the older patient and that in younger ones is the increased frequency in older patients of the expression of proteins involved in drug transport. These are associated with chemoresistance to some of the drugs used in AML, such as anthracyclines and etoposide. Expression also tends to be associated with a stem cell phenotype and adverse cytogenetics. The most widely studied is P glycoprotein (P-gp), which is an energy-dependent transporter protein product of the *MDR1* gene on chromosome 7 and which belongs to the ATP-binding cassette (ABC) transporter family. AML in older patients frequently overexpresses this protein, which has been shown to be predictive for inferior rates of remission and remission durations. The expression levels reported may vary in different series because of differences in techniques of measurement. Quantitative flow cytometry has brought a degree of consistency to measurement, but a functional assessment (of dye efflux) and blockage with P-gp inhibitor is also recommended. *In vitro* preclinical studies have demonstrated that available agents such as cyclosporin or its analogue PSC-833 can block P-gp function; however, only one trial to date has so far shown that using such agents has a clinical benefit. This may be because P-gp is not the only mechanism of chemoresistance.

MRP1 (multidrug resistance protein 1) is another ABC transporter family gene and is located on chromosome 16. Lung resistance protein (LRP) is a subunit of the major vault protein which has been identified in some anthracycline-resistant cell lines and appears to be involved in drug transport. LRP expression has been reported in 30–50% cases of AML in different series, but the majority of studies have been unable to show a correlation with response. MRP expression above normal can be found in 50% of patients with untreated AML, but there is no consensus on its impact on survival (see also Chapter 35).

The impact of prognostic factors on treatment choice

It is becoming routine to take into account the risk of relapse, as defined by some of the factors described, in order to target treatment. The most obvious example is the growing acceptance that transplantation is not required for patients with good-risk disease. Poor-risk patients must be identified promptly and offered either transplantation or some experimental approach since currently available chemotherapy is inadequate. Further data need regarding whether transplant, sibling or unrelated,

significantly benefits high-risk patients are needed. Similar information is also required about the significance of FLT-3 status with respect to the impact of transplantation. Children respond very well to intensive chemotherapy, with the majority enjoying prolonged remissions. Only the small number of children with high-risk features require a first-line transplant approach.

In older patients (> 60 years) either patients or doctors make a judgement at diagnosis as to whether intensive chemotherapy will be beneficial. Prognostic factors such as cytogenetics and performance score can inform this choice. Very poor-risk cytogenetics (e.g. complex changes) carries such a low prospect of success that the question arises as to whether such patients should receive intensive treatment even though they are considered fit enough.

Acute promyelocytic leukaemia

Acute promyelocytic leukaemia (APL) is a special case in which the presence of the t(15;17) predicts sensitivity to treatment with all-*trans*-retinoic acid (ATRA). It has been recognized for more than 20 years that this leukaemia subtype is sensitive to anthracyclines. Experience recently has clearly demonstrated that the combination of ATRA with chemotherapy has made a dramatic improvement, with survival now expected to exceed 80%. Even better prospects are becoming apparent when an anthracycline (idarubicin) and ATRA used together form the backbone of treatment. Simple maintenance with courses of ATRA with orally available agents such as methotrexate and 6-mercaptopurine has been shown in some studies to provide additional benefit. Since the molecular consequences of the t(15;17) are known, evaluation of the role of molecular monitoring is most developed in APL and provides a model for disease monitoring in AML.

Treatment in the older patient

Improvement in survival in older patients over the last 20 years has been much more elusive. With better supportive care, intensive chemotherapy can expect to achieve remission in 50–60% of cases. However, 80% of cases will relapse by 2 years. This result has been achieved with various combinations of induction and consolidation schedules and is not improved by maintenance to any great extent. There will be a greater interest in maintenance in future studies. Because the outcome is poor, two issues arise. Are there prognostic factors which confirm which patients will benefit from an intensive treatment approach? The data are less convincing than in younger patients, but younger age (60–70 years), higher performance score and favourable cytogenetic risk group can identify a minority of patients with a better than average outcome. However, several patients have adverse factors – older age, poorer performance score, complex cytogenetics or a chemoresistant phenotype. These patients will have a worse prognosis, which raises the issue of whether they should receive palliative care from the start. One modestly sized study compared a palliative treatment approach with conventional chemotherapy. It demonstrated that the use of intensive chemo-therapy, because it achieved remission, was more beneficial in older patients, but to date no study has been large enough to ask that question within the risk groups.

One strategy for improvement is to target the function of P-gp. Only one out of several studies using cyclosporin or its analogue has managed to improve survival in relapsed disease, but other studies combining it with first-line treatment have been unsuccessful. This may be because P-gp is not the only resistance mechanism present in leukaemic cells, and once a cell has become resistant by one mechanism there are already other resistance routes.

Minimal residual disease detection (see also Chapter 34)

The assumption behind assessing minimal residual disease is that it will add greater definition to risk prediction by the prog-nostic factors already recognized. However, early detection will first have to be validated clinically and then interventions in these situations proved to be superior to intervention at the time of haematological relapse.

Morphology, cytogenetics and fluorescence *in situ* hybri-dization (FISH) are relatively insensitive techniques to detect residual disease. It is possible, using a large panel of monoclonal antibodies, to delineate in 85% of cases an 'aberrant' immuno-phenotype at diagnosis. This will be overexpression of an antigen, co-expression of antigens normally associated with different stages of maturation which does not occur in novel haemo-poiesis, absence of myeloid antigen expression or expression of non-myeloid antigens.

This is complex and quite expensive technology, but it has been shown in modestly sized series that detection of cells with these phenotypes at a sensitivity of 1 in 10^4 or 1 in 10^5 is possible and can be predictive of relapse. That is, the persistent expres-sion of the aberrant phenotype found at diagnosis is associated with a higher relapse risk. Up to about half of remission cases can have aberrant expression, which trebles the risk of relapse.

Nucleic acid-based approaches involving RT-PCR have been used particularly in APL. The cloning of a number of break-points (Table 31.1) provides the opportunity to utilize a PCR-based approach. Most experience has been gained in APL cases using the PML–RAR-α hybrid protein as the target, with assays with a sensitivity of 1 in 10^4. A number of conclusions have emerged which currently influence clinical practice. If the RT-PCR remains positive after consolidation chemotherapy, the risk of relapse is high (> 70%). However, most of the relapses that subsequently occur are in patients who were found to be negat-ive after consolidation. The majority of patients are molecularly negative at this time point, but 20% will nevertheless relapse.

A strategy of regular monitoring of bone marrow (e.g. 3-monthly) is capable of detecting reappearance of molecular positivity about 3–6 months before haematological relapse. No randomized studies have compared the strategy of retreatment at the time of molecular relapse with intervention at the time of haematological relapse. As the risk of haematological relapse in a patient who was RT-PCR negative but then becomes positive is very high, early intervention in this disease seems justified.

Anecdotal evidence suggests that intervention at molecular relapse has a better outcome than intervention at haematolo-gical relapse. Less information is available about monitoring of the *AML–ETO* or *CBFβ–MYH11* fusion genes associated with the t(8;21) and inv(16) translocations. Longitudinal studies using the *AML–ETO* fusion have demonstrated that patients in long-term remission may have molecularly detectable 'disease'. This has been attributed to the presence of transcript in other lin-eages, e.g. monocytes. It seems probable that molecular data will have to be accumulated for each transcript before firm clinical decisions can be based on this information. The transcripts most amenable to monitoring occur in 20–25% of cases which have favourable-risk cytogenetics with fewer relapses, so large pro-spective trials will be required to accumulate enough patients, with enough events to clarify the situation. More sensitivity may be added to this approach using quantitative RT-PCR.

Although several other molecular targets are available, they individually represent small numbers of patients. It may be pos-sible to use a more ubiquitously available molecular target. The Wilms' tumour (*WT1*) gene is overexpressed in the majority of AML cases compared with normal haemopoiesis and has been reported to have potential for molecular monitoring in the majority of cases. Mutations of the *RAS* or *FLT-3* genes are not likely to be useful in this context because some cases which have the mutation at diagnosis lose it at relapse and vice versa.

The management of relapse

The majority of patients will relapse. If this happens after a stem cell transplant procedure, the benefit of further therapy is questionable. This is, however, dependent on when the relapse occurs. Within 1 year, further treatment is unlikely to have sus-tained benefit and retransplantation is usually associated with a very high complication rate. If the relapse occurs later, further chemotherapy with retransplantation may save a few patients. The development of donor lymphocyte infusions has been a very effective approach for the treatment of post-allograft relapse in chronic myeloid leukaemia, but has a low rate of success in AML.

For patients who relapse after chemotherapy, three factors will dictate the clinical outcome – duration of first remission, age and cytogenetic risk group. Patients with good-risk disease have a high (75–80%) rate of second remission. Patients who are young with a long CR1 will have a reasonable survival, whereas older patients with a short CR1 will do poorly (Table 31.5). Since the second remission rate in good-risk disease defined by cytogenetics is relatively good, transplant is usually delayed till second remission. There is no clear 'best choice' chemotherapy for other risk groups, so this is often the setting for experimental therapy development.

Acute promyelocytic leukaemia is again a special case. Pati-ents can respond again to retinoic acid and chemotherapy, but

Table 31.5 Outcome of relapse in patients over 60 years receiving reinduction treatment (*n* = 1529).

(a) Remission rate.

	15–59 years (%)	60–69 years (%)	> 70 years (%)
CR1 (months)			
< 6	15	11	13
6–12	33	29	26
> 12	56	67	53

(b) Survival from relapse at 2 years.

	< 35 years (%)	35–60 years (%)	60 + years (%)
CR1 (months)			
< 6	10	7	4
6–12	16	14	8
>12	41	27	16

recently arsenic trioxide and the CD33-directed immunoconjugate (gemtuzumab ozogamicin) have been found to be effective. Remission rates of > 80% have been reported and, interestingly, following consolidation therapy, a similar proportion can be returned to RT-PCR negativity. This opens up the opportunity of autologous transplantation, the successful outcome of which depends on the autograft, and preferably the patient being molecularly negative. For patients who remain molecularly positive after reinduction, an allogeneic transplant is indicated.

For non-APL patients, whatever treatment is used to re-establish remission, it is unlikely to be durable without a transplant. Although prospective studies are rare, transplant registry data suggest that about 30% of patients can be salvaged with a transplant with little overall difference whether the source of stem cell is allogeneic or autologous.

Future developments

Classification

The classification of this disease will no doubt continue the trend of taking into account genetic and clinical features as well as

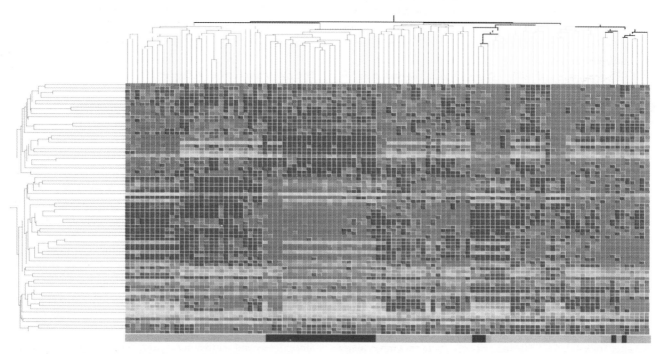

Figure 31.9 A gene and experiment cluster of AML samples. A gene list was identified from the 22 283-gene probe set on the Affymetrix U133A gene chip, which was capable of predicting cytogenetic risk group. This list was used to cluster the samples into similar groups and cluster genes showing similar expression profiles (within the cluster, red indicates high expression whereas green is low or absent expression). One group for each of the good- and poor-risk groups was obtained, but several clusters of standard-risk patients were identified, which may correlate with the diverse nature of this subgroup. Blue, good-risk patients; pink, standard-risk patients; yellow, poor-risk patients. Note that the right-hand cluster contains patients with good, standard and poor risk.

morphology. The technology could eventually allow subgroups to be identified on the basis of a gene expression signature such as is seen in Figure 31.9. High-density microarray chips representing genes can already distinguish major cytogenetic and FAB groups and the presence of a *FLT-3* mutation. This currently offers no advantage over currently available methods but is only at the developmental stage. It will throw light on associated molecular abnormalities which may eventually become targets for drug design and may be capable of predicting disease or toxicity response. The bioinformatics challenges are considerable given the enormous amount of information that these data produce.

Therapeutics

There is general acceptance that little further progress will be made by simply shuffling currently available drugs with respect to either scheduling or dosage. There may still need to be refinements with respect to toxicity. There is much interest in targeting treatment either by matching the treatment approach to the patient based on prognostic factors or by immunologically directing treatment to leukaemic cells and thereby enhancing the selectivity of treatment. Gemtuzumab ozogamicin is an immunotoxin which is being extensively explored in this respect. This is an immunoconjugate combining an IgG_4 anti-CD33 humanized monoclonal antibody with the highly potent anti-tumour antibiotic calicheamicin. The key to its utility is that, when the antibody combines with CD33 antigen, the complex is rapidly internalized to the cell, where the chemical linker between drug and antibody is lysed. A crucial property is that the linker is lysed only intracellularly and not in the circulation. CD33, although expressed on 90% of cases of AML, is not leukaemia specific. There is expression on haemopoietic precursors but not on stem cells or, as far as is known, other tissues. The conjugate is clearly active. As a single agent, it can achieve complete remission in relapse or as first-line treatment in older patients. Pancytopenia is not avoided and transient hepatotoxicity will be seen in some patients. It does not result in the alopecia or mucositis usually associated with chemotherapy. There are a number of areas for its use under investigation in AML, e.g. use in induction in older patients before chemotherapy; for induction in patients unfit for chemotherapy; as maintenance of remission; as first-line and relapse treatment in APL; as part of transplant conditioning; and in simultaneous combination with conventional chemotherapy. All of these approaches are still experimental.

Allogeneic transplant has proved over the years to be a highly effective immunological approach. However, as previously pointed out, the overall survival advantage is not always clear. Part of the reason is that, because it is only safely applicable to younger patients, it is competing with the group of patients with the most favourable responses to chemotherapy. Non-intensive transplants have demonstrated that it is feasible to achieve full chimeric status, i.e. 100% donor cells in the bone marrow, without using intensive chemoradiotherapy. This can be done safely in older patients, but there remain concerns about the balance between avoiding relapse on the one hand and GvHD on the other. This could represent a consolidation option for older patients for whom conventional chemotherapy is less successful and where there is an anti-leukaemic effect of standard allograft. The approach presumes that there will be a significant GVL effect operating in AML. There are only preliminary data on this approach in AML, which is still experimental; assessment in a prospective clinical trial is required.

Many small molecules – particularly tyrosine kinase inhibitors – are becoming available for cancer treatment. So far none has matched the impact of Glivec in chronic myeloid leukaemia. The recognition of the *FLT-3* mutation as a common mutation in AML, which autophosphorylates the receptor and downstream molecules, has led to the discovery of a few agents with powerful – but not specific – FLT-3 inhibition. Preclinical models provide considerable encouragement for efficacy. Initial clinical studies show a response in about 50% of patients with relapsed disease, with occasional complete remissions. Because of lack of specificity, it is likely that these agents will need to be used in combination with each other, or with chemotherapy. Inhibitors of the RAS pathway molecules have also had preliminary assessments. Some responses have been seen, but it is also clear that the agents tested are not specific. Since many small molecules will be available for testing novel approaches to clinical trials will need to develop. Either a much greater international collaboration is needed to provide sufficient numbers of the patient subgroups or different statistical methods will be required.

Selected bibliography

Bullinger L, Dohner K, Bair E *et al.* (2004) Use of gene-expression profiling to identify prognostic subclasses in acute myeloid leukemia. *New England Journal of Medicine* **350**: 1605–16.

Burnett AK (2002) Acute myeloid leukemia: treatment of adults under 60 years. *Reviews in Clinical and Experimental Hematology* **6**: 26–45.

Burnett AK (2002) Transplantation in adults with AML: a clinician's perspective. *British Journal of Haematology* **118**: 1–8.

Caligiuri MA, Strout MP, Gilliland G (1997) Molecular biology of acute myeloid leukemia. *Seminars in Oncology* **24**: 32–44.

Grimwade D, Haferlach T (2004) Gene-expression profiling in acute myeloid leukemia. *New England Journal of Medicine* **350**: 1676–8.

Grimwade D, Walker H, Oliver F *et al.* (1998) The importance of diagnostic cytogenetics on outcome in AML: analysis of 1612 patients entered into the MRC AML: 10 trial. *Blood* **92**: 2322–3.

Grimwade D, Walker H, Harrison G *et al.* (2001) The predictive value of hierarchical cytogenetic classification in older adults with AML: analysis of 1065 adults entered ino the MRC AML11 Trial. *Blood* **98**: 1312–20.

Kottaridis PD, Gale RE, Frew ME *et al.* (2001) The presence of a FLT3 internal tandem duplication in patients with acute myeloid leukemia (AML) adds important prognostic information to cytogenetic risk group and response to the first cycle of chemotherapy: analysis of 854 patients from the United Kingdom Medical Research Council AML 10 and 12 Trials. *Blood* **98**: 1752–9.

Levis M, Small D (2003) FLT3: IT does matter in leukemia. *Leukemia* **17**: 1738–52.

Lowenberg B, Burnett AK, Downing JR (1999) Acute myeloid leukaemia. *New England Journal of Medicine* **341**: 1051–62.

Sonneveld P, List AF (2001) Chemotherapy resistance in acute myeloid leukaemia. *Clinical Haematology Best Practice and Research* **14**: 211–33.

Valk PJM, Verhaak RGW, Beijen MA *et al.* (2004) Prognostically useful gene-expression profiles in acute myeloid leukemia. *New England Journal of Medicine* **350**: 1617–28.

CHAPTER 32

Adult acute lymphoblastic leukaemia

32

Dieter Hoelzer and Nicola Gökbuget

Introduction

Acute lymphoblastic leukaemia (ALL) is a malignant disease characterized by the accumulation of lymphoblasts. In recent adult ALL trials – published between 1999 and 2002 – a trend towards higher complete remission (CR) rates of 80–85% and leukaemia-free survival (LFS) rates of 30–40% has been observed. Intensified consolidation, the extended use of stem cell transplantation (SCT), improvement in supportive care and more experience in treatment centres could have contributed to better outcome. Furthermore, a number of promising new treatment and management modalities for ALL came up including molecular targeting with BCR–ABL kinase inhibitors, antibody therapy and new approaches in SCT. In addition, risk-adapted treatment strategies have been developed over many years and risk models are continuously amended by new prognostic factors, e.g. by evaluation of minimal residual disease (MRD).

Diagnosis

Classification of blast cell phenotype in adult ALL requires morphological and cytochemical evaluation, immunophenotyping, cytogenetic and molecular genetic analysis. Morphology remains the method by which acute leukaemia is initially detected and, together with cytochemical reactions, is the major aid in distinguishing between ALL and acute myeloid leukaemia (AML). For more precise subclassification of ALL into B or T lineages, immunological techniques must be used to detect lineage-specific antigens as well as surface or intracytoplasmic molecules. Cytogenetic analysis is still a prerequisite for diagnosis of ALL because it has prognostic value, but molecular genetic techniques for identification of particular subsets of ALL (e.g. *BCR–ABL*-positive ALL) are of increasing importance. Molecular markers, particularly rearrangements of T-cell receptor (TCR) and immunoglobulin heavy-chain (IgH) genes, are presently used to evaluate therapeutic efficacy in individual patients by detection of MRD (see Chapter 34).

Morphology

The cytological features of leukaemic blast cells in ALL and their division into L1 to L3 according to the French–American–British (FAB) classification are discussed in Chapter 29. The distribution of L1 and L2 subtypes is of minor relevance for prediction of outcome in ALL. The subtype L3, observed in approximately 5% of adult ALL patients, should, however, be identified because it is indicative for mature B-cell ALL, which is subject to different treatment. The diagnosis should be confirmed by surface marker analysis.

Cell surface marker analysis

Acute lymphocyte leukaemia is divided into subtypes by immunological criteria based on the presence of specific receptors or antigens on the cell surface of leukaemic blast cells. Within the B- or T-lineage ALL, the subtypes are defined according to their stage of differentiation. For more details on the immunological

Table 32.1 Immunological classification, corresponding cytogenetic and molecular aberrations and frequencies in adult ALL.

	Adults (%)*	Surface marker	Cytogenetics**	Molecular genetics**
B-lineage		HLA-DR$^+$, TdT$^+$, CD19$^+$ and/or CD79a$^+$ and/or CD22$^+$		
Pro B-ALL	11	No further differentiation markers	t(4;11)	ALL1(MLL)-AF4
Common-ALL	50	CD10$^+$	t(9;22)	BCR-ABL
Pre B-ALL	12	CD10$^{+/-}$, cytoplasmic immunoglobulin (cyIgM$^+$)	t(9;22), t(1;19)	BCR-ABL; E2A-PBX1
B-ALL	5	CD10$^{+/-}$, surface immunoglobulin (sIgM$^+$)	t(8;14)	CMYC-IgH
T-lineage		TdT$^+$, cytoplasmic CD3 (cyCD3)$^+$ or surface CD3 (sCD3)$^+$		
Early T-ALL	6	cyCD3$^+$, CD7$^+$, CD5 $^{+/-}$, CD2 $^{+/-}$	t(11;14)	LMO1/–TCRa/d
Cortical T-ALL (Thy ALL)	10	cyCD3$^+$, CD7$^+$, CD1a$^+$, sCD3$^{+/-}$	t(10;14)	HOX-11-TCRa/d
Mature T-ALL	6	sCD3$^+$, CD1a$^-$		

*Frequencies according to central immunophenotyping of the GMALL Study group; personal communication of Professor E.Thiel and Dr S. Schwartz, Free University of Berlin, Germany.
**Most frequent, typical aberrations.

classification of ALL, see Chapter 29. The frequency and definition of subtypes in adult ALL is given in Table 32.1. The European Group for the Immunological Characterization of Acute Leukaemia (EGIL) has proposed a unified classification for ALL immunophenotypes.

B-lineage ALL

Pro-B ALL, also termed *pre-pre-B ALL* or early pre-B, is CD10 negative and lacks specific B- or T-cell differentiation markers but expresses human leukocyte antigen (HLA)-DR, TdT and CD19, and has rearranged immunoglobulin genes (Table 32.1). It occurs in approximately 9–11% of adult ALL.

Common ALL (c-ALL) is the major immunological subtype in adult ALL. It constitutes > 50% of cases of adult ALL. C-ALL is characterized by the presence of CD10 (Table 32.1). Blast cells do not express markers that characterize relatively mature B cells such as cytoplasmic or surface membrane immunoglobulins. The blast cells are positive for CD19 and TdT.

Pre-B ALL is characterized by the expression of cytoplasmic immunoglobulin, which is absent in common ALL, but is identical to common ALL with respect to the expression of all other cell markers (Table 32.1).

Mature B-cell ALL is found in approximately 5% of adult ALL patients. The blast cells express surface antigens of mature B cells, including surface membrane immunoglobulin. CD10 may be present, as well as, occasionally, cytoplasmic immunoglobulin (Table 32.1).

T-lineage ALL

Approximately 22% of adult ALL cases have blast cells with a T-cell phenotype. All cases express the T-cell antigen gp40 (CD7), and they may, according to their degree of T-cell differentiation,

express other T-cell antigens [e.g. the E rosette receptor (CD2) or the cortical thymocyte antigen T6 (CD1)] (Table 32.1). A minority of T-cell ALL blast cells expresses CD10 together with T-cell antigens. In most cases of T-cell ALL, one or more of the T-cell receptor genes are rearranged. These properties make it possible to classify T-cell ALL according to their stage of differentiation.

Early T-precursor ALL accounts for 6% of adult ALL. It shows characteristic T-cell markers (cyCD3 and CD7) but no further differentiation markers.

Thymic (cortical) T-ALL is the most frequent subtype of T-ALL (10%). It is characterized particularly by the expression of CD1a. Surface CD3 may be present. Since this subtype is associated with a better prognosis, its identification is of particular importance.

Mature T-ALL has a frequency of 6%. The blast cells do not express CD1a but they are positive for surface CD3.

Clinical relevance of cytogenetic and molecular genetic analysis in adult ALL

Cytogenetic abnormalities are independent prognostic variables for predicting the outcome of adult ALL. In three multicentre studies, clonal chromosomal aberrations could be detected in approximately 62–85% of adult ALL patients.

The Ph chromosome t(9;22)(q34;q11) results from a translocation involving the breakpoint cluster region of the *BCR* gene on chromosome 22 and the *ABL* gene on chromosome 9. PCR analyses revealed an incidence of 20–30% *BCR–ABL*+ ALL in adult compared with 3% in childhood ALL patients. One-third of adult ALL patients with a Ph chromosome show M-*BCR* rearrangements (resulting in a 210-kDa protein), similar to patients with chronic myeloid leukaemia (CML), whereas two-thirds have m-*BCR* rearrangements (resulting in a 190-kDa protein). It is noteworthy that *BCR–ABL* is more frequently detected than the corresponding chromosome abnormality t(9;22) because of occasional difficulties in obtaining adequate material for cytogenetic analysis (see also Chapter 30).

The most frequent form of 11q23 abnormalities in ALL is t(4;11)(q21;q23). The translocation is frequently detected in infant leukaemia and in patients with the pro-B ALL subtype (CD10 negative). The overall incidence in adults is approximately 5%. Typical molecular aberrations in ALL with associated cytogenetic translocations and immunological subtypes are summarized in Table 32.1.

The role of cytogenetic analysis in adult ALL has to be re-evaluated critically. The most frequent cytogenetic aberrations and those with the largest prognostic impact can also be detected by the corresponding molecular genetic abnormalities, as mentioned above. These techniques are more reliable and have a greater sensitivity, e.g. a detection level of more than 10^{-6} for BCR–ABL. They are, therefore, more useful for initial detection of the aberrations and for follow-up analysis of minimal residual disease (see below). In addition, the observed incidence of the majority of cytogenetic aberrations is very low and therefore a correlation to clinical outcome and even more therapeutic consequences are limited. Nevertheless, cytogenetic analysis is still recommended as a routine diagnostic method in ALL.

Clinical manifestation

Most adult ALL patients initially present with clinical symptoms resulting from bone marrow failure. Physical findings such as pallor, tachycardia, weakness and fatigue are due to anaemia; petechiae or other haemorrhagic manifestations are attributable to thrombocytopenia; infectious complications are due to neutropenia. Clinical signs of leukaemia related directly to infiltration of typical organs with leukaemic blasts, such as lymphadenopathy, splenomegaly, and hepatomegaly, are present in most patients but are infrequently the problems for which the patient first seeks medical advice.

Symptoms and clinical manifestations of adult ALL patients, 15–65 years of age, entering two consecutive German multicentre trials are given in Table 32.2 according to their appearance in the different immunological subtypes. One-third had infection or fever at presentation, and one-third presented with haemorrhagic episodes. Weight loss was observed only occasionally. Approximately one-half of the patients presented at diagnosis with lymphadenopathy, splenomegaly and hepatomegaly, and hilar lymph node enlargement or a thymic mass (detected on chest radiographs or computerizd tomography scans) in approximately 14% of patients. Most patients (85%) with mediastinal masses had T-cell ALL. Massive thymic enlargement can cause dyspnoea, especially when associated with pleural effusions. Although 7% of ALL patients at presentation had central nervous system (CNS) involvement (as demonstrated by leukaemic blast cells in the cerebrospinal fluid), only 4% of these initially had CNS symptoms such as headache, vomiting, lethargy, nuchal rigidity and cranial or peripheral nerve dysfunction.

Virtually any organ can be infiltrated by ALL blast cells, and approximately one-tenth of the patients had such organ involvement but with a wide variation between subtypes (Table 32.2). Most often a pleural effusion was observed, and this occurred almost exclusively in those patients with mediastinal enlargement and T-cell ALL. Some of those patients also had a

Table 32.2 Symptoms and clinical signs at diagnosis in adult ALL patients*.

		T- lineage (%)	B- precursor (%)	Mature B (%)
Gender	Male	73	54	78
	Female	27	46	22
Age	15–20 years	22	19	8
	20–50 years	67	58	64
	> 50 years	11	24	27
Bleeding		28	28	30
Infections		22	29	37
Lymphadenopathy		77	40	61
Hepatomegaly		45	41	56
Splenomegaly		55	43	47
Mediastinal tumour		62	1	5
CNS involvement		8	3	13
Other organ involvement		15	4	32

*n = 640 patients of GMALL studies 03/87 and 04/89.

		T- lineage (%)	B- precursor (%)	Mature B (%)
Leucocytes or WBC	$< 10 \times 10^9$/L	18	40	37
	$10–50 \times 10^9$/L	36	31	42
	$> 50 \times 10^9$/L	46	29	20
Granulocytes	$< 0.5 \times 10^9$/L	13	28	3
	$> 0.5 \times 10^9$/L	87	72	97
Platelets	$< 25 \times 10^9$/L	21	32	29
	$> 25 \times 10^9$/L	79	68	71
Hb	< 8 g/dL	16	29	17
	> 8 g/dL	84	71	83

Table 32.3 Blood counts at the time of diagnosis in adult ALL*.

*$n = 640$ patients of GMALL studies 03/87 and 04/89.

pericardial effusion. Bone or joint pain was rarely observed compared with childhood ALL; bone lesions could be found in only 1% of cases. Initial involvement of the testis was very rare (< 1%). Leukaemic infiltration of retina, skin, tonsils, lung, or kidney was observed only occasionally, particularly in mature B-cell ALL and to a lesser extent in T-cell ALL, all of them associated with a poorer outcome.

Laboratory evaluation

The peripheral blood cell values at diagnosis of the same cohort of patients are given in Tables 32.3 and 32.4, which again shows differences between the subtypes of adult ALL. Overall, the leucocyte count was elevated in 59% of the cohort, 14% had normal counts and 27% had leucopenia. In 92% of the patients, leukaemic blast cells were seen in the blood film. Thus, 'aleukaemic' leukaemias account for only a small proportion of cases of adult ALL. With automated blood counting, the diagnosis may be missed in patients with normal or decreased white blood cell (WBC) counts and with low or zero blast cells in peripheral blood. In any case, but also for this reason, microscopic examination of blood films in people suspected of having acute leukaemia is an absolute requirement. An elevated blood count $> 100 \times 10^9$/L was observed in 16% of the patients, and occasionally WBC counts $> 500 \times 10^9$/L occurred. In general, a high WBC count is found more frequently in T-cell ALL patients compared with those with B-lineage ALL (Table 32.3).

Neutrophils $< 500 \times 10^6$/L were seen overall in 23% of the patients. Severe neutropenia at diagnosis is observed more often in B-precursor ALL (28%). Thrombocytopenia $< 25 \times 10^9$/L occurred in one-third of adult ALL patients, corresponding roughly with the symptoms of infection and bleeding present at diagnosis. Anaemia at diagnosis is observed in most adult ALL patients, but only in a small proportion is it severe with haemoglobin < 8 g/dL (Table 32.3).

Bone marrow aspiration or biopsy is mandatory for diagnosis of ALL. In < 15% of patients, the bone marrow cannot be aspirated and a biopsy must be performed. Dry taps are due to densely packed blast cells, fibrosis, or inadequate technique; the first two resolve after therapy. Most patients have > 50%, or even > 90%, of blast cells in the bone marrow. In < 3% of cases, the blast cells constitute < 50% of the nucleated marrow cells.

A lumbar puncture should be done to determine whether the CNS is involved. If there is a risk of bleeding as a result of a very low platelet count, or of blast cell contamination due to a high leukaemic blast content in the peripheral blood, lumbar puncture should be postponed. When the leucocyte count in the spinal fluid is low or the morphological detection of blasts is inconclusive, demonstration of an immunologically defined blast cell population can confirm a diagnosis of CNS involvement.

The most frequent metabolic abnormality is an increased serum uric acid level in approximately one-half of the patients;

Table 32.4 Coagulation parameters at the time of diagnosis in adult ALL*.

	Value	Patients (%)
Fibrinogen (g/L)	< 1	4
	> 1	96
Prothrombin time (%)	< 50	7
	50–75	34
	75–100	34
	> 100	25
Partial thromboplastin time (sec)	< 30	33
	30–40	53
	40–50	11
	> 50	3

*$n = 640$ patients of GMALL studies 03/87 and 04/89.

hypercalcaemia is rare. Serum lactate dehydrogenase (LDH) is often elevated as a result of cell destruction in patients with a large tumour mass. In a small proportion of patients (Table 32.4), the initial fibrinogen level was < 1 g/L. Disseminated intravascular coagulation in ALL was rarely observed at diagnosis.

Differential diagnosis

Difficulty is rarely experienced in establishing the diagnosis of ALL. The differentiation from lymphocytosis, lymphadenopathy and hepatosplenomegaly in viral infections and other acute or chronic leukaemias can usually be done by lymphocyte surface markers.

Aleukaemic pancytopenic ALL patients without blast cells in peripheral blood (< 10%) have to be distinguished from those with aplastic anaemia, which may also be a preleukaemic syndrome. In contrast to ALL, in aplastic anaemia the bone marrow is hypocellular. In rare cases with low bone marrow infiltration, an arbitrary distinction between ALL and lymphoblastic NHL is usually chosen according to the degree of infiltration, above or below 25%.

Mixed or hybrid leukaemias are those in which blast cells express lymphoid as well as myeloid antigens; they may also be termed biphenotypic or bilineage leukaemias. Biphenotypic leukaemias are defined as those in which markers of lymphoid and myeloid lineages are co-expressed on the same leukaemic cells. The European Group for the Immunological Characterization of Leukemia (EGIL) has suggested a scoring system which is helpful for definition of biphenotypic leukaemia depending on the type and degree of expression of lymphoid and myeloid markers. Bilineage leukaemias are those with two populations of blast cells that have either lymphoid or myeloid antigens and might be allocated to a treatment strategy either for ALL or for AML. After start of therapy with either regimen, one population may disappear whereas the other is maintained and may require a shift of therapy (see also Chapter 31).

Occasionally, difficulties can occur in distinguishing Ph/ BCR–ABL-positive ALL from primary lymphoid blast crisis of CML. Sometimes final diagnosis can be done only after treatment initiation. In ALL patients achieving complete clinical remission (CR), the peripheral blood count shows normal values, whereas CML cases may revert to a chronic phase with pathological leftshift.

Initial evaluation and supportive therapy

Speed in clinical evaluation and diagnosis is important in order to initiate supportive measures and to decide on appropriate therapy. In only a few cases is the leukaemic process so advanced that immediate treatment is necessary (e.g. in patients with symptoms due to a large mediastinal mass and pleural effusion, a very high WBC or a rapidly progressing B-cell ALL).

A few general measures should be initiated at once. Sufficient fluid intake to guarantee urine production of 100 mL/h throughout induction therapy should be maintained to reduce the danger of uric acid formation. Patients should also receive allopurinol to reduce the formation of uric acid and avoid the danger of urate nephropathy. Allopurinol blocks the enzyme xanthine oxidase, which mediates the generation of uric acid from xanthine as a product of purine catabolism. Allopurinol should be given at a dose of 300 mg/day, which may be increased to 600 mg/day if high leucocyte counts or organomegaly persist. The dose of allopurinol has to be reduced when 6-mercaptopurine is given because it potentiates the action of 6-mercaptopurine. Rasburicase is a new recombinant uratoxidase enzyme which catalyses the oxidation of uric acid to allantoin. Rasburicase can reduce high uric acid faster and more safely than allopurinol, thereby preventing a tumour lysis syndrome in almost all cases. It might therefore be an alternative in patients with high risk of tumour lysis syndrome.

Parenteral fluid administration may be required when the patient's oral intake is inadequate because of nausea or difficulty in swallowing. Placement of an implantable port system is advantageous when anticipating a long period of induction therapy or when part of the therapy will be carried out on an outpatient basis (see also Chapter 36).

Blood substitution

In general, platelet transfusions should be given in response to bleeding episodes and to prevent bleeding when platelet counts fall to < 10×10^9/L and to < 20×10^9/L when there is a bleeding tendency or the patient is febrile. Most often, 4–8 units of platelets are given daily until bleeding ceases. HLA-matched platelets are given to patients who become refractory to random donor platelets. The incidence of fatal haemorrhage during induction therapy has been significantly lowered by these measures. Red cell transfusions have a lower priority than platelet substitution. They should be given according to haemoglobin value (always if haemoglobin below 8 g/dL) but depending on age, comorbidity (e.g. cardiac) and clinical symptoms. The clinical benefit of granulocyte transfusions in patients with severe infections is under investigation.

Infection management

The use of more intense cytostatic regimens has resulted not only in improved response rates of malignancies but also in higher infection-associated morbidity and mortality. Long-term neutropenia is the most important risk factor, but CD4 lymphopenia, antibody deficiency and multiple immunosuppression in allogeneic stem cell transplantation also lead to severe and lethal infections. Whereas formerly Gram-negative microorganisms were the leading cause of febrile neutropenia, in the last decade Gram-positive bacterial infections, mostly caused by staphylococci, have increased and are frequently correlated with indwelling central venous access. Invasive fungal infections are, however, the most dangerous development, with increasing frequency particularly of mould infections. The successful management of febrile neutropenia is based on hygienic procedures including body hygiene, germ-reduced food, reverse isolation or high-efficiency particulate air filtration, antibiotic prophylaxis, sufficient diagnostics, and consequent empirical antimicrobial therapy.

For antibacterial prophylaxis, cotrimoxazole or fluorochinolones, both mainly directed against Gram-negative organisms, have mostly been used. Cotrimoxazole also reduces the incidence of *Pneumocystis carinii* pneumonia, which occurs in approximately 20% of ALL patients without prophylaxis. Although antifungal prophylaxis with oral amphotericin B solution or triazoles may successfully reduce *Candida* colonization and prevent local *Candida* infections, the prophylactic procedures for reducing systemic mycoses are disappointing. Fluconazole has been reported to reduce only systemic *Candida albicans* infections in SCT patients, but non-*albicans* infections, especially by fluconazole-resistant *Candida krusei*, are emerging. Because of its high mortality and difficulty in diagnosis, *Aspergillus* infection is a particular problem. Attempts to prevent aspergilloses have included prophylaxis with itraconazole, intravenous low-dose amphotericin B, liposomal amphotericin B and inhalation of aerosolized amphotericin B, but in randomized studies no clear benefit could be shown. In febrile neutropenia, early diagnostic procedures are necessary. They include physical examination, microbiological investigations, imaging procedures and biopsies. Cultures of blood, urine, sputum and other infected areas are mandatory. *Aspergillus* galactomannan antigen test (Platelia) may aid diagnostic efforts in suspected aspergillosis. Furthermore, PCR methods are investigated for early detection of fungal infections. Imaging procedures such as chest radiography and abdominal ultrasound are routine diagnostic tools. High-resolution computerized tomography of the lungs is one of the most important diagnostic steps for the early diagnosis of *Aspergillus* pneumonia. Fungal pneumonias also may be microbiologically proven with bronchoalveolar lavage or biopsy.

Successful treatment of febrile neutropenia is based on immediate empirical administration of broad-spectrum antibiotics. As initial therapy, combinations such as β-lactam antibiotics plus aminoglycosides or monotherapy (e.g. with carbapenems, piperacillin-tazobactam or cephalosporins of class 3 and 3a) are standard. In view of the increasing problems of invasive fungal infections, empiric antifungal treatment with amphotericin B or fluconazole for patients with refractory fever or pulmonary infiltration has been established. So far, conventional amphotericin B, amphotericin lipid formulations, 5-flucytosine, fluconazole and itraconazole represented antimycotic standard treatment in proven or suspected invasive mycoses. This standard, however, is nowadays changing by introduction of high-potency new antimycotics such as voriconazole (particularly effective in the treatment of aspergillosis, but also of fluconazole-resistant candidosis or fusariosis) and caspofungin (successful treatment for candidoses and aspergilloses).

Haemopoietic growth factors

The use of haemopoietic growth factors such as granulocyte colony-stimulating factor (G-CSF) is a valuable component of supportive therapy during the treatment of ALL (Table 32.5). There is no indication so far that these CSFs stimulate leukaemic cell growth in a clinically significant manner.

Most clinical trials demonstrate that the prophylactic administration of G-CSF significantly accelerates neutrophil recovery, and several prospective, randomized studies also show that this is associated with a substantially reduced incidence and duration of febrile neutropenia and of severe infections in ALL, and also reduced induction mortality.

The scheduling of G-CSF is of great importance. When G-CSF is first given at the end of a 4-week induction chemotherapy regimen, potential benefits are limited. Therefore, it is noteworthy that G-CSF may even be given in parallel with chemotherapy without aggravating the myelotoxicity of these specific regimens and that this scheduling is an important determinant of the clinical efficacy. On the other hand, after short consolidation cycles G-CSF treatment may be postponed.

A closer adherence to the dose and schedule of chemotherapeutic regimens should be theoretically possible by the use of G-CSF. A benefit in terms of long-term outcome by increased dose intensity achieved by the use of G-CSF has not yet been demonstrated in any trial.

Chemotherapy

Chemotherapy of ALL is usually divided into several phases, beginning with remission induction. The objective of induction chemotherapy is to achieve CR, i.e. eradication of leukaemia as determined by morphological criteria and, more recently, also by molecular markers. The post-remission therapy usually consists of intensification or consolidation cycles and maintenance treatment. Most often specific prophylactic CNS treatment is added (Table 32.6).

Remission induction therapy

Correct diagnosis and management of the initial complications are the prerequisites for successful induction therapy. A cautious cell reduction phase is often recommended for patients with a large leukaemic cell burden or a high leucocyte count. Patients with extreme leucocytosis ($> 100 \times 10^9$/L) have been treated initially with leukapheresis, but these patients can also be managed with steroids in combination with vincristine or cyclophosphamide. For mature B-cell ALL, initial treatment with

Table 32.5 Trials of G-CSF in adult ALL.

Reference	Patients	Chemotherapy	Growth factor	n	Days until ANC > 0.5×10^9/L or > 1.0×10^9/L *		Incidence of infections	Early death (%)
Kantarjian *et al.* (1993)	CR1	Consolidation	G-CSF	14	14	< 0.001	2	0
			Histological control	14	18		4	14
Ottmann *et al.* (1995)	CR1/PR	Induction II	G-CSF	37	8		43	0
			Randomised control	39	12.5		56	3
Geissler *et al.* (1997)	*De novo*	Induction I	G-CSF	23	16	< 0.005	40	4
			Randomised control	22	24		77	9
Larson *et al.* (1997)	*De novo*	Induction I	G-CSF	102	16	< 0.001	NR	4
			Placebo	93	22*			11

NR, no response.

cyclophosphamide and prednisone for 1 week usually results in a safe reduction of large tumour masses, in most cases without tumour lysis syndrome.

Standard induction therapy for ALL includes prednisone, vincristine, anthracyclines (mostly daunorubicin) and also L-asparaginase. Further drugs, such as cyclophosphamide, cytarabine (either conventional or high dose), mercaptopurine and others, are added in many protocols, sometimes named as early intensification.

Prednisone and prednisolone have been most frequently administered, although *dexamethasone* shows a higher anti-leukaemic activity *in vitro* and a better penetration of the cerebrospinal fluid. Extensive use of dexamethasone may, however, be associated with an increased risk of septicaemias and fungal infections which may be circumvented if treatment time and dose is reduced.

Anthracycline dose intensity and schedule may play an important role in induction therapy of ALL. In the past daunorubicin was mostly administered at a weekly schedule, but recently many trials include dose intensification with doses of 30–60 mg/m^2 at a 2–3 day schedule. Intensive anthracycline therapy may be associated with a higher induction mortality. Therefore, intensive supportive care and probably the use of growth factors is recommended with these types of protocols.

Asparaginase (A) does not affect the CR rate but improves LFS. If not used during induction therapy, it is often included as part of the consolidation treatment. Three different A preparations with significantly different half-lives are available: native *E. coli* A (1.2 days), *Erwinia* A (0.65 days) and PEG-L-A (5.7 days). The availability may vary between different countries. In order to reach equal efficacy, the application schedule has to be adapted and is generally daily for *Erwinia*, every second day for *E. coli* and 1–2 weekly for PEG-L-A.

The role of *cyclophosphamide* (C) – generally administered at the beginning of induction therapy – has been evaluated in several studies. A randomized study by the Italian GIMEMA group comparing a three-drug induction with or without C did not show a difference in terms of CR rate (81% vs. 82%). However, in several non-randomized trials, high CR rates (85–91%) were achieved with regimens including C pretreatment, particularly in adult T-ALL.

High-dose treatment

A more recent strategy is to add high-dose cytarabine (HDAC) before or after the standard induction therapy. This approach has resulted in a median CR rate of 79%, which is not superior to that obtained with conventional treatment, and it remains uncertain whether, and for which subgroups, it may be beneficial for LFS. Up-front treatment before conventional chemotherapy yielded higher CR rates than treatment afterwards, which was in part related to a higher induction mortality (reviewed in Gökbuget and Hoelzer 2002). Furthermore, any type of induction therapy with HDAC may lead to an increased incidence of severe neutropenias after subsequent chemotherapy cycles. The relatively high early mortality rate is now decreasing with better handling and improved supportive care. Overall, the aim of HDAC treatment is not only to improve the CR rate but, even more, to increase the quality of remission. This means that a lower tumour load should lead to a better LFS. So far, however, no convincing results are available to support this hypothesis.

In conclusion, all approaches for induction therapy including high-dose treatment result in a CR rate of approximately 80% in adult ALL. However, the molecular CR rate is clearly lower and the addition of new therapeutic approaches – other than chemotherapy – such as molecular targeting or antibody

Table 32.6 Overall treatment results in adult ALL in larger studies*.

Group	n	Age	Induction	Consolidation	Maintenance	CR (%)	LFS
GATLA (Lluesma-Gonalons et al. 1991)	137	30	V, P, D	–	MP, M, V, P	80	20% at 5 years
GATLA (Lluesma-Gonalons et al. 1991)	145	29	V, P, D, A, C, AC, MP	AD, V, DX, A, AC, C, MP	M, MP, V, P	78	34% at 6 years
CALGB 8011 (Ellison et al. 1991)	277	33	V, P, A, D	MP, M, [AC, D]	MP, M, V, P	64	29% at 9 years
CALGB 8513 (Cuttner et al. 1991)	164	32	V, P, Mi/D, HdM	V, P, Mi/D, HdM, AC, MP, A	–	64	18% at 3 years
USCF (Linker et al. 1997)	109	15–50	V, P, D, A	V, P, A, D, IdM, VM, AC	M, MP	88	42% at 5 years
EORTC (Stryckmans et al. 1992)	106	27	V, P, AD, [HdAC]	A, HdC, [M, TG, AC]	MP, M, P, V, AD, BCNU, C	74	40% at 8 years
L+B+VOPAL/HEAVD (Bassan et al. 1992)	212	27	V, P, A, AD, [C; HdAC]		MP, M, C	71	32% at 10 years
GMALL 01 (Hoelzer et al. 1993)	368	25	V, P, A, D, C, AC, M, MP	V, DX, AD, AC, C, TG	MP, M	74	35% at 10 years
GMALL 02 (Hoelzer et al. 1993)	562	28	V, P, A, D, C, AC, M, MP	V, DX, AD, AC, C, TG, VM, AC	MP, M	75	39% at 7 years
UKALL IX (Durrant et al. 1993)	266		V, P, A, (MP, M)/D		MP, M, V, P	68	22% at 8 years
FGTALL (Fiere et al. 1993)	581	33	V, P, D/R, C, [amsa, AC]	D/R, AC, A	MP, M, V, C, P, D/R, DT, BCNU	76	17% at 5 years
SAKK (Wernli et al. 1994)	140	31	V, P, D, M, A, HdAC, VP	allo/auto BMT; > 50 years: HDC	–	69	21% at 5 years
Lyon + other (Attal et al. 1995)	135	31	V, P, A, D, C, AC, MP	HdM, AC, allo/auto BMT	[Il-2]	93	44% at 3 years
CALGB 8811 (Larson et al. 1995)	197	32	V, P, A, D, C	C, MP, AC, V, A, M, AD, DX, TG	MP, M, V, P	85	30% at 5 years
GIMEMA 0183 (Mandelli et al. 1996)	358	31	V, P, A, D	V, IdM, IdAC, P, VM, AC	MP, M, V, P, [A, AC, VM, IdAC]	79	25% at 10 years
HOVON (Dekker et al. 1997)	130	35	V, P, A, D	HdAC, amsa, MP, VP	–	73	28% at 5 years
UKALL XA (Durrant et al. 1997)	618	>15	V, P, D, A	[AC, VP, D, TG]	MP, MTX, V, P	82	28% at 5 years
PETHEMA (Ribera et al. 1998)	108	28	V, P, D, A, C	HdM, V, D, P, A, C, VM, AC	MP, M, [VD, P, Mi, A, C, VM, AC]	86	41% at 4 years
CALGB (Larson et al. 1998)	198	35	C, D, V, P, A	C, MP, AC, V, A, MP, M, AD, DX, TG, P	MP, M, V, P	85	40% at 3 years
MD Anderson (Kantarjian et al. 2000)	204	39	V, AD, DX, C	HdM, HdAC, P	M, MP, V, P	91	38% at 5 years
SWEDEN (Hallbook et al. 2002)	120	44	HdAC, C, D, V, BM	amsa, HdAC, V, BM, C, D, VP +/– SCT	MP, M, D, V, P, AC, TG	86	36% at 3 years
GIMEMA (Annino et al. 2002)	794	28	V, P, A, D, C, [HdAC, Mi]	V, HdM, HdAC, DX, VM	MP, M, V, [AC, Mi, VM, HdAC, HdM, DX]	82	29% at 9 years

*Since 1990, > 100 patients, follow-up > 3 years.

[x, y], with or without; x/y, either/or; CR, rate of clinical remission; LFS, leukaemia-free survival.

V, vincristine; P, prednisone; amsa, amsacon; A, L-asparaginase; BM, betamethasone; D, daunorubicin; M, methotrexate; MP, 6-mercaptopurine; AC, cytosine arabinoside; C, cyclophosphamide; DX, dexamethasone; TG, thioguanine; AD, doxorubicin; DT, dactinomycin; BCNU, carmustine; R, rubidazone; Mi, mitoxantrone; HdM, high-dose M; IdM, intermediate-dose M; HdAC, high-dose AC; IdAC, intermediate-dose AC; VM, teniposide; VP, etoposide; VD, vindesine.

treatment may be the future approach to increase the molecular CR rate.

Failure of induction therapy

Twenty per cent of adult ALL patients do not achieve CR after induction therapy, in contrast to < 3% of children with ALL. Mortality during induction is age dependent, increasing with age from < 3% in adolescents to 20% in patients > 60 years of age. The main cause of death in approximately two-thirds of the patients is infection, in part fungal infection. The remaining non-responders may achieve a partial remission or may be refractory to standard treatment. These patients have an extremely poor prognosis. They are therefore candidates for experimental treatment approaches or consideration for a SCT, even if not in CR but in good partial remission.

Consolidation therapy

Consolidation therapy refers to high-dose chemotherapy, to the use of multiple new agents, or to readministration of the induction regimen. These measures are aimed at eliminating residual leukaemia after induction chemotherapy and thereby preventing relapse as well as emergence of drug-resistant cells.

In adult ALL, intensification therapy can prolong LFS (see Table 32.6). Intensification schedules include teniposide, etoposide, m-amsacrine, mitoxantrone, idarubicin and HDAC, or intermediate- or high-dose methotrexate (HDMTX). Allogeneic SCT from sibling or unrelated donors or autologous SCT is now the major approach for intensive post-induction therapy in high-risk patients. But also, before SCT, consolidation therapy is usually given to achieve a CR of good quality.

High-dose chemotherapy

High-dose chemotherapy in consolidation has been used mainly to overcome drug resistance or to achieve therapeutic drug levels in the cerebrospinal fluid.

High-dose cytarabine

Although there is considerable experience with high-dose cytarabine (HDAC) for the treatment of ALL, it remains uncertain what dose is optimal; usually doses ranging from $1–3 \, \text{g/m}^2$ every 12 h for 4–5 days are given within several combinations. HDAC has been included in several trials in adult *de novo* ALL as part of consolidation therapy or during induction and consolidation treatment. With a weighted mean for the LFS of 30% (26–50%), the results are not superior to trials without HDAC.

It seems that specific subgroups of ALL benefit from a HDAC treatment; thus, encouraging results are achieved for paediatric B-cell ALL. It remains uncertain to what extent HDAC contributes to the effects of HDMTX in these patients. Apparently also for adult pro-B ALL, HDAC is beneficial, since cure rates of 50% can be achieved. For other adult poor-risk groups, particularly Ph+ ALL, HDAC is apparently not improving the outcome.

An additional argument for the use of HDAC might be its effectiveness in treating CNS leukaemia. There is evidence that in ALL and NHL, higher levels of AC triphosphate can be reached with $3 \, \text{g/m}^2$ than with the lower dose of $1 \, \text{g/m}^2$ AC; in addition, with the higher dose, the cerebrospinal fluid can be cleared of blast cells.

High-dose methotrexate (HDMTX)

The use of HDMTX has been extensively studied for the treatment of childhood ALL and, to a lesser extent, adult ALL. A wide range of doses ($0.5–8 \, \text{g/m}^2$) has been used. HDMTX appears to be effective in preventing systemic and testicular relapses.

The effect of HDMTX on CNS leukaemia may contribute to the favourable results reported with its use. Overall, the intensive use of HDMTX may have had a major in improvement of outcome in paediatric B-lineage ALL.

Several studies have investigated the efficacy of HDMTX in adult ALL – as consolidation or during consolidation and induction treatment. The weighted mean for LFS of six studies, which also comprised a variety of other drugs, is 41%, with a wide range (31–56%). Most favourable results have been achieved in small trials with HDMTX as part of intensive multidrug consolidation regimens.

The combination of cycles having HDAC with cycles having HDMTX during consolidation was reported from six trials with a weighted mean for LFS of 32% (17–48%). Thus, there is some evidence that the inclusion of HDAC and HDMTX as part of multidrug consolidation treatment may improve overall results.

Maintenance therapy

The aim of maintenance or continuation therapy is to eliminate minimal residual disease (MRD). The optimal form and duration of maintenance therapy remains open but can hopefully be better defined by tailoring according to MRD.

Currently maintenance therapy in adult ALL is being revised; according to MRD (e.g. none for MRD-negative patients), to ALL subtype (e.g. none for mature B-ALL) and including new therapeutic options (e.g. a tyrosine kinase inhibitor for BCR–ABL-positive ALL).

Prophylaxis of central nervous system leukaemia

Central nervous system leukaemia occurs in 6% (1–10%) of patients with adult ALL at diagnosis, with a higher incidence in T-cell ALL (8%) and mature B-cell ALL (13%).

Treatment and prophylaxis of CNS leukaemia may consist of intrathecal methotrexate alone or in combination with AC or prednisone, an intraventricular therapy, systemic treatment with HDAC or HDMTX or cranial irradiation.

Adult ALL patients who did not receive specific prophylactic CNS treatment in earlier trials have a CNS relapse rate of 30% (29–32%), similar to that observed in children without CNS prophylaxis. With intrathecal chemotherapy alone, the rate of isolated and combined CNS relapses could be reduced to 13% (8–19%). Intermittent injections during maintenance therapy improves the efficacy compared with only a few doses during induction treatment. In most adult ALL trials, additional prophylactic CNS irradiation (24 Gy) has been included. Long-term toxicities are apparently less severe than in paediatric patients. This combined approach further reduces the CNS relapse rate to 9% (3–19%). There is some evidence that early irradiation after remission induction is superior to delayed irradiation during consolidation treatment. It is questionable whether systemic high-dose treatment alone provides sufficient CNS prophylaxis because the CNS relapse rate is approximately 14% (10–16%). In many recent trials, combined treatment approaches have shown high efficacy. For high-dose chemotherapy together with intrathecal therapy, the rate of CNS relapses was 7% (2–16%); with additional CNS irradiation, the relapse rate was 6% (1–13%). The efficacy of intensified CNS prophylaxis was also demonstrated in a retrospective analysis from the MD Anderson Cancer Center, where the lowest CNS relapse rate (2%) was achieved in a trial with early high-dose chemotherapy and intrathecal therapy for all patients.

Because the risk for CNS relapse is associated with other prognostic factors such as T-cell ALL, B-cell ALL, extreme leucocytosis, high leukaemia cell proliferation rate, high serum LDH levels, and extramedullary organ involvement, a risk-adapted CNS prophylaxis has been suggested. This approach, however, in contrast to childhood ALL, is not widely used in adults.

Therapy for relapsed and resistant leukaemia

Patients who fail to achieve CR or those who relapse subsequently have been treated with a variety of protocols. The use of regimens including vincristine, anthracyclines, and steroids, similar to standard induction treatment, led to CR rates of approximately 60% in earlier studies but these patients generally had no intensive first-line treatment.

High-dose AC has been extensively studied in relapsed adult ALL. From several small pilot studies comprising < 100 patients, the weighted mean CR rate was 37%. Higher CR rates (50–60%) were achieved with combination regimens that included HDAC and mitoxantrone, amsacrine or vincristine plus steroids. Because HDAC is increasingly administered during front-line treatment, its efficacy during relapse treatment may be impaired. Therefore, new combinations with idarubicin (46–64% CR rate) or fludarabine (67–83% CR rate) or other agents have been evaluated. Median remission duration did not exceed 5 months.

The most significant predictive factor for treatment response in relapsed patients is the duration of first remission. Patients with longer previous remission (> 18 months) have a higher CR rate and longer remission duration than those with a short previous remission (< 18 months).

For all chemotherapy regimens, the duration of second remission is usually short (< 6 months), and the long-term survival rate with chemotherapy alone is < 5%. Thus, the only

curative chance for adult patients with relapsed or resistant ALL is SCT, and the major aim of relapse treatment is the induction of a second remission with sufficient duration to prepare SCT.

Stem cell transplantation

Stem cell transplantation (SCT) from peripheral blood and to a lesser extent from bone marrow is the major post-remission strategy for eradication of residual disease in adult ALL. Prognostic factors for remission duration after chemotherapy (i.e. age, WBC count, immunophenotype, BCR–ABL status) are also predictive for the outcome after SCT (see also Chapter 25).

Allogeneic SCT from sibling donors

The outcome of allogeneic SCT for ALL depends on the age and remission status of the patient. The best results have been obtained with patients transplanted during first remission, among whom the probability of survival is approximately 50% (Table 32.7). After allogeneic SCT in second remission, the LFS rate is 34% and in advanced ALL (refractory or in relapse), allogeneic SCT results in an 18% long-term survival rate (Table 32.7).

There is evidence that a graft-versus-leukaemia (GvL) effect is also present in ALL, as indicated by several observations, such as lower relapse rates in patients with acute and/or chronic GvHD, lower recurrence rates after matched unrelated donor (MUD) SCT, induction of remission by withdrawal of prophylaxis against GvHD or donor lymphocyte infusions (DLI) in single patients with relapsed ALL. However, DLI applied in patients with relapse after SCT in order to induce GvL have a response rate of only 15% in ALL, which is much lower than the 40% in AML or 70–80% in CML.

Matched unrelated SCT

The use of SCT from MUDs has constantly increased in recent years in order to overcome the limitations of sibling donor, but also to exploit GvL effects. It can result in long-term survival of about 40% for patients transplanted in first CR and 25% for patients in CR2 (Table 32.7). The low relapse rate of 10% for patients in CR1 strengthens the hypothesis of a GvL effect. The high rate of transplant-related mortality (TRM) of approximately 40% in CR1 patients is still the major obstacle in MUD SCT. This might be reduced by improved donor selection, less toxic preparative regimens, better management of GvHD and improved supportive care.

Overall, the results of MUD SCT in ALL seem encouraging, and it has become the treatment of choice for high-risk patients in CR1 if a sibling donor is not available. For patients with BCR–ABL-positive ALL the results of MUD SCT are already approaching those of sibling SCT. Mismatched or haploidentical

Table 32.7 Recent results of stem cell transplantation in adult ALL.

Stem cell transplant	Disease stage	n	LFS/OS* (%)	Relapse incidence* (%)	TRM* (%)
Allogeneic	CR1	1100	50 (21–71)	24 (10–50)	27 (12–42)
	CR2	1019	34 (13–60)	48 (62–71)	29 (40–75)
	Relapsed/refractory	216	18 (8–33)	75 (60–77)	47 (46–47)
Autologous	CR1	1369	42 (15–65)	51 (27–68)	5 (0–8)
	CR2	258	24 (20–27)	70 (59–75)	18[‡]
MUD	CR1	318	39 (32–51)	10 (6–19)	47 (32–54)
	≥ CR2	231	27 (17–28)	8[†]	75[†]
	Relapsed/refractory	47	5[†]	31[†]	64[†]
NMSCT	All stages	132	23 (0–50)	47 (30–56)	42 (10–72)

*Weighted mean and range of published studies.

[†]One study (Cornelissen *et al.* 2001).

[‡]One study.

OS, overall survival; MUD, matched unrelated donor; TRM, transplant related mortality; NMSCT, non-myeloablative SCT.

SCT in adult ALL is still experimental and an option only for rare cases; it is explored by few very experienced SCT centres.

Autologous SCT

The results for autologous SCT in first remission in adult ALL are surprisingly good, with an LFS of 42% and a low TRM of < 5%. Similar results with an LFS rate of 42% in standard-risk ALL (*n* = 280) and 40% in high-risk ALL (*n* = 174) have been reported for a large series from the European Bone Marrow Transplant Group (EBMT).

This type of SCT is associated with a higher relapse risk (> 50%) because of the risk of reinfusing residual leukaemic cells and even more so because of the lack of a GvL effect. Purging of bone marrow or peripheral blood to eliminate or reduce remaining leukaemic blast cells is feasible but has not become a routine measure. Maintenance treatment after autologous SCT may contribute to a reduction of relapse risk but is not widely used. With new treatment options available, such as molecular targeting with BCR–ABL kinase inhibitors or monoclonal antibodies, maintenance treatment after autologous SCT may be revisited.

With the increasing number of MUD transplants and the advantage of GvL effects, the role of autologous SCT may decrease. However, because of the low TRM, this is still a reasonable approach for elderly patients. In addition, autologous SCT can shorten overall treatment in adult ALL to 3 months instead of 2 years of chemotherapy and maintenance treatment. This approach is also supported by several prospective randomized trials in adult ALL showing equal outcome for chemotherapy consolidation and autologous SCT.

Non-myeloablative SCT

Non-myeloablative SCT or reduced-intensity conditioning regimens (NMSCT) are new approaches which deserve evaluation in ALL and may lead to an extension of indications for allogeneic SCT (see Chapter 25). In contrast to conventional SCT, which mainly relies on cell kill by high-dose chemotherapy and total body irradiation (TBI), NMSCT relies on the use of GvL effects. Immunosuppression, e.g. with purine analogues, other cytostatic drugs and/or low-dose TBI, is followed by the infusion of donor stem cells from siblings or MUD with adapted immunosuppression to establish host tolerance.

So far, in more than 100 adult ALL patients with high median age and poor prognostic features, the probabilities for survival after NMSCT was around 23% with relapse rate of 47% and TRM of 42 (Table 32.7). Overall, it seemed to be of some benefit in patients in CR1. In patients with advanced refractory or relapsed ALL, this form of SCT is at present not successful due to a high TRM rate.

Role of SCT in adult ALL

The question of whether all patients in first CR with suitable sibling donor should receive allogeneic SCT or whether it should be reserved for patients with high-risk features remains controversial. Several recent studies include early SCT (mainly from matched related donors), but so far it has not been demonstrated that this approach has a favourable impact on overall outcome. In addition, quality of life of transplanted patients has to be considered. There is agreement that all high-risk patients are candidates for SCT in first CR, including sibling and

Table 32.8 Outcome of adult ALL according to subgroups.

Subgroup	Incidence (%)	n	CR rate (%)*	MDR* (months)	LFS (%)*
Overall		4474	75 (63–86)	23 (11–41)	31 (13–44)
Age (years)					
15–20			82–95		32–65**
20–50			80		35–40
50–60			40–70		20–30
>60			20–60		10–20
Subtype					
T-ALL	24	621	65–85	25	30–50
Thymic			90		50–60
Early/mature			70–80		30
Pro-B-ALL	11	57	75		40–50
Common ALL	57	881	80	22	30–40
B-ALL	3	89	77		> 50
Cytogenetics					
Ph/BCR–ABL+ ALL	24	352	66	9	15–20

*Pooled data from published studies.
**Results from paediatric studies.
CR, complete remission; MDR, median duration of remission; LFS, leukaemia-free survival.

matched unrelated allogeneic SCT. Ongoing studies investigate whether allogeneic sibling SCT is also superior for standard-risk ALL; however, for this comparison, selection mechanisms, e.g. for age and comorbidity, have to be considered. The analysis of patients with and without donor may be a reasonable approach. Autologous SCT seems to be equal to chemotherapy, and whether the argument of shorter treatment duration compared with chemotherapy is valid remains to be determined. The role of new approaches such as NMSCT or new conditioning regimens remains open.

Outcome of ALL subtypes and prognostic factors

Major adverse prognostic factors for attaining a CR are advanced age and Ph+ ALL. Prognostic factors are of greater importance for duration of remission and survival (Table 32.8). Appreciation of the impact of such risk factors (Table 32.9) can result in the generation of risk-adapted treatment protocols for adult ALL.

Age

There is a continuous decline in the CR rate from 95% in children to 40–60% in patients > 50–60 years of age. Most trials demonstrate that increasing age is also associated with a shorter survival (median 3–14 months) and a LFS of only 10–20%.

It is difficult to define an age limit where a change in prognosis

Table 32.9 Adverse prognostic factors for remission duration in adult ALL*.

Clinical characteristics	Higher age (> 50 years, > 60 years) High WBC (> 30 000/µL in B-lineage)
Immunophenotype	Pro B Early T Mature T
Cytogenetics/molecular genetics	t(9;22)/BCR-ABL or t(4;11)/ALL1-AF4
Treatment response	Late achievement of CR (> 3, 4 weeks) MRD positivity

*As they emerged from more than 3000 adult ALL patients treated in the GMALL (German Multicenter Studies for Adult ALL) trials.

occurs, but in almost all studies LFS is inferior in patients older than 50–60 years of age. This age limit seems to be practical because patients below this age are candidates for intensified treatment approaches such as SCT, whereas, for the older group, new strategies need to be explored, carefully weighing the gain in survival against quality of life. Thus, elderly patients > 50–55 years of age who have achieved a CR and are in good clinical condition are potential candidates for autologous SCT or NMSCT. One promising new strategy is to treat elderly patients with Ph/BCR–ABL-positive ALL with the BCR–ABL kinase inhibitor imantinib during induction to avoid the complications of chemotherapy.

Adolescent patients (15–20 years) with ALL are treated either according to protocols for paediatric ALL or in adult ALL trials. There is increasing evidence that results with paediatric protocols are superior, albeit in these retrospective analyses it remains open whether identical adolescent cohorts were treated and particularly whether dose intensity of protocols was similar.

Immunophenotype and cytogenetics

The immunophenotype is an important independent prognostic variable in ALL. In ongoing trials, it is used to adjust treatment regimens accordingly, e.g. separate regimens for mature B-cell ALL. A further example for clinical application is the identification of patients for antibody therapy, e.g. anti-CD20 (Rituximab) in CD20-positive B-lineage ALL or B-cell ALL or anti-CD52 (Campath-1h) in CD52-positive ALL.

T-lineage ALL

Results for T-cell ALL have substantially improved compared with survival rates of < 10% 20 years ago. There is, however, a substantial difference in outcome for the T-ALL subtypes. Thymic T-ALL, which accounts for half of the adult T-ALL patients, has a favourable outcome, with CR rates of 85–90% and survival > 50% at 5 years. Early T-ALL and mature T-ALL have a poorer outcome, with CR rates of 70% and LFS rates of approximately 30%.

The addition of cyclophosphamide and cytarabine to the usual drugs for ALL is mainly responsible for this improvement. HDMTX contributed to the improvement of survival in children, as did HDAC. HDAC improved the prognosis for adult ALL patients with high WBC counts and T-cell ALL. For adults, the benefit of HDMTX in T-cell ALL has to be confirmed in larger trials. New treatment approaches in adult T-ALL include purine analogues such as cladribine and compound GW506U78 (nelarabine) or antibody therapy, e.g. anti-CD52. Also, SCT for early/mature T-ALL patients in CR 1 seems promising.

B-lineage ALL

In *common and pre-B-ALL*, CR rates in adult trials have improved to 80% or more, but patients in most studies still relapse over a period of up to 5–6 years, and only one-third survive. Within B-precursor ALL, prognostic factors are decisive for outcome; high-risk patients with adverse prognostic features such as high WBC ($> 30 \times 10^9$/L) and/or late achievement of CR (> 3–4 weeks) (Table 32.8) have a survival of 25% or less, whereas standard-risk patients without any of those features have a 5-year survival of > 50%.

Philadelphia chromosome/BCR–ABL-positive ALL has the worst prognosis in children as well as in adults. In adults, however, the adverse impact is much greater as the incidence in children is only 3% compared with 25% in adults or even > 40% in elderly

ALL patients. In 13 studies with a total of 384 patients, the weighted mean CR rate is 67% (44–76%). The median remission duration in all series is short (5–11 months) and the survival rate, from 0% to 16% at 3–5 years, is extremely poor.

Treatment options for Ph/*BCR–ABL*-positive ALL in adults include HDMTX or HDAC; so far, no convincing progress for this subgroup of patients has been reported. The only curative chance for adult Ph/*BCR–ABL*-positive ALL patients is therefore SCT. A promising new treatment modality for Ph/*BCR–ABL*-positive ALL is the use of the ABL tyrosine kinase inhibitor imantib (see also Chapter 37).

In the past, adults with the subtype *pro-B ALL* or the *t(4;11)* translocation had a poor prognosis, as did infant ALL patients. With intensive regimens including HDAC and mitoxantrone as consolidation therapy, the results in adults seem to have improved. Pro-B-ALL patients also benefit from allogeneic SCT in CR1, with survival rates of 60%, as well as from autologous SCT. The adverse impact of the translocation t(4;11) seems to have changed as well with new treatment modalities.

In *mature B-cell ALL*, CR remission rates were low (40%) two decades ago, and remission duration was short (11 months). A change was brought about by innovative childhood B-cell ALL studies that significantly improved outcome. The drugs responsible for the improvement were high doses of fractionated cyclophosphamide, ifosfamide, HDMTX ($0.5–8$ g/m^2) and HDAC in conjunction with the conventional drugs for remission induction in ALL, given in short cycles at frequent intervals over a period of 6 months.

The application of these childhood B-cell ALL protocols in original or modified form also brought a substantial improvement for adult patients with B-cell ALL. CR rate is now approximately 75% (62–83%) and the LFS 55% (20–71%). Adverse prognostic factors are late CR (more than two cycles of chemotherapy), high WBC ($> 30 \times 10^9$/L) and age > 50 years. Patients with these high-risk features are probably candidates for SCT. B-cell ALL has a higher incidence of CNS involvement at diagnosis, and of CNS relapse. Therefore, effective measures against CNS disease, such as HDMTX and HDAC as well as intrathecal therapy, are important components of treatment regimens. On the other hand, maintenance treatment has been omitted. Because relapses occur almost exclusively within the first year in childhood as well as in adult B-cell ALL studies, patients thereafter can be considered as cured. Recent treatment protocols include antibody therapy with anti-CD20 (rituximab) since more than 80% of the patients are CD20-positive, with quite promising preliminary results.

Minimal residual disease – practical application in adult ALL

In childhood ALL, it has been demonstrated that level and course of MRD are independent prognostic factors (Chapter 34). These results have been confirmed by a considerable number of mainly retrospective studies in adult ALL. There are, however, some important differences. A very good response, as indicated by an early and rapid decrease of MRD during induction, may be associated with a very low relapse risk. However, in general, the decrease in MRD occurs more slowly in adults, and fewer patients reach a negative MRD status. This applies particularly for patients with low MRD immediately after induction, who still show a considerable relapse rate of approximately 50%. Thus, in adult ALL, MRD analysis immediately after induction provides a good tool for identification of high relapse risk but not of those with low risk. The longitudinal course of MRD may be more important in adults than in children. High MRD at any time-point after induction is associated with a higher relapse risk, and the predictive value increases at later time-points (months 6–9).

The predictive value of MRD evaluation depends on the technical quality, such as sensitivity (10^{-4} for negative results), number of targets (at least two) and the frequency of evaluations (3 monthly) in individual patients. In a retrospective study of the GMALL (German Multicenter Studies for Adult ALL), a broad spectrum of target genes (IgH, IgK and TCR rearrangements) was measured quantitatively with high sensitivity ($< 10^{-4}$). Based on these results, MRD-based risk groups could be defined; MRD low risk was defined as MRD negative at all time-points after induction therapy confirmed with two markers and a sensitivity $> 10^{-4}$. MRD high risk was defined as MRD above 10^{-4} at two time-points after induction therapy without subsequent decrease. There was, however, a surprisingly large intermediate-risk group of patients who could not be allocated to either subset. The major reasons for allocation to the MRD-based intermediate-risk group were lack of a second marker (58%), insufficient sensitivity (51%) and inconclusive course of MRD (28%). However, most patients in this group had combinations of several reasons, e.g. only one marker and insufficient sensitivity, which made a reasonable assessment of the relapse risk impossible. Fifty per cent of the patients were allocated to this group, which is also large in paediatric ALL. In the ongoing GMALL study in patients with low-risk MRD, treatment is stopped after 1 year, whereas in high-risk MRD patients, intensification with stem cell transplantation or experimental treatment is intended. It is unclear at present how to proceed with intermediate-risk MRD patients. In an ongoing GMALL trial, these patients receive maintenance therapy with six intensification cycles for 1 year or more.

Overall, in adult ALL, a variety of potential clinical applications for MRD evaluation are already apparent. One of them is the new definition of CR, which considers the molecular remission status in addition to remission status assessed by morphology. Another important issue is the definition of new MRD-based prognostic factors in addition to conventional risk factors and the definition of MRD-based treatment decisions as described for the GMALL study above. Finally, MRD analysis may be used for molecular monitoring of new treatment ele-

ments such as chemotherapy, antibody treatment, molecular therapy, SCT and others.

Treatment with monoclonal antibodies

Targeted therapy with monoclonal antibodies (MAbs) is a new treatment option in adult ALL. ALL blasts express a variety of specific antigens such as CD19, CD20, cyCD22 for B-lineage ALL or CD25, CD/CD3 for T-lineage ALL and CD52 or CD33 for both, which may serve as targets for treatment with monoclonal antibodies. The presence of the target antigen on at least 20–30% of the blast cells is generally considered as a prerequisite for MAb therapy. Anti-CD20 (rituximab) and anti-CD52 (Campath-1) are currently being explored in adult ALL. First results with the combination of chemotherapy and Rituximab are promising in mature B-ALL.

Other MAbs, such as B43(anti-CD19)–genistein, B43(anti-CD19)–PAP and anti-B4-bR(anti-CD19) in B-lineage ALL and anti-CD7–ricin in T-lineage ALL, have been investigated in phase I–II pilot trials in ALL.

Anti-CD20

Rituximab is a chimeric MAb to CD20 which is expressed on normal and malignant B lymphocytes. It exerts significant anti-tumour activity and has led to an improvement of results in B-cell non-Hodgkin's lymphoma (NHL). CD20, defined as expression on more than 20% of the blast cells, is, however, also present on one-third of B-precursor ALL blasts, particularly in the elderly patients (40–50%), and the majority of mature B-ALL blast cells (80–90%).

This provides a rationale to explore rituximab in B-precursor ALL, mature B-ALL and Burkitt's lymphoma. Favourable results were observed in two trials in which rituximab was used in combination with intensive chemotherapy. Nineteen patients with newly diagnosed Burkitt's NHL or mature B-ALL received anti-CD20 together with the hyper-CVAD regimen for a total of eight doses. Eighty-nine per cent complete remission (CR) was observed. In a GMALL study with 53 patients (mature B-ALL, Burkitt's and other high-grade NHL) the remission rate was 91% in mature B-ALL and in Burkitt's NHL a response rate of 96% (partial or CR) was achieved after two cycles. Although preliminary, these studies indicate that there was apparently no additional toxicity compared with the previous protocol with chemotherapy only. The GMALL study group has recently started prospective trials with a combination of anti-CD20 and chemotherapy also in patients with B-precursor ALL.

Anti-CD52

The CD52 antigen is expressed in most lymphatic cells and to a higher degree in T compared with B lymphoblasts. CD52 antibodies were first used for *ex vivo* T-cell depletion of allogeneic bone marrow grafts in order to prevent GvHD. The humanized antibody Campath-1H showed anti-tumour activity in CLL, T-PLL and other T-NHL. In a few cases of relapsed adult ALL, clinical effects were observed, with reduction of WBC, clearance of peripheral blast cells and partial remission (PR). Although the experience with Campath-1H in overt relapse of ALL is limited, several studies are ongoing, in relapse (also in combination with chemotherapy), in CR with positive MRD or even in *de novo* ALL as consolidation treatment.

ABL tyrosine kinase inhibitors in Ph/BCR–ABL-positive ALL

In *Ph/BCR–ABL*-positive (Ph$^+$) leukaemia the *BCR–ABL* fusion gene is causally involved in leukaemogenesis and is considered to be essential for leukaemic transformation. With a selective inhibitor of the ABL tyrosine kinase (STI571, imatinib, Gleevec®), cellular proliferation of *BCR–ABL*-positive CML and ALL cells can be inhibited selectively (see Chapter 37).

Clinical experience with imatinib in advanced Ph$^+$ ALL

In a study of relapsed or refractory Ph$^+$ ALL patients, monotherapy with imatinib at a daily dose of 600 mg orally produced a haematological response in 60%. A complete haematological remission with normalization of peripheral blood counts (ANC > 1.5/nL, platelets > 100/nL) was noted in 19% of patients. Rapid blast cell clearance occurred within 1 week of treatment in the majority of patients, but this peripheral blood response did not necessarily correspond with a bone marrow response. Median estimated time to progression for ALL patients was 2.2 months.

Haematological toxicity of grades III and IV was frequent but was rarely associated with serious infectious or haemorrhagic complications. Non-haematological toxicity attributed to imatinib consisted primarily of mild to moderate gastrointestinal discomfort, peripheral and facial oedema and muscle cramps, and was readily manageable. No patient discontinued therapy because of non-haematological adverse events and there were no imatinib-related deaths. Thus, imatinib was well tolerated even in heavily pretreated patients.

Imatinib and allogeneic stem cell transplantation in Ph$^+$ ALL

The efficacy of imatinib was also explored in patients with Ph$^+$ ALL who relapsed after allogeneic SCT. Twenty consecutive Ph$^+$ ALL patients received single-agent imatinib (600 mg/day orally) after relapse subsequent to allogeneic SCT. Complete remission was seen in approximately 50%. Donor cell chimerism increased to above 96% in both bone marrow and peripheral blood within the first 4 weeks of imatinib in responding patients, indicating a selective expansion of Ph-negative donor cells over the leukaemic clone. Disease-free survival after 2 years was approximately 20% and overall survival 40%, owing to subsequent salvage therapy. Thus, imatinib as a single agent induces remissions in a substantial proportion of patients relapsing after allogeneic SCT, and in a few cases even a molecular remission can be achieved.

Current concepts for imatinib treatment in *de novo* Ph$^+$ ALL

As a consequence of the encouraging results in relapsed/refractory ALL, imatinib soon entered trials in *de novo* ALL. Imatinib at a dose of 600 mg/day orally was given for 4 weeks after induction therapy in *de novo* Ph$^+$ ALL with CR. The BCR–ABL level after induction therapy decreased by more than 0.5 log in half of the cases, remained unchanged or increased in 40% and approximately 10% of the patients achieved molecular CR. In a subsequent study, imatinib is now given in parallel to the second phase of induction therapy.

Preliminary encouraging results of a combination regimen have also been shown by the group at MD Anderson. Patients with Ph$^+$ ALL received imatinib in parallel with intensive chemotherapy (HyperCVAD regimen) for several cycles without serious unexpected toxicity. Imatinib as 'up-front' therapy in patients with newly diagnosed Ph$^+$ ALL is also currently being tested by the GMALL Study Group in a randomized trial in elderly (> 65 years) patients with *de novo* Ph$^+$ ALL. First results show that this combination is safe, that complete remissions can be achieved by a imatinib monotherapy and that the combination of imatinib and chemotherapy is feasible.

The list of novel compounds that show activity against BCR–ABL expressing cell lines is rapidly growing, including new anti-leukaemic agents that translate insights from basic science into clinical application. Hopefully, these new modalities of molecular targeted therapies will soon improve the outcome of the so far worst ALL subtype – the Ph$^+$ ALL.

Selected bibliography

Annino L, Gökbuget N, Delannoy A (2002) Acute lymphoblastic leukemia in the elderly. *Hematology Journal* 3: 219–23.

Annino L, Vegna ML, Camera A *et al.* (2002) Treatment of adult acute lymphoblastic leukemia (ALL): long-term follow-up of the GIMEMA ALL 0288 randomized study. *Blood* 99: 863–71.

Arnold R, Beelen D, Bunjes D *et al.* (2003) Phenotype predicts outcome after allogeneic stem cell transplantation in adult high risk ALL patients. *Blood* 102: abstract #1719.

Arnold R, Massenkeil G, Bornhauser M, Ehninger *et al.* (2002) Nonmyeloablative stem cell transplantation in adults with high-risk ALL may be effective in early but not in advanced disease. *Leukemia* 16: 2423–8.

Attal M, Blaise D, Marit G et al. (1995) Consolidation treatment of adult acute lymphoblastic leukemia: a prospective, randomized trial comparing allogeneic versus autologous bone marrow transplantation and testing the impact of recombinant interleukin-2 after autologous bone marrow transplantation. Blood 86: 1619–28.

Bassan R, Battista R, Rohatiner et al. (1992) Treatment of adult acute lymphoblastic leukaemia (ALL) over a 16 year period. Leukemia 6 (Suppl. 2): 186–90.

Bassan R, Lerede T, Barbui T (1996) Strategies for the treatment of recurrent acute lymphoblastic leukemia in adults. Haematologica 81: 20–36.

Brueggemann M, Raff T, Gökbuget N et al. (2003) Early tumor kinetics in adult acute lymphoblastic leukemia (ALL) has high prognostic impact. Blood 102: 11 (Abstract #215).

Buchheidt D, Skladny H, Baust C, Hehlmann R (2000) Systemic infections with Candida sp. and Aspergillus sp. in immunocompromised patients with hematological malignancies: current serological and molecular diagnostic methods. Chemotherapy 46: 219–28.

Cornelissen JJ, Carston M, Kollman C et al. (2001) Unrelated marrow transplantation for adult patients with poor-risk acute lymphoblastic leukemia: strong graft-versus-leukemia effect and risk factors determining outcome. Blood 97: 1572–7.

Cornely OA, Ullmann AJ, Karthaus M (2003) Evidence-based assessment of primary antifungal prophylaxis in patients with hematologic malignancies. Blood 101: 3365–72.

Cortes J, O'Brien SM, Pierce S et al. (1995) The value of high-dose systemic chemotherapy and intrathecal therapy for central nervous system prophylaxis in different risk groups of adult acute lymphoblastic leukemia. Blood 86: 2091–7.

Cuttner J, Mick R, Budman DR et al. (1991) Phase III trial of brief intensive treatment of adult acute lymphocytic leukemia comparing daunorubicin and mitoxantrone: a CALGB study. Leukemia 5: 425–31.

Dekker AW, van't Veer MB, Sizoo W et al. (1997) Intensive post-remission chemotherapy without maintenance therapy in adults with acute lymphoblastic leukemia. Journal of Clinical Oncology 15: 476–82.

Durrant IJ (1993) Results of Medical Research Council trial UKALL IX in acute lymphoblastic leukaemia in adults: report from the Medical Research Council Working Party on Adult Leukaemia. British Journal of Haematology 85: 84–92.

Durrant IJ, Prentice HG, Richards SM (1997) Intensification of treatment for adults with acute lymphoblastic leukaemia: results of UK Medical Research Council randomized trial UKALL XA. British Journal of Haematology 99: 84–92.

Ellison RR, Mick R, Cuttner J et al. (1991) The effects of postinduction intensification treatment with cytarabine and daunorubicin in adult acute lymphocytic leukemia: a prospective randomized clinical trial by Cancer and Leukemia Group B. Journal of Clinical Oncology 9: 2002–15.

European Group for the Immunological Characterization of Leukemia (EGIL), Bene MC, Castoldi G et al. (1995) Proposals for the immunological classification of acute leukemias. Leukemia 9: 1783–6.

Fiere D, Lepage E, Sebban C et al. (1993) Adult acute lymphoblastic leukemia: a multicentric randomized trial testing bone marrow transplantation as postremission therapy. Journal of Clinical Oncology 11: 1990–2001.

Geissler K, Koller E, Hubmann E et al. (1997) Granulocyte colony-stimulating factor as an adjunct to induction chemotherapy for adult acute lymphoblastic leukemia–a randomized phase-III study. Blood 90: 590–6.

Gökbuget N, Hoelzer D (1998) Meningeosis leukaemia in adult acute lymphoblastic leukaemia. Journal of Neuro-Oncology 38: 167–80.

Gökbuget N, Hoelzer D (2002) The role of high-dose cytarabine in induction therapy for adult ALL. Leukemia Research 26: 473–6.

Gökbuget N, Hoelzer D (2003) Non-myeloablative conditioning before allogeneic stem cell transplantation in adult acute lymphoblastic leukemia. Haematologica 88: 484–6.

Gökbuget N, Hoelzer D (2004) Treatment with monoclonal antibodies in acute lymphoblastic leukemia: current knowledge and future prospects. Annals of Hematology 83: 201–5.

Gökbuget N, Kneba M, Raff T et al. (2002) Risk-adapted treatment according to minimal residual disease in adult ALL. Best Practice and Research in Clinical Haematology 15: 639–52.

Gökbuget N, Raff T, Brueggemann M et al. (2003) prospective risk stratification based on minimal residual disease (MRD) Is feasible in adult ALL but limited by a high proportion of MRD-intermediate risk. Blood 102: Abstract #1373.

Hallbook H, Simonsson B, Ahlgren T et al. (2002) High-dose cytarabine in upfront therapy for adult patients with acute lymphoblastic leukaemia. British Journal of Haematology 118: 748–54.

Hoelzer D, Arnold R, Freund M et al. (1999) Characteristics, outcome and risk factors in adult T-lineage acute lymphoblastic leukemia (ALL). Blood 94: 2926a.

Hoelzer D, Baur K-H, Giagounidis A et al. (2003) Short Intensive chemotherapy with rituximab seems successful in Burkitt NHL, mature B-ALL and other high-grade B-NHL. Blood 102: Abstract #236.

Hoelzer D, Ludwig W-D, Thiel E et al. (1996) Improved outcome in adult B-cell acute lymphoblastic leukemia. Blood 87: 495–508.

Hoelzer D, Thiel E, Ludwig WD et al. (1993) Follow-up of the first two successive German multicentre trials for adult ALL (01/81 and 02/84). Leukemia 17 (Suppl. 2): 130–4.

Hughes WT, Armstrong D, Bodey GP et al. (2002) Guidelines for the use of antimicrobial agents in neutropenic patients with cancer. Clinical Infectious Diseases 34: 730.

Kantarjian HM, Estey E, O'Brien S et al. (1993) Granulocyte-stimulating factor supportive treatment following intensive chemotherapy in acute lymphocytic leukemia first remission. Cancer 72: 2950–5.

Kantarjian HM, O'Brien S, Smith TL et al. (2000) Results of treatment with hyper-CVAD, a dose-intensive regimen, in adult acute lymphocytic leukemia. Journal of Clinical Oncology 18: 547–61.

Kurtzberg J, Keating M, Moore JO et al. (1996) 2-amino-9-B-D-arabinosyl-6-methoxy-9H-guanine (GW506U; Compound 506U) is highly active in patients with T-cell malignancies: Results of a phase I trial in pediatric and adult patients with refractory hematological malignancies. Blood 88: 2666a.

Labopin M, Gorin NC (1992) Autologous bone marrow transplantation in 2502 patients with acute leukemia in Europe: a retrospective study. Leukemia 6: 95–9.

Larson RA, Dodge RK, Burns CP *et al.* (1995) A five-drug remission induction regimen with intensive consolidation for adults with acute lymphoblastic leukemia: Cancer and Leukemia Group B study 8811. *Blood* 85: 2025–37.

Larson RA, Dodge RK, Linker CA *et al.* (1998) A randomized controlled trial of filgrastim during remission induction and consolidation chemotherapy for adults with acute lymphoblastic leukemia: CALGB study 9111. *Blood* 92: 1556–64.

Lee EJ, Petroni GR, Schiffer CA *et al.* (2001) Brief-duration high-intensity chemotherapy for patients with small noncleaved-cell lymphoma or FAB L3 acute lymphocytic leukemia: results of cancer and leukemia group B study 9251. *Journal of Clinical Oncology* 19: 4014–22.

Linker CA (1997) Risk-adapted treatment of adult acute lymphoblastic leukemia (ALL). *Leukemia* 11: S24–7.

Lluesma-Gonalons M, Pavlovsky S, Santarelli MT *et al.* (1991) Improved results of an intensified therapy in adult acute lymphocytic leukemia. *Annals of Oncology* 2: 33–9.

Ludwig W-D, Rieder H, Bartram CR *et al.* (1998) Immunophenotypic and genotypic features, clinical characteristics, and treatment outcome of adult pro-B acute lymphoblastic leukemia: results of the German multicenter trials GMALL 03/87 and 04/89. *Blood* 92: 1898–1909.

Mandelli F, Annino L, Rotoli B (1996) The GIMEMA ALL 0183 trial: analysis of 10-year follow-up. *British Journal of Haematology* 92: 665–72.

Martino R, Giralt S, Caballero MD *et al.* (2003) Allogeneic hematopoietic stem cell transplantation with reduced-intensity conditioning in acute lymphoblastic leukemia: a feasibility study. *Haematologica* 88: 555–60.

Ottmann OG, Druker BJ, Sawyers CL *et al.* (2002) A phase II study of imatinib mesylate (Glivec) in patients with relapsed or refractory Philadelphia chromosome-positive acute lymphoid leukemias. *Blood* 100: 1965–71.

Ottmann OG, Hoelzer D, Gracien E *et al.* (1995) Concomitant granulocyte colony-stimulating factor and induction chemoradiotherapy in adult lymphoblastic leukemia: a randomized phase III trial. *Blood* 86: 444–50.

Ottmann OG, Wassmann B, Gökbuget N *et al.* (2003) A randomized trial of imatinib versus chemotherapy induction followed by concurrent imatinib and chemotherapy as first-line treatment in elderly patients with *de novo* Philadelphia-positive acute lymphoblastic leukemia. *Blood* 102: Abstract #791.

Ribera JM, Ortega JJ, Oriol A *et al.* (1998) Late intensification chemotherapy has not improved the results of intensive chemotherapy in adult acute lymphoblastic leukemia. Results of a prospective multicenter randomized trial (PETHEMA ALL-89) Spanish Society of Hematology. *Haematologica* 83: 222–30.

Rowe JM, Richards S, Wiernik PH *et al.* (1999) Allogeneic bone marrow transplantation (BMT) for adults with acute lymphoblastic leukemia (ALL) in first complete remission (CR): Early results from the international ALL trial (MRC UKALL/ECOG E2993). *Blood* 94: 732a.

Ruhnke M, Maschmeyer G (2002) Management of mycoses in patients with hematologic disease and cancer – review of the literature. *European Journal of Medical Research* 7: 227–35.

Slavin S, Nagler A, Naparstek E *et al.* (1998) Nonmyeloablative stem cell transplantation and cell therapy as an alternative to conventional bone marrow transplantation with lethal cytoreduction for the treatment of malignant and nonmalignant hematologic disorders. *Blood* 91: 756–63.

Stryckmans P, de Witte T, Marie JP *et al.* (1992) Therapy of adult ALL: overview of 2 successive EORTC studies: (ALL-2 and ALL-3). *Leukemia* 6: 199–203.

Thiebaut A, Vernant JP, Degos L *et al.* (2000) Adult acute lymphocytic leukemia study testing chemotherapy and autologous and allogeneic transplantation. A follow-up report of the French protocol LALA 87. *Hematology/Oncology Clinics of North America* 14: 1353–66.

Thomas DA, Cortes J, Giles FJ *et al.* (2002) Rituximab and hyper-CVAD for adult Burkitt's (BL) or Burkitt's-like (BLL) leukemia or lymphoma. *Blood* 100: 3022.

Thomas DA, Cortes J, O'Brien S *et al.* (1999) Hyper-CVAD program in Burkitt's-type adult acute lymphoblastic leukemia. *Journal of Clinical Oncology* 17: 2461–70.

Thomas DA, Faderl S, Cortes J *et al.* (2003) Treatment of Philadelphia chromosome-positive acute lymphocytic leukemia with hyper-CVAD and imatinib mesylate. *Blood* 102: Abstract #790.

Todeschini G, Tecchio C, Meneghini V *et al.* (1998) Estimated 6-year event-free survival of 55% in 60 consecutive adult acute lymphoblastic leukemia patients treated with an intensive phase II protocol based on high induction dose of daunorubicin. *Leukemia* 12: 144–9.

Wassmann B, Scheuring UJ, Pfeifer H *et al.* (2003) Imatinib mesylate induces sustained molecular remissions in philadelphia-chromosome positive acute lymphoblastic leukemia (Ph ALL) following molecular relapse after stem cell transplantation (SCT). *The Hematology Journal* 4: 146 (Abstract 474).

Welborn JL (1994) Impact of reinduction regimens for relapsed and refractory acute lymphoblastic leukemia in adults. *American Journal of Hematology* 45: 341–4.

Wernli M, Tichelli A, von Fliedner V *et al.* (1994) Intensive induction/consolidation therapy without maintenance in adult acute lymphoblastic leukaemia: a pilot assessment. *British Journal of Haematology* 87: 39–43.

CHAPTER 33

Childhood acute lymphoblastic leukaemia

Der-Cherng Liang and Ching-Hon Pui

Introduction

Acute lymphoblastic leukaemia (ALL) is the most common childhood cancer. Remarkable progress has been achieved in its treatment such that the 5-year event-free survival rates in the most successful clinical trials now range from 75% to 83% (Table 33.1). With retrieval therapy for those who suffer a relapse, approximately 80% of patients can be cured (i.e. no evidence of disease for 10 or more years). This advance can be attributed to the risk-directed therapies developed through well-designed clinical trials and improved supportive care. Current efforts to further improve the cure rate include minimal residual disease detection, molecular genetic studies of lymphoblasts, pharmacogenetics studies, pharmacodynamic studies of anti-leukaemic agents, gene expression profiling and the development of targeted therapies. These studies promise to increase the precision of risk assessment, to optimize therapy, to circumvent drug resistance and to elucidate the mechanisms of leukaemogenesis. In this chapter, we review the current status of the

Table 33.1 Results of selected clinical trials in patients with acute lymphoblastic leukaemia.

Study	Years	No. of patients	Age (years)	% 5-year event-free survival ($\pm$ SE)	Reference
BFM 90	1990–95	2178	0–18	78 $\pm$ 1.0	Schrappe *et al.* (2000a)
CCG-1800	1989–95	5121	0–21	75 $\pm$ 1.0	Gaynon *et al.* (2000)
COALL-92	1992–97	538	1–18	76.9 $\pm$ 1.9	Harms and Janka-Schaub (2000)
DFCI-91–01	1991–95	377	0–18	83 $\pm$ 2	Silverman *et al.* (2001)
NOPHO ALL-92	1992–98	1143	0–15	77.6 $\pm$ 1.4	Gustaffson *et al.* (2000)
SJCRH XIII	1991–94	165	0–18	80.2 $\pm$ 9.2	Pui *et al.* (1998a)

BFM, Berlin–Frankfurt–Münster; CCG, Children's Cancer Group; COALL, Cooperative Study Group of Childhood Acute Lymphoblastic Leukaemia; DFCI, Dana-Farber Cancer Institute; NOPHO, Nordic Society of Paediatric Haematology and Oncology; SJCRH, St Jude Children's Research Hospital.

biological studies and treatment of childhood ALL and suggest future directions.

Epidemiology

The incidence of ALL is higher in boys than in girls, except during infancy, when there is a slight female predominance. Age-specific incidence patterns are characterized by a peak between the ages of 2 and 5 years, followed by falling rates during later childhood, adolescence and young adulthood. There are substantial geographic differences in the incidence of ALL. The rates are higher among populations in northern and western Europe, North America and Oceania and lower among those in Asia, South America and Africa. In the industrialized countries, the incidence is higher among children of European descent than among those of African descent. In this regard, the annual rates (per million population) of childhood ALL from birth to 19 years of age for US whites, US blacks, UK and India are 32.9, 14.8, 29.7 and 11.0 respectively.

Only a small proportion (< 5%) of patients with childhood ALL have underlying hereditary genetic abnormalities. Children with Down's syndrome have a 10- to 20-fold increased risk of developing ALL. Other genetic disorders associated with an increased incidence of ALL include ataxia telangiectasia and Bloom's syndrome. The association between ALL and congenital immunodeficiencies, such as X-linked agammaglobulinaemia and common variable immunodeficiency, is not well established.

Fraternal twins of patients have a two- to fourfold increased risk of ALL during the first decade of life compared with that of unrelated children. When ALL occurs in one identical twin, the other twin has a 20% chance of developing the disease. If ALL is diagnosed in the index twin during infancy, the other twin almost invariably will develop leukaemia within a few months. Molecular studies have demonstrated that intrauterine metastasis of ALL from one twin to the other, via the shared placental circulation, is responsible for the concordant leukaemia.

Aetiology and pathogenesis

The causes of the vast majority of cases remain to be clarified but likely involve an interaction between the host inherited susceptibility, environment, haemopoietic development and chance.

Primary genetic abnormalities and cooperative mutations

Acquired genetic changes are considered to be central to the development of leukaemia. These changes affect the number (ploidy) and/or the structure of chromosomes, such as trans-

locations, inversions, deletions, point mutations, and amplifications. Transformation of haemopoietic stem cells requires subversion of the controls of normal proliferation, a block in differentiation, resistance to death signals (apoptosis) and enhanced self-renewal. The primary mechanisms of leukaemia induction include aberrant activation of proto-oncogenes (e.g. MYC, TAL1, LYL1, LMO2 and HOX11) and generation of fusion genes encoding active kinases (e.g. BCR–ABL) or transcription factors (e.g. TEL–AML1, E2A–PBX1 and MLL linked to one of many fusion partners).

Current multistep models of carcinogenesis predict that the oncogenic events triggered by chromosomal rearrangements are not sufficient by themselves to induce overt leukaemia. The spectrum of secondary mutations involved in the development of leukaemia and their role in the clinical heterogeneity of specific leukaemia subtypes remain to be clarified. These mutations involve both genetic and epigenetic changes in key growth regulatory pathways, including those controlled by the tumour suppressors RB (the retinoblastoma protein and related family members, p130 and p107) and p53. RB plays a critical role in controlling cell cycle entry. The hypophosphorylated RB inhibits the ability of the E2F family of transcription factors to induce the transcription of genes necessary for S-phase entry. Mitogenic signals induce the formation of active cyclin D-dependent kinases, which, together with cyclin E–Cdk2, phosphorylate RB and abolish its growth-inhibitory functions. The activity of cyclin D-dependent kinases is in turn regulated by the INK4 proteins (p16^{INK4a}, p15^{INK4b}, p18^{INK4c} and p19^{INK4d}), which specifically inhibit the activity of cyclin D-dependent kinases and prevent the phosphorylation of RB. Inactivating mutations or deletions of RB are rare in ALL. By contrast, functional silencing of p16^{INK4a} and p15^{INK4b} occurs in almost all cases of childhood T-cell ALL and in a small proportion of B-lineage ALLs. Although the loss of p16^{INK4a} and p15^{INK4b} expression may play a role in the development of leukaemia, it has no independent prognostic significance.

The p53 transcription factor functions as a sensor of aberrant cellular proliferation, DNA damage and hypoxia, and its activation results in either cell cycle arrest or apoptosis. The activity of p53 is negatively regulated by HDM2 (the human homologue of mouse Mdm2), which directly binds to p53 and induces its degradation. The p14^{ARF} tumour suppressor in turn binds HDM2 to antagonize its ability to negatively regulate p53. Silencing of p14^{ARF} is a frequent event in ALL, and overexpression of HDM2 or silencing of the p53 transcriptional target p21^{CIP1} is observed in approximately 50% of ALL cases. Importantly, p16^{INK4a} and p14^{ARF} are encoded by alternative reading frames in the same genetic locus. The high frequency of homozygous deletions that eliminate the expression of both gene products suggests that alterations of both the RB and p53 pathways collaborate in the pathogenesis of ALL. However, it is likely that additional key regulators will be identified as targets for genetic or epigenetic alterations in ALL.

Prenatal origin of some leukaemias

The retrospective identification of leukaemia-specific fusion genes (e.g. *MLL–AF4*, *TEL–AML1*) in the neonatal blood spots and the development of concordant leukaemia in identical twins indicate that some leukaemias have a prenatal origin. ALL with the t(4; 11)/*MLL–AF4* has a high concordance rate in identical twins (nearly 100%) and a very short latency period (a few weeks to a few months), suggesting that this fusion alone is either leukaemogenic or requires only a small number of cooperative mutations to cause leukaemia. By contrast, the concordance rate in twins with the *TEL–AML1* fusion or T-cell phenotype is lower, and the postnatal latency period is longer, suggesting that additional postnatal events are required for leukaemic transformation. This concept is supported by the identification of rare cells expressing *TEL–AML1* fusion transcripts in approximately 1% of cord blood samples from newborns, a frequency 100-fold higher than the incidence of ALL defined by this fusion transcript. However, clearly, not all childhood cases develop *in utero*. For example, the t(1;19)/*E2A–PBX1* ALL appears to have a postnatal origin in most cases.

Environmental factors and host pharmacogenetics

The *MLL* gene, located on chromosome 11q23, is frequently involved in infant leukaemias and in therapy-related acute myeloid leukaemia (AML) after treatment with topoisomerase II inhibitors. It is possible that transplacental fetal exposure to topoisomerase II inhibitors, such as flavonoids in food and drink, quinolone, benzene metabolites, catechins, podophyllin resin, and even estrogens, is a critical event in the generation of leukaemias with *MLL* rearrangements. A case–control study disclosed significant associations between *in utero* exposure to DNA-damaging drugs, herb medicines or pesticides and the development of infant leukaemias with *MLL* rearrangements. Conceivably, a reduced ability of fetuses or their mothers to detoxify these agents could underlie an enhanced susceptibility to ALL.

Genetic polymorphisms of carcinogen-detoxifying enzyme have been variously associated with the development of leukaemia. For example, deficiency of glutathione S-transferases (GST-M1 and GST-T1), enzymes that detoxify electrophilic metabolites by catalysing their conjugation to glutathione, is associated with infant leukaemias without *MLL* rearrangement and with ALL in black children. Polymorphisms of another enzyme, reduced nicotinamide adenine dinucleotide phosphate:quinone oxidoreductase, which converts benzoquinones to less toxic hydroxyl metabolites, has been associated with the development of infant and childhood ALL. Cytochrome P-450 CYP1A1*2A genotype has also been linked to an increased risk of childhood ALL. Recent studies suggest that folate pathways may play a role in the susceptibility to ALL, and that folate supplement may reduce the risk, observations warranting additional studies for confirmation.

Although environmental factors such as chemical mutagens have been implicated in the aetiologies of leukaemia, solid evidence is lacking. Previous studies have largely excluded residential exposure to magnetic fields as a major instigating factor in leukaemogenesis. Two hypotheses have suggested that abnormal response to common infections plays an important role in the development of childhood ALL. Because high socioeconomic status and social isolation are associated with an increased risk of childhood B-precursor ALL, one hypothesis proposes that many such cases, especially those diagnosed between 2 and 5 years of age, are the consequence of a delayed exposure to common infections to a time when there is increased lymphoid cell proliferation and hence increased chance of leukaemogenic genetic mutations. The other hypothesis suggests that transiently increased rates of leukaemia, sometimes in clear geographic clusters, are due to population mixing, resulting in infection in previously unexposed and hence susceptible individuals.

Clinical presentation

The presenting symptoms and signs are quite variable (Table 33.2). Most patients have an acute onset, while in others the initial signs and symptoms appear insidiously. Fever occurs in approximately 50–60% of patients. In at least two-thirds of these patients, fever is due to leukaemia and will resolve within 72 h after the start of induction therapy. Fatigability and malaise are common. Over one-third of the patients may present with a limp, bone pain, arthralgia, or refusal to walk due to leukaemic infiltration of the periosteum, bone or joint or to expansion of marrow by leukaemic cells. Children with prominent bone pain sometimes have nearly normal blood counts, which can lead to a delay in diagnosis. Many patients have manifestations of bleeding, especially epistaxis or oozing from gum. Occasionally, patients present with life-threatening infection or bleeding. Less common symptoms and signs include headache, vomiting, respiratory distress and anuria. Rarely, ALL is detected during routine examination.

Physical examination often reveals pallor, petechiae and ecchymoses in the skin or mucous membranes, and bone tenderness. Liver, spleen and lymph nodes are the most common sites of extramedullary involvement and are enlarged in more than half the patients. Facial and/or abducens nerve palsies are occasionally seen. Ocular involvement can manifest as leukaemic infiltration of the orbit, optic nerve, retina or anterior chamber of the eye (hypopyon). Epidural spinal cord compression is a rare but serious presenting finding and requires immediate treatment to prevent permanent sequelae.

Overt testicular involvement occurs in only 2% of patients, mostly infants or adolescents with T-cell ALL. Less common presenting features include subcutaneous nodules (leukaemia

Table 33.2 Presenting clinical and laboratory features of children with newly diagnosed ALL.

Feature	Percentage of white children (SJCRH)	Percentage of total (BFM)
Age (years)		
≤ 1	2.7	2.7
2–9	71.6	79.6
≥ 10	25.7	17.7
Male	56.0	57.9
Liver edge below costal margin > 4 cm	31.6	30.9
Spleen edge below costal margin > 4 cm	30.4	27.0
Mediastinal mass	10.4	8.1
Central nervous system leukaemia (CNS 3)*	2.7	2.5
Leucocyte count × 10⁹/L		
< 10	46.2	45.9
10–50	29.3	31.8
≥ 50	24.5	22.3
Haemoglobin < 8 g/dL	51.8	53.7
Immunophenotype		
Early pre-B	53.7	69.3
Pre-B	24.9	17.0
T-cell	15.4	13.5
Transitional pre-B	4.0	
B	2.0	
DNA index ≥ 1.16	22.1	25.7
t(1;19)/E2A–PBX1	2.9	2.1
t(9;22)/BCR–ABL	2.4	2.2
t(4;11)/MLL–AF4	3.0	2.9
t(12;21)/TEL–AML1	18.9	

BFM, Berlin–Frankfurt–Münster 90 (1990–95, not including B-ALL; Schrappe *et al.* 2000b); SJCRH, St Jude Children's Research Hospital (1979–2002).
*CNS 3 status denotes the presence of leukaemic cells in a cerebrospinal fluid that contains ≥ 5 WBC/μL with identifiable blasts.

cutis), enlarged salivary glands and priapism. Finally, in some patients, infiltration of the tonsils, adenoids, appendix or mesenteric lymph nodes leads to a surgical intervention before leukaemia is diagnosed.

Patients with cerebellar ataxia who develop a lymphoid neoplasm should be suspected of having ataxia telangiectasia. Increased serum alpha-fetoprotein is a useful aid in the diagnosis. Recognition of ataxia telangiectasia is important because these patients have excessive and sometimes fatal complications from treatment with irradiation (leukoencephalopathy) and cyclophosphamide (haemorrhagic cystitis).

Laboratory findings

Anaemia, abnormal leucocyte and differential counts, and thrombocytopenia are usually present at diagnosis. The initial leucocyte counts range from 0.1 to 1500 × 10⁹/L (median 12 × 10⁹/L) and

are increased (> 10 × 10⁹/L) in slightly over one-half of patients. Hyperleucocytosis (> 100 × 10⁹/L) occurs in 10–15% of patients. Profound neutropenia (< 0.5 × 10⁹/L) occurs in 40% of patients, rendering them at high risk of infection. The majority of circulating leucocytes are lymphocytes or lymphoblasts. In patients with low initial counts (< 2 × 10⁹/L), often there are no circulating lymphoblasts in blood smears. Hypereosinophilia, generally reactive, may be present at diagnosis.

Thrombocytopenia (median count 50 × 10⁹/L) is usually present at diagnosis and severe haemorrhage is uncommon, even when platelet counts are as low as 20 × 10⁹/L, provided that infection and fever are absent. Coagulopathy, usually mild, may occur in T-cell ALL and is only rarely associated with severe haemorrhage. More than 75% of patients present with anaemia; haemoglobin is commonly < 8 g/dL. Anaemia or thrombocytopenia is often mild (or even absent) in patients with T-cell ALL. Rarely, pancytopenia followed by a period of spontaneous haemopoietic recovery may precede the diagnosis of ALL.

Elevated serum uric acid levels are common in patients with a large leukaemic cell burden. Increased serum phosphorus or potassium or water retention may occur and is aggravated by renal impairment. Leukaemic cell lysis (or tumour lysis) syndrome occurs most frequent in mature B-cell ALL, but it may also happen in T-cell ALL or B-precursor ALL with large leukaemic cell burden. Although an enlarged kidney can be detected in 30–50% of patients, kidney size at diagnosis lacks prognostic or therapeutic implications. Approximately 0.5% of patients have hypercalcaemia because of the release of parathyroid hormone-like protein from lymphoblasts. Hypercalcaemia generally resolves rapidly with hydration and chemotherapy. Liver dysfunction due to leukaemic infiltration occurs in 10%–20% of patients, is usually mild and has no important clinical or prognostic consequences. The serum lactate dehydrogenase level is frequently elevated and correlates with the leukaemic cell burden and prognosis. Serum immunoglobulin levels are modestly low (mostly IgA and IgM) in approximately one-third of patients.

Betweeen 50% and 60% of cases with T-cell ALL present with an anterior mediastinal mass. Chest radiography is needed to detect a mediastinal mass or pleural effusion. A bulky mass that compresses the great vessels and trachea can lead to superior vena cava syndrome. Patients with this syndrome tolerate anaesthesia poorly. Abnormalities of the bone, such as metaphyseal banding, periosteal reactions, osteolysis, osteosclerosis or osteopenia, can be revealed by radiography in one-half of the patients. As these changes do not affect treatment and outcome, routine bone radiography is not indicated. Spinal radiography is helpful in patients suspected of having vertebral collapse.

Cerebrospinal fluid should be carefully examined. Lymphoblasts can be identified in as many as one-third of patients at diagnosis, the majority of whom lack neurological symptoms. Traditionally, central nervous system (CNS) leukaemia is defined by the presence of at least five leucocytes per microlitre of cerebrospinal fluid plus lymphoblasts in a cytocentrifuged smear, or by the presence of cranial nerve palsies. However, we contend that the presence of any amount of lymphoblasts in cerebrospinal fluid (even due to iatrogenic introduction from a traumatic lumbar puncture) at diagnosis portends an increased risk of relapse and should be treated with intensive intrathecal therapy. However, the presence of blasts cells in cerebrospinal fluid with a normal cell count during treatment may not be predictive of CNS relapse.

Diagnosis

Virtually all patients have abnormal physical finding(s), abnormal blood counts and/or differential counts, or both. With a clinical suspicion of leukaemia, bone marrow aspiration should be performed. Bone marrow biopsy is occasionally needed in patients with a very packed bone marrow or marrow fibrosis,

leading to difficulty in bone marrow aspiration. Touch preparations should be made from all specimens, to provide air-dried materials for stainings.

Differential diagnosis

Bone pain, arthralgia and occasionally arthritis may mimic juvenile rheumatoid arthritis, rheumatic fever, other collagen diseases or osteomyelitis. Infectious mononucleosis and other viral infections can be confused with ALL; detection of atypical lymphocytes or elevated viral titres aid in the diagnosis. ALL can be readily distinguished from immune thrombocytopenic purpura, as isolated thrombocytopenia is rare in leukaemia. Aplastic anaemia may also present with pancytopenia and complications associated with bone marrow failure, but rarely with hepatosplenomegaly and lymphadenopathy. Paediatric small round cell tumours, when they invade bone marrow, may mimic ALL. However, tumour cells often form clumps in marrow, and tumour can be found by imaging studies.

Morphology and cytochemistry

Morphological analysis of leukaemic cells in smears stained with Romanowsky stain distinguishes three subtypes (L1, L2 and L3) as classified by the French–American–British (FAB) cooperative group. Myeloperoxidase, Sudan black B and ASD-chloroacetate esterase are specific for myeloblasts and α-naphthyl butyrate (or acetate) esterase is specific for monoblasts, while periodic acid–Schiff reagent reacts positively in over 70% of ALL cases. Because of the subjective nature of distinction between L1 and L2 subtypes, and the poor correlation of these subtypes with immunological and genetic features, morphological classification system has not been useful in the clinical management of ALL. Contemporary classification of ALL relies on immunophenotyping, cytogenetics and molecular analyses.

Immunophenotyping

Table 33.3 summarizes antigen expression profiles that distinguish different subtypes of ALL. The most commonly used system divides ALL into early pre-B, pre-B, B-cell and T-cell subtypes. For therapeutic purposes, one needs only to distinguish B-cell and T-cell ALL from all other B-lineage (B-cell precursor) ALL (see also Chapter 29).

Early pre-B ALL

About 60% of ALL patients have an early pre-B immunophenotype. Although immunoglobulin heavy-chain genes are usually rearranged in these cells, immunoglobulins are not detectable.

Table 33.3 Immunological classification of childhood acute lymphoblastic leukaemia.

SJCRH classification		EGIL classification	
Immunological subgroup	Immunophenotypic profile	Immunological subgroup	Immunophenotypic profile
B-lineage ALL	CD19$^+$/CD22$^+$/cyCD3$^-$/MPO$^-$	B-lineage ALL	CD19$^+$ and/or CD79α$^+$ and/or CD22$^+$
Early pre-B	CD79α$^±$/CD10$^+$/Igμ$^-$	B-I (pro-B)	No B-cell differentiation antigens
		B-II (common B)	CD10$^+$
Pre-B ALL	CD79α$^+$/CD10$^+$/cyIgμ$^+$	B-III (pre-B)	cyIgμ$^+$
Transitional (late) pre-B	CD79α$^+$/CD10$^+$/cyIgμ$^+$/sIgμ$^+$		
Mature B	CD79α$^+$/CD10$^±$/cyIgμ$^+$/sIgμ$^+$/sIgλ$^+$ or sIgκ$^+$	B-IV (mature B)	cyIg$^+$ or sIgκ+ or λ+
T-lineage ALL	CD7$^+$/cyCD3$^+$/CD22$^-$/CD79a$^±$/MPO$^-$	T-lineage ALL	Cytoplasmic/surface CD3$^+$
Pre-T	sCD3$^-$/CD5$^-$/CD1$^-$/CD4$^-$/CD8$^-$/CD10$^-$	T-I (pro-T)	CD7$^+$
Early-T	sCD3$^-$/CD5$^+$/CD1$^-$/CD4$^-$/CD8$^±$/CD10$^-$	T-II (pre-T)	CD2$^+$ and/or CD5+ and/or CD8+
Common-T	sCD3^{lo}/CD5$^+$/CD1$^±$/CD4$^±$/CD8$^±$/CD10$^±$	T-III (cortical T)	CD1a$^+$
Late-T	sCD3^{hi}/CD5$^+$/CD1$^-$/CD4+ or CD8+/CD10$^-$	T-IV (mature T)	Surface CD3$^+$, CD1a–
		α/β (group a)	TCRα/β$^+$
		γ/δ (group b)	TCRγ/δ$^+$

EGIL, European Group for the Immunological Characterization of Leukemia; Ig, immunoglobulin; cyIg, cytoplasmic immunoglobulin; sIg, surface immunoglobulin; SJCRH, St Jude Children's Research Hospital; TCR, T-cell receptor.

The blasts always express CD19. Almost all cases have cytoplasmic CD22 and CD79a; weak surface CD22 expression is also evident in many cases. CD10 and terminal deoxynucleotidyl transferase (TdT) are detectable in 90% of cases, and more than 75% of cases express CD34. CD20 is present on a minor proportion of blasts in one-half of cases. In 10–15% of cases, CD45 is very weakly expressed or undetectable; leukaemic cells with this feature are usually hyperdiploid. Early pre-B ALL includes patients with a wide variety of genetic abnormalities (discussed later).

Pre-B ALL

About 20–25% of ALL patients have a pre-B immunophenotype with cytoplasmic immunoglobulin mu heavy chains and no detectable surface immunoglobulins. Like early pre-B, this subtype expresses CD19, CD22 and CD79a. Rearrangement of immunoglobulin light-chain genes is evident in some cases, but kappa and lambda proteins are not detectable. More than 95% of cases express CD10 and TdT. Only two-thirds express CD34. In many cases, surface CD20 is absent or is weakly expressed. Between 20% and 25% of pre-B ALL patients exhibit the t(1;19)(q23;p13) or the der(19)t(1;19)(q23;p13) genotype.

Transitional (or late) pre-B ALL

Approximately 3% of ALL patients have this phenotype. The blasts express both cytoplasmic and surface immunoglobulin mu heavy chains without kappa or lambda light chains. The blasts express CD10, usually TdT, and sometimes CD34. Except for a

high frequency of hyperdiploidy, > 50 chromosomes, there is no characteristic chromosomal abnormality in this subtype of ALL.

B-cell ALL

In 2% of ALL cases, blasts express surface immunoglobulin mu heavy chains plus either kappa or lambda light chains. L3 morphology is typical of, but not diagnostic of, B-cell ALL. Blasts express CD19, CD22, CD20 and frequently CD10; CD34 is negative. In rare cases, TdT is expressed. Often, these cases represent the leukaemic phase of Burkitt's lymphoma (see also Chapter 29).

The genetic abnormality of this subtype is the reciprocal translocation of chromosome 8 with one of the three chromosomes (most commonly number 14) containing an immunoglobulin gene. The critical event in these translocations, t(8;14)(q24;q32), t(2;8)(p12;q24) and t(8;22)(q24;q11), is the juxtaposition of the *MYC* proto-oncogene (at 8q24) with the mu (at 14q32), kappa (at 2p12) and lambda (at 22q11) genes respectively. These rearrangements dysregulate the expression of c-*MYC* encoding a transcription factor, resulting in altered cell proliferation and survival. Dysregulation of c-*MYC* expression, in the presence of other genetic alterations, resulted in B-lineage leukaemia/lymphoma in mice.

It should be noted that occasional patients with the t(8;14) and L3 morphology display a less differentiated B-precursor immunophenotype or lack surface or cytoplasmic immunoglobulin. Even less common is B-cell ALL with L1 or L2 morphology, expression of TdT, CD34 and CD20 (weakly) and no t(8;14), t(2;8) or t(8;22). Clinically, the presence of the specific translocation is of greatest importance for assigning patients to receive therapy for B-cell ALL. Patients without the specific translocation can be treated with therapy for B-cell precursor ALL.

T-cell ALL

T-cell ALL accounts for 12–15% of ALL cases. Blasts express surface CD7 and cytoplasmic CD3 (cCD3). More than 90% of blasts express CD2, CD5 and TdT. Surface CD1a, CD3, CD4 and CD8 are detected in fewer than 45% of cases. HLA-DR is not commonly expressed, and 40–45% of cases are positive for CD 10 and/or CD21.

T-cell ALL can be subdivided according to the distinct stages of T-cell ontogeny: pro-T (CD7$^+$), pre-T (CD2$^+$ and/or CD5$^+$ and/or CD8$^+$), cortical T (CD1a$^+$), and mature T (membrane CD3$^+$, CD1a$^-$). However, as many as 25% of cases do not conform to any of these stages. Moreover, several studies have yielded conflicting results about the prognostic significance of the antigen(s) expression.

T-cell receptor (TCR) proteins are heterogeneously expressed in T-cell ALL. In approximately two-thirds of T-cell cases, membrane CD3 and TCR proteins are absent. In half of these cases, however, TCR proteins (TCRβ, TCRα, or both) are present in the cytoplasm. Most cases with membrane CD3 and TCR chains express the αβ form of the TCR, whereas a minority express TCRγδ proteins. T-cell cases can also be subdivided into prognostically distinct genetic subtypes (see below).

ALL with aberrant antigen expression

Many leukaemias express antigens associated with multiple haemopoietic lineages. There is no uniform terminology or diagnostic criteria for these type of leukaemias. They have been variously termed acute mixed-lineage, hybrid, chimeric or biphenotypic leukaemia. 'Biclonal' or 'oligoclonal' leukaemia, which consists of two or more morphologically or immunophenotypically distinct leukaemic cell populations, is very rare.

Expression of myeloid antigens in ALL has no prognostic significance but can be of value for assessing minimal residual disease by multiparameter flow cytometry. Cases with myeloid antigen expression have a higher frequency of *MLL* rearrangement or *TEL–AML1* (also termed *ETV6–CBFA2*) fusion than do other cases.

Cytogenetic and molecular classification

Leukaemia arises from a haemopoietic progenitor cell that has sustained specific genetic damage leading to malignant transformation and proliferation. Classification based on genetic abnormalities yields clinically and biologically more relevant information than other approaches. To date, 75% of childhood

ALL cases have specific genetic abnormalities with therapeutic and prognostic significance. Karyotypically, ALL cases can be classified according to chromosome number (ploidy) or specific rearrangements. We will only review briefly here the most common abnormalities (see also Chapter 30).

Ploidy groups

Commonly recognized ploidy groups are hyperdiploidy > 50 chromosomes, hyperdiploidy 47–50, normal karyotype, pseudodiploidy (normal number of chromosomes with structural changes), hypodiploidy 45, hypodiploidy < 45 (including near-haploidy 24–28 chromosomes), near-triploidy (69–81 chromosomes) and near-tetraploidy (82–94 chromosomes). Hyperdiploidy > 50 is associated with an age of 1–10 years, a low median leucocyte count, a tendency to accumulate increased amounts of methotrexate polyglutamates, increased sensitivity to antimetabolites, a marked propensity for spontaneous apoptosis *in vitro* and a favourable prognosis, even with treatment based on antimetabolites. Trisomies of chromosomes 4, 10 and 17 have been correlated with the most favourable outcome, but no distinguishing biological features have been identified in this subset.

Cases with near-triploidy have treatment response similar to that of non-hyperdiploid ALL; those with near-tetraploidy have a higher frequency of T-cell immunophenotype. Among cases with hypodiploidy < 45, there is a significant trend for progressively worse outcome with decreasing chromosome number, such that cases with near-haploidy have the worst prognosis.

t(12;21)(p13;q22)/*TEL–AML1* fusion

TEL–AML1 fusion from a cryptic t(12;21) is the most common specific genetic rearrangement in childhood ALL, and can be identified only by molecular analysis. It is identified in 20–25% of Caucasian patients in the USA and Western Europe but in only 15% of Chinese patients in Taiwan and 15% of Japanese patients. The prognosis of this genetic abnormality depends on the treatment. While it is generally associated with a good prognosis, it has no prognostic impact in some studies. ALL cells bearing this abnormality have an increased sensitivity to asparaginase *in vitro*. It has been postulated that increased expression of CD40 and HLA-DR may render these cells more susceptible to immune surveillance.

The *TEL* gene on chromosome 12 belongs to the *ETS* family of transcription factors. *TEL* functions as a sequence-specific DNA-binding transcription regulator. It is normally widely expressed and appears to have an essential role in yolk sac angiogenesis, neuronal development and the establishment of bone marrow haemopoiesis. *AML1* (*CBFA2*) on chromosome 21 encodes a transcription factor that binds DNA as a heterodimer with CBFB and is essential for development of definitive haemopoiesis. The TEL–AML1 protein represses AML1-mediated transcriptional activation through a dominant negative mechanism. The non-translocated *TEL* allele is frequently deleted in cases with the t(12;21); this deletion seems to be crucial for leukaemogenesis.

E2A–PBX1 and *E2A–HLF* fusion

The t(1;19)(q23;p13) with *E2A–PBX1* fusion, found in 5–6% of childhood ALL, is one of the most common translocations and is primarily seen in patients with pre-B ALL. The negative prognostic impact once associated with this karyotype has been abolished with contemporary treatment. The affected genes are those encoding the E2A transcription factor on chromosome 19 and the PBX1 homeodomain-containing transcription factor on chromosome 1. The resulting E2A–PBX1 fusion protein contains the transactivation domains of *E2A* linked to the DNA-binding homeodomain of *PBX1*. *PBX1* is required for the maintenance of definitive haemopoiesis and contributes to the growth of subsets of haemopoietic progenitors through its inter-action with major HOX proteins. Ectopic expression of the E2A–PBX1 chimeric protein in mice leads to the development of leukaemia. The leukaemogenic effect of E2A–PBX1 is mediated, at least in part, by the induction of cell differentiation arrest.

A second *E2A* fusion gene, identified in 0.5–1% of cases with early pre-B immunophenotype, is created by the t(17;19)(q22;p13), in which *E2A* is fused to the gene that encodes hepatic leukaemia factor (*HLF*) on chromosome 17. The E2A–HLF fusion protein contains the transactivation domains of E2A linked to the DNA-binding and protein–protein interaction motifs of HLF. This fusion protein appears to inhibit apoptosis. Though relatively infrequent, these cases are easily recognized by their association with hypercalcaemia and disseminated intravascular coagulation at diagnosis. The prognosis of this genetic subtype appears to be poor.

BCR–ABL fusion

The t(9;22)(q34;q11), found in approximately 3% of childhood ALL, encodes a chimeric gene consisting of the 5′ portion of *BCR* fused to the 3′ portion of *ABL*. In chronic myeloid leukaemia, breaks occur most often within the major breakpoint cluster region (BCR) and encode a 210-kDa BCR–ABL chimeric tyrosine kinase (see also Chapter 37). In ALL, breaks occur most often within the minor breakpoint cluster regions, forming a 190-kDa BCR–ABL. In each fusion protein, N-terminal sequences of ABL are replaced by BCR sequences. This alteration results in a constitutively active ABL tyrosine kinase that induces aberrant signalling and activates multiple cellular pathways. Expression of either chimeric protein results in malignant transformation of haemopoietic cells and causes leukaemia in murine models. As a group, ALL with *BCR–ABL* fusion has been consistently associated with poor response to therapy; allogeneic haemopoietic stem cell transplantation is the treatment of choice if there is a suitable donor.

MLL gene rearrangements

Translocations affecting 11q23 chromosomal region occur in 8% of childhood ALL and in 70–80% of infant cases. The gene involved at the 11q23 region is *MLL* (mixed-lineage leukaemia or myeloid–lymphoid), also known as *HRX*, *ALL1* or *HTRX1*. More than 40 chromosomal loci are known to participate in *MLL* rearrangements. The most common translocation is the t(4;11)(q21;q23), which produces a chimeric protein that contains the N-terminal portion of *MLL* linked in-frame to the C-terminal portion of *AF4*.

MLL is crucial for embryonic development and haemopoiesis. *MLL* normally maintains expression of specific *HOX* genes by binding to DNA and recruiting a histone acetylase that keeps chromatin in an open conformation, accessible to transcriptional activators. In addition to interacting with DNA, *MLL* also directly interacts with the antiphosphatase SBF1, which positively regulates kinase signalling pathways. The leukaemia-associated alterations in *MLL* directly disrupt both of these important activities.

MLL rearrangements are associated with a young age, large leukaemic cell burden and central nervous system (CNS) involvement. The blast cells usually have CD10-negative B-cell precursor immunophenotype and expression of myeloid-associated antigens such as CD13, CD15 and CD33 is frequent. However, cases with the t(11;19)(q23;p13.3) with *MLL–ENL* fusion may have a T-cell phenotype. Age is the most important prognostic factor: infants younger than 1 year fare significantly worse than patients 1 year of age or older. Among infants with the t(4;11), a poor prednisone response and age < 3 months confer an especially poor prognosis; a poor prednisone response also appears to be associated with a poor response in older children with the t(4;11). Among patients with the t(11;19) and *MLL–ENL* fusion, those with a T-lineage immunophenotype, who are generally over 1 year of age, have a better outcome than patients over 1 year of age with B-cell precursor ALL. Haemopoietic stem cell transplantation failed to improve outcome in patients with the t(4;11). Two large cooperative group studies are evaluating the efficacy of intensified therapy that includes high-dose cytarabine, which appears to be particularly effective *in vitro* for leukaemic cells with the t(4;11). The finding of high levels of *FLT-3* expression in *MLL*-rearranged leukaemic cells has led to an ongoing phase I trial of FLT-3-targeted tyrosine kinase inhibitors.

Genetic abnormalities in T-cell ALL

Up to a quarter of patients with T-cell ALL lack detectable cytogenetic abnormalities. The most common specific translocations involve T-cell receptor alpha/delta gene loci on chromosome 14q11 and beta locus on 7q32–36. The translocations juxtapose enhancer elements responsible for the expression of T-cell receptor genes next to a variety of oncogene loci, leading to overexpression of specific genes and disruption of transcriptional pathways involved in normal T-cell development and survival. Genes that are dysregulated in T-cell ALL include *SCL(TAL1)*, *LMO1(TTG-1)*, *LMO2(TTG-2)* and *HOX11*. As a result of the t(1;14)(p33;q11), *SCL* (a gene involved in early haemopoiesis) is inserted next to the *TCRAD* loci; *SCL* expression is associated with *TALd* rearrangement, a cryptic abnormality resulting in an internal deletion of a 90- to 100-kb DNA in the 5′-untranslated region of *SCL*, in an additional 25% of T-cell ALL cases. This deletion juxtaposes the promoter sequences of a nearby gene (*SIL*, for *SCL*-interrupting locus) with the *SCL* coding region, resulting in the expression of a fused *SIL–SCL* transcript that encodes a normal SCL protein. However, misexpression of *SCL* has been detected in up to 60% of T-cell ALL cases, a frequency far exceeding that predicted by karyotype or *TALd* rearrangement.

The t(11;14)(p15;q11) and t(11;14)(p13;q11) inserts *LMO1* and *LMO2* into the *TCRAD* loci, leading to inappropriate expression of the respective LMO1 and LMO2 proteins, which contain two zinc-binding domains and participate in multi-protein DNA-binding complexes. *LMO2*, like *SCL*, plays an essential role in the development of primitive and definitive haemopoiesis. *LMO1* is normally expressed in CNS development and its misexpression is thought to contribute to the development of T-cell ALL in much the same way as for *LMO2*.

Another change found in T-cell ALL is the deletion from chromosome 9p21 of the *INK4a* and *INK4b* genes, which encode the p16^{INK4a} and p15^{INK4b} inhibitors of the Cdk4 cyclin D-dependent kinase. This locus, which is deleted in more than 50% of cases, also encodes a cell cycle regulatory protein, p19^{ARF}, which arrests cell cycle progression through p53.

A recent study using gene expression-profiling technology grouped T-cell ALL cases based on overexpression of the oncogenes *HOX11L2*, *LYL1*, *HOX11*, *TAL1* and *MLL-ENL*. Only one of the oncogenic transcription factors was highly expressed in most of the cases. Overexpression of *LMO1* or *LMO2* was found in most cases overexpressing *TAL1*, and high levels of *LMO2* were noted in *LYL1*$^+$ cases. Microarray analysis revealed that *LYL1*$^+$ cases showed an expression of the genes corresponding to an undifferentiated stage of thymocyte development, *HOX11*$^+$ cases showed a pattern reflecting the early thymocytic differentiation, and *TAL1*$^+$ cases had late thymocytic differentiation. A very favourable prognosis was observed in *HOX11*$^+$ cases, whose cells also have gene expression associated with a propensity to apoptosis. Expression of *HOX11L2*, a transcriptional regulator closely related to *HOX11*, is frequently found in T-cell ALL. The prognosis of this subset depends on treatment and was poor in some studies (Ballerini *et al.*, 2002; Ferrando *et al.*, 2002).

Subtypes of B-cell precursor ALL defined by global gene expression

Using oligonucleotide microarrays, Yeoh *et al.* (2002) identi-fied gene expression patterns that distinguished B-lineage ALL from T-cell ALL, confirming the results of a smaller series (Golub *et al.*, 1999). Moreover, expression profiles clearly identified each of the prognostically important subgroup of B-cell precursor ALL, including hyperdiploidy > 50 chromosomes, *BCR–ABL*, *E2A–PBX1*, *TEL–AML1* and *MLL* gene rearrangement. Examination of the genes constituting the expression signatures provides important insights into the biology of the leukaemia subgroups. For example, dysregulation of *HOX* gene family members has been identified as a dominant mechanism of leukaemic transformation in *MLL*-rearranged leukaemia. Microarray analysis also demonstrated that lymphoid leukaemic cells of different molecular subtypes share common pathways of genomic response to same treatment, and that changes in gene expression are treatment specific, suggesting that gene expression profiling can serve as a new tool for assessing the interaction of anti-cancer agents and providing a basis for optimizing combination chemotherapy.

Prognostic factors and risk groups

Assessment of the relapse risk is an integral part of the approach to ALL therapy. Only high-risk cases are treated intensively, with less toxic therapy reserved for cases at lower risk of treatment failure. Treatment is the single most important prognostic factor. For example, T-cell ALL, B-cell ALL and B-precursor ALL with the t(1;19), once associated with a very poor prognosis, now have a cure rate of 70% or more in some treatment protocols. Likewise, the poor prognosis of adolescence and black race can be abolished with effective contemporary therapy, although in most studies black race is still associated with a poor prognosis.

Age and leucocyte count

In B-cell precursor ALL, age and leucocyte count are consistent prognostic factors. Based on the Rome/US National Cancer Institute criteria, among B-cell precursor ALL cases, the two-thirds with presenting age of 1–9 years and initial leucocyte count < 50 × 10^9/L are classified to have standard-risk ALL, and the other one-third high-risk. However, this classification has limited value because one-third of the standard-risk patients may relapse, while patients at very high risk cannot be reliably distinguished from the high-risk patients. Moreover, the prognostic impact of age and, to a lesser extent, leucocyte count can be explained partly by their association with specific genetic abnormalities. For example, the overall poor prognosis of infant ALL is due to the very high frequency of *MLL* rearrangement (70– 80%) in this age group, whereas the favourable outcome of patients aged 1–9 years is related to the fact that 70% of them have hyperdiploidy > 50 chromosomes or *TEL–AML1* fusion, both favourable genetic features.

Table 33.4 Current ALL risk classifications of childhood acute lymphoblastic leukaemia.

Risk group	Features
St Jude Children's Research Hospital Low	B-cell precursor phenotype and age 1–9 years with leucocyte count < 50 × 10⁹/L, DNA index ≥ 1.16 and < 1.60, or *TEL–AML1* fusion; without CNS or testicular leukaemia, or a t(1;19), t(4;11), t(9;22), or *MLL* rearrangement; level of minimal residual leukaemia < 0.01% at the end of 6-week remission induction
Standard	T-cell phenotype and B-cell precursor cases not classified as low or high risk
High	t(9;22) or *BCR–ABL* fusion, induction failure, or blasts 1% or more (by flow cytometry or polymerase chain reaction) at the end of 6-week remission induction
Children's Oncology Group (B-lineage cases) Low	1–9 years with leucocyte count < 50 × 10⁹/L, have either trisomies 4, 10 and 17 or *TEL–AML1* fusion, rapid early response, without CNS or testicular leukaemia, or a *E2A–PBX1* fusion, *BCR–ABL* fusion or *MLL* rearrangement
Standard	1–9 years with leucocyte count < 50 × 10⁹/L, without trisomies 4, 10 and 17 or *TEL–AML1* fusion, and those with one of these genetic features but slow early response
High	The remaining cases who have no features of very-high risk
Very high-risk	*BCR–ABL* fusion, hypodiploidy, DNA index < 0.81 or initial induction failure
Berlin–Frankfurt–Münster Consortium* Standard	Prednisone good response; molecular remission at the end of induction; no t(9;22)/*BCR-ABL* or t(4;11)/*MLL–AF4*
Medium	Prednisone good response; morphological remission on day 33; no t(9;22)/*BCR–ABL* or t(4;11)/*MLL–AF4*; not fulfil other standard- or high-risk criteria
High	Prednisone poor response; M2 or M3 marrow on day 33; presence of t(9;22)/*BCR–ABL* or t(4;11)/*MLL–AF4*; or ≥ 0.1% leukaemic cells at the end of induction

*M Schrappe, personal communication.

Genetic abnormalities and immunophenotypes

Leukaemic cell genetic abnormality and immunophenotype (T-cell, B-cell and B-precursor) have been incorporated into most classification systems (Table 33.4). Although *HOX11* over-expression confers a favourable prognosis in T-cell ALL, this genetic feature has yet to be included in the current risk classifications.

Even genetic abnormalities can only account partly for the prognosis. For example, up to 20% of patients with hyper-diploidy > 50 chromosomes or *TEL–AML1* fusion relapse. On the other hand, a substantial proportion of the patients with *BCR–ABL* who are 1–9 years old and have low leucocyte counts or who have good early response to prednisone may be cured with intensive chemotherapy alone. Similarly, among patients

with *MLL* rearrangements, those 1–9 years of age with good early response to prednisone, or with *MLL–ENL* fusion and a T-cell phenotype, respond well to chemotherapy.

Pharmacodynamic and pharmacogenetics factors

One plausible reason for the unpredictable relation between biological features of leukaemic cells and response to therapy is that pharmacodynamic and pharmacogenetic factors can exert a crucial influence on the effectiveness of treatment. There is a wide variation in the rate of metabolism of anti-leukaemic agents. Low systemic exposure to methotrexate and low-dose intensity of mercaptopurine have each been associated with a poor treatment outcome. Thus, treatment is unsuccessful in some patients because they have received inadequate doses of drugs, and not because their leukaemia is resistant to therapy. Some anticonvulsants, such as phenytoin, phenobarbital and carbamazepine, can induce cytochrome P450 enzymes, thereby increasing the systemic clearance of a number of anti-leukaemic agents and leading to a poor treatment outcome. In patients who require anticonvulsants, we recommend the use of gabapentin and valproic acid, which are less likely to induce the activity of drug metabolism enzymes.

Patients who have deficiency of thiopurine methyltransferase (TPMT), the enzyme that catalyses the S-methylation (inactivation) of mercaptopurine, tend to have better leukaemia-free survival, probably because they receive a higher dose intensity of mercaptopurine. The null genotype (absence of both alleles) for GSTM1 or GSTT1 and for GSTP1 Val_{105}/Val_{105} has also been linked with lower risk in some treatment protocols, probably because of the reduction in detoxification of cytotoxic chemotherapy.

Early response to therapy

Because response to therapy is determined by both leukaemic cell genetics and host pharmacogenetics, measurements of this response *in vivo* should have a better prognostic strength than that of any other individual biological or host-related feature. The independent prognostic significance of the early response to induction therapy, as measured by the initial decrease of blasts in blood or bone marrow, was first recognized by the investigators of the Berlin–Frankfurt–Münster (BFM) Study Group and the Children's Cancer Group. However, neither measure has great precision, since 20% of patients with a good initial response eventually relapsed, while a third of patients with a poor response survived.

Recent development of assays to measure minimal residual disease by polymerase chain reaction of clonal antigen–receptor gene rearrangements, or by flow cytometry of aberrant immunophenotype, has greatly improved the sensitivity and specificity of assessment of early treatment response. Patients who attain a molecular or immunophenotypic remission, defined as leukaemic involvement of less than 10^{-4} nucleated bone marrow cells after induction therapy, have a significantly more favourable prognosis than those who do not; patients who are in morphological remission but have a post-induction residual leukaemia of 1% or more fare as poorly as those who do not achieve morphological remission. Half the patients show a disease reduction to 10^{-4} or lower after only 2 weeks of induction therapy, and they have an exceptionally good prognosis. Sequential monitoring can further improve the precision. The persistence of minimal residual disease (MRD) is associated with an estimated 70% cumulative risk of relapse. Patients with residual leukaemia of 0.1% or more at 4 months have an especially dismal outcome. Tandem application of flow cytometry and polymerase chain reaction testing has allowed us to study MRD successfully in virtually 100% of cases. We have therefore incorporated MRD detection into our current risk classification system (Table 33.4) (see also Chapter 34).

Other factors

Leukaemia cell growth in model systems, such as mice with severe combined immunodeficiency, cultures on stromal cell layers, or semisolid/liquid culture system, correlates with an adverse prognosis and with resistance to chemotherapy. Other factors related to a poor prognosis include male gender, malnutrition and expression of transporters of xenobiotics of the adenosine triphosphate-binding cassette protein superfamily.

Supportive care

At diagnosis, all febrile patients should be given empiric broad-spectrum antibiotics until an infection can be excluded. Most patients require packed red blood cell transfusions. We transfuse patients who have circulating leukaemic blasts with platelets to keep count close to $100 \times 10^9/L$ before diagnostic lumbar puncture to reduce the risk of traumatic tap. Patients with a traumatic tap and leukaemic blasts in cerebrospinal fluid require intensified intrathecal therapy. After the clearance of circulating blasts, intrathecal therapy can be safely performed without prophylactic platelet transfusion, especially during vincristine–prednisone–asparaginase induction therapy, which is associated with a hypercoagulable state. All blood products should be irradiated in patients who are receiving chemotherapy to prevent graft-versus-host disease.

Careful attention to fluid and electrolyte balance is essential, both at diagnosis and for 48–72 hours after the start of chemotherapy. All patients require intravenous hydration. Specific measures to treat or prevent hyperuricaemia include allopurinol (a xanthine oxidase inhibitor that can prevent uric acid formation) and rasburicase (a recombinant urate oxidase that breaks down uric acid to allantoin – a readily excretable metabolite with 5- to 10-fold higher solubility than uric acid). Rasburicase is a more effective agent than allopurinol, and also facilitates the excretion of phosphorus, partly because of its potent uricolytic effect, obviating the need to alkalinize urine, and partly because of improved renal function with its use. Rasburicase is contraindicated in patients with glucose-6-phosphate dehydrogenase deficiency because hydrogen peroxide, a byproduct of uric acid breakdown, can cause haemolysis or methaemoglobinaemia in these patients. In many patients, a phosphorus binder is needed to treat or prevent hyperphosphataemia and corresponding hypocalcaemia. Rarely, dialysis is needed for acute renal failure.

For patients with extreme hyperleucocytosis, some investigators have advocated the use of leukapheresis or exchange transfusion (in small children) to reduce the morbidity and mortality from leukostasis or leukaemic cell lysis, whilst others questioned the need for these measures.

Other important supportive care measures include prophylactic use of trimethoprim–sulphamethoxazole or atovaquone (in patients with poor tolerance to trimethoprim–sulphamethoxazole) for *Pneumocystis carinii* pneumonitis, the placement of indwelling catheters and psychosocial support. Prophylactic use of granulocyte colony-stimulating factor after induction or during consolidation therapy shortened the duration of severe neutropenia but failed to reduce episodes of febrile neutropenia or improve treatment outcome. In one study, the growth factor appeared to increase the risk of therapy-related AML in the context of epipodophyllotoxin-based therapy. The role of colony-stimulating factors and granulocyte transfusion in the treatment of neutropenia in children with cancer was discussed in a recent review (Liang, 2003).

Principles of treatment

The identification of reliable prognostic factors in ALL and the recognition of ALL as a heterogeneous disease have led to the use of risk-directed therapy. B-cell ALL cases are treated separately with short-term intensive therapy including high doses of methotrexate, cytarabine and cyclophosphamide, as well as anthracycline and intensive intrathecal therapy. For all other patients, specific approaches to therapy differ but consistently emphasize remission induction followed by intensification or consolidation therapy to eliminate residual leukaemia, eradication of CNS leukaemia, and treatment to ensure continuation of remission. The major advances established and some lessons

learned from the recently completed clinical trials are summarized in Tables 33.5 and 33.6. In most studies, patients are divided into three risk groups, even though there has not been a consensus on the most useful criteria or on the terminology. The Children's Oncology Group recently proposed a four-group classification: low risk, standard risk, high risk, and very high risk (Table 33.4).

Induction therapy

The goal of remission induction therapy is to induce a complete remission by eradicating more than 99% of leukaemic burden, and by restoring normal haemopoiesis. Induction therapy typically includes a glucocorticoid (prednisone, prednisolone or dexamethasone), vincristine and at least a third agent (asparaginase, anthracycline, or both). There are several forms of asparaginase, each with a different half-life and hence potency. Two preparations were derived from *Escherichia coli*: Leunase (Kyowa Hacco Kogyo, Japan) is more potent and toxic than Elspar (Merck Sharp & Dohme, USA). Elspar has a half-life of 1.28 ± 0.35 days (SD); when it is covalently bound to monomethoxypolyethylene glycol (PEG), it has a half-life of 5.73 ± 3.24 days. There is another product, derived from *Erwinia chrysanthemi*, with a short half-life of 0.65 ± 0.13 days.

The reported differences in efficacy and toxicity of the various preparations can be attributed to the use of unequivalent doses. In the randomized EORTC 58881 trial, children received *Erwinia* asparaginase had a poorer event-free survival than

Table 33.5 Major advances established from the recently completed clinical trials.

Advance established	Reference
CNS-directed treatment	
1 Early intensification of intrathecal therapy improved outcome	Pui *et al.* (1998)
2 Traumatic lumbar puncture with blasts at diagnosis was associated with an inferior outcome	Gajjar *et al.* (2000), Bürger *et al.* (2003)
3 Cranial irradiation 12 Gy provided adequate CNS prophylaxis	Schrappe *et al.* (2000a,b)
4 Extended intrathecal therapy could replace cranial irradiation in intermediate-risk cases	Pui *et al.* (1998), Conter *et al.* (2000)
5 Omission of cranial irradiation for all patients may be feasible	Manera *et al.* (2000), Vilmer *et al.* (2000)
Intensification/reinduction chemotherapy	
1 Prolonged asparaginase intensification and dexamethasone improved outcome.	Silverman *et al.* (2000, 2001)
2 Intensive asparaginase consolidation benefited T-cell ALL	Maloney *et al.* (2000)
3 Double reinduction improved outcome for high-risk or intermediate-risk cases	Lange *et al.* (2002), Aricò *et al.* (2002)
4 Prolonged reinduction/intensification (augmented BFM therapy) improved outcome of high-risk cases with poor early response	Nachman *et al.* (1998)
High-dose methotrexate	
1 High-dose methotrexate was superior to fractionated oral methotrexate for intensification	Mahoney *et al.* (1998), Harris *et al.* (2000), Mahoney *et al.* (2000)
2 Very high-dose methotrexate (5 g/m^2) benefited T-cell ALL	Schrappe *et al.* (2000a,b)

Table 33.6 Lessons learned from the recently completed clinical trials.

Lesson learned	Reference
Intensive chemotherapy blocks resulted in inferior outcome in high-risk cases	Schrappe *et al.* (2000a,b)
High-dose intravenous mercaptopurine failed to improve outcome	Mahoney *et al.* (2000), Vilmer *et al.* (2000), Silverman *et al.* (2001), Bostrom *et al.* (2003)
High-dose cytarabine given in limited doses failed to improve outcome	Millot *et al.* (2001)
Allogeneic transplantation did not benefit t(4;11) cases	Pui *et al.* (2003b)
Thioguanine treatment did not improve outcome and was associated with hepatic veno-occlusive disease and thrombocytopenia	Harms *et al.* (2003)
Intensive mercaptopurine therapy may potentiate the risk of cranial irradiation-associated brain tumour or epipodophyllotoxin-related acute myeloid leukaemia, especially in patients with thiopurine methyltransferase deficiency	Relling *et al.* (1999b), Pui and Relling (2000)
Erwinia asparaginase at the same dose was inferior to *E. coli* asparaginase	Duval *et al.* (2002)
Hyperfractionated cranial irradiation may be inferior to conventional cranial irradiation	Silverman *et al.* (2001)

those who received *E. coli* preparation at the same dosage of 10 000 IU/m^2 twice weekly. In the Dana-Farber Consortium Protocol 1991–2001, no difference in event-free survival was noted between patients randomly allocated to receive *E. coli* asparaginase 25 000 IU/m^2 weekly for 30 weeks and those who received PEG-asparaginase 2500 IU/m^2 every other week for 30 weeks. Notably, patients who received fewer than 25 weeks of asparaginase therapy had a worse outcome than those who received 25 or more weeks of treatment. In the Pediatric Oncology Group 9310 study of relapsed ALL, the reinduction rate was significantly higher in patients who received 4-weekly doses of PEG-asparaginase than in those who received two doses given every other week. In one randomized trial, one dose of PEG-asparaginase at 2500 IU/m^2 produced more rapid clearance of lymphoblasts in day 7 and day 14 bone marrow and more prolonged asparaginase activity than five doses of native asparaginase at 6000 IU/m^2 on days 3, 5, 8, 10 and 12.

Collectively, the data suggested that PEG-asparaginase at 2500 IU/m^2 for one dose, *E. coli*-derived preparation at 25 000 IU/m^2 per week for 2 weeks or 10 000 IU/m^2 three times a week for 2 weeks, and *Erwinia* product at 25 000 IU/m^2 twice a week for 2 weeks appear to be equally effective. In terms of leukaemia control, the dose intensity and duration of asparaginase treatment are more important than the type of asparaginase used. *Erwinia* asparaginase should be used in patients with allergic reactions to *E. coli* preparation because antibodies against *E. coli* asparaginase cross-react with PEG-asparaginase.

Although asparaginase is an indispensable agent in the treatment of ALL, its use in remission induction is being challenged. In one randomized trial comparing the relative efficacy and toxicity of asparaginase and epirubicin as a third remission-induction agent in patients with standard-risk (low-risk) ALL, patients treated with Leunase 10 000 three times a week for 3 weeks had a significantly lower induction rate owing to a

higher rate of fatal infection. Reducing the dose of Leunase to 5000 IU/m^2 improved the remission induction rate. Dana-Farber Consortium protocols and COALL studies using asparaginase in the post-induction phase had an excellent long-term outcome with low morbidities (especially in terms of thrombotic complications and hyperglycaemia). Hence, additional studies are needed to determine the optimal timing of asparaginase treatment.

Dexamethasone has substituted for prednisone or prednisolone in induction and/or continuation treatment in some regimens because of its better penetrance into cerebrospinal fluid and its longer half-life. Although this substitution improved outcome in one randomized trial, it has also been implicated with excessive life-threatening infections and septic deaths in another. A number of major randomized clinical trials are evaluating the efficacy and toxicities of dexamethasone treatment during remission induction. To this end, higher dose of corticosteroid was shown to abrogate relative drug resistance in an upfront single-agent window study.

An intensified induction therapy is generally used in high-risk and very high-risk cases on the premise that a more rapid and profound reduction of leukaemic burden may forestall the development of drug resistance. Intensive induction therapy, however, may not be necessary for standard-risk (low-risk) cases, provided that patients receive post-induction intensification therapy. Moreover, intensive induction therapy may lead to a poor overall outcome because of an increase in early morbidity and mortality.

With modern chemotherapy and supportive care, 97–99% of children attained complete remission. Approximately 1% of the failures are due to toxic deaths during remission induction and another 1% to drug-resistant leukaemia. Patients who fail to achieve remission have a short survival and, if remission is eventually achieved, a higher rate of relapse. Therefore, most investigators offer these patients the option of allogeneic transplantation after extended induction treatment. As mentioned earlier, patients with 1% or more residual leukaemia at the end of induction had an outcome as poor as those with induction failure and may also be candidates for allogeneic transplantation.

Intensive chemotherapy has been associated with the development of sepsis, disseminated fungal infection and typhlitis. Oral candidiasis occurs frequently. For oropharyngeal candidiasis, it is preferable to use poorly absorbed clotrimazole than other azole compounds to avoid inhibiting cytochrome P450 enzymes, resulting in excessive vincristine toxicities. Foods that may be contaminated with pathogens should be avoided. Glucose intolerance should be monitored in patients at increased risk of hyperglycaemia – adolescents, obese patients and Down's syndrome patients – during early remission induction with asparaginase. Too much salt intake may cause hypertension and seizure, especially in patients with severe constipation. Patients with Charcot–Marie–Tooth hereditary neuropathy are at particularly high risk for vincristine-induced profound neuropathy. Behaviour changes are common owing to the prolonged hospitalization, disease and glucocorticoid treatment, especially dexamethasone.

Intensification (consolidation) and reinduction

Once normal haemopoiesis is restored, patients can tolerate intensification (consolidation) therapy. There is no consensus on the best regimens and their duration. Delayed intensification (or reinduction), pioneered by investigators in the BFM group, is perhaps the most widely used regimen. It is basically a repetition of the induction therapy at 3 months after remission induction. Investigators of the Children's Cancer Group confirmed its efficacy and subsequently showed that double delayed intensification started at week 32 further improved outcome of patients with high-risk (or so called intermediate-risk) ALL. Extended and more intensive intensification therapy also significantly benefited patients with high-risk ALL and a slow response to initial induction therapy, especially in younger children. Whether this approach will benefit standard-risk cases is now under investigation. Hence, reinduction or delayed intensification appears to be beneficial to all patients, whereas double or prolonged intensification appears to be beneficial to patients with high-risk or very high-risk ALL.

Effective components of intensification treatment include the intensive use of asparaginase and high-dose methotrexate. The need for very high-dose methotrexate (5 g/m^2) in T-cell ALL is consistent with the finding that T-lymphoblasts accumulate methotrexate and its active polyglutamates metabolites less avidly than do B-lineage blasts, so that higher serum concentrations of methotrexate are needed for adequate response. The optimum dose of methotrexate for various genetic subtypes of B-precursor ALL remains to be determined, but a dose of 2.5 g/m^2 should be adequate in most cases.

The most successful post-remission intensification regimens generally feature continuous therapy, whereas high-dose pulse therapy with long rest periods due to myelosuppression appears to be less effective. This observation is consistent with the concept of metronomic dosing for solid tumours, based on the idea that continuous or frequent administration of cytotoxic drugs may improve outcome by abrogating the ability of slowly proliferating endothelial cells, essential for survival of tumour cells, to repair and recover during the usual rest period. Angiogenesis has also been seen in ALL, and chemotherapy could affect the recovery of bone marrow mesenchymal and endothelial cells that provide essential survival factors for leukaemic cells.

CNS-directed therapy

Treatment for subclinical or overt CNS leukaemia is an integral part of successful therapy for ALL. Patients with one or more of the following features are at increased risk of CNS relapse and require more intensive CNS-directed therapy: large leukaemic cell burden, T-cell ALL, high-risk genetic abnormality, and the presence of leukaemic cells in cerebrospinal fluid, even if caused by iatrogenic introduction from a traumatic lumbar puncture.

Dexamethasone and intrathecal therapy were shown to improve CNS control. Whether triple (methotrexate, hydrocortisone and cytarabine) intrathecal therapy is more efficacious than intrathecal methotrexate alone remains to be determined. High-dose methotrexate is useful for preventing haematological or testicular relapse, but has only a marginal effect on controlling CNS leukaemia.

Cranial irradiation is effective CNS therapy. However, it can cause substantial neurotoxicity, endocrinopathy and occasional brain tumours. In a study with extended follow-up, prior cranial irradiation (18–24 Gy) was associated with a $20.9 \pm 3.9\%$ (SE) cumulative risk of second neoplasm at 30 years from remission induction, higher mortality rate than that of the general population, and increased unemployment rate. Although 12 Gy cranial radiation together with intrathecal methotrexate and effective systemic chemotherapy can provide adequate CNS control, the long-term sequelae of this approach is unknown. Three clinical trials tested the feasibility of omitting cranial irradiation. In one study, the omission of cranial irradiation was implicated with increased CNS and haematological relapse in T-cell ALL with a presenting leucocyte count of more than $100 \times 10^9/\text{L}$. The inadequate systemic chemotherapy may have contributed to the increased rate of relapse. Two other studies omitted cranial irradiation for all patients. The cumulative risks of isolated CNS relapse were 4.2% and 3.0%, and rates of any CNS relapse were 8.3% and 6.0% respectively. CD10-negative B-cell precursor (pro-B) phenotype, CNS2 or CNS3 status and a leucocyte count of greater than $100 \times 10^9/\text{L}$ conferred an increased risk of CNS relapse. It should be noted that patients with isolated CNS relapse who had previously not received cranial irradiation have a very high retrieval rate. Dutch and St Jude Children's Research Hospital investigators are testing the hypothesis that, in the context of intensive systemic and intrathecal therapy, cranial irradiation can be omitted for all patients. In these studies, cranial irradiation is now reserved for salvage therapy, thus sparing the vast majority of patients from its toxicities.

Continuation treatment

Children with ALL, except those with B-cell leukaemia, require long-term continuation treatment. Attempts to shorten the duration of treatment to 24 months or less resulted in a high rate of relapse. A study which intensified early therapy but shortened total treatment duration to 1 year also resulted in poor overall result. Many investigators prefer to extend treatment for boys to 3 years because of their generally poorer outcome compared with girls, although the benefit of this approach remains to be determined. There is no advantage to prolonging treatment beyond 3 years.

The standard 'backbone' of continuation treatment is the combination of methotrexate given weekly and mercaptopurine given daily. By its inhibiting effect on *de novo* purine synthesis, methotrexate is synergistic with mercaptopurine, enhancing the conversion of mercaptopurine to thioguanine nucleotide, the active metabolite. Pharmacokinetic studies of methotrexate and mercaptopurine have revealed wide intrapatient and interpatient variability in drug disposition. Accumulation of higher intracellular levels of the active metabolites, methotrexate polyglutamates and thioguanine nucleotides, has led to a better outcome. Taking mercaptopurine at bedtime with an empty stomach is advisable for good efficacy. Mercaptopurine should not be taken together with milk or milk products which contain xanthine oxidase, which can degrade the drug. Tailoring dose as indicated by neutrophil count has led to a better outcome. However, overzealous use of mercaptopurine, so that neutropenia precludes further use of chemotherapy and thus reduces overall dose intensity, is counterproductive.

Rare patients (1 in 300) are homozygous deficient for thiopurine-S-methyltransferase and have extreme sensitivity to mercaptopurine, requiring marked reduction in dosage. Approximately 10% of patients have heterozygous deficiency, and may also need dose reduction. Molecular diagnosis can identify the patients who have the enzyme deficiency and allow selective dose reduction of the responsible agent in patients with poor tolerance to antimetabolite-based therapy, leaving the other drugs in full doses. Patients with the enzyme deficiency are also at greater risk of developing radiation-induced brain tumours and therapy-related acute myeloid leukaemia.

The parenteral administration of methotrexate affords a way to overcome decreased bioavailability and poor compliance.

Adjusting the dose of intravenous high-dose methotrexate to account for the patient's ability to clear the drug improves the outcome of B-precursor ALL. Multiple fractionated lower dose oral methotrexate and high-dose intravenous mercaptopurine are ineffective. Notably, methotrexate may induce encephalopathy, even when given orally, when treatment is intensive and leucovorin rescue is insufficient. Patients with Down's syndrome tolerate methotrexate poorly. By inhibiting enzymes involved in folate homeostasis and by depleting cellular reduced folates, high-dose methotrexate treatment may cause transient hyperhomocysteinaemia, which may be responsible for the neurotoxicity.

The addition of intermittent pulses of vincristine and a glucocorticoid to the continuation treatment regimens improves results. Dexamethasone has been substituted for prednisone during continuation therapy in many clinical trials. However, studies to determine the optimum dose and duration of dexamethasone therapy are needed. Glucocorticoid treatment, especially with dexamethasone, often causes behaviour changes; the dose occasionally needs to be reduced or even held because of psychotic reactions. Extended use of glucocorticoid may result in stunted growth, obesity, osteoporosis and avascular necrosis of bone which can be debilitating. Several studies will determine if interrupted use of glucocorticoid, e.g. administration for 1 week and then discontinuation for 1 week during reinduction therapy, can reduce the side-effects but maintain the efficacy.

Allogeneic haemopoietic stem-cell transplantation

Because improvements in transplantation and chemotherapy are occurring in parallel, the indications for transplantation in newly diagnosed and relapsed ALL patients should be re-evaluated periodically. At present, Philadelphia-positive ALL, induction failure and early marrow relapse are clear indications for transplantation. Transplantation has not been shown to improve outcome in other types of very high-risk ALL, such as infant ALL with *MLL* rearrangement, whose outcome may be improved by intensive therapy containing high-dose cytarabine.

Future directions

The trend towards increasingly aggressive therapy is likely to reach a point of diminishing returns. The hope for the future probably is the development of therapies that target the fundamental biological processes. Advances in the molecular classification of ALL, through use of DNA microarrays or proteomic techniques, will almost certainly identify targets for more specific treatments. One precedent is imatinib mesylate (Glivec, Gleevec) for *BCR–ABL*-positive ALL. This agent, which inhibits the BCR–ABL oncoprotein and Kit tyrosine kinases, has induced transient remissions of *BCR–ABL*-positive ALL, as well as partial responses in patients with other malignancies, and is regarded as the forerunner of a new generation of molecularly targeted anti-cancer drugs (see also Chapter 37). Other potentially useful agents still in development include inhibitors of FLT-3 tyrosine kinase for leukaemias having activating mutations of this kinase, and histone deacetylase inhibitors for leukaemias such as *TEL–AML1*-positive ALL. Further refinements in the molecular classification of ALL, together with the identification of genetic features that affect the efficacy and toxicity of anti-leukaemic therapy, will afford unique opportunities to devise treatment plans for individual patients, and thus to realize the ultimate goal of curing all children with ALL.

Selected bibliography

Abshire TC, Pollock BH, Billett AL *et al.* (2000) Weekly polyethylene glycol conjugated L-asparaginase compared with biweekly dosing produces superior induction remission rates in childhood relapsed acute lymphoblastic leukemia: a Pediatric Oncology Group Study. *Blood* **96**: 1709–15.

Alessandri AJ, Reid GS, Bader SA *et al.* (2002) ETV6 (TEL)-AML1 pre-B acute lymphoblastic leukaemia cells are associated with a distinct antigen-presenting phenotype. *British Journal of Haematology* **116**: 266–72.

Aricò M, Valsecchi MG, Camitta B *et al.* (2000) Outcome of treatment in children with Philadelphia chromosome-positive acute lymphoblastic leukaemia. *New England Journal of Medicine* **342**: 998–1006.

Aricò M, Valsecchi MG, Conter V *et al.* (2002) Improved outcome in high-risk childhood acute lymphoblastic leukaemia defined by prednisone-poor response treated with double Berlin–Frankfurt–Münster protocol II. *Blood* **100**: 420–6.

Armstrong SA, Staunton JE, Silverman LB *et al.* (2002) *MLL* translocations specify a distinct gene expression profile that distinguishes a unique leukemia. *Nature Genetics* **30**: 41–7.

Avramis VI, Sencer S, Periclou AP *et al.* (2002) A randomized comparison of native *Escherichia coli* asparaginase and polyethylene glycol conjugated asparaginase for treatment of children with newly diagnosed standard-risk acute lymphoblastic leukaemia: a Children's Cancer Group study. *Blood* **99**: 1986–94.

Ballerini P, Blaise A, Busson-Le Coniat M *et al.* (2002) HOX11L2 expression defines a clinical subtype of pediatric T-ALL associated with poor prognosis. *Blood* **100**: 991–7.

Batova A, Shao L, Dicciani MB *et al.* (2002) The histone deacetylase inhibitor AN-9 has selective toxicity to actue leukaemia and drug-resistant primary leukaemia and cancer cell lines. *Blood* **100**: 3319–24.

Bhatia S, Sather HN, Heerema NA *et al.* (2002) Racial and ethnic differences in survival of children with acute lymphoblastic leukemia. *Blood* **100**: 1957–64.

Bostrom BC, Sensel MR, Sather HN *et al.* (2003) Dexamethasone versus prednisone and daily oral versus weekly intravenous mercaptopurine for patients with standard-risk acute lymphoblastic leukemia: a report from the Children's Cancer Group. *Blood* **101**: 3809–17.

Bürger B, Zimmermann M, Mann G *et al.* (2003) Diagnostic cerebrospinal fluid (CSF) examination in children with acute lymphoblastic leukemia (ALL): significance of low leukocyte counts with blasts or traumatic lumbar puncture. *Journal of Clinical Oncology* **21**: 184–8.

Calero Moreno TM, Gustafsson G, Garwicz S *et al.* (2002) Deletion of the Ink4-locus (the p16ink4a, p14ARF and p15ink4b genes) predicts relapse in children with ALL treated according to the Nordic protocols NOPHO-86 and NOPHO-92. *Leukemia* **16**: 2037–45.

Chauvenet AR, Shashi V, Selsky C *et al.* (2003) Vincristine-induced neuropathy as the initial presentation of Charcot-Marie-Tooth disease in acute lymphoblastic leukemia: a Pediatric Oncology Group study. *Journal of Pediatric Hematology and Oncology* **25**: 316–20.

Cheok MH, Yang W, Pui C-H *et al.* (2003) Treatment-specific changes in gene expression discriminate *in vivo* drug response in human leukemia cells. *Nature Genetics* **34**: 85–90.

Clarke M, Gaynon P, Hann I *et al.* (2003) CNS-directed therapy for childhood acute lymphoblastic leukemia: Childhood ALL Collaborative Group overview of 43 randomized trials. *Journal of Clinical Oncology* **21**: 1798–1809.

Conter V, Schrappe M, Aricò M *et al.* (1997) Role of cranial radiotherapy for childhood T-cell acute lymphoblastic leukemia with high WBC count and good response to prednisone. *Journal of Clinical Oncology* **15**: 2786–91.

Conter V, Aricò M, Valsecchi MG *et al.* (2000) Long-term results of the Italian Association of Pediatric Hematology and Oncology (AIEOP) acute lymphoblastic leukemia studies, 1982–1995. *Leukemia* **14**: 2196–204.

Coustan-Smith E, Sancho J, Behm FG *et al.* (2000) Prognostic importance of measuring early clearance of leukemic cells by flow cytometry in childhood acute lymphoblastic leukemia. *Blood* **100**: 52–8.

Dash A, Gilliland DG (2001) Molecular genetics of acute myeloid leukemia. *Best Practice and Research in Clinical Haematology* **14**: 49–64.

Druker BJ, Sawyers CL, Kantarjian H *et al.* (2001) Activity of a specific inhibitor of the BCR-ABL tyrosine kinase in the blast crisis of chronic myeloid leukemia and acute lymphoblastic leukemia with the Philadelphia chromosome. *New England Journal of Medicine* **344**: 1038–42.

Duval M, Suciu S, Ferster A *et al.* (2002) Comparison of *Escherichia coli*-asparaginase with *Erwinia*-asparaginase in the treatment of childhood lymphoid malignancies: results of a randomized European Organization for Research and Treatment of Cancer – Children's Leukemia Group phase 3 trial. *Blood* **99**: 2734–9.

Ernst P, Wang J, Korsmeyer SJ (2002) The role of *MLL* in hematopoiesis and leukemia. *Current Opinions in Hematology* **9**: 282–7.

Evans WE, McLeod HL (2003) Pharmacogenomics – drug disposition, drug targets, and side-effects. *New England Journal of Medicine* **348**: 538–49.

Ferrando AA, Neuberg, DS, Staunton J *et al.* (2002) Gene expression signatures define novel oncogenic pathways in T cell acute lymphoblastic leukemia. *Cancer Cell* **1**: 75–87.

Ferrando AA, Armstrong SA, Neuberg DS *et al.* (2003) Gene expression signatures in *MLL*-rearranged T-lineage and B-precursor acute leukemias: dominance of *HOX* dysregulation. *Blood* **102**: 262–8.

Gajja A, Harrison PL, Sandlund JT *et al.* (2000) Traumatic lumbar puncture at diagnosis adversely affects outcome in childhood acute lymphoblastic leukemia. *Blood* **96**: 3381–4.

Gaynon PS, Trigg ME, Heerema NA *et al.* (2000) Children's Cancer Group trials in childhood acute lymphoblastic leukemia (1983–1995). *Leukemia* **14**: 2223–33.

Gilliland DG (2002) Promise and challenge of molecularly targeted therapy in hematologic malignancy. *Current Opinions in Hematology* **9**: 265–7.

Goldman SC, Holcenberg JS, Finklestein JZ *et al.* (2001) A randomized comparison between rasburicase and allopurinol in children with lymphoma or leukaemia at high risk for tumor lysis. *Blood* **97**: 2998–3003.

Golub TR, Slonim DK, Tamayo P *et al.* (1999) Molecular classification of cancer: class discovery and class prediction by gene expression monitoring. *Science* **286**: 531–7.

Greaves MF, Maia AT, Wiemels JL *et al.* (2003) Leukemia in twins: lessons in natural history. *Blood* **102**: 2321–33.

Gustafsson G, Schmiegelow K, Forestier E *et al.* (2000) Improving outcome through two decades in childhood ALL in the Nordic countries: the impact of high-dose methotrexate in the reduction of CNS irradiation. *Leukemia* **14**: 2267–75.

Hanahan D, Bergers G, Bergsland E *et al.* (2000) Less is more, regularly: metronomic dosing of cytotoxic drugs can target tumor angiogenesis in mice. *Journal of Clinical Investigation* **105**: 1045–7.

Harms DO, Janka-Schaub GE (2000) Co-operative study group for childhood acute lymphoblastic leukemia (COALL): long-term follow-up of trials 82, 85, 89 and 92. *Leukemia* **14**: 2234–9.

Harms DO, Göbel U, Spaar HJ *et al.* (2003) Thioguanine offers no advantage over mercaptopurine in maintenance treatment of childhood ALL: results of the randomized trial COALL-92. *Blood* **102**: 2736–40.

Harris MB, Shuster JJ, Pullen J *et al.* (2000) Treatment of children with early pre-B and pre-B acute lymphocytic leukemia with antimetabolite-based intensification regimens: A Pediatric Oncology Group Study. *Leukemia* **14**: 1570–6.

Heath JA, Steinherz PG, Altman A *et al.* (2003) Human granulocyte colony-stimulating factor in children with high-risk acute lymphoblastic leukemia: a Children's Cancer Group Study. *Journal of Clinical Oncology* **21**: 1612–17.

Howard SC, Gajjar A, Ribeiro RC *et al.* (2000) Safety of lumbar puncture for children with acute lymphoblastic leukemia and thrombocytopenia. *JAMA* **284**: 2222–4.

Hurwitz CA, Silverman LB, Schorin MA *et al.* (2000) Substituting dexamethasone for prednisone complicates remission induction in children with acute lymphoblastic leukemia. *Cancer* **88**: 1964–9.

Kamps WA, Bökkerink JPM, Hakvoort-Cammel FGAJ *et al.* (2002) BFM-oriented treatment for children with acute lymphoblastic leukemia without cranial irradiation and treatment reduction for standard risk patients: results of DCLSG protocol ALL-8 (1991–1996). *Leukemia* **16**: 1099–111.

Kishi S, Griener J, Cheng C *et al.* (2003) Homocysteine, pharmacogenetics, and neurotoxicity in children with leukemia. *Journal of Clinical Oncology* **15**: 3084–91.

Krajinovic M, Labuda D, Mathonnet G *et al.* (2002) Polymorphisms in genes encoding drugs and xenobiotic metabolizing enzymes, DNA repair enzymes, and response to treatment of childhood acute lymphoblastic leukemia. *Clinical Cancer Research* **8**: 802–10.

Lange BJ, Bostrom BC, Cherlow JM *et al.* (2002) Double-delayed intensification improves event-free survival for children with intermediate-risk acute lymphoblastic leukemia: a report from the Children's Cancer Group. *Blood* **99**: 825–33.

Levis M, Allebach J, Tse KF *et al.* (2002) A FLT3-targeted tyrosine kinase inhibitor is cytotoxic to leukemia cells *in vitro* and *in vivo*. *Blood* **99**: 3885–91.

Liang D-C (2003) The role of colony-stimulating factors and granulocyte transfusion in treatment options for neutropenia in children with cancer. *Pediatric Drugs* **5**: 673–84.

Liang D-C, Hung I-J, Yang C-P *et al.* (1999) Unexpected mortality from the use of *E. coli* L-asparaginase during remission induction therapy for childhood acute lymphoblastic leukemia: a report from the Taiwan Pediatric Oncology Group. *Leukemia* **13**: 155–60.

Loh ML, Rubnitz JE (2002) TEL/AML1-positive pediatric leukemia: prognostic significance and therapeutic approaches. *Current Opinions in Hematology* **9**: 345–52.

Lorsbach RB, Downing JR (2001) The role of the AML1 transcription factor in leukemogenesis. *International Journal of Hematology* **74**: 258–65.

MacBeath G (2002) Protein microarrays and proteomics. *Nature Genetics* **32**: 526–32.

Mahoney DH, Shuster JJ, Nitschke R *et al.* (1998) Acute neurotoxicity in children with B-precursor acute lymphoid leukemia: an association with intermediate-dose intravenous methotrexate and intrathecal triple therapy – a Pediatric Oncology Group Study. *Journal of Clinical Oncology* **16**: 1712–22.

Mahoney DH Jr, Shuster JJ, Nitschke R *et al.* (2000) Intensification with intermediate-dose intravenous methotrexate is effective therapy for children with lower-risk B-precursor acute lymphoblastic leukemia: A Pediatric Oncology Group Study. *Journal of Clinical Oncology* **18**: 1285–94.

Maia AT, Ford AM, Jalali GR *et al.* (2001) Molecular tracking of leukemogenesis in a triplet pregnancy. *Blood* **98**: 478–82.

Maloney KW, Shuster JJ, Murphy S *et al.* (2000) Long-term results of treatment studies for childhood acute lymphoblastic leukemia: Pediatric Oncology Group studies from 1986–1994. *Leukemia* **14**: 2276–85.

Manera R, Ramirez I, Mullins J *et al.* (2000) Pilot studies of species-specific chemotherapy of childhood acute lymphoblastic leukemia using genotype and immunophenotype. *Leukemia* **14**: 1354–61.

Melnick A, Licht JD (2002) Histone deacetylases as therapeutic targets in hematologic malignancies. *Current Opinions in Hematology* **9**: 322–32.

Millot F, Suciu S, Philippe N *et al.* (2001) Value of high-dose cytarabine during interval therapy of a Berlin–Frankfurt–Munster-based protocol in increased-risk children with acute lymphoblastic leukemia and lymphoblastic lymphoma: results of the European Organization for Research and Treatment of Cancer 58881

Randomized Phase III Trial. *Journal of Clinical Oncology* **19**: 1935–42.

Mori H, Colman SM, Xiao Z *et al.* (2002) Chromosome translocations and covert leukemic clones are generated during normal fetal development. *Proceedings of the National Academy of Sciences of the USA* **99**: 8242–7.

Nachman JB, Sather HN, Sensel MG *et al.* (1998) Augmented post-induction therapy for children with high-risk acute lymphoblastic leukemia and a slow response to initial therapy. *New England Journal of Medicine* **338**: 1663–71.

Panzer-Grümayer ER, Schneider M, Panzer S *et al.* (2000) Rapid molecular response during early induction chemotherapy predicts a good outcome in childhood acute lymphoblastic leukemia. *Blood* **95**: 790–4.

Patte C, Auperin A, Michon J *et al.* (2001) The Société Française d'Oncologie Pédiatrique LMB98 protocol: highly effective multi-agent chemotherapy tailored to the tumor burden and initial response in 561 unselected children with B-cell lymphomas and L3 leukemia. *Blood* **97**: 3370–9.

Petricoin EF, Zoon KC, Kohn EC *et al.* (2002) Clinical proteomics: translating benchside promise into bedside reality. *Nature Review of Drug Discovery* **1**: 683–95.

Pui C-H, Campana D (2000) New definition of remission in childhood acute lymphoblastic leukaemia. *Leukemia* **14**: 783–5.

Pui C-H, Evans WE (1998) Acute lymphoblastic leukaemia. *New England Journal of Medicine* **339**: 605–15.

Pui C-H, Relling MV (2000) Topoisomerase II inhibitor-related acute myeloid leukaemia. *British Journal of Haematology* **109**: 13–23.

Pui C-H, Carroll AJ, Head D *et al.* (1990) Near-triploid and near-tetraploid acute lymphoblastic leukaemia of childhood. *Blood* **76**: 590–6.

Pui C-H, Raimondi SC, Hancock ML *et al.* (1994) Immunologic, cytogenetic, and clinical characterization of childhood acute lymphoblastic leukaemia with the t(1;19) (q23;p13) or its derivative. *Journal of Clinical Oncology* **12**: 2601–6.

Pui C-H, Mahmoud HH, Rivera GK *et al.* (1998) Early intensification of intrathecal chemotherapy virtually eliminates central nervous system relapse in children with acute lymphoblastic leukaemia. *Blood* **92**: 411–15.

Pui C-H, Campana D, Evans WE (2001a) Childhood acute lymphoblastic leukaemia – current status and future perspectives. *Lancet Oncology* **2**: 597–607.

Pui C-H, Mahmoud HH, Wiley JM *et al.* (2001b) Recombinant urate oxidase for the prophylaxis or treatment of hyperuricaemia in patients with leukaemia or lymphoma. *Journal of Clinical Oncology* **19**: 697–704.

Pui C-H, Cheng C, Leung W *et al.* (2003) Extended follow-up of long-term survivors of childhood acute lymphoblastic leukaemia. *New England Journal of Medicine* **349**: 640–9.

Pui C-H, Chessells JM, Camitta B *et al.* (2003) Clinical heterogeneity in childhood acute lymphoblastic leukemia with 11q23 rearrangements. *Leukemia* **17**: 700–6.

Pui C-H, Sandlund JT, Pei D *et al.* (2003) Results of therapy for acute lymphoblastic leukemia in black and white children. *JAMA* **290**: 2001–7

Pui C-H, Relling MV, Downing JR (2004) Acute lymphoblastic leukaemia. *New England Journal of Medicine* **350**: 1535–48.

Relling MV, Dervieux T (2001) Pharmacogenetics and cancer therapy. *National Reiew of Cancer* **1**: 99–108.

Relling MV, Hancock ML, Rivera GK *et al.* (1999a) Mercaptopurine therapy intolerance and heterozygosity at the thiopurine S-methyltransferase gene locus. *Journal of the National Cancer Institute* **91**: 2001–8.

Relling MV, Rubnitz JE, Rivera GK *et al.* (1999b) High incidence of secondary brain tumors after radiotherapy and antimetabolites. *Lancet* **354**: 34–9.

Relling MV, Boyett JM, Blanco JG *et al.* (2003) Granulocyte colony-stimulating factor and the risk of secondary myeloid malignancy. *Blood* **101**: 3862–7.

Schrappe M, Reiter A, Ludwig WD *et al.* (2000a) Improved outcome in childhood acute lymphoblastic leukaemia despite reduced use of anthracyclines and cranial radiotherapy: results of trial ALL-BFM 90. German-Austrian-Swiss ALL-BFM Study Group. *Blood* **95**: 3310–22.

Schrappe M, Reiter A, Zimmermann M *et al.* (2000b) Long-term results of four consecutive trials in childhood ALL performed by the ALL-BFM study group from 1981 to 1995. *Leukemia* **14**: 2205–22.

Schwartz CL, Thompson EB, Gelber RD *et al.* (2001) Improved response with higher corticosteroid dose in children with acute lymphoblastic leukemia. *Journal of Clinical Oncology* **19**: 1040–6.

Seeger K, Stackelberg AV, Taube T *et al.* (2001) Relapse of TEL-AML1–positive acute lymphoblastic leukemia in childhood: a matched-pair analysis. *Journal of Clinical Oncology* **19**: 3188–93.

Sherr CJ, McCormick F (2002) The RB and p53 pathways in cancer. *Cancer Cell* **2**: 103–12.

Silverman LB, Declerck L, Gelber RD *et al.* (2000) Results of Dana-Farber Cancer Institute Consortium protocols for children with newly diagnosed acute lymphoblastic leukemia (1981–1995). *Leukemia* **14**: 2247–56.

Silverman LB, Gelber RD, Dalton VK *et al.* (2001) Improved outcome for children with acute lymphoblastic leukemia: results of Dana-Farber Consortium Protocol 91–01. *Blood* **97**: 1211–18.

Stanulla M, Schrappe M, Brechlin AM *et al.* (2000) Polymorphisms within glutathione S-transferase genes (GSTM1, GSTT1, GSTP1) and risk of relapse in childhood B-cell precursor acute lymphoblastic leukemia: a case-control study. *Blood* **95**: 1222–8.

Szczepanski T, Orfão A, van der Velden VHJ (2001) Minimal residual disease in leukaemia patients. *Lancet Oncology* **2**: 409–17.

Taub JW, Konrad MA, Ge Y *et al.* (2002) High frequency of leukemic clones in newborn screening blood samples of children with B-precursor acute lymphoblastic leukemia. *Blood* **99**: 2992–6.

Toyoda Y, Manabe A, Tsuchida M *et al.* (2000) Six months of maintenance chemotherapy after intensified treatment for acute lymphoblastic leukemia of childhood. *Journal of Clinical Oncology* **18**: 1508–16.

Venkatakrishnan K, von Moltke LL, Greenblatt DJ (2000) Effects of the antifungal agents on oxidative drug metabolism: clinical relevance. *Clinical Pharmacokinetics* **38**: 111–80.

Vilmer E, Suciu S, Ferster A *et al.* (2000) Long-term results of three randomized trials (58831, 58832, 58881) in childhood acute lymphoblastic leukaemia: A CLCG-EORTC report. *Leukemia* **14**: 2257–66.

Wiemels JL, Smith RN, Taylor GM *et al.* (2001) Methylene-tetrahydrofolate reductase (MTHFR) polymorphisms and risk of molecularly defined subtypes of childhood acute leukemia. *Proceedings of the National Academy of Sciences of the USA* **98**: 4004–9.

Wiemels JL, Leonard BC, Wang Y *et al.* (2002) Site-specific translocation and evidence of postnatal origin of the t(1;19) E2A-PBX1 fusion in childhood acute lymphoblastic leukemia. *Proceedings of the National Academy of Sciences of the USA* **99**: 15101–6.

Yeoh EJ, Ross ME, Shurtleff SA *et al.* (2002) Classification, subtype discovery, and prediction of outcome in pediatric acute lymphoblastic leukemia by gene expression profiling. *Cancer Cell* **1**: 133–43.

CHAPTER 34

Minimal residual disease in acute leukaemia

34

Letizia Foroni, Paula M Gameiro and A Victor Hoffbrand

Basic aspects of detection of minimal residual disease in acute leukaemia

Patients with acute lymphoblastic or acute myeloid leukaemia may harbour up to 10^{12} malignant cells at presentation. With chemotherapy, the majority of both children and adults (below the age of 65 years) achieve complete clinical remission (CCR) following the first course of induction therapy. However, even in CCR, patients can still have as many as 10^{10} malignant cells in the marrow, and this is responsible for relapse in 15–20% of children and 50–60% of adults with acute lymphoblastic leukaemia (ALL) and in a varying proportion of patients with acute myeloid leukaemia (AML).

A variety of methods have been developed to detect malignant cells in patients in CCR, i.e. to detect 'minimal residual disease' (MRD) with higher sensitivity than morphology. This conventionally defines CCR by the presence of less than 5% blasts in the bone marrow. The goal of more sensitive techniques for MRD detection is to adjust patients' therapy in order to reduce both the risk of relapse and of overtreatment, particularly in children. It is also aimed at determining the quality of stem cell harvests for autologous stem cell transplantation (SCT) and prediction of early relapse in patients following allogeneic SCT, e.g. when donor leucocyte infusion may be particularly effective at eliminating residual disease.

MRD is defined as the lowest level of disease detectable in patients in CCR by the methods available. A reliable technique for MRD detection should be specific (discriminate malignant from normal cells), sensitive (able to detect up to one leukaemic cell in at least 10^4 normal cells), reproducible (widely applicable in different laboratories) and quantitative (provide a numerical estimate of positive cells).

Several tests have been developed. Among these, the detection of tumour-associated aberrant immunophenotypic patterns by flow cytometry and leukaemic cell DNA or RNA by the polymerase chain reaction (PCR) have become the two most extensively used (Figure 34.1). They combine the highest levels of sensitivity and specificity. Other techniques, including

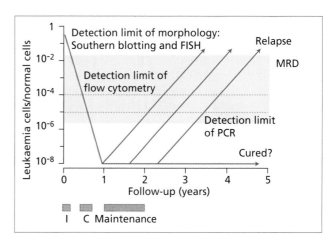

Figure 34.1 Relation between MRD level, stage of treatment and clinical status.

cytogenetics, fluorescence *in situ* hybridization (FISH) and Southern blotting lack the sensitivity required for detection of MRD.

Minimal residual disease detection by immunology and flow cytometry

Acute lymphoblastic leukaemia

The use of muliparameter flow cytometry for the immunological measurement of MRD requires the identification of a leukaemic-specific pattern of antigen expression (or profile) at presentation which is then sought at follow-up. The various phenotypes that can be used for MRD detection have been summarized (Table 34. 1).

Table 34.1 Main marker combinations used to study MRD in childhood ALL and AML.

Cell lineage	Marker combination	Applicability (%)*
T-lineage ALL	TdT/CD5/CD3	90–95
	CD34/CD5/CD3	20–25
B-lineage ALL	CD19/CD34/CD10/CD38	40–60
	CD19/CD34/CD10/CD58	40–60
	CD19/CD34/CD10/CD45	40–60
	CD19/CD34/CD10/TdT	40–50
	CD19/CD34/CD10/CD66c	30–40
	CD19/CD34/TdT/IgM	10–20
	CD19/CD34/CD10/CD22	10–15
	CD19/CD34/CD10/CD13	10–15
	CD19/CD34/CD10/CD15	10–15
	CD19/CD34/CD10/NG-2	5–10
AML	CD33/CD34/CD117/CD15	20–40
	CD33/CD34/CD117/CD13	20–40
	CD13/CD33/CD34/CD56	20–30
	CD13/CD33/CD34/CD133	20–30
	CD13/CD33/CD34/CD7	20–30
	CD13/CD33/CD34/CD38	15–20
	CD33/CD34/CD117/HLA-Dr	15–20
	CD13/CD33/CD34/CD15	15–20
	CD33/CD34/CD117/CD11b	10–15
	CD13/CD33/CD34/CD19	5–10

*Percentage of patients with each type of leukaemia in whom MRD could be studied with the listed antibody combination. Percentages were calculated by including only cases in which intensity of antigen expression was sufficiently different from that of normal bone marrow cells to afford a sensitivity of detection of 1 in 10^4 or greater for ALL and 1 in 10^3 or greater in AML (table kindly provided by D. Campana, Professor of Paediatrics, University of Tennessee College of Medicine, Memphis, USA).

The method requires fresh material for analysis and operators skilled in flow cytometry to achieve the identification of rare leukaemic cells in the background of normal bone marrow cells. In competent hands, it can achieve sensitivity of 1 in 10^4 and a result can be obtained in 2–3 hours.

In T cell precursor ALL (T-ALL) patients, for instance, the double expression of terminal deoxynucleotidyl transferase (TdT) and cytoplasmic CD3 (cCD3) antigens makes the identification of leukaemic cells reliable up to 1 in 10^4 since normal bone marrow does not contain cells of this phenotype. Flow cytometry tests in childhood T-ALL show that the test is a good prognostic indicator of outcome with comparable levels of MRD in peripheral blood and BM samples, suggesting that monitoring of T-ALL patients can be done using peripheral blood samples.

In B-precursor ALL, distinction of leukaemic cells from normal regenerative post-chemotherapy cells is more difficult and may vary with the stage of treatment. In childhood B-precursor ALL patients, flow cytometry shows that MRD at < 0.01% as early as day 19 post induction identifies patients with high leukaemic cytoreduction and high frequency of subsequent CCR (> 97%). By contrast, MRD between > 0.1% and 1% at week 14 post induction identifies patients with a poor outcome (> 68% relapse incidence compared with 7% in patients MRD negative at this stage). High relapse rates are also observed in patients with MRD at any level in bone marrow samples beyond 3 months from presentation. Peripheral blood is approximately 10-fold less sensitive than bone marrow in B-precursor ALL, so a positive MRD test in PB identifies patients at higher risk of relapse than patients with MRD only in the bone marrow.

Acute myeloid leukaemia

Multiparameter flow cytometry has also been extensively applied to AML. Cross-lineage antigen expression and ectopic expression or abnormal light scatter patterns identify up to 50% of AML cases suitable for MRD investigation with a sensitivity of 1 in 10^4 (Table 34.1). MRD levels post induction identify four groups of patients. Patients with MRD < $1:10^4$ show no relapse while relapse rates increase to 14% with MRD at $1:10^3$–10^4, 50% for MRD levels between $1:10^2$ and $1:10^3$ and 84% with MRD above $1:10^2$. These higher MRD values are more frequent in patients with other adverse prognostic factors such as unfavourable cytogenetics and high white blood cell counts. Nevertheless, MRD detection remains independently prognostic in a multivariate analysis.

Flow cytometry offers several advantages since it provides a direct measurement of the number of leukaemic cells present. It is rapid, measures size of cells and distinguishes between viable and dead cells. Immunophenotypic change of the leukaemic cells may give negative results. Complete phenotypic switches are, however, rare.

Minimal residual disease detection by polymerase chain reaction

Acute lymphoblastic leukaemia

Minimal residual disease investigation in ALL using PCR relies on the detection of one or other of two molecular targets that distinguish the leukaemic cell from normal lymphoid cells: (i) junctional regions that result from clonal immunoglobulin and T-cell receptor gene rearrangement and (ii) fusion transcripts due to specific chromosomal translocations. Antigen receptor gene rearrangements occur naturally in B and T cells as part of normal lymphocyte development (see Chapter 20) and, because their sequences are unique in each precursor cell, can be considered as cell/patient-specific targets. The fusion transcripts resulting from chromosomal translocations are leukaemia but not patient specific. The two targets have different biological, technical and clinical aspects and are discussed separately. The results are available in 24–72 h, depending on the technique used.

Antigen receptor gene targets for MRD detection

Both B and T cells have highly specific cell-surface receptors, the immunoglobulin (Ig) or B-cell antigen receptor (BCR) and the T-cell receptor (TCR) respectively, for structure, organization and gene rearrangement of IgH and TCR molecules.

PCR-based MRD detection using antigen receptor genes

Identification of a clonal marker in B-precursor ALL and T-ALL

The process of Ig and TCR rearrangement gives rise to a unique rearrangement in each B cell (involving the genes for Ig production) and T cell (involving the genes for TCR production). The Ig gene rearrangement for the heavy chain is illustrated in Figure 34.2. The same process of rearrangement applies for the TCR-β and -δ genes. For the Ig light-chain k and λ, TCR-λ and TCR-α genes, no D elements are present. Because of its unique size and basepair combination, the complementarity determining region (CDR) 3 segment is the unique element that distinguishes the rearranged IgH gene in different B cells. All the cells derived from a single B-cell precursor carry the same rearrangement.

Since ALL is a clonal proliferation of precursor lymphoid cells, all leukaemic cells in each patient share the same Ig rearrangement (in B-precursor ALL) or TCR rearrangement (in T-ALL).

The presentation bone marrow or peripheral blood samples are processed for DNA extraction and the unique Ig or TCR gene rearrangement is identified using a combination of primers for the V, D and J segments of the different Ig heavy, Ig light genes and TCR-γ, TCR-β, TCR-δ and TCR-α genes. The primers are usually designed from regions of homology in the V or J segments to avoid having to use one primer for each one of the V,

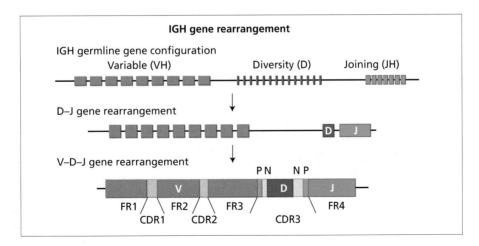

Figure 34.2 VDJ gene rearrangement and identification of framework (FR), complementarity determining region (CDR), P and N nucleotides. FR and CDR regions are defined by the absence of contact with the antigen and lower mutation rate (FR) or direct contact with the antigen and higher incidence of mutations in the functional Ig protein (CDR). P nucleotides are novel basepairs complementary to the last germline nucleotides of the V and J elements while N nucleotides are *de novo* nucleotides added by terminal deoxynucleotidyl transferase (TdT) during the process of rearrangement. The joining element is referred to as FR4 region in the completed VDJ rearranged segment.

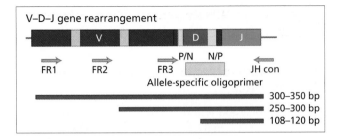

Figure 34.3 PCR strategy for the identification of clonal IGH gene rearrangement in B-precursor ALL. Family primers homologous to the FR1 or FR2 or FR3 regions are used in conjunction with a JH consensus primer. The primers are chosen from these regions which are less prone to be somatically mutated following the VDJ rearrangement (see legend to Figure 34.2). Different size fragments can be identified depending on the set of primers used.

D or J segments, which would be very labour intensive. An example of the strategy used for the amplification of the IgH genes is illustrated in Figure 34.3. The same strategy can be applied to TCR and Ig light-chain genes.

An example of amplification of clonal IgH rearrangement using primers for the FR1 and JH segments is illustrated in Figure 34.4.

The use of Ig and TCR gene rearrangements as MRD targets in precursor B- and T-cell ALL has the advantage of being widely applicable and being informative in 95–99% of patients (Table 34.2). Immunoglobulin genes are rearranged in more than 95% of precursor-B ALL cases: 98% for IgH (V_H–J_H and D_H–V_H), 50% for IgK (Vκ–Jκ and IgK–Kde) and 20% for IgL (Vλ–Jλ). In 5–10% of T-ALL cases, IgH genes are also rearranged. TCR-δ, TCR-γ and TCR-β clonal rearrangement occur

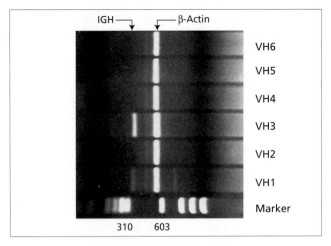

Figure 34.4 Example of a VH3 clonal population in a B-precursor ALL patient. DNA from a B-precursor ALL patient was screened with each of the FR1 primers for the six major VH family of genes (VH1 to VH6) and a JH primer, as illustrated in Figure 34.2. The major VH3 clonal marker can be easily seen as a specific band in the VH3 lane of approximately 350 bp size product. In this case a minor VH1 clonal band can also be seen. Amplification of the β-actin gene was carried out to control for quality and quantity of DNA loading. A PCR product of approximately 600 bp is visible in each lane.

in 70%, 90% and 50%, respectively, of the T-lineage ALL and also, as cross-lineage TCR gene rearrangements, in 50%, 70% and 10% of B-precursor ALL respectively (Table 34.2). Consequently, at least one (in 75% of patients), but often two (in 50% of cases) or three (in 40% of cases), rearrangements can

Gene rearrangement	Precursor B-ALL (%)		Precursor T-ALL (%)	
	Adult	Childhood	Adult	Childhood
IgH	75–80	90–95	5–10*	5–10*
D_H–J_H	20		10	
V_H–D_H–J_H	>95		~2	
Igκ	40–50		0	
Vκ–Jκ	30			
Vκ–Kde	50			
Igλ	20		0	
TCR-β	10		50	
TCR-γ	70		60–70	>90
TCR-δ	50†		~70‡	

Table 34.2 Frequency of Ig and TCR gene rearrangements in precursor B- and T-lineage ALL.

*Lineage IgH gene rearrangements in T-ALL are mainly incomplete D_H–J_H rearrangements and occur more frequently in CD3⁻ T-ALL (~20%) and TCR-γδ⁺ T-ALL (50%) compared with TCR-αβ⁺ T-ALL cases (< 5%).
†Predominantly Vδ2–Dδ3 and Dδ2–Dδ3 rearrangements.
‡Predominantly Vδ1–Jδ1 complete rearrangements and Dδ2–Jδ1 rearrangements.

be identified as molecular targets in ALL and used for MRD assessment.

The patient's leukaemic clone is then sequenced and the sequence of the CDR3 region identified. This region is unique for each patient and an oligoprimer is designed from its unique sequence and used in allele-specific oligonucleotide (ASO)-based MRD analysis (Figure 34.3 and text below).

PCR-based MRD detection

Fingerprinting gene analysis

Fingerprinting PCR-based MRD tests identify in remission marrow DNA the patient's original clone based on its unique size and migration mobility (Figure 34.5). Identification of residual leukaemia is carried out using the same combination of primers that yielded a signal in the presentation sample (for instance, VH3/JH and VH1/JH in Figure 34.4). The PCR reaction, however, is spiked with radiolabelled nucleotide ($[\alpha\text{-}^{32}P]dCTP$) and the PCR product is then separated on a high-density acrylamide gel and autoradiographed to pick up the radiolabelled signal of the PCR product. In normal bone marrow, a 'ladder' of fragments is detected corresponding to the various IgH rearrangements in the heterogeneous B-cell population. In the follow-up sample, a signal identical in size to that from the original leukaemic presentation bone marrow sample will be observed if residual cells are present (Figure 34.5).

Alternatively, a fluorescence assay can be used (gene scanning analysis; Figure 34.6). Both techniques provide sensitivity of detection up to 1:10^3.

Allele-specific oligonucleotide (ASO) MRD detection

The ASO, designed from the CDR3 region (Figure 34.3), can be used to increase the sensitivity of MRD detection up to 1:10^4 or 1:10^5. The increase in sensitivity is due to the specificity for the leukaemic cell that this primer carries since the CDR3 region is unique to each rearrangement. Technically, the increase in sensitivity can be achieved by a variety of methods: (i) the ASO can be used in a radiolabelled PCR reaction as antisense primer (in place of the JH primer) in combination with the V family primer identified in the presentation sample (for instance a VH3 for the case in Figure 34.4); (ii) the ASO primer can be labelled and used as a probe in a hybridization experiment when the follow-up sample DNA is deposited on a filter paper (by dot-blot); or (iii) use as a sense or antisense primer in a quantitative PCR test using TaqMan or LightCycler technology (as described later) in combination with a JH or VH primer respectively. This is the most advanced technique and is replacing other approaches in many laboratories.

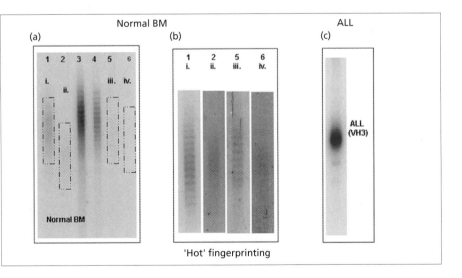

Figure 34.5 Example of fingerprinting analysis. A ladder of fragments corresponding to the various IGH rearrangements in polyclonal B cells is illustrated in (a) and (b) for DNA from normal bone marrow. This can be compared with the unique strong band detected in the bone marrow DNA of a patient with B-precursor ALL (c). The number above each lane in (a) and (b) indicates the VH gene family used for the PCR amplification (VH1 to VH6). (b) represents a longer exposure of (a), lanes 1, 2, 5 and 6.

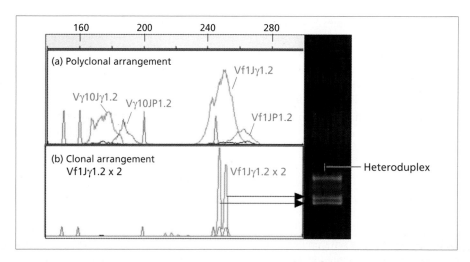

Figure 34.6 Analysis of multiplex TCR-γ rearrangement by PCR from DNA using fluorescent primers and Genescan evaluation (left) compared with non-denaturing PAGE analysis of heteroduplex (HD) PCR products (right). (a) Polyclonal rearrangements. (b) Clonal biallelic rearrangement in a B-cell precursor ALL, analysed by gene scanning or heteroduplex. Slow-migrating clonal heteroduplexes are seen when both alleles undergo rearrangement with the same Vγ and Jγ segments. Homoduplexes are indicated by arrows. The use of differently labelled primers allows identification of the V and J segments used, as shown. Size markers are in red (diagram kindly provided by Kheïra Beldjord and Professor E. Mackintyre, Laboratoire d'Hématologie, Hôpital Necker Tour Pasteur, Paris, France).

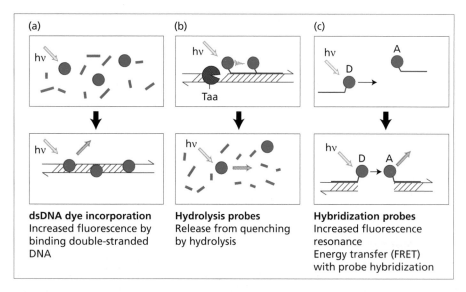

Figure 34.7 Real-time PCR techniques. (a) Incorporation of SyberGreen fluorescent dye as the PCR develops. (b) The hydrolysis probes are the basis for the TaqMan technology. (c) Hybridization probed with fluorescence resonance energy transfer (Roche) (courtesy of Dr Andreas Hochhaus, Heidelberg University, Mannheim, Germany).

Increased sensitivity can be achieved using cellular enrichment of lymphoid cells prior to PCR amplification or the amplification of multiple aliquots of DNA from remission BM samples.

Real-time PCR MRD detection

Real-time quantitative PCR (RQ-PCR) has been applied for the detection of *Ig/TCR* gene rearrangements in ALL. Whether using SYBR Green I hydrolysis probes or fluorescence resonance energy transfer (FRET), this technology provides rapid, repro-ducible and quantitative results for both *Ig/TCR* and gene fusion RT-PCR targets. The strategy used is illustrated in Figure 34.7.

Equipment and probe costs are becoming cheaper for application to large-scale studies. An extensive review of this technology has been published and we refer the reader to this for further information (Van der Velden *et al.*, 2003).

The technique of real-time PCR was pioneered in 1992 to detect PCR products as they accumulated by measuring the intercalation of ethidium bromide and hence increased fluorescence as the reaction proceeded (Figure 34.7a). The method was subsequently improved by changing to a probe-based rather than intercalation-based detection system (Figure 34.7b). The probe carries a quencher that prevents the reporter dye fluorescing unless it is separated by the activity of the *Taq* polymerase as DNA is synthesized. Finally, the hybridization probe makes use of two sequence-specific oligonucleotides labelled with different fluorescent dyes. The light excites one primer which then transfers energy to the second oligoprimer and it is then converted into a quantified signal (FRET) (Figure 34.7c).

Quantitative PCR is visualized as the PCR cycles take place. It provides a signal comparison between different amounts of substrate and several samples can be tested simultaneously.

Clinical value of monitoring for antigen receptor gene rearrangements by PCR in ALL

Molecular investigation of antigen receptor gene rearrangements shows that targets for MRD can be identified in over 90% of childhood ALL and in 75–85% of adult ALL. These techniques are valuable for risk stratification of patients, based on their levels of residual disease at different time points.

Childhood ALL

In childhood ALL, single-point MRD assessment at day 28 post induction is a useful test for the identification of patients at increased risk of relapse. MRD PCR-based quantitative tests carried out as early as day 15 during induction therapy can identify patients with rapid molecular responses and an excellent prognosis, similar to flow cytometry tests on day 19, when lack of detectable residual leukaemic cells is associated with long-term disease-free survival.

At day 28, depending on the MRD level, patients fall within a high-, intermediate- or low-risk group. MRD $\geq 10^2$ identifies the group at highest risk of relapse. MRD level between 10^3 and 10^4 defines an intermediate-risk group and further monitoring should be performed to ensure complete conversion to MRD-negative tests in the following months. Sequential quantitative measurements of residual disease (at 12 and 20 weeks) identify patients with a fast decline in disease to undetectable levels that strongly correlate with durable CCR. Patients with no detectable disease or levels $< 10^4$ at day 28 represent a low-risk group and have the best outcome.

Any level of detectable disease beyond 3 months identifies patients at high risk. Examples of correlation between MRD tests and disease-free survival for samples collected during the first 24 months of treatment at our institution are illustrated in Figure 34.8. PCR-based MRD tests carry the most significant predictive value when compared with other criteria such as immunophenotype, age, sex, WBC count and cytogenetics. Tests in B- and T-lineage childhood ALL provide highly significant prediction of

outcome. MRD studies by PCR (but not by flow cytometry) show a higher incidence of disease in childhood T-ALL in remission than in B-precursor ALL, and this correlates with a poorer outcome of T-compared with B-precursor ALL in this age group.

Adult ALL

Results from the largest cohort (85 patients) so far studied showed, as observed in childhood, that MRD-PCR positivity at early time-points is predictive of outcome. The higher the level of MRD, the greater the chance of relapse (Figure 34.9). Over 50% of patients have detectable residual disease post induction, and residual disease decreases with time in patients destined to remain in CCR. In patients who eventually relapse, the disease is never fully eradicated and, in a proportion of patients (15–20%), relapse is associated with re-emergence of disease detected by PCR between 6 and 9 months post consolidation and during maintenance (Figure 34.9).

In T-ALL adult patients, data are more limited. In contrast to the strong predictive value of MRD tests in childhood T-ALL, in adults MRD tests appear to be best at predicting outcome only when carried out during maintenance therapy, i.e. beyond 6–9 months from presentation, rather than during the induction and consolidation phase, as seen in adult B-precursor ALL.

MRD detection at the end of treatment

Conversion from negative to positive MRD or the persistence of MRD-positive results to the end of treatment is associated with relapse in ALL patients irrespective of age. The aim must be to treat such patients before clinical relapse, as already practised in acute promyelocytic leukaemia (APL) and in chronic myeloid leukaemia (CML) post allogeneic SCT.

MRD detection in stem cell transplant ALL patients

In adult B-precursor ALL group, a close correlation has been observed between level of disease in harvested stem cells and clinical outcome in patients receiving autologous SCT (Figure 34.10). Similar observations have been made in non-Hodgkin's lymphoma and chronic lymphocytic leukaemia. On the other hand, outcome of adult ALL patients receiving allogeneic stem cell transplants appears to correlate with whether or not residual disease can be detected in the bone marrow after, rather than before, the procedure.

In childhood ALL, it is the MRD status before allo-BMT that affects outcome. This is probably because most children receiving SCT have extremely resistant disease and only the minority without such disease prior to SCT do well. In adults, SCT is often carried out in patients in first clinical remission, who may well also be in molecular remission.

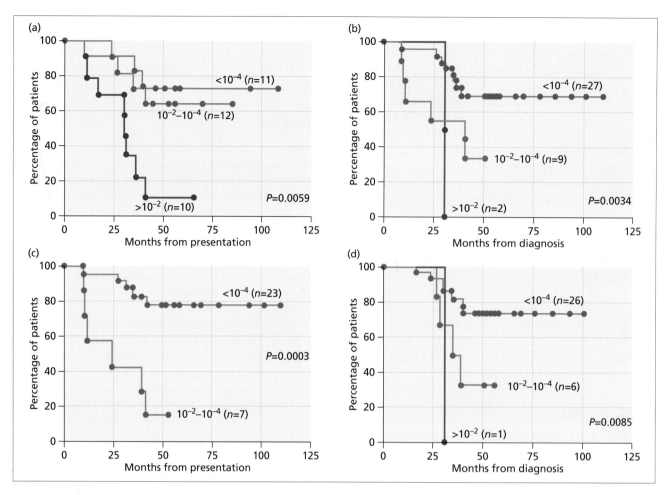

Figure 34.8 Survival curves for childhood ALL patients according to MRD status and clinical outcome (from Gameiro *et al.*, 2002). The best survival is observed in patients with negative MRD at all time-points analysed. The higher the level of residual, the greater is the occurrence of clinical relapse. (a) Disease-free survival (DFS): day 28. (b) DFS: 2–5 months. (c) DFS: 6–9 months. (d) DFS: 10–24 months.

False-negative and false-positive MRD tests

Although PCR technology can in theory be sensitive to $1:10^5$ (Figure 34.1), false-negative results can still occur in ALL. First, they can arise when intervals between BM assessments are long, e.g. greater than 5 months. Monitoring at 3-month intervals (or more frequently) is recommended. Second, clonal evolution at relapse can result in negative tests. In rare patients, new clones emerge post treatment; this is associated with the emergence of resistant disease and, almost invariably, with poor outcome. Third, the presence of multiple (usually between two and six) B or T subclones at presentation (referred to as oligoclonality) can cause subsequent false-negative MRD tests. Oligoclonality arises primarily because the gene rearrangement machinery (i.e. TdT and recombination-activating genes, RAGs) is still active and functioning in precursor-B and T-cell leukaemia. Oligoclonality is seen in 20–30% of B-precursor ALL and 10–20% of T-ALL. It is, therefore, recommended that all B-cell subclones should be clearly identified at presentation and monitored during CCR. Fourth, PCR-negative tests in the bone marrow can in some cases accompany extramedullary relapses in the central nervous system, skin and testis. More frequently, extramedullary relapses are accompanied by positive MRD tests in the bone marrow. Finally, there may be heterogeneous distribution of the leukaemic cells in the bone marrow after treatment or patchy disease that may lead to false-negative tests. To avoid false-negative results during MRD-PCR monitoring in ALL, it is preferable that at least two molecular targets are used, and one of them, if possible, should be a gene fusion transcript.

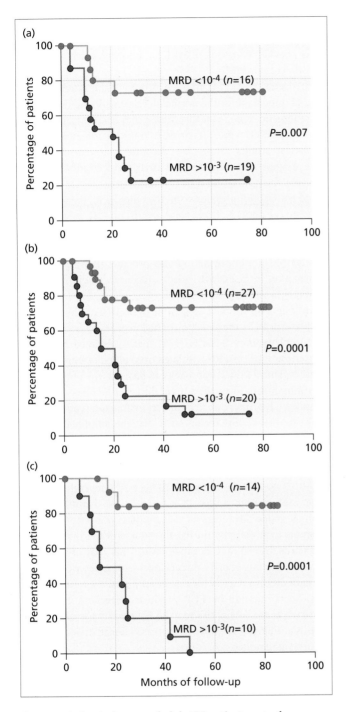

Figure 34.9 Survival curves of adult ALL patients up to the beginning of maintenance therapy. (a) DFS: 0–2 months. (B) DFS: 3–5 months. (c) DFS: 6–9 months. MRD analysis of adult ALL patients reveals a strong correlation with clinical outcome, with the strongest correlation observed at 3–5 and 6–9 months (Mortuza *et al.*, 2002).

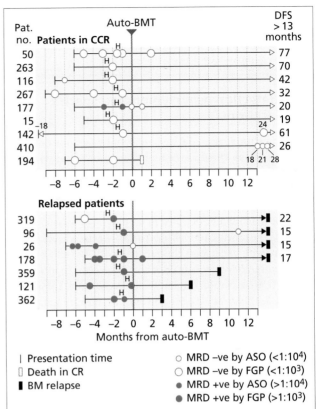

Figure 34.10 MRD analysis in patients receiving autologous SCT. A clear circle indicates a negative MRD test. A red circle indicates a positive MRD test, with a higher level (10^{-2} to 10^{-3}) being indicated by larger circles, while smaller circles illustrate levels at 10^{-4}. A black bar indicates haematological relapse and DFS is expressed in months from presentation. The vertical bar across the figure shows the time of SCT. The patients are separated into those who stayed in CCR (upper part of the figure) and patients who relapsed (lower part of the figure). The figure illustrates that residual disease prior to autologous SCT is associated with high incidence of relapse (cases in the lower part of the figure).

MRD detection in other lymphoid malignancies

MRD detection using antigen receptor genes

Non-Hodgkin's lymphoma (NHL) of B lineage is characterized by the clonal expansion of a lymphoid cell that has progressed through the B-cell development pathway. The clonal cells carry complete and functional IgH and IgL chain gene rearrangements. Clonal analysis of Ig genes and, in the cases of T-cell lymphomas, TCR genes can be used for monitoring residual disease in lymphoma patients following the identification of a B-cell clonal Ig or TCR rearrangement at presentation. Indeed, in lymphoma patients the clone identified in the original lymph node biopsy can be sought in the peripheral blood and bone marrow for further staging of the disease.

MRD detection using lymphoma-specific translocations

In different histological subgroups of lymphomas, other markers can be identified. These derive from chromosomal translocations such as t(14;18) in follicular NHL, t(11;14) in mantle cell lymphoma, t(2;5) in anaplastic large-cell NHL or t(8;14) in Burkitt's lymphoma. The most frequent and widely investigated marker is t(14;18), which can be detected in up to 85% of follicular NHL patients. The translocation brings the *Bcl-2* gene adjacent to the IgH locus with breakpoint cluster regions (BCRs) either within the 3′-untranslated sequences of the *Bcl-2* gene (major BCR) or 20 kb downstream (minor BCR). As the breakpoints are localized within a restricted region of DNA, they are suitable for amplification by PCR for both the diagnostic and follow-up bone marrow or peripheral blood samples. Sensitivity up to 1:10^5 cells can easily be achieved. It is particularly clinically important for patients to achieve molecular remission post SCT. As the translocation can be detected in lymphocytes of normal individuals, however, accurate quantification and time-point analysis is required, which will make future clinical studies more relevant.

There is at present limited information on the use of MRD for the monitoring of patients carrying t(11;14), t(2;5) and t(8;14). The heterogeneity of the breakpoints over a region sometimes larger than several thousand basepairs (bp) precludes the use of genomic DNA PCR for monitoring of MRD in these patients. In general, Ig and TCR rearrangement analysis, although rather more laborious, provides the most useful method for MRD investigation in lymphoma patients. The t(11;14) resulting in increased expression of cyclin D1 (on 11q13) can be detected using RT-PCR on RNA prepared from mantle cell lymphoma patients and is used for confirmation in diagnostic material.

Finally, although detectable in 65% of lymphoma patients, in 30–40% of CLL and multiple myeloma patients, Bcl-6 mutations (in the 5′ region of the gene, particularly 3′ of exon 1) have little or no application in the monitoring of MRD in patients with lymphoproliferative diseases.

Chromosomal translocations as molecular targets for MRD analysis

In acute leukaemias, chromosomal translocations result in two types of alteration, the production of gene fusions and the relocation of oncogenes to the vicinity of the transcription control elements of the Ig or TCR genes (see Chapter 30). Although both types of translocation result in the production of novel molecular targets, in practice only the gene fusions are suitable for the investigation of MRD. Moreover, the detection of fusion genes provides a method of MRD monitoring widely applicable in both ALL and AML.

The genes involved in these acquired aberrations are in general important for the normal development and function of haemopoietic cells. Typically, these genes encode transcription factors, cell cycle regulators or signal transduction molecules.

Clinical studies show that chromosomal rearrangements have prognostic value and can be used for risk stratification. For example, the t(9;22) and t(4;11) translocations in ALL are associated with a poor prognosis. On the other hand, the t(12;21) in ALL and the t(15;17), t(8;21) and inv(16) in AML are associated with a good prognosis. Therefore, the identification of such translocations at the molecular level not only identifies targets for MRD monitoring but also provides useful prognostic information in cases with failed cytogenetic analysis (see also Chapters 31 and 33).

Although, for Ig and TCR gene analysis, DNA is the preferred template for PCR, the detection of fusion genes relies exclusively on complementary DNA (cDNA) that is obtained by reverse transcription (RT) of RNA isolated from blood or bone marrow samples. This RT-PCR approach can be used when breakpoints lie within introns or small exons of the genes involved. Oligonucleotide PCR primers are designed from the exon sequences that flank the breakpoint region such that the amplified product contains the leukaemia-specific fusion sequence.

RT-PCR for MRD detection is quick (24–72 h), readily applicable to a wide range of patients, highly reproducible and very sensitive. Sensitivities average 1:10^4 to 1:10^6, depending on the target and whether nested PCR or real-time quantification is used. A major advantage in using fusion transcripts as PCR targets is their stability during the course of the disease. This safeguards against false-negative results that may arise in ALL due to continuing Ig or TCR rearrangement, as described above. Its main disadvantage is the risk of false-positive results due to cross-contamination by PCR products, especially if a nested approach is used. This risk may be reduced by the use of real-time quantitative PCR since its increased sensitivity can obviate the need for a nested procedure.

Acute lymphoblastic leukaemia

Approximately 40% of the ALL patients are positive for a recurrent chromosomal translocation. The most frequent chromosomal translocations and deletions in ALL are listed in Table 34.3.

t(1;19)(q23;p13): E2A-PBX1
The t(1;19)(q23;p13), resulting in the production of a chimeric basic helix–loop–helix (bHLH) transcription factor (E2A) – homeodomain (PBX1) protein – is most frequent in pre-B ALL expressing cytoplasmic Ig but is also sporadically detected in cytoplasmic Ig-negative B-precursor ALL, CD10$^+$ cALL or even

Table 34.3 Fusion genes suitable for MRD analysis in adult and childhood ALL.

Chromosomal translocation	Fusion gene	Relative frequency per type of leukaemia			
		Precursor B-ALL (%)		T-ALL (%)	
		Children	Adults	Children	Adults
t(1;19)(q23;p13)	E2A–PBX1	5–8	3–4	–	–
t(4;11)(q21;q23)	MLL–AF4	3–5*	3–4	–	–
t(9;22)(q34;q11)	BCR–ABL p190	3–5	15–30	< 1	< 1
t(9;22)(q34;q11)	BCR–ABL p210	1–2	10–15	< 1	< 1
t(12;21)(p13;q22)	ETV6–AML1	25–30	< 2	–	–
Del(1)(p32;p32)	SIL–TAL1	–	–	10–25	~10
Total		40–50	40–50	10–25	~10

*In infant ALL, the frequency of t(4;11) can be as high as 70% (adapted from van Dongen *et al.*, 1999).

T-ALL and AML. In most cases, the fusion transcript results from the splicing of exon 13 of *E2A* to exon 2 of *PBX1*. A variant fusion transcript is found in about 5–10% of the positive cases, owing to an additional stretch of 27 nucleotides in the junctional region resulting from alternative splicing.

Using a nested RT-PCR method, the *E2A–PBX1* transcript can be detected with a sensitivity of $1:10^4$ to $1:10^5$. MRD analysis using *E2A–PBX* fusion genes shows that persisting negative MRD predicts for CCR. Positive results, however, do not necessarily predict for future relapse. Whether quantification of MRD would have greater predictive value remains to be tested in a larger number of patients.

t(12;21)(p13;q22): ETV6-AML1

The t(12;21)(p13;q22) is a cryptic translocation not readily observed by conventional cytogenetics and the ETV6(TEL)–AML1(CBFA2) fusion transcript can be detected in patients with and without a cytogenetically visible chromosome 12 and/or 21 abnormality. FISH and PCR are therefore important techniques employed for its detection.

The t(12;21) is usually associated with a precursor cALL and more rarely pre-B ALL phenotype. It is rarely seen in adult ALL although it is the commonest translocation in childhood ALL (Table 34.3), with a peak incidence in the 2–5 year age group. The breakpoint region usually lies between exons 5 and 6 of the *ETV6* gene and between exon 1 and 3 of *AML1*. Fusion transcripts resulting from splicing of *ETV6* exon 5 to other AML1 exons can also be formed. The majority of the positive patients have the *ETV6* gene deleted on the non-translocated allele. It has been proposed that the translocation occurs during fetal development. The *ETV6–AML1* fusion transcript can be identified with a sensitivity of $1:10^{-4}$ to $1:10^{-5}$ using a nested RT-PCR approach. Accurate quantification of *ETV6–AML1* has shown that MRD measurements are a good prognostic indicator of future outcome.

11q23 abnormalities

Rearrangements involving the *MLL* (mixed leukaemia lymphoma) gene (also called *ALL1*, *HRX* or *Htrx1*) on chromosome 11q23 and multiple partner genes are found in precursor B-ALL, T-ALL, AML, myelodysplastic syndrome (MDS) and secondary leukaemia. The presence of *MLL* rearrangements is usually associated with a poor prognosis.

In ALL, the most common translocation partner of *MLL* is the *AF4* (*FEL*) gene on chromosome 4q21. Fifty to seventy per cent of infant ALL cases and approximately 5% of paediatric and adult ALL cases are *MLL–AF4* positive and associated with a pro-B-ALL ('null') phenotype (CD19+, CD34+, TdT+, cytoplasmic CD79+, CD10−). There is also frequent expression of myeloid antigens (CD15 and/or CD65).

The *MLL* and *AF4* genes are composed of 37 and 20 exons respectively, and at least 10 different fusion transcripts have been identified as a result of translocation breakpoints occurring in different introns of both genes. Breakpoints downstream of the *MLL* exon 9 in adult and paediatric ALL, but downstream of exon 11 in infant ALL and upstream of exon 4 of the AF4 gene, are commonly detected by PCR. Differential splicing is a common finding leading to more than one fusion transcript in some patients. All t(4;11)-positive cases transcribe the *MLL–AF4* fusion gene, whereas only 70% of cases transcribe the reciprocal, *AF4–MLL*, product. Interestingly, low levels of the *MLL1–AF4* transcript have been detected in some ALL cases without cytogenetically detectable t(4;11) and in haemopoietic tissues of healthy individuals.

Using a nested PCR strategy, the various *AF4–MLL* transcripts can be identified with a detection limit of $1:10^4–1:10^5$. MRD studies have shown that early conversion and persisting MRD negativity is consistently associated with CCR.

t(9;22)(q34;q11): BCR-ABL (p210 and p190)

The derivative chromosome 22, or Philadelphia chromosome

Chromosomal translocation	Subtype	Fusion gene	Relative frequency (%)	
			Children	Adults
t(8;21)(q22;q22)	M2	AML1–ETO	10–14	6–8
t(15;17)(q22;q21)	M3	PML–RARα	8–10	5–15
inv(16)(p13;q22)	M4Eo	CBFβ–MYH11	5–7	5–6
t(6;11)(q27;q23)		MLL–AF6	22	2–3†
t(9;11)(p22;q23)	M4, M5a/b	MLL–AF9		
t(10;11)(p11;q23)		MLL–AF10		
t(6;9)(p23;q34)	M1, M2, M4, M7	DEK–CAN		
t(9;22)(q34;q11)	M0, M1	BCR–ABL	Rare	Rare
Total			25–30	20–25*

Table 34.4 Fusion genes suitable for MRD analysis in AML.

*In AML patients > 60 years the total frequency of detectable fusion genes is only 10–15%.
†This frequency is higher in therapy related AML (~9%).

(Ph), of the t(9;22)(q34;q11) carries the BCR–ABL fusion gene encoding a chimeric protein of 190, 210 or 230 kDa, depending on the location of the breakpoint. This is the well-known hallmark of chronic myeloid leukaemia (CML) (see Chapter 37) but also occurs in 5–30% of ALL (Table 34.3) and rare cases of AML (Table 34.4).

Conventional nested RT-PCR can detect this transcript with a sensitivity of up to 1:10⁻⁵. Importantly, low levels of BCR–ABL transcripts have been detected in peripheral blood samples of a sizeable proportion of healthy individuals.

Quantitative monitoring of MRD shows that in PH⁺ childhood ALL, a group of patients who are good responders clear residual disease during the first 5 months of treatment, whereas the poor responders have high levels of MRD and progress to haematological relapse. In adult ALL, persisting high levels of residual disease are usual and associated with haematological relapse. In the majority of cases, allogeneic transplant is the only treatment that achieves long-term molecular remission.

del(1)(p32;p32): SIL-TAL1

The SIL–TAL1 fusion gene results from a site-specific deletion on chromosome 1 between the TAL1 and SIL genes. As a result, in T cells, a normal TAL1 protein is expressed but under the control of the SIL gene promoter. SIL–TAL1 transcripts are exclusively found in cases of T-ALL and the detection of TAL1 deletions at the genomic level is not associated with particular clinical features. RT-PCR amplification of SIL–TAL1 transcripts can reach the sensitivity of 1:10⁵, making it an excellent target for MRD investigation.

Acute myeloid leukaemia

Immunoglobulin and TCR rearrangements are rare in AML and therefore chromosome translocations provide the most important targets for MRD analysis by PCR. The most common chromosomal translocations, detected in approximately 30–40% of AML patients, and their corresponding fusion transcripts are listed in Table 34.4 (see also Chapter 30).

t(8;21)(q22;q22): AML1-ETO

The t(8;21)(q22;q22) fuses the AML1 (CBFA2) gene on chromosome 21 with the ETO (MTG8) gene on chromosome 8. Breakpoints localize between exons 5 and 6 of AML1 and upstream of exon 2 of ETO. The translocation occurs mainly in de novo AML of FAB M2 subtype but may be seen also in AML cases with FAB M1 or M4 morphology.

Quantitative assessment of the AML1–ETO fusion gene shows a linear decrease (at least 2–4 logs) in copy number in most patients as a result of remission induction. The majority of patients remain positive at a low level during consolidation therapy. In patients destined to relapse, higher levels of MRD are observed before starting consolidation. Prior to relapse, an increase in level of MRD is observed in approximately 75% of patients. Patients with persisting level of MRD for many years have been identified but the incidence of relapse is not increased in a steady-state MRD status.

t(15;17)(q22;q21): PML-RARA

The t(15;17)(q22;q21) translocation, associated with acute promyelocytic leukaemia (APL)(FAB M3), fuses the PML gene, on 15q22, to the RARA gene on 17q21. The breakpoint cluster region on chromosome 17 localizes within RARA intron 2. Within PML there are three breakpoint cluster regions: breakpoint cluster region 3 (BCR 3) in intron 3, BCR2 in exon 6 (rarely in intron 5) and BCR1 in intron 6. At the messenger RNA level, BCR1, BCR2 and BCR3 are also called the long (L), variant (V) and short (S) isoforms, respectively. Alternative splicing within PML transcripts and the alternative use of two RARA polyadenylation sites are responsible for the production of additional PML-RARA transcripts of different sizes.

There are at least four variant translocations involving the *RARA* gene, with the same breakpoint, associated with the APL phenotype. These fusion partners are the *NPM* at 5q35, *PLZF* at 11q23, *NuMA* at 11q13 and *STAT5b* at 11q11.

As a consequence of the t(15;17)(q22;q21) translocation, both *PML–RARA* and *RARA–PML* fusions can be transcribed. While *PML–RARA* is consistently found in APL patients, *RARA–PML* is detectable in only 70% of cases. Thus, *PML–RARA* is most widely used for diagnosis and MRD monitoring in APL. This transcript can be detected by RT-PCR with a sensitivity of $1:10^4$.

At least 50% of patients with APL are MRD positive after the first cycle of chemotherapy. Most positive patients show a progressive decrease in MRD during the four or five chemotherapy blocks. Patients post consolidation who are in molecular remission have a high probability of CCR. Patients who revert to PCR-positive tests after the end of treatment, however, have a high probability of relapse. Patients with a low MRD level ($< 10^{-5}$) at the end of consolidation include a large proportion of relapse cases and monitoring should therefore continue at 2- to 3-month intervals for 1–2 years after completion of treatment.

The *PML–RARA* transcript can be detected with increased sensitivity by RQ-PCR compared with semiquantitative nested/two-round PCR techniques. Accurate quantification can identify patients with an increasing number of transcripts preceding haematological relapse. Patients treated at the time of molecular relapse have 2-year event-free survival (EFS) rates superior to those treated at the time of haematological relapse.

Inv(16)(p13;q22) and t(16;16)

The pericentric inversion of chromosome 16, inv 16(p13;q22), and the rarer t(16;16)(p13;q22) are recurrently associated with AML of the FAB subgroup M4 with abnormal eosinophils (M4Eo). These aberrations fuse the *CBFB* (*PEBP2b*) gene at 16q22 to the *MYH11* gene at 16p13. There is marked heterogeneity in the resulting *CBFB–MYH11* fusion transcripts owing to variability of genomic breakpoints in both *CBFB* and *MYH11* and to alternative splicing. Ten different types of fusion transcripts have been identified so far. The most common (> 85% of positive patients) is type A, resulting from ligation of *CBFB* exon 5 to exon 12 of *MYH11*. Although closely associated with AML M4Eo, the *CBFb–MYH11* fusion transcript has also been detected in AML patients in whom the cytogenetic abnormality could not be detected, including patients with AML M4 without eosinophils, M2, M5 and, less frequently M1, M6 and M7. The *CBFβ–MYH11* can be detected by RT-PCR with a sensitivity of $1:10^5$.

MRD monitoring shows that the mean *CBFB–MYH11* fusion transcript copy number is significantly higher in patients destined to relapse than in patients remaining in CCR. Moreover, in CCR patients, the copy number drops below the detection threshold after the treatment protocol is completed and MRD remains undetectable in subsequent analyses. In contrast, in patients who relapse, the copy number in CR never declines below the detection threshold. Both accurate quantification and a cut-off value for positive tests (as predictive of relapse) need to be established in large-scale studies in this group of patients.

FLT-3 internal tandem repeats, c-KIT mutations and WT1 levels

Additional changes in AML cells include the recently described internal tandem repeats (ITDs) and point mutations in both the *FLT-3* and *c-KIT* genes. *FLT-3* ITDs and mutations occur in up to 30% of some AML subtypes (most frequently in M3/APL, but also in 35% of patients with a normal karyotype). They identify a poor prognostic group, except when detected in APL. Unfortunately, they are a poor target for MRD monitoring in AML because they are frequently associated with subclones at presentation and may appear *de novo* at relapse or vice versa.

Mutations in *c-KIT* (exon 8 and Asp816) are detected in 10–15% of AML patients with inv(16) and t(8;21), are mutually exclusive with *FLT-3* mutations and are associated with a poor prognosis. *C-KIT* mutations carry only a limited practical use for MRD detection, however, since they seem to be a secondary event in the disease progression and can be lost at time of relapse.

WT1 is overexpressed in over 60–70% of AML cases and in 50–60% of ALL regardless of the presence of other fusion transcripts. Quantitative analysis of *WT1* at presentation and during remission (fewer than 10^3 copies post induction and second consolidation) significantly correlates with better DFS and overall survival (OS). A rise in *WT1* levels and persistently high levels are associated with poorer outcome.

Conclusions

The application of flow cytometry and molecular techniques (including real-time quantification) has enabled us to detect and quantify MRD in acute leukaemia to levels of sensitivity of $1:10^4$ to 10^5. PCR techniques can be used to detect leukaemic cells among normal counterparts using both clonal changes in antigen receptor genes (IgH and TCR) and leukaemic-specific changes (translocations, point mutations). The predictive value of these tests has been found to be independent of other risk factors such as age, sex and presenting leucocyte count. Quantitative and semiquantitative assessment of MRD is becoming important in defining relapse risk as a function of MRD level immediately post induction and at later time points.

For both children and adults the challenge is to incorporate MRD analysis into prognostic indices in large randomized trials. Some studies have recently been initiated in Europe and the UK using MRD values at day 28 and during the first 3 months of treatment for ALL for risk stratification and change in treatment. The potential benefit would seem to be largest in 'standard-risk'

ALL as judged by conventional criteria (age, sex, presenting leucocyte count, chromosomal translocations). In this the largest category of patients, overall benefit has been obtained by treatment intensification, but this is at the expense of overtreating a substantial number of patients, especially children, who may be cured with less intensive protocols. A large number of adults appear to be cured by standard chemotherapy and could be spared invasive SCT procedures. The corollary to this is the potential for detecting a new group of high-risk patients, both adults and children, on the basis of slow MRD clearance. These could be candidates for further treatment intensification including SCT in first CR or alternative targeted treatment.

Selected bibliography

Bader P, Hancock J, Kreyenberg H et al. (2002) Minimal residual disease (MRD) status prior to allogeneic stem cell transplantation is a powerful predictor for post-transplant outcome in children with ALL. Leukemia 16: 1668–72.

Brisco MJ, Condon J, Hughes E et al. (1994) Outcome prediction in childhood acute lymphoblastic leukaemia by molecular quantification of residual disease at the end of induction. Lancet 343: 196–200.

Campana D (2003) Determination of minimal residual disease in leukaemia patients. British Journal of Haematology 121: 823–38.

Campana D, Coustan-Smith E (2002) Advances in the immunological monitoring of childhood acute lymphoblastic leukaemia. Best Practice and Research in Clinical Haematology 15: 1–19.

Cave H, Bosch v.d.Wt, Suciu S et al. (1998) Clinical significance of minimal residual disease in childhood acute lymphoblastic leukemia. European Organization for Research and Treatment of Cancer–Childhood Leukemia Cooperative Group. New England Journal of Medicine 339: 591–8.

Diverio D, Rossi V, Avvisati G et al. (1998) Early detection of relapse by prospective reverse transcriptase-polymerase chain reaction analysis of the PML/RARalpha fusion gene in patients with acute promyelocytic leukemia enrolled in the GIMEMA-AIEOP multicenter 'AIDA' trial. GIMEMA-AIEOP Multicenter 'AIDA' Trial. Blood 92: 784–9.

Foroni L, Harrison CJ, Hoffbrand AV, Potter MN (1999) Investigation of minimal residual disease in childhood and adult acute lymphoblastic leukaemia by molecular analysis. British Journal of Haematology 105: 7–24.

Gameiro P, Mortuza FY, Hoffbrand AV, Foroni L (2002) Minimal residual disease monitoring in adult T-cell acute lymphoblastic leukemia: a molecular-based approach using T-cell receptor γ and δ gene rearrangements. Haematologica 87: 1126–34.

Gribben JG (2002) Monitoring disease in lymphoma and CLL patients using molecular techniques. Best Practice and Research in Clinical Haematology 15: 179–95.

Grimwade D, Lo Coco F (2002) Acute promyelocytic leukemia: a model for the role of molecular diagnosis and residual disease monitoring in directing treatment approach in acute myeloid leukemia. Leukemia 16: 1959–73.

Mortuza FY, Papaioannou M, Moreira I et al. (2002) Minimal residual disease (MRD) tests provide an independent predictor of clinical outcome in adult acute lymphoblastic leukemia. Journal of Clinical Oncology 20: 1094–104.

San Miguel JF, Ciudad J, Vidriales MB et al. (1999) Immunophenotypical detection of minimal residual disease in acute leukemia. Critical Review of Oncology and Hematology 32: 175–85.

Szczepanski T, Beishuizen A, Pongers-Willemse MJ et al. (1999) Cross-lineage T cell receptor gene rearrangements occur in more than ninety per cent of childhood precursor-B acute lymphoblastic leukemias: alternative PCR targets for detection of minimal residual disease. Leukemia 13: 196–205.

Szczepanski T, Langerak AW, Wolvers-Tettero IL et al. (1998) Immunoglobulin and T cell receptor gene rearrangement patterns in acute lymphoblastic leukemia are less mature in adults than in children: implications for selection of PCR targets for detection of minimal residual disease. Leukemia 12: 1081–8.

Szczepanski T, Orfao A, van der Velden VH et al. (2001) Minimal residual disease in leukaemia patients. Lancet Oncology 2: 409–17.

Tonegawa S (1983) Somatic generation of antibody diversity. Nature 302: 575–81.

van der Velden VH, Hochhaus A, Cazzaniga G et al. (2003) Detection of minimal residual disease in hematologic malignancies by real-time quantitative PCR: principles, approaches, and laboratory aspects. Leukemia 17: 1013–34.

van der Velden VH, Joosten SA, Willemse MJ et al. (2001) Real-time quantitative PCR for detection of minimal residual disease before allogeneic stem cell transplantation predicts outcome in children with acute lymphoblastic leukemia. Leukemia 15: 1485–7.

van Dongen JJ, Macintyre EA, Gabert JA et al. (1999) Standardized RT-PCR analysis of fusion gene transcripts from chromosome aberrations in acute leukemia for detection of minimal residual disease. Report of the BIOMED-1 Concerted Action: investigation of minimal residual disease in acute leukemia. Leukemia 13: 1901–28.

van Dongen JJ, Seriu T, Panzer-Grumayer ER et al. (1998) Prognostic value of minimal residual disease in acute lymphoblastic leukaemia in childhood. Lancet 352: 1731–8.

CHAPTER 35

Multidrug resistance in leukaemia

Jean-Pierre Marie and Ollivier Legrand

35

Introduction

Chemotherapy is particularly effective in acute leukaemia, as is demonstrated by the detection of minimal residual disease: in childhood acute lymphoblastic leukaemia (ALL), the fraction of leukaemic cells that survive per week was estimated at 0.008 during the first 14 days of treatment, and, with an estimated number of leukaemic cells at diagnosis of 10^{12}, the mean size of the resistant population can be estimated as 10^7 cells at the end of induction treatment. These cells will be responsible for relapse if no further treatment (or despite this treatment) within 1–3 years.

Farber *et al.* (1948) were the first to describe drug resistance in ALL 55 years ago, and this obstacle is still the major cause of death in all types of acute leukaemia.

Mechanisms of drug resistance

Thirty-five years ago, Goldie and Coldman (1979) proposed a mathematical model for drug resistance, assuming that selected subclones of cancer cells eventually became resistant to chemotherapeutic drugs, owing to a high spontaneous mutation rate. These cells could escape the effect of cytotoxic drugs, through decreased uptake, increased catabolism, decreased transformation of a prodrug, modification of drug target, increase in DNA repair or resistance to drug-induced apoptosis.

Over the last 20 years, experimental models and clinical research have identified several causes of drug resistance in tumours. The most frequently observed phenomenon is the appearance of a broad spectrum of resistance, called 'multidrug resistance', or MDR.

Multidrug resistance

It was clinically observed that tumour cells resistant to a class of drug, are usually also cross-resistant to chemotherapy with a different target. This phenomenon, called MDR, was described *in vitro* by Biedler and Riehm during the 1970s in Chinese hamster ovary cells and is now recognized as a most frequent phenotype developed in cultured tumour cells exposed to anthracyclines or vinca alkaloids.

This MDR phenotype confers to the cells cross-resistance to a broad range of structurally and functionally unrelated cytotoxic agents, sharing common properties: all are plant or microbial products, known as xenobiotics. The resistant tumour cells maintain lower intracellular drug concentrations than do their sensitive counterparts, and in the large majority of cases express transport proteins of the ABC (ATP-binding cassette) superfamily, responsible for the active efflux of these drugs.

More recently, other mechanisms of resistance to a broad spectrum of drugs have been described: increase in DNA repair, and defects of drug-induced apoptosis, either due to strong survival signals delivered to the tumoral cells by microenvironment, or because of a defect in the apoptosis pathway (Figure 35.1). Unfortunately, very few confirmed data are available concerning these mechanisms in leukaemia, and the focus of this chapter will be on the ABC proteins.

ABC proteins

These transmembrane proteins are specialized in energy-dependent cellular transport. The encoding *MDR* genes are highly conserved between species, from bacteria to man. The

575

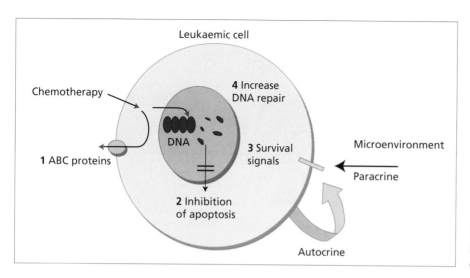

Figure 35.1 Mechanisms responsible for multidrug resistance in leukaemic cells.

Table 35.1 Classes of cytotoxic drugs expelled by P-gp. All of these drugs are from natural origin (xenobiotics).

Sources of cytotoxic drugs	Drugs expelled by P-gp
Streptomyces	Anthracyclines
	Daunorubicin,
	THP-adriamycin
	Idarubicin
	Mitoxantrone
	Amsacrine
Cantharanthus roseus	Vinca alkaloids
	Vinblastine
	Vincristine
	Navelbine
Taxus brevifolia	Taxanes
	Paclitaxel
	Taxotere
Mandrake plant	Epipodophyllotoxin:
	VP16
	VM26

role of these proteins is mainly protection against xenobiotics, including many hydrophobic cytostatics of natural origin (Table 35.1). The minimum structure of the protein is an ABC unit of 200–250 amino acids, consisting of consensus Walker A and B motifs and the ABC signature, located between the two Walker domains, for ATP binding, and six transmembrane domains (TMDs) (such as ABCG2). The more common structure consists of two ABC and 12 transmembrane domains (ABCB1 or P-glycoprotein), and a few members have five more transmembrane domains, with an external N-termination (ABCC1–2–3) (Figure 35.2).

A new classification of this family, with eight subgroups, is now adopted (see www.humanabc.org). The members responsible for drug efflux belong to several classes (Table 35.2), i.e. ABCB (P-gp), ABCC (MRPs family), ABCG (BCRP), the evidence for this being that the transfection of their cDNA in sensitive cell lines gives rise to the MDR phenotype. These proteins share resistance to anthracyclines, but have a variable spectrum of resistance to other natural compounds (vinca alkaloids, epipodophillotoxines, taxanes) (Table 35.3). Recently, it was shown that the presence of single-nucleotide polymorphisms in P-gp

Table 35.2 Classification of ABC proteins involved in multidrug resistance in cancer.

Nomenclature	Name	Localization/structure	Chromosomal location	MDR phenotype after transfection
ABCB1	P-gp/MDR1	Plasma membrane (TMD–ABC)2	7q21	++
ABCC1	MRP1	Plasma membrane TMD0(TMD–ABC)2	16q13.1	+ (if GSH)
ABCC2	MRP2(cMOAT)	Plasma membrane TMD0(TMD–ABC)2	10q24	+/− (if GSH)
ABCG2	BCRP/MXR1/ABCP	Plasma membrane (works as dimer) (TMD–ABC)	4q22	+

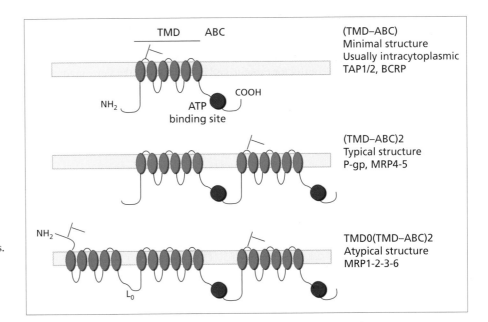

Figure 35.2 Structure of ABC proteins. TMD, transmembrane domain; ABC, ATP-binding cassette; TAP1/2, transporters associated with antigen processing.

Table 35.3 Spectrum of drug resistance of the main ABC proteins involved in drug resistance.

Drug sensitivity	P-gp	MRP1–MRP2 (if GSH)	BCRP
Anthracyclines	Resistant (R)	R	R
Mitoxantrone	R	Sensitive (S)	R
Vinca alkaloids	R	R	S
Taxanes	R	S	S
VP16	R	R	R
Methotrexate	S	R	S
Other		Cisplatin	Topotecan

(C3435T) or in BCRP (T/G482A) results in modification of drug efflux.

At present, the exact mechanism of drug binding to ABC pumps is unknown. In P-gp, mutagenesis showed that transmembrane domains 5, 6, 11 and 12 are crucial for drug efflux. It is suggested that a drug-induced conformational change creates a hydrophobic pocket, able to bind and transport the substrate out of the cell.

The ABC proteins are expressed in tissues that are highly exposed to xenobiotics, e.g. the gastrointestinal tract and the lung mucosa, and in organs involved in secretion processes like liver and kidneys. The presence of the three main ABC proteins involved in drug transport – P-gp, MRP1 and BCRP on endothelial cells – deserves attention: a blockade of these pumps would cause increased uptake of drugs from the bloodstream, decreasing the efficiency of the blood–brain barrier.

P-glycoprotein

The first – and probably most important – protein described in cell models of MDR resistance by Juliano and Ling in 1976 is P-glycoprotein (P-gp), encoded by the *ABCB1* (*MDR1*) gene. This heavily glycosylated protein of 170 kDa is expressed in many tissues which filter or expel toxins: gut, hepatocytes and renal tubules. It also protects the brain and testes (expressed on endothelial capillary cells of these organs). Progenitor cells (CD34+) expressed P-gp, as well as lymphocytes (NK > CD8 > CD4).

After several years of contradictory results concerning the frequency and value of P-gp expression in tumours, several workshops proposed a consensus on technical recommendations for measuring P-gp. Protein detection and, more importantly, functional tests by flow cytometry are recommended for leukaemic samples. Several monoclonal antibodies, recognizing an external epitope, are available for protein expression, and several fluorescent probes could be used (mainly Rhodamine 123), with and without specific inhibitors, for measuring the drug efflux.

The main recommendations are the following:
1 The tumour cell population in the sample must be as pure as possible, especially if 'bulk' techniques are used (RT-PCR).
2 Two different techniques should be used for validation, preferably with single-cell detection methods; protein detection and functional testing by flow cytometry are recommended for leukaemic samples.
3 Calibration controls (all assays must be positive, including one cell line with a low level of positivity, comparable to clinical leukaemic samples) and negative controls must be used. The same control cell lines have to be used by all centres working together.

4 A major confounding factor is the use of an arbitrary minimal cut-off for classifying samples as 'positive' or 'negative'. It is recommended that the data be reported as continuous variables, expressed as a ratio of MAb/control for protein, and as probe + inhibitor/probe alone for function.

P-gp in AML

Many studies have reported a high frequency of *MDR1* gene expression in adult acute myeloid leukaemia (AML). In large multicentre studies between one-third and one-half of cases are 'positive' at diagnosis, whatever the technique used, and usually a higher proportion of positive cases are described in elderly patients. The MDR phenotype is associated with poor prognosis, such as CD34 or CD7, and is more often expressed in AML with 'poor' cytogenetic features, as –7 or complex karyotype. In multivariate analysis, P-gp and karyotype have independent prognostic value.

Except for the promyelocytic subtype (AML M3), which is devoid of P-gp expression, all other AML subtypes are able to express the MDR phenotype. In the majority of cases, functional tests (dye efflux) correlate with P-gp expression, except in CD34⁻ cells, such as myelomonocytic and monoblastic leukaemias. For this reason, dye efflux appears to be more informative than quantification of P-gp itself in AML.

The correlation between *MDR1* gene expression and treatment outcome is well documented in AML: many studies have reported a relationship between either the absence of remission (refractory disease and death during aplasia) and the overexpression of P-gp, or between the overexpression of P-gp and refractory disease (Table 35.4).

Few studies are published on childhood AML. The global incidence of MDR1/P-gp (+) is lower than in adult AML (13–30%),

and no study has shown a correlation between MDR1/P-gp and prognosis (complete remission, overall survival, disease-free survival). Thus, it seems that P-gp expression does not have the same predictive value in childhood AML as it does in adult AML.

P-gp in childhood ALL

The main prognostic factor for long-term survival in childhood acute lymphoblastic leukaemia (ALL) is the sensitivity to corticosteroids. The cellular mechanisms of this resistance are not known, but the *in vivo* corticosensitivity test is highly predictive for long-term survival.

The incidence of *MDR1* overexpression in untreated patients with ALL is generally found to be low (< 10%) at diagnosis and even at relapse, except during the most advanced stage of the disease, when clinical drug resistance is usually observed. The MDR1 phenotype is not predictive for induction treatment failure, whatever the method of detection used.

P-gp in adult ALL

Few studies of ALL are conducted exclusively in adults, unlike AML. The frequency of positive cases is roughly 15–20%, and no studies have demonstrated a correlation between P-gp function and treatment failure.

The MDR phenotype in ALL is found only in ALL subgroups, such as CD7⁺ CD4⁻ CD8⁻ ALL, which are thought to originate from a haemopoietic stem cell, and has a worse prognosis.

In addition, half of all cases of adult T lymphoma–leukaemia (ATL) are positive for P-gp at diagnosis, and all patients with relapsed disease refractory to polychemotherapy are positive for P-gp. In this disease, the P-gp positivity could be due to the 'tax'

Table 35.4 Correlations between P-gp expression and clinical outcome in adult AML treated with standard chemotherapy (anthracycline + 100–200 mg/m² of Ara-C for 7–10 days with or without another drug).

Reference	Number of patients	Techniques	CR/resist.	DFS
Campos *et al.* (1992)	150	Flow cytometry (MRK16)	CR: $P = 0.00001$*	$P = 0.05$*
Nüssler *et al.* (1996)	166	Flow cytometry (C219/4E3)	CR: $P = 0.002$*	NT
Del Poeta *et al.* (1996)	158	Flow cytometry (C219+JSB1)	CR: $P = 0.001$*	$P = 0.02$
Hunault *et al.* (1997)	110	ARN/MRK16	Resist: $P = 0.00001$*	NT
VdHeuvel *et al.* (1997)	130	Immunocytochemistry	CR: $P = 0.01$*	NT
According to consensus (two techniques)				
Leith *et al.* (1997)	211(> 55 years old)	Flow cytometry (MRK16) + function	CR: $P = 0.004$*; Resist: $P = 0.0007$*	NS
Willman (1997)	352(< 55 years old)	Flow cytometry (MRK16) + function	CR: $P = 0.012$*; Resist: $P = 0.0007$*	NT
Legrand *et al.* (2001)	129	Flow cytometry (UIC2) + function	Resist: $P = 0.002$	$P = 0.005$

*Multivariate analysis.
Consensus: see Beck *et al.* (1996) and Marie *et al.* (1997).
CR, complete remission; DFS, disease-free survival; NT, not tested.

protein of HTLV1, which is able to promote MDR1 expression in cells transfected with the viral gene.

P-gp in chronic lymphocytic leukaemia (CLL)

In CLL, several authors have described a large majority of patients expressing a low level of P-gp, either before or after chemotherapy. The MDR phenotype is also detected in normal B lymphocytes, and therefore is probably constitutively moderately expressed in CLL, but with no implication in clinical drug resistance.

P-gp in chronic myeloid leukaemia (CML)

During the chronic phase, P-gp expression does not differ from that in normal counterpart cells in CML. Blast cells of the acute phase could express P-gp, with the same prognostic value as in other acute leukaemias. Interestingly, imatinib mesylate (Gleevec®) is a substrate of P-gp.

MRP family (ABCC1–6)

The members of the ABCC family (*MRP1–6*; 'multidrug resistance-associated protein') have low homology (15%) with *MDR1*, and mainly act together with glutathione.

MRPs (but not P-gp) are transporters of organic anions such as methotrexate (itself an organic anion) and of neutral organic drugs conjugated to acidic ligands (GSH), such as cisplatin (MRP2) and arsenite (MRP1). Anthracyclines and vinca alkaloids, both weak organic bases, are conjugated with GSH, but are transported together with free GSH (Figure 35.3). MRP1 and -2 are particularly involved in the transport of chemotherapeutic

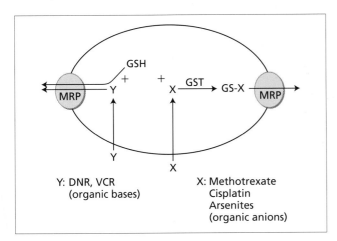

Y: DNR, VCR (organic bases)

X: Methotrexate
Cisplatin
Arsenites
(organic anions)

Figure 35.3 MRP1 and -2 mediated drug efflux. Two modalities of drug transport are shown: (i) the GS–X complex is expelled by MRP: organic anions such as methotrexate and cisplatin; (ii) Y is cotransported by MRP in the presence of GSH: organic bases such as anthracyclines and vinca alkaloids.

agents in human cancer cells. In leukaemia, monoclonal antibodies are used for measurement of MRP expression, and MRP1–2 efficiency could be checked by cytofluorimetry with a functional test, using calcein-AM as a probe and MK571 or probenicid as inhibitors.

Only MRP1 expression has been investigated on a large enough scale to generate enough data for objective analysis. In AML, compared with P-gp, discordant results have been published concerning the incidence of MRP1 expression; the range of MRP expression is narrow compared with P-gp, and a basal expression is found in all cases. One-third of the patients present with high expression. The prognostic value of MRP itself is not yet clearly determined, but both P-gp and MRP1 functions are of prognostic importance in adult AML. The role of other MRPs is still under investigation.

Few publications have concerned MRP in ALL, but all showed a measurable level of this protein at diagnosis, comparatively higher than in AML, and some cases showed an increase after treatment.

CLL cells express variable levels of MRP at diagnosis and after treatment, but the amount of MRP does not influence the course of the disease.

ABCG2 (Table 35.2)

Recently, a small ABC protein, ABCG2 (or BCRP), was described simultaneously by three different groups. It was described as a 'specific' ABC protein of the placenta (ABCP), as a new ABC protein expressed in a MDR1(–) MRP1(–) breast-resistant cell line (MCF7/Adr/Vp) ('BCRP'), and in a colon carcinoma cell line resistant to mitoxantrone (MXR1). This small protein, working as a dimer, is particularly active to efflux mitoxantrone, but also the other anthracyclines, bisantrene, and topotecan. It is expressed on side population (SP) cells, the pluripotent stem cells able to efflux the dye Hoescht 33342.

ABCG2 is expressed in a subset of leukaemic cells, but its role in clinical drug resistance is, to date, unknown.

Lung resistance protein/major vault protein

A wide variety of P-gp-negative multidrug-resistant cancer cell lines expressed the 'lung resistance-related protein' (LRP), identified as the major vault protein (MVP). Vaults are not ABC proteins, and are supposed to mediate the bidirectional transport of a variety of substrates between the nucleus and the cytoplasm. Until now, proof of the involvement of LRP/MVP in the MDR phenotype could not be demonstrated by transfection or antisense experiments.

In the majority of cases of AML, LRP/MVP is low, but detectable by RT-PCR, and the clinical significance of LRP

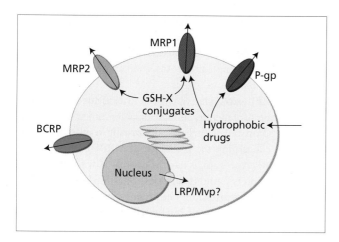

Figure 35.4 Efflux pumps involved in drug efflux in leukaemic cells. For LRP/MVP, the demonstration of drug efflux was, until now, not proven by transfection or antisense experiments.

expression is unclear. In relapsed childhood ALL, LRP expression (but not P-gp) was associated with an increased *in vitro* resistance to daunorubicin.

In summary, at least four ABC pumps and one non-ABC protein are able to expel several non-related cytotoxic drugs from the leukaemic cells, with probable redundancy (Figure 35.4).

Resistance to drug-induced apoptosis

The final effect of cytotoxic agents is apoptosis. Any factor able to reduce the amount of drug-induced apoptosis will increase cell survival, and therefore could be responsible for multidrug resistance. According to the known pathway of apoptosis involved in drug resistance (Figure 35.5), the role of several molecules has been investigated.

p53

p53 is activated in response to DNA damage, and stops the cell in the G_1 phase (via p21), permitting DNA repair, whereas apoptosis can be considered to be a failsafe mechanism to rid the organism of cells with severely damaged DNA. In cases of non-functional p53, the threshold of DNA damage leading to apoptosis increases, and this could contribute to drug resistance. In haematological malignancies, p53 is usually functional at diagnosis, but mutations have been described during progression of the disease in both lymphoid (mainly CLL) and myeloid leukaemias, and this progression corresponds mainly to highly resistant tumours.

Inhibitors of the cell cycle

Genetic alterations affecting the INK4 cell cycle inhibitors, p16^{INK4a} and p15^{INK4b}, which govern phosphorylation of the retinoblastoma protein (pRb) and control exit from the G_1 phase of the cell cycle, are frequently mutated in ALL (~ 30%), are present in high-risk ALL (relapse, T subtype), and are associated with an aggressive course of the disease.

In CLL, a high cell content of p27, a universal cyclin-cdk inhibitor, is correlated with a poor survival and an increased *in vitro* survival in the presence of a drug such as fludarabine.

Bcl-2 family

The anti-apoptotic properties of Bcl-2 and Bcl-x_L are well demonstrated *in vitro*, and their overexpression has been shown to protect tumour cell lines from the toxicity of several chemotherapeutic agents. AML cells with high Bcl-2 content correlated with a lower rate of complete remission. On the other hand, bax expression correlates with drug sensitivity to doxorubicin, cyclophosphamide and chlorambucil in CLL, and relapse in

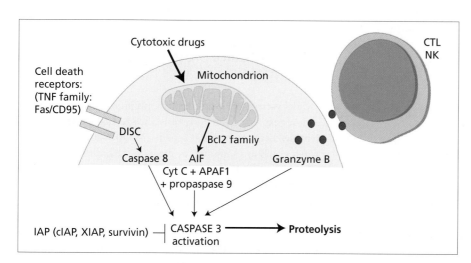

Figure 35.5 Scheme of apoptosis. The cytotoxic drugs act mainly through mitochondria. AIF, apoptosis inducing factor; APAF1, apoptotic protease activating factor 1; Cyt C, cytochrome C; DISC, death-inducing signalling complex; IAP, inhibitor of apoptosis.

childhood ALL is associated with a decrease of the bax/Bcl-2 ratio.

BCR–ABL

The chimeric protein BCR–ABL, specific to CML and frequent in adult ALL, has been shown to confer resistance to genotoxic agent-induced apoptosis (Ara-C, daunorubicin, VP-16, etc.) *in vitro*, via a prolongation of cell cycle arrest at the G_2/M restriction point, without altering either the p53 pathway or DNA repair.

Imatinib, a specific anti-thyrosine kinase drug, is a very potent inhibitor of BCR–ABL effects, but resistance to this drug was quickly described in patients, due mainly to mutations in the chimeric BCR–ABL protein (see also Chapter 37).

Reversal of multidrug resistance

P-gp inhibition

Since the first observation of *in vitro* modulation of MDR phenotype by verapamil in 1981, it was recognized that several drugs already in use in the clinic inhibit P-gp efflux, and reverse MDR phenotype in experimental systems. This perspective to overcome clinical multidrug resistance has led to the strategy of concomitant administration of chemotherapy and a 'MDR modulator'. These compounds act mainly as competitive or non-competitive inhibitors, by competition with the drug for the binding site, or by binding to other P-gp sites that cause allosteric changes of the molecule, resulting in a decrease of cytotoxic drug binding.

Phase I and II trials

Several phase I and II trials were conducted in leukaemia, multiple myeloma, lymphoma and solid tumours using verapamil, amiodarone, quinine or cyclosporin A together with an anthracycline, VP16 or a taxane. These trials were not restricted to MDR(+) tumours, and it was difficult to know the benefit of these associations for the patients. The pharmacokinetics performed during these trials suggested evidence that verapamil and amiodarone had a minimum toxic dose (MTD) below the required dose for *in vivo* P-gp inhibition, and that quinine and cyclosporin A could be used as P-gp modulators with acceptable toxicity. Another interesting finding was the dramatic decrease of anti-cancer drug clearance when cyclosporin A was coadministered. This pharmacokinetic interaction led to a prolonged terminal half-life, and an increased area under the concentration curve (AUC) of the cytostatic, and therefore an increased toxicity. This interaction is less pronounced for quinine, probably because of the absence of inhibition of P450-mediated metabolism, observed when cyclosporin A is administered.

Phase III trials with quinine and cyclosporin A

To confirm the interest of such association, several randomized phase III trials, with or without these modulators, were tested (Tables 35.5 and 35.6). In the four trials published so far, the chemotherapy used as the reference (with or without modulator) included cytosine arabinoside (Ara-C), a non-P-gp substrate, at high dose, together with daunorubicin or idarubicin, or mitoxantrone. The use of these high doses of Ara-C, able to eradicate positive P-gp cells, reduced the chance of observing a difference between the two regimens. It is important to note that in none of these trials were the doses of anthracyclines reduced.

When quinine (30 mg/kg/day, given by continuous intravenous infusion) was added to an anthracycline and Ara-C, either in poor-prognosis adult leukaemia cases (relapsing/refractory/secondary) or in untreated *de novo* AML, global results (rate of complete remission, overall survival) did not show any difference from the 'control' arm (same chemotherapy without quinine). It was noted that, in poor-prognosis patients: (i) clinical drug resistance was higher in the control group; and (ii) toxic death rate was higher in the quinine group, counteracting the potential benefit of MDR reversal. In *de novo* untreated patients, the addition of quinine benefited only the patients with functionally P-gp-positive AML cells, but did not influence the overall survival of such patients.

The addition of cyclosporin A at high dose (16 mg/kg/day) during the 3 days of continuous infusion of daunorubicin and high doses of Ara-C in relapsing/refractory AML patients significantly reduced the frequency of resistance and increased the relapse-free survival and the overall survival. The effect of cyclosporin A on survival was greater in the patients with P-gp(+) leukaemic cells than in the others. This interesting result could not be reproduced, with the same schedule, in patients experiencing a blast crisis of CML.

Quinine and cyclosporin A, molecules already on the market for a long time, were chosen for their ability to inhibit *in vivo* P-gp efflux. This was demonstrated by the potency of the serum from patients treated with high doses of these drugs to circumvent P-gp efflux in cell lines exposed to this serum.

Trials with PSC833 and other modulators in leukaemia

Several drugs were developed for the unique purpose of MDR reversal. The most advanced P-gp modulator is PSC-833, an analogue of cyclosporin D, 10-fold more potent than cyclosporin A, without any renal or immunosuppressive toxicity.

Extensive dose-finding trials of coadministered cytotoxic drugs (anthracyclines, VP16, and taxol in solid tumours) were conducted with this modulator used at the fixed dose of 10 mg/kg/day, continuous intravenous infusion, after a loading dose of 2 mg/kg over 2 h. These phase I studies concluded that it was necessary to reduce the daily dose of mitozantrone by 30–50%,

Table 35.5 Published randomized phase III trials testing quinine in adult AML.

Modulator	Chemotherapy	Disease	Selection	No. of patients	Criteria	+ Modulator	Control	P	Reference
Quinine 30 mg/kg/day Continuous i.v. infusion	Ara-C 1 g/m^2 × 10 Mitox 12 mg/m^2 × 4	Relapsing/ refractory/ secondary AML	No	318	CR rate	52.8%	45.5%	NS	Solary *et al.* (1996)
					Refractoriness	28%	40%	0.04	
					Death during TT	13%	4%	0.02	
			P-gp(+)	80	CR rate	62%	40%	0.05	
Quinine 30 mg/kg/day Continuous i.v. infusion	Ara-C 1 g/m^2 × 10 Mitox 12 mg/m^2 × 4	High-risk myelodysplastic syndrome	No	131	CR rate	47%	41%	NS	Wattel *et al.* (1998)
					Refractoriness	28%	40%	0.04	
					Death during TT	13%	4%	0.02	
					Median survival	13 months	11 months	NS	
			P-gp(+)	42	CR rate	52%	18%	0.02	
					Median survival	13 months	8 months	0.01	
			P-gp(−)	49	CR rate	35%	49%	NS	
					Median survival	14 months	14 months	NS	
Quinine 30 mg/kg/day Continuous i.v. infusion	Ara-C 200 mg/m^2 × 7 Ida. 8 mg/m^2 × 5	*De novo* AML dysplastic syndrome	No	425	CR rate	68.1%	65.9%	NS	Solary *et al.* (2003)
					Median DFS	45.3 months	41.1 months	NS	
			Rho123(+)	54	CR rate	82.8%	48%	0.01	
			Rho123(−)	106	CR rate	77.4%	86.8%	NS	

NS, not significant; TT, transfusion therapy.

Table 35.6 Published randomized phase III trial testing cyclosporin A or PSC833 in elderly patients with untreated AML and blast crisis of CML.

Modulator	Chemotherapy	Disease	Selection	No. of patients	Criteria	+ Modulator	Control	P	Reference
Cyclosporin 16 mg/kg/day Continuous i.v. infusion	Ara-C 3 g/m^2 × 5 days DNR 45 mg/m^2 × 3 Continuous i.v. infusion	Relapsing/ refractory/ secondary AML	No	226	CR rate	45%	36%	NS	List et al. (2001)
					Refractoriness	31%	47%	0.008	
					Death during TT	18%	22%	NS	
					Survival at 2 years	22%	12%	0.046	
			P-gp(+)	68	CR rate	46%	26%	NS	
			P-gp(−)	129	CR rate	39%	34%	NS	
Cyclosporin 16 mg/kg/day Continuous i.v. infusion	Ara-C 3 g/m^2 × 5 days DNR 45 mg/m^2 × 3 Continuous i.v. infusion	Myeloid Blast crisis of CML	No	77	CR rate	5%	18%	NS	List et al. (2002)
					Refractoriness	68%	53%	NS	
					Survival at 6 months	32%	47%	NS	
PSC833 10 mg/kg/day Continuous i.v. infusion	Ara-C 100 mg/m^2 × 7 DNR 60 mg/m^2 × 3 VP 1660 mg/m^2 × 3	Untreated AML > 60 years old	No	120	CR rate	39%	46%	⎫ 0.008	Baer et al. (2002)
					Refractoriness	26%	34%	⎬	
					Death during TT	44%	20%	⎭	
			P-gp(+)	43	CR rate	48%**	41%*	*0.03	
					Refractoriness	19%**	41%*	**NS	
					Death during TT	33%**	18%*		
			P-gp(−)	23	CR rate	50%**	91%*		
					Refractoriness	17%**	9%*		
					Death during TT	33%**	0%*		

*Patients treated with chemotherapy and modulator; **patients treated with chemotherapy alone.

the dose of daunorubicin by one-third, and the dose of VP16 by 40–60%, depending on the associations tested. When such adaptations of dose are used, the AUCs of these drugs are similar in both arms, and toxicities related to the cytostatics are also equivalent. The limiting toxicity of PSC833 alone was reversible ataxia and dysmetria, suggestive of a cerebellar dysfunction, possibly due to the inhibition of blood–brain barrier.

Several randomized phase III trials in AML (in elderly untreated patients and in relapsed/refractory younger patients) compared chemotherapy alone with chemotherapy (with lowered doses of anthracyclines and VP16) and PSC833, given intravenously by 24-h infusion during the administration of the anthracyclines and VP16. A higher rate of early mortality (despite the cytostatic dose reduction) was observed in the elderly patients treated with the addition of PSC833 (Table 35.6), raising the question of the consequences of the P-gp inhibition in normal tissues. The trial was stopped prematurely, but it is interesting to see that, in P-gp (+) patients, the increased number of toxic death due to the addition of PSC833 was compensated for by a particularly low proportion of resistant disease (19% vs. 41% without PSC833). Several large multicentre phase III trials testing PSC833 have been completed in relapsed and *de novo* AML, but not yet published, waiting for longer follow-up. Concerning the complete remission (CR) rate, no striking differences were observed between the two arms, tempering enthusiasm concerning the concept of P-gp inhibitors in drug-resistant leukaemia.

The failure of PSC833 to increase the CR rate in the whole population of AML patients could be explained, if higher toxicity is excluded, by the dramatic reduction of cytotoxic drugs, leading to a reduction of the maximum and/or steady-state concentration, detrimental to anti-cancer efficacy. The redundant role of the three major ABC pumps, often present together on the leukaemic cell surface, could also be explained.

The other drugs engineered for P-gp inhibition are less advanced, still in phase I and II, mainly in solid tumours. LY335979 is a quinoline derivative, specific to P-gp, and delivered orally, with a low effect on the pharmacokinetics of coadministered drugs. XR9576, an anthranilic acid derivative, delivered orally, is also being tested.

Reversion of other ABC pumps

Because of the failure of P-gp inhibitors to increase significantly the CR rate and overall survival in AML, and the putative role of other ABC pumps in drug resistance, it will be interesting to test inhibitors of several pumps. Two drugs are interesting in this setting: GG120918, a derivative of acridone carboxamide, that was developed as an inhibitor of P-gp, but was also described as a potent inhibitor of BCRP; and VX-710 (Biricodar®), a pipecolinate derivative, a modulator of P-gp and MRP1. The decision to develop GG120918 was, until now, not a priority, and Vertex Pharmaceutical is developing a phase II trial for Biricodar®.

Restoration of drug-induced apoptosis

Restoration of drug-induced apoptosis could be obtained *in vitro* with Bcl-2 antisense. The G3139, an 18-mer oligonucleotide complementary to the first codons of *Bcl-2*, was given subcutaneously during phase I, permitting the setting of the dose at a level able to give a high concentration of circulating Bcl-2 antisense without major toxicity, and a phase II trial is now completed in AML, together with chemotherapy. A randomized phase III trial is now running in untreated elderly patients with AML.

Ras inhibition

The membrane-associated G proteins encoded by the *ras* family of proto-oncogenes are potential targets for new therapeutic agents. Ras proteins are activated downstream of protein tyrosine kinases and, in turn, trigger a cascade of phosphorylation events through sequential activation of Raf, MEK-1 and ERKs. To be active, ras has to be farnesylated. Therefore, several inhibitors of farnesyl transferase (FTI) have recently been developed to counteract drug resistance due to activation of the phosphorylation cascade. A phase I trial with R115777 demonstrated a significant inhibition of ERK phosphorylation in blasts from acute leukaemia after treatment, and clinical responses, including few complete remissions, were observed. Several FTIs are now under investigation in AML and in CML.

Future directions

We have seen that a single mechanistic pathway cannot explain the genesis of resistance in leukaemia. Rather, drug resistance probably involves the altered expression of a diverse group of genetic factors influencing various biochemical pathways.

To determine the up- and downregulated genes responsible for drug resistance, the DNA microarray technology is particularly useful. Its capacity for simultaneous probing of the genome on high-density microarrays has enabled the analysis of the expression profiles of thousands of genes.

Such an analysis was conducted in doxorubicin-sensitive and -resistant cell lines and in clinical samples of AML, permitting the selection of cell cycle, signal transduction genes and transcription factor genes. The differential expression of only 28 genes (out of 23 040 tested) was the core of a 'drug response scoring' in adult AML set by Okutsu *et al.* (2002), allowing the prediction of the good and poor responders to a 'classical' induction therapy with 7 days of Ara-C (100 mg/m^2/day) and 3 days of anthracycline (idarubicin).

These analyses may ultimately enable us to use the signature expression profiles of drug-resistant leukaemia to predict response to drugs and to design targeted therapeutic regimens to circumvent drug resistance.

Selected bibliography

Baer MR, George SL, Dodge RK *et al.* (2002) Phase 3 study of the multidrug resistance modulator PSC-833 in previously untreated patients 60 years of age and older with acute myeloid leukemia: Cancer and Leukemia Group B Study 9720. *Blood* **100**: 1224–32.

Beck W, Grogan T, Willman C *et al.* (1996) Methods to detect P-glycoprotein-associated multidrug resistance in patients' tumors: consensus recommendations. *Cancer Research* **56**: 3010–20.

Biedler J, Riehm H (1970) Cellular resistance to actinomycin D in Chinese hamster *in vitro*: cross resistance, radioautographic and cytogenetic studies. *Cancer Research* **30**: 1174–80.

Borst P, Evers R, Kool M *et al.* (2000) A family of drug transporters: the multidrug resistance-associated proteins. *Journal of National Cancer Institute* **92**: 1295–302.

Brisco MJ, Sykes PJ, Dolman G *et al.* (2000) Early resistance to therapy during induction in childhood acute lymphoblastic leukemia. *Cancer Research* **60**: 5092–6.

Campos L, Guyotat D, Archimbaud E *et al.* (1992) Clinical significance of multidrug resistance P-glycoprotein expression on acute nonlymphoblastic leukemia cells at diagnosis. *Blood* **79**: 473–6.

Del Poeta G, Stasi R, Aronica G *et al.* (1996) Clinical relevance of P-glycoprotein expression in *de novo* acute myeloid leukemia. *Blood* **87**: 1997–2004.

Farber S, Diamond L, Mercer R *et al.* (1948) Temporary remission in acute leukemia in children produced by folic acid antagonist 4-aminopteroyl-glutamic acid (aminopterin). *New England Journal of Medicine* **238**: 787–93.

Goldie J, Coldman A (1979) A mathematical model for relating the drug sensitivity of tumors to their spontaneous mutation rate. *Cancer Treatment Research* **63**: 1727–31.

Hunault M, Zhou D, Delmer A *et al.* (1997) Multidrug resistance (MDR1) gene expression in acute myeloid leukemia: major prognosis significance for the *in vivo* drug resistance to induction treatment. *Annals of Hematology* **74**: 65–71.

Imamura J, Miyishi I, Koeffler H (1994) p53 in hematologic malignancies. *Blood* **84**: 2412–21.

Johnston SRD (2001) Farnesyl transferase inhibitors: a novel targeted therapy for cancer. *Lancet Oncology* **2**: 18–26.

Juliano RL, Ling V (1976) A surface glycoprotein modulating drug permeability in Chinese hamster ovary cell mutants. *Biochimica Biophysica Acta* **455**: 152–62.

Klein I, Sarkadi B, Varadi A (1999) An inventory of the human ABC proteins. *Biochimica Biophysica Acta* **1461**: 237–62.

Kohn K (1996) Regulatory genes and drug sensitivity. *Journal of the National Cancer Institute* **88**: 1255–6.

Kudoh K, Ramanna M, Ravatn R *et al.* (2000) Monitoring the expression profiles of doxorubicin-induced and doxorubicin-resistant cancer cells by cDNA microarray. *Cancer Research* **60**: 4161–6.

Legrand O, Perrot J, Baudard M *et al.* (2001) JC-1: a very sensitive fluorescent probe to test Pgp activity in adult acute myeloid leukemia. *Blood* **97**: 502–8.

Leith C, Kopecky K, Godwin J *et al.* (1997) Acute myeloid leukemia in the elderly: assessment of multidrug resistance (MDR1) and cytogenetics distinguishes biologic subgroups with remarkably distinct responses to standard chemotherapy. A Southwest Oncology Group study. *Blood* **89**: 3323–29.

List AF, Kopecky KJ, Willman CL *et al.* (2001) Benefit of cyclosporine modulation of drug resistance in patients with poor-risk acute myeloid leukemia: a Southwest Oncology Group study. *Blood* **98**: 3212–20.

List AF, Kopecky KJ, Willman CL *et al.* (2002) Cyclosporine inhibition of P-glycoprotein in chronic myeloid leukemia blast phase. *Blood* **100**: 1910–12.

Marcucci G, Byrd JC, Dai G *et al.* (2003) Phase 1 and pharmacodynamic studies of G3139: a Bcl-2 antisense oligonucleotide, in combination with chemotherapy in refractory or relapsed acute leukemia. *Blood* **101**: 425–32.

Marie JP, Huet S, Faussat AM *et al.* (1997) Multicentric evaluation of the MDR phenotype in leukemia. *Leukemia* **11**: 1086–94.

Marie JP (2001) Drug resistance in hematological malignancies. *Current Opinion in Oncology* **13**: 463–9.

Nimmanapalli R, Bhalla K (2002) Mechanisms of resistance to imatinib mesylate in Bcr-Abl-positive leukemias. *Current Opinion in Oncology* **14**: 616–20.

Nüssler V, Pelka-Fleischer R, Zwierzina H *et al.* (1996) P-glycoprotein expression in patients with acute leukemia – clinical relevance. *Leukemia* **10** (Suppl. 3): S23–S31.

Okutsu J, Tsunoda T, Kaneta Y *et al.* (2002) Prediction of chemosensitivity for patients with acute myeloid leukemia, according to expression levels of 28 genes selected by genome-wide complementary DNA microarray analysis. *Molecular Cancer Therapy* **1**: 1035–42.

Reed J (1995) Bcl-2: prevention of apoptosis as a mechanism of drug resistance. *Hematological and Oncological Clinics of North America* **9**: 451–73.

Scheffer GL, Schroeijers AB, Izquierdo MA *et al.* (2000) Lung resistance-related protein/major vault protein and vaults in multidrug-resistant cancer. *Current Opinion in Oncology* **12**: 550–6.

Sherr C (1996) Cancer cell cycles. *Science* **274**: 1672–7.

Sikic BI, Fisher GA, Lum BL *et al.* (1997) Modulation and prevention of multidrug resistance by inhibitors of P-glycoprotein. *Cancer Chemotherapy and Pharmacology* **40** (Suppl.): S13–19.

Solary E, Drenou B, Campos L *et al.* (2003) Quinine as a multidrug resistance inhibitor: a phase III multicentric randomized study in adult *de novo* acute myelogenous leukemia. *Blood* **102**: 1202–10.

Solary E, Witz B, Caillot D *et al.* (1996) Combination of quinine as a potential reversing agent with mitoxantrone and cytarabine for the treatment of acute leukemias: a randomized multicentric study. *Blood* **88**: 1198–205.

van den Heuvel-Eibrink MM, van der Holt B, te Boekhorst PA *et al.* (1997) MDR 1 expression is an independent prognostic factor for response and survival in *de novo* acute myeloid leukaemia. *British Journal of Haematology* **99**: 76–83.

Willman CL (1997) The prognostic significance of the expression and function of multidrug resistance transporter proteins in acute myeloid leukemia: studies of the Southwest Oncology Group Leukemia Research Program. *American Seminars in Hematology* **34** (Suppl. 5): 25–33.

Zhou S, Schuetz JD Bunting KD *et al.* (2001) The ABC transporter Bcrp1/ABCG2 is expressed in a wide variery of stem cells and in a molecular determinant of the side-population phenotype. *Nature Medicine* **7**: 1028–34.

CHAPTER 36

Supportive care in the management of leukaemia

36

Archibald G Prentice and J Peter Donnelly

Introduction

The outlook for patients with acute and chronic leukaemias has improved considerably in the past 40 years, mainly because of more effective therapy. Better understanding and management of the complications have also improved survival and quality of life. These complications vary with the pace of the disease (acute or chronic), with specific subtypes of myeloid and lymphoid leukaemias, and with the intensity and duration of therapy.

The effectiveness of support depends on the coordinated work of specialist doctors, nurses, therapists and pharmacists, working in facilities dedicated to the care of these patients. In the intensive care of patients with acute leukaemia, it is especially important that there should be clear rules about when and why nurses should ask medical staff to review their observations and equally clear rules about the doctors' responses. Timely and accurate communication between professional groups is essential, and all should be working to agreed written standards. Management of all the complications requires careful and regular recording of basic observations by nurses, most of whom should be registered and experienced in leukaemia care. This team needs a high skill mix, and an overall nurse–patient ratio above 1 to allow internal shift rotation that provides a continuous level of expertise.

Whatever the type of leukaemia, patients should be treated according to protocols as part of well-designed, multicentre, controlled trials.

The management of each group of complications is described both in general and with reference to specific types of leukaemia and forms of therapy. Complications requiring supportive care can be classified as:

1 psychological, due to loss of performance and self-determination and protracted treatment-related complications, such as the need for isolation as protection against infection;

2 reproductive due to the need to prevent pregnancy in female patients during intensive cytotoxic exposure and to preserve fertility in patients of childbearing age;

3 anaemia, due to failure of red cell production, bleeding or haemolysis;

4 bleeding, due to thrombocytopenia and lack of clotting factors, through either failure of production or excessive consumption (disseminated intravascular coagulation);

5 infections, due to failure of production of adequate numbers of functionally normal neutrophils, and monocytes/macrophages and failure of other components of the immune response, including the gut mucosal barrier;

6 metabolic, due to disturbances in fluid and electrolyte and acid–base balance, related to the disease or the treatment or both;

7 nutritional, when oral intake fails and loss of lean body mass is significant;

8 nausea and vomiting, due to chemotherapy and other drugs;

9 pain, due to involvement of specific anatomical sites in the disease or as a result of specific therapies;

10 palliative supportive care, necessary when cytotoxic therapy fails to induce or maintain lasting, complete remission; this does not exclude further cytotoxic therapy as part of other efforts to control distressing symptoms.

Psychological support

Regardless of the subtype of disease and form of therapy, this support starts with an explanation of the diagnosis and treatment by a senior haematologist accompanied by a specialist nurse, both of whom should be active and experienced in this type of care and communication. It is essential to gain the trust of the patients and their immediate families or partners from the outset so that they can understand and accept the need for the proposed intensity and duration of treatment and the risks of complications. As well as needing support for their distress on learning the diagnosis, most will also ask for detailed information including prognosis. Any relevant clinical trial can be described, and informed consent obtained for enrolment and randomization between different treatment options. A relationship of mutual and complete openness should be established as soon as possible, and questions and discussion encouraged.

Most patients may appear to be psychologically able to deal with these illnesses and all of their complications. But many patients find that loss of control of their normal daily activity is difficult to manage, particularly prolonged stays in hospital, including periods in protective isolation. Nearly all will suffer some loss of self-assurance and self-esteem, particularly if they fall ill at the peak of their responsibilities and abilities in their domestic and working lives. Fear of failure of therapy may be lessened if remission is achieved, but the patients' anticipation of the complications of subsequent cycles of therapy may add to their psychological problems.

Having little control over this cumulative experience, patients can develop significant neurotic or psychotic pathology, sometimes well after therapy is finished and as they attempt to resume a normal life. The clinical team must be alert to the development of any signs that such problems are impending and deal with them before patients suffer significant and lasting harm. In dealing with these problems, it is difficult for professional carers to maintain a balanced approach that suits each patient. It is as easy to be too intrusive with those patients who can cope without help as it is to fail to detect psychopathology in those who cannot. This area of supportive care underlines the need for integrated teamwork.

Regardless of age and subtype, patients with acute leukaemias present with a short history, are often seriously unwell due to acute marrow failure and require immediate admission to a haematology unit for intensive therapy. Their psychological complications are often more intensely expressed and require equally intensive support because their loss of function is so acute and severe. This type of supportive care should be an integral part of any therapy, whether it is given with the intention to achieve complete remission in younger patients or as palliation in the elderly and frail.

Reproductive issues

Before any chemotherapy is given to adolescents and young men, they should be counselled about the possibility of loss of fertility and offered the opportunity to store sperm. If therapy cannot be delayed, sperm should be collected as soon as possible to minimize the risk of damage to sperm already formed and stored and because of the potential infertility induced by any cytotoxic therapy, particularly intensive chemotherapy. Patients who opt to store sperm need expert counselling in all of the associated ethical issues before collection, particularly their wish to destroy or preserve the collection should the patient die. They and their partners may wish to conserve the sperm for future fertilization after the patient's death. Loss of fertility due to chemotherapy is much less likely in women, who should avoid falling pregnant while receiving such therapy because of likely damage to the embryo and fetus. Preservation *in vitro* of unfertilized ova is not yet possible and not undertaken routinely.

Impaired sexual function can be a problem in both sexes following intensive chemotherapy. Patients and their partners are often reluctant to discuss these problems with their specialist carers and are more likely to discuss them with nursing colleagues. Expert counselling or psychological care can be effective in restoring potency.

Anaemia and thrombocytopenia

In all types of leukaemias, and with all types of treatment, there is a risk of marrow failure leading to anaemia and thrombocytopenia. The pace at which they develop and their severity vary with the type of leukaemia and therapy, and many of the complications are seen whatever the intensity of therapy. As these causes and effects are most marked in the acute leukaemias, the support needed in that context is described in greater detail. By the time most patients present, their ability to produce red cells and platelets will be severely impaired and they will need regular and frequent transfusions of both. Administration of a wide range of intravenous therapies, including blood products, may be necessary simultaneously. Long-lasting, tunnelled, multilumen, central venous catheters (CVCs) facilitate rapid intravenous access for such multiple therapies, and also reduce the risk of blood-borne infection by reducing the need for multiple and repeated peripheral venous access. Sterile handling of these lines is therefore essential at all times. It is not necessary to transfuse either whole or fresh blood but there are some simple basic rules that should be followed regarding red cell and platelet transfusion (Table 36.1).

Table 36.1 Ten rules for transfusion and coagulation failure in acute leukaemia.

Rule	Reason	Exceptions
1 In younger patients use CMV-negative blood until CMV status known	High transplant-related CMV death risk	No transplant planned
2 Transfuse if Hb < 8 g/dL	Symptom control	Cardiac failure
3 Delay if white count > 100×10^9/L	Hyperviscosity risks bleeds and clots	None
4 Give platelets priority	Red cells dilute low count	Big bleeds; give both
5 Big volumes need diuretics	Circulatory overload	None but plan K^+ and Na^+ infusions too
6 Keep platelets > 10×10^9/L	Prevent bleeding	> 20×10^9/L during sepsis
7 Use ABO-identical platelets	Maximize effect	No clinical harm if only non-identical available
8 HLA-restricted platelets if refractory to donations	Loss of effect	May resolve allowing use of non-restricted donations
9 Use pethidine for allergic/febrile reactions	Avoid undetected cumulative steroid immunosuppression	None
10 Use only ABO-compatible plasma-derived products to correct clotting times	Avoid ABO haemolytic reactions	None; therapy determined by specific bleeding problems

Cytomegalovirus-negative blood products

As transfusion of both red cells and platelets may be required at the outset, it is important to establish immediately whether elective allogeneic stem cell transplantation (SCT) is likely as part of the care plan. If it is, those patients should always be transfused with blood products that are less likely to increase the risk of cytomegalovirus (CMV) transfusion, using leucodepleted or filtered donor blood or blood only from known CMV-negative donors until the patient's own CMV status is known. This applies to all patients under the age of 55 years who have potential sibling donors. CMV infection is a major cause of morbidity and mortality in allogeneic SCT and prevention is more effective than treatment.

Acute anaemia

Onset of anaemia is often rapid in patients with acute leukaemia so they are unable to compensate haemodynamically as in anaemia of slower onset. Because of their acutely reduced red cell mass and hence oxygen-carrying capacity, they are likely to be symptomatic and should be transfused as soon as they have been assessed clinically and the result of their blood count is known. This rule may need to be modified in the presence of symptomatic or treated cardiac disease (see Planning large volume transfusions, below). With chemotherapy red cell production remains suppressed and the patient remains dependent on repeated transfusions.

Conventional teaching is to try to maintain the haemoglobin level above 10 g/dL. This has been challenged recently and the Adult Leukaemia Working Party of the UK National Cancer Research Institute is planning a randomized trial to determine the risks and benefits of lowering the threshold of the haemo-

globin level at which red cell transfusion is indicated. There is evidence that patients in other critically ill categories will tolerate much lower levels (as low as 6 g/dL) and that transfusing at higher levels may be harmful. In practice, many leukaemia and transplant units already withhold red cell transfusion until the haemoglobin drops to 8 g/dL for patients whose cardiorespiratory function is not compromised.

Excessive red cell transfusion may lead to alloimmunization, with red cell blood group and white cell HLA antigens potentially creating difficulties for future transfusion and SCT. In the transplant patient (autologous and allogeneic), there is also the risk of iron overload, but this appears unlikely to be a problem with conventional chemotherapy.

Hyperviscosity of high white counts

Patients who present with acute leukaemias with very high white blood cell (WBC) counts, particularly over 100×10^9/L, should be given blood only if it is not possible to wait for reduction of the WBC either by leucapheresis or chemotherapy. These patients are already at risk of thrombotic and haemorrhagic events due to hyperviscosity, and transfusion will increase that risk, even if it is slow. It is probably safe to allow such patients to start their chemotherapy with a haemoglobin level as low as 8 g/dL. Patients with high WBCs in chronic myeloid leukaemia (CML) may develop hyperviscosity problems, but these are rare in chronic lymphocytic leukaemia (CLL).

Planning large-volume transfusions

When planning a large red cell transfusion, it is essential to estimate in advance the total intravenous fluid load these patients will receive over any following 24-h period. Most patients with acute leukaemia are elderly and will already have some degree of cardiovascular pathology. Some chemotherapy, such as the anthracyclines commonly used in the remission induction of acute myeloblastic leukaemia (AML) and acute lymphoblastic leukaemia (ALL), are also unpredictably cardiotoxic below a total cumulative dose in individual patients. If a large intravenous fluid load is unavoidable and intravascular overload is likely, elective diuretic therapy should be prescribed, usually with small doses (20 mg) of intravenous furosemide (frusemide) at planned intervals throughout a prolonged infusion. The use of diuretics in this way may lead to electrolyte depletion, which requires correction (see Metabolic support, below). Careful observation of basic vital signs, more simply daily weights, will indicate whether there is an excessive intravascular fluid load contributing to compromised cardiac and respiratory function.

Platelets take priority

When these patients require both red cell and platelet transfusions, platelets should always be given first. Platelet production is compromised to such a degree that a large red cell transfusion will dilute the platelet count to a potentially dangerously lower level. Platelets for transfusion are provided in single packs known as an 'adult therapeutic dose' (ATD), which contains approximately 10^{11} platelets. These are obtained either by apheresis from a single donor or by pooling platelets harvested from the buffy coats of packs of blood from six donors.

Platelets can be given so quickly through a CVC, such that even with sudden and heavy bleeding it is seldom necessary to give red cells first, and red cells and platelets can be given simultaneously.

Minimum platelet level

The planned trial of restriction of red cell transfusions is partly based on the evidence that the previous threshold for the transfusion of platelets at 20×10^9/L or less was overcautious and a threshold of 10×10^9/L is equally unlikely to lead to significant bleeding. Platelet transfusions may also alloimmunize against red cell and HLA antigens.

In general, platelets are not given until the count falls below the lower limit, but there are exceptions to this rule. It is important to remember that a count just over this lower threshold is often obtained early in the morning and the count may drop below it within the following 24 h before a further count is undertaken. So the rate of fall in previous counts should prove a useful guide as to when platelet concentrate should be infused. Platelet function and survival may both be compromised in the presence of sepsis and some systemic antibiotics (particularly penicillins in high dose), so the higher threshold of 20×10^9/L should be used in patients with these risk factors. Whenever possible, platelet infusions should not be given temporally close to infusions of amphotericin B (see Infections, below) because of

the evidence that this drug will interfere with platelet function and thus reduce the effectiveness of the donation.

It has been suggested that patients who are stable and not infected may tolerate platelet counts as low as 5×10^9/L, provided the count is unlikely to fall further. This policy requires considerable faith in the accuracy and reproducibility of the laboratory technology of counting platelets.

'Compatible' platelets

Whenever possible, platelet concentrate of a red cell ABO group that is identical to that of the patient should be transfused. If non-identical platelets are used, there may be loss of platelet function and an inferior increment in the recipient's count. Whether this technical benefit is ever clinically significant has never been proven conclusively, but it seems reasonable to give patients the theoretical best possible donation if they need platelets at all, especially if one applies the policy of only transfusing at the lower count of 10×10^9/L.

Platelet 'increments'

Regular platelet counts are needed to plan platelet transfusions and will also reveal failure to obtain a satisfactory increment in the patient's platelet count following transfusion of an ATD. Such patients are described as 'refractory' to platelet transfusion because of the development of alloantibodies to the HLA antigens borne by platelets, and may manifest bleeding or bruising even before a failure of increment is detected. This refractory state should be confirmed with two platelet counts, one pretransfusion and one taken 30-min post transfusion. On confirmation of this problem, the patient's HLA type should be determined immediately if this has not already been performed for the purposes of subsequent transplantation. The National Blood Service will then supply HLA-restricted, if not -identical, platelet donations until such time as a trial of HLA-unrestricted donations can be safely given again. Platelet refractoriness need not be permanent but can recur and is not necessarily heralded by a febrile reaction to transfusion.

Febrile reactions

During the course of treatment, patients will experience many episodes of fever for which there will be many potential explanations. Febrile reactions to blood and blood products are usually easy to identify as they occur during or immediately after the transfusion and should not be confused with the fever of infection (see Infections, below). If the reaction occurs during transfusion, transfusion should be slowed at first, or stopped if this does not reduce the severity of symptoms and signs. If that fails to abort the first febrile reaction, only then should a single intravenous injection of an antihistamine be given, such as chlorpheniramine 25 mg. If that is insufficient, many haematologists will give hydrocortisone 100 mg intravenously, and some will give both hydrocortisone and chlorpheniramine simultaneously.

The frequency and severity of these reactions may lead to the prescription of these two drugs either 'as required' or as prophylaxis for these reactions, which leads, in turn, to their uncontrolled use by inexperienced junior doctors and nurses. The total cumulative dose of immunosuppressive steroids may go unseen, and the use of hydrocortisone in the management of these febrile reactions should be discouraged. Whether these reactions are due to blood products or drugs such as amphotericin B, the most effective treatment or prophylaxis is pethidine 12.5 mg intravenously. This drug is not immunosuppressive and this dose is neither sedating nor, on repetition, addictive, but it should not be used in fever that is probably due to infection.

Specific bleeding problems

In addition to the risk of bleeding because of low platelets, there are further specific coagulation problems that require early detection and planned management. Patients should be monitored for evidence of failure of coagulation, even when they are receiving regular platelet infusions. Clinical observation should include regular fundoscopy for retinal bleeding and testing for haematuria. During remission induction and consolidation therapy for acute leukaemia, platelet transfusion is unavoidable. Fresh-frozen plasma and cryoprecipitate are needed infrequently and should only be used for specific indications and in the absence of virally inactivated products. When correcting coagulation deficiency with plasma-derived products, ABO red cell group-compatible donations should be used to avoid ABO haemolytic reactions. The use of any blood products should follow best practice guidelines provided at present.

Asparaginase in the remission induction phase of the treatment of ALL can inhibit synthesis of coagulation factors, particularly fibrinogen, which should be replaced using fresh-frozen plasma or cryoprecipitate. Very rarely, asparaginase may cause superior sagittal vein thrombosis without warning, but especially in children with unsuspected genetic thrombophilia, for example factor V Leiden.

The hypergranular variant of acute promyelocytic leukaemia (M3) carries a very high risk of bleeding because of disseminated intravascular coagulation (DIC) or fibrinolysis. This can be present at diagnosis or is precipitated by chemotherapy, in either case because of the systemic prothrombotic action of the cytoplasmic granules released by the malignant blasts. The treatment, as in all cases of DIC, is to deal with the primary cause, in this case to lower the blast count as soon after diagnosis as possible. It may be accompanied by microangiopathic haemolytic anaemia. All-*trans*-retinoic acid (ATRA) is now a standard part of initial chemotherapy for these patients, as it induces maturation of granulocytes, reducing release of the prothrombotic contents of their granules and lowering the risk of DIC.

Many older adult patients are now anticoagulated with warfarin, aspirin and clopidogrel, or a combination of these, to lessen their risk of acute myocardial infarction or stroke. The physician who initiated this therapy should be identified, if possible, to discuss the risks of stopping these immediately after diagnosis and throughout the treatment of the leukaemia. All anti-platelet therapy should be stopped because protracted and severe thrombocytopenia will recur during the course of therapy. The long action of aspirin and clopidogrel make rapid reversal of their anti-platelet effect impossible if the platelet count drops suddenly. Low-molecular-weight heparin (LMWH) should replace warfarin in those patients who have a high risk of arterial or venous thrombosis, and should be stopped once the platelet count falls below 50×10^9/L. Long-term anticoagulation should not be restarted until all chemotherapy is finished and the patient is in a stable remission.

In patients with chronic and relapsed or refractory leukaemia, there may be chronic mucosal blood loss due to persistent and severe thrombocytopenia, which may be refractory to donor platelet transfusions. Oral tranexamic acid can reduce such blood loss and hormonal suppression can prevent endometrial bleeding. Persistent marrow failure without overt blood loss may require repeat red cell transfusions in patients with chronic leukaemias, particularly chronic lymphocytic leukaemia (CLL). These should be given to relieve symptoms and not according to any set level of haemoglobin. Red cell alloantibodies and iron overload complicate repeated transfusion. CLL patients can develop autoimmune haemolysis and thrombocytopenia. The management of these complications is described in Chapter 38. Erythropoietin is of little value in the treatment of chronic anaemia associated with chronic and relapsed/refractory acute leukaemias but may occasionally be of value following SCT if engraftment is slow.

In all SCT patients, all blood products must be irradiated before transfusion to avoid the risk of graft-versus-host disease (GvHD) mounted by donor lymphocytes against the immunocompromised host. The risk of transfusion-related GvHD is much lower in autografts than in allografts. Any transfusion given to those patients whose peripheral blood stem cells (PBSCs) are to be collected within the subsequent 2–3 weeks must also be irradiated, as transfused donor lymphocytes in the PBSC collection may remain alloreactive until post autograft, and lead to clinically significant GvHD.

Infections

Some infections occur with all types of leukaemia and therapy, whereas others show more specific associations. As a general rule, the greater the duration and severity of immunosuppression, the greater is the risk of life-threatening infection with a bigger range of organisms. During chemotherapy, patients with acute leukaemia have a high risk of life-threatening infections

Table 36.2 Origins of common potential bacterial pathogens.

	Endogenous	*Exogenous*
Gram-negative bacilli	*Escherichia coli*	*Pseudomonas aeruginosa*
	Klebsiella pneumoniae	*Enterobacter cloacae*
Gram-positive bacilli	*Corynebacterium* species	*Bacillus* species
	Clostridium species	
	e.g. *C. septicum*	
Gram-positive cocci	*Staphylococcus aureus*	*Enterococcus faecium*
	Coagulase-negative staphylococci	
	e.g. *Staphylococcus epidermidis*	
	Viridans streptococci	
	e.g. *Streptococcus mitis*	
	Enterococcus faecalis	
	Stomatococcus mucilaginosus	

because of the combination of neutropenia due to the disease and the chemotherapy, which also suppresses both humoral (B cell) and cell-mediated (T cell) immunity and worsens an already poor nutritional state. The risk is greatest with the profound and protracted immunosuppression required in allogeneic SCT from an unrelated donor.

Common causes of bacterial infection are depicted in Table 36.2. This limited range of bacteria accounts for most of the opportunistic infections identified during the course of neutropenia, despite the fact that the body is colonized with so many more. Strictly anaerobic bacteria are rarely the cause of systemic infection, although they outnumber other bacteria by several billion. Fungal infections tend to occur after bacterial infections. The body's surfaces, particularly in the oral cavity and gut, are inhabited by billions of bacteria spread over many hundreds of genera, and our environment contains hundreds more bacteria and fungi. But most remain harmless, or at least undetected as causes of fever during profound immunosuppression, despite leukaemic patients' close encounter with them.

All protocols for prophylaxis, investigation and treatment of infection should be agreed by haematologists and microbiologists. These protocols should be supplemented with regular discussion of individual patients' investigations and results, and by audits of responses to results and of effectiveness of the protocols.

Fever as evidence of infection during chemotherapy and stem cell transplantation

Although repeatedly neutropenic for prolonged periods, most patients with acute leukaemia will become febrile at some point. A minority of these episodes will be accompanied by symptoms and signs of localizing infection, such as dysuria and urinary frequency or inflammation of the CVC tunnel. Because of the perceived need to treat presumed bacteraemia promptly in most cases, the fever will be, at least initially, of unknown ori-

gin (FUO). This empiric approach may have some unfavourable consequences of excessive treatment, such as insufficient microbiological diagnosis, more adverse drug reactions, emergent bacterial resistance and increased costs. There are many other causes of fever in these patients, including blood products, drugs (chemotherapy and antibiotics), tumour lysis syndrome (TLS), DIC and, in SCT, total body irradiation (TBI) and GvHD. It is sometimes possible to identify one or more of these as the cause(s) of fever and thus avoid unnecessary antibiotic therapy.

Infections can go unnoticed because the inflammatory response is muted and no pus is formed because of neutropenia. Foci of infections can also be easily overlooked unless physical examination is frequent. Infections may start as fever with or without bacteraemia, followed by clinical evidence of localized infection, and constant vigilance is needed to detect the sequential development of systemic infection (Figure 36.1). Despite the meagre signs and symptoms of infection in an immunocompromised patient, it is still essential to conduct a careful physical examination, paying particular attention to the oropharynx, including the dentition, the lungs, the skin and exit sites of venous access devices, and the perianal region. Rectal examination is inadvisable in the severely neutropenic and thrombocytopenic patient because of the risk of bacteraemia. The most common sites of infection when present are the oral cavity, the lung and the skin, with its underlying soft tissues. Clinically detectable sources of infections occur in up to one in five cases and tend to be those in the skin and its structures or in the mucosal barrier, including the respiratory tract (Figure 36.2).

Microbiological proof of infection is found in only 20–30% of cases of neutropenic fever and a further 10–20% of cases can be defined as clinical infections.

All units treating these patients must have a clear written protocol that balances the risks and benefits of exact diagnosis against empiric therapy by making good use of all available evidence at the onset of FUO. This protocol must include a description of the specimens to be obtained by the microbiology

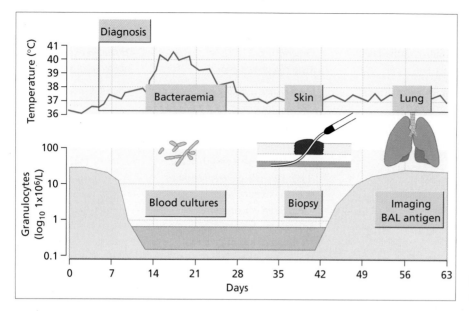

Figure 36.1 Common infections during neutropenia.

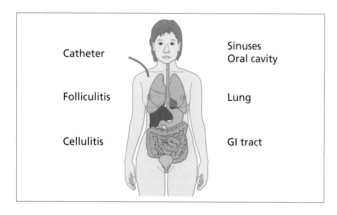

Figure 36.2 Sources of infection – the role of mucositis.

laboratory. Many diagnostic opportunities are missed if the laboratory is not clear about what is to be done with samples from these patients, and how results should be interpreted and reported. Obtaining specimens from some infectious foci may be difficult if this requires aspiration or biopsy during severe thrombocytopenia. Even when a specimen is obtained from a normally sterile site, the yield of pathogens is usually low,

interpretation is difficult and the results may not influence management. Failure to identify a focus of infection and to obtain appropriate samples may leave the fever unexplained. In most cases, microbiological diagnosis depends on identification of pathogens in blood cultures.

Laboratory investigation of neutropenic fever of unknown origin

Blood cultures

The utility of blood cultures depends on adherence to a few simple rules (Table 36.3). The specificity of blood cultures is increased if samples are taken from at least two separate sites, preferably including all lumina of a CVC. Blood should be drawn from a peripheral vein and from the CVC to confirm the significance of growing skin commensals in the culture medium, such as the Gram-positive coagulase-negative staphylococci. Other isolates including Gram-negative bacilli and viridans streptococci seldom colonize the lumen of a CVC. The total amount of blood sampled at any one time constitutes a single blood culture. Sensitivity and specificity are increased if at least 20 mL of blood taken from each sampling site at each time is

Table 36.3 Blood cultures.

When	At onset of fever
How	A sample of 20 mL blood from a peripheral vein and, when present, samples of 20 mL from each lumen of an indwelling vascular catheter
Method	Each sample divided between an aerobic and an anaerobic bottle
Time to positivity	Most organisms are detected within 24 h and 50% within 12 h
Time to identity	24–48 h, i.e. within the empirical phase
Utility	Identifies cause of fever in 20–30% of cases

divided between an aerobic and an anaerobic bottle to detect the majority of common pathogens.

Oral/rectal swabs

Viridans streptococci of the *mitis* group (*Streptococcus mitis* and *S. oralis*) are universal residents of the oral cavity and, with the exception of bacterial endocarditis, are seldom associated with infectious diseases. However, in the last two decades, these bacteria have been causing bacteraemia regularly in patients with severe oral mucositis. Similarly, *Clostridium* spp., for example *C. septicum*, are also normal commensal bacteria of the large bowel but can cause bacteraemia in patients suffering from a particularly severe form of gut mucositis, namely neutropenic enterocolitis (typhlitis). Given their presence in most individuals as part of the normal flora, it is pointless to obtain specimens from the oral cavity or rectum to detect these bacteria.

Specimens for pulmonary infection

Investigating pulmonary infection has become more demanding and involves obtaining blood samples as well as specimens from the respiratory tract. Bronchoalveolar lavage (BAL) specimens are advised for patients with pulmonary infiltrates and can yield the pathogen in 30–50% of cases. There are no standards for handling such specimens in the laboratory or in the diagnostic tests themselves. The residue of BAL samples after centrifugation is examined for *Pneumocystis jirovecii* (formerly *carinii*), the acid-fast bacilli and *Nocardia* spp., common bacteria, and moulds (*Aspergillus* spp.) and is subjected to culture for fungi and bacteria, including *Legionella* spp. and *Mycobacterium* spp. BAL may also be examined for the presence of *Aspergillus* galactomannan antigen, which is found frequently in cases of invasive pulmonary aspergillosis, and microbial DNA may be detected by PCR techniques.

Standards for virological investigations vary, but the influenza and parainfluenza viruses, adenovirus, respiratory syncytial virus and CMV may also be detected. When superficial pulmonary lesions are present, specimens might be obtained by percutaneous or open lung biopsy, provided that the benefit outweighs the risk, diagnosis is uncertain and treatment is not working. Although neutropenic patients do not produce sputum, they frequently expectorate mucous secretions, which should be sent for microscopy and culture. Recovery of moulds including *Aspergillus* on two or more consecutive occasions suggests that they are causative organisms from a patient with pulmonary infiltrates. The common practice of microbiology laboratories in discarding expectorated secretions without pus cells should not apply to these patients.

Skin lesions

Identifying the cause of a skin or soft-tissue infection is difficult because culturing superficial swabs of lesions rarely discriminates between pathogens and commensal flora. Culture and histological examination of skin punch-biopsy specimens is very helpful in diagnosing disseminated infections due to *Candida* spp., *Trichosporon* spp. and *Fusarium* spp., but aspiration of skin lesions is seldom successful as pus is usually absent.

Gut investigations

In oesophagitis, endoscopy occasionally distinguishes infection due to herpes simplex from that due to *Candida* spp. but clinical suspicion of infective oesophagitis rarely leads to endoscopy because appearances are usually non-specific and the procedure is hazardous. Persistent diarrhoea or abdominal pain requires a cytotoxicity assay on a stool sample for *C. difficile* toxin, and patients with right lower quadrant pain suggestive of typhlitis should have blood cultures taken to exclude the presence of *C. septicum* or *C. tertium*, as recovery of these bacteria usually indicates neutropenic enterocolitis. Although infections due to *Candida* spp., the Gram-negative bacilli, *Escherichia coli*, *Klebsiella pneumoniae*, and *P. aeruginosa*, *Clostridium* spp. and enterococci, including vancomycin-resistant enterococci (VRE), usually originate from the large bowel, there is no value in culturing faeces as there are many more patients colonized than infected.

Urinary tract

Urine should be obtained for standard culture when there are signs or symptoms of a urinary tract infection but not otherwise. Urine from SCT recipients with haemorrhagic cystitis should be tested for adenovirus and BK virus.

Non-cultural techniques

The role of non-cultural methods for diagnosis is small but expanding. *Legionella* antigen detection in urine is specific but detects only *L. pneumophila* type 1. Detection of CMV DNA by quantitative PCR may replace detection of the pp65 antigen in peripheral blood neutrophils among SCT recipients, and there is increasing expertise in using PCR to detect fungal DNA in blood and urine, but these remain investigational. Kits for the detection of *Aspergillus* antigen in serum, plasma and other sterile body fluids using an enzyme-linked immunosorbent assay (ELISA) are commercially available and can be used to screen patients at risk of aspergillosis. The specificity is generally high but the sensitivity has varied considerably, depending upon the nature of the specimen (blood, bronchial material, cerebral spinal fluid), the threshold employed (0.5–1.5), the frequency of sampling (once or twice weekly or less) and the prevalence of the disease in the population under study. Unlike PCR, the detection of the *Aspergillus* antigen by ELISA is considered equivalent to recovery by culture as mycological evidence.

Surveillance cultures

There is no point in undertaking surveillance cultures unless the results are used to guide therapeutic or prophylactic choice. Surveillance cultures of faeces are used if there is risk of emergent ciprofloxacin-resistant *Escherichia coli* or *Pseudomonas aeruginosa* when the drug is being used for prophylaxis. Testing faeces for carriage of these bacteria is a prudent form of surveillance to permit early detection of rising resistance before there is a corresponding rise in the infections caused by resistant bacteria. Detection of *Candida* carriage can be used to start prophylaxis and, conversely, failure to detect the yeast or opportunistic Gram-negative bacilli in oral samples or faeces suggests that infection is highly unlikely as the negative predictive value of these cultures exceeds 95%.

Proven systemic infection during neutropenia

Surveys show that the rate of proven bacteraemia during periods of neutropenia has remained between 20% and 25% over many years. In adults, the range of bacteria identified has also altered very little but the ratio of Gram-positive to Gram-negative organisms has varied. In the 1970s, there were two to three times as many Gram-negative as -positive infections, in the late 1980s and early 1990s, this ratio was reversed and now the risks of Gram-negative and -positive infection are approximately equal. It is not entirely clear why this has happened, and it is important to emphasize that individual units can have a pattern of causative organisms that is unique and unlike this international spectrum. Therefore, it is important for each unit to monitor local rates of isolation of bacterial (and other) pathogens and their patterns of antibiotic susceptibility in liaison with the microbiologists, who should be members of the multidisciplinary team.

There have been changes in practice that have been widely applied and are blamed for the changing Gram-negative and -positive rates. For example, in the management of adult acute leukaemia there has been a trend towards more intensity of therapy, with an increasing risk of gut mucositis. In the presence of this complication, the use of blockade of gastric acid production increases the risk of streptococcal bacteraemia. The widespread use of indwelling CVC provides another portal of entry for Gram-positive staphylococci. The cause of greatest concern has been the indiscriminate use of oral quinolone antibacterials (ofloxacin, ciprofloxacin) as prophylaxis against Gram-negative bacteraemia, which has not reduced the overall risk rate but simply shifted towards the Gram-positive organisms. Such prophylaxis is justifiable in allogeneic SCT recipients, but it may not be appropriate in lower-risk patients who are receiving chemotherapy.

Recent studies suggest that the risk of Gram-negative bacteraemia has not diminished in many single centres and is on the increase in centres that have never used quinolones as prophylaxis, in those which have recently discontinued this use and even in those in which this use continues (Figure 36.3). The latest European data show that the risk of proven bacteraemia is now up to 28%, mainly due to a significant doubling of the risk of Gram-negative infections.

It is difficult to reconcile these data with a unifying explanation. But it does seem clear that, despite a relatively high risk of bacteraemia, there is insufficient evidence to support continuous prophylaxis against bacterial infections with broad-spectrum antibiotics during conventional chemotherapy. It is doubtful that this will substantially reduce the risk of such infections and may compromise the efficacy of these antibiotics when they are needed.

In bacteraemia associated with onset of fever, the most commonly identified organisms are the Gram-negative bacilli *E. coli*, *P. aeruginosa*, *Proteus*, *Klebsiella* and Enterobacter spp. and the Gram-positive cocci *Staphylococcus epidermidis*, *Staph. aureus* (increasingly the methicillin-resistant strains, MRSA), the viridans streptococci belonging to the *mitis* group *S. mitis* and *S. oralis*. Other species such as *Enterococcus faecalis* and *Clostridium* spp. occur only after 7–10 days' therapy with broad-spectrum

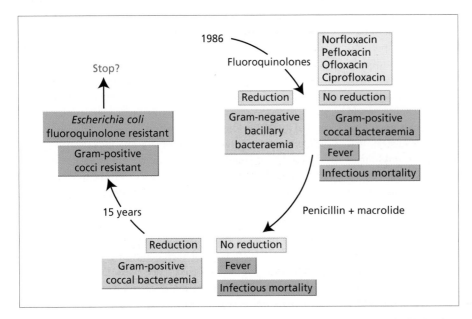

Figure 36.3 The life cycle of fluoroquinolone prophylaxis.

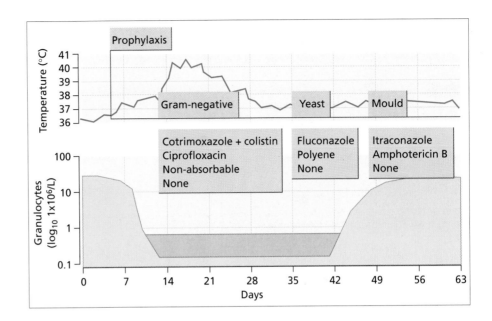

Figure 36.4 Antibiotic choices for prophylaxis during neutropenia.

antibiotics, in association with gut mucositis, including neutropenic enterocolitis (typhlitis).

The reported incidence of proven systemic fungal infection (SFI) is around 15% in SCT, and the risk rises in severe chronic GvHD requiring prolonged immunosuppression with steroids. The majority of these infections are now due to *Aspergillus* spp. and are seen more than 100 days after engraftment. The mortality rate of SFI is high in these patients. The rate of SFI during conventional chemotherapy is less clear but it is still a significant risk, particularly if T-cell suppression is induced by potent purine analogues such as fludarabine and high-dose cytosine arabinoside. The risk is low in the predictably brief duration of neutropenia with autologous SCT.

In allogeneic SCT, the rate of CMV seropositivity and clinical CMV infection vary according to the pre-transplant status of the donor and recipient. The post-transplant CMV-associated fatality rate is around 40%.

Prophylaxis of infections

Given that some infections occur frequently and arise from body sites harbouring an abundant normal commensal flora, it is not surprising that antimicrobial prophylaxis is advocated and adopted by many centres treating patients with acute leukaemia. Essentially, when adopted, prophylaxis is started just before chemotherapy is begun with the aim of suppressing or eradicating potentially opportunistic pathogens ahead of the anticipated neutropenia (Figure 36.4).

The early cocktails of non-absorbable antibiotics, such as framycetin, colistin and nystatin (FRACON) or gentamicin, vancomycin and nystatin (GVN), were superseded by cotrimoxazole and colistin and later by the fluoroquinolones, norfloxacin, pefloxacin, ciprofloxacin and ofloxacin. The need for antibacter-

ial prophylaxis is still in doubt. As described above, antibacterial prophylaxis had no impact on the overall incidences of fever or mortality over many years, and almost all patients given such prophylaxis will also be given further broad-spectrum antibiotics for FUO. Some institutes are now faced with patients harbouring fluoroquinolone-resistant *E. coli*, causing them to have to abandon prophylaxis altogether.

The risk of SFI varies with the intensity of therapy and its complications and is greatest in SCT patients with protracted GvHD. Non-absorbable polyenes, such as amphotericin B and nystatin, do not provide systemic protection. Fluconazole reduces the risk of *C. albicans* significantly in SCT, but not in conventional chemotherapy; it is not effective against certain yeasts, including *C. krusei* and *C. glabrata*, and it is inactive against moulds (e.g. *Aspergillus* spp.). Itraconazole is active against a broader spectrum of fungi than fluconazole. With the availability of interchangeable oral solution and intravenous formulations, this triazole is more effective than fluconazole in preventing a range of *Candida* spp. and *Aspergillus* SFI in SCT and conventional chemotherapy, provided that sufficient drug is given to achieve protective systemic levels. There is no evidence that newer triazoles (e.g. posaconazole and voriconazole) or lipid formulations of polyenes (e.g. liposomal amphotericin B) are as effective as itraconazole in prophylaxis of SFI.

There is no evidence to support antiviral prophylaxis during neutropenia that is induced by conventional chemotherapy, except in patients with CLL and a strong past history of herpes infection if they are given fludarabine. In allogeneic SCT, all patients are given aciclovir prophylaxis to reduce their risk of infection with a range of viruses, particularly CMV, which has a high fatality rate. Post-SCT CMV is best prevented by transplantation from a negative donor to a negative recipient, with exclusive use of leucodepleted blood products.

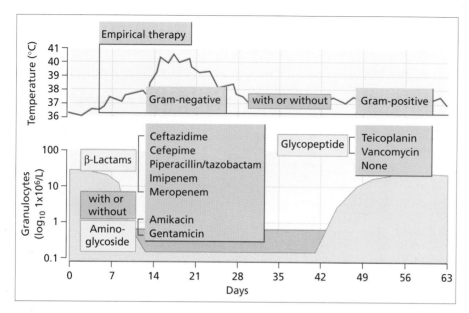

Figure 36.5 Initial empirical antibiotic options during neutropenia.

Empiric therapy of fever of unknown origin

In the 1960s, the combined mortality rate from Gram-negative and -positive bacteraemia during neutropenia induced by therapy for acute leukaemia was estimated at 90%. The introduction of the rapid, empiric use of broad-spectrum antibiotics with the onset of FUO was a major advance in supportive care. Now that this is routine practice (usually with a β-lactam and an amino-glycoside or else a β-lactam alone: see Figure 36.5). The mortality rate from proven bacterial infections is 7% overall, 10% for Gram-negative organisms and 6% for Gram-positive organisms at 30 days from onset of fever.

Each unit should establish and audit the application of rules for the use of these antibiotics in the treatment of FUO. Other causes of fever have been described above and the likelihood of them being the cause of any FUO should be carefully considered before antibiotics are given. There should be a working defini-tion of when a FUO is likely to be due to bacteraemia or other systemic infection to justify systemic antibiotic therapy, includ-ing degree of neutropenia and height and duration of fever. A review of the literature shows wide variation in such definitions as they are applied to clinical trials. For patients receiving conventional chemotherapy for acute leukaemia, one practical suggestion is that once the neutrophil count drops below 0.5×10^9/L and the temperature reaches 38°C twice in 1 h despite the use of paracetamol, empiric antibiotic therapy should be given. Clearly, if the patient is shocked or shows early signs of haemo-dynamic and respiratory instability, a single temperature reading of 38°C is sufficient. The peripheral temperature may be normal or the patient may even be hypothermic on development of shock due to sepsis. Blood cultures should always be taken from both any CVC and a peripheral vein, and always before anti-biotics are started.

Despite the dramatic reduction in mortality associated with the use of broad-spectrum antibiotics, they have their limita-tions. They have relatively poor activity against staphylococci (including MRSA) and streptococci, β-lactams must be given in multiple daily infusions occupying considerable access time through CVC, and the rate of Gram-negative organisms is in-creasing. The emergence of VRE associated with increased use of third-generation cephalosporins (e.g. ceftazidime) suggests that this class of antibiotics may not be appropriate for empirical therapy. The toxicity of the aminoglycosides requires frequent monitoring of levels and adjustment of dose or timing of administration.

Several randomized controlled trials have now shown that the rate of response of FUO is around 50%, whether an amino-glycoside is used in addition to a β-lactam or not. So initial empiric mono-therapy is sufficient using ceftazidime, cefepime, piperacillin–tazobactam, imipenem or meropenem. There is no need to add vancomycin or teicoplanin into the initial empirical regimen as no study to date has shown any difference in outcome or in the rate of defervescence, subsequent infections, use of additional antimicrobial agents or mortality.

Subsequent antimicrobial therapy

In some patients, when fever persists there may be no growth from culture samples, other microbiological results may be uninformative and there may be no clinical evidence that in-dicates the need for a switch to an alternative antibiotic. The assumption is often made that such patients have CVC-related staphylococcal infections, and vancomycin or teicoplanin is added empirically. Recent randomized placebo-controlled trials have shown that this makes no significant difference to response rates or mortality. This practice also encourages the emergence of VRE, so the value of such 'second-line' antibacterial empiric therapy is unclear and only justifiable when there is clinical evidence of infection of the line tunnel.

Subsequently, antibiotic therapy may be modified, depending on the results of initial blood cultures or specimens taken from other sites or the development of new infections defined clinically or microbiologically. The empirical regimen should be continued and complemented with other drugs such as a glycopeptide (e.g. vancomycin) or an antifungal agent. There are individual infections which may be proven microbiologically (e.g. *Candida* in blood cultures) or may be suspected clinically or radiologically (e.g. invasive pulmonary aspergillosis or *Pneumocystis jirovecii* pneumonitis), which justify switching to alternative therapies or adding them to existing antibiotics. A willingness to perform early computerized tomography (CT) scanning of the chest may shorten the time to starting systemic antifungal therapy in suspected invasive pulmonary aspergillosis. Plain chest radiography is notoriously unreliable and should not be used to confirm or exclude this diagnosis.

Each unit should devise a protocol in which the criteria for adding subsequent therapy are defined, based on clinical and microbiological findings (Table 36.4) either given on the basis of the organism causing a microbiologically defined infection (Figure 36.6) or on the basis of the site involved in a clinically defined infection (Figure 36.7). There is little evidence to support precise times when additional or substitute antibiotics should be introduced. The superiority of any one therapeutic agent over any other active against proven *Aspergillus* spp. SFI or probable or possible SFI is based on relative toxicity. In presumed or proven *Pneumocystis* pneumonitis, the drug of choice is high-dose cotrimoxazole, with steroids to reduce the risk of postinfective fibrosis.

Table 36.4 Rules for additional therapy.

Related to primary infective event
- Clinical deterioration
- Progression or persistence
- Initial bacterial pathogen resistant
- Non-bacterial infection
- > 5 days' fever

Related to subsequent infective event
- New microbiologically defined infection
    bacterial
    fungal
    viral
- New clinically defined infection
- New fever

Allogeneic stem cell transplantation patients

The febrile SCT recipient represents a special case of neutropenic FUO because of the increased risk of opportunistic infection with viruses, particularly those of the herpes group, herpes simplex and CMV. The procedures involved in SCT are very similar across units, as are the infective risks. Hence prophylaxis is very similar, e.g. valaciclovir or aciclovir for herpesviruses and a fluoroquinolone to suppress Gram-negative organisms.

An alternative approach is to only give these agents for prophylaxis when the patient is known to be a carrier of the particular organism. SCT recipients predictably develop fever shortly after the time of transplant and it is essential not to treat the immediate fever of total body irradiation with broad-spectrum

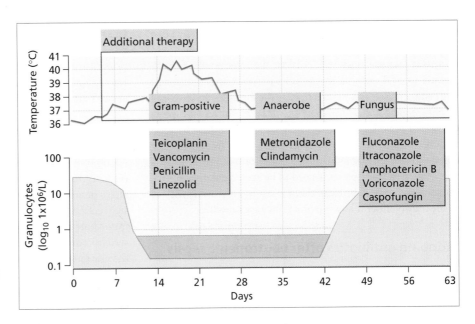

Figure 36.6 Microbiologically directed antibiotic treatment during neutropenia.

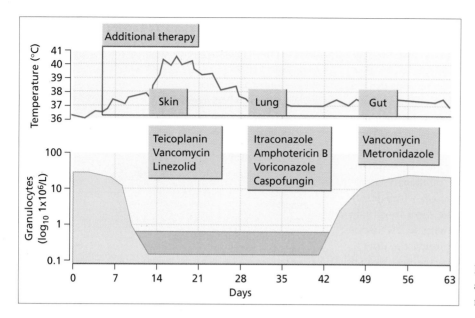

Figure 36.7 Clinically directed antibiotic treatment during neutropenia.

antibiotics. There is disagreement about whether broad-spectrum therapy should be started at a predetermined time post transplant on the assumption that FUO is imminent, or empirically at the onset of FUO. Whichever approach is followed, the pattern of infection during the neutropenia of SCT is predictable, justifying screening for CMV using a pp65 antigen ELISA or PCR, and *Aspergillus* infection using a galactomannan ELISA or PCR. Treatment may be pre-emptive if these organisms are detected.

By contrast with other neutropenic patients, the risk of infection to SCT recipients extends long after the neutropenia has resolved, particularly with chronic and severe GvHD treated with corticosteroids. These are now the major risk factors for SFI due to *A. fumigatus*, most cases occurring after 100 days, possibly as community acquired infections. These have a high case fatality rate, justifying prolonged prophylaxis. Bacteraemia due to certain Gram-negative bacilli, including *P. aeruginosa*, also occurs at this late stage. In addition, the hypogammaglobulinaemia of SCT persists for months or years after transplant with an increased risk of infection by the encapsulated bacteria *S. pneumoniae* and *Haemophilus influenza*. During the post-transplant period, prolonged prophylaxis against these bacteria may be justified as diagnosis and appropriate treatment may come too late, but there is limited evidence that prophylaxis is cost-effective. These patients need to be seen regularly and frequently, and have to be clear about when to present themselves to the transplant or follow-up unit if they are unwell.

Stopping antibiotics after neutropenic sepsis

Provided that fever has resolved and the temperature has been normal for at least 5 days, antibacterials can be stopped if there has been no bacterial growth on cultures. However, if significant organisms are grown on blood cultures antibiotics should be given for at least 10 days following lysis of fever. Systemic infections (bacterial or yeast) related to colonization or infection of a CVC or the tunnel may require removal of the CVC to reduce the risk of recurrence. It is less clear when systemic antifungal therapy can be safely stopped in invasive aspergillosis, as radiological changes may persist well after eradication of the causative organism.

Infections specific to childhood and adult acute lymphoblastic leukaemia

The significant additional risk in these patients is *Pneumocystis jirovecii* pneumonitis, which may be lessened by cotrimoxazole 960 mg b.d. orally, twice weekly. The infection has a characteristically rapid onset and presentation with marked hypoxia, relatively few abnormal physical signs apart from increased respiratory effort and extensive pulmonary shadowing on chest radiography. Confirmation of the diagnosis is difficult as there are no reliable objective tests.

Growth factors and granulocyte infusions

Recombinant human granulocyte colony-stimulating factor (G-CSF) may reduce the severity and duration of neutropenia after chemotherapy or SCT, but only if the patient has enough stem cells that are able to be stimulated. The response will not be immediate and it is not clear that this reduces the risk of serious systemic infection, the mortality rate from these infections or the mortality rate overall. Infusion of high-dose granulocyte collections from donors stimulated by G-CSF may be indicated if infection is resistant to antimicrobials and delayed neutrophil recovery is expected. But there is little evidence to support their use, and they should be avoided in patients with pre-existing HLA alloimmunization or requiring mechanical ventilation.

Infection risks in chronic leukaemias

In the CLLs there is a wide range of suppression of both humoral and cell-mediated immunity and, consequently, a wide spectrum of potential infecting organisms from the relatively low-risk superficial herpetic infection to potentially fatal bacterial pneumonia. These risks increase with progression of disease and intensity of therapy. The use of the more potent purine analogues, fludarabine and cladribine, intensify these risks not only by inducing short-term neutropenia, but also by profound suppression of T-cell function. Atypical infections such as *P. jeroveci* pneumonitis, *Listeria* and fungal infections have been reported, and prophylactic cotrimoxazole is indicated during and for 6 months after these drugs are given, to allow sufficient recovery of T-cell function. In hairy cell leukaemia, there is often neutropenia and monocytopenia with a major bacterial infection at presentation. These patients require the same prophylaxis as other CLLs if treated with purine analogues.

The infection risks of CML are similar to those of the acute leukaemias, although less severe in chronic stable phase. Since the introduction of imatinib, which induces rapid, smooth and lasting control of the disease, the risk of infection has been greatly reduced.

Metabolic complications

Fluid balance

Fluid intake and output must be monitored carefully in patients treated intensively. Accurate observation and recording of these data is the task of specialist nurses, and medical staff must review these regularly. Maintenance of fluid balance is a continuous problem in these patients, particularly the elderly, who have an increased risk of renal and congestive heart failure. The delivery of chemotherapy, blood and blood products, antibiotics and parenteral feeding needs large volumes which may exceed physiological requirements without oral intake. Fluid overload happens relatively quickly if monitoring is overlooked and it should be anticipated and avoided (Anaemia and thrombocytopenia, Planning large volume transfusions, above).

Vomiting, diarrhoea, sweating and insensible respiratory loss may singly, or in combination, lead steadily, sometimes rapidly, to dehydration. The vasodilatation and hypotension of sepsis will exacerbate hypovolaemia, which should be anticipated. Replacement of volume is achieved with normal saline solution alternating with 5% dextrose solution. Acute onset of these complications can require rapid infusion of colloid (polysaccharide solutions such as gelofusin) for expansion of intravascular volume particularly when a shift of body fluid is suspected from the intravascular space into tissues as can occur in septic shock. However, polysaccharide solutions are metabolized quickly and solutions of albumin are preferable when loss of plasma osmotic pressure is due to chronic hypoalbuminaemia. Fresh-frozen plasma should not be used for this indication. Prolonged hypovolaemia will result in acute renal tubular necrosis (ATN), therefore an early decision is needed about the likely cause of oliguria, in case this is due to a 'renal' rather than the 'pre-renal' hypovolaemic cause of acute renal failure (ARF). Supporting a balanced throughput of volume of fluid is complicated by a number of electrolyte and metabolic problems.

Hyperuricaemia and tumour lysis syndrome

The rapid rate of cell proliferation and death in acute leukaemia increases the catabolism of nucleic acids, which terminates with the excess production of uric acid. Therefore, patients may present with biochemical hyperuricaemia (HU) or its clinical consequences or develop these once treatment starts. The most extreme form of this is the tumour lysis syndrome (TLS), in which severe HU, hyperphosphataemia, hyperkalaemia and hypocalcaemia are associated with supersaturation of the urine with uric acid, which is then deposited in crystals in the renal tubules and distal collecting system. These biochemical abnormalities result in a major increase in the morbidity and mortality of patients, including ARF, which requires haemodialysis.

Tumour lysis syndrome is a frequent complication of advanced stage Burkitt's lymphoma and B-cell ALL in childhood and of any adult leukaemia with a very high presenting blast count and, despite attempts to manage the metabolic problems, as many as 25% of such children develop ARF on starting chemotherapy. The precise incidence of clinical and subclinical TLS are not known. Subclinical TLS could cause unrecognized morbidity and adversely affect the efficacy and safety of other therapies, some of which are also nephrotoxic.

The standard management for HU is allopurinol (300 mg daily orally), hydration and attempted urinary alkalinization. Hydration is technically easy with CVCs, but the complexities of maintaining fluid balance and avoiding overload are described above. Urinary alkalinization is achievable but complicates the management of fluid and electrolyte balance and, in practice, it is difficult to maintain the urinary pH above 8. Allopurinol blocks the formation of uric acid by inhibition of xanthine oxidase, increasing plasma and urinary concentrations of hypoxanthine and xanthine. Xanthine is less soluble than uric acid in urine and occasional cases of nephropathy are described as a consequence of this therapy. Patients have a backlog of excess uric acid that they must excrete, particularly those with a high tumour burden, and allopurinol has no effect on that. Hypersensitivity to allopurinol is well recognized, especially in the elderly, and causes distressing allergic dermatitis that may exfoliate. Interaction with other medications (warfarin, thiazide diuretics, antibiotics such as ampicillin and amoxycillin and chemotherapy such as mercaptopurine and azathioprine) is well described. Many patients have difficulty taking the drug orally; this may not be widely recognized and the alternative intravenous (i.v.) formulation is not sufficiently prescribed. Allopurinol reduces or makes normal the serum uric acid level in the great majority of adult and paediatric patients. The recombinant enzyme, rasburicase, produces a fall in uric acid concentrations within 1 h and is a safe and effective alternative for those patients who require rapid control of HU or cannot tolerate allopurinol. At present, recommended dosage schedules may be excessive and the drug is expensive, but rasburicase also avoids the need for hyperhydration and urinary alkalinization (see also Chapter 33).

Abnormalities of renal function and electrolyte balance

The hyperphosphataemia, hyperkalaemia and hypocalcaemia associated with TLS are described above, but other electrolyte problems occur more commonly. Hypokalaemia and hyponatraemia are the most frequent, and require regular intravenous supplements. Prolonged and copious diarrhoea will also result in hypokalaemia. Both hypokalaemia and hyponatraemia are also intrinsic to the disease owing to high plasma levels of lysosyme (particularly in the monocytic FAB subtypes M4 and 5), which interferes with proximal tubular function. Intravenous amphotericin B also induces renal tubular wasting of potassium and magnesium. This can be at least partially blocked by the diuretic amiloride (20 mg daily orally) but intravenous supplements of potassium, and less often of magnesium, are usually also required in patients receiving intravenous conventional amphotericin B. Oral replacement of these electrolytes is ineffective. Liposomal amphotericin B is less likely to create these electrolyte problems.

It is common practice to estimate urea and electrolyte levels daily during the aplastic phase of intensive chemotherapy, and magnesium levels should be estimated twice weekly. Otherwise, hypomagnesaemia may not be appreciated as the cause of confusion, neuropathy assumed to be due to hypocalcaemia and unexplained arrhythmia. Aminoglycosides and vancomycin are also toxic to renal tubules and can exacerbate these problems. Cyclosporin A therapy in SCT is also nephrotoxic. Regular and frequent monitoring of the levels of all of these drugs will reduce the risk of renal damage.

The same problems with electrolyte balance may occur in the ATN which results from hypotension due to sepsis, major blood loss and pulmonary capillary leak syndrome in acute respiratory distress syndrome (ARDS). ATN is accompanied by failure of glomerular filtration, with oliguria or anuria, and a rise in the levels of serum creatinine and urea. In these patients, if the primary insult is treated successfully, then ATN resolves with a compensatory diuretic phase and full recovery of renal function. It is important to keep pace with the diuresis with adequate fluid replacement.

Amphotericin B is also toxic to glomeruli and it should be discontinued or switched to the liposomal form once the creatinine has exceeded twice the level on starting the drug, assuming that was a normal figure. The renal toxicity of amphotericin B is almost always reversible and should not exclude its use if there is no pre-existing renal pathology or toxicity related to another drug. Before liposomal preparations were available, intravenous sodium loading was recommended to lessen the renal and electrolyte problems of amphotericin B. This is seldom used now although it has never been compared prospectively against liposomal amphotericin B.

Liver function abnormalities

In patients presenting with acute leukaemia, raised levels of lactate dehydrogenase are common because this is derived from bone marrow as well as liver. Some will also have non-specific elevation of alkaline phosphatase and transaminase levels. About one-half will develop abnormally high levels of one or all of these measures of liver function owing to the direct hepatocellular toxicity of chemotherapy with increased levels of serum bilirubin sufficient to cause clinical jaundice. It is seldom necessary to modify doses of remission induction drugs because of these abnormalities but, recently, there has been some concern about the hepatotoxicity of the antimetabolite purine analogue thioguanine, which is no longer available. Cytosine arabinoside, another purine analogue, also induces cholestasis and this hepatotoxicity may have been underestimated in the past.

Hyperbilirubinaemia with clinical jaundice is a frequent and sometimes overlooked complication of red cell transfusion which does not of itself indicate liver disease but is more obvious if liver function is impaired for any other reason. The hepatotoxicity of most chemotherapy is transient and resolves spontaneously with regeneration of normal marrow and induction of remission. It is usually asymptomatic and seldom progresses to severe liver failure, ascites, cirrhosis or portal hypertension except in specific cases described below. However, even minor impairment of liver function will affect other drugs that are dependent on liver metabolism to a degree that may require modification of doses.

Severe and fatal liver damage may occur with veno-occlusive disease in allogeneic SCT, which is described in detail in Chapter 24. This is thought to be a complication of preparatory or conditioning therapies prior to infusion of stem cells. A similar syndrome is seen with the new drug, mylotarg, which is now part of remission induction in the latest MRC AML 15 trial in adults. Mylotarg consists of the cytotoxic antibiotic, ozogamicin, which is linked to an anti-CD33 monoclonal antibody and is activated by hydrolysis once it is internalized following attachment of the antibody to leukaemic myeloblasts. The preceding phase II pilot study of this agent, given in association with therapy for induction and consolidation of remission, revealed the dose-limiting hepatic toxicity of this 'magic bullet'. As with the simultaneous use of nephrotoxic drugs, careful monitoring of all potentially hepatotoxic drugs or any drugs which are metabolized by the liver will be necessary if they are used simultaneously. These drugs include the triazole antifungal group (fluconazole, itraconazole, voriconazole, posaconazole and ravuconazole), all of which impair liver function to variable degrees.

Chronic liver damage, including cirrhosis and the greatly increased risk of hepatocellular carcinoma, is now a well-recognized late effect of blood transfusion owing to infection with the hepatitis C virus. Attempts to eradicate or reduce the viral load of these patients, using ribavarine and interferon, have met with limited success. As UK blood donors are routinely screened for this virus, the problem should become less prevalent in the future among multiply transfused patients.

The iron overload of multiple transfusion during therapy for acute leukaemias appears to cause clinical liver problems only in transplanted patients and can be reduced subsequently by venesection with or without iron chelation. In patients who are transfusion dependent due to marrow failure associated with chronic leukaemias, myelodysplasia or failure of therapy for any form of leukaemia the inconvenience and side-effects of iron chelation usually outweigh any potential benefit, especially when life expectancy is short.

Nutritional support

During intensive therapy, anorexia persists, even if nausea and vomiting and the pain of mucositis can be controlled. Loss of total body mass is inevitable, the extent of which depends on the duration of anorexia and the impact of additional catabolic insults such as severe infection. All dietary supplementation should be managed by dietitians and pharmacists in order to calculate accurately the contents of the supplements, on the basis of regular blood results. Oral supplementation may be sufficient to maintain an adequate caloric intake in less severe cases. For patients with a predictable or actual 10% or greater reduction in pre-treatment weight, total nutrition is indicated. This is likely in the majority of patients receiving allogeneic haemopoietic stem cell transplantation (HSCT). This can be given through a nasojejunal, fine, silastic tube, provided that this is inserted before the onset of mucositis, otherwise nutritional support must be given by indwelling intravenous catheter. As soon as patients recover the will to eat, all such dietary supplements can be cautiously withdrawn.

Nausea and vomiting

There is a high risk of severe and acute emesis with intensive chemotherapy. Every effort should be made to prevent this distressing complication and to avoid the development of anticipatory emesis should prophylaxis be ineffective. If control fails early then the chances of later successful control are reduced. It must be remembered that emesis may be due to other drugs (e.g. analgesics and antimicrobials), to acute infection and to other complications of leukaemia and its treatment such as meningeal relapse, intestinal obstruction (e.g. secondary to hypokalaemia and gut or retroperitoneal bleeding) or intracranial bleeding.

There are three major groups of antiemetic drugs, the serotonin antagonists (e.g. ondansetron and granisetron), the steroids (mainly dexamethasone) and a wide range of drugs that are sedative as well as antiemetic (e.g. metoclopramide, domperidone, haloperidol, lorazepam, cannabinoids and phenothiazines). Of these three classes, the serotonin antagonists will control emesis induced by intensive chemotherapy completely in about two-thirds of patients. Additional dexamethasone may benefit a further 10–20% of patients. All the sedating antiemetic agents are of second choice in intensive therapy. Their dosage, route of administration and scheduling should be strictly controlled and they should not be given on an uncontrolled or 'as required' basis. Cumulative oversedation is a major risk in these patients, particularly if they need simultaneous opiates for mucositis and antihistamines for allergic reactions to blood and drugs and develop hypoxia of infection or heart failure. Many of these drugs can also cause distressing dyskinesias.

For nausea due to less intensive oral therapy of CLL oral or hydoxyurea for CML metaclopramide may suffice and many patients do not need any antiemetic drug. There is a very low risk of nausea with imatinib.

Pain

Bone pain is an uncommon presenting feature of acute leukaemia, is due to an expanded marrow cavity packed with blasts and can occur or recur on relapse. Such pain is relieved by remission induction but may need temporary control with opiates. G-CSF and granulocyte–macrophage colony-stimulating factor (GM-CSF) can cause the same problem by expansion of normal marrow cells due to excessive stimulation.

Avascular necrosis of bone is seen in less than 5% of patients with ALL and lymphomas, particularly in association with high-dose steroids and cyclophosphamide. It usually affects younger patients, involves the ends of long bones and can cause permanent bone death requiring subsequent joint replacement. The diagnosis is elusive and requires magnetic resonance image (MRI) scanning. The pain is often severe enough to need relief with opiates. High-dose cytosine arabinoside can cause a painful vasculitis severe enough to lead to necrosis of soft tissue and skin. The neuropathy of the vinca alkaloids (usually vincristine but occasionally vinblastine) may present as limb pain or as painful constipation. The serotonin antagonists may cause headache in susceptible individuals and headache may also be due to intracranial bleeding or infection. Any bleed in any confined compartment will be painful, for example chest wall pain following haemorrhagic insertion of a CVC.

In SCT, the use of TBI and high-dose chemotherapy make gut mucositis inevitable. The extent, duration and severity vary but most patients will need some level of opiate relief. In most patients, this starts in the second week after therapy and resolves spontaneously without lasting sequelae from the third to fourth week onwards. As with all causes of pain, this requires whatever level of controlled drug analgesia is necessary to make the symptoms bearable without inducing brain or respiratory failure. Continuous i.v. infusion of an opiate is often required in severe mucositis and additional continuous anti-emetic may be needed in the same infusion. Palifermin (recombinant human keratinocyte growth factor) has been shown to reduce oral mucositis after intensive chemotherapy. All units should have a written protocol for pain control, which is similar to that used by the local palliative care team.

Palliation

The above account of supportive care of the patient with leukaemia describes an holistic approach. It is common for patients who have experienced this to wish to remain with the same haematology team for their terminal care when there is no further prospect of control of their underlying disease. There should be choices at this stage, which include the transfer of the patient to the palliative care team and joint management by them with haematology in whichever unit the patient and their family feel most suits the patient's needs. These choices should include dying at home, an option that requires some help from the acute care unit to mobilize the resources available in some communities to support this option. Most of the issues which arise in this palliative phase of care are described above. There can be much more flexibility in the frequency and choice of blood support, in pain control and in the use of antibiotics. Wherever palliative care is given, the patient and family should not feel abandoned by the team who supported them during previous periods of treatment.

Selected bibliography

Caillot D, Casasnovas O, Bernard A et al. (1997) Improved management of invasive pulmonary aspergillosis in neutropenic patients using early thoracic computed tomographic scan and surgery. Journal of Clinical Oncology 15: 139–47.

Cometta A, Calandra T, Gaya H et al. (1996) Monotherapy with meropenem versus combination therapy with ceftazidime plus amikacin as empiric therapy for fever in granulocytopenic patients with cancer. The International Antimicrobial Therapy Cooperative Group of the European Organization for Research and Treatment of Cancer and the Gruppo Italiano Malattie Ematologiche Maligne dell'Adulto Infection Program. Antimicrobial Agents Chemotherapy 40: 1108–15.

Cometta A, Kern WV, De Bock R et al. (2003) Vancomycin versus placebo for treating persistent fever in patients with neutropenic cancer receiving piperacillin–tazobactam monotherapy. Clinical Infectious Diseases 37: 382–9.

Cruciani M, Rampazzo R, Malena M et al. (1996) Prophylaxis with fluoroquinolones for bacterial infections in neutropenic patients: a meta-analysis. Clinical Infectious Diseases 23: 795–805.

Donnelly JP (2001) Infection in bone marrow transplant patients. In: Pathology and Immunology of Transplantation and Rejection (S Thiru, H Waldmaan, eds), pp. 526–66. Blackwell Science, Oxford.

Donnelly JP (2001) Prophylaxis of infections. In: Textbook of Febrile Neutropenia (KVI Rolston, EB Rubenstein, eds), pp. 215–43. Martin Dunitz, London.

Doyle D, Hanks GW, Macdonald N (eds) (1993) Oxford Textbook of Palliative Care. Oxford University Press, Oxford.

Engels EA, Lau J, Barza M (1998) Efficacy of quinolone prophylaxis in neutropenic cancer patients: a meta-analysis. Journal of Clinical Oncology 16: 1179–87.

Feusner J, Farber MS (2000) Role of intravenous allopurinol in the management of acute tumour lysis syndrome. Seminars in Oncology 28 (Suppl. 5): 13–8.

Furno P, Bucaneve G, Del Favero A (2002) Monotherapy or aminoglycoside-containing combinations for empirical antibiotic treatment of febrile neutropenic patients: a meta-analysis. Lancet Infectious Diseases 2: 231–42.

Glasmacher A, Prentice AG, Gorschluter M et al. (2003) Itraconazole prevents invasive fungal infections in neutropenic patients treated for haematological malignancies; evidence from a meta-analysis of 3597 patients. Journal of Clinical Oncology 21: 4616–26.

Maertens J, Van Eldere J, Verhaegen J et al. (2002) Use of circulating galactomannan screening for early diagnosis of invasive aspergillosis in allogeneic stem cell transplant recipients. Journal of Infectious Diseases 186: 1297–306.

McClelland B (2001) Effective use of blood components. In: Practical Transfusion Medicine (MF Murphy, DH Pamphilon, eds), pp. 65–76. Blackwell Science, Oxford.

Murphy MF (2001) Haematological disease. In: Practical Transfusion Medicine (MF Murphy, DH Pamphilon, eds), pp. 108–18. Blackwell Science, Oxford.

Paul M, Soares-Weiser K, Leibovici L (2003) Beta lactam monotherapy versus beta lactam-aminoglycoside combination therapy for fever with neutropenia: systematic review and meta-analysis. British Medical Journal 326: 1111.

Pui C-H, Mahmoud HH, Wiley JM et al. (2001) Recombinant urate oxidase for the prophylaxis and treatment of hyperuricaemia in patients with leukaemia and lymphoma. Journal of Clinical Oncology 19: 697–704.

Spielberger R, Stiff P, Bensinger W et al. (2004) Palifermin for oral mucositis after intensive therapy for hematologic cancers. New England Journal of Medicine 351: 2590–8.

Twycross R, Wilcock A (eds) (2001) Symptom Management in Advanced Cancer. Radcliffe Medical Press, Oxford.

CHAPTER 37

Chronic myeloid leukaemia

37

John M Goldman and Tariq I Mughal

Introduction

Chronic myeloid leukaemia (CML) (also known as chronic myelogenous leukaemia, chronic granulocytic leukaemia) is a clonal disease that results from an acquired genetic change in a pluripotential haemopoietic stem cell. This altered stem cell proliferates and generates a population of differentiated cells that gradually displaces normal haemopoiesis and leads to a greatly expanded total myeloid mass. One important landmark in the study of CML was the discovery of the Philadelphia (Ph) chromosome in 1960; another was the characterization in the 1980s of the *BCR–ABL* chimeric gene and associated oncoprotein and a third was the demonstration that introducing the *BCR–ABL* gene into murine stem cells in experimental animals caused a disease simulating human CML.

Until the 1980s, CML was generally assumed to be incurable and was treated palliatively – in the early days with radiotherapy, and more recently with alkylating agents, notably busulphan. CML can be permanently eradicated in the majority of patients who survive after haemopoietic stem cell transplantation (SCT), but the proportion of patients eligible for SCT is still relatively small. The introduction into clinical practice of imatinib in 1998 was an important therapeutic advance, as with this agent most patients achieve a complete cytogenetic response and may expect prolongation of survival compared with other methods of treatment.

Classification

The majority of patients with CML have a relatively homogeneous disease characterized at diagnosis by splenomegaly, leucocy-
tosis and the presence of a Ph chromosome in all leukaemic cells. A minority of patients have a less typical disease that may be classified as atypical CML, chronic myelomonocytic leukaemia or chronic neutrophilic leukaemia. Children may have a disease referred to as juvenile chronic myelomonocytic leukaemia. In none of these variants is there a Ph chromosome.

Epidemiology, aetiology and natural history

The incidence of CML appears to be constant worldwide. It occurs in about 1.0–1.5 per 100 000 of the population per annum in all countries where statistics are adequate. CML is rare below the age of 20 years but occurs at all decades of life, with a median age of onset of 50–60 years. The incidence is slightly higher in males than in females.

The risk of developing CML is slightly but significantly increased by exposure to high doses of irradiation, as occurred in survivors of the atomic bombs exploded in Japan in 1945, and in patients irradiated for ankylosing spondylitis but, in general, almost all cases must be regarded as 'sporadic' and no predisposing factors are identifiable. In particular, there is no familial predisposition and no definite association with HLA genotypes has been recognized. No contributory infectious agent has been incriminated.

Clinically, CML is a biphasic or triphasic disease that is usually diagnosed in the initial 'chronic', 'indolent' or 'stable' phase and then spontaneously evolves after some years into an advanced phase, which can sometimes be subdivided into an earlier accelerated phase and a later acute or blastic phase. There has been much debate about the duration of disease before the diagnosis is established, a question that is essentially unanswerable. If it is assumed that the disease starts with a 'transforming event' occurring in a single stem cell, it could be 5–10 years before the disease becomes clinically manifest. This estimate depends on the assumption that the leucocyte doubling time in the prediagnosis phase is not fundamentally different from the doubling time after diagnosis (which may not be the case), and the observation that the latent interval between exposure to irradiation from atomic bombs and the earliest identifiable increased incidence of CML was about 7 years. One study concluded that a routine blood count might have identified CML on average 6 months before it was actually diagnosed in individual patients.

Patients are usually in the 'chronic' phase when CML is diagnosed. This chronic phase lasts typically 2–7 years but it may, in rare cases, last more than 15 or even 20 years. Even more rarely, spontaneous remissions have been described. In about one-half of cases the chronic phase transforms unpredictably and abruptly to a more aggressive phase that used to be referred to as 'blastic crisis' and is now usually described as acute or blastic transformation. In the other half of cases, the disease evolves somewhat more gradually, through an intermediate phase described as 'accelerated' phase, which may last for months or years, before frank blastic transformation supervenes, which may have myeloblastic or lymphoblastic features. Occasional patients have a disease that progresses gradually to a myelofibrotic or osteomyelosclerotic picture that is characterized by extensive marrow fibrosis and sometimes gross overgrowth of bony trabeculae; the clinical problems are then usually due to failure of haemopoiesis rather than to blast cell proliferation, but a predominantly blastic disease can still supervene. The duration of survival after onset of transformation is usually 2–6 months.

Staging

Many attempts have been made to subclassify or 'stage' chronic-

Table 37.1 Sokal index for predicting survival.

Prognostic indices

Good prognosis	< 0.8
Moderate prognosis	0.8–1.2
Poor prognosis	> 1.2

Mathematical expression

Exp.[0.0116(age – 43.4)] + + 0.0345 (spleen size – 7.51)
+ 0.188 [(platelet count/700)2 – 0.563]
+ 0.0887 (percentage of blasts – 2.10)

phase CML at diagnosis, in a manner that would permit some prediction of the duration of chronic phase in individual patients. The most commonly used classification, devised by Sokal and colleagues (1984), is based on a formula that takes account of the patient's age, blast cell count, spleen size and platelet count at diagnosis (Table 37.1). A similar classification, which may or may not prove more useful than that of Sokal, was introduced by Hasford (1999), called the Hasford or Euro score (Figure 37.1), which makes use of eosinophil and basophil numbers in addition to the values included in the Sokal system.

In practice, patients who have a low leucocyte doubling time probably survive longer than those with more rapid doubling times. Moreover, the patient's response to initial treatment does give some information about duration of survival; for example, a relatively low requirement for cytotoxic drugs to control the leucocyte count in the first year after diagnosis or a complete cytogenetic response to interferon α (IFN-α) are both good prognostic factors. Conversely, other possible adverse prognostic factors, such as the presence of deletions in the der9q+ chromosome and a rapid rate of shortening of telomeres in the leukaemia cell population, may in the future be integrated into systems for

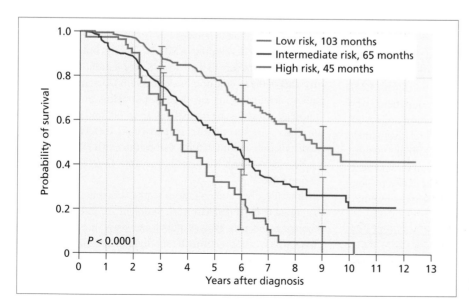

Figure 37.1 Probability of survival and median survival values for a population of CML patients classified into three prognostic categories according to the Euro score devised by Hasford *et al.* (1999).

staging patients with CML. It is likely, however, that the results of gene expression profiling will eventually be the most informative approach for predicting overall duration of disease.

Cytokinetics

It is presumed that the leukaemic stem cell replicates and that its progeny give rise to increased numbers of myeloid progenitor cells and also of differentiated progeny. Thus, the normal marrow is gradually replaced by a leukaemic myeloid mass that expands to fill normal fat spaces and encroaches on areas of long bones that are normally devoid of haemopoiesis in the adult. The increased myelopoiesis involves primarily the granulocyte series, but megakaryocyte and platelet numbers are also usually increased. Obvious erythroid hyperplasia and polycythaemia occur only rarely.

In the absence of a convincing assay for human haemopoietic stem cells, a number of efforts have been made to quantify *in vitro* its nearest counterpart, variously designated 'long-term culture-initiating cells', 'high-proliferative capacity progenitor cells' or 'blast colony-forming cells'. In general, the numbers of such cells seem to be moderately increased (e.g. 3- to 10-fold) in CML marrow compared with normal marrow, but results are inconsistent. In contrast, the numbers of committed progenitors, i.e. CFU-GEMM, BFU-E and CFU-GM, are clearly increased compared with normal, and this increase is proportionately much larger in the blood than in the marrow of untreated CML patients. BFU-E and CFU-GM numbers in the blood are significantly correlated with the leucocyte count; their numbers are restored to normal or subnormal levels by appropriate treatment.

Theoretically, an apparently autonomous proliferation of myeloid progenitors could be due to increased responsiveness to one or more physiological stimulators of haemopoiesis or to loss of sensitivity to a normal inhibitor. As a consequence of this, many efforts have been directed to assessing the response of CML progenitors to haemopoietic growth factors, notably granulocyte colony-stimulating factor (G-CSF), granulocyte–macrophage colony-stimulating factor (GM-CSF), interleukin 3 (IL-3), stem cell factor (SCF) and erythropoietin. There is some evidence that the autonomous proliferation could be due to an autocrine loop involving G-CSF and IL-3. It may also be due to increased production of elastase by the leukaemia cells that inhibit the response of normal but not leukaemia cells to G-CSF.

CML progenitors in *in vitro* culture systems adhere less well to preformed marrow stromal layers than their normal counterparts. This may be due to an abnormality of an integrin or absence of a glycophosphatidyl inositol-anchored protein that has not yet been defined. Thus, it is possible that the excessive proliferation of CML progenitors is due in part to their premature escape from physiological inhibitory influences in the stem cell 'niche'.

Cytogenetics

The Philadelphia (originally designated Ph[1], now der22q[-] or Ph) chromosome (see Chapter 29) is an acquired cytogenetic abnormality that characterizes all leukaemic cells in CML. It is formed as a result of a reciprocal translocation of chromosomal material between the long arms of one chromosome 22 and one chromosome 9, an event referred to as t(9;22)(q34;q11) (Figure 37.2). The (9;22) translocation generates the *BCR–ABL* fusion gene on the Ph chromosome (see below) and also a 'reciprocal' fusion gene, designated *ABL–BCR*, on the derivative 9q[+] chromosome. Such translocations involving just two chromosomes are described as 'simple', whereas about 10% of patients have 'complex' translocations involving chromosomes 9, 22 and one or sometimes two other chromosomes.

In CML patients, the Ph chromosome is present in all myeloid cell lineages, in some B cells and in a very small proportion of T cells. It is found in no other cells of the body. This distribution is not altered by traditional treatment with busulphan or hydroxyurea. Although valuable since the 1960s as a marker of the leukaemic cell, its true pathogenetic significance remained uncertain until the identification of the *BCR–ABL* chimeric gene in the 1980s. About 15% of patients have small deletions of chromosomal material on der9q[+], which usually include the reciprocal *ABL–BCR* gene. Such deletions are thought to occur contemporaneously with the formation of the *BCR–ABL* gene on the Ph chromosome and denote a relatively poor overall prognosis. A small proportion of patients with clinically classical CML lack the Ph chromosome; however, some of these also have a typical *BCR–ABL* gene expressed as a p210 oncoprotein (see below).

Some, but not all, patients acquire additional clonal cytogenetic abnormalities during the course of the chronic phase. There was suspicion that some such changes might be caused in part by administration of alkylating agents, but they can undoubtedly occur spontaneously. The observation of non-random changes, typically +8, +Ph, iso-17q or +19, sometimes means that such new clones will expand and that blastic transformation will manifest itself within weeks or months, but these new clones (other than iso-17q) can remain clinically unimportant for many years. In overt blastic transformation, 80% of patients have clonal cytogenetic changes in addition to the Ph translocation.

Molecular biology

It was shown in the early 1980s that the *ABL* proto-oncogene, which encodes a non-receptor tyrosine kinase, was located normally on chromosome 9 but was translocated to chromosome 22 in CML patients. In 1984 the precise positions of the genomic breakpoint on chromosome 22 in different CML patients were found to be 'clustered' in a relatively small 5.8-kb region to

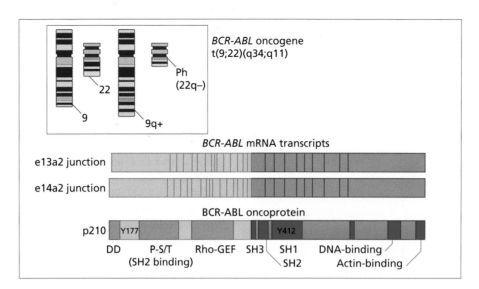

Figure 37.2 The t(9;22) translocation and its products: the *BCR–ABL* oncogene on the Ph chromosome and the reciprocal *ABL–BCR* on the derivative 9q⁺ chromosome. In classic CML, *BCR–ABL* is transcribed into mRNA molecules with e13a2 or e14a2 junctions, which are then translated into the p210^BCR–ABL oncoprotein. This oncoprotein is a hybrid containing functional domains from the N-terminal end of BCR [dimerization domain (DD)], SRC-homology 2 (SH2)-binding and the Rho GTP–GDP exchange-factor (GEF) domains and the C-terminal end of ABL. [Only SRC-homology regions 2, 3 and 1 (SH2, SH3 and SH1 respectively) and the DNA- and actin-binding domains are shown.] Tyrosine 177 (Y177) in the *BCR* portion of the fusion gene and tyrosine 412 (Y412) in the ABL portion are important for the docking of adapter proteins and for BCR–ABL autophosphorylation respectively. P-S/T denotes phosphoserine and phosphothreonine.

which the name 'breakpoint cluster region' (BCR) was given. Later, it became clear that this region formed the central part of a relatively large gene now known as the *BCR* gene, whose normal function is not well defined, and the breakpoint region was renamed '*major* breakpoint cluster region' (M-BCR). In contrast, the position of the genomic breakpoint in the *ABL* gene is very variable, but it always occurs upstream of the second (common) exon (a2). Thus, the Ph translocation results in juxtaposition of 5′-sequences from the *BCR* gene with 3′-ABL sequences derived from chromosome 9 (Figure 37.3). It produces a chimeric gene, designated *BCR–ABL* that is transcribed as an 8.5-kb mRNA and encodes a protein with a molecular weight of 210 kDa. This p210^BCR–ABL oncoprotein has far greater tyrosine kinase activity than the normal *ABL* gene product.

In CML, there are two variants of the BCR–ABL transcript, depending upon whether the break in M-BCR occurs in the intron between exons e13 and e14, or in the intron between exons e14 and e15. A break in the former intron yields an e13a2 mRNA junction and a break in the latter intron yields an e14a2 junction. (It should be noted that exon e13 was previously termed exon b2 and exon e14 was previously b3; thus the two RNA junctions were known until recently as b2a2 and b3a2 respectively.) Most patients have transcripts with features of either e13a2 or e14a2, but occasional patients have both transcripts present in their leukaemia cells. The precise type of *BCR–ABL* transcript has no prognostic significance for CML

patients. Moreover, the reciprocal *ABL–BCR* gene on der9q⁺ is expressed in about 70% of patients, but its expression or lack of expression does not have prognostic significance.

A minority of patients with Ph-positive acute lymphoblastic leukaemia (ALL), more often adults than children, also have *BCR–ABL* fusion genes in their leukaemia cells (see Chapters 29 and 31). In about one-third of Ph-positive ALL patients, the molecular features of the *BCR–ABL* gene are indistinguishable from those of CML; in the remaining two-thirds the genomic breakpoint occurs in the first intron of the *BCR* gene (a zone designated 'minor breakpoint cluster region' or m-BCR) and the *BCR–ABL* gene results from fusion of the first exon (designated e1) of the *BCR* gene with the second exon (a2) of the *ABL* gene. The mRNA is designated e1a2 and encodes a protein of 190 kDa (p190^BCR–ABL). Very rare patients with CML have a p190 protein instead of the usual p210. Equally rare is the finding of a Ph chromosome in association with chronic neutrophilic leukaemia. Such patients may have an mRNA formed from an e19a2 fusion gene associated with a p230^BCR–ABL oncoprotein.

The *BCR–ABL* gene has been cloned and inserted into a retroviral vector that has been used to transfect murine haemopoietic stem cells; these transduced stem cells can generate a disease resembling human CML in mice. Thus, the *BCR–ABL* gene is thought to play a pivotal role in the genesis of chronic-phase CML.

The mechanism by which the BCR–ABL oncoprotein alters stem cell kinetics remains ill-defined. It undoubtedly aberrantly

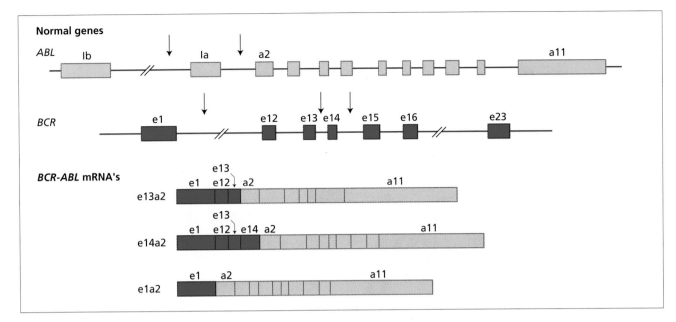

Normal genes

Figure 37.3 The structure of the normal *BCR* and *ABL* genes and the fusion transcripts found in CML and Ph-positive ALL. The ABL gene contains two alternative 5'-exons (named Ib and Ia) followed by 10 'common' exons numbered a2 to a11 (orange boxes). Breakpoints in CML and Ph-positive ALL usually occur in the introns between exons Ib and Ia or between exons Ia and a2 (as shown by vertical arrows). The *BCR* gene comprises a total of 23 exons, 11 exons upstream of the M-BCR region, five exons in the M-BCR that were originally termed b1 to b5 and are now renamed e12 to e16, and seven exons downstream of M-BCR.

For convenience, only exons e1, e12 to e16 and e23 are shown. Breakpoints in CML usually occur between exons e13 (b2) and e14 (b3) or between exons e14 (b3) and e15 (b4) of the M-BCR (as shown by two vertical arrows placed centrally). The majority of patients with Ph-positive ALL have breakpoints in the first intron of the gene (between e1 and e2 (not shown), arrow at left). Three possible BCR–ABL mRNA transcripts are shown below. The first two (e13a2 and e14a2 respectively) are characteristic of CML. The bottom mRNA (e1a2) is found in the majority of patients with Ph-positive ALL (see text).

autophosphorylates and also phosphorylates a wide range of intracellular proteins that would not normally be phosphorylated, Crkl, Mek 1/2, Rac and Jnk. It may act by activating the RAS or STAT signal transduction pathways. Alternatively, it may activate the p13 kinase–AKT pathway involved in facilitating apoptosis (Figure 37.4). As an activated ABL opposes cellular apoptosis, the *BCR–ABL* gene might act by impeding 'programmed cell death' in target stem cells.

The molecular basis of disease progression is still obscure, but it seems reasonable to infer that one or more probably a sequence of additional genetic events occurs in the Ph-positive clone. When the critical combination of additional events is achieved, clinically definable transformation ensues. At this stage, the leukaemia cells usually harbour one or other of the additional cytogenetic changes referred to above. About 20% of patients with CML in myeloid transformation have point mutations or deletions in the coding sequence of the *p53* tumour-suppressor gene, a gene implicated in progression of a variety of solid tumours, notably colonic carcinoma. The retinoblastoma (*RB*) gene is deleted in rare cases of CML in megakaryoblastic transformation, and changes in the *LYN*, *EVI-1* and *MYC* genes are described. About one-half of the patients with lymphoid

blast transformations have homozygous deletions in the p16 gene, whose normal function is to inhibit cyclin-dependent kinase 4. Molecular changes underlying the non-random cytogenetic changes described above have not been identified.

Clinical features

In the past, the majority of patients presented with symptoms, usually attributable to splenomegaly, haemorrhage or anaemia. In recent years, CML has been diagnosed in almost 50% of patients before the onset of symptoms as a result of 'routine' blood tests performed as part of medical examinations in healthy persons, for pregnancy, before blood donation or in the course of investigation for unrelated disorders. When present, symptoms may include lethargy, loss of energy, shortness of breath on exertion or weight loss or haemorrhage from various sites. Increased sweating is characteristic. Spontaneous bruising or unexplained bleeding from gums, intestinal or urinary tract are relatively common. Visual disturbances may occur. Fever and lymphadenopathy are rare in chronic phase. The patient may have severe pain or discomfort in the splenic area, often

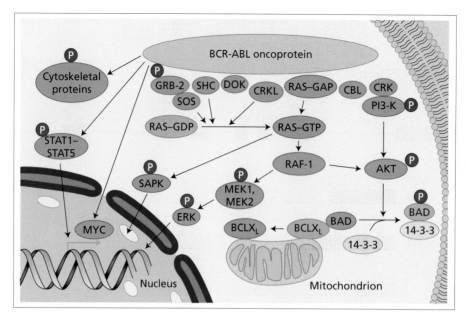

Figure 37.4 Signal transduction pathways affected by BCR–ABL. The cellular effects of BCR–ABL are exerted through interactions with various proteins that transduce the oncogenic signals responsible for the activation or repression of gene transcription, of mitochondrial processing of apoptotic responses, of cytoskeletal organization and of the degradation of inhibitory proteins. The key pathways implicated so far are those involving RAS, mitogen-activated protein (MAP) kinases, signal transducers and activators of transcription (STAT), phosphatidylinositol 3-kinase (PI 3-K) and MYC. Most of the interactions are mediated through tyrosine phosphorylation and require the binding of BCR–ABL to adapter proteins such as growth factor receptor-bound protein 2 (GRB-2), DOK, CRK, CRK-like protein (CRKL), SRC homology-containing protein (SHC) and casitas B-lineage lymphoma protein (CBL). As we start to dissect these various interactions, we can now design drugs aimed at disrupting specific branches of these pathways in an attempt either to kill the CML cell or to cause its phenotype to revert to normal. It is obvious that the best target is BCR–ABL proper, as this is the only protein that is exclusive to the leukaemic clone. The second-best approach is to target key downstream effectors of BCR–ABL; however, this approach might, in principle, adversely affect normal haemopoiesis as well. P denotes phosphate.

associated with splenic infarction, or may have noticed a lump or mass in the right upper abdomen. Visual disturbances may be due to retinal haemorrhages. Sudden hearing loss occurs very rarely. Patients may present with features of gout or priapism in males, both of which are also rare.

At diagnosis, 50–70% of patients have splenomegaly. The spleen varies from just palpable to being so large that it occupies all the left side of the abdomen and is palpable also in the right iliac fossa. The liver is frequently also enlarged but with a soft edge that is difficult to define. There may be no other abnormal findings. Ecchymoses of varying sizes and ages may be present and may form discoloured subcutaneous lumps. Some patients have asymptomatic retinal haemorrhages. Patients with very high leucocyte counts may have features of leucostasis, with retinal vein engorgement and respiratory insufficiency.

Patients presenting with more advanced disease nearly always have some of the features described above. In addition, they may have bone tenderness or signs of infection. In established blastic transformation, the spleen is frequently enlarged and may be painful. The liver may become very large. Patients may develop fever, lymphadenopathy or very rarely lytic lesions of bone.

Haematology

Chronic phase

Patients with splenomegaly are usually anaemic, while the haemoglobin concentration may be normal in patients with 'early' disease. The leucocyte count at diagnosis is usually in the range of $20–200 \times 10^9/L$, but the diagnosis of CML can be established by appropriate investigations in patients with persistent leucocytosis in the range $10–20 \times 10^9/L$; at the other extreme occasional patients may present with leucocyte numbers in the range $200–800 \times 10^9/L$. The blood film shows a full spectrum of cells in the granulocyte series, ranging from blast forms to mature neutrophils, with intermediate myelocytes and neutrophils predominating (Figure 37.5). The percentage of blast cells is loosely related to the absolute number of leucocytes, but a value higher than 12% suggests that the patient may already be in acceleration or transformation. The percentages of eosinophils and basophils are usually increased, and the absence of basophilia casts doubt on the diagnosis. Absolute numbers of lymphocytes and monocytes are slightly increased, but both are

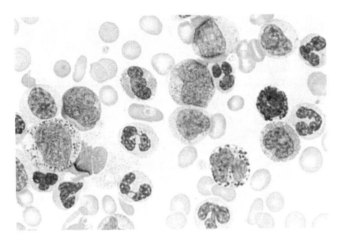

Figure 37.5 Peripheral blood appearances of a patient with CML at diagnosis. Note increased numbers of leucocytes including immature granulocytes and occasional blast cells.

reduced as percentages in the differential count. Platelet numbers are usually increased in the range of $300-600 \times 10^9$/L but may be normal or even reduced. Occasional nucleated red cells are present in the circulation in some patients. The alkaline phosphatase content of the neutrophil cytoplasm is diminished or absent. BCR–ABL transcripts can be demonstrated in the blood with ease, using the reverse transcription polymerase chain reaction (RT-PCR). In a minority of patients, the leucocyte count, if left untreated, shows a cyclical variation, but the overall trend is upwards.

Examination of the bone marrow by aspiration or trephine biopsy is not necessary to confirm the diagnosis of CML, but is usually carried out to assess the degree of marrow fibrosis, to perform cytogenetic analysis and to exclude incipient transformation. The marrow aspirate may show multiple small hypercellular fragments or may be so hypercellular that fragments cannot easily be discerned. The trails show a cellular composition resembling that of the CML blood. Blast cells in chronic phase number from 2% to 10%. Eosinophils and basophils are usually prominent; megakaryocytes are small, hypolobated and very numerous. Occasionally, Gaucher-like cells are present. The marrow biopsy shows complete loss of fat spaces with dense hypercellularity. The reticulin content may be normal or modestly increased.

Advanced phases

The haematological picture in acceleration is very variable. It may differ little from chronic phase but blast cell numbers may be increased disproportionately (Table 37.2). There may be anaemia in the presence of a normal leucocyte count. Platelet numbers may be greatly increased ($> 1000 \times 10^9$/L) or reduced (below 100×10^9/L) in a manner not accounted for by treatment. The marrow also shows a picture no longer consistent with chronic-phase disease, often with increased numbers of blast cells or promyelocytes and/or increased fibrosis.

Blastic transformation is defined by the presence of more than 30% blasts or blasts plus promyelocytes in the blood or marrow. Frequently, this criterion is irrelevant because blast cell numbers

Table 37.2 Criteria to distinguish the chronic, accelerated and blastic phases of CML based on proposals published by the World Health Organization (2001).

Chronic phase
Ability to reduce spleen size and restore and maintain a 'normal' blood count with appropriate therapy

Accelerated phase
(defined by one or more of the following features)
- Blasts 10–19% of white blood cells in peripheral blood and/or of nucleated bone marrow cells
- Peripheral blood basophils ≥ 20%
- Persistent thrombocytopenia ($< 100 \times 10^9$/L) unrelated to therapy, or persistent thrombocytosis ($> 1000 \times 10^9$/L) unresponsive to therapy
- Increasing spleen size and increasing white blood cell count unresponsive to therapy
- Megakaryocyte proliferation in sheets or clusters in association with marked reticulin or collagen fibrosis

Blastic phase
(defined by one or more of the following features)
- Blasts > 20% of peripheral blood leucocytes or of nucleated bone marrow cells
- Extramedullary blast proliferation
- Large foci or clusters of blasts in the bone marrow biopsy

Note: In this classification, unlike some other classifications, the acquisition of new cytogenetic abnormalities in addition to the Ph chromosome is not by itself a criterion for 'promoting' a chronic phase patient to accelerated phase.

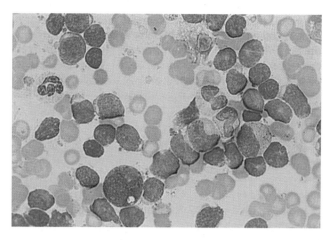

Figure 37.6 Peripheral blood appearances of a patient with CML in lymphoid blast cell transformation.

in both sites have risen abruptly to exceed 80%. Their morphology is very variable. About 70% of patients have blasts classifiable generally as myeloid, which resemble to a degree the cells that characterize acute myeloid leukaemia (AML) (see Chapter 29). Such cells may be predominantly myeloblastic, monoblastic, erythroblastic or megakaryoblastic, and blast cells of different myeloid lineages frequently co-exist. These cells are best defined by their cytochemical and immunophenotypic characteristics though they do not usually fit neatly into the FAB classification for AML. About 20% of patients have lymphoid blast cells; these may resemble the FAB-L1 cells that typify childhood acute lymphoblastic leukaemia (ALL) or, more commonly, have L2 appearances (Figure 37.6). Immunophenotyping shows the typical membrane markers of a precursor B-cell ALL, namely CD10 (CALLA) and CD19 positivity, and further studies may show nuclear positivity for terminal deoxynucleotidyl transferase (TdT). Molecular studies show clonal rearrangement of immunoglobulin (Ig) chains and occasionally of TCR genes. The remaining 10% of blast cell transformations have mixed myeloid and lymphoid characteristics.

The clinical features associated with advanced disease are quite variable. In some cases, the patient is initially entirely asymptomatic and the diagnosis is based entirely on blood and marrow findings. In other cases, the patient may develop fevers, excessive sweating, anorexia and weight loss or bone pain. Rarely, there are localized lytic lesions of bone, which may be single or multiple. Occasionally, patients present with generalized lymphadenopathy; biopsy shows nodal infiltration with blast cells that may be myeloid or lymphoid. Localized skin infiltrates may be seen. Discrete masses of immature leukaemia cells may develop at almost any site; these are sometimes referred to as 'chloromas' or 'granulocytic sarcomas'. Patients with lymphoid blast cells in the blood and marrow may have involvement of the cerebrospinal fluid at the same time, or central nervous system (CNS) involvement may become symptomatic only at a later stage.

Biochemical changes

The biochemical changes seen in CML are non-specific. Patients diagnosed in chronic phase may have a slightly raised serum uric acid but the level is frequently normal. The serum alkaline phosphatase is usually normal or slightly raised. The lactate dehydrogenase (LDH) is usually raised. Serum K^+ may be spuriously raised due to leakage of intracellular potassium from platelets or, less commonly, from leucocytes after the blood is drawn. In such cases, the K^+ level in freshly drawn citrated blood is usually normal, as is the electrocardiogram. The serum vitamin B_{12} and B_{12} binding capacity are greatly increased due to raised levels of transcobalamin I.

In transformation, the serum uric acid may be raised, sometimes substantially, and tests of liver function are usually moderately abnormal. Hypercalcaemia is present occasionally and is usually due to bone destruction; very rarely, it may be attributable to a parathormone-like material ectopically produced by the blast cells.

Management of chronic myeloid leukaemia in chronic phase

The management of the newly diagnosed CML patients has changed very greatly in the last few years. In the 1970s, it was conventional for the physician to start treatment soon after diagnosis with busulphan and then to await further developments. The patient received little information about prognosis. Today, in most, but not all, countries, the patient is informed of the diagnosis and given as much information as possible about the disease and its prognosis. The various options for treatment are usually discussed at this stage, which, for the younger patient, include the possible need for allogeneic SCT at some stage in the disease. This means that the patient, all siblings and other family members should be HLA typed. The issue of gonadal function is important and men who have not completed their families should be offered semen cryopreservation before any treatment is started.

There is no urgency to start treatment immediately in asymptomatic patients with leucocyte counts below 100×10^9/L. This means that leucapheresis with cryopreservation of blood stem cells can be performed before anti-leukaemia treatment is instituted. Such stored cells may be used for autografting at a later date. However, drug treatment should ideally be started soon after the diagnosis is confirmed. The best single agent at present for patients in chronic phase not destined for allogeneic SCT is imatinib, but a number of combinations of imatinib with other agents are being tested. Hydroxyurea is a reasonable alternative in the short term if imatinib is not immediately available. IFN-α, until recently the treatment of choice, and busulphan should both be reserved for special indications.

Imatinib mesylate

Imatinib mesylate (Glivec or Gleevec; previously known as STI571 or CGP 57148B), a 2-phenylaminopyrimidine compound, is an ABL tyrosine kinase inhibitor that entered clinical trials in 1998. It was thought originally to act by occupying the ATP-binding pocket of the Abl kinase component of the BCR–ABL oncoprotein, and thereby blocking the capacity of the enzyme to phosphorylate downstream effector molecules; it is now thought to act by binding to an adjacent domain in a manner than holds the Abl component of the BCR–ABL oncoprotein molecule in an inactive configuration (Figure 37.7). The drug rapidly reverses the clinical and haematological abnormalities and induces major cytogenetic responses in over 80% of previously untreated chronic phase patients. It is usually administered orally at a dose of 400 mg per day, although pilot studies suggest that initial treatment with 600 mg or even 800 mg daily may give better results.

Side-effects include nausea, headache, rashes, infraorbital oedema, bone pains and, sometimes, more generalized fluid retention. The rashes can from time to time be treated by temporarily interrupting imatinib and then re-instituting it under short-term corticosteroid cover. Hepatotoxicity characterized by raised serum transaminases is occasionally seen and may necessitate stopping the drug. Some caution must be also exercised in the light of a recent report of potentially fatal cerebral oedema. An interesting non-sinister effect, hair repigmentation, has been reported in a small group of responders. The toxicity in general seems to be appreciably less than that associated with IFN-α.

A significant minority of patients experience neutropenia and/or thrombocytopenia within the first few months of starting treatment with imatinib at standard dosage (i.e. 400 mg per day). In some cases, isolated neutropenia may be managed simply by adding G-CSF (e.g. 300–480 μg subcutaneously on alternate days or less often) for a finite period, after which it may be possible to reduce or stop the drug. In other cases, G-CSF works less well and it may be necessary to reduce or stop imatinib. If thrombocytopenia develops, it may be necessary to reduce the dose, although some believe that the drug is relatively ineffective at daily doses below 300 mg. Conversely, thrombocytosis sometimes persists in a patient whose leucocyte count is well controlled by imatinib; in such cases, the addition of hydroxyurea or anagrelide usually controls the platelet count.

The issue of how long to continue imatinib remains unresolved. For the patient who has achieved a complete cytogenetic remission, available evidence suggests that stopping the drug leads to recurrence of Ph positivity and eventually leucocytosis in the majority of cases, although on occasion the cytogenetic remission continues without treatment for many months or even longer. At present, the best advice for the responding patient is to continue the drug indefinitely. Conversely, for the patient who has failed to achieve a major cytogenetic response (> 66% Ph negativity in the bone marrow) after 1 year of treatment, the case for continuing treatment with imatinib is weak and alternative approaches should be considered.

Even in patients who achieve complete cytogenetic remission, low numbers of BCR–ABL transcripts can usually be detected by RT-PCR, which means that one cannot conclude that imatinib as a single agent eradicates all evidence of CML. A prospective randomized phase III trial designed to compare imatinib as a single agent with the combination of IFN-α with cytarabine in previously untreated patients started in June 2000. The interim results showed that 74% of the patients treated with imatinib achieved a complete cytogenetic remission compared with 14% of those in the control arm. Progression-free survival was significantly better in the imatinib-treated cohort than in the IFN-α and cytarabine group (97.2% versus 90.3%; $P < 0.001$). It is still too early to ascertain whether patients treated with imatinib have superior overall survival but the impressive numbers of complete cytogenetic responses and low levels of residual BCR–ABL transcripts achievable in many patients mean that this agent is now the treatment of choice for all or almost all newly diagnosed patients.

Response to imatinib is best monitored by regular cytogenetic studies or bone marrow analysis, supported, if necessary, by fluorescence *in situ* hybridization studies for the *BCR–ABL* gene for patients not yet in complete cytogenetic remission. For patients who have achieved cytogenetic remission, a quantitative

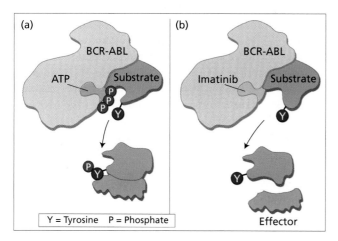

Figure 37.7 The presumed mechanism of action of imatinib. The phosphorylation of a substrate is shown schematically in (a). ATP occupies the pocket in the ABL component of the BCR–ABL oncoprotein, whence it donates a phosphate (P) group to a tyrosine (Y) residue on an unspecified substrate. The substrate then detaches itself from the BCR–ABL oncoprotein and makes functional contact with a further downstream effector molecule. In (b) imatinib occupies the ATP binding site and thereby prevents phosphorylation of the substrate. This molecule in turn fails to make contact with the effector protein and the signal transduction pathway that would otherwise transmit the 'leukaemia signal' is interrupted.

RT-PCR for BCR–ABL transcripts is the only approach that can assess the degree of response and recognize incipient relapse, which may indicate the need for a revised therapeutic strategy, including in some cases allogeneic SCT.

The acquisition of resistance to imatinib appears to be rare in patients with CML in chronic phase within the first 2 years of diagnosis. It is more common in patients who start imatinib in 'late chronic phase' after prior treatment with other agents. Resistance to imatinib has been seen in up to 70% of those treated in myeloid blast crisis, and all of those in lymphoid blast crisis relapse within 6 months of their initial response. Resistance appears to result from a variety of diverse mechanisms, including the 'acquisition' of point mutations in the ABL kinase domain, overexpression of the BCR–ABL oncoprotein and overexpression of P-glycoprotein, which accelerates exit of the drug from individual cells. Thus far at least 20 point mutations have been identified in leukaemia cells obtained from patients with variable degrees of resistance to imatinib. They each code for different amino acid substitutions in the Abl kinase component of the BCR–ABL oncoprotein. Cells with one such substitution, the replacement of a threonine by an isoleucine at position 315 (referred to as the T315I mutation), seem to be especially resistant to the inhibitory action of imatinib. Cells with other substitutions are relatively less resistant. Recent evidence suggests that the finding of amino acid substitutions in one particular part of the Abl kinase domain, the phosphate-binding loop (the so-called P-loop), may predict for disease progression and thus relatively poor survival. It is probable that these subclones pre-exist the administration of imatinib but are allowed to expand when the wild-type molecule is inhibited by imatinib.

Hydroxyurea

Hydroxyurea is a ribonucleotide reductase inhibitor that targets relatively mature myeloid progenitors in proliferative cycle. Its pharmacological action is rapid and readily reversible. Treatment for patients in chronic phase is usually started with 1.0–2.0 g daily by mouth and continued indefinitely. The leucocyte count starts to fall within days and the spleen reduces in size. It is usually possible to reverse all features of CML within 4–8 weeks of starting treatment with hydroxyurea. The dosage can then be titrated against the leucocyte count, the usual maintenance dose being between 1.0 and 1.5 g daily. In a patient whose leucocyte count is controlled, any reduction in the dose leads to a rapid increase in the leucocyte numbers, a phenomenon that disturbs the patient but has no ominous significance. The drug has relatively few side-effects. At high dosage it may cause nausea, diarrhoea or other gastrointestinal disturbance. Some patients get ulcers of the buccal mucosa. Skin rashes are seen. Most patients develop megaloblastic changes in the marrow with macrocytosis in the blood. The drug remains useful today for rapid cytoreduction in the newly diagnosed patient and may also be useful in patients unable to tolerate imatinib.

Interferon-α

Interferon-α is a member of a large family of glycoproteins of biological origin with antiviral and antiproliferative properties. Studies in the early 1980s using material purified from human cell lines showed that it was active in reducing the leucocyte count and reversing all features of CML in 70–80% of CML patients. Of particular interest at the time was the observation that 5–15% of patients achieved major reduction in the percentage of Ph-positive marrow metaphases with restoration of Ph-negative (putatively normal) haemopoiesis. It raised the important question of whether these 'cytogenetic responders' would have their life prolonged by treatment with IFN-α, and prospectively randomized controlled studies were initiated. Compared with hydroxyurea, IFN-α offered a survival advantage that was maximal for those who achieved complete cytogenetic remissions. These observations meant that IFN-α replaced hydroxyurea and busulphan in the 1980s as primary treatment for CML in chronic phase, and remained so until the introduction of imatinib.

Interferon-α must be administered by subcutaneous injection at daily doses ranging from 3 to 5 megaunits per/m². There is no good evidence that the higher doses are clinically superior. Toxicity is common in older patients, but is generally mild and reversible. Almost all patients experience fevers, shivers, muscle aches and general 'flu-like' features on starting the drug; these last usually 2–3 weeks but may be alleviated by paracetamol. They recur when dosage is increased. A significant minority of patients cannot tolerate the drug on account of lethargy, malaise, anorexia, weight loss, depression and other affective disorders or alopecia. Autoimmune syndromes, such as thyrotoxicosis, may also occur. A long-acting form of IFN-α, pegylated IFN-α, has been introduced recently, but, other than ease of administration, it seems to have little advantage over conventional formulations.

Busulphan

Busulphan (1,4-dimethanesulphonyloxybutane) is a polyfunctional alkylating agent that is now infrequently used (except as conditioning before transplant procedures). It targets a relatively primitive stem cell and the effects of administration are prolonged for some weeks after stopping the drug. It was the mainstay of treatment for CML in the period 1960–80. Treatment was conventionally started with 8 mg daily by mouth and the dosage was reduced as the leucocyte count began to fall. It was essential to reduce the dosage substantially or to stop the drug before the leucocyte count fell below 20×10^9/L because profound and prolonged leucopenia might otherwise be produced.

Busulphan could be administered either in finite courses lasting up to 4 weeks or continuously at a maintenance dose between 0.5 and 2.0 mg per day. Occasional patients were 'hypersensitive' to the effects of busulphan and developed severe, sometimes irreversible, pancytopenia with marrow hypoplasia on standard dosage. Overdosage could achieve the same effect in any patient. Gonadal failure (as mentioned above) invariably occurred within a few months of starting treatment and was almost always irreversible. Other toxic effects included cutaneous pigmentation, pulmonary fibrosis and a wasting syndrome resembling hypoadrenalism. These points notwithstanding, the drug may be useful in older patients whose compliance is uncertain as it can also be given orally in the clinic as a single dose of 50 or 100 mg, to be repeated as necessary after 4 weeks or longer.

Homoharringtonine

Another drug of interest for CML in chronic phase is homoharringtonine, a semisynthetic plant alkaloid that enhances apoptosis of CML cells. It produces haematological responses in 60–70% of patients and major cytogenetic responses in 25% in small series of patients in chronic phase. The results appear to improve with the addition of IFN-α. For the moment, it remains an investigational agent.

Allogeneic stem cell transplantation

Younger patients with HLA-identical sibling donors may be offered the option of treatment by allogeneic SCT (see Chapter 24). Most specialist centres exclude from consideration patients who are over the age of 50 or 55 years. The major factors influencing survival are patient age, disease phase at time of SCT, disease duration, degree of histocompatibility between donor and recipient, and gender of donor. In general, patients are 'conditioned' for transplant with cyclophosphamide at high dosage followed by total body irradiation, or with the combination of busulphan and cyclophosphamide at high dosage. If all goes well, reasonable marrow function is achieved in 3–4 weeks

after the infusion of donor haemopoietic stem cells and the patient leaves the hospital.

The possible major complications include graft-versus-host disease, reactivation of infection with cytomegalovirus or other viruses, idiopathic pneumonitis and veno-occlusive disease of the liver. For patients with CML treated by SCT with marrow from HLA-identical siblings, the overall leukaemia-free survival at 5 years is now 60–80% (Figure 37.8). There is a roughly 20% chance of transplant-related mortality and a 15% chance of relapse. Patients surviving without haematological evidence of disease can be monitored by serial cytogenetic studies and by use of the much more sensitive RT-PCR, which can detect very low numbers of BCR–ABL transcripts in the blood or marrow. These studies suggest (but do not prove) that in the majority of long-term survivors the CML may truly have been eradicated.

The recognition that the graft-versus-leukaemia (GvL) effect plays a major role in eradicating CML after allografting led to the concept that the toxicity of the transplant procedure could be substantially reduced by decreasing the intensity of the pretransplant conditioning. The strategy is thus to focus predominantly on the use of immunosuppressive rather than myeloablative agents, to maximize the numbers of haemopoietic stem cells transfused and to exploit the GvL effect mediated by donor alloreactive immunocompetent cells to eliminate the leukaemia cells. Such procedures have been termed variously non-myeloablative SCTs (NSCTs), reduced-intensity conditioning SCTs or mini-SCTs, and reflect advances in our understanding of how SCT actually works (see Chapter 24). It is still too early to say whether such NSCTs will prove superior to conventional transplants in the longer term, but the technique could make SCT more widely available to higher risk and perhaps also to older patients.

The qualified success of conventional SCTs using matched siblings led in the late 1980s to increasing use of 'matched' unrelated donors for SCT for patients with CML. At present,

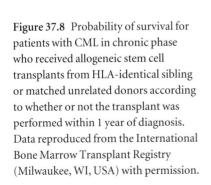

Figure 37.8 Probability of survival for patients with CML in chronic phase who received allogeneic stem cell transplants from HLA-identical sibling or matched unrelated donors according to whether or not the transplant was performed within 1 year of diagnosis. Data reproduced from the International Bone Marrow Transplant Registry (Milwaukee, WI, USA) with permission.

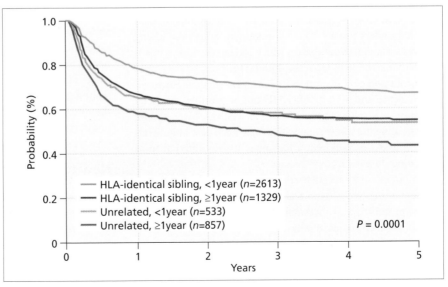

serologically matched unrelated donors can be identified for about 50% of white patients and for lower percentages of patients of other ethnic origins. However, molecular methods for typing HLA class I and II have now largely superseded serological techniques, and complete matches for a given patient for five gene pairs, HLA-A, -B, -C, -DR and -DQ, are relatively rare. Thus, in the absence of a 'perfect match' the clinician has to decide what degree of mismatch may be acceptable for a given transplant. In general, the results of transplants using such unrelated donors are less good at present than results of using HLA-identical siblings, but some patients will probably prove to be cured.

About 10–30% of patients submitted to allogeneic SCT relapse within the first 3 years post transplant. The relapse in usually insidious and characterized first by rising levels of BCR–ABL transcripts, then by increasing number of Ph-positive marrow metaphases and, finally (if untreated), by haematological features of chronic-phase disease. This provides some rationale for the recommendation that patients should be monitored post-transplant by regular RT-PCR and cytogenetic studies. Rare patients in cytogenetic remission relapse directly to advanced-phase disease without any identified intervening period of chronic-phase disease.

There are various options for the management of relapse to chronic-phase disease, including use of IFN-α, hydroxyurea, imatinib, a second transplant using the same or another donor or lymphocyte transfusions from the original donor. Such donor lymphocyte transfusions (donor lymphocyte infusion, DLI) have gained popularity in recent years, and are believed to reflect the capacity of lymphoid cells collected from the original transplant donor to mediate a 'GvL' effect, even although they may have failed to eradicate the leukaemia at the time of the original transplant. In practice, mononuclear cells are collected from the transplant donor in one or two leucapheresis procedures and transfused to the patient (who receives no other conditioning and usually no prophylaxis for GvHD). Within 3–6 months the leukaemia is restored to complete cytogenetic remission in about 80% of CML patients treated in this way and these responders also achieve PCR negativity. Some responding patients sustain marrow aplasia, which can be reversed by transfusion of marrow cells from the donor. However, severe GvHD may occur and can, on rare occasions, prove lethal. However, the incidence and severity of GvHD can be greatly reduced by starting the lymphocyte transfusions at relatively low cell dose and repeating the transfusion with a higher cell dose at intervals of 4–12 weeks as required, a technique usually referred to as 'escalating-dose' DLI.

At present, opinions are evenly divided on the optimal management of the patient who relapses with increasing BCR–ABL transcript numbers or increasing Ph positivity after allogeneic SCT. Some feel that escalating-dose DLI is the best approach, whereas others prefer to resume treatment with imatinib. It may be possible to resolve this issue with a suitably designed prospective study.

Treatment decisions for newly diagnosed patients in chronic phase

The success of imatinib has made it extremely difficult to decide how best to treat the newly diagnosed patient, especially a patient for whom a suitable donor for allogeneic SCT is available and who would routinely have been advised to proceed to transplant in the 'pre-imatinib era'. The problem is due quite simply to two facts: first, although a successful transplant can cure CML, the outcome for an individual patient cannot reliably be predicted and, second, though the short-term results of treating patients with imatinib look excellent, the extent to which this agent will in general prolong life is not yet clear. Moreover, it is likely that results of transplant will improve in the foreseeable future, and likely also that some of the newer agents now in development may be able to control CML in patients resistant to imatinib. For the present one may consider initial treatment by allogeneic stem cell transplant for any young patient with an optimal donor, but unquestionably the great majority of patients should start treatment with imatinib or with a trial combination including imatinib. Patients with possible transplant donors who fail imatinib should be considered for all-SCT (Figure 37.9).

For patients for whom transplant would not have been considered in the 1990s, initial treatment should be with imatinib or an imatinib-containing combination. Those who respond should presumably continue the drug indefinitely. Those who do not respond or who, having initially responded, then lose their response should be considered for alternative therapy, e.g. the substitution or addition of other agents or perhaps autografting. Some such patients could be suitable for a reduced-intensity conditioning allo-SCT.

The decision-making process is especially complicated when CML is diagnosed in an asymptomatic patient presenting to an antenatal clinic. For a woman in the first trimester of pregnancy it is probably best to delay treatment, avoiding if possible all forms of chemotherapy, including imatinib. Leucapheresis and/or blood transfusion could be undertaken if essential. The same might apply to patients in the second trimester of pregnancy, but administration of interferon-α is probably safe at this stage. The safety of imatinib is not yet established. In the third trimester the objective should be maintain the platelet count in the normal range, and this should be achievable with apheresis or interferon-α.

New therapeutic approaches

The demonstration that imatinib durably blocks the kinase activity of the BCR–ABL oncoprotein has provided a major incentive for the development of a second generation of kinase inhibitors. One such agent, BMS354825, has a chemical structure rather different from that of imatinib and appears to inhibit the kinase activity of both the *ABL* and *SRC* gene products.

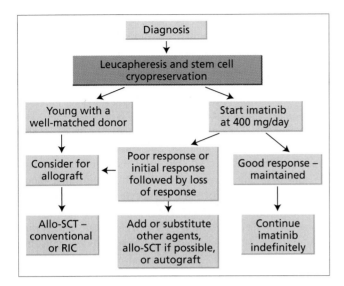

Figure 37.9 Algorithm showing a possible approach to the management of a patient with newly diagnosed CML in chronic phase. A minority of young patients with HLA-identical siblings (or possibly well-matched unrelated donors) may be eligible for initial treatment by allografting. The great majority of newly diagnosed patients, including those with possible transplant donors, should probably be treated first with imatinib. Those who respond well and maintain their response should continue on the drug indefinitely. Patients who respond less well or who lose their response should be considered for other therapy. SCT, stem cell transplantation; RIC, reduced intensity conditioning.

Preliminary clinical experience suggests that it may be active against leukaemia cells from patients who have developed resistance to imatinib as a consequence of expanded clones with kinase domain mutations. Similarly, the new ABL/SRC inhibitor currently designated AMN107 (Novartis Pharma) may prove to be equally active in imatinib-resistant cell lines. It is likely that other analogous kinase inhibitors will become available before long. It would be logical to test such new agents in combination with imatinib.

The demonstration of a powerful GvL effect in CML has renewed interest in the possibility that some form of immunotherapeutic manipulation could be effective in CML. Some evidence suggests that patients vaccinated with oligopeptides corresponding to the junctional region of the BCR–ABL protein may generate immune responses that may be of clinical benefit. Other targets for vaccine therapy now under study include the Wilms tumour-1 protein and proteinase-3, both of which are overexpressed in CML cells.

Autografting in chronic phase

Because only a minority of patients are eligible for allogeneic SCT, much interest has focused on the possibility that life may

be prolonged and some cures effected by autografting CML patients still in chronic phase. It is possible that the pool of leukaemic stem cells can be substantially reduced by an autograft procedure, and autografting may confer a short-term proliferative advantage on Ph-negative (presumably normal) stem cells. In practice, some patients have achieved temporary Ph-negative haemopoiesis after autografting. Preliminary studies have been reported in which patients have been autografted with Ph-negative stem cells collected from the peripheral blood in the recovery phase following high-dose combination chemotherapy; some such patients achieved durable Ph negativity.

Management of chronic myeloid leukaemia in advanced phase

Accelerated-phase disease

It is difficult to make general statements about the optimal management of patients in accelerated-phase disease as the criteria for this diagnosis are so very varied. Some patients can be managed merely with a minor alteration in their cytotoxic drugs regimen. Those who have not been treated previously with imatinib may obtain benefit from the introduction of this agent. Other patients may benefit from splenectomy or regular red cell transfusion. Patients whose disease seems to be moving towards overt blastic transformation may benefit from appropriate cytotoxic drug combinations. Allogeneic SCT should certainly be considered for younger patients if suitable donors can be identified. Reduced-intensity conditioning allografts are probably not indicated, as the efficacy of the GvL effecting advanced-phase CML is not clearly established.

Blastic transformation

Patients in blastic transformation may be treated with combinations of cytotoxic drugs in the hope of prolonging life but cure can no longer be a realistic objective. Conversely, it is not unreasonable to use a relatively innocuous drug such as hydroxyurea at higher dosage to restrain blast cell numbers and maintain the patient at home for as long as possible. If the patient has a myeloid transformation, he or she can be treated with drugs that are appropriate to the induction of remission in AML, namely daunorubicin, cytosine arabinoside with or without 6-thioguanine, or etoposide. The blast cell numbers will be reduced substantially in most cases but their numbers usually increase again within 3–6 weeks. Perhaps 20% of patients are restored to a situation resembling chronic phase disease and this benefit may last for 3–6 months. A very small minority, probably less than 10%, may achieve substantial degrees of Ph-negative haemopoiesis. This is most likely in patients who entered blastic transformation very soon after diagnosis.

Patients in lymphoid transformation may be treated, with a

little more optimism, with drugs applicable to the management of adult ALL (e.g. prednisolone, vincristine, daunorucibin and methotrexate with or without L-asparaginase). More than 50% of patients will be restored to 'second' chronic phase, at which point this status can be maintained with daily 6-mercaptopurine and weekly methotrexate. Because leukaemia involving the CNS is so relatively common in responding patients, those who achieve second chronic phase should have neuroprophylaxis with intrathecal methotrexate weekly for six consecutive weeks, but the administration of cranial irradiation is probably excessive. Some patients treated for lymphoid transformation of CML may sustain long periods of apparent 'remission'.

Imatinib may be remarkably effective in controlling the clinical and haematological features of CML in advanced phases in the very short term. In some patients in established myeloid blastic transformation, who received 600 mg daily, massive splenomegaly was entirely reversed and blast cells were eliminated from the blood and marrow, but such responses are almost always short-lived. Thus, imatinib should be incorporated into a programme of therapy that involves also use of conventional cytotoxic drugs and possibly also allogeneic SCT.

Allogeneic SCT using HLA-matched sibling donors can be performed in accelerated phase; the probability of leukaemia-free survival at 5 years is 30–50%. SCT performed in overt blastic transformation is nearly always unsuccessful. The mortality resulting from GvHD is extremely high and the probability of relapse in those who survive the transplant procedure is very considerable. The probability of survival at 5 years is consequently 0–10%. However, patients who can be restored to 'second' chronic phase by combination chemotherapy or by imatinib may have a relatively low risk of transplant-related mortality and may therefore be considered for allogeneic SCT with a view to eliminating both chronic disease and residual blastic disease provided that a suitable donor can be identified.

Variants of chronic myeloid leukaemia

Ph-negative chronic myeloid leukaemia

About 6% of patients with haematologically acceptable CML lack the Ph chromosome (see above). About one-half of these patients have a BCR–ABL gene that is molecularly identical to the BCR–ABL gene of Ph-positive CML; this gene is usually on the morphologically normal chromosome 22q but may occasionally be found on chromosome 9q. Such patients have a clinical course similar to those with Ph-positive disease. Conversely, the patients with no BCR–ABL gene frequently have haematological features that are subtly different from Ph-positive disease. They may lack basophilia, lack blast and myelocyte peaks in the leucocyte differential, or show dysplastic features. They are more likely to have some degree of monocytosis. These patients

respond poorly to imatinib, IFN-α or hydroxyurea, and overall their survival is inferior to that of Ph-positive patients.

Chronic myelomonocytic leukaemia

This is a rare myeloproliferative condition affecting predominantly elderly men but found at all ages (see Chapter 39). The patient may present with features of anaemia or haemorrhage. The spleen is typically enlarged and thus the clinical picture superficially resembles CML. However, the blood and marrow are quite different. Marrow cells lack a Ph chromosome. Blood monocytosis is prominent and monocyte numbers may be as high as 50×10^9/L. Thrombocytopenia is common. Basophilia and eosinophilia are absent. Dysplastic changes are usually present in the granulocyte and erythroid series. Consequently, the disease is included in the FAB classification of the myelodysplastic syndromes (see Chapter 39).

Very rare patients have been described with a chronic myelomonocytic leukaemia (CMML)-like blood picture associated with a consistent cytogenetic abnormalities in their leukaemia cells other than t(9;22). Most of these patients have either a t(5;12) associated with fusion of the *ETV* and *PDGFRB* genes or a t(8;13) associated with fusion of *ZNF198* and *FGFR1* genes but, in fact, other fusion partners have also been reported (Table 37.3). PDGFRB and FGFR1 are both receptor tyrosine kinases that are presumably 'activated' by mechanisms analogous to those that activate ABL gene in *BCR–ABL*-positive CML. The t(5;12) and t(8;13) leukaemias are both characterized by prominent eosinophilia but basophilia is usually absent. The t(5;12) leukaemias respond extremely well to low doses of imatinib but the t(8;13) leukaemias do not.

Chronic neutrophilic leukaemia

This is an exceedingly rare disorder that is usually diagnosed incidentally. The patient has a raised blood neutrophil count without immature granulocytes, and without basophilia or eosinophilia. The level of neutrophil alkaline phosphatase is usually raised. The marrow is hypercellular but cytogenetic studies are usually normal. The diagnosis is based largely on exclusion of other identifiable causes for the leucocytosis. Most patients have no symptoms referable to the neutrophilia and no physical signs, although some have minor degrees of splenomegaly. Treatment may not be required (see also Chapter 45).

Eosinophilic leukaemia

Most cases of raised eosinophil counts without identifiable primary cause have in the past been classified as examples of the 'hypereosinophilic syndrome' (HES) (see Chapter 45). However, it has been shown recently that some such patients respond well to treatment with imatinib, and some of these responding

Table 37.3 Cytogenetic abnormalities associated with deregulated tyrosine kinases in chronic myeloproliferative disorders.

Cytogenetic abnormality	Fusion protein	Leukaemia
t(9;22)(q34;q11)	BCR–ABL	CML or acute lymphoblastic leukaemia
t(8;22)(p11;q11)	BCR–FGFR1	BCR–ABL-negative CML
t(4;22)(q12;q11)	BCR–PDGFRA	Atypical CML
t(8;13)(p11;q12)	ZNF198–FGFR1	8p Myeloproliferative syndrome
t(6;8)(q27;p11)	FOP–FGFR1	8p Myeloproliferative syndrome
t(8;9)(p12;q33)	CEP110–FGFR1	8p Myeloproliferative syndrome
t(8;19)(p12;q13)	HERV/K–FGFR1	8p Myeloproliferative syndrome
t(5;12)(q31–33;p13)	TEL–PDGFRB	CMML/atypical CML
t(5;7)(q33;q11)	HIP1–PDGFRB	CMML/atypical CML
t(5;17)(q33;p13)	RAB5–PDGFRB	CMML/atypical CML
t(5;10)(q33;q21)	H4–PDGFRB	CMML/atypical CML
t(9;12)(q34;p13)	TEL–ABL	Atypical CML/BCR–ABL-negative CML
t(9;12)(p24;p13)	TEL–JAK2	Atypical CML/BCR–ABL-negative CML
t(9;22)(p24;q11)	BCR–JAK2	Atypical CML/BCR–ABL-negative CML
del(4)(q12)	FIP1L1–PDGFRA	Hypereosinophilic syndrome

CML, chronic myeloid leukaemia; CMML, chronic myelomonocytic leukaemia.

patients have evidence of a new fusion gene designated *FIP1L1–PDGFRA*, resulting from an interstitial deletion on chromosome 4 in their myeloid cells (see Table 37.3). In other cases in which no fusion gene has been identified, the number of immature cells in the blood and marrow is increased and the finding of a clonal cytogenetic abnormality in myeloid cells is strong evidence for a diagnosis of eosinophilic leukaemia (EL). It seems likely therefore that many, if not all, cases previously classified as HES may turn out to be due to a fusion gene and thus be classified more correctly as examples of EL. Occasional patients with EL progress to blastic transformation in a manner similar to Ph-positive CML. Patients with the *FIP1L1–PDGFRA* fusion gene usually respond well to relatively low does of imatinib.

Juvenile myelomonocytic leukaemia

Juvenile myelomonocytic leukaemia (JMML) is a rare disease affecting children under the age of 12 years. It represents about 2% of all childhood leukaemias. It includes a heterogeneous spectrum of myelodysplastic/myeloproliferative diseases that may be difficult to classify. Patients usually have symptoms of anaemia with lymphadenopathy and hepatosplenomegaly. There is a variety of skin rashes. Leucocyte numbers are increased with variable numbers of blast cells in the peripheral blood. Such cells are hypersensitive to GM-CSF *in vitro*. The haemoglobin F level may be elevated. The marrow is hypercellular but usually lacks chromosomal abnormalities, although monosomy 7 may be present. The disease responds poorly to standard cytotoxic drugs but patients may benefit from allogeneic SCT. Relapse after SCT is relatively common but relapses may be treated successfully with DLI.

Selected bibliography

Arico M, Biondi A, Pui C-H (1997) Juvenile myelomonocytic leukemia. *Blood* **90**: 479–88.

Bain B (2003) Cytogenetic and molecular genetic aspects of eosinophilic leukaemias. *British Journal of Haematology* **122**: 173–9.

Barrett AJ (2003) Allogeneic stem cell transplantation for chronic myeloid leukemia. *Seminars in Hematology* **40**: 59–71.

Branford S, Rudzki Z, Walsh S *et al.* (2003) Detection of BCR–ABL mutations in patients with CML treated with imatinib is virtually always accompanied by clinical resistance, and mutations in the ATP phosphate binding loop (P-loop) are associated with a poor prognosis. *Blood* **102**: 276–83.

Carella AM, Beltrami G, Corsetti MT (2003) Autografting in chronic myeloid leukemia. *Seminars in Hematology* **40**: 72–86.

Cools J, DeAngelo DJ, Gotlib J *et al.* (2003) A tyrosine kinase created by fusion of the PDGFRA and FIP1L1 genes as a therapeutic target of imatinib in idiopathic hypereosinophilic syndrome. *New England Journal of Medicine* **348**: 1201–14.

Druker BJ, Talpaz M, Resta DJ *et al.* (2001) Efficacy and safety of a specific inhibitor of the BCR-ABL tyrosine kinase in chronic myeloid leukemia. *New England Journal of Medicine* **344**: 1031–7.

Goldman JM (2005) Monitoring minimal residual disease in BCR-ABL-positive chronic myeloid leukemia in the imatinib era. *Current Opinion in Haematology* (in press).

Goldman JM, Druker B (2001) Chronic myeloid leukemia: current treatment options. *Blood* **98**: 2039–42.

Goldman JM, Melo JV (2003) Chronic myeloid leukemia: advances in biology and new approaches to treatment. *New England Journal of Medicine* **349**: 1449–62.

Gratwohl A, Hermans J, Goldman JM *et al.* (1998) Risk assessment for patients with chronic myeloid leukaemia before allogeneic bone marrow transplantation. *Lancet* **352**: 1087–92.

Guilhot F, Chastang C, Michallet M *et al.* (1977) Interferon alfa-2b combined with cytarabine versus interferon alone in chronic myelogenous leukemia. *New England Journal of Medicine* **337**: 223–9.

Hasford J, Pfirrmann M, Hehlmann R *et al.* (1998) A new prognostic score for survival of patients with chronic myeloid leukemia treated with interferon alfa. Writing Committee for the Collaborative CML Prognostic Factors Project Group. *Journal of National Cancer Institute* **90**: 850–8.

Hughes TP, Kaeda J, Branford S *et al.* (2003) Frequency of major molecular responses to imatinib or interferon alfa plus cytarabine in newly diagnosed chronic myeloid leukemia. *New England Journal of Medicine* **349**: 1421–30.

Melo JV (1996) The molecular biology of chronic myeloid leukaemia. *Leukemia* **10**: 751–6.

Mughal TI, Yong A, Szydlo R *et al.* (2001) The probability of long-term leukaemia free survival for patients in molecular remission 5 years after allogeneic stem cell transplantation for chronic myeloid leukaemia in chronic phase. *British Journal of Haematology* **115**: 569–74.

Niemeyer CM, Fenu S, Hasle H *et al.* (1998) Differentiating juvenile myelomonocytic leukemia from infectious disease – response. *Blood* **91**: 366–7.

O'Brien SG, Guilhot F, Larson RA *et al.* (2003) Imatinib compared with interferon and low dose cytarabine for newly diagnosed chronic-phase chronic myeloid leukemia. *New England Journal of Medicine* **348**: 994–1004.

Sawyers CL (1999) Chronic myeloid leukemia. *New England Journal of Medicine* **340**: 1330–40.

Shah NP, Nicholl JM, Nagar B *et al.* (2002) Multiple BCR–ABL kinase domain mutations confer polyclonal resistance to the tyrosine kinase inhibitor imatinib (STIS71) in chronic phase and blastic crisis chronic myeloid leukemia. *Cancer* **2**: 117–25.

Shannon KM (2002) Resistance in the land of molecular therapeutics. *Cancer Cell* **2**: 99–102.

Sokal JE, Cox EB, Baccarani M *et al.* (1984) Prognostic discrimination in 'good risk' chronic granulocytic leukemia. *Blood* **63**: 789–99.

World Health Organization (2001) *World Health Organization Classification of Tumours. Tumours of the Haemopoietic and Lymphoid Tissues* (ES Jaffe, NL Harris, H Stein *et al.*, eds), pp. 20–6. IARC Press, Lyon.

CHAPTER 38

Chronic lymphocytic leukaemia and other B-cell disorders

Daniel Catovsky

38

Introduction

Within the broad term of B-cell lymphoproliferative disorders we include a number of disease entities arising from mature B lymphocytes and which involve primarily the blood, bone marrow and other lymphoid organs such as the spleen. All of them are classified within the World Health Organization (WHO) proposals (see Chapter 43) on the basis of their histopathological appearances as this is often the key for their diagnosis. Their clinical course is often chronic and they affect mainly adults. All show, early in their course, circulating leukaemic cells in various degrees. Some of these conditions could be considered as primary leukaemias and these will be dealt with in this chapter. Others represent the leukaemic phase of low-grade non-Hodgkin's lymphomas (NHL) and their recognition is important for the purpose of differential diagnosis and patient management.

The study of lymphoid leukaemias has been enriched with the advent of monoclonal antibodies (MAbs) which define antigenic determinants that are specific for the B- and T-cell lineages. Characterization of these malignancies is not possible without the use of these reagents and/or other membrane markers which define the cell lineage and the maturation stage of the leukaemic cell. DNA analysis for the detection of immunoglobulin and T-cell receptor gene rearrangements has been incorporated as another diagnostic test for cell lineage and clonality and for monitoring minimal residual disease (MRD) after therapy. Chromosome abnormalities which characterise some of the genetic changes in the lymphoid leukaemias are now also important for diagnostic and prognostic purposes and are rout-inely studied by fluorescence *in situ* hybridization (FISH) as it is not easy to obtain metaphases in slowly dividing lymphocytes.

The primary B-cell leukaemias include chronic lymphocytic leukaemia (CLL), which is by far the most common, the rare B-prolymphocytic leukaemia (B-PLL) and hairy cell leukaemia (HCL). The B-NHLs which most frequently affect the blood and bone marrow include splenic marginal zone lymphoma (SMZL) or splenic lymphoma with circulating villous lymphocytes (SLVL), mantle cell lymphoma (MCL), which not infrequently has lymphocytosis, particularly in the splenomegalic or nonnodal form, and follicular lymphoma which, in its generalized or systemic form (stage IV), regularly affects the bone marrow and may spill over to the peripheral blood.

Methodology for diagnosis

Examination of the morphology of leukaemic cells in well-prepared peripheral blood and bone marrow films stained with Romanowsky dyes is the first diagnostic procedure. Details which are helpful in the analysis of cell types are: cell size, nucleo-cytoplasmic (N/C) ratio, regularity or irregularity of the nuclear outline, the characteristics of the cytoplasm such as the presence and length of any villus formations, the degree of basophilia, the presence or absence of cytoplasmic granules, the degree of nuclear chromatin condensation and its pattern, and the prominence, frequency and localization of the nucleolus.

The second crucial element for the diagnosis of any type of lymphocytosis is to use a small battery of membrane markers to

Table 38.1 The immunophenotype of CLL: tests used as basis for a scoring system.

Marker (result)	Score
SmIg (weak)	1
CD5 (+)	1
CD23 (+)	1
FMC7 (−)*	1
CD79b (− or −/+)	1
Total	5

*Epitope of CD20 but CD20 not useful for scoring.

define the immunophenotype (B or T) and whether the process is clonal or polyclonal. Once a monoclonal B-cell proliferation is established by light-chain restriction, e.g. kappa or lambda, one can clarify the problem further by using a restricted panel of monoclonal antibodies to define a particular disease immunophenotype. Our group has, over a number of years, worked out a panel of reagents that help define the typical immunophenotype of CLL (Table 38.1). The original proposal by Matutes et al. (1994) was revised by replacing CD22 with CD79b, which is one of the components of the B-cell antigen receptor molecule. Table 38.1 indicates in brackets after each of the five markers used the expected result in CLL. Figure 38.1 illustrates the contrast between the flow cytometry profile of a case of CLL which scores 5 and one of follicular lymphoma presenting with lymphocytosis which scores 0.

Table 38.2 summarizes the results of applying the panel of markers of the CLL score to the B-cell disorders. High scores are, by definition, expected in CLL; low scores are the feature in the other B-cell leukaemias and B-cell NHL. The data refer mainly to results in peripheral blood samples. Figure 38.2 illustrates the almost complete lack of overlap between CLL and the B-NHLs evolving with lymphocytosis. There are, however, a number of issues which may present problems. First, as shown in Table 38.2, some cases of CLL with atypical morphology, e.g. clefted or cleaved nucleus, plasmacytoid features, and cases with more than 10% prolymphocytes (CLL/PL) may have scores lower

Table 38.2 CLL score in B-cell disorders.

Disease	Score
CLL	
Typical	4–5
Atypical; CLL/PL	3–5
B-prolymphocytic leukaemia	0–1
Hairy cell leukaemia	0–1
NHL with leukaemia*	0–2

*Follicular, mantle, splenic marginal zone.

than 4 or 5. Rare cases of NHL may approach scores of 2 or 3; thus, reliance only on the immunophenotype may be misleading. Second, the important distinction between CLL and MCL, another CD5-positive disease, may require other tests, e.g. FISH (see below). In our experience of 60 cases of MCL with lymphocytosis studied with this panel of MAb, the highest score was 2. Recently, we have also identified a group of patients with CD5-positive leukaemia in which MCL was excluded by FISH and which also gave scores of 1 or 2. We have provisionally described them as very atypical CLL as we are not sure of the exact nature of this condition.

An important consideration when using membrane markers is the distinction between CD20 and FMC7. FMC7 has now been recognized as binding to a conformational epitope of the CD20 molecule. Despite this, FMC7 does not correlate with CD20 staining in CLL. Most cases of CLL and other B-cell disorders express CD20, hence its value as a pan-B-cell marker and as a target for the monoclonal antibody rituximab. We have reexamined the possible use of CD20 instead of FMC7 for the scoring of CLL (as suggested by some authors) in close to 1000 cases and concluded that FMC7 is of greater diagnostic value to distinguish CLL (where it is negative) from the other B-cell disorders in which it is strongly expressed. The findings with CD20 and FMC7 are very similar only in the non-CLL B-cell disorders.

When considering the possibility of a diagnosis of NHL, it is essential to obtain tissue for histology to confirm this suspicion and facilitate the classification of the disease. When the WBC is high (e.g. above 50×10^9/L) and the blood film shows unequivocal features of CLL or B-PLL, lymph node histology may not be essential, and not infrequently it is not available.

Bone marrow trephine biopsies are always required as they provide important diagnostic and prognostic information. The pattern of bone marrow infiltration – paratrabecular, diffuse, nodular or interstitial – the cell morphology, the status of the normal haemopoietic elements, the presence of fibrosis, proliferation centres, etc., are all features which can help to confirm a diagnosis of CLL or NHL, provide indications about the mechanism of anaemia or thrombocytopenia and help predict the outcome of splenectomy. The pattern and degree of lymphocytic infiltration in CLL have been considered an important prognostic variable independent of the clinical stage. For disorders with an enlarged spleen, e.g. B-PLL, HCL, splenic lymphoma with circulating SLVLs and some forms of MCL, spleen histology is often of diagnostic value.

The difficulties in eliciting metaphases for cytogenetic analysis in CLL and other small lymphocytic disorders has emphasized the value of FISH analysis which can be assessed on interphase cells. There is, however, no specific genetic abnormality in CLL and the current FISH studies are valuable as prognostic indicators (see below). FISH is important to exclude the two NHLs which have characteristic abnormalities, MCL with t(11;14)(q13;q32) and follicular lymphoma with t(11;14)(q32;q21). Other abnormalities, e.g. deletions 6q21, 11q23, 13q14 and 17p21 (the p53

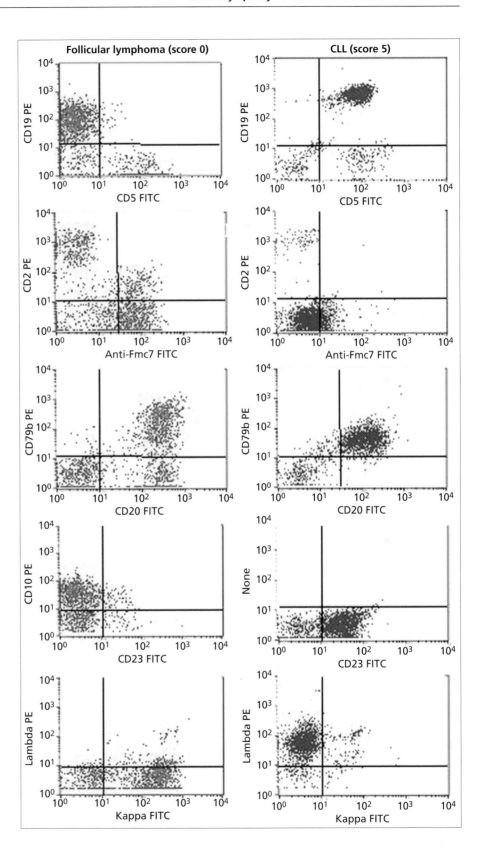

Figure 38.1 Flow cytometry analysis of peripheral blood samples from a case of follicular lymphoma with lymphocytosis (score 0) compared with a case of CLL (score 5) using the antibodies listed in Table 38.1.

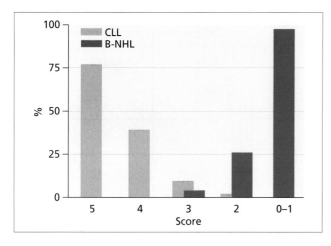

Figure 38.2 Distribution frequency of scores in CLL (high scores) compared with cases of B-cell non-Hodgkin's lymphoma (B-NHL) with circulating lymphoma cells (low scores).

locus) and trisomy 12, are seen in variable degree in most types of B-cell NHL as well as in CLL.

Chronic lymphocytic leukaemia

Chronic lymphocytic leukaemia accounts for about 25% of all leukaemias. In adults over the age of 50 years it is the most common form, particularly in the West. In the Far East, its incidence is low. In our series of over 2000 samples with B-cell lymphocytosis, CLL represented two-thirds of cases and close to one-third were represented by NHL in leukaemic phase (or 'spillover'). CLL affects twice as many males as females, with a peak incidence between 60 and 80 years. In the MRC CLL trials, 70% of patients entered were aged 60 years or over, and 15% were below 50 years. There is a tendency for older patients to present with less advanced disease. CLL is rarely diagnosed below the age of 40 years and is even more rare below 30. In the last 10 years, we have seen several patients in their late 20s. In such cases, a diagnosis of follicular lymphoma needs to be excluded. Of all the leukaemias, CLL has the highest familial incidence, which can be documented in 5–10% of patients (see below).

Pioneering work by Dameshek and Galton in the 1960s introduced the concept of CLL as a progressive accumulation of lymphocytes, starting in lymph nodes and/or the bone marrow and gradually expanding to most haemopoietic organs. This concept of slow progression was the basis of the clinical staging system proposed by Rai et al. (1975) and will explain the progressive abnormalities of the immune system which result in hypogammaglobulinaemia and, not infrequently, autoimmune complications. The bone marrow, viewed by detailed histology, also reflects the progression of CLL from early interstitial and nodular infiltration to late diffuse lymphocytic replacement of normal haemopoietic elements.

Several factors may be involved in the pathogenesis of CLL, including antigen stimulation within specific microenvironments and failure to undergo apoptosis. The protein BCL2 is consistently overexpressed and prevents or delays the death of CLL lymphocytes. Stromal cells and activated CD4$^+$ T lymphocytes may favour proliferation within tissue pseudofollicles (these are called proliferating centres and are the tissue hallmark of CLL).

Clinical and laboratory features

In approximately 50% of patients, the disease is diagnosed by chance following blood examination. In others, the presentation is prompted by symptoms of anaemia or by the discovery of painless lymph node enlargement. Systemic symptoms such as pyrexia, sweating or weight loss are rare. Not infrequently, prolonged chest infection or pneumonia is the first manifestation of CLL.

Lymph node enlargement is symmetrical and involves the neck, axillae and inguinal regions. Splenomegaly of variable degree is present in two-thirds of cases. Significant hepatomegaly is less frequent. It is possible to document lymph node enlargement in the hilar regions on routine radiographs, or in the retroperitoneal regions by ultrasound or computerized tomography (CT) scanning procedures. Although the latter investigations may not add significant prognostic information and are not used for staging purposes (see below), they are often useful for follow-up after treatment. An abdominal CT scan is important to document the extent of abdominal lymphadenopathy in patients presenting with palpable nodes. It is rare to find large para-aortic nodes in patients presenting without peripheral lymphadenopathy. Late in the disease process, however, this is not uncommon, and abdominal CT scans may be necessary to document progression.

The diagnosis of CLL requires evidence of lymphocytosis, at least 10×10^9/L, and lymphocytic infiltration in the bone marrow of at least 40%. With immunological methods, particularly the detection of monoclonal B-cell populations by light-chain restriction, it is possible to diagnose the disease with lymphocyte counts below this threshold. Morphologically, the lymphocytes in blood films are small and show scanty cytoplasm and a characteristic pattern of nuclear chromatin clumping; the nucleolus is inconspicuous and azurophil granules are seen only in a minority of normal T cells (Figure 38.3). The presence of smear cells, which correlates with the level of WBC, is of diagnostic value. A proportion of prolymphocytes (1–5%) are nearly always seen with counts $> 30 \times 10^9$/L. If the proportion of prolymphocytes is greater than 10%, it represents a variant designated CLL/PL (Figure 38.4). As reported by the French–American–British (FAB) group, some patients have a mixed pattern of small and large cells and others have lymphoplasmacytoid features or even cells with nuclear clefts. These are often associated with other atypical features (see below).

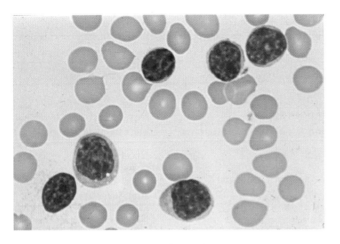

Figure 38.3 Blood film of a typical case of CLL.

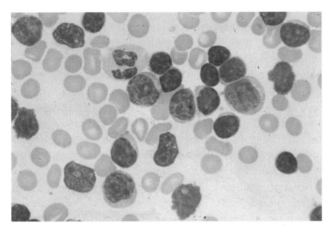

Figure 38.4 Blood film from a case of CLL/PL. Note the dual population of small lymphocytes and larger nucleolated prolymphocytes.

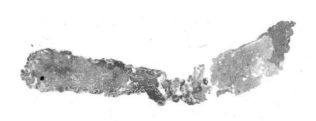

Figure 38.5 Low magnification of a trephine biopsy from a patient with CLL and heavy (packed) lymphocytic infiltration.

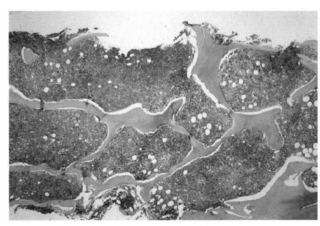

Figure 38.6 Higher magnification of the same case as Figure 38.5 showing scanty fat spaces and diffuse lymphocytic infiltration.

As stated above (Table 38.1), a combination of membrane markers is often diagnostic of CLL, distinguishing it not only from T-cell disorders but also from other B-lymphoproliferative disorders (Table 38.2). The diseases which are often confused with CLL are follicular lymphoma, splenic marginal zone lymphoma or SLVL and MCL when they present with lymphocytosis.

Anaemia and thrombocytopenia are important prognostic features in CLL and form part of the information used for staging. In advanced CLL, there is heavy lymphocytic infiltration resulting in bone marrow failure. The trephine biopsy shows heavy replacement of fat spaces and haemopoietic cells by lymphocytes (Figures 38.5 and 38.6). In an ageing population it is important always to exclude nutritional deficiencies (iron, folate), which can easily be corrected by appropriate supplements. The possible causes of anaemia in CLL are listed in Table 38.3. The current staging systems do not clearly distinguish the causes of anaemia as having different prognostic significance. This is

probably because marrow failure is by far the most common cause and there is an assumption that most haematologists will be able to detect the nutritional deficiencies. There is evidence, however, that autoimmune complications, e.g. anaemia or thrombocytopenia, which are rare at presentation, 7% and 1% respectively, do not necessarily confer a poor prognosis if adequately treated. It is important always to carry out the direct antiglobulin (Coombs) test at diagnosis in each patient. In a proportion of patients, autoimmune complications follow the initiation of therapy with alkylating agents or, as more recently recognized, after fludarabine. Therefore, the importance of the direct antiglobulin test is twofold: to document autoimmune haemolytic anaemia (AIHA) and to detect the triggering of AIHA after therapy. Not infrequently, patients have a positive Coombs test at presentation without overt haemolysis (e.g. no reticulocytosis or raised bilirubin). The documentation of autoimmune thrombocytopenic purpura (ITP) requires the demonstration of platelet-associated immunoglobulin. If this is not possible, one can still suspect peripheral destruction of platelets by examination of the bone marrow (see below).

Table 38.3 Causes of anaemia in CLL and their management.

Cause	Diagnostic test	Treatment	Significance
Bone marrow (BM) failure	BM aspirate and/or trephine biopsy	Corticosteroids; CLL therapy	Advanced CLL; stage III (Ral); C (Binet)
Haemolytic anaemia	Coombs test	Corticosteroids; immunosuppression; splenectomy	Does not affect prognosis but more frequent in active CLL
Red cell aplasia	BM examination	(See text)	Uncertain
Hypersplenism	BM; spleen size	Splenectomy; CLL therapy	Prognosis depends on stage after splenectomy
Fotate or iron deficiency	Indices, Fe and folate levels	Appropriate supplements	None; restage when anaemia corrected

Hypogammaglobulinaemia is the rule in advanced CLL and is responsible for the high incidence of upper respiratory tract infections. Small monoclonal (M) bands, often immunoglobulin M (IgM), are seen in less than 10% of cases. The appearance of an M band during the evolution of the disease or the discovery of free light chains in the urine (Bence Jones proteinuria) may indicate transformation.

Bone marrow examination (Table 38.4)

After the examination of peripheral blood films and the five markers for defining the immunophenotype, a bone marrow examination is the next most important test in CLL. Although it is common practice to perform an aspirate and a trephine biopsy, the latter is probably more informative. Aspirates are useful to confirm the cell morphology, to assess residual haemopoiesis and to ascertain any myelodysplastic features (in heavily treated patients). They are, however, not as informative as the core biopsy regarding overall cellularity and degree of infiltration.

The value of the biopsy is fourfold. The degree of infiltration is an important prognostic feature: a densely packed bone marrow (or diffuse pattern) with little or no residual fat spaces (Figure 38.6) correlates with advanced CLL – stage C (Binet) or III–IV (Rai) (see below). A trephine needs to be at least 2 cm in length (Figure 38.5) to be informative. Other bone marrow patterns are interstitial, with relatively abundant fat spaces (Figure 38.7), and nodular (Figure 38.8). Both of these are seen alone or in combination (mixed pattern) in relatively early stages of the disease. A second value of bone marrow is to clarify the nature of the cytopenia. For example, an increased number of megakaryocytes in the presence of low platelets may suggest ITP (Figure 38.9). Absence of red cell precursors and a low reticulocyte count suggest red cell aplasia. When this is due to parvovirus infection, large basophilic erythroid precursors can be seen in the bone marrow aspirates. The pattern of bone marrow infiltration may also help in the differential diagnosis with other lymphomas. For example, true paratrabecular deposits are common in follicular lymphoma and may be seen in SLVL and MCL, but not in CLL. Proliferation centres, a classic feature of

Table 38.4 The value of bone marrow trephine biopsies in CLL.

- Prognostic feature
  Diffuse = packed BM has poor prognosis
- Clarify the nature of cytopenias
  Low platelets > megakaryocytes
  Red cell aplasia
- Differential diagnosis with low-grade NHL
  Paratrabecular pattern not seen in CLL
  > Proliferation centres in CLL/PL
- To assess response to treatment
  Nodular PR seen only on biopsy

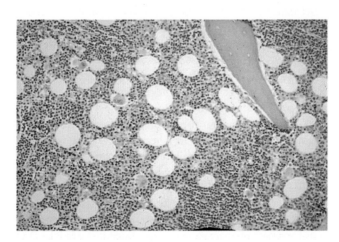

Figure 38.7 Interstitial lymphocytic infiltration in a case of early CLL with preserved haemopoiesis and abundant fat spaces.

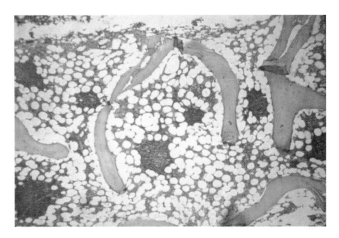

Figure 38.8 Nodular pattern of infiltration in CLL, early in the disease. A similar pattern described as nodular partial remission may be seen after chemotherapy in patients with previously diffuse involvement.

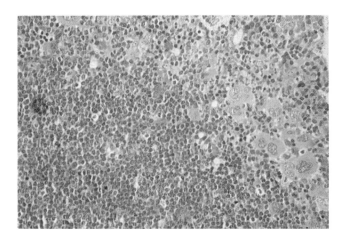

Figure 38.9 Diffuse infiltration in the bone marrow in a patient with CLL, a large spleen and thrombocytopenia. Note the large number of megakaryocytes which indicated that splenectomy will improve the low platelet count.

CLL and small lymphocytic lymphoma (SLL), are seen in lymph node biopsies, and in very active CLL also in bone marrow biopsies, not infrequently associated with an increased proportion of prolymphocytes (CLL/PL) in blood and bone marrow films. The proliferating centres have a high proliferation index as detected by immunocytochemistry staining for Ki-67 or MIB-1 and show prolymphocytes and blasts (para-immunoblasts). There is also a high expression of CD23 in the proliferating centres of lymph nodes and spleen greater than in the small lymphocytes. This may explain the high levels of soluble CD23 in the serum of patients with active CLL and its correlation with adverse prognosis. Proliferation centres are unique to CLL and SLL and are absent in NHL, particularly cases of MCL, which may otherwise resemble CLL.

With advances in treatment and with current targets aiming at maximum response, bone marrow biopsies are crucial to assess response. In particular, a nodular partial remission (PR), which is a very good clinical response, can only be defined by a bone marrow biopsy and not an aspirate. In such cases, the bone marrow aspirate may show less than 30% lymphocytes which, by the old criteria of response, could have been considered complete remission (CR). Immunostaining of the nodules is also important to assess response. If they are composed mainly of B cells (stained with CD20), they reflect residual CLL. If they are mainly T cells (stained with CD3) or a mixture, they may not represent residual CLL and are consistent with a true CR.

In patients with very early CLL with minimal lymphocytosis and otherwise normal blood counts, a bone marrow test may not be necessary and could be delayed until such a time when there is a suspicion of disease progression. Still, this information could be used to compare with a new bone marrow done when progression is suspected and the changes (e.g. greater infiltration) may facilitate a decision about the need to start therapy. Similarly, when assessing treatment responses, it is always useful to compare the pre-treatment bone marrow with the one at the end of therapy.

Staging systems

The two widely accepted systems are those of Rai *et al.* (1975) and Binet *et al.* (1981). Rai's staging system takes the view that CLL cells accumulate first in the blood and bone marrow, then in lymph nodes and spleen, finally leading to bone marrow failure. The chances of a patient surviving will depend largely on the stage at which he/she presents to the physician's attention. The Rai system has five stages: 0, no anaemia, thrombocytopenia or physical signs; I, lymphadenopathy only; II, splenomegaly and/or hepatomegaly with or without lymph node enlargement and without anaemia or thrombocytopenia; III, anaemia below 11 g/dL, irrespective of physical signs; and IV, thrombocytopenia below 100×10^9/L, with or without any of the above features. Binet modified this system following extensive multivariate analysis from two French studies. This system is simpler, has only three stages (A, B and C) and is probably more accurate with respect to the prognosis for patients with Rai stages I and II. For these patients, a subdivision according to the number of involved sites (as in Binet's staging) shows prognostic advantages over the subdivision in I and II. The Binet system groups together patients with anaemia (Hb < 10 g/dL) and thrombocytopenia (platelets $< 100 \times 10^9$/L) as group C. The remainder of patients are staged according to the number of lymphoid organs involved, considering as one each of the following areas: neck, axillae and inguinal regions, spleen and liver. Group A patients have no organ enlargement or up to two areas; group B patients have 3–5 involved areas. The International Workshop on CLL proposed to retain the Rai stages as substages for group A, as A(0), A(I) and A(II), mainly with a view to preserving the identification of the most benign group of Rai stage 0. From several studies, including early MRC trials, it appears that there is a distinct trend favouring A(0) compared with A(I) and A(II). More recently, the Rai staging has also been simplified and used in USA trials as follows: stages 0 (low grade), I and II (intermediate) and III and IV (advanced stage). Except for the difference in the level of haemoglobin (Hb) (10 or 11), Rai stages III and IV are the same as Binet C.

In practice, staging is necessary to predict prognosis, make decisions about which patients need treatment and facilitate allocation in randomized trials. There is little argument that stage C patients need therapy and also those with stage B, the majority of whom show features of disease progression – upward trend in the WBC, greater lymph node enlargement leading to symptoms of sweating and weight loss if the disease becomes bulky. There are also now conclusive data from several randomized trials that patients with stage A do not benefit from early treatment with chlorambucil. If anything, the approach of treating asymptomatic patients seems to have a deleterious effect.

The distribution of patients in the various stages, although variable, depending on whether from a retrospective study or a prospective randomized trial, is more or less as follows: A, 50%; B, 30%; and C, 20%. For both sexes, the proportion of stage A patients increases with age, with the highest proportion recorded over the age of 70 years. One of the important issues regarding which patients to treat is that staging, in particular stage A, appears to be a static definition and does not clearly predict whether patients will progress or not. The Spanish group has shown that a short lymphocyte doubling time (less than 12 months) in stage A correlates with poor prognosis. Similarly, the French group showed that those with Hb < 12 g/dL and/or lymphocyte count greater than 30×10^9/L (called A″) fared worse than those with Hb > 12 and lymphocytes < 30×10^9/L (A′). We examined both these factors in an observational study, MRC CLL3A, and found that both were strong indicators of prognosis and that the two criteria were independent of each other. We currently use a definition for stage A progressive for patients with short doubling times, downward trend in Hb and/or platelets, increasing organomegaly and systemic symptoms. Using these criteria, we have shown in both the CLL3 and CLL4 trials that stage A progressive fared the same as those with stage B, confirming the validity of the clinical criteria used. Both A progressive and B fared better than stage C.

New prognostic factors are now emerging in CLL (see below), and these will need to be tested against the relatively simple and well-established parameters. These will be relevant in particular to stage A but also perhaps to identify prognosis and good responders in the other stages. While these new tests are incorporated and tested in the clinic, the simple clinical observations, blood counts, symptoms and physical examination will remain as the best guideline on outcome. Stage is still very important as a starting point and, when considering the whole population with CLL, remains the best prognostic indicator. However, for randomized trials in which stage A non-progressive patients will not be entered, the prognostic value of staging loses its strength and other measures which assess the biology of the disease may become more relevant.

Prognostic factors

In a disease with such a variable pattern of survival it is important to examine critically the factors which determine survival. Most studies have shown that the best prognostic feature is the stage of the disease by either system. Individual features such as Hb, platelets, spleen size and number of lymph nodes enlarged are all important but are already incorporated in the stages. Now new categories of factors seem to add important prognostic information in addition to stage, age, sex and response to therapy. These reflect important biological features of the disease as assessed by molecular and flow cytometry methods. A number of studies have shown that some of these prognostic factors are independent of staging. Of the laboratory features, the level of the WBC, e.g. lymphocytes > 30×10^9/L in stage A, the proportion of prolymphocytes and the pattern of bone marrow involvement, e.g. diffuse involvement, have been shown to be important by several groups. Similarly, response to treatment seems to be an important independent feature. Although patients with early disease respond better than those with late disease, within each stage those who respond better will have a longer survival. Age is relevant in as much as, in the CLL age group, causes of death other than the disease itself are also very important. The influence of age is greater in stage A, in which up to 50% of patients may die of causes unrelated to CLL. Overall, one-third of patients may die of causes other than CLL, such as other neoplasms or cardiovascular accidents, and these are significantly influenced by age.

One biological factor which has emerged in all UK CLL trials for the last 25 years is sex. Female patients survive significantly longer than males and tend to respond better to treatment. In addition, females have a lower incidence of the disease and the M/F ratio is 2.5:1; this is higher in younger patients and lower in older ones. The M/F ratio is 3:1 in patients entered into treatment trials. The proportion of patients with stage A disease is higher in women than in men, i.e. 41% vs. 27%, whilst more men have stages B and C, i.e. 36% vs. 28%. When these favourable factors are taken into account and one considers that women tend to be older, sex remains as a prognostic factor independent of age, stage and response to treatment. The biology behind the better prognosis of women is not as yet obvious. The proportion of those with mutated immunoglobulin V_H genes is higher (see below), and this may provide a possible explanation.

Response to treatment has also emerged as an important prognostic variable. However, and disappointingly, large randomized trials have as yet failed to show a survival advantage for those treatments with higher response rates, e.g. fludarabine. One likely reason is that although treatment response matters, a patient not responding to treatment A, e.g. chlorambucil, may then respond to treatment B, e.g. fludarabine (as shown in the MRC CLL3NR study) and, therefore, the patient changes from non-responder to responder. Only those non-responders to all treatments fare particularly badly.

The study of prognostic factors in CLL is currently undergoing a major revolution as new objective variables emerging from laboratory research may redefine more objectively the disease categories. The new prognostic factors include genetic markers, mutational status of the IgV$_H$ gene and surrogate markers such as CD38 and ZAP-70, the latter measured by flow cytometry. Other laboratory studies have been shown to have prognostic value but they were not easy to perform or were not shown consistently by all groups to have clinical value. This includes morphology, lymphocyte count, serum levels of β$_2$-microglobulin, lactate dehydrogenase (LDH), thymidine kinase and soluble CD23. It seems that the focus now is on new reproducible markers which relate to the underlying biology, proliferative potential and responsiveness to therapy.

Cytogenetics

It was known for many years that analysis of the karyotype of CLL lymphocytes stimulated to divide by a variety of mitogens elicited positive results in less than 50% of cases. This was due to two main reasons: the frequent observation of normal metaphases, which reflected the karyotype of the normal T cells, and the frequent lack of metaphases in cases with high WBC. Nevertheless, these early studies were important in identifying the abnormalities which can be found in CLL and which can now be studied more extensively by FISH analysis. This technique uses specific probes to detect these genetic changes on interphase cells. There is now a panel of at least five probes to study the most frequent abnormalities which can be detected in 80% of cases. Thus, we are now in a position in CLL similar to that of the acute leukaemias in which distinct chromosome abnormalities of prognostic significance can be detected in most patients. However, it is important to state that none of the abnormalities found are unique or specific for CLL and can be found in other B-cell leukaemias and NHL.

The most important contribution to the subject has been that of Dohner *et al.* (2000), who, in a study of 325 patients, proposed a hierarchical model for prognosis based on the genetic aberrations found in CLL (Table 38.5). This model is based on the prognostic value of such markers and it is necessary because some patients have more than one abnormality but the one which counts is the one listed higher in the table. It should be noted that deletions of 13q14 (Figure 38.10) confer a good prognosis (even better than no abnormality), but only provided they are found as a single change. Table 38.5 also shows that the incidence of the abnormalities is similar in cases entered thus far in the CLL4 trial. Of note is that there are few, if any, chromosome translocations in CLL; most changes are deletions or trisomy 12.

Table 38.5 Hierarchical model of chromosomal abnormalities in CLL.

Karyotype	Döhner	CLL4
No. of patients	352	223
17p deletion	7%	7%
11q deletion	17%	17%
12q trisomy	14%	10%
Normal karyotype	18%	26%
13q del as sole abnormality	36%	35%
Other abnormalities	8%	5%*

*6q21 deletion.

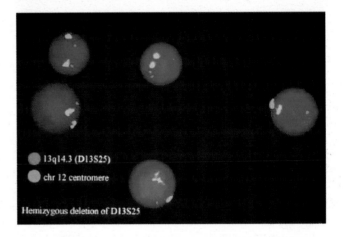

Figure 38.10 FISH analysis with a 13q14 probe showing missing red dots in several cells denoting 13q deletion; all the cells are disomic for chromosome 12 (normal pattern).

Table 38.6 Genetic abnormalities associated with progression and poor prognosis in CLL.

11q23 deletions (20% of cases)	• Younger age • Lymphadenopathy • Short survival
Trisomy 12 (15% of cases)	• CLL/PL • Disease progression • High proliferation rate
Abnormal 17p13 (p53 mutations/deletions 7% of cases)	• CLL/PL • Poor response to therapy • Transformation

Table 38.6 summarizes the main clinical and prognostic features associated with the three abnormalities which confer poor prognosis in CLL. The 17p deletion (Figure 38.11) has a much higher incidence (three or four times) in patients with advanced CLL, particularly after multiple treatments, than in those requiring treatment for the first time. The result of the 17p21 deletion

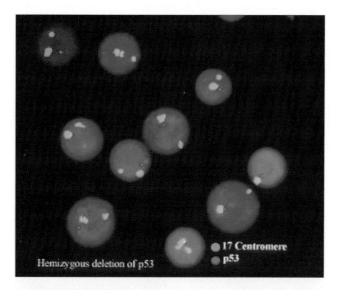

Figure 38.11 FISH analysis with a p53 probe (red) and a control 17 probe. Note many cells with only one (instead of two) red dot, indicating p53 deletion.

Table 38.7 Mutational status of IgV$_H$ genes in CLL.

	Unmutated	*Mutated*
Incidence	45%	55%
M:F ratio	11:1	1.1:1
Morphology	Atypical	Typical
Trisomy 12	Frequent	Infrequent
Abnormal 13q14	Rare	Common
Stage (BiNet)	B&C (2/3)	Stage A (2/3)
Disease course	Progressive	Stable
CD38/ZAP70	Expressed	Negative
Therapy	Required	Not needed
Response	Poor	Normal
Survival	Short	Long

at the p53 locus often correlates with a point mutation in the other allele and this results in the total inactivation of the *p53* suppressor gene, the most common molecular change in cancer patients. Although the usual method for detecting p53 abnormalities is to use FISH to detect deletion of 17p, overexpression of the *p53* gene can be demonstrated by flow cytometry, immunocytochemistry and immunohistochemistry. The significance of *p53* overexpression is probably the same: although both abnormalities are not always detected at the same time, both tend to correlate with *p53* mutations.

The group with other abnormalities (Table 38.5) includes cases with deletion of 6q21 which, both in Dohner's series and in our current series, represents 6% of cases. These patients tend to present with high lymphocyte counts but apparently have an overall good prognosis. A rare translocation, t(14;19)(q23;q13), is found in less than 1% of cases. Although these patients were reported as having CLL, they seem to have atypical features and poor prognosis. This abnormality cannot, at present, be detected by FISH. In half of the cases, t(14;19) is associated with trisomy 12. We found two such cases within those described as very atypical CLL with scores of 1. Despite being CD5$^+$, MCL was excluded by FISH and cyclin D1 staining.

The analysis of results of the CLL4 trial may clarify further the prognostic value of the five genetic markers in CLL and whether other features such as response to therapy can be predicted by means of FISH analysis.

VH mutations, CD38 and ZAP-70

The most interesting and exciting new findings relating to prognosis and which may underlie the clinical heterogeneity of CLL

are the mutational status of the IgV$_H$ gene, and the expression of CD38 and of ZAP-70. Somatic hypermutation is a process by which B cells, after the initial recombination of the Ig genes, undergo further change in order to produce high-affinity antibodies. This event occurs within the germinal centre and gives rise to memory B cells and plasma cells.

CLL was, for many years, thought to be a disease of early or immature CD5$^+$ B cells with unmutated IgV$_H$ genes. A similar hypothesis was made with MCL. More recent studies showed heterogeneity, and this was consolidated by two landmark papers in 1999 by Damle *et al.* and Hamblin *et al.* and demonstrated that just over half of the patients had mutated V$_H$ genes (Table 38.7), defined as < 98% homology to the nearest germline sequence, although in some studies < 97% is used as the cut-off level.

Many studies have confirmed the original finding, which suggested initially that there were two types of CLL: the unmutated type, associated with all the features of poor prognosis, and the mutated type, associated with stable disease and good prognosis (Table 38.7). Of interest is the finding that many of the features known to be of poor prognosis, such as stages B and C, male sex, atypical morphology, trisomy 12, 11q deletion, etc., are seen predominantly in unmutated cases whereas the opposite is true for the mutated ones. The early studies also showed that unmutated cases correlated with higher expression of the transmembrane glycoprotein CD38. This correlation is seen, however, in only two-thirds of cases. Therefore, and contrary to early speculation, CD38 could not be regarded as a surrogate marker for V$_H$ mutational status. Nevertheless, many studies have now shown that CD38 is an important prognostic marker. Low percentages correlate with stable disease, while a high percentage of CD38$^+$ cells predicts a short time to disease progression and worse overall survival.

There are several caveats on the determination of CD38. Although assessed by flow cytometry and simpler than PCR and sequencing, which are used for V$_H$ mutations, CD38 testing should be only on the CLL B cells and exclude T cells which

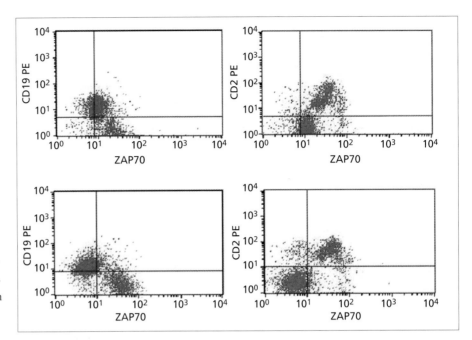

Figure 38.12 Flow cytometry plots of ZAP70 in CLL Top left: ZAP70+, CD19+ lymphocytes; top right: control ZAP70+ T and NK lymphocytes (CD2+). Bottom left: a ZAP70− case and the positive control T/NK cells (bottom right).

strongly express this antigen. This is currently done by triple labelling with CD5, CD19 and CD38 and appropriate gating. Another issue is the best threshold for CD38 positivity. The early reports suggest 30%, but more recent studies and our own experience suggest a lower figure, 7%, as being more likely to be accurate. In some reports, CD38 has prognostic value independently of V_H status, but it is likely that this relatively simple determination adds to the constellation of markers useful to assess prognosis in individual patients.

The heterogeneity in mutational status, which is, in fact, not unique to CLL, suggested two distinct origins for the disease: from unmutated naive B cells and from memory B cells. Subsequent data based on gene expression profiling showed unequivocally that CLL has a characteristic pattern of expression (or signature) which is independent of IgV_H mutation and is distinct from that of other B-cell lymphomas such as MCL, follicular lymphoma and diffuse large-cell B-cell NHL. The genotype of CLL was defined by a common pattern of expression of 12 000 genes, with only between 23 and 200 differentially expressed in mutated vs. unmutated cases. One notable difference is the high expression (four to five times higher) of ZAP-70 in unmutated cases. ZAP-70 encodes a protein tyrosine kinase and is of relevance in T-cell signalling. ZAP-70 can be demonstrated by flow cytometry, immunocytochemistry and Western blotting, and several studies have now shown a high concordance with the mutation status (~90%). Thus, ZAP-70 may be a better surrogate marker than CD38 to establish V_H mutational status without having recourse to molecular methodology. Studies using ZAP-70 have confirmed its prognostic value, particularly in patients with stage A disease, in whom an early assessment of the need for future therapy may be desirable. The

assessment of ZAP by flow cytometry (Figure 38.12) requires the exclusion not only of T cells (as for CD38) but also of NK cells, as both cell types express this cytoplasmic protein strongly. Thus, the determination of ZAP-70 requires cell permeabilization procedures and staining for CD3 and CD56 (for T and NK cells), CD19 and CD5 (for CLL cells) and ZAP-70 (Figure 38.12). Details are given in the report by Crespo *et al.* (2003).

The conclusion, from the gene expression profile and other studies, is that CLL derives from an activated, antigen-experienced B cell which resembles memory B cells and has a common pathogenetic pathway. The lack of balanced translocations which occur during Ig recombination and is seen in other B-cell NHL, e.g. MCL, follicular lymphoma, suggests that the mechanism of transformation in CLL is different and may not involve changes resulting from antigen exposure in germinal centres. A clear explanation for the differences in mutational status has not yet emerged.

Differential diagnosis

This was partly discussed in methodology for diagnosis. The main problem is when CLL has atypical features, more commonly morphology, less commonly immunophenotype, and, very rarely, both. We have provisionally described the latter situation as very atypical CLL. The most common change is the increased proportion of larger nucleolated lymphocytes or prolymphocytes. When there are more than 10% of these cells in blood films, the designation CLL/PL is used.

CLL/PL is a proliferative form of CLL, not infrequently associated with trisomy 12 or p53 deletion, high rate of cell divisions (as shown with the antibody Ki-67) and histologically by proliferating centres in lymph nodes and bone marrow sections. Occasionally, lymph nodes seem totally replaced by prolymphocyte-like cells and we have used the term accelerated CLL. However, the peripheral blood films always show a dual population of small lymphocytes and larger prolymphocytes. CLL does not transform to B-PLL, which is a distinct clinico-pathological entity (see below).

When atypical features are present, including those of CLL/PL, it is important to consider the differential diagnosis with NHL in leukaemic phase, notably MCL which, like CLL, is CD5 positive. The best method to exclude (or confirm) MCL is to test for t(11;14) by FISH and/or to demonstrate expression of cyclin D1. Other NHLs can be excluded by histological criteria and the combination of immunophenotype and peripheral blood morphology.

Large-cell transformation or Richter's syndrome

'Immunoblastic' transformation or Richter's syndrome is well recognized in CLL. The change occurs usually in one or several lymph nodes which, when examined histologically, show the features of large-cell lymphoma. Richter's syndrome is associated with systemic symptoms (fever and weight loss) and with unexpected unilateral lymph node enlargement, not rarely in the retroperitoneal area. Richter's occurs in 3–5% of CLL cases, but the incidence may be higher if lymph node biopsies are performed when clinical changes with systemic symptoms develop in a patient with previously well-controlled disease. In rare cases, the transformation takes place in the bone marrow and is therefore seen in trephine biopsies and, rarely, is associated with 'spillover' to the blood. In such cases, the morphology resembles that of an acute leukaemia, with large blasts which are SmIg positive and some of the CLL markers (Figure 38.13). Richter's syndrome is often associated with monoclonal proteins in the serum or free light chains in the urine. Studies with Ig gene re-

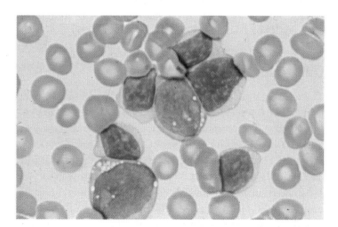

Figure 38.13 Blood film of a patient with Richter's syndrome with circulating large blast cells.

arrangements are useful to demonstrate if the new malignant clone arose from a pre-existing CLL B cell or whether it is a new clone. The latter is seen in at least one-third of cases. Genetic imbalances are frequent in Richter's syndrome, the most common being p53 abnormalities (17p deletion, overexpression and/or mutation).

Current evidence suggests that intense immunosuppression with agents such as fludarabine and the subsequent CD4 lymphopenia may trigger Richter transformation in some cases, and, not infrequently, evidence of involvement of the Epstein–Barr virus (EBV) in the pathogenesis has been shown by demonstration of the EBV latent membrane protein (LMP), by immunohistology or of EBV-encoded RNA (EBER) by *in situ* hybridization. A role for EBV in the pathogenesis of Richter's syndrome has been reported in close to 15–20% of cases. In a minority of cases, the large-cell transformation induced by EBV has Reed–Sternberg-like cells, and in others the histology is identical to that of Hodgkin's disease. It is debatable whether cases of classic Hodgkin's disease should be considered a true transformation or a new event triggered, but not always, by EBV.

Hypercalcaemia with or without obvious osteolytic lesions is a well-recognized finding in very advanced CLL. It does not represent, in itself, transformation to a large-cell lymphoma as, often, the histology is that of heavy infiltration by small lymphocytes. Not infrequently, hypercalcaemia is a terminal event.

Familial CLL

Evidence from epidemiological and family studies supports the view that there is inherited susceptibility to CLL in a significant subset of patients. Case reports of leukaemia families, case–control and case cohort studies all showed that the relative risk of developing CLL in patients' relatives is 3–5 times higher than in the normal population.

A number of features seem to characterize the disease in familial CLL. One is the phenomenon of anticipation, manifested by early onset and more severe disease in successive generations. Several studies, including our own, have shown that the age at diagnosis of offspring is approximately 20 years earlier than in their parents. The phenomenon of anticipation is known in other hereditary conditions and is due to the expansion of trinucleotide repeats. However, this mechanism does not appear to be the case in CLL. Recent studies have also demonstrated a higher incidence of subclinical CLL, that is the detection of small B-cell clones by a very sensitive flow cytometry assay using CD5, CD19, CD20 and CD79b, in 'normal' relatives, with an incidence four times greater than in the general population. This incidence is even higher when looking at individuals under 40 years of age.

The search for CLL predisposition genes has been active in the last few years with the possibility of collecting DNA samples of familial cases. Figure 38.14 illustrates families with several affected members ascertained during our current study which

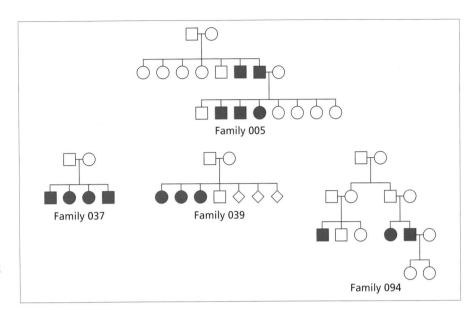

Figure 38.14 Four pedigrees of familial CLL cases with 3 or more affected per family.

has identified several families with three, four or five affected individuals. Through a family history questionnaire, we have determined that, in addition to CLL, other leukaemias and low-grade NHL can be found in such families. No clear-cut candidate gene has yet emerged, and several genes have been excluded as candidates. One of those excluded is the ataxia telangiectasia mutated (*ATM*) gene, which is mutated in ~20% of CLL samples, including some germline mutations. Other genes unlikely to play a role in linkage are the major histocompatibility complex (chromosome 6p21.3) and those in the pseudo-autosomal region (chromosomes Y and X). It will be possible in the next few years, through genome-wide linkage and association studies, to identify the gene(s) responsible for the inherited form of CLL. Most studies have suggested the vertical transmission of an autosomal gene with pleiotropic effects. A positive identification will also provide insights into the pathogenesis of the disease in general.

Monoclonal and polyclonal B-cell lymphocytosis

Improved flow cytometry technology has allowed the detection of small B-cell clones in 2.7% of normal individuals, particularly those over the age of 60 years. The significance of these clones which share immunophenotypic features with those of CLL is unknown. As mentioned above, such clones are found with higher frequency in healthy relatives of patients with CLL and an analogy has been made with the concept of MGUS (monoclonal gammopathy of unknown significance), therefore suggesting that some individuals with monoclonal B-cell lymphocytosis (MBCL) may evolve to CLL, but in others it may remain quiescent and not progress. It is also possible that MBCL may be the precursor state for other B-cell disorders, not just CLL.

In distinct contrast to MBCL, a rare abnormality described as polyclonal B-cell lymphocytosis (PBCL) has now been recognized. In affected patients, the absolute number of B cells is increased, not subclinical, but staining with anti-light chain antibodies shows lack of clonality and normal proportions of kappa- and lambda-staining cells. For several reasons, this entity, which appears not to be malignant in nature, needs to be recognized, not least because in some patients it may mimic CLL or other B-cell disorders. Features of PBCL are median age 40 years, lymphocyte count 3–15 (median 6.5), splenomegaly (15%) and mild BM infiltration. Ninety-five per cent of patients are smokers and 90% have HLA-DR7 in their genotype. The cell markers are non-clonal, CD19- and FMC7-positive, CD5 and CD23 are not expressed, and the patients have elevated levels of serum IgM (polyclonal). Despite the benign and non-clonal nature, a distinct abnormality has been shown in the B-lymphocytes: an extra copy of the long arm of chromosome 3 in the form of iso(3q). The blood picture is pleomorphic and frequently shows binucleated lymphocytes (Figure 38.15) which are characteristic of this condition. It is important to follow these patients closely and it is even more important not to institute any treatment.

Management

The indications for active treatment depend on the stage of the disease. For patients with stage A (Binet) or stages 0, I and II (Rai), a period of observation may be necessary to decide whether the pattern of the disease is stable or progressive. Most patients with stage B and two-thirds of those with Rai stage II will show progression within the first year or two after diagnosis. This is manifested by further organ enlargement, a downward trend in the Hb and/or platelets and a slowly rising WBC. As

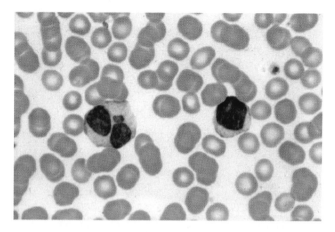

Figure 38.15 Blood film from a case of polyclonal B-cell lymphocytosis showing a binucleated cell characteristic of this condition.

responses are better with less disease, some trials have compared early versus delayed therapy to see whether survival improves. Both a French trial and an MRC trial showed that early treatment with chlorambucil was, if anything, deleterious, with more deaths due to progression in the group treated early. This was confirmed in a large overview. Thus, the old wisdom of wait and see should continue to prevail for stage A patients, at least for the time being.

Nevertheless, the issue of early treatment in stage A patients with stable disease may now need to be revised, for two main reasons. First, it is now possible to identify better the patients likely to progress through some of the new prognostic factors defined above, e.g. unmutated V_H genes, CD38/ZAP70 expression, short doubling time, 17p or 11q deletions. It is in this group that randomized studies should be carried out to see whether early therapy may improve survival. Second, the purine analogues, alone or in combination, increase the proportion of remitters and the quality of the responses; therefore, there may be a potential benefit of their use early in high-risk cases. It should be remembered that most patients with stage A progressive can be identified by simple criteria: lymphocyte doubling time less than 12 months, downward trend in Hb and/or platelets, 50% or more increase in organomegaly and constitutional symptoms. In the CLL3 and CLL4 trials, the survival of these patients (who entered with the above criteria) was similar to that of patients with stage B disease. It is also likely that in this group of patients one will find the poor prognostic factors defined by laboratory studies.

We should be aware that spontaneous clinical remissions may occur in CLL but these are not complete. We reported 10 patients (eight with stage A and two with stage B disease) who achieved remission without any therapy. Two had trisomy 12. Based on patients entered in MRC CLL trials, 1.5% of stage A patients may undergo a spontaneous reduction of the lymphocyte count greater than 50%.

Criteria for response

The definitions of response used in the UK for CLL3 and CLL4 trials are broadly similar to the National Cancer Institute (NCI) guidelines used in the USA. A bone marrow biopsy is required to define the new category of nodular partial remission (PR) by the presence of discrete or moderately large nodules of residual CLL. In this context, it is important to carry out immunohistochemistry as in some patients the nodules may contain mainly T cells rather than B cells. The former cases should be defined as achieving complete remission (CR). CR requires normalization of blood counts and the bone marrow whereas a PR requires the regression of at least 50% of organomegaly and lymphocyte counts (in the UK trials the requirement is a lymphocyte count less than 15×10^9/L). The NCI identifies rare groups of patients who may fulfil the criteria of CR except for persistent anaemia or thrombocytopenia. This may be due to persistent myelotoxicity or autoimmune phenomena. The NCI proposed that such cases be included as PRs. Another criterion for response proposed originally by the International Workshop on CLL but not widely used now is the downgrading of stages B or C to stage A for CR and from stage C to B for PR.

It has been shown recently that refinements in flow cytometry may contribute to defining minimal residual disease (MRD) with the same level of sensitivity or even greater than molecular methods (e.g. PCR). Flow cytometry requires at least two antibodies, CD5 and CD19, and gating on the B cells (CD19+). A more sensitive quantitation can be achieved by means of four antibodies: CD5, CD19, CD20 and CD79b. This improves the criteria for CR which can now be subclassified as MRD+ or MRD−. MRD positivity, i.e. more than 0.05% bone marrow cells, predicts for a short event-free survival. Flow cytometry is also useful to monitor peripheral blood counts when lymphocyte counts are less than 1×10^9/L after therapy. The detection of MRD+ cells in the PB usually correlates with persistence of at least 5% CLL lymphocytes in the bone marrow.

Treatment

Table 38.8 lists all the agents which can be used alone or in combination for the treatment of CLL. The list has been enriched with three nucleoside analogues and two monoclonal antibodies and illustrates the greater potential that now exists for achieving a greater number of good responses when these are used as first-, second- or even third-line therapy.

The role of corticosteroids as initial treatment for stage C patients is generally accepted. Platelets rise within 4–6 weeks; the Hb also rises; the WBC follows a characteristic curve, rising after 3 or 4 weeks, sometimes doubling the initial count and then gradually coming down. This is nearly always accompanied by a decrease in size and softening of lymph nodes and spleen. This beneficial effect facilitates the subsequent measures which employ agents having an effect on normal haemopoietic cells,

Table 38.8 Agents used alone or in combination for the treatment of CLL.

- Chlorambucil (oral)
- Cyclophosphamide (oral/i.v.)
- Prednisolone (standard/high dose)
- Fludarabine (oral/i.v.)
- Cladribine (2-CdA; i.v./s.c.)
- Pentostatin (DCF; i.v.)
- Rituximab (anti-CD20)
- Campath-1H (anti-CD52; i.v./s.c.)
- Genasense (BCL2 antisense)
- Zevalin (rituximab + yttrium-90)

and it seems more important when used before chlorambucil. Because of the side-effects associated with their use, it is advisable to retain steroids only for the early treatment of bone marrow failure and for autoimmune complications.

There is no evidence that chlorambucil given monthly in higher doses is more effective than a low dose administered continuously. However, the intermittent dose achieves the same effect with a smaller amount of the alkylating agent, and there is no evidence that adding prednisolone to the monthly courses of chlorambucil increases response rate or prolongs survival. It should be noted that the doses of chlorambucil (and of cyclophosphamide) have varied widely in different studies and there is clear indication of a dose–response curve. For example, the CALGB trial and the German CLL5 trial used chlorambucil at a dose equivalent to 40 mg/m^2 monthly and the reported CR rates were 3% and 5%, whereas the CLL3 trial used 60 mg/m^2 and the CR rate was 19%. In CLL4, the dose has been increased to 70 mg/m^2 (given as 10 mg/m^2 for 7 days every 4 weeks).

There have been several trials comparing chlorambucil with the combination COP (cyclophosphamide, oncovin and prednisolone); none showed an advantage for COP. It is apparent that the antimitotic agent oncovin (vincristine) has little role in CLL and in other similarly slowly progressive diseases. The value of prednisolone given monthly in COP is no better than when used with chlorambucil. Cyclophosphamide has no advantage over chlorambucil although it may be better as an immunosuppressive agent used continuously in patients with AHA.

The role of anthracyclines in the treatment of CLL is not clear but it is likely to be small. The combination of epirubicin with chlorambucil in CLL3 did not show an improved survival and only a marginally higher CR rate (22%). When used as the combination cyclophosphamide, doxorubicin, oncovin and prednisone (CHOP), it may be useful for patients with progressive disease who are poor responders to chlorambucil or fludarabine and for those who developed Richter's syndrome. The French version, or 'mini'-CHOP, uses more cyclophosphamide and half the dose of doxorubicin and in their large randomized trial proved better than the combination CAP (standard doses

as CHOP but minus oncovin). The complete haematological responses with mini-CHOP in previously untreated CLL were almost as good (33%) as with fludarabine (40%), but patients treated with the latter had a longer disease-free interval.

CLL lymphocytes are very sensitive to low-dose irradiation; splenic irradiation has been used in the early MRC trials and its general effect is sometimes manifested by a reduction in peripheral lymphadenopathy. The spleen size often regresses to become unpalpable and there is a dramatic fall in the WBC. This modality is now rarely used but the effect of irradiation is still exploited in transplantation protocols as total body irradiation (TBI).

Of the new generation of nucleoside analogues in the last decade, fludarabine has shown greatest promise for the treatment of CLL and low-grade NHL. Fludarabine has several modes of action which include inhibition of DNA synthesis and DNA repair and activation of the apoptotic pathways. These mechanisms enhance significantly the effect of this agent when used in combination with other drugs, e.g. cyclophosphamide and mitozantrone, and antibodies, e.g. rituximab. The main work carried out by Keating *et al.* in the 1990s at the MD Anderson Cancer Center showed that fludarabine has a high CR rate (~33%) in previously untreated patients, and still has high responses (15–20%) in those previously treated. This latter experience has been confirmed in the UK with evidence of lack of cross-resistance with chlorambucil or anthracycline-containing combinations. In the non-responders to chlorambucil or chlorambucil plus epirubicin in CLL3, the CR rate of single-agent fludarabine was 17%, with 64% PR.

The issue of first-line fludarabine and/or its combination with cyclophosphamide is currently being assessed in CLL4. Two large trials, French and American, showed a high response and prolonged disease-free survival but no overall survival advantage using first-line fludarabine against CAP or chlorambucil. Of interest is that the crossover of non-responders to chlorambucil in the CALGB study achieved 40% responses with fludarabine but, of the non-responders to fludarabine, only 7% responded to chlorambucil.

Using fludarabine in combination with other agents the CR rates have increased, e.g. from 20–35% when used alone in previously untreated patients to 30–45% with cyclophosphamide, 45% with rituximab and 65% with the combination FCR (fludarabine, cyclophosphamide and rituximab) in the MD Anderson experience. FCMR (adding mitozantrone) may be an even more powerful combination, but it has been used only in the salvage setting to improve on the already good responses achieved with FCM (without rituximab).

The downside of using strong combinations with fludarabine is that they are more myelotoxic (manifested as neutropenia) and immunosuppressive (manifested as lymphopenia) and care should be taken to take prophylactic measures such as using cotrimoxazole to prevent *Pneumocystis carinii* pneumonia (PCP) and aciclovir to prevent herpesvirus reactivations. On the positive side is that responses may last longer and flow cytometry now shows many cases with negative MRD.

New studies will show whether patients with poor prognostic features also benefit from these more intensive regimens. Those in the worse category, represented by those with p53 abnormalities, do not respond to alkylating agents but may respond to high-dose methylprednisolone (HDMP) given in 5-day pulses monthly at 1 g/m^2 intravenously or by mouth and may respond to Campath-1H, a monoclonal antibody with activity against B and T cells. In our studies with HDMP, we relied on the prediction assessed by an *in vitro* cytotoxicity assay, or DiSC assay, and we observed good responses in 50% of cases with p53 abnormalities.

The introduction of Campath-1H (alemtuzumab) and rituximab has opened the door of more targeted biological agents with little or no myelotoxicity. Campath-1H (anti-CD52) acts through antibody- and complement-mediated cytotoxicity and can be used intravenously or by subcutaneous injection. It has potent activity in previously untreated CLL but requires prolonged periods (18 weeks) of treatment to achieve CR, according to a Swedish study, when given subcutaneously. In previously treated and fludarabine-resistant CLL the CR rate is 2%, but 31% achieve a PR. Its role in the management of CLL continues in active investigation, whether as first line, as consolidation to improve the quality of remission and MRD and/or as salvage therapy to rescue resistant cases. Currently, too, Campath is being tested in combination with fludarabine and with rituximab. The combination of Campath-1H with rituximab has been reported to achieve 8% CR and 44% PR (including 40% nodular PR) in relapsed and refractory CLL. The rationale is based, in addition to lack of overlapping toxicities, on the greater effect of Campath-1H in clearing blood, bone marrow and spleen and the greater effect of rituximab in reducing nodal masses.

Rituximab (anti-CD20) has potent activity in high- and low-grade NHL and CLL when used in combination with fludarabine, FC, FCM, chlorambucil and HDMP. Its mechanism of action is by complement-dependent cytotoxicity, activation of the intrinsic pathway of apoptosis and membrane-associated kinases. The lack of T-cell immunosuppression and its good tolerability makes it ideal for older individuals. Several studies are ongoing but it is likely that all will be positive, the limiting factor remaining its high cost. Different from Campath, too, is that rituximab has limited activity on its own, unless used in very high doses, therefore remaining as an effective potentiator of apoptosis in combination with cytotoxic drugs.

Two other purine analogues with good activity in CLL are cladribine (2-chlorodeoxyadenosine or 2-CDA) and pentostatin (2-deoxycoformycin or DCF). Cladribine, in particular, can achieve as good responses as fludarabine and, in previously untreated CLL, the CR rate of the combination cladribine plus cyclophosphamide has been reported as 29% and nodular PR 24%. Although cladribine and fludarabine have not been compared directly, cladribine appears to be the more myelotoxic of the two agents.

The role of splenectomy

Splenectomy is indicated for patients with a large spleen and in whom the initial treatment achieves only a moderate reduction of the spleen size. Patients with features of hypersplenism (peripheral cytopenias and an active bone marrow) benefit from splenectomy. Splenectomy is indicated for patients with autoimmune thrombocytopenia (ITP) or haemolytic anaemia (AHA) refractory to corticosteroids. In our experience, this procedure has been associated with no mortality and seems to have been of great benefit to patients with a large spleen and blood counts consistent with stage C disease. Provided patients are given long-term penicillin, this operation often has a beneficial effect on the disease, even if only as part of a debulking procedure. Prophylaxis with pneumococcal vaccines may not be effective in advanced CLL where antibody formation is reduced, although there is evidence of antibody responses to *Haemophilus influenza* B (HiB) vaccinations. Even in patients with very advanced CLL, splenectomy improves quality of life by raising Hb levels and improving platelet counts in about 50% of them. This operation generally prolongs life and facilitates the subsequent use of further chemotherapy. A rise in the lymphocyte count is often seen after splenectomy, but still one-third of patients do not require therapy for long periods. The post-splenectomy survival was 4.7 years in our series of 47 cases of CLL.

Stem cell transplantation (SCT)

The possibility of achieving a higher rate of CR in CLL and the fact that 15% of patients are diagnosed before the age of 50 years led investigators to explore ways of improving the duration of remission or even attempting a cure by means of high-dose therapy and SCT rescue. The number of autologous and allogeneic transplants for CLL has increased dramatically in Europe in the last decade. Three modalities are currently considered: autologous SCT, conventional allogeneic with high-intensity therapy and allogeneic with low-intensity procedures, or 'mini' allografts. There are no published randomized trials, but the overall picture is reflected in the statistics collected by the European Bone Marrow Transplant (EBMT) Organization.

The feasibility of autologous SCT in CLL was tested in the MRC pilot study, which registered just over 100 patients between 1996 and 2001. After remission with fludarabine and priming with cyclophosphamide, a peripheral blood stem cell harvest was planned in the good remitters (CR, nodular PR). Only two-thirds of patients were transplanted after high-dose cyclophosphamide and TBI. Failure to do so was because of inadequate remission in 20% and failure to harvest enough stem cells (CD34$^+$ cells) in those achieving remission. What is clear, from this and other autograft studies, is that high-dose therapy may prolong remission duration with little or no transplant-related mortality (TRM). The question of long-term benefits is currently being tested in a European intergroup study, which in the

UK is MRC CLL5. It is clear that this therapy does not provide a cure as ~50% relapse in the first 5 years. A German study showed that patients with unmutated V_H genes do significantly less well than those with mutated V_H genes. Comparison of unmutated cases with a matched group treated without autograft suggests that this therapy may, in fact, be more beneficial to the unmutated or poor prognostic cases than to the mutated ones.

Allogeneic transplants in CLL may offer the chance of a cure in a minority of patients. However, the TRM of conventional allografts is ~40% in the EBMT database. Even if these figures improve in selected centres, the high mortality is unacceptable. The new modality of 'mini' allograft has lower TRM of around 18%, which is still higher than with autografts (~5%). Long-term results are not available with mini allografts, but figures of overall survival at 3 years are encouraging, though no better than with autografts. The use of unrelated donors is still experimental, but currently the TRM is high, even with the low-intensity procedures.

Management of autoimmune complications

The most common immune complications in CLL are AHA, ITP and pure red cell aplasia (PRCA). Control of haemolysis can be achieved by corticosteroids (prednisolone or dexamethasone), but long-term management requires the direct antiglobulin test to become negative. This can be achieved with the addition of another agent, usually daily cyclophosphamide (e.g. 100 mg/day), cyclosporin A (e.g. 150 mg twice a day) or mycophenolate mofetil (e.g. 1 g twice a day). Rarely, in resistant cases, these agents may be used in combination. The advantage of cyclophosphamide is that it may provide a degree of control of the CLL. Rituximab has been reported to have beneficial effect when used in combination with cyclophosphamide and dexamethasone. AHA often needs long-term treatment and may require a splenectomy. When the direct antiglobulin test remains positive, the risk of haemolysis remains.

Immune thrombocytopenia, although less common, also requires active treatment as for AHA. High-dose gammaglobulin infusions over 5 days may improve the platelet count and are often a good guide as to the subsequent benefit of splenectomy. Cyclosporin A and rituximab are both effective in refractory ITP. Slow infusions of vinca alkaloids, e.g. 1 mg of vincristine, and danazol have been useful in some cases. ITP is usually more difficult to manage than AHA and, more often than in the latter, one needs to resort to splenectomy.

Pure red cell aplasia is an uncommon but well-recognized complication. Some cases are secondary to a parvovirus B19 infection. Rituximab and Campath-1H have been reported to be able to reverse this process which is sometimes very acute. It is paradoxical that rituximab and Campath-1H have occasionally been reported to facilitate parvovirus infection and cause PRCA. Rituximab has also been associated with delayed-onset neutropenia. On the other hand, fludarabine can occasionally induce remission of PRCA and refractory ITP, although more commonly it has the opposite effect. The exact mechanism of the immune complications in CLL is still poorly understood and this explains the unusual, but well-documented, reports of the same agents causing or correcting these complications.

Supportive care

The main objective of treatment for CLL is to prolong survival with a good quality of life; therefore, care should be taken to prevent and/or treat promptly any complications arising from the immunodeficiency associated with the disease or its treatment. Thus, prompt antibiotic treatment for seemingly benign upper respiratory tract infections and antiviral measures to prevent the spread of herpetic infections are as important as the specific treatment for the disease. Patients with repeated infections and very low gammaglobulin levels may benefit from courses of intravenous gammaglobulin injections, e.g. 400 mg/kg every 4 weeks, particularly during the winter. Additional measures are the administration of allopurinol when starting therapy with a WBC > 50×10^9/L, oral antifungals and H_2 blockers or proton pump inhibitors when using corticosteroids.

Causes of infection in CLL are multifactorial. Neutropenic episodes during chemotherapy require the use of G-CSF. Patients with long-term respiratory infections may require active prophylactic measures such as nebulized antibiotics to prevent Gram-negative infections. Cotrimoxazole is mandatory to prevent infections, particularly PCP, when fludarabine or Campath-1H are used. The latter requires regular monitoring for cytomegalovirus (CMV) and prompt treatment when such immunosuppressed patients, usually lymphopenic, become symptomatic and positive for CMV. The main factors predisposing to infections in CLL are the number of chemotherapy regimens and the activity of the disease more than the levels of serum immunoglobulins.

Erythropoietin (Epo) is now an accepted treatment for anaemia associated with cancer therapy. Patients with CLL and persistent anaemia (Hb < 10 g/dL) will benefit from Epo given three times a week or 40 000 units weekly. There is strong evidence for benefits, particularly an improvement in quality of life. Epo should be given for a minimum of 4 weeks before deciding that there is no response, and iron deposits need to be adequate. There is no evidence that Epo is useful in PRCA. Folic acid supplements are often useful in patients with macrocytic indices resulting from low folate levels. They should always be given in AHA.

Secondary MDS/AML

The increased intensity of treatments, in particular combinations of alkylating agents and purine analogues, may be responsible for an increased incidence of secondary myelodysplasia and acute myeloid leukaemia in CLL. Combinations with mitozantrone and the use of TBI for stem cell transplants are also major risk factors for these secondary events. Single-agent therapy with chlorambucil or fludarabine is rarely associated with MDS/AML.

Prolymphocytic leukaemia

Prolymphocytic leukaemia (B-PLL) was considered a variant of CLL since its description by Galton *et al.* in 1974. In the last decade it has become apparent that there are important clinical and laboratory differences between these two disorders which, despite the existence of the group with CLL/PL discussed above, suggest that B-PLL is a distinct, but rare, disorder. This is supported by differences in the morphology and cell markers (Table 38.2), physical signs (almost exclusively splenomegaly in PLL) and clinical evolution. The key for diagnosis is the recognition of the prolymphocyte as the predominant cell in well-prepared peripheral blood films. The mean age of patients presenting with B-PLL is 70 years, which is 5 years older than the main age of CLL patients.

The main features of B-PLL are splenomegaly without lymphadenopathy, and a high WBC, usually over 100×10^9/L at the time of presentation. Anaemia and thrombocytopenia (as for stage C CLL) are seen in at least 50% of cases. Other laboratory findings are no different from high-count CLL – increased uric acid, low serum immunoglobulins – but the incidence of a monoclonal band appears to be higher than in CLL.

Differential diagnosis

The main diagnostic criterion is the identification of prolymphocytes as the predominant population in blood films. Usually, 55% prolymphocytes is the figure that discriminates B-PLL from CLL and CLL/PL, although the percentage of prolymphocytes in B-PLL is usually greater than 70%. The prolymphocyte is twice the size of a small CLL lymphocyte, has moderately condensed nuclear chromatin, a prominent central nucleolus and a lower nucleolus:cytoplasmic ratio than CLL cells (Figure 38.16). B prolymphocytes are more uniform and have a more regular nuclear outline than those of CLL/PL. They are larger and have clearer cytoplasm and a lower nucleolus:cytoplasmic ratio than T prolymphocytes. Using the scoring system depicted in Table 38.1, most B-PLL scored 0–1 and, rarely, 2 or 3. One-third of cases of B-PLL may be CD5 positive; this and other features may present a diagnostic problem with MCL with leukaemia.

The distinction from HCL variant is based mainly on the appearances of the cytoplasm; in HCL variant the cytoplasm is more abundant and distinctly villous, whereas in B-PLL it is generally smooth.

The issue of MCL was reviewed recently by us in eight cases diagnosed in the past as B-PLL but bearing the translocation t(11;14)(q13;32) characteristic of MCL. Detailed histology review and comparison with 13 cases of B-PLL without t(11;14) led us

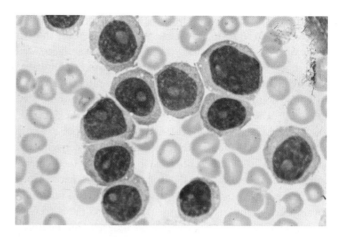

Figure 38.16 Typical blood film from a case of B-prolymphocytic leukaemia with the characteristic large size, abundant cytoplasm and prominent nucleolus.

to the conclusion that the cases with t(11;14) and which over-express cyclin D1 represent a splenomegalic form of MCL.

Treatment

Alkylating agents, e.g. chlorambucil or the combination COP, are of little value in the management of B-PLL. Response rates (partial responses and rare CRs) to splenic irradiation and/or the combination cyclophosphamide, doxorubicin, oncovin and prednisone (CHOP) have been recorded in up to one-third of cases. Splenectomy is often useful to remove a major proliferative focus which represents a considerable part of the tumour mass in this disease, to relieve hypersplenism and facilitate further therapy. Considering the older age group affected by B-PLL, splenectomy is not a practical proposition in some patients. Preliminary data suggest that 50% of patients may respond with partial or complete remission to fludarabine. There are insufficient data on the use of fludarabine combinations (FC, FCM, FCR) in B-PLL. One of the reasons for the poor response to therapy in this disease is the high frequency of p53 abnormalities, documented in 50–60% of cases.

Hairy cell leukaemia

Hairy cell leukaemia (HCL) is a well-recognized clinicopathological entity which affects males more frequently than females (M/F ratio 4:1), usually over the age of 40 years. The disease has, historically, elicited great interest, for different reasons: in the 1960s, in order to establish the diagnostic features of the newly described entity and subsequently, in the 1970s and 80s, advances in immunology led to the identification of the hairy cell as a B cell and demonstrated rearrangement of the heavy- and light-chain immunoglobulin genes. In the 1980s and 1990s,

HCL attracted considerable attention because of the significant advances in its treatment, first with alpha-interferon (IFN-α) and later with the purine analogues pentostatin and cladribine.

Clinical and laboratory findings

The main disease features result from the pancytopenia affecting most patients. HCL patients are moderately neutropenic and severely monocytopenic; thus, bacterial and opportunistic infections do occur. There is evidence that the incidence of typical and atypical mycobacterial infections is increased, but this was seen more frequently before the current treatments became available.

The main physical signs are splenomegaly and hepatomegaly. Lymphadenopathy is rare, but we have reported cases with massive abdominal lymphadenopathy and morphological features suggestive of transformation. A survey by routine CT scan showed a higher incidence than hitherto suspected of enlarged abdominal nodes. This is seen more often in relapsed patients and those with long-standing HCL and it tends to correlate with bulky disease.

Anaemia results from reduced bone marrow production and splenic pooling. Haemolysis is exceptional. The WBC may be low, normal or high (rarely above 20×10^9/L), but neutropenia and monocytopenia are constant. Some patients have no detectable hairy cells on blood films; two-thirds have 10–15% and others more than 50%. Patients with low WBC and no circulating hairy cells present diagnostic problems. Platelet counts are below 100×10^9/L in most cases.

Diagnosis

The recognition of typical hairy cells in peripheral blood films is useful for establishing or suggesting this diagnosis. Hairy cells are large – twice the size of a normal lymphocyte – and have abundant cytoplasm (low N/C ratio) which is characteristically villous in its outline (Figure 38.17). The nucleus is round, oval or slightly indented, and occasionally bilobed. A smooth nuclear chromatin, absence of a visible nucleolus and low N/C ratio are landmarks of typical hairy cells. Cells from the rare HCL variant have similar cytoplasmic features but have a round nucleolus with more condensed chromatin and a distinct nucleolus resembling prolymphocytes (Figure 38.18).

Bone marrow aspirates are, as a rule, unsuccessful as no fragments and few cells are obtained. Therefore, a trephine biopsy is essential. This shows diffuse interstitial infiltration of variable degree; occasionally the infiltration is focal. A typical feature is the arrangement of the cellular infiltrate, which is loose, leaving plenty of space between cells, often with a clear zone around each cell which is unique to this condition (Figures 38.19 and 38.20). This contrasts with the more dense infiltration in CLL and PLL or the paratrabecular involvement in NHL. Reticulin is always increased (Figure 38.21) and the cells stain strongly with

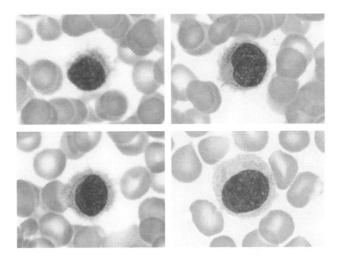

Figure 38.17 Individual hairy cells from blood films from two patients with HCL.

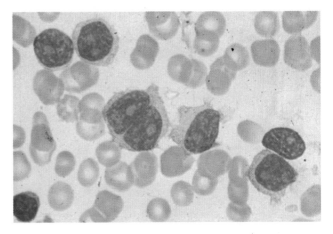

Figure 38.18 Blood film from a case of HCL variant showing large nucleolated villous cells, one of them binucleated.

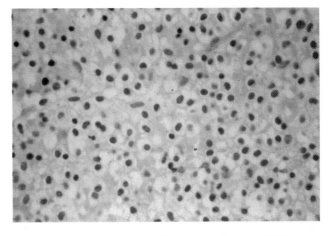

Figure 38.19 Bone marrow trephine section of a case of HCL showing the typical clear zone around the hairy cells in a paraffin embedded section.

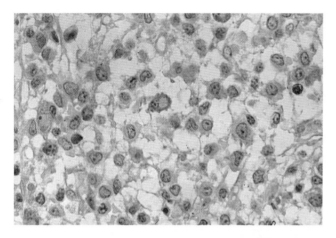

Figure 38.20 Bone marrow trephine from a case of HCL embedded in methacrylate giving good morphological detail of the hairy cells.

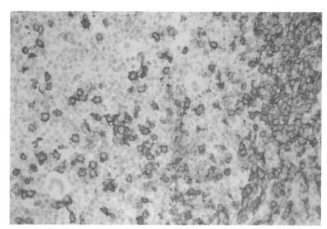

Figure 38.22 Staining for CD20 in a bone marrow section from HCL before treatment.

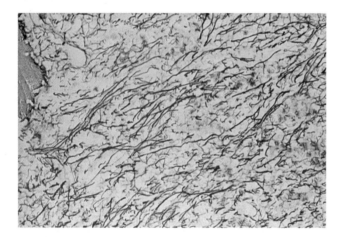

Figure 38.21 Increased reticulin pattern in a case of HCL.

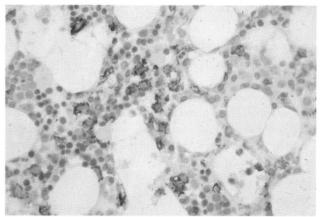

Figure 38.23 Staining for CD20 in a patient treated for HCL showing a cluster of residual CD20$^+$ cells, suggesting that the remission is incomplete.

anti-CD20 (Figure 38.22). The immunocytochemical staining for CD20 is crucial to demonstrate clusters of hairy cells following therapy, suggesting residual disease. This is otherwise difficult to assess on conventional sections (Figure 38.23).

Spleen histology, when available, shows distinct diagnostic features: infiltration by mononuclear cells with a blunt nucleus in the red pulp with little residual white pulp, and formation of pseudosinuses filled with erythrocytes ('red cell lakes'). Tartrate-resistant acid phosphatase (TRAP) demonstrated on hairy cells corresponds to a unique isoenzyme 5 and is specific for HCL. This enzyme is now tested by means of a MAb. Electron microscopy reveals ribosome–lamella complexes in one-third of the cases. Rarely, this intracytoplasmic inclusion can be seen on light microscopy.

Hairy cells are considered activated B cells with features of late maturation stages. SmIg is usually strong and characteristically shows several heavy-chain isotopes, often including IgA and

IgG and sharing a single heavy chain. The cells of most cases of HCL variant express IgG as a single heavy chain. HCL cells are strongly FMC7, CD20 and CD22 positive but, in contrast to other B-cell disorders, they consistently express CD25, CD103 and CD123. In contrast to CLL, hairy cells are always CD5 negative and their score using the CLL panel is very low (Table 38.2).

The HCL variant is very rare and is characterized by high WBC ($50-80 \times 10^9$/L) and splenomegaly. The cells do not express CD25 and CD123. They are often CD11c positive and, in half of the cases, CD103 is also positive. The bone marrow and spleen histology of the HCL variant closely resemble the typical disease. The main diagnostic difficulty in HCL variant is with splenic marginal zone lymphoma (or SLVL), except for the spleen histology which, in the former is mainly red pulp and in the latter predominantly white pulp.

Treatment

Many modalities have been tried in the past to improve the bone marrow function of patients with HCL. The prime objective of treatment should be the normalization of blood counts, as pancytopenia is the main source of complications, and to induce prolonged remissions. There are now two main agents, cladribine and pentostatin, which are widely used. In the past, only moderate success was seen with low-dose chlorambucil, splenic irradiation or even anthracyclines, and these are no longer indicated in HCL. Other treatments still used but for specific indications are splenectomy and IFN-α.

Splenectomy is a well-established treatment and has been shown to improve the quality of life and prolong survival in this disease. It should now be reserved for patients with very large spleens and some bone marrow reserve. In about 20% of successfully splenectomized patients, the counts remain normal for many years and no other therapy is thus indicated; some of them may never relapse although they may remain with little bone marrow involvement.

Interferon-α was used widely since the first report by Quesada in 1984. IFN-α induces a gradual normalization of blood counts, reduction of hairy cells in the blood and gradually from the bone marrow, return of monocytes and improvement of neutropenia. The improvements in the blood are not associated with a clearance in the bone marrow, and CRs are seen in only 20–30% of cases. The duration of response once IFN-α is discontinued is relatively short (median 15–18 months), although blood counts may remain normal for well over a year. The tendency once therapy has ceased is to relapse slowly. IFN-α is now reserved for problem cases and to help initial treatment in patients with severe cytopenias.

The two agents currently used in HCL, pentostatin (deoxycoformycin) and cladribine (2-chlorodeoxyadenosine), achieve CR in 80–85% of patients, with the remainder being partial responders. True resistance is seldom seen at first treatment. Long-term results are excellent, with very few patients actually dying of HCL. Ninety per cent of all patients and 95% of those with CR are alive at 10 years if one excludes non-HCL causes of death. About 30–40% tend to relapse once treatment is discontinued in the first 5–10 years (Figure 38.24). Relapses after 10 years are rare. Second CRs are obtained in 75% of patients and there is no evidence of cross-resistance between these agents. Despite this, a small group of patients tend to relapse every 2 or 3 years. For this group, plus the rare non-responders to purine analogues and those who achieve only PR, who in our experience have poorer survival than complete remitters, new modalities need to be developed.

Monoclonal antibodies against CD20 (rituximab) and CD22 (coupled with an immunotoxin) have now shown activity in HCL. Hairy cells express strongly CD20 and CD22, and these antibodies seem to achieve good responses in the group of relapsing patients, although, when rituximab is used alone in

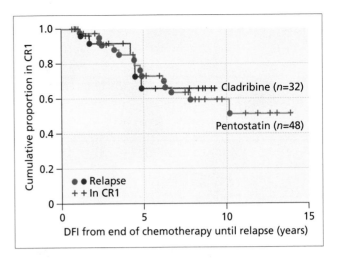

Figure 38.24 Disease-free interval (DFI) in previously untreated patients with HCL treated with pentostatin or cladribine, showing a median DFI close to 10 years in those achieving a complete remission (CR1).

cladribine relapses, the CR rate is low (~15%). Its main role may be, as in other B-cell disorders, when used in combination with one of the purine analogues.

Patients with HCL variant respond less well to cladribine and pentostatin and not at all to IFN-α. Good palliation of symptoms and improvement of blood counts can be achieved with splenectomy which, in our experience, has been the most successful modality in this relatively resistant disease.

Supportive care for HCL is confined to patients undergoing therapy with nucleoside analogues, which can cause transient neutropenia in the early phases and prolonged lymphopenia later on. Long-term cotrimoxazole until lymphocyte counts rise above $1 \times 10^9/L$ and also long periods on aciclovir are recommended. Major infections are only seen in untreated patients or those responding poorly to therapy.

The leukaemic phase of low-grade NHL

There are three types of NHL which not infrequently evolve with lymphocytosis which mimics and can be confused with, CLL. These are follicular lymphoma (FL), splenic marginal zone lymphoma or splenic lymphoma with circulating villous lymphocytes (SLVL) and mantle cell lymphoma (MCL).

Follicular lymphoma

Fifteen per cent of FL patients may have circulating lymphoma cells ($5–20 \times 10^9/L$), and this correlates with bone marrow involvement. A minority may present with WBC $> 40 \times 10^9/L$ (up to $200 \times 10^9/L$) and extensive disease, generalized lymphadenopathy and hepatosplenomegaly. Usually the circulating cells

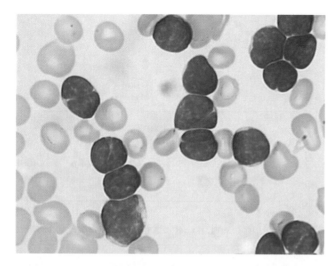

Figure 38.25 Blood film of a patient with follicular lymphoma presenting with significant lymphocytosis (55×10^9/L). The cells show a cleaved nucleus, angular shape, homogeneous chromatin pattern, high N/C ratio and small size.

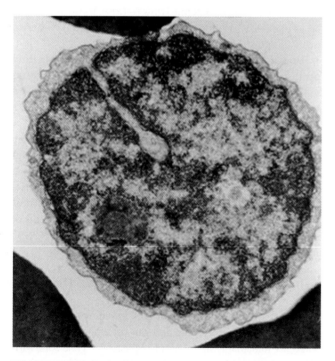

Figure 38.26 Electron microscopy of a circulating follicular centre lymphocyte showing a deep nuclear cleft.

are very small with almost no visible cytoplasm, the nuclear chromatin is smooth without clumps of heterochromatin and no visible nucleolus, and the nuclear shape is angular and has a small cleft (Figure 38.25). This is seen also at ultrastructural level (Figure 38.26). The differential diagnosis from CLL is supported by the immunophenotype. FL cells usually score 0 or

1 (Figure 38.1). Lymph node histology is essential to confirm a diagnosis of FL. Only patients with very high WBC may have poor prognosis; cases with a minor degree of spillover respond as cases without circulating cells. It is important to recall that late-stage FL may have circulating blasts (centroblasts) characterized by a peripherally located nucleolus and this corresponds with transformation to a large-cell lymphoma.

Splenic lymphoma

Splenic lymphoma with villous lymphocytes has now been recognized by the WHO classification as a distinct pathological entity described as splenic marginal zone lymphoma (SMZL). It is likely that at least two-thirds of patients with this lymphoma have circulating villous lymphocytes. A minority do not have frankly villous cells despite being clonal and in some the diagnosis can be suspected without circulating lymphocytes but can only be established after splenectomy. Therefore, the true incidence of this condition without circulating villous cells is unknown. A Spanish study of 60 patients, all splenectomized, described > 5% circulating abnormal cells in 68%, with a WBC greater than 4×10^9/L in 70%; their median lymphocyte count was ~8×10^9/L. Our own data on 129 patients with SLVL showed a median WBC of 16×10^9/L, median Hb of 11.8 g/dL and platelets 145×10^9/L.

Splenic lymphoma with villous lymphocytes is an indolent form of NHL. The median age of patients is 69 years and the majority present with splenomegaly. There is a slight female predominance. Anaemia and/or thrombocytopenia are seen in 40% of cases. One-third of patients have a serum monoclonal band, usually IgM below 30 g/L. Diagnosis is suspected on a typical blood film (Figure 38.27) showing small lymphocytes with an irregular membrane outline and short villi, often confined to

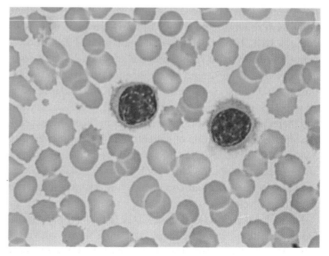

Figure 38.27 Lymphocytes from a case of splenic lymphoma with circulating villous lymphocytes.

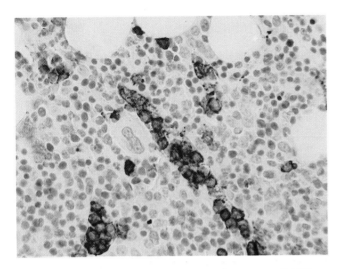

Figure 38.28 Bone marrow trephine biopsy from a case of SLVL showing the characteristic intrasinusoidal infiltration seen in this disease highlighted by the anti-CD20 antibody.

one pole of the cells. A nucleolus is visible in half of the cases. Cytoplasmic basophilia is seen in ~10% of lymphocytes. The immunophenotype (Table 38.2) is different from CLL. SLVL cells can be distinguished from HCL and the HCL variant because they are negative with CD103 and CD123; they express CD25 and are always CD11c positive.

Bone marrow aspirates may show the same cells as in the blood, with variable degrees of infiltration. It has become apparent in the last few years that a distinct pattern of intrasinusoidal infiltration (Figure 38.28) is characteristic of SLVL and is highlighted with anti-B-cell antibodies (CD20, CD79a). This pattern of infiltration is rare in other types of NHL. In addition, the pattern of bone marrow infiltration can be nodular, interstitial and/or paratrabecular.

The spleen histology shows a characteristic bizoned pattern in the white pulp with a central zone of small lymphocytes with scanty cytoplasm and a peripheral zone of larger cells with more dispersed chromatin and more abundant cytoplasm. The red pulp is always infiltrated by both the smaller and larger cells. Plasmacytic differentiation may be seen.

There is no unique cytogenetic abnormality in SLVL but unbalanced translocations and deletions of 7q22–32 have been described in ~30%; 50% of cases have a monoallelic deletion at 13q14 but, in contrast to CLL, it affects mainly the RB1 locus. Trisomy 3, an abnormality seen in extranodal marginal zone lymphoma, has been found in 17% of cases. Abnormalities of p53 (mainly deletions) are found in 17% of cases and are associated with worse prognosis. Studies of the IgV$_H$ genes shows a heterogeneous pattern of mutations. Two-thirds of cases show V$_H$ mutations and one-third of cases are unmutated, currently without any apparent clinical or prognostic implications. Ongo-

ing mutations, a feature also seen in FL, has been observed in some cases.

An association with hepatitis C has been reported but the incidence of this event is unknown. Of interest is that IFN-α has been reported to induce CR in hepatitis C-positive SLVL patients. An association in hyper-reactive malaria and tropical splenomegaly has been described in African cases. Large-cell transformation is seen in 10% of cases, and this is related to p53 abnormalities.

Splenectomy is the treatment of choice in this disease, with splenectomized patients faring significantly better than those treated with chemotherapy only. Conventional therapies with alkylating agents and the combination CHOP are not very effective. Fludarabine has been recently reported to induce a high rate of complete remissions. The median survival in our series is 13 years, with 72% of patients alive at 5 years. Anaemia and lymphocytosis greater than 16×10^9/L seem to be associated with worse outcome.

Mantle cell lymphoma

Mantle cell lymphoma has been recognized as a distinct pathological entity for the last 12 years. Blood and bone marrow involvement are common. Possibly 40–50% of cases of MCL evolving with splenomegaly (non-nodal form) have significant lymphocytosis, sometimes mimicking CLL, CLL/PL or B-PLL (see above).

Morphologically, the cells are of medium size with a variable amount of cytoplasm, an irregular nucleus with nuclear cleft, a distinctly stippled chromatin pattern and an indistinct nucleolus (Figure 38.29). When the latter is seen in many cells, B-PLL is suspected. If the small lymphocytes predominate or if there is a mixture of small and large cells, CLL/PL is suspected. Rare cases, in our experience, have a high WBC count with cells resembling

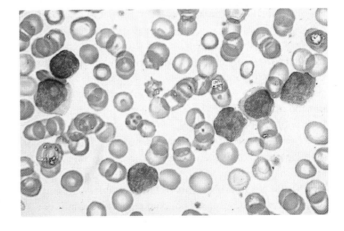

Figure 38.29 Blood film from a patient with mantle cell lymphoma and lymphocytosis. The cells are medium size, slightly irregular in shape and have a speckled nuclear chromatin pattern.

those of SLVL. A lymphoblastoid form with blast-like cells has also been recognized.

Marker studies show that MCL cells are always CD5$^+$, CD19$^+$, CD20$^+$, thus raising the issue of CLL. In a series of over 60 cases which we studied, the majority (68%) scored 1, being CD5$^+$ but CD23$^-$ (in contrast to CLL), 17% scored 0 (CD5$^-$, CD23$^-$) and 15% scored 2 or 3 (CD5$^+$, CD23$^+$).

The bone marrow trephine biopsy shows a rather monotonous infiltration by slightly irregular cells. Crucially, and in contrast with CLL and particularly CLL/PL, no proliferating centres are seen in MCL (nor in the lymph node biopsies). The pattern of bone marrow infiltration is often diffuse in advanced cases, but in other cases is nodular and/or paratrabecular.

The characteristic translocation t(11;14)(q13;q32) is demonstrated in all cases by conventional cytogenetics or more easily by FISH analysis. The rearrangement of the Bcl-1/PRAD-1 gene at 11q13 results in the overexpression of cyclin D1, one of the proteins that controls the cell cycle. Cyclin D1 can be demonstrated in histological sections. Techniques for its demonstration by flow cytometry or by detecting cyclin D1 mRNA are also available but are less simple.

The correlation between cyclin D1 overexpression and t(11;14) is very high, in our experience. Studies on the mutational status of the IgV$_H$ genes has demonstrated, as in CLL and SLVL, molecular heterogeneity. About 30% of patients showed a mutated pattern and biased use of specific V$_H$ segments, particularly V$_H$3–21 and V$_H$3–34, which are seen also in mutated cases of CLL. A UK study showed different patterns of V$_H$ mutations in MCL presenting with lymphocytosis. Among a group described as non-nodal (76% had splenomegaly), 56% of patients had mutated V$_H$ genes, while 90% of the group with peripheral lymphadenopathy, described as nodal, had unmutated V$_H$ genes. There was a significant survival difference between these two groups: the non-nodal group had a median survival of 79 months whilst in the nodal group it was 30 months. Although the mutational status did not affect survival per se, a small group of long survivors were seen in the mutated group.

Therapy in MCL has been unsatisfactory, although improvements have recently been reported using fludarabine combinations such as fludarabine, cyclophosphamide and mitozantrone plus rituximab, as reported by a German study. A significant proportion of MCL patients have p53 abnormalities which underlie their poor response to therapy.

We reported good responses to splenectomy in MCL patients with leukaemia and splenomegaly. The average weight of the spleen in this group was 2.6 kg. Two-thirds of the patients benefited, with improvements in blood counts. A minority of the patients (4 out of 16) did not require further therapy for relatively prolonged periods, with improvements in the pre-existing cytopenias. It is possible that the group which most benefits from splenectomy is the one with mutated V$_H$ genes and described as non-nodal in the study by Orchard et al. (2003).

Selected bibliography

Bennett JM, Catovsky D, Daniel MT et al. (1989) Proposals for the classification of chronic (mature) B and T lymphoid leukaemias. French–American–British (FAB) Cooperative Group. Journal of Clinical Pathology 42: 567–84.

Binet JL, Auquier A, Dighiero G et al. (1981) A new prognostic classification of chronic lymphocytic leukemia derived from a multivariate survival analysis. Cancer 48: 198–206.

Bosanquet AG, Johnson SA, Richards SM (1999) Prognosis for fludarabine therapy of chronic lymphocytic leukaemia based on ex vivo drug response by DiSC assay. British Journal of Haematology 106: 71–7.

Caligaris-Cappio F (2003) Role of the microenvironment in chronic lymphocytic leukaemia. British Journal of Haematology 123: 380–8.

CLL Trialists' Collaborative Group (1999) Chemotherapeutic options in chronic lymphocytic leukemia: a meta-analysis of the randomized trials. Journal of the National Cancer Institute 91: 861–8.

Cheson BD, Bennett JM, Grever M et al. (1996) National Cancer Institute-sponsored Working Group guidelines for chronic lymphocytic leukemia: revised guidelines for diagnosis and treatment. Blood 87: 4990–7.

Crespo M, Bosch F, Villamor N et al. (2003) ZAP-70 expression as a surrogate for immunoglobulin-variable-region mutations in chronic lymphocytic leukemia. New England Journal of Medicine 18: 1764–75.

Damle RN, Wasil T, Fais F et al. (1999) Ig V gene mutation status and CD38 expression as novel prognostic indicators in chronic lymphocytic leukemia. Blood 94: 1840–7.

Del Giudice I, Matutes E, Morilla R et al. (2004) The diagnostic value of CD123 in B-cell disorders with hairy or villous lymphocytes. Haematologica 89: 303–8.

Delgado J, Matutes E, Morilla AM et al. (2003) Diagnostic significance of CD20 and FMC7 expression in B-cell disorders. American Journal of Clinical Pathology 120: 754–9.

Dewald GW, Brockman SR, Paternoster SF et al. (2003) Chromosome anomalies detected by interphase fluorescence in-site hybridization: correlation with significant biological features of B-cell chronic lymphocytic leukaemia. British Journal of Haematology 121: 287–95.

Dyer MJ, Oscier DG (2002) The configuration of the immunoglobulin genes in B cell chronic lymphocytic leukaemia. Leukemia 16: 973–84.

Franco V, Florena AM, Iannitto E (2003) Splenic marginal zone lymphoma. Blood 101: 2464–72.

Galton DAG, Goldman JM, Wiltshaw E et al. (1974) Prolymphocytic leukaemia. British Journal of Haematology 27: 7–23.

Garcia-Marco JA, Price CM, Ellis J et al. (1996) Correlation of trisomy 12 with proliferating cells by combined immunocytochemistry and fluorescence in situ hybridization in chronic lymphocytic leukemia. Leukemia 10: 1705–11.

Giles FJ, Bekele BN, O'Brien S et al. (2003) A prognostic model for survival in chronic lymphocytic leukaemia based on p53 expression. British Journal of Haematology 121: 578–85.

Hamblin TJ, Davis Z, Gardiner A, Oscier D, Stevenson FK (1999) Unmutated Ig V_H genes are associated with a more aggressive form of chronic lymphocytic leukemia. *Blood* **94**: 1848–54.

Hedenus M, Adriansson M, San Miguel J *et al.* (2003) Efficacy and safety of darbepoetin alfa in anaemic patients with lymphoproliferative malignancies: a randomized, double blinded placebo-controlled study. *British Journal of Haematology* **122**: 394–403.

Houlston RS, Sellick G, Yuille M, Matutes E, Catovsky D (2003) Causation of chronic lymphocytic leukemia–insights from familial disease. *Leukemia Research* **27**: 871–6.

Jaffe ES, Harris NL, Stein H *et al.* (eds) (2001) *Pathology and Genetics of Tumours of Haematopoietic and Lymphoid Tissues. World Health Organization Classification of Tumours.* IARC Press, Lyon.

Keating MJ, Kantarjian H, O'Brien S *et al.* (1991) Fludarabine: a new agent with marked cytoreductive activity in untreated chronic lymphocytic leukemia. *Journal of Clinical Oncology* **9**: 44–9.

Krober A, Seiler T, Benner A *et al.* (2002) V_H mutation status, CD38 expression level, genomic aberrations, and survival in chronic lymphocytic leukemia. *Blood* **100**: 1410–16.

Lampert IA, Wotherspoon A, Van Noorden, Hasserjian RP (1999) High expression of CD23 in the proliferation centres of chronic lymphocytic leukaemia in lymph nodes and spleen. *Human Pathology* **30**: 648–54.

Matutes E, Owusu-Ankomah K, Morilla R *et al.* (1994) The immunological profile of B-cell disorders and proposal of a scoring system for the diagnosis of CLL. *Leukemia* **8**: 1640–5.

Matutes E, Parry-Jones N, Brito-Babapulle V *et al.* (2004) The leukemic presentation of mantle-cell lymphoma: disease features and prognostic factors in 58 patients. *Leukemia and Lymphoma* **45**: 2007–15.

Moreau EJ, Matutes E, A'Hern RP *et al.* (1997) Improvement of the chronic lymphocytic leukemia scoring system with the monoclonal antibody SN8 (CD79b). *American Journal of Clinical Pathology* **108**: 378–82.

Orchard J, Garand R, Davis Z *et al.* (2003) A subset of t(11;14) lymphoma with mantle cell features displays mutated IgV_H genes and includes patients with good prognosis, nonnodal disease. *Blood* **101**: 4975–81.

Parry-Jones N, Matutes E, Gruszka-Westwood AM *et al.* (2003) Prognostic features of splenic lymphoma with villous lymphocytes: a report on 129 patients. *British Journal of Haematology* **120**: 759–64.

Rai KR, Sawitsky A, Cronkite E *et al.* (1975) Clinical staging of chronic lymphocytic leukemia. *Blood* **46**: 219–34.

Rawstron AC, Yuille MR, Fuller J *et al.* (2002) Inherited predisposition to CLL is detectable as subclinical monoclonal B-lymphocyte expansion. *Blood* **100**: 2289–90.

Ruchlemer R, Wotherspoon AC, Thompson JN *et al.* (2002) Splenectomy in mantle cell lymphoma with leukaemia: a comparison with chronic lymphocytic leukaemia. *British Journal of Haematology* **118**: 952–8.

Staudt LM (2003) Molecular diagnosis of the hematologic cancers. *New England Journal of Medicine* **348**: 1777–85.

Thomas R, Ribeiro I, Shepherd P *et al.* (2002) Spontaneous clinical regression in chronic lymphocytic leukaemia. *British Journal of Haematology* **116**: 341–5.

Thornton PD, Gruszka-Westwood AM, Hamoudi RA *et al.* (2003) Characterization of TP53 abnormalities in chronic lymphocytic leukaemia. *The Haematology Journal* **5**: 47–54.

Wiestner A, Rosenwald A, Barry TS *et al.* (2003) ZAP-70 expression identifies a chronic lymphocytic leukemia subtype with unmutated immunoglobulin genes, inferior clinical outcome, and distinct gene expression profile. *Blood* **101**: 4944–51.

CHAPTER 39

T-cell lymphoproliferative disorders

Estella Matutes

Introduction and classification

The chronic or mature T-cell lymphoproliferative disorders comprise a variety of disease entities which result from the clonal proliferation of post-thymic T lymphocytes. They should be distinguished from the immature or thymic derived T-cell neoplasms, i.e. T-cell acute lymphoblastic leukaemia (T-ALL) and lymphoblastic lymphomas as the disease course and therapeutic approaches are very different. The distinction between these two groups of T-cell malignancies is made on clinical grounds, immunophenotype and cell morphology [terminal transferase (TdT)-positive blasts in T-ALL compared with TdT-negative mature T lymphocytes in chronic T-cell disorders].

The incidence of the T-cell disorders varies around the world. Overall they are more common in Eastern and rare in Western countries, where they account for 10–15% of lymphoid malignancies. This different distribution may relate to both host and environmental factors. Advances in immunophenotyping and molecular cytogenetics together with a detailed analysis of the cell morphology and histopathology have significantly contributed to a more precise classification of the T-cell neoplasms. Further, the role of viruses in T-cell malignancies, essentially the Epstein–Barr virus (EBV) and the human T-cell leukaemia lymphoma virus type I (HTLV-I), has been well recognized. HTLV-I is the primary aetiological agent of adult T-cell leukaemia lymphoma (ATLL), and EBV has been shown to be involved in the pathogenesis of certain lymphomas such as the extranodal nasal angiocentric lymphomas.

These advances have not only shed some light onto the pathogenesis of these diseases but have also resulted in better approaches to managing these patients. Information on the gene profiles assessed by microarray analysis is scanty and still in its infancy. However, it is likely that in the near future they will have a major impact by allowing the devising of novel targeted therapies as well as helping to elucidate new genes or oncogenes involved in the pathogenesis of these disorders.

For classification purposes of the T-lymphoproliferative disorders, it is essential to compound the clinical features with laboratory investigations. The latter should include (i) lymphocyte morphology; (ii) histology of bone marrow and lymphoid tissues; (iii) immunological markers; (iv) cytogenetics using standard techniques or fluorescence *in situ* hybridization (FISH); (v) analysis of the T-cell receptor (TCR) chain genes by Southern blot or polymerase chain reaction (PCR) to demonstrate clonality of the T-cell population; and (vi) serology for HTLV-I and, if needed, DNA analysis to document the clonal integration of this retrovirus. Some of these investigations are key diagnostic tests while others may have prognostic or therapeutical implications. In addition, molecular analysis to search for certain oncogenes such as *TCL-1*, *p53*, etc. is relevant by giving some clues in the pathogenesis and/or progression of the disease.

On the basis of the clinical manifestations and origin of the neoplasm, the T-lymphoid disorders can be classified in three main groups: (i) primary leukaemias which arise in the bone marrow and evolve with a leukaemic picture; (ii) leukaemia/lymphoma syndromes or the leukaemic phase of T-cell lymphomas (T-NHL) in which the tumour arises in lymphoid tissues but a leukaemic picture is very common; and (iii) T-NHL, which originate in peripheral lymphoid tissues and very rarely involve the blood. Each of these groups includes disease entities distinguishable by their clinical and laboratory features and the majority have been recognized as such by the WHO classification (Table 39.1).

The disease features of the T-cell malignancies, the basis for diagnosis, their prognosis and management as well as the pathogenic events involved in disease initiation and/or progression will be described.

Primary leukaemias

This group includes two diseases: T-prolymphocytic leukaemia (T-PLL) and T-cell large granular lymphocyte leukaemia (T-LGL leukaemia).

Table 39.1 Classification of T-cell lymphoproliferative disorders.

Primary leukaemias
T-cell prolymphocytic leukaemia (T-PLL)
T-cell large granular lymphocyte (LGL) leukaemia

Leukaemia/lymphoma syndromes
Sézary's syndrome (SS)/mycosis fungoides (MF)
Adult T-cell leukaemia lymphoma (ATLL)

Peripheral T-cell lymphomas (T-NHL)
Unspecified
Specific variants
   Hepatosplenic γ/δ T-NHL
   Subcutaneous panniculitis-like T-NHL
   Angioimmunoblastic (AIL)
   Extranodal T/NK, nasal type
   Enteropathy T-NHL (intestinal)
   Anaplastic large-cell lymphoma (ALCL)

T-prolymphocytic leukaemia (T-PLL)

T-prolymphocytic leukaemia was first documented in a patient presenting with clinical features similar to B-PLL but in whom the cells had a T-cell phenotype. T-PLL is recognized in the WHO classification as a distinct T-cell disorder with three morphological variants. Despite the morphological heterogeneity, all these variants have a similar clinical course and identical molecular genetics.

Aetiology

T-prolymphocytic leukaemia is a rare disease and together with B-cell PLL accounts for around 2% of all mature lymphoid leukaemias. It is overall more frequent than B-cell PLL. T-PLL has been described in the West and East without a geographical or racial clustering. There is no evidence that radiation, carcinogenic agents and/or viruses play a role in the pathogenesis of T-PLL. However, there is a prevalence of T-PLL in patients with ataxia telangiectasia (AT) and it has been speculated, but not yet proven, that the AT mutated gene (*ATM*) may play a role in the development of T-PLL (see Pathogenesis).

Clinical features

T-PLL affects adults (median age 65 years) and is more frequent in males. Patients manifest with widespread disease and close to one-third with skin lesions. Main physical signs are hepatosplenomegaly and lymphadenopathy. Effusions are seen in 15% of patients but are frequent at a terminal and/or relapse phase of the disease; central nervous system (CNS) involvement is rare (Table 39.2). A few patients are asymptomatic and they manifest with non-specific symptoms and a slowly progressive lymphocytosis resembling the picture seen in stage A chronic lymphocytic leukaemia (CLL). This 'smouldering' form of T-PLL progresses in terms of months or rarely years. Lymphocyte counts range from 35 to 1000×10^9/L and a third of the cases have anaemia and/or thrombocytopenia. Serology and/or DNA analysis for HTLV-I/II are consistently negative. Liver function tests may be impaired and urate and sodium lactate dehydrogenase (LDH) raised. Bone marrow shows a variable degree of involvement and the most common pattern of lymphoid infiltration in the trephine biopsy is mixed (interstitial plus diffuse) or diffuse with reticulin fibrosis.

Diagnosis

Cell morphology and immunological markers are the key diagnostic tests. In two-thirds of cases, the lymphocytes have condensed chromatin, regular or irregular nuclear outline, prominent nucleolus and a deeply basophilic cytoplasm with

Table 39.2 Disease features of mature T-cell disorders.

Disease	Spleen/liver	Nodes	Skin	Others
T-PLL	+++/++	++	++	Effusions
T-cell LGL leukaemia	++/+	–	+	Cytopenias, PRCA
Sézary syndrome	–/–	+	+++	
ATLL	++/++	+++	+	Hypercalcaemia, HTLV-I
γ/δ T-NHL	+++/++	–	+	Extranodal sites
Subcutaneous panniculitic-like	–	–	+++	
AIL	++/++	+++	++	AHA, dysproteinemia
Extranodal nasal	+/+	+	+	Nasal, extranodal sites
Intestinal	–/–	+	–	Bowel
ALCL	+/+	++	+	

+++, > 70% of cases; ++, 40–70% of cases; +, 20–40% of cases; –, < 20% of cases.
AHA, autoimmune haemolytic anaemia; HTLV-I, human T-cell leukaemia lymphoma virus I; PRCA, pure red cell aplasia.

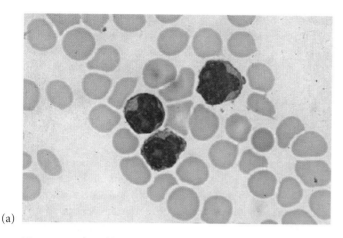
(a)

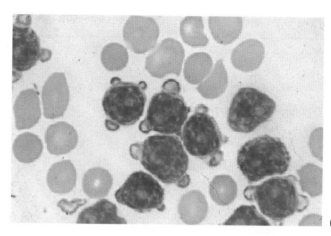
(b)

Figure 39.1 (a and b) Peripheral blood films from two cases of T-PLL showing medium-size lymphoid cells with prominent nucleolus and basophilic cytoplasm.

protrusions or blebs (typical T-PLL) (Figure 39.1). In the remaining, the lymphocytes are smaller in size and the nucleolus is small or not visible by light microscopy (small-cell variant of T-PLL) and/or have a cerebriform nucleus resembling Sézary cells (cerebriform variant). Although the small-cell T-PLL has been referred to as 'T-CLL', such designation may lead to confusion as these patients with small-cell T-PLL have an aggressive disease course and the immunophenotype and cytogenetics are similar to typical T-PLL. The two morphological T-PLL variants are formally recognized as T-PLL in the WHO classification.

Tissue histology is not essential for the diagnosis of T-PLL. The tissues which are more frequently available for review are spleen and skin. The spleen histology shows expansion of the white pulp extending to the red pulp and thus is different from T-cell LGL leukaemia. Skin histology is different from Sézary's syndrome (SS) and shows dermal infiltration preferentially around the appendages without epidermotropism.

Immunological markers show that T-prolymphocytes, unlike T-lymphoblasts, are negative with TdT and the cortical thymic marker CD1a while expressing CD2, CD5 and CD7, the latter with strong intensity. CD3 and anti-TCR-α/β are negative in the cell membrane from 20% of patients but are always expressed in the cytoplasm. The most common phenotype is CD4+CD8– (65% of cases), in ~ 10% cells are CD8+CD4–, and in 25% the cells co-express CD4 and CD8 (Table 39.3). T-prolymphocytes are negative with monoclonal antibodies (McAb) against natural killer (NK) cells, TIA-1 and HLA-DR; CD25 is negative or weak and CD52w (Campath-1H) is strongly expressed.

Pathogenesis

Chromosomal abnormalities are complex and essentially involve chromosomes 14, 8 and 11. The abnormality inv(14)(q11;q32) is characteristic of T-PLL and is detected in greater than two-thirds of the cases. This juxtaposes the TCR-α gene (14q11) to the oncogen TCL-1 (14q32.1) Few cases have rearrangement of

the TCL-1 gene and most have TCL-1 overexpression, supporting the theory that this oncogen plays a role in the pathogenesis of this disease (Table 39.3). In some cases, the *TCR-α* gene (14q11) is juxtaposed to the *MTCP-1* gene (Xq28), resulting in the t(X;14)(q28;q11). The *MTCP-1* gene has homology with *TCL-1* and it has been shown to be expressed in two T-PLL patients who developed the leukaemia following a preceding phase of AT. Abnormalities of chromosome 8 involving both arms of this chromosome are frequent; although the c-*myc* oncogene (8q24) is not rearranged, overexpression of c-*myc* is found in cases with iso8q. 11q23 abnormalities are rarely detected by cytogenetics, but involvement of the *ATM* gene (11q23) by molecular analysis is common. There are genetic similarities between the sporadic T-PLL form and circulating T-lymphocytes from AT patients. These patients are at risk of developing lymphoid malignancies including T-PLL. T-cell clones in AT carry similar abnormalities to leukaemic T-prolymphocytes, and expression of TCL-1 transcripts occurs in both the preleukaemic and leukaemic phases in AT patients, as it does in the sporadic T-PLL phases. Further, mutations of the *ATM* gene (11q23) responsible for AT have been well documented in T-PLL. All these findings stress the close relationship between the sporadic form of T-PLL and the leukaemia that develops in AT patients.

Differential diagnosis

The differential diagnosis of T-PLL arises with B-PLL, T-ALL and other mature T-cell leukaemias and lymphomas. Distinction between T- and B-PLL and T-ALL can be made by immunophenotyping. The differential diagnosis between T-PLL and T-cell LGL leukaemia is not problematic except in cases of smouldering small-cell variant T-PLL. Immunophenotype and cytogenetics together with cell morphology allow the distinction between these two conditions. Cell morphology, clinical features, skin histology and HTLV-I status will differentiate T-PLL from T-cell lymphomas in the leukaemic phase, such as ATLL and SS.

Table 39.3 Immunophenotype and genotype in T-cell disorders.*

Disease	Immunophenotype	Genotype
T-PLL	CD7^{++}, CD4$^+$ or CD4$^+$/CD8$^+$	inv (14), iso 8q ATM, TCL-1
T-cell LGL leukaemia	CD7$^{+/-}$, CD8$^+$, CD57$^+$, CD16$^+$	Unknown
Sézary syndrome	CD7$^{+/-}$, CD4$^+$, CD8$^-$	Aneuploidy
Adult T-cell leukaemia lymphoma	CD7$^-$, CD4$^+$, CD25$^+$	HTLV-I
γ/δ hepatosplenic T-NHL	TCR-γ/δ$^+$, CD16+, CD56$^+$, TIA-1$^+$	iso7q
Subcutaneous panniculitic-like	CD3$^+$, CD8$^+$, TIA-1$^+$	Unknown
Angioimmunoblastic T-NHL	CD3$^+$, CD5$^+$, CD10$^+$	+8, +5, del6q
Extranodal T/NK, nasal type	CD3epsilon$^+$, CD56$^+$, LMP-1$^+$	EBV
Enteropathy-type T-NHL	CD3$^+$, CD8$^+$, CD103$^+$	?EBV
Anaplastic large-cell lymphoma	CD30$^+$, CD3$^+$, CD25$^+$, EMA$^+$	t(2;5) NPM-ALK

*Refers only to the most relevant and distinct features.
ATM, ataxia telangiectasia mutated gene; EBV, Epstein–Barr virus; HTLV, human T-cell leukaemia/lymphoma virus; LMP-1, latent membrane protein; NPM-ALK, nucleolar phosphoprotein–anaplastic lymphoma tyrosine kinase.

Disease course and therapy

T-prolymphocytic leukaemia has an aggressive course and survival is short, estimated to be around 7 months in the historical series. Patients are resistant or achieve transient responses to most chemotherapies. A decade ago we showed that 2′-deoxycoformycin is effective in this disease with response rates of 45%, 10% of which were complete responses (CRs); this resulted in a survival improvement. Recently, we have documented the remarkable activity of the monoclonal antibody (MAb) Campath-1H either used as a first-line therapy or following 2′-deoxycoformycin. Over two-thirds of patients respond to this agent, and most achieve a CR. However, most patients following Campath-1H, eventually relapse, and therefore responses need to be consolidated with high-dose therapy and stem cell transplant. Such a schedule has been successfully used in some patients with encouraging results. A chart illustrating the response to Campath-1H in a T-PLL patient is shown in Figure 39.2.

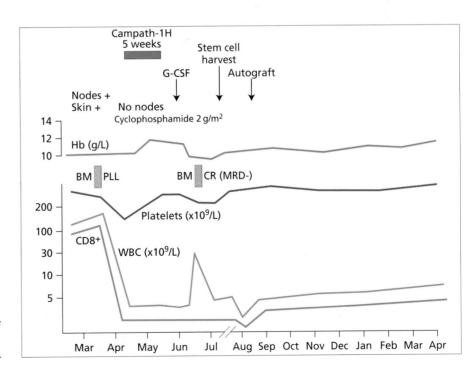

Figure 39.2 Flow chart from a T-PLL patient illustrating a complete response to Campath-1H and subsequent consolidation with stem cell transplant.

Large granular lymphocyte leukaemia (LGL leukaemia)

Large granular lymphocyte leukaemia was described three decades ago and was at that time designated T-CLL, to contrast with B-cell CLL. A variety of designations, such as Tγ lymphoproliferative disorder, chronic T-cell lymphocytosis with neutropenia, T8+ T-CLL, natural killer (NK), cytotoxic and/or suppressor T-cell CLL, were used until Loughran (1993) coined the term of LGL leukaemia for this disease. Depending on the origin of the LGL cells, LGL leukaemia can be subdivided into two main groups: one group which is derived from T cells (CD3+) and another, more uncommon, group derived from NK cells (CD3−). However, in the WHO classification, only the T-cell LGL is considered as LGL leukaemia, while NK-LGL is included within the spectrum of the NK neoplasms. Therefore, we will strictly refer here to the T-cell LGL leukaemia.

Aetiology

The aetiology of T-cell LGL leukaemia is unknown. This disorder is more frequently seen in patients with autoimmune diseases, in particular those with rheumatoid arthritis and Felty's syndrome. The latter patients, as those with T-cell LGL leukaemia, have, with a high frequency, the DR4 haplotype. This suggests a common immunogenetic basis for all these conditions. In contrast, it is unlikely that DNA or RNA viruses play a major pathogenic role in T-cell LGL leukaemia. Although some reports have documented the presence of HTLV-I/II antibodies in a few cases, the data are questionable and have not been confirmed by molecular studies. Similarly, only occasional cases, particularly derived from NK cells, have been linked to EBV infection.

Clinical features

T-cell LGL leukaemia affects adults and is rare in children; it is slightly more frequent in females. Patients are asymptomatic or manifest with symptoms derived from cytopenias, essentially recurrent infections, autoimmune disease or rarely present as pure red cell aplasia; the disease may evolve as a pure lymphomatous form in a minority of cases. Physical examination shows splenomegaly in close to two-thirds of patients and hepatomegaly in one-half; skin lesions may be present but lymphadenopathy is exceedingly rare (Table 39.2). The lymphocyte count is normal or slightly raised, usually under 15×10^9/L, with the majority of cells being LGL; neutropenia is very common, and one-third of patients have anaemia and/or thrombocytopenia. In a few cases, a Coombs-positive haemolytic anaemia and autoimmune thrombocytopenia have been documented. Some patients test positive for rheumatoid factor (RA), antinuclear antibodies, circulating immune complexes and hypo- or hypergammaglobulinaemia. Bone marrow shows mild lymphoid infiltration, often with an interstitial pattern. It is not rare that marrow involvement is missed in both the aspirates and trephine biopsies but can be revealed by membrane markers or immunohistochemistry respectively. There may be erythroid and myeloid hyperplasia with maturation arrest.

Diagnosis

Cell morphology, immunological markers and molecular analysis investigating the configuration of the TCR-β or -γ chain genes are the key diagnostic tests. The circulating lymphocytes are medium in size, and have an eccentric nucleus with mature chromatin, no visible nucleolus and abundant pale cytoplasm with azurophilic granulation (Figure 39.3). The granules contain acid hydrolases, in particular acid phosphatase, perforin

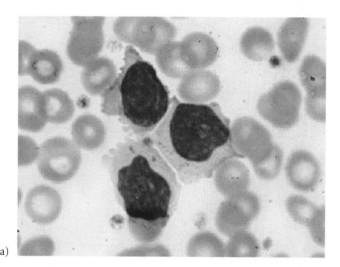
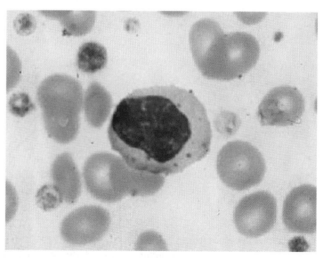

(a)

(b)

Figure 39.3 (a and b) Peripheral blood film from patients with T-cell LGL leukaemia showing lymphocytes with an eccentric nucleus, condensed chromatin and abundant pale cytoplasm with azurophilic granules.

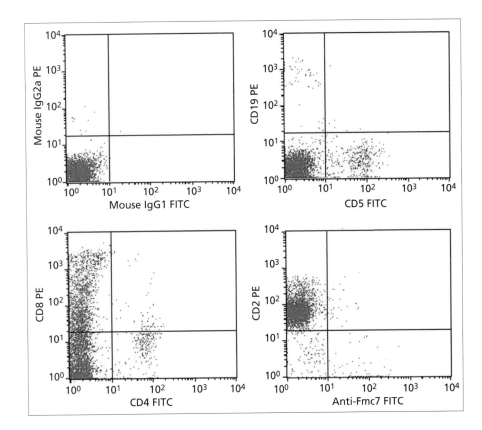

Figure 39.4 Flow cytometry plots of lymphocytes from a T-cell LGL leukaemia illustrating that most cells are CD2$^+$ and CD8$^+$, but are CD4$^-$ and CD5$^-$.

and cytokines involved in the cytotoxic function of these lymphocytes. At the ultrastructural level, some of these granules may display a special configuration and are designated parallel tubular arrays (PTAs). Morphologically, the lymphocytes in T-cell LGL leukaemia cannot be distinguished from the minor circulating LGL population present in the blood from normal individuals.

Tissue histology is only available in some cases and is rarely essential for diagnosis. The spleen histology shows red pulp expansion with atrophic or a reactive white pulp resembling the pattern seen in hairy-cell leukaemia; however, pseudolake formation is not seen and the infiltrating cells have, unlike in hairy cell leukaemia, a T-cell phenotype. Sarcoid-like granulomas may be present in a few cases. The liver histology shows sinusoidal infiltration extending to the portal tracts.

Membrane markers in T-cell LGL leukaemia show that cells from most cases are CD2$^+$, CD3$^+$ TCR-α/β^+ whereas CD5 and CD7 are negative in around half of the cases. The most common phenotypic profile is CD8$^+$ CD4$^-$ CD57$^+$ CD16$^+$ TIA-1$^+$ (Table 39.3, Figure 39.4). A few cases have unusual phenotypes such as co-expression of CD4 and CD8 or a CD4$^+$ CD8$^-$ phenotype with or without co-expression of NK-associated markers. T-cell activation markers such as HLA-DR determinants and CD38 are expressed in a variable number of cases. Although the p55 α-chain of the interleukin 2 (IL-2) receptor (CD25) is usually absent in the cell membrane, LGL cells express the p75 inter-

mediate-affinity IL-2 receptor β-chain. LGL cells express both Fas (CD95) and its ligand but are resistant to apoptosis due to an impairment of the Fas apoptotic-induced pathway.

Southern blot and/or polymerase chain reaction (PCR) studies using primers specific for the variable regions of the TCR-β or -γ chain genes are essential to demonstrate the clonal nature of the expanded LGL population and distinguish them from reactive non-clonal LGL proliferations. In the majority of T-cell LGL leukaemia cases, the cells have a rearranged TCR-β chain gene, and only a few have rearrangements of the TCR-γ chain gene (Figure 39.5). It is now possible to demonstrate clonality by flow cytometry using a wide range of MAbs against the different variable regions of the TCR-β chain gene. Unlike in reactive LGL proliferations, in which different proportions of cells will stain with the various MAbs, in LGL leukaemia, cells will stain only with one of them.

Pathogenesis

There is no evidence for a recurrent chromosomal abnormality in T-cell LGL leukaemia. A number of cases may show normal karyotypes despite being clonal by DNA analysis. As outlined earlier, it is likely that T-cell LGL leukaemia has an immune or autoimmune basis. This hypothesis is supported not only by its association with autoimmune diseases but also by the evidence that immunosuppressive agents may control the disease manifestations in some patients. In addition, the cytopenias

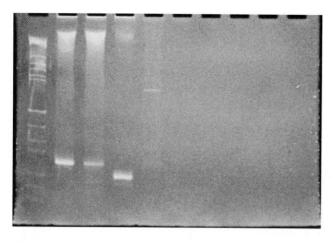

Figure 39.5 PCR analysis on a case of T-cell LGL leukaemia showing a single rearranged band for the TCR-γ chain gene in the blood (second row) and bone marrow (third row). The first row is 1 kb ladder, the fourth a positive control and the fifth a negative control.

seem to be unrelated to bone marrow infiltration and/or hypersplenism and instead derived from an inhibitory effect of the LGL on the haemopoietic differentiation and maturation interfering with and/or arresting the physiological differentiation process.

Differential diagnosis

The differential diagnosis of T-cell LGL leukaemia arises with polyclonal T-cell lymphocytosis following splenectomy or reactive to viral infections, B-cell CLL and with other T-cell disorders. DNA analysis will allow to distinguish reactive from clonal LGL proliferations as in the former the TCR chain genes will be in germline configuration. Morphology and membrane markers distinguish T-cell LGL leukaemia from other B- and T-cell disorders.

Prognosis and therapy

The clinical course of T-cell LGL leukaemia is often stable or slowly progressive; only a few patients present with widespread and progressive disease. It has been suggested that cases whose cells express CD56 and/or CD26 behave more aggressively. Transformation into a large-cell lymphoma, a phenomenon similar to Richter's syndrome in CLL, is exceedingly rare.

The prognosis of LGL leukaemia is difficult to ascertain but overall is good compared with the other T-cell malignancies. Thus, data based on relatively large series of patients show that 80% of them survive at 4 years and the overall median survival is greater than 10 years. The main causes of death are infections and only in a few patients is death associated with progressive disease.

A substantial proportion of patients, e.g. those without cytopenias and stable blood counts, do not require treatment and only monitoring, e.g. 'watch and wait', a policy similar to that adopted in stage A B-CLL. Treatment is indicated in those with severe cytopenias, recurrent infections and/or progressive lymphocytosis or organomegaly. There is no gold-standard therapy to be used in LGL leukaemia. Overall, therapeutic strategies are based on the use of immunosuppressive agents as there is no evidence that high-dose therapy will benefit these patients by eradicating the clone. These treatments include cyclosporin A, low-dose cyclophosphamide (e.g. 200–300 mg/week) or weekly pulses of methotrexate (10 mg/m^2). There are no data concerning the disease features which will predict response to one or another immunosuppressive drug (Figure 39.6). There is limited experience of the use of haemopoietic growth factors, e.g. GM-CSF, G-CSF or erythropoietin. However, in the author's

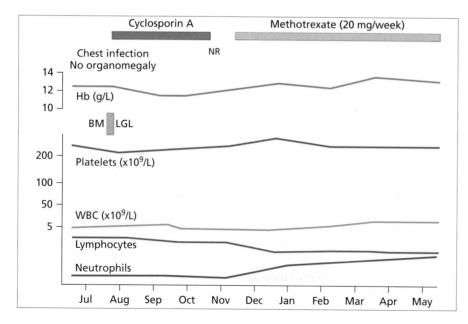

Figure 39.6 Flow chart from a patient with T-cell LGL leukaemia with profound neutropenia (neutrophils: 0.1×10^9/L). The patient did not respond to cyclosporin A, but the neutropenia improved (neutrophils: 1×10^9/L) with weekly pulses of methotrexate.

experience, these may be considered as adjuvants to maintain or improve the blood cell counts. Few patients respond to 2′-deoxycoformycin, but this drug has not been extensively used in LGL leukaemia. Splenectomy does not correct the neutropenia or cytopenias and usually results in an increase of circulating LGL. Still, in patients with bulky spleen, this procedure may help by removing tumour burden. Patients with widespread disease, e.g. skin lesions, hepatosplenomegaly, rising WBC, should be managed with combination chemotherapy.

Leukaemia/lymphoma syndromes
(Table 39.1)

The leukaemia/lymphoma syndromes or leukaemic phase of T-NHL comprise T-cell neoplasms that arise in peripheral lymphoid tissues but with a high frequency present with blood involvement mimicking T-cell leukaemias. These include two diseases: Sézary's syndrome (SS) and adult-T-cell leukaemia lymphoma (ATLL).

Sézary's syndrome (SS)/mycosis fungoides (MF)

Aetiology

These are cutaneous T-cell lymphomas (CTCLs), with SS being considered the leukaemic manifestation of MF. Their aetiology is unknown. Although some studies have suggested a link between SS/MF with HTLV-I/II on the basis of the detection of retroviral sequences in the tumour cells, other studies have not confirmed these findings. In addition, HTLV-I antibodies are not detected in the patient's serum and a clonal integration of HTLV-I in the tumour cells has not been demonstrated in any case with 'bona fide' SS/MF. A cooperative study in more than 100 cases of CTCL using sensitive molecular tests, serology and cell culture has failed to show a single CTCL harbouring HTLV-I/II. Therefore, there is no robust evidence for the involvement of these retroviruses in SS/MF.

A relationship between MF and other T-cell conditions, chiefly lymphomatoid papulosis, has been entertained. Lymphomatoid papulosis is a recurrent skin eruption characterized by the presence of nodules with evidence by histology of anaplastic Reed–Sternberg-like cells infiltrating the skin. Although in the past its neoplastic nature had been debated, this issue was later settled as clonal. TCR rearrangements were documented in some patients. Such conditions may precede not only CTCL but also anaplastic lymphoma (ALCL) and/or Hodgkin's disease. The association between lymphomatoid papulosis and CTCL has been established in a case that presented with lymphomatoid papulosis and subsequently developed Hodgkin's disease and MF with evidence of the same clone in the three tumours. Currently, lymphomatoid papulosis is included in the group of primary cutaneous T-NHL by the WHO (see below).

Clinical features

Sézary's syndrome and MF affect elderly patients and are more common in males. Patients present with pruritus, and skin lesions either localized, e.g. nodules or plaques, or a generalized rash (Table 39.2). In patients with early-stage disease, the correct diagnosis is not always made at presentation and the manifestations are considered as reactive dermatitis even when skin histology is available. Physical examination shows generalized erythrodermia and/or nodules; organomegaly is rare. In SS, the WBC count is normal or raised with circulating atypical lymphocytes. Anaemia and thrombocytopenia are uncommon and bone marrow is usually not involved. Serology for HTLV-I is consistently negative even in cases originating from regions in which this virus is endemic.

Diagnosis

The diagnosis is based on cell morphology, skin histology and immunological markers.

The circulating blood lymphocytes are small to large size and exhibit a cerebriform nucleus often seen as a hyperchromatic nucleus (Figure 39.7); the cytoplasm is scanty or medium size and, in some cases, vacuolation is prominent. According to the cell size, two variants of SS had been recognized, the small- and large-cell variants. Small cells and/or a mixture of small and large cells are the predominant type in the peripheral blood. The nuclear configuration of the Sézary cells is best defined by ultrastructural analysis that reveals a serpentine nucleus with multiple narrow indentations.

Skin histology is a key diagnostic test in SS and in MF. This shows the presence of dermal lymphoid infiltrates which characteristically extend into the epidermis, a phenomenon designated epidermotropism; in some cases the infiltrates involve the subcutaneous fat. Pautrier microabcesses are typical but not unique to these conditions as they may be seen in T-NHL and ATLL.

Histology of other tissues is rarely available at diagnosis. The enlarged lymph nodes may show a reactive lymphadenitis or infiltration by lymphoma (Figure 39.8). Bone marrow, when involved, shows a mild interstitial infiltration.

Immunophenotyping demonstrates that the circulating neoplastic Sézary cells are positive for CD2, CD3 and CD5 whilst CD7 is negative in ~50% of cases (Table 39.3). The most common phenotype is CD4+ CD8−, but other unusual phenotypes, e.g. CD8+ CD4− or co-expression of CD4/CD8, may be seen in a minority of cases. NK-associated markers are, as a rule, negative while expression of T-cell activation markers is variable. Unlike in ATLL, CD25 is rarely expressed in Sézary cells and, when positive, the reactivity is weaker than in ATLL cells. In the skin, the interdigitating Langerhans cells admixed with the neoplastic lymphocytes are CD1a+ and S-100+. Cases transforming into a large T-cell lymphoma display aberrant phenotypes with loss of pan-T markers and often expression of T-cell activation antigens such as CD30, CD25 and HLA-DR.

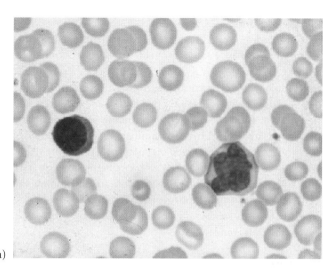
(a)

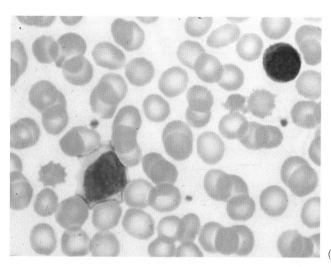
(b)

Figure 39.7 (a and b) Peripheral blood films from a patient with Sézary's syndrome showing large and small cells with a convoluted hyperchromatic nucleus.

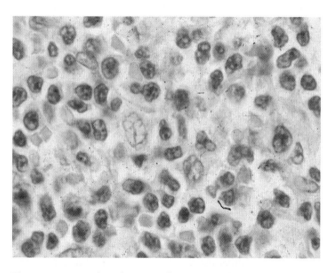

Figure 39.8 Lymph node section from a patient with Sézary's syndrome showing diffuse infiltration by lymphoid cells, some with an irregular nucleus.

Pathogenesis

Chromosomal abnormalities are complex and have variable ploidy. Hyperploidy is frequent in the large-cell variant and aneuploidy or hypoploidy in the small-cell form. There are also differences in the DNA content between these two forms when analysed by flow cytometry. There is no evidence for a recurrent chromosomal abnormality in SS, but chromosomes 6, 2, 1 and 17q are the most commonly involved. Clonal evolution may be seen in some cases, particularly those transforming into large cell. Abnormalities of chromosome 17p have been documented in some cases, as well as p53 protein overexpression and p53 gene deletion; however, p53 mutations are rare in SS and there-fore it has been postulated that the *mdm-2* gene may be, to some extent, responsible for the p53 inactivation in SS.

Differential diagnosis

The differential diagnosis arises with reactive dermatitis, T-PLL presenting with skin lesions, ATLL and cutaneous B-cell lymphomas. Cell morphology and immunological markers allow the distinction between SS and T-PLL and cutaneous B-NHL HTLV-I serology is the key test to distinguish SS from ATLL, essentially in cases presenting primarily with cutaneous forms of ATLL. The pattern and extent of skin infiltration and histochemistry usually allows the differentiation of SS from reactive dermatitis. However, in problematic cases, PCR analysis investigating the configuration of the TCR chain genes is needed; in SS this will show a rearranged T-cell band, unlike in reactive dermatitis where the pattern is polyclonal.

Clinical course, prognosis and treatment

The clinical course of MF/SS is usually relatively chronic. Thus, 87% of MF patients survive 5 years, whereas SS follows a more progressive course with shorter survival. The outcome for patients with abnormal clones seems to be worse than those with random heteroploidy. Transformation of SS or MF into a large-cell T-NHL is uncommon but has been documented in 8–19% of cases in retrospective studies. Transformation may be localized or systemic and chiefly is associated with advanced stages and a short survival. Only in a few cases has it been demonstrated that the tumour in the phase of transformation arises from the original clone. This is essential as SS/MF patients have an increased risk of secondary malignancies and, thus, the non-haemopoietic nature of the tumour needs to be excluded.

A variety of treatments, including topical and systemic agents, have been used in SS/MF. In patients, particularly the elderly and those with localized skin disease, PUVA (psoralen with UVA irradiation), electron-beam and/or topical BCNU and steroids may alleviate and control the skin symptoms. Local radiotherapy is useful in patients with localized plaques. Systemic therapy is particularly indicated in young patients and/or those with widespread disease. This is based on either single-agent therapy with methotrexate, cyclophosphamide or etoposide or combination of drugs, e.g. CHOP (cyclophosphamide, hydroxydaunorubicin, oncovin and prednisolone). Over the last decade, new therapies have been employed, such as purine analogues, interferons, retinoids and immunotherapy with an anti-IL-2 MAb conjugated with the diphtheria toxin. Responses to purine analogues, either 2′-deoxycoformycin, 2-chlorodeoxyadenosine or fludarabine, range from 30% to 62%. Interferon-α alone or combined with retinoids (etretinate) is effective in cases with cutaneous disease but not in systemic disease. The MAb Campath-1H has been used in some patients with relapsed and refractory disease with encouraging results.

Adult T-cell leukaemia lymphoma (ATLL)

Aetiology and epidemiology

Adult T-cell leukaemia lymphoma is a unique malignancy in which the primary aetiological agent has been well established. This disease is caused by a retrovirus, HTLV-I, which is almost universally detected in all the patients. ATLL was first described as a distinct clinical entity in 1977. Its association with HTLV-I was demonstrated in the early 1980s almost simultaneously in USA and Japan, based on seroepidemiological studies and the isolation of HTLV-I from ATLL cells. ATLL is clustered in HTLV-I endemic areas such as Japan, the Caribbean, Africa, South America and the Middle East, and among immigrants from these countries to Europe and USA. In the UK, this disease is seen in immigrants of Afro-Caribbean descent. Familial cases of ATLL have been documented, and it has been suggested that a shared environment and perhaps a genetic background influence the development of ATLL in these families.

Clinical features

Adult T-cell leukaemia lymphoma affects adults without sex predominance. The disease manifests with leukaemia in over two-thirds of cases (leukaemia form), whereas approximately 25% have no blood involvement (lymphoma form). Within the leukaemia form, three subtypes are distinguished: acute, chronic and smouldering. Acute ATLL is the most common, accounting for 65% of cases. Patients present acutely with widespread disease, leucocytosis, opportunistic infections and/or hypercalcaemia. Physical examination shows lymphadenopathy, skin lesions and/or hepatosplenomegaly (Table 39.2). Chronic ATLL (5% of cases) presents with stable or slowly progressive lymphocytosis with the presence of atypical lymphocytes and minor or no lymphadenopathy or skin involvement. Smouldering ATLL (5% of cases) is characterized by normal blood counts with less

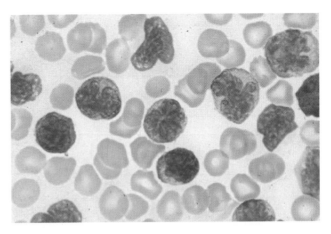

Figure 39.9 Peripheral blood film from a patient with ATLL showing lymphocytes with a polylobed nucleus (flower cells).

than 4% atypical lymphocytes and recurrent skin lesions or lung infiltrates. Hypercalcaemia by definition is not detected in chronic and smouldering ATLL. Both these forms progress in terms of months or rarely years into acute ATLL. A few ATLL patients have manifestations of conditions linked to HTLV-I infection such as tropical spastic paraparesis, arthritis, uveitis, etc. These either manifest concomitantly with, or precede the onset of, the T-cell neoplasm. Peripheral blood counts show a raised WBC with lymphocytosis in the acute and chronic leukaemia forms. Anaemia and thrombocytopenia is seen in close to a third of cases. Biochemistry shows a markedly raised LDH and the liver function tests may be abnormal. Hypercalcaemia is the most distinct biochemical abnormality, seen in 50% of cases at presentation and in up to two-thirds during the disease course. Rarely, it is associated with osteolytic lesions. The pathogenesis responsible for the hypercalcaemia is described below.

Diagnosis

The diagnosis of ATLL is based on cell morphology, immunophenotype and essentially by the demonstration of HTLV-I antibodies on the patient's serum or retrovirus sequences into the cell's DNA.

Morphological analysis of the peripheral blood films shows a pleomorphic picture with the presence of cells of different size and degree of nuclear irregularities in the acute and chronic leukaemia ATLL subtypes. The prototype cell, designated 'flower cell', is a medium-size lymphocyte with condensed chromatin and a convoluted or polylobated nucleus (Figure 39.9); a few cells may have a cerebriform nuclei and a minority show features of immunoblasts.

Immunological markers show that ATLL cells have a mature T-cell phenotype CD2+, CD5+. CD3 is expressed in the cytoplasm but, in some cases, cells lack expression of CD3 and TCR-α/β in the membrane. It has been suggested that the decreased

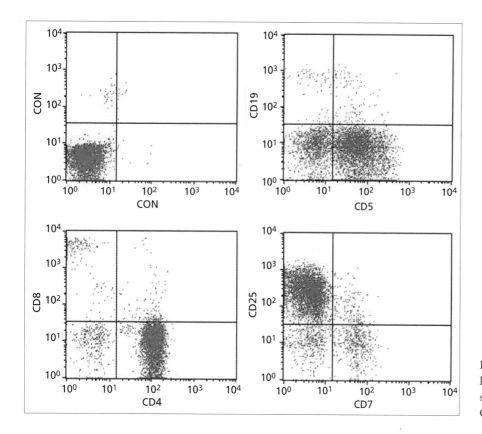

Figure 39.10 Flow cytometry plots of lymphocytes from an ATLL patient showing reactivity with CD5, CD4 and CD25 while CD7 is negative.

numbers of CD3 and TCR molecules in ATLL cells results from the cell activation by the retrovirus and that might play a role in the disease pathogenesis. Most ATLL cases have a CD4+ CD8− phenotype. Unusual cases with uncommon phenotypes such as co-expression of CD4 and CD8, or a CD8+ CD4− phenotype have been reported in Japan and appear to have a more aggressive disease. A distinct feature of ATLL cells is the strong expression of the p55 alpha chain of the IL-2 receptor (CD25) in the cell membrane (Figure 39.10). Soluble IL-2 receptors are detected in the patient's serum and the levels correlate with tumour burden and response to therapy. The possible role of the IL-2 and IL-2 receptor system has been entertained for a number of years and is discussed later. Other markers linked to T-cell activation such as HLA-DR determinants and CD38 are expressed in a variable proportion of cases.

Lymphoid tissue histology is not essential for diagnosis in patients presenting with leukaemia. In the lymphoma forms, tissue histology is an important diagnostic test; however, the histological pattern by itself does not allow the making of a diagnosis of ATLL as the pattern of infiltration might be similar to the other post-thymic T-NHL. Often, there is diffuse infiltration by pleomorphic lymphoid cells of different size, similar to what is seen in non-HTLV-I unrelated T-NHL; in a few cases, the pattern of involvement mimics AIL T-NHL or Hodgkin's disease. ATLL does not fit in a single category in the revised European-American classification of lymphoid neoplasms (REAL) and WHO classifications and it is only defined by the presence of HTLV-I. The pattern of skin infiltration is not specific either, as in half of ATLL cases it is identical to that of SS, with evidence of epidermotropism. Bone marrow biopsy shows mild or no lymphoid infiltration but bone resorption and proliferation of osteoclasts is not rare, particularly in patients with hypercalcaemia.

Demonstration of HTLV-I is the key test for the definitive diagnosis of ATLL. Serum antibodies to HTLV-I can be detected by ELISA or Western blot in virtually all ATLL patients. In a small minority of patients who have a clinical and laboratory picture characteristic of ATLL, the retrovirus cannot be detected by either serology or molecular analysis. This suggests that, in a few cases, the initiating event responsible for the development of ATLL is not HTLV-I, a scenario similar to that seen with EBV in endemic and non-endemic Burkitt's lymphomas. Still, when findings are negative for HTLV-I, one should question the diagnosis of ATLL.

Pathogenesis

Chromosome abnormalities with complex karyotypes and clonal evolution are frequent. Rearrangements of chromosome 14 at breakpoints q11 and q32, characteristic of T-PLL, are rare. In smouldering ATLL, clonal and non-clonal abnormalities have been documented and occasional cases show clonal evolution from the smouldering to the acute phase. Sequential cytogenetic studies at the various phases of HTLV-I infection from carrier to acute ATLL might give some clues in the steps involved in the leukaemogenesis of HTLV-I-induced malignancy as the secondary factors involved in the neoplastic transformation of HTLV-I-infected lymphocytes are largely unknown.

The pathogenic role of IL-2 and its receptor had been suggested in the past on the basis of the independent growth of some HTLV-I-positive cell lines, the continuous transcription of the IL-2 receptor gene, the increased levels of IL-2 receptor mRNA and the fact that HTLV-I induces IL-2 receptor expression in normal T-lymphocytes when infected by this retrovirus. However, definitive evidence has not been proven as ATLL cells do not secrete IL-2, nor have increased mRNA levels for this cytokine.

The mechanism of hypercalcaemia seems to relate to the release of cytokines, chiefly a parathyroid-like hormone, IL-1 and tumour necrosis factor β by the tumour cells. These lead to bone resorption and release of calcium into the serum.

It is well established that HTLV-I is the primary aetiological agent of ATLL, shown by the presence of a mono-/oligoclonal integration of HTLV-I sequences into the leukaemic cell's DNA. Although HTLV-I infection constitutes the first step in the development of ATLL, it is not enough by itself to cause malignancy as only 0.5% of HTLV-I carriers will develop the disease and the life risk to develop the malignancy in a carrier is estimated to be around 5%. Infection in early life seems to be a risk factor. Concerning pathogenesis, HTLV-I does not carry an oncogene and the sites of integration vary from tumour to tumour. However, the retrovirus harbours various regulatory genes, e.g. *tax*, which code for proteins responsible for cell immortalization by activating some cellular genes relevant for proliferation and differentiation (trans-activation pathway). It is likely that disruption of other genes such as mutations of the tumour-suppressor genes *p53*, *p16* and *p15* are also implicated in the development of the neoplasm.

Differential diagnosis

The differential diagnosis of ATLL arises with primary T-cell leukaemias and T-NHL not associated to HTLV-I. In addition, smouldering ATLL raises diagnostic problems with carriers of the retrovirus. T-cell leukaemias and T-NHL can be distinguished from ATLL by clinical features, morphology and, essentially, by the presence or absence of HTLV-I. The HTLV-I test is essential, as the lymphoma. ATLL type or its cutaneous form cannot be distinguished, respectively, from pleomorphic T-NHL or MF/SS when only histology is considered. Further, in endemic areas and when the picture is not typical of ATLL, DNA analysis in addition to serology is needed to confirm that HTLV-I is clonally integrated in the leukaemic cells. Distinction between smouldering ATLL and carriers of the retrovirus is based on molecular analysis with probes specific for HTLV-I that will show a mono-/oligoclonal pattern of retroviral integration in smouldering ATLL versus a polyclonal pattern in the carriers.

Clinical course and therapy

Adult T-cell leukaemia lymphoma is an aggressive malignancy for which no successful treatment is yet available. Patients are refractory or transiently respond to chemotherapy or purine analogues. Survival ranges from 5 months to 13 months. Smouldering and chronic ATLL pursue an indolent course until the disease progresses and becomes refractory to therapy. The poor outlook of ATLL relates to both chemotherapy resistance and complications (hypercalcaemia and opportunistic infections) that make management difficult. Most patients have been treated with CHOP, similar schedules and/or single-agent therapy. Although partial remission (PR) or clinical complete responses have been achieved in some patients, these are short-lived. Results are not superior with immunotherapy with MAb against the IL-2 receptor. A combination of α-interferon and zidovudine seems to be effective, particularly when used after or combined with chemotherapy. Schedules combining chemotherapy plus anti-T-cell MAb may improve the outcome of these patients.

T-cell non-Hodgkin's lymphomas (T-NHL)

The tissue-based T-cell NHL encompasses a variety of entities that essentially affect lymphoid tissues and/or extranodal sites. Some of them are frequent in the East while very uncommon in the western countries. A minority of patients may develop or manifest with a leukaemic picture and, when the circulating cells are large blasts (Figure 39.11), present problems of differential diagnosis with acute leukaemias. According to the REAL and WHO, the T-NHL are classified as shown in Table 39.1.

Peripheral T-NHL (unspecified)

This term includes T-NHL difficult to classify by histology and molecular genetics. Problems in classifying these lymphomas

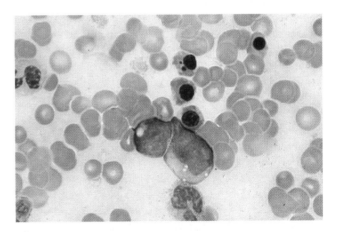

Figure 39.11 Bone marrow aspirate from a patient with T-NHL showing two large blasts.

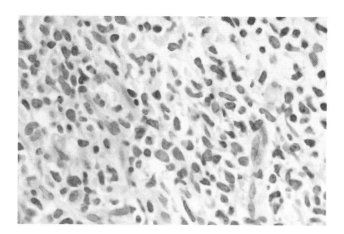

Figure 39.12 Bone marrow trephine biopsy from a patient with peripheral T-cell lymphoma (unspecified) showing diffuse infiltration by pleomorphic lymphoid cells.

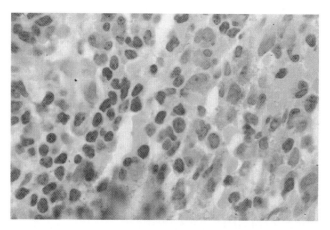

Figure 39.13 Bone marrow trephine showing infiltration by lymphoid cells with marked eosinophilia in a patient with T-NHL.

result from their rarity and the lack of objective criteria to better define them. Most peripheral T-NHLs are referred to as non-lymphoblastic TdT-negative T-NHL. Patients present with organomegaly, 'B' symptoms and some with extranodal disease; haemophagocytosis and/or impairment of the immune system are not uncommon. The term 'peripheral T-NHL with haemophagocytic syndrome' has been used to designate cases with prominent haemophagocytosis.

Lymph node histology shows diffuse effacement of the architecture by atypical lymphocytes (Figure 39.12), or infiltration may be confined to interfollicular areas (T-zone variant) and/or the paracortical zone. There may be a background of eosinophils and histiocytes (Figure 39.13). The neoplastic cells express several T-cell markers CD2, CD3, CD5, CD7 with variable expression of CD4 and CD8. Aberrant phenotypes with lack of expression of pan-T markers are common. Bone marrow rarely is involved. There is no consistent chromosomal abnormality but complex

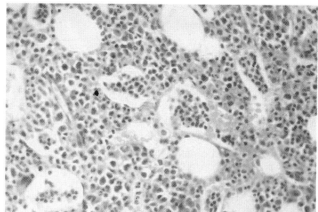

Figure 39.14 Bone marrow trephine section from a patient with hepatosplenic Tγ/δ lymphoma showing intrasinusoidal infiltration.

karyotypes are common. Most peripheral T-NHL should be considered high to intermediate grade. Treatment modalities based on combinations of agents such as CHOP, intensified CHOP plus etoposide or given at shorter intervals (e.g. every 2 weeks), followed or not by stem cell transplant, still remains the gold standard.

Peripheral T-NHL-specific variants (Table 39.1)

Six T-NHL have been considered by the WHO as distinct entities on the basis of the clinical and laboratory features. The most relevant features of these lymphomas are described below.

Hepatosplenic γ/δ T-NHL

This tumour derives from TCR-γ/δ^+ T-cells and affects preferentially young males. It is more common in immunocompromised patients. Hepatosplenomegaly is the main feature, but extranodal sites (e.g. skin) may be involved (Table 39.2). The histology is distinct, with an intrasinusoidal pattern of infiltration in all tissues affected such as spleen, liver and bone marrow (Figures 39.14 and 39.15). This mimics the pattern of distribution of normal Tγ/δ lymphocytes which home preferentially in the spleen sinusoids while R-α/β lymphocytes migrate to the periarteriolar sheets. The neoplastic cells have a CD2$^+$ CD7$^+$ CD3$^{+/-}$ TCR-γ/δ+ phenotype (Figure 39.16) and are usually negative with MAbs against TCR-α/β, CD5, CD4 and CD8 or expression of CD8 is weak. Often, the cells are positive with the NK-associated markers CD16 and CD56. A consistent feature is the expression of TCR-γ/δ and TIA-1, a MAb that identifies cytotoxic granule-associated proteins. Molecular studies show rearrangement of the TCR-γ/δ chain genes whilst the TCR-α/β are in the germ line. Cytogenetics have shown that some cases have iso7q and it has been suggested that this is a recurrent abnormality in this lymphoma (Table 39.3). EBV seems not to play a major pathogenic role. The clinical course is aggressive and median survival is less than 2 years despite intensive therapy.

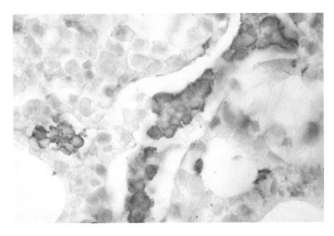

Figure 39.15 Immunohistochemistry on the bone marrow from Figure 39.14 showing that most lymphocytes in the sinusoids express cytoplasmic CD3.

Subcutaneous panniculitis-like T-NHL

This manifests with skin nodules resembling a benign panniculitis; haemophagocytic syndrome is frequent and may be fatal. Skin histology shows lymphoid infiltrates admixed with adipocytes in the subcutaneous tissue with extension to the dermis. Fat and connective tissue necrosis and granulomas are common; angiocentricity unlike in angiocentric T-NHL is not seen. The mitotic rate is high. The neoplastic cells are CD2⁺, CD3⁺, often CD8⁺ and express granzyme B, perforins and TIA-1 suggesting that this lymphoma arises from cytotoxic T-cells. Molecular analysis shows rearrangement of the TCR-β chain gene. There are limited data on outcome and response to therapy but prognosis seems poor.

Angioimmunoblastic (AIL) T-NHL

Angioimmunoblastic (AIL) T-NHL had already been described in the 1970s. It affects adults and has an acute onset. 'B' symptoms, pruritus, cutaneous rash, organomegaly, effusions and immune disturbance either autoimmune phenomena, immunodeficiency and/or dysproteinemia are common (Table 39.2). Although the neoplastic nature of this lymphoma had been debated in the past, this issue has been settled by the demonstration of clonality by cytogenetics and DNA analysis. Cases of clonal AIL T-NHL evolving from reactive hyperplasia have been described, and this change may correlate with clinical progression. The diagnosis is based on clinical features and histology. The lymph node shows a diffuse pleomorphic infiltrate composed by lymphocytes, plasma cells, immunoblasts and eosinophils; proliferation of epithelioid post-capillary venules and increased numbers of dendritic cells is common. There is obliteration of the follicular structure described as 'burned-out' follicular centres. The bone marrow is often involved on the trephine biopsy and the aspirates may show reactive features with increase in

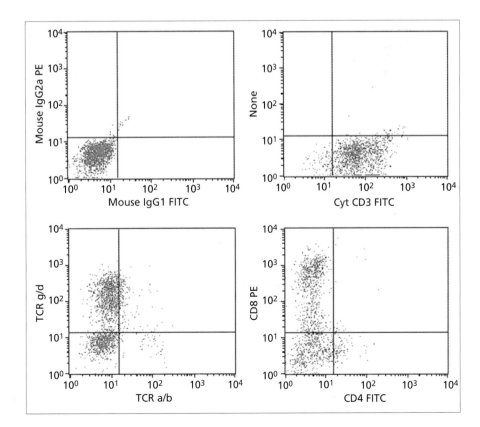

Figure 39.16 Flow cytometry plots of bone marrow cells from a patient with hepatosplenic γ/δ T-NHL showing that the lymphocytes express in the membrane TCRγ/δ, cytoplasmic CD3 and CD8 and are negative with anti-TCR-α/β and CD4.

polyclonal plasma cells. The lymphoma cells have a T-cell phenotype (CD2+ CD5+ CD3+), and often are CD10+; the proliferative rate is high. Complex karyotypes with multiple clones involving trisomy 3 or iso3q, trisomy 5 and del6q are common. DNA analysis of the TCR genes has firmly confirmed the T-cell clonality in AIL T-NHL. Most cases have rearrangement of the TCR-β and/or -γ chain genes and in a few cases, both immunoglobulin and TCR chain genes are rearranged. The pathogenic role of EBV is uncertain in this lymphoma, and it is likely that the presence of this virus in the tissues represents an epiphenomenon reflecting the polyclonal expansion of B-cells in an immunocompromised host. The clinical course is acute and prognosis is poor. Although transient spontaneous remissions have been documented, the lymphoma always recurs. Some patients initially respond to corticosteroids or combination chemotherapy but most relapse. A few reports on single cases have documented responses to fludarabine. The median survival ranges from 13 to 17 months. It is likely that more aggressive regimens including stem cell transplantation and/or combinations of chemotherapy with anti-T-cell monoclonal antibody will improve the dismal outcome of this lymphoma.

Extranodal T/NK lymphoma, nasal type

This type is significantly more frequent in China and Central/South America. Other designations for this lymphoma include lymphomatoid granulomatosis, polymorphic reticulosis, angiocentric immunoproliferative lesion or NK lymphoma. A workshop on angiocentric T-NHL outlined its peculiarities and stressed the differences between angiocentric nasal T/NK lymphomas and lymphomatoid granulomatosis. Lymphomatoid papulosis is now a well-recognized entity considered within cutaneous T-NHL. The term 'angiocentric' lymphoma was coined to define what represents different disease manifestations of related entities and to emphasize the angiocentricity of the lesions. Although the clonal T-cell nature of the lymphoid cells is not always demonstrated, the clinical course suggests that this is a neoplastic process. Patients present with extranodal disease, particularly a nasal mass; other tissues involved may be skin, testes, CNS, lung, bowel, bone, etc. The tumour histology shows lymphoid infiltrates admixed with histiocytes with a marked angiocentricity and angiodestruction (Figure 39.17).

It has been suggested that necrosis relates to the release of tumour necrosis factor overexpressed by the tumour cells and likely induced by EBV. Three grades (I–III) have been recognized on the basis of the cell size and degree of atypia and necrosis; it has been suggested that these histological subtypes may correlate with the clinical course, the best for the small-cell type. Immunophenotype shows that a proportion of cases have a T-cell phenotype often CD4+ CD8− while the remaining have an NK phenotype with lack of specific T-cell markers and expression of CD56 (Figure 39.18); these later cases still express in the cytoplasm the epsilon chain of the CD3. HLA-DR determinants, CD38, CD30 and CD25 may be positive, indicating that the

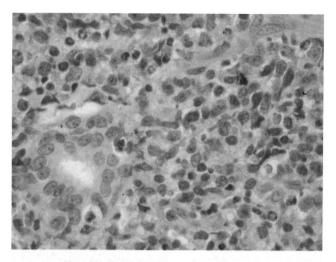

Figure 39.17 Section from a nasal mass of a patient with extranodal T/NK lymphoma, nasal type, showing infiltration by lymphoid cells with angiocentricity.

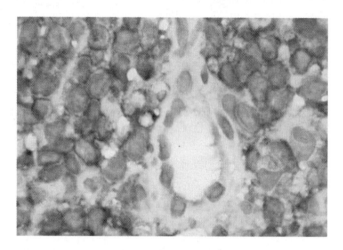

Figure 39.18 Immunohistochemistry of the tissue from Figure 39.17 showing a strong reactivity with CD56.

tumour cells are activated lymphocytes. The latent membrane protein (LMP-1) of EBV can be demonstrated by immunohistochemistry in most cases. Cytogenetic information is scanty, but abnormalities involving iso6p, del(6q), iso1q, are common. Rearrangement of the TCR-chain genes has been documented in only a minority of cases, while most have germline TCR genes despite the fact that the features are of a malignant neoplasm and the epsilon chain of the CD3 is expressed. This has led to the speculation that the nature of the neoplastic cells is close to the NK lineage. The pathogenic role of EBV in this lymphoma has been well established by both serology and molecular analysis, the latter showing single clonal episomal bands in the tumour cells and, thus, demonstrating the clonal nature of the cells despite the germline configuration of the TCR-chain genes. Therefore, detection of EBV RNA (EBERs) is useful to distinguish this lymphoma from cases with benign or inflammatory nasal lymphoid infiltrates. Patients with stage I/II grade lesions may respond to single agents or combination chemotherapy, but those with more extensive disease or grade III pursue an aggressive course. Prognosis is poor when dissemination occurs.

Enteropathy-type T-NHL (intestinal)

Intestinal lymphomas are often B-cell derived but a minority have a T-cell phenotype. This lymphoma seems to arise from a CD3+ CD8+ CD103+ T lymphocyte present in the normal epithelial intestinal mucosa. Some of these patients have a previous history of coeliac disease and/or a gluten-sensitive enteropathy. The relationship between intestinal T-NHL and coeliac disease is supported by the higher frequency of this lymphoma in geographical regions where gluten enteropathy is common; diet may improve symptoms and patients have the HLA genotype seen in coeliac disease. The main manifestations are abdominal pain, chronic diarrhoea and/or weight loss; rarely bowel perforation or obstruction is the first manifestation. Histology shows intraepithelial and subepithelial lymphoid infiltration of the mucosa and villous atrophy with reactive eosinophils and histiocytes. Three histological subtypes considering the presence or not of enteropathy have been documented. These appear to correlate with outcome, the worst for patients with enteropathy associated T-NHL. The lymphoma cells express T-cell markers (CD7+, CD3+/−) and rarely are CD8 or CD4 positive. The expression of HML-1 (CD103), a marker present in normal intestinal lymphocytes, is a consistent finding supporting the theory that this lymphoma arises from the intraepithelial mucosa T-cells. The TCR-β/γ chain genes are rearranged. A high prevalence of EBV has been documented in Mexican but not in European patients. The clinical course is aggressive, with survival estimated to be less than 1 year. Patients with localized bowel disease have longer survival than those with generalized disease. Surgery is often the diagnostic procedure and the first therapeutical approach. Problems in the patient's management are the intolerance to chemotherapy due to poor nutrition, low performance status and low albumin. The outcome is significantly worse than that of low-grade intestinal B-NHL, in which the disease is controlled with minor intervention.

Anaplastic large-cell lymphoma (ALCL)

Anaplastic large-cell lymphoma was first recognized by Stein and is now considered as a distinct clinicobiological entity with characteristic molecular features and expression of Ki-1 (CD30), a marker also present in Reed–Sternberg cells. Because of the undifferentiated morphology, it was originally designated ALCL. It has a bimodal age of presentation (childhood and elderly) without clear sex predominance. Lymphadenopathy and cutaneous lesions are the most frequent manifestations while extranodal disease is rare (Table 39.2). There are two forms – systemic and primarily cutaneous ALCL – and it is controversial whether

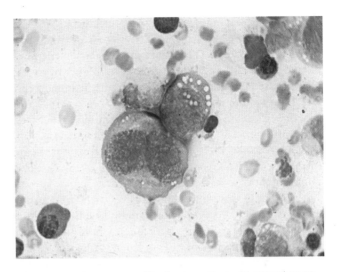

Figure 39.19 Bone marrow film from a patient with CD30+ ALCL showing infiltration by large bizarre anaplastic cells.

these forms are biologically different. In the WHO classification, the cutaneous CD30+ ALCL is considered within the group of primary cutaneous T-NHL together with lymphomatoid papulosis and 'borderline lesions'. In addition, there is a secondary ALCL which develops in patients with lymphomatoid papulosis, MF and Hodgkin's disease and the prognosis in this group is worse than in *de novo* ALCL.

Lymph node histology shows lymphoid infiltration of the T zone and paracortical areas, with or without intrasinusoidal involvement. Capsular thickening and fibrous tissue deposition are common. The skin shows infiltration of the dermis and subcutaneous tissue but epidermotropism is rare. Morphologically, ALCL is heterogeneous. The typical morphology is that of very large lymphoid cells, sometimes multinucleated, resembling Reed–Sternberg cells (Figure 39.19). Several morphological variants of ALCL have been recognized: monomorphic, Hodgkin's-like, histiocytic rich or small cell. Despite this morphological heterogeneity, all these variants bear the t(2;5). Most cases have a T-cell phenotype and often lack expression of some T-cell markers; a few cases have a 'null' (non-B, non-T) phenotype.

ALCL cells universally express CD30 (Ki-1), the hallmark of this lymphoma (Table 39.3). Lymphocyte activation markers such as CD25, HLA-DR determinants and CD71 and the epithelial membrane antigen (EMA) are often positive while the cells are cytokeratin negative. Unlike Reed–Sternberg cells, ALCL cells are, as a rule, CD15 negative. This is important to consider as diagnostic problems of this lymphoma frequently arise with Hodgkin's disease. Recent studies have shown that ALCL cells express perforin and granzyme B, molecules present in cytotoxic and NK cells, and thus suggested that ALCL cells derive from activated cytotoxic T cells. The chromosomal abnormality t(2;5)(p23;q35) is characteristic of ALCL. This leads to the rearrangement of the nucleolar phosphoprotein gene (*NPM*) on 5q35 with the anaplastic lymphoma tyrosine kinase (*ALK*) gene on 2p23 (Table 39.3). This fusion generates a chimeric transcript, NPM–ALK, which can be detected by FISH or by reverse transcriptase PCR using specific primers and by immunohistochemistry with an antibody against the *ALK*-encoded p80 protein. The expression or absence of p80 protein appears to have a prognostic impact. The NPM–ALK transcripts are detectable in most cases of nodal Ki-1[+] ALCL, but in only a few with the pure cutaneous form. This reinforces the fact that the latter represent a different entity, as regarded by the WHO.

It is unlikely that viruses such as EBV or HTLV-I play a pathogenic role in the development of this lymphoma. All the studies documenting the presence of these viruses are not solid and probably included some cases with other diagnosis.

The clinical course of ALCL is variable. Patients with early stages (I/II) and/or primary ALCL fare relatively well compared with those with advanced stages, bulky disease and/or secondary ALCL. The main prognostic factor in multivariate analysis is advanced stage (III/IV). There is no gold standard therapy for ALCL, and therapy should be tailored considering age, performance status and extent of the disease. Localized skin lesions may respond to radiotherapy but in advanced stages combination chemotherapy should be recommended. Unlike other T-NHL, ALCL patients have sensitive disease and usually respond to chemotherapy with an overall response rate of 55–100% in different series reported; however, most patients relapse. Autologous transplant has been successful in relapsed or newly diagnosed patients and this is the choice for young patients with advanced stages.

Differential diagnosis of peripheral T-NHL

The differential diagnosis arises with: (i) B-cell lymphomas, essentially T-cell rich B-NHL; (ii) reactive non-neoplastic lymphadenitis; and (iii) rarely, with Hodgkin's disease or acute leukaemias. Histology and immunohistochemistry allow distinguishing B- from T-cell lymphomas. In difficult cases, markers should be complemented with TCR and immunoglobulin chain gene analysis. The latter, in addition, will exclude cases of reactive lymphadenitis with difficult histology. Immunophenotype allows the distinction between large-cell T-NHL and acute myeloid leukaemia.

Diagnostic problems with other diseases may also arise with specific T-NHL subtypes. For instance, subpanniculitis-like T-NHL should be distinguished from benign skin conditions or histiocytosis, AIL T-NHL from reactive disorders, CD30[+] ALCL from Hodgkin's disease, and peripheral T-NHL, with marked haemophagocytic component, from histiocytic tumours or a reactive haemophagocytic syndrome. In such a setting, it is important to compound clinical features with the histopathology and, if required, with molecular analysis of the TCR chain genes.

Conclusions

The mature or chronic T-cell lymphoproliferative disorders comprise a variety of disease entities with distinct clinical and laboratory features. They can be classified on the basis of the clinical presentation and disease manifestations into primary leukaemias, leukaemia/lymphoma syndromes and T-cell lymphomas. The precise diagnosis is important in terms of patient management, prognosis and therapy. Most of these disorders have an aggressive clinical course and are considered as high- to intermediate-grade lymphomas. The application of molecular techniques together with immunological markers has greatly helped the understanding of their pathogenesis by the identification of genes or oncogenes responsible for disease initiation or progression and has allowed defining disease entities. This, in turn, has provided the basis for the development of novel and specific therapies for certain conditions, with improvement in survival. However, further research is needed to define a number of disorders which at present have not emerged as distinct entities. In this context, gene microarray analysis may allow us to establish new lymphoma entities, shed further light on their pathogenesis and devise gene-targeted therapies.

Acknowledgements

We thank Ricardo Morilla for providing the flow cytometry figures and Lok Lam for providing the PCR figure for the TCR.

Selected bibliography

Bazarbachi A, Soriano V, Pawson R *et al.* (1997) Mycosis fungoides and Sézary syndrome are not associated with HTLV-I infection: an international study. *British Journal of Haematology* **98**: 927–33.

Brito-Babapulle V, Pomfret M, Matutes E, Catovsky D (1987) Cytogenetic studies on prolymphocytic leukaemia. II T cell prolymphocytic leukemia. *Blood* **70**: 926–31.

Brouet JC, Flandrin G, Sasprotes M *et al.* (1975) Chronic lymphocytic leukaemia of T-cell origin. Immunological and clinical evaluation in eleven patients. *Lancet* ii: 890–3.

Catovsky D, Galetto J, Okos A *et al.* (1973) Prolymphocytic leukaemia of B- and T-cell type. *Lancet* 2: 232–234.

Catovsky D, Matutes E (2001) Leukemias of mature T cells. Chapter 43. In: *Neoplastic Hematopathology*, 2nd edn (D M Knowles, ed.), pp. 1589–902. Lippincott Williams and Wilkins, Philadelphia.

Chan WC, Casey JH (1995) Lymphoma of mucosa-associated lymphoid tissue. In: *Haematological Oncology, Volume 4* (J Armitage, A Newland, A Keating, A Burnett, eds), p. 78. Cambridge University Press, Cambridge.

Dearden CE, Matutes E, Cazin B *et al.* (2001) High remission rate in T-cell prolymphocytic leukemia with Campath-1H. *Blood* **98**: 1721–6.

Gallo RC (1995) Surprising advance in the treatment of viral leukemia. *New England Journal of Medicine* **332**: 1783–4.

Harris NL, Jaffe ES, Stein H *et al.* (1994) A revised European-American classfication of lymphoid neoplasms: A proposal from the International Lymphoma Study Group. *Blood* **84**: 1361–92.

Jaffe ES, Chan JKC, Su I-J *et al.* (1996) Report of the Workshop on nasal and related extranodal angiocentric T/Natural killer cell lymphomas. *American Journal of Surgery and Pathology* **20**: 103–11.

Jaffe ES, Harris NL, Stein H, Vardiman JW (2001) *World Health Organization (WHO) Classification of Tumours. Tumours of Haematopoietic and Lymphoid Tissues*, pp. 189–230. IARC Press, Lyon.

Lamy T, Loughran TP Jr. (1999) Current concepts: large granular lymphocyte leukemia. *Blood Reviews* **13**: 230–40.

Langerak AW, van den Beemd R, Wolvers-Tettero ILM *et al.* (2001) Molecular and flow cytometric analysis of the Vβ repertoire for clonality assessment in mature TCRαβ T-cell proliferations. *Blood* **98**: 165–73.

Loughran TP (1993) Clonal diseases of large granular lymphocytes. *Blood* **82**: 1–14.

Lundin J, Hagberg H, Repp R *et al.* (2003) Phase 2 study of alemtuzumab (anti-CD52 monoclonal antibody) in patients with advanced mycosis fungoides/Sézary syndrome. *Blood* **101**: 4267–72.

Marks DI, Vonderheid EC, Kurz BW *et al.* (1996) Analysis of p53 and mdm-2 expression in 18 patients with Sézary syndrome. *British Journal of Haematology* **92**: 890–9.

Matutes E, Brito-Babapulle V, Swansbury J *et al.* (1991) Clinical and laboratory features of 78 cases of T-prolymphocytic leukemia. *Blood* **78**: 3269–74.

Matutes E, Catovsky D (1998) Adult T-cell leukaemia lymphoma. In: *Leukemia*, 3rd edn (JA Whittaker, ed.), Chapter 18. Blackwell Scientific Publications, Oxford.

Matutes E (1999) *T-cell Lymphoproliferative Disorders. Classification, Clinical and Laboratory Aspects.* Harwood Academic Publishers, Amsterdam.

Matutes E, Brito-Babapulle V, Dearden C *et al.* (2001) Prolymphocytic leukemia of B- and T-cell types: biology and therapy. In: *Chronic Lymphoid Leukemias*, 2nd edn (B Cheson, ed.), Chapter 24. Marcel Dekker, New York.

Matutes E, Taylor GP, Cavenagh J *et al.* (2001) Interferon alpha and Zidovudine therapy in adult T-cell leukaemia lymphoma: response and outcome in 15 patients. *British Journal of Haematology* **113**: 779–84.

Matutes E, Wotherspoon AC, Parker NE *et al.* (2001) Transformation of T-cell granular lymphocyte leukaemia into a high grade large T-cell lymphoma. *British Journal of Haematology* **115**: 801–6.

Matutes E (2003) Chronic T-cell lymphoproliferative disorders. *Reviews in Clinical and Experimental Hematology* **6**: 401–20.

Mercieca J, Matutes E, Dearden C *et al.* (1994) The role of pentostatin in the treatment of T-cell malignancies: Analysis of response rate in 145 patients according to disease subtype. *Journal of Clinical Oncology* **12**: 2588–93.

Pawson R, Schulz TF, Matutes E, Catovsky D (1997) The human T-cell lymphotropic virus type I/II are not involved in T-prolymphocytic leukaemia and large granular lymphocyte leukemia. *Leukemia* **11**: 1305–11.

Shiota M, Nakamura S, Ichinohasama R *et al.* (1995) Anaplastic large cell lymphomas expressing the novel chimeric protein p80 NPM/ALK: A distinct clinicopathologic entity. *Blood* **86**: 1954–60.

Thangavelu M, Finn WG, Yelavarthi KK *et al.* (1997) Recurring structural chromosome abnormalities in peripheral blood lymphocytes of patients with mycosis fungoides/Sézary syndrome. *Blood* **89**: 3371–7.

Tien H-F, Su I-J, Tang J-L *et al.* (1997) Clonal chromosome abnormalities as direct evidence for clonality in nasal T/natural killer lymphomas. *British Journal of Haematology* **97**: 621–5.

Waldmann TA (1994) New approaches to the treatment of ATLL In: *Adult T-cell Leukaemia* (K Takatsuki, ed.), pp. 238–62. Oxford University Press, Oxford.

Zaja F, Russo D, Silvestri F *et al.* (1997) Retrospective analysis of 23 cases with peripheral T-cell lymphoma, unspecified: clinical characteristics and outcome. *Hematologica* **82**: 171–7.

CHAPTER 40

The myelodysplastic syndromes

40

David G Oscier and Sally B Killick

Introduction

The myelodysplastic syndromes (MDS) are clonal disorders of haemopoiesis. They share characteristic morphological abnormalities of the blood and bone marrow and a risk of evolution to acute leukaemia which varies depending on the subtype of MDS. The majority of patients are elderly and present with symptoms of marrow failure despite increased marrow cellularity. The nomenclature used to describe this syndrome has changed over the last 70 years. In the 1930s, the term 'refractory anaemia' was used to describe anaemic patients who were unresponsive to iron, vitamin B_{12} or folic acid. While some had 'anaemia of chronic disorders' others had features typical of MDS. A subgroup of patients with refractory anaemia was subsequently shown to have ring sideroblasts in the bone marrow. In the 1950s, it was appreciated that acute leukaemia in the elderly was often preceded by a 'pre-leukaemic' phase of peripheral blood cytopenia associated with either normal or a slightly increased percentage of bone marrow blasts. In 1982, the French–American–British (FAB) group proposed a morphological classification based on the percentage of blasts and ringed sideroblasts in the bone marrow and the presence or absence of a peripheral blood monocytosis which divided MDS into five subgroups. Patients with > 30% blasts in the bone marrow were considered to have acute leukaemia. In 2001, the World Health Organization (WHO) published a new classification of MDS incorporating morphological, genetic and clinical features; key differences from the FAB classification were the lowering of the blast threshold for the diagnosis of acute myeloid leukaemia (AML) to 20% and the

creation of a new category of mixed myelodysplastic and myeloproliferative diseases for patients with both proliferative features and dysplastic morphology. This chapter will utilize the WHO classification but includes a separate section on childhood MDS, which has some distinctive features.

Adult myelodysplastic syndromes

Incidence

Data on the incidence of MDS classified according to FAB criteria are derived mainly from European studies. Overall annual incidence rates are 3–4 per 100 000, but the rate increases dramatically with age, exceeding 30 per 100 000 for patients over the age of 80 (Figure 40.1). Data from the Italian registry show that 60% of patients are over the age of 70 years at diagnosis. The male to female ratio is 1.4:1. The most accurate epidemiological data on MDS come from the town district of Dusseldorf, where the incidence of MDS rose from 1.0 to 4.1 per 100 000 per year between 1976 and 1986. Subsequently, the incidence has remained stable and the early rise in incidence almost certainly reflected improvements in the diagnosis of MDS and an increasing tendency to investigate elderly cytopenic patients.

Aetiology

The aetiology of most cases of primary MDS remains unknown. Data from case–control studies are not always consistent but suggest modest associations with ionizing radiation, exposure to

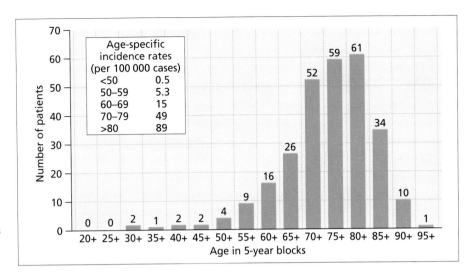

Figure 40.1 Age distribution of patients presenting with MDS in Bournemouth, 1981–1990.

benzene, solvents and pesticides, and with smoking. There is current interest in the possibility that polymorphisms in genes which encode proteins which interact with environmental factors may be associated with an increased susceptibility to MDS. Examples include enzymes responsible for the metabolism of carcinogens, defence against oxidative stress and DNA repair. In approximately 15% of patients, secondary or therapy-related MDS (TR-MDS) develops after exposure to cytotoxic chemotherapy and/or wide-field radiotherapy. The cytotoxic agents most commonly implicated are alkylating agents, nitrosoureas and procarbazine but not topoisomerase II inhibitors. The maximum incidence of TR-MDS occurs 5–7 years, with a range of 1–10 years, following exposure to chemotherapy. The risk increases with age and with prolonged exposure to low-dose chemotherapy. The risk of developing TR-MDS or acute myeloid leukaemia (AML) following autologous transplantation for lymphoma, myeloma or solid tumours varies widely between series (1–12%). Most cases develop within 5 years of transplantation and risk factors include increasing age, the duration and quantity of pretransplant chemotherapy and the use of total body irradiation as part of the conditioning regimen.

As discussed below, TR-MDS is associated with a higher incidence of trilineage dysplasia, genetic abnormalities, evolution to AML and poor response to treatment than is primary MDS.

Clinical and laboratory features

Clinical features

Twenty per cent of primary adult MDS patients are diagnosed from an incidental blood count, but the majority of the remainder present with features of bone marrow failure; 80% complain of fatigue due to anaemia while 20% present with infections or bleeding. Bacterial pneumonias and skin abscesses are the most common infections, occurring particularly in patients with a neutrophil count $< 1 \times 10^9$/L. Lymphadenopathy, hepatomegaly and splenomegaly are rarely found. There is an association

between MDS and several rare disorders that seem to have an immunological basis. These include febrile neutrophilic dermatosis (Sweet's syndrome), pyoderma gangrenosum, cutaneous vasculitis and relapsing polychondritis.

Blood count

Most patients are anaemic at presentation; 30–50% are pancytopenic, while 20% have anaemia in combination with either neutropenia or thrombocytopenia. Approximately 5% have isolated neutropenia or thrombocytopenia. Rarely, the diagnosis of MDS may be suspected because of macrocytosis or abnormalities in the blood film in the presence of a normal blood count. Parameters such as the myeloperoxidase index of granulocytes (MPXI), erythrocyte distribution width (RDW) and platelet distribution width (PDW) generated by automated cell counters are frequently abnormal and may become useful as markers for early MDS.

Blood and marrow morphology

The ability to diagnose MDS is critically dependent on optimal staining of blood and marrow slides with a Romanowsky stain. The accuracy of the marrow differential increases with the number of cells counted, which should be a minimum of 500. Less than 0.5 ml of marrow should be aspirated for morphological assessment to avoid excessive dilution with peripheral blood cells. The main morphological abnormalities found in MDS are summarized in Table 40.1 and examples are shown in Figure 40.2. The presence of hypochromic red cell fragments, particularly when accompanied by basophilic stippling, is strongly suggestive of refractory anaemia with ring sideroblasts. Rarely, male patients may present with or develop a pronounced dimorphic picture due to acquired haemoglobin H disease. Interobserver variation is a problem in diagnosis of MDS and is lowest for the detection of ring sideroblasts, micromegakaryocytes and increased blasts, and highest for mild dyserythropoiesis and neutrophil hypogranularity. It is important to recognize that

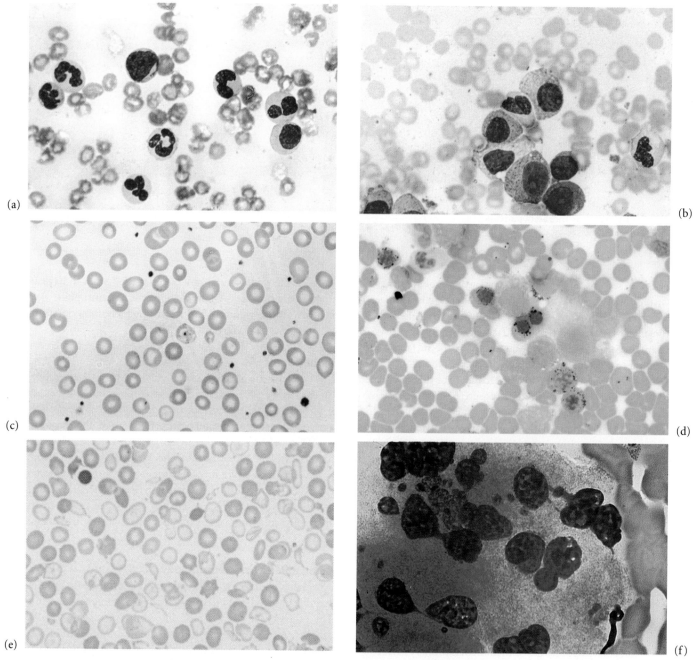

(a)

(b)

(c)

(d)

(e)

(f)

Figure 40.2 (a) Peripheral blood showing hypogranular and Pelger neutrophils and a single blast. (b) Marrow aspirate showing dysplastic granulopoiesis and a type I and a type II blast. (c) Peripheral blood from a patient with RARS showing a red cell with basophilic stippling and a central Howell–Jolly body. (d) Marrow aspirate stained with Perls' stain from a patient with RARS, showing ring sideroblasts. (e) Peripheral blood from a patient with RAEB, ring sideroblasts and acquired haemoglobin H, showing a grossly dimorphic picture. (f) Dysplastic megakaryocyte with widely separated nuclei. (g) Large mononuclear megakaryocyte.

(h) Micromegakaryocyte. (i) Marrow trephine biopsy showing an abnormal localization of immature precursors (ALIP) (courtesy of Dr Bridget Williams, Department of Histopathology, Royal Victoria Infirmary, Newcastle upon Tyne). (j) Marrow trephine stained for neutrophil elastase showing a 'true ALIP' (courtesy of Dr Bridget Wilkins, Department of Histopathology, Royal Victoria Infirmary, Newcastle upon Tyne). (k) Peripheral blood from a patient with CMML showing monocytes and promonocytes. (l) CMML marrow showing immature myeloid and monocytic cells.

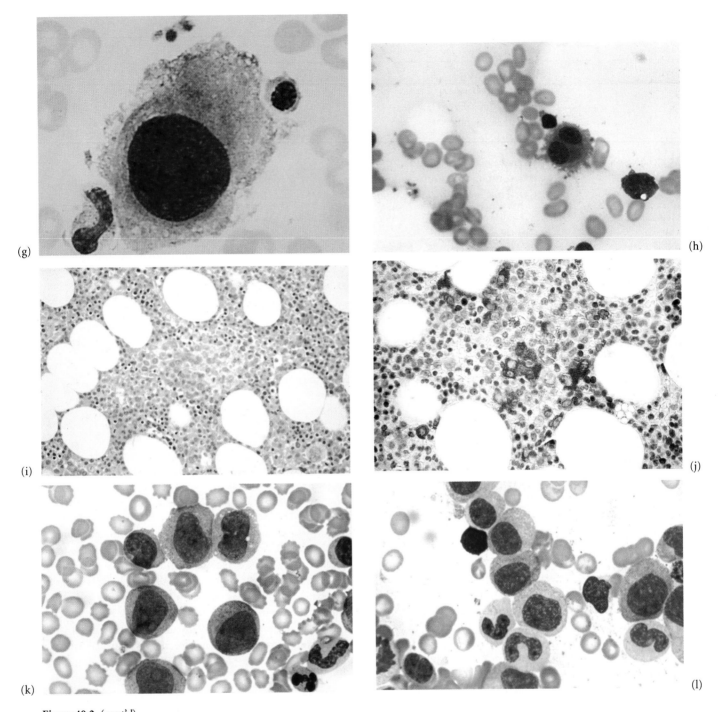

Figure 40.2 (*cont'd*)

dysplastic morphology may also be seen in healthy elderly individuals (affecting < 10% of marrow cells) and in a variety of non-clonal disorders including vitamin B_{12} and folic acid deficiency, heavy metal and alcohol poisoning, HIV and parvovirus infections and exposure to treatments such as anti-tuberculous therapy and granulocyte colony-stimulating factor (G-CSF).

Marrow histology

Bone marrow histology can provide additional diagnostic and prognostic information not obtainable from a marrow aspirate alone and should be routinely undertaken whenever bone marrow examination is performed in proven or suspected cases of MDS. Although the marrow is frequently hypercellular in MDS,

Table 40.1 Morphological abnormalities in MDS.

Lineage	Blood	Bone marrow
Erythroid	Oval macrocytosis	Erythroid hypoplasia
	Aniso-poikilocytosis	Multinuclearity
	Hypochromic red cell fragments	Dyskaryorrhexis
	Basophilic stippling	Cytoplasmic vacuolation
	Nucleated red cells	Ringed sideroblasts
Myeloid	Hypogranular neutrophils	Hypogranularity
	Hypolobation of neutrophil nuclei (Pelger cells)	Increased eosinophils and/or basophils
	Coarse nuclear chromatin clumping	Increased blasts
Megakaryocytes	Agranular platelets	Micromegakaryocytes
	Giant platelets	Large mono- or binuclear megakaryocytes
		Megakaryocytes with widely dispersed nuclei

hypocellularity, defined as cellularity < 30% of normal by reference to age-matched control subjects, is found in between 10% and 20% of cases. The precise incidence of hypocellularity is difficult to define since studies using magnetic resonance imaging have shown that marrow cellularity may be patchy, particularly in cases with no increase in marrow blasts. A slight increase in reticulin is seen in 50% of MDS cases, but marked fibrosis occurs in < 10%. Marrow hypocellularity, increased fibrosis and an inflammatory infiltrate comprising plasma cells, eosinophils, lymphoid aggregates and areas of oedema are more common in TR-MDS than in primary cases.

Marrow topography is frequently abnormal in MDS. In health, immature myeloid precursors are seen close to bony trabeculae and around blood vessels, whereas developing erythroid cells and megakaryocytes are seen in intertrabecular spaces. In MDS, myeloid precursors are displaced from trabecular margins and small clusters of myeloblasts and promyelocytes are sometimes seen in intertrabecular spaces. The clusters are called ALIPS (abnormal localization of immature precursors) and may develop due to autocrine production of vascular endothelial growth factor. The presence of ALIPS is considered to be an adverse prognostic factor in patients with less than 5% marrow blasts, but they are difficult to recognize and quantify and their presence is not specific to MDS. Clustering of megakaryocytes and the presence of both erythroid cells and megakaryocytes in paratrabecular areas are also features of MDS.

Cytogenetic, genetic and epigenetic abnormalities

Clonal cytogenetic abnormalities are found on direct or short-term culture of bone marrow in between 10% and 50% of cases of primary MDS, depending on the subtype, and 90% of cases of TR-MDS; the most common abnormalities are shown in

Table 40.2 Incidence (%) of chromosome abnormalities in MDS.

Abnormality	Primary MDS	TR MDS
del 5q/monosomy 5	10–20	30
del 7q/monosomy 7	10	40
trisomy 8	10	10
t(11q23)	6	3
del 17p	3	8
del 20q	5	< 1
Complex karyotype	10–20	90

Table 40.2. The use of fluorescence *in situ* hybridization (FISH) in interphase cells, using probes to detect the common cytogenetic abnormalities in MDS, enables clonal abnormalities to be detected in up to 10% of patients with a normal karyotype. Patients with higher blasts counts are more likely to have complex karyotypic abnormalities. Serial studies show that karyotypic evolution occurs in approximately 15% of cases. Apart from the 5q-minus syndrome, which is discussed in more detail later, cytogenetic abnormalities are not specific for particular subtypes of MDS. In contrast to *de novo* AML, chromosome translocations are rare in MDS and most cytogenetic abnormalities involve the gain or loss of genetic material. Although the genetic consequences of the common cytogenetic abnormalities remain unknown, minimally deleted regions have been defined for the deletions associated with the 5q-minus syndrome, for 5q deletions occurring in TR-MDS and AML, and for the deletion on chromosome 20q. A number of separate deleted regions have been identified on chromosome 7q. Deletions of classical tumour-suppressor genes are accompanied by mutations or epigenetic silencing of the remaining allele. There is no evidence for mutation or loss of function of any gene on the remaining allele within the minimally deleted regions on chromosomes 5, 7

and 20, suggesting that a dosage effect resulting from the loss of a single allele (haploinsufficiency) may contribute to the malignant phenotype.

Further progress in defining key genes in the pathogenesis of MDS should come from genetic engineering studies in which the common chromosomal deletions in MDS are reproduced in mice.

Gene expression profiling using cDNA microarray analysis has been performed on both purified CD34-positive cells and neutrophils from patients with MDS. A characteristic expression profile has been identified for patients with trisomy of chromosome 8 and differences have been observed between myelodysplastic and normal CD34-positive cells and between patients with good-risk and poor-risk MDS.

Mutations of oncogenes and tumour-suppressor genes important in other haematological malignancies and in solid tumours have also been identified in MDS. RAS mutations, usually involving N-RAS, are found in up to 20% of cases depending on the subtype. Mutations of RAS may occur early in MDS and persist throughout the course of the disease or may be lost or first appear at the time of leukaemic transformation. Mutations of the p53 gene, CSF-1R gene and AML1 gene and internal duplication of the FLT-3 gene are found in less than 10% of cases. It is increasingly recognized that methylation of CpG islands in the promoter region of genes may result in gene silencing in malignancy in the absence of mutation or deletion. Hypermethylation of the p15 gene, which encodes an inhibitor of cell cycle progression, is found in 50% of patients with MDS, particularly in patients with raised blast cell counts. There is a correlation between clinical response to both 5-azacytidine

and 5-aza-2-deoxycytidine, both potent inhibitors of cytidine methylation, and demethylation of the p15 gene.

Shortened telomeres, increased telomerase activity and microsatellite instability have also been described in MDS.

Detailed cytogenetic and genetic studies of patients with TR-MDS have identified patterns of associated abnormalities. Patients with monosomy 5 or deletion of 5q frequently have complex karyotypic abnormalities, a high incidence of p53 mutations and a very poor prognosis. Abnormalities of chromosome 7 are associated with hypermethylation of the p15 gene while tandem duplications of the FLT-3 gene are most commonly found in the minority of patients with a normal karyotype.

Other investigations

Immunophenotyping of blood or bone marrow cells is not routinely performed in MDS, but abnormalities such as low sidescatter, downregulation of antigens normally expressed on myeloid cells, and abnormal patterns of cell marker expression are commonly found in MDS. In addition, blast cells are more frequently CD34-positive and myeloperoxidase-negative than in de novo AML and the expression of additional markers on blast cells such as CD7 may have prognostic significance. In vitro colony growth is frequently defective in MDS, particularly in patients with increased marrow blasts, but the techniques are too cumbersome and poorly standardized for routine use.

Further laboratory tests frequently abnormal in MDS are shown in Table 40.3.

Table 40.3 Laboratory findings in MDS.

Investigation	Abnormality
Ferrokinetics	Ineffective erythropoiesis
Haemoglobin F	Frequently raised in JMML
Haemoglobin H	Raised in acquired haemoglobin H disease
Ham's test	Rarely positive
NAP score	Frequently low
Serum lysozyme	Increased in CMML
Granulocyte function	Reduced motility, adherence phagocytosis and bacterial killing
Platelet function	Prolonged bleeding time, reduced aggregation with adrenaline and collagen
Platelet-associated immunoglobulin	May be raised in the absence of immune-mediated thrombocytopenia
Lymphocyte populations	Reduced CD4 and natural killer cells
Immunoglobulins	Polyclonal gammopathy in 30%
	Hypogammaglobulinaemia in 20%
	Paraprotein in 5–10%
Autoantibodies	Found in 50% of cases of CMML

Table 40.4 The FAB classification of MDS.

Subtype	Blood	Bone marrow
Refractory anaemia (RA)	< 1% blasts	Dysplasia < 5% blasts
Refractory anaemia with ringed sideroblasts (RARS)	< 1% blasts	As for RA and > 15% ringed sideroblasts
Refractory anaemia with excess blasts (RAEB)	< 5% blasts	Dysplasia 5–19% blasts
Refractory anaemia with excess blasts in transformation (RAEBt)	< 5% blasts	Dysplasia 20–29% blasts or Auer rods
Chronic myelomonocytic leukaemia (CMML)	> 1×10^9/L monocytes	Dysplasia < 30% blasts

Table 40.5 The WHO classification of MDS.

Subtype	Blood	Bone marrow
Refractory anaemia (RA)	Anaemia	Erythroid dysplasia only
Refractory anaemia with ringed sideroblasts (RARS)	Anaemia	Erythroid dysplasia only > 15% ringed sideroblasts
Refractory cytopenia with multilineage dysplasia (RCMD)	Bi- or pancytopenia	Dysplasia in > 10% of cells in two or more cell lineages
Refractory cytopenia with multilineage dysplasia and ringed sideroblasts (RCMD-RS)	Bi- or pancytopenia	Dysplasia in > 10% of cells in two or more cell lineages > 15% ringed sideroblasts
Refractory anaemia with excess blasts-1 (RAEB-1)	Cytopenias; < 5% blasts	Uni- or multilineage dysplasia 5–9% blasts
Refractory anaemia with excess blasts-2 (RAEB-2)	Cytopenias or 5–19% blasts or Auer rods	Uni- or multilineage dysplasia 10–19% blasts or Auer rods
Myelodysplastic syndrome unclassified (MDS-U)	Cytopenias	Myeloid or megakaryocytic dysplasia
MDS associated with isolated del (5q)	Anaemia; normal or increased platelets	Megakaryocytes with hypolobated nuclei < 5% blasts

Classification of MDS

The FAB and WHO classifications of MDS and their interrelationship are shown in Tables 40.4–40.6.

The FAB classification (Table 40.4)

The FAB classification divides MDS into five subgroups with differing prognoses. The typical case of refractory anaemia (RA) presents with anaemia and a hypercellular marrow showing dyserythropoiesis but minimal granulocytic or megakaryocytic abnormalities. However, this group is clinically heterogeneous and includes patients with varying degrees of dysplasia and also patients with neutropenia and/or thrombocytopenia without anaemia. The diagnosis of refractory anaemia with ring sideroblasts (RARS) is made when ring sideroblasts forming a complete or partial ring around the nucleus make up more than 15% of erythroid cells, although small numbers of ring sideroblasts are found in over 60% of cases of MDS regardless of the subtype. Patients with an increase in marrow blasts are subdivided into those with refractory anaemia with excess blasts (RAEB) when the marrow blasts range between 5% and 19% and those with refractory anaemia with excess blasts in transformation (RAEBt) with a blast percentage between 20% and 29%. The latter term was introduced in recognition of the minority of patients with an increase in marrow blasts whose disease follows a more indolent course than is typically seen in AML. Chronic

Table 40.6 Relationship between the FAB and WHO classifications.

FAB	WHO
RA	RA (unilineage)
	RCMD
	5q− syndrome
RARS	RARS (unilineage)
	RCMD-RS
RAEB	RAEB-1
	RAEB-2
RAEBt	AML with multilineage dysplasia
	AML and MDS, therapy related
CMML	Myelodysplastic/myeloproliferative diseases

myelomonocytic leukaemia (CMML) encompasses all cases with more than 1×10^9/L circulating monocytes. This subgroup was also recognized to be heterogeneous and includes patients with a high monocyte count and splenomegaly more typical of a myeloproliferative disorder as well as patients with a modest monocytosis and a clinical course similar to that seen in refractory anaemia or refractory anaemia with excess blasts.

The WHO classification (Table 40.5)

The WHO classification is a modification of the FAB classification incorporating more recent clinical and genetic data. Following the observation that patients with less than 5% marrow blasts had a poorer prognosis if multilineage dysplasia was present, the terms refractory anaemia and refractory anaemia with ring sideroblasts are confined to patients with unilineage erythroid dysplasia. New terms, refractory cytopenia with multilineage dysplasia(RCMD) and refractory cytopenia with multilineage dysplasia and ring sideroblasts, have been introduced for cases with bi- or pancytopenia and dysplastic features in more than 10% of cells in two or more myeloid lineages. It is recognized that patients with unilineage erythroid dysplasia, or in whom dysplasia is seen in < 10% of cells in two lineages, may be difficult to diagnose as having MDS in the absence of a clonal karyotypic abnormality. It is recommended that such patients are re-evaluated at 6 months. MDS associated with an isolated deletion of chromosome 5q is considered to be a separate subgroup based on the uniformity of clinical and laboratory features of cases with this cytogenetic abnormality. The majority of patients are elderly women who present with a macrocytic anaemia, normal white cell count and a normal or raised platelet count. The marrow aspirate shows erythroid hypoplasia and large mono- or binuclear megakaryocytes. Most patients present with or develop a red cell transfusion requirement and the risk of leukaemic transformation is low.

The WHO classification recognizes the prognostic importance of the percentage of bone marrow blasts in MDS and includes myeloblasts, monoblasts, promonocytes and megakaryoblasts, but not erythroblasts, within the definition of a blast cell. CD34-positive cells defined immunophenotypically are not considered to be synonymous with the blast cells.

The term refractory anaemia with excess blasts is retained but subdivided into two subgroups based on the previous observation that patients with 10–19% of marrow blasts or more than 5% of circulating blasts (RAEB2) had a poorer prognosis than patients with < 10% of marrow blasts or fewer than 5% circulating blasts (RAEB1) (Table 40.6). The significance of Auer rods within blast cells remains uncertain in MDS, but all patients in whom Auer rods are seen are categorized as having RAEB2. In view of clinical and biological similarities, such as cytogenetic abnormalities, a high expression of multidrug-resistant glycoprotein and poor response to chemotherapy, between patients with dysplastic features and 20–29% marrow blasts and those with 30% or more blasts, the term refractory anaemia with excess blasts in transformation was abolished and all cases with dysplasia and more than 20% of blasts are classified as acute myeloid leukaemia with multilineage dysplasia. In addition, cases with the typical chromosome translocations found in *de novo* AML such as the t(15:17), t(18:21) and in(16) are considered to have AML regardless of the percentage of marrow blasts.

A new subgroup of MDS unclassified has also been introduced specifically for patients with unilineage, myeloid or megakaryocytic dysplasia and not as a depository for inadequately investigated cases.

Chronic myelomonocytic leukaemia is now included in a new classification of mixed myeloproliferative and myelodysplastic disorders.

Although the various WHO subgroups have differing clinical and biological features (Table 40.7), the use of quantitative criteria such as marrow blast percentage to define subgroups is of necessity arbitrary, and while some patients may remain within a single WHO subgroup others may progress through two or more subgroups during the course of their disease. It cannot be assumed that the clinical course of a patient presenting with RAEB will be the same as that of a patient with a preceding history of RCMD.

Pathogenesis

The pathogenesis of primary adult MDS is poorly understood. Genetic and functional abnormalities of haemopoietic stem cells, immunological abnormalities and increased apoptosis of bone marrow cells are all well documented, as discussed below (Figure 40.3).

Subtype	% of MDS	Cytogenetic abnormalities (%)	Median survival (months)
RA	5–10	25	66
RARS	10	< 10	72
RCMD	24	50	33
RCMD-RS	15	50	33
RAEB	40	30–50	10 (RAEB-1)
			18 (RAEB-2)
Isolated del 5q	5	100	116

Table 40.7 WHO classification – clinical and laboratory features.

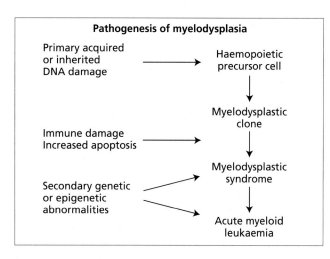

Figure 40.3 Pathogenesis of myelodysplasia.

MDS: a stem cell disorder

The presence of trilineage dysplasia and cytogenetic abnormalities provides irrefutable evidence for involvement of a multipotent haemopoietic stem cell in MDS. The nature of the initiating event is unknown but is likely to be heterogeneous and include both inherited and acquired DNA damage. Insight into the nature of the target cell in MDS has come from recent studies utilizing interphase FISH. In normal marrow, haemopoietic stem cells reside in the CD34-positive, CD38-negative cell fraction. Interphase FISH studies in patients with the 5q-minus syndrome show that this cytogenetic abnormality is found in both CD34-positive, CD38-negative and CD34-positive, CD19-positive pro-B cells, suggesting that the disease originates in a lymphomyeloid stem cell. Similar studies in patients with trisomy 8 show that this abnormality originates in a more mature myeloid stem cell but CD34-positive, CD38-negative cells which lack trisomy 8 are still functionally defective, implying that trisomy 8 is not an initiating event in the pathogenesis of MDS. It is currently unclear whether cases in which morphological abnormalities are confined to a single lineage arise in a lineage-committed or multipotent stem cell. The frequent finding of multiple cytogenetic abnormalities, point mutations in oncogenes and epigenetic abnormalities, particularly in TR-MDS but also in primary MDS, clearly demonstrates the multistep pathogenesis of MDS.

In addition to abnormalities of the nuclear genome, mitochondrial DNA mutations are also found in up to 50% cases. In patients with ringed sideroblasts, iron deposition occurs within mitochondria, and it has been suggested that mitochondrial DNA mutations may impair the function of the mitochondrial respiratory chain, leading to oxidation of ferrous to ferric iron with the consequent accumulation of ferric iron within mitochondria. Support for this model comes from the study of Pearson's syndrome, which is a rare congenital disorder characterized by large lesions of mitochondrial DNA and a refractory anaemia with ringed sideroblasts in the bone marrow.

Immunological abnormalities in MDS

Aplastic anaemia and hypocellular MDS have many features in common. Both disorders are characterized by a clonal expansion of T cells (the clones are antigen driven and not neoplastic), over-representation of HLA-DR15, the presence of mutations in the PIG-A gene characteristic of paroxysmal nocturnal haemoglobinuria (PNH) and clinical response to immunosuppressive therapy. In addition, patients with aplastic anaemia frequently present with a macrocytosis and dyserythropoiesis. Clonal cytogenetic abnormalities are occasionally found at presentation but develop in up to 30% of patients within 3 years of follow-up, and, following successful immunosuppressive therapy, 12% of patients develop MDS within 12 years. A current hypothesis suggests that aplastic anaemia and hypocellular MDS are closely related disorders (Figure 40.4) in which damage to a haemopoietic stem cell results in an immune response directed against both transformed and normal haemopoietic stem cells. The clinical outcome depends on the vigour of the immune response and the resistance of the neoplastic clone to immune-mediated damage. PNH clones, which are present in small numbers in normal marrows, appear able to expand in marrows rendered hypocellular by T-cell mediated damage. The expanded T cells in MDS may occasionally become neoplastic, resulting in T-cell large granular lymphocytic leukaemia.

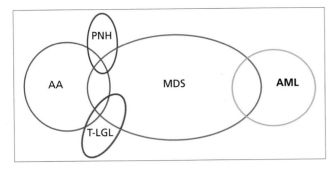

Figure 40.4 Interrelationship between aplastic anaemia, myelodysplasia, paroxysmal nocturnal haemaglobinuria and T-cell large granulocytic leukaemia.

Apoptosis in MDS

A long-recognized paradox in MDS has been the association between a hypercellular bone marrow and peripheral blood cytopenias. In patients undergoing leukaemic transformation, cytopenias probably result from a failure of maturation of the neoplastic clone. However, there is increasing evidence that the ineffective haemopoiesis seen in patients without increased blasts is due to an increased susceptibility of CD34-positive MDS cells to apoptosis. Apoptosis is more prominent in early MDS (RA, RARS) than in advanced MDS (RAEBt and AML). In keeping with this finding, small studies have shown that Bcl-2 expression is lower in early MDS than with disease progression to AML, and patients with early MDS seem to have higher ratios of proapoptotic than of antiapoptotic proteins. There does not seem to be a correlation between CD34$^+$ apoptosis and age, subtype of MDS, peripheral cytopenias or marrow cellularity. Apoptosis may be triggered by a variety of factors, including intrinsic DNA damage, mitochondrial dysfunction, cytotoxic T cells, overexpression of the cytokine TNF-α with subsequent upregulation of the FAS/FASL pathway and abnormalities of marrow stromal cells. A recent study has shown that erythroid precursors in MDS spontaneously release cytochrome C from mitochondria, leading to activation of caspase 9 and apoptosis. G-CSF inhibits cytochrome C release, and this may provide an explanation for the use of G-CSF in conjunction with erythropoietin in treating the anaemia of patients with RA, RARS and RCMD. Other agents targeted at proapoptotic pathways, e.g. amifostine or pentoxifylline, have not fulfilled their early promises.

Natural history and prognostic factors

The median survival of adult patients with primary MDS is approximately 20 months and the prognosis for each WHO subgroup is worse than for age- and sex-matched control subjects. The marked heterogeneity in outcome in MDS was illustrated by

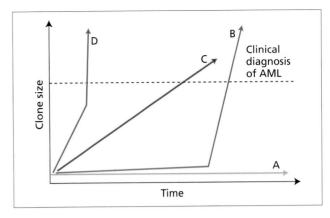

Figure 40.5 Hypothetical model of evolution patterns in patients with MDS, based on growth advantage instability of the malignant clone (from Tricot *et al.* 1985, with permission).

a study of 46 patients, which correlated the morphological and cytogenetic changes that occurred during the course of the disease with survival (Figure 40.5). Forty-eight per cent of patients (group A) had a stable course over many years. The initial FAB diagnosis in these cases was RA, RARS or CMML, and the majority were ALIP negative. Additional chromosome abnormalities rarely occurred during the course of the disease, and many patients died from incidental causes. Twenty-four per cent of patients (group C) had a gradual increase in the percentage of marrow blasts. These patients were often ALIP-positive at diagnosis and rarely showed karyotypic evolution. They frequently succumbed to infections or haemorrhagic complications with or without evolution to acute leukaemia. A further type of evolution (group B or D), found in 28% of patients, was characterized by a rapid increase in blast cells. The majority of these patients already had an abnormal karyotype at presentation, and most were ALIP positive. The sudden increase in blasts was frequently accompanied by additional chromosomal abnormalities. Another form of evolution not shown in Figure 40.5 is characterized by increasing pancytopenia without an increase in marrow blasts. Dysplastic changes may become more pronounced, and occasionally increasing anaemia may be due to red cell aplasia. It is unclear whether these changes reflect clonal expansion or clonal evolution.

This heterogeneity in clinical course has stimulated an ongoing quest for prognostic factors. A list of factors with adverse prognostic significance is shown in Table 40.8. Since the WHO classification incorporates known prognostic factors such as cytopenias, increased marrow blasts, the presence of trilineage dysplasia and the isolated loss of chromosome 5q, it is not surprising that it has prognostic significance. A different approach has been to devise prognostic scoring systems incorporating a number of known prognostic factors, and is suitable for use in all patients with MDS regardless of their subtype. In 1997, an International Prognostic Scoring System (IPSS) was published

Table 40.8 Adverse prognostic factors in MDS.

Clinical
Therapy-related MDS

Blood
Severe cytopenias
Raised LDH or β_2-microglobulin

Marrow morphology
Increased blasts
Trilineage dysplasia
Presence of ALIPS

Chromosome abnormalities
Loss of chromosome 5 or 7
Deletion of chromosome 3q, 5q (excluding 5q syndrome), 7q, 17p
Structural abnormality of chromosome 11q23
Complex chromosome abnormalities
Karyotypic evolution

Genetic/epigenetic abnormalities
P53, RAS mutations
Overexpression of WT1
p15 hypermethylation
Telomere shortening
Gene expression profile

Immunophenotype
CD7-positive blasts

In vitro *colony growth*
Leukaemic growth pattern

based on the retrospective evaluation of a clinical, morphological and cytogenetic data from 816 patients who were either untreated or had received only short courses of low-dose oral chemotherapy or haemopoietic growth factors. The study included patients classified as having MDS according to the FAB criteria except that patients with proliferative CMML with a white blood count of $> 12 \times 10^9$/L were excluded. The IPSS is shown in Table 40.9, and patients may be allocated into one of four risk groups – low,

intermediate I, intermediate II or high – whose median survival according to age at diagnosis is shown in Table 40.10. The clinical value of a single prognostic factor or a scoring system is critically dependent on the type of treatment a patient receives. The IPSS has been validated in patients undergoing allogeneic transplantation, but the outcome of patients receiving intensive chemotherapy is more dependant on cytogenetic data than the percentage of marrow blasts and the IPSS appears to be less useful in this setting. Different sets of predictive factors for response to haemopoietic growth factors and to immunosuppressive therapy have also been developed and these are discussed later.

It is likely that newer prognostic factors, including data from gene expression profiling, will be incorporated into scoring systems and will improve the prognostic power.

Management

The management of MDS is generally unsatisfactory. The literature abounds with small uncontrolled studies, usually detailing the short-term response to a wide variety of agents. There is also a dearth of randomized trials such that the relative merit of various forms of treatment remains unclear. This lack of good trial data in a relatively common disorder with a short median survival reflects both the difficulty of trial design and the disappointing preliminary results obtained with most currently available treatments but is largely due to the advanced age of most of the patients, whose general health, social situation and own wishes and expectations are major factors in determining appropriate treatment. Management options range from observation only, supportive care, a variety of treatments (cytotoxics, transplantation, growth factors, immunosuppression), to only symptom relief for patients whose general health is so poor that an improvement in their haematological status would confer no corresponding improvement in quality of life. Identification of risk factors for disease progression and use of the IPSS score to predict outcome may help guide the clinician in deciding patient management. However, there are two caveats: in asymptomatic patients, a period of observation to determine the rate of disease progression can be helpful before formulating a management plan, and it is unwise to base treatment on the results of blood

Table 40.9 International Prognostic Scoring System (IPSS).

Score value	0	0.5	1.0	1.5	2.0
BM blasts (%)	<5	5–10	–	11–20	21–30
Karyotype*	Good	Intermediate	Poor		
Cytopenias	0/1	2/3			

*Good: normal, −Y, del(5q), del(20q); poor: complex (> 3 abnormalities) or chromosome 7 anomalies; intermediate: other abnormalities.
Cytopenias defined as haemoglobin concentration < 10 g/dL, neutrophils < 1.5 × 10^9/L and platelets < 100 × 10^9/L.

Table 40.10 Median survival of primary myelodysplastic syndrome using the IPSS score.

Risk group	IPSS score	Median survivial			
		< 60 years	> 60 years	< 70 years	> 70 years
Low	0	11.8	4.8	9	3.9
Intermediate 1	0.5–1.0	5.2	2.7	4.4	2.4
Intermediate 2	1.5–2.0	1.8	1.1	1.3	1.2
High	> 2.5	0.3	0.5	0.4	0.4

and marrow findings taken during an acute infective episode as transient increases in the neutrophil count and percentage of marrow blasts may be seen.

Supportive care

The mainstay of supportive care is the use of red cell transfusions in patients who are symptomatically anaemic. Blood transfusions, however, do have certain risks associated, including iron overload in multitransfused patients. Although iron chelation, with desferrioxamine, is generally recommended in good-risk MDS, there are few data in the literature to suggest that this expensive and inconvenient treatment improves overall survival. Recommendations on when to commence chelation are therefore difficult. It would be reasonable to consider chelation once a patient has received 5 g iron (approximately 25 units of red cells), but limited to those patients with a good prognosis according to the IPSS score, have no other significant comorbidities and are at an age that would clinically benefit. Vitamin C in low dose increases iron excretion and should be started after 4 weeks of commencing chelation. Desferrioxamine is generally given as a subcutaneous infusion over 10–12 h; alternatively, it can be given via an indwelling catheter. The use of oral iron chelators have not been routinely used in MDS.

Platelet transfusions are indicated in thrombocytopenic patients in the treatment of acute bleeding episodes, or as prophylaxis prior to surgery or following chemotherapy. However, their long-term use, for example in the prevention of recurrent epistaxis or mouth bleeding in elderly patients with persistent thrombocytopenia, presents major logistic (and financial) problems. The potential clinical importance of platelet and neutrophil dysfunction in patients whose counts may be normal or minimally depressed should not be forgotten when deciding on the need for platelet support prior to surgery or the choice between oral and intravenous antibiotics in an infected patient. The potential role of growth factors in supportive care is discussed below.

Growth factors

Erythropoietin (Epo)

Anaemia represents one of the major clinical problems for patients with MDS. The aim of recombinant Epo is to improve the overall quality of life by avoiding fluctuations in the haemo-globin concentration. It also has the added benefit of avoiding the risks associated with red cell transfusions. Unfortunately, those who would benefit most are least likely to respond. Predictors of response include low serum Epo level of < 200 U/L (usually raised in MDS), non-RARS subtype and no or low transfusion requirements (two or less units/month). It is generally well tolerated and studies have shown a benefit of Epo over placebo, with overall response rates (100% reduction in transfusion requirements) of 16–24%.

There is some synergism between Epo and granulocyte colony-stimulating factor (G-CSF). The effect is most marked in patients with RARS (approximately 50% response rates), who have a very low response rate to Epo alone (approximately 8% response). In some patients the response to combination therapy can be maintained with Epo alone, whereas others require both Epo and G-CSF. A prototype predictive model for response to Epo + G-CSF has been described (Figure 40.6), based on the serum Epo level and pretreatment transfusion need. This approach could be useful to the clinician when deciding whether or not to embark on this treatment to avoid unnecessary cost and patient inconvenience. It is thought that growth factors in MDS work by reducing haemopoietic progenitor cell apoptosis, leading to more effective erythropoiesis.

Granulocyte colony-stimulating factor (G-CSF)

Over 90% of MDS patients receiving short-term G-CSF show a dose-dependent neutrophilia, with an improvement in neutrophil function but no increase in eosinophils, monocytes or lymphocytes. In a minority of patients the haemoglobin and/or platelet count is increased. Its use is usually reserved for patients with severe sepsis or as part of intensive chemotherapy.

Immunosuppression

Accumulating evidence suggests that there is an immunological process involved in the pathogenesis of MDS. For this reason, as in aplastic anaemia, several groups have had success in treating 'low-risk' MDS (RA, RARS) with anti-thymocyte globulin. It is expected that 30–50% of patients will have a response to treatment, evident by an improvement in blood counts and a reduction or cessation of blood products. There seems to be a trend towards better response rates in those patients with hypocellular MDS or who have HLA-DR15. The treatment is not curative

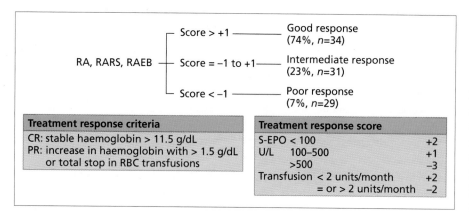

Figure 40.6 Predictive model for response rates to therapy with Epo plus GCSF based upon pretreatment Epo concentration and transfusion need (reproduced with permission from Hellstrom-Lindberg *et al.*, *British Journal of Haematology* 2003; 120: 1037–46).

but durable responses have been noted. Cyclosporin, probably acting by a similar mechanism, has also been shown to have an effect in one small study. The results of large randomized trials of immunosuppression in MDS are awaited.

Intensive chemotherapy

Typically, treatment of MDS with intensive chemotherapy is marked by low remission rates and high relapse rates, often complicated by prolonged chemotherapy induced hypoplasia. The reason that the disease is difficult to treat is thought to be the high drug resistance of the malignant clone. Complete remission (CR) rates are generally accepted as being lower than in patients with *de novo* AML; however, these comparisons are valid only if the patient groups are of similar age and those with apparently *de novo* AML are rigorously assessed for the presence of trilineage dysplasia.

The CR rates for high-risk MDS from studies in the mid- to late 1990s are 38–79%. Factors associated with a higher chance of CR include early treatment (within 3 months of diagnosis), young age (< 50 years), normal karyotype and the presence of Auer rods (Table 40.11). Remissions are typically short-lived (5–15 months), which provides the rationale for consolidating induction chemotherapy with transplantation in suitable patients. It is now generally accepted that among those MDS patients with complex karyotypes, particularly involving loss of chromosome 5 or 7, the CR rate is lower and remission duration even shorter. These factors should be borne in mind when deciding whether a patient should receive intensive chemotherapy.

Table 40.11 Positive predictors for response to intensive chemotherapy.

Age < 50 years
Normal karyotype
Auer rods
Treatment within 3 months of diagnosis

In vitro studies have shown that fludarabine is an effective DNA terminator and increases the intracellular concentration of Ara-C; this is the rationale behind the combination FLA. The addition of G-CSF (FLAG) is thought to increase the sensitivity of the blasts to Ara-C; however, this observation has not been translated into a clinical benefit as CR rates are similar with FLAG and FLA. Overall, studies have shown CR rates of approximately 66% with the two regimens.

Finally, patients with treatment-related MDS have a particularly poor prognosis. CR rates are lower and duration of remissions shorter.

Stem cell transplantation (SCT)

It is apparent that intensive chemotherapy alone in high-risk patients with MDS does not produce durable remissions and therefore consolidation is needed. This can be either allogeneic or autologous SCT. There is no place for SCT in patients who do not achieve CR with induction chemotherapy. Transplantation is also offered to appropriate patients with early MDS, although these patients do not usually require chemotherapy before transplant (if marrow blasts < 5%).

Allogeneic SCT

Data from the International BMT Registry (IBMTR) show that the best results following allo-SCT occur in patients under 40 years old with short disease duration and < 5% bone marrow blasts. Patients with RA/RARS receiving an HLA-identical sibling SCT have an overall 3-year survival of 53%, compared with 36% 3-year survival in those with RAEB, RAEBt or CMML (1991–1997). Data from the European BMT group (EBMT) show similar results (1983–1998), with 3-year actuarial disease-free survival of untreated RA/RARS and RAEBt/sAML of 55% and 28% respectively. Thus, the status of the underlying disease is a major contributing factor to disease-free survival (Table 40.12).

The value of giving pretransplant chemotherapy in advanced MDS remains debatable. European BMT centres favour intensive chemotherapy prior to SCT in an attempt to reduce relapse rates,

Table 40.12 Poor prognostic factors for outcome following allo-SCT in MDS.

Older age
Poor-risk cytogenetics
High IPSS score
Advanced disease (RAEB, RAEBt)
Treatment-related MDS
Prolonged disease duration
Marrow fibrosis

whereas most patients in North America are transplanted without induction chemotherapy. Pretransplant chemotherapy has the added advantage of selecting out those who do not enter CR, as these will have a worse overall survival following transplantation.

As MDS is more common with advancing age and transplant-related mortality (TRM) is high in this group of patients, interest has been shown in non-myeloablative SCT. Conditioning (fludarabine, busulphan, Campath) is highly immunosuppressive but not myeloablative, so TRM is reduced. Disease control depends on a graft-versus-MDS effect and donor lymphocyte infusions can be given post transplant in patients with a mixed chimera. Early results suggest that TRM is significantly reduced when compared with standard SCT, but this benefit is offset by high relapse rates seen 1–2 years post transplant. Longer follow-up and larger numbers of patients are needed to establish whether this will be an effective form of treatment in MDS.

Autologous SCT

For those patients ineligible for allo-SCT, autologous SCT (bone marrow or PBSCs) may be a viable alternative. Polyclonal $CD34^+$ progenitors can be harvested from the blood of MDS patients in the recovery phase of intensive chemotherapy and used to achieve rapid and stable engraftment following high-dose chemotherapy. Although the feasibility of autologous bone marrow and PBSC SCT in MDS is well established, the efficacy remains to be determined. Data from EBMT on autologous BMT in first CR show 2-year survival, disease-free survival and relapse rates of 39%, 34% and 64% respectively. MDS patients have higher relapse rates than matched AML controls, suggesting higher residual disease burden in the graft.

Novel therapies

Improvement in our understanding of the underlying mechanisms in the pathogenesis of MDS has led to identification of a variety of potential therapeutic targets.

Thalidomide and its analogues

Exactly how thalidomide acts in MDS is unclear, but it is thought that it inhibits TNF-α production, has an antiangiogenic effect and modulates the immune system. There have now been many small studies, particularly in low-risk MDS. Response rates have been described in up to half the patients treated, although only a minority of these patients have become independent of transfusions. The use of thalidomide has been limited by unacceptable toxicities. Considering that many of these patients are elderly and quality-of-life issues are paramount, it is interesting to note that even patients having a major haematological response (off transfusions) have elected to come off treatment due to side-effects. Thalidomide analogues are now in trial (CC-5013, Revimid). CC-5013 seems to have a lower toxicity profile, and response rates (transfusion independence) have been seen in about one-third of non-5q− patients. Those with the 5q− syndrome have higher response rates and this may represent an effective new treatment option for this subgroup of patients.

Demethylation agents

Methylation in MDS was discussed in detail earlier in the chapter. The epigenetic therapeutic approach with either 5-azacytidine or 5-aza-2'-deoxycytidine induces demethylation of hypermethylated genes. Silverman's group has investigated 5-azacytidine, a pyrimidine nucleoside cytosine analogue. The results of a randomized study of azacytidine versus observation in MDS patients show an overall response rate of 63% in the azacytidine arm; 6% achieved a complete response and median time to leukaemic progression was 22 months (compared with 12 months in the observational arm). A significant improvement in median survival has not been shown, although quality of life in the treatment group was reported as better.

Therapeutic strategy

Deciding the best approach for the treatment of patients with MDS can be difficult. It is helpful to use the IPSS score to guide treatment, in addition to the patient's age, performance status and, most importantly, the patient's own wishes.

Management of anaemia

Red cell transfusions should be given to any patient with symptomatic anaemia. Alternatives to blood transfusions should be considered in suitable patients, including growth factors, immunosuppression and newer agents such as the thalidomide analogues. Figure 40.7 outlines a reasonable approach.

IPSS low

As the median survival without treatment is 4.8 years (> 60 years) to 11.8 years (< 60 years), the morbidity and mortality from intensive chemotherapy or SCT cannot be justified. It is more appropriate to monitor these patients for disease progression.

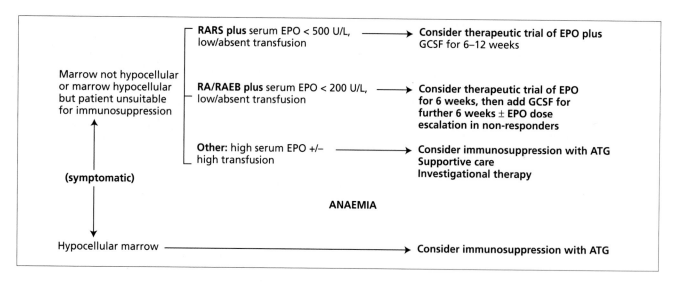

Figure 40.7 Guidelines for the management of symptomatic anaemia in MDS patients (reproduced with permission from Bowen *et al.*, *British Journal of Haematology* 2003; **120**: 187–200).

IPSS Intermediate-1

It is reasonable to consider SCT in this group of patients, particularly in those < 50 years with a sibling donor available, as the outcome after SCT is improved if performed early in the disease. However, with the median survival for patients < 60 years being 5.2 years, and a known significant TRM, the decision to transplant these patients is difficult, particularly in those with mild cytopenias and a normal karyotype. These patients could be left under close observation. Patients < 65 years with severe cytopenias or showing disease progression should be discussed with the local transplant unit.

IPSS Intermediate-2/High

Patients in this poor prognostic group who are less than 65 years should be considered for chemotherapy plus SCT. When making this decision, it is useful to consider the predictive factors for response to chemotherapy (Table 40.11) and outcome following SCT (Table 40.12). In addition, SCT should be performed only in those patients who achieve a complete or good partial response to chemotherapy. The flow chart in Figure 40.8 gives an overview of recommendations for SCT consolidation by the UK MDS guideline group.

It is difficult to give recommendations for the treatment of patients with high-risk MDS over the age of 65 years. These patients are eligible for the elderly NCRI AML trial (AML 14); however, much will depend on patients' performance status, comorbidities and own wishes. It is reasonable to await the result of the karyotype before deciding on treatment, as patients with poor-risk karyotypes have low response rates to intensive AML-type induction.

The place for novel therapies

With the advent of more new agents for the treatment of MDS, such as the thalidomide analogues and azacytidine, the decisions become even more complex. However, as with all investigational therapies, patients should be treated within clinical research protocols.

Myelodysplastic/myeloproliferative diseases

The WHO classification of myelodysplastic/myeloproliferative diseases (MDS/MPD) is shown in Table 40.13 and includes patients with both proliferative features characterized by marrow hypercellularity and increased numbers of circulating cells in one or more lineages, as well as dysplastic features characterized by abnormal cell morphology and cytopenia(s).

Chronic myelomonocytic leukaemia

Chronic myelomonocytic leukaemia (CMML) constitutes 15–20% of cases of MDS, defined according to FAB criteria. There is

Table 40.13 WHO classification of myelodysplastic/myeloproliferative diseases.

Chronic myelomonocytic leukaemia	CMML
Atypical chronic myeloid leukaemia	aCML
Juvenile myelomonocytic leukaemia	JMML
Myelodysplastic/myeloproliferative disease	Unclassifiable

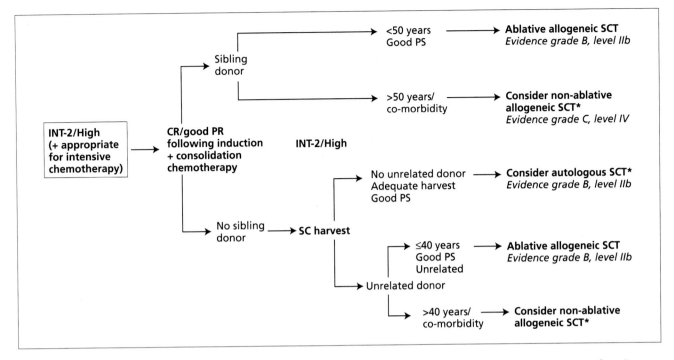

Figure 40.8 Guidelines for SCT in the management of IPSS INT-2/high MDS patients ≤ 65 years (reproduced with permission from Bowen et al., *British Journal of Haematology* 2003; **120**: 187–200). *Within CRP where available.

Table 40.14 Diagnostic criteria for CMML.

Persistent monocytosis of $> 1 \times 10^9$/L
No BCR-ABL fusion gene
< 20% blasts in blood or marrow
Dysplasia in one or more lineages

a male predominance and median age of presentation is 72 years. Only 10% of cases present under the age of 60. The aetiology is unknown and therapy-related CMML is extremely rare.

The diagnostic criteria are shown in Table 40.14. If dysplastic features are minimal or absent, the diagnosis of CMML is still tenable if a clonal cytogenetic abnormality is present or if monocytosis persists for at least 3 months in the absence of other causes of monocytosis.

Clinical and laboratory features

Approximately 50% of patients have splenomegaly at presentation. Patients with high monocyte counts may develop a maculopapular skin infiltrate or monocytic pleural or pericardial effusions. Mild anaemia and thrombocytopenia are common and the white cell count may vary from normal to over 80×10^9/L. Monocytes may have normal morphology or may have agranular cytoplasm and/or abnormal nuclear lobation. The bone marrow is usually hypercellular and typical trilineage dysplastic

features are found in over 80% of cases. Cytochemical studies may aid the distinction between monocyte and granulocyte precursors. Cytogenetic abnormalities are found in 30–40% of cases and are not specific for CMML. Deletions of 5q are rare in CMML. The incidence of *RAS* mutations is higher than in other forms of myelodysplasia and is found in up to 40% of cases. Hypermethylation of the *p15* gene and reduced expression of p15 protein in marrow trephines is found in approximately 50% of patients with CMML. A minority of patients with either CMML or atypical chronic myeloid leukaemia present with chromosome translocations which disrupt either the fibroblast growth factor receptor-1 gene on chromosome 8p11 or the platelet-derived growth factor receptor B gene on chromosome 5q31. These translocations involve multiple partners and result in the expression of tyrosine kinase fusion proteins. These patients usually present with marked eosinophilia and are important to identify as they respond well to imatinib mesylate but not to conventional chemotherapy.

Natural history and prognosis

CMML has been subdivided into dysplastic and proliferative subtypes, but there are no clinical, morphological or biological features which reliably separate the two groups, and patients presenting with low monocyte counts and dysplastic features may subsequently acquire proliferative features during the course of the disease. The clinical course is variable, with a median survival of approximately 2 years. Adverse prognostic features include

	CML	CMML	Atypical CML
Dysplasia	< 10% except in transformation	+	++
Monocytosis	Absolute monocytosis but < 3%	+	+
Immature granulocytes	Myelocyte peak	< 15%	> 15%
Basophilia	+	–	±
BCR–ABL rearrangement			
± Ph chromosome	Yes	No	No
RAS mutations	No	40%	?

Table 40.15 Differential diagnosis of proliferative MDS.

CML, chronic myeloid leukaemia; CMML, chronic myelomonocytic leukaemia.

anaemia, thrombocytopenia, lymphocytosis, a raised serum lactate dehydrogenase (LDH) and an increased percentage of bone marrow blasts. The importance of the marrow blast percentage in predicting outcome is highlighted in the WHO classification which subdivides CMML into cases with < 10% marrow blasts (CMML-I) and those with 10–19% blasts (CMML-II).

Treatment

The majority of patients with CMML are elderly (> 60 years), and when the proliferative phase prevails oral chemotherapy with hydroxyurea would be the treatment of choice. In a multicentre European randomized trial of hydroxyurea versus etoposide in adult CMML, the response rate and median survival was 60% and 20 months for hydroxyurea, and 36% and 9 months for etoposide.

Younger patients with adverse features should be considered for more intensive treatment. The EBMT data for allogeneic (related and unrelated) SCT in adult patients with CMML, however, show poor long-term outcomes, with 5-year estimated overall survivals of only 21%. As with other types of MDS, patients have a better outcome if transplanted early in their disease. Alternatively, AML-type induction can be given, consolidated with autologous SCT.

Particularly in young patients, treatment options for CMML are not optimal, and, therefore, wherever possible, patients should be put into clinical trials .

Atypical chronic myeloid leukaemia

Atypical chronic myeloid leukaemia (aCML) is a poorly defined entity characterized by a leucocytosis, more than 10% circulating immature myeloid cells that are rarely more than 5% blasts, and prominent dysgranulopoiesis. A subset is characterized by neutrophils and myeloid precursors with pronounced clumping of nuclear chromatin. The distinguishing features between CMML, aCML and CML are shown in Table 40.15.

Most patients present with anaemia and/or thrombocytopenia and splenomegaly is common. Eighty per cent of cases have a cytogenetic abnormality but, as with CMML, none is specific for aCML. The prognosis is poorer than for CMML,

with a median survival of < 20 months. The response to intensive chemotherapy is generally poor (see also Chapter 37).

Myelodysplastic/myeloproliferative disease, unclassifiable

This category includes patients with one or more myelodysplastic features, less than 20% blasts in the bone marrow and either a platelet count of more than 600×10^9/L or a white cell count of more than 12×10^9/L with or without splenomegaly. There should be no preceding history of a well-defined chronic myeloproliferative disorder and patients should lack a BCR–ABL fusion gene, a deletion of chromosome 5q or a translocation of chromosome 3q21.

Within this subgroup are patients who present with both a thrombocytosis and more than 15% of ringed sideroblasts in the bone marrow.

Paediatric myelodysplasia

Myelodysplastic syndromes are rare in childhood, with an overall incidence between 1.35 and 3.6 per million, making up less than 5% of childhood malignancies. In contrast to adult MDS, which is commoner in the elderly, most cases of paediatric MDS develop in children less than 5 years old. A classification based on the WHO classification has recently been proposed by an international working group and is shown in Table 40.16.

Juvenile myelomonocytic leukaemia

Juvenile myelomonocytic leukaemia (JMML) is a disorder with both myelodysplastic and myeloproliferative features. The incidence is 1.2 per million per year and the median age at presentation is 1.8 years. Ninety-five per cent of cases occur in children under 5 years old. The condition is twice as common in boys. The incidence of JMML is increased in children with neurofibromatosis type I (NFI) and with Noonan's syndrome. Diagnostic criteria for JMML are shown in Table 40.17. Typically, there is a leucocytosis comprising neutrophils, immature myeloid cells

Table 40.16 Classification of paediatric MDS.

Juvenile myelomonocytic leukaemia (JMML)

Down's syndrome (DS)
    Transient abnormal myelopoiesis (TAM)
    Myeloid leukaemia of DS

Myelodysplastic syndrome (MDS)
    Refractory cytopenia (RC)
    Refractory anaemia with excess blasts (RAEB)
    RAEB in transformation

Table 40.17 Diagnostic guidelines for JMML.

Suggestive clinical features
Hepatosplenomegaly
Lymphadenopathy
Pallor
Skin rash

Laboratory features
Essential
    No *BCR–ABL* fusion gene
    Monocytes $> 1 \times 10^9$/L
    Marrow blasts $< 20\%$

Plus at least two of the following
    Increased HbF
    Circulating myeloid precursors
    WBC $> 10 \times 10^9$/L
    Clonal cytogenetic abnormality
    Hypersensitivity of myeloid precursors to GM-CSF

and monocytes. Blasts usually constitute less than 5% of blood cells. The marrow is hypercellular and dysplastic features are often minimal. Approximately 30% of patients have monosomy 7, and 10% have other chromosomal abnormalities, whereas chromosome analysis is normal in 60% of cases.

Monocyte–macrophage colonies derived from either blood or bone marrow from patients with JMML are characterized by hypersensitivity to granulocyte–monocyte colony-stimulating factor (GM-CSF). This hypersensitivity is due to defects in the RAS–MAP kinase signalling pathway resulting from mutations in either a *RAS* gene, the *NFI* gene (the cause of neurofibromatosis type I) or the *PTPNII* gene (the cause of Noonan's syndrome).

The prognosis of JMML is variable, with survival ranging from 5 months to 4 years without treatment. Poor prognostic factors include age of more than 2 years, thrombocytopenia and elevated haemoglobin F levels. Blast transformation occurs in 10–20% of cases, and most patients die from organ failure, espe-cially respiratory failure, due to leukaemic infiltration. Although responses may be achieved with regimens containing cytosine arabinoside and/or *cis*-retinoic acid, the only curative therapy is allogeneic transplantation. The relapse rate following transplanta-tion approaches 50% in some series, but further responses have been obtained with donor lymphocyte infusions. Novel therapies targeting the RAS–MAP kinase pathway are currently in trial (see also Chapter 37).

Myeloid leukaemia in Down's syndrome

Ten per cent of children with Down's syndrome develop a tran-sient abnormal myelopoiesis neonatally. The majority of cases spontaneously remit by 3 months, but 25% develop megakar-yoblastic leukaemia 1–3 years later. Dysplastic features are com-mon and the percentage of marrow blasts has no biological or prognostic significance. These patients respond well to intensive chemotherapy.

Myelodysplastic syndromes

Myelodysplastic syndromes may develop in previously healthy children, in association with congenital bone marrow failure syndrome such as Fanconi's anaemia, following chemother-apy and/or radiotherapy, or be familial. Most patients present with pancytopenia, and the marrow shows characteristic dys-plastic features with or without an increase in blasts. Ringed sideroblasts are extremely rare in a child with MDS, and their presence should instigate a search for other causes of sideroblas-tic anaemia, such as a mitochondrial DNA defect or a disorder of haem synthesis. An abnormal karyotype is found in 60–70% of cases, the commonest abnormality being monosomy 7, found in 30% of cases. Patients presenting with refractory cytopenia may pursue an indolent course for several years, but disease progres-sion is inevitable. The value of prognostic scoring systems is less clear than in adult MDS. Allogeneic transplantation is the treat-ment of choice for all forms of childhood MDS, but there is still debate whether patients with increased blasts should receive prior intensive chemotherapy.

Selected bibliography

Barrett J, Saunthararajah Y, Molldrem J (2000) Myelodysplastic syn-drome and aplastic anaemia: distinct entities or diseases linked by a common pathophysiology. *Seminars in Hematology* 37: 15–29.

Bennett JM (ed.) (2002) *The Myelodysplastic Syndromes Pathobiology and Clinical Management.* Marcel Dekker, New York.

Bowen D, Culligan D, Jowitt S *et al.* (2003) Guidelines for diagnosis and therapy of adult myelodysplastic syndrome. *British Journal of Haematology* 120: 187–200.

De Witte T, Hermans J, Vossen J *et al.* (2000) haematopoietic stem cell transplantation for patients with myelodysplasia and sec-ondary acute myeloid leukaemia: a report on behalf of the

Chronic Leukaemia Working Party of the EBMT. *British Journal of Haematology* 110: 620–30.

Greenberg P, Cox C, LeBeau MM *et al.* (1997) International Scoring System for evaluating prognosis in myelodysplastic syndromes. *Blood* 89: 2079–88.

Hasle H, Niemeyer CM, Chessells JM *et al.* (2003) A paediatric approach to the WHO classification of myelodysplastic and myeloproliferative diseases. *Leukaemia* 17: 277–82.

Hellstrom-Lindberg E, Gulbrandsen N, Lindberg G *et al.* (2003) A validated decision model for treating the anaemia of myelodysplastic syndrome with erythropoietin and granulocyte colony-stimulating factor: significant effects on quality of life. *British Journal of Haematology* 120: 1037–46.

Jaffe ES, Harris NL, Stein H, Vardiman JW (eds) (2001) *WHO Classification Tumours of Haematopoietic and Lymphoid Tissues.* IARC Press, Lyons.

Killick SB, Mufti G, Cavenagh JD *et al.* (2003) A pilot study of antithymocyte globulin (ATG) in the treatment of patients with 'low risk' myelodysplastia. *British Journal of Haematology* 120: 679–84.

Pedersen-Bjergaard J, Andersen MK, Christiansen DH *et al.* (2002) Genetic pathways in therapy-related myelodysplasia and acute myeloid leukaemia. *Blood* 99: 1909–12.

Rowe JM (ed.) (2004) Myelodysplastic syndromes: etiology, natural history, current and future therapies. *Clinical Haematology* 17: 535–661.

Silverman LR, Demakos EP, Peterson BL *et al.* (2002) Randomized controlled trial of azacytidine in patients with the myelodysplastic syndrome: a study of the Cancer and Leukaemia Group. *Journal of Clinical Oncology* 20: 2429–40.

CHAPTER 41

Myeloma

41

Evangelos Terpos and Amin Rahemtulla

Definition and epidemiology

Multiple myeloma is a B-cell malignancy characterized by a monoclonal expansion and accumulation of abnormal plasma cells in the bone marrow compartment. The clinical manifestations of myeloma are heterogeneous, and include bone complications, symptoms of impaired haemopoiesis and hyperviscosity, renal dysfunction, infections, peripheral neuropathy and extramedullary disease.

Myeloma belongs to a group of disorders called plasma cell dyscrasias that also include benign monoclonal diseases such as monoclonal gammopathy of undetermined significance (MGUS), indolent lymphomas such as lymphoplasmacytic lymphoma (Waldenström's macroglobulinaemia), and rare, biologically interesting disorders, such as heavy-chain diseases. All disorders share common plasma cell morphological features and most are associated with the production of abnormal immunoglobulins. Indolent/smouldering or asymptomatic myeloma has an intramedullary tumour cell content of > 10% but none of the other complications, such as lytic lesions, characteristic of multiple myeloma, nor symptoms from any complications. Myeloma may rarely involve extramedullary sites, such as blood, pleural fluid and skin. Extramedullary myeloma seems to be more aggressive, and when plasma cells are present in the blood at a proportion of greater than 20% of the white blood cells the condition is known as plasma cell leukaemia. Table 41.1 summarizes the criteria for the definition of multiple myeloma, indolent or asymptomatic myeloma and MGUS.

Myeloma constitutes 1% of all cancers, but it is the second most common blood cancer after lymphomas and accounts for 10% of haematological malignancies. Myeloma has an annual incidence in the UK of 60 per million; at any one time there will be 10–15 000 patients with the condition. Cancer Research UK statistics show that there were 3730 new cases of myeloma in the UK in 2000 and there were 2600 deaths from this condition in 2002. The median age at diagnosis is 60–65 years; fewer than 2% of myeloma patients are under 40 years old at diagnosis. There are various theories about the age at onset and these include: (i) a reduction in ability of immune system of the elderly to eliminate potential myeloma precursors; (ii) the cumulative impact of environmental exposures with age; and (iii) hormonal effects of ageing. However, recent statistics indicate that myeloma is increasing in incidence and occurring more frequently in individuals aged below 55 years. Myeloma seems to be more common in men than women. The reasons for this are unclear but may include both hormonal effects and job-related exposure. Myeloma has a higher incidence in Afro-Caribbean ethnic groups compared with Caucasians in the UK, and in the USA the incidence also varies by race: from about 1/100 000 population/year for Asians, to about 4/100 000 population/year for Caucasians and 8–10/100 000 population/year for Afro-Americans.

Table 41.1 Criteria for the diagnosis of multiple myeloma, indolent myeloma and MGUS.

(A) Multiple myeloma

Major	I	Plasmacytoma on tissue biopsy
criteria	II	Bone marrow infiltration with > 30% plasma cells
	III	Monoclonal globulin spike (paraprotein) on serum electrophoresis (IgG > 35 g/L, IgA > 20 g/L), or on concentrated urine electrophoresis (> 1g/24 h of κ or λ light chains)
Minor	a	Bone marrow infiltration with 10–30% plasma cells
criteria	b	Paraprotein less than the level defined above
	c	Lytic bone lesions
	d	Normal IgM < 0.5 g/L, IgA < 1 g/L or IgG < 6 g/L

The diagnosis of multiple myeloma requires a minimum of two major criteria or one major criterion + one minor criterion, or three minor criteria always including a and b.

(B) Indolent (or asymptomatic) multiple myeloma

Same as multiple myeloma except:

No bone lesions or one asymptomatic lytic lesion (X-ray survey)

Paraprotein level: IgG < 70 g/L and IgA < 50 g/L

No symptoms:

Haemoglobin > 10 g/dL

Serum calcium normal

Serum creatinine < 170 μmol/L

No infections

(C) MGUS

Paraprotein present, but at levels IgG < 35 g/L, IgA< 20 g/L, Urinary light chains < 1 g/24h

Furthermore:

Normal level of residual polyclonal immunoglobulins

Bone marrow plasma cells < 10% (and without cytological abnormalities)

No bone lesions

No symptoms

No evidence of other B-cell proliferative disorder

A variety of genetic and environmental factors have been proposed to explain the increased incidence in individuals of African descent. Differences in hormone receptors, immune reactivity and toxin metabolism have been evaluated. The diversity of possible exposures and genetic susceptibility factors make proof difficult. Although there is a tendency for myeloma to occur in families (3–5%), the likelihood of inheritance is low and no inherited genes have been identified.

Pathogenesis

Origin of the malignant plasma cell

Multiple myeloma is a malignant condition caused by clonal proliferation of plasma cells. These plasma cells are usually confined to the bone marrow but may be seen in the peripheral blood in end-stage myeloma (Figure 41.1). The precise stage at which malignant change occurs in myeloma cells has not yet been clarified. Current evidence suggests, however, that myeloma cell is a long-lived plasma cell, which has been exposed to antigen having undergone the B-cell maturation processes. Maturation of normal B-cell precursors to mature plasma cells involves rearrangement of the immunoglobulin (Ig) genes with subsequent somatic mutation of the variable (V) region. The myeloma cell is a post-germinal centre plasma cell which has undergone immunoglobulin gene recombination, class-switching and somatic hypermutation, and homes to the bone marrow (see Chapter 20). Molecular analysis of the peripheral blood mononuclear cells in myeloma has clearly demonstrated the presence of circulating clonal B cells with the same Ig gene rearrangement and the same somatic hypermutation as the marrow malignant plasma cells.

Myeloma cells proliferate at a low rate. The plasma cell labelling index typically detects less than 1% of tumour cells that are actively synthesizing DNA until late in the course of the disease, and is a better prognostic indicator than plasma cell infiltration of the bone marrow. Plasma cells may be identified by high CD38, high CD138 and low CD45 expression by flow cytometry. Myeloma cells are also CD19⁻ or CD19⁺/CD56⁺, whereas normal plasma cells are consistently CD19⁺/CD56⁻. In myeloma, the proliferative cells usually express CD45 and the level of expression of this gene is higher than that observed in the non-proliferative compartment. Better clarification of the myeloma cell compartments will help to better understand the biology of the disease.

Environmental exposure

The cause of myeloma is unknown as no single factor has been consistently associated with it. Exposure to chemicals, such as dioxins, solvents and cleaners, and to radiation may be associated with the development of myeloma in predisposed individuals. Studies of atomic bomb survivors have shown an increased incidence of myeloma 15–20 years after exposure to radiation. Viral infections have also been implicated in the pathogenesis of myeloma. Several studies have suggested a link between myeloma

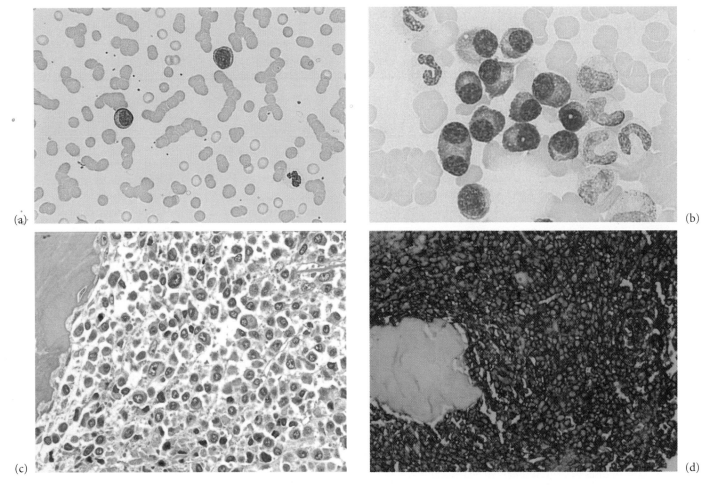

Figure 41.1 (a) Photomicrograph of peripheral blood film in myeloma. Note the marked rouleaux and a plasma cell. (b) Film of bone marrow aspirate in myeloma. The cluster of plasma cells shows abnormal morphology. (c) Bone marrow trephine showing infiltration with plasma cells (haematoxylin and eosin stain). (d) Bone marrow trephine showing massive infiltration with plasma cells (immunoperoxidase stain for CD-138) (trephine biopsies kindly provided by Professor K Naresh).

and herpesvirus infections (especially herpesvirus 8), Epstein–Barr virus, human immunodeficiency virus, hepatitis viruses, as well as to new 'stealth adapted' viruses such as mutated cytomegalovirus. However, epidemiological studies attempting to establish definite associations between myeloma and certain infections or autoimmune diseases have, so far, remained inconclusive.

Increased karyotypic instability

Increasing evidence suggests that the development of myeloma is a multistep process that includes the progressive occurrence of multiple structural chromosomal changes. Karyotypes of myeloma are more similar to those of epithelial tumours and the blast phase of chronic myeloid leukaemia than to those of other haemopoietic malignancies. However, the number of unbalanced translocations (translocations that generate a derivative chromosome(s) that has lost sequences from the involved chromosomes) is greatly increased in myeloma compared with epithelial tumours, as revealed by comparative genomic hybridization (CGH).

Monosomy 13, translocations into the switch regions of the IgH genes involving a large array of chromosomal partners (switch translocations), chromosome 8q (c-*myc* oncogene) abnormalities, and other numerical chromosomal changes (monosomy, trisomy) are detected in up to 80–90% of myeloma cases. Monosomy 13 is discussed below, while the common chromosomal partners in switch translocations and the involved candidate oncogenes in the pathogenesis of myeloma are shown in Table 41.2. Hyperdiploidy, with chromosome counts of greater than 50, has been reported in 30–45% of abnormal cases by conventional cytogenetics and CGH. Deletions of chromosome

Table 41.2 Frequent chromosomal partners and candidate oncogenes in switch translocations [t(partner chromosome;14) (involved region;q32)] involved in the pathogenesis of multiple myeloma.

Chromosomal partners	Frequency in myeloma patients	Candidate oncogene	Localization	Distance between breakpoints and oncogenes	Function
11q13	15–20%	Cyclin D1	der(14)	100–330 kb	Cell cycle regulator
		Myeov	der(11)		Unknown
4p16	12–17%	FGFR3	der(14)	50–100 kb	Growth factor receptor tyrosine kinase
		MMSET/WHSC1	der(4)		Chromatin remodelling
16q32	5–10%	c-maf	der(14)	550–1350 kb	Transcription factor
6p21	5%	Cyclin D3	der(14)	65 kb	Cell cycle regulator
6p25	< 5%	MUM1/IRF4	der(14)	Immediately adjacent	Transcriptional regulator of IFN and IFN-stimulated genes

FGFR3, fibroblast growth factor receptor 3; MMSET/WHSC1, multiple malformation syndrome/Wolf–Hirschhorn syndrome gene 1; MUM1/IRF4, multiple myeloma oncogene 1/interferon-responsive factor 4.

13q, 6q and 16q have also been described. Hypodiploidy is also a common finding, with loss of chromosomes 8, 13, 14 and X observed by conventional cytogenetics.

Chromosome 13q loss

Monoallelic loss of 13q sequences is one of the most frequent abnormalities in myeloma. Monosomy of chromosome 13 occurs more commonly (92%), while the interstitial deletion or translocation of 13q occurs less frequently. Loss of 13q is detected in 15–20% of cases by conventional cytogenetics and in 50% of cases using interphase fluorescence *in situ* hybridization (FISH) analysis. Chromosome 13q loss has also been detected in 20–40% of MGUS cases. There seems to be a higher incidence of monosomy 13 in myeloma patients with pre-existing MGUS (70%) than in those patients without such a history. Moreover, the frequency of chromosome 13q loss increases with disease stage, reaching 70% in plasma cell leukaemia. On the other hand, in most MGUS patients, only a subset of myeloma cells have the 13q abnormality, while in multiple myeloma almost all tumour cells have this defect. Thus, these data raise the possibility that monosomy 13 is an early event in the pathogenesis of the disease. The genes that are located on chromosome 13 and implicated in the pathogenesis of myeloma have not yet been recognized.

Prognostic significance of cytogenetic abnormalities

Several studies have demonstrated that monosomy 13, detected by conventional cytogenetics, is a predictor for survival. However, the high incidence of this cytogenetic abnormality in MGUS patients and its co-existence in many cases with a large variety of other chromosomal aberrations, revealed by molecular

cytogenetics, makes the prognostic value of monosomy 13 alone difficult to ascertain. Conventional karyotyping has also demonstrated a poor prognosis associated with chromosome 11q translocations, including t(11;14) and reciprocal translocations with chromosomes 8, 9 and 12. However, this was not confirmed by molecular cytogenetics, and the possibility that conventional karyotyping technique has selected cases which are hyperproliferative must be considered. Gene expression profile from microarray technology may provide a more accurate and comprehensive assessment of molecular changes, and is currently used to characterize myeloma at a molecular level and correlate with response rates in trials of novel agents.

Bone marrow microenvironment in myeloma

The pathogenesis of multiple myeloma is complex and includes mutual interactions that affect the number and function of both malignant cells and normal bone marrow stromal cells (BMSCs). Bone marrow microenvironment includes the extracellular matrix and at least five types of stromal cells: fibroblasts, osteoblasts, osteoclasts, vascular endothelial cells and lymphocytes. Reciprocal positive and negative interactions among these cells are mediated by a variety of cytokines and adhesion molecules. The homing of myeloma cells to the bone marrow seems to involve selective adhesion to bone marrow endothelial cells, transendothelial migration and adhesion to stromal cells through the production of stromal-derived factor 1 (SDF-1) and insulin-like growth factor 1 (IGF-1), which are secreted by bone marrow endothelial and stromal cells and have a chemoattractant effect on myeloma cells. Adhesion of myeloma cells to BMSCs, through the $\alpha_4\beta_1$-integrin/vascular cell adhesion molecule 1 (VCAM-1) interaction, induces the paracrine secretion of cytokines such as interleukin 6 (IL-6), IL-1β, IL-11, tumour necrosis factors (TNFs), transforming growth factor-

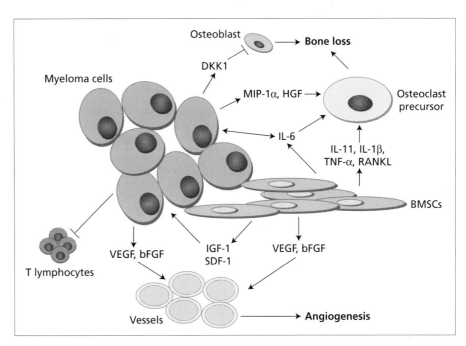

Figure 41.2 The bone marrow microenvironment in multiple myeloma. The multiple interactions between myeloma, stromal and endothelial cells and osteoclasts reflect the vital role of the bone marrow microenvironment in the biology of the disease. The production of different cytokines by both stromal and myeloma cells enhances myeloma proliferation and growth, osteoclast activation and vessel formation. Furthermore, the inhibition of T-lymphocytes, through mechanisms which are unclear, increases the immunodeficiency in myeloma, while the suppression of osteoblasts in combination with osteoclast activation leads to bone loss.

beta (TGF-β) and receptor activator of nuclear factor-kappa B ligand (RANKL) by BMSCs (Figure 41.2). The production of IL-6 by BMSCs, which is via activation of the nuclear factor-kappa B (NF-κB), triggers the proliferation of myeloma cells, and protects them against dexamethasone-induced apoptosis. The activation of NF-κB, which is a transcriptional factor, is responsible for the production of other growth factors and adhesion molecules, such as vascular endothelial growth factor (VEGF), VCAM-1 and E-selectin, by the BMSCs and myeloma cells. Inactivated NF-κB is located in the cytoplasm of the cell bound to its inhibitor IκB The activation of NF-κB involves the following sequence of events: activation of IκB-kinase → IκB phosphorylation → ubiquitination and degradation of IκB by the proteasome → dissociation of NF-κB from IκB → nuclear translocation of NF-κB → production of molecules that are crucial for myeloma survival. The value of this pathway for myeloma cell growth is evident by the anti-myeloma effect of drugs, such as dexamethasone, thalidomide and bortezomib (proteasome inhibitor), which inhibit NF-κB.

Angiogenesis is also increased in some cases of myeloma and correlates with disease activity and survival. Secreted VEGF from myeloma cells interacts with receptors on endothelial cells to enhance their migration and proliferation. Additional factors, such as the basic fibroblast growth factor (bFGF), produced by either myeloma or stromal cells, also induce angiogenesis (Figure 41.2). However, the precise role of angiogenesis in myeloma remains to be established. In myeloma, there is also an inhibition of T-lymphocyte function through mechanisms, which are not clear but may include production of inhibitory molecules, such as interferon-alpha (IFN-α) at high concentrations and reduction of interferon-gamma (IFN-γ).

Biology of bone disease

Bone destruction in myeloma is related to increased osteoclastic activity which is not accompanied by a comparable increase in osteoblast formation. This uncoupling of resorption and formation leads to rapid bone loss, osteoporosis, lytic lesions and fractures. The enhanced and uncontrolled osteoclastic activity has been confirmed consistently in several animal models and is also reflected by the increase in markers of bone resorption, including N- or C-terminal cross-linking telopeptide of type I collagen (NTX or ICTP/CTX respectively) and tartrate-resistant acid phosphatase type 5b (TRACP-5b), in the serum of myeloma patients. A number of cytokines and growth factors that are produced by either myeloma cells or BMSCs have been implicated in the increased osteoclast formation and activity in myeloma. These cytokines include IL-6, IL-1β, IL-11, TNF-α, TNF-β, bFGF, IGF and, more recently, macrophage inflammatory protein 1 alpha (MIP-1α), hepatocyte growth factor and the RANKL pathway. The recently characterized RANKL interacts with a cellular receptor activator of NF-κB (RANK), and a soluble decoy receptor of RANKL, named osteoprotegerin (OPG). Following activation of RANK on osteoclasts by its ligand, RANKL, differentiation, proliferation, and survival of osteoclasts is enhanced. OPG is reduced in patients with myeloma, while the levels of soluble RANKL (sRANKL) are increased; thus, the ratio sRANKL/OPG is increased, allowing greater interaction between RANKL and RANK. This correlates not only with the extent of lytic lesions but also with survival in myeloma. The induction of release of the different cytokines, such as IL-6 and IL-1β, TNFs, bFGF and IGFs, due to the adherence of myeloma cells to stromal cells, modifies the bone marrow microenvironment, enhancing

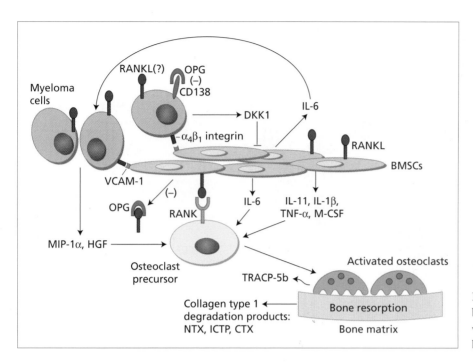

Figure 41.3 The interactions in the bone marrow microenvironment, which influence the development of bone disease in multiple myeloma.

RANKL expression by osteoblasts. IL-6 also acts as a growth factor for osteoclasts, and as survival factor for myeloma cells. In addition, IL-11 is also produced by both myeloma and stromal cells and exerts its effect through RANKL/RANK/OPG pathway, inducing osteoclastogenesis while inhibiting osteoblast formation. More recently, gene expression profiling studies have revealed that myeloma cells produce dickkop-1 protein, which inhibits Wnt-mediated osteoblast differentiation, leading to reduced bone formation. MIP-1α, a low-molecular-weight chemokine which belongs to the RANTES family, is also produced by myeloma cells and activates the osteoclasts. MIP-1α levels are elevated in bone marrow plasma of patients with myeloma and correlate with the presence of lytic lesions. Figure 41.3 summarizes the currently available data about osteoclast activation in myeloma, reflecting the role of the bone marrow microenvironment in the development of myeloma-related bone disease.

Clinical features

Plasma cell infiltration of bone marrow results in bone marrow failure and bone lesions. Patients therefore present with symptoms due to bone disease, hypercalcaemia, impaired haemopoiesis, immune paresis and renal failure. In a minority of patients, plasma cell infiltration of soft tissues is seen at presentation. Plasmacytomas may spread extradurally or may cause spinal cord compression. High serum paraprotein may result in hyperviscosity, and high levels of light chains (Bence Jones protein) in the urine may result in renal failure. The clinical features may be due to the following.

Bone disease

Bone pain is the most common symptom and results from osteolytic lesions and pathological fractures – mainly wedging or collapse of vertebral bodies with or without osteoporosis (Figure 41.4). In advanced disease, pathological fractures of the long bones, ribs and sternum may occur. Skull lesions, in general, very rarely cause pain.

Immune paresis and impaired haemopoiesis

A large proportion of patients with multiple myeloma have reduced serum levels of normal immunoglobulins. In some of these patients, the immune paresis is severe enough to make them susceptible to bacterial infections, and levels of immunoglobulin rarely return to normal levels following chemotherapy even if the disease has responded well and paraprotein levels have fallen. Immune paresis, renal failure, neutropenia and antimyeloma therapy can combine to cause severe immunodeficiency, and infections are a major cause of death in these patients.

Normochromic, normocytic anaemia is a common finding in myeloma, and symptoms related to this may be a presenting feature at diagnosis. Anaemia may be due to the infiltration of the bone marrow by myeloma cells, due to chronic inflammation or the use of cytotoxic drugs. Serum erythropoietin levels are usually appropriately raised in those patients with good renal function and inappropriately low in those patients with poor renal function. Thrombocytopenia and neutropenia may also occur due to bone marrow infiltration by malignant plasma cells or to the use of chemotherapy.

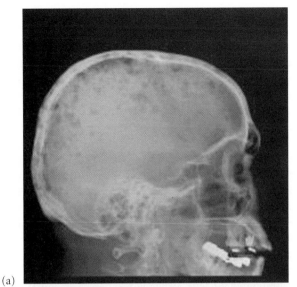

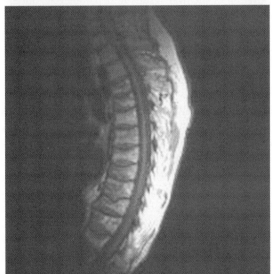

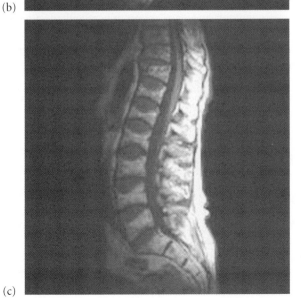

(a)

(b)

(c)

Hypercalcaemia

There is an imbalance between bone formation and bone destruction resulting in a continuing loss of calcium from the skeleton. At presentation, around a quarter of all patients have hypercalcaemia with associated lytic bone lesions and/or osteoporosis. Patients may be symptomatic, with polydypsia, polyuria and constipation. Hypercalcaemia may be severe enough to cause life-threatening dehydration and renal failure.

Nephropathy

Patients with multiple myeloma may present with uraemia which may or may not be corrected by rehydration and chemotherapy. Renal dysfunction occurs when the tubular absorptive capacity of light chains is exhausted, resulting in interstitial nephritis with light-chain casts. Other causes of renal dysfunction are hypercalcaemia with hypercalciuria, amyloid light-chain (AL) amyloidosis associated with λ-light-chain disease, immunoglobulin light-chain deposition, infection, hyperuricaemia and the use of anti-inflammatory drugs. The infiltration of the kidneys by myeloma cells may also occur but is rare.

Neurological complications

Neurological abnormalities are mainly caused by tumour growth compressing the spinal cord or cranial nerves. Peripheral neuropathy is frequently due to perineuronal amyloid deposition. Polyneuropathy may also be observed as a part of POEMS syndrome (polyneuropathy, organomegaly, endocrinopathy, monoclonal gammopathy and skin changes). Plasma cell leukaemia may involve the meninges, while intracerebral mass lesions are very rare.

Hyperviscosity

Hyperviscosity occurs in less than 10% of patients and usually associated with an IgM paraprotein. The intrinsic viscosity of IgM, which usually exists as a 900-kDa pentamer, is relatively high compared with IgA or IgG, and the hyperviscosity syndrome therefore occurs at relatively lower concentrations, typically 40–50 g/L. Patients with IgA myeloma present more often with hyperviscosity syndrome than those with IgG myeloma because of the greater tendency of IgA to form multimers. Among patients with IgG myeloma, those who have IgG3 subclass paraprotein are more likely to develop this syndrome. It leads to

Figure 41.4 (*left*) Characteristic bone lytic lesions and pathological fractures in multiple myeloma. (a) Typical 'punched-out' lytic lesions in the skull (plain radiograph). (b and c) Magnetic resonance imaging in multiple myeloma; mixed diffuse/focal abnormalities and fractures involving the thoracic and lumbar spine.

cerebral, pulmonary and renal dysfunction as well as a haemorrhagic tendency. Patients may present with visual, cardiovascular and neurological symptoms, often accompanied by fatigue, malaise and weight loss. Visual dysfunction may range from mild visual disturbance to sudden loss of vision. Fundoscopy may show progression from retinal vein distension to increasing vessel tortuosity, with arteriovenous 'nipping', areas of beading and dilatation of small venules ('string of sausages' appearance) to full-blown retinopathy with florid haemorrhages and exudates. The neurological symptoms of hyperviscosity syndrome include headache, fluctuating level of consciousness, mental slowing, dizziness, ataxia, vertigo, neuropathies, convulsion and coma. The increased viscosity also increases plasma volume and may compromise cardiac function.

Coagulopathy

Coagulopathy in multiple myeloma is well documented but is rarely a clinical problem. Bleeding may be the result of hyperviscosity, perivascular amyloidosis, acquired coagulopathy, or thrombocytopenia. An acquired coagulopathy due to interference of fibrin aggregation by the paraprotein or an acquired inhibitor of factors VIII or X has been documented. The bleeding tendency may also be due to the coating of platelets by the paraprotein. This may result in chronic, recurrent bleeding of the gums and the upper respiratory and gastrointestinal tracts. The bleeding time is usually prolonged and *in vitro* platelet function is abnormal. Some patients may develop thrombosis as a result of hyperviscosity or secondary to acquired deficiency of protein C or due to lupus anticoagulant.

Amyloidosis (see also Chapter 42)

Amyloidosis results from the abnormal extracellular deposition and accumulation of protein and protein derivatives and is clinically evident in around 5% of patients with multiple myeloma. The amyloid deposit shows green birefringence when stained with Congo red and viewed under polarized light. The disease becomes clinically significant when its diffuse form affects organ function by replacing the normal cells. The extracellular deposit is invariably made up of three components. The fibrillar protein is the component that defines the type of amyloidosis and depends on the underlying disease. It is made of fibrils arranged primarily in a β-pleated sheet secondary structure. The other two components are the serum amyloid P and charged glycosaminoglycans, which are ubiquitous in all types of amyloidosis and probably contribute to the formation of the β-pleated sheet structure. In primary amyloidosis, which is usually associated with multiple myeloma, the characteristic fibrillar protein is a fragment of the variable immunoglobulin light (and/or rarely heavy) chain and thus is different from patient to patient. This type of amyloidosis is referred to as AL amyloidosis.

The common presentations of AL amyloidosis include carpal tunnel syndrome, congestive cardiac failure, macroglossia, gastrointestinal disturbances, neuropathies (peripheral and autonomic) and lesions of the skin, subcutaneous tissues, tendon sheaths and fasciae. The most commonly involved organ system in AL amyloidosis is the gastrointestinal system, with the colon being the most frequently involved organ. Oesophageal and gastric involvement usually manifests as dysmotility, wall thickening and gastro-oesophageal reflux disease. These result from amyloid infiltration of the muscularis and/or destruction of the Auerbach plexus. When the small intestine is involved, the most common finding is diffuse or nodular wall thickening. Abdominal pain, malabsorption, haemorrhage and perforation are rare complications. Colonic biopsy specimens are positive in 80% of patients with systemic amyloidosis. Splenomegaly is the only finding associated with splenic involvement. This causes increased fragility, and spontaneous rupture may occur. Diffuse infiltration of the liver results in hepatomegaly, but abnormal liver function is rare. If liver dysfunction is present then the prognosis is very poor. Macroglossia may result from amyloid infiltration of the intrinsic muscles and could interfere with swallowing and respiration.

Cardiac involvement is common in AL amyloidosis and can remain silent until it manifests as progressive cardiac failure exacerbated by conduction disturbances and coronary arterial insufficiency. Pulmonary involvement in amyloidosis is relatively rare. Patients present with recurrent pneumonia which is responsive to antibiotic treatment. This is due to obstruction of the associated bronchus or bronchiole either by interstitial thickening, resembling bronchiolitis obliterans or, more rarely, a focal amyloidoma. Renal infiltration may also occur but renal dysfunction is rare, usually manifesting as nephrotic syndrome. Peripheral neuropathy with autonomic failure may also occur in primary amyloidosis. Initial neuropathic symptoms include distal sensory loss with elevated temperature thresholds. Autonomic symptoms and signs are prominent and affect multiple systems. Orthostatic symptoms with near-syncope or syncope are quite common. Constipation alternating with diarrhoea is due to infiltration of the myenteric and submucosal plexus. Infiltration of the oesophagus causes dysphagia. Widespread anhidrosis with compensatory sweating is commonly observed. Impotence is frequent in men.

Laboratory findings

Diagnosis

The criteria for the diagnosis of multiple myeloma are shown in Table 41.1, while the work-up for the diagnosis of myeloma is described in Table 41.3. The diagnostic work-up may reveal a normochromic, normocytic anaemia, hypercalcaemia, hyper-

Table 41.3 The work-up for myeloma.

Full blood count, film and ESR

Evaluation of kidney function, serum calcium, CRP, β_2-microglobulin, LDH, uric acid levels and liver function tests.

Protein electrophoresis and paraprotein quantitation

Quantitative analysis of the normal immunoglobulins

24-hour urine collection for light chain (Bence Jones protein) excretion

Coagulation screen

Bone marrow aspiration and trephine biopsy for morphology, immunophenotyping (CD 138, CD79a, kappa, lambda, CD20) and cytogenetics

A complete skeletal survey. Patients with symptoms or signs of cord compression would require further investigation with computerized tomography (CT) or magnetic resonance imaging (MRI)

Table 41.4 The Durie–Salmon staging system.

I	*All of the following*
	Haemoglobin > 10.5 g/dL
	Serum calcium normal
	X-rays show normal bone structure or solitary bone plasmocytoma only
	Low paraprotein levels
	IgG < 50 g/L
	IgA < 30 g/L
	Urinary light chain < 4 g/24 h
II	*Fitting neither stage I nor stage III*
III	*One or more of the following*
	Haemoglobin < 8.5 g/dL
	Serum calcium > 3 mmol/L
	Advanced lytic bone lesions (> three lytic lesions)
	High paraprotein levels
	IgG > 70/L
	IgA > 50 g/L
	Urinary light chain > 12 g/24 h

Subclassification

A	Serum creatinine < 170 μmol/L
B	Serum creatinine ≥ 170 μmol/L

uricaemia, low serum albumin or abnormal coagulation. In most patients with myeloma, the malignant plasma cells secrete an abnormal immunoglobulin (paraprotein), but around 1% of patients have non-secretory disease. Nearly 60% of the patients have detectable IgG paraprotein, 20% have IgA paraprotein, 15–20% light-chain only paraprotein, and less than 1% have IgD or IgE paraprotein. Suppression of the normal immunoglobulins is a typical finding in most cases. Other biochemical findings include increased levels of urea and creatinine in renal dysfunction, elevated serum levels of C-reactive protein and β_2-microglobulin, which are associated with poor prognosis, increased levels of lactate dehydrogenase, increased levels of markers of bone resorption (TRACP-5b and collagen degradation products: NTX, ICTP, CTX), and decreased levels of markers of bone formation (bone alkaline phosphatase and osteocalcin). Skeletal survey would indicate the extent of lytic bone lesions. If there are symptoms or signs of spinal cord compression then further imaging with computerized tomography (CT) or magnetic resonance imaging (MRI) is recommended. Isotope bone scans are of limited value because of decreased osteoblast function. Positron emission tomography (PET) is not useful because of the small size of the infiltrates in the bone marrow and lower metabolic rate of the tumour compared with normal tissue but may be useful in cases of macroscopic plasmacytomas. Measurement of bone density with DEXA scan may be useful to monitor progress of the disease in patients with osteoporosis.

The differential diagnosis includes MGUS, which is associated with lower paraprotein levels, less plasmacytosis in the bone marrow, and no anaemia, renal dysfunction or lytic lesions (see Table 41.1). Patients with solitary plasmacytoma may have no evidence of systematic disease, while AL amyloidosis can be dis-

tinguished by renal or rectal biopsy, or fine-needle aspiration of subcutaneous fat and staining the tissue with Congo red. Amyloidosis may be suspected in cases with carpal tunnel syndrome, macroglossia, renal dysfunction, or cardiomegaly associated with arrhythmias, low-voltage and conduction defects on electrocardiogram. Scintigraphy with radiolabelled serum amyloid P component (SAP) scan can be used to quantitate and document the distribution of amyloid.

Staging and prognosis

Once the diagnosis of multiple myeloma has been established, staging of the disease should be performed. Salmon–Durie staging system is the standard system for staging a myeloma patient and is shown in Table 41.4. A number of prognostic indices have been proposed to date using different risk factors. In all these indices, β_2-microglobulin remains the most powerful prognostic marker, while CRP, albumin, LDH, and chromosome 13q loss have also been shown to be of prognostic value. Recently, the International Myeloma Working Group has proposed a novel prognostic index (International Prognostic Index; IPI) for the staging of multiple myeloma. This system, based on almost 8500 patients, includes only two parameters, β_2-microglobulin and albumin, and is described in Table 41.5.

Table 41.5 International Prognostic Index for multiple myeloma.

Staging	Parameters	Number of patients	Median survival (months)
Stage 1	β_2-m < 3.5 ALB ≥ 35	2401	62
Stage 2	β_2-m < 3.5 ALB < 35 or β_2-m 3.5–5.5	3278	44
Stage 3	β_2-m > 5.5	2770	29

β_2-m, serum β_2-microglobulin (mg/L); ALB, serum albumin (g/L).
Factors that predict for lower risk:
Age < 60 + β_2-m < 3.5 mg/L + ALB > 35 g/L
Factors that predict for higher risk:
β_2-m > 10 mg/L + ALB < 35 g/L
Low platelet count
Cytogenetics do influence outcome; however, chromosome 13 deletion and complex chromosome abnormalities do not seem to add to the impact of age, β_2-m and ALB.

Treatment

Asymptomatic/indolent multiple myeloma

Patients with no symptoms, normal renal function and absence of bone lesions, classified as stage I (according to Salmon–Durie criteria), may remain stable for a long time without any chemotherapy. These patients account for about 20% of myeloma patients, and have a median time to disease progression of 2–3 years. The survival is similar when treatment (melphalan and prednisolone) is administered just after diagnosis or at disease progression in stage I patients. However, the disease needs to be evaluated at regular intervals (every 2–3 months) to separate the stable, asymptomatic patients who do not need treatment from patients with progressive, symptomatic disease. Signs of disease progression, such as rising paraprotein levels, falling haemoglobin levels, radiological evidence of bone disease, or an increase in bone marrow infiltration in non-secretory myeloma, are indications to start treatment. Asymptomatic patients with at least one lytic lesion visible on radiographs have a median time to progression of 8 months, whereas abnormal marrow appearance on magnetic resonance imaging (MRI) is also associated with higher risk of disease progression.

Conventional chemotherapy (Table 41.6)

Conventional doses of chemotherapy rarely result in complete remission (CR) and cure is not achieved. Initial chemotherapy

for patients with symptomatic multiple myeloma includes melphalan and prednisolone (MP), vincristine, doxorubicin and dexamethasone (VAD), alkylator-based combinations, cyclophosphamide with or without prednisolone, dexamethasone alone, idarubicin with dexamethasone and many other steroid-containing regimens. The response to treatment is assessed by a number of criteria described in Table 41.7.

Melphalan and prednisolone

This classical anti-myeloma regimen includes melphalan given at a dose of 6–8 mg/m^2/day combined with prednisolone at a dose of 40–60 mg/day for 4–7 days at 4- to 6-week intervals. It induces partial remission (PR) in approximately 50% patients, while CR is very rare. Patients who respond to treatment show a progressive fall in the paraprotein until a plateau phase (stable paraprotein level for at least 3 months together with transfusion independency and minimal symptoms) is reached. Further treatment of these patients with conventional doses of drugs does not result in improvement of outcome. The median duration of survival is around 3 years in most series, and the plateau phase usually has a duration of 18–24 months before progression. The role of prednisolone in the MP regimen is controversial. A number of trials have shown that the addition of standard dose of prednisolone to oral melphalan is not superior to melphalan alone with respect to overall survival, although the response rates may be higher with the combination. This should be kept in mind, particularly when dealing with patients who are at a high risk of steroid-related side-effects. Melphalan alone is usually given at a dose of 7–12 mg/m^2/day for 4 days every 3–4 weeks. Melphalan alone and MP are usually well tolerated and side-effects include mild nausea and myelosuppression, while alopecia is rare.

Various combination regimens, described below, have been used in an attempt to improve the outcome in myeloma patients. A meta-analysis of 6633 patients in 27 randomized trials comparing combination chemotherapy with MP confirmed that outcome after treatment with these regimens is very similar and they offer no advantage over MP. However, MP must be avoided in patients who are going to be treated with autologous stem cell transplantation (ASCT) owing to its toxicity to bone marrow stem cells. Previous treatment with melphalan is associated with a significantly lower yield of CD34$^+$ cells.

VAD and VAD-associated regimens

The combination of vincristine and doxorubicin administered by continuous 4 days infusion with the addition of high-dose oral dexamethasone is the most frequently used first-line chemotherapy regimen for myeloma. This regimen produces quick and high response rates (up to 80%) with a CR rate of 10–25%. The administration of liposomal doxorubicin (40 mg/m^2 intravenously, over 1 h, on day 1 only) instead of the 'classical' doxorubicin in the VAD regimen produces similar efficacy with fewer episodes of alopecia, and less frequent hospitalization. The

Table 41.6 Regimens for treatment of myeloma.

Drug regimen	Dose	Days
MP (many variations)		
M = Melphalan	7 mg/m²/day p.o.	1–5
P = Prednisolone	60 mg/day p.o.	1–5
Cyclophosphamide	400 mg/m² p.o. once a week for 12 weeks	Weekly
Prednisolone	60 mg p.o. alternate days for 6 weeks	Alternate days
VAD regimen (28-day cycle)		
V = Vincristine	0.4 mg/day c.i.v.	1–4
A = Doxorubicin (adriamycin)	9 mg/m²/day c.i.v.	1–4
D = Dexamethasone	40 mg/day p.o.	1–4 (and 9–12, 17–20 in the first cycle)
VAMP (28-day cycle)		
V = Vincristine	0.4 mg/day c.i.v.	1–4
A = Doxorubicin (adriamycin)	9 mg/m²/day c.i.v.	1–4
MP = Methylprednisolone	1.5 g i.v./p.o.	1–5
C-VAMP (28-day cycle)		
C = Cyclophosphamide	500 mg i.v	1, 8, 15
V = Vincristine	0.4 mg/day c.i.v.	1–4
A = Doxorubicin (adriamycin)	9 mg/m²/day c.i.v.	1–4
MP = Methylprednisolone	1.5 g i.v./p.o.	1–5
Z-Dex (21-day cycle)		
Z = Idarubicin (Zavedos)	10 mg/m²/day p.o.	1–4
Dex = Dexamethasone	40 mg/day p.o.	1–4 (and 8–11, 15–18 in the first cycle)
VMCP (21-day cycle)		
V = Vincristine	1 mg i.v.	1
M = Melphalan	5 mg/m²/day p.o.	1–4
C = Cyclophosphamide	110 mg/m²/day p.o.	1–4
P = Prednisolone	60 mg/m²/day p.o.	1–4
VBAP (21-day cycle)		
V = Vincristine	1 mg i.v.	1
B = Carmustine	30 mg/m² i.v.	1
A = Doxorubicin (adriamycin)	30 mg/m² i.v.	1
P = Prednisolone	60 mg/m²/day p.o.	1–4
ABCM (28-day cycle)		
A = Doxorubicin	30 mg/m² i.v.	
B = BCNU	30 mg/m² i.v.	1
C = Cyclophosphamide	100 mg/m²/day p.o.	22–25
M = Melphalan	6 mg/m²/day p.o.	22–25
Thalidomide	100–600 mg/day p.o.	Daily
CTD (21-day cycle)		
C = Cyclophosphamide	500 mg p.o.	1, 8, 15
T = Thalidomide	100–200 mg/day p.o.	Daily
D = Dexamethasone	40 mg/day p.o.	1–4 and 12–15
CVAD (21-day cycle)		
C = Cyclophosphamide	500 mg p.o. or i.v.	1, 8, 15
V = Vincristine	0.4 mg/day c.i.v.	1–4
A = Doxorubicin (adriamycin)	9 mg/m²/day c.i.v.	1–4
D = Dexamethasone	40 mg/day p.o.	1–4 and 12–15

Continued on next page

Table 41.6 (cont'd)

Drug regimen	Dose	Days
Thal/Dex (28-day cycle) (many variations)		
Thal = Thalidomide	100–200 mg/day p.o.	Daily
Dex = Dexamethasone	40 mg/day p.o.	1–4 (and 14–18) or once a week
DT-PACE (28- to 42-day cycle)		
D = Dexamethasone	40 mg/day p.o.	1–4
T = Thalidomide	400 mg/day p.o.	Daily
P = cis-Platinum	10 mg/m^2/day c.i.v.	1–4
A = Doxorubicin (adriamycin)	10 mg/m^2/day c.i.v.	1–4
C = Cyclophosphamide	400 mg/m^2/day c.i.v.	1–4
E = Etoposide	40 mg/m^2/day c.i.v.	1–4
G-CSF	300 µg/day s.c. until neutrophil recovery	
DCEP (28-day cycle)		
D = Dexamethasone	40 mg/day p.o.	1–4
C = Cyclophosphamide	750 mg/day c.i.v.	1–4
E = Etoposide	75 mg/day c.i.v.	1–4
P = cis-Platinum	25 mg/day c.i.v.	1–4
G-CSF	300 µg/day s.c. until neutrophil recovery	
TCED (28-day cycle)		
T = Thalidomide	400 mg/day p.o.	Daily
C = Cyclophosphamide	400 mg/m^2/day c.i.v.	1–4
E = Etoposide	40 mg/m^2/day c.i.v.	1–4
D = Dexamethasone	40 mg/day p.o.	1–4
Bortezomib (21-day cycle × 8 then 35-day cycle × 3)	1.3 mg/m^2 i.v.	1,4,8,11 (in the 21-day cycle) 1,8,15,22 (in the 35-day cycle)

c.i.v., continuous intravenous infusion; i.v., intravenous; p.o., per os.

replacement of dexamethasone with methylprednisolone (VAMP) and the addition of cyclophosphamide to this regimen (C-VAMP) results in the same response rate as the VAD regimen. However, there are no randomized trials comparing VAMP and C-VAMP with VAD chemotherapy. All these regimens produce no durable remissions and they offer no advantage in overall survival over MP. They are suitable for patients in whom high-dose chemotherapy (HDT) and ASCT are planned as the treatment does not damage the haemopoietic stem cells. These regimens may also be used in patients with renal failure as they do not cause increased toxicity in such patients. There is evidence that high-dose dexamethasone is responsible for much of the efficacy of VAD chemotherapy. Intermittent courses of dexamethasone produce an overall response rate of near 45%, similar overall survival as with VAD chemotherapy, and less serious complications (4% vs. 27% for patients receiving dexamethasone alone or VAD respectively). These results suggest that dexamethasone alone, 40 mg daily for 4 days every 2 weeks until response and then monthly, offers advantages over other regimens in respect of the absence of myelotoxicity, simplicity, suitability in pati-

ents with renal failure or in patients who require simultaneous radiotherapy. The addition of oral idarubicin to high-dose dexamethasone for 4 days every month, for 4 months (Z-Dex), produces an overall response rate of 75–80%, with 17% of patients achieving CR. Myelosuppression is seen in 70% of the patients while gastrointestinal toxicity and alopecia are infrequently reported. Furthermore, stem cells can still be harvested after treatment with this regimen. However, randomized trials comparing Z-Dex with VAD have not been carried out.

Alkylator-based combination regimens

These regimens generally include a combination of steroids (mainly prednisolone; P), cyclophosphamide (C) and melphalan (M) with agents such as vincristine (V), doxorubicin (A) and carmustine (BCNU; B). There is no advantage of these regimens over MP, even in patients with a poor prognosis. Furthermore, alkylator-based combination chemotherapy regimens are more myelotoxic than MP, affect subsequent stem cell mobilization and frequently cause vomiting, alopecia, cardiotoxicity and infection.

Table 41.7 EBMT criteria or response to anti-myeloma treatment.

Response	Criteria for response
Complete remission (CR)	*Requires all of the following* • Disappearance of the original monoclonal protein from the blood and urine on at least two determinations for a minimum of 6 weeks by immunofixation studies • < 5% plasma cells in the bone marrow on at least two determinations for a minimum of 6 weeks • No increase in the size or number of lytic bone lesions • Disappearance of soft tissue plasmacytomas for at least 6 weeks
Partial remission (PR)	*Requires all of the following* • ≥ 50% reduction in the level of serum monoclonal protein for at least two determinations 6 weeks apart • If present, reduction in 24-h urinary light-chain excretion by either 90% or to < 200 mg for at least two determinations 6 weeks apart • ≥ 50% reduction in the size of soft tissue plasmacytomas (by clinical or radiographic examination) for at least 6 weeks • No increase in the size or number of lytic bone lesions
Minimal response (MR)	*Requires all of the following* • 25–49% reduction in the level of serum monoclonal protein for at least two determinations 6 weeks apart • If present, a 50–89% reduction in 24-h urinary light-chain excretion, which still exceeds 200 mg/24 h for at least two determinations 6 weeks apart • 25–49% reduction in the size of soft-tissue plasmacytomas (by clinical or radiographic examination) for at least 6 weeks • No increase in the size or number of lytic bone lesions
No change (NC)	Not meeting the criteria for MR or PD
Progressive disease (PD) (for patients not in CR)	*Requires one or more of the following* • > 25% increase in the level of serum monoclonal paraprotein, which must also be an absolute increase for at least 5 g/L and confirmed on a repeat investigation • > 25% increase in 24-h urinary light-chain excretion, which must also be an absolute increase of at least 200 mg/24 h and confirmed on a repeat investigation • > 25% increase in plasma cells in a bone marrow aspirate or on trephine biopsy, which must also be an absolute increase of at least 10% • Definite increase in the size of existing lytic bone lesions or soft-tissue plasmacytomas • Development of new bone lesions or soft tissue plasmacytomas • Development of hypercalcaemia (corrected serum calcium > 2.8 mmol/L not attributable to any other case)
Relapse from CR	*Requires one or more of the following* • Reappearance of serum or urinary paraprotein on immunofixation or routine electrophoresis confirmed by at least one follow-up and excluding oligoclonal immune reconstitution • < 5% plasma cells in a bone marrow aspirate or on trephine biopsy • Definite increase in the size of residual lytic bone lesions or soft-tissue plasmacytomas • Development of new bone lesions or soft tissue plasmacytomas • Development of hypercalcaemia (corrected serum calcium > 2.8 mmol/L not attributable to any other case)

Induction chemotherapy plus interferon-alpha

Interferon-alpha (IFN-α) alone is not effective as part of induction therapy in myeloma patients. Two large meta-analyses studies of 4802 patients showed a slight benefit in both progression-free survival and overall survival (6 and 2 months respectively) in patients treated with chemotherapy plus IFN-α. However, the Nordic Myeloma Study Group has shown no benefit in survival in patients treated with IFN-α during induction chemotherapy, while there is a significant reduction in quality of life for patients receiving IFN-α during the first year of treatment. Therefore, it seems that there is no role for IFN-α in induction treatment.

Thalidomide and dexamethasone

The combination of thalidomide and dexamethasone produces response rates up to 65% in newly diagnosed patients, which is similar to VAD-like regimens. Unfortunately, venous thromboembolism is seen in 10% of patients, a side-effect that suggests that this combination is not suitable for induction treatment. Trials studying the effect of thalidomide and dexamethasone in combination with chemotherapeutic agents, including cyclophosphamide, are being carried out at present.

Autologous stem cell transplantation

In the absence of any significant progress in conventional chemotherapy, HDT with ASCT has become one of the most widely explored strategies to improve anti-myeloma treatment. ASCT has become the treatment of choice for symptomatic eligible patients with multiple myeloma. It is usually given after initial cytoreduction with VAD-related regimens. Peripheral blood stem cells (PBSCs) are harvested after mobilization with a combination of chemotherapy and growth factors.

High response rates with CR up to 30% can be achieved after ASCT, even in patients refractory to conventional treatment, leading to longer progression-free and overall survival. Two large randomized trials have been carried out to study the role of HDT and ASCT in myeloma. The first was conducted by the Inter-Groupe Francophone du Myélome (IFM 1996) in newly diagnosed patients with stage II or III myeloma. Patients received four to six cycles of VMCP/BVAP induction followed by randomization to additional conventional chemotherapy for a total of 18 cycles or high-dose melphalan and total body irradiation followed by ASCT. ASCT was superior to chemotherapy in terms of response rate (38% CR plus good PR vs. 14%), the 6-year event-free survival (25% vs. 14%) and overall survival (43% vs. 28%). This result was confirmed by a large MRC trial (2003) in which 407 patients with previously untreated myeloma received either standard conventional chemotherapy alone or conventional chemotherapy followed by HDT and ASCT. The CR rate was higher in the transplant group (44% vs. 8%) and so was the overall survival (54 vs. 42 months) and progression-free survival (32 vs. 20 months). Therefore, HDT and ASCT is considered the treatment of choice for patients below 70 years of age. Although some elderly patients may also benefit from the procedure, ASCT is not recommended for elderly myeloma patients who are not fit.

The median overall survival from the time of ASCT is approximately 50 months. The procedure is safe, and the transplantation-related mortality (TRM) is below 2%. The recommended dose of melphalan is 200 mg/m^2. Addition of total body irradiation does not lengthen progression-free or overall survival but adds significantly to toxicity. Low levels of β_2-microglobulin at diagnosis, and the achievement of CR post ASCT, are associated with a better prognosis and seem to be the most important factors in predicting the final outcome.

The issue of early versus late ASCT has been studied and, although there is no difference in overall survival between these treatment modalities, patients who receive an early ASCT have a longer period without symptoms, treatment and treatment-related toxicity. CD34 selection or purging of harvested stem cells does not influence survival and the role of tandem transplants remains unclear. A recent randomized IFM trial showed better survival in those patients with myeloma who were treated with tandem transplants than in those treated with a single transplant. Unfortunately, the patients in the single transplant group received HDT with 140 mg/m^2 melphalan and 8 Gy total body irradiation. This combination has already been shown to result in inferior survival when compared with HDT with 200 mg/m^2 melphalan alone. Future trials will need to compare tandem transplants with single transplants after HDT with 200 mg/m^2 melphalan. HDT may also be carried out in patients with renal failure if they are otherwise fit. The TRM for patients with creatinine levels of above 170 μmol/L is around 6% and the probability of survival at 5 years is 55%.

Allogeneic stem cell transplantation

Allogeneic bone marrow transplantation is too risky to be considered for most patients, but the possibility of a potentially curable graft-versus-myeloma (GvM) effect gives this procedure the best chance for long-term disease control. Registry data show that in patients who have undergone allogeneic matched sibling-donor transplantation, the long-term survival is around 25%. However, the median survival is similar to that in patients who receive ASCT, mainly because of the high TRM rate of between 20% and 40%, which seems to be higher in male patients. Allogeneic transplantations with matched unrelated donors have an even higher TRM and may be considered only in exceptional cases and carried out at specialist centres in the context of a clinical trial. Patients who survive the procedure have a 60% chance of achieving CR and a 50% possibility of achieving molecular remission compared with 7% of patients who have a molecular remission after ASCT. However, only around 20% of allografted patients are in continued CR 5 or more years post transplant. Chronic graft-versus-host disease (GvHD) correlates with CR in allotransplant patients and provides further evidence of an allogeneic GvM effect. There are a number of small studies in the literature showing a direct GvM effect of donor lymphocyte infusions (DLIs). The GvM effect of DLI is often accompanied by severe GvHD. In order to harness this GvM effect, current research is focused on allogeneic transplantation from HLA identical sibling after conditioning with a non-myeloablative or reduced-intensity conditioning regimens followed by DLI to eradicate residual tumour. These 'mini-transplants' have the theoretical advantage of low TRM (near 20%) while maintaining the GvM effect. However, further studies are required to fully evaluate this procedure.

Maintenance therapy

Interferon-alpha

Interferon-α as maintenance therapy following induction chemotherapy results in a slight improvement in progression-free and overall survival of nearly 5–7 months. The addition of chemotherapy (VAD, MP, CP) to the IFN-α maintenance does not seem to improve survival when compared with IFN-α alone. Meta-analysis by the Myeloma Trialists' Collaborative Group showed slightly increased survival in myeloma patients who were given IFN-α as maintenance treatment after conventional chemotherapy but not in those who had undergone ASCT. Taking into consideration the benefit of IFN-α and considerable toxicity, consisting mainly of flu-like symptoms and malaise, the decision to treat individual patients would depend on how well IFN-α is tolerated. The dose of IFN-α has varied among different studies, ranging between 1.5–3 MU/m^2, subcutaneously, three times per week.

Other regimens

Dexamethasone alone, 20 mg/m^2 orally each morning for 4 days, monthly until relapse, offers no advantage over IFN-α. The role of new agents, such as thalidomide or bortezomib, as maintenance treatment post ASCT is under investigation.

Treatment of refractory and relapsed disease

Primary refractory disease

Patients with disease refractory to VAD may respond to alkylating agents and vice versa. Patients with alkylating agent- or VAD-refractory disease may still respond to high-dose melphalan followed by ASCT. Refractory patients have a better outcome after transplantation than after chemotherapy, although patients with prolonged (> 1 year) primary resistant disease gain only minimal benefit from HDT and ASCT.

Relapsed disease

The therapeutic options include repeating initial chemotherapy or, alternatively, using another combination of chemotherapeutic agents mentioned above, followed by HDT and ASCT. Patients who have been treated with MP initially may respond well to the same treatment (response of about 50%) or to VAD-related regimens. Weekly oral or intravenous cyclophosphamide may also be effective. A second ASCT may be performed in patients who relapse after an initial autograft. In these patients, β_2-microglobulin levels, the disease status at transplantation and bone marrow plasma cell infiltration correlate with response and overall survival. Allogeneic transplantation may be an option in some patients, with response rates of around 40% but confers no advantage in term of overall survival compared with ASCT.

Thalidomide

Thalidomide, which was removed from widespread clinical use in 1962 because of severe teratogenicity, has been shown to produce response rates of 30% in patients with refractory or relapsed disease. In the first report by Singhal et al. (1999), thalidomide was given at a starting dose of 200 mg/day, increasing in 200-mg increments every 2 weeks to a maximum dose of 800 mg/day. However, the optimal dose of thalidomide remains uncertain, and this issue can be resolved only by appropriate prospective clinical trials. The combination of thalidomide with dexamethasone seems to increase the response rate to around 50%. The combination of thalidomide with chemotherapy and dexamethasone (CDT: cyclophosphamide, dexamethasone and thalidomide; hyper-CDT: cyclophosphamide, dexamethasone, and thalidomide; TCED: thalidomide, cyclophosphamide, etoposide, and dexamethasone; DT-PACE: dexamethasone, thalidomide, cisplatin, doxorubicin, cyclophosphamide and etoposide) has produced overall response rates of 30–80% in patients with advanced myeloma. The precise role of these combinations in the management of myeloma has not yet been clarified.

Venous thromboembolism has emerged as the single most important complication of thalidomide. The frequency of thromboembolic disease is less than 5% when thalidomide is used alone but is increased to near 15% when thalidomide is given with dexamethasone and almost to 30% when thalidomide is given in combination with chemotherapy. To date, no identifiable prothrombotic abnormality has been found to be predictive of thrombosis in these patients. Other side-effects of thalidomide include peripheral neuropathy, somnolence, constipation, tremor, xerostomia, neutropenia, hypothyroidism, rash and bradycardia. Peripheral neuropathy is a major potential problem with thalidomide as it can be irreversible if the drug is not promptly withdrawn. Thus, patients need to be followed up very closely for the first few months of thalidomide administration.

Bortezomib

Bortezomib (formerly PS341) is a small molecule that is a potent and selective inhibitor of the 26S proteasome, which is the primary component of the protein degradation pathway of the cell. Bortezomib inhibits proliferation and induces apoptosis of human myeloma cell lines. It also inhibits the NF-κB activation, overcomes drug resistance and adds to the anti-myeloma activity of dexamethasone in vitro. In a recent trial of 202 refractory myeloma patients who had received more than three lines of previous treatment, the response rate to bortezomib was 35% (CR and very good PR almost 10%). The median overall survival was 16 months, with a median duration of response of 12 months. A phase III trial comparing bortezomib and high doses of dexamethasone is in progress. This drug has recently been approved by the United States Food and Drug Administration on the basis of the encouraging phase II results and the UK licence application is pending.

Revimid

Revimid is an immunomodulatory agent that exhibits no sedative side-effects but occasionally causes neurotoxic side-effects. Responses have been reported in one-third of patients with advanced and refractory myeloma. Many of these patients had been previously exposed to thalidomide, although true thalidomide resistance was infrequently established. Unlike thalidomide, Revimid causes myelosuppression, which in the setting of compromised bone marrow reserve due to extensive prior cytotoxic drug exposure, may not be fully reversible. Trials are currently under way to investigate the dosing schedules and responses in combination with dexamethasone.

Management of bone disease and hypercalcaemia

The clinical manifestations of myeloma include osteolytic bone destruction and hypercalcaemia. The initial therapy of patients with hypercalcaemia consists of vigorous hydration with intravenous saline and diuresis with frusemide once the patient is rehydrated. Corticosteroids are very effective in hypercalcaemia through their anti-tumour effect, anti-osteoclast activity and reduction of gastrointestinal absorption of calcium. If the patient remains hypercalcaemic after rehydration and diuresis, a specific intravenous anti-osteoclast agent such as pamidronate or zoledronic acid should be used. The majority of the patients achieve normal serum calcium levels within 7 days. In resistant cases, parenteral mithramycin or calcitonin may be indicated. Calcitonin causes a reduction in calcium levels within 12–24 h, but the response is moderate and brief. Mithramycin is effective but toxic, causing myelosuppression, hepatitis and renal damage. Progression of skeletal disease is often not affected by chemotherapy even in patients who seem to be responding. Therapeutic options include the use of bisphosphonates with or without local radiotherapy or surgery.

Bisphosphonates

Bisphosphonates inhibit osteoclast activity by preventing the osteoclast differentiation, inducing osteoclast apoptosis and interrupting their attachment to the bone. They also induce apoptosis of human myeloma cells *in vitro*, reduce IL-6 secretion by bone marrow stromal cells and cause expansion of $\gamma\delta$ T-cells with anti-myeloma activity, suggesting a possible anti-tumour effect of these agents. The effects of bisphosphonates have been evaluated in randomized trials. Oral clodronate (1600 mg, orally, daily) reduces skeleton-related events (SREs), such as pathological fractures, surgery for fracture or impending fracture, radiotherapy to the bone, spinal cord compression and hypercalcaemia. Patients without overt skeletal disease at diagnosis benefit the most, an observation that supports the use of bisphosphonates early in the management of the disease. The second-generation aminobisphosphonate pamidronate, given monthly at a dose of 90 mg intravenously, also reduces SREs and

improves pain and quality of life. It may also extend survival in a subgroup of patients with advanced disease, while it decreases paraprotein, IL-6 and bone resorption markers in myeloma patients, including those in plateau phase. A large meta-analysis, which included 11 randomized trials with 2183 patients, showed that the addition of bisphosphonates (pamidronate or clodronate) to the specific anti-myeloma treatment reduces pathological vertebral fractures and pain. However, there is no effect on mortality, the incidence of non-vertebral fractures or the incidence of hypercalcaemia. No randomized trials have been carried out between the different doses of clodronate or between clodronate and pamidronate to evaluate the differences between these two efficacious bisphosphonates in the management of myeloma bone disease. Ibandronate, a new third-generation bisphosphonate, does not seem to be effective at the doses of 2 mg and 4 mg. Zoledronic acid is a novel third-generation bisphosphonate, which produces the greatest osteoclast inhibition *in vitro*, inhibits the development of osteolytic bone disease and increases progression-free survival in murine myeloma models. It is administered intravenously, in a 15-min infusion, at a dose of 4 mg, and is superior to pamidronate in the treatment of hypercalcaemia of malignancy. However, no superiority over pamidronate has been established in terms of SREs in myeloma. Evidence suggests that long-term bisphosphonate treatment with pamidronate, zoledronic acid or clodronate is necessary for all myeloma patients with lytic bone disease.

Radiotherapy

Radiotherapy may be required in patients who have extramedullary plasmacytoma, in those who have painful destruction of a vertebral body or a pathological fracture, or in whom there is computerized tomography (CT) or MRI evidence of spinal cord compression. Percutaneous vertebroplasty has only recently been introduced as a treatment for osteolytic lesions and osteoporotic compression fractures of the vertebrae. Early results in 187 patients with metastases, myeloma or osteoporotic compression fractures are very promising as approximately 80% of patients with pain unresponsive to medical treatment experience a significant degree of pain relief.

Surgery

Surgery has a role in the management of selected myeloma patients with spinal cord compression or those with unstable vertebral fractures.

Drug resistance

Drug resistance is a major obstacle to successful drug treatment of multiple myeloma. Several mechanisms of drug resistance have been identified (see also Chapter 35). Previous studies had suggested that P-glycoprotein overexpression was responsible for chemotherapy resistance in myeloma cells. Attempts in many clinical studies to reverse multidrug resistance by downregulating P-glycoprotein have not been successful so far.

Another mechanism is related to resistance to apoptosis (programmed cell death), induced by cytotoxic drugs or radiation, of myeloma cells. The proteins involved in this mechanism include B-cell leukaemia/lymphoma protein 2 (Bcl-2), Bcl-XL, Mcl-1 and mutations in the p53 protein. Although switch translocations leading to the activation of multiple partners play an important part in the pathogenesis of myeloma, these translocations do not involve Bcl-2 family members. However, Bcl-2 is expressed in many myeloma cell lines and plasma cells from myeloma patients. Bcl-XL is expressed more often at the time of patient relapse and correlates with resistance to chemotherapy. Mcl-1 is expressed in virtually all cell lines and patient samples examined thus far. Whether these proteins have overlapping functions or work independently to promote myeloma cell survival is unclear. Investigators have started to target these proteins to overcome drug resistance. Some laboratories have been able to correlate induction of apoptosis with decreased expression of Mcl-1. *In vitro* studies have shown that inhibition of Mcl-1 expression with antisense oligonucleotide results in rapid apoptosis and this killing is potentiated by the addition of dexamethasone.

More recently, increased activity of the transcription factor nuclear factor kappa B (NF-κB) has been implicated in the mechanism of chemotherapy resistance of myeloma cells. NF-κB activity protects cells from apoptosis induced by cytotoxic drugs, TNF, IL-1 and many other stimuli. It can activate the expression of TNF receptor-associated factors (TRAF) 1 and 2 and cellular inhibitors of apoptosis genes (cIAP), thereby inhibiting caspase-8 activation and apoptosis. It also inhibits apoptosis by activating cFLIP as well as Bcl-XL and XIAP. Inhibition of C activity in both melphalan-sensitive and melphalan-resistant myeloma cell lines resulted in increased apoptosis. Newer agents such as bortezomib have, therefore, been specifically designed to block NF-κB activation and thus promote apoptosis in chemotherapy-resistant myeloma cells.

Future drug development will likely result in drugs which, either alone or in combination with chemotherapy and radiation, lower the threshold for apoptosis of myeloma cells and overcome chemotherapy resistance.

Supportive therapy

Anaemia

Traditionally, symptomatic anaemia has been managed by red cell transfusion. There is now increasing evidence that recombinant human erythropoietin (rHuEpo) is useful in the management of anaemia in myeloma. In a randomized trial that included 121 transfusion-dependent patients with low-grade non-Hodgkin's lymphoma or myeloma without renal impairment, a response rate of 60% was achieved when a daily dose of 5000 U was given s.c. (subcutaneously). Another double-blind, placebo-controlled trial in 145 anaemic myeloma patients with normal renal function showed that rHuEpo at a dose of 150 IU/kg, s.c., three times weekly, produces a reduction in transfusion requirements, a mean increase in haemoglobin of 1.8 g/dL and an improvement in quality of life. Although there are no reliable predictors of response to rHuEpo, low endogenous erythropoietin concentration seems to be the most helpful predictive factor for response. These data suggest that a therapeutic trial of rHuEpo should be considered in any myeloma patient with symptomatic anaemia.

Renal failure

A degree of renal impairment occurs in up to 50% of myeloma patients at some stage of their disease, while advanced renal failure requiring haemodialysis occurs in 3–12%. In the majority of the patients, renal function will improve in response to simple measures such as rehydration, correction of hypercalcaemia with bisphosphonates, fluid rehydration and administration of glucocorticoids, or discontinuation of nephrotoxic drugs such as non-steroidal anti-inflammatory drugs (NSAIDs) and treatment of any infections. The risk of renal failure, which may be precipitated by the use of intravenous X-ray contrast media, can be reduced by ensuring adequate hydration and by using dyes of reduced osmolality. Allopurinol should be prescribed with the cytotoxic chemotherapy. Half of those who recover do so in the first 6 weeks but late recovery is still possible. Renal impairment is most likely to be reversed in patients with mild impairment, independently of the underlying myeloma.

The efficacy of plasma exchange in patients with hyperviscosity is well established. However, evidence of its usefulness in the treatment of cast nephropathy is equivocal, and therefore it should be used only in the context of a clinical trial. Plasma exchange is effective at removing light chains from the blood, and one retrospective case study suggests that plasma exchange may offer some benefit in preventing initiation of dialysis, as well as preventing acute renal failure progressing to chronic renal failure. It may be necessary to biopsy the kidney to differentiate between cast nephropathy, amyloidosis, light-chain deposition disease and acute tubular necrosis. Renal dialysis may be required to manage the renal failure in some patients. Both peritoneal and haemodialysis have been used successfully in newly diagnosed patients presenting with acute renal failure. Dialysis should be offered to patients in renal failure to allow time for a trial of anti-myeloma chemotherapy. It is the control of the underlying disease rather than the reversal of renal failure, which determines survival benefit. VAD chemotherapy or dexamethasone alone is recommended for initial treatment of patients with renal impairment. Cyclophosphamide is excreted in the urine and therefore a dosage reduction is needed. Patients with multiple myeloma and renal failure have been treated with high-dose therapy with melphalan with some success. There is no consensus concerning the dosage of melphalan in patients with impaired renal function. Melphalan undergoes spontaneous degradation in the blood, and most of the inactive metabolites are excreted in the faeces and some in the urine. Some case reports suggest that the dose of melphalan should be reduced to prevent severe mucositis while others found no change in the pharmacokinetics of high-dose melphalan in patients with renal failure. Patients treated with standard-dose melphalan even when they were on haemodialysis had a treatment-related mortality of less than 5%.

Conclusion and future prospects

Figure 41.5 summarizes the management of patients. The use of HDT and ASCT has improved quality of life and survival and is now considered the standard therapy after initial chemotherapy with VAD or VAD-related regimen. For patients not suitable for ASCT, MP remains the treatment of choice. Unfortunately, most patients die from their disease, and strategies to improve the outcome of ASCT such as tandem transplantation and manipulation of the graft have not been helpful. Allogeneic SCT may be curative in a proportion of patients and should be considered in younger patients with HLA-compatible siblings. Current transplantation trials involve 'debulking' with an ASCT followed by reduced-intensity conditioned allogeneic sibling transplant. This strategy is aimed at harnessing the GvM of the donor graft while maintaining a low TRM. Further progress in management may come from clinical trials which are currently being carried out with other potential agents, including thalidomide analogues [selected cytokine inhibitory drugs (SelCIDs) and immunomodulatory drugs (IMiDs)], arsenic trioxide and proteasome inhibitors, such as bortezomib.

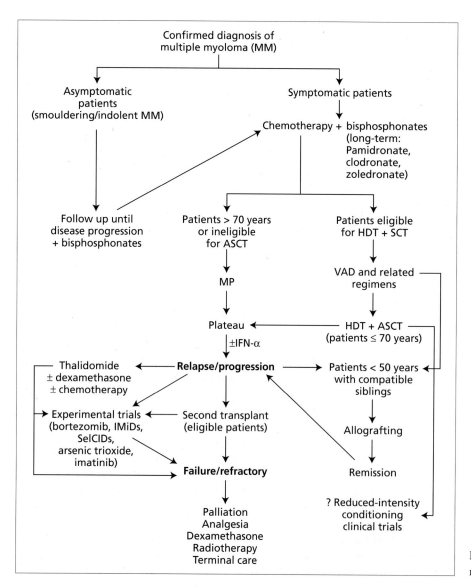

Figure 41.5 Algorithm for the management of patients with myeloma.

Monoclonal gammopathy of uncertain significance

The term 'monoclonal gammopathy of undetermined significance' (MGUS) indicates the presence of a paraprotein in patients without evidence of multiple myeloma, Waldenström's macroglobulinaemia, AL amyloidosis or a related plasma cell proliferative disorder. MGUS is characterized by the following: a serum paraprotein concentration less than 35 g/L; less than 10% plasma cells in the bone marrow; or no Bence Jones protein in the urine; absence of lytic bone lesions; and no related anaemia, hypercalcaemia or renal insufficiency (see Table 41.1). Paraproteins occur without myeloma or Waldenström's macroglobulinaemia in approximately 3% of persons older than 70 years. A monoclonal increase in immunoglobulins results from a clonal process that is malignant or potentially malignant, whereas a reactive or inflammatory process causes a polyclonal increase in immunoglobulins. It is, therefore, essential to distinguish between monoclonal and polyclonal proliferation of plasma cells. It is important to determine whether the monoclonal gammopathy remains stable and benign or progresses to myeloma or a related disorder. Long-term follow-up of a group of 1384 MGUS patients from Minnesota showed that 8% of patients developed myeloma, primary AL amyloidosis, lymphoma with an IgM paraprotein, Waldenström's macroglobulinaemia, plasmacytoma or chronic lymphocytic leukaemia. The cumulative probability of progression to one of these disorders was 10% at 10 years, 21% at 20 years and 26% at 25 years. Although the risk of progression was only 1% per year, patients were at risk of progression even after 25 years or more of stable MGUS.

The sequence of events responsible for malignant transformation of MGUS to myeloma or a related plasma cell proliferative disorder is poorly understood. Alterations, including cytogenetic changes, expression of cytokines and expression of adhesion molecules, occur in both the myeloma cell and the bone marrow microenvironment during this transformation, but the specific pathogenetic role of these alterations is unclear. FISH studies show that 60% of patients with myeloma have IgH (14q32) translocations. Of note, these studies have indicated that these translocations are not unique to myeloma but are also present in MGUS. In one series, 46% of patients with MGUS had IgH translocations, with t(11;14)(q13;q32) being the most common. Because IgH translocations occur in both MGUS and myeloma, their primary role probably lies in the initiation of the clone rather than progression of MGUS to myeloma. Deletions of chromosome 13, which have been in myeloma also occur in MGUS. However, it is not clear if this accelerates the rate of progression from MGUS to myeloma. Aneuploidy appears to occur in some patients with MGUS. Hyperdiploidy has also been noted in bone marrow plasma cells of patients with MGUS.

Changes in the bone marrow microenvironment have also

been described. Angiogenesis increases progressively along the spectrum of plasma cell disorders, from the more benign MGUS stage to advanced myeloma, suggesting that angiogenesis may be related to disease progression. It is likely that progression of MGUS to myeloma involves the dysregulation of various cytokines in plasma cells and stromal cells, leading to osteoclast activation and lytic bone lesions. However, none of the findings, including plasma cell morphology, made at diagnosis of MGUS distinguishes between patients whose condition will remain stable and those in whom a malignant condition will develop. When multiple myeloma or Waldenström's macroglobulinaemia develops, the type of paraprotein is the same as that of the MGUS. The initial concentration of paraprotein is an important risk factor for progression to a plasma cell disorder. In one study, the risk of transformation to myeloma or a related disorder 20 years after the diagnosis of MGUS was 14% for patients with an initial paraprotein level of 5 g/L or less, 16% for 10 g/L, 25% for 15 g/L, 41% for 20 g/L, 49% for 25 g/L and 64% for 30 g/L. There is no significant difference in survival between patients with MGUS and age-matched control subjects. No one factor can differentiate a patient with a benign monoclonal gammopathy from one in whom a malignant plasma cell disorder subsequently develops although attempts are currently being made, through gene expression profiling, to determine if a pattern of gene expression can be identified to predict progression to myeloma. These patients need to be followed up regularly and serum paraprotein level must be measured every 6–12 months to determine whether their condition has transformed.

Lymphoplasmacytic lymphoma/ Waldenström's macroglobulinaemia

Lymphoplasmacytic lymphoma/Waldenström's macroglobulinaemia (LPL) is a B-cell lymphoma that shows maturation to plasmacytoid lymphocytes and plasma cells and is associated with an IgM paraprotein with hyperviscosity or cryoglobulinaemia. It is discussed in greater detail in Chapter 45.

Solitary plasmacytoma

Solitary bone and extramedullary plasmacytomas are rare. Their diagnosis is based on histological confirmation of monoclonal plasma cell infiltration of a single disease site and on the exclusion of multiple myeloma. The treatment of choice for both entities is localized radiotherapy. Using modern radiotherapy and at a total dose of 4000–5000 cGy, the risk for local recurrence is less than 5%. There is no role for systemic chemotherapy in the management of these disorders. The prognosis of patients with solitary extramedullary plasmacytoma appears to be better than for patients with solitary bone plasmacytoma, as approximately 70% of patients with solitary extramedullary plasmacytoma remain disease free at 10 years compared with 30% of patients with bone plasmacytoma.

Plasma-cell leukaemia

In 2% of the cases of myeloma, plasma cells may be present in peripheral blood. Plasma cell leukaemia is defined as a level of plasma cells in the peripheral blood that exceeds 2×10^9/L or > 20% of the white cells. It may occur at the time of diagnosis, when it is known as primary plasma cell leukaemia, or evolve as a terminal complication during the course of multiple myeloma, when it is called secondary plasma cell leukaemia. Plasma cell leukaemia is more frequent in light-chain (Bence Jones protein) or IgD myeloma. It is seen less frequently in IgA or IgG myeloma. Osteolytic lesion and bone pain are less frequent and lymphadenopathy, organomegaly and renal failure more frequent in plasma cell leukaemia. It is an aggressive disease associated with short survival.

Non-secretory myeloma

About 1% of multiple myeloma patients have plasma cells that synthesize but do not secrete immunoglobulin molecules, resulting in absence of paraprotein. Monoclonal cytoplasmic immunoglobulin is demonstrated in the malignant plasma cells by immunohistochemistry. In rare cases, no cytoplasmic immunoglobulin is detected. The clinical features are very similar to secretory multiple myeloma except for a lower incidence of renal complications. The diagnosis can be missed because of the lack of serum or urine monoclonal immunoglobulin unless bone marrow biopsy with immunohistochemistry is carried out.

Osteosclerotic myeloma (POEMS syndrome)

Osteosclerotic myeloma is often a component of the rare POEMS syndrome, which includes polyneuropathy (sensorineural demyelination), organomegaly (hepatomegaly, splenomegaly), endocrinopathy (diabetes, gynaecomastia, testicular atrophy, impotence), monoclonal gammopathy and skin changes (hyperpigmentation, hypertrichosis). It is characterized by a plasma cell infiltrate in the marrow accompanied by thickened bone trabeculae and often lymph node changes resembling the plasma cell variant of Castleman's disease. Patients may present with polyneuropathy and symptoms related to endocrinopathy, skeletal lesions or lymphadenopathy. They usually have either IgAλ or IgGλ paraprotein. The level of paraprotein in the serum and urine is usually low. Anaemia, hypercalcaemia, renal dysfunction and pathological fractures are rare. Bone marrow trephine shows a characteristic osteosclerotic plasmacytoma which may occur singly or multiply. The lesion shows thickened trabecular bone with closely associated peritrabecular fibrosis with entrapped plasma cells. The rest of the bone marrow away from the lesions is relatively normal with less than 5% plasma cells. Lymph node biopsy shows a follicular proliferation with regressed and reactive follicles and interfollicular plasma cell accumulation, consistent with the plasma cell variant of Castleman's disease. One study showed that the survival may be better than that for typical multiple myeloma.

Heavy-chain diseases

These are B-cell neoplasms that produce monoclonal heavy chains but no light chains. There is considerable heterogeneity in the morphology and clinical features. The heavy chain is either a μ or γ or α which is truncated and not capable of full assembly and would therefore be of varying size. The deletions are located mainly in the Fab fragment with a normal Fc portion. It may therefore not have the characteristic 'spike' on serum electrophoresis and requires immunoelectrophoresis or immunofixation to confirm heavy-chain specificity. These diseases probably represent variants of lymphoma. In γ-heavy-chain disease (γ-HCD) and α-HCD there is a reduction in the synthesis of light chains, whereas in μ-HCD, light chains are produced in moderate quantities but are not incorporated into immunoglobulin molecules.

α-Heavy-chain disease is a variant of extranodal marginal zone B-cell lymphoma of the mucosa-associated lymphoid tissue (MALT) type in which defective α-chains are secreted. It occurs in young adults with a peak incidence in the second and third decades. It is endemic in areas bordering the Mediterranean, including Israel, Egypt, Saudi Arabia and North Africa. It is associated with low socioeconomic status and consequential poor hygiene, malnutrition and frequent intestinal infections. It involves the gastrointestinal tract, mainly the small intestine and mesenteric nodes, resulting in malabsorption, diarrhoea, hypocalcaemia, abdominal pain, wasting, fever and steatorrhoea. It is also known as immunoproliferative small intestinal disease (IPSID). The serum protein electrophoresis is usually normal because of the variation in the IgA molecular forms or it shows hypogammaglobulinaemia. Anti-IgA antibody is therefore required to make the diagnosis by immunofixation. Serial studies of patients who are diagnosed early in the course of their disease suggest that the lamina propria of the duodenum and jejunum and regional mesenteric nodes and retroperitoneal nodes are initially infiltrated by small lymphocytes and plasma cells. As the disease progresses, the lamina propria becomes more heavily infiltrated with plasma cells with extension into the submucosa and the muscularis mucosa. Further progression results in the appearance of immunoblastic tumours of the small bowel and mesenteric nodes. Initially the entire length of the small intestine is diffusely involved, but later on in the course of the disease pleomorphic immunoblastic tumours may develop with intestinal obstruction, intussusception or perforation. The plasma cells and marginal zone cells express monoclonal cytoplasmic α heavy-chain without light chains, express pan-B-cell antigens but not CD5 or CD10. If α-HCD is treated with antibiotics at an early stage of disease, then complete remission may be achieved. Many patients may undergo transformation to large B-cell lymphoma with fatal result.

μ-Heavy-chain disease is an extremely rare disease of adults resulting from a B-cell neoplasm resembling chronic lymphocytic leukaemia (CLL) and involving the spleen, liver, bone marrow and peripheral blood, in which a defective μ-chain lacking a variable region is produced. Most patients present with a slowly progressive chronic lymphocytic leukaemia. μ-HCD can be differentiated from CLL by the high frequency of hepatosplenomegaly and absence of lymphadenopathy. Routine serum protein electrophoresis is usually normal but immunoelectrophoresis may show m-polymers of varying sizes. Light chains, particularly κ-chains, are commonly found in the urine. Bone marrow biopsy shows a mixture of characteristic vacuolated plasma cells and small, round lymphocytes similar to CLL cells. The cells show monoclonal cytoplasmic m-chain without light chain, express pan-B cell antigens but do not express CD5 or CD10.

γ-Heavy-chain disease is a lymphoplamacytic lymphoma that produces a truncated γ-chain, which does not bind to light chains to form a complete immunoglobulin molecule. It is a rare disease with a median age of onset at 60. Most patients have systemic symptoms such as anorexia, weakness, fever, weight loss and recurrent bacterial infections or may exhibit autoimmune processes such as haemolytic anaemia, autoimmune thrombocytopenia. These patients have lymphadenopathy, splenomegaly, hepatomegaly and peripheral eosinophilia. Serum protein electrophoresis may be normal, but the diagnosis may be made by demonstration of IgG without light chains by immunofixation. There is usually very little light chain production with urinary light chain less than 1 g/24 h. Lymph nodes show a mixture of lymphocytes, plasmacytoid lymphocytes, plasma cells, immunoblasts and eosinophils. When plasma cells predominate, it may resemble multiple myeloma. The neoplastic cells have monoclonal cytoplasmic γ-chains and express pan-B cell markers, but do not express CD5 or CD10. The clinical course is variable but it can be rapidly progressive with a median survival of 12 months.

Selected bibliography

Attal M, Harousseau JL, Facon T et al. (2003) Single versus double autologous stem-cell transplantation for multiple myeloma. New England Journal of Medicine 349: 2495–502.

Attal M, Harousseau JL, Stoppa AM et al. (1996) A prospective, randomized trial of autologous bone marrow transplantation and

chemotherapy in multiple myeloma. Intergroupe Francais du Myelome. New England Journal of Medicine 335: 91–7.

Bataille R, Harousseau JL (1997) Multiple Myeloma. New England Journal of Medicine 336: 1657–64.

Berenson JR, Hillner BE, Kyle RA et al. (2002) American Society of Clinical Oncology clinical practice guidelines: the role of bisphosphonates in multiple myeloma. Journal of Clinical Oncology 20: 3719–36.

Blade J, Samson D, Reece D et al. (1998) Criteria for evaluating disease response and progression in patients with multiple myeloma treated by high-dose therapy and haemopoietic stem cell transplantation. Myeloma Subcommittee of the EBMT. British Journal of Haematology 102: 1115–23.

Cavenagh JD, Oakervee H for the UK Myeloma Forum and the BCSH Haematology/Oncology Task Forces (2003) Thalidomide in multiple myeloma: current status and future prospects. British Journal of Haematology 120: 18–26.

Child JA, Morgan GJ, Davies FE et al. (2003) High-dose chemotherapy with hematopoietic stem-cell rescue for multiple myeloma. New England Journal of Medicine 348: 1875–83.

Dimopoulos MA, Moulopoulos LA, Maniatis A, Alexanian R (2000) Solitary plasmacytoma of bone and asymptomatic multiple myeloma. Blood 96: 2037–44.

Durie BGM, Kyle RA, Belch A et al. (2003) Myeloma management guidelines: a consensus report from the Scientific Advisors of the International Myeloma Foundation. The Haematology Journal 4: 379–98.

Gahrton G, Svensson H, Cavo M et al. (2001) Progress in allogeneic bone marrow and peripheral blood stem cell transplantation for multiple myeloma: a comparison between transplants performed 1983–93 and 1994–8 at European Group for Blood and Marrow Transplantation centres. British Journal of Haematology 113: 209–16.

Greipp PR, San Miguel JF, Fonseca R et al. (2003) Development of an International Prognostic Index (IPI) for myeloma: report of the International Myeloma Working Group. The Hematology Journal 4 (Suppl 1): S42–S44.

Harousseau JL (2002) High-dose therapy in multiple myeloma. Annals of Oncology 13 (Suppl 4): 49–54.

Hayashi T, Hideshima T, Anderson KC (2003) Novel therapies for multiple myeloma. British Journal of Haematology 120: 10–17.

Jaffe ES, Harris NL, Stein H, Vardiman JW (eds) (2001) World Health Organization Classification of Tumours. Pathology and Genetics of Tumours of Haematopoietic and Lymphoid Tissues. IARC Press, Lyon.

Kuehl WM, Bergsagel PL (2002) Multiple myeloma: evolving genetic events and host interactions. Nature Reviews Cancer 2: 175–87.

Kumar A, Loughran T, Alsina M et al. (2003) Management of multiple myeloma: a systematic review and critical appraisal of published studies. Lancet Oncology 4: 293–304.

Kyle RA, Therneau TM, Rajkumar SV et al. (2002) A long-term study of prognosis in monoclonal gammopathies of undetermined significance. New England Journal of Medicine 346: 564–9.

Moreau P, Facon T, Attal M et al. (2002) Comparison of 200 mg/m^2 melphalan and 8 Gy total body irradiation plus 140 mg/m^2 melphalan as conditioning regimens for peripheral blood stem cell transplantation in patients with newly diagnosed multiple myeloma: final analysis of the Intregroupe Francophone du Myelome 9502 randomized trial. *Blood* **99**: 731–5.

Myeloma Trialists' Collaborative Group (1998) Combination chemotherapy vs. melphalan plus prednisone as treatment for multiple myeloma: an overview of 6633 patients from 27 randomized trials. *Journal of Clinical Oncology* **16**: 3832–42.

Myeloma Trialists' Collaborative Group (2001) Interferon as therapy for multiple myeloma: an individual patient data overview of 24 randomized trials and 4012 patients. *British Journal of Haematology* **113**: 1020–34.

Rajkumar SV, Kyle RA, Gertz MA (2002) Myeloma and the newly diagnosed patient: a focus on treatment and management. *Seminars in Oncology* **29** (6 Suppl 17): 5–10.

Rawstron AC, Davies FE, DasGupta R *et al.* (2002) Flow cytometric disease monitoring in multiple myeloma: the relationship between normal and neoplastic plasma cells predicts outcome after transplantation. *Blood* **100**: 3095–100.

Riccardi A, Mora O, Tinelli C *et al.* (2000) Long-term survival of stage I multiple myeloma given chemotherapy just after diagnosis or at progression of the disease: a multicentre randomized study. *British Journal of Cancer* **82**: 1254–60.

Richardson PG, Barlogie B, Berenson J *et al.* (2003) A phase 2 study of bortezomib in relapsed, refractory myeloma. *New England Journal of Medicine* **348**: 2609–17.

Singhal S, Mehta J, Desikan R *et al.* (1999) Antitumor activity of thalidomide in refractory multiple myeloma. *New England Journal of Medicine* **341**: 1565–71.

Terpos E, Szydlo R, Apperley JF *et al.* (2003) Soluble receptor activator of nuclear factor kappa-B ligand/osteoprotegerin ratio predicts survival in multiple myeloma: proposal for a novel prognostic index. *Blood* **102**: 1064–9.

Terpos E, Politou M, Rahemtulla A (2003) New insights into the pathophysiology and management of bone disease in multiple myeloma. *British Journal of Haematology* **123**: 758–69.

Tian E, Zhan F, Walker R *et al.* (2003) The role of the Wnt-signaling antagonist DKK1 in the development of osteolytic lesions in multiple myeloma. *New England Journal of Medicine* **349**: 2483–94.

UK Myeloma Forum Guidelines Working Group (2001) Guidelines on the diagnosis and management of multiple myeloma. *British Journal of Haematology* **115**: 522–40.

UK Myeloma Forum AL Amyloidosis Guidelines Working Group (2004) Guidelines on the diagnosis and management of AL amyloidosis. *British Journal of Haematology* **125**: 671–700.

CHAPTER 42

Amyloidosis

Hugh JB Goodman and Philip N Hawkins

Introduction

Amyloidosis is a disorder of protein folding in which normally soluble proteins are deposited in the extracellular space as insoluble fibrils that progressively disrupt tissue structure and function. Some 20 different unrelated proteins can form amyloid *in vivo*, and clinical amyloidosis is classified according to the fibril protein type (Table 42.1). Although the term amyloid is derived from the Greek for starch-like, the misnomer was recognized over 100 years ago and has remained unchallenged.

Amyloid deposition may be systemic or localized, hereditary or acquired, life-threatening or an incidental finding. Organ involvement varies within and between fibril types and clinical phenotypes overlap greatly. Systemic amyloidosis may involve virtually any tissue and is often fatal, although its prognosis has been improved by haemodialysis, kidney, liver and heart transplantation, and by increasingly effective treatment of the various conditions that underlie it. Localized amyloid deposits are confined to specific foci or to a particular organ or tissue, and can be clinically silent through to causing serious disease such as haemorrhage in local respiratory or urogenital tract AL amyloid. In addition to the amyloidoses *per se*, local amyloid deposition is a hallmark pathological feature of uncertain significance in other important diseases including Alzheimer's disease, the prion disorders and type II diabetes mellitus.

The chapter is devoted mainly to describing the clinical features, diagnosis and management of AL (monoclonal immunoglobulin light chain) amyloidosis, which is the most common and serious form of systemic amyloidosis in industrialized societies. The differential diagnosis and other amyloid fibril types that can mimic AL type are also discussed.

Pathogenesis of amyloid

Amyloidosis breaks the dogma that tertiary structure of proteins is determined solely by their primary amino acid sequence. Amyloid-forming proteins can exist in two completely different stable structures, the transformation evidently involving massive refolding of the native form into one that can autoaggregate in a highly ordered manner to produce the characteristic predominantly β-sheet, rigid, non-branching fibrils of 10–15 nm in diameter and of indeterminate length. Acquired biophysical properties common to all amyloid fibrils include insolubility in physiological solutions, relative resistance to proteolysis, and ability to bind Congo red dye in an ordered manner that gives the diagnostic green birefringence under cross-polarized light.

Amyloid deposition can occur in three circumstances. The first is when there is a sustained abnormally high concentration of certain normal proteins, such as serum amyloid A protein (SAA) in chronic inflammation and β_2-microglobulin in renal failure, which underlie susceptibility to AA and Aβ_2M amyloidosis respectively. The second situation is when there is a normal concentration of a normal, but inherently amyloidogenic, protein over a very prolonged period, such as transthyretin in senile amyloidosis (ATTR) and β-protein in Alzheimer's disease. The third situation is the production of an acquired or inherited variant protein with an abnormal structure, such as amyloidogenic monoclonal immunoglobulin light chains or the amyloidogenic variants of transthyretin, lysozyme, apolipoprotein AI, fibrinogen Aα chain, etc. The genetic and environmental factors that influence individual susceptibility to and timing of amyloid deposition are unclear, but once the process has begun amyloid deposition is unremitting as long as the supply of the respective precursor protein remains undiminished.

Table 42.1 Classification of amyloidosis.*

Type	Fibril precursor protein	Clinical syndrome
AA	Serum amyloid A protein	Systemic amyloidosis associated with acquired or hereditary chronic inflammatory diseases. Formerly known as secondary or reactive amyloidosis
AL	Monoclonal immunoglobulin light chains	Systemic amyloidosis associated with myeloma, monoclonal gammopathy, occult B cell dyscrasia. Formerly known as primary amyloidosis
ATTR	Normal plasma transthyretin	Senile systemic amyloidosis with predominant cardiac involvement
ATTR	Genetic variants of transthyretin (e.g. ATTR Met30, Ala60, Ile122)	Familial amyloid polyneuropathy (FAP), with systemic amyloidosis and often prominent amyloid cardiomyopathy
$A\beta_2M$	β_2-Microglobulin	Dialysis related amyloidosis (DRA) associated with renal failure and long-term dialysis. Predominantly musculoskeletal symptoms
$A\beta$	β-Protein precursor (and rare genetic variants)	Cerebrovascular and intracerebral plaque amyloid in Alzheimer's disease. Occasional familial cases
AApoAI	Genetic variants of apolipoprotein AI (e.g. AApoAI Arg26, Arg60)	Autosomal dominant systemic amyloidosis. Predominantly non-neuropathic with prominent visceral involvement, especially nephropathy. Minor wild-type ApoAI amyloid deposits may occur in the aorta
AFib	Genetic variants of fibrinogen α chain (e.g. AFib Val526)	Autosomal dominant systemic amyloidosis. Non-neuropathic usually with prominent nephropathy
ALys	Genetic variants of lysozyme (e.g. ALys His67)	Autosomal dominant systemic amyloidosis. Non-neuropathic with prominent renal and gastrointestinal involvement
ACys	Genetic variant of cystatin C (Gln68)	Hereditary cerebral haemorrhage with cerebral and systemic amyloidosis
AGel	Genetic variants of gelsolin (e.g. Asn187)	Autosomal dominant systemic amyloidosis. Predominant cranial nerve involvement with lattice corneal dystrophy
AIAPP	Islet amyloid polypeptide	Amyloid in islets of Langerhans in type II diabetes mellitus and insulinoma

*Amyloid composed of peptide hormones, prion protein, and unknown proteins, not included.

Amyloid deposits consist mainly of amyloid fibrils, but they also contain some common minor constituents, including certain glycosaminoglycans (GAGs) and the normal circulating plasma protein serum amyloid P component (SAP), as well as various other trace proteins. SAP binds in a specific calcium-dependent manner to a ligand that is present on all amyloid fibrils but not on their precursor proteins, and studies in knock-out mice indicate that SAP contributes to amyloidogenesis.

Amyloid fibril-associated GAGs mainly comprise heparan and dermatan sulphates. Their universal presence, restricted heterogeneity and intimate relationship with the fibrils suggest that they may also contribute to the development or stability of amyloid deposits, a possibility that has lately been supported by the inhibitory effect of low-molecular-weight GAG analogues on the experimental induction of AA amyloidosis in mice.

Many of the pathological effects of amyloid can be attributed to its physical presence. Extensive deposits, which may amount to kilograms, are structurally disruptive and incompatible with normal function, as are strategically located smaller deposits, for example in glomeruli or nerves. Amyloid fibrils may also be cytotoxic. However, the relationship between the quantity of amyloid and degree of associated organ dysfunction differs greatly between individuals, and there is a strong impression that the rate of new amyloid deposition may be as important a determinant of progressive organ failure as the amyloid load itself.

Systemic AL amyloidosis

Systemic AL (formerly known as 'primary') amyloidosis occurs in a small proportion of individuals with monoclonal B-cell dyscrasias. AL fibrils are derived from monoclonal immunoglobulin light chains, which are unique in each patient, underlying the remarkably broad clinical picture in this particular form of amyloidosis. Virtually any organ or combination of organs other than the brain may be directly affected, commonly including the heart. However, symptoms are often non-specific and screening techniques frequently fail to detect the underlying monoclonal gammopathies leading to delayed diagnosis, by which time the deposits are often very extensive and the prognosis poor.

AL fibrils and monoclonal light chains

AL fibrils are composed of part or sometimes the whole of the variable (V_L) domain of monoclonal immunoglobulin light chains. The molecular weight of the fibril subunit protein therefore varies between about 8000 and 30 000 Da. The inherent 'amyloidogenicity' of certain monoclonal light chains has been elegantly demonstrated in an *in vivo* model in which purified Bence Jones proteins were injected into mice. Animals receiving light chains from patients with AL amyloid developed typical amyloid deposits composed of the human protein, whereas animals receiving light chains from myeloma patients without amyloid did not. AL fibrils are more commonly derived from λ than κ light chains, despite the fact that κ isotypes predominate among both normal immunoglobulins and monoclonal gammopathies. Some amyloidogenic light chains have distinctive amino acid replacements or insertions compared with non-amyloid monoclonal light chains, including replacement of hydrophilic framework residues by hydrophobic ones, changes that can promote aggregation and insolubility. Certain light-chain isotypes, notably $V_{\lambda VI}$, are especially amyloidogenic, and there is a degree of concordance between some isotypes and their tropism for being deposited as amyloid in particular organ systems. For example, the $V_{\lambda VI}$ isotype often presents with dominant renal involvement whereas the $V_{\lambda II}$ isotype frequently involves the heart.

The plasma cell dyscrasia

Although almost any dyscrasia of differentiated B lymphocytes, including multiple myeloma, Waldenström's macroglobulinaemia and other malignant lymphomas/leukaemias, may produce a monoclonal immunoglobulin that can sometimes form AL amyloid, well over 80% of cases are associated with low-grade and otherwise 'benign' monoclonal gammopathies. Histological studies indicate that amyloid deposition occurs in up to 15% of cases of myeloma, but usually in small and clinically insignificant amounts, and that it probably occurs in less than 5% of patients with 'benign' monoclonal gammopathy of undetermined significance (MGUS).

Clinical features

AL amyloidosis accounts for more than 1 in 1500 deaths in Britain and occurs equally in men and women. The median age at presentation is 65 years, but it can occur in young adults and is

probably much underdiagnosed in the elderly, in whom it would be expected to have the highest incidence. It is the most serious and commonly diagnosed form of systemic amyloidosis, and presently outnumbers referrals of AA amyloidosis to the UK National Amyloidosis Centre by a factor of 8:1.

Common organ-related features at presentation are proteinuria and nephrotic syndrome, renal impairment, symptomatic cardiac involvement, neuropathy and hepatomegaly. Dysfunction of a single organ may dominate the clinical picture. Fatigue, weight loss and malaise are frequent. The heart is affected pathologically in up to 90% of patients, in 30% of whom restrictive cardiomyopathy is a presenting feature, and in up to half of whom it is fatal. Rarer cardiac presentations include arrhythmias and angina, the latter sometimes due to coronary amyloid angiopathy. Dominant renal amyloid is the presenting feature in one-third of patients, typically presenting with nephrotic syndrome and/or renal impairment. Gut involvement may cause motility disturbances, which can also be secondary to autonomic neuropathy, and malabsorption, perforation, haemorrhage or obstruction. Macroglossia occurs in 5–10% but is almost pathognomonic of AL amyloidosis (Figure 42.1). Hyposplenism is not infrequent in both AA and AL amyloidosis but is rarely documented. Painful sensory polyneuropathy with early loss of pain and temperature sensation followed later by motor deficits occur in 10–20% of cases and carpal tunnel syndrome occurs in 20%. Autonomic neuropathy leading to impotence, orthostatic hypotension and gastrointestinal disturbances may

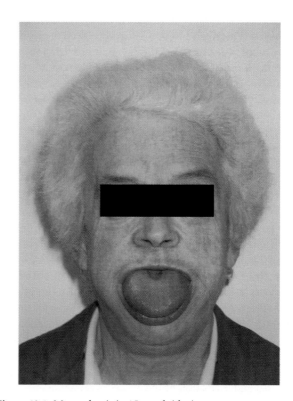

Figure 42.1 Macroglossia in AL amyloidosis.

occur alone or together with peripheral neuropathy, and has a poor prognosis. Involvement of dermal blood vessels is common and may cause purpura, most distinctively in a periorbital distribution ('raccoon eyes'). Direct skin involvement takes the form of papules, nodules and plaques, usually on the face and upper trunk. Articular amyloid is rare but the symptoms can be severe and superficially mimic an inflammatory polyarthritis. Soft-tissue infiltration may occur, characteristically involving the lower face or the glenohumeral joints and surrounding tissues to produce the 'shoulder pad' sign. An uncommon but serious manifestation of AL amyloid is an acquired bleeding diathesis that may be associated with deficiency of factor X and sometimes also factor IX, or with increased fibrinolysis. It does not occur in other amyloidoses, although in both AL and AA disease there may be serious bleeding in the absence of any identifiable factor deficiency.

Natural history/prognosis

Systemic AL amyloidosis is a progressive systemic disease with a prognosis far worse than AA and hereditary types. Median survival in historical series is only 12–15 months. Half of deaths are due to cardiac involvement, and in patients in whom heart failure is evident at presentation median survival is only about 6 months. Autonomic neuropathy and liver involvement with hyperbilirubinaemia are also associated with a very poor prognosis, whereas dominant renal involvement or peripheral neuropathy has a better outlook.

The traditional impression that amyloid deposition is irreversible and inexorably progressive largely reflects the persistent nature of the acquired or hereditary conditions that underlie it. It is now clear that amyloid deposits generally exist in a slowly dynamic state, and that they often gradually regress if the amyloid fibril precursor protein supply can be reduced. Under favourable circumstances organ function may improve and prolonged survival can occur. This knowledge has encouraged a much more aggressive approach to patient management in recent years.

Diagnosis and investigation of AL amyloidosis

Amyloid should be considered in the differential diagnosis of renal failure, nephrotic syndrome, restrictive cardiomyopathy, peripheral or autonomic neuropathy and hepatomegaly, etc., but early symptoms are often very non-specific and insidious, such as malaise or weight loss. The index of suspicion should be high in patients known to have clonal B-cell dyscrasias, but in practice the diagnosis of amyloidosis is usually an unexpected finding following biopsy of an organ with disturbed function. The approach to diagnosis is outlined in Table 42.2, and essentially comprises confirmation of the presence of amyloid, determination of fibril type, characterization of the underlying plasma cell dyscrasia, and evaluation of the extent, distribution and function of involved organs.

Confirming the presence of amyloid

Histology

In systemic forms of amyloidosis, deposits occur in blood vessels and as small interstitial foci throughout the body, providing the basis for 'screening' biopsies of abdominal fat or rectum which are diagnostic in 50–80% of cases. Diffuse parenchymal amyloid deposits may occur in few or many organs, and biopsy of a clinically affected organ, for example of kidney, heart, liver or gastrointestinal tract, is likely to give positive results in more than 95% of cases. The appearance on H&E-stained tissue of pink amorphous material should raise suspicion of amyloid and prompt further more specific stains. Many cotton dyes, fluorochromes and metachromatic stains are used, but Congo red staining giving green birefringence under cross-polarized light is generally accepted to be the diagnostic gold standard in amyloidosis (Figure 42.2). False-positive and -negative interpretation of the Congo red stain is not rare but can be minimized by using the alkaline–alcohol method (Puchtler et al., 1962), fresh reagents, tissue sections of optimal 5–10 μm thickness, inclusion of positive control tissue and high-quality polarizing filters. Some Congo red techniques stain connective tissues quite strongly and produce white or very pale-green birefringence that can cause diagnostic errors.

Electron microscopy

Amyloid fibrils cannot always be convincingly identified ultrastructurally, and a diagnosis of amyloidosis made through electron microscopy alone should be regarded with caution since other pathological processes involve deposition of fibrillar material.

SAP scintigraphy

Radiolabelled SAP scintigraphy is a specific nuclear medicine imaging technique that demonstrates the presence and distribution of amyloid deposits in vivo in a quantitative manner. It was developed and is used routinely at the UK National Amyloidosis Centre, but is not available commercially. ^{123}I-SAP localizes rapidly and specifically to amyloid deposits, of all fibril types, in proportion to the amount of amyloid present. SAP scintigraphy confirms the presence of amyloid in most patients with AL type, and virtually all with AA type. The scans provide information that is different and complementary to biopsy histology, notably including data on the whole body and individual organ amyloid load in serial follow-up studies, for example following chemotherapy in AL amyloidosis (Figure 42.3). The organ distribution of amyloid on SAP scintigraphy can be indicative of the fibril type, for example bone uptake occurs only in AL amyloidosis. Unfortunately, amyloid in the moving heart and in small or diffuse hollow structures such as nerves and the gut is not adequately visualized by SAP scintigraphy. Various other tracers, including conventional bone-seeking agents and radiolabelled aprotinin, sometimes localize non-specifically to amyloid deposits but do not have any defined clinical role.

Table 42.2 Approach to the investigation and monitoring of suspected AL amyloidosis.

	Confirmation of amyloid	Determination of amyloid type	Evaluation of organ involvement	Investigation of Plasma cell dyscrasia	Monitoring
Pathology	Biopsy and Congo red histology of affected organ, screening tissue (e.g. fat aspirate or rectum) or any available specimen	Immunohistochemical staining of tissue sections with a panel of antibodies to amyloid fibril proteins (often not definitive in AL) amyloidosis)	Biopsy of affected organ (but subsequent biopsies merely to determine the extent of amyloid involvement are not recommended)	Bone marrow aspirate and biopsy with light-chain immunophenotyping	Follow-up biopsies usually not helpful in monitoring amyloid load
Haematology, biochemistry, immunology		Identification of a monoclonal gammopathy supports AL type but may be an incidental finding	Serum creatinine and creatinine clearance, albumin, 24-h urine protein Liver function tests Coagulation screen	Full blood count, urea and electrolytes, creatinine, calcium Immunoglobulins Electrophoresis and immunofixation of serum and urine Quantitative serum free light chain assay	Serum free light chain and paraprotein concentration
Imaging	SAP scintigraphy	SAP scintigraphy (evidence of marrow involvement is indicative of AL type)	Echocardiogram, ECG SAP scintigraphy	Skeletal survey	SAP scintigraphy
Other		DNA analysis Amyloid fibril protein sequencing	As otherwise indicated, e.g. nerve conduction studies		Serial assessment of organ function, e.g. liver and renal function tests, echocardiogram and other investigations as indicated

Identifying fibril type

It has been common practice to diagnose apparently 'primary' cases of amyloidosis as AL type, especially when a monoclonal gammopathy can be demonstrated. However, the underlying chronic inflammatory disease process is clinically covert in 5–10% of patients with AA amyloidosis, and a family history is quite often absent in patients with hereditary amyloidosis caused by variant forms of fibrinogen Aα chain and transthyretin, due to low penetrance and late onset of symptoms. The coincidental presence of a monoclonal gammopathy can therefore be gravely misleading and lead to inappropriate use of cytotoxic agents. The combination of immunohistochemical staining and DNA analysis usually allows confirmation of fibril type or exclusion of hereditary forms.

Immunohistochemistry

Immunohistochemical staining of amyloid containing tissue sections using a panel of antibodies against known amyloid proteins is the most accessible method for characterizing fibril type. However, definitive results often cannot be obtained in AL amyloid due to a combination of background staining of normal immunoglobulin and failure of antibodies to bind to κ or λ light chains in their abnormal amyloid conformation. In contrast, antibodies against serum amyloid A protein can confirm or exclude AA amyloid in virtually all cases, and, with optimization, antibodies are similarly useful in most hereditary forms. Reliable interpretation of immunohistochemical stains is not possible unless positive and negative controls have been used, and the specificity of staining by absorption with appropriate antigens has been demonstrated in each run.

DNA analysis

Sequencing of the genes associated with hereditary amyloidosis is now performed routinely in our centre to exclude hereditary amyloidosis when presumed AL type cannot be confirmed definitively, as well as in all patients in whom familial disease is suspected. Corroboration by other methods (e.g. immunohistochemistry)

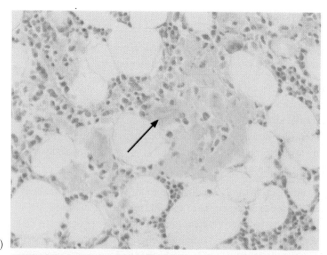

(a)

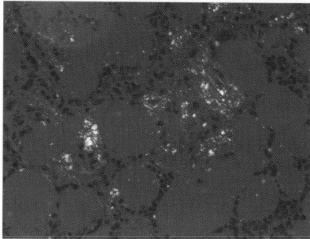

(b)

Figure 42.2 Appearance of amyloid in a bone marrow biopsy (×40, 6-μm section). (a) Congo red stain showing amorphous pink material in the interstitium and small blood vessel (arrow). (b) Same section under high-intensity cross-polarized light showing diagnostic apple-green birefringence.

is necessary to confirm that identified mutations are indeed the cause of the amyloid.

Assessment of the plasma cell dyscrasia

A monoclonal whole paraprotein or free light chains can be identified by electrophoresis and immunofixation of serum and urine in only 80% of patients with AL amyloid. However, a new fully quantitative high-sensitivity immunoassay (Freelite™, The Binding Site, Birmingham, UK) can demonstrate and monitor a clonal excess of serum free light chains in about 98% of cases.

Bone marrow aspiration and trephine biopsy are required to characterize the underlying B-cell dyscrasia, which comprises a subtle plasma cell infiltrate in about 80% of cases. The presence of amyloid in a bone marrow specimen is highly suggestive of AL

type. Immunophenotyping and cytogenetic findings in AL amyloidosis are similar to those in myeloma, which can be diagnosed concurrently according to standard criteria (e.g. Jaffe *et al.*, 2002). Immune paresis occurs frequently in AL amyloidosis, but lytic lesions or hypercalcaemia are strongly suggestive of myeloma.

Assessment of organ involvement

Organ involvement by amyloid can be ascertained clinically, histologically, according to function and by SAP scintigraphy, but the clinical significance of these findings may differ substantially. Various criteria and methods for evaluating organ involvement are presently in use (Table 42.3). ECG and two-dimensional Doppler echocardiography are vital tools for evaluating cardiac involvement, and variously show reduced standard lead voltages, poor R-wave progression in the chest leads ('pseudo-infarct' pattern) along with small, concentrically thickened ventricular walls, dilated atria and homogeneously thickened and echogenic valves. Cardiac amyloidosis is a restrictive cardiomyopathy and diastolic dysfunction is easily missed and difficult to quantify. The status of other organs can be assessed either through routine tests of liver and renal function, etc., or by specialist investigations as indicated, for example autonomic function and nerve conduction tests, high-resolution pulmonary CT scanning, etc.

Differential diagnosis

Alternative diagnoses that frequently need to be considered include amyloidosis of non-AL types, principally AA and hereditary forms, localized forms of AL amyloidosis, non-amyloid light chain deposition disease, and non-amyloid paraprotein-associated neuropathies.

Management of AL amyloidosis

Therapy is not yet available that can specifically inhibit the formation of amyloid or enhance its clearance, although both strategies are being pursued experimentally. The objective of treatment at present is to suppress production of the amyloidogenic monoclonal light chains in the hope that progression of the disease will be slowed down, halted or reversed. However, few clinical trials have been performed, clinical benefit is typically much delayed, and many patients have advanced multisystem disease at diagnosis and therefore tolerate chemotherapy poorly. Quantitative measurements of circulating free immunoglobulin light chains are often the most effective means for guiding treatment in individual patients, and, although it is generally desirable to suppress the underlying clonal disease as rapidly as possible, reduction in the concentration of the amyloidogenic class of free light chain by just 50–75% is often sufficient to confer substantial survival benefit, regardless of the type of chemotherapy used. More intensive suppression of the clonal disease may be unneces-

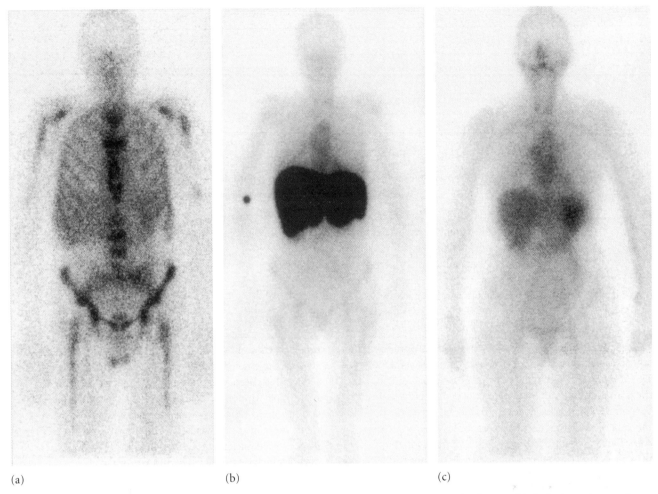

(a)   (b)   (c)

Figure 42.3 Radiolabelled ^{123}I-SAP whole-body scintigraphy, anterior images. (a) The tracer has localized virtually exclusively to amyloid deposits in the bones in this particular patient, a distribution that is pathognomonic for amyloid of AL type. (b) and (c) Serial scintigraphs in a 56-year-old woman with AL amyloidosis. At presentation in 1998 (b) she had massive uptake in the spleen and liver, obscuring any renal signal. She underwent high-dose chemotherapy, and the follow-up scan in 2002 (c) shows that the deposits have regressed very substantially.

sary, and efforts to minimize toxicity from chemotherapy should be paramount.

Certain organs affected by amyloid tend to fare better than others following treatment. Kidney function, particularly proteinuria, in the absence of renal impairment often improves when the clonal disease is adequately suppressed, whereas cardiac and peripheral nerve function tend to improve extremely slowly if at all.

Melphalan and prednisolone

Efficacy of cyclic oral melphalan with or without prednisolone has been demonstrated in a randomized controlled trial in which colchicine was effectively used as a placebo. However, benefits of treatment were very slow and were substantial in only 20% of cases, and one-fifth of responders developed myelodysplasia or leukaemia. Although dose-intensive chemotherapy regimens have not been tested as rigorously as low-dose oral melphalan and prednisolone, the evidence that they may be much more efficacious is compelling.

Vincristine, doxorubicin (Adriamycin) and dexamethasone (VAD)

VAD and similar regimens are well established as infusional induction regimens in myeloma, associated with response rates of 60–80%, complete response rates of 10–25% and rapid reduction in tumour burden. They do not deplete stem cell reserve, keeping open the option for subsequent PBSCT. Problems with the use of VAD/C-VAMP (see also Chapter 41) in AL amyloidosis include exacerbation of peripheral and autonomic neuropathy by vincristine, induction or worsening of fluid retention in renal

Table 42.3 Non-invasive diagnostic criteria of amyloid-related major organ involvement.*

Organ involvement	Comenzo et al. (1998)	Dispenzieri et al. (2001)
Heart	Mean left ventricular wall thickness on echocardiography > 11 mm with no history of hypertension or valvular heart disease *or* Unexplained low voltage (< 0.5 mV) on ECG	Cardiac interventricular septum > 12 mm and/or infiltrative cardiomyopathy and/or diastolic dysfunction determined by echocardiography
Kidney	Proteinuria > 0.5 g/24 h	Proteinuria > 0.5 g/24 h
Liver	Hepatomegaly with an alkaline phosphatase > 200 U/L	Hepatomegaly (> 4 cm below costal margin) with an alkaline phosphatase > 1.5 × upper limit of normal
Nerve	Based on clinical history, autonomic dysfunction with orthostasis, gastric atony by gastric emptying scan or abnormal sensory and/or motor findings on neurological examination	Peripheral neuropathy (other than carpal tunnel syndrome) or autonomic neuropathy

*In patients in whom a positive diagnosis has been made by tissue biopsy.

or cardiac amyloidosis by dexamethasone/methylprednisolone, which can also cause bone fractures and vertebral collapse. Doxorubicin has not been shown to exacerbate amyloid cardiomyopathy, but caution is recommended. There have been no randomized controlled trials of VAD in AL amyloidosis, but in our experience the clonal disease response rate is approximately 63% (based on a fall in the aberrant serum free light-chain values by > 50%), and organ function improves in about half of VAD-treated patients.

Intermediate-dose intravenous melphalan (IDM)

The variable absorption of melphalan from the gastrointestinal tract led investigators to trial intravenous intermediate-dose melphalan (25 mg/m^2) and oral dexamethasone in patients with untreated multiple myeloma. This regimen has been used as first-line therapy in patients with AL amyloidosis at the National Amyloidosis Centre, who were selected on the basis that they were not fit enough to receive VAD-based treatment, because of age, poor performance status, severe amyloid cardiomyopathy or neuropathy. Dexamethasone was omitted in patients with significant fluid retention. Efficacy, in terms of both clonal disease and organ response, was similar to VAD. It is prudent to harvest stem cells from patients who might subsequently benefit from PBSCT since IDM depletes stem cell reserve.

Autologous peripheral blood stem cell transplantation (PBSCT) (see also Chapter 41)

Use of high-dose melphalan therapy (HDT) and PBSCT in AL amyloidosis was first reported in 1996, and several series have

reported clinical benefit in up to about 60% of patients who survive the procedure. However, treatment-related mortality (TRM) has been consistently and substantially higher than in multiple myeloma, ranging from 14% to 39%, reflecting the compromised function of multiple organ systems by amyloid. Refinement of patient selection and improvement of peritransplantation management are therefore urgent priorities. Causes of death include cardiac arrhythmias, intractable hypotension, multiple organ failure and gastrointestinal bleeding. Measures that can reduce morbidity and mortality of PBSCT in AL amyloidosis include omitting substantial prehydration, administering the melphalan in two divided doses, and not using granulocyte colony-stimulating factor (G-CSF) to enhance engraftment. TRM is higher in patients with clinical involvement of three or more organ systems, those aged above 55–65 years and those with chronic renal failure. Even stem cell mobilization has significant risks in AL amyloidosis.

The efficacy of PBSCT in AL amyloidosis has not been determined in any controlled comparative study, and its apparently good outcome may reflect selection of fitter good-prognosis patients (Dispenzieri, 2001). The role of PBSCT therefore remains unclear, and because of its special problems in AL amyloidosis it is recommended that such patients are treated in units with expertise of this particular disease. It seems reasonable to restrict PBSCT to younger patients with one or two involved organs who have not had previous amyloid-related gastrointestinal bleeding and who do not have severe cardiomyopathy, advanced renal failure or are dialysis dependent. Our own practice is rarely to recommend PBSCT as first-line therapy, but to consider its role in patients who have not responded adequately to VAD and/or IDM in terms of their clinical status or serum free light-chain values.

Allogeneic bone marrow transplantation

Successful allogeneic BMT for AL amyloidosis was reported in 1998 and 3 years post BMT was associated with complete clinical recovery. TRM in this setting would probably be inordinately high, and there are currently no data on reduced-intensity conditioning in AL amyloid.

Thalidomide

Early impressions on the potential role of thalidomide in AL amyloidosis are that the degree and rate of response of the underlying clonal plasma cell disease are similar to those in multiple myeloma. Adverse effects including somnolence, constipation, development of irreversible neuropathy and risk of venous and arterial thrombosis limit its application to AL amyloidosis.

Supportive treatment and organ transplantation

Supportive therapy remains a critical component of management, whereas therapy directed against the underlying clonal disease can be instituted. Renal dialysis may be necessary, and is usually both feasible and well tolerated. Renal, cardiac and other transplants have a role in selected patients who have otherwise well-preserved organ function and in whom adjunctive chemotherapy before or after surgery has either already been successful or remains realistic. Rigorous control of hypertension is vital in renal amyloidosis. Surgical resection of amyloidotic tissue is occasionally beneficial but, in general, a conservative approach to surgery, anaesthesia and other invasive procedures is advised. Should any such procedure be undertaken, meticulous attention to blood pressure and fluid balance is essential, especially in patients with renal and/or cardiac involvement. Amyloidotic tissues may heal poorly and are liable to haemorrhage. Diuretics are the mainstay of treatment in cardiac amyloidosis, and vasodilating drugs are generally best avoided. Dysrhythmias may respond to conventional pharmacological therapy or to pacing.

Localized AL amyloidosis

Localized deposits of AL amyloid can occur almost anywhere in the body, characteristic sites including the skin, airways, conjunctiva and urogenital tract. They may be nodular or confluent and are associated with a usually inconspicuous focal infiltrate of clonal B-cell producing amyloidogenic light chains. Local AL amyloid rarely progresses into a truly systemic disease, and conservative management is usually appropriate. Orbital AL amyloid presents as mass lesions which can disrupt eye movement and the structure of the orbit. Localized laryngeal AL

amyloidosis is a well-recognized syndrome that is often amenable to direct or laser excision, but hereditary systemic ApoAI amyloidosis can also present in this manner. Amyloidosis in the bronchial tree is virtually always of localized AL type, as are solitary or multiple amyloid nodules within the lung tissue. In contrast, diffuse alveolar septal parenchymal deposition is commonly a manifestation of systemic AL amyloidosis. Lichenoid and macular forms of cutaneous amyloid are thought to be derived from keratin or related proteins, whereas nodular cutaneous amyloidosis deposits are generally of AL type, and can sometimes be a manifestation of systemic AL amyloidosis. Localized urogenital AL deposits usually present with haematuria or, less commonly, obstruction, and can occur anywhere from the renal collecting system to the urethra.

Other forms of systemic amyloidosis

Among more than 1500 patients with systemic amyloidosis who have been referred for evaluation at the National Amyloidosis Centre, approximately 80% have had AL type, 10% AA (reactive systemic) type, and the remainder have had a variety of hereditary, localized and other types. Although some features of systemic AL amyloidosis are very characteristic of this particular type, such as macroglossia, periorbital purpura and certain permutations of organ involvement, the clinical phenotypes of AA, AL and hereditary systemic amyloidosis can be completely indistinguishable. Furthermore, the underlying chronic inflammatory disease process is clinically covert in 5–10% of patients with AA amyloidosis, and a family history is often absent in patients with hereditary TTR and fibrinogen Aα chain amyloidosis, which are the most common familial forms.

AA amyloidosis

Reactive systemic AA (secondary) amyloidosis occurs in 1–5% of patients with chronic inflammatory diseases that evoke a substantial acute phase response, after a median latency of about 10 years. AA amyloid fibrils are derived from the circulating acute phase reactant, serum amyloid A protein (SAA), the serum concentration of which can increase from the healthy reference range of less than 10 mg/L to over 1000 mg/L during active inflammation. The commonest associated diseases in the developed world include rheumatoid arthritis, juvenile idiopathic arthritis and Crohn's disease. Familial Mediterranean fever (FMF) and chronic infections remain important causes in some parts of world. Castleman's disease of the solitary plasma cell type is probably the commonest underlying condition that can remain clinically covert.

Most patients present with nephropathy, particularly proteinuria, but liver and gastrointestinal involvement may occur at a late stage. Clinical involvement of the heart and nerves occurs very rarely. Diagnosis of AA amyloid is usually achieved by rectal or renal biopsy, and the AA fibril type can be confirmed immunohistochemically using anti-SAA antibodies in most cases. SAP scintigraphy virtually always shows involvement of the spleen and kidneys; hepatic involvement is a late feature associated with a poor prognosis. Treatment in AA amyloidosis should be guided by frequent estimation of SAA concentration and will depend on the nature of the underlying inflammatory disease, ranging from anti-TNF agents in rheumatoid arthritis and colchicine in FMF to surgical resection of Castleman's disease tumours. Any therapy that reduces SAA production to healthy baseline levels prevents further deposition of AA amyloid, frequently leads to the regression of existing amyloid deposits with improvement in amyloid-related organ dysfunction, and significantly improves long-term survival.

β_2-Microglobulin amyloidosis (Aβ_2M)

β_2-Microglobulin amyloidosis, also known as dialysis-related amyloidosis (DRA), occurs due to the accumulation of β_2-microglobulin in renal failure and predominantly affects articular and periarticular structures in patients with end-stage renal failure who have been on dialysis for at least 7–10 years. Susceptibility factors include older age and the use of 'non-biocompatible' dialysis membranes. Carpal tunnel syndrome is often the first clinical manifestation, and large joint arthralgias, tenosynovitis, spondyloarthropathies and periarticular bone cysts are common. Although Aβ_2M is a systemic form of amyloidosis, deposits outside the musculoskeletal system are seldom of clinical significance. The disabling arthralgia may respond partially to non-steroidal anti-inflammatory drugs or corticosteroids, but the only really effective treatment for this condition is normalization of β_2-microglobulin levels through renal transplantation. Carpal tunnel syndrome is amenable to surgery but may recur.

Transthyretin amyloidosis

Normal transthyretin (TTR) is inherently but weakly amyloidogenic, and minor TTR amyloid (ATTR) deposits are common in elderly individuals. Clinically significant involvement is almost completely restricted to the heart, and senile cardiac amyloid derived from wild-type TTR occurs in up to 25% subjects over 80 years of age. This syndrome is extremely rare before 65 years of age. There is no specific treatment but patients may survive for many years with reasonably good quality of life managed with diuretics alone.

Hereditary systemic amyloidoses

Hereditary systemic amyloidosis is caused by deposition of genetically variant proteins as amyloid fibrils, and is associated with mutations in the genes for transthyretin, fibrinogen Aα chain, cystatin C, gelsolin, apolipoprotein AI, apolipoprotein AII, and lysozyme. These disorders are all inherited in an autosomal dominant manner with variable penetrance, and usually present in adult life.

Familial amyloidotic polyneuropathy (FAP) associated with mutations in the gene for TTR is the most common type of hereditary amyloidosis. It is characterized by progressive and disabling peripheral and autonomic neuropathy, often along with cardiac involvement; vitreous amyloid deposits may also occur and are virtually pathognomonic of the syndrome. Symptoms typically present between the third and seventh decades. More than 80 TTR variants are associated with FAP, the most frequent of which is the substitution of methionine for valine at residue 30 (TTR Met30). There are well-recognized foci of this in Portugal, Japan and Sweden, but FAP has been reported in most ethnic groups. TTR Ala60 is the most frequent cause of FAP in the British population, typically presenting after age 50 years and usually with marked cardiac involvement. TTR Ile122 occurs in 3–4% of black Africans and is associated with a phenotype indistinguishable from senile (wild type) cardiac amyloidosis other than often presenting about 10 years earlier. The majority of TTR is produced by hepatocytes, and liver transplantation is the only effective treatment for this disorder. Although the visceral amyloid deposits frequently regress following liver transplantation, the neuropathy is often irreversible and established cardiac amyloidosis may paradoxically progress due to on-going fibril formation by wild-type TTR in this particular organ. Combined heart and liver transplantation has been performed successfully in a small number of cases.

The syndrome of non-neuropathic hereditary systemic amyloidosis is caused by mutations in the genes for fibrinogen Aα chain, lysozyme, apolipoprotein AI and AII. Most such patients present with renal impairment and/or proteinuria, but substantial deposits in the liver and spleen are frequent in hereditary lysozyme and apolipoprotein AI amyloidosis, and the heart may be involved in hereditary apolipoprotein AI amyloidosis. Prominent neuropathy occurs in some patients with apolipoprotein AI Arg26. Although kindreds with hereditary amyloidosis are rare, 10% of patients referred to the National Amyloidosis Centre with apparently sporadic amyloidosis do in fact have hereditary forms of the disease. About half of these are associated with TTR mutations, and most of the remainder are associated with variant fibrinogen Aα chain Val526. Penetrance of this particular mutation is extremely low in most families, thus obscuring the genetic aetiology, but the renal histology is characteristic showing substantial accumulation of amyloid within enlarged glomeruli, but none in blood vessels or the interstitium. Hereditary cystatin C amyloidosis manifests in Icelandic families as cerebral amyloid angiopathy with recurrent cerebral haemorrhage, and gelsolin variants are associated with predominant cranial neuropathy, most often in Finnish patients.

DNA analysis is now performed routinely at the UK National Amyloidosis Centre on patients with systemic amyloidosis in whom AA or AL fibril type cannot be definitively verified.

Conclusion and future directions

Improved understanding of the aetiology and pathogenesis of amyloid has led to numerous recent improvements in the characterization and management of amyloidosis. Chemotherapy in systemic AL amyloidosis can now be guided by its early effect on serum free light-chain concentration, and routine DNA analysis can prevent patients with otherwise unrecognized hereditary amyloidosis from receiving inappropriate cytotoxic treatment. Clinical improvement following successful treatment of the various conditions that underlie amyloidosis is always delayed, and supportive measures are of great importance.

Novel therapeutic strategies include small molecules, peptides and GAG analogues that bind to fibril precursors and stabilize their native fold, or interfere with refolding and/or aggregation into the common amyloid conformation. Immunotherapy approaches and SAP depletion are being explored as specific therapies directed at promoting regression of amyloid. Several of these new therapeutic approaches are already being tested in patients with the hope that they may be effective in a diverse spectrum of amyloid related disorders.

Selected bibliography

Benson MD, Uemichi T (1996) Transthyretin amyloidosis. *Amyloid: the International Journal of Experimental and Clinical Investigation* 3: 44–56.

Booth DR, Sunde M, Bellotti V *et al.* (1997) Instability, unfolding and aggregation of human lysozyme variants underlying amyloid fibrillogenesis. *Nature* 385: 787–93.

Botto M, Hawkins PN, Bickerstaff MCM *et al.* (1997) Amyloid deposition is delayed in mice with targeted deletion of the serum amyloid P component gene. *Nature Medicine* 3: 855–9.

Comenzo RL, Gertz MA (2002) Autologous stem cell transplantation for primary systemic amyloidosis. *Blood* 99: 4276–82.

Comenzo RL, Vosburgh E, Falk RH *et al.* (1998) Dose-intensive melphalan with blood stem-cell support for the treatment of AL (amyloid light-chain) amyloidosis: survival and responses in 25 patients. *Blood* 91: 3662–70.

Dispenzieri A, Lacy MQ, Kyle RA *et al.* (2001) Eligibility for hematopoietic stem-cell transplantation for primary systemic amyloidosis is a favorable prognostic factor for survival. *Journal of Clinical Oncology* 19: 3350–6.

Drüeke TB (1998) Dialysis-related amyloidosis. *Nephrology, Dialysis, Transplantation* 13 (Suppl. 1): 58–64.

Dubrey SW, Cha K, Anderson J *et al.* (1998) The clinical features of immunoglobulin light-chain (AL) amyloidosis with heart involvement. *Quarterly Journal of Medicine* 91: 141–57.

Dubrey SW, Burke MM, Khaghani A *et al.* (2001) Long term results of heart transplantation in patients with amyloid heart disease. *Heart* 85: 202–7.

Gertz MA, Lacy MQ, Dispenzieri A *et al.* (2002) Stem cell transplantation for the management of primary systemic amyloidosis. *American Journal of Medicine* 113: 549–55.

Gillmore JD, Lovat LB, Persey MR *et al.* (2001) Amyloid load and clinical outcome in AA amyloidosis in relation to circulating concentration of serum amyloid A protein. *Lancet* 358: 24–9.

Hawkins PN (2002) Serum amyloid P component scintigraphy for diagnosis and monitoring amyloidosis. *Current Opinion in Nephrology and Hypertension* 11: 649–55.

Hawkins PN, Lavender JP, Pepys MB (1990) Evaluation of systemic amyloidosis by scintigraphy with ^{123}I-labelled serum amyloid P component. *New England Journal of Medicine* 323: 508–13.

Jaffe ES, Harris NL, Stein H, Vardiman JW (eds) (2001) *World Health Organization Classification of Tumours. Pathology and Genetics of Tumours of Haematopoietic and Lymphoid Tissues.* IARC Press, Lyon.

Kyle RA, Gertz MA (1995) Primary systemic amyloidosis: clinical and laboratory features in 474 cases. *Seminars in Hematology* 32: 45–59.

Kyle RA, Gertz MA, Greipp PR *et al.* (1997) A trial of three regimens for primary amyloidosis: colchicine alone, melphalan and prednisone, and melphalan, prednisone, and colchicine. *New England Journal of Medicine* 336: 1202–7.

Lachmann HJ, Hawkins, PN (2001) Amyloidosis, familial renal. www.emedicine.com/med/topic3379.htm.

Lachmann HJ, Booth DR, Booth SE *et al.* (2002) Misdiagnosis of hereditary amyloidosis as AL (primary) amyloidosis. *New England Journal of Medicine* 346: 1786–91.

Lachmann HJ, Gallimore R, Gillmore JD *et al.* (2003) Outcome in systemic AL amyloidosis in relation to changes in concentration of circulating free immunoglobulin light chains following chemotherapy. *British Journal of Haematology* 122: 78–84.

Pepys MB, Herbert J, Hutchinson WL *et al.* (2002) Targeted pharmacological depletion of serum amyloid P component for treatment of human amyloidosis. *Nature* 417: 254–9.

Puchtler H, Sweat F, Levine M (1962) On the binding of Congo red by amyloid. *Journal of Histochemistry and Cytochemistry* 10: 355–64.

Samson D, Gaminara E, Newland A *et al.* (1989) Infusion of vincristine and doxorubicin with oral dexamethasone as first-line therapy for multiple myeloma. *Lancet* ii: 882–5.

Sanchorawala V, Wright DG, Seldin DC *et al.* (2001) An overview of the use of high-dose melphalan with autologous stem cell transplantation for the treatment of AL amyloidosis. *Bone Marrow Transplantation* 28: 637–42.

Schey SA, Kazmi M, Ireland R, Lakhani A (1998) The use of intravenous intermediate dose melphalan and dexamethasone as induction treatment in the management of *de novo* multiple myeloma. *European Journal of Haematology* 61: 306–10.

Solomon A, Weiss DT, Kattine AA (1991) Nephrotoxic potential of Bence Jones proteins. *New England Journal of Medicine* 324: 1845–51.

Sunde M, Serpell LC, Bartlam M *et al.* (1997) Common core structure of amyloid fibrils by synchrotron X-ray diffraction. *Journal of Molecular Biology* 273: 729–39.

UK Myeloma Forum AL Amyloidosis Guidelines Working Group (2004) Guidelines on the diagnosis and management of AL amyloidosis. *British Journal of Haematology* 125: 671–700.

CHAPTER 43

The classification of lymphoma

Peter G Isaacson

Introduction

The aim of any lymphoma classification is to provide an international language allowing communication between those with a special interest in this group of diseases. The classification must be reproducible and clinically relevant, so that treatment results can be compared world-wide, and sufficiently flexible to permit the incorporation of new data. Finally, the classification must be histopathologically based since it is the histopathologist who, in most instances, makes the initial diagnosis. Traditionally, Hodgkin's disease (Hodgkin's lymphoma) and non-Hodgkin's lymphomas have been classified separately. This is a reflection of the specific identifying cell and limited morphological range of Hodgkin's disease together with its distinctive clinical features. In comparison, the clinicopathological features of the non-Hodgkin's lymphomas are much more wide-ranging and less distinct for any given entity. Not surprisingly, therefore, there have been only two classifications of Hodgkin's disease proposed since 1925, whereas more than 25 classifications of non-Hodgkin's lymphoma have appeared in the same period.

To the early pathologists the histological appearances of all non-Hodgkin's lymphomas were alike, consisting of replacement of the normal lymph node architecture by sheets of small or sometimes larger dark-staining cells. However, it was quite clear that not all cases behaved the same; the survival of patients with non-Hodgkin's lymphoma varied from a few months to many years. Pathologists were, therefore, increasingly asked by their clinical colleagues whether they could predict the natural course of an individual case. Following the emergence of therapeutic successes with Hodgkin's disease, more effective means of

therapy for the non-Hodgkin's lymphomas began to be developed. The effectiveness of these therapies was not homogeneous within the non-Hodgkin's lymphomas as a whole but clearly varied with the histology and, consequently, clinicians began to demand much more precise and clinically relevant histological diagnoses. In response to this, Rappaport (1966) formulated the first clinically relevant histological classification of the non-Hodgkin's lymphomas. The Rappaport classification, broadly speaking, divided lymphomas into those composed of small cells and large cells, each of which could be further subdivided into those with a follicular (or nodular) growth pattern and those that were diffuse. The follicular and small-cell tumours were clinically less aggressive; a better survival could, therefore, be expected and, importantly, less potent and less toxic therapy was suitable for these cases. The converse applied to cases with a diffuse growth pattern especially if composed of large cells.

As histological techniques improved, allowing finer morphological discrimination between cells, so more detailed classifications emerged. In parallel with these improvements it was becoming possible to establish the phenotype of the lymphoma cells using immunological techniques. It soon became evident that the lymphoma cells were closely related to normal lymph node cells and that the cells of many non-Hodgkin's lymphomas recapitulated the cytology of normal lymphocytes, particularly the B cells of the follicle centre. It was also clear, however, that there were an alarmingly wide variety of lymphoid neoplasms, and a whole host of classifications based on these new concepts sprung up. This caused so much confusion that a series of special international meetings was convened to decide on a single clinically relevant classification that could be used throughout the world. In the absence of any consensus, The United States

National Cancer Institute convened a study to evaluate the competing classifications and the result was the compromise 'Working Formulation for Clinical Use' (Non-Hodgkin's Lymphoma Classification Project, 1982). It was stressed at the time that this 'formulation', although based on histopathological appearances, was a language for translation between the competing classifications and not a classification in its own right. However, it was rapidly accepted as such by pathologists, particularly in the USA, where it became the classification of choice. The working formulation divided lymphomas into three grades based on their clinical behaviour, assessed using therapy current in the late 1960s and early 1970s, and thereafter used imprecise collective morphological terms such as 'large cell' and 'mixed small and large cell' to characterize individual entities. The result was that different clinicopathological entities were lumped together and as new entities were described, they merely became absorbed into this inflexible system. The Working Formulation was incapable of incorporating the rapidly expanding amount of immunophenotypic data on which pathologists were increasingly relying for lymphoma diagnosis. The Working Formulation thus soon lost its main reason for existence, namely its clinical relevance.

The majority of European pathologists never accepted the Working Formulation and preferred to use the Kiel classification. This classification and its updated editions (Stansfeld et al., 1988) was based on modern immunophenotypic data dividing lymphomas into B and T-cell types and, thereafter, into individual entities based largely on the similarity of their cells to normal lymphocyte variants. According to their cytological characteristics, rather than their predetermined clinical behaviour and in keeping with established schemes for other tumours, the lymphomas were designated low or high grade. Unlike the Working Formulation, the Kiel classification had a sound biological basis and could easily be updated, thus maintaining its clinical relevance. Criticisms that could be levelled at the Kiel classification included its over-reliance on establishing the normal cell counterpart for each type of lymphoma, illogical over-splitting of some entities, and its failure to take into account the extranodal lymphomas.

The use of different lymphoma classifications on either side of the Atlantic, and the inherent defects in each, defied the basic requirement of a classification, namely that of providing a language for international communication, and threatened a return to the chaos of the 1970s. Moreover, new techniques and new concepts were emerging that urgently needed to be incorporated into the principles underlying lymphoma classification. Developments in immunohistochemistry meant that a cell lineage could confidently be assigned to most lymphomas and that many distinctive functional properties of the neoplastic cells could be determined. Distinctive molecular genetic properties of the different disorders also began to emerge, and some of these could be identified using simple immunohistochemical techniques. Another important development was the recognition that many lymphomas arose in extranodal sites and that site of origin was often a significant clinical determinant.

The Revised European American Lymphoma (REAL) classification

In 1991, a group of pathologists from both sides of the Atlantic and the Far East formed an International Lymphoma Study Group (ILSG) which met annually to discuss research. Not surprisingly, this group soon found itself addressing the problems of lymphoma classification as outlined above and the need for a new approach to these problems soon became evident. Of the three alternative approaches that emerged, namely to update either the Working Formulation or the Kiel classification or to produce an entirely new classification, a decision was made to adopt the latter course. The basis for what was to become the Revised European American Lymphoma (REAL) Classification was the construction of a list of neoplastic lymphoproliferative disorders each defined as far as possible according to a set of five properties, namely morphology (histology), immunophenotype, genotype, normal cell counterpart and clinical features. The degree to which these properties contribute to the classification of each entity varies. For some such as mantle cell lymphoma each property is highly distinctive, perhaps reflecting its basic distinctive genotype, while for others such as nasal type NK-cell lymphoma clinical features together with immunophenotype are the most important.

The World Health Organisation (WHO) classification

In 1995, under the auspices of the WHO, the (American) Society for Hematopathology and the European Association for Haematopathology undertook a joint project to produce a comprehensive classification of all haematological neoplasms including those of myeloid lymphoid and histiocytic lineage. Recognizing that the REAL classification had only recently been proposed and was in the process of clinical evaluation, the brief for lymphoid neoplasms was to update and revise the REAL classification with input from additional experts in order to broaden the consensus. The formation of the steering committee and 10 subcommittees, each charged with the review of a specific group of neoplasms, involved 52 expert histopathologists and haematologists. In recognition of the importance of clinical relevance, a clinical advisory committee of 35 experts in the fields of leukaemia and lymphoma from around the world was convened. The subcommittees and the clinical advisory committee met separately, the former on many occasions, and recommendations were fed to the steering committee prior to a joint meeting of all committee members that was held in November 1997 at Airlie House in Virginia. The purposes of this final 'grand' meeting were to iron out particular controversies, most of which had arisen consequent to actual use or, in effect, field testing of the REAL classification, to ensure that there was common ground between pathologists and clinicians and to agree on the final format. The agenda of the Airlie House meeting comprised a series of topics and questions that had been proposed by members of the subcommittee and the clinical advisory committee. In the case of the lymphomas, discussion of these topics served to refine and update the REAL classification which could then be subsumed into the WHO scheme.

The basis of the REAL and WHO classifications

Morphology

Morphology is, in effect, the collective expression of the immunophenotype, genotype and normal cell counterpart and as such remains the mainstay of lymphoma diagnosis. Once an entity has been defined on the basis of its collective properties, morphology on its own is often sufficient for a definitive diagnosis. However, lymphomas of identical morphology, but arising in different sites, may constitute different disease entities and some single disease entities may be morphologically heterogeneous. For example, anaplastic large-cell lymphoma (ALCL) arising in lymph nodes behaves much more aggressively than the morphologically identical tumour arising in the skin while the cytological features of enteropathy-type T-cell lymphoma are highly variable and do not influence its clinical behaviour. Histological grade alone, which should not be confused with clinical aggressiveness, is no longer considered a basis for the separation of lymphomas into broad groups. Many entities may transform from low- to high-grade disease as part of their natural history and can present *de novo* as either low- or high-grade lesions.

Immunophenotype

The immunophenotype of lymphomas was first used for broad grouping of lymphomas into B-cell and T-cell types in the Kiel classification. With the specific inclusion of the natural killer (NK) cell phenotype into the T-cell group, this distinction remains a fundamental consideration in the REAL classification and serves as a primary step in the separation of the lymphomas into two broad groups. Within these broad groupings the detailed immunophenotype is useful in helping to define individual entities but in only a few instances does a combination of immunophenotypic properties alone serve to define an entity that cannot be distinguished by other means. This is true of mantle cell lymphoma where the defining genotype, t(11;14), results in expression of cyclin D1, the defining immunophenotype.

Genotype

With increasing recognition that cancer is a genetic disease, the genotype of lymphomas is assuming greater significance in their classification. For some entities, such as follicular lymphoma, [t(14;18)] and mantle cell lymphoma [t(11;14)], the genotype is indeed the defining property. However, genotyping is beyond the capability of most laboratories and, fortunately, the genotype finds expression as reproducible morphological and/or immunophenotypic features that allow confident and reproducible diagnoses.

Normal cell counterpart

The normal cell counterpart, when known, is a useful aid to classification as it helps to characterize the morphology and phenotype of the lymphoma and, importantly, to understand its clinical behaviour, which may relate to the physiological pathways of the normal cell. This property has more significance for B-cell than T-cell lymphomas, largely because more is known about the B-cell subtypes and their functional characteristics.

Clinical features

The inclusion of clinical features, including site of origin, aggressiveness and prognosis, as an integral and practical part of the definition of lymphomas as distinct diseases is one of the more novel aspects of the REAL and WHO classifications.

Site of origin

Neither the Working Formulation nor the Kiel classification acknowledged the fact that a high percentage of lymphomas do not arise in lymph nodes. In the USA extranodal lymphoma accounts for some 25% of all cases, while in the Far East the percentage is much higher, amounting to 45% in Japan and 60% in Korea. The importance of the site of origin of lymphomas should not be underestimated. The distribution of lymphoma types shows a markedly different bias in different sites. Thus, extranodal Hodgkin's lymphoma is altogether rare, and follicular lymphoma, one of the commonest lymph node tumours, occurs only infrequently as a primary tumour in the gastrointestinal tract despite its high content of native lymphoid tissue. In some organs and/or tissues, such as the skin, gastrointestinal tract and, to a lesser extent, the spleen, lymphomas more or less specifically characteristic of that site alone occur. Examples include cutaneous follicle centre cell lymphoma, enteropathy-type T-cell lymphoma and splenic marginal zone lymphoma. For clinical purposes it is sometimes useful to group together the lymphomas that arise in specific sites and to approach the diagnosis of lymphoma arising in those sites in this way rather than in the purest sense of an overall lymphoma classification. This is best exemplified by lymphomas arising in the gastrointestinal tract and the skin. However, the use of entirely separate classifications for lymphomas arising at different extranodal sites is to be discouraged.

Clinical aggressiveness

The REAL and WHO classifications make a clear distinction between histological or cytological grade and clinical aggressiveness. Histological grade is based on cell and especially nuclear size, density of nuclear chromatin and the proliferation fraction as assessed by the number of mitotic figures or the proliferation fraction determined by Ki-67 immunostaining. Thus, low-grade lymphomas are composed of small cells with dense nuclear chromatin and a low proliferation fraction; the converse is true for high-grade tumours. The REAL and WHO classifications, unlike the Kiel classification, do not separate lymphomas according to grade in recognition of the fact that low-grade lymphomas may transform to a high-grade tumour without changing the disease 'entity'. By and large, histological grade correlates with clinical aggressiveness but this is not always the case. Mantle cell lymphoma is histologically low grade but clinically aggressive, as are some T-cell lymphomas such as angioimmunoblastic T-cell lymphoma. Both the Working Formulation and the Kiel classification stressed the fundamental importance of 'grade', although using the term in a different sense, in determining treatment. The REAL and WHO classifications instead lay stress on the disease entity. Thus, not all 'low-grade' B-cell lymphomas are necessarily treated alike as exemplified by hairy cell leukaemia for which highly specific therapy has evolved (see also Chapter 38). It is likely that as the different entities are better defined and recognized clinically, more disease specific therapies will emerge.

Prognosis

Clinical aggressiveness is not the same as prognosis, with which it is often confused. For example, ALCL, a high-grade neoplasm, is clinically aggressive but has a good prognosis since it responds excellently to therapy. A variety of prognostic factors within each disease influence the clinical outcome. One of these is histological grade but clinical features are also important. The more important of these have been collected together to form the International Prognostic Index (IPI), the measurement of which is a powerful predictor of clinical outcome in any given patient.

The structure of the WHO classification
(Table 43.1)

Like the Kiel classification, the lymphomas, defined according to the principles described above, are primarily divided broadly into B- and T-cell groups. A modification is the inclusion of lymphomas with a natural killer (NK)-cell phenotype in the T-cell group. In each group the precursor cell, or lymphoblastic, lymphomas are separated from the larger group of peripheral

Table 43.1 The World Health Organization classification of lymphoid malignancies.

B-cell neoplasms
Precursor B-cell neoplasm
B-cell lymphoblastic lymphoma/leukaemia

Mature B-cell neoplasms
Chronic lymphocytic leukaemia/small lymphocytic lymphoma
Prolymphocytic leukaemia
Lymphoplasmacytic lymphoma
Splenic marginal zone lymphoma
Hairy cell leukaemia
Plasma cell myeloma
Monoclonal gammopathy of undetermined significance (MGUS)
Solitary plasmacytoma of bone
Extraosseus plasmacytoma
Primary amyloidosis
Heavy chain diseases
Extranodal marginal zone lymphoma of mucosa-associated lymphoid tissue (MALT lymphoma)
Nodal marginal zone lymphoma
Follicular lymphoma
Mantle cell lymphoma
Diffuse large B-cell lymphoma
Mediastinal (thymic) large B-cell lymphoma
Intravascular large B-cell lymphoma
Primary effusion lymphoma
Burkitt's lymphoma

B-cell proliferations of uncertain malignant potential
Lymphomatoid granulomatosis
Post-transplant lymphoproliferative disorder, polymorphic

T- and putative NK-cell neoplasms
Precursor T-cell neoplasm
T-lymphoblastic lymphoma/leukaemia

Mature T-cell and NK-cell neoplasms
T-cell prolymphocytic leukaemia
T-cell large granular lymphocytic leukaemia
Aggressive NK-cell leukaemia
Adult T-cell lymphoma/leukaemia (HTLV-1+)
Mycosis fungoides
Sézary's syndrome
Primary cutaneous CD30-positive lymphoproliferative disorders
Extranodal T/NK-cell lymphoma, nasal type
Enteropathy-type T-cell lymphoma
Angioimmunoblastic T-cell lymphoma
Peripheral T-cell lymphoma unspecified
Hepatosplenic T-cell lymphoma
Subcutaneous panniculitis-like T-cell lymphoma
Blastic NK-cell lymphoma
Angioimmunoblastic T-cell lymphoma
Anaplastic large-cell lymphoma

Table 43.1 (*cont'd*)

Hodgkin's lymphoma
Nodular lymphocyte predominance
Classical
Nodular sclerosis
Lymphocyte rich (nodular)
Mixed cellularity
Lymphocyte depletion

cell tumours. The order in which the different entities are cited is not fixed and can be changed according to the convenience of the user. The B-cell lymphomas are grouped into those with peripheral blood involvement, plasma cell neoplasms, extranodal lymphomas, nodal lymphomas and lymphoproliferative disorders of uncertain malignant potential. The T/NK-cell lymphomas are similarly grouped into those that tend to involve the peripheral blood, cutaneous lymphomas, other extranodal lymphomas, nodal lymphomas and a single entity of uncertain lineage.

Hodgkin's lymphoma

Breaking with tradition, the authors of the REAL classification took the decision to include Hodgkin's disease in the lymphoma classification albeit as a separate table. This concept was continued in the WHO classification with the modification that Hodgkin's disease is designated as Hodgkin's lymphoma (HL), in recognition of the compelling evidence for the B-cell derivation of Hodgkin's disease. Despite this evidence, there is still preference for maintaining the 'Hodgkin' eponym. In this way the unique features of HL, including, importantly, its specific therapy and good prognosis, will continue to be recognized. Not surprisingly, the classification of this disorder is little changed from those of 1947 and 1966. The only changes in its classification are the implicit recognition that lymphocyte-predominant HL is a different disorder from classical HL and the addition of the category 'lymphocyte-rich HL'. It is hoped that the inclusion of this new category will serve to prevent misdiagnosis of these cases as lymphocyte-predominant HL, especially when they present with nodular or follicular histology. It could be argued that Hodgkin's lymphoma eventually will be listed in the table of B-cell lymphomas.

Reproducibility and clinical relevance

The value of any lymphoma classification is only as good as its histopathological reproducibility and its clinical relevance. In this respect, the validity of the REAL and WHO classifications had already been tested to a certain extent prior to their publication since many of the entities had been subject to detailed clinicopathological analysis in the medical literature. Shortly after its publication, moreover, the reproducibility and clinical relevance of the REAL classification were formally evaluated.

The Lymphoma Classification Project
(Lymphoma Classification Project, 1997)

Following its publication, an international study was convened to determine whether the REAL classification could be readily applied by a group of six expert haematopathologists, who, with one exception, were not associated with the original proposal. The specific aims of the project were to judge whether the classification could be used in practice, to test its inter-observer reproducibility, to assess the need for immunophenotyping in making a diagnosis (one of the criticisms following its publication having been that the REAL classification was not cost-effective in this respect!), to determine whether the constituent diseases were clinically distinctive either at presentation or in terms of clinical outcome, and to determine the relevant frequency of these diseases in the study populations. The participating pathologists, assisted by clinicians and statisticians, studied 1400 cases of lymphoma comprising 80–210 cases in each of eight centres in North America, Europe, Asia and Africa.

The participants found that the REAL classification was highly practical, allowing the ready classification of 95% of cases. Inter-observer reproducibility was greater than 85% for most categories, which was a substantial improvement over previous studies using other classifications, in which reproducibility was frequently in the region of only 60% or less. Immunophenotyping was not necessary for the classification of certain diseases including follicular lymphoma and lymphocytic lymphoma/chronic lymphocytic leukaemia but essential for the classification of T-cell lymphomas and particularly helpful for some B-cell disorders, including mantle cell lymphoma and diffuse large B-cell lymphoma.

In making clinicopathological correlations, the Lymphoma Classification Project showed that the different diseases recognized by the REAL classification did indeed differ in terms of clinical presentation and survival supporting the contention that they were distinct biological entities. However, an important finding of the study was that classification is not the only predictor of clinical outcome of any individual case. In this respect, the power of the IPI was confirmed. For example, patients with follicular lymphoma and an IPI score of 1–3 have a median survival of 7–10 years, while the median survival for the minority with an IPI of 4 or 5 is significantly reduced to 1.5 years.

The relative frequency of the different lymphomas

When discussing lymphoma classification there tends, inevitably, to be greater emphasis on the rare and difficult conditions than is necessarily warranted by their frequency. Because of epidemiological differences and regional bias, it is difficult to generalize about the distribution of the different lymphomas. However, extrapolating from previous studies that preceded the REAL classification, and the results of the Lymphoma Classification Project it possible to obtain some sort of perspective. Thus, in North America and Europe B-cell lymphomas account for some 85% of all lymphomas. The Lymphoma Classification Project found that, together, large B-cell lymphoma (30.6%), follicular lymphoma (22.1%), MALT lymphoma (7.6%), lymphocytic lymphoma/chronic lymphocytic leukaemia (6.7%) and mantle cell lymphoma (6.0%) constituted 73% of all lymphomas. Given that Asian and African patients were represented by only two of the eight centres, these relative incidence figures are less valid for Asia or Africa, where overall there is a much lower frequency of follicular lymphoma, and in parts of Asia, a higher frequency of T-cell lymphoma.

Updating the classification

Previous experience, especially with the Working Formulation, has shown the folly of considering any lymphoma classification a permanent entity. New concepts and consequently newly recognized diseases are constantly arising and demand to be included in any classification. The REAL classification recognized this both tacitly and overtly by the inclusion of provisional entities. The question of how to address the problem of updating the classification was left hanging, however. In this respect it was a fortunate coincidence that, shortly after the publication of the REAL classification, the WHO commenced the ambitious project with the aim of formulating a new comprehensive classification of both lymphoma and leukaemia. In terms of the lymphomas, the WHO classification project has essentially addressed the immediate problem of updating and refining the REAL classification. However, the problem of continuous updating of the WHO classification still remains to be addressed.

Issues relating to individual entities in the WHO classification

As with any new classification, when the WHO lymphoma classification was presented to the haematologists and oncologists who would be using it in the clinic, several contentious issues arose that deserve special consideration and clarification.

Precursor cell neoplasms

With respect to the relationship of the solid precursor cell tumours with the leukaemias, the FAB terms L1, L2 and L3 are no longer relevant since L1 and L2 do not predict immunophenotype or clinical behaviour and L3 is equivalent to Burkitt's lymphoma in a leukaemic phase. Lymphoblastic lymphomas

and leukaemias are the same disease in different stages (see also Chapters 29, 32 and 33).

The mature B-cell leukaemias

The term 'mature' is preferable to 'peripheral' to describe the majority of the lymphomas. Chronic lymphocytic leukaemia and lymphocytic lymphoma are clearly the same disease although they tend to be seen by different clinicians. However, prolymphocytic leukaemia is distinctly different (see also Chapter 38).

Follicular lymphoma

Grading of follicular lymphoma is a contentious issue, but it is now agreed that grading should be carried out according to the method proposed by Mann and Berard (1982), who described three grades based on the number of large cells (centroblasts) per high-power field. Grade 3 follicular lymphoma is divided into 3a and 3b, the latter used for tumours comprising sheets of centroblasts. In practice, only grade 3 (more than 15 centroblasts per high-power field) is clinically significant, being indicative of more aggressive disease that may require doxorubicin-containing therapy. The presence and percentage of diffuse areas should also be commented on, although the clinical significance of this point is not yet clear.

Cutaneous follicle centre lymphoma

This rather poorly defined skin tumour tends to occur in the upper half of the body and appears to be unrelated to follicular lymphoma but rather a variant of diffuse large B-cell lymphoma. Its importance lies in its remarkably indolent clinical behaviour.

Marginal zone lymphomas

Three separate entities constitute this group of lymphomas. The first two, marginal zone lymphoma of mucosa-associated lymphoid tissue (MALT lymphoma) and nodal marginal-zone lymphoma +/− monocytoid B-cells are closely related, but the third, splenic marginal-zone lymphoma is a quite different disease.

Marginal zone lymphoma of mucosa-associated lymphoid tissue (MALT lymphoma)

This type of lymphoma arises in extranodal sites and recapitulates the histology of the Peyer's patch. The stomach is the commonest site. MALT lymphomas are, by definition, low grade. Transformation to a diffuse large B-cell (high-grade) lymphoma can occur, and this phenomenon is clinically significant and should be documented in the histology report. However, the term 'high-grade MALT lymphoma' should not be used for these cases. In particular, diffuse large B-cell lymphomas arising *de novo* at extranodal sites where MALT lymphomas occur, such as the stomach, should not be called high-grade MALT lymphomas since this terminology may bias the clinician towards inappropriate therapy.

Nodal marginal zone lymphoma with or without monocytoid B-cells

The lymph node histology of this entity is identical to that of lymph node involvement by MALT lymphoma so that the possibility of a cryptic MALT lymphoma should always be borne in mind when a diagnosis of nodal marginal zone lymphoma is entertained.

Splenic marginal zone lymphoma (SMZL)

The constituent cells of SMZL bear only passing resemblance to splenic marginal zone cells and do not share their immunophenotype. Patients typically present with splenomegaly, often accompanied by anaemia and thrombocytopenia. Peripheral blood involvement is often, but not always, present, and in some of these cases the circulating neoplastic lymphocytes have a villous appearance. These cases were previously termed 'splenic lymphoma with villous lymphocytes'. The use of this somewhat imprecise term will not only fail to include those cases without circulating villous lymphocytes but, more importantly, tends to include other cases of B-cell lymphoma with peripheral blood spillover since the cells of various lymphomas may sometimes adopt a villous appearance, either real or artefactual, in the peripheral blood. This is an important consideration since SMZL tends to respond favourably to splenectomy alone in contrast to its poor response to chemotherapy (see also Chapter 38).

Diffuse large B-cell lymphoma (DLBCL) and Burkitt-like lymphoma

The classification of large B-cell lymphomas as a single group has been controversial. Various morphological subtypes have been recognized, including centroblastic, immunoblastic and T-cell rich, but the clinical significance of subclassifying DLBCL in this way is of doubtful significance and they do not appear to constitute separate diseases. There are, however, three rare large B-cell lymphomas that do appear to merit the designation as distinct diseases, namely primary mediastinal (thymic) large B-cell lymphoma, intravascular lymphoma and primary effusion lymphoma. There is little doubt that within the category of DLBCL there are at least several more distinct entities that might benefit from different therapies. Their recognition is one of the challenges facing haematopathologists and several promising approaches, including gene profiling, have already been identified.

The borderline between DLBCL and Burkitt's lymphoma (BL) is not always clear-cut. The WHO clinical advisory meeting took the decision that those DLBCL with Burkitt-like morphology, c-*myc* rearrangement and a proliferation fraction of 100% are best described as having 'atypical Burkitt lymphoma' and should receive therapy tailored for BL. Thus, they represent a subtype of BL, the others being endemic BL, non-endemic BL and immunodeficiency-associated BL.

Mature T- and NK-cell lymphomas

Clinical syndromes rather than cytomorphological features form the principal basis for the identification of real diseases within this difficult group. Several provisional disorders listed in the REAL classification are now recognized as defined entities but, despite many attempts to recognize distinct diseases, most T-cell lymphomas end up being classified as 'T-cell lymphoma unspecified'. This is clearly unsatisfactory and is partly due to the rarity of T-cell lymphomas as a whole. It is to be hoped that the adoption of the new principles of classification will, as new data accumulate, lead to the rationalization of this group.

Anaplastic large-cell lymphoma

Previously defined on the basis of its cytology and expression of CD30 (Stein *et al.*, 1985), it has become clear that more than one 'real' disease can exhibit these features. The discovery of the t(2;5) translocation, which results in the expression of anaplastic lymphoma kinase (ALK) protein, has helped to define a form of T/null-cell ALCL that tends to occur in children and young adults and which, although aggressive, carries a good prognosis with appropriate therapy. It seems likely that the somewhat similar, but t(2;5) (ALK)-negative, cases are a different disorder, but this awaits confirmation. It is clear, however that primary cutaneous ALCL which is always ALK negative and, moreover, lacks a cytotoxic phenotype, is an entirely different entity. Cutaneous ALCL is closely related to the benign disorder lymphomatoid papulosis, and the term 'cutaneous lymphoproliferative disorder' has been suggested for those cases with overlapping features. Whether such a term is appropriate in a lymphoma classification is a moot point.

Conclusions

The WHO classification of lymphoid neoplasms represents a major step forward in our understanding of these tumours. Moreover, in building on the REAL classification it has pointed the way to practical methods of further updating which will be essential if the classification is to endure and to continue to serve the needs of clinicians. Implicit in the classification are signposts for further research, particularly with respect to diffuse large B-cell lymphoma and T-cell lymphoma, unspecified. The formulation of the WHO classifications must be counted as a considerable achievement. By contrast with previous attempts to classify this difficult group of tumours, a large number of pathologists, 19 for the REAL classification and over 50 for the WHO scheme, has been involved and to have achieved consensus within this group is remarkable! Perhaps even more remarkable is to have maintained this consensus in presenting such radically new concepts to the clinicians who treat patients with lymphoma.

Selected bibliography

Aisenberg AC (1999) Primary large cell lymphoma of the mediastinum. *Seminars in Oncology* **26**: 251–8.

Ashton-Key M, Thorpe PA, Allen JP, Isaacson PG (1995) Follicular Hodgkin's disease. *American Journal of Surgical Patholgy* **19**: 1294–9.

Banks P, Chan J, Cleary M *et al.* (1992) Mantle cell lymphoma: a proposal for unification of morphologic, immunologic, and molecular data. *American Journal of Surgical Pathology* **16**: 637–40.

Campo E, Raffeld M, Jaffe ES (1999) Mantle-cell lymphoma. *Seminars in Hematology* **36**: 115–27.

Catovsky D, Matutes E (1999) Splenic lymphoma with circulating villous lymphocytes/splenic marginal zone lymphoma. *Seminars in Hematology* **36**: 148–54.

Chan JK, Ng CS, Isaacson PG (1990) Relationship between high-grade lymphoma and low grade B-cell mucosa-associated lymphoid tissue lymphoma (MALToma) of the stomach. *American Journal of Pathology* **136**: 1153–64.

de Bruin PC, Beljaards RC, van Heerde P *et al.* (1993) Differences in clinical behaviour and immunophenotype between primary cutaneous and primary nodal anaplastic large cell lymphoma of T-cell or null cell phenotype. *Histopathology* **23**: 127–35.

Estalilla OC, Koo CH, Brynes RK, Medeiros LJ (1999) Intravascular large B-cell lymphoma. A report of five cases initially diagnosed by bone marrow biopsy. *American Journal of Clinical Pathology* **112**: 248–55.

Falini B, Bigerna B, Fizzotti M *et al.* (1998) ALK expression defines a distinct group of T/null lymphomas ('ALK lymphomas') with a wide morphological spectrum. *American Journal of Pathology* **153**: 875–86.

Harris NL, Jaffe ES, Stein H *et al.* (1994) A revised European-American Classification of lymphoid neoplasms: A proposal from the International Lymphoma Study Group. *Blood* **84**: 1361–92.

Isaacson PG (1992) Extranodal lymphomas: the MALT concept. *Verhandlungen der Deutschen Gesellschaft für Pathologie* **76**: 14–23.

Isaacson PG (1997) Primary splenic lymphoma. *Cancer Surveys* **30**: 193–212.

Isaacson PG (1999) Gastrointestinal lymphomas of T- and B-cell types. *Modern Pathology* **12**: 151–58.

Jackson H, Parker H (1947) *Hodgkin's Disease and Allied Disorders. Classification and Characterization of Lymphadenopathies.* Oxford University Press, New York.

Jaffe ES, Harris NL, Stein H, Vardiman JW (2001) *World Health Organization Classification of Tumours: Pathology and Genetics of Tumours of Haematopoietic and Lymphoid Tissues.* IARC Press, Lyon.

Jaffe ES, Chan JKC, Su IJ *et al.* (1996) Report of the workshop on nasal and related extranodal angiocentric T/NK cell lymphomas: definitions, differential diagnosis, and epidemiology. *American Journal of Surgical Pathology* **20**: 103–11.

Knowles DM (1999) Immunodeficiency-associated lymphoproliferative disorders. *Modern Pathology* **12**: 200–17.

Kuppers R, Rajewsky K, Zhao M *et al.* (1995) Hodgkin's disease: clonal Ig gene rearrangements in Hodgkin's and Reed–Sternberg cells picked from histological sections. *Annals of the New York Academy of Sciences* **764**: 523–4.

Lukes RJ, Craver LF, Hall TC *et al.* (1996) RYE classification of Hodgkin's disease. *Cancer Research* **26**: 1311.

Lymphoma Classification Project (1997) A clinical evaluation of the International Lymphoma Study Group classification of non-Hodgkin's lymphoma. *Blood* **89**: 3909–18.

Mann R, Berard C (1982) Criteria for the cytologic subclassification of follicular lymphomas: a proposed alternative method. *Hematological Oncology* **1**: 187–92.

Marafioti T, Hummel M, Anagnostopoulos I *et al.* (1997) Origin of nodular lymphocyte-predominance Hodgkin's disease from a clonal expansion of highly mutated germinal-center B cells. *New England Journal of Medicine* **337**: 453–8.

Martin AR, Weisenberger DD, Chan WC *et al.* (1995) Prognostic value of cellular proliferation and histologic grade in follicular lymphoma. *Blood* **85**: 3671–8.

Mollejo M, Menarguez J, Lloret E *et al.* (1995) Splenic marginal zone lymphoma: a distinctive type of low-grade B-cell lymphoma. A clinicopathological study of 13 cases. *American Journal of Surgical Pathology* **19**: 1146–57.

Nizze H, Cogliatti SB, von Schilling C *et al.* (1991) Monocytoid B-cell lymphoma: morphological variants and relationship to low grade B-cell lymphoma of the mucosa-associated lymphoid tissue. *Histopathology* **18**: 403–14.

Non-Hodgkin's Lymphoma Pathologic Classification Project (1982) National Cancer Institute sponsored classifications of non-Hodgkin's lymphomas: summary and description of a Working Formulation for clinical usage. *Cancer* **49**: 2112–35.

Paulli M, Bert E, Rosso R *et al.* (1996) CD30/Ki-1 positive lymphoproliferative disorders of the skin. Clinicopathologic correlation and statistical analysis of 86 cases: A multicentric study from the EORTC cutaneous lymphoma project group. *Journal of Clinical Oncology* **13**: 1343.

Rappaport H (1966) *Tumors of the Hematopoietic System. Atlas of Tumor Pathology*, Section III. Armed Forces Institute of Pathology, Washington, DC.

Shipp MA (1994) Prognostic factors in aggressive non-Hodgkin's lymphoma: who has 'high-risk' disease? *Blood* **83**: 1165–73.

Stansfeld, A, Diebold, J, Kapanci, Y *et al.* (1988) Updated Kiel classification for lymphomas. *Lancet* **1**: 292.

Stein H, Mason DY, Gerdes J *et al.* (1985) The expression of the Hodgkin's disease associated antigen Ki-1 in reactive and neoplastic lymphoid tissue: evidence that Reed–Sternberg cells and histiocytic malignancies are derived from activated lymphoid cells. *Blood* **66**: 848–58.

Willemze R, Beljaards RC (1993) Spectrum of primary cutaneous CD30 (Ki-1)-positive lymphoproliferative disorders. A proposal for classification and guidelines for management and treatment. *Journal of American Academy of Dermatology* **28**: 973–80.

Willemze R, Meijer CJLM, Sentis HJ *et al.* (1987) Primary cutaneous large cell lymphomas of follicular center cell origin. *Journal of American Academy of Dermatology* **16**: 518.

Willemze R, Kerl H, Sterry W *et al.* (1997) EORTC Classification for primary cutaneous lymphomas: A proposal from the Cutaneous Lymphoma Study Group of the European Organization for Research and Treatment of cancer. *Blood* **90**: 354–71.

Wright DH (1997) Enteropathy associated T cell lymphoma. *Cancer Surveys* **30**: 249–61.

CHAPTER 44

Hodgkin's lymphoma

Lynny Yung and David Linch

Introduction

Hodgkin's lymphoma is an uncommon tumour, although it is one of the more frequent malignancies in young people. Traditionally, radiation therapy was the primary treatment agent, and the first successful combination chemotherapy regimen was introduced in the 1960s. Since then, combined-modality therapy has developed allowing reduction of both chemotherapy and radiation doses. The outcome of patients with Hodgkin's lymphoma has improved greatly over the last few decades such that is should now be considered curable in the large majority of cases. With the excellent cure rates now attainable, the late effects of treatment have become more apparent. Current therapeutic strategies must aim to maintain the high cure rates while minimizing these late effects.

Epidemiology

Hodgkin's lymphoma is relatively uncommon with an incidence of approximately 2.3/100 000 per annum. Hodgkin's lymphoma is a disease of young adults, and in the 15–34 years age group it is the second most common malignancy in men and the fourth most common in women. The incidence in women peaks in the third decade and then falls, but in men the incidence remains fairly constant thereafter. The overall incidence is stable, which contrasts with the non-Hodgkin's lymphomas, whose incidence appears to be rising.

Histological classification (see also Chapter 43)

The diagnosis of Hodgkin's lymphoma (HL) is based on the finding of Hodgkin/Reed–Sternberg cells in an appropriate cel-

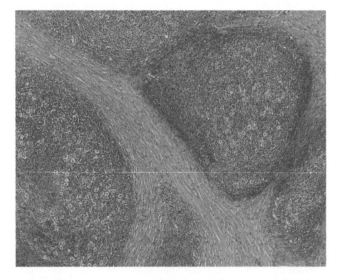

Figure 44.1 Low-power view of lymph node biopsy of classical Hodgkin's lymphoma showing nodularity and sclerosis.

lular background of reactive T cells and eosinophils with varying degrees of fibrosis. Hodgkin's lymphoma is broadly classified into two distinct entities, nodular lymphocyte predominant Hodgkin's lymphoma (NLPHL) and classical Hodgkin's lymphoma (Figures 44.1–44.8). NLPHL represents about 5% of all cases of Hodgkin's lymphoma. It is more common in males and frequently presents with limited nodal disease of the neck without constitutional symptoms.

Classical Hodgkin's lymphoma is divided into four subtypes (Table 44.1). In the developed world nodular sclerosing Hodgkin's lymphoma accounts for the majority of cases. 'Diffuse lymphocyte-predominant Hodgkin's disease' is now known as

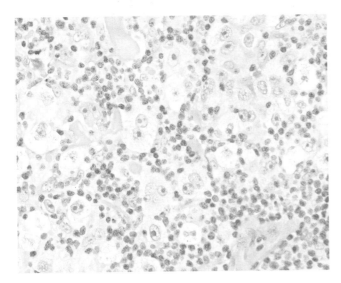

Figure 44.2 High-power view of classical Hodgkin's lymphoma showing abundant Reed–Sternberg cells and occasional eosinophils.

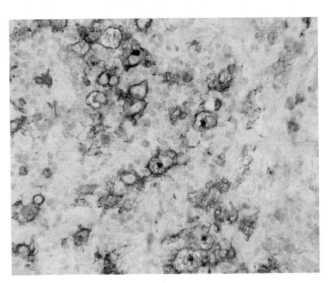

Figure 44.4 CD15 immunostain of classical Hodgkin's lymphoma.

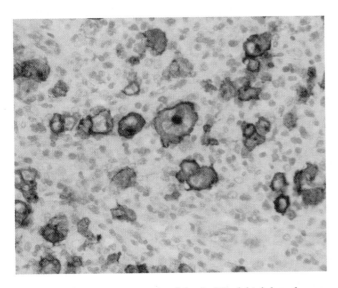

Figure 44.3 CD30 immunostain of classical Hodgkin's lymphoma showing clear membranous and Golgi apparatus staining of the Hodgkin/Reed–Sternberg cells.

Figure 44.5 Low-power view of lymph node biopsy of nodular lymphocyte predominant Hodgkin's lymphoma showing nodular features and slight mottled appearance of the follicles.

lymphocyte-rich classical HL, and most cases of lymphocyte-depleted Hodgkin's lymphoma have been reclassified as cases of nodular sclerosing disease or anaplastic large-cell lymphomas. Histological appearances have been studied in relation to prognosis. A new grading system for advanced-stage disease with nodular sclerosis in which risk is assigned on the basis of four histological features (eosinophilia, lymphocyte depletion, cellular atypia and necrosis) has been proposed. This system requires validation as currently all subtypes of classical Hodgkin's lymphoma are treated in the same way.

Pathogenesis

The pathogenesis of Hodgkin's lymphoma is not yet fully understood; however, the nature of the Hodgkin/Reed–Sternberg (H/RS) cell has now been elucidated. The pathognomonic H/RS cell is derived from a B lymphocyte with clonal rearrangements in the V, D and J segments of the IgH chain locus in the majority of patients. The malignant cells in NLPHL have both the immunophenotype and genotype of post-germinal centre B-cells

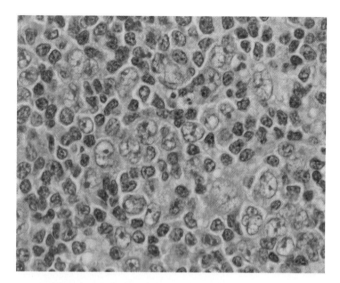

Figure 44.6 High-power view of nodular lymphocyte-predominant Hodgkin's lymphoma showing many convoluted lymphocytic and histiocytic (L&H) or 'popcorn' cells.

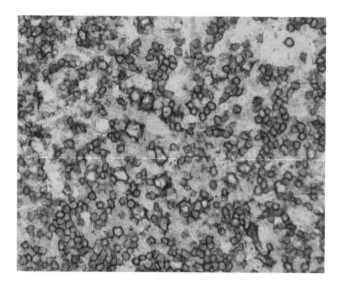

Figure 44.7 CD20 staining of nodular lymphocyte predominant Hodgkin's lymphoma. Note that the L&H cells are typically surrounded by a rosette of CD20 negating, reactive T-cells.

including immunoglobulin production and high expression of pan-B cell antigens such as CD20 (Table 44.2 and Figures 44.7 and 44.8).

In classical Hodgkin's lymphoma, however, mature B-cell antigen expression may be low or absent and there is no immunoglobulin production despite the immunoglobulin gene rearrangements and subsequent somatic mutations. In some cases the lack of immunoglobulin production is due to crippling mutations in the immunoglobulin gene (e.g. creation of stop codons), but in other cases there is dysregulation of the transcriptional machinery involved in immunoglobulin gene expression.

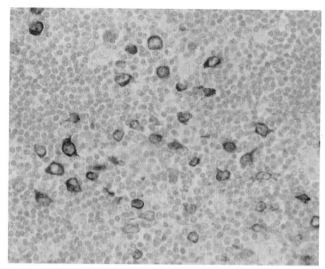

Figure 44.8 J-chain immunostaining of nodular lymphocyte predominant Hodgkin's lymphoma demonstrating immunoglobulin production of L&H cells, a feature not seen in classical Hodgkin's lymphoma.

Table 44.1 WHO classification of Hodgkin's lymphoma.

Nodular lymphocyte-predominant Hodgkin's lymphoma
Classical Hodgkin's lymphoma
    Nodular sclerosis classical Hodgkin's lymphoma
    Mixed-cellularity classical Hodgkin's lymphoma
    Lymphocyte-rich classical Hodgkin's lymphoma
    Lymphocyte-depleted classical Hodgkin's lymphoma

The octamer motif is an important element in the regulation of immunoglobulin promoter and enhancer function. The absence of the transcription factor Oct2 or its coactivator BOB1/OBF1 from Reed–Sternberg cells has been demonstrated in cases of classical Hodgkin's lymphoma, whereas Oct2 was found to be highly expressed in the malignant cells of NLPHL.

It seems likely that the Hodgkin/Reed–Sternberg cell has mechanisms in place that protect it from apoptosis. The immunoglobulin receptor complex provides important survival signals to developing B cells and the absence of immunoglobulin expression could put Hodgkin's cells at a survival disadvantage. Hypermutation of rearranged immunoglobulin genes is characteristic of normal germinal centre activity. B-cells that acquire unfavourable mutations are negatively selected and thus eliminated, primarily via Fas-mediated apoptosis. Constitutive expression of C-FLIP, a downregulator of Fas, has been detected in Hodgkin/Reed–Sternberg cells and may represent an antiapoptotic pathway.

The NF-κB pathway is another mechanism by which H/RS cells might escape apoptosis. NF-κB is a family of transcription factors involved in the regulation of multiple processes including

Table 44.2 Comparison of phenotypes of classical and lymphocyte-predominant Hodgkin's lymphoma.

	Classical Hodgkin's lymphoma, Reed–Sternberg cells	Nodular lymphocyte-predominant Hodgkin's lymphoma, atypical lymphocytic and histiocytic (L&H) cells
CD30	Positive	Negative
CD15	Usually positive	Negative
Immunoglobulin expression	Absent	Present
CD20	Negative	Positive
Other B-cell antigens	Usually negative	Usually positive

apoptosis and oncogenesis; NF-κB itself is regulated via a number of upstream elements including CD40 ligand and TNF receptor-associated factors. In resting cells NF-κB resides in the cytoplasm bound to its inhibitor IκB. Activation of the cell by various routes such as via CD40 ligand or LMP1, leads to the activation of Iκkinase and the phosphorylation of IκB and subsequent ubiquitination with degradation by the 26S proteasome. The liberated NF-κB is then able to move into the nucleus, where it activates transcription of a number of target genes involved in the prevention of apoptosis. NF-κB activity has been shown to be upregulated in H/RS cells of the majority of cases of classical Hodgkin's lymphoma, and mutations of the *IKK* gene family have been detected and are associated with nuclear translocation of NF-κB, thus leading to upregulation of its target genes.

There are several other events such as infection by the Epstein–Barr virus (EBV) which may be important in the survival of the H/RS cell. EBV nuclear proteins such as EBNA and LMP1 have been detected in around 40% of cases of classical Hodgkin's lymphoma, with the highest frequency in mixed cellularity disease. LMP1 is known to have oncogenic potential by triggering Bcl-2 expression and acting via the CD40 cell signalling pathway, thus allowing cells to evade apoptosis. The association with EBV varies with age; the majority of childhood and elderly Hodgkin's lymphoma is EBV associated however, around only 25–50% of young adults have EBV-positive tumours. This age group (15–34 years) represents the peak incidence of the disease, and the possibility of alternative lymphotropic viruses being involved in the pathogenesis of EBV-negative cases has been suggested but not yet demonstrated. It is well recognized that the incidence of Hodgkin's lymphoma in HIV-positive patients is increased by around sevenfold and almost all cases are associated with EBV infection. Hodgkin's lymphoma associated with organ and bone marrow transplantation and with congenital immunodeficiency syndromes has also been shown to be usually EBV associated.

Clinical presentation

The presenting features of Hodgkin's lymphoma are numerous. The majority of patients present with an enlarged but otherwise

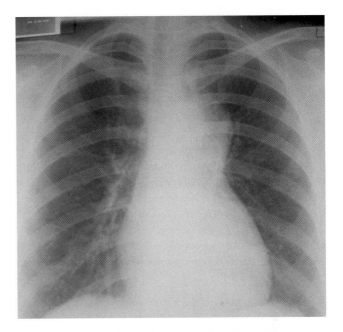

Figure 44.9 Chest radiograph showing enlarged superior mediastinum.

asymptomatic lump(s), most often in the lower neck or supraclavicular region. Mediastinal masses are frequent and are sometimes discovered after routine chest radiography (Figure 44.9). Less commonly, patients complain of chest discomfort with a cough or dyspnoea. Around 25% of patients will have systemic symptoms at presentation. Typical symptoms are fatigue, fever, weight loss and night sweats. Pruritus and intermittent fevers (so-called Pel–Ebstein fever) often associated with night sweats are classical symptoms of Hodgkin's lymphoma.

An important feature of Hodgkin's lymphoma is contiguous spread, with disease most commonly starting above the diaphragm in the cervical nodes and spreading to involve adjacent nodes and less commonly non-lymphoid tissue.

Splenomegaly may occur without involvement by disease; however, hepatosplenomegaly invariably indicates disease infiltration. Peripheral blood manifestations are common but non-specific, with lymphocytopenia and anaemia being indicators of advanced disease. Eosinophilia is frequently reported, although opinion differs as to whether this has prognostic significance.

Staging

The Ann Arbor staging system was developed over 30 years ago to define those patients who could be treated by radiotherapy, and it is still valuable in defining the extent of therapy even though radiation alone is less frequently employed. The Cotswolds modification (Table 44.3) made in 1989, takes into account the importance of bulky disease and the fact that laparotomy and splenectomy are no longer recommended as staging procedures as they have been shown to have no effect on overall survival, and are associated with significant morbidity and occasionally mortality.

Lymphangiography is now rarely performed and computerized tomography (CT) scanning is the major means of staging both intrathoracic and intra-abdominal disease (Figure 44.10). Magnetic resonance imaging (MRI) scanning is largely restricted to the evaluation of specific situations such as bony involvement and spinal cord compression. Fluorodeoxyglucose positron emission tomography (FDG-PET) scanning may also have a role, relying on the uptake of 2-fluoro-2-deoxy-D-glucose by metabolically active tissues possibly revealing disease in sites difficult to image by CT scanning (Figure 44.11). Current practice, however, does not include PET scanning as part of the staging investigations although this may change with the increased availability of this technology.

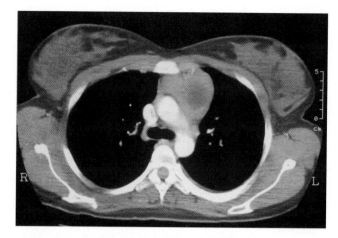

Figure 44.10 CT scan of the chest showing large anterior mediastinal mass with area of probable necrosis.

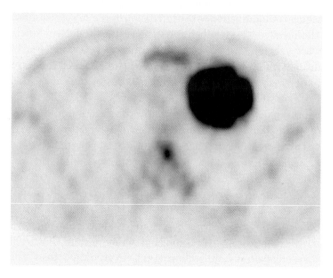

Figure 44.11 FDG-PET scan showing FDG-avidity of large mediastinal mass.

Table 44.3 Ann Arbor staging system with Cotswolds modifications for Hodgkin's lymphoma.

Stage

I	Involvement of a single lymph-node region or lymphoid structure (e.g. spleen, thymus, Waldeyer's ring)
II	≥ 2 lymph node regions on the same side of the diaphragm
III	Lymph nodes on both sides of the diaphragm
III1	With splenic hilar, coeliac or portal nodes
III2	With para-aortic, iliac, mesenteric nodes
IV	Involvement of extranodal site(s) beyond that designated 'E'

Modifying features

A	No symptoms
B	Fever, drenching night sweats, weight loss > 10% in 6 months
X	Bulky disease: > one-third widening of mediastinum > 10 cm maximum diameter of nodal mass
E	Involvement of single, contiguous or proximal extranodal site
CS	Clinical stage
PS	Pathological stage

Prognostic factors

In 1985, the British National Lymphoma Investigation (BNLI) published a prognostic index in localized Hodgkin's lymphoma which was based on an analysis of over 2000 patients. This was a complex index and therefore was not widely adopted, although risk stratified therapy is now an established principle of management. The EORTC (European Organization for Research and Treatment of Cancer) have identified a number of features indicative of a worse prognosis in stage I and II disease and used these to stratify therapy (Table 44.4). In more advanced disease the International Prognostic Score (or Hasenclever index) was developed (Table 44.5) based on an analysis of over 5000 patients treated initially with an anthracycline-containing

Table 44.4 EORTC risk factors in localized disease.

Favourable
Patients must have *all* of the following features
    Clinical stage I and II
    Maximum of three nodal areas involved
    Age < 50 years
    ESR < 50 mm/h without B symptoms or ESR < 30 mm/h with
      B symptoms
    Mediastinal/thoracic ratio < 0.35.

Unfavourable
Patients have *any* of the following features
    Clinical stage II with involvement of at least four nodal areas
    Age > 50 years
    ESR > 50 mm/h if asymptomatic or ESR > 30 mm/h if
      B symptoms
    Mediastinal/thoracic ratio > 0.35

Table 44.5 Hasenclever index.

Age > 45 years
Male gender
Serum albumin < 40 g/L
Haemoglobin level < 10.5 g/dL
Stage IV disease
Leucocytosis (white cell count $\geq 15 \times 10^9$/L)
Lymphopenia ($< 0.6 \times 10^9$/L or < 8% of the white cell count)

chemotherapy regimen. Seven factors were identified, each of which reduced the predicted 5-year freedom from progression rate by around 8%.

Response assessment

Complete response (CR) following therapy is often difficult to determine in patients with Hodgkin's lymphoma as residual masses are very common (Figure 44.12). The entity of CRu (unconfirmed/uncertain) was therefore introduced, and refers to those patients in whom there is uncertainty about the remission status due to persisting radiological abnormalities particularly in the mediastinum. Gallium scanning techniques have been used in the assessment of residual masses and comparative studies between gallium scanning and PET are under way. Gallium is predominantly excreted via the gastrointestinal tract which may limit its use in the assessment of abdominal disease.

PET scanning is likely to play an important role in clarifying remission status in this group of patients as the 2-fluoro-2-deoxy-glucose is taken up by residual metabolically active

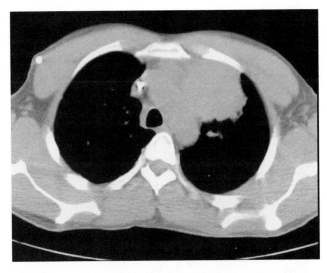

Figure 44.12 CT scan of the chest showing large residual mass at end of treatment.

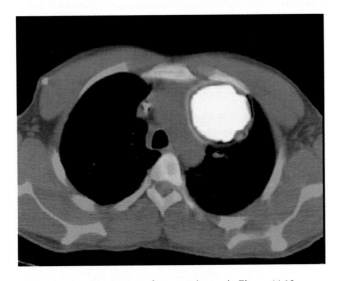

Figure 44.13 PET-CT scan of same patient as in Figure 44.12 showing FDG avidity of large residual mass.

tumour cells and not fibrotic tissue. FDG-PET has higher sensitivity, specificity, positive and negative predictive values for disease-free survival (DFS) than CT scanning. In some centres, PET-CT is available to produce images which enable comparison of areas of FDG avidity with lesions seen on the CT scan (Figures 44.13 and 44.14). The optimal timing of a PET scan has yet to be determined as recent chemotherapy may result in a positive scan due to ongoing macrophage activity. Patients with suspicious symptoms or a residual mass at the end of treatment may be monitored with PET scans and offered further therapy as indicated. However, PET may be less discriminating in the evaluation of inflammatory or extranodal disease and it is currently recommended that unusual lesions are biopsied.

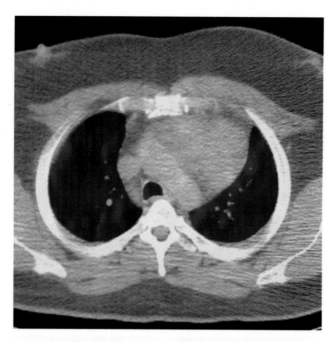

Figure 44.14 PET-CT scan showing FDG-'cold' residual mass.

Therapy

The outcome in both localized and advanced Hodgkin's lymphoma has improved greatly over the last 30 years such that the disease is now considered curable in the large majority of cases. Unlike many other forms of cancer, it is often possible to effect a cure even if first-line treatment fails and this creates the dilemma of whether it is better to use more extensive/intensive therapy initially to cure the maximum number of individuals possible with that course of therapy, or whether it is better to use lesser therapy initially and rely on more intensive salvage therapy in a greater proportion of patients. The decision must be based on the analysis of long-term survival rates with the different strategies and the consideration of short- and long-term side-effects of treatment including the psychological trauma associated with relapse when a less intensive initial therapy is used.

Nodular lymphocyte predominant Hodgkin's lymphoma

NLPHL is a distinct entity and needs to be considered separately from the therapeutic standpoint.

There have been no prospective randomized trials carried out specifically in NLPHL. As the disease is usually localized, it is most often treated with surgical excision and involved-field radiotherapy, although if the surgical excision is complete the radiotherapy may be unnecessary. Complete response rates of 96% with 8-year disease-free survival of 99% or 98% in stage I and II, respectively, have been reported by the European Task

Force on Lymphoma. The treatment of advanced disease is generally the same as for classical Hodgkin's lymphoma, i.e. combination chemotherapy. However, NLPHL tends to relapse as a large-cell lymphoma and relapse may occur 10–15 years after the initial diagnosis. It is important therefore to correctly diagnose and stage this entity accurately as the outcome in patients with advanced-stage NLPHL approaches that of patients with classical disease.

Recently, groups from Stanford, USA, and Germany have reported the use of the CD20 monoclonal antibody rituximab in patients with NLPHL The therapy is well tolerated and results have been encouraging. Longer follow-up is required, but rituximab should certainly be considered for patients failing combination chemotherapy.

Classical Hodgkin's lymphoma

All forms of classical Hodgkin's lymphoma are usually treated in the same way, with anatomical stage being the most important factor in determining therapy. In some centres specific histological subtypes are used as prognostic factors and could therefore modify the risk group and the therapy prescribed.

Localized disease, i.e. stage I and stage IIA

A plethora of trials have been conducted in localized Hodgkin's lymphoma but it is difficult to compare directly the results from different trials. Entry criteria vary, with some groups stratifying localized disease into a number of different risk groups. The EORTC, for instance, has considered localized disease in two risk groups (favourable and unfavourable, see Table 44.4). In the UK, the usual practice is to have only one category of localized disease, and patients with stage IIB or IIIA disease are considered as having advanced disease.

The traditional therapy for localized disease was radiotherapy alone. This resulted in high rates of complete remission but relapse was frequent. The more extensive the radiation fields, the lower the relapse rate; this has been shown in a randomized trial conducted by the BNLI in which 'mantle' or 'inverted Y' radiation fields resulted in an approximately 11% higher time to treatment failure rate than involved-field radiotherapy. In Europe, even more extended radiation fields have been routinely used, but despite this, the relapse rate is still of the order of 20–30%. Interestingly, more extensive radiation fields have not translated into improved survival attesting to the success of chemotherapy in those patients relapsing after radiation. Nonetheless, such high relapse rates are now considered to be unacceptable.

The relapse risk can be reduced by the use of combined-modality therapy (CMT) incorporating both chemotherapy and radiotherapy. There is little evidence again that this improves survival, but within the context of CMT it is possible to use shorter courses of chemotherapy than are used in advanced disease and more restricted radiation fields. In unfavourable risk disease, the EORTC H7 CMT trial showed that four cycles of chemotherapy were as effective as six and involved-field radiation as effective as subtotal nodal irradiation (STNI). Even in this poor-risk group the 6-year failure-free survival and overall survival rates were 89% and 90% respectively. Even shorter courses of chemotherapy are adequate in patients with better-risk disease. Three cycles of a MOPP/ABV hybrid regimen plus involved-field radiotherapy have been shown to be more effective than STNI, resulting in a 4-year event-free survival of 99% in the EORTC/GELA H8F trial. Three cycles of combination chemotherapy (usually ABVD) plus involved-field radiotherapy should thus be considered the standard for treatment in favourable-risk localized disease. A number of even shorter chemotherapy regimens have been combined with involved-field radiotherapy and, although they may be less efficacious than three cycles of MOPP/ABV or equivalent, they probably have less short- and long-term toxicity. As well as reducing the radiation field and dose in CMT, it may also be possible to reduce the amount of chemotherapy. In the German HD8 trial for intermediate-stage patients (stage I or II disease with at least one risk factor) treated with four courses of alternating COPP and ABVD, no difference in survival or freedom from treatment failure rates were shown between those receiving involved-field radiotherapy and those receiving extended-field radiotherapy; however, side-effects were more common in patients receiving extended-field radiotherapy. The current HD10 trial explores the use of reduced doses of radiation as well as restricted fields.

Concern over radiation-induced second malignancies has raised the issue of whether localized disease should be treated with chemotherapy alone, and this issue is addressed in the current Canadian National Cancer Institute HD6 phase III study which randomizes patients with clinical stage I–IIA to ABVD chemotherapy or STNI.

It may be that shorter courses of chemotherapy alone are adequate, especially when the length of chemotherapy is guided by interval PET scanning, and this will be tested in the forthcoming UK NCRI trial.

Advanced disease

The introduction of the MOPP (mustine, vincristine, procarbazine and prednisolone) combination chemotherapy regimen was a major landmark in the treatment of advanced Hodgkin's lymphoma. In the following few years a number of modifications to this regimen were made which maintained the efficacy but reduced the toxicity associated with MOPP. The next most important step was the development in the 1970s of the ABVD regimen (doxorubicin, bleomycin, vinblastine and dacarbazine). This was originally introduced as a salvage regimen for patients who had failed MOPP chemotherapy and was designed as far as possible to contain non-cross-resistant drugs to those in MOPP. This was later used as first-line therapy, particularly because the

drugs in ABVD were far less likely to induce infertility and secondary leukaemia than those in MOPP. ABVD was also combined with MOPP or MOPP-like therapy in either alternating or hybrid regimens so as to introduce a large number of drugs over a short time period in the hope of reducing the development of tumour resistance. A seminal trial was reported in 1992 by the Cancer and Leukaemia Group B (CALGB) comparing MOPP, ABVD and alternating MOPP/ABVD as the first chemotherapy in patients with stage III and IV disease. This showed that ABVD and alternating MOPP/ABVD were superior to MOPP in terms of response rate and failure-free survival (Table 44.6). Several studies compared MOPP alternating with ABVD with a MOPP/ABV hybrid and showed no significant differences. The CALGB trial had been too small to determine whether MOPP alternating with ABVD was superior to ABVD alone, but ABVD became widely accepted as the treatment of choice because of its lesser long-term toxicity. This practice was substantiated in the follow-up CALGB 8952 trial, which compared a MOPP/ABV hybrid against ABVD in patients with stage III or IV disease or after radiotherapy failure. At 5 years, the failure-free survival in the two arms was 63% and 66% respectively, with an overall survival of 81% and 82%. This trial was stopped after 856 patients had been randomized because of an excess of treatment-related deaths and second malignancies in the hybrid arm (Table 44.6).

Encouraging results have been reported using some alternative regimens. The Stanford V regimen is a 12-week regime of seven active agents with radiotherapy to sites of initial bulk; this is summarized in Table 44.6. A small randomized Italian study, however, found the Stanford V regimen to be inferior to ABVD and randomized trials comparing Stanford V against ABVD therapy are still ongoing.

A new hybrid regimen BEACOPP (bleomycin, etoposide, doxorubicin, cyclophosphamide vincristine, procarbazine, and prednisone) developed by the German Hodgkin's Study Group has been compared with their standard alternating regimen (COPP/ABVD) and a dose-intensified version of BEACOPP (escalated BEACOPP). The escalated BEACOPP requires the routine administration of G-CSF. The COPP/ABVD arm was closed early because it was found to result in a significantly inferior freedom from treatment failure (FFTF) compared with the BEACOPP arms at the first interim analysis. The final analysis has revealed significant improvement in the FFTF at 5 years in the BEACOPP arm compared with the COPP/ABVD arm (76% vs. 69%) and a further significant improvement in the escalated BEACOPP arm, in which the FFTF at 5 years is 87%. Both BEACOPP arms showed an advantage in overall survival at 5 years over the standard COPP/ABVD arm; however, there was no significant difference between baseline BEACOPP and escalated BEACOPP. The rate of early disease progression was lower in the escalated dose BEACOPP arm than in the baseline BEACOPP and COPP-ABVD arms. The initial concern of an increased incidence of AML/MDS in the escalated dose arm has not been confirmed in later analyses. In addition, it must be noted that

Table 44.6 Selected randomized trials in advanced disease.

Group (reference)	Disease stage and treatment	Number of patients	Failure-free survival (FFS) %	Overall survival (OS) %	Time (years)
Chemotherapy only CALGB (Canellos *et al.*, 1992)	III, IV MOPP MOPP/ABVD ABVD	361	 50 65 61 $P < 0.05$	 66 75 76	5
INT Milan (Viviani *et al.*, 1996)	I_B–IV MOPP/ABVD alternating MOPP/ABV hybrid (RT to initial bulk in both arms)	427 (415 evaluable)	 67 69	 74 72	10
*CALGB 8952 (Duggan *et al.*, 2003)	III–IV or after RT failure MOPP/ABV ABVD	856	 67 65	 85 87	3
Stanford (Horning *et al.*, 2002)	III, IV or locally extensive I or II Stanford V ± RT	142	 89	 96	5
Intergruppo Italiano (Levis *et al.*, 2002)	II_B–IV ABVD MOPP-EBV-CAD Stanford V	355 (272 evaluable)	 81 85 57 $P < 0.01$	 95 96 91	4
†German Hodgkin's Study Group HD9 (Diehl *et al.*, 2003)	II_B–III_A with risk factors or III/IV A: COPP/ABVD B: BEACOPP (baseline) C: BEACOPP (escalated) RT permitted to sites of initial bulk	1201 (1195 evaluable)	 69 76 87 $P < 0.001$	 83 88 91 A and B $P = 0.16$ B and C $P = 0.06$ A and C $P = 0.002$	5
BNLI (Hancock *et al.*, 2001)	II_B–IV ChLVPP/PABLOE IPS 0–3 IPS 4–7	326	 77 71	 88 74	5
Chemotherapy and radiotherapy GELA H89 (Ferme *et al.*, 2000)	III_B–IV MOPP/ABV×6 + STNI MOPP/ABV×8 ABVPP×6 +STNI ABVPP×8	559 (418 evaluable)	 82 80 75 68 $P = 0.01$	 88 85 78 94 $P = 0.02$	5
EORTC 20884 (Aleman *et al.*, 2003)	III–IV MOPP/ABV to CR + IFRT MOPP/ABV to CR, no IFRT	739 421 in CR	 79 84 $P = 0.35$	 85 91 $P = 0.07$	5

CALGB, Cancer and Leukaemia Group B; EORTC, European Organization for the Research and Treatment of Cancer; GELA, Groupe d'Etudes de Lymphomes d'Adulte; IFRT, involved-field radiotherapy; IPS, International Prognostic Score; RT, radiotherapy.
*This trial was closed early due to an excess of treatment-related deaths and second malignancies in the hybrid arm.
†Escalated BEACOPP therapy requires the routine administration of G-CSF.

there is considerably more chance of infertility with a pro-carbazine-containing regimen than with ABVD. At the very least this study demonstrates that there is a clear dose–response relationship within the dose range possible without haemopoietic stem cell support. Selected studies of treatment of advanced disease are summarized in Table 44.6.

There is an argument that high-risk patients may benefit from more intensive regimens such as BEACOPP. In the UK, the ChlVPP/PABLOE alternating regimen has been widely used, and an analysis of 326 patients is summarized in Table 44.6. This study also suggests that a significant proportion of the patients failing alternating therapy could be rescued with alternative approaches. In the approximately 20% of patients with an IPS of 4–7, the FFS at 5 years was expectedly lower at 71% and fewer failures were rescued so that the OS was only 74%. It may therefore be that regimens such as escalated BEACOPP may be most beneficial in high-risk patients and this will be explored in a European Intergroup trial. The strategy of high-dose therapy with stem cell transplantation in first remission has also been tested in a randomized trial, which failed to show any benefit of early high-dose therapy. It should be noted that in this trial the patients receiving continued conventional dose therapy had an excellent 5-year failure-free survival of 83%, thus illustrating the difficulty in defining a poor-prognosis group once a good response to initial therapy has been obtained.

Radiotherapy in advanced Hodgkin's lymphoma

The use of consolidation radiotherapy in patients with advanced Hodgkin's lymphoma is common, especially if a CRu is attained and there was bulky disease at presentation. The evidence for this practice is not strong. The Groupe d'Etude des Lymphomes de L'Adulte (GELA) designed a complex study (H89) comparing six cycles of two different chemotherapy regimes with a second randomization to two more cycles of the same chemotherapy or to subtotal or total nodal irradiation (Table 44.6). There was no advantage to radiotherapy consolidation when a doxorubicin-containing regimen had been used. The EORTC 20884 trial of involved-field radiotherapy in patients with advanced Hodgkin's lymphoma showed no advantage to consolidation radiotherapy for those achieving CR after MOPP/ABV chemotherapy. Interestingly, however, patients only achieving a partial remission after MOPP/ABV had a similar overall outcome if they were given additional radiotherapy (Table 44.6). A meta-analysis comparing chemotherapy with combined-modality therapies concluded that, providing the amount of chemotherapy was adequate, the addition of radiotherapy did not improve tumour control and might be associated with a reduced survival attributable to long-term effects of treatment. Despite these negative conclusions about consolidation radiotherapy it must be noted that two of the most recent regimens reported to date both use radiotherapy consolidation in the majority of patients.

In Stanford V, 85% of patients received radiotherapy and in escalated BEACOPP radiotherapy was given to the majority of patients.

Treatment of childhood Hodgkin's lymphoma

Hodgkin's lymphoma in children and adolescents is curable in over 90% of cases. With rising numbers of long-term survivors, the impact of long-term effects becomes increasingly important. A number of specific childhood regimens have been developed which aim to maintain these excellent remission rates but reduce the likelihood of developing late effects. These regimens encompass the same general principles, namely avoidance of laparotomy staging to reduce the risk of fulminant sepsis, risk-adjusted therapy to avoid overtreatment of favourable-risk patients, combined modality treatment at all stages of the disease, avoidance of procarbazine in boys to protect future fertility and minimization of radiation dose and field and anthracycline dose. Many of these principles are now also being applied in adult patients with Hodgkin's lymphoma.

Relapsed disease

A proportion of patients receiving chemotherapy, either *de novo* or after radiation failure, will have refractory disease or will relapse from remission. Occasional patients can be cured by radiotherapy if the persistent or relapsed disease is localized, but the majority of patients will require systemic therapy. In patients with long first remissions, a significant proportion of patients may be cured by further standard dose chemotherapy, but the results of such approaches are poor if the remission has been short or the disease was refractory to initial chemotherapy. In the report of the long-term follow-up of the initial cohort of patients treated with MOPP at the NCI, there were no survivors beyond 10 years in those who had not achieved a remission.

High-dose chemotherapy and autologous stem cell transplantation was first pioneered in relapsed Hodgkin's lymphoma over 40 years ago, but it is only in the last two decades that it has become an established modality of treatment. In the last decade peripheral blood stem cells have replaced the use of bone marrow as the source of haemopoietic stem cells. In the early 1980s the procedure-related mortality associated with an autograft was in the order of 10%, but with improved patient selection and better supportive care this has fallen to 3% or less. In large single-centre series and in registry reviews, the overall survival rates of patients receiving autologous transplantation for relapsed or resistant disease are approximately 40–50%. A number of different conditioning regimens have been used, and high-dose chemotherapy is generally preferred to total body irradiation (TBI). This is because chemotherapy is logistically easier to administer, appears as effective as TBI and may be associated with less pneumonitis, although high-dose chemotherapy is also associated with pneumonitis, particularly in patients who have received mediastinal radiation in the preceding year. Following high-dose therapy it is common practice to irradiate persistent masses or sites of previous large volume disease, although there are no trial data to substantiate this practice.

Prior to high-dose therapy, standard-dose chemotherapy is usually given to reduce disease bulk and demonstrate chemosensitivity. In patients with progressive disease despite standard-dose chemotherapy, or who have persistent B symptoms or a raised lactate dehydrgenase (LDH), the results of high-dose therapy are probably too poor to justify proceeding to this course of action. It must be noted, however, that in some cases a mass will not immediately shrink in size and failure to achieve a formal response (complete or partial remission) should not disqualify a patient from receiving an autograft.

The BNLI carried out a small randomized trial of BEAM (carmustine, etoposide, cytarabine and melphalan) followed by autologous stem cell transplantation or mini-BEAM (the same drugs at lower doses) in patients with refractory or relapsed disease. There was a highly significant progression-free survival advantage in the high-dose therapy arm, and similar results have subsequently been reported from a larger German study. Neither study demonstrated an overall survival benefit and this may, in part, be due to the small size of these trials, but may also be because some patients failing standard dose salvage therapy can still be rescued by high-dose therapy at a later time. This raises the issue of when is the optimal time to consider an autograft procedure. It is widely recommended for all patients below the age of 65 years who fail first-line chemotherapy, although this may not be appropriate if there has been a first complete remission lasting more than 3 years.

The value of allogeneic transplantation in Hodgkin's lymphoma is unclear. High transplant-related mortality rates have been reported in several series. However, there may be a reduced relapse rate in those patients surviving an allogeneic transplant, suggesting a graft-versus-lymphoma effect. There is current interest in the use of less toxic non-myeloablative allogeneic transplants in Hodgkin's lymphoma, particularly in patients who have failed a previous autograft, and in a UK study involving 24 patients with relapsed or refractory HL there were only two procedure-related deaths. Interestingly, several patients who subsequently relapsed responded to donor lymphocyte infusions. Further follow-up and larger trials will be required to ascertain the role of this modality of therapy.

Late effects of Hodgkin's lymphoma and its treatment

As the cure rate for Hodgkin's lymphoma has increased and longer-term follow-up data have become available, the significance of the late effects of treatment have become more apparent (Table 44.7). In a study of young adults aged 29 years or less at diagnosis, and who achieved a stable complete remission after

Table 44.7 Late effects of Hodgkin's lymphoma and its treatment.

Second malignancies
Cardiac disease
Endocrine dysfunction
Psychological trauma
Lung damage (usually subclinical)
Hyposplenism (following splenectomy or splenic irradiation)

first- or second-line therapy, the actuarial overall survival at 20 years was 93% and 85% respectively, compared with 98.5% in the age-matched general population. In some patients treated for favourable-risk disease it has been shown that, at 12–15 years after therapy, the mortality risk related to therapy exceeds the risk of dying from Hodgkin's lymphoma. The two most frequent causes of excess deaths are second malignancies and ischaemic heart disease.

The commonest second malignancy is lung cancer. This is mainly attributable to radiotherapy, although chemotherapy also contributes to the risk. Patients who have had thoracic irradiation must be warned of the risk of developing secondary lung cancer and must be strongly discouraged from smoking. The risk of developing secondary myeloid leukaemia is related to the cumulative dose of alkylating agents received and, therefore, occurs predominantly in patients who have had remitting and relapsing disease. The risk of secondary breast cancer is greatest in adolescent females or young women who received mediastinal or axillary irradiation. There is a clear dose–response relationship, which emphasizes the use of the minimal radiation dose required for tumour control. The risk in such patients of ever developing breast cancer is in the region of 1 in 4, and patients at such high risk must be made aware of this fact and offered access to a screening programme. Other malignancies that occur in excess in patients treated for Hodgkin's lymphoma include non-Hodgkin's lymphomas, cancers of the colon, stomach, head and neck and thyroid, and malignant melanoma. Advice should be given regarding early consultation for suspicious symptoms and the avoidance of sunburn.

The Stanford group reported a threefold increase in relative risk of cardiac death in Hodgkin's lymphoma survivors representing a major risk as the incidence of cardiac disease in the general population is so high. The major contributory factor is mediastinal irradiation, especially if a dose in excess of 30 Gy is used. Whether the increasing use of anthracyclines will have a long-term impact on cardiac disease is not yet clear.

The most common endocrine disorders are hypothyroidism following radiotherapy to the lower neck and infertility. Around half of patients receiving neck radiation will develop hypothyroidism, and these patients should be monitored accordingly. Infertility is caused by irradiation of the gonads and the use of drugs such as procarbazine and alkylating agents. It is their repeated use that is most damaging, and young female patients receiving an autologous transplant will often remain fertile if they are still menstruating prior to the high-dose therapy. Sperm cryopreservation prior to chemotherapy should be offered to men who have not completed their families. Artificial insemination has a relatively low success rate per cycle; however, intracytoplasmic sperm injection may be more successful. Hodgkin's lymphoma may often be slow growing, and this permits the harvesting of eggs, *in vitro* fertilization and embryo storage in those young women who have an established partner. Oocyte cryopreservation and ovarian tissue banking are currently in development and remain experimental.

The psychological trauma associated with contracting a malignant disease, receiving radiotherapy and chemotherapy and coping with the risk or eventuality of relapse is considerable. A significant proportion of patients report lower perceived levels of overall health, dissatisfaction in their personal relationships and difficulties in obtaining life assurance and financial loans as a result of the disease and/or its treatment.

Current strategies must therefore aim to give the minimal therapy without jeopardizing the high rates of cure that are now possible with front-line therapy. This will require large randomized trials with long follow-up.

Novel therapies

Cytotoxic drugs

Gemcitabine, an analogue of cytarabine, has been found to have anti-tumour activity in Hodgkin's lymphoma. It is well tolerated with a favourable toxicity profile, and response rates in excess of 35% in heavily pretreated patients can be achieved. Future studies will explore the use of gemcitabine in combination with other active cytotoxic agents.

As NF-κB has been shown to be activated in Hodgkin's lymphoma cells, this pathway is an important target for new drug development. Particular attention is focused on proteasome inhibitors which prevent degradation of IκB and thus minimize the liberation of active NF-κB.

Immunotherapy

Limited success has been seen following the reinfusion of EBV-specific cytotoxic T lymphocytes (CTLs) in patients with Hodgkin's lymphoma. H/RS cells have been shown to evade destruction by EBV-specific CTLs by downregulating the T-cell receptor response and by the secretion of cytokines, which may prevent the generation of an effective cell-mediated response. Strategies aiming to generate LMP-selective CTLs, possibly with the use of autologous dendritic cells may prove more efficacious.

One of the most promising antigens for targeted immunotherapy is the CD30 antigen. Studies investigating anti-tumour activity of an anti-CD30 monoclonal antibody and radioimmunotherapy with ^{131}I-labelled anti-CD30 antibody are ongoing.

Use of bispecific antibodies such as CD30/CD25 and CD30/CD3 are currently the subject of phase I/II trials and may be more effective than the single agent alone.

Conclusion

Much progress has been made in recent years regarding both the cellular aspects of the Hodgkin/Reed–Sternberg cell and the treatment of the resultant tumour. The results of therapy are extremely good, and attention must be paid to minimizing late effects of treatment. In many cases the same ultimate survival can be achieved using different therapeutic approaches. The choice of approach depends on an appreciation of short- and long-term side-effects, and increasingly the patient must be involved in an informed decision-making process.

Acknowledgements

Acknowledgements are made to the Department of Imaging, University College Hospitals, London, and Department of Nuclear Medicine, Middlesex Hospital, London, for the radiological slides, and to the Department of Histopathology, University College London, for the histopathology slides.

Selected bibliography

Aleman BM, Raemaekers JM, Tirelli U *et al.* (2003) Involved-field radiotherapy for advanced Hodgkin's lymphoma. *New England Journal of Medicine* 348: 2396–406.

Annunziata CM, Safiran YJ, Irving SG, Kasid UN, Cossman J (2000) Hodgkin's disease: pharmacologic intervention of the CD40-NF kappa B pathway by a protease inhibitor. *Blood* 96: 2841–8.

Bhatia S, Robison LL, Oberlin O *et al.* (1996) Breast cancer and other second neoplasms after childhood Hodgkin's disease. *New England Journal of Medicine* 334: 745–51.

Bonadonna G, Zucali R, Monfardini S *et al.* (1975) Combination chemotherapy of Hodgkin's disease with adriamycin, bleomycin, vinblastine, and imidazole carbomoxide versus MOPP. *Cancer* 36: 252–259.

Bonfante V, Santoro A, Viviani S *et al.* Outcome of patients with Hodgkin's disease failing after primary MOPP-ABVD. *Journal of Clinical Oncology* (1997) 15: 528–34.

Canellos GP, Anderson JR, Propert KJ *et al.* (1992) Chemotherapy of advanced Hodgkin's disease with MOPP, ABVD, or MOPP alternating with ABVD. *New England Journal of Medicine* 327: 1478–84.

Chen Fei, Castronova Vince, Shi Xianglin (2001) New insights into the role of nuclear factor-κB in cell growth regulation. *American Journal of Pathology* 159: 387–97.

Chopra R, McMillan AK, Linch DC *et al.* (1993) The place of high-dose BEAM therapy and autologous bone marrow transplantation in poor risk Hodgkin's disease. A single-center eight-year study of 155 patients. *Blood* **81**: 1137.

DeVita VT, Jr, Serpick AA, Carbone PP (1970) Combination chemotherapy in the treatment of advanced Hodgkin's disease. *Annals of Internal Medicine* **73**: 881–95.

Diehl V, Franklin J, Pfreundschuh M *et al.* (2003) Standard and increased-dose BEACOPP chemotherapy compared with COPP-ABVD for advanced Hodgkin's disease. *New England Journal of Medicine* **348**: 2386–95.

Duggan DB, Petroni GR, Johnson JL *et al.* (2003) Randomised comparison of ABVD and MOPP/ABV hybrid for the treatment of Advanced Hodgkin's disease: report of an intergroup trial. *Journal of Clinical Oncology* **21**: 607–14.

Ferme C, Sebban C, Hennequin C *et al.* (2000) Comparison of chemotherapy to radiotherapy as consolidation of complete or good response after six cycles of chemotherapy for patients with advanced Hodgkin's disease: results of the Groupe d'Etudes des Lymphomes de l'Adulte H89 trial. *Blood* **95**: 2246–52.

Hancock BW, Gregory WM, Cullen MH *et al.* (2001) ChlVPP alternating with PABlOE is superior to PABlOE alone in the initial treatment of advanced Hodgkin's disease: results of a British National Lymphoma Investigation/Central Lymphoma Group randomized controlled trial. *British Journal of Cancer* **84**: 1293–300.

Hasenclever D, Diehl V (1998) A prognostic score for advanced Hodgkin's disease. International Prognostic Factors Project on Advanced Hodgkin's Disease. *New England Journal of Medicine* **339**: 1506–14.

Horning SJ, Hoppe RT, Breslin S *et al.* (2002) Stanford V and radiotherapy for locally extensive and advanced Hodgkin's disease: mature results of a prospective clinical trial. *Journal of Clinical Oncology* **20**: 630–7.

Linch DC, Winfield D, Goldstone AH *et al.* (1993) Dose intensification with autologous bone-marrow transplatntaion in relapsed and resistant Hodgkin's disease: results of a BNLI randomized trial. *Lancet* **341**: 1051–4.

Linch DC, Goldstone AH (1999) High-dose therapy for Hodgkin's disease. *British Journal of Haematology* **107**: 685–690.

Loeffler M, Brosteanu O, Hasenclever D *et al.* (1998) Meta-analysis of chemotherapy versus combined modality treatment trials in Hodgkin's disease. International Database on Hodgkin's Disease Overview Study Group. *Journal of Clinical Oncology* **16**: 818–29.

Longo DL, Young RC, Wesley M *et al.* (1986) Twenty years of MOPP therapy for Hodgkin's disease. *Journal of Clinical Oncology* **4**: 1295–306.

Majolino I, Pearce R, Taghipour G, Goldstone AH (1997) Peripheral blood stem cell transplantation versus autologous bone marrow transplantation in Hodgkin's and non-Hodgkin's lymphomas: a new matched-pair analysis of the European Group for Blood and Marrow Transplantation Registry Data. Lymphoma Working Party of the European Group for Blood and Marrow Transplantation. *Journal of Clinical Oncology* **15**: 509–17.

Ng AK, Bernardo MP, Weller E *et al.* (2002) Long-term survival and competing causes of death in patients with early-stage Hodgkin's disease treated at age 50 or younger. *Journal of Clinical Oncology* **20**: 2101–8.

Schellong G, Potter R, Bramswig J *et al.* (1999) High cure rates and reduced long-term toxicity in pediatric Hodgkin's disease: the German–Austrian multicenter trial DAL-HD-90. The German–Austrian Pediatric Hodgkin's Disease Study Group. *Journal of Clinical Oncology* **17**: 3736–44.

Schmitz N, Pfistner B, Sextro M *et al.* (2002) Aggressive conventional chemotherapy compared with high-dose chemotherapy with autologous haemopoietic stem-cell transplantation for relapsed chemosensitive Hodgkin's disease: a randomized trial. *Lancet* **359**: 2065–71.

Specht L, Gray RG, Clarke MJ, Peto R (1998) Influence of more extensive radiotherapy and adjuvant chemotherapy on long-term outcome of early-stage Hodgkin's disease: a meta-analysis of 23 randomized trials involving 3 888 patients. International Hodgkin's Disease Collaborative Group. *Journal of Clinical Oncology* **16**: 830–43.

Stein H, Marafioti T, Foss HD *et al.* (2001) Down-regulation of BOB1.OBF1 and Oct2 in classical Hodgkin's disease but not in lymphocyte predominant Hodgkin's disease correlates with immunoglobulin transcription. *Blood* **97**: 496–501.

Viviani S, Bonadonna G, Santoro A *et al.* (1996) Alternating versus hybrid MOPP and ABVD combinations in advanced Hodgkin's disease: ten-year results. *Journal of Clinical Oncology* **14**: 1424–30.

Von Wasielewski S, Franklin J, Fischer R *et al.* (2003) Nodular sclerosing Hodgkin's disease: new grading predicts prognosis in intermediate and advanced stages. *Blood* **101**: 4063–9.

CHAPTER 45

Aetiology and management of non-Hodgkin's lymphoma

45

Irit Avivi and Anthony H Goldstone

Epidemiology

Frequency

The incidence of non-Hodgkin's lymphoma (NHL) has dramatically increased since the 1950s, in both the UK and the USA (from 6.9 per 100 000 person-years in 1947–50, up to 17.4 per 100 000 in 1984–88), becoming the fifth most common cancer in the USA. This is only partially accounted for by HIV-related lymphomas, and there is suggestive, although not definitive, evidence that the role of environmental factors may be also essential.

Non-Hodgkin's lymphoma is slightly more common in males than in females, and in the USA it is more common in white people than in black people. Although NHL can occur at any age, the incidence rises considerably with age.

Geographical variations

Proportions of cases in different histological categories vary markedly from one country to another and among different racial groups. Although some of these variations may be spurious, reflecting local specifics of medical practice, real differences undoubtedly exist. For example, follicular lymphoma (FL), one of the most common NHLs in Europe and the USA, is rare in Japan and other Far Eastern countries. In contrast, HTLV-1 is much more common in the Far East (Japan) and in the Caribbean islands than Western countries.

These differences are perhaps not surprising, given the role of the immune system (from which these neoplasms arise) in constantly monitoring and reacting to antigenic factors in the environment. This must cause variations between different parts of the world in the degree to which individual cell populations in lymphoid tissue are activated, which is likely to be reflected in the frequency variations of different lymphomas.

Aetiology

In the majority of cases of NHL, the cause is not identified, although several factors are known to play a role in lymphomagenesis. A small number of lymphomas originate from chronic antigenic stimulation; for example, *Helicobacter pylori* (HP) infection appears to be a possible causative agent for the development of gastric mucosa-associated lymphoid tissue (MALT) lymphoma. Eradication of HP with antibiotics appears to be initial effective therapy for localized gastric MALT lymphoma. Similarly, infection with *Campylobacter jejuni* has been suggested recently to be associated with the development of immunoproliferative small intestinal disease (IPSID).

Viruses

Several viruses have been implicated in lymphoma pathogenesis, although none of them is directly causative in the way similar to that of the oncogenic virus inducing neoplasia in animals.

Epstein–Barr virus

Epstein–Barr virus (EBV) was first thought to be associated with lymphomagenesis following its isolation from endemic Burkitt's lymphoma tissue, but it is now known to be a major factor causing development of NHL in immunosuppressed individuals [e.g. HIV patients or those post solid-organ/allogeneic stem cell transplantation (SCT), in whom it is called post-transplant lymphoproliferative disease]. There are two forms of cellular infection by EBV: latent and replicative. In latent infection, the virus enters the cell and remains in the DNA; B cells become immortalized and acquire neoplastic potential. In replicative infection, viral particles are released from cells, whereas the cells themselves die.

It is the latent type of infection that transforms infected resting B cells into proliferating blasts. The mechanism of this remarkable effect depends on the expression of several viral latent proteins that are under control of a master transcription factor, EBV nuclear antigen 2 (EBNA-2). The pattern of viral gene expression that derives this process is called the growth programme (Table 45.1).

This process can happen in the presence of the following conditions: first, the EBV-infected cells that express the growth programme must be unable to exit the cell cycle and become resting memory B cells, and second, the cytotoxic T-cell response must be impeded, so that lymphoblasts would not be killed. Post-transplant lymphoproliferative disease (PTLD) may therefore develop when B cells (other than naive B cells) become infected and express the growth programme without being able to exit it, and continue to proliferate in the absence of effective cytotoxic T-cell response.

Epstein–Barr virus is also associated with the development of the endemic (African) type of Burkitt's lymphoma (BL), in which it is expressed by 98%. However, the exact mechanism of EBV involvement in BL development is unclear. None of the growth promoting latent genes is expressed, whereas the only detected latent protein of the virus is EBNA-1. Burkitt's lymphoma is characterized by deregulated activation of c-*MYC* oncogene (Table 45.2), resulting in a sustained proliferation mode, in which cells express EBNA-1 only. EBV may therefore have a role in the development of BL. However, given the multistep process of tumorigenesis, it is actually impossible to be sure whether the final cellular or viral phenotype of BL is related to the original infected precursor.

Human T-cell leukaemia virus type I

Adult T-cell leukaemia/lymphoma (ATLL) is a T-cell malignancy that occurs after a 40- to 60-year period of clinical

Table 45.1 Transcriptional programmes used by EBV to establish and maintain infection.

Type of infected B cells*	Programme	Genes expressed	Function of the programme
Naive cell	Growth	EBNA-1 through EBNA-6, LMP-1, LMP-2A, LMP-3B	Activated B cell
Germinal centre cell	Default	EBNA-1, LMP-1, LMP-2A	Differentiate activated B cells into memory cells
Peripheral blood memory cell	Latency	None	Allows lifetime persistence
Dividing peripheral blood memory cell		EBNA-1 only	Allows viral DNA in latency programme cell to divide
Plasma cell	Lytic	All lytic genes	Replicates virus in plasma cell

*Except where indicated, the types of cell are primarily restricted to the lymphoid tissues of Waldeyer's ring.

EBNA, EBV nuclear antigen; LMP, latent membrane protein.

From Thorley-Lawson DA, Gross A (2004), Persistence of the Epstein–Barr virus and the origins of associated lymphomas. *New England Journal of Medicine* **350**: 1328–37 with permission.

Table 45.2 Chromosomal translocations found in non-Hodgkin's lymphoma.

Translocation	Gene involved	Type of lymphoma
t(8;14)(q24;q32)	c-*MYC* and IgH	Burkitt's lymphoma
t(8;2)(p11/2;24)	c-*MYC* and Igκ	Burkitt's lymphoma
t(8;22)(q24;q11)	c-*MYC* and Igλ	Burkitt's lymphoma
t(11;14)(q24;q32)	*BCL-1* (cyclin D1) and IgH	Mantle cell
t(14;18)(q32;q21)	*BCL-2* and IgH	Follicular lymphoma
t(3;4)(q27;q32) and variants	*BCL-6* and various partners	Large B cell
t(2;5)(p23;q35)	*NPM* and *ALK*	T-cell anaplastic large cell

latency in about 3–5% of human T-cell leukaemia virus type I (HTLV-1)-infected individuals. ATLL cells are monoclonally expanded and harbour an integrated provirus. A persistent oligo/polyclonal expansion of HTLV 1-bearing cells has been shown to precede ATLL, supporting the fact that in ATLL tumour cells arise from a clonally expanding non-malignant cell.

Tax protein, encoded and expressed by an activated form of HTLV-1, rescues virus-expressing T cells from apoptotic death. This suggests that Tax protein can rescue the host cells of the activated virus from the ultimate apoptotic death, contributing to tumorigenesis.

Kaposi sarcoma-associated virus

Kaposi sarcoma-associated virus (KSHV) is the causative agent of both Kaposi sarcoma (KS) and primary effusion lymphoma (PEL). KSHV, called also HHV-8, appears to have an important role in the pathogenesis of both KS and primary effusion lymphoma (PEL), elaborating growth factors and cytokines that promote tumour growth. It encodes putative oncogenes and genes that stimulate angiogenesis and cell proliferation, including G-protein-coupled receptor-promoting cell transformation and angiogenesis and 'interleukin 6 (IL-6) homologous cytokine', preventing cell apoptosis in IL-6-dependent cell lines.

The KSHV G-protein-coupled receptor (vGPCR) is a homologue of the human IL-8 receptor that signals constitutively, activates mitogen- and stress-activated kinases, and induces transcription via multiple transcription factors, including AP-1 and nuclear factor kappa B (NF-κB). Furthermore, vGPCR causes cellular transformation *in vitro* and leads to KS-like tumours in transgenic mouse models.

KSHV also encodes a cyclin D homologue, K cyclin, which is thought to promote viral oncogenesis. The expression of K cyclin in cultured cells not only triggers cell cycle progression, but also engages the p53 tumour-suppressor pathway, which probably restricts the oncogenic potential of K cyclin.

Immunosuppression

Lymphomas, almost always of the histologically aggressive variety, have become more common in immunosuppressed patients with the discovery of AIDS and increase in solid organ

and SCT. Lymphoma has been reported to occur in 4–10% of patients with AIDS and the pathogenesis is almost certainly multifactorial. The increased risk of infections with viruses such as EBV, chronic antigen exposure and cytokine stimulation arising from repeated infections result in polyclonal B-cell activation and, therefore, a greater chance of mutations that develop randomly during mitosis. Almost all cases of central nervous system (CNS) lymphomas and Hodgkin's lymphoma diagnosed in immunosuppressed patients are EBV+.

Lymphomas develop in < 1% of allogeneic SCT recipients, although the risk is higher in the patients receiving rigorous T cell-depleted transplants followed by heavy post-graft immunosuppression (e.g. anti-thymocyte globulins, applied for graft-versus-host disease). In heart or lung transplants, the incidence of lymphomas is as high as 4–7%. Most post-transplant lymphomas are EBV related (see previous discussion on EBV-related lymphomas). At early stages, they may be polyclonal or oligoclonal and only later become monoclonal, but the clonal nature of the proliferation does not appear to predict closely the response to immunosuppression withdrawal, which may result in spontaneous remission.

Genetic and occupational factors

Several studies reported an increased risk of NHL in first-degree relatives of lymphoma (HD/NHL) probands compared with the general population. The temporal proximity of HD/HD and NHL/NHL sibling pairs argues for environmental as well as genetic aetiology.

An increased incidence of NHL has been reported in people working in agriculture, forestry, logging industries, as well as in those involved in metalworking machinery, printing and publishing industry, motor vehicles and telephone communications. The risk seems to increase with employment duration and vary by histological type.

Occupational exposure to specific chemicals, such as benzidine, mineral, cutting or lubricating oil, pesticides, herbicides and wood dust seem to play an important role in the development of NHL. However, the exact impact of these factors is still debated and their contribution to pre-existing genetic factors is not totally clear.

Cytogenetics and oncogenes

Cytogenetic analysis in non-Hodgkin's lymphoma can be difficult, given the problem of isolating neoplastic cells from tissue biopsy samples for karyotypic analysis. However, several large studies suggest that nearly all cases have a cytogenetic abnormality. It may be either numerical or structural but a number of translocations are particularly interesting because of their association with specific types of lymphoma and the insights they have provided into the process of lymphomagenesis. Rearrangements frequently involve T-cell receptor (TCR) or immunoglobulin (Ig) genes, which rearrange as part of the normal process of lymphoid differentiation (Chapter 28). In some cases, the aberrant recombination may be due to structural similarities between the regions close to the breakpoints and the heptamer/ nonamer recombinase-recognition sequences bordering the normally rearranging genes. The rearrangements typically cause deregulation (usually upregulation) of oncogenes brought under the influence of immunoglobulin TCR promoter and enhancer sequences (see Table 45.2).

There is some disagreement concerning the frequency of the t(14;18) in FLs, but most studies report its presence in about 85% of patients. Some of the discrepancies may reflect true geographical variation; for instance, in Japan the reported incidence is only 33%. The breakpoints on chromosome 18 occur at two sites, approximately 20 kb apart, within or near the transcriptional unit of the *BCL2* gene. Approximately two-thirds of the breakpoints occur within 150 basepairs, known as the 'major breakpoint region', in the 5′-untranslated region of the *BCL-2* gene, and most of the remaining breakpoints occur 3′ to this in the 'minor cluster region'. The *BCL-2* gene codes for a protein localized in the inner mitochondrial membrane, which is involved in the inhibition of apoptosis rather than the induction of proliferation. This blockage of cell death in neoplastic germinal centre cells may account for the fact that the FLs are, at least initially, slow growing.

The usual cytogenetic abnormality in Burkitt's lymphoma is a translocation involving the c-*MYC* gene on chromosome 8 and the Ig heavy-chain gene on chromosome 14, which is found in over 80% of cases. Although both the endemic and sporadic forms of Burkitt's lymphoma have the same gross translocations, there are subtle differences at the molecular level. Variant translocations involve chromosome 8 and either chromosome 2 or 22, where the breakpoints involve, respectively, kappa and lambda light-chain genes. In all cases, there is upregulation of c-*MYC*, a nuclear transcription factor involved in cell proliferation and the control of apoptosis.

The t(11l;14) translocation is found in mantle cell lymphomas. The oncogene on chromosome 11 is known as *BCL-l* or *PRAD-l*, and encodes a D-cyclin involved in cell cycle control (Table 45.2).

The *BCL-6* gene is a transcription factor of the zinc finger family, whose precise function is unknown. It has recently been suggested to maintain B cells in a germinal centre-like state, inhibiting B-cell differentiation. Rearrangements of *BCL-6* occur in over one-third of large-cell lymphomas and in an even higher number of cases mutations within the gene are found. The presence of BCL6 rearrangement has been suggested to predict favourable prognosis, although not confirmed in all studies (Table 45.2).

T-cell lymphomas are less frequent than B-cell lymphomas and have been less extensively studied at the molecular level. T-cell lymphoblastic lymphomas may have abnormalities similar to those found in T-cell acute lymphoblastic leukaemia (ALL), such as abnormalities of the *TAL-1* gene on chromosome 1, the *HOX11* gene on chromosome 10 and the *RHOMB2* gene on chromosome 11.

Anaplastic Ki-1 (CD30)-positive large-cell lymphomas are usually of T-cell origin, and in at least one-half of the cases there is a t(2;5)(p23;q35) translocation (see Figure 45.1 and Table 45.2). The genes involved in this translocation encode a receptor tyrosine kinase called anaplastic lymphoma kinase (ALK) on chromosome 2, and nucleophosmin on chromosome 5. The resulting hybrid gene encodes a hybrid protein in which about 40% of nucleophosmin is fused to the entire cytoplasmic portion of ALK. The nucleophosmin moiety not only induces ALK expression (as nucleophosmin is a ubiquitously expressed nuclear protein), but also activates the kinase through cross-linking.

Figure 45.1 Anaplastic large-cell lymphoma of T-cell type.

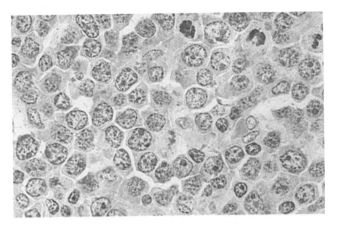

Figure 45.2 Large B-cell lymphoma. The cells are larger than normal lymphocytes and have a round nucleus with prominent nucleoli, some adjacent to the nuclear membrane ('centroblasts').

When a chromosomal translocation is frequently found in a particular lymphoma type, e.g. t(14;18) in FL, and if the breakpoint falls within a well-defined and limited region(s), polymerase chain reaction (PCR) analysis may be used either to assist in diagnosis or to detect minimal residual disease. However, the clinical significance and value of such studies have yet to be determined, as it is not completely clear what the prognostic importance may be of small numbers of cells carrying this translocation in patients who are in clinical remission.

Recently, DNA microarray technology has opened new avenues for the understanding of lymphomas. By hybridization of cDNA to arrays containing > 10 000 different DNA fragments, this approach allows simultaneous evaluation of the mRNA expression of thousands of genes in a single experiment. These data can then be used for identification of lymphoma subgroups, with a defined gene expression pattern, not previously identified by morphology, cytogenetics or molecular techniques.

This approach has already provided novel insights into different entities of B-cell NHLs; measurement of the expression of only six genes was found to be predictive of overall survival in diffuse large B-cell lymphoma (Figure 45.2) and the prognosis of FL has been related to the molecular features of tumour-infiltrating cells.

Clinical features

The median age of presentation of low-grade lymphomas and large-cell lymphomas is around 55–60 years, with a slight male predominance. In FL (Figure 45.3), the marrow is involved in about 50% of cases at diagnosis (Figure 45.4). Burkitt's lymphoma often presents with extranodal disease, appearing in the jaw in Africa, and as gastrointestinal disease or in other intra-abdominal sites in the West. Hypercalcaemia is frequent.

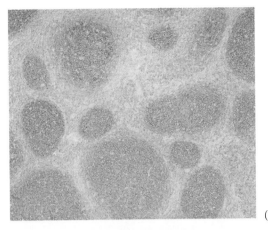

(a)

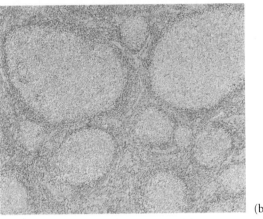

(b)

Figure 45.3 Immunostaining of follicular lymphoma showing its typical nodular appearance: (a) CD20 is expressed by the tumour cells, whereas (b) CD3 is confined to reactive T cells. (Paraffin sections: APAAP immunoalkaline phosphatase stain.)

Widespread painless lymphadenopathy is more common at presentation in NHL than in Hodgkin's disease (HD) and contiguous spread is not so apparent. Superior vena cava syndrome caused by a bulky mediastinal mass is also more frequent in NHL than in Hodgkin's lymphoma. Hepatosplenomegaly is frequent at diagnosis.

Patients with indolent histology are less likely to have B symptoms (unexplained fever of 38°C or higher, night sweats and loss of more than 10% of body weight in 6 months) than those with an aggressive histology, but this is not invariable. Some patients present with systemic symptoms without peripheral lymphadenopathy, which can result in considerable delays in diagnosis. Symptoms and signs may be due to the involvement of particular organs (e.g. skin, gastrointestinal tract, salivary glands, lungs, renal tract and central nervous system).

Lymphoblastic lymphoma usually occurs in children and young adults, often with thymic mass, systemic symptoms and bone marrow failure.

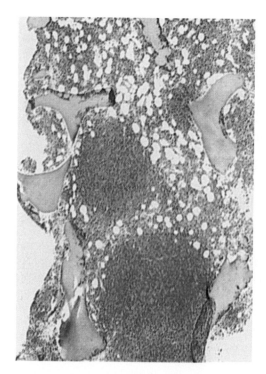

Figure 45.4 Non-Hodgkin's lymphoma in the marrow: paratrabecular localization.

Table 45.3 Prognostic factors for aggressive lymphoma: International Prognostic Index (IPI) (reproduced from *New England Journal of Medicine* (1993) **329**: 987 with permission).

Age > 60 years
Ann Arbor stage III or IV
Increased lactate dehydrogenase concentration
Performance score of > 2
Involvement of more than one extranodal site

Table 45.4 Ann Arbor staging system.

Stage I	Involvement in a single lymph node region or single extralymphatic site
Stage II	Involvement of two or more lymph node regions on the same side of the diaphragm; localized contiguous involvement of only one extralymphatic site and lymph node region (stage IIE)
Stage III	Involvement of lymph node regions on both sides of the diaphragm; may include spleen
Stage IV	Disseminated involvement of one or more extralymphatic organs with or without lymph node involvement

Laboratory investigations

Histological diagnosis from biopsy of a lymph node, bone marrow or extranodal mass is essential (Figures 45.1–45.8). Fine-needle aspiration may help to exclude or suggest lymphoma, but histological examination is essential to complete the diagnosis. Immunocytochemistry is now performed and, in specialized units, cytogenetic and immunoglobulin or TCR rearrangement analysis, as well as, more recently, DNA microarray testing.

Anaemia at diagnosis is usually indicative of widespread disease and may reflect a non-specific manifestation of malignancy. However, it can also be due to hypersplenism or bone marrow infiltration. Occasional patients, most often those with indolent histology, have an autoimmune haemolysis. The white count is variable. Overspill of lymphoma cells into the blood is relatively frequent in late stages of indolent lymphoma and can infrequently be seen by light microscopy at diagnosis. It can be detected much more frequently using PCR technique. Hypo-albuminaemia is another non-specific feature associated with a systemic disturbance and is indicative of a poor prognosis. A raised level of lactate dehydrogenase (LDH) is usually associated with advanced disease and is an important independent prognostic factor (Table 45.3). Paraproteins are found in about 15% of indolent lymphomas and in a little less than 5% of histologically aggressive lymphomas.

Staging

The Ann Arbor staging system, initially developed for Hodgkin's disease, is used in adults with NHL (Table 45.4). Inspection of Waldeyer's ring is particularly important, and a bone marrow biopsy should be performed in all patients. Although a laparotomy may sometimes be required to relieve a gut obstruction, stop a GI haemorrhage or make a diagnosis of a disease restricted to the abdomen, there is widespread agreement that a staging laparotomy is not justified. In children, the St Jude staging system is usually used. Radiography, computerized tomography (CT), magnetic resonance imaging (MRI) or positron emission tomography (PET) scanning are used for initial staging of the disease and are of value in monitoring response to therapy and detection of residual disease or relapse.

Treatment

Treatment of NHL is mainly based on the histological findings, dividing patients into two major groups: patients with indolent versus aggressive NHL. However, therapeutic decisions are also taken with regard to patient's age, performance status and disease extension (Table 45.3). There are also some special subtypes of lymphoma (e.g. CNS lymphoma, MALT lymphoma) that will be discussed separately.

Follicular lymphoma

Localized disease

Approximately 20% of follicular lymphoma (FL) patients present with non-bulky localized disease. Almost one-half of them may be cured with localized radiotherapy. MacManus and colleagues from Stanford University reviewed in 1996 the outcome of 177 FL stage I/II patients treated with radiotherapy only: 64% of these patients approached 10-year actuarial survival, whereas 44% remained disease free. Similar results were reported by the MD Anderson group, in which tumour size and Ann Arbor stage have significantly affected progression-free survival (PFS) (15-year PFS = 49% for tumour < 3 cm versus 29% for mass 3.0 cm, $P = 0.04$, and Ann Arbor stage; 66% versus 26% for stages I and II, respectively, $P = 0.006$). Ann Arbor stage has also affected the cause-specific survival ($P = 0.01$), but overall survival was apparently unaffected by the extent of the radiation field. It seems that radiotherapy can cure approximately one-half of patients with stage I and one-quarter of those with stage II FL. Patients with localized disease should therefore receive involved-field radiation without undue delay, aiming not only to eliminate their symptoms, but also to achieve disease cure.

Adding adjuvant chemotherapy to radiotherapy for localized disease

As most relapses following radiotherapy occur outside the radiation field, a reasonable approach would be to combine radiotherapy with systemic chemotherapy, aiming to reduce relapse risk and improve cure rate.

The British National Lymphoma Investigation (BNLI) has prospectively compared the outcome of 148 patients with localized low-grade lymphoma, treated with radiotherapy, with/without adjuvant continuous chlorambucil (CHL). There were no significant differences either in overall survival (OS) or in disease-free survival (DFS) between the two treatment groups (maximal follow-up = 18 years). Intensification of chemotherapy (e.g. CHOP, Table 45.5) also failed to improve patients' outcome.

However, there were some retrospective and prospective non-randomized trials that reported an improved PFS in patients treated with combined modality treatment compared with radiotherapy alone. In the MD Anderson Cancer Center, patients with low-grade lymphoma, stage I/II, were treated with 10 cycles of COP–Bleo/CHOP–Bleo (Table 45.5), followed by involved-field radiation. The 10-year PFS and OS approached 76% and 82%, respectively, which were higher than previously reported results with involved-field radiotherapy alone (Seymour *et al.*, 2003). These findings have encouraged the development of a joint phase III study by the Trans Tasman Radiation Oncology Group (TROG) and the Australasian Leukaemia and Lymphoma Group (ALLG) in which patients with clinical stage I/II FL are randomized to involved-field radiotherapy with or without six cycles of cytotoxic chemotherapy (TROG 99.03 trial – started recruitment in early 2000). However, at present there are no proven data to support the addition of chemotherapy; chemotherapy should therefore be used in such patients after relapse.

Table 45.5 Chemotherapy protocols used in NHL.

CVP	Cyclophosphamide, vincristine, prednisolone
FMC	Fludarabine/cyclophosphamide/mitoxantrone
CHOP	Cyclophosphamide, doxorubicin, vincristine, prednisolone
MACE–CYTABOM	Doxorubicin, etoposide, prednisolone, cytarabine, bleomycin, vincristine, methotrexate
MACOP B	Methotrexate, doxorubicin, cyclophosphamide, vincristine, bleomycin
m-BACOD	Methotrexate, bleomycin, doxorubicin, cyclophosphamide, vincristine, dexamethasone
ESHAP	Etoposide, cytarabine, methylprednisolone, cisplatin
Mini-BEAM	BCNU, etoposide, cytarabine, melphalan
ICE	Ifosfamide, carboplatin, and etoposide
DHAP	Dexamethasone, high-dose cytarabine and cisplatin
DVIP	Dexamethasone, etoposide, ifosfamide and cisplatin
CODOX–M/IVAC	Cyclophosphamide, doxorubicin, high-dose methotrexate/ifosfamide, etoposide and high-dose cytarabine
Hyper CVAD	Hyperfractionated cyclophosphamide, vincristine, doxorubicin and dexamethasone
ACVBP	Doxorubicin, cyclophosphamide, vindesine, bleomycin, prednisolone

Is there any place for radiotherapy in relapsed disease?

Low-dose (4 Gy) involved-field radiotherapy appears to provide a high response rate (92% overall response rate, with 61% complete responses) with durable remissions (> 1 year) in patients with relapsed disease. Low-dose radiotherapy should therefore be considered in patients with recurrent, localized disease, irrespective of their initial presentation.

Advanced disease

Patients with FL tend to have a highly variable outcome. Although some patients experience early progression and die of their disease in less than 5 years, others may have an indolent course and live for 15 years or longer. Conventional chemotherapy is, however, unable to prolong long-term survival compared with observation. In the absence of a specific therapy for an indolent disease (50% survival at 10 years), management is mainly targeted to reduce symptoms and prolong time to progression (TTP), rather than prolong survival.

Patients' quality of life and treatment-related side-effects should be carefully considered, especially in the background of an incurable disease, which occurs mainly in elderly patients whose life expectancy irrespective of diseases may be less than 20 years.

Management therefore ranges from a 'watch-and-wait' approach through different kinds of chemotherapy regimens (monoclonal antibodies applied in symptomatic patients) as far as experimental intensive therapies (autologous/allogeneic SCT) considered in younger patients aiming to prolong survival and achieve cure.

What is required is a series of complementary structured randomized studies that will give proper data over a number of years. Unfortunately, newer modalities such as monoclonal antibodies with some sort of stem cell transplant will inevitably be introduced during the lifetime of an incidental patient's disease and 'skew' the findings. It is almost impossible to study a patient over 10–15 years without allowing him/her to potentially benefit from new treatments emerging during that period.

Chemotherapy for follicular lymphoma

As mentioned above, historically treatment has been unable to prolong long-term survival. Therefore, it is mainly offered to reduce symptoms and signs of the disease and improve quality of life.

A large number of patients are asymptomatic at diagnosis. Deferral of treatment in such patients seems to have no adverse impact on survival. The BNLI has recently reported the outcome of 309 patients with asymptomatic advanced stage III/IV low-grade lymphoma, who were randomly assigned to receive oral chlorambucil 10 mg/m^2 continuously ($n = 158$) versus observation until disease progression ($n = 151$) (local radiotherapy to symptomatic enlarged lymph nodes was permitted in both arms). There was no significant difference in OS and cause-

specific survival (CSS) between the two arms. However, age below 60 years and stage III versus IV conferred a significant survival advantage. The actuarial chance of not requiring chemotherapy at 10 years was almost 20%, supporting the strategy of 'watch and wait' in these 'advanced' patients. Similarly, the Groupe d'Étude des Lymphomes Folliculaires (GELF) found no differences in overall survival between low-tumour burden patients randomized to prednimustine/interferon versus observation only. As a rule, conservative management should be considered in asymptomatic patients, keeping their quality of life without having unnecessary toxicity.

Alkylating agents

Those individuals who have symptoms can receive either oral or intravenous therapies.

Oral chlorambucil and cyclophosphamide, both alkylating agents, remain good therapies for those who do not need rapid debulking of their tumour mass. Combination chemotherapy with CVP (cyclophosphamide, vincristine, prednisolone – see Table 45.5) does not improve either overall survival or TTP compared with chlorambucil. However, with chlorambucil, response is faster, making this regimen a preferable option for patients with large tumour mass and/or significant symptoms.

Doxorubicin-containing regimens

The role of doxorubicin-containing regimens for indolent lymphoma remains unproven. The Southwestern Oncology Group (SWOG) reviewed survival data of 415 low-grade lymphoma patients treated with CHOP (see Table 45.5). Median survival in these patients approached 6.9 years, which was not higher than reported previously with less aggressive therapies. However, although several studies suggest that patients with high-grade histology (> 15 centroblasts per high-power field) do benefit from doxorubicin-containing regimens, achieving a prolonged TTP with improved overall survival, others failed to confirm this strategy.

It should be noted that part of these inconclusive results reflects changes in definitions in lymphoma grading over the last three decades, making these studies difficult to compare.

Nevertheless, there are still some patients for whom doxorubicin-containing regimens may be appropriate, although the data to support this approach remain controversial. Patients with grade III FL and those presented with constitutional symptoms, high tumour burden and elevated LDH (all parameters suggesting a more aggressive disease, despite the indolent histology) may be more appropriate for doxorubicin-containing combination.

Purine analogues

The more recent purine analogues – fludarabine, 2-chlorodeoxyadenosine (cladribine) and deoxycoformycin (pentostatin) – present a group of potently lymphotoxic antimetabolite agents, non-cross-resistant to alkylating agent therapy. Their activity in the indolent NHLs, particularly in the follicular subtype, may be due to their unique ability as antimetabolites to inhibit resting as well as dividing cells.

Several retrospective studies suggested a higher response rate with single-agent fludarabine (FLU) compared with alkylating agent-based regimens. However, prospective randomized trials failed to confirm these results, suggesting CVP/CHVP interferon to be as good as single-agent fludarabine.

Several retrospective/phase I studies have suggested that fludarabine-containing combinations (e.g. FC, fludarabine, cyclophosphamide; FND, fludarabine, mitoxantrone, dexamethasone) are superior to traditional alkylating regimens or fludarabine only, providing a higher complete response (CR) rate in both therapy-naive and relapsed patients. Other studies, however, failed to repeat these results, emphasizing the need for prospective randomized trials.

The Bologna prospective randomized trial compared the outcome of 'treatment-naive' LGL/MCL patients, treated with FLU for 5 days versus fludarabine–idarubicin (FLU–ID) (FLU for 3 days, idarubicin, ID, 12 mg/m^2 on day 1). There was no difference in response rate between the two arms, but remission duration was significantly longer in those who received FLU–ID therapy ($P = 0.021$). However, it is unclear if this improvement translates into an improved survival, and it may increase treatment-related toxicity, particularly opportunistic infections that may sometimes be extremely severe. A phase III ECOG trial comparing fludarabine (25 mg/m^2, days 1–5) and cyclophosphamide (1000 mg/m^2, day 1) with CVP was prematurely closed as a result of excess deaths in the fludarabine arm.

Fludarabine does cause immunosuppression – resulting in increased incidence of opportunistic infection necessitating prophylaxis against *Pneumocystis carinii*. It may also cause myelosuppression and adversely affect stem cell harvesting. However, it is usually well tolerated and, as the introduction of an oral formulation, its use has become much easier. Several studies performed in patients with chronic lymphocytic leukaemia (CLL) and low-grade lymphoma, confirmed oral fludarabine to be as effective as the intravenous formulation.

Side-effects of chemotherapy

Chemotherapy-related side-effects should be seriously considered, taking into account the historical inability of chemotherapy to improve patients' survival. Chemotherapy may adversely affect quality of life, causing myelosuppression and immunosuppression with increased risk of infections. Myelodysplastic changes and increased risk of leukaemia were mainly reported with alkylating agents; however, these may also be associated with fludarabine. For young patients, infertility may be a primary concern of treatment.

Interferon

Recombinant interferon-alpha (IFN-α) has been used simultan-

eously with initial cytotoxic chemotherapy or as a maintenance therapy in patients who responded to initial chemotherapy aiming to enhance immunological response and prolong survival.

Interferon with induction chemotherapy

Several prospective randomized trials have compared the activity of IFN-α-containing regimens versus chemotherapy. Two studies only, both using anthracycline-containing regimens, revealed a statistically significant improved time to treatment failure (TTF) and DFS in those who received IFN as part of induction chemotherapy. A meta-analysis presented at the meeting of the American Society of Clinical Oncology in 1998 showed a statistically significantly longer survival in patients with high tumour mass, treated with anthracycline-containing regimens and high-dose IFN (5 megaunits, three times per week).

Interferon maintenance therapy

Although several prospective trials failed to show any survival advantage with IFN-α maintenance therapy, two observed a significantly prolonged remission duration ($P > 0.001$) and improved OS in patients who received IFN compared with those who had no maintenance treatment ($P > 0.001$). Both of these studies used a relatively high dose of IFN (5 megaunits, three times per week) for at least 1 year, suggesting that high-dose and long maintenance therapy is effective. IFN therefore remains a consideration for therapy but the optimal dose and duration of treatment are still unclear and, given the potential side effects, usage at present may be less attractive than other options.

Monoclonal antibodies

Although response rates and PFS may have improved slightly, the overall survival has not increased, and advanced indolent NHL remains essentially incurable without allogeneic bone marrow transplant. A number of new ways of outcome improvement are being investigated, including monoclonal antibodies (MAbs) targeted against specific antigens expressed by lymphoma cells (Table 45.6).

The cell-surface antigen CD20 is in many ways an ideal target as it is expressed by 95% of B-cell NHL cases but not on haemopoietic stem cells; it has a functional role in B-cell growth and also does not normally circulate as a free antigen in plasma, so the free antigen does not compete for antibody binding.

Rituximab is an anti-CD20 chimeric MAb which was the first approved for NHL treatment. Response is achieved through several mechanisms, including complement-dependent cytotoxicity (CDC), antibody-dependent cellular cytotoxicity (ADCC) and induction of apoptosis. Rituximab is also able to sensitize lymphoma cells to the cytotoxic activity of chemotherapy.

Previously untreated low-grade lymphoma

Single-agent therapy with rituximab appears to be effective in previously untreated low-grade NHL patients, yielding a high response rate of 62–73%, including 20–44% CRs.

Table 45.6 Monoclonal antibodies in NHL.

Antibody	Antigen	Conjugate
Rituximab (IDEC-C2B8: rituxan)	CD20	None
Alemtuzumab (Campath-1H)	CD52	None
HII2 (Epratuzumab)	CD22	None
Hu1D10 (Apolizumab Remitogen)	HLA-DR	None
Ibritumomab tiuxetan (IDEC-Y2B8: Zevalin)	CD20	^{90}Y
Tositumomab (Bexxar)	CD20	^{131}I
Immunotoxins	CD19, CD22	*Pseudomonas*
Ricin A, Shiga toxin		Exotoxin A (PE38)

Extended therapy has been suggested to be better than rituximab induction alone. A phase III trial comparing rituximab maintenance therapy with observation only (following rituximab induction) showed a significantly improved PFS in those who received rituximab maintenance, with no increase in treatment-related adverse events (Gianni *et al.*, 2003). Whether maintenance with rituximab to these complete responders can prolong survival remains to be seen.

The single-agent activity of rituximab, coupled with its distinct mechanisms of action, non-overlapping toxicity and ability to sensitize lymphoma cells to cytotoxic activity, has encouraged researchers to evaluate its combinations with chemotherapy. In a phase II trial, rituximab plus chemotherapy (CHOP or CVP) has demonstrated significant activity, achieving a high response rate of 97% (including 57% CR) in 82 patients with previously untreated FL.

A characteristic chromosomal translocation t(14;18), leading to an overexpression of *bcl-2*, an anti-apoptotic gene that may serve as a survival factor for lymphoma cells, is carried by 85% of patients with FL, and it can be detected by PCR. Achievement of molecular remission post therapy (clearance of *bcl-2*$^+$ cells) appears to be associated with prolonged PFS and may even predict a longer OS. Various chemotherapy regimens (e.g. FND–R, fludarabine, novantrone, dexamethasone; CHOP–R) have yielded similar results, reporting molecular remissions with prolonged PFS. Rituximab-containing chemotherapy regimens appear to increase both clinical and molecular remission rates when compared with those usually achieved with chemotherapy only, giving grounds for optimism.

An open multicentre randomized phase III study, comparing CVP (cyclophosphamide, vincristine, prednisolone) with CVP–rituximab (R-CVP) in previously untreated patients with FL stage III/IV, has recently confirmed R-CVP to be superior to CVP only, providing a significantly higher overall response rate (81% versus 57%, with 40% CRs versus 10% respectively: $P < 0.0001$) and prolonged TTF and TTP compared with CVP alone ($P < 0.0001$ for both parameters).

Relapsed low-grade lymphoma

Single-agent rituximab is also effective in relapsed disease, providing responses in 38–59% of patients, including CR in up to 28%. The pivotal trial in this setting reported an overall response rate (ORR) of 48%, with a median TTP of 13 months in responders (McLaughlin *et al.*, 1998). Nevertheless, responses are not durable and patients eventually relapse. Attempts to improve PFS by extending rituximab treatment or combining rituximab with chemotherapy are being undertaken at present. A study by the German Low-Grade Lymphoma Study Group is comparing the combination of fludarabine, cyclophosphamide and mitoxantrone (FCM) with rituximab plus FCM in patients with relapsed follicular and mantle cell lymphoma (MCL). Interim analyses showed an ORR of 83% in the immunochemotherapy arm compared with 53% for FCM alone, indicating that combined modality treatment may be superior to chemotherapy alone.

Many studies now suggest that combination immunochemotherapy may be more effective than single-agent rituximab or chemotherapy alone and thus this treatment may be offered to patients with relapsed disease who can tolerate a combined regimen. Results of prospective comparative trials are still needed, however, to confirm the superiority of this strategy.

New unconjugated antibodies and combinations of monoclonal antibodies

New MAbs directed at different antigens expressed by lymphoma cells are being investigated at present (anti-CD22, hLL2, epratuzumab; anti-DR, Hu1D10, remitogen, apolizumab and anti-CD19 MAbs; see Table 45.6). Hu1D10 is a humanized MAb, directed at a polymorphic determinant (1D10 antigen) on the HLA-DR β-chain expressed by normal and malignant B cells. A recent study found that it was well tolerated and effective in some patients with FL who did not respond to rituximab. Response occurred on day 100+ and was occasionally accompanied by development of new anti-lymphoma antibodies, detected months after Hu1D10 had cleared.

Alemtuzumab (Campath-1-H), directed against CD52, may be used in both B- and T-cell NHL. An increased risk of opportunistic infection (related to T-cell depletion) may limit its use.

Combination of monoclonal antibodies

Combined MAbs directed at different antigens may have a synergistic effect, leading to increased response rate. Various combinations are being investigated (e.g. rituximab and alemtuzumab, rituximab and anti-CD22: epratuzumab). Data are still too limited to draw final conclusions about their potential toxicity and efficacy. In summary, there is little doubt about the efficacy of rituximab in FL, but there is still doubt as to whether

Table 45.7 Characteristics of currently available radioimmunoconjugates used in NHL.

Characteristics	^{131}I	^{90}Y
Emission	β and γ	β
Half-life	8 days	2.5 days
Energy	–	× 5
Imaging	Can be used for radioimmunoscintigraphy	Cannot be used for radioimmunoscintigraphy by conventional methods*
Stability	Rapid degradation after endocytosis	Retained stable by tumour cells after endocytosis
Hospitalization	Hospitalization	Outpatient*

*As a result of having no γ emission.

Table 45.8 Potential problems for using radioimmunoconjugates.

Needs a special knowledge and can be given by an expert only
Treatment with ^{131}I (emitting γ-particles) hospitalization for isolation
Accumulative toxicity may limit future stem cell harvesting
Long-term toxicity unknown (possibility of secondary malignancies)

any treatment significantly modifies the ultimate duration of disease.

Radiolabelled monoclonal antibodies (radioimmunoconjugates)

Lymphoma cells are sensitive to radiation, which makes them an ideal target for immunoradiotherapy. The radioimmunoconjugates kill tumour cells predominantly by radioactive emission and can therefore be effective in patients who do not respond to unconjugated antibodies (e.g. rituximab). The β-particles emitted by ^{131}I and ^{90}Y radioisotopes have high penetration (over many cell diameters), allowing eradication of tumour cells that are not expressing the targeted antigen but are adjacent to target CD20+ cells; this is known as 'crossfire' effect.

The most common radioisotopes are ^{131}I (β/γ-emitter) and ^{90}Y (a pure β-emitter) (Table 45.7). Although ^{131}I is inexpensive and easily conjugated, ^{90}Y has five times more energy, a longer path length and a shorter half-life than ^{131}I (2.5 days versus 8 days). A potential problem with pure β-emitters (e.g. ^{90}Y) is that dosimetry is relatively complicated. However, pure β-emitters can be given to outpatients, as there is no radiation risk for those who come into contact with them. This risk is substantially higher with γ-particles (^{131}I) (Table 45.8).

Radioimmunoconjugates in patients with relapsed disease

During the past decade, two products directed against CD20 antigen – ^{131}I-labelled tositumomab and ^{90}Y-labelled ibritumomab tiuxetan – have been studied. Both products have produced response rates of 70–80% in patients with relapsed/

treatment-naive low-grade lymphoma, and 50–60% in low-grade lymphoma that has transformed into an intermediate or high-grade lymphoma. Median duration of response to a single course of treatment approached 1 year. The treatment was well tolerated. However, prolonged myelosuppression with a potential risk of long-term myelodysplastic syndrome/myelogenous leukaemia was noted (Witzig et al., 2003). A phase III trial, comparing rituximab with ^{90}Y-labelled ibritumomab tiuxetan in patients with relapsed/refractory low-grade lymphoma/transformed B-cell NHL, confirmed the efficacy of radioimmunoconjugates, showing a higher response rate in those who received ^{90}Y-labelled ibritumomab tiuxetan. There was no difference in median TTP, but durable responses (≥ 6 m) were more frequent in the radioimmunotherapy arm. Radioimmunoconjugates can even be effective in those who failed to respond to non-conjugated MAbs.

Radioimmunoconjugates in therapy-naive patients

The Southwest Oncology Group (SWOG) has recently reviewed the outcome of 90 previously untreated FL patients (Press et al., 2003), treated with six cycles of CHOP followed by tositumomab/^{131}I-tositumomab (SWOG, Phase II trial, S9911). ORR was 90% (including 67% CRs) and 2-year PFS and OS were 81% and 97% respectively. Based on these encouraging results, SWOG has recently conducted a phase III prospective randomized trial, comparing CHOP–R with CHOP–tositumomab/^{131}I-tositumomab (S0016, ongoing trial).

Immunotoxins

Immunotoxins are specific antibodies connected to toxins through a linker that is easily cleavable on the malignant cell surface but stable while the toxin circulates in the blood. For the immunotoxin to be effective, the antigen should be expressed extensively on the surface of the targeted cell, and should be able to be internalized in response to antibody binding so that the toxin can kill the cell. The most commonly used toxins – ricin A, diphtheria, *Pseudomonas* exotoxin A (PE) and Shiga-like toxin-1 – kill by inhibiting protein synthesis. The efficacy and safety of most of these immunotoxins have yet to be proven. However, an anti-CD22 immunotoxin (RFB4 (dsFv)-PE38 (BL22)) has been recently reported to be extremely potent in hairy cell leukaemia (HCL) patients who failed 2-CDA. As CD22 antigen is expressed by other lymphoproliferative disorders (i.e. MCL and DLCL), BL22 immunotoxin may also be applied in these patients.

Stem cell transplantation in low-grade non-Hodgkin's lymphoma

Autologous stem cell transplantation

There are increasing data suggesting autologous stem cell transplantation (ASCT) to be valuable in FL patients beyond CR1. The only prospective trial that compared SCT with observation in patients who obtained CR/PR following second-line chemotherapy, revealed an improved PFS and OS in transplanted patients (Schouten et al., 2003). Bierman and colleagues (2003), on behalf of the EBMT/EBMTR and ABMTR, have recently reported increased survival in NHL patients treated with syngeneic SCT compared with allogeneic transplantation, suggesting high-dose therapy (HDT) to be highly effective. Furthermore, FL patients who received unpurged autografts had a five-times higher risk of relapse ($P = 0.008$) than recipients of syngeneic transplants, and recipients of unpurged autografts had a significantly increased relapse risk ($P = 0.0009$) compared with patients who received purged autografts, indicating SCT purging to be potentially valuable in these patients. DFS and OS were significantly better with purged versus unpurged autograft, $P = 0.003$ and $P = 0.04$ respectively.

Despite these encouraging results, there is still need for data from prospective randomized trials to confirm the beneficial effect of HDT and SCT purging on OS and DFS. The optimum timing of SCT (CR1 or beyond) remains to be determined by the ongoing randomized multicentre trial of the German Low-grade Lymphoma Study Group.

Non-conjugated monoclonal antibodies, radioimmunoconjugates and autologous stem cell transplantation

It is well established that conventional chemotherapy does not prolong survival in patients with low-grade lymphoma. However, ASCT may improve PFS, and most FL patients will eventually relapse due to contamination of the harvest product with lymphoma cells or re-growth of malignant cells that survived the HDT. Molecular remission before transplant appears to be linked to increase PFS. Therefore, it is tempting to try to purge the stem cells before transplantation, to minimize harvest contamination and reduce relapse risk. Similarly, it might be a reasonable approach to add rituximab post transplant (mopping up), aiming to eradicate residual cells that survived high-dose chemotherapy (ongoing EBMT Lym1 study). The efficacy of both stem cell purging/post-transplant 'mopping-up' is still debated, and results from prospective randomized trials are awaited.

Radioimmunoconjugates may also be used as part of ASCT in NHL, enabling the delivery of higher radiotherapy doses without significantly increasing treatment-related toxicity. Major studies were mainly performed in patients with high-grade lymphoma. However, there will be a role in low-grade lymphoma if proven to be effective and safe.

Allogeneic stem cell transplantation in low-grade lymphoma

Advanced low-grade lymphomas are usually incurable with conventional-dose chemotherapy. It is uncertain whether cures are possible with HDT and bone marrow transplant from a human leucocyte antigen (HLA)-identical sibling. Recent data from several studies suggest that allogeneic SCT is potentially curative (Bierman et al., 2003), although the existence of a strong graft-versus-leukaemia (GvL) effect remains uncertain and treatment-related mortality (TRM) remains high.

Low-intensity stem cell transplantation (LI SCT) is being increasingly used for various kinds of haematological malignancies, aiming to exploit the curative potential of ASCT by inducing graft-versus-tumour effect without the morbidity and mortality associated with conventional transplantation. Several studies have recently suggested this approach to be less toxic and potentially curable in patients with low-grade lymphoma. However, data are still premature and need further evaluation with a longer follow-up.

Suggested algorithm for therapy of low-grade non-Hodgkin's lymphoma (mostly follicular lymphoma)

At diagnosis
Localized disease
Use of involved-field radiation.

Disseminated disease (stage III/IV)
Asymptomatic patient In asymptomatic patients a 'watch and wait' policy is generally appropriate. Younger patients with advanced asymptomatic disease my be considered for clinical trials (e.g. BNLI trial: rituximab in patients with stage III/IV asymptomatic FL).

Symptomatic patient Use of chemotherapy and/or immunotherapy to relieve symptoms. Treatment regimen should be chosen according to patient's performance status and age. Data regarding upfront SCT (performed in CR1) are still scanty, but there is some evidence to suggest that it may have a role, although this has to be confirmed in prospective randomized trials.

Relapsed disease At the time of relapse it is important to evaluate patients' symptoms and rule out biological progression as identified by histological evidence of progression, asynchronous growth in prior disease sites, appearance of B symptoms and high LDH. Patients who have previously achieved a prolonged response to alkylating agents may be retreated, whereas those who failed to respond or progressed quickly may benefit from purine analogue-based therapies. The addition of MAbs may improve results even further. Histological evidence of transformation or clinical suspicion of more aggressive disease indicates the need for anthracycline-containing regimens.

Further intensification of treatment ASCT should be particularly considered in those who have an histological evidence of transformation. ASCT may be valuable in patients beyond CR1, providing a prolonged DFS and OS. Younger patients with progressive disease may be considered for allogeneic SCT, the only potentially curative therapy for patients with advanced disease. Useful outcomes have been seen in patients undergoing allogeneic SCT after failure of autograft but TRM remains an issue.

Marginal zone B-cell lymphoma (Figure 45.5)

The term 'marginal zone lymphoma' (MZL) is actually referring to three closely related lymphoma subtypes, including nodal, primary splenic and extranodal lymphomas of mucosa-associated lymphoid tissue (MALT) (see Chapter 43).

These lymphomas are characterized by mature B cells, lacking expression of CD5 and CD10. MALT lymphoma is described below in 'extranodal disease' (Figure 45.5).

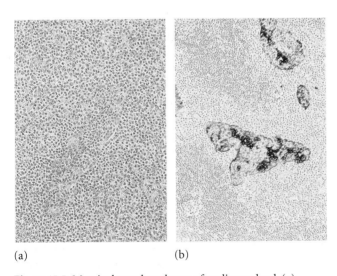

(a)   (b)

Figure 45.5 Marginal zone lymphoma of a salivary gland. (a) Sheets of marginal zone B cells and formation of a lymphoepithelial lesion. (b) Immunoperoxidase stain for low molecular weight cytokeratin (MNF116) shows positive staining of normal epithelial cells infiltrated by lymphoma.

Splenic marginal zone lymphoma (with or without villous lymphocytes) and nodal variant

Splenic MZL often presents as splenomegaly with bone marrow and peripheral blood involvement, whereas lymph nodes/extranodal sites are usually spared. Splenic MZL is characterized by micronodular infiltration of the spleen with marginal-zone differentiation; the immunophenotype is usually IgM^+ $IgD^{+/-}$ cytoplasmic$^-$ $Ig^{-/+}$ pan B antigens$^+$ $CD5^-$ $CD10^-$ $CD23^-$ $CD43^{-/+}$ cyclin $D1^-$. It generally tends to have an indolent course; however, autoimmune complications are often associated with tumour progression, with increase of blastic forms and shorter survival. To date, no definitive curative therapy has been established.

Splenectomy is considered to be the treatment of choice for symptomatic patients (pain, cytopenias), resulting in correction of pancytopenia and improvement of life quality (see Chapter 38).

The utility of purine analogues and anti-CD20 antibodies has to be clarified in prospective trials, although retrospective data suggest those modalities to be effective.

Waldenström's macroglobulinaemia

Waldenström's macroglobulinaemia (WM) represents a clonal expansion of post-germinal centre lymphoid cells expressing IgM, CD19 and CD20. High IgM levels may cause hyperviscosity syndrome, manifested with shortness of breath.

Patient management ranges from 'wait and see' for asymptomatic patients, through various types of chemotherapy agents (e.g. alkylating agents with/without steroids, purine nucleoside analogues), monoclonal antibodies (e.g. rituximab) and immunomodulators (e.g. thalidomide), to autologous/allogeneic SCT. Patients presenting with hyperviscosity also need adjuvant plasmapheresis.

Chemotherapy of Waldenström's macroglobulinaemia

Treatment of WM has been dependent on alkylating agents (e.g. chlorambucil) for years, resulting in 60% response rate with a median survival of about 60 months. Purine analogues (e.g. fludarabine and cladribine) appear to be active in both previously untreated patients and those who fail to respond to alkylating agents/relapsed disease, providing response rates of 38–85% and 30–50% respectively.

The only prospective randomized trial comparing an alkylating containing regimen (cyclophosphamide, doxorubicin, prednisolone – CAP) with fludarabine for patients with relapsed/primary refractory disease, observed an improved PFS in those who received fludarabine. There are still no prospective randomized data comparing these strategies as first-line therapy.

Monoclonal antibodies

Waldenström's macroglobulinaemia is a low-grade lymphoplasmacytoid lymphoma characterized by CD20 expression on malignant cells. Several studies have shown rituximab to be active in WM, providing responses in up to 35% of previously untreated patients. However, rituximab can cause a sudden rise in serum IgM and viscosity levels in certain patients, which may lead to complications; therefore, close monitoring of these parameters and symptoms of hyperviscosity is recommended during therapy. Similarly, Zevalin (^{90}Y-ibritumomab tiuxetan) is likely to be effective and a phase I trial evaluating this MAb in patients with WM is ongoing.

Stem cell transplantation for Waldenström's macroglobulinaemia

Several small studies reported encouraging results with ASCT in heavily pretreated patients, providing high response rates (95%), with improved PFS in some patients. Allogeneic SCT does produce prolonged remissions with potential cures compared with autograft, but TRM approaches 40%. Future strategies in WM will include a plan to evaluate the role of HDT along with biological agents (e.g. rituximab purging), maintenance strategies (including immunotherapy) and evaluation of non-myeloablative regimens containing fludarabine to achieve higher response rates and improve survival.

Novel therapies

The accumulating evidence regarding the efficacy of thalidomide in myeloma encouraged investigators to explore its activity in WD. Dimopoulos and colleagues reported a response rate of 25% in heavily pretreated patients, treated with thalidomide, whereas combination therapy with thalidomide, dexamethasone and clarithromycin resulted in a higher response rate, approaching 40–83% (Coleman et al., 2003).

The potential role of immune modulatory drugs (revimid, actimid) is being investigated at present. However, the number of patients included in these studies was small and further studies are needed to confirm thalidomide activity in WM. Several emerging therapies, including the proteasome inhibitor PS-341; inhibitors of the heatshock protein 90 (hsp90) molecular chaperone (e.g. geldanamycin and its analogues); histone deacetylase inhibitors (e.g. suberoylanilide hydroxamic acid) are all being explored as potential agents for WM. These agents induce growth arrest and apoptosis of WM cells. A combination of these agents with chemotherapy may increase treatment efficacy, inhibiting diverse pathways that are important for tumour growth and survival.

Guidelines for Waldenström's macroglobulinaemia

The International Workshop on WM has recently published its recommendations for the treatment of patients with WM (Gertz et al., 2003).

1 Alkylating agents, nucleoside analogues (e.g. cladribine and fludarabine) and rituximab are reasonable choices for first-line therapy of WM. Combinations of alkylating agents, nucleoside analogues or rituximab should at this time be encouraged in the context of a clinical trial.

2 Patients with relapsed disease can be treated with an alternative first-line agent or re-use of the same agent. Thalidomide with/without chemotherapy can also be considered at relapse.

3 ASCT may be considered for patients with refractory or relapsing disease. (However, patients considered for ASCT may fail mobilization following treatment with alkylator or nucleoside analogue.)

4 Allogeneic transplantation should only be undertaken in the context of a clinical trial. Plasmapheresis should be considered as interim therapy until definitive therapy can be initiated.

5 Splenectomy is rarely indicated but has been used to manage painful splenomegaly and hypersplenism.

Hairy cell leukaemia (see also Chapter 38)

Hairy cell leukaemia (HCL) is an uncommon B-cell chronic lymphoproliferative disorder characterized by an indolent course. The majority of patients do require therapy, having life-threatening infections due to pancytopenia or symptomatic splenomegaly. During the last 20 years, remarkable progress has been made in the treatment of HCL. Splenectomy, which used to be the treatment of choice, is rarely being used since the introduction of interferon alpha (IFN-α) in 1984. However, most interferon-induced responses are partial and not durable.

Purine analogues (cladribine, pentostatin) provide durable complete responses in the majority of patients, making these agents the treatment of choice, whereas IFN-α is reserved at present for those who fail to respond to purine analogues. Purine analogues are capable of re-inducing complete remissions in many of those who relapse.

Patients who fail to respond to purine analogues/IFN can be successfully treated with unconjugated/conjugated MAbs (recombinant immunotoxins), targeted against various antigens expressed by tumour cells. Rituximab has been recently shown to have variable activity in patients with relapsed/refractory HCL, providing responses in 25–80% of them. Two recombinant immunotoxins, BL22 and LMB-2, targeting CD22 and CD25 respectively, have demonstrated to be active in patients with HCL resistant to purine analogues. BL22 was reported to induce complete remissions (CRs) in the majority of patients with cladribine-resistant HCL.

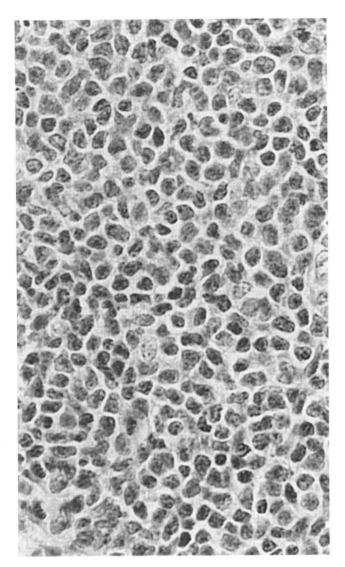

Figure 45.6 Irregular small lymphoid cells (small cleaved cells; centrocytes) typical of mantle cell lymphomas.

Mantle cell lymphoma (Figure 45.6)

Conventional chemotherapy regimens do improve PFS, but can rarely lead to cure. None of the following chemotherapeutic regimens – CVP, CHOP, fludarabine – seems to be significantly better than any other, providing an OS of only 3–4 years. The addition of rituximab to these regimens appears to result in increased remission rate. In a recent publication, CHOP–rituximab yielded a response rate of more than 90%, including 48% CR rate. However, PFS remains unsatisfactory, similar to that reported with CHOP.

Autologous ASCT in first CR may be beneficial, although a high proportion of patients will still relapse following trans-

plant. Pretransplant immunological *ex vivo* purging has been suggested to improve patient outcome. Results were disappointing and the chances for patients to achieve molecular remission (MR) in the bone marrow harvest product were less than 15%.

Magni and colleagues (2000) have reported encouraging results with *in vivo* purging in mantle cell lymphoma (MCL) patients. Fifteen patients with NHL (including seven with newly diagnosed MCL and eight with relapsed FL/other low-grade lymphoma) were prospectively treated with two cycles of intensive chemotherapy, each one followed by two doses of rituximab. This regimen included two sessions of stem cell harvest and four sessions of stem cell re-infusion, carried out between chemotherapy courses. Results were compared with those of 10 matched patients who were treated concurrently with the same regimen, but without rituximab; 14 out of 15 patients in the 'high-dose rituximab' group achieved PCR-negative harvests, compared with 40% in the control group ($P = 0.007$). A recent update of this study (Gianni *et al.*, 2003) confirmed durable remissions (median follow up at 54 months), with an OS and EFS of 89% and 79%, respectively, compared with 42% and 18% in 35 age-matched historical control subjects, treated with chemotherapy only. Other groups have reported similar results.

Mopping up post transplant may also be useful, increasing the MR rate achieved with an autograft. The feasibility of both methods is being studied at present, with newly diagnosed MCL treated with CHOP–rituximab, followed by an autograft with post-transplant rituximab. An update of this ongoing phase II study has suggested increased molecular remission (MR) rate following rituximab maintenance (Mangel *et al.*, 2002). Pre- and post-transplant rituximab increases the MR rate obtained with autograft; however, the follow-up is still too short to confirm any survival advantage with both strategies.

The optimal timing for pretransplant purging/post-transplant rituximab, as well as the duration of the treatment are under investigation. New intensified chemotherapy regimens that include rituximab but preclude HDT–autograft, may provide the same response rate as observed with 'rituximab–HDT' regimens. Longer follow-up is needed to confirm the role of rituximab–HDT as part of the management of MCL.

Aggressive B-cell NHL

Treatment of diffuse large-cell lymphoma (DLCL) is mainly based on anthracycline-containing combinations, with or without adjuvant radiotherapy. However, there are some variations in treatment related to patient's age, performance status, number of poor prognostic factors at presentation (Table 45.3) and the presence of extranodal involvement (e.g. testis, Waldeyer's ring, bone marrow).

A large international trial suggested that in patients under 60 years of age, the presence of two of the following risk factors – raised LDH, stage III or IV and poor performance status

– predicts a lower chance to achieve CR and increased risk of relapse (Table 45.5).

Stage I disease

Overall survival in patients with 'laparotomy-confirmed' non-bulky localized disease (stage I/II) approaches 80% at 10 years from diagnosis. Local radiotherapy can be curative in up to 90% of patients with 'laparotomy-confirmed' stage I/IE disease. The majority of patients with 'clinically confirmed stage I/IE' do have occult disease in other areas (undetected without laparotomy), however, causing disease relapse outside the radiation field. The British National Lymphoma Investigation (BNLI) reported a 10-year DFS and OS of 45% and 67% respectively, in 243 patients who were treated with local radiotherapy for stage I/IE disease. In patients younger than 60 years ($n = 140$), the actuarial cause specific death approached 80%. It is therefore quite clear that local radiotherapy is insufficient and systemic treatment such as chemotherapy is necessary.

Shenkier and colleagues (2002) have suggested treating such patients with a brief chemotherapy course (three cycles of anthracycline-containing regimen) followed by radiotherapy, reporting a 10-year actuarial overall and progression-free survival rates of 63% and 74%, respectively, which is higher than previously reported with radiotherapy only. A prospective randomized trial, comparing both strategies, has also reported a significantly improved DFS and OS in patients who received combined modality treatment.

Stage II–IV disease

Patients with more advanced stages of disease should receive combination chemotherapy. It is now over 30 years since the doxorubicin-containing CHOP regimen was first introduced. Despite a CR rate of 60–70%, less than 40% remain disease free at 5 years from diagnosis. Since that time, different chemotherapy regimens have been introduced (e.g. MACOP–B, m-BACOD; Table 45.5), however, none of them has proved to be superior to CHOP. Several prospective studies have failed to show any advantage of intensified regimens over CHOP, supporting the continued usage of CHOP in B-cell DLCL. A study performed by the Eastern Cooperative Oncology Group (ECOG), comparing CHOP with m-BACOD in patients with stage III/IV disease, showed no difference in CR rate or OS between the two arms, whereas m-BACOD was more toxic. Similarly, a collaborative study of the Southwestern Oncology Group/Eastern Cooperative Oncology Group, comparing CHOP with three different intensified regimens (MACOP–B, m-BACOD and Pro–MACECytabom) showed no survival advantage of any of these regimens compared with CHOP.

Mature data from the BNLI trial, comparing CHOP with PACEBOM, have shown a survival advantage of PACEBOM in patients younger than 50 years ($P = 0.002$) and in those who had stage IV disease ($P = 0.02$), suggesting that an etoposide-containing multiagent weekly regimen may be superior to CHOP (Linch et al., 2000).

However, it should be noted that most of these phase III studies compared CHOP with various chemotherapy regimens that contained a lower dose of doxorubicin and/or cyclophosphamide – two of the most potent drugs in diffuse large B-cell lymphoma (DLCL) therapy, which may partially explain the inferiority of these combinations.

In contrast, intensified CHOP (escalated dose of cyclophosphamide/doxorubicin and/or shorter duration between cycles, with/without additional drugs; e.g. MTX/cytarabine) appears to increase CR rate and improve DFS. Several phase II studies have recently suggested these regimens to be highly potent and well tolerated, indicating the need for a phase III study to confirm its superiority compared with conventional CHOP. It is still unclear whether biweekly CHOP is preferable to dose-escalated CHOP; however, recent data from the Japanese Clinical Oncology Group prospective trial suggest both variants to be effective, but biweekly CHOP may be less toxic (Itoh et al., 2002).

Adjuvant immunotherapy has been suggested to improve patients' outcome. A prospective randomized trial in 399 elderly patients with previously untreated DLCL demonstrated a significant advantage for CHOP–R over CHOP alone (Coiffier et al., 2002). Patients in the CHOP–R group had a higher CR rate (75% versus 63%, $P = 0.005$), improved PFS (2-year disease progression of 9% versus 22%, $P = 0.007$; 2-year relapse rate of 14% versus 25%, $P = 0.002$) and increased OS (2-year OS 70% versus 57%, $P = 0.007$), with no significant increase in treatment-related toxicity. This study identified CHOP–R as the gold standard therapy in elderly patients with DLCL.

In contrast, the intergroup 4944 trial, comparing CHOP–R versus CHOP followed by rituximab (R) maintenance for elderly patients with DLCL, failed to show any differences in overall response rate or in early progression (6 months) between the two arms of induction (CHOP and CHOP–R). However, induction with CHOP–R (followed by R maintenance or observation) significantly prolonged time to treatment failure (TTF), whereas R maintenance also significantly prolonged TTF in responders. This advantage appeared limited to patients induced with CHOP alone. There was no significant difference in OS at 2.7 years' follow-up. It should be noted that this trial, in contrast to the GELA study, was not designed to directly compare CHOP–R with CHOP. Furthermore, rituximab in induction was applied differently, which might explain the differences between the two studies. Results of a similar ongoing study, comparing CHOP with CHOP–R in younger patients, are awaited.

Prophylactic therapy to the central nervous system

Patients with DLCL who present with a high International Prognostic Index (IPI) (particularly those with high LDH and/or extranodal disease) are at higher risk for CNS relapse and should therefore receive CNS prophylactic therapy (see CNS prophylaxis, below).

Adjuvant radiotherapy

The role of adjuvant radiotherapy in DLCL remains controversial. Although this kind of radiotherapy is recommended at present for patients with stage I/II disease, it is unclear if adjuvant radiotherapy has any benefit in patients with advanced (stage III–IV) bulky disease, who had completed six to eight cycles of systemic combination chemotherapy. Several retrospective and one prospective randomized study, addressing this issue, suggested that adjuvant radiotherapy may be valuable, providing that an improved DFS and OS compared with chemotherapy alone.

Nieder and colleagues (2003) have recently proposed guidelines for radiotherapy in DLCL, based both on their experience and on the available literature. According to their recommendations, a tumour of less than 3.5 cm (possibly < 6 cm) can be treated with 30 or 30.6 Gy after achieving CR. Tumours of 7–10 cm may need a higher dose, i.e. 40 Gy, whereas larger masses may need up to 45 Gy. Adjuvant radiotherapy may improve both PFS and OS, reducing relapse rate in the irradiated field. Radiation may cause short/long-term side-effects; therefore, minimal effective doses should be delivered, aiming to minimize toxicity (salivary glands, orbital structures, lung, heart, etc.).

'Up-front' autologous stem cell transplantation

The role of up-front ASCT (performed in CR1 in patients with very high risk DLCL) is still controversial. The UKLG LY02 prospective randomized trial compared the outcome of poor-risk DLCL patients, treated with three courses of CHOP followed by BEAM/ASCT versus further cycles of CHOP. There was no significant difference in OS between the two arms. In contrast, the LNH87–2 prospective randomized trial observed improved survival in high-risk patients treated with up-front transplantation (with ASCT, 8-year DFS and OS were 55% and 64% versus 39% and 49% with conventional consolidation respectively). Improved results with ASCT were recently reported by another French group (Milpied *et al.*, 2004). Tandem transplant does not appear to add any survival advantage compared with a single transplant. Today, the potentially improved response to CHOP of adding rituximab, must cast future doubts on the value of up-front ASCT as consolidation.

Autologous stem cell transplantation in relapsed and primary refractory disease

Once a patient has failed initial chemotherapy, the prognosis is poor and long-term overall survival is less than 10%. High-dose therapy followed by ASCT is effective only in those who have shown some response to conventional dose second-line chemotherapy prior to ASCT (PR or responsive relapse). Patients who progressed on first-line salvage therapy have a very low chance of responding to a second-line salvage regimen and should therefore be considered for experimental therapies, whereas those who respond could go ahead and have an ASCT. The prospective randomized multinational Parma trial confirmed the superiority of intensified treatment in patients with sensitive relapse, providing a significantly longer event-free survival.

The subgroup of patients that fails to respond to induction is defined as 'primary refractory disease'. Attempts to overcome this biological resistance, by early ASCT, have failed to achieve better results than conventional chemotherapy. ASCT should therefore be limited to those who respond to second-line chemotherapy.

Allogeneic stem cell transplantation in aggressive non-Hodgkin's lymphoma

Some patients are likely to have a very poor prognosis with conventional therapy, including those who failed ASCT, those presenting with a very high IPI and those with special subtypes of aggressive NHL (e.g. γδ T-cell NHL). Such patients may be considered for allogeneic SCT.

Several reports suggested allogeneic SCT to be potentially curative in high-risk patients with chemosensitive disease. There is no certainty regarding the existence of a strong graft-versus-leukaemia (GvL) effect in intermediate/high grade of the disease, whereas mortality following transplantation remains high, indicating that this treatment should be reserved for selected patients only. Data available at present regarding the role of low intensity SCT in aggressive NL appear to be even less promising because of a high relapse rate and a relatively high TRM (37%). The majority of patients included in these studies had very advanced disease, which might have adversely affected study results. Further studies that explore low-intensity SCT in earlier stages are awaited.

Aggressive T-cell lymphoma

Peripheral T-cell non-Hodgkin's lymphoma otherwise unspecified (Figure 45.7)

Peripheral T cell lymphomas (PTCL) derive from post-thymic T cells at various stages of differentiation. Several studies have suggested T-cell phenotype to be an independent prognostic factor associated with decreased DFS and OS. Treatment of T-cell lymphomas is based on multi-agent chemotherapy (e.g. CHOP); however, patients' outcome remains disappointing and the majority of patients die of their disease. At present, no chemotherapy regimens have been found to be superior to CHOP. The

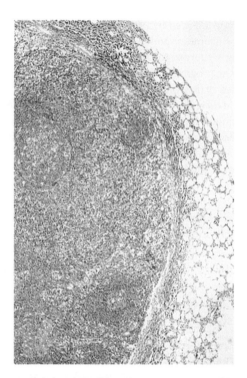

Figure 45.7 Peripheral T-cell lymphoma. Expansion of the paracortical region of a lymph node, with wide separation of germinal follicles.

ability of upfront ASCT (performed in CR1) to improve long-term outcome remains controversial. Further studies evaluating new combination chemotherapies, HDT (both up-front ASCT and allogeneic SCT) are required.

CD30⁺ anaplastic large-cell lymphoma

Two entities of systemic ALCL have been identified: ALCL ALK (anaplastic lymphoma kinase)⁺ and ALCL ALK⁻. ALK expression is caused by chromosomal translocations, most commonly t(2;5), causing the *NPM* gene, located at 5q35 to fuse with gene at 2p23⁻ encoding the receptor tyrosine kinase ALK. The *ALK* gene comes under the control of the *NPM* promoter, resulting in a permanent transcription of the *NPM–ALK* hybrid gene into a 80-kDa chimeric protein named NPM–ALK or p80. The new protein appears to have mitogenic activity, promoting T-cell transformation and tumour growth.

Systemic ALCL ALK⁺ occurs mainly in young males and is characterized by an aggressive course without therapy. Combination chemotherapy (e.g. CHOP) does improve survival; however, long-term outcome in those who present with intermediate/high-risk IPI is disappointing (5-year OS: 41% versus 94% in patients with low-risk IPI), emphasizing the need for new therapeutic modalities in this subgroup of patients. These patients should probably be enrolled into clinical trials, looking

at the value of more intensified regimen with or without up-front ASCT. Specific therapies such as MAbs directed against CD30 and/or specific inhibitors of NMP–ALK (Bonvini *et al.*, 2002) should also be explored.

Unfortunately, patients with ALCL ALK⁻ appear to be less responsive to combination chemotherapy, achieving a 5-year OS of less than 50% (15–45%). The role of HDT followed by up-front autologous/allogeneic SCT is under investigation.

Secondary central nervous system lymphoma in aggressive non-Hodgkin's lymphoma

It is established that less than 2% of low-grade lymphoma patients develop CNS involvement, compared with 5% in DLCL patients and 80% in those who have Burkitt's/Burkitt-like/lymphoblastic lymphoma and do not receive prophylactic therapy.

Secondary central nervous system lymphoma in patients with diffuse large-cell lymphoma

About 5% of DLCL patients may develop CNS relapse within 1 year, with or without a simultaneous systemic relapse. Several risk factors for CNS involvement have been suggested, which include advanced stage of disease (III, IV), elevated LDH, involvement of more than one extranodal site, involvement of testis/bone marrow/paranasal sinuses/Waldeyer ring, B symptoms and high IPI (Table 45.9).

Haioun and colleagues (2000) from the Groupe d'Etudes des Lymphomes de l'Adulte have reported the outcome of 1373 patients with aggressive NHL (excluding patients with lymphoblastic/Burkitt's lymphoma), treated with chemotherapy regimen including CNS prophylactic therapy with IT MTX with each cycle and two pulses of 2 g/m² of MTX. Despite receiving CNS prophylactic therapy, 22 patients developed CNS relapses (16 isolated). Multivariate analysis showed increased LDH and more than one extranodal involvement to be independent risk factors for CNS relapse.

Table 45.9 Risk factors for CNS involvement.

High IPI score

Extranodal sites involved (0 or 1 versus > 1)

Raised LDH level

Age < 60 years

Specific involvement of the following organs: bone marrow, testis, paranasal sinuses and Waldeyer's ring

Low albumin level

Retroperitoneal glands

Further analysis proved high IPI to be the only independent parameter associated with increased risk for CNS disease (low and low-intermediate versus high-intermediate and high IPI, relative risk = 7). The outcome of those who developed CNS relapse was extremely poor, with a median survival of less than 6 months.

The Norwegian study, which is the largest study ever published on CNS involvement in patients with DLCL, confirmed high IPI to be strongly associated with increased risk for CNS relapse (Hollender et al., 2002).

What is the best prophylactic therapy and who should receive it?

Patients with FL or other lymphocytic lymphoma, having a very low risk to develop CNS relapse (< 1%), should not receive any CNS prophylactic therapy. Patients with DLCL and those with 'peripheral T-cell lymphoma not otherwise specified' (PCTL-NOS) appear to have a higher risk for CNS relapse and may therefore need CNS prophylactic therapy. Patients presenting with a high IPI score (particularly those who have a high LDH level or involvement of more than one extranodal site) have the highest risk for CNS relapse.

The question of the best CNS prophylactic therapy remains unclear. It seems that CNS prophylactic therapy based on intrathecal therapy (IT) only should be relatively prolonged (> 6 ITs), otherwise it is unable to eliminate relapse risk completely, but can only reduce it.

The efficacy of systemic methotrexate (MTX) in the absence of IT MTX is being investigated at present by the joint study of Southwestern Oncology Group and Eastern Cooperative Oncology Group (SWOG/ECOG), which compares m-BACOD, MACOP–B CHOP and PROMACE–CYTABOM, using different doses of MTX (200 mg/m^2, 400 mg/m^2 and 1500 mg/m^2). It is worth noting that the highest dose only has a significant CNS efficacy.

High-dose cytarabine (10 g/m^2 or higher) may also be a reasonable option for CNS prophylaxis, reducing CNS relapse rate in ALL patients (who are at higher risk for CNS involvement). Incorporation of high-dose cytarabine/MTX (> 2–3 g/m^2) may be particularly useful in patients with a high IPI. Further studies evaluating prospectively long-term toxicity and efficacy of each of these strategies are required.

Suggested algorithm for therapy of aggressive non-Hodgkin's lymphoma (summary)

At diagnosis
• Anthracyclines containing combination chemotherapy, with/ without rituximab (CHOP–rituximab) are already proven to be superior to CHOP in patients who are more than 60 years old).
• Patients with intermediate-high/high IPI (particularly those

who present with raised LDH and/or extranodal involvement) should receive CNS prophylactic therapy.
• Adjuvant radiotherapy may be considered in patients with bulky disease.
• No clear role for up-front ASCT (performed in CR1).

At relapse
• Second-line regimens (e.g. ESHAP, DVIP, DHAP, mini-BEAM), followed by ASCT.
• Allogeneic SCT may be considered in patients who failed ASCT/special subtypes of NHL (e.g. γδ lymphoma).

High-grade lymphoma

Burkitt's lymphoma and small non-cleaved Burkitt's-like lymphoma (Figure 45.8)

These are highly aggressive forms of non-Hodgkin's lymphoma, frequently involving extranodal organs (e.g. CNS, in 20%) but usually without tumour cells detected in the peripheral blood and characterized by dysregulation of c-MYC oncogene.

Treatment of these patients is based on multidrug combination chemotherapy, including drugs which highly penetrate CNS (e.g. CODOX–M/IVAC regimen, hyper CVAD) (Table 45.5). Approximately 50–80% of adult patients can be cured with these intensive chemotherapy regimens, and in paediatric populations the cure rate is even higher.

The risk for tumour lysis syndrome (TLS), especially after initiating chemotherapy, is relatively high, reflecting the high proliferation rate of tumour cells. Vigorous hydration with alkalinization, accompanied by administration of uric acid synthesis inhibitor (e.g. allopurinol)/recombinant urate oxidase (rasburicase), are very important in preventing/reducing the severity of this complication (see also Chapter 36). Hypercalcaemia is also frequent at presentation and needs appropriate therapy with, for example, hydration and biphosphonate.

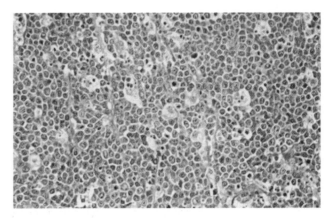

Figure 45.8 Burkitt's lymphoma. Sheets of lymphoblasts and 'starry sky' tangible body macrophages.

Lymphoblastic lymphoma

These are actually derived from early B/T cells, and should therefore be treated as ALL (see Chapters 32 and 33). High-dose therapy with total body irradiation–autograft in first remission gives as good an outcome as extended chemotherapy, whereas the role of allogeneic SCT is probably spared for the relapsed patients. Allogeneic SCT provides a lower relapse rate compared with autograft; however, long-term survival is not necessarily higher due to increased TRM as observed with allograft.

Extranodal lymphomas

At least 25% of NHLs arise from tissues other than lymph nodes, including sites that normally contain no lymphatic tissue. The incidence of NHL, particularly primary extranodal lymphoma (ENL), is gradually increasing (e.g. primary CNS/gastrointestinal/breast), most probably due to the increase in viral infections, especially HIV, and exposure to environmental factors.

Primary gastrointestinal lymphoma

Gastrointestinal (GI) lymphoma is the most common form of extranodal lymphoma, accounting for 30–40% of cases.

Mucosa-associated lymphoid tissue and marginal zone lymphoma

Helicobacter pylori infection appears to be a possible causative agent for development of gastric malt lymphoma. Eradication of *H. pylori* with antibiotics appears to be initial effective therapy for localized gastric mucosa-associated lymphoid tissue (MALT) lymphoma. Preliminary analysis of the LY03 trial (International Extranodal Lymphoma Study Group, the United Kingdom Lymphoma Group and the Groupe d'Etude des Lymphomes de l'Adulte) confirmed that at least one-half of the cases treated with antibiotics achieve histological CR (Zucca *et al.*, 2002). Median time for optimal response is 6 months, but some patients require even 24 months to achieve CR. Response rate is the highest in those whose disease is restricted to mucosa (78%), and in those who have no nodal involvement by endoscopic ultrasonography. The extent of tumour penetration into the gastric wall is inversely correlated with CR rate.

Based on these data it seems reasonable to treat localized disease with antibiotic therapy, followed by a strict endoscopic follow-up, including multiple biopsies 2 months after therapy to confirm eradication of bacteria, with repeated endoscopies and biopsies at least twice per year for 2 years to confirm histological regression of the tumour.

Histological complete remission (hCR) does not necessarily predict cure: PCR for the detection of monoclonality remains positive in approximately one-half of those who achieved hCR, suggesting a suppression, but not eradication, of the lymphoma clone. In cases of unsuccessful eradication of *H. pylori* (PR/resist-

ance disease), a second-line high-dose anti-*H. pylori* therapy should be addressed, containing three or four drugs, omeprazole being one of them (e.g. omeprazole, bismuth citrate, metronidazole, tetracycline). Those patients whose tumour fails to regress despite second-line therapy frequently express t(11;18) and those who present with *H. pylori*-negative localized gastric lymphoma may still respond to chemotherapy (e.g. oral cyclophosphamide/chlorambucil), radiotherapy, surgery or combinations of these treatments (e.g. surgery with chemotherapy). At present there are no prospective randomized trials comparing these modalities. Recent data suggest low-dose radiotherapy to be effective for patients with stage I/II disease, providing a 5-year DFS of 93%.

Surgery may offer excellent control of disease, but without a total gastrectomy, there is no guarantee for cure, as disease tends to be multifocal, involving areas that may look macroscopically normal. Patients with advanced-stage disease are unlikely to be cured with antibiotics only and are therefore treated with systemic chemotherapy/immunotherapy up front.

Diffuse large-cell lymphoma of the stomach

Advanced gastrointestinal DLCL tends to behave like a primarily nodal advanced disease. These tumours were traditionally treated with gastrectomy, however, recent data suggest that this strategy is unnecessary in most cases, where combination chemotherapy with or without adjuvant radiotherapy provides high response and cure rates. At present, the International Extranodal Lymphoma Study Group is investigating the role of short-course chemotherapy, followed by involved-field radiotherapy, in patients with localized gastric DLCL.

In some cases, histological transformation of mucosa-associated lymphoid tissue (MALT) lymphoma might occur and therefore it may be reasonable to add an anti-*H. pylori* therapy, aiming to eradicate the bacteria and avoid potential relapses. Furthermore, anti-*H. pylori* therapy applied in these 'H. pylori-positive cases' yielded a high response rate, indicating a 'pathogenic dependency' on *H. pylori* infection.

Diffuse large-cell lymphoma of the intestine

At present, there are no studies that demonstrate surgery to be unnecessary, and management is therefore based on surgical resection followed by systemic chemotherapy.

Immunoproliferative small intestinal disease

Immunoproliferative small intestinal disease (IPSID) (also known as α-chain disease) arises in small intestinal mucosa-associated lymphoid tissue (MALT) and is characterized by the expression of a monotypic truncated Ig α-heavy chain without an associated light chain. IPSID is mostly found in young adults of low socioeconomic class in developing countries. The aetiology of this disease is unclear, although various causative pathogens (e.g. *Campylobacter jejuni*), and genetic and toxic mechanisms have been proposed.

One-half of all IPSID patients present with concurrent intestinal B-cell lymphoma, whereas most of the remaining patients develop frank lymphoma within a few years. Whereas patients with early-stage disease may respond to antibiotics, those who present with more advanced disease should be treated with chemotherapy.

Enteropathy-associated T-cell lymphoma

Enteropathy-associated T-cell lymphoma (EATCL) arises in the setting of gluten-induced enteropathy and evolves from reactive intraepithelial lymphocytes through a low-grade lymphocytic neoplasm to a high-grade tumour, which is usually the cause of the presenting symptoms. A gluten-free diet appears to markedly reduce the risk for lymphoma; those who have already developed EATCL should receive specific therapy (e.g. CHOP), although there are no specific guidelines on how to treat these patients.

Non-gastric mucosa-associated lymphoid tissue lymphoma (non-gastric MALT)

Mucosa-associated lymphoid tissue (MALT) lymphoma can also occur in salivary glands, skin, thyroid, conjunctiva, orbit, larynx, lung, breast, kidney, liver and prostate; in these cases it tends to have an indolent course. Treatment should be 'patient-tailored', considering the site of disease and the patient's symptoms. Management therefore ranges from a 'watch and wait' policy, through various kinds of therapy, including chemotherapy, monoclonal antibodies (e.g. rituximab) to radiotherapy and surgery.

Primary cutaneous lymphoma

Primary cutaneous B and T lymphomas represent a heterogeneous group, characterized by isolated accumulation of malignant lymphocytes originating in the skin, without extracutaneous manifestations at presentation and during the first 6 months thereafter.

Cutaneous T-cell lymphoma

Cutaneous T-cell lymphoma represents a group of skin lymphomas, characterized by a dominant filtration of clonal T cells (see also Chapter 39).

Mycosis fungoides (MF), the most common form of CTCL, has an indolent course, unless nodal/visceral involvement exists. The treatment is mainly palliative and is based on 'skin targeted modalities', including PUVA, electron beam radiation, narrowband UVA (NB-UVA), topical steroids, nitrogen mustard, carmustine and vitamin D. PUVA and NB-UVA remain the gold standard therapy at early stages (IA/IIA), whereas systemic therapies are reserved for more advanced stages. Treatment options in these cases may include chlorambucil, methotrexate, doxorubicin, etoposide, retinoids, rexinoids, interferon, extracorporal photopheresis, interferon alpha/gamma, or conjugated monoclonal antibodies (e.g. anti-CD52) and immunotoxins (e.g. IL-2 receptor-specific fusion protein combined with diphtheria toxin, which selectively target the IL-2 receptor on malignant and activated T cells). Systemic therapies are frequently combined with topical agents. INF-α with or without phototherapy appears to be highly effective in advanced disease, providing responses in up to 80% of patients. Other immunomodulatory agents, such as recombinant human IL-2, anti-adiotype vaccines and gene therapies, are under investigation.

Young patients with biologically aggressive disease who failed conventional therapies may be considered for allogeneic SCT.

Sézary's syndrome

Sézary's syndrome (SS) is an aggressive CTL, characterized by erythrodema, lymphadenopathy and circulating malignant T cells with ceribriform nuclei. Therapy is usually based on a combination of systemic and topical therapy; chemotherapy agents (e.g. alkylators, including temozolomide), IL-2 diphtheria toxin, retinoids/rexonoid, accompanied with topical steroids or PUVA. Extracorporal photopheresis may also be effective, especially in those who present with a low number of circulating Sézary cells. Several groups have recently reported a dramatic response to anti-CD52 MAbs.

CD30+ large-cell lymphoma is the most common form of non-MF primary CTLC that appears to have an indolent course, with a 5-year survival in 90% of cases. These patients are usually treated successfully with spot radiation or surgical excision, and only those who progress are considered for systemic treatment. On the other hand, patients with CD30− T-cell large-cell lymphoma tend to have aggressive disease with poor prognosis and should therefore receive multi-agent systemic chemotherapy at diagnosis, irrespective of disease stage.

Cutaneous B-cell lymphoma

Primary cutaneous B-cell lymphoma (CBCL) presents a group of lymphomas characterized by dominant infiltration of clonal B cells in the skin. Follicle centre lymphoma (FCL), the most frequent CBCL, is characterized by a localized slowly progressive lesion in the neck/head or trunk and is associated with an excellent prognosis (5-year OS > 90%). Local radiation remains the preferred therapy for patients with localized disease (localized with regional satellites), whereas those who present with disseminated skin disease may be observed or treated with systemic chemotherapy with or without MoABs (e.g. rituximab).

Immunocytoma (marginal zone lymphoma), the second most common CBCL, is also considered to have an indolent course with a 5-year OS approaching 97%. Patient management is similar to that of patients with FCL. A more aggressive type of CBCL, represented with nodules/tumours on one or both legs, is called *'large-cell lymphoma of the leg'*. Despite its less indolent nature, the treatment of choice for early stages remains local (local radiation or excision), whereas those who present with disseminated disease are treated with systemic chemotherapy with or without adjuvant MAbs.

In summary, primary cutaneous lymphomas present a heterogeneous group of B- and T-cell lymphomas with a variety of clinical presentations and prognoses. Accurate diagnosis and assessment of prognostic factors determine patients' management. The majority of patients should be considered for conservative palliative therapy (e.g. local or topical treatments), unless they present with histologically aggressive lymphoma (e.g. large-cell CTCL) or disseminated stage of an 'indolent' disease (extracutaneous involvement), for which they should receive systemic therapy. New emerging therapies (MAbs, topical and systemic rexinoids, recombinant toxins and immunomodulators) may succeed in improving long-term outcome; however, further studies are needed.

Primary central nervous system lymphoma

Primary CNS lymphoma is defined as lymphoma arising in the cranial–spinal axis (brain, spinal cord, leptomeninges and eye). It is usually disseminated within the nervous system at presentation (in 50% of immunocompetent patients and in nearly 100% of AIDS patients). The histology in most cases is compatible with DLCLs (90%) or non-cleaved cell lymphoma.

Age, poor performance status, involvement of deep structures, high LDH level and a high protein level in cerebrospinal fluid (CSF) appear to predict poor prognosis. Until recently, the traditional therapy was based on whole-brain radiation. Unfortunately, the relapse rate within/outside the radiation field approached 90% and 5-year survival was less than 10%, suggesting that radiotherapy is insufficient. Combination therapy, however (chemotherapy with radiotherapy), appears to be more effective, providing a 5-year OS of 30–50%, but may cause delayed neurotoxicity, especially in patients older than 60 years. Several studies suggested 'high-dose methotrexate (MTX)-containing regimens' to be as good as combined modality treatment, but less neurotoxic. Therefore, chemotherapy should become the standard therapy in elderly patients, whereas radiotherapy should be reserved for those who relapse or fail to respond to chemotherapy.

Chemoradiotherapy is at present the standard treatment in younger patients. However, further attempts to reduce long-term neurotoxicity in this group, delivering lower doses of radiotherapy/ omitting radiotherapy, but providing intensified chemotherapy regimens such as up-front ASCT, should be explored.

Lymphoma in the immunocompromised patient

Most frequently the disease is diagnosed in patients with *acquired* immunodeficiency, caused by HIV infection (AIDS-related lymphoma) or immunosuppresive drugs (e.g. post-transplant lymphoproliferative disorder).

Post transplant lymphoproliferative disorders (PTLDs) range from polyclonal plasmacytic hyperplasia, up to monoclonal B-cell proliferation, polymorphic hyperplasia/lymphoma, immunoblastic lymphoma or myeloma. EBV virus causes the majority of these disorders: impaired T-cell function leads to proliferation of EBV latently infected polyclonal B cells, whereas subsequent genomic mutations result in monoclonal PTLD.

Prevention of EBV infection/reactivation may therefore be essential. Antiviral agents (e.g. aciclovir, ganciclovir), passive immunotherapy and pre-emptive immunotherapy, using cytotoxic T lymphocytes targeted against EBV, are all applied to prevent PTLDs, with variable success. Patients who develop PTLD may respond to reduction in immunosuppressive therapy, especially those who develop PTLD within 1 year from transplant (ORR = 80% versus 10% in patients who developed PTLD beyond 1 year).

Anti-B cell MAbs (e.g. anti-CD20, anti-CD21 and anti-CD24) are also effective, providing responses in 65% of patients. IFN-α, being an antiviral and anti-tumour agent, was shown to induce prolonged remissions when combined with reduction in immunosuppression. Chemotherapy is usually reserved for those patients who have failed to respond to previous modalities. Lower doses of chemotherapy (e.g. reduced CHOP) appear to be highly effective but less toxic than conventional regimens. Adoptive immunotherapy following allogeneic SCT may also be effective. Donor lymphocyte infusion (DLI) may cause severe GvHD, limiting their use. In contrast, antiEBV cytotoxic T lymphocytes do provide a more specific effect, but are less available, being produced over weeks to months by expert laboratories.

AIDS-related non-Hodgkin's lymphoma

The histological diagnosis in the majority of such patients is DLCL (60%) or Burkitt's lymphoma (30%). Combination chemotherapy is the treatment of choice. Treatment-related toxicity might be higher than observed in non-HIV patients, especially in those with advanced AIDS disease. Therapy should be individually tailored; therefore, those who have advanced AIDS and limited anti-retroviral therapeutic options should receive a palliative chemotherapy (e.g. oral prednisolone, bleomycin)/ radiotherapy, whereas those who have early disease/good performance status may tolerate curative chemotherapy regimens (e.g. reduced dose/conventional dose of CHOP/m-BACOD/ CDE/EPOCH/CODOX–M/IVAC) with or without rituximab. Recent publications indicate that concurrent treatment with highly active anti-retroviral therapy (HAART) significantly improves the outcome of HIV-related NHL, providing an OS and DFS similar to that of non-HIV patients.

Lymphoma in elderly patients

DLCL accounts for 50% of lymphomas in patients older than 60 years. Unfortunately, the outcome in this population is worse than that observed in younger adults, partly because of the high incidence of co-existing medical problems, affecting organ function. Attempts to improve patients' outcome, providing intensified chemotherapy regimens (compared with CHOP), ended with increased toxicity without improvement in survival, whereas less toxic regimens were often less effective. However, the prospective randomized GELA study, comparing CHOP with CHOP–rituximab (CHOP–R), has recently reported an improved DFS and OS in elderly patients (> 60 years) treated with CHOP–R, with no increase in treatment-related toxicity.

The addition of granulocyte colony-stimulating factors (G-CSF) can shorten duration of neutropenia, enabling the delivery of chemotherapy at the planned time and dose intensity. Several studies have recently reported encouraging results with HDT/ASCT in patients older than 60 (4-year OS in patients with chemosensitive relapsed disease approached 40%), indicating the feasibility of this treatment in selected patients.

Selected bibliography

Abrey LE, Yahalom J, DeAngelis LM. (2000) Treatment for primary CNS lymphoma: the next step. *Journal of Clinical Oncology* **18**: 3144–50.

Anagnostopoulos A, Aleman A, Giralt S. (2003) Autologous and allogeneic stem cell transplantation in Waldenstrom's macroglobulinemia: review of the literature and future directions. *Seminars in Oncology* **30**: 286–90.

Ardeshna KM, Smith P, Norton A *et al.* (2003) British National Lymphoma Investigation: Long-term effect of a watch and wait policy versus immediate systemic treatment for asymptomatic advanced-stage non-Hodgkin's lymphoma: a randomised controlled trial. *Lancet* **16**: 516–22.

Bais C, Santomasso B, Coso O *et al.* (1998) G-protein-coupled receptor of Kaposi's sarcoma-associated herpesvirus is a viral oncogene and angiogenesis activator. *Nature* **391**: 86–9.

Balzarotti M, Spina M, Sarina B *et al.* (2002) Intensified CHOP regimen in aggressive lymphomas: maximal dose intensity and dose density of doxorubicin and cyclophosphamide. *Annals of Oncology* **3**: 1341–6.

Bertoni F, Conconi A, Capella C *et al.* (2002) International Extranodal Lymphoma Study Group; United Kingdom Lymphoma Group Molecular follow-up in gastric mucosa-associated lymphoid tissue lymphomas: early analysis of the LY03 cooperative trial. *Blood* **99**: 2541–4.

Bierman PJ, Sweetenham JW, Loberiza FR Jr *et al.* (2003) Syngeneic hematopoietic stem-cell transplantation for non-Hodgkin's lymphoma: a comparison with allogeneic and autologous transplantation – The Lymphoma Working Committee of the International Bone Marrow Transplant Registry and the European Group for Blood and Marrow Transplantation. *Journal of Clinical Oncology* **21**: 3744–53.

Blayney DW, LeBlanc ML, Grogan T *et al.* (2003) Dose-intense chemotherapy every 2 weeks with dose-intense cyclophosphamide, doxorubicin, vincristine, and prednisone may improve survival in intermediate- and high-grade lymphoma: a phase II study of the Southwest Oncology Group (SWOG 9349). *Journal of Clinical Oncology* **21**: 2466–73.

Boogaerts MA, Van Hoof A, Catovsky D *et al.* (2001) Activity of oral fludarabine phosphate in previously treated chronic lymphocytic leukemia. *Journal of Clinical Oncology* **19**: 4252–8.

Caballero MD, Perez-Simon JA, Iriondo A *et al.* (2003) High-dose therapy in diffuse large cell lymphoma: results and prognostic factors in 452 patients from the GEL-TAMO Spanish Cooperative Group. *Annals of Oncology* **14**: 140–51.

Chen LT, Lin JT, Shyu RY *et al.* (2001) Prospective study of *Helicobacter pylori* eradication therapy in stage I(E) high-grade mucosa-associated lymphoid tissue lymphoma of the stomach. *Journal of Clinical Oncology* **19**: 4245–51.

Chiarion-Sileni V, Bononi A, Fornasa CV *et al.* (2002) Phase II trial of interferon-alpha-2a plus psolaren with ultraviolet light A in patients with cutaneous T-cell lymphoma. *Cancer* **95**: 569–75.

Coiffier B, Lepage E, Briere J *et al.* (2002) CHOP chemotherapy plus rituximab compared with CHOP alone in elderly patients with diffuse large-B-cell lymphoma. *New England Journal of Medicine* **346**: 235–42.

Coleman M, Leonard J, Lyons L *et al.* (2003) Treatment of Waldenstrom's macroglobulinemia with clarithromycin, low-dose thalidomide, and dexamethasone. *Seminars in Oncology* **30**: 270–4.

Colombata P, Salles G, Brousse N *et al.* (2001) Rituximab (anti-CD20 monoclonal antibody) as single first-line therapy for patients with follicular lymphoma with a low tumor burden: clinical and molecular evaluation. *Blood* **97**: 101–6.

Cortes J, Thomas D, Rios A *et al.* (2002) Hyperfractionated cyclophosphamide, vincristine, doxorubicin, and dexamethasone and highly active antiretroviral therapy for patients with acquired immunodeficiency syndrome-related Burkitt lymphoma/leukemia. *Cancer* **94**: 1492–9.

Dave SS, Wright G, Tan B *et al.* (2004) Prediction of survival in follicular lymphoma based on molecular features in tumour-infiltrating cells. *New England Journal of Medicine* **351**: 2159–69.

Davis TA, White CA, Grillo-Lopez AJ *et al.* (1999) Single-agent monoclonal antibody efficacy in bulky non-Hodgkin's lymphoma: results of a phase II trial of rituximab. *Journal of Clinical Oncology* **17**: 1851–7.

Decaudin D, Lepage E, Brousse N *et al.* (1999) Low-grade stage III–IV follicular lymphoma: multivariate analysis of prognostic factors in 484 patients. *Journal of Clinical Oncology* **17**: 2499–505.

Desikan R, Dhodapkar M, Siegel D *et al.* (1999) High-dose therapy with autologous haemopoietic stem cell support for Waldenstrom's macroglobulinaemia. *British Journal of Haematology* **105**: 993–6.

Dimopoulos MA, Zomas A, Viniou NA *et al.* (2001) Treatment of Waldenstrom's macroglobulinemia with thalidomide. *Journal of Clinical Oncology* **19**: 3596–601.

Dimopoulos MA, Fountzilas G, Papageorgiou E *et al.* (2002) Hellenic Cooperative Oncology Group Primary treatment of low-grade non-Hodgkin's lymphoma with the combination of fludarabine and mitoxantrone: a phase II study of the Hellenic Cooperative Oncology Group. *Leukaemia and Lymphoma* **43**: 111–14.

Eucker J, Schille C, Schmid P *et al.* (2002) The combination of fludarabine and cyclophosphamide results in a high remission rate with moderate toxicity in low-grade non-Hodgkin's lymphomas. *Anti-cancer Drugs* 13: 907–13.

Faderl S, Thomas DA, O'Brien S *et al.* (2003) Experience with alemtuzumab plus rituximab in patients with relapsed and refractory lymphoid malignancies. *Blood* 101: 3413–5.

Falini B, Pulford K, Pucciarini A *et al.* (1999) Lymphomas expressing ALK fusion protein(s) other than NPM-ALK. *Blood* 94: 3509–15.

Ferreri AJ, Abrey LE, Blay JY *et al.* (2003) Summary statement on primary central nervous system lymphomas from the Eighth International Conference on Malignant Lymphoma Lugano Switzerland June 12 to 15 2002. *Journal of Clinical Oncology* 21: 2407–14.

Fisher RI, Gaynor ER, Dahlberg S *et al.* (1993) Comparison of a standard regimen (CHOP) with three intensive chemotherapy regimens for advanced non-Hodgkin's lymphoma. *New England Journal of Medicine* 328: 1002–6.

Forrest DL, Thompson K, Nevill TJ *et al.* (2002) Allogeneic hematopoietic stem cell transplantation for progressive follicular lymphoma. *Bone Marrow Transplant* 29: 973–8.

Frankel AE, Neville DM, Bugge TA *et al.* (2003) Immunotoxin therapy of hematologic malignancies. *Seminars in Oncology* 30: 545–57.

Freedman AS, Neuberg D, Mauch P (1999) Long-term follow-up of autologous bone marrow transplantation in patients with relapsed follicular lymphoma. *Blood* 94: 3325–33.

Gertz MA, Anagnostopoulos A, Anderson K *et al.* (2003) Treatment recommendations in Waldenstrom's macroglobulinemia: consensus panel recommendations from the Second International Workshop on Waldenstrom's Macroglobulinemia. *Seminars in Oncology* 30: 121–1.

Ghetie MA, Bright H, Vitetta ES (2001) Homodimers but not monomers of Rituxan (chimeric anti-CD20) induce apoptosis in human B-lymphoma cells and synergize with a chemotherapeutic agent and an immunotoxin. *Blood* 97: 1392–8.

Gianni AM, Magni M, Martelli M *et al.* (2003) Long-term remission in mantle cell lymphoma following high-dose sequential chemotherapy and in vivo rituximab-purged stem cell auto-grafting (R-HDS regimen). *Blood* 102: 749–55.

Gobbi PG, Ghirardelli ML, Cavalli C *et al.* (2000) The role of surgery in the treatment of gastrointestinal lymphomas other than low-grade MALT lymphomas. *Haematologica* 85: 372–80.

Gopal AK, Gooley TA, Golden JB *et al.* (2001) Efficacy of high-dose therapy and autologous hematopoietic stem cell transplantation for non-Hodgkin's lymphoma in adults 60 years of age and older. *Bone Marrow Transplant* 27: 593–9.

Guitart J, Wickless SC, Oyama Y *et al.* (2002) Long-term remission after allogeneic hematopoietic stem cell transplantation for refractory cutaneous T-cell lymphoma. *Archives of Dermatology* 138: 1359–65 (Review).

Haas RL, Poortmans de Jong D *et al.* (2003) High response rates and lasting remissions after low-dose involved field radiotherapy in indolent lymphomas. *Journal of Clinical Oncology* 21: 2474–80.

Hainsworth JD, Litchy S, Burris III *et al.* (2002) Rituximab as first-line and maintenance therapy for patients with indolent non-Hodgkin's lymphoma. *Journal of Clinical Oncology* 20: 4261–7.

Haioun C, Besson C, Lepage E *et al.* (2000) Incidence and risk factors of central nervous system relapse in histologically aggressive non-Hodgkin's lymphoma uniformly treated and receiving intrathecal central nervous system prophylaxis: a GELA study on 974 patients. *Annals of Oncology* 11: 685–90.

Haioun C, Lepage E, Gisselbrecht C *et al.* (2000) Survival benefit of high-dose therapy in poor-risk aggressive non-Hodgkin's lymphoma: final analysis of the prospective LNH87–2 protocol. *Journal of Clinical Oncology* 18: 3025–30.

Haque T, Wilkie GM, Taylor C *et al.* (2002) Treatment of Epstein-Barr-virus-positive post-transplantation lymphoproliferative disease with partly HLA-matched allogeneic cytotoxic T cells. *Lancet* 360: 436–42.

Hess G, Flohr T, Huber C *et al.* (2003) Safety and feasibility of CHOP/rituximab induction treatment followed by high-dose chemo/radiotherapy and autologous PBSC-transplantation in patients with previously untreated mantle cell or indolent B-cell-non-Hodgkin's lymphoma. *Bone Marrow Transplant* 31: 775–82.

Hiddemann W, Dreyling M, Unterhalt M (2003) Rituximab plus chemotherapy in follicular and mantle cell lymphomas. *Seminars in Oncology* 30 (Suppl 2):16–20.

Ho AY, Devereux S, Mufti GJ *et al.* (2003) Reduced-intensity rituximab-BEAM-CAMPATH allogeneic haematopoietic stem cell transplantation for follicular lymphoma is feasible and induces durable molecular remissions. *Bone Marrow Transplant* 31: 551–7.

Hochster HS, Oken MM, Winter JN *et al.* (2000) Phase I study of fludarabine plus cyclophosphamide in patients with previously untreated low-grade lymphoma: results and long-term follow-up-a report from the Eastern Cooperative Oncology Group. *Journal of Clinical Oncology* 18: 987–94.

Hoffmann C, Wolf E, Fatkenheuer G *et al.* (2003) Response to highly active antiretroviral therapy strongly predicts outcome in patients with AIDS-related lymphoma *AIDS* 17: 1521–9.

Hollender A, Kvaloy S, Nom O *et al.* (2002) Central nervous system involvement following diagnosis of non-Hodgkin's lymphoma: a risk model. *Annals of Oncology* 13: 1099–107.

Howard OM, Gribben JG, Neuberg DS *et al.* (2002) Rituximab and CHOP induction therapy for newly diagnosed mantle-cell lymphoma: molecular complete responses are not predictive of progression-free survival. *Journal of Clinical Oncology* 20: 1288–94.

Howden CW, Hunt RH (1998) Guidelines for the management of *Helicobacter pylori* infection Ad Hoc Committee on Practice Parameters of the American College of Gastroenterology. *American Journal of Gastroenterology* 93: 2330–8.

Itoh K, Ohtsu T, Fukuda H *et al.* (2002) Randomized phase II study of biweekly CHOP and dose-escalated CHOP with prophylactic use of lenograstim (glycosylated G-CSF) in aggressive non-Hodgkin's lymphoma. *Annals of Oncology* 13: 1347–55.

Kaminski MS, Estes J, Zasadny KR *et al.* (2000) Radioimmunotherapy with iodine (131) I tositumomab for relapsed or refractory B-cell non-Hodgkin's lymphoma: updated results and long-term follow-up of the University of Michigan experience. *Blood* 96: 1259–66.

Kennedy GA, Seymour JF, Wolf M *et al.* (2003) Treatment of patients with advanced mycosis fungoides and Sezary syndrome with alemtuzumab. *European Journal of Haematology* 71: 250–6.

Klasa RJ, Meyer RM, Shustik C *et al.* (2003) Randomised phase III study of fludarabine phosphate versus cyclophosphamide vincristine and prednisone in patients with recurrent low-grade non-Hodgkin's lymphoma previously treated with an alkylating agent or alkylator-containing regimen. *Journal of Clinical Oncology* 21: 2626.

Ladetto M, Corradini P, Vallet S *et al.* (2002) High rate of clinical and molecular remissions in follicular lymphoma patients receiving high-dose sequential chemotherapy and autografting at diagnosis: a multicenter prospective study by the Gruppo Italiano Trapianto Midollo Osseo (GITMO). *Blood* 100: 1559–65.

Lecuit M, Abachin E, Martin A *et al.* (2004) Immunoproliferative small intestinal disease associated with *Campylobacter jejuni*. *New England Journal of Medicine* 350: 239–48.

Levine JE, Harris RE, Loberiza FR Jr *et al.* (2003) Lymphoma Study Writing Committee International Bone Marrow Transplant Registry and Autologous Blood and Marrow Transplant Registry A comparison of allogeneic and autologous bone marrow transplantation for lymphoblastic lymphoma. *Blood* 101: 2476–82.

Linch DC, Smith P, Hancock BW *et al.* (2000) A randomized British National Lymphoma Investigation trial of CHOP vs a weekly multi-agent regimen (PACEBOM) in patients with histologically aggressive non-Hodgkin's lymphoma. *Annals of Oncology* 11 (Suppl 1): 87–90.

Little RF, Pittaluga S, Grant N *et al.* (2003) Highly effective treatment of acquired immunodeficiency syndrome-related lymphoma with dose-adjusted EPOCH: impact of antiretroviral therapy suspension and tumor biology. *Blood* 101: 4653–9.

Loren AW, Porter DL, Stadtmauer EA *et al.* (2003) Post-transplant lymphoproliferative disorder: a review. *Bone Marrow Transplant* 31: 145–55 (Review).

Lossos IS, Czerwinski DK, Alizadeh AA *et al.* (2004) Prediction of survival in diffuse large-B-cell lymphoma based on the expression of six genes. *New England Journal of Medicine* 350: 1828–37.

Lundin J, Hagberg H, Repp R *et al.* (2003) Phase 2 study of alemtuzumab (anti-CD52 monoclonal antibody) in patients with advanced mycosis fungoides/Sezary syndrome. *Blood* 101: 4267–72.

MacManus MP, Hoppe RT (1996) Is radiotherapy curative for stage I and II low-grade follicular lymphoma? Results of a long-term follow-up study of patients treated at Stanford University. *Journal of Clinical Oncology* 14: 1282–90.

MacManus MP, Seymour JF (2001) Management of localized low-grade follicular lymphomas. *Australasian Radiology* 45: 326–34.

Magni M, Di Nicola M, Devizzi L *et al.* (2000) Successful in vivo purging of CD34⁻ containing peripheral blood harvests in mantle cell and indolent lymphoma: evidence for a role of both chemotherapy and rituximab infusion. *Blood* 96: 864–9.

McLaughlin P, Grillo-Lopez AJ, Link BK *et al.* (1998) Rituximab chimeric anti-CD20 monoclonal antibody therapy for relapsed indolent lymphoma: half of patients respond to a four-dose treatment program. *Journal of Clinical Oncology* 16: 2825–33.

Micallef IN, Lillington DM, Apostolidis J *et al.* (2000) Therapy-related myelodysplasia and secondary acute myelogenous leukemia after high-dose therapy with autologous hematopoietic progenitor-cell support for lymphoid malignancies. *Journal of Clinical Oncology* 18: 947–55.

Milpied N, Deconinck E, Gaillard F *et al.* (2004) Initial treatment of aggressive lymphoma with high-dose chemotherapy and autologous stem-cell support. *New England Journal of Medicine* 350: 1287–95.

Mounier N, Simon D, Haioun C *et al.* (2002) Impact of high-dose chemotherapy on peripheral T-cell lymphomas. *Journal of Clinical Oncology* 20: 1426–7.

Multani P (2002) Development of radioimmunotherapy for the treatment of non-Hodgkin's lymphoma. *International Journal of Hematology* 76: 401–10.

Munshi NC, Barlogie B (2003) Role for high-dose therapy with autologous hematopoietic stem cell support in Waldenstrom's macroglobulinemia. *Seminars in Oncology* 30: 282–5.

Nakamura T, Inagaki H, Seto M *et al.* (2003) Gastric low-grade B-cell MALT lymphoma: treatment response and genetic alteration. *Journal of Gastroenterology* 38: 921–9.

Peniket AJ, Ruiz de Elvira MC, Taghipour G *et al.* (2003) European Bone Marrow Transplantation (EBMT) Lymphoma Registry. An EBMT registry matched study of allogeneic stem cell transplants for lymphoma: allogeneic transplantation is associated with a lower relapse rate but a higher procedure-related mortality rate than autologous transplantation. *Bone Marrow Transplant* 31: 667–8.

Press OW, Unger JM, Braziel RM *et al.* (2003) A phase 2 trial of CHOP chemotherapy followed by tositumomab/iodine I 131 tositumomab for previously untreated follicular non-Hodgkin's lymphoma. *Blood* 102: 1606–12.

Robinson SP, Goldstone AH, Mackinnon S *et al.* (2002) Lymphoma Working Party of the European Group for Blood and Bone Marrow Transplantation Chemo resistant or aggressive lymphoma predicts for a poor outcome following reduced-intensity allogeneic progenitor cell transplantation: an analysis from the lymphoma. *Blood* 100: 4310–6.

Rodriguez J, Munsell M, Yazji S *et al.* (2001) Impact of high-dose chemotherapy on peripheral T-cell lymphomas. *Journal of Clinical Oncology* 19: 3766–70.

Schouten HC, Qianm W, Kvaloym S *et al.* (2003) High-dose therapy improves progression-free survival and survival in relapsed follicular non-Hodgkin's lymphoma: results from the randomized European CUP trial. *Journal of Clinical Oncology* 21: 3918–27.

Seropian S, Bahceci E, Cooper DL (2003) Allogeneic peripheral blood stem cell transplantation for high-risk non-Hodgkin's lymphoma. *Bone Marrow Transplant* 32: 763–9.

Seymour JF, McLaughlin P, Fuller LM *et al.* (1996) High rate of prolonged remissions following combined modality therapy for patients with localized low-grade lymphoma. *Annals of Oncology* 7: 157–63.

Seymour JF, Pro B, Fuller LM *et al.* (2003) Long-term follow-up of a prospective study of combined modality therapy for stage I–II indolent non-Hodgkin's lymphoma. *Journal of Clinical Oncology* 1: 2115–22 (Review).

Shenkier TN, Voss N, Fairey R *et al.* (2002) Brief chemotherapy and involved-region irradiation for limited-stage diffuse large-cell lymphoma: an 18-year experience from the British Columbia Cancer Agency. *Journal of Clinical Oncology* 20: 197–204.

Smalley RV, Weller E, Hawkins MJ *et al.* (2001) Final analysis of the ECOG I-COPA trial (E6484) in patients with non-Hodgkin's lymphoma treated with interferon alfa (IFN-alpha2a) plus an anthracycline-based induction regimen. *Leukemia* 15: 1118–22.

Suryanarayan K, Natkunam Y, Berry G *et al.* (2001) Modified cyclophosphamide hydroxydaunorubicin vincristine and prednisone therapy for post-transplantation lymphoproliferative disease in pediatric patients undergoing solid organ transplantation. *Journal of Pediatric Hematology and Oncology* **23**: 452–5.

Thieblemont C, Berger F, Dumontet C *et al.* (2000) Mucosa-associated lymphoid tissue lymphoma is a disseminated disease in one third of 158 patients analyzed. *Blood* **95**: 802–6 (Review).

Thomas DA, O'Brien S, Bueso-Ramos C *et al.* (2003) Rituximab in relapsed or refractory hairy cell leukemia. *Blood* **102**: 3906–11.

Thorley-Lawson DA, Gross A (2004) Persistence of the Epstein–Barr virus and the origins of associated lymphomas. *New England Journal of Medicine* **350**: 1328–37 (Review).

Tilly H, Lepage E, Coiffier B *et al.* (2003) Intensive conventional chemotherapy (ACVBP regimen) compared with standard CHOP for poor-prognosis aggressive non-Hodgkin's lymphoma. *Blood* **102**: 4284–9.

Tirelli U, Spina M, Jaeger U *et al.* (2002) Infusional CDE with rituximab for the treatment of human immunodeficiency virus-associated non-Hodgkin's lymphoma: preliminary results of a phase I/II study. Recent results. *Cancer Research* **159**: 49–53.

Tomita N, Kodama F, Kanamori H *et al.* (2002) Prophylactic intrathecal methotrexate and hydrocortisone reduces central nervous system recurrence and improves survival in aggressive non-Hodgkin's lymphoma. *Cancer* **95**: 576–80.

Tournilhac O, Leblond V, Tabrizi R *et al.* (2003) Transplantation in Waldenstrom's macroglobulinemia: the French experience. *Seminars in Oncology* **30**: 291–6.

Tsimberidou AM, McLaughlin P, Younes A *et al.* (2002) Fludarabine mitoxantrone dexamethasone (FND) compared with an alternating triple therapy (ATT) regimen in patients with stage IV indolent lymphoma. *Blood* **100**: 4351–7.

Vaccher E, Spina M, Talamini R *et al.* (2003) Improvement of systemic human immunodeficiency virus-related non-Hodgkin's lymphoma outcome in the era of highly active antiretroviral therapy. *Clinical Infectious Diseases* **37**: 1556–64.

Van Besien K, Loberiza FR Jr, Bajorunaite R *et al.* (2003) Comparison of autologous and allogeneic hematopoietic stem cell transplantation for follicular lymphoma. *Blood* **102**: 3521–9.

Villela L, Sureda A, Canals C *et al.* (2003) Low transplant-related mortality in older patients with hematologic malignancies undergoing autologous stem cell transplantation. *Haematologica* **88**: 300–5.

Wang ES, Straus DJ, Teruya-Feldstein J *et al.* (2003) Intensive chemotherapy with cyclophosphamide doxorubicin high-dose methotrexate/ifosfamide etoposide and high-dose cytarabine (CODOX-M/IVAC) for human immunodeficiency virus-associated Burkitt lymphoma. *Cancer* **98**: 1196–205.

Wilder RB, Jones D, Tucker SL *et al.* (2001) Long-term results with radiotherapy for Stage I–II follicular lymphomas. *International Journal of Radiation Oncology* Biology *and Physics* **51**: 1219–27.

Witzig TE, Flinn IW, Gordon LI *et al.* (2002) Treatment with ibritumomab tiuxetan radioimmunotherapy in patients with rituximab-refractory follicular non-Hodgkin's lymphoma. *Journal of Clinical Oncology* **20**: 3262–9.

Witzig TE, White CA, Gordon LI *et al.* (2003) Safety of yttrium-90 ibritumomab tiuxetan radioimmunotherapy for relapsed low-grade follicular or transformed non-Hodgkin's lymphoma. *Journal of Clinical Oncology* **21**: 1263–70.

Wotherspoon AC, Doglioni C, Diss TC *et al.* (1993) Regression of primary low-grade B-cell gastric lymphoma of mucosa-associated lymphoid tissue type after eradication of *Helicobacter pylori*. *Lancet* **342**: 575–7.

Wunderlich A, Kloess M, Reiser M *et al.* (2003) Practicability and acute haematological toxicity of 2- and 3-weekly CHOP and CHOEP chemotherapy for aggressive non-Hodgkin's lymphoma: results from the NHL-B trial of the German High-Grade Non-Hodgkin's Lymphoma Study Group (DSHNHL). *Annals of Oncology* **14**: 881–93.

Ye H, Liu H, Raderer M *et al.* (2003) High incidence of t(11;18)(q21;q21) in *Helicobacter pylori*-negative gastric MALT lymphoma. *Blood* **101**: 2547–50.

Young RC, Longo DL, Glatstein E *et al.* (1988) The treatment of indolent lymphomas: watchful waiting v aggressive combined modality treatment. *Seminars in Hematology* **25** (Suppl 2): 11–6.

Zinzani PL, Magagnoli M, Moretti L *et al.* (2000) Randomized trial of fludarabine versus fludarabine and idarubicin as frontline treatment in patients with indolent or mantle-cell lymphoma. *Journal of Clinical Oncology* **18**: 773–9.

Zucca E, Bertoni F, Roggero E *et al.* (2000) The gastric marginal zone B-cell lymphoma of MALT type. *Blood* **96**: 410–9.

Zucca E, Conconi A, Cavalli F (2002) Treatment of extranodal lymphomas. *Best Practice and Research in Clinical Haematology* **15**: 533–47.

CHAPTER 46

Myeloproliferative disorders

46

George Vassiliou and Anthony R Green

Introduction

For the purposes of this chapter, the term myeloproliferative disorders (MPDs) will refer to clonal disorders of haemopoiesis that lead to an increase in the numbers of one or more mature blood cell progeny. The chronic myeloid leukaemias would fit this definition and share pathogenetic features with some of the MPDs, but have, historically (since the discovery of the Philadelphia chromosome), been studied separately from the MPDs and are described in Chapter 37. The myelodysplastic syndromes (MDS) can also, in a minority of cases, fit our working definition of MPD, in being associated with increased numbers of mature cell progeny, but dysplasia is a major feature and there are, usually, co-existing cytopenias. Not surprisingly, a small number of patients do not fit neatly into a single category and exhibit features of both MPD and MDS (see also Chapter 40).

This chapter will focus on the classical MPDs: polycythaemia (rubra) vera (PV), essential thrombocythaemia (ET) and idiopathic myelofibrosis (IMF), three related disorders originally grouped together by Dameshek in 1951. They share clinical, morphological and molecular features and can transform, in their course, into one another. They are believed to be clonal disorders of the pluripotent haemopoietic stem cell and have, to varying degrees, the potential to transform into acute myeloid leukaemia (AML). Secondary (non-clonal) polycythaemias and thrombocytoses will also be discussed in this chapter, as they often enter the differential diagnosis of their clonal counterparts.

In addition, some of the less common MPDs will be described, namely mastocytosis and its variants, the clonal eosinophilic syndromes and chronic neutrophilic leukaemia (CNL) (see also Chapter 37). The ontogeny of the target cell for transformation is less well established in these disorders, but there is accumulating evidence implicating the pluripotent haemopoietic stem cell in at least some cases.

The polycythaemias

True polycythaemia refers to an absolute increase in total body red cell volume (or mass), which usually manifests itself as a raised haemoglobin concentration (Hb) and/or packed cell volume (PCV). A raised Hb (or PCV) can also be secondary to a reduction in plasma volume, without an increase in total red cell volume; this is known as apparent (or relative) polycythaemia.

True polycythaemia is further subdivided into primary polycythaemia (polycythaemia vera), a clonal haematological disorder, and secondary polycythaemia, which results from an increased erythropoietin drive, either in the presence or in the absence of hypoxia (Figure 46.1).

Polycythaemia vera

The central pathological feature of PV is an expansion in the total red cell mass, although elevations in the platelet and/or neutrophil counts are relatively common. The first description

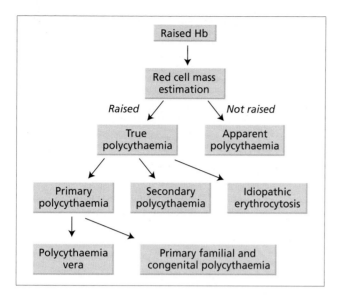

Figure 46.1 An aetiological classification of polycythaemia.

of PV was by Vaquez in 1892. Osler, in 1903, published the first series of patients, identifying salient clinical features setting PV apart from other erythrocytoses. Considerable information has been gathered about PV since the work of these pioneers, much of it due to the work of the Polycythaemia Vera Study Group (PVSG), which was set up in 1967 with the aim of optimising diagnosis and management of PV. The recent discovery of the V617F mutation in the pseudokinase domain of the tyrosine kinase JAK2, in nearly all cases of PV, represents a major advance in our understanding of this disorder.

Pathophysiology

PV is a stem cell disorder characterised by hyperplasia of all three major myeloid cell lineages. The first line of evidence in support of the stem cell origin of PV came in the form of clonality studies. Using X-chromosome inactivation patterns (XCIPs) in the mid-1970s Fialkow and colleagues showed that neutrophils, erythrocytes and platelets originated from the same clone. Large studies have since confirmed these findings.

Erythropoiesis in PV is autonomous and does not rely on erythropoietin (EPO). Plasma levels of this hormone are reduced in PV patients and PV progenitor cells, unlike normal ones, can survive in vitro and give rise to erythroid colonies (BFU-E) in the absence of added erythropoietin (endogenous erythroid colonies, EECs). PV erythroid progenitors show an increased sensitivity to EPO but also to several other growth factors including insulin-like growth factor-1, thrombopoietin, interleukin-3, and granulocyte/monocyte colony-stimulating factor. Germline mutations in the erythropoietin receptor (EPOR) are known to occur in inherited polycythaemia, but such mutations are absent in patients with PV.

In 2005, several groups identified a unique acquired mutation in the cytoplasmic tyrosine kinase JAK2 in myeloid cells from the great majority of patients with PV. JAK2 lies downstream of several cell surface receptors including EPOR. Upon EPO binding to EPOR, JAK2 becomes phosphorylated and in turn phosphorylates downstream targets, most important of which are the STATs (signal transducers and activators of transcription), leading to stimulation of erythropoiesis. Valine 617 is located in the JH2 domain of JAK2, which acts to repress its kinase activity (Figure 46.2). The V617F mutation leads to increased kinase activity, confers cytokine independence and results in erythrocytosis in a mouse transplant model. The mutation appears to be fairly specific to the classical MPD and although it has been reported in small numbers of patients with related myeloid neoplasms, it is not present in lymphoid or non-haemopoietic cancers. Intriguingly, the mutation is homozygous in a proportion of patients with PV and IMF but this is rare in ET.

The significance of a number of observations made prior to the discovery of JAK2V617F remains unclear, although most are likely to represent secondary phenomena. Such observations include (i) over-expression of the mRNA of the gene PRV-1 in granulocytes from PV patients when compared to normal controls or patients with secondary erythrocytoses, (ii) over-expression of the anti-apoptotic protein Bcl-xL in PV erythroid progenitors and (iii) reduced expression of the thrombopoietin receptor (c-mpl) in platelets from patients with PV, ET and IMF. The recurrent chromosomal abnormalities present in about 20–30% of patients with PV may represent mutations co-operating with JAK2V617F.

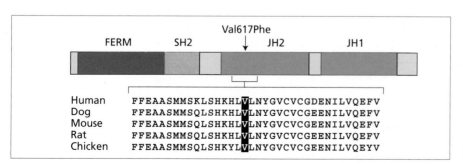

Figure 46.2 Diagrammatic representation of JAK2 indicating the location of valine 617 and the very high degree of cross-species aminoacid homology in its JH2 domain. The JH2 domain normally acts to repress the kinase activity of JAK2, but its ability to do so is impaired in the presence of the JAK2 V617F mutation (Modified from Baxter et al., 2005).

Clinical features

Epidemiology

The annual incidence of PV is reported to be around 2–3 per 100 000 of the population with a male–female ratio of 1.2:1. The median age at onset is 55–60 years and although incidence increases with age, PV can occur at any age even, rarely, in childhood.

Thrombotic complications

Thrombosis is the most common serious complication of PV. Untreated PV patients run a greatly increased risk of thrombosis, which can be arterial, venous or microvascular. The increased PCV leads to an increased blood viscosity, rheological abnormalities and abnormal platelet–endothelial contact. Additionally, procoagulant changes in platelets (e.g. decreased response to prostaglandin D_2), thrombocytosis and pre-existing vascular disease can all conspire to dramatically increase thrombotic risk.

Arterial occlusions can lead to myocardial infarcts, strokes, transient ischaemic attacks, amaurosis, scotomata, mesenteric and limb ischaemia. Less commonly, microvascular occlusions affecting the extremities and erythromelalgia can occur.

In the venous circulation, unusual sites such as the splanchnic vessels can be involved. As a result, mesenteric, splenic and hepatoportal thromboses (Figure 46.3) are recognised presenting features of PV. Superficial thrombophlebitis, conventional deep venous thromboses and pulmonary emboli are also seen.

Neurological features

Over and above the consequences of occlusive vascular lesions,

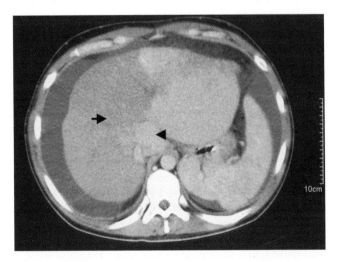

Figure 46.3 Polycythaemia vera presenting with the Budd–Chiari syndrome in a 28-year-old man: contrast computerized tomography showing reduced enhancement of the right lobe of the liver (arrow) with characteristic sparing of the caudate lobe (arrowhead). On this occasion, the left lobe was also relatively spared. Marked ascites and a bulky spleen are also seen.

the sluggish cerebral blood flow secondary to the increased PCV is thought to underlie features such as headaches, drowsiness, insomnia, amnesia, tinnitus, vertigo, chorea and even depression. Transient visual disturbances also occur.

Pruritus

This symptom occurs in about one-quarter of PV patients and in some it may be severe. It is characteristically aquagenic, precipitated by warm baths and can be associated with erythema, swelling or even pain. Pruritus is often relieved by controlling the PCV, but its aetiology remains elusive. Hyperhistaminaemia and iron deficiency may have a role and there is an increased incidence in patients with a lower mean corpuscular volume (MCV).

Skin

Plethora, dilated conjunctival vessels and rosacea-like facial skin changes are not uncommon at presentation. Brown discoloration of the skin, erythromelalgia and, rarely, Sweet's syndrome may be seen.

Splenomegaly

Palpable splenomegaly is seen in 30–50% of cases of PV. It is unclear if its presence affects prognosis, but it may be associated with an increased risk of progression to myelofibrosis.

Hypertension and gout

Hypertension is probably more common in patients with PV as is hyperuricaemia, with gout seen in about 5% of cases.

Leukaemic transformation

This is perhaps the most feared complication of PV, but the risk of developing acute leukaemia in PV patients treated only with venesection is very small (1–3%). This risk, however, increases dramatically (more than 10-fold) when radioactive phosphorus (^{32}P), chlorambucil or irradiation are used as treatment. The median time interval between first starting such therapy and developing acute leukaemia is 5–8 years.

Myelofibrosis

Progression to myelofibrosis (Figure 46.4) occurs in around 10–20% of PV cases at 15 years after diagnosis. This figure is approximate, not least because different studies have used distinct criteria to define myelofibrotic transformation. Transformation often occurs gradually over many years and is thought to be associated with an increased risk of leukaemic conversion. The management of these patients is similar to that of IMF.

Investigations

The diagnosis of PV requires both the identification of features in support of this diagnosis as well as the exclusion of secondary and apparent polycythaemia. The original set of diagnostic criteria was formulated by the PVSG in the 1970s. Based on these

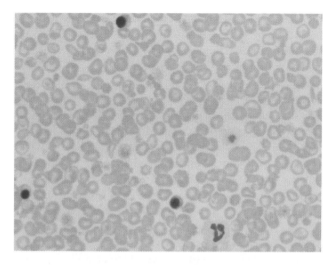

Figure 46.4 Blood film from a case of post-polycythaemic myelofibrosis after splenectomy. Note the presence of nucleated erythrocytes, giant platelets and features of splenectomy including target cells, spherocytes and acanthocytes (×20).

Table 46.1 Diagnostic criteria for polycythaemia vera.

A1.	Raised red cell mass (> 25% above predicted, or PCV ≥ 0.60 in men or ≥ 0.56 in women)*
A2.	Absence of causes of secondary erythrocytosis (normal arterial oxygen saturation and no elevation of serum erythropoietin)
A3.	Palpable splenomegaly
A4.	Presence of JAK2 V617F mutation or other cytogenetic abnormality (excluding *BCR-ABL*) in haemopoietic cells
B1.	Thrombocytosis (platelets > 400×10^9/L)
B2.	Neutrophilia (neutrophils > 10×10^9/L; > 12.5×10^9/L in smokers)
B3.	Radiological splenomegaly
B4.	Endogenous erythroid colonies or low serum erythropoietin

A1 + A2 + either another A or two B criteria establishes PV.
*These PCV values are invariably associated with a raised red cell mass in an adult population.
Modified from Pearson *et al.* (2000).

and taking into account recent developments in the field an up-to-date set of diagnostic criteria is given in Table 46.1.

Establishing the presence of a true erythrocytosis remains the cornerstone of diagnosis, and usually requires demonstration of a raised red cell mass, although this can be assumed to be present when the PCV is ≥ 0.6 in men or ≥ 0.56 in women. It is likely that, with the establishment of PCR-based methods for detecting the JAK2 V617F mutation, this tool will become routinely available in laboratories offering molecular diagnostic services. This will allow most patients to be diagnosed on the basis of a raised red cell mass, normal O_2 saturations and the presence of JAK2 V617F. It is also important to emphasize that the V617F

mutation has been identified in a small proportion of other hematological malignancies (for example, acute myeloid leukemia, chronic myelomonocytic leukemia and myelodysplasia). However, none of these disorders is associated with a raised red cell mass and clinical distinction from PV is rarely an issue.

A minority of patients with clinical PV is negative for the V617F mutation, even when tested using sensitive detection methods. In these patients, the diagnosis of PV can be made if the other criteria set out in Table 46.1 are met. Alternative diagnostic criteria have been proposed recently as part of the 'WHO classification of tumours'. However, these criteria have been criticised on a number of grounds and particularly for the suggestion that a haemoglobin concentration of > 18.5 g/dl for men or > 16.5 g/dl for women is equivalent to a raised red cell mass.

Treatment

Identification of the JAK2 V617F mutation has generated a lot of interest into the development of therapeutic JAK2 inhibitors. However, as patients with PV currently have a very good prognosis new agents will have to display an excellent safety profile. For the time being, the treatment of PV should employ existing treatment modalities whose effectiveness has been validated; as described below.

In the absence of thrombocytosis, regular venesection remains the mainstay of treatment for PV in patients who can tolerate it. A target haematocrit of < 0.45 is widely used, following the demonstration that, in patients with PV, higher haematocrits are associated with a significantly increased risk of thrombosis. With repeat venesections, iron deficiency often ensues, which reduces the frequency of further venesections but may be associated with a reactive thrombocytosis.

Cytoreductive therapy is recommended for patients with thrombocytosis, in view of the probable increased risk of thrombosis, as well as for patients unable to undergo venesection. Hydroxyurea (hydroxycarbamide) is the most commonly used drug. It is orally bioavailable and generally very well tolerated. It will reduce both the haematocrit and the platelet count. The commonest complications are leucopenia or thrombocytopenia, which are dose dependent and can usually be avoided by close monitoring of the blood count when the drug is first introduced. In susceptible patients it can cause photosensitivity, painful leg ulcers and gastrointestinal side-effects. The usual dose is 1–2 g daily.

It has been suggested that hydroxyurea may increase the inherent leukaemogenic risk associated with PV. This concern is largely based on studies involving small numbers of patients or patients who have also required other cytotoxic agents (and may therefore represent a subgroup with more aggressive disease). At present, there are no convincing data to show that hydroxyurea, when used as a single agent, significantly increases the risk of leukaemia, although a small effect cannot be excluded. Preliminary data from studies of hydroxyurea in sickle cell disease are reassuring, but longer follow-up is required.

Interferon-alpha (IFN-α) is effective in controlling both the platelet count and the PCV. It is not widely used because of its cost, route of administration (subcutaneous injection) and its side-effects (including fatigue, flu-like symptoms, depression). It can be useful, however, in young patients who are reluctant to take other cytotoxic agents, in pregnancy and in patients with intractable pruritus. The usual dose range is 3–5 mU three times per week.

Anagrelide is a newer agent that lowers the platelet count by inhibiting megakaryocyte differentiation. It can be useful in controlling the platelet count of patients being treated with venesection and can also be combined with hydroxyurea to allow the use of lower doses of both agents. Approximately 10% of patients are completely refractory to anagrelide. The usual dose is 1–2 mg daily, but occasional patients may require doses of up to 8 mg daily. Its side-effects are mainly secondary to its inotropic and vasodilatory properties and include headaches, palpitations and fluid retention.

Busulphan is sometimes used in elderly patients or when all other treatments are not tolerated. It is very convenient as it need only be administered intermittently, but may increase the risk of leukaemia. The usual dosage is 25–75 mg as a single dose every 2–3 months.

Low-dose aspirin (100 mg daily) reduces thrombotic complications in PV and is used in most patients without contraindications to this drug.

Pruritus often improves with control of the PCV but paroxetine, antihistamines and aspirin (in some cases) can help. There is also evidence that IFN can be useful in intractable cases.

In view of the age of most patients and the relatively benign natural history of treated PV, bone marrow transplantation is not advocated for stable disease. The role, if any, of transplants employing reduced-intensity conditioning regimes is not yet clear.

Prognosis

In the first half of the twentieth century, untreated polycythaemia had a dismal prognosis with a 50% survival of less than 2 years. However, adequately treated PV now has a relatively benign natural history with a life expectancy of over 11 years, bearing in mind that the average age of onset is 60 years.

Other causes of polycythaemia

All disorders with an increased red cell mass which are not due to a clonal proliferation of haemopoietic progenitors are included under this heading. They are most conveniently subclassified into primary and secondary causes. In primary polycythaemia, the defect is intrinsic to the red cell precursors, which are hypersensitive to erythropoietin. In secondary polycythaemia, the defect is upstream of the red cell precursors. The latter group can be further subdivided into polycythaemias in the presence or in the absence of systemic hypoxia. A small group of patients do not fall into any of these categories and are given the diagnosis of idiopathic erythrocytosis (IE) (Table 46.2). The clinical management of many of these syndromes is not well defined.

The term apparent polycythaemia refers to a raised haematocrit in the absence of a raised red cell mass and is discussed later in this chapter.

Primary polycythaemia

Primary familial and congenital polycythaemia

Primary familial and congenital polycythaemia (PFCP) is a rare disorder in which erythropoiesis is intrinsically overactive. The disorder is usually transmitted in an autosomal dominant manner with some cases appearing sporadically. Clinical features include the presence of isolated erythrocytosis without evolution into leukemia or other myeloproliferative disorders, absence of splenomegaly, normal white blood cell and platelet counts, low or normal plasma erythropoietin (Epo) levels, normal haemoglobin–oxygen dissociation curve/P_{50}, and hypersensitivity of erythroid progenitors to Epo. Mutations in the gene encoding the erythropoietin receptor (EpoR) have been described in several (but not all) families with PFCP. In most cases, the mutations lead to a C-terminal truncation of the EpoR protein, with increased sensitivity to Epo.

Secondary polycythaemia

Polycythaemias in the presence of systemic hypoxia

Chronic lung disease and hypopnoea

Lung disease is the predominant cause of chronic systemic hypoxia at sea level. Hypoxaemic chronic obstructive pulmonary disease (COPD) is the commonest syndrome, but any lung–airway disease leading to chronic hypoxia could cause polycythaemia. Syndromes such as obstructive sleep apnoea and hypoventilation due to muscle weakness or paralysis can also occasionally be associated with secondary polycythaemia.

Where possible, hypoxia should be ameliorated by treating the lung disease or with home oxygen therapy. Polycythaemia has opposing effects on oxygen delivery as it increases the oxygen-carrying capacity while also increasing blood viscosity. Unfortunately, there is little evidence from clinical trials to guide management. In practice, many specialists suggest that venesection should be performed for haematocrits above 0.55.

High altitude

Residents at altitudes above 4000 m compensate for the ambient hypoxia by multisystem adaptation, including mild polycythaemia, increase in capillary perfusion and lung diffusion capacity as well as biochemical changes in metabolic enzymes and myoglobin. Cardiac work does not need to increase in most well adapted

Table 46.2 Causes of polycythaemia other than polycythaemia vera.

Primary polycythaemia (intrinsic defect in red cell progenitors)	Primary familial and congenital polycythaemia		
Secondary polycythaemia	Polycythaemia in the presence of systemic hypoxia	Chronic hypoxia	Lung disease
			Hypopnoea
			High altitude
			Congenital cyanotic heart disease
		Defective oxygen transport	High-affinity haemoglobins
			Red cell metabolic defects (low 2,3-BPG)
			Methaemoglobinaemia
			Heavy smoking (carboxyhaemoglobinaemia)
	Polycythaemia in the absence of systemic hypoxia	Inherited/congenital polycythaemia	Chuvash polycythaemia
		Abnormal erythropoietin secretion	Renal tumours
			Cystic/polycystic kidney disease
			Renal transplantation
			Renal hypoxia (e.g. renal artery stenosis)
			Cerebellar haemangioma
			Hepatocellular carcinoma
		Endocrine syndromes	Administration of androgenic steroids
			Cushing's syndrome
			Conn's syndrome
			Phaeochromocytoma (rarely)
			Bartter's syndrome
Idiopathic erythrocytosis			

individuals. Excessive altitude polycythaemia (PCV > 0.65) is seen in a proportion of cases and is often accompanied by hyperuricaemia and proteinuria. Some of these individuals eventually decompensate and develop chronic mountain sickness (Monge's disease). Such people deteriorate steadily and develop extreme polycythaemia (sometimes PCV > 0.75), arterial desaturation and right heart failure. Symptoms range from mental slowing, headaches and lethargy to breathlessness, dry cough and signs of right heart failure. Many of the cases described were miners with coincidental pulmonary disease and the latter may play a significant role in the process of decompensation. Resettlement at lower altitudes halts disease progression and can partly reverse it.

Treatment with angiotensin-converting enzyme (ACE) inhibitors has been shown in randomized studies to reduce the PCV and proteinuria seen in excessive altitude polycythaemia.

Congenital cyanotic heart disease

Congenital heart defects leading to a right-to-left shunt can cause dramatic polycythaemia (up to PCV > 0.80). Surgery to correct the cardiac defect should be undertaken when possible. A few inoperable patients survive to adulthood and the management of their polycythaemia is not straightforward. As in patients with chronic lung disease, the increase in oxygen-

carrying capacity afforded by polycythaemia is countered by an increased viscosity and associated haemodynamic changes. Here, however, we are often dealing with young patients with responsive vasculatures, which can usually accommodate such changes. Some experts advocate venesection when the PCV is greater than 0.60, whereas others allow the haematocrit to rise further and venesect for symptoms such as recurrent haemoptysis, marked fatigue or deteriorating exercise tolerance.

High-affinity haemoglobins

High-affinity haemoglobins release less oxygen for a given oxygen partial pressure, and may thus give rise to tissue hypoxia. This leads to an erythropoietin-driven polycythaemia, which tends to re-normalize erythropoietin levels. The pathognomonic anomaly is a left shift in the oxygen dissociation curve (Figure 46.5). The precise variant can be identified by mutational screening of DNA or by protein mass spectrometry.

There are over 40 haemoglobin variants with an increased affinity for oxygen, all dominantly inherited. Most are due to mutations in β-globin, with a small number due to mutations in α-globin. Mutations are clustered in regions of the globin chains involved in the regulation of the transition between tense (T) and relaxed (R) states of haemoglobin. Normally, oxy-HbA is in

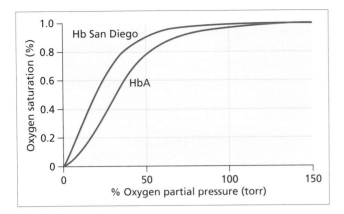

Figure 46.5 Haemoglobin–oxygen dissociation curves from a 27-year-old man with a raised red cell mass and a normal person (HbA) showing the presence of a high-affinity Hb ('left shift'). Mass spectrometric analysis showed the man to be heterozygous for Hb San Diego, a high-affinity β-chain variant.

the T state and has low affinity for oxygen, and deoxy-HbA is in the R state and has a high affinity for oxygen. Thus, mutations at the αβ contact site (e.g. Hb San Diego), the C-terminus (e.g. Hb Bethesda) and the 2,3-BPG (2,3-bisphosphoglycerate) binding site (e.g. Hb Helsinki) are the commonest.

Most people with a high-affinity Hb are in good health and are either diagnosed coincidentally or after being noticed to be plethoric. Some experience excessive muscle fatigue after vigorous exercise. Hyperviscosity is rarely a problem and surveys have failed to identify increased cardiovascular morbidity or mortality. Pregnancy is not adversely affected, even in mothers with haemoglobin affinity that exceeds that of HbF.

Red cell metabolic defects

Very rare cases of polycythaemia are due to abnormalities in red cell metabolism that lead to a reduction in intra-erythrocytic 2,3-BPG. The best characterized defect is a mutant 2,3-BPG mutase. The only well characterized family with this disorder showed an autosomal recessive inheritance, although heterozygous family members had a decreased P_{50} and, in some cases, a moderate polycythaemia. This disorder is excluded by the finding of a normal P_{50} in a fresh blood sample.

Methaemoglobinaemia

Oxidation of haem iron converts it from its normal ferrous (Fe^{2+}) to the ferric (Fe^{3+}) form and, correspondingly, haemoglobin (HbA) becomes methaemoglobin (Met-HbA). This constitutes an important antioxidant mechanism for the red cell, and conversion of Met-HbA back to HbA requires the generation of NADH from glycolysis. The rate of HbA auto-oxidation is about 20 times slower under normal circumstances than the rate of Met-HbA reduction, thus preventing Met-HbA accumulation.

Methaemoglobin has an increased affinity for oxygen and a left-shifted oxygen dissociation curve. Pathological acquired methaemoglobinaemia can result from exposure to strong oxidants (e.g. dapsone, paraquat, benzocaine) and can be life-threatening when severe but is rarely sufficiently long-lived to give rise to polycythaemia.

Hereditary methaemoglobinaemias can be due to haemoglobin mutations involving amino acids around the haem pocket (haemoglobin M disease), or secondary to enzymatic deficiencies that interfere with the generation of NADH which is required for day-to-day methaemoglobin reduction (namely NADH reductase and cytochrome $b5$ reductase). In view of the chronic nature of the methaemoglobinaemia in these disorders, secondary erythrocytosis can develop in the same manner as for high-affinity haemoglobin mutants.

Heavy smoking

Heavy smoking can lead to mild polycythaemia in the absence of hypoxic lung disease. The underlying cause of this is a raised carboxyhaemoglobin (CO-Hb) level resulting from chronically raised carbon monoxide (CO) levels. CO-Hb levels in urban dwelling non-smokers are rarely higher than 2%, with levels ranging from 3% to 20% in smokers. The short half-life of CO in the body (3–5 h) leads, in smokers, to a rise in CO-Hb during the day and a fall during sleep, making it difficult to compare measurements taken at different times. Binding of CO to Hb, as well as displacing O_2, leads to a conformational change similar to that seen in methaemoglobinaemia, with a similar left shift in the oxygen dissociation curve and a fall in P_{50}.

Polycythaemia in the absence of systemic hypoxia

Inherited/congenital polycythaemia

Chuvash polycythaemia

Chuvash polycythaemia (CP) is an autosomal recessive condition that is endemic in the Russian mid-Volga river region of Chuvashia. Patients have increased levels of circulating erythropoietin but do not carry mutations of the Epo receptor. CP was recently shown to be associated with a C → T mutation at nucleotide 598 (leads to an Arg200Trp substitution) in the von Hippel–Lindau (VHL) gene. The *VHL* gene is pivotal for ubiquitination and subsequent degradation of HIF-1 transcription factor, which is central to the oxygen-sensing pathway. This *VHL* mutant leads to a reduced rate of degradation of HIF1 and upregulation of downstream targets including Epo, leading to polycythaemia. Recently, some of the rare non-Russian families with inherited polycythaemia were also shown to carry *VHL* mutations.

Abnormal erythropoietin secretion

Abnormal Epo secretion is a well-recognized cause of secondary polycythaemia and is most commonly secondary to renal pathologies such as renal tumours (benign and malignant), polycystic kidney disease and diseases associated with local hypoxia such as renal cysts, hydronephrosis and renal artery stenosis. The polycythaemia usually responds to treatment of the underlying renal pathology.

Erythrocytosis occurs in 20–30% of patients after renal transplantation. The biggest risk to such patients is hypertension, strokes and cardiovascular complications. In many cases, the erythrocytosis and associated hypertension respond to ACE inhibitors. Theophylline may also be effective in some cases. Patients who remain polycythaemic despite such treatments should be treated with repeated venesections to maintain their haematocrit below 45%; 30–40% of cases resolve spontaneously.

Non-renal tumours can rarely be associated with polycythaemia. The commonest reported ones are hepatocellular carcinoma, cerebellar and other haemangiomata and large uterine fibromyomata. Polycythaemia responds to removal of the tumour in most of these cases.

Endocrine disorders

The mechanism underlying the development of polycythaemia in most endocrine disorders lies in the overproduction of androgens, which can produce polycythaemia by increasing Epo levels and also, probably, through a direct action on bone marrow progenitors.

Idiopathic erythrocytosis

In a small proportion of patients with polycythaemia the criteria for the diagnosis of PV are not met and no other aetiology for the raised red cell mass can be identified. This group is heterogeneous and likely to include patients with germline mutations causing polycythaemia as well as some that will go on to develop overt PV. With the advent of increasingly sophisticated diagnostic tests and the identification of the molecular lesions in many inherited forms of polycythaemia, idiopathic erythrocytosis is becoming a rare entity.

Apparent polycythaemia

Apparent polycythaemia refers to a raised PCV (> 0.51 in males, > 0.48 in females) in the presence of a normal red cell volume (less than 25% above the predicted mean normal value). The raised haematocrit is due to a reduction in the plasma volume. Smoking, hypertension, obesity, excessive alcohol and diuretic therapy have all been associated with apparent polycythaemia. Pathogenesis is uncertain and almost certainly heterogeneous. Some cases of high-affinity Hbs have been reportedly associated with apparent rather than true polycythaemia, but this may simply reflect the moderate nature of the elevation in red cell volume in such cases.

It is not clear whether apparent polycythaemia is associated with increased rates of thrombosis, but it seems sensible to encourage affected individuals to avoid known predisposing factors. There are no convincing data that routine venesection is beneficial but some authorities advocate venesection at PCV > 0.55, particularly for those at risk of vaso-occlusive events.

Essential thrombocythaemia

The fundamental pathological feature of essential thrombocythaemia (ET) is a persistent elevation in the platelet count to above $600 \times 10^9/l$. However, ET has been poorly understood largely because of a lack of positive diagnostic criteria together with the fact that cases labelled as ET are likely to be pathogenetically heterogeneous. In 1934 Epstein & Goedel first described a patient with persistent elevation of the platelet count in association with megakaryocyte hyperplasia and tendency for venous thromboses and haemorrhage. Subsequently Ozer and Gunz independently described two series of patients in 1960 thus confirming ET as a specific clinical entity. The recent discovery that approximately half the cases of ET carry the JAK2V617F mutation as do half the cases of IMF and nearly all cases of PV, has enhanced our understanding of the relationship between the three disorders.

Pathophysiology

X-chromosome inactivation patterns (XCIP) provided the first evidence that ET may be a clonal stem cell disorder involving granulocytes, platelets and red cells but not T-cells. The hope that this finding could provide a much-needed diagnostic tool has been confounded by two observations: Firstly the fact that around 25% of normal elderly females have acquired skewing of XCIP in myeloid cells. Secondly the evidence that myelopoiesis can be polyclonal in many cases of ET. Taken together, these findings demonstrate that XCIP analysis cannot be used as a routine diagnostic test in ET.

Clinical and pathological features vary significantly between patients with ET suggesting that the disease is heterogeneous. Prospective data from over 800 patients with ET has demonstrated that the presence or absence of the JAK2 V617F mutation divide ET into two biologically distinct disorders. Mutation-positive ET exists along a continuum with PV as it displays multiple features of the latter, with significantly increased haemoglobin levels, neutrophil counts and bone marrow erythropoiesis, more venous thromboses and a higher incidence of polycythaemic transformation. Mutation-negative patients do nonetheless exhibit many clinical and laboratory features characteristic of a myeloproliferative disorder including the presence of endogenous erythroid colonies and a risk of transformation to acute leukaemia.

Clinical features

Epidemiology
The annual incidence of ET is similar to that of PV at around 1.5–2.0 cases per 100 000 of the population. The median age at onset is 50–55 years and, although it can occur at any age, it is rare in childhood.

Thrombotic complications
As with PV, thrombotic complications are the main cause of morbidity and mortality in ET. Thromboses are present in around 15–20% of patients at presentation and may be arterial or venous. The range of clinical syndromes is similar to PV, but the frequency of splanchnic thromboses is probably lower.

A number of risk factors are associated with an increase in the risk of thrombosis in patients with ET. The best characterized are age over 60 years and a prior history of thrombosis. Other risk factors for thrombosis in ET are likely to include high platelet count (> 1000), hyperlipidaemia, hypertension and cigarette smoking. More recently, provisional data suggest that male gender, monoclonal haemopoiesis, the presence of antiphospholipid antibodies, spontaneous megakaryocyte or erythroid colonies and inheritance of the factor V Leiden polymorphism may also increase the risk of thrombosis. Platelet function abnormalities do not correlate with thrombotic risk.

Haemorrhagic complications
Bleeding is less common and less well studied than thrombosis in ET, but can be dramatic when it happens. Efforts to correlate the thrombotic risk to platelet function abnormalities have generally been fruitless and this investigation is also unable to predict haemorrhagic risk. Bleeding is, however, more common in patients with platelet counts above 1000 and, in at least some cases, this is due to an acquired von Willebrand disease, with a decrease in high-molecular-weight multimers.

Splenomegaly and hyposplenism
Splenomegaly is present in about 20–25% of ET patients at diagnosis and it is rarely more than moderate. Progressive enlargement of the spleen during the course of ET should raise suspicion of evolving myelofibrosis. It has been suggested that over time, some patients with ET develop splenic atrophy secondary to silent microinfarcts in the splenic microcirculation. Frank hyposplenism and its complications are rare however.

Transformation to myelofibrosis or polycythaemia vera
Transformation to myelofibrosis and, more rarely, to PV, are recognized complications of ET. Some, but not all, cases of apparent polycythaemic transformation may represent resolution of prior iron deficiency, as can happen with iron supplementation and after the menopause. The insidious onset of myelofibrotic transformation and the reluctance to serially study bone marrow

trephine biopsies have hampered attempts to define its nature and frequency. From the limited available data, myelofibrotic transformation occurs in less than 10% and polycythaemic transformation in less than 1–2% of ET patients over 10 years.

Leukaemic transformation
ET can evolve into a myelodysplastic syndrome (MDS) or AML even in untreated cases, but only rarely. The presence of cytogenetic abnormalities and treatment with alkylating agents increase this risk. Approximately 3% of patients treated with hydroxyurea alone develop MDS or AML if followed for a median time of 8 years. As with PV, there are no data that demonstrate that hydroxyurea as a single agent significantly increases the risk of leukaemia inherent to this disease, but a small effect cannot be excluded.

Investigations

The lack of pathognomonic features and the existence of many other causes of a raised platelet count have posed significant hurdles in the diagnosis of ET. The identification of the JAK2 V617F mutation now provides a very useful positive diagnostic criterion for approximately 50% of ET patients. However, for V617F negative patients ET remains a diagnosis of exclusion and can only be made after other clonal blood disorders and reactive thrombocytosis have been ruled out. A proposed diagnostic schema for ET, based on the original criteria set out by the PVSG, is given in Table 46.3.

An alternative set of diagnostic criteria, which include salient bone marrow morphological features, have been proposed as part of the 'WHO classification of tumours'. It is not yet clear, however, whether these are sufficiently robust to be used in routine diagnosis. Nevertheless, bone marrow histological features such as giant, multilobated megakaryocytes and megakaryocyte clustering (Figure 46.6) can be of value in making the diagnosis of ET, although the relationship of this histological feature to the presence or absence of JAK2 V617F has not yet been examined.

Reactive thrombocytosis
Thrombocytosis is most commonly reactive and secondary to increased levels of circulating cytokines that stimulate thrombopoiesis. Inflammatory, vasculitic and allergic disorders, acute and chronic infections, malignancies, haemolysis, iron deficiency and blood loss can all lead to an increased platelet count (Table 46.4). Reactive thrombocytosis can sometimes be marked and, occasionally, the platelet count can be greater than 1000×10^9/L. There is usually evidence of on-going inflammation in the form of a raised erythrocyte sedimentation rate (ESR) or C-reactive protein but this is not always the case.

Other clonal thrombocytoses
A number of other haematological malignancies can be associated

Table 46.3 Proposed diagnostic criteria for essential thrombocythaemia (ET).

A1.	Platelet count $> 600 \times 10^9$/L for at least 2 months
A2.	Acquired JAK2 V617F mutation
B1.	No cause for a reactive thrombocytosis
	– e.g. normal inflammatory indices
B2.	No evidence of iron deficiency
	– stainable iron in the marrow or normal red cell MCV *
B3.	No evidence of PV
	– hematocrit < midpoint of normal range or normal red cell mass in presence of normal iron stores
B4.	No evidence of chronic myeloid leukemia
	– no Philadelphia chromosome or *bcr-abl* fusion
B5.	No evidence of myelofibrosis
	– no collagen fibrosis and ≤ grade 2 reticulin fibrosis (using 0–4 scale)
B6.	No evidence of a myelodysplastic syndrome[†]
	– no significant dysplasia
	– no cytogenetic abnormalities suggestive of myelodysplasia

Diagnosis of ET requires A1 + A2 + B3 − 6 or A1 + B1 − 6

*If these measurements suggest iron deficiency, PV cannot be excluded unless a trial of iron therapy fails to increase the red cell mass into the polycythaemic range (patients need to be monitored closely since a rapid rise in hematocrit can precipitate thrombosis).
[†]Less than 5% of patients with myelodysplastic syndrome carry the V617F JAK2 mutation.

Table 46.4 Causes of a reactive thrombocytosis.

Iron deficiency
Blood loss (acute or chronic)
Hyposplenism/splenectomy
Surgery
Chronic inflammation
   Vasculitides
   Inflammatory bowel disease
   Connective tissue disorders
   Rheumatoid arthritis
   Chronic infections
Malignancies
Rebound thrombocytosis
   Following treatment of immune thrombocytopenic purpura
   Recovery from chemotherapy
Drugs
   Vincristine

with thrombocytosis. Chronic myeloid leukaemia (CML) can be excluded by demonstrating the absence of the bcr-abl fusion transcript. If the haemoglobin or haematocrit are near the upper limit of normal it is useful to measure the red cell mass in order to exclude PV, remembering that iron deficiency can mask a raised red cell mass. Screening for the JAK2 V617F mutation can be particularly useful in this setting since the vast majority of patients with PV are mutation positive. Established IMF can be excluded by the absence of significant bone marrow fibrosis.

Lastly, myelodysplastic syndromes can also be associated with a thrombocytosis in a minority of cases, but there are usually coexisting cytopenias, dysplastic features or specific cytogenetic abnormalities (e.g. deletion 5q).

Treatment

When considering the management of patients with ET, it is helpful to stratify patients into risk groups, according to their risk of vascular complications, and take treatment decisions on this basis. Patients may be assigned to a high-, intermediate- or low-risk category.

High-risk patients

High-risk patients are those over 60 years old and those with one or more high-risk features, i.e. a platelet count $> 1500 \times 10^9$/L, a prior history of thrombosis or significant thrombotic risk factors such as diabetes or hypertension. In high-risk patients control of the platelet count with hydroxyurea reduces thrombotic events. The MRC PT-1 trial has recently compared treatment with hydroxyurea plus low-dose aspirin to anagrelide plus low-dose aspirin. Patients receiving anagrelide plus aspirin were significantly more likely to reach the composite primary

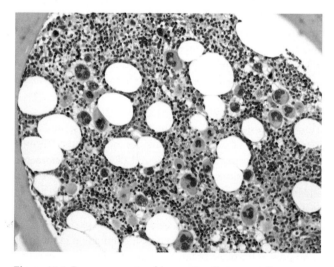

Figure 46.6 Bone marrow trephine section (haematoxylin and eosin, H&E) from a 60-year-old man with essential thrombocythaemia. Note the hypercellularity and marked increase in megakaryocyte numbers, consisting largely of clusters of mature, multilobated forms.

endpoint (arterial thrombosis, venous thrombosis or major haemorrhage) and more likely to discontinue their allocated treatment. Compared to hydroxyurea plus aspirin, treatment with anagrelide plus aspirin was associated with a significantly increased rate of arterial thrombosis, major haemorrhage and myelofibrotic transformation, but a decreased rate of venous thromboembolism. These results suggest that hydroxyurea plus aspirin should remain first line therapy for high-risk patients. Anagrelide is a useful second line agent but the decision to use concurrent aspirin should depend on the relative risks of arterial thrombosis and haemorrhage in the individual patient.

Analysis of patients from the PT-1 trial according to JAK2 status has shown that compared with V617F negative patients, mutation positive patients share many features with PV including a higher risk of venous thrombosis. Moreover V617F positive patients were more sensitive to hydroxyurea than anagrelide, raising the possibility that hydroxyurea is particularly effective in these patients.

IFN-α can give good control of the platelet count in ET, but as discussed under PV, its significant side-effect profile, subcutaneous administration and cost prevent its widespread use. It has a clearer role in the management of ET in pregnancy (vide infra) and some favour it in young patients. Busulphan can achieve good control of the platelet count but is only rarely used because of concerns over its long-term leukaemogenic potential. This is true for other alkylating agents and for radioactive phosphorus (^{32}P).

Intermediate-risk patients

Intermediate-risk patients are those between 40 and 60 years old who lack any of the high-risk features listed above. It is not clear whether it is beneficial to lower the platelet count in this group. Most receive either aspirin alone, or hydroxyurea and aspirin.

Low-risk patients

Low-risk patients are those younger than 40 years old who lack any high-risk features. Low risk patients are usually given low-dose aspirin alone unless there is a contraindication such as previous peptic ulceration, ET-associated haemorrhage or allergy to salicylates. Anti-platelet agents such as dipyridamole, ticlopidine or clopidogrel should be considered in these cases.

Prognosis

Few studies have directly addressed survival in ET and these have reached different conclusions. Some suggest that mortality at 10 years is that of age-matched controls, whereas others found it to be worse. In high-risk patients, hydroxyurea reduces vaso-occlusive events from 10.7 to 1.6 per 100 patient-years.

Essential thrombocythaemia and pregnancy

ET is the MPD encountered most frequently in women of childbearing age. Fertility is probably reduced in women with ET, but data are lacking on this. In pregnancy, the commonest complication of ET is first-trimester miscarriage, which occurs in up to 30% of pregnancies. This is thought to be secondary to placental microinfarcts and insufficiency. The reported increased incidence of antiphospholipid antibodies in ET may contribute to this. Other less frequent complications include intrauterine death, growth retardation, premature delivery and pre-eclampsia. The risk of maternal thrombosis and haemorrhage is higher than in normal pregnancy, nonetheless a successful outcome (live birth) is achieved in around 60% of cases and no maternal deaths were seen in a recent review of 220 pregnancies.

The optimal management of ET in pregnancy has not yet been fully defined. There is conflicting evidence about the effectiveness of aspirin but, given the good documentation of its safety in a large unrelated study of pre-eclampsia, it should probably be given to most patients who are pregnant or planning a pregnancy. Pregnancies deemed at high risk of thrombosis either on the basis of a prior history of thrombosis or a platelet count of over 1000×10^9/L should be considered for therapy with a combination of IFN and aspirin. Hydroxyurea and anagrelide should not be used on account of their teratogenic potential. In addition to lowering the platelet count, cases at the highest risk of thrombosis, such as those with previous thrombosis, hypertension or diabetes, should be considered for antithrombotic prophylaxis normally in the form of low-molecular-weight heparin.

The platelet count may rise dramatically in the post-partum period but can normally be controlled with hydroxyurea or anagrelide. Hydroxyurea and anagrelide are excreted in breast milk so that breast-feeding is contraindicated while a patient is receiving either of these agents. Although IFN-α is also excreted in breast milk, it is unlikely to be absorbed intact by the baby and there are anecdotal reports of successful breast-feeding while the mother was receiving IFN.

Idiopathic myelofibrosis

Also known as agnogenic myeloid metaplasia, idiopathic myelofibrosis (IMF) has the poorest prognosis of the MPDs. PV and ET can develop into a condition that resembles IMF, usually after a latency of many years. The first reported case of IMF is probably that reported by Hueck in 1879 as a 'peculiar leukaemia'. It was not until Dameshek's seminal work in 1951 that IMF was recognised as a myeloproliferative disorder. The identification of the JAK2 V617F mutation in approximately half the cases of IMF and ET and nearly all cases of PV, has revolutionised our understanding of the relationship between the three disorders.

Pathophysiology

Idiopathic myelofibrosis is a clonal myeloproliferative disorder of the pluripotent haemopoietic stem cell, in which the proliferation of multiple cell lineages is accompanied by progressive bone marrow fibrosis. This is true for both JAK2 V617F positive and negative cases whilst the precise effect of the mutation on the IMF phenotype awaits further studies.

Marrow fibrosis is thought to be secondary to the release of pro-inflammatory cytokines from abnormal clonal cells (primarily megakaryocytes), which act to stimulate fibroblast proliferation and fibrosis. In support of this premise, transgenic mice expressing high levels of TPO rapidly develop myelofibrosis in association with increased megakaryocyte numbers. Additionally mice expressing reduced levels of the transcription factor GATA-1, which impairs the ability of their megakaryocytes to differentiate into platelets, also develop myelofibrosis in association with increased expression of cytokines such as transforming growth factor-β1, platelet-derived growth factor and vascular endothelial growth factor in the bone marrow.

In the peripheral circulation there is an increase in the number of CD34-positive cells together with increased numbers of progenitors capable of giving rise to a variety of haemopoietic colonies. As with PV and ET, erythroid and megakaryocytic colonies can also be derived in the absence of exogenous growth factors.

Cytogenetic abnormalities are commoner in IMF than in other MPDs and are found in up to 60% of cases. The commonest are deletions of 20q and 13q, trisomy 8, and abnormalities of chromosomes 1, 5, 7 and 9. These may co-operate with JAK2 V617F in producing the IMF phenotype. Oncogene mutations are rare and include point mutations in N-RAS, c-KIT and P53.

Clinical features

Epidemiology

The estimated annual incidence of IMF is around 0.5–1.5 per 100 000 of the population, with most patients diagnosed in the sixth decade and roughly equal involvement of the two sexes. Up to a third of patients are asymptomatic at diagnosis and many of these are discovered after unrelated blood tests show modest abnormalities such as anaemia and thrombocytopenia.

Splenomegaly

An enlarged spleen is found in almost all patients at presentation and splenic pain/discomfort is a common presenting symptom of IMF. Most cases develop moderate to marked splenomegaly during the course of the disease and about 10% of cases develop massive splenomegaly, with the spleen extending to the right iliac fossa (Figure 46.7). This dramatic increase in splenic mass (up to 20–30 times normal) can lead to a substantial increase in splenic blood flow which, in the most severe cases, can lead to portal hypertension with oesophageal varices and ascites. Painful and painless splenic infarcts are common sequelae of splenomegaly in IMF.

Extramedullary haemopoiesis

The spleen is the commonest site of extramedullary haemopoiesis

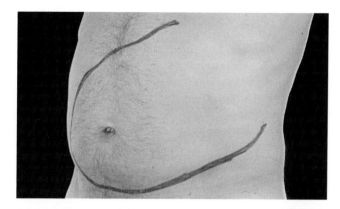

Figure 46.7 Massive splenomegaly in a 53-year-old man with an 8-year history of idiopathic myelofibrosis (IMF).

in IMF. The liver is also usually involved and this can lead to significant hepatomegaly. Unusual sites can sometimes be affected, leading to haemopoietic tumours surrounded by a capsule of connective tissue. Such sites include lymph nodes, central nervous system, skin, pericardium, peritoneum, pleura, ovaries, kidneys, adrenals, gastrointestinal tract and lungs. Many such cases remain asymptomatic, but involvement of the central nervous system can be a cause of serious morbidity. Treatment with radiotherapy or surgery, when required, almost always leads to resolution of these masses.

Systemic symptoms

A hypermetabolic state presenting with fevers, anorexia, weight loss and night sweats develops in many cases of IMF, sometimes early on in the disease. The presence of such symptoms is associated with a poor prognosis.

Anaemia

Mild to moderate anaemia is found in most patients at presentation and worsens as myelofibrosis progresses. The anaemia is in large part due to reduced erythropoiesis, but may be compounded by hypersplenism, bleeding and iron or folate deficiency. Acquired HbH disease is a rare complication.

Platelet abnormalities

Platelet counts are raised in up to one-half of the cases at presentation and can be associated with thrombotic complications. However, progressive thrombocytopenia is a frequent occurrence and becomes increasingly troublesome as the disease progresses. Dysmegakaryopoiesis and abnormal platelet function further add to the risk of haemorrhagic complications.

White cells and leukaemic transformation

The presence of immature myeloid as well as erythroid progenitors is a characteristic feature of IMF (Figure 46.8). Neutrophilia is common, as are modest elevations in basophil and eosinophil counts. As the disease progresses, leucopenia increases in fre-

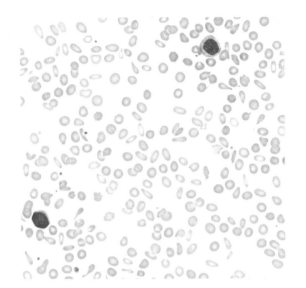

Figure 46.8 Peripheral blood film in IMF, showing a blast, an abnormal myelocyte, teardrop red cells and marked anisopoikilocytosis.

quency and is believed to be secondary to progressive hypersplenism, dysmyelopoiesis and progressive replacement of the bone marrow by fibrotic tissue. In end-stage IMF, myeloid precursors become increasingly common relative to mature cells, as do circulating blasts. Transformation to AML occurs in 5–10% of cases of IMF and is usually rapidly fatal.

Investigations

Diagnostic criteria for IMF are shown in Table 46.5 (the role of JAK2 V617F. Other causes of bone marrow fibrosis are listed in Table 46.6.

Peripheral blood

The presence of myeloid and erythroid precursors in the peripheral blood (leucoerythroblastic blood picture) is common in IMF (see Figure 46.8). Other causes of a leucoerythroblastic blood film include bone marrow infiltration, severe sepsis, severe haemolysis and a sick neonate. Teardrop poikilocytes (dacryocytes), basophilic stippling, macrocytosis (which may or may not be secondary to folate deficiency), giant platelets and megakaryocyte fragments may also be present.

Bone marrow

Attempts at bone marrow aspiration often yield a dry-tap or a haemodilute sample, making aspirate morphology of limited diagnostic value. Sufficient material can often be obtained from either bone marrow or peripheral blood to assess the karyotype, which can help exclude diagnoses such as CML. Other chromosomal abnormalities may be found in up to 60% of cases as detailed above. Abnormalities of chromosomes 5 and

Table 46.5 Diagnostic criteria for idiopathic myelofibrosis.

A1	Diffuse bone marrow fibrosis*
A2	No Philadelphia chromosome or BCR–ABL rearrangement
B1	Acquired JAK2 V617F mutation
B2	Splenomegaly
B3	Anisopoikilocytosis with tear-drop poikilocytes
B4	Circulating immature myeloid cells
B5	Circulating erythroblasts
B6	Myeloid metaplasia

Both A criteria and B1+B2 *or*
Both A criteria and at least four B criteria make the diagnosis of IMF when B1 or B2 absent.
*Requires microscopic evidence of grade III or IV fibrosis.
Modified from Barosi *et al.* (1999).

Table 46.6 Differential diagnosis of marrow fibrosis.

Haematological malignancies	Drugs/toxins
Idiopathic myelofibrosis	Benzene
Chronic myeloid leukaemia	Thorotrast
Acute myelofibrosis (AML M7)	Irradiation
Myelodysplasia	
Myeloma	Bone disease
Hairy-cell leukaemia	Paget's disease
Non-Hodgkin's lymphoma	Osteopetrosis
Hodgkin's disease	Hyperparathyroidism
Systemic mastocytosis	Hypoparathyroidism
Metastatic carcinoma	Inflammatory diseases
	Systemic sclerosis
Infections	Systemic lupus
Tuberculosis	erythematosus
Leishmaniasis	
	Other
	Grey platelet syndrome

7 are usually found in patients with prior exposure to genotoxic agents and are associated with a poor prognosis.

Bone marrow trephine biopsy is essential to make a diagnosis of IMF. Initial stages are characterized by an increase in bone marrow cellularity in association with a disorganization of marrow architecture and the presence of abnormal large megakaryocytes often occurring in clusters (Figure 46.9). Bone marrow fibrosis becomes increasingly dominant and progressively replaces haemopoiesis. Intrasinusoidal haemopoiesis can sometimes be seen at this stage (Figure 46.10). The degree of fibrosis is best demonstrated using silver impregnation, which stains reticulin fibres (see Figure 46.9). Collagen fibres are best demonstrated using a trichrome stain. The degree of fibrosis can be graded

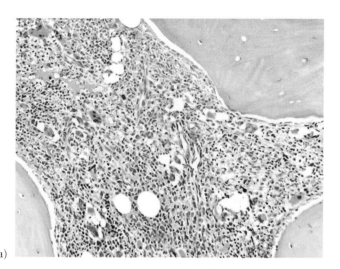
(a)

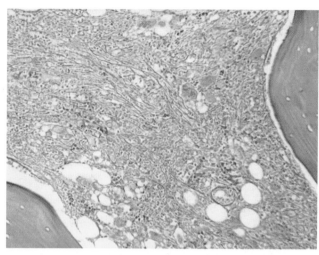
(b)

Figure 46.9 Bone marrow trephine sections from a patient with early-stage IMF. The H&E stain (a) shows hypercellularity, disorganized architecture, increase in megakaryocyte numbers and prominent sinusoids. The silver stain (b) also shows a marked increase in reticulin fibres.

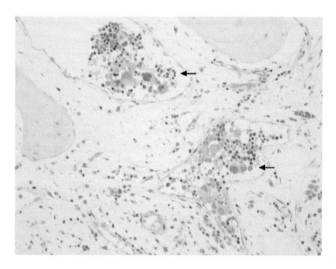

Figure 46.10 Bone marrow trephine section in IMF (H&E). Note the presence of two dilated sinusoids (arrows) containing immature haemopoietic cells, including megakaryocytes.

from I to IV according to severity. In a minority of cases of advanced IMF (less than 10%), osteosclerosis ensues with thickening of the trabecula and extensive deposition of osteoid. Such changes may be evident on plain radiography.

Treatment

The only curative treatment for IMF is allogeneic stem cell transplantation, but this is only appropriate for a small proportion of patients. In the remaining cases therapy remains supportive and aimed at alleviating symptoms, but has little impact on the relatively poor survival of IMF patients. It is for this reason that the

future development of therapeutic JAK2 inhibitors is most eagerly awaited for these patients rather than those with PV or ET who have a much better prognosis.

Conventional allogeneic bone marrow transplantation is only a realistic option in young patients who represent perhaps 10% of all cases. The decision to proceed to transplantation should always be made in light of the patient's specific prognosis, age and general fitness. Only small series have been reported and the long-term survival of patients < 45 years is approximately 50%, with a 30% transplant-related mortality. For patients > 45 years, outcomes are much worse, with long-term survival of 10–20%. Small numbers of reduced-intensity transplants have been reported, which show that this modality is feasible and safe in patients over 50 years old, although its efficacy is not yet clear.

Anaemia responds to treatment with androgens in up to one-third of cases, with the best responses seen in patients without massive splenomegaly and with a normal karyotype. The drugs most commonly used are oxymethalone (50–150 mg daily) and danazol (400–600 mg daily). Both of these can have virilizing effects and can lead to abnormal liver function. Patients with a reduced red cell survival may respond to treatment with corticosteroids. Human recombinant erythropoietin has recently shown promise in small clinical studies of anaemia in IMF. Splenectomy also has a role (see below). Despite these treatments, most patients become transfusion dependent eventually.

Cytoreductive therapy can be useful in the management of some aspects of IMF, such as hepatosplenomegaly, constitutional symptoms and troublesome thrombocytosis. Hydroxyurea is the most widely used agent but anagrelide has also been used for thrombocytosis.

The indications for splenectomy include splenic pain, constitutional symptoms, portal hypertension and transfusion-dependent anaemia. In contrast, there is no good evidence that

Table 46.7 Prognostic scoring systems in myelofibrosis: the Lille scoring system.

Number of adverse prognostic factors	Risk group	Cases (%)	Median survival (months)
0	Low	47	93
1	Intermediate	45	26
2	High	8	13

Adverse prognostic factors: Hb 10 g/dL, WBC < 4 or > 30 × 10^9/L.
From Dupriez et al. (1996).

thrombocytopenia responds to splenectomy. The procedure has significant mortality (around 10%) and morbidity, particularly in elderly patients. Problems include perioperative bleeding, infection and thrombosis as well as rebound thrombocytosis and progressive hepatomegaly. It is particularly important to correct any coagulation abnormalities prior to surgery.

Splenic irradiation is an alternative to splenectomy in some cases and it can significantly reduce splenic size, albeit transiently. This procedure is not without complications as it can lead to life-threatening cytopenias. Radiotherapy can also be useful for treating pockets of extramedullary haemopoiesis involving vital organs or bodily cavities.

The antiangiogenic drug thalidomide has been reported to improve anaemia, thrombocytopenia or splenomegaly in approximately one-half of the patients, but these changes are clinically significant only in a small proportion (< 20%). Thalidomide is poorly tolerated at conventional doses (> 100 mg per day) with more than one-half of the patients being unable to tolerate it beyond 3 months and it increases the risk of extreme thrombocytosis and probably that of venous thrombosis. Trials of lower doses of the drug alone or in combination with prednisolone are under way and preliminary data suggest that such doses are better tolerated and may be similarly efficacious.

Imatinib mesylate has at most a modest effect in reducing splenic size in IMF, but other tyrosine kinase inhibitors are under investigation. Bisphosphonates can help with bone pain.

Prognosis

The median survival is 3–5 years, but the range is very wide. As a result, efforts have been made to devise algorithms to individualize prognosis. The two most widely used algorithms are shown in Tables 46.7 and 46.8. Recently, an elevated blood CD34$^+$ cell count > 300 × 10^6/L and the presence of JAK2 V617F, were also identified as adverse prognostic features.

Mastocytosis

Mastocytosis comprises a rare group of disorders characterized by a pathological increase in mast cells in tissues, including the

Table 46.8 Prognostic scoring systems in myelofibrosis: The Sheffield prognostic system.

Age (years)	Hb (g/dL)	Karyotype	Median survival months (95% CI)
< 68	> 10	Normal	180 (6–354)
		Abnormal	72 (32–112)
	≤ 10	Normal	54 (46–62)
		Abnormal	22 (14–30)
> 68	> 10	Normal	70 (61–79)
		Abnormal	78 (26–130)
	≤ 10	Normal	44 (31–57)
		Abnormal	16 (5–27)

From Reilly et al. (1997).

Table 46.9 Classification of mastocytosis.

Cutaneous mastocytosis	Urticaria pigmentosa and variants
	Mastocytoma of the skin
Systemic mastocytosis	Indolent
	Aggressive
Systemic mastocytosis with associated haematological non-mast cell disorder	
Mast cell leukaemia	
Mast cell sarcoma	

Modified from Valent et al. (2001).

skin, bone marrow, liver, spleen, lymph nodes and gastrointestinal tract. Mastocytosis can be an isolated finding or can form part of other haematological disorders, including myelodysplastic syndromes, myeloproliferative disorders or AML. Some cases involve just the skin (cutaneous mastocytosis) whereas others involve multiple tissues and are associated with systemic symptoms (systemic mastocytosis). A proposal for the classification of mast cell diseases was recently put forward (Table 46.9).

The first case of urticaria pigmentosa (a form of cutaneous mastocytosis) was described in 1869 by Nettleship, and systemic disease due to increased mast cells was first documented by Ellis in 1949. The observation that stem cell factor (SCF) is an essential growth factor for mast cell development has led to significant advances in our understanding of this group of diseases.

Pathophysiology

After a search for abnormalities of SCF failed to identify any pathological changes, researchers turned to c-Kit, the tyrosine kinase receptor for SCF. A c-*kit* point mutation leading to a single amino acid substitution (Asp816Val) was thus identified. This mutation leads to ligand-independent phosphorylation of c-Kit and a consequent clonal expansion of mast cells.

Asp816Val was originally identified in cases of mastocytosis with associated haematological disorders but is now known to be present in the majority of adults presenting with urticaria pigmentosa or indolent systemic mastocytosis. More recently, other activating mutations affecting the same codon have been identified in a minority of adult cases of cutaneous mastocytosis (Asp816Tyr, Asp816Phe). A different mutation has been reported in a small number of cases of paediatric mastocytosis, namely Lys839Glu, which surprisingly gives rise to a dominant-negative (inactivating) form of c-Kit; the significance of this observation remains unresolved.

Recent reports have suggested that in some cases of mastocytosis the c-*kit* mutation is found in other haemopoietic cells such as B cells, myeloid cells and T cells. These results suggest that mastocytosis, as with the classical MPDs, may be a clonal disorder of the haemopoietic stem cell.

Clinical features

Cutaneous manifestations

Urticaria pigmentosa is the usual presenting feature in children and adults with isolated mastocytosis. Yellowish-brown lesions, usually macular and sometimes papular, appear in a patchy distribution. Less commonly, there is diffuse involvement of the skin, which becomes thickened and darker brown (Figure 46.11). Pruritus is common, as is flushing, and some cases develop haemorrhagic bullous disease. Whealing of lesions upon rubbing is known as Darier's sign.

Systemic disease

Systemic manifestations are very heterogeneous and are thought to be largely secondary to mast cell mediator release. Episodes of flushing, angioedema, or even anaphylaxis with or without any specific trigger, can arise as a result of systemic histamine release. Gastrointestinal symptoms include abdominal pain, diarrhoea, nausea and vomiting. Gastritis and peptic ulceration may occur secondary to hyperhistaminaemia and severe cases may develop malabsorption. Osteoporosis is well recognized

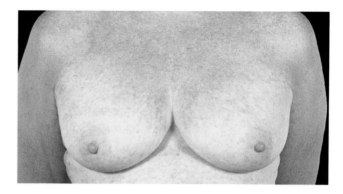

Figure 46.11 Urticaria pigmentosa in a 55-year-old woman. Note the widespread pink or brownish macules that become confluent in areas.

and can sometimes lead to pathological fractures. Peripheral blood cytopenias may arise secondary to mast cell infiltration of the bone marrow. Hepatosplenomegaly is more common in cases associated with another clonal haematological disorder. Fever, fatigue and weight loss can sometimes ensue and may result from the release of cytokines such as tumour necrosis factor-alpha (TNF-α) and IL-1.

Symptoms of organ failure due to infiltration are characteristic of aggressive systemic mastocytosis. Depending on the organs involved, cytopenias, pathological fractures, impaired liver function, ascites and malabsorption can all be seen.

Investigations

Clinical features of mastocytosis can be highly suggestive of the disease but diagnosis usually requires histological and biochemical confirmation. An algorithm has been proposed for the diagnosis of systemic mast cell disease and is shown in Table 46.10.

Table 46.10 Criteria for the diagnosis of systemic mast cell disease.

Major
Multifocal dense infiltrates of mast cells in bone marrow and/or other extracutaneous tissues

Minor
More than 25% of mast cells on bone marrow smears or tissue biopsies are atypical or spindle-shaped

Identification of a codon 816 c-*kit* point mutation in blood, bone marrow or lesional skin

Mast cells in bone marrow, blood or other lesional tissues expressing CD25 or CD2

Baseline total serum tryptase greater than 20 ng/mL

Major and one minor, or three or more minor criteria needed for diagnosis.

Modified from Valent *et al.* (2001).

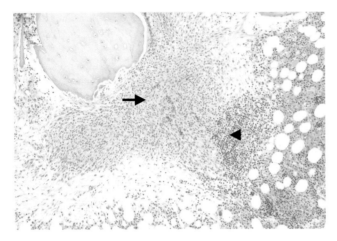

Figure 46.12 Systemic mastocytosis involving the bone marrow (H&E). Malignant whorls of rounded and spindle-shaped mast cells are seen infiltrating the bone marrow in a paratrabecular distribution (arrow). A lymphoid aggregate and areas of hypocellularity are seen interspersed between the mast cell infiltrate and neighbouring haemopoietic islands (arrowhead) (courtesy of Dr Wendy Erber).

Routine investigations should include a full blood count, liver function tests and a random serum tryptase. Tests for histamine metabolites in 24-h urine specimens are probably no more useful than measurements of serum tryptase. Plasma levels of soluble CD25 and CD117 (kit) have shown promise as novel markers of mast cell disease.

Bone marrow aspiration and trephine biopsy allow assessment of bone marrow involvement. Mast cell aggregates can be visualized on conventional haematoxylin and eosin-stained sections (Figure 46.12) but stand out much more clearly with stains such as toluidine blue (Figure 46.13). Immunochemistry using antitryptase antibodies can also be very useful, being highly specific for mast cells. Flow cytometry to look for expression of CD2 and CD25 in bone marrow mast cells may be useful as this phenotype is not seen in normal mast cells.

Abdominal ultrasound or computerized tomography should be performed to look for hepatosplenomegaly and lymphadenopathy. Plain radiography and bone densitometry can be used to look for bone involvement and osteoporosis. Endoscopy and biopsy can be useful if gut involvement is suspected.

Treatment

Despite significant advances in the understanding of its pathophysiology, no curative treatment exists for mastocytosis, the management of which remains symptomatic.

There are four main components to the management of mastocytosis:
1 avoidance of factors that can trigger mediator release from mast cells;
2 treatment of acute mediator release;

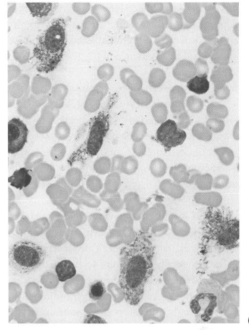
(a)

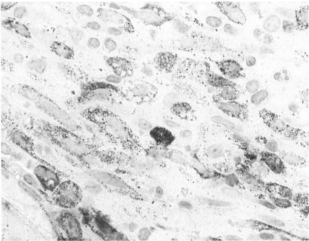
(b)

Figure 46.13 Toluidine blue stain of bone marrow aspirate (a) and trephine biopsy section (b) in systemic mastocytosis. Abnormal spindle-shaped mast cells containing metachromatic granules are seen.

3 treatment of chronic mediator release;
4 reduction of the mast cell burden/organ infiltration.

Avoidance of triggers of mast cell mediator release is primarily an exercise in patient education. Severe reactions due to systemic mast cell mediator release are difficult to predict in patients with mastocytosis and do not correlate well with disease category, mast cell burden or severity of other symptoms. All patients and relevant health-care workers should be warned of particular triggers, including general anaesthesia, contrast radiography and insect stings. Known mast cell activators such as morphine and dextran should only be introduced with great caution. Patients with previous anaphylaxis or severe hypotension should carry injectable adrenaline and they, their family and friends should be instructed in its intramuscular administration. Local mediator release in cutaneous mastocytosis can be moderated by avoidance of triggering factors such as friction and heat.

Acute systemic mast cell mediator release should be treated in much the same way as other forms of anaphylaxis. Treatment with adrenaline and intravenous fluids should be started as soon as possible, with early involvement of intensive care specialists in severe cases. Antihistamines (H_1 and H_2 blockers) should be introduced and continued long-term if the episode was particularly severe or recurrent.

Symptoms of chronic mediator release are the commonest clinical problem in mastocytosis. Symptomatic cutaneous disease should be managed with the help of a dermatologist. Treatments include H_1 and H_2 blockers, topical corticosteroids and PUVA for severe disease. Non-life threatening systemic symptoms such as flushing, abdominal pain and diarrhoea should be treated with H_1 and H_2 blockers, sodium cromoglycate and corticosteroids. Inhibitors of prostaglandin synthesis, such as aspirin and non-steroidal anti-inflammatory drugs, can also be useful. Aspirin should always be started with caution as it can initially lead to acute mediator release. Such drugs can be used prophylactically if symptoms recur frequently. Gastrointestinal disease usually responds to the drugs used to treat chronic systemic symptoms. Leukotriene antagonists anecdotally help with abdominal cramps and diarrhoea. Peptic ulcer and reflux disease should be treated with proton pump inhibitors. Osteoporosis should be treated with bisphosphonates and may be prevented with bisphosphonates or calcium and vitamin D supplementation. Bone density should be recorded and monitored according to the severity of osteoporosis. Radiotherapy can help with severe localized pain.

For patients in whom adequate symptomatic control cannot be achieved and for those with aggressive mastocytosis, IFN-α, usually given in combination with oral corticosteroids, should be considered. Splenectomy may help reduce the mast cell burden and associated systemic symptoms. Cladribine has been found effective in isolated cases of systemic mastocytosis.

Treatment with chemotherapy is usually reserved for cases of rapidly progressive aggressive mastocytosis, mast cell leukaemia and mast cell sarcoma, but published data are not encouraging. Mast cell sarcoma may also respond to local radiotherapy when appropriate. Allogeneic bone marrow transplantation should also be considered. Treatment of any associated haematological disorder should be undertaken as appropriate for that disorder and the overall prognosis is usually that of the latter.

Future treatments

Treatments that target the mutant c-kit tyrosine kinase have attracted a lot of interest recently. Imatinib was known to inhibit wild-type c-kit in *in vitro* studies and be active against juxtamembrane mutants of c-kit found in gastrointestinal stromal tumours. By contrast, the drug does not have the same effect on malignant mast cells carrying codon 816 mutations, probably because the mutant c-kit does not allow access of imatinib to the site, hence conferring resistance to this drug in a similar way to acquired imatinib resistance in CML (see also Chapter 37). In keeping with this, there have been early reports of its lack of efficacy in the presence of codon 816 mutations. A recent report showing that imatinib was effective in patients with mastocytosis with associated eosinophilia but without demonstrable c-kit mutations awaits confirmation, particularly as these cases may represent variants of chronic eosinophilic leukaemia (CEL). Novel tyrosine kinase inhibitors, which can inhibit the Asp816Val mutant c-*kit in vitro*, are under investigation at present.

Prognosis

Age and disease category are the most important determinants of outcome. The most benign syndrome is paediatric mastocytoma, which disappears with time in over 50% of cases. Paediatric urticaria pigmentosa also has a good prognosis and resolves in about one-half of the cases.

In adult mastocytosis, urticaria pigmentosa is usually associated with mast cell deposits in the marrow or other tissues, making this a systemic syndrome. Indolent systemic mastocytosis carries a favourable prognosis and usually persists as a chronic low-grade disorder, although it rarely progresses to aggressive mastocytosis or mastocytosis associated with another haematological malignancy. Aggressive systemic mastocytosis can show a slowly progressive or a rapid clinical course but its overall prognosis has not been well defined in clinical studies. Mast cell leukaemia is rare but has a grave prognosis with a median survival of less than 6 months.

Clonal hypereosinophilic syndromes

Eosinophilia is aetiologically diverse, with helminthic infections being its commonest cause worldwide and atopic disease its commonest cause in the industrialized world. Paul Ehlrich was first to describe the eosinophil in 1879. Based on his and others' observations, it was realized that eosinophilia occurred in helminthic infections, tumours and allergic disorders such as asthma. A case of myeloid leukaemia with marked blood eosinophilia was described by Stillman in 1912. The term hypereosinophilic syndrome (HES) was coined by Hardy and Anderson in 1968, who gave it the definition that is still in use to date. Recently, major progress has been made in elucidating the molecular pathogenesis of clonal eosinophilia as described below.

Pathophysiology

Eosinophilia can be divided into three categories: reactive, idiopathic and clonal (Table 46.11). In reactive eosinophilia, which

Table 46.11 Causes of eosinophilia.

Reactive eosinophilia	Infections	Parasitic
		Others (rarely)
	Vasculitides	Polyarteritis nodosa
		Churg–Strauss syndrome
	Connective Tissue Disorders	Rheumatoid arthritis
		Systemic sclerosis
		Systemic lupus erythematosus
	Allergic and inflammatory disorders	Asthma
		Eczema
		Bullous skin diseases
		Inflammatory bowel disease
	Drug reactions	Hypersensitivity
		L-Tryptophan (eosinophilia–myalgia syndrome)
	Immunodeficiencies	Wiskott–Aldrich Syndrome
		Job's syndrome (hyper-IgE syndrome)
	Neoplasia	Hodgkin's disease
		Non-Hodgkin's lymphoma
		Peripheral blood T-cell clones
		Some cases of acute lymphoblastic leukaemia
		Non-haematological cancers (rarely)
Clonal eosinophilia	Chronic eosinophilic leukaemia	
	Atypical chronic myeloid leukaemia (*PDGFRβ* fusions)	
	8p11 Myeloproliferative syndrome (*FGFR1* fusions)	
	Chronic myeloid leukaemia (*BCR–ABL* fusion)	
	Acute myeloid leukaemia, e.g. carrying inv(16)	
	Acute lymphoblastic leukaemia (occasionally)	
Idiopathic eosinophilia	Hypereosinophilic syndrome	

is by far the most common, the eosinophil count is thought to reflect release of a number of growth factors including IL-3, IL-5 and granulocyte–macrophage colony-stimulating factor (GM-CSF). A large number of diseases can result in the release of these cytokines, including parasitic infections, allergic diseases, vasculitides, drug reactions and malignancies.

Idiopathic eosinophilias are those in which the cause is obscure. Within this category, HES describes patients with an unexplained elevation of peripheral blood eosinophils ($> 1.5 \times 10^9$/L) for more than 6 months associated with end-organ damage.

Clonal eosinophilias are those in which the eosinophilia is part of a clonal haematological malignancy. CEL is defined as an eosinophil count $> 1.5 \times 10^9$/L, with evidence of eosinophil clonality or an increased blast account in blood or bone marrow. The distinction between this entity and HES is blurred as it relies on the availability of a clonal marker. Indeed it has been shown recently that 25–50% of cases labelled as HES in fact have a microdeletion on chromosome 4, which results in the fusion of

the *FIP1L1* and *PDGFRα* genes and the generation of a constitutively active tyrosine kinase. Importantly, patients carrying this fusion respond well to the tyrosine kinase inhibitor imatinib. Some patients with HES that do not carry this fusion gene also respond to imatinib, suggesting that in such cases other tyrosine kinases may be dysregulated.

In addition to CEL, a number of other haematological malignancies may be associated with increased numbers of clonal eosinophils, and in many cases, this reflects tyrosine kinase dysregulation. *PDGFRβ* rearrangements (e.g. *TEL–PDGFRβ*) may present as chronic myelomonocytic leukaemia (CMML) or atypical CML. The 8p11 myeloproliferative syndrome (EMS) is associated with rearrangements in the *FGFR1* gene (e.g. *ZNF198–FGFR1*) and leads to a chronic myeloproliferative disorder that frequently presents with eosinophilia and associated T-cell lymphoblastic lymphoma. CML, a consequence of the *BCR–ABL* tyrosine kinase fusion protein, may also be associated with clonal eosinophilia (see also Chapter 37).

Eosinophilia as part of the malignant clone also occurs in patients with AML associated with inversion of chromosome 16 and the *SMMHC–CBFβ* rearrangement. It has been reported that rare cases of acute lymphoblastic leukaemia (ALL) may be associated with clonal eosinophilia but in this disease the eosinophilia is more usually secondary to growth factor release. Growth factor release is also believed to underlie the reactive eosinophilia seen in Hodgkin's disease and in cases with clonal T cells in the peripheral blood.

Sustained hypereosinophilia can lead to symptomatology and end-organ damage regardless of its aetiology, but does not always do so. The reasons for this are unclear but may lie in the heterogeneity of eosinophilia and genetic differences between individuals that affect the propensity of eosinophils and other granulocytes to inflict tissue damage.

Clinical features

Much of the tissue damage in eosinophilia is believed to be secondary to eosinophil degranulation and release of mediators such as eosinophil cationic protein and major basic protein. Eosinophil mediators act mainly locally in tissues infiltrated by eosinophils to cause tissue damage. The recent finding that a raised serum tryptase in a subset of cases with clonal eosinophilia hints at a role for other cells (mast cells) in some cases.

Patients can present with constitutional symptoms such as fatigue, muscle aches or fevers. Pruritus, angioedema, diarrhoea and cough may also be present. Many tissues can be involved, but cardiac disease is the major cause of mortality. The heart can be affected by endomyocardial fibrosis, pericarditis, myocarditis and intramural thrombus formation. Death is usually due to dilated cardiomyopathy.

Involvement of the central and peripheral nervous systems can result in mononeuritis multiplex, paraparesis, encephalopathy and even dementia. Pulmonary involvement can take the form of pulmonary infiltrates, fibrosis or pleural disease with effusions. Gastrointestinal involvement can manifest as diarrhoea, gastritis, colitis, hepatitis or the Budd–Chiari syndrome. The skin can be affected by pruritus, angioedema, papules or plaques. Rarely, other tissues such as the kidneys and bones can be involved.

Investigations

There are two aims in the investigation of eosinophilia, one is to establish its aetiology and the other to look for evidence of end-organ damage. As regards the former, given the diverse nature of the aetiologies of eosinophilia, a full history including family history, drug history and travel history can provide valuable clues. Investigations will usually aim to exclude reactive causes and will be guided by the clinical picture.

Bone marrow aspiration will reveal morphological abnormalities associated with haematological malignancies and allows

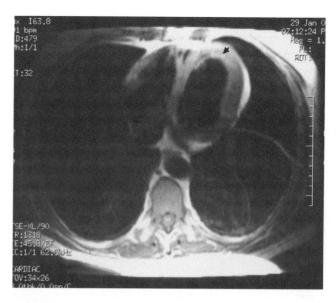

Figure 46.14 Cardiac magnetic resonance imaging scan in a 65-year-old man with HES, showing a rim of subendocardial fibrosis (arrow).

cytogenetic analysis. It is also important to look for clonal T-cell receptor (TCR) gene rearrangements, the *FIPIL1–PDGFRα* and *BCR–ABL* fusion genes, as well as rearrangements of the *PDGFRβ* and *FGFR1* genes. It has been reported that serum tryptase is raised in patients with the *FIPIL1–PDGFRα* fusion.

Investigations to assess end-organ damage will depend on the clinical presentation. However, echocardiography should be performed and repeated annually in patients with sustained eosinophilia, particularly as cardiac disease correlates poorly with the eosinophil count. If there is strong clinical suspicion of cardiac damage then cardiac magnetic resonance imaging (MRI) can be useful, as this is more sensitive in detecting early disease (Figure 46.14). If there is doubt as to the aetiology of cardiac disease, endomyocardial biopsy may demonstrate eosinophil infiltration. Serial monitoring of pulmonary function may be required if there is evidence of lung involvement.

Treatment

Treatment should be used to halt or reverse organ damage. Eosinophilia without evidence of end-organ damage does not usually require treatment. When underlying clonal or non-clonal disorders are identified they should be treated appropriately.

Patients with rearrangements of the *PDGFRα* or *PDGFRβ* genes, respond well to imatinib, with normalization of eosinophil counts within weeks. A trial of imatinib is also reasonable in patients with HES who lack a clonal marker, as a proportion of these patients also respond.

For patients who do not respond to imatinib, prednisolone is the initial treatment of choice. Steroids reduce blood eosinophilia and the inflammation resulting from tissue infiltration. Cardiac disease may respond even in the absence of a significant reduction in the eosinophil count. Hydroxyurea and IFN-α may benefit patients resistant to steroids. Cladribine and cyclosporin were also found to be of use in some cases.

Prognosis

The reported prognoses of CEL and HES are highly variable, with estimates of 3-year survival ranging from 23% to 96%. This is likely to reflect heterogeneity within these two categories of patients. In patients with HES, indicators of a poor prognosis include lack of response to steroids, a markedly elevated eosinophil count, normal IgE levels, splenomegaly, dysplastic features and male sex. Many of these adverse prognostic indicators may simply be markers of clonal (versus reactive) eosinophilia.

Chronic neutrophilic leukaemia

Chronic neutrophilia is a very common entity, and is usually secondary to chronic infections, chronic inflammation or malignancy. A very small subgroup of patients with chronic neutrophilia have chronic neutrophilic leukaemia (CNL), a clonal haematological disorder (Figure 46.15). Given the absence of a specific marker for this disease, CNL, like ET, is a diagnosis of exclusion.

The first description of CNL was probably that by Tuohy in 1920. In the ensuing 75 years, a total of less than 100 cases have been reported in the literature, mostly as isolated case reports. This rarity has hampered progress in the understanding of its pathogenesis (see also Chapter 37).

Pathophysiology

Isolated mild to moderate neutrophilia is commonly seen in many clinical contexts associated with inflammation, ranging from infections to tissue trauma/infarction, haemorrhage, arthritis, inflammatory bowel disease and many other ailments. Additionally, it can be seen in smokers, after vigorous exercise and in patients taking corticosteroids. In these contexts, the aetiology is usually apparent and such cases are rarely referred to a haematologist.

Marked chronic neutrophilia (neutrophils $\geq 20 \times 10^9$/L) is usually secondary to a chronic infection or an underlying malignancy. Neutrophilia is particularly common in metastatic cancer but can pre-date overt malignancy by months or years. Such leukaemoid reactions are thought to reflect the release of cytokines such as granulocyte colony-stimulating factor (G-CSF) and granulocyte–macrophage colony-stimulating factor (GM-CSF) from tumour cells.

Neutrophilia is clonal in a small number of cases. These cases can be subdivided into two main groups: 'true' CNL and neutrophilic chronic myeloid leukaemia (N-CML). The two groups

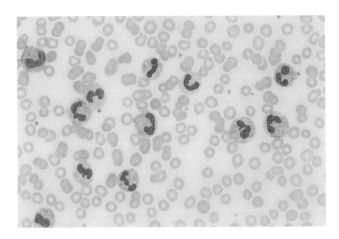

Figure 46.15 Abundance of mature neutrophils and band forms in a blood film from a patient with chronic neutrophilic leukaemia.

are only distinguishable by the presence in the latter of a rare type of *BCR–ABL* rearrangement that produces a 230-kDa fusion protein (p230). In addition, rare patients with a myelodysplastic syndrome can closely mimic CNL but exhibit dysplastic features and there are anecdotal reports of PV evolving into a disorder indistinguishable from CNL. The literature also includes reports of what was thought to be clonal chronic neutrophilia in association with plasma cell dyscrasias. However, data are accumulating that this type of neutrophilia is non-clonal and probably a result of cytokine release from clonal plasma cells.

Diagnostic features of CNL are shown in Table 46.12. N-CML usually exhibits these features, save for its association with the p. 230 *BCR–ABL* rearrangement.

Table 46.12 Diagnostic features of chronic neutrophilic leukaemia.

Peripheral blood leucocytosis > 25×10^9/L
Segmented neutrophils and bands > 80% of white blood cells
Immature granulocytes < 10% of white blood cells
Myeloblasts < 1% of white blood cells
Hypercellular bone marrow biopsy
Neutrophilic granulocytes increased in percentage and number
Myeloblasts < 5% of nucleated marrow cells
Normal neutrophil maturation pattern
Hepatosplenomegaly
No identifiable cause of reactive neutrophilia
No evidence of another haematological malignancy
No Philadelphia chromosome or *BCR–ABL* fusion
No evidence of another myeloproliferative disorder (i.e. normal PCV, platelets < 600, no bone marrow fibrosis or other features of IMF)
No evidence of a myelodysplastic syndrome (i.e. no dysplasia, monocytes < 1×10^9/L)

Modified from Vardiman *et al.* (2001).

Clinical features and treatment

A recent review of the literature identified only 33 cases that fulfilled criteria for CNL. These cases exhibited a 2:1 male–female ratio and a median age at diagnosis of 62.5 years (range 15–86 years). The median survival was 30 months, with only 28% of cases surviving to 5 years. Transformation to AML ensued in 21% (7 out of 33) and this was invariably lethal. Other causes of death included sepsis and haemorrhage.

Hb was normal and platelet counts above 100×10^9/L in most cases. The mean leucocyte count at diagnosis was 54.3×10^9/L. Vitamin B_{12} levels were raised and neutrophil alkaline phosphatase (NAP) levels were not low in most cases. Hyperuricaemia and gout were common. Bone marrow biopsies were markedly hypercellular and showed a marked granulocytic proliferation, as did the bone marrow aspirates. Cytogenetic abnormalities were seen in about a third, with deletion of 20q being the only recurrent abnormality identified thus far. In a small number of cases, XCIP studies were used to demonstrate the clonal nature of CNL in patients lacking a cytogenetic marker.

The optimal treatment of CNL remains unclear. Oral cytoreductive agents such as hydroxyurea and busulphan can control the neutrophil count, as can IFN. The only potentially curative modality is allogeneic bone marrow transplantation and this option should be considered in younger patients.

Neutrophilic chronic myeloid leukaemia

This entity is probably even more rare than CNL, with only a handful of documented cases in the literature. The reported cases followed a more benign course than conventional CML, with a lower white cell count, lower proportion of immature granulocytes, milder anaemia, less marked splenomegaly and a lower propensity to acute transformation. Given recent advances in the treatment of bcr–abl-related diseases, it is important to consider and exclude neutrophilic chronic myeloid leukaemia (N-CML) during the investigation of chronic neutrophilia.

Selected bibliography

Barosi G, Ambrosetti A, Finelli C et al. (1999) The Italian Consensus Conference on Diagnostic Criteria for Myelofibrosis with Myeloid Metaplasia. British Journal of Haematology 104: 730–7.

Baxter EJ, Scott LM, Campbell PJ et al. (2005) Acquired mutation of the tyrosine kinase JAK2 in human myeloproliferative disorders. Lancet 365: 1054–61.

Brito-Babapulle F (2003) The eosinophilias, including the idiopathic hypereosinophilic syndrome. British Journal of Haematology 121: 203–23.

Campbell PJ, Scott LM, Buck G et al. (2005) JAK2 V617F mutation identifies a biologically distinct subtype of essential thrombocythaemia which resembles polycythaemia vera. Lancet (in press).

Dupriez B, Morel P, Demory JL et al. (1996) Prognostic factors in agnogenic myeloid metaplasia: a report of 195 cases with a new scoring system. Blood 88: 1013–18.

Finazzi G, Caruso V, Marchioli R et al. (2005) Acute leukemia in polycythemia vera: an analysis of 1638 patients enrolled in a prospective observational study. Blood 105: 2664–2670.

Harrison CN, Campbell PJ, Buck G et al. (2005) Hydroxyurea compared with anagrelide in high-risk essential thrombocythemia. New England Journal of Medicine 353: 33–45.

Harrison CN (2002) Current trends in essential thrombocythaemia. British Journal of Haematology 117: 796–808.

James C, Ugo V, Le Couedic JP et al. (2005) A unique clonal JAK2 mutation leading to constitutive signalling causes polycythaemia vera. Nature 434: 1144–8.

Kralovics R, Passamonti F, Buser AS et al. (2005) A gain-of-function mutation of JAK2 in myeloproliferative disorders. New England Journal of Medicine 352: 1779–90.

Levine RL, Wadleigh M, Cools J et al. (2005) Activating mutation in the tyrosine kinase JAK2 in polycythemia vera, essential thrombocythemia, and myeloid metaplasia with myelofibrosis. Cancer Cell 7: 387–97.

Messinezy M, Pearson TC (1993) Apparent polycythaemia: diagnosis, pathogenesis and management. European Journal of Haematology 51: 125–31.

Pearson TC, Treacher DF (1990) Polycythaemia in systemic disease II. In: Haematological Aspects of Systemic Disease, pp. 67–119. Baillière Tindall, London.

Pearson TC, Messinezy M, Westwood et al. (2000) A polycythaemia vera update: diagnosis, pathobiology and treatment. Hematology (American Society of Hematology Education Program), pp. 51–68.

Reilly JT (2002) Chronic neutrophilic leukaemia: a distinct clinical entity? British Journal of Haematology 116: 10–18.

Reilly JT, Snowden JA, Spearing RL et al. (1997) Cytogenetic abnormalities and their prognostic significance in idiopathic myelofibrosis: a study of 106 cases. British Journal of Haematology 98: 96–102.

Tefferi A (2000) Myelofibrosis with myeloid metaplasia. New England Journal of Medicine 342: 1255–65.

Valent P, Horny HP, Escribano L et al. (2001) Diagnostic criteria and classification of mastocytosis: a consensus proposal. Leukaemia Research 25: 603–25.

Valent P, Akin C, Sperr WR et al. (2003) Diagnosis and treatment of systemic mastocytosis: state of the art. British Journal of Haematology 122: 695–717.

Vardiman JW, Pierre R, Thiele J et al. (2001) Chronic myeloproliferative disorders. In: World Health Organization Classification of Tumours: Tumours of the Haematopoietic and Lymphoid Tissues, pp. 15–44.

CHAPTER 47

Normal haemostasis

47

Geoffrey Kemball-Cook, Edward GD Tuddenham and John H McVey

Introduction

Haemostasis is one of a number of protective processes that have evolved in order to maintain a stable physiology. It has many features in common with (and to some extent interacts with) other defence mechanisms in the body, such as the immune system and the inflammatory response. These links are most clearly seen in ancient species such as the horseshoe crab (*Limulus polyphemus*), where a primitive 'coagulation' pathway is initiated by entry of endotoxin into the haemolymph. Vestiges of this process still exist in humans and may give rise to serious clinical consequences. For example, disseminated intravascular coagulation (DIC) can be initiated by Gram-negative septicaemia (see Chapter 51). However, consequent upon the development of a high-pressure blood circulatory system, extra components have evolved and have resulted in a complex, highly integrated process in all vertebrates (Figure 47.1). Indeed, recent analysis of the haemostatic network in bony fish suggests that the network in its entirety evolved over 430 million years ago, prior to the divergence of bony fish from tetrapods.

The high blood pressure generated on the arterial side of vertebrate circulation requires a powerful, almost instantaneous but strictly localized *procoagulant* response in order to minimize blood loss from sites of vascular injury without compromising blood flow generally. Systemic *anticoagulant* and clot-dissolving components have also evolved to prevent extension of the procoagulant response beyond the vicinity of vascular injury resulting in unwanted thrombus formation in the slow, sometimes intermittent, blood flow in the veins. The resultant haemostatic system is thus a complex mosaic of activating or inhibitory feedback or feed-forward pathways, integrating its five major components (blood vessels, blood platelets, coagula-tion factors, coagulation inhibitors and fibrinolytic elements). Furthermore, links between haemostasis and other elements of the body's overall defence response, such as the complement and kinin-generating processes and phagocytosis, must also be considered.

This chapter reviews current concepts of haemostasis in humans and is aimed at providing a background for the understanding of the haemostatic disorders described in succeeding chapters. Attempting to understand these complex events is a considerable task, even to the expert; for the relative newcomer to the subject, it may first be useful to present an overview of events that follow damage to a blood vessel, leading to effective haemostasis and subsequent restoration of vessel patency. Following this introduction, each of five main areas will be examined in relative isolation, while at the same time acknowledging points of interaction and overlap.

Overview of haemostasis

In the most simplistic terms, blood coagulation occurs when the enzyme thrombin is generated and proteolyses soluble plasma fibrinogen, forming the insoluble fibrin polymer, or clot; this provides the physical consolidation of vessel wound repair following injury. 'Haemostasis' refers more widely to the process whereby blood coagulation is initiated and terminated in a tightly regulated fashion, together with the removal (or fibrinolysis) of the clot as part of vascular remodelling; as such, haemostasis describes the global process by which vessel integrity and patency are maintained over the whole organism, for its lifetime.

Although it is pedagogically convenient to present the subsystems of haemostasis as if they operate independently, the whole

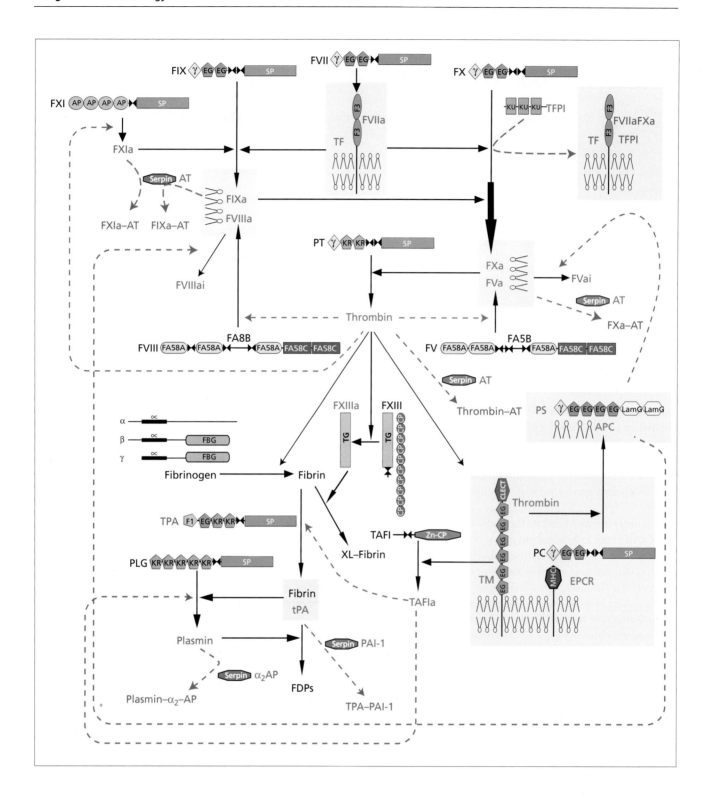

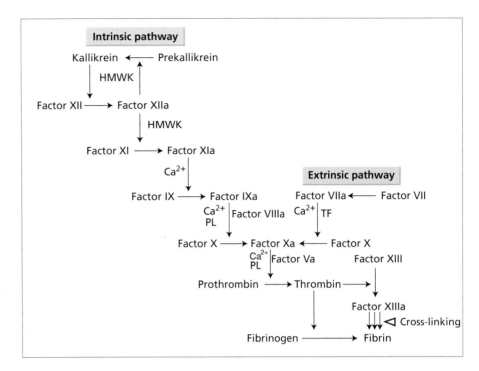

Figure 47.2 The coagulation cascade. The traditional concept of blood coagulation with separate intrinsic and extrinsic pathways converging in the generation of FXa. HMWK, high-molecular-weight kininogen; PL, phospholipid.

haemostatic mechanism is integrated *in vivo* so that thrombin generation is localized, limited and followed by fibrinolysis and tissue remodelling, which are also localized and limited. Furthermore, thrombin generation is not a simple exponential 'cascade' as was originally envisaged, but a complex network of interactions with positive and negative feedback loops, thus the effects of varying the concentration of any component in such a system is not intuitively obvious. Figure 47.2 presents a version of the earlier 'cascade' concept for intrinsic and extrinsic pathways of thrombin generation.

Although a tremendous improvement over previous ideas, obvious deficiencies of such a scheme include:
• no explanation for the absence of a clinical bleeding tendency in deficiencies of factor (F) XII, prekallikrein or high-molecular-

weight kininogen, even though these deficiencies markedly prolong surface-activated coagulation assays for haemostasis *in vitro*;
• no explanation for why factor FVIII or FIX deficiency cause clinically severe bleeding, as the extrinsic pathway ought to bypass the need for FVIII and FIX;
• no explanation for bleeding in FXI deficiency less severe than seen with FVIII and FIX deficiency;
• no explanation for the lag phase followed by explosively rapid thrombin generation observed experimentally;
• no appreciation of the overriding importance of tissue factor (TF) in the initiation of all coagulation processes, both in normal haemostasis and pathological situations such as thrombosis;
• no appreciation of the complex role of platelets, other than as provision of a 'procoagulant surface' (see Chapter 47).

Figure 47.1 (*opposite*) The haemostasis network. The network includes elements of coagulation initiation via TF–FVIIa interaction, amplification via the FX-ase and prothrombinase complexes, feedback inhibition through specific inhibitors and clot dissolution by fibrinolysis. Module organization of proteins is indicated (see Figure 47.8) as proposed by Bork and Bairoch (www.bork.embl-heidelberg.de/modules/) and all abbreviations are given in the text. Protein names are coloured as follows: functionally active proteins, red; inactivated or inhibited proteins, blue; precursors and fibrinogen-derived components, black. Lines and arrows are coloured thus: dashed red lines, positive procoagulant feedback loops; dashed blue lines, negative feedback and inhibitory loops; solid black lines, interactions or processes. Cream boxes indicate assembly of macromolecular complexes on a cellular phospholipid surface. The process of blood coagulation is

initiated by the exposure of cells expressing TF to flowing blood. Thrombin generation is propagated by a series of positive feedback loops, leading to fibrin deposition. This process is controlled by a series of negative feedback steps: the initiation complex is inhibited by the formation of the quaternary complex TF–FVIIa–FXa–TFPI and the active proteases FIXa, FXa and thrombin are inactivated by the serpin AT. In addition, thrombin initiates a negative feedback pathway by activating PC, leading to the inhibition of FVa and FVIIIa. The generation of fibrin leads to activation of the fibrinolytic pathway through binding of tPA, which leads to plasminogen activation and fibrin degradation. This pathway is also subject to inhibition through the binding of the serpins PAI-1 and α_2-AP to tPA and plasmin respectively. All these processes, plus platelet activation occur simultaneously or with short lag times.

Table 47.1 Role of 'contact factors' in integrating body defence mechanisms.

Pathway involved	Function	Comment
Coagulation	Prevention of blood loss	Not essential for normal haemostasis
Fibrinolysis	Maintenance of vessel patency	May be important
Complement	Contribution to immune response	Not essential
Kinin generation	Pain, capillary permeability, cardiovascular effects	May be important *in vivo*
Renin–angiotensin system	Blood pressure control	No demonstrated role *in vivo*
Chemotaxis	Phagocytosis, bactericidal activity	May be important *in vivo*

Tissue factor initiates blood coagulation

A major development over the past 10 years has been the realization that exposure of blood to cells expressing TF on their surface is both necessary and sufficient to initiate blood coagulation *in vivo*. The contact system ('intrinsic' pathway, see Figure 47.2) therefore does not appear to have a physiological role in haemostasis. Table 47.1 presents some other putative roles for the 'contact factors' in body defence. TF is constitutively expressed at biological boundaries such as skin, organ surfaces, vascular adventitia and epithelial–mesenchymal surfaces, where it functions as a 'haemostatic envelope'. This ensures that following disruption of vascular integrity blood is immediately exposed to cells expressing TF, leading to the initiation of blood coagulation. The primary control of haemostasis is therefore the anatomical segregation of cells expressing functional TF from other components of the coagulation network present in blood.

Amplification of the initial stimulus

An updated concept of TF-initiated thrombin generation, including the important feedback reactions of thrombin, is shown in Figure 47.3. As stated above, it is now clear from various *in vitro* and *in vivo* experiments that the physiological initiator of blood coagulation is the exposure of the circulating zymogen FVII to membrane-bound TF. Activation of FVII to the protease FVIIa and formation of a very high affinity complex of TF with FVIIa results in the activation of factors IX (FIX) and X (FX) by the TF–FVIIa complex. In the absence of its activated cofactor FVa, FXa generates only trace amounts of thrombin from prothrombin. Although insufficient to initiate significant fibrin polymerization, thrombin formed in this 'initiation' stage of coagulation is able to back-activate FV and FVIII by limited proteolysis. In the 'amplification' phase of coagulation FVIIIa forms a complex with FIXa, the 'FX-ase' complex (FVIIIa–FIXa) and activates sufficient FXa that in complex with FVa forms the 'prothrombinase' complex (FVa–FXa), resulting in the explosive generation of thrombin that ultimately leads to generation of a fibrin clot.

A key feature of these processes is the assembly of multiprotein complexes on a phospholipid (PL) surface provided *in vivo* by cell surfaces; for procoagulant complexes such as FX-ase and prothrombinase, this surface is provided by activated platelets (see Chapter 48). Each of these complexes consist of a cofactor (TF, FVa, FVIIIa), an enzyme (FVIIa, FIXa, FXa) and a substrate that is a zymogen (FIX, FX and prothrombin) of a serine protease. The product of one reaction becomes the enzyme in the next complex. The cofactors FV and FVIII are themselves activated by limited proteolytic digestion.

Feedback inhibition of the procoagulant response

This process of 'amplification' occurs independently of the TF–FVIIa complex, which is rapidly inactivated by tissue factor pathway inhibitor (TFPI) by forming a quaternary inhibited complex (Figure 47.4). This explains the requirement for indirect activation of FX via FIXa–FVIIIa, and back-activation of FXI by thrombin, to permit further activation of FIX. Figure 47.4 also indicates the role of one of the other important inhibitors of the network, antithrombin (AT), which generally damps down thrombin generation by forming inactive complexes with FIX, FX, FXI and thrombin. The rate of inhibition by AT is substantially increased by binding glycosaminoglycans (GAGs) on the surface of endothelial cells.

Thrombin also proteolytically activates an anticoagulant pathway (Figure 47.5; protein C (PC) pathway). Thrombomodulin (TM), an endothelial cell (EC) surface receptor, plays a pivotal role in the activation of this anticoagulant pathway. TM binds thrombin and, by an allosteric mechanism, alters its substrate specificity. The procoagulant substrates of thrombin, including FV, FVIII and fibrinogen, are no longer efficiently proteolysed. The preferred substrate of the thrombin–TM complex is PC, a zymogen that is proteolysed to activated PC (APC). The activation of PC is augmented by another cellular receptor, endothelial cell protein C receptor (EPCR), which provides a direct EC binding site for PC and thus increases the apparent affinity of the thrombin–TM complex for PC. In complex with its cofactor, protein S (PS), APC rapidly inactivates the procoagulant cofac-

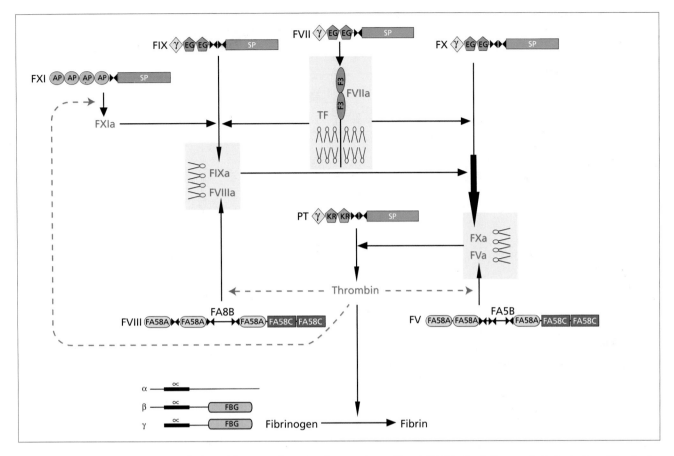

Figure 47.3 The haemostasis network: thrombin generation. Blood coagulation is initiated by exposure of FVII to cells expressing the integral membrane protein TF. Activation of FVII to the protease FVIIa results in the activation of FIX and FX by the TF–FVIIa complex. In the absence of its activated cofactor FVa, FXa generates only trace amounts of thrombin. Although insufficient to initiate significant fibrin polymerization, trace amounts of thrombin formed in this 'initiation' stage of coagulation are able to back-activate FV and FVIII by limited proteolysis. In the 'amplification' phase of coagulation, FVIIIa forms a complex with FIXa, activating sufficient FXa (in complex with FVa) to lead to the explosive generation of thrombin, ultimately leading to generation of a fibrin clot. The FX-ase (FVIIIa–FIXa) and prothrombinase (FVa–FXa) complexes assemble on phospholipid surfaces. Colours and symbols as in Figure 47.1.

tors FVa and FVIIIa by specific proteolysis, forming a negative-feedback loop. The PC pathway assembles on the EC surface and is most active in the microvasculature, where the relative EC surface area is highest.

Fibrinolysis

The final step in the regulation of fibrin deposition is the prevention and/or rapid removal of insoluble fibrin by the fibrinolytic system (Figure 47.6) described more fully later in the chapter. Briefly, generation of fibrin and its binding of tissue plasminogen activator (tPA) leads to an increase in the affinity of tPA for and action upon plasminogen (PLG). This results in generation of plasmin at the site of the fibrin clot, leading to generation of soluble fibrin degradation products (FDPs). The fibrinolytic sys-

tem is also subject to inhibition through the action of inhibitors of tPA and plasmin, namely plasminogen activator inhibitor 1 (PAI-1) and α_2-antiplasmin (α_2-AP) respectively.

Blood vessels

Blood vessel structure

The basic structure of blood vessels can be broken down into three layers (Figure 47.7a): the intima, the media and the adventitia. It is the materials that make up these layers and the size of these layers themselves that differentiate arteries from veins, and indeed one artery or one vein from another artery or vein. The intima is the innermost layer and the surface is covered with a

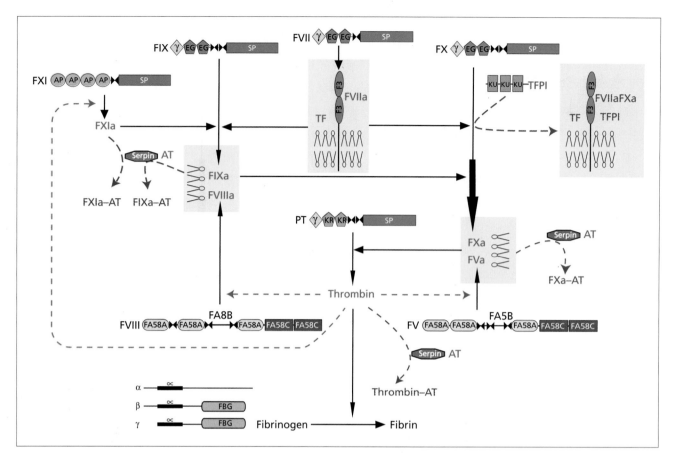

Figure 47.4 The haemostasis network: inhibitors of thrombin generation. The 'initiation' of blood coagulation via generation of FIXa and FXa by TF–FVIIa is shut down by the action of TFPI, which forms a quaternary complex with TF–FVIIa–FXa. Further generation of FIXa occurs following back activation of FXI by thrombin. The serine proteases FIXa, FXa, FXI and thrombin are all inhibited by antithrombin (AT). Colours and symbols as in Figure 47.1.

single layer of ECs (the endothelium), which rest on a basement membrane of subendothelial microfibrils that are composed of collagen fibres and some elastin. The media or middle layer contains mainly circularly arranged smooth muscle cells and collagenous fibrils, and is divided from the adventitia by the external elastic lamina. The muscle cells contract and relax, whereas the elastin allows vessels to stretch and recoil. The adventitia or outermost layer is composed of collagen fibres and fibroblasts that protect the blood vessel and anchor it to surrounding structures.

The endothelium

The endothelium functions in a multitude of physiological processes including the control of cellular trafficking, the regulation of vasomotor tone and maintenance of blood fluidity. ECs possess surface receptors for a variety of physiological substances, for example thrombin and angiotensin II, which may influence vascular tone directly or indirectly through various haemostasis-related events. Once activated, ECs express at their surface, and in some cases release into the plasma, a variety of intracellular adhesion molecules (e.g. vascular cell adhesion molecule, E-selectin, P-selectin and von Willebrand factor, vWF), which modulate leucocyte and platelet adhesion, inflammation, phagocytosis and vascular permeability.

However, the endothelium should not be regarded as a simple homogeneous cell type. It would appear that EC phenotypes are differentially regulated; at any given point in time, structural and functional phenotypes may vary between segments of the vascular tree and at any given location, the endothelial phenotypes may change from one moment to the next. EC heterogeneity occurs between different organs, within the vascular loop of a given organ, and even between neighbouring ECs of a single vessel.

Endothelial cell activities affecting platelet–vessel wall interaction

Intact ECs exert a powerful inhibitory influence on haemostasis by virtue of the factors that they synthesize and release or express

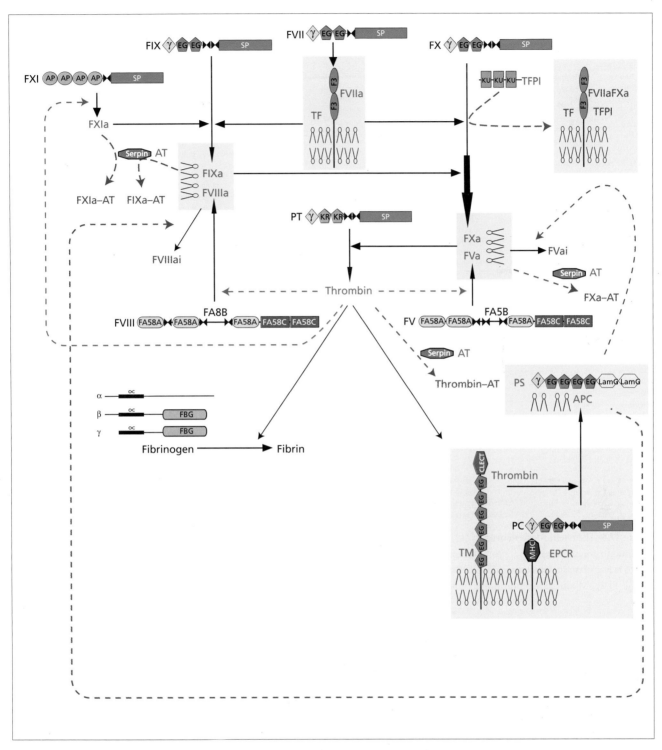

Figure 47.5 The haemostasis network: protein C pathway. Thrombin bound to TM on endothelial cell surfaces activates PC bound to its receptor EPCR. APC in complex with its cofactor PS inactivates FVa and FVIIIa by further proteolytic cleavages. Colours and symbols as in Figure 47.1.

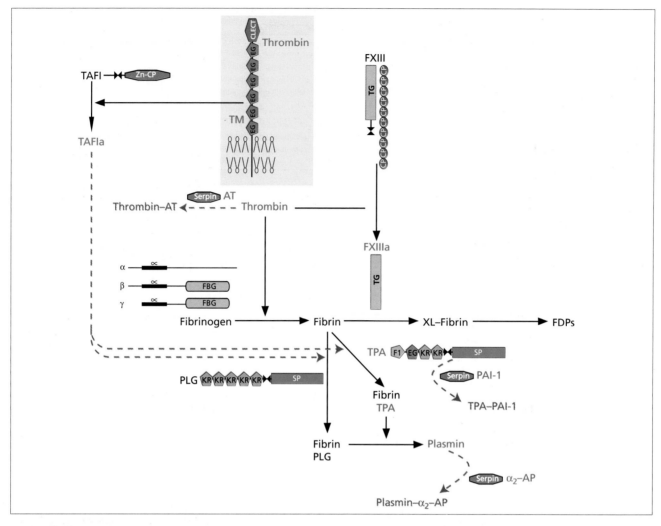

Figure 47.6 The haemostasis network: fibrinolysis. Both PLG and tPA bind to polymerized fibrin, promoting the cleavage of PLG by tPA to active plasmin, which then degrades cross-linked fibrin to soluble FDPs. Modulation of fibrinolysis is achieved by serpin inhibition: PAI-1 inactivates tPA, while α_2-AP inhibits plasmin. In addition, TAFIa removes Lys residues from fibrin, removing PLG and tPA binding sites. Colours and symbols as in Figure 47.1.

on their surface (see Figure 47.7b). Two of these, prostaglandin I_2 (PGI$_2$, or prostacyclin) and nitric oxide (NO), also known as endothelium-derived relaxing factor (EDRF), have powerful vasodilator activity, acting on smooth muscle cells in the vessel wall (basal-directed secretion) and hence modulating blood flow. Both substances inhibit aggregation of platelets and leucocytes (luminal-directed secretion) by raising intraplatelet levels of cyclic adenosine monophosphate (cAMP) and cyclic guanosine monophosphate (cGMP) respectively (see below).

PGI$_2$ is the major prostaglandin synthesized by ECs, a small amount also being produced by fibroblasts and smooth muscle cells. Its action on platelets involves binding to a specific G-protein coupled receptor (PTGIR) that activates adenylate cyclase, which increases the intraplatelet cAMP concentration. This pro-

motes Ca^{2+} uptake into the dense tubular system and inhibits phosphatidylinositol metabolism, both of which prevent platelet aggregation and the consequent release of storage granules containing procoagulant molecules, for example vWF and FV. The effect of PGI$_2$ on the vessel wall (where the target cell is the smooth muscle cell) is vasodilatation.

The precursor of PGI$_2$ is arachidonic acid, derived from EC membrane phospholipids by phospholipases. Arachidonic acid is first converted to prostaglandins PGG$_2$ and PGH$_2$, the so-called cyclic endoperoxides, by cyclo-oxygenase, and then to PGI$_2$ by prostacyclin synthetase. Thrombin and other agents (see above) that are generated at the site of injury stimulate the synthesis of PGI$_2$ by adjacent ECs, which counteracts the platelet-aggregating activity of the protease and thereby helps to

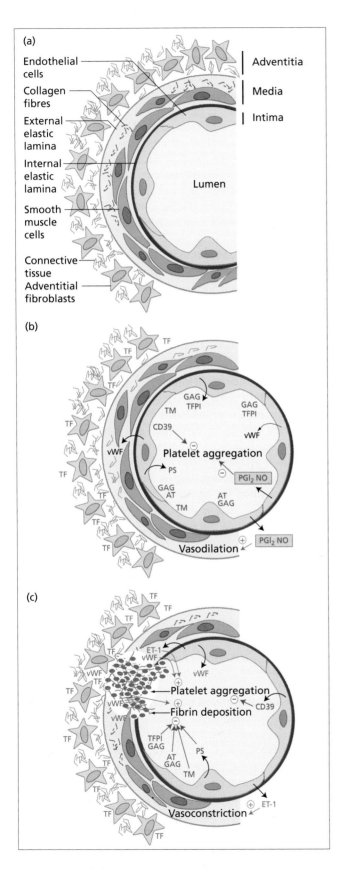

localize platelet plug formation. Elevation of intravascular pressure and trauma, including venepuncture, also increase PGI_2 production and may be a source of artefactually high plasma levels. PGI_2 is rather unstable and largely degrades spontaneously to 6-keto $PGF_1\alpha$, with a half-life of only a few minutes in whole blood. 6-keto $PGF_1\alpha$ is biologically inert, but in some tissues a variable proportion of PGI_2 may be enzymatically converted to other prostaglandins such as 6-keto $PGF_1\alpha$ or di-hydro di-keto $PGF_1\alpha$, which retain some platelet-inhibitory activity.

The once-held belief that PGI_2 is a circulating hormone with limited platelet–platelet interactions within the bloodstream is probably false, as plasma levels of PGI_2 are at least two orders of magnitude below that needed to inhibit platelet aggregation. Although in some settings, such as following severe trauma, it is possible that markedly raised systemic levels could occur transiently, it is more likely that PGI_2 serves mainly as a local hormone, principally concerned with vascular tone, but possibly also inhibiting the extension of the platelet plug beyond the immediate vicinity of any endothelial damage.

NO is synthesized in smooth muscle cells, macrophages and activated platelets, as well as by ECs. Its synthesis and secretion may be constitutive (when it serves as a local hormone to 'fine-tune' blood flow). Stimulated (inducible) synthesis of NO also occurs in ECs exposed to cytokines (interleukin 1, IL-1, tissue necrosis factor, TNF, or endotoxin for example), is slower but long lasting, and can have undesirable side-effects such as inflammation, cytotoxicity or prolonged hypotension. Like PGI_2, it has a very short half-life (3–5 s), being rapidly oxidized to the inactive nitrite (NO_2^-) or nitrate (NO_3^-) forms.

In addition to PGI_2 and NO, ECs also express an ecto-ADPase (CD39) on their cell surface, which rapidly metabolizes ATP and ADP that is released from activated platelets to AMP, thereby drastically reducing or abolishing platelet recruitment and aggregation.

The 21-amino-acid peptide endothelin-1 (ET-1) is the predominant isoform of the endothelin peptide family, which includes ET-2, ET-3 and ET-4. It exerts various biological effects,

Figure 47.7 (*left*) Blood vessel architecture and functions in haemostasis. (a) Anatomy of a generic blood vessel, not to scale, as layer thicknesses vary widely between arterial and venous sides, and between large and small vessels. The main three layers (intima, media and adventitia) are shown. (b) Role of the endothelium in maintaining vessel patency through general anticoagulant and anti-platelet mechanisms. In the absence of vessel damage, TF cannot contact plasma components, coagulation inhibitors are present on the endothelial surface and platelet aggregation is inhibited. (c) Localized haemostatic response to vessel injury, through initiation of coagulation by TF exposure and platelet activation/aggregation by exposure of extravascular collagen to plasma vWF. Procoagulant responses away from lesion site are damped down by anticoagulant and anti-platelet factors derived from endothelium.

including vasoconstriction and the stimulation of cell proliferation in tissues both within and outside of the cardiovascular system. In the endothelium, ET-1 is predominantly released abluminally towards the vascular smooth muscle, where it acts as a potent vasoconstrictor and mitogen for smooth muscle cells. In addition, ET-1 stimulates the production of cytokines and growth factors. Furthermore, it stimulates neutrophil adhesion and platelet aggregation and is chemotactic for macrophages.

vWF is a multimeric adhesive glycoprotein that plays an important role in primary haemostasis by promoting platelet adhesion to subendothelium at sites of vascular injury and platelet–platelet interaction under high shear-rate conditions. It is also a carrier of FVIII and this association protects FVIII from rapid proteolysis. Failure of FVIII to bind vWF, as occurs in the 'Normandy' variant of von Willebrand disease (see Chapter 49), leads to its rapid turnover and resulting FVIII deficiency. vWF is synthesized by ECs, megakaryocytes and platelets. It is secreted via constitutive and regulated pathways, the latter involving storage and release following stimulation. The constitutive secretion pathway is active only in ECs. The storage granules found in cells that synthesize vWF are the Weibel–Palade body in ECs and the α-granule in megakaryocytes and platelets.

Mature vWF is composed of identical disulphide-linked subunits, each comprising 2050-amino-acid residues and up to 22 carbohydrate chains with a mass of approximately 278 kDa of which 10–19% is carbohydrate. Two subunits joined at the C-termini form dimers that are the building blocks of larger multimers ranging in size from approximately 500 kDa to in excess of 10 000 kDa. The ultra-large vWF multimers secreted by ECs may appear as thin filaments that are several microns long or as globular molecules. Under conditions of high shear stress, these globular molecules may be unwound, especially if platelets are available to bind. These ultra-large vWF multimers can only be detected transiently in normal plasma because they are cleaved by a plasma metalloproteinase (ADAMTS 13). Deficiency of ADAMTS 13 results in accumulation of ultra-large vWF multimers in plasma, leading to enhanced shear-induced platelet aggregation; this is responsible for the microvascular thrombosis seen in patients with thrombotic thrombocytopenic purpura (TTP; see Chapter 52). The adhesion of platelets to vWF is mediated through the binding of the platelet receptor GPIbα to the A1 domain of vWF immobilized on exposed subendothelial matrices. Mutations in the genes encoding the GPIbα complex lead to the bleeding disorder Bernard–Soulier syndrome.

Thrombospondin 1 (TSP1) is an abundant constituent of the platelet α-granules of platelets and Weibel–Palade bodies of ECs. TSP1 was first identified as a thrombin-sensitive protein (TSP) that was released in response to activation of platelets by thrombin. Upon release from platelets, TSP1 binds to the platelet surface in a Ca^{2+}-dependent manner and interacts with integrins $\alpha_{IIb}\beta_3$ and $\alpha_v\beta_3$, CD36 and the integrin-associated protein

(IAP), integrin-bound fibrinogen and fibronectin. TSP1 activates $\alpha_{IIb}\beta_3$ through its binding to IAP. This results in spreading of platelets and aggregation.

Endothelial cell anticoagulant activities

ECs express two cellular receptors, TM and EPCR, which regulate the anticoagulant pathway initiated by thrombin (protein C pathway). TM is constitutively expressed on all ECs with the exception of the brain. EPCR is expressed strongly in the ECs of arteries and veins in heart and lung, less intensely in capillaries in the lung and skin, and not at all in the endothelium of small vessels of the liver and kidney. In addition, ECs synthesize and secrete PS, the cofactor for APC inactivation of FVa and FVIIIa.

TFPI is synthesized and secreted by ECs. TF–FVIIa activity is controlled by TFPI, which forms a quaternary inhibited complex TF–FVIIa–FXa–TFPI. The vast majority of TFPI is associated with the vascular endothelium, binding GAGs on the surface of ECs. The GAGs are also important in binding and modulating the activity of AT, which inhibits FIXa, FXa, FXIa and thrombin.

Endothelium and vessel injury

Disruption of the vessel wall following injury leads to exposure of procoagulant stimuli (see Figure 47.7c). Cells of the adventitia or epithelial cells of the surrounding tissues express TF constitutively on their surfaces. Formation of a complex between TF and FVII present in blood flowing from the injured vessel initiates coagulation, resulting in fibrin generation. Exposure of collagen within the subendothelial layers of the vessel wall leads to immobilization of plasma vWF triggering platelet adhesion, aggregation and activation. Release of the contents of platelet α-granules increases the local vWF concentration and activation of ECs results in release of Weibel–Palade bodies, further increasing the local concentration of vWF and expression of the cell adhesion molecule, P-selectin, leading to further recruitment of platelets. In addition, release of ET-1 from the endothelium stimulates platelet aggregation and vasoconstriction, limiting blood loss. The anticoagulant activities of the ECs discussed above serve to limit fibrin deposition and prevent vascular occlusion.

Endothelial cell-derived fibrinolytic factors

Three important fibrinolytic factors are detectable in the vessel wall: tissue plasminogen activator (tPA) and plasminogen activator inhibitor type 1 (PAI-1) are synthesized primarily by ECs, whereas urinary plasminogen activator (uPA, urokinase) is mainly derived from fibroblast-like cells in the kidney and gut. Unlike vWF and P-selectin, tPA and PAI-1 are not stored in the Weibel–Palade bodies and, in the resting state, synthesis and secretion are slow, resulting in low circulating levels. However, stimulated synthesis and release occur in response to a variety of stimuli.

Platelets

Platelets play a vital role both in the formation of an aggregate or primary plug that stems blood loss at the site of injury, but also by supplying a cellular surface, which is tailored to the assembly of procoagulant complexes such as FX-ase and prothrombinase. Chapter 48 gives details of platelet biogenesis and function, including their specific roles in haemostasis.

The following three sections of this chapter give an overview of the genetics, biochemistry, structure and physiology of the proteins involved in haemostasis. The first section (Coagulation factors) deals largely with the proteins that are required to generate and amplify the procoagulant stimulus, resulting in the formation of a stable fibrin clot. The following two sections (Naturally occurring inhibitors of blood coagulation, and Fibrinolysis) treat the regulatory pathways that delimit and control this powerful procoagulant response, and ultimately participate in remodelling of tissues following trauma.

Coagulation factors

Almost certainly, all the major soluble protein components of the thrombin-generating pathways, the PC pathway, the fibrinolytic pathway and their respective inhibitors have now been identified. In addition, a number of cell surface receptors relevant to these pathways have also been identified, but new receptors are still being discovered; the last word on the physiology of these systems certainly remains to be written.

Coagulation factor modules

The haemostatic proteins are generally assembled from a small number of modules or domains; indeed, the coagulation zymogens were the first family of proteins in which modular assembly was recognized (Figure 47.8). Although differing in exact amino acid sequence in different proteins, a module always adopts the same three-dimensional structure or *fold*. Here these modules will be introduced, following which the proteins themselves will be described briefly.

Gamma-carboxyglutamic acid module

The defining feature of this module is the presence of a number (9–12) of glutamic acid residues that are post-translationally modified by the addition of a carboxyl group to the γ-carbon by a vitamin K-dependent carboxylase: the gamma-carboxyglutamic acid (GLA) domain is usually N-terminal and confers affinity to negatively charged phospholipid (PL) membranes such as those of activated platelets or ECs, promoting the assembly of functional multiprotein complexes on these surfaces. Proteins containing GLA modules are commonly referred to as 'vitamin K-dependent factors' as this vitamin is a cofactor in the carboxylation reaction: they include prothrombin, FVII, FIX, FX, PC, PS and protein Z.

In the absence of Ca^{2+} ions, the module is partially disordered, but the crystal structure of several GLA-containing factors in the presence of Ca^{2+} ions reveals a fold in which the GLA residues are directed inwards towards a row of these ions; as blood contains approximately 1 mmol/L free Ca^{2+} ions it is expected that GLA modules will be in this functional form *in vivo*. The mechanism whereby the Ca^{2+} ion-dependent fold leads to the property of binding to PL probably involves the exposure of hydrophobic residues (an 'omega-loop') on the surface of the folded GLA module.

Amphipathic helix modules

These modules are also known as aromatic amino acid stacks and frequently occur immediately C-terminal to GLA modules. They consist of three turns of α-helix, one face of which has hydrophilic residues and the opposite face hydrophobic aromatic side chains. In prothrombin, the helix is folded along the top edge of the GLA module, whereas in the TF–FVIIa complex the module is stretched out so that its hydrophobic face interacts with the membrane proximal module of TF, its cellular receptor.

Epidermal growth factor-like module

These modules are widely dispersed in nature and are often involved in protein–protein interaction. The typical structure is a β-pleated sheet maintained by a characteristic 1–3, 2–4, 5–6 arrangement of three disulphide bonds. Haemostatic proteins contain one (tPA, pro-urokinase), two (FVII, FIX, FX, PC), four (PS) or six (TM) EGF modules. The N-terminal epidermal growth factor (EGF) modules of PC, FVII, FIX and FX contain a high-affinity Ca^{2+} ion binding site.

Kringle module

Found first in prothrombin (two modules) and named for the resemblance of the two-dimensional disulphide bond structure to a type of pastry, these modules also appear in fibrinolytic proteins (pro-urokinase, plasminogen and tPA) and in apolipoprotein(a). The three-dimensional fold brings into close apposition the sulphur atoms of two disulphide bonds to create a compact ellipsoidal structure that is often involved in protein–protein interaction (e.g. kringle 2 of prothrombin with FVa).

Apple module

Also known as PAN modules, these are found in the haemostatic proteins only in FXI and prekallikrein (four each) and they mediate protein interactions. In FXI, binding to high-molecular-weight kininogen (HMWK) is via apple 1, FIX via apples 2 and 3 and homodimerization via apple 4. The complete three-dimensional fold is unknown although that of a submodule has been reported.

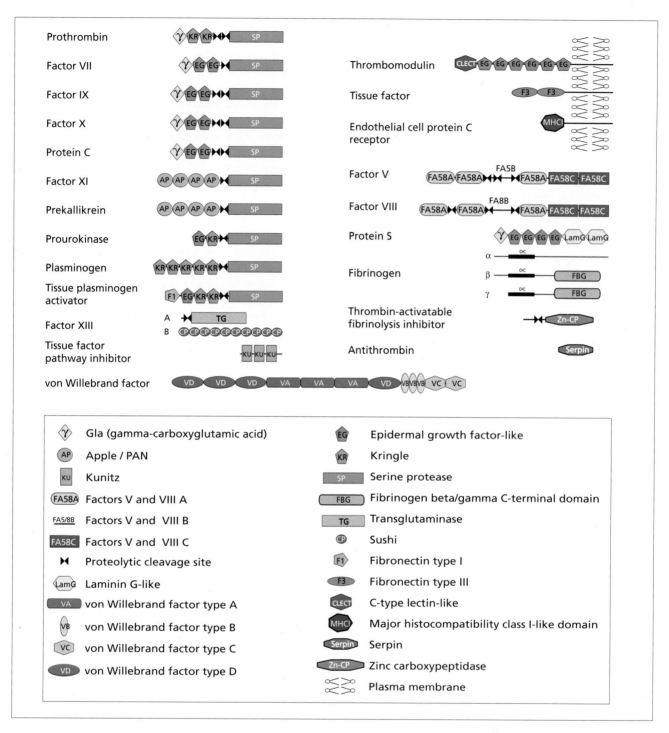

Figure 47.8 Modular organization of haemostasis proteins. Evolutionary relationship of many factors is suggested by their modular organization of proteins, represented as proposed by Bork and Bairoch (www.bork.embl-heidelberg.de/modules/).

Serine protease module

Chymotrypsin-like serine protease modules carry out many of the specific proteolytic steps in haemostasis. The core of these modules shows remarkable conservation with the structure of chymotrypsin, with three residues forming the canonical catalytic triad (His57, Asp102, Ser195; chymotrypsin numbering). All the protease modules circulate as part of a multidomain inactive zymogen, and are activated by cleavage of an interdomain connecting peptide at an Arg–Val or Arg–Ile bond. The neo-N terminus then folds into a cleft in the globular protease module to ion-pair with an invariant Asp residue adjacent to the active site Ser, creating an oxyanion hole essential for substrate accommodation and catalytic function. These modules are always found at the C-terminus of the multidomain proteases, apart from thrombin, which consists of a single protease domain after activation of prothrombin.

Serine protease inhibitor (serpin) module

The serpins are a family of single-module proteins that have evolved to neutralize (more or less specifically) individual serine proteases, although some cross-specificity is seen. The general mechanism seems to be as follows (although in specific instances it may vary). The β-pleated sheet structure of the serpin presents a bait loop that enters the active site of its protease target; the protease cleaves the bait loop but remains covalently tethered to one end of it via its active site Ser, moves to the opposite end of the serpin molecule by a form of 'spring mechanism' and is subsequently degraded.

Glycosaminoglycans (GAGs) such as heparin or heparan sulphate accelerate the inhibition process in some serpins by converting a latent form of the serpin to an active form, through binding to a region of β-sheet strands 3 and 5, forcing the bait loop into an active conformation; this is at least a major part of the explanation for the anticoagulant action of clinical heparin administration. GAGs may also accelerate serpin inhibition of specific proteases by a 'template' mechanism, whereby both proteins bind to the same GAG chain. The detailed structure of the trimeric complex of thrombin, antithrombin and heparin has recently been determined by X-ray crystallography.

Kunitz module

Kunitz domains are found throughout nature in a large number of proteins, generally inhibitors of specific serine proteases. The canonical Kunitz inhibitor is bovine pancreatic trypsin inhibitor (BPTI), which has been closely studied. The Kunitz fold contains three disulphide bridges and structural analysis of protease inhibitor pairs shows that the general mechanism of inhibition involves insertion of a loop containing the module's Arg15 side chain (BPTI numbering) into the enzyme's serine protease module, where it occupies and disrupts the active site. Crucial for the modulation of activity of TF–FVIIa, the coagulation initiation complex, is tissue factor pathway inhibitor (TFPI), a three-Kunitz module protein found predominantly on the EC surface, tethered by affinity to cell surface GAGs.

FV and FVIII A module

Three of these (A1, A2 and A3) are each present in FV and FVIII. Each A module consists of two plastocyanin-like 'Greek key' β-barrels, which, in the blue proteins, coordinate type-I copper ions. They are involved in the multiple protein–protein interactions that permit assembly of the FX-ase and prothrombinase complexes. From the crystal structure of ceruloplasmin, it is predicted that the three modules are arranged in a triangular

structure in the two coagulation factors. The anticoagulant action of the protease activated protein C (APC) is mediated via specific cleavages in the N-terminal A1 and A2 domains of the activated cofactors.

FV and FVIII C module

Two of these (C1 and C2) are each present in FV and FVIII (and also milk fat-binding globule proteins among others). The C-terminal C2 domains of each have been implicated in PL binding, and the crystal structures of both FV C2 and FVIII C2 reveal a β-sandwich core and a possible mode of this binding, via insertion of hydrophobic amino-acid side chains into the PL bilayer, together with the close approach of positively charged Arg and Lys side-chains to negatively charged PL head groups. In FVIII, the C1 domain may have a role in vWF interaction. In addition, a recent partial structure for APC-cleaved FVa suggests that C1 may also be involved in PL binding.

FV and FVIII B sequences

Both FV and FVIII contain large heavily glycosylated sequences that have been termed 'B domains' as they lie between the A and C modules (although it is uncertain whether these fold as distinct modules). The B domains of FV and FVIII share little sequence identity with each other. They lack procoagulant function as B-domainless versions of these factors retain full activity; there is some evidence that these sequences interact with chaperone/quality-checking proteins during synthesis.

Fibronectin module types I and III

These modules are named for their appearance in the matrix protein fibronectin. An FN-I module is found in tPA and two FN-III modules in TF: the TF modules bind FVIIa in a similar manner to that in which growth hormone receptor binds its hormone ligand. The underlying fold of FN-III is a flattened β-barrel and also occurs in cytokine receptors, immunoglobulins and related proteins such as CD2 and CD4.

von Willebrand factor modules

vWF contains several types of repeated module (A, B, C and D: unrelated to A, B and C found in FV and FVIII), some of which are shared with other multimeric adhesive proteins. So far, structures have been obtained for A1 (implicated in platelet interaction) and A3 (which contains a major site for interaction with collagen fibres).

LamG module

The vitamin-K dependent PS acts as a cofactor in the APC inactivation of FVa and FVIIIa, and has two C-terminal laminin G-like modules where most other vitamin K-dependent haemostatic proteins have a serine protease module. Previously this structure was termed the steroid hormone binding-globulin domain.

MHC class I/CD1 family module

The endothelial protein C receptor (EPCR) is a transmembrane receptor whose external structure is homologous with that of the MHC class I/CD1 family: this MHC/CD1 module interacts with the GLA domain of PC.

Lectin-like module

This module is found at the N-terminus of the anticoagulant protein TM, the EC receptor responsible for binding to thrombin and altering its substrate specificity. The lectin-like module has recently been shown to be responsible for inhibition of leucocyte adhesion to activated endothelium.

Factor XIII modules

FXIII, the transglutaminase that cross-links newly formed fibrin to generate a stable clot, is a non-covalently assembled tetramer consisting of 2 FXIII A and 2 FXIII B modules. Each A module contains four domains (the enzymatic core, two β-barrels and a β-sandwich), whereas the B module consists of ten consecutive Sushi domains (also called glycoprotein-1 or CP domains).

Transmembrane and cytoplasmic modules

Transmembrane modules are hydrophobic segments of variable sequence found in the cell surface membrane-anchored proteins TF, TM, EPCR and thrombin receptors such as the protease-activated receptors (PARs), and which usually adopt an α-helical fold. Some transmembrane cellular receptors, such as TF, also have a cytoplasmic module: these may play a role in cell signalling.

Proteins of the coagulation network

Table 47.2 gives a summary of characteristics of the proteins discussed, including gene location, number of exons, molecular mass, circulating concentration, plasma half-life and presumed function.

Tissue factor

Tissue factor is unambiguously regarded as the sole initiator of coagulation in both normal and pathological coagulation. The processed mature protein is 263 amino acids in length after signal peptide cleavage. The 219-residue extracellular region consists of two FN-III modules anchored into the cell membrane by a 23-residue transmembrane sequence: the extracellular region binds tightly to FVIIa to form a highly active procoagulant complex after exposure of cell surface TF to plasma FVIIa. The 21-residue cytoplasmic module has been implicated in intracellular signalling, however transgenic experiments in mice have shown that this module is not required either for development or coagulant function, so the function of this module is still unclear.

Vascular adventitial cells, neuroglia, vascular smooth muscle and epidermal cells express TF constitutively. It therefore forms a protective envelope around blood vessels and organs, ready to initiate clotting as soon as blood leaks out of vessels. TF is also expressed by monocytes and endothelium after activation by inflammatory cytokines or by endotoxin, for example in sepsis, and on cancerous tissues. Intravascular exposure of TF by any route, but particularly after atherosclerotic plaque rupture (releasing TF-bearing monocytes), can result in thrombosis. Recent work has also focused on the novel hypothesis that functionally active TF can circulate in flowing blood on small procoagulant particles, which may also be transferred from one blood cell type to another via specific receptor-mediated interactions.

Factor VII

Plasma FVII binds to TF, for example after vessel trauma or plaque rupture, to form a complex that initiates coagulation by directly activating FX and to a lesser extent FIX. The FVII gene lies adjacent to the factor X gene, suggesting gene duplication during evolution, and close to that of protein Z. In common with other GLA module-containing proteins, a propeptide sequence encoded by exon 2 directs the GLA module, coded by exon 3, for γ-carboxylation at 10 Glu residues. The two EGF modules are encoded by exons 4 and 5. Exon 6 encodes the connecting or activation peptide, and exons 7 and 8 the serine protease module. FVII is activated by cleavage between residues Arg152 and Ile153, yielding a two-chain disulphide-linked FVIIa molecule; however, this has little catalytic activity until it is bound to TF. The half-life of FVII zymogen in plasma is 3 h and, exceptionally, the half-life of the FVIIa enzyme is 2.5 h, probably because there is no plasma inhibitor capable of effectively neutralizing free FVIIa. In recent years, recombinant FVIIa has entered clinical use as a treatment, first, for haemophiliacs with inhibitors to exogenous FVIII, and, second, for a wider range of bleeding problems and general surgical intervention.

Factor X

The gene and protein structures of FX closely resemble those of FVII. Unlike FVII, zymogen FX circulates as a two-chain, disulphide-linked heterodimer due to excision of a tribasic peptide (Arg–Lys–Arg) at residues 139–141 during synthesis. The light chain of FX therefore consists of the GLA module with 11 γ-carboxyglutamate residues, the amphipathic helix, and two EGF modules. The half-life of FX in plasma is 36 h. FX is activated by either FIXa–FVIIIa or TF–FVIIa, on PL surfaces in the presence of Ca^{2+} ions. FXa forms a PL-bound complex with FVa, which efficiently activates prothrombin (prothrombinase complex).

Factor IX

The FIX gene is located at band Xq26, about 15.2 Mbp from the FVIII gene, thus deficiencies of both factors are X-linked disorders. Deficiency of either FVIII or FIX results in clinical haemophilia (A or B respectively), as the main function of FIX is to participate in the FX-ase complex FIXa–FVIIIa. The FIX

Table 47.2 Key proteins involved in the haemostatic network.

Common name	Abbreviation	Subunit	Gene symbol	Gene location	No. of exons	Amino acids (mature)	M_r of monomer (kDa)	Plasma level (µg/mL)	Plasma level (nmol/L)	$T_{1/2}$ (h)	Main action
Tissue factor	TF		F3	1p13	6	263	44	NA	NA	NA	Cofactor for FVII/FVIIa
Prothrombin	FII		F2	11p11.1	14	579	72	90	1400	65	Clots FBG, activates PC, FXI, TAFI
Factor V	FV		F5	1q23	25	2196	330	10	30	15	Cofactor for FXa
Factor VII	FVII		F7	13q34	8	416	50	0.5	10	3	Activates FIX and FX
Factor VIII	FVIII		F8	Xq28	26	2332	330	0.1	0.3	10	Cofactor for FIXa
Factor IX	FIX		F9	Xq27	8	415	56	5	90	25	Activates FX
Factor X	FX		F10	13q34	8	445	59	8	135	40	Activates prothrombin
Factor XI	FXI		F11	4q35	15	607	80*	5	30	45	Activates FIX
Prekallikrein	PK		KLKB1	4q35	15	638	86	50	580	35	Antiangiogenic, profibrinolytic
Factor XIII† (A chain)‡	FXIII	A	F13A1	6p25	15	731	75†	10	30	200	Crosslinks fibrin
Factor XIII† (B chain)	FXIII	B	F13B	1q31	12	641	80†	10	30	200	Crosslinks fibrin
Fibrinogen (α chain)‡	FGN	α	FGA	4q32	6	866	68‡	3000	9000	90	Mechanical stabilization of clot
Fibrinogen (β chain)‡	FGN	β	FGB	4q32	8	491	52‡	3000	9000	90	Mechanical stabilization of clot
Fibrinogen (γ chain)‡	FGN	γ	FGG	4q32	10	453	49‡	3000	9000	90	Mechanical stabilization of clot
von Willebrand factor	VWF		VWF	12p13	52	2050	255	10	40	12	Cell adhesion and FVIII carrier
Thrombomodulin	TM		THBD	20p11.1	1	557	60	NA	NA	NA	Cofactor in PC/TAFI activation
Endothelial protein C receptor	EPCR		PROCR	20q11.1	7	220	27	NA	NA	NA	Cofactor in PC activation
Protein C	PC		PROC	2q14.2	9	419	62	4	65	6	Inactivation of FVa and FVIIIa
Protein S	PS		PROS1	3q11.2	15	676	69	10 (free)	145	?	Inactivation of FVa and FVIIIa
Tissue factor pathway inhibitor	TFPI		TFPI	2q33	12	304	42	0.08	2.5	?	Inhibition of coagulation initiation
Antithrombin	AT		SERPINC1	1q23	9	464	58	140	2400	5	Inhibits thrombin, FIX, FX, FXI
Heparin cofactor II	HCII		SERPIND1	22q11	5	499	66	90	1200	60	Prevention of arterial thrombosis?
Plasminogen	PLG		PLG	6q27	14	791	92	200	2000	50	Dissolution of clot in wound repair
Tissue plasminogen activator	TPA		PLAT	8p11.1	14	562	69	0.005	0.07	0.03	Plasma activator of plasminogen
Prourokinase	UK		PLAU	10q22	11	431	54	0.0015	0.04	0.03	Tissue activator of plasminogen
Plasminogen activator inhibitor 1	PAI-1		SERPINE1	7q22	9	379	52	10	200	0.1	Inhibition of TPA and UPA
Alpha2-antiplasmin	α2-AP		SERPINF2	17p13	9	452	67	70	1000	72	Inhibition of plasmin
Thrombin-activatable fibrinolysis inhibitor	TAFI		CPB2	13q14	11	401	60	5	75	0.2	Inhibition of fibrinolysis

*Factor XI circulates as a 160-kDa homodimer of two 80-kDa monomers.

†Factor XIII circulates as a 326-kDa tetramer of two A- and two B-chains.

‡Fibrinogen circulates as a 340-kDa complex of two each of A-, B- and C-chains.

promoter has been extensively studied and includes sites for liver-specific transcription factors and an androgen-responsive promoter element, which accounts for the haemophilia B Leiden phenotype (FIX deficiency which corrects spontaneously at puberty). The plasma half-life of FIX is 18 h.

The mature protein consists of 415 amino acids and the GLA module contains 12 γ-carboxylated residues. Either TF–FVIIa or FXIa cleaves FIX within the connecting peptide (between residues 145–146 and 180–181), releasing an activation peptide to achieve full activation of FIX.

Factor XI

The protein circulates as a homodimer, linked through a di-sulphide bridge located in apple module 4. Activation of FXI is by a single cleavage performed by thrombin; FXIa then activates FIX directly in free solution. FXI activation by the contact pro-tein FXIIa was originally thought to be a relevant step in 'intrin-sic' or contact-activated coagulation, but it is now considered that the feedback activation of FXI by trace thrombin provides a physiologically relevant route for generation of increased amounts of FIXa to assemble FX-ase during the amplification of the initial TF stimulus.

Factor XIII

FXIII circulates as a tetramer of two A-chains and two B-chains. The B-chains function as carrier for the A-chains, which, after activation by thrombin, function as a transglutaminase to cross-link fibrin and other proteins in the clot, resulting in a stable structure. FXIIIa contains a free sulphydryl group at the active site. Platelets also contain FXIII A-chain dimers, which are fully functional after thrombin activation.

von Willebrand factor

The vWF mRNA encodes a large propeptide essential for multi-merization and the mature protomer, totalling 2813 amino acids, which is formed of four repeating modules termed A, B, C and D. During post-translational processing, the protomers dimerize then multimerize with excision of the propeptide. vWF is synthesized in ECs (where it is stored in Weibel–Palade bod-ies) and in megakaryocytes, where it is stored in the α-granules of platelets. Both Weibel–Palade body and α-granule vWF are released on stimulation by various agonists, including throm-bin. Plasma also contains vWF, which is released from ECs via a constitutive pathway. vWF serves two unique functions in haemostasis, as a carrier for FVIII and as the bifunctional ligand mediating platelet GPIb α adhesion to collagen.

Factor VIII

The FVIII gene spans 187 kb of the X chromosome (Xq28) and encodes a protein of 2351 amino acids. After removal of the 19-amino-acid signal sequence, a single chain of 2332 amino acids is transiently formed but is subsequently further processed prior to release as a series of heterodimers, due to variable cleavage within the B-domain sequence. Owing to internal homology, the FVIII module structure can be represented as A1–A2–B–A3–C1–C2. FVIII also has three short acidic inter-module peptides (*a1, a2* and *a3*) that are closely implicated in FVIII function.

FVIII is the essential cofactor for activation of FX by FIXa in the 'FX-ase' complex. It has no function until proteolysed to FVIIIa by thrombin or FXa at Arg372–Ser373 and Arg1689–Ser1690. FVIIIa is directly inactivated by APC cleavage at Arg336–Ser337 and Arg562–Ser563, however, functional activ-ity of FVIIIa also decays rapidly by dissociation of the A2 subunit from FVIIIa. The structure and function of FVIII have recently been reviewed (Saenko *et al.,* 2002).

Factor V

The mature protein product is 2196 amino acids in length after cleavage of a 28-amino-acid signal peptide. The structure of FV, like that of FVIII, can be represented as Al–A2–B–A3–C1–C2. However, the B-domain sequences of FV and FVIII share little sequence identity with each other, although their lengths are similar and both are heavily glycosylated. FV also differs from FVIII in that it lacks the three short acidic intermodule peptides (*a1, a2* and *a3*) implicated in FVIII function.

FV is the cofactor for the activation of prothrombin by FXa. It has no cofactor activity until proteolysed by thrombin or FXa at Arg709–Ser710, Arg1018–Thr1019 and Arg1545–Ser1547. FVa is inactivated by APC through cleavages at Arg506–Ser507 and Arg1765–Leu1766. The initial (and rate limiting) cleavage is at Arg506. This is the site of the mutation in FV Leiden (FV Arg506 → Gln), which is resistant to APC, leading to the most common form of familial thrombophilia.

Fibrinogen

The fibrinogen gene cluster is located on chromosome 4 (q32) in the order β-α-γ, with β transcribed in the opposite direction to α and γ. The three chains of fibrinogen are disulphide cross-linked and folded together in an intricate manner. The overall structure of fibrinogen is a symmetrical dimer α2-β2-γ2. Viewed by electron microscopy, the molecule is trinodular, with the outer two globular modules (fragments D) containing the C-termini of all three chains connected to the central globular module (fragment E), which contains the N-termini of all six chains tethered together by disulphide bonds. Coiled coil regions, forming α-helical ropes, connect the lateral and central globular modules.

Polymerization of fibrinogen occurs when thrombin cleaves two short negatively charged fibrinopeptides A and B from the N-termini of the α- and β-chains respectively. This reveals new N-terminal sequences in the fragment E region (called knobs) that fit into holes in the fragment D regions. Polymerization then occurs spontaneously in a staggered half-overlap array, which can elongate indefinitely in either direction. Electron microscopy studies were and still are important in resolving the molecular architecture of fibrillar fibrin formation, but from 1997 elegant crystal structures of parts of the fibrin(ogen) molecule were successfully produced in a number of laboratories. These structures are revealing the elegant mechanisms of fibrin polymerization.

Prothrombin

The mDNA encodes a preproleader sequence similar to that found in other vitamin K-dependent proteins, followed by a GLA module, two kringle modules, an activation peptide and a serine protease module. FXa complexed with FVa activates prothrombin zymogen to thrombin on a phospholipid surface ('prothrombinase'), upon cleavage of two peptide bonds. The first between Arg271 and Thr272 releases the protease module from the GLA and kringle modules; the second at Arg320–Ile321 generates the catalytic site of thrombin by a typical trypsin-like conformational rearrangement. Fully cleaved thrombin is termed α-thrombin, and is active in free solution against many substrates including fibrinogen, FV, FVIII, FXI (acting as a procoagulant), PC (acting in complex with TM as an anticoagulant) and a range of cellular transmembrane protease-activated receptors or PARs. Thrombin also activates thrombin-activated fibrinolytic inhibitor (TAFI) (in complex with TM), inhibiting fibrinolysis.

Naturally occurring inhibitors of blood coagulation

In common with other defence mechanisms, such as those resulting in kinin release and complement activation, the blood coagulation process can be activated very rapidly when the need arises. This involves the generation of proteolytic enzymes, such as thrombin, which are potentially lethal if their action is not limited. For example, 10 mL of plasma can generate, in theory, sufficient thrombin to clot all of the fibrinogen in the body in 30 s. That it does not normally do so is due in part to the fact that the procoagulant response is most pronounced in the vicinity of the platelet plug forming at the point of vascular injury, while, elsewhere, coagulation is inhibited by substances in plasma or on the vascular surface that exhibit anticoagulant activity.

Classification of physiological anticoagulants

Physiological anticoagulants fall into two main groups: those that inhibit the serine proteases of the coagulation cascade (both Kunitz-type and serpins), and those involved in destruction of the activated coagulation cofactors FVa and FVIIIa (components of the PC system). These inhibitors assume great physiological significance: relatively minor deficiencies (50–70% of average levels) of some of these inhibitors, such as might be found in individuals heterozygous for a genetic defect, are associated with an increased incidence of thrombosis, and homozygous deficiencies are frequently either fatal in the first few years of life unless prophylactic replacement therapy is instituted, or are not found in nature, suggesting early fetal loss.

In addition to the specific inhibitors, there are some other inhibitory mechanisms that do not fit into either of the above categories, one of these being the detoxifying property of the liver, which plays an important role in removal of activated clotting factors, both directly and after their combination with natural inhibitors. Furthermore, the removal of free thrombin occurs as a result of its adsorption on to fibrin or on to fibrin(ogen) degradation products (FDP). The latter, which cannot themselves take part in a clot, may interfere with normal fibrin polymerization. Although less well-defined than the others, this group appears to be physiologically important, as qualitative defects of fibrinogen (dysfibrinogenaemias) that result in reduced thrombin binding may be associated with a thrombotic disorder (see Chapter 53).

Tissue factor pathway inhibitor – a Kunitz-type inhibitor

The various serpins found in blood (see below) probably play no role in the inhibition of FVIIa in the initiating TF–FVIIa complex. Instead, the action of this serine protease–cofactor complex is modulated by tissue factor pathway inhibitor (TFPI), which is largely found non-covalently associated with GAGs on the EC surface. TFPI structure comprises N- and C-terminal sequences (the latter probably responsible for interaction with GAGs), between which are found three Kunitz-type modules, K1, K2 and K3. The isolated protein has little effect on FVIIa alone, but can form a 1:1 complex with FXa, probably through specific interaction with the K2 module. This TFPI–FXa complex interacts effectively with the TF–FVIIa complex through a specific interaction between TFPI K1 and the FVIIa protease domain, forming a four-member TFPI–FXa–TF–FVIIa complex in which both proteases are inhibited.

Most TFPI in the vasculature (approximately 90%) is associated with (and thought to be synthesized by) ECs, particularly in the microcirculation, with a smaller amount (5–10%) being found in platelets and the rest in plasma. Virtually all circulating TFPI is associated with lipoproteins. Heparin therapy induces a large increase (up to 10-fold) in the plasma concentration of TFPI, suggesting that TFPI binding to ECs is mediated by surface GAGs and that this is reversed by heparin.

Disruption of the murine TFPI gene is incompatible with normal development, suggesting that a deficiency of functional TFPI might lead to clinical thrombosis. However, as the bulk of intravascular TFPI is associated with the EC surface, simple measurement of plasma TFPI levels is not a clear indicator of a deficiency state. Moderately low plasma levels can occur in DIC, septicaemia and following major surgery, possibly due to increased utilization, but heparin infusion increases plasma TFPI in such patients. Whether or not congenital deficiency of TFPI is a risk factor for thrombosis remains uncertain: after several negative studies in this area, recently a case–control study found a relationship between low levels of TFPI and enhanced risk of deep vein thrombosis.

Serine protease inhibitors (serpins) and heparin

Human plasma contains at least seven inhibitors of serine protease coagulation factors. Apart from α2-macroglobulin, all are single-chain serpins of molecular mass 40–65 kDa. Specificity is imparted by their tertiary structure, which engenders high affinity for a defined substrate or small range of substrates. Of this group, only antithrombin (AT) and heparin cofactor II (HCII) assume haemostatic significance, acting predominantly on proteases generated late in the coagulation cascade (i.e. thrombin and FXa). A deficiency of any of the other serpins (although sometimes giving rise to a clinical disorder due to the failure of neutralization of a serine protease not involved in coagulation pathways) is asymptomatic in terms of haemostasis and will not be treated in detail below.

Several serpins contain GAG binding sites, which, particularly in the case of AT and HCII, but to a lesser extent for PAI type 1 (PAI-1) and APC inhibitor, greatly enhance the rate of interaction with (although not the affinity for) their specific protease(s). As a major source of heparin-like material is heparan sulphate on the EC surface, another possible function of the heparin binding site of these inhibitors (especially AT and HCII) might be to allow them to exert a general and constitutive anticoagulant effect on intact vessels; this may also act to prevent extension of a procoagulant response beyond an area of damaged endothelium.

Antithrombin

Antithrombin (formerly antithrombin III) is a 58-kDa serpin that is synthesized principally in the liver, with a high plasma concentration of 2.4 μmol/L. The turnover of AT *in vivo* is complex, with a rapid initial clearance ($T_{1/2}$ = 10 min) due to equilibration with EC-bound AT, a slower ($T_{1/2}$ = 3 h) clearance rate due to equilibration with the extravascular compartment, and a much slower linear phase with an overall $T_{1/2}$ of 90 h.

Disruption of the murine AT gene results in death of all embryos shortly before birth, with extensive evidence of subcutaneous haemorrhage. In humans, heterozygous AT deficiency is associated with familial thrombosis.

AT forms a stable 1:1 complex with several serine protease coagulation factors, predominantly thrombin but also to some extent FIXa, FXIa, FXIIIa and kallikrein. Initially, the serine at the active centre of the protease cleaves a peptide bond (involving Arg393) in the 'bait loop' near the C-terminus of AT: a large conformational change in the serpin ensues, with the protease still attached to the loop moving to the opposite end of the serpin. The inactivated enzyme-serpin complex is now cleared

rapidly. Complex formation is progressive and only with thrombin and FXa is it rapid enough to be of physiological significance. In purified *in vitro* systems, the $T_{1/2}$ is around 30 s for free thrombin, 90 s for FXa, and 10–25 min for the other enzymes. In each case, the inhibitor–protease complex is rapidly cleared ($T_{1/2}$ = 3 min) from the circulation by the liver.

Heparin, without altering the stoichiometry, induces a > 2000-fold increase in the rate of thrombin inactivation by AT, such that its action becomes almost instantaneous ($T_{1/2}$ < 0.01 s). The unique mechanism of this activation involves release of the 'bait loop' from partial insertion in the β-sheet core of the molecule following heparin binding to AT. Heparin also strongly enhances AT neutralization of FXa and, to a lesser extent FIXa, particularly in the presence of Ca^{2+}, but at therapeutic concentrations it is without significant effect on AT inhibition of contact factors.

Anti-angiogenic and anti-tumour activities have also been described for the cleaved serpin in mouse models. This finding provides further evidence for the inter-relationship of coagulation and angiogenic pathways.

Heparin cofactor II

This serpin (M_r 65 000) is present in plasma at a high concentration of 90 μg/mL (1.2 μmol/L). It appears to be a specific 1:1 inhibitor of thrombin and to have little or no anti-FXa activity. The rate of thrombin neutralization by HCII is increased approximately 1000-fold by heparin, although because of its lower heparin affinity it requires 5–10 times more heparin than does AT. Interaction seems to depend largely on the high anionic charge of heparin and related GAGs. Details of the molecular mechanism of HCII interaction with thrombin have recently been elucidated by X-ray crystallography.

That HCII has some physiological significance is suggested by the fact that it falls in parallel with AT in DIC. However, as AT is in a twofold molar excess over HCII, the latter cannot altogether compensate for a deficiency of AT, which, as stated above, is a well-established cause of a thrombotic tendency. Whether or not HCII deficiency leads to a similar clinical picture remains to be established, as few cases have yet been described and only occasionally has concomitant thrombotic disease been present. HCII mouse knockout animals develop normally and do not show spontaneous thrombosis; however, they show an enhanced propensity to carotid occlusion after deliberate injury to the endothelium, corrected by infusion of purified HCII, suggesting that HCII has a role in prevention of arterial thrombosis.

Heparin and heparin-like substances in plasma

Heparin belongs to the group of polysulphated mucopolysaccharides known as glycosaminoglycans (GAGs), the major commercial source being porcine intestinal mucosa. By virtue of its strong positive charge, heparin combines non-specifically with a number of cationic proteins such as albumin and reacts in a highly specific way with β-lipoproteins, fibrinogen, HCII and

AT. It also mobilizes platelet PF4 and TFPI, which are bound to GAGs on the surface of ECs, and releases lipoprotein lipase into plasma.

Unfractionated heparin (UFH) is an extremely heterogeneous polymer, being composed of between 10 and 100 saccharide units. Only about one-quarter of UFH has any anticoagulant activity *in vitro*, the remainder possibly being responsible for some of its deleterious side-effects, the most important of which is heparin-induced thrombocytopenia. In recent years, UFH has been subjected to various fractionation procedures (including cleavage by nitrous acid, heparinase and oxidizing agents), yielding a number of low-molecular-weight heparin preparations. These low-molecular-weight heparins contain 10–20 saccharide units (M_r 4–6 kDa) and are less often associated with thrombocytopenia. In addition, a minimal pentasaccharide with anticoagulant activity has been identified.

Unfractionated and low-molecular-weight heparin differ in their affinities for the plasma factors with which they interact and in the specific serine proteases that they inhibit; this, together with the dosage administered, must be taken into account when selecting laboratory tests to monitor their therapeutic effect (see Chapter 55). The major anticoagulant activity of both UFH and low-molecular-weight heparin is attributed to the pentasaccharide sequence containing at its centre a 2,3,6 (3-O-sulpho) trisulphated glucosamine group. It is this that binds to lysyl or tryptophan residues in AT in the region of the D helix, inducing the conformational change in the inhibitor. A second anticoagulant action of UFH (at least 20 saccharide units are required) involves direct binding between thrombin (but not FXa or other proteases) and a heparin sequence adjacent to the pentasaccharide. This property of UFH, which brings thrombin and AT into close proximity of each other, explains the greater thrombin-neutralizing activity of UFH compared with low-molecular-weight heparin.

There is of course no detectable heparin in normal plasma. However, endogenous heparin-like molecules (e.g. dermatan sulphate and heparan sulphate), are present on the surface of ECs and, by enhancing the action of AT and HCII, these would have antithrombotic effects. Such mechanisms seem to be of clinical importance, as recurrent thromboses have been reported in association with several dysfunctional AT molecules that inhibit thrombin normally in the absence of heparin but which do not show enhanced reactivity in its presence, presumably due to defects at the heparin binding sites. At points of vascular injury, local accumulation of activated platelets provides a source of heparin-neutralizing activity (PF4) that could overcome the anticoagulant effects of EC-bound heparinoids and permit the procoagulant response to proceed.

Protein Z and protein Z-dependent inhibitor

Protein Z (PZ) is a 62-kDa vitamin K-dependent plasma protein that serves as a cofactor for the inhibition of FXa by PZ-dependent protease inhibitor (ZPI). Although PZ was first described in the 1970s, ZPI is a recently identified 72-kDa member of the serpin superfamily.

The organization of the PZ gene and the structure of the molecule are very similar to those of coagulation factors FVII, FIX, FX and protein C; however, the PZ 'serine protease' module lacks the canonical active site His and Ser residues and therefore cannot function as a protease. PZ circulates in plasma in a complex with ZPI. Inhibition of factor Xa by ZPI in the presence of PL and Ca^{2+} ions is enhanced 1000-fold by PZ, but ZPI also inhibits FXIa in a process that does not require PZ, PL or Ca^{2+}. ZPI activity is consumed during coagulation through proteolysis mediated by FXa (with PZ) and FXIa. PZ may serve to dampen the procoagulant response *in vivo* as PZ deficiency dramatically increases the severity of the prothrombotic phenotype of FV Leiden mice. Studies to determine the potential roles of PZ and ZPI deficiency in human thrombosis are in progress.

Alpha-1-antitrypsin

This is a serpin whose primary targets are predominantly pancreatic and leucocyte elastases. In addition, it is reported to be responsible for about 70% and 35%, respectively, of the FXIa- and FXa-neutralizing activity in plasma, but it has little effect on overall thrombin inhibition and a straightforward deficiency of α_1-antitrypsin (α_1-AT) is not associated with hypercoagulability.

An abnormal molecular form of α_1-AT in which there is a Met → Ser substitution at the active centre (antitrypsin Pittsburgh) has been described, rendering it functionally identical to AT with a high affinity for thrombin. At a plasma concentration of 25 μmol/L, the variant circulates at a 10-fold higher level than AT, and gives rise to a clinical bleeding tendency. It is, however, unaffected by heparin.

C1-esterase inhibitor

The primary target of this serpin is the activated form of the first component of complement, but it also contributes in a minor way to neutralization of FXIa and plasmin. A deficiency of C1-esterase inhibitor, although of no haemostatic consequence, causes angioneurotic oedema, the characteristic lesions of which may sometimes be confused with haematomas.

α_2-Antiplasmin

This serpin is the principal inhibitor of the fibrinolytic enzyme plasmin. It also has weak activity against several coagulation proteases, especially the contact factors. However, any anticoagulant action against proteases late in the coagulation cascade (e.g. FXa) is only apparent at concentrations well in excess of those in normal plasma. Its mechanism of action and clinical importance are discussed further in the section on fibrinolysis below.

α_2-Macroglobulin

α_2-Macroglobulin (α_2-MG) (M_r 740 000) is composed of four identical chains, is not a member of the serpin superfamily and its effects are not restricted to serine proteases. It binds to coagulation factors at a site away from the serine-active centre, the interaction involving the formation of a bond between cysteine and glutamate residues in the inhibitor and a lysyl group in the protease. Inhibition is produced by steric hindrance rather than by active site inactivation and, indeed, the proteases retain some esterolytic and amidolytic activity, particularly against small peptides, a fact that should be borne in mind when using chromogenic substrates to assay coagulation inhibitors. It is responsible for approximately 50%, 20% and 10% of the inhibition of kallikrein, thrombin and FXa respectively.

A deficiency of α_2-MG is not associated with a thrombotic tendency. It is, however, an acute phase reactant and it is possible that, when elevated under conditions of stress, or when the other major antithrombins or antiplasmins are overwhelmed, it might become a significant inhibitor of coagulation or fibrinolysis. Moreover, it has been suggested that the raised level of α_2-MG that exists in children (150–200% of adult values) may compensate for a low level of AT, and explain why thrombotic episodes do not usually occur before puberty in congenitally AT-deficient patients.

The protein C pathway – inhibition of cofactors FVa and FVIIIa

The activated forms of coagulation cofactors FV and FVIII (FVa and FVIIIa) are potent procoagulants that enormously enhance the activity of serine protease factors in the 'FX-ase' and 'prothrombinase' complexes (see above). It is not unexpected that these cofactors should be subject to a negative feedback mechanism that limits their procoagulant activity. This is achieved by a complex series of reactions collectively referred to as the 'protein C pathway'. Four key factors (Table 47.2) are now known to be involved, the interactions as shown in Figure 47.5.

Protein C

This vitamin K-dependent serine protease has an identical module composition to the procoagulant factors FVII, FIX and FX. In order to exert its anticoagulant effect, PC must first be activated to APC. This is achieved by the action of thrombin which cleaves the heavy chain, releasing a 12-residue (Gly158–Arg169) activation peptide and revealing the active site by the usual chymotrypsin-like mechanism. Thrombin activation of PC is slow in free solution but is markedly accelerated by specific EC receptors for both thrombin (TM) and PC (EPCR), which coordinate the assembly of a membrane complex for PC activation.

Once generated, APC interacts with PS bound to the phospholipid surface of activated platelets, enhancing APC's anticoagulant activity (see below) against FVa and FVIIIa. These procoagulant cofactors are inactivated by APC on the platelet surface by specific cleavage in their A domains, terminating the activity of FX-ase and prothrombinase by disrupting their binding sites for FIXa and FXa respectively; in the absence of PS,

this reaction is inefficient. It appears that APC inactivation of FVa is dominant *in vivo* compared with that of FVIIIa, as the most common form of familial thrombosis is found in individuals with FV Leiden, a mutation of Arg506 in FV, the most important APC cleavage site; however, no corresponding incidence of thrombosis has been associated with mutations at APC sites in the FVIII molecule.

PC is synthesized in the liver, and, being vitamin K dependent, is often low in the newborn. However, such deficiency is compensated for by the reduction in plasma of the vitamin K-dependent procoagulant factors (prothrombin, VII, IX and X), even though its substrates (FV and FVIII) are normal at birth (see Chapter 60). Disruption of the murine PC gene results in lethal perinatal consumptive coagulopathy, whereas in humans homozygous PC deficiency is associated with lethal purpura fulminans (in the absence of PC replacement therapy) and heterozygous individuals have a high risk of venous thrombosis. These observations underlie the crucial importance of the PC pathway for control of normal haemostasis, as well as other pathological states such as sepsis.

Thrombomodulin

Thrombomodulin (TM) is an integral transmembrane receptor found on ECs (in which it is probably synthesized) in virtually all body tissues. It appears to be absent in the brain vasculature and in hepatic sinusoids and lymph node venules. TM is essential for normal fetal development as shown by mouse knockout studies, although $TM^{+/-}$ heterozygous mice appear to be completely healthy.

The protein has an extracellular region composed of an N-terminal lectin-like or CLECT domain and six EGF modules, a transmembrane sequence and a small cytoplasmic region. TM forms a 1:1 complex with thrombin (via the protease's anion-binding exosite I and TM EGF modules 4–6), preventing binding of the protease to its various procoagulant substrates (fibrinogen, FV, FVIII, FXIII and platelet receptors involved in aggregation). TM also plays a part in binding of PC zymogen and, after formation of the TM–thrombin complex on the cell surface, there is a 20 000-fold increase in the rate of activation of PC, so that thrombin effectively becomes an anticoagulant. Binding of PC to TM is also enhanced by EPCR.

The TM–thrombin complex is short-lived, being endocytosed by ECs, where the thrombin is taken up and degraded by the lysosomes while TM recirculates to the cell membrane.

Endothelial protein C receptor

Endothelial protein C receptor (EPCR) was cloned in 1994 as a novel transmembrane receptor on ECs that was able to bind PC and promote its activation by the thrombin–TM complex. The extracellular portion of EPCR is related to the MHC class-I/CD1 proteins, however it lacks the α-3 domain found in the extracellular portion of most of the family: there is good evidence that the α-1 and -2 extracellular modules of EPCR interact with the

PC GLA module. EPCR may function by localizing the PC molecule to the EC surface, moving laterally on the cell surface to locate a thrombin–TM complex, then presenting the PC molecule optimally for thrombin cleavage to form APC.

The essential role of EPCR was demonstrated recently by targeted deletion of the murine EPCR gene, resulting in early fetal death with evidence of thrombosis at the maternal–fetal interface. Abrogation of EPCR function *in vitro* reduces the rate of PC activation by thrombin–TM, whereas blockage of EPCR action by a specific anti-EPCR monoclonal antibody in baboons given thrombin resulted in reduced APC levels amid evidence of excessive coagulopathy. Blockage of EPCR on challenge with *Escherichia coli* also led to worse outcomes in an animal model of sepsis, whereas administration of APC improved survival in experimental sepsis. Evidence supporting a role of the APC system has been provided *in vitro* by studies implicating the APC–EPCR complex in cleavage of PAR-1, leading to induction of protective genes against sepsis; however, most recently clinical trials of APC in patients with sepsis have shown no clear overall benefit.

Protein S and C4b-binding protein

Protein S is a single-chain vitamin K-dependent glycoprotein, although unlike the other vitamin K-dependent coagulation proteins it is not a serine protease, having two C-terminal LamG modules rather than a serine protease module, following an N-terminal GLA and four EGF modules rather than two. It is chiefly synthesized in the liver by ECs. About 40% of the PS in plasma is in the free form, whereas the remaining 60% is associated in a 1:1 complex with C4b-binding protein (C4bBP). Both forms bind strongly via the PS GLA module to negatively charged PLs exposed on the surface of activated platelets. Free PS (although having no strong inhibitory effect on FVa or FVIIIa itself) forms a Ca^{2+} ion-dependent complex with APC, helping to orient the APC active site above the PL surface and enhancing its anticoagulant activity against both proteins. However, C4bBP-bound PS does not enhance protein C function against FVa, suggesting a role for C4bBP in modulation of the APC pathway. Free thrombin cleaves PS N-terminal to the GLA domain, removing its ability to bind to both PL and protein C and thereby abolishing its protein C cofactor activity.

C4bBP is a large molecule containing seven α-chains (each of which binds one molecule of the C4b component of complement), and a single β-chain (to which one molecule of PS attaches). It is an acute-phase reactant, which can increase by up to fourfold in severe inflammatory states. It is likely that such raised levels would disturb the equilibrium between free and bound PS, and result in a fall in the free (biologically active) form, predisposing to a hypercoagulable state.

Many haemostatic factors change during pregnancy. Free PS falls during pregnancy (Table 47.3) and to a lesser extent in women receiving oestrogen supplements, but it is disputed whether this results from altered reactivity with C4bBP or if it contributes to hypercoagulability in pregnancy or during

Table 47.3 Haemostasis changes during pregnancy.

Platelet count	No consistent change but often falls
Platelet volume	Slight progressive increase
Platelet aggregation	Progressive enhancement
Bleeding time	Unchanged
Fibrinogen	Progressive rise up to 400% basal
Prothrombin	No consistent change
Factor V	No consistent change
Factor VII	Progressive rise up to 300% basal
Factor VIII	Progressive rise up to 200% basal
von Willebrand factor	Progressive rise up to 250% basal
Factor IX	Variable, no consistent change
Factor X	No consistent change
Factor XI	Progressive fall to 50% basal
Factor XII	No consistent change
Factor XIII	Progressive fall to 50% basal
Antithrombin	No consistent change
Heparin cofactor II	No consistent change
Tissue factor pathway inhibitor	Progressive rise
α_1-Antitrypsin	Progressive rise up to 300% basal
α_2-Macroglobulin	No consistent change
Protein C	No consistent change
Protein S	Progressive fall to 50% basal
C4b-binding protein	No consistent change
Protein C inhibitor	Progressive fall to 30% basal
Plasminogen	Progressive rise up to 300% basal
tPA	No consistent change
α_2-Antiplasmin	Progressive rise up to 300% basal
PAI-1	Progressive rise up to 300% basal
PAI-2	Progressive marked rise
TAFI	No change
FDP	Slight increase
Crosslinked FDP	Slight increase
Fibrinopeptide A	Progressive rise up to 300% basal
Euglobulin lysis time	Progressive prolongation up to 600% basal

oestrogen therapy. Total PS, like other vitamin K-dependent factors, is reduced in the newborn; levels as low as 20% of adult values can occur. However, this is compensated for by a marked reduction in C4bBP at birth (5–20% of adult levels), so that a relatively normal level of functional (free) PS is maintained.

Protein C inhibitors

As with other serine proteases, APC is subject to inhibition by serpins (the $T_{1/2}$ of APC in plasma is 15–20 min), including APC inhibitor or PCI, plasminogen activation inhibitor type-1 (PAI-1) and α_1-AT. The relative contributions of these *in vivo* is difficult to assess. PCI slowly but progressively blocks the action of APC (and to a much lesser extent, thrombin and FXa), in each case forming a 1:1 complex: in addition PCI action is enhanced 20-fold by heparin and more weakly by other GAGs, but the physiological significance of this is uncertain. Despite the name, disruption of the murine PCI gene leads not to coagulopathy but to infertility due to lack of inhibition of another protease target of the serpin, the sperm protein acrosin.

Fibrinolysis

It is widely acknowledged that the principal functions of the fibrinolytic system are to ensure that fibrin deposition in excess of that required to prevent blood loss from damaged vessels is either prevented or rapidly removed (i.e. that a localized pro-coagulant response is achieved without compromising blood circulation generally) and, following re-establishment of hae-mostasis, an existing fibrin mesh is later removed as part of the process of tissue remodelling. The system of pro- and anti-fibrinolytic factors that has evolved to meet these requirements is closely coupled to that which results in fibrin clot formation. Fibrinolysis is essentially a localized, surface-bound phenomenon, with most events being catalysed by the presence of cross-linked fibrin itself, i.e. 'fibrin orchestrates its own destruction'. For this reason, the assays of fibrinolytic factors carried out in the soluble phase, in particular in systemic blood, may be misleading and should be interpreted with great caution.

Components of the fibrinolytic system

These include plasminogen (PLG) and plasmin, several endogen-ous (tissue or plasma-derived) or exogenous (e.g. bacterial or venom derived) PLG activators, and a number of inhibitors of plasmin or of the PLG activators. Some basic features of the endogenous factors are shown in Table 47.2, and a simplified representation of their interaction in Figure 47.6. Both endogen-ous and exogenous fibrinolytic factors have been used clinically to treat venous and arterial thrombosis, with varying degrees of success (see Chapter 58).

Plasminogen and plasmin

PLG is a single-chain glycoprotein zymogen of the serine pro-tease plasmin, which carries out the enzymatic degradation of cross-linked fibrin. Besides its active site serine, plasmin con-tains five kringle modules, four of which have a lysine binding site, through which the molecule interacts with lysine residues in its substrates (e.g. fibrin), its activators (e.g. tissue PLG activator and urinary PLG activator) and its inhibitors (principally PLG activation inhibitor type 1). In its native form, it has a glutamic acid residue at its N-terminus and is known as Glu-PLG. Conversion of PLG to plasmin can proceed via two routes. Most PLG activators (see below) cleave the Arg561–Val562 bond to

form Glu-plasmin, a disulphide-linked two-chain molecule. The heavy chain is derived from the N-terminal region and bears the lysine binding sites, whereas the C-terminal light chain con-tains the serine active centre. Glu-plasmin, despite being a serine protease, is functionally ineffective as its lysine binding sites remain masked. It is converted autocatalytically to Lys-plasmin by N-terminal cleavage, chiefly between Lys76 and Lys77, which exposes the lysine binding sites and thus markedly enhances its interaction with fibrin.

Both Glu- and Lys-plasmin also attack the same Lys76–Lys77 bond in Glu-PLG to form the zymogen Lys-PLG. This binds to fibrin before activation to the protease and is thus brought into close proximity with the physiological PLG activators (which also bind to fibrin) that convert it to Lys-plasmin. As a con-sequence, the conversion of PLG to plasmin by tPA is enhanced by two to three orders of magnitude; this serves to localize the fibrinolytic response to the fibrin clot, where plasmin is to some extent protected from the effects of circulating antiplasmins, which (as indicated below) would otherwise neutralize plasmin extremely rapidly (< 50 ms). The fact that Lys-PLG is potentially a much more effective agent in fibrinolysis than Glu-PLG is reflected in its half-life, which is around 20 h compared with 50 h for the latter.

Action of plasmin on fibrin and fibrinogen

Plasmin can hydrolyse a variety of substrates including factors V and VIII, but its major physiological targets are fibrin and fibrinogen, which are split progressively into a heterogeneous mixture of small soluble peptides (plasmin attacks at least 50 cleavage sites in fibrinogen) known collectively as fibrin de-gradation products (FDPs). The first stage in the proteolysis of fibrinogen involves the removal of several small peptides (fragments A, B and C) from the C-terminus of the A α-chains, each involving cleavage after a lysine residue. This is rapidly followed by removal of the first 42 amino acids from the N-terminal end of the B β-chain (the Bβ1–42 fragment). The large residual portion, which is known as fragment X, and which still contains fibrinopeptide A, remains thrombin-clottable and will agglutinate some *Staphylococcus* spp. Assaying of the Bβ1–42 fragment released from fibrinogen by plasmin gives a sensitive index of fibrinogenolytic activity.

Asymmetrical digestion of all three pairs of chains of fibrin or fibrinogen then occurs with the release of the D fragment, in which the chains remained linked by disulphide bonds. The residue, known as fragment Y, is again attacked by plasmin, cleaving a second fragment D and leaving the disulphide-linked N-terminal ends of all six chains, which are referred to as frag-ment E. Fragments Y, D and E are not thrombin-clottable and do not agglutinate staphylococci. Their presence can be detected immunologically using an antibody-coated latex bead agglutina-tion assay, which provides a simple test for most FDPs, although carefully prepared serum must be used to prevent cross-reactivity of the antibody with fibrinogen in plasma. These assays detect both fibrin and FDPs indiscriminately.

Following thrombin generation and consequent activation of FXIII, inter- or intramolecular transamidation of the α- or γ-chains by FXIIIa occurs and then the action of plasmin yields characteristic D-dimer, D-dimer-E fragments and oligomers of fragments X and Y (collectively known as cross-linked FDP or XDP), in addition to X, Y, D and E. These XDPs can be detected very simply using monoclonal antibody-coated latex beads. Because the monoclonal antibodies to XDPs do not cross-react with fibrinogen, they can be detected directly in citrated plasma. The presence of D-dimers in blood samples can be used in a clinical algorithm that predicts the likelihood of the presence of venous thrombosis (see Chapter 55).

Furthermore, plasmin-induced cleavage of the N-terminal end of the β-chain of fibrin (the Bβ1–14 fibrinopeptide B fragment having been removed by thrombin) produces a β15–42 fragment, the detection of which indicates fibrin (as opposed to fibrinogen) degradation. Consequently, assays for the Bβ1–42 and β15–42 fragments used in combination, may be clinically useful by indicating whether fibrinogen or fibrin has been degraded, and thus whether fibrinolytic activity is primary or secondary to fibrin formation. However, clinically, FDP assays are used to detect disseminated intravascular coagulation, when mixed fibrin/fibrinogen degradation products appear in the circulation (see Chapter 51).

Plasminogen activators

Tissue plasminogen activator

Tissue plasminogen activator (tPA) is a serine protease secreted by ECs. It is not synthesized by the liver or kidney but is found in most extravascular body fluids, including saliva, milk, bile, cerebrospinal fluid and urine. Intravascular tPA is quickly cleared by the liver or inactivated by the fast-acting tPA inhibitor (see below), the half-life of tPA in plasma being approximately 2 min. The resting level of tPA in plasma is around 70 pmol/L, most of which is in an inactive complex with tPA inhibitors (see below).

Several physical and biochemical stimuli, including venous occlusion, strenuous exercise, thrombin, adrenaline and vasopressin or its analogues such as DDAVP (see Chapter 49) markedly increase the rate of tPA release, although its biological activity remains negligible until it becomes bound to fibrin, whereupon its affinity for and action upon PLG is greatly potentiated. The activity of tPA is further enhanced by plasmin itself, which cleaves tPA at Arg275–Ile276 into a two-chain molecule, whose binding sites are exposed, thus enabling it to form a complex with PLG and fibrinogen more readily. The ability of venous occlusion to stimulate tPA release from ECs forms the basis of a test of fibrinolytic activity known as the 'cuff test'.

Both single-chain tPA and the two-chain form possess very little serine protease activity until they bind to fibrin, whereupon tPA affinity for and activation of fibrin-bound PLG is increased at least 100-fold. The principal interactions involve binding between the second kringle module of tPA and lysine residues on the α- and β-chains of fibrin (and, in particular Lys157 on the α-chain of partly degraded fibrin). This association enhances the cleavage of the Arg561–Val562 bond in adjacent PLG molecules, forming active plasmin.

Urinary plasminogen activator

So called because it was first extracted from urine, urinary plasminogen activator (uPA) is synthesized chiefly by the tubules and collecting ducts in the kidney and by fibroblast-like cells in the gastrointestinal tract. It is a serine protease secreted as an inactive single-chain zymogen (pro-urokinase) that is cleaved by activators in plasma (including kallikrein and plasmin) at Lys158–Ile159 to produce active, two-chain uPA. The protease activity of uPA is associated with the heavy chain, which may dissociate from the light chain carrying the PLG binding site. The isolated heavy chains, which are also known as low-molecular-weight urokinase, are therefore poorer PLG activators than the two-chain form.

uPA cleaves the same Arg561–Val562 bond in PLG as tPA. Although uPA contains a kringle module, this does not impart high affinity for fibrin and it binds instead (via its EGF module) to its cell-associated receptor; thus it has been proposed that uPA may be preferentially involved in cellular events (such as differentiation and mitogenesis) rather than with dissolution of fibrin clots.

Exogenous plasminogen activators

These are derived from non-human sources, including animals (e.g. vampire bat saliva and some snake venoms) and certain plants and micro-organisms. The best known of these is streptokinase (SK), which is derived from some strains of β-haemolytic streptococci and which has for many years been used, with moderate success, as a fibrinolytic agent for the treatment of life-threatening thrombotic states (see Chapter 58). SK is a non-enzymatic polypeptide, which forms a stable 1:1 complex with PLG as a result of which the latter undergoes a conformational change, unmasking its serine-active centre. The 'plasmin' that is formed remains associated with SK but can convert free PLG to plasmin.

Inhibitors of fibrinolysis

The plasmin-generating potential of plasma is sufficient to degrade completely all of the fibrinogen in the body in a very short period of time. It is prevented from doing so by the PLG activator inhibitors or PAIs, most of which belong to the serpin family, and by a number of circulating inhibitors of plasmin itself (the antiplasmins).

Inhibitors of plasminogen activation

Plasminogen activator inhibitor type 1

Plasminogen activator inhibitor type 1 (PAI-1) is an important, fast-acting serpin inhibitor of tPA, uPA and, to a small extent, plasmin, which is secreted by ECs. It is also found in platelet α-granules. In plasma, it occurs in two forms: a functionally active 'free' form (that is stabilized by association with vitronectin) and as an inactive complex with tPA. Basal PAI-1 concentration in plasma is low at 0.5 nmol/L, of which at least 80% is in complex with tPA or uPA). It follows a diurnal rhythm, with an early morning peak that is around twice that in the late afternoon, and its activity is also increased by heparin. There is growing evidence that elevated levels of PAI-1 are associated with an increased incidence of venous and arterial thrombosis, and there is a suggested association between the early morning peak level of PAI-1 and a higher incidence of myocardial infarction at that time, the extent of this diurnal variation being associated with polymorphisms in the PAI-1 gene.

The three main profibrinolytic serine proteases (tPA, uPA and plasmin) all cleave the same bond (Arg346–Met347) in the reactive serpin loop of PAI-1, and are thus inhibited by formation of a 1:1 complex. PAI-1 binds non-covalently to fibrin, but, although it can then complex with and inhibit fibrin-bound tPA (with most of the complexes remaining bound to the fibrin), it does so less effectively than with free tPA. Soluble tPA–PAI-1 complexes are rapidly removed by the liver ($T_{1/2}$ = 4 min), as are uPA–PAI-1 complexes that have dissociated from fibrin.

Plasminogen activator inhibitor type 2

This serpin inhibitor of tPA is mainly produced by the placenta and may thus contribute to the inhibition of fibrinolysis which occurs during pregnancy. It is also synthesized in monocytes and epidermal cells, but is not usually found in the plasma of non-pregnant subjects. It is detectable in plasma from about the eighth week of pregnancy, rising to a peak at around 33 weeks and falling only slowly after delivery, the half-life being around 24 h. Paradoxically, levels are often low in pre-eclampsia due to placental insufficiency. The inhibitory action of plasminogen activator inhibitor type 2 (PAI-2) involves its Arg380–Thr381 residues and it is more effective against uPA than tPA, although for both the potency is at least 10-fold less than that of PAI-1.

Similarly, other protease inhibitors such as α_1-AT, C1-esterase inhibitor, α_2-AP (see below), α_2-MG and protease nexin 1 (one of a group of cell membrane-bound, heparin-potentiated serpins) also neutralize tPA, but at a rate that is probably too slow to be of physiological significance. α_2-MG is, however, thought to be the major inhibitor of the SK–PLG complex.

Inhibitors of plasmin

As they do with thrombin and tPA, a number of the broad-spectrum inhibitors contribute to neutralization of plasmin. By far the most potent plasmin inhibitor is the serpin α_2-AP, a single-chain glycoprotein synthesized by the liver, which has a half-life of about 60 h and shows considerable sequence identity with antithrombin and α1-antitrypsin. Its physiological importance is supported by the fact that a congenital deficiency (known as Miyasato disease) is associated with a clinically significant bleeding disorder due to uncontrolled fibrinolytic activity, and that levels are reduced in disseminated intravascular coagulation (DIC) and during thrombolytic therapy.

α_2-Antiplasmin

This serpin is the predominant plasmin inhibitor. It forms a stable 1:1 complex with plasmin, in which the protease is completely inactivated. The reaction appears to involve the cleavage by plasmin of a specific leucine–methionine bond in the inhibitor, exposing the reactive loop Arg364–Met365 peptide bond to the serine-active centre on the light chain of plasmin. Plasmin-modified α_2-AP can also bind to native Glu-PLG and to fibrin, the latter reaction being mediated by FXIIIa-mediated cross-linking. Thus, in addition to inactivating preformed plasmin, α_2-AP retards fibrinolysis by reducing PLG activation and by 'masking' the lysine binding sites through which plasmin(ogen) interacts with fibrin. However, these subsidiary mechanisms for inhibiting fibrinolysis are to some extent overcome by any Lys-plasmin(ogen) present, which has a higher affinity than Glu-PLG for fibrin, and is thus less susceptible to the action of α_2-AP.

In plasma (as opposed to on fibrin strands), although the concentration of PLG (~2 µmol/L) exceeds that of α_2-AP (~1 µmol/L), basal fibrinogenolytic activity is minimal because the tiny amounts of plasmin normally generated under physiological conditions are rapidly neutralized by the inhibitor. However, in certain pathological conditions (e.g. obstetric emergencies or snake bite) where extreme activation of fibrinolysis occurs, the latter may be swamped. Under these circumstances, other inhibitors, in particular α_2-MG and histidine-rich glycoprotein (HRG), may become clinically important. The action of α_2-MG on plasmin is similar to its effect on thrombin. Following the plasmin-induced cleavage of a specific arginine–leucine bond in the inhibitor, the latter forms a 1:1 complex with the light chain of plasmin. The serine-active centre of plasmin is not involved and the complex retains weak biological activity, albeit only briefly, until it is removed in the liver. HRG inhibits fibrinolysis by blocking the lysine binding sites of PLG, thus preventing its interaction with fibrinogen.

Lipoprotein A

The protein portion of lipoprotein A is termed apo(a). It is synthesized in the liver and circulates in plasma, has considerable structural homology with PLG, possessing serine protease and kringle modules. It can compete with PLG for binding sites on fibrin(ogen) or tPA, and may also increase PAI-1 expression, both actions potentially inhibiting fibrinolysis. That lipoprotein A has some clinical importance is indicated by the finding that raised levels are associated with an increased incidence of thrombosis.

Thrombin-activated fibrinolytic inhibitor

In the presence of thrombomodulin, thrombin activates carboxypeptidase B, also called TAFI, and TAFIa in turn inhibits fibrinolysis; this provides another link between coagulation and the fibrinolytic pathway. TAFI removes the C-terminal lysine residues formed by limited plasmin proteolysis of fibrin, removing the binding-sites for PLG and tPA. Thus the fibrin cofactor function in PLG activation is reduced, downregulating fibrinolysis. Murine TAFI knockout animals have defective wound repair and data from backcrossing against heterozygous PLG-deficient mice showed that TAFI modulates both fibrinolysis and cell migration *in vivo*.

Selected bibliography

Aird WC (2003) Endothelial cell heterogeneity. *Critical Care Medicine* 31: S221–S30.

Bajaj MS, Birktoft JJ, Steer SA *et al.* (2001) Structure and biology of tissue factor pathway inhibitor. *Thrombosis and Haemostasis* 86: 959–72.

Bouma BN, Meijers, JC (2003) Thrombin-activatable fibrinolysis inhibitor (TAFI, plasma procarboxypeptidase B, procarboxypeptidase R, procarboxypeptidase U). *Journal of Thrombosis and Haemostasis* 1: 1566–74.

Colman RW (1999) Biologic activities of the contact factors *in vivo* potentiation of hypotension, inflammation, and fibrinolysis, and inhibition of cell adhesion, angiogenesis and thrombosis. *Thrombosis and Haemostasis* 82: 1568–77.

Dahlback B, Villoutreix BO (2003) Molecular recognition in the protein C anticoagulant pathway. *Journal of Thrombosis and Haemostasis* 1: 1525–34.

Esmon CT (2000) The endothelial cell protein C receptor. *Thrombosis and Haemostasis* 83: 639–43.

Huntington JA (2003) Mechanisms of glycosaminoglycan activation of the serpins in hemostasis. *Journal of Thrombosis and Haemostasis* 1: 1535–49.

Morrissey JH (2001) Tissue factor: an enzyme cofactor and a true receptor. *Thrombosis and Haemostasis* 86: 66–74.

Ruggeri ZM (2003) Von Willebrand factor, platelets and endothelial cell interactions. *Journal of Thrombosis and Haemostasis* 1: 1335–42.

Saenko EL, Ananyeva NM, Tuddenham EG *et al.* (2002) Factor VIII – novel insights into form and function. *British Journal of Haematology* 119: 323–31.

Schmaier AH (2000) Plasma kallikrein/kinin system: a revised hypothesis for its activation and its physiologic contributions. *Current Opinion in Hematology* 7: 261–5.

Weiler H, Isermann BH (2003) Thrombomodulin. *Journal of Thrombosis and Haemostasis* 1: 1515–24.

CHAPTER 48

The vascular function of platelets

Stephen P Watson and Paul Harrison

Introduction

Platelets are small, anucleate cells that play a critical role in haemostasis and thrombosis. Platelets ordinarily circulate in the bloodstream in a quiescent state but undergo 'explosive' activation following damage to the vessel wall, leading to rapid formation of a platelet aggregate or vascular plug and occlusion of the site of damage. In simple terms, the more rapidly that platelets can achieve this, the lower the amount of blood that is lost. Platelets are therefore enriched in signalling proteins and surface receptors that enable them to achieve a rapid response, whereas major defects in platelet function or platelet number are associated with an excessive loss of blood. Significantly, disorders associated with vessel damage or a marked increase in platelet number or reactivity lead to thrombus formation in intact vessels and vascular occlusion and can cause arterial thrombotic disorders such as stroke and myocardial infarction, two of the major causes of morbidity and mortality in the Western world.

It is essential that platelets are able to achieve this interplay between quiescence and 'explosive' activation in high-pressure arteries and arterioles and in the low-pressure venous system. To achieve this interplay, platelet reactivity is strictly controlled by a series of positive feedback signals, when needed, or inhibitory signals that counter activation in intact vessels. Key factors that support rapid activation at sites of vessel injury include thrombogenic components of the subendothelial matrix, the release of positive feedback signals from the platelet, the generation of thrombin by the coagulation cascade and activation of platelet

integrins, enabling them to bind to their ligands within the bloodstream. Factors that oppose activation in the intact vasculature include the constitutive release of a gaseous transmitter, nitric oxide, from the endothelial cells that make up the vessel wall and the anti-platelet activity of the endothelial cell membrane itself.

The role of platelets in haemostasis is intimately linked to the coagulation cascade. Activated platelets provide a negatively charged lipid surface that supports the generation of thrombin, which reinforces platelet activation and other processes as discussed in the preceding chapter. The major platelet integrin $\alpha_{IIb}\beta_3$ (also known as GPIIb–IIIa) also forms a bridge between the platelet cytoskeleton and the polymerized fibrin that is generated by the coagulation cascade. Outside-in signals through $\alpha_{IIb}\beta_3$ promote 'clot retraction', which serves to strengthen the thrombus and thereby prevent embolization, even in the presence of the very high shear forces that exist within small arterioles and capillaries. Thus, the processes of platelet activation and coagulation are part of an intertwined biological programme that gives rise to the orchestrated formation of a haemostatic plug.

The role of platelets is also far wider than that of simply supporting thrombus formation. Platelet dense and α-granules are packed with a rich diversity of small molecules and proteins that play fundamental roles in other aspects of haemostasis and also in host defence. For example, platelets release agents that promote vessel constriction, vessel repair and leucocyte recruitment. In particular, there is growing recognition of the role of platelets in inflammatory responses in the vasculature. Platelets have been proposed to play a key role in the onset and progression of vascular inflammatory disorders such as atherosclerosis and vascular infections such as endocarditis.

It is important to consider why platelets release such a diverse library of biological molecules. The cell most closely linked to platelet function in invertebrates, the haemocyte, had a far wider spectrum of actions than the platelet, supporting both inflammatory processes and aggregatory events. In higher organisms, two distinct sets of nucleated cells can be found, namely thrombocytes and leucocytes, whose primary roles are to support haemostasis and inflammatory responses respectively. Mammals, on the other hand, are the only animal to have anucleated platelets. Given this route of evolution, it is not surprising that platelets have retained many of the features of inflammatory cells, especially given that they are the first and most abundant cell that accumulates at sites of vascular infection. The challenge is to establish the significance of the non-haemostatic molecules in platelets in health and disease.

Platelets are one of the major targets for the prevention and treatment of thrombotic and, to a lesser extent, vascular inflammatory disorders. Careful attention, however, should be given to the case as to whether a patient should receive anti-platelet therapy, and the nature that this therapy should take, bearing in mind that such treatment always carries a risk, albeit usually minor, of increased bleeding. For the majority of individuals receiving the major orally active anti-platelet drugs, aspirin or clopidogrel (a $P2Y_{12}$ ADP receptor antagonist), this risk is extremely low, unless otherwise contraindicated by conditions such as peptic ulcer. But, the risk is not zero. In this context, the growing tendency of otherwise healthy passengers to take aspirin as an anti-platelet therapy in long-haul flights should be viewed with concern. The major risk in long-haul flights is venous rather than arterial thrombosis through stasis in peripheral veins. Venous thrombosis is minimally inhibited by treatment with aspirin, whereas this treatment does lead to a small increase in risk of bleeding, which exceeds the benefit. Heparin would be a far better alternative therapy, but has the drawback that it is only delivered by injection.

The decision on whether a patient should receive anti-platelet therapy is based on the net sum of risk factors for arterial thrombosis, such as age, weight, lifestyle, cholesterol, smoking and family history, and the potential of excessive bleeding. It is now accepted that individuals who are considered to be at a medium to high risk of thrombosis should receive some form of anti-platelet therapy (unless otherwise contraindicated), usually low-dose aspirin or clopidogrel, in combination with other treatments such as statins or blood pressure-lowering drugs. Stronger inhibitors of platelet function, namely blockers of the major platelet integrin, $\alpha IIb\beta3$, are used only in acute situations of thrombotic risk such as unstable angina or during surgical procedures such as angioplasty and stenting because of problems arising from excessive blood loss.

The aim of this short review is to describe the features of platelets that enable them to perform their physiological roles in the vasculature. More extensive information on platelets can be found in two excellent books that cover all aspects of platelet function in health and disease (Gresele et al., 2002; Michelson, 2002).

Platelet structure and organelles

Platelets have several unique features that enable them to efficiently perform their primary function, namely the rapid formation of a vascular plug following vessel injury. Platelets are extremely small and discoid in shape, with dimensions of approximately 3.0 μm by 0.5 μm, and a mean volume of 7–11 fL. This shape and small size enables the platelets to be pushed to the edge of the vessel, placing them next to the endothelial cells and in the right place to respond to vascular damage. They are present at a high level in the human circulation, usually between 150 and 400×10^9 platelets/L. This level of expression appears to represent a considerable degree of redundancy, as individuals with platelet counts as low as 10×10^9 platelets/L tend to exhibit only occasional, major spontaneous bleeds, although they are at considerable risk of bleeding during major trauma.

The discoid shape of the platelet is formed by the platelet cytoskeleton, which consists of a spectrin-based membrane skeleton; circumferential bands of single microtubule that lies beneath the plasma membrane; and a rigid actin filament network that fills the cytoplasm of the cell. The disc shape is not essential for platelet function, as murine platelets that lack β_1-tubulin, the major component of the microtubules, are spherical and yet undergo normal aggregation and secretion responses. Much of the rigid structure and platelet strength results from the 2 million copies of actin per platelet, of which approximately 40% are assembled into actin polymers. These polymers connect with each other and with the cyosolic tail of the membrane glycoprotein (GP) Ibα via filamin in a lattice-like structure.

A further illustration of the way that platelets have evolved to form their specialized function is the absence of a nucleus, which is consistent with their short lifespan of 10 days and their acute role in haemostasis, which does not allow sufficient time for de novo protein synthesis. In other words, when incorporated into a thrombus and having undergone activation (including secretion), the role of the platelet is simply to serve as part of a haemostatic plug. It is now recognized that stimulated platelets possess a very limited capacity for protein synthesis, as the result of residual mRNA that has been carried over from their precursor cell, the megakaryocyte. However, there is little evidence to suggest that the capacity to make new proteins is of functional relevance. Nevertheless, this does provide the opportunity to perform a limited repertoire of molecular biological approaches, although the very low levels of mRNA, its poor quality and issues concerning contamination from other cells necessitates considerable caution and care in their application and interpretation. Despite this, several groups are using genomic approaches, often in combination with proteomics, to determine the composition of the platelet in order to gain new insights into platelet regulation. It is essential in these cases to also use other experimental approaches to confirm new findings and observations.

Platelets contain three main types of storage granules: dense, α-granules and lysosomes, each of which rapidly release their contents upon activation. α-Granules are the most numerous, with about 80 per platelet, and contain a rich diversity of proteins and membrane receptors that support many processes in haemostasis and in host defence. Dense granules contain high levels of small molecules that support platelet activation and mediate vasoconstriction. They are present at a 10-fold lower level that for α-granules, with approximately seven per platelet. Lysosomes also release their contents on activation, although the significance of this is unclear.

Platelets are particularly rich in signalling and cytoskeletal proteins. The high level of signalling proteins supports the rapid switch from quiescence to activation that occurs following damage to the vasculature. For example, it has been estimated that 0.1% of platelet protein is the tyrosine kinase Src, which is two to three orders of magnitude higher than in most other cells. The high cytoskeletal protein content is required for the dramatic change in morphology that occurs upon platelet activation and for securing the thrombus at the site of vascular damage, even in the presence of the very high shear forces. Platelets have a dense network of intracellular membranes known as the dense tubular system, which rapidly liberate their stores of the intracellular messenger Ca^{2+} in response to the generation of the second messenger, inositol 1,4,5-trisphosphate (IP3). Platelets also have a dense network of invaginations of the surface membrane known as the surface-connected canalicular system, which serves to increase the surface area of the plasma membrane and thereby provide more sites for release of intracellular granules and interactions with other surfaces. Platelets contain several mitochondria that generate energy during their short lifespan (Figure 48.1).

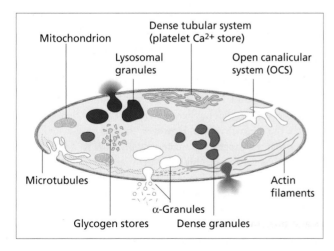

Figure 48.1 Platelet ultrastructure.

Murine platelets

The uniquely small size of the platelet and absence of a nucleus restricts the application of many of the modern day molecular and cell biology technologies in the dissection of platelet regulation and function. As a consequence, genetically modified mice are being increasingly used to provide a genetic means to address protein function within the platelet, although this approach must be adopted with the very real concern of species differences both with respect to role of specific proteins and vascular rheology. The former is illustrated by the nature of the receptors for one of the major platelet agonists, thrombin. Human platelets express PAR_1 and PAR_4 receptors, whereas murine platelets express PAR_3 and PAR_4. There are also fundamental issues in rheology between human and murine vessels, as well as in platelet size and number. These are likely to have significant implications for factors such as affinities of ligand for their receptors and receptor number. Nevertheless, despite these concerns, the fundamental aspects of the processes that govern platelet activation in the mouse appear to be shared with human, and the value of murine models in analysing haemostasis and thrombosis is immense.

Platelet formation

Platelets are formed from megakaryocytes in the bone marrow. Megakaryocytes are one of the largest cells in the body, reaching up to 50 μm in diameter, and are characterized by a large nuclear content. The nucleus of the megakaryocyte undergoes a process known as endomitosis that involves nuclear replication without cellular division, giving rise to DNA ploidy values that range from 4 n to 64 n. The reason why endomitosis occurs is not fully understood, but it may simply reflect the need to increase the DNA content to enable the cell to expand its protein synthesis capacity to generate 2000–3000 platelets per megakaryocyte. In addition, it allows cell growth and differentiation to occur without interruption by nuclear and cell divisions.

The differentiation of bone marrow progenitor cells along the megakaryocyte lineage is regulated by the cytokine thrombopoietin (TPO), which was first identified in 1995. TPO regulates megakaryocytopoiesis through a single receptor, c-Mpl, which signals through the JAK–STAT family of kinases and transcription factors respectively. The circulating free level of TPO is controlled by the number of circulating platelets and bone marrow megakaryocytes and their precursors through binding to c-Mpl on their surface. This provides a simple elegant means to tightly control the circulating platelet count. TPO binds to c-Mpl, signals and is then internalized and degraded. Thus, if the platelet count decreases, the free level of TPO rises and there is an increase in megakaryocytopoiesis. TPO offers great hope as a form of treatment for patients with thrombocytopenia and is the focus of a number of ongoing clinical trials.

Recent reviews provide further information on megakaryocytopoiesis and platelet formation (Caen *et al.*, 1999; Italiano and Shivdasani, 2003). The study of Italiano and colleagues (1999) shows a remarkable time-lapse video of platelet generation from megakaryocytes *in vitro*.

Platelet function

The responses associated with platelet activation and their roles in haemostasis are discussed below.

Adhesion

The initiating event following vascular damage is platelet adhesion to exposed subendothelial matrix proteins. The platelet glycoprotein (GP) receptors which mediate adhesion are dependent on the rate of shear. Under the intermediate to high shear conditions found in arterioles, this event is strictly dependent on von Willebrand factor (vWF) and its receptor, the GPIb–IX–V complex. However, at the lower rates of shear found in the venous circulation and in the static conditions frequently used for experimental purposes, adhesion can occur directly to other subendothelial matrix proteins such as collagen and fibrinogen, although vWF also supports this event in these vessels. In both cases, adhesion is strengthened considerably through activation of platelet surface integrins, which leads to an increase in affinity for their adhesive ligands.

Adhesion applies also to recruitment of circulating platelets into the thrombus. vWF, exposed on the surface of the growing thrombus, also plays a fundamental role in this process, most notably at the high rates of shear that exist within arterioles and in diseased vessels. The platelet-bound vWF that supports these events is derived from plasma and via secretion from platelet α-granules. Adhesion to the growing thrombus is supported by binding of fibrinogen to the integrin $\alpha_{IIb}\beta_3$, a process that is more correctly termed aggregation.

Shape change and spreading

Upon activation, platelets become spherical and extend pseudopodia to enable them to attach to other platelets and to the vessel wall. The transition to a sphere increases their optical density, a process that can be readily followed in a Born aggregometer and which precedes aggregation. This increase in optical density is termed 'shape change', although this term should be used with caution unless supported by scanning electron microscopy, as an increase in density can also be brought about in other ways. Shape change is mediated by phosphorylation of myosin light chains, either as a consequence of elevation in intracellular Ca^{2+} ions, which activate myosin light chain kinase, or through inhibition of myosin light chain phosphatase, which is regulated downstream of Rho kinase.

Adhesion of platelets to a reactive surface, such as collagen or fibrinogen, is also first characterized by transition from a discoid to a more rounded form, but this is then followed by formation of filopodia, which grow from the periphery of the cell, and lamellipodia, which fill in the area between adjacent filopodia. Stress fibres can also be seen with strong agonists. As the platelet flattens and spreads, granules and organelles are squeezed into the centre of the cell, resulting in a characteristic fried egg appearance. Granules are secreted from the centre of the cell directly into the surface open canalicular system before release into the surrounding medium. These dramatic changes in morphology are brought about by a powerful severing and reassembly of the actin cytoskeleton through regulation of a number of actin regulatory proteins.

Aggregation

Aggregation is used to describe cross-linking of platelets through binding of fibrinogen, or other bivalent or multivalent ligands such as vWF to the integrin $\alpha_{IIb}\beta_3$ on adjacent cells. In resting platelets, the integrin $\alpha_{IIb}\beta_3$ exists in a low-affinity conformation that is unable to bind to vWF or fibrinogen at the concentrations found within plasma (although it is able to bind to immobilized forms of these two ligands under static or low shear conditions). Upon platelet activation, so-termed 'inside-out' signals from other receptors cause $\alpha_{IIb}\beta_3$ to undergo a conformational change that increases its affinity for fibrinogen, vWF and other RGD (arginine–glycine–aspartate)-containing ligands, including fibronectin and CD40 ligand (CD40L). In turn, binding of fibrinogen and other ligands to $\alpha_{IIb}\beta_3$ promotes 'outside-in' signals that reinforce platelet activation. Although fibrinogen is considered to be the major ligand for $\alpha_{IIb}\beta_3$, thrombus formation has been reported, albeit after a considerable delay, in mice deficient in both fibrinogen and vWF, bringing other RGD-containing ligands into consideration as potential regulators of aggregation, most notably fibronectin, which is also present in plasma.

The events that give rise to activation of αIIbβ3 remain poorly understood. The integrin can be activated through elevation of Ca^{2+} and by activation of protein kinase C, rapIb and phosphatidylinositol 3-kinase (PI3 kinase), although it is unclear whether these act through separate pathways or target a common regulatory protein. Elevation of Ca^{2+} is required for rapid activation of $\alpha_{IIb}\beta_3$ and plays an essential role in thrombus formation *in vivo*. Increasing evidence implicates the cytoskeleton-binding protein talin in the regulation of $\alpha_{IIb}\beta_3$, although the molecular basis of its action remains to be determined.

A deficiency or mutation in $\alpha_{IIb}\beta_3$ gives rise to the bleeding disorder Glanzmann's thrombasthenia. Although extremely rare, there are upwards of 300 patients who have been identified with this condition. Surprisingly, given the severity of the effect on platelet aggregation, these patients have relatively few bleeding problems, provided that they avoid unnecessary risk of trauma and are moved to a hospitalized environment following injury.

Secretion

The three types of platelet granules contain a distinct set of contents that play varying roles in haemostasis. Platelet-dense granules contain the adenine nucleotides ADP and ATP, the amine 5-HT and Ca^{2+}. The rapid release of ADP from dense granules plays a major positive feedback role in promoting platelet activation (see below).

Platelet α-granules and their membranes contain a wide variety of proteins that support a multitude of processes during haemostasis (Table 48.1). Many of these proteins are made *de novo* in the megakaryocyte such as platelet factor 4 and vWF, whereas others are taken up from the plasma by receptor-mediated endocytosis (e.g. fibrinogen) or by fluid-phase pinocytosis.

Platelet α-granules contain the adhesive proteins fibrinogen and vWF. α-Granule release of vWF is critical for normal thrombus formation at intermediate and high rates of flow. The membrane of platelet α-granules also contains the major platelet integrin $α_{IIb}β_3$. Resting platelets express 50 000–80 000 molecules of $α_{IIb}β_3$ on their surface and this number increases to greater than 100 000 molecules following fusion of α-granules with the plasma membrane. This serves as a positive feedback signal and is also of clinical significance with respect to the action of many $α_{IIb}β_3$ agents, which are unable to block the

Table 48.1 Platelet α-granule constituents.

Physiological role	Constituent
Angiogenesis	VEGF-A, VEGF-C
Antibodies	IgG
Coagulation cascade	FV, FVIII
Endothelial cell activation	TGF-β
Fibrinolysis	Plasminogen, PAI-1, $α_2$-antiplasmin
Growth factors	PDGF; FGF; HGF; IGF-1; EGF
Leucocyte recruitment	Chemokines: platelet factor 4, RANTES; β-thromboglobulin, ENA-78
Matrix breakdown	Hydrolytic enzymes
Membrane proteins	$α_{IIb}β_3$, P-selectin
Miscellaneous	Amyloid β-protein precursor
Platelet activation	Gas6
Proteases	Protease nexin II
Thrombus formation	Fibrinogen, fibronectin, vWF
Unknown	Thrombospondin

Examples of platelet α-granule constituents and their physiological roles are shown. Several other molecules have also been reported to be present in α-granules and to be released upon activation.

integrin on α-granules until expressed on the cell surface. P-selectin is also found in α-granule membranes. P-selectin helps to stabilize the thrombus through capture of tissue factor-rich microparticles that support the coagulation cascade, and mediates leucocyte recruitment through P-selectin glycoprotein ligand-1 (PSGL-1) on the leucocyte surface. P-selectin is frequently used to monitor platelet α-granule secretion by flow cytometry using a labelled antibody.

Platelet α-granules contain a number of coagulation factors, including factor V, factor VIII, protein S and PAI-1, which play key roles in the coagulation process as discussed in the previous chapter. α-Granules also contain chemokines, such as platelet factor 4, β-thromboglobulin, ENA-78 and RANTES, which attract circulating leucocytes. They also contain platelet-derived growth factor (PDGF), which supports smooth muscle proliferation and vascular endothelial growth factor (VEGF) A and C, which support tumour angiogenesis. The role of many of the other platelet α-granule contents, such as thrombospondin-1, in thrombus formation is unclear.

Recently, a component of platelet α-granules, the vitamin K-dependent protein, Gas6, has been proposed to play a major role in supporting platelet aggregation, through activation of its surface receptors, Axl, Mer and Sky. Gas6 is of particular interest in the context of development of novel antithrombotics, as blocking antibodies prevent thrombus growth but do not have a significant effect on bleeding. The molecular basis of this action and its significance remain to be established.

Lysosomes are part of the host defence mechanism against invading organisms. They contain a variety of hydrolytic enzymes that target invading organisms and also breakdown extracellular matrix proteins. Lysosomes remove phagocytosed particulate matter and bacteria.

A deficiency in dense or α-granules is the basis of a heterogeneous group of secretory disorders that are associated with excessive bleeding. These disorders include grey platelet syndrome, which is associated with α-granule storage pool deficiency, and Hermansky–Pudlak and Chédiak–Higashi syndromes, which are associated with dense granule storage pool deficiency. The last two disorders often have characteristic pigment defects and deficiencies in lysosomes in other cells.

Phospholipase A$_2$

TxA_2 is one of the two major platelet positive feedback agonists. TxA_2 is generated *de novo* upon activation of cytosolic PLA_2, which liberates arachidonic acid from the 2-position of membrane phospholipids. The term *cytosolic PLA$_2$* is used to distinguish the phospholipase from the structurally distinct class of soluble PLA_2s, which mediate their actions through an extracellular action. Arachidonic acid is metabolized by cyclo-oxygenase (COX-1) and lipoxygenase enzymes to endoperoxides/thromboxanes and leukotrienes respectively. Endoperoxides and TxA_2 regulate platelets through activation of thromboxane (or TP) receptors. Leukotrienes are not thought to play a major role in regulating platelets, with their primary actions being mediated on other vascular cells.

Cytosolic PLA_2 is regulated by translocation to platelet membranes founding response to elevation of cytosolic Ca^{2+}. PLA_2 is constitutively active and so translocation is sufficient to bring about lipid hydrolysis. In addition, the activity of PLA_2 is marginally increased upon phosphorylation by mitogen-activated protein kinases, although in the absence of translocation, this does not lead to activation as the lipase is unable to access its substrates.

Procoagulant activity

A critical function of platelet activation is to provide a negatively charged phospholipid surface for the assembly of two multiprotein complexes that form a vital part of the coagulation cascade, namely the tenase and prothrombinase complexes as discussed in Chapter 46. A complex of FIXa–FVIIIa on the negatively charged lipid surface converts factor X to factor Xa (tenase complex) which, in turn, forms a complex with FVa on the same surface to efficiently convert prothrombin to thrombin (prothrombinase complex). In this way, a large amount of thrombin is generated in the vicinity of the platelet surface to convert fibrinogen to fibrin and to further enhance platelet activation. The newly generated thrombin is also able to diffuse to the surface of intact endothelial cells where it binds to thrombomodulin and activates protein C, which itself is bound to the endothelial surface via endothelial cell protein C receptor (EPCR). Once generated, activated protein C (APC) interacts with phosphatidylserine on the surface of activated platelets to prevent assembly of the tenase and prothrombinase complexes through cleavage of FVa and FVIIIa (see Chapter 46). Thus, the negatively charged platelet surface also supports the protein C pathway that serves to limit the coagulation cascade. The 'compartmentalization' of reactions to lipid surfaces in this way ensures that thrombin is generated at the place that it is required during haemostasis.

The formation of the negatively charged lipid surface on activated platelets is commonly described as aminophospholipid exposure or procoagulant activity. It is formed by the movement of phosphatidylserine from the inner to the outer leaflet of the platelet membrane. The movement of phosphatidylserine can be monitored experimentally by flow cytometry or fluorescent microscopy through the binding of annexin V, factor V or factor VIII, using either fluorescently labelled secondary antibodies or by direct labelling with a fluorescent group such as fluorescein isothiocyanate (FITC).

The molecular basis of the procoagulant response, including the identity of the enzyme (or 'flipase') that promotes the translocation of phosphatidylserine across the membrane, is not established. It is recognized, however, that the response is elicited only by powerful platelet agonists and that it requires Ca^{2+} entry across the plasma membrane. Platelets from four patients have been reported to be unable to undergo a procoagulant response. This clinical condition has been termed Scott syndrome and is associated with significant bleeding, although, if managed, does not appear to have an effect on life expectancy.

Platelet-derived microparticles

Platelet-derived microparticles are generated during platelet activation and are usually seen together with an increase in procoagulant activity. The formation of platelet microparticles also requires Ca^{2+} entry and is readily seen in response to stimulation by Ca^{2+} ionophore but requires high agonist concentrations and favourable conditions for them to be formed upon receptor activation. The functional role of platelet-derived microparticles is unclear, although they have been proposed to play a number of critical roles in supporting thrombus formation by serving as a surface for the tenase and prothrombinase complexes. They may also play a role in promoting thrombotic disease.

The study of platelet-derived and other types of circulating microparticles is a highly active area of research. Recent evidence suggests that activated platelets and microparticles can interact with monocytes via a P selectin-dependent pathway to induce tissue factor synthesis and further release of monocyte-derived microparticles. It has been proposed that these tissue factor-positive microparticles provide a source of circulating tissue factor, which is incorporated into growing thrombi, reinforcing thrombus formation through activation of the coagulation cascade and leading to formation of fibrin. This therefore explains the ability of P-selectin and its receptor, PSGL-1, to stabilize thrombus formation.

Clot retraction

It has been known for more than two centuries that blood clots retract over a time course of minutes to hours, a process that is termed clot retraction. This event helps platelet-rich thrombi to withstand the high shear forces found in small arterioles and in other vessels. Platelets are the force-generating components of clot retraction, with the integrin $\alpha_{IIb}\beta_3$ playing a fundamental role by linking the cytoplasmic actin filaments to surface-bound fibrin polymers. In addition, the integrin generates the intracellular signals that underlie clot retraction through activation of tyrosine kinases and PI3 kinase. This cascade leads to the assembly of an intracellular complex of a number of actin-binding proteins including talin, filamin, zyxin, α-actinin, moeisin and vinculin, which interacts with the integrin tail and with actin. Once tethered in this way, platelet myosin serves as a motor to drive the process of clot retraction.

Clot retraction can be readily measured in thrombin-stimulated platelet-rich plasma by taking aliquots of the volume of plasma over time after the addition of thrombin. Thrombin rapidly generates a blood clot that fills an aggregometer tube but which gradually reduces to almost 20% of its original volume (i.e. clot retraction) over a course of 60 min.

Late events in platelet aggregation/thrombus formation

There is increasing evidence that stabilization of the platelet plug requires delayed intracellular signals from receptors that function only when platelets make persistent contact with other platelets. This process has been termed as the 'late-events of platelet activation' or the perpetuation phase of activation. Several recently discovered platelet receptors have been implicated in these 'late-events' (as discussed in Other platelet ligands and their receptors, below).

Thrombus formation in arterioles

The molecular basis of thrombus formation *in vivo* in vascular beds at intermediate and high rates of shear is made up of a number of phases, namely tethering, adhesion, thrombus formation and thrombus stabilization (Figure 48.2). Subendothelial collagen plays a key role in this set of events through direct and indirect mechanisms. Collagen binds plasma vWF, which mediates platelet tethering at intermediate and high rates of flow because of its fast on-rate of association to platelet GPIb–IX–V. The fast off-rate of this interaction, however, and the weak nature of the signals from GPIb–IX–V (see below), means that other subendothelial proteins and soluble platelet agonists are

required to generate the signals required for integrin activation and stable adhesion. Collagen is the most thrombogenic component of the subendothelial matrix, mediating activation via the immunoglobulin receptor, GPVI. Signals from GPVI lead to activation of platelet integrins, including $\alpha_{IIb}\beta_3$ and $\alpha_2\beta_1$ (also known as GPIa–IIa), which support stable adhesion. Adhesion of platelets to vWF and collagen also has the effect of reinforcing platelet activation as a result of a net increase in binding to GPVI (the so-termed, two-site, two-state model of platelet–collagen interaction). Signals from GPVI, as well as from integrins $\alpha_{IIb}\beta_3$ and $\alpha2\beta1$, stimulate platelet spreading, thereby strengthening attachment to the exposed subendothelium and increasing the surface area for thrombus growth. The intracellular signals also lead to the release of the positive feedback mediators ADP and TxA_2, which, along with GPIb–IX–V and $\alpha_{IIb}\beta_3$, help to recruit additional circulating platelets into the developing thrombus via tethering and aggregation. Signals from $\alpha_{IIb}\beta_3$ and other receptors serve to stabilize thrombus formation through processes such as clot retraction.

The glycoproteins GPIb–IX–V and $\alpha_{IIb}\beta_3$ are essential for thrombus formation, whereas other receptors can be by-passed to varying extents because of their overlapping roles. In this context, the relatively mild bleeding disorder that has been reported in genetically modified mice and human patients who are deficient in GPVI is particularly interesting, and gives rise to speculation that the subendothelium may express other adhesive proteins that are able to promote powerful platelet activation. In this context, it is interesting to speculate whether the events that underlie thrombus formation vary with the composition of the

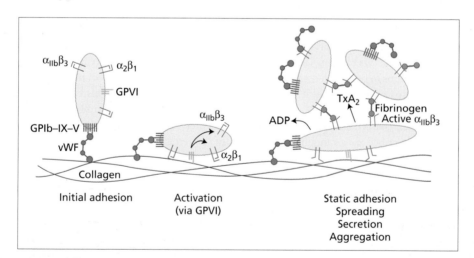

Figure 48.2 Thrombus formation at medium and high rates of shear. Platelets are initially captured (tethered) by vWF bound to immobilized collagen. Collagen activates platelets via GPVI leading to an increase in affinity of the integrins $\alpha_{IIb}\beta_3$ and $\alpha_2\beta_1$ for vWF/fibrinogen and collagen respectively. This mediates stable adhesion and potentiates activation through further activation of

GPVI and also release of ADP and TxA_2. The formation of a procoagulant surface also supports formation of thrombin. vWF and fibrinogen, in combination with ADP, TxA_2 and thrombin, mediate thrombus formation (aggregation) and stabilization (clot retraction). Platelet spreading also serves to stabilize the thrombus on the subendothelium.

subendothelial matrix. Connective tissue contains many other proteins whose role on platelets has been poorly characterized, and which may play a role in supporting thrombus formation. This is illustrated by recent reports of platelet activation by decorin, which signals via the integrin $\alpha_2\beta_1$.

Stimulatory agonists and their receptors

Platelets express surface receptors for a remarkable number and wide diversity of extracellular ligands, including adhesive ligands, amines, chemokines, cytokines, lipids, nucleotides, proteases and transmembrane proteins (Table 48.2). It is important therefore to determine which of these have significant roles in regulating haemostasis and thrombosis in vivo. There is a considerable redundancy between many of these stimuli and several others also induce only weak activation, questioning their functional relevance. This section focuses on those receptors and their ligands that are recognized to play important roles in platelet regulation. Many of these receptors are important targets for anti-thrombotic drugs.

ADP and ATP

ADP was first recognized as a major regulator of platelets in the early 1960s but it is only within the last few years that its importance as a positive feedback agonist has been fully established. ADP, along with ATP, is stored in dense granules and released rapidly upon platelet activation. ADP supports platelet activation through two G-protein-coupled, seven transmembrane receptors, $P2Y_1$ and $P2Y_{12}$. ATP activates the structurally distinct, $P2X_1$ receptor, which contains an intrinsic ion channel.

The $P2Y_{12}$ receptor is coupled to the G_i family of G-proteins, which, among other actions, inhibit adenylyl cyclase and activate PI3 kinase. On its own, the $P2Y_{12}$ receptor has a minimal effect on platelet activity, but it undergoes a remarkable synergy with G_q-coupled and tyrosine kinase-linked receptors to induce powerful platelet activation. Thus, the major feature of ADP's positive-feedback action is its ability to synergize with signals from other receptors, a fact that had been overlooked until the late 1990s. Significantly, the $P2Y_{12}$ receptor is unique in the context that it is the only receptor that activates the G_i family of G-proteins at sites of damage to the vasculature. The α_{2A}-adrenoceptor also activates G_i family proteins, but this is not thought to play a role in normal haemostasis, although this may be of relevance under conditions that lead to release of adrenaline. This unique role of the $P2Y_{12}$ receptor explains why it is presently considered to be the most attractive target for development of novel anti-thrombotic agents. The $P2Y_{12}$ receptor antagonist, clopidogrel, is a billion dollar-selling drug in the USA and sales are increasing rapidly. There is intense activity within the pharmaceutical sector towards development of further $P2Y_{12}$ receptor antagonists.

The $P2Y_1$ receptor is coupled to the G_q and $G_{12/13}$ families of G-proteins, which regulate PLCβ and rho kinase respectively. The $P2Y_1$ receptor is expressed at a very low level, in the order of 150 sites per platelet, and undergoes rapid desensitization during platelet preparation unless reagents such as apyrase are included used to prevent accumulation of adenine nucleotides. These two features have meant that its role has also been underestimated until the last few years. There is now a growing recognition of the role of the $P2Y_1$ receptor in the *early* events that initiate haemostasis and thrombosis through studies in $P2Y_1$-deficient mice and use of $P2Y_1$ receptor antagonists. Of particular importance is the ability of the $P2Y_1$ receptor to synergize with the $P2Y_{12}$ receptor in promoting platelet activation. The $P2Y_1$ receptor is also a potential target for novel antithrombotics, although this is unlikely to be realized because of its expression on other tissues. At later times of stimulation, the activation of G_q and $G_{12/13}$ families of G-proteins by thrombin and TxA_2 masks the role of the $P2Y_1$ receptor.

Increasing evidence suggests that the significance of the $P2X_1$ receptor has also been overlooked. As for the $P2Y_1$ receptor, it is expressed at a low level and undergoes rapid desensitization. Further, it has only recently been recognized to be a receptor for ATP, rather than for ADP. The particular significance of the $P2X_1$ receptor in mediating platelet activation is its ability to promote entry of Ca^{2+} through its intrinsic channel, a process that takes place far more rapidly than IP3-mediated Ca^{2+} release. This generates very high concentrations of Ca^{2+} close to the plasma membrane, enabling it to regulate distinct intracellular events.

TxA_2

TxA_2, along with ADP, is a major positive feedback mediator. TxA_2 regulates platelet activation through the G_q- and $G_{12/13}$-coupled thromboxane (TP) receptor. TxA_2 is rapidly metabolized to the inactive metabolite TxB_2, which prevents its use in functional studies, where the stable mimetic, U46619, is preferred. Additionally, TxB_2 is used to monitor activation of this pathway in platelets by radioimmunoassay. The TP receptor activates platelets through a pathway that is dependent on the $P2Y_{12}$ receptor, further emphasizing the importance of the latter in regulating platelet function.

The clinical importance of the TxA_2 pathway in platelet activation is illustrated by the antithrombotic action of aspirin, which inhibits platelet cyclo-oxygenase. The irreversible nature of aspirin, in combination with the inability of platelets to synthesize significant levels of new proteins, means that the effective therapeutic concentration of aspirin is considerably lower than that required to target cyclo-oxygenase in other cells. Large-scale clinical trials have shown that aspirin reduces the mortality of myocardial infarction by approximately 25% and the number of vascular events in individuals at risk by about one-third. The clinical effectiveness of low-dose aspirin is similar to that of the $P2Y_{12}$ receptor antagonist, clopidogrel, making it the drug of

Agonist	Receptor	Effect and physiological role
Adhesion molecules		
Collagen	GPVI	Major signalling receptor for collagen
	$\alpha_2\beta_1$	Supports adhesion by collagen
Fibrinogen	$\alpha_{IIb}\beta_3$	Aggregation, spreading and clot retraction
Fibronectin	$\alpha_5\beta_1$, $\alpha_{IIb}\beta_3$	$\alpha_5\beta_1$ mediates adhesion
Laminin	$\alpha_6\beta_1$	Adhesion
von Willebrand factor	GPIb–IX–V, $\alpha_{IIb}\beta_3$	Platelet tethering (see also fibrinogen)
Amines		
Adrenaline	α_2 and β_2	
5-HT	5-HT_{2A}	Mediates vasoconstriction
Chemokines		
SDF-1	$CXCR_4$	Maturation of megakaryocytes
MDC and TARC	CCR_4	Platelet–monocyte interactions?
RANTES	CCR_1 and CCR_3	
Cytokines		
TPO	c-Mpl	Maturation of megakaryocytes
Hormones		
Insulin		
Leptin		
PDGF		
Immune complexes		
Fc portion of antibodies	FcγRIIA	Immune-based platelet activation
Lipids		
Lysophospholipids		
PAF	PAF	
Prostacyclin	IP	Endothelium-mediated inhibition
Sphingosine 1-phosphate		
Thromboxanes	TP	Major positive feedback agonist
Nucleotides		
Adenosine	A_{2A}	
ADP	$P2Y_1$	Early role in platelet activation
	$P2Y_{12}$	Major positive feedback receptor
ATP	$P2X_1$	Possible early role in platelet activation
Peptides		
Endothelin	ET	
Vasopressin	VP_1	
Proteases		
Thrombin	PAR_1, PAR_4	Coagulation-dependent platelet activation
Surface molecules		
CD40 ligand	CD40 and $\alpha_{IIb}\beta_3$	
Tyrosine kinase receptors		
Angiopoietin 1 and 2	Tie-1	
EphrinB1	EphA4 and EphB1	Late events in platelet activation?
Vitamin K-dependent		
Gas6	Sky, Axl and Mer	Supports platelet activation?

Table 48.2 Platelet agonists and their surface receptors.

Platelets express a remarkable number and variety of receptors for a wide range of ligands. For many of these receptor–ligand combinations, however, the effect on platelet activation is weak and of uncertain significance. Moreover, several of the examples shown have only been the subject of a handful of publications and require independent confirmation. Examples of these include functional roles for Gas6, insulin, PDGF, ephrins and Eph kinases and leptin. Shear forces of 1500 s^{-1} and above should also be considered to be an agonist, although the basis of this is not known.

choice unless otherwise contraindicated (e.g. peptic ulcer) on consideration of cost. Aspirin and clopidogrel are sometimes used in combination, although this carries a major risk of excessive bleeding, most notably in surgery.

Thrombin

The serine protease thrombin is the major product of the coagulation cascade (see Chapter 46). Thrombin regulates several key pathways in haemostasis, including fibrin formation, the protein C pathway and platelet activation. These diverse actions of thrombin are regulated by a series of binding proteins that target the protease to the appropriate region of the haemostatic cascade.

Thrombin activates human platelets through the proteolytic cleavage of the G-protein-coupled, seven transmembrane receptors, PAR_1 and PAR_4. Thrombin releases a short peptide from the N-terminal region of each receptor, thereby exposing a new N-terminal sequence that functions as a tethered ligand by binding to the receptor and promoting activation. Synthetic peptides corresponding to this newly exposed sequence induce receptor activation in the absence of receptor cleavage. These thrombin receptor-activating-peptides (TRAPs) are powerful tools to study the roles of PAR_1 and PAR_4 receptors. In human platelets, PAR_1 mediates rapid activation in response to low concentrations of thrombin, whereas PAR_4 is activated by higher concentrations of the protease. PAR_1 and PAR_4 receptors induce activation through G_q- and $G_{12/13}$-families of G-proteins, both of which synergize with the $P2Y_{12}$ ADP receptor.

Platelets express a third, high-affinity binding site for thrombin on the GPIbα subunit of the GPIb–IX–V. Binding of thrombin to GPIbα positions the protease in the vicinity of the PAR_1 and PAR_4 receptors, facilitating their activation. In addition, binding of thrombin to GPIbα has been proposed to generate intracellular signals through a pathway that requires cleavage of GPV. The ability of this pathway to activate platelet is controversial because it is inconsistent with reports of abolition of platelet activation by thrombin in mice deficient in PAR_4 receptors.

Collagen

Collagen is a major component of the subendothelial matrix and is recognized as one of the *initial* ligands that mediate platelet adhesion and platelet activation following damage to the vasculature. Nine forms of collagen have been described within the vessel wall, with types I and III being the predominant ones in the deeper layers of the vessel wall, whereas type VI predominate in more superficial layers. All vascular collagens bind to the receptors GPVI and $\alpha_2\beta_1$. In addition, there are reports of the presence of additional receptors for collagen on platelets, although these need to be confirmed and their role determined.

Collagen is composed of three helical chains, which interact together to form a superhelical structure that is interrupted by non-helical regions. The presence of glycine (G) at every third position is essential to form the helical structure. In addition, the amino acids proline (P) and hydroxyproline (O) make up approximately 10% of the helical backbone. Synthetic collagen peptides based on these three amino acids have been shown to bind selectively to GPVI or integrin $\alpha_2\beta_1$. Peptides that are specific to GPVI have a backbone of GPO residues, whereas peptides that bind to $\alpha_2\beta_1$ have a backbone of GPP residues interspersed with at least one or more GER motifs, usually GFOGER. The GER sequence confers binding to $\alpha_2\beta_1$, whereas GPP is unable to bind to $\alpha_2\beta_1$ (or GPVI) but is required to present GER in a helical conformation. Many snake toxins also target GPVI, such as C-type lectin, convulxin, which was instrumental in the original cloning of the receptor. Convulxin, a tetramer composed of distinct α- and β-subunits, induces powerful activation of GPVI through cross-linking.

Collagen stimulates platelet activation through the immunoglobulin receptor, GPVI, which is associated with the Fc receptor (FcR) γ-chain. The GPVI–FcR γ-chain complex signals through a tyrosine kinase-based pathway that shares many of the features used by antigen (e.g. TCR) and Fc receptors. All of these receptor complexes contain one or more immunoreceptor tyrosine-based activation motif (ITAMs) in their cytosolic tails. In the case of GPVI receptor complex, the FcR γ-chain is a disulphide-linked homodimer, with each chain possessing one ITAM sequence. GPVI signals through tyrosine phosphorylation of the FcR γ-chain ITAM by the Src family kinases, Fyn and Lyn. This leads to recruitment of Syk through its SH2 domains, which bind to the ITAM phosphotyrosines. Syk regulates a downstream signalling cascade that is composed of a series of adapter proteins and effector enzymes. Adapters form an intracellular scaffold that is now recognized to be critical in the regulation of effector proteins such as PLCγ2, PI3 kinase and Tec family tyrosine kinases. A general and more detailed scheme of signalling by GPVI is shown in Figure 48.3a and b. The general mechanism of inhibition by PECAM-1 (see PECAM-1 (CD31), below) and comparison with thrombin signalling are shown in Figure 48.3a and b respectively.

GPVI can be considered to be unique among platelet glycoprotein receptors in that it is the only one that signals through an ITAM pathway at sites of damage to the vasculature. The low-affinity platelet immune receptor, FcγRIIA, also signals through this pathway but is not thought to play a role in haemostasis. GPVI synergizes with the $P2Y_{12}$ receptor to mediate platelet activation.

The primary role of the second major collagen receptor, $\alpha_2\beta_1$, is to promote platelet adhesion, although it is also able to support limited platelet activation. The physiological significance of $\alpha_2\beta_1$, in supporting thrombus formation *in vivo*, however, remains unclear because both of these roles are redundant with those of other platelet integrins, most notably $\alpha_{IIb}\beta_3$. Interestingly, polymorphisms in the α_2 subunit can lead to a three- to fivefold increase in expression. A weak correlation has been found between polymorphic forms that increase expression and thrombotic disease, most notably in younger individuals. These observations

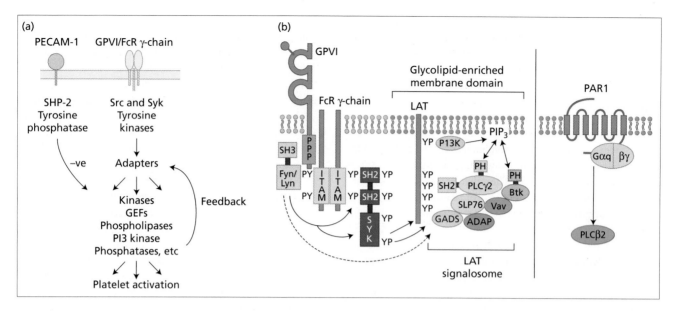

Figure 48.3 GPVI signalling. (a) The signalling events mediated through GPVI and their regulation by PECAM-1 are shown. GPVI signalling is mediated by sequential activation of Src and Syk tyrosines. Syk regulates a number of adapter proteins that form a signalling scaffold for the regulation of effector enzymes including phospholipase (e.g. PLCγ2), kinases (e.g. a third family of tyrosine kinases, known as the Tec family which includes Btk) and GTP exchange factors (GEFs), which regulate small G-proteins. The GPVI signalling cascade is selectively inhibited by activation of another member of the superimmunoglobulin family of proteins, PECAM-1, through recruitment of the tyrosine phosphatase,

SHP-2. (b) The regulation of PLCγ2 and PLCβ2 by the collagen receptor GPVI and the thrombin receptor PAR$_1$ respectively. The binding of the following domains is shown: SH3 domains bind to proline rich sequences, SH2 domains bind to phosphotyrosine groups and PH domains to the 3-phosphorylated lipid, PIP3. The following proteins are adapters: ADAP, GADS, LAT and SLP-76. Vav is a GTP exchange factor (GEF); Fyn and Lyn are Src family tyrosine kinases; Syk and Btk are members of two different families of tyrosine kinases. Signalling by GPVI and by PAR$_1$ takes place in cholesterol-rich regions of the membrane known as Gems or lipid rafts.

suggest that the integrin is a target for antithrombotics, although this is unlikely to be realized because of side-effects resulting from expression on other cells.

A handful of patients have been described with low or undetectable levels of GPVI. Surprisingly, these patients have only a mild bleeding disorder, suggesting that the role of the glycoprotein can be bypassed by other signalling receptors. The three patients that have been described with deficiency of $\alpha_2\beta_1$ also have other vascular complications that hamper the drawing of conclusions on the *in vivo* significance of the integrin.

Fibrinogen

Plasma fibrinogen is widely recognized as a major mediator of platelet aggregation and is vital for fibrin formation. Fibrinogen is composed of three, disulphide-linked chains in a symmetrical structure as discussed in Chapter 46. The two heads of fibrinogen cross-link adjacent, activated platelets by binding to the activated (or high-affinity) form of the major platelet integrin, $\alpha_{IIb}\beta_3$. Fibrinogen is the precursor of the insoluble fibrin polymer that is formed following proteolytic cleavage by thrombin.

Thus, fibrinogen plays a central role in the coagulation cascade and in platelet activation.

Studies on platelets *in vitro* have provided abundant evidence for the critical role of fibrinogen in supporting aggregation. However, several other ligands also bind to $\alpha_{IIb}\beta_3$, including the adhesive proteins vWF, fibronectin and vitronectin, and CD40L which is expressed and released from the platelet surface during activation. All of these ligands support platelet aggregation under appropriate circumstances, although their precise role in supporting haemostasis and thrombosis is unclear. Fibrinogen is also able to support platelet adhesion at low rates of shear, even in the absence of a conformational change in the integrin $\alpha_{IIb}\beta_3$. However, at higher rates of shear, it requires vWF to promote platelet tethering before it can support adhesion as discussed above.

Binding of fibrinogen and other ligands to $\alpha_{IIb}\beta_3$ is promoted by inside-out signals from various G-protein-coupled and tyrosine kinase-linked receptors as a result of a conformational change in the integrin. The binding of ligands to $\alpha_{IIb}\beta_3$, in turn, generates outside-in signals that stimulate spreading and support other responses through a synergistic interaction with the P2Y$_{12}$ ADP receptor. Thus, $\alpha_{IIb}\beta_3$ plays a direct role in regulating platelet activity, as well as in supporting adhesion and aggregation.

Integrin $\alpha_{IIb}\beta_3$ is a major target for the acute treatment of patients with coronary artery disease undergoing procedures such as coronary angioplasty and stenting. The powerful action of the $\alpha_{IIb}\beta_3$ antagonists, however, means that excessive bleeding is a major side-effect and that therapy must be restricted to the hospitalized environment. The prototype drug in this class is the humanized antibody F(ab) fragment abciximab, which was introduced in the mid-1990s and has now been given to more than 2 million patients worldwide. Two peptide $\alpha_{IIb}\beta_3$-blocking agents, integrilin and tirofiban, are also used in the clinic. Clinical trials with orally acting active $\alpha_{IIb}\beta_3$ antagonists have been stopped, however, due to their limited efficacy and side-effects, and there now seems little prospect of this class of anti-platelet drug entering the market in this form.

von Willebrand factor

The glycoprotein vWF is made up of a series of multimers that vary in size in plasma from 0.5 to 20 million daltons, giving rise to the characteristic vWF ladder when analysed by gel chromatography. Larger multimers of vWF are more effective in mediating platelet tethering at high rates of flow. vWF is stored and released from endothelial cell Weibel–Palade bodies as an ultra-large multimer, that is greater than 20 million daltons. The released vWF is broken down into the smaller multimers by the specific metalloproteinase, ADAMTS13. Deficiencies in ADAMTS13 leads to the persistence of ultra-large vWF multimers in the circulation and a thrombotic microangiopathy, known as thrombotic thrombocytopenic purpura (TTP), which is characterized by vWF-rich platelet aggregates in skin and vital organs.

At intermediate and higher rates of shear, vWF undergoes a conformational change from a closed structure to an extended form that can reach several microns in length and which has multiple platelet and collagen binding sites. vWF can also self-associate when extended to form very large filaments on the surface of endothelial cells and on collagen. In this extended form, vWF is able to bind platelets through the GPIb–IX–V complex and thereby support thrombus formation, even at very low rates of shear when immobilized on a surface. This extended form of vWF can also be induced using the antibiotic ristocetin or the snake venom toxin botrocetin. These tools are routinely used in experimental laboratories to promote the interaction of vWF with GPIb–IX–V in the absence of shear. Ristocetin is used in clinical laboratories to promote platelet agglutination through GPIb–IX–V as a test for patients with mutations in the receptor complex, known as Bernard–Soulier syndrome (BSS).

The critical role of vWF in mediating platelet tethering during thrombus formation is discussed above. vWF's role in this process is dependent on the fast on-rate of association to the GPIbα subunit in the GPIb–IX–V complex. The stable recruitment of platelets into the thrombus, however, requires interaction with other platelet agonists or very high rates of shear (which is also able to act as an agonist) to activate platelet integrins. This dependency on multiple interactions prevents thrombus formation occurring when platelets are exposed to vWF in the absence of other stimuli, such as may occur on the surface of endothelial cells during release of the adhesive protein. The large multimeric structure enables it to interact with many other proteins involved in the coagulation cascade, including factor VIII, as discussed in Chapter 46.

GPIb–IX–V has been shown to generate weak intracellular signals that promote spreading and activation of $\alpha_{IIb}\beta_3$ through a pathway that is dependent on Src kinases and PLCγ2, but which is distinct from that used by the collagen receptor GPVI (see below). GPIb–IX–V, however, is a relatively weak stimulus and the significance of its ability to activate $\alpha_{IIb}\beta_3$ is uncertain, bearing in mind that it is unable to support stable adhesion under high shear conditions in the absence of other receptor stimuli. A full evaluation of the importance of GPIb–IX–V signalling is hampered, however, by its critical role in platelet tethering; nevertheless, the redundancy with the more powerful signals from other platelet glycoproteins suggests that its importance is likely to be relatively minor.

GPIb–IX–V binds to a number of other ligands. GPIb–IX–V binds to the integrin $\alpha_M\beta_2$ (also known as Mac-1 or CR3) on the surface of leucocytes, and this interaction, along with binding of platelet P-selectin to PSGL-1, is implicated in the attachment and transmigration of leucocytes through a mural thrombus. GPIb–IX–V also binds to P-selectin and this has been shown to support rolling of platelets with activated endothelium in low-pressure vessels, although the physiological significance of this is unclear. GPIb–IX–V binds to $\alpha_M\beta_2$ receptors in the liver and it has recently been proposed that this is responsible for the clearance of platelets that have been stored at 4°C as a result of clustering of the GPIb–IX–V complex on the platelet surface. Preliminary data suggest that modification of GPIb enables the storage of platelets at 4°C, thereby avoiding many of the lability problems that result from their storage at room temperature.

Mutations in GPIbα, GPIbβ and GPIX give rise to the bleeding disorder BSS, which is characterized by macrothrombocytopenia and fragile platelets. BSS is an extremely rare disorder, with just over 100 cases described worldwide. The reduction in platelet count and change in morphology in BSS platelets is a consequence of the pivotal role of GPIb–IX–V in platelet formation. GPIb–IX–V forms a lattice like structure on the platelet surface mediated through its interaction with the cytoskeleton via the actin-binding protein filamin. This interaction is vital for platelet generation as described in the recent reviews by Hartwig and Italiano (2003) and Italiano and Shivdasani (2003).

Other platelet ligands and their receptors

Table 48.2 lists other receptors that have been described on the platelet surface. Many of these have a minimal effect on platelet activity, whereas others are not exposed to their endogenous ligands during normal haemostasis, although this may not be the case in thrombosis. In many of these cases, therefore, the physiological role of the receptor in regulating platelet function is negligible.

There are several reasons why platelets express receptors that do not appear to have a physiological role. Some of these receptors may regulate platelet activity in lower organisms or they may support megakaryocytopoiesis and platelet formation. The latter may explain, for example, the presence of receptors for chemokines and the cytokine thrombopoietin on platelets, which have critical roles in megakaryocytopoiesis but cause only weak potentiality of platelet activation.

Many of the receptors in Table 48.2 are activated by agonists that are released during platelet activation. The action of many of these agonists on platelets is weak, with only ADP and thromboxanes being recognized as major feedback regulators of platelet activation. However, several of these mediators play important roles in other vascular processes. For example, 5-HT mediates powerful vasoconstriction, thereby limiting blood loss.

It is of interest that platelets express low levels of the integrins $\alpha_5\beta_1$, $\alpha_6\beta_1$ and $\alpha_v\beta_3$, which support platelet adhesion to a number of subendothelial matrix proteins, including fibronectin, laminin and vitronectin respectively (see Table 48.2). The role of these integrins in supporting adhesion, however, is masked to a large extent *in vivo* by the presence of the major platelet integrin, $\alpha_{IIb}\beta_3$, and also by the presence of each other.

An emerging theme in our understanding of the events that underlie platelet activation is the role of surface proteins in 'late events' that help to stabilize the thrombus and minimize embolization. These include outside-in signals from platelet integrins as discussed above but, in addition, several recently discovered receptors on platelets have been implicated at this stage in platelet activation, including ephrins and Eph kinases, the cell adhesion molecule L1 and the α-granule membrane protein CD40L. Eph kinases are cell-surface receptor tyrosine kinases and their ligands, the ephrins and L1, are also transmembrane proteins. Potentially, both Eph kinases and ephrins can generate intracellular signals when platelets come into contact with each other. CD40L binds to its receptor CD40, which is expressed on platelets, and the integrin $\alpha_{IIb}\beta_3$. Mice deficient in CD40L have a delayed occlusion time and a reduction in thrombus stability, which is thought to be mediated through loss of the interaction with the integrin, as mice that lack CD40 do not have the same phenotype. This emerging field promises to shed new light into the mechanisms of platelet regulation and may identify new targets for development of novel antithrombotics.

Platelets express many other membrane proteins whose function is unknown. This includes CD36, which was originally thought to be a receptor for collagen and thrombospondin. CD36 is absent in 3% of the Asian population but, as these individuals do not have major haemostatic problems, it is not thought to play a major role in supporting platelet activation. Platelets also express high levels of the immunoglobulin superfamily member, JAM-1; the tetraspanin proteins, CD9 and CD63 and the integrin-associated protein, CD48. The role of these and other proteins in platelet activation is unknown.

One receptor that is worthy of special mention is the platelet low-affinity receptor, FcγRIIA. FcγRIIA stimulates powerful activation of platelets through the same signalling pathway as that used by collagen. Although FcγRIIA does not appear to be required for haemostasis, it plays a role in immunological defence against bacteria, viruses and parasites. The low affinity immune receptor also plays a critical role in a variety of immune or autoimmune and alloimmune disorders involving antibody–antigen clustering, which results in platelet activation. This is of particular relevance to heparin-induced thrombocytopenia, which is a major complication of treatment of some patients with the anticoagulant.

Inhibitory agonists and their receptors

It is essential for platelets to have powerful inhibitory mechanisms that prevent activation in intact, healthy vessels and which limit thrombus growth during haemostasis. Perhaps surprisingly, therefore, a relatively small number of pathways have been shown to mediate platelet inhibition. This is related to the antithrombotic nature of the endothelial cell surface and the presence of effective mechanisms for removal of platelet stimulatory agonists in the circulation. Additionally, platelet integrins are unable to bind to circulating adhesive proteins such as vWF, fibrinogen and fibronectin in their inactive state. The major pathways mediating platelet inhibition are discussed below. These four pathways interact in a coordinated way, together with endothelial thrombomodulin, which regulates the level of thrombin, to prevent platelet activation on the endothelial surface.

Nitric oxide

Nitric oxide (NO) is the most important inhibitor of platelet function. It is constitutively released from endothelial cells that surround the vasculature, and is made in minor levels in macrophages and in stimulated platelets. It can also be inducibly upregulated in endothelial cells. NO has a short half-life in the vasculature, in the order of 3–5 s, which means that the highest concentration of the gaseous transmitter is found in the vicinity of the endothelial cell, a key site of inhibition of platelet function.

NO mediates powerful inhibition of platelet activation and also promotes vasodilatation. These effects are mediated through direct activation of guanylate cyclase, leading to the generation of cGMP and activation of protein kinase G (PKG). The substrates for PKG in platelets include type III phosphodiesterase

(PDE), which hydrolyses cAMP, which itself is inhibitory. The inhibition of type III phosphodiesterase by cGMP leads to elevation in cAMP and activation of PKA. PKA and PKG inhibit platelet activation through a number of shared pathways, including inhibition of phosphoinositide metabolism and through Ca^{2+} extrusion. The anti-platelet function of NO is likely to contribute in part to the efficacy of cGMP-elevating drugs such as nitrites, which are used in the treatment of unstable angina.

Prostacyclin

Prostacyclin (prostaglandin I_2 or PGI_2) is the major prostaglandin synthesized by endothelial cells. It is synthesized from arachidonic acid through the sequential actions of cyclo-oxygenase and prostacyclin synthetase. Prostacyclin exerts a powerful inhibitory effect on platelets and also promotes vasodilatation through elevation of cAMP. Prostacyclin activates the Gs-coupled, seven transmembrane IP (or prostacyclin) receptor, which regulates adenylyl cyclase. cAMP inhibits platelet activation through a number of pathways, as discussed above.

The concentration of prostacyclin in the bloodstream is too low to mediate a widespread inhibition of platelet activation. Instead, the anti-platelet action of prostacyclin is thought to be of primary significance in inhibiting activation at the edge of damaged vessels, when the growing thrombus comes into contact with the endothelium. This action is facilitated by the liberation of arachidonic acid from the platelet, which is converted to prostacyclin by the endothelial cells.

Platelets express low levels of several other receptors that are coupled to Gs, most notably the adenosine A_{2A} receptor. Although the A_{2A} receptor inhibits platelet reactivity under certain experimental paradigms, it is expressed at a low level and is not considered to be a major route of inhibition.

PECAM-1 (CD31)

Recent studies have demonstrated that the transmembrane protein PECAM-1 plays an important role in inhibiting platelet function. PECAM-1 is expressed in high levels in the platelet surface membrane, with about 10 000 copies per cell. It is a member of the immunoglobulin (Ig) superfamily of surface receptors and is characterized by the presence of six extracellular Ig domains and an immunoreceptor tyrosine-based inhibition motif (ITIM) in its cytosolic tail. Increasing evidence suggests that PECAM-1 is its own ligand, and that binding to PECAM-1 molecules on other cells mediates inhibition. Cross-linking of PECAM-1 using specific antibodies or recombinant PECAM-1 selectively inhibits the activation of platelets by the collagen receptor GPVI and by FcγRIIA through the recruitment of the tyrosine phosphatase, SHP-2 (Figure 48.3). The primary role of this inhibitory action may be to prevent platelet activation on endothelial cells, which express more than 1 million copies of PECAM-1 per cell. Thus, the interaction of platelets with endo-

thelial cells generates inhibitory signals that prevent the activation of platelets by collagen and possibly also agonists.

Ecto-ADPase (CD39)

Platelets and endothelial cells express an ecto-ADPase (CD39) on their cell surface that rapidly metabolizes ATP and ADP to AMP. This prevents activation of platelets by low levels of the nucleotides in the circulation or on the endothelial surface.

Signalling pathways underlying platelet activation

The major receptor types that mediate platelet activation can be broadly divided into those that initiate activation through tyrosine kinase-linked and G-protein-dependent pathways. The former includes the major platelet adhesive ligands, namely collagen, vWF and fibrinogen, whereas, G-protein-coupled receptors are activated by 'soluble' ligands, such as thrombin, thromboxanes and ADP. These two distinct pathways undergo synergy with each other and regulate a number of closely related effector proteins, including isoforms of PLC and PI3 kinase. In addition, Ca^{2+} plays a critical role in platelet activation by both groups of receptors. Indeed, from the point of the cell, there may be little difference between activation of distinct isoforms of effector enzymes that liberate the same second messengers such as IP3, 1,2-diacylglycerol and phosphatidylinositol 3,4,5-trisphosphate (PI 3,4,5-P3). This section broadly outlines the pathways that underlie platelet activation by these two groups of receptors.

Tyrosine kinase-linked receptors

Platelets express three distinct families of surface glycoproteins that signal through Src family tyrosine kinases that lie upstream of PLCγ2 and PI3 kinase. These are the ITAM receptors, GPVI and FcγRIIA, platelet integrins, including $\alpha_{IIb}\beta_3$ and $\alpha_2\beta_1$, and the leucine-rich repeat protein, GPIb–IX–V. These three groups of receptors differ, however, in the mechanism and magnitude of regulation of PLCγ2. GPVI and FcγRIIA induce powerful activation of PLCγ2 through sequential activation of Src and Syk family kinases. Pivotal in their signalling cascades is phosphorylation of two tyrosines in the conserved ITAM sequence, which leads to recruitment and activation of Syk which, in turn, regulates downstream effector proteins. The major platelet integrin, $\alpha_{IIb}\beta_3$, also signals via sequential activation of Src and Syk family kinases, although in contrast with the above, this pathway is ITAM independent. In addition, $\alpha_{IIb}\beta_3$ induces a much lower level of activation of PLCγ2, and also activates the tyrosine kinase, focal adhesion kinase (FAK) through a pathway that is dependent on actin polymerization. The activation of Syk and PLCγ2 by $\alpha_{IIb}\beta_3$ supports platelet spreading. GPIb–IX–V also regulates Src kinases and PLCγ2 through an ITAM-independent pathway; however, GPIb–IX–V, is an extremely weak stimulus and the importance of this supporting thrombus formation *in vivo* is unclear (see above).

G-protein-coupled receptors

The major G-protein-coupled receptors that underlie platelet activation can be divided into two groups on the basis of their associated G-proteins. The largest group is coupled to the G_q and $G_{12/13}$ families of G-proteins, and includes the $P2Y_1$ ADP receptor, the PAR_1 and PAR_4 thrombin receptors and the TP thromboxane receptor. The extent to which these receptors induce platelet activation varies according to their levels of expression. Thus, for example, the $P2Y_1$ ADP receptor is present at a very low density and so is only able to stimulate aggregation through synergy with the $P2Y_{12}$ ADP receptor. The two thrombin receptors are present in higher levels and are able promote aggregation on their own, although they also undergo synergy with the $P2Y_{12}$ ADP receptor. G_q regulates PLCβ and is thought to be the primary basis of platelet activation by these receptors. $G_{12/13}$ G-proteins activate the small G-protein Rho that lies upstream of Rho kinase, which mediates shape change (see above). Activation of $G_{12/13}$ G-proteins is also able to undergo synergy with ADP to promote aggregation, although the basis of this is not established.

G_i-coupled G-proteins inhibit adenylyl cyclase and activate PI3 kinase, among other actions. The $P2Y_{12}$ ADP receptor is the major regulator of this family of G-proteins in platelets. The $P2Y_{12}$ ADP receptor undergoes marked synergy with other stimulatory receptors leading to powerful aggregation and secretion as illustrated above. The molecular basis of this synergy is mediated in part through activation of the PI3 kinase pathway, but is independent of inhibition of adenylyl cyclase.

Ca²⁺ and protein kinase C

Ca^{2+} plays a critical role in nearly all aspects of platelet activation, including aggregation and secretion. An increase in Ca^{2+} is brought about by its release from intracellular stores by the action of IP3 or by entry through the plasma membrane, either as a consequence of depletion of intracellular stores, a process known as capacitative entry, or by direct opening of membrane Ca^{2+} channels. Given the importance of Ca^{2+} in regulating platelet activity, we still know surprisingly little about the mechanisms that control Ca^{2+} entry into the cell, although it seems likely that these involve membrane TRP channels.

The majority of the actions of Ca^{2+} are dependent on the calcium-binding protein calmodulin. In addition, however, many Ca^{2+}-dependent responses also require activation of other signalling pathways, such as protein kinase C, which regulates secretion through phosphorylation of SNARE proteins and SNARE regulatory proteins. Fluorometric ratio dyes such as Fura2 or Oregon green have revolutionized the study of Ca^{2+} in platelets and have recently demonstrated the critical role of the cation in nucleating thrombus formation on immobilized ligands. Agents that block Ca^{2+} elevation and protein kinase C represent potential novel antithrombotics, but are also likely to have many other actions.

Phosphatidylinositol 3-kinase

The phosphatidylinositol 3-kinase (PI3 kinase) second-messenger pathway generates the 3-phosphorylated membrane lipids, PI 3,4,5-P3 and PI 3,4-P2. These lipid-based messengers are implicated in the regulation of over 200 proteins in the genome that contain pleckstrin homology (PH) domains. The binding of PH domains to the 3-phosphorylated lipids enables their recruitment to the plasma membrane. Examples of proteins that have PH domains are PLCβ and -γ isoforms and Tec family kinases, such as Btk, which regulate Ca^{2+} entry in platelets and phosphorylate PLCγ2. PI3 kinases isoforms are regulated by G-protein-coupled and tyrosine kinase-linked receptors. There are many potential routes through which activation of PI3 kinases can give rise to platelet activation and underlie synergy between receptors.

Platelet function testing in the clinic

Platelet-based bleeding problems

Platelet function tests are primarily utilized to aid in the diagnosis and management of patients presenting with bleeding problems rather than thrombosis. Before any platelet function test is requested a full clinical and family history is always taken to determine the underlying cause of the bleeding problem. This includes studying the pattern of bleeding, whether it is lifelong or recent, triggered by trauma (e.g. dentistry, surgery or accident), is present within other family members and associated with any medication the patient may be taking. If a platelet defect is suspected then there are now a variety of tests available that can be utilized to diagnose any underlying cause of the bleeding problem. The investigation of platelet function is often affected by the collection and processing of blood samples. Platelets are not only prone to artefactual *in vitro* activation, but also to desensitization. Most functional tests therefore have to be performed relatively quickly (e.g. < 2 h from sampling). Also normal platelet function is highly dependent upon Ca^{2+} concentration and so the choice of anticoagulant is important. Any obvious defect in platelet number should of course always be first excluded by performing a full blood count.

The bleeding time was the first *in vivo* test of platelet function and is performed by timing the arrest of bleeding from standard-sized cuts that are made within the skin of the forearm. Although the test is clinically useful and has been refined, most clinicians consider the test to be poorly reproducible, invasive, insensitive (particularly to mild platelet defects) and time consuming. Despite these drawbacks, the test is still widely utilized as a first-line screening tool and can identify patients with severe platelet defects. In the 1960s, platelet aggregation quickly became the gold standard of platelet function testing and revolutionized our ability to identify and diagnose many platelet defects. Most aggregometers monitor the changes in light transmission that occur in a suspension of platelets that are stimulated with different concentrations of various agonists (e.g. ADP, collagen, adrenaline, ristocetin, etc.). The pattern of responses obtained enables the experienced operator to quickly diagnose whether there are defects in various platelet receptors, platelet granules and downstream signalling or metabolic pathways. These two techniques coupled with measurement of platelet adenine nucleotides remained the mainstay of platelet function testing until the late 1980s.

The introduction of flow cytometry into haematology laboratories provided an exquisite, sensitive and powerful tool for studying platelets. Flow cytometric analysis of platelets is usually performed in fresh whole blood and the technique can also be used with very small quantities of blood, even in thrombocytopenia. The major diagnostic use of this technique is to determine the copy density of platelet membrane glycoproteins and receptors. This method is therefore useful for confirming the absence of various glycoproteins or receptors in disease. Platelet function testing can also be performed and the ability of platelets to degranulate, express activation markers (e.g. P-selectin) and negatively charged phospholipid in response to agonists can all be studied.

A major limitation in the above tests is that they are performed at low shear conditions and therefore do not mimic accurately many of the important physiological processes of platelet adhesion, activation and aggregation that occur at higher shear rates *in vivo*. Given this and the problems faced with the *in vivo* bleeding time, a number of *in vitro* tests that attempt to accurately simulate platelet function have been developed. These include the PFA-100 (platelet function analyzer) and CPA (cone and plate analyzer) devices. These simulate high-shear platelet adhesion to foreign surfaces (e.g. collagen) and either monitor the drop in flow rate as an aperture is closed by platelet adhesion/aggregation or study the degree of platelet aggregation and surface coverage respectively. The PFA-100 instrument has been widely utilized for the last 6 years and provides a potential replacement of the bleeding time as a screening test, as it is more sensitive to certain platelet defects and von Willebrand disease. The CPA device has been commercialized only recently as the IMPACT device, so experience is still very limited. However, it is highly likely that these types of instruments will be increasingly utilized in the future and may prove to be useful not only as aids in diagnosing platelet defects and monitoring anti-platelet therapy, but also in predicting bleeding and thrombosis in various patient groups.

Advances in genetic testing of platelet defects coupled with the impending definition of the platelet transcriptosome should also facilitate the use of microarray technology to rapidly diagnose defects and receptor polymorphisms in both health and disease. This area, however, is still in its infancy.

There is clearly still no gold standard for platelet testing, and indeed there may never be. It is likely that a variety of approaches will always be required to confirm a platelet-based bleeding disorder and that the most important of these may remain as clinical history and the ruling out of obvious alternative explanations. It is also likely that specialist test centres will be required for the identification of rare and new platelet-based defects.

Platelets and thrombosis

It is important to consider whether patients with arterial thrombotic conditions have over-reactive platelets or whether the platelets are simply doing what they normally do within an abnormal environment. Given the link between arterial thrombosis with age and the environment, it is highly likely that the vast majority of cases fall into the latter group and that little would be gained by analysing their platelets for 'hyper-reactivity' through platelet function testing, without additional information. Individuals with a high platelet count ($> 600 \times 10^9$/L), such as that found in essential thrombocythaemia, are at increased risk of thrombosis, although many remain symptomless. An important area of research in thrombosis is the influence of inherited platelet receptor polymorphisms. These studies, although interesting, are still often limited by low sample numbers and conflicting data, most likely reflecting the complex nature of the disease, which is influenced by many factors.

Future developments

The last few years have seen remarkable advances in our understanding of the regulation and role of platelets in haemostasis and in inflammatory disorders. Many of these advances in our understanding of platelet function are the result of the impact of new technologies and experimental approaches.

The sequencing of the genome and the use of mass spectrometry in protein identification have led to attempts to map the platelet transcriptosome and proteome respectively, although these fields remain in their infancy because many modern-day molecular techniques are more difficult to apply to these anucleate cells.

An increasing emphasis is being placed by many laboratories upon the analysis of platelets from mutant mice, and many important new observations on platelet function have been made and are likely to continue to be made in this way over the coming years, many of which may stem from the unexpected observation of a platelet-based bleeding problem. Nevertheless, this approach must be used with the caveat 'mice are not men', even although the fundamental basis of haemostasis in the two species seems to be the same. The continuing elucidation of the molecular basis of patients with novel platelet-based bleeding problems is anticipated to play a major role in our understanding of the events that govern platelet regulation, although the rarity of these patients severely hampers progress in this area.

Imaging techniques are providing remarkable new insights into the complexity and dynamics of the processes that underlie all aspects of platelet activation both *in vitro* and *in vivo*. Although these techniques are hampered by the small size of the platelet, the field is young, and many new and exciting observations are being discovered through application of this technology. This is further enhanced by its application to mouse models, which is beginning to reveal new insights into the biochemical and cytoskeletal events that underlie real time *in vivo* thrombus formation.

With all these developments and information, the student is left with a bewildering complexity and a feeling of 'where will it all end'? In considering this, it is important to recognize that, perhaps surprisingly, many of the proteins in platelets appear to have minor or negligible roles in regulating activation. The number of major proteins and pathways that play major roles in regulating platelet activation is a much smaller number.

The goal remains to develop improved antithrombotic agents that provides effective treatment without an increased risk of bleeding. Although it may never be possible to attain this goal, as we begin to understand more about the events that underlie thrombus formation, there will be increased opportunity for discovery of more rational forms of therapy. New medicines may be targeted at the very early stages of platelet activation and may be more effective in preventing thrombosis without significantly disturbing normal haemostasis.

Acknowledgements

S.P.W. is a British Heart Foundation Chair. Dr Watson gratefully acknowledges the support of the British Heart Foundation, Wellcome Trust and BBSRC, and all the past and present members of his laboratory who have contributed much to the ideas and thoughts that have formed the basis of this chapter. We thank Drs Yotis Senis and Ben Atkinson for preparing the figures.

Selected bibliography

Andre P, Prasad KS, Denis CV *et al.* (2002) CD40L stabilizes arterial thrombi by a β3 integrin-dependent mechanism. *Nature Medicine* **8**: 247–52.

Angelillo-Scherrer A, de Frutos P, Aparicio C *et al.* (2001) Deficiency or inhibition of Gas6 causes platelet dysfunction and protects mice against thrombosis. *Nature Medicine* **7**: 215–21.

Bhatt DL, Topol EJ (2003) Scientific and therapeutic advances in anti-platelet therapy. *Nature Drug Discovery* **2**: 15–18.

Caen JP, Han ZC, Bellucci S *et al.* (1999) Regulation of megakaryocytopoiesis. *Haemostasis* **29**: 27–40.

Falati S, Liu Q, Gross P *et al.* (2003) Accumulation of tissue factor into developing thrombi in vivo is dependent upon microparticle P-selectin glycoprotein ligand 1 and platelet P-selectin. *Journal of Experimental Medicine* **197**: 1585–98.

George JN (2000) Platelets. *Lancet* **355**: 1531–9.

Gresele P, Page C, Fuster V *et al.* (eds) (2002) *Platelets in Thrombotic and Non-thrombotic Disorders*. Cambridge University Press, Cambridge.

Hartwig J, Italiano J Jr (2003) The birth of the platelet. *Journal of Thrombosis and Haemostasis* **1**: 1580–6.

Huo Y, Schober A, Forlow SB *et al.* (2003) Circulating activated platelets exacerbate atherosclerosis in mice deficient in apolipoprotein E. *Nature Medicine* **9**: 61–7.

Italiano JE, Shivdasani RA (2003) Megakaryocytes and beyond: the birth of platelets. *Journal of Thrombosis and Haemostasis* **1**: 1174–82.

Italiano JE, Lecine P, Shivdasani RA *et al.* (1999) Blood platelets are assembled principally at the ends of proplatelet processes produced by differentiated megakaryocytes. *Journal of Cell Biology* **147**: 1299–1312.

Jackson SP, Schoenwalder SM (2003) Anti-platelet therapy: in search of the magic bullet. *Nature Drug Discovery* **2**: 775–89.

Michelson AD (ed.) (2002) *Platelets*. Academic Press, San Diego, CA.

Nieswandt B, Watson SP (2003) Platelet-collagen interaction: is GPVI the central receptor? *Blood* **102**: 449–61.

Prevost N, Woulfe D, Tognolini M *et al.* (2003) Contact-dependent signaling during the late events of platelet activation. *Journal of Thrombosis and Haemostasis* **1**: 1613–27.

Ruggeri ZM (2002) Platelets in atherothrombosis. *Nature Medicine* **8**: 1227–34.

CHAPTER 49

Inherited bleeding disorders

Michael A Laffan and Christine A Lee

49

Introduction

The existence of lifelong bleeding disorders and their familial occurrence was noted in the medical literature as early as the sixteenth century. No doubt this was because the clinical syndrome of haemophilia is highly distinctive. Early writers were impressed by the helplessness of the physician in the face of such extreme haemophilic bleeding. A full understanding of the pathophysiology and genetics of these disorders was long delayed because of the complexities of the clotting mechanism. Advances in protein chemistry and recombinant DNA technology have now produced a comprehensive account both of normal coagulation and of the molecular genetics of haemophilia. An earlier chapter outlines the coagulation mechanism. In this chapter, the clinical features of inherited bleeding disorders will be described, together with a summary of the genetic lesions identified in the various coagulation factor deficiency states. Table 49.1 summarizes inherited bleeding disorders, their mode of inheritance, the molecular genetic basis where known and the incidence.

Advances in molecular biology have enabled more precise diagnosis and reduced the dependence on plasma-derived concentrates, at least in the economically rich countries. Direct identification of the mutation responsible for the factor deficiency in an individual kindred has now superseded the use of restriction fragment length polymorphisms (RFLPs). This can remove the uncertainty from carrier detection in many cases. The methodology for these analyses is now a crucial part of haemophilia care and will be discussed in full.

Haemophilia A

Clinical features

The majority of patients are male, but haemophilia can occur very rarely in females (see below). The severity and frequency of bleeding in X-linked factor VIII deficiency are inversely correlated with the residual factor VIII level. Table 49.2 summarizes this relationship and gives the relative frequency of categories, based on UK national data. The main load- or strain-bearing joints – ankles, knees and elbows – are most affected but any joint can be the site of bleeding. If untreated, this intracapsular bleeding causes severe swelling, pain, stiffness and inflammation, which gradually resolves over days or weeks. It is not clear why bleeding in haemophilia shows a predilection for joints, but it has been suggested recently that synthesis of tissue factor pathway inhibitor (TFPI) in synovial tissue may be at least part of the explanation.

Blood is highly irritant to the synovium and causes synovial overgrowth, with a tendency to rebleed from friable vascular tissue, thus setting up a vicious circle. It is probably through the accumulation of iron in chondrocytes that a rapid degenerative arthritis occurs, leading to an irregularity of articular contour, then thinning of the cartilage, bony overgrowth and subchondral cysts, and, finally, ankylosis (Figure 49.1). As a result of the vicious circle of bleeding and synovial hypertrophy, a particular joint tends to become the 'target joint' in an individual, whereas other joints may be relatively spared.

Muscle bleeding can be seen in any anatomical site, but it most

Table 49.1 Inherited bleeding disorders.

Disorder (synonym)	Pathophysiology	Mode of inheritance	Molecular genetics	Approximate incidence per 10^6 population[†]
Common group				
Haemophilia A (classical haemophilia)	Factor VIII deficient or defective	XL	Deletions, inversions, missense, nonsense, insertions, splicing	100
von Willebrand's disease	von Willebrand factor deficient or defective	AD or AR	Deletions, missense nonsense	AD: 100 or more* AR: 1
Haemophilia B (Christmas disease)	Factor IX deficient or defective	XL	Deletions, missense nonsense, splicing	20
Haemophilia C (PTA deficiency)	Factor XI deficient	AD or R	Missense, nonsense splicing	5% in Ashkenazi Jews, others rare
Rare group				
Factor X deficiency		AR	Deletions, missense	1
Factor V deficiency		AR	?	1
Factor VII deficiency		AR	Missense, nonsense, deletion, splicing	
Factor II (prothrombin) deficiency		AR	?, missense	1
Afibrinogenaemia		AR		
Dysfibrinogenaemia		AD	Missense	1
Factor XIII deficiency		AR	Missense, deletion	1
Factor V plus VIII deficiency		AR	Missense, nonsense, deletion, insertion	1
Hyperplasminaemia α_2-antiplasmin deficiency		AR	Missense, insertion	Very rare

XL, X-linked recessive; AD, autosomal dominant; AR, autosomal recessive.
*Recent population surveys indicate much higher incidence of mild von Willebrand's disease.
[†]Figures applicable to developed countries; incidence is lower in developing countries due to very high early mortality and low reproductive fitness of suffers.

Table 49.2 Haemophilia A*: clinical severity.

Factor VIII U/dL	Bleeding tendency	Relative incidence (% of cases)
< 2	Severe: frequent spontaneous[†] bleeding into joints, muscles and internal organs	50
2–10	Moderately severe: some 'spontaneous bleeds', bleeding after minor trauma	30
>10–30	Mild: bleeding only after significant trauma, surgery	20

*This table is also applicable to factor IX, X and II deficiencies, but not to factors VII, XI, V, XIII or von Willebrand factor deficiencies (see text).
[†]'Spontaneous' bleeding refers to those episodes in which no obvious precipitating event preceded the bleed. No doubt, minor tissue damage consequent on everyday activities actually initiates bleeding.

often presents in the large load-bearing groups of the thigh, calf, posterior abdominal wall and buttocks. Local pressure effects often cause entrapment neuropathy, particularly of the femoral nerve, with iliopsoas bleeding. This causes a common symptom triad of groin pain, hip flexure and cutaneous sensory loss over the femoral nerve distribution. Bleeding into the calf, forearm or peroneal muscles can lead to ischaemic necrosis and contracture.

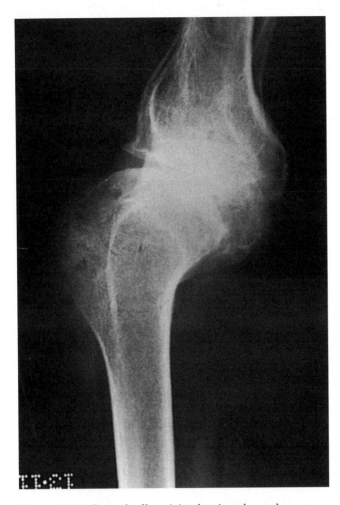

Figure 49.1 Radiograph of knee joint showing advanced haemophilic arthropathy. Note the loss of cartilage, eburnation, deformity subluxation, osteophytes, subchondral cysts and irregularity of joint contours.

Haematuria is less common than joint or muscle bleeding in individuals with haemophilia, but the most severely affected patients have one or two episodes per decade. These may be painless and resolve spontaneously, but, if bleeding is heavy, it can produce clot colic. Usually, no anatomical abnormality is found to account for the haematuria on radiological investigation.

Central nervous system bleeding is uncommon but can occur after a slight head injury and was formerly the most common cause of death in haemophilia A. Intestinal tract bleeding usually presents as obstruction due to intramural haemorrhage, but haematemesis and melaena also occasionally occur and should be routinely investigated, as they may be due to peptic ulcer or malignancy.

Oropharyngeal bleeding, although uncommon, is clinically dangerous, as extension through the soft tissues of the floor of the mouth can lead to respiratory obstruction. Bleeding from the tongue after laceration can be very persistent and troublesome due to fibrinolytic substances in saliva and the impossibility of immobilizing the tongue.

Surgery and open trauma invariably lead to dangerous haemorrhage in the untreated individual with haemophilia. There may be persistence of haemorrhage often after an initial short-lived period of haemostasis. Clots, if formed, are bulky and friable and break off, with renewed haemorrhage occurring intermittently over days and weeks. This is only seen today in patients who are resistant to conventional replacement therapy, and is due to the presence of inhibitors (see below) or when patients with mild or moderate haemophilia present after their first surgical or dental procedure.

Bruising is a feature of haemophilia A, but it is usually only of cosmetic significance as it remains superficial and self-limiting. Large extending ecchymoses may occasionally require treatment.

Presentation

When a woman is known to be a carrier or at high risk, the cord blood factor VIII level will establish the diagnosis in the infant. However, the haemophilia may be sporadic with no family history and, in such cases, the haemophilic condition may come to light in the neonatal period with cephalohaematoma or prolonged bleeding from the cord. In cultures where early circumcision is the rule, this will cause prolonged haemorrhage, as was noted in the Babylonian Talmud almost 2000 years ago. Quite often, the diagnosis is delayed until it is noticed that the infant has many large bruises from hand pressure when being picked up or from minor knocks on the cot. These sometimes cause diagnostic confusion and the erroneous label of 'battered baby syndrome' may be applied, with needless psychological trauma to the parents. As soon as the infant starts to crawl actively, joint bleeding will begin to appear. In other children, excessive bleeding from the eruption of primary dentition, or from lacerations, leads to the performance of diagnostic tests. Mild cases may only present in later life when severe trauma or surgery provokes unusual bleeding.

Pathophysiology

All the clinical features of haemophilia A are due directly or indirectly to lack of the clotting factor VIII. The gene for this protein cofactor is located near the tip of the long arm of the X chromosome (Xq 2.8ter), which accounts for the sex-linked pattern of inheritance. Individuals with haemophilia are unable to produce factor VIII due to various mutations (see below) at the factor VIII locus. A lack of factor VIII as a cofactor drastically slows the rate of generation of factor Xa, despite the presence of all other coagulation factors and platelets in normal amounts. Conversely, replacement by intravenous infusion of factor VIII can normalize the haemostatic mechanism of the haemophilic individual.

Laboratory diagnosis

Screening tests show a long activated partial thromboplastin time (APTT), normal prothrombin time (PT), thrombin clotting time (TCT) and bleeding time, and a normal platelet count. Specific assays show factor VIII clotting activity below 50 U/dL, with all other factors normal, and also normal von Willebrand factor (VWF) antigen and ristocetin cofactor. A test for antibodies to factor VIII should always be performed.

Treatment

Clotting factor concentrates

The discovery that factor VIIIC (FVIIIC) was concentrated in cryoprecipitate and the subsequent description of the production of antihaemophilic globulin in a closed bag system made more specific replacement therapy for people with haemophilia possible. Home treatment for the majority of patients became feasible and, with the advent of *lyophilized* concentrates prepared from the plasma from many thousands of donors, the prospect of a normal life for the severely affected haemophilic individual was brought very close. Until virucidal methods were applied to such concentrates from 1985 onwards, many individuals with haemophilia contracted hepatitis, chronic liver disease and AIDS. However, clotting factor concentrates are now virucidally treated and are very safe, particularly with the advent of recombinant clotting factor concentrates. The plasma-derived clotting factor concentrates in use at present are high-purity products with a high specific activity. They are prepared by monoclonal immunoabsorption and other techniques, which result in a pure final product of high specific activity. In the case of FVIII concentrate, this may be purified using a monoclonal antibody specific for the von Willebrand protein or a monoclonal antibody specific to FVIIIC itself. Other techniques of fractionation use chromatographic purification.

Viral infections were a major complication of replacement therapy before adequate inactivation steps were applied. There are three main virucidal methods:

1 terminal heating of the lyophilized product at 80°C (dry heating);

2 heating in solution at 60°C (pasteurization) in the presence of stabilizers or in moisture with hot vapour under high pressure;

3 adding a solvent–detergent mixture during the manufacturing process.

The risk of HIV infection in virally inactivated concentrates is very small, probably as low as 1:200 000–1:300 000. The risk of transmission of hepatitis B and C has also been dramatically reduced. However, there remains the problem of transmission of hepatitis A and parvovirus, which can break through solvent–detergent sterilization and, for this reason, many inactivation processes involve more than one virucidal method. For FIX concentrate, the process of nanofiltration has been used, which can prevent transmission of hepatitis A and parvovirus. It is probable that the fractionation processes used to produce plasma-derived concentrates also overcome the theoretical risk of prion transmission.

Recombinant factor VIII

The structure of the FVIII gene and the isolation of cDNA clones encoding the complete FVIII sequence in the *in vitro* expression of human factor VIII in tissue culture were described in 1984. As a result, it has been possible to develop a recombinant FVIII product: two full-length recombinant products, *Kogenate* (Bayer)–*Helixate* (Aventis) and *Recombinate* (Baxter), and one which is B domainless known as rVIIISQ with the trade name of *Refacto* (Wyeth).

Kogenate–Helixate was made by transfecting cDNA for FVIII into an established mammalian cell line of baby hamster kidney. The secreted protein was purified by multiple purification steps, including ion exchange chromatography and immunoaffinity chromatography with murine monoclonal antibody. The first-generation Kogenate requires albumin as a stabilizer but, more recently, this recombinant FVIII is stabilized using sucrose, avoiding the need for the addition of human albumin.

Recombinate was manufactured by introducing the human FVIII and the von Willebrand factor DNA into Chinese hamster ovary cells.

Refacto is a B domain-depleted recombinant FVIII – the domain is dispensable for the haemostatic activity of VIII. The B domain-depleted molecule is much more stable and albumin is not necessary for stabilization.

More recent formulations of recombinant FVIII are devoid of animal products such as albumin (Table 49.3).

The assay of recombinant clotting factors

In pharmacokinetic studies, it was found that the chromogenic assay produced considerably higher levels than one-stage assays. The influence of phospholipids was studied on these discrepancies. It was found that when the APTT reagent was replaced by platelets in the one-stage assays the results of the chromogenic assay and the one-stage assay were similar (Figure 49.2). Furthermore, using the basic principle of 'like *versus* like', this discrepancy between chromogenic and one-stage methods could be eliminated by using the recombinant product diluted in haemophilic plasma as a standard reference (Figure 49.2).

Treatment on demand

Since the development of replacement therapy, the goal of treatment for haemophilia patients has been the prevention of haemorrhagic episodes. Based on studies from haemophilia carriers and patients with mild haemophilia, we assume that a level of between 5% and 30% is probably adequate to overcome mild bleeds, but certainly not adequate for major surgery or trauma. We know that the severity and the frequency of haemarthrosis is

Table 49.3 Summary of recombinant products available.

	Cell line	Gene	Protein in culture medium	Murine MAbs	Human albumin as stabilizer	Viral inactivation removal	Generation
Recombinate	CHO	VIII VWF	Bovine albumin insulin, aprotinin	Yes	Yes	No	1
Helixate/kogenate	BHK	VIII	Human albumin	Yes	No	SD	2
Refacto	CHO	B domain-deleted VIII	Human albumin	Yes	No	SD	2
NovoSeven	BHK	VII	Bovine serum	Yes	No	SD	2
Benefix	CHO	IX	No	No	No	NF	3

BHK, baby hamster kidney; CHO, Chinese hamster ovary; MAbs, monoclonal antibodies; NF, nanofiltration; SD, solvent detergent.
Reproduced from UKHCDO guidelines (2003), with permission.

Table 49.4 Indications and guidelines for factor replacement in haemophilia A and B.

Site of haemorrhage	Dose (U/kg body weight)			
	Optimal factor level (%)	FVIII	FIX	Duration in days
Joint	30–50	20–30	30–50	1–2
Muscle	30–50	20–30	30–40	1–2
Gastrointestinal tract	40–60	30–40	40–60	7–10
Oral mucosa	30–50	20–30	30–40	Until healing
Epistaxis	30–50	20–30	40–60	Until healing
Haematuria	30–100	25–50	70–100	Until healing
Central nervous system	60–100	50	80–100	7–10
Retroperitoneal	50–100	30–50	60–100	7–10
Trauma or surgery	50–100	30–50	60–100	Until healing

Reproduced from Escobar (2003), with permission.

directly related to the degree of deficiency of the clotting factor, but the precise plasma level needed to prevent haemarthrosis is still unknown.

Therapeutic infusion of replacement factor should be administered as early as possible and to a haemostatic level to stop haemorrhagic events. The dosing factor replacement is still based on theoretical calculations and clinical experience.

Guidelines for the treatment of haemorrhagic episodes in haemophilia are given in Table 49.4. Different levels of clotting factor have been proposed, depending on the type and severity of bleed: thus, 12–35% for major bleeding episodes, 12–17% for minor bleeding events, 40–50% for severe trauma and 30% for minor events and 10–20% for spontaneous bleeding episodes.

Formulae based on plasma volume and expected recovery give a rough guide to dosage, but, where the level is critical, as for surgery or when there is serious bleeding, it should always be checked by assay after infusion. On average, factor VIII infusion produces a plasma increment of 2 U/dL per unit infused per kilogram of body weight. From this, a simple formula can be derived as follows: dose to be infused (units) = [weight (kg) × increment needed (U/dL)]/2. Assessing the period of treatment required is a matter of clinical judgement of the individual episode or lesion.

Cover for surgery, other than very minor procedures, requires maintenance of normal factor VIII levels for approximately 1 week, followed by a period at reduced dosage during convalescence. This can be achieved either by repeated bolus injections every 8–12 h (paying particular attention to the trough levels) or by continuous infusion. It must be noted that the doses required during the immediate post-operative period may be considerably more than expected.

Prophylaxis

There is a long tradition of giving prophylaxis to young boys with haemophilia. This was begun in 1958 for boys with haemophilia A. The rationale for the prophylactic model was the observation that chronic arthropathy was seen less frequently and less severely in individuals with a FVIII level of 1–4 IU/dL.

Prophylaxis was developed at Malmö, Sweden, and based on the pharmacokinetic modelling; regular prophylactic treatment is begun at 1–1.5 years before the onset of joint bleeds.

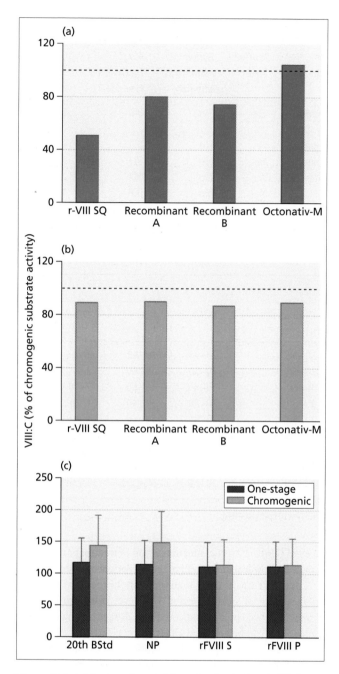

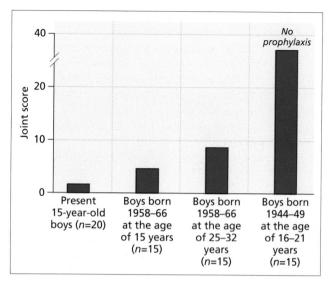

Figure 49.3 Orthopaedic joint scores for the present intensively treated. A 15-year-old group compared with a less intensively treated group at different ages, and to patients not receiving prophylaxis (historical control subjects) (UKHCDO (2003)).

Figure 49.2 (a) Activated partial thromboplastin time (APTT)-based one-stage assays (reproduced from Mikaelsson *et al.* (1998), with permission). (b) Platelet-based one-stage assays (reproduced from Mikaelsson *et al.* (1998), with permission). (c) FVIII recovery levels – ratio of one-stage APTT–chromogenic (reproduced from Lee *et al.* (1999), with permission).

Ideally, FVIII is administered every second day at a dose of 20–40 IU/kg. The goal is to achieve a trough level of > 1 IU/dL. There is good evidence that the Malmö model is effective in preventing haemophilic arthropathy. For the youngest cohort of

boys born in 1981–90, who began prophylaxis between 1–2 years with 4000–9000 IU/kg annually, both the orthopaedic and radiological scores were zero (Figure 49.3).

The use of the peripheral vein is the most preferred approach when beginning prophylactic treatment. However, if this is not possible then the implantation of a Port-a-Cath may be necessary. Substantial experience with Port-a-Caths has been published. Although the advantages of such devices are recognized, septic complications remain a challenge. A number of studies have been published, which show an infection rate ranging from 0.2 to 3.4 infections per 1000 catheter-days.

DDAVP

The non-blood-derived alternative, DDAVP® (1-deamino-8-D-arginine vasopressin) can be used to treat mild haemophilia. This synthetic analogue of vasopressin retains the antidiuretic action of the natural hormone and also stimulates the release of tissue plasminogen activator. In practice, these effects can be used to elevate the plasma factor VIII level two- to fourfold above the baseline, presumably by its release from storage site(s). Patients are advised to restrict their fluid intake after DDAVP. This is especially important in children in whom unrestricted fluid intake may result in hyponatraemia and convulsions. DDAVP is contraindicated in elderly patients and those with vascular disease, because arterial thrombosis is a theoretical risk and has been reported following DDAVP in these circumstances.

DDAVP can correct the haemostatic defect in mild haemophilia A or von Willebrand disease (VWD) sufficiently to cover minor surgery or treat a minor bleeding episode. A typical regimen would be to give 0.3 μg/kg body weight by slow intravenous infusion over 20 min (or by subcutaneous injection), together with 1 g of tranexamic acid.

The effect is maximal at 30 min for an intravenous dose and 1 h following a subcutaneous dose. The factor VIII rises three-fold on average. The half-life of the endogenously released factor VIII is about 8 h and the dose can be repeated. Although tachyphylaxis occurs and the second dose may produce a rise 30% of the first, there is often no further drop with succeeding doses. It is customary to advise that no more than three infusions should be given within 48 h because the reserves will be exhausted.

Complications of therapy

Inhibitors

Antibodies to factor VIII (inhibitors) are most common in patients with severe rather than mild haemophilia and are most likely to develop during childhood, but, rarely, inhibitors may develop after years of treatment. Prospective studies have shown that in the past the incidence of inhibitors in patients with haemophilia has generally been underestimated and that virtually all inhibitors occur within 25 treatment days. Studies to determine the true incidence are fraught with difficulty owing to bias in patient selection, frequency and sensitivity of testing and previous treatment. It is impossible at present to give a definitive figure for the incidence of inhibitor development, but overall studies have reported a cumulative risk for severe haemophilia to be approximately 20% by the age of 5–8 years. There is also a genetic component and inhibitors are found six times more often in pairs of brothers than would be expected by chance. One important determinant is the genetic lesion responsible for the factor VIII deficiency. Patients with large deletions or stop codons in the light chain appear to be particularly prone to inhibitor development. Approximately 25% of patients with the common intron 22 inversion develop inhibitors. These figures apply to the high-responding inhibitors that are clinically troublesome. Close monitoring may reveal low-level and transient inhibitors in a further 20% or so of patients. As more is learned of the molecular bases for factor VIII deficiency, it should be possible, perhaps in association with human leucocyte antigen typing, to define more precisely the individual risk. Because the development of inhibitors is unpredictable, it is important to test for their emergence at clinic visits and before operations.

Antibodies to FVIII are typically time independent in their action and therefore an incubation time of 2–4 h is required to measure the effect of the antibody. The Bethesda assay is the most commonly used. An inhibitor is defined as low titre < 5 BU and high titre > 5 BU. A low-responding antibody remains at a low or moderate level, whereas in high responders, treatment with FVIII elicits a sharp anamnestic rise after 5–8 days.

Low responders can be treated repeatedly with high doses of factor VIII concentrate. However, high responders are refractory to treatment with FVIII concentrate and therefore alternative therapies have been developed.

Inhibitors – treatment of bleeding

Porcine FVIII or 'bypassing agents' may be used to treat acute haemorrhage. Plasma-derived porcine FVIII is unavailable at present and a recombinant porcine FVIII is entering clinic trial.

The most common available 'bypassing agents' are human recombinant FVIIa or plasma-derived concentrates that contain activated coagulation factors such as FEIBA and Autoplex.

Recombinant FVIIa was developed specifically as treatment for bleeding episodes in individuals with haemophilia complicated by inhibitor antibodies. Activated FVII is not proteolytically active itself and does not therefore produce systemic activation of coagulation when infused. The FVIIa complexes with tissue factor at the site of the injury and, as it is not neutralized by circulating antithrombin, infused FVIIa can reach the site of injury where it complexes with the tissue factor exposed at the site, inducing local haemostasis. The process is independent of the presence of FVIII or FIX and is not affected by inhibitors to FVIII or FIX.

Human FVIIa was cloned in the mid-1980s and was expressed in baby hamster kidney cells. The baby hamster kidney cells were capable of γ-carboxylation and the FVII is secreted in the single-chain form. The amino acid sequence has been shown to be identical to the human form.

The advantages of recombinant FVIIa include viral safety, low systemic activation of coagulation, effectiveness independent of inhibitor titre and an excellent overall safety profile allowing for home use and ease of administration. The main disadvantage is the short half-life and therefore the need for frequent administration.

The activated coagulation factors, FEIBA and Autoplex, work by activating the coagulation cascade at levels below the action of the inhibitor. Conventional factor IX concentrate (prothrombin complex concentrate) can also be used as a bypassing agent.

Treatment of inhibitors – immune tolerance

Immune tolerance regimens can be used to eradicate high-titre antibodies. It is best to allow the inhibitor to fall to a titre < 10 BU by using bypassing agents. The success is greatest in younger patients (< 7 years) and with a historic peak titre < 200 BU. At present, there is an international study comparing a dose of 50 or 200 IU/kg three times per week for 6 months. Success is defined as normalization of the FVIII recovery. The success rate using varying regimens has been reported as 70–90%.

Successful eradication of the inhibitor has also been reported with a combination regimen of cyclophosphamide, intravenous immunoglobulin, high-dose factor VIII and immunoadsorption.

Molecular genetics of haemophilia A

The factor VIII gene (Figure 49.4) spans 190-kb pairs of the X chromosome. The protein-coding regions (exons) are separated by 25 introns, some of very large size (e.g. intron 22 is over 35 kb). The processed mRNA specifies a protein of 2351 amino acids, which is synthesized in the liver, spleen and lymph nodes,

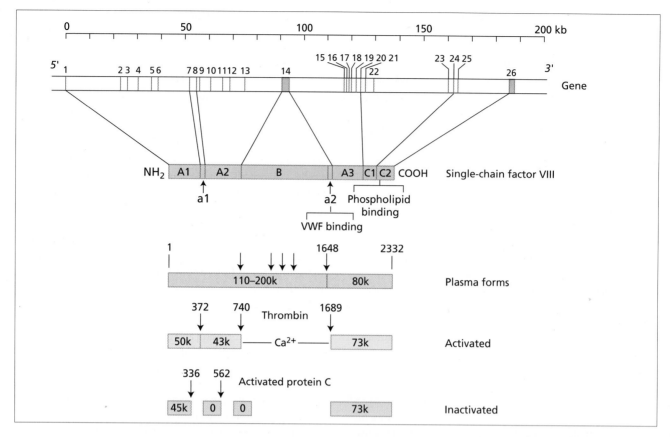

Figure 49.4 The factor VIII gene and protein. Top line, scale for gene in kilobase pairs of DNA; second line, location of exons (protein coding segments) of the factor VIII gene shown as solid bars; second to third line, corresponding domains of factor VIII gene and protein; fourth line, plasma factor VIII is heterogeneous due to cleavage at various points within the B domain during synthesis and secretion, yielding heterodimers in which the heavy chain (N-terminal segment) pairs from 740 to 1648 amino acids; fifth line, thrombin activation releases the a_2-segment from the light chain, the B domain from the heavy chain and cleaves between the A1 and A2 domains; bottom line, inactivation of factor VIIa by activated protein C is accompanied by cleavages at 336, releasing the a1-domain and 562 in the middle of the A2 domain.

and from which a 19-amino-acid N-terminal leader sequence is cleaved upon secretion. The mature plasma protein initially consists of a single chain of 2332 amino acids, but partially proteolysed derivatives are present in plasma as well. The sequence contains a triplicated region (A1, A2, A3 in Figure 49.4), whose elements are more than 30% homologous with each other and with similar regions of ceruloplasmin (the copper transport enzyme). This indicates only common ancestry, as function has diverged markedly for these two plasma proteins. A second duplicated homology region (C1, C2) bears resemblance to a lectin from the slime mould and to milk fat globule-binding protein. The third type of sequence in the protein is the heavily glycosylated B domain, which is coded entirely within exon 14, connects A2 and A3, and is removed upon thrombin activation of factor VIII. After thrombin activation, the cofactor consists of a heterotrimer: the N-terminal heavy chain corresponding to region A1, the domain isolated by cleavages at 372/373 and 740/741, which is held by a divalent cation-independent linkage

to the C-terminal light chain corresponding to part of A3 plus C1 and C2 (see Figure 49.4). The B-domain is discarded by cleavages at 740/741 and 1689/1690.

Protein C cleaves at 336/337 and 562/563, totally inactivating the cofactor. Binding to VWF is partly via the light chain, but other structure–function relationships, such as factor IXa, factor X and phospholipid binding sites, have not yet been resolved. However, quite small regions of this large protein are critical for function, as it can be totally inactivated by certain monoclonal antibodies whose binding epitopes are restricted in size. Antibodies to the B domain have no effect on function.

Thanks to the development of the PCR-based rapid screening and sequencing methods, the mutations in nearly all patients with haemophilia A can be identified. Consequently, a large database of mutations has accumulated. These include large deletions and missense mutations, as well as nonsense, frameshift splicing (affecting mRNA processing) and insertional mutations. Surprisingly, about one-half of all severe haemophilia is due to

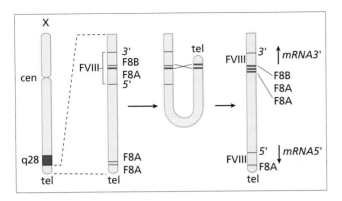

Figure 49.5 How the tip flips: the mechanism of inversion through intron 22. The mutation is responsible for up to one-half of all cases of severe haemophilia A. During spermatogenesis, at meiosis the single X pairs with the Y chromosome in the homologous regions, but there is nothing to pair with most of the long arm of X. Unfortunately, the possibility of intrachromosomal pairing and crossover exists because there are three copies of a gene designated F8A, one lying within intron 22, and two in the opposite orientation situated 400 kb telomeric to the factor VIII gene. Crossover with either the distal or the proximal F8A copy divides the factor VIII gene in two, such that separately transcribed mRNAs are produced, neither of which encodes functional factor VIII.

major inversion (Figure 49.5) that occurs quite frequently during male gametogenesis (approximately 1 in 10 000 spermatozoa).

Carriers of haemophilia A have on average 50% of the normal mean level of the clotting factor (or its antigen VIII: Ag). However, owing to the wide scatter of normal values (50–150%), an individual will often be within the normal range. By measuring the level of von Willebrand factor antigen (VWF:Ag), the autosomally coded carrier protein for factor VIII, it is possible to improve discrimination as the carriers will tend to have lower levels of VIII than VWF. Even so, there is still some overlap (about 15%) where the carriers fall into the normal ratio. This is due to the 'lyonization' effect, whereby random X inactivation can predominantly cause the X chromosome bearing the mutant allele to be inactivated. In brief, one can obtain very strong evidence for carriership by this method but never definitely rule it out.

Haemophilia A in females

True homozygous haemophilia A is rare, but well described, being due to the marriage of a carrier to an affected male, usually a cousin. Severe menstrual haemorrhage occurs but responds to factor VIII infusion. About 50% of carriers have a low enough factor VIII level to be classified as mild haemophilia, requiring precautions to cover surgery and occasionally experiencing traumatic bleeding. Due to sperm mutation in the father, especially in the prevalent inversion, a carrier can present *de novo* with no family history of haemophilia. Acquired autoantibodies

to factor VIII arise in previously normal people, sometimes in association with rheumatoid arthritis or in the puerperium. This is acquired haemophilia but has no genetic basis. Treatment resembles that described above under 'Inhibitors'. Haemophilia A has been described in a female with Turner's syndrome. Translocation through the factor VIII locus has given rise to severe haemophilia in an affected female due to exclusive inactivation of the normal X chromosome. The most usual reason for finding a low factor VIII in a female if the above has been excluded is VWD. This should usually be evident from assays of VWF and a prolonged bleeding time. Of course, VWD and haemophilia A can co-exist in the same family, which makes carrier detection difficult. Type 2N VWD (see below) may also be confused with mild haemophilia A.

Haemophilia B

Inheritance and diagnosis

Haemophilia B is an X-linked deficiency of FIX and behaves clinically like haemophilia A. FIX is responsible for the activation of FX in the presence of activated FVIII, calcium and phospholipid. FIX is synthesized in the liver and is a vitamin K-dependent protease that is similar to prothrombin, FVII, FX and protein C. The FIX protein consists of 454 amino acids. The FIX gene is contained on the long arm of the X chromosome and contains eight exons. The complete sequence of the gene has been determined. As the FIX gene is a simple gene, it has been possible to perform detailed analysis using polymerase chain reaction (PCR)-based analysis. In this way, virtually all cases of haemophilia B genetic mutations have been established. A haemophilia database is also available on the internet at http://www.unds.ac.uk/molgen/.

It is possible to perform mutational analysis to establish carriership because the complete DNA sequence of the gene is known. Isolated factor IX deficiency is always hereditary and the clinical severity of haemophilia B shows the same relationship with the residual factor level as for factor VIII in haemophilia.

Treatment

The mainstay of treatment is factor IX concentrate. Previously intermediate-purity prothrombin complex concentrates containing all the vitamin K dependent factors were used. However, these concentrates were associated with the risk of thrombosis, particularly when used repeatedly, for example in surgery. High-purity factor IX concentrates are now available, which are produced either by monoclonal antibody or improved affinity column methods. Factor IX concentrates are prepared from the same screened plasma pools as factor VIII and undergo similar viral inactivation procedures, although for FIX concentrate the process of nanofiltration has been used, which can prevent transmission of hepatitis A and parvovirus. Although the FIX gene was cloned in 1982, the development of recombinant FIX, Benefix, was more difficult because of the post-translational modification that is required. Clinical trials of the pharmacokinetics and treatment in previously treated and untreated patents were begun in 1995. Although the clinical effect was good, the recovery was only 72% of that observed with the monoclonal purified plasma-derived FIX.

Dosage calculation in the treatment of haemophilia B follows the same principles as set out for factor VIII deficiency, except that a higher initial dosage is required, owing to a lower recovery. Thus: dose to be infused (units) = [weight (kg) × increment needed (u/dL)]/0.9 or 0.8 for recombinant FIX. Also, the longer half-life (18 h) means that daily infusions often suffice to maintain good levels after surgery. Severely affected patients are usually maintained on once- or twice-weekly prophylaxis to prevent spontaneous bleeds. This is practicable because of the better supply and the longer half-life of the factor.

Gene therapy

Haemophilia is an excellent model for gene therapy because the clinical manifestation is the result of a deficiency of the single gene product and only a low amount of protein is required to ameliorate symptoms. At the present time there are three gene transfer trials in patients with haemophilia A and B, and two are ongoing (Table 49.5).

The preliminary data from these phase I trials are encouraging. However, the plasma levels of FVIII or FIX attained is less than in the animal models and is certainly insufficient to free patients from treatment with clotting factor concentrates. Also, there has been a short duration of the transgene activity. Although no inhibitors have been documented, this remains a theoretical risk. Furthermore, the detection of small amounts of viral vector genome in the semen continues to raise the possibility of the risk of germline integration. Insertional mutagenesis has occurred in a phase I trial of Moloney retrovirus carrying

Table 49.5 Clinical trials of gene therapy in patients with haemophilia.

Company	Started	Type of haemophilia	Vector and method of gene transfer	Safety	Efficacy	Current status
Transkaryotic therapies	November 1998	A	Non-viral plasmid DNA/ex vivo, modification of autologous fibroblasts	No inhibitor	FVIII levels up to 4% transiently in 4 out of 12 subjects; reduced factor requirement	Completed and published; phase II trial starting soon
Avigen	June 1999	B	Adeno-associated virus/in vivo, intramuscular	No Inhibitor	FIX levels up to 1.6% transiently in 3 out of 8 subjects; reduced factor requirement	Completed and published
Chiron	June 1999	A	Replication – deficient retrovirus/in vivo, intravenous	No inhibitor; transient positive semen signal in one patient	FVIII levels up to 6.1% transiently in 6 out of 12 subjects or 5 more days after replacement therapy	Completed and published
GenStar	June 2001	A	'Gutted' adenovirus driven to liver-specific expression/in vivo, intravenous	First patient had abnormalities of transaminases thrombocytopenia and inflammatory symptoms	FVIII levels 1%	Second patient started on trial with a lower dose
Avigen	June 2001	B	Adeno-associated virus driven to liver-specific expression through hepatic artery infusion	Positive semen signals in the first three patients	No FIX levels with the low dose, data not available for mid-dose	Trial on hold

From Mannuccio (2003), with permission.

the interleukin receptor, and this has been a cause for concern for all of those involved in gene therapy.

The ethics of gene therapy for haemophilia are complex – it could be argued that for young patients with haemophilia, regular prophylactic factor infusions already deliver a near-normal life. The financing of a genetic 'cure' for haemophilia is another complicating concern. The money spent at present buys viral safety, musculoskeletal and surgical prophylaxis, inhibitor eradication and rapid treatment for acute bleeding for the haemophilia community. Gene transfer experimentation in haemophilia has played an integral role in furthering the science of gene therapy in general but it is likely to be a long time before it becomes the routine therapy for children with haemophilia.

General organization of haemophilia care

As these are relatively uncommon disorders, with many and varied effects on patients and families at all stages of life, who require care and support services across the whole field of medicine and social services, it is now accepted that this care can best be delivered comprehensively by referral centres. The staff of a major comprehensive care centre will include physicians, nurses, social workers, laboratory scientists and physiotherapists, devoting all or a substantial part of their time to haemophilia care. An orthopaedic surgeon prepared to see haemophilic patients regularly in a clinic set aside for their problems is a vital addition to this team. In the UK, there is now a national service specification produced by the Haemophilia Alliance for haemophilia and related conditions, which sets out the standards of care to be provided through the haemophilia centre network originally set up in the 1960s and early 1970s. It is recognized that not every centre can provide every facility and that there should be a fairly wide distribution according to population density, which determines numbers of patients. As defined by the national specification, the functions of a centre are to provide a 24-h emergency treatment for the haemophilic patients and their families and a full range of diagnostic tests for identifying new patients and monitoring treatment. Full records should be kept of all treatments, whether given in hospital or as home therapy. Progress should be monitored through regular follow-up, with paediatric, dental and orthopaedic referrals being organized by the centre as necessary. (Many centres are, in fact, in paediatric departments or run by paediatricians.) Genetic counselling, including carrier detection and antenatal diagnosis, must be available for families of haemophilic patients. Large centres providing all these facilities and treating at least 40 patients with severe haemophilia will be designated comprehensive care centres. It is envisaged that all patients will have access to a comprehensive care centre, either directly or via their smaller local centre. A part- or full-time social worker should be part of the team, able to review the wider problems of living that affect the haemophilic patient at school, home and work.

Centres provide access to specialized care for monitoring patients with HIV and HCV infection. Upon diagnosis, all patients are issued with a special medical card indicating laboratory test results, inhibitor status, main centre and local centre for treatment.

Caring for haemophilic patients and their families is demanding, but rewarding. Until the recent setbacks, the trend has been towards an ever-improving life expectancy and social participation, based on continuing medical progress and the skill and devotion of many professionals. It is both tragic and ironic that the main foundation upon which this progress rested (factor concentrate) has also been the route in which life-threatening infections have been introduced to about one-half of the most severely affected patients with haemophilia A. However, there are now excellent therapies for both HIV and HCV infection.

Of course, the younger generation of haemophiliacs are now treated with virus-safe concentrates and have escaped both HIV and liver disease, and lead virtually normal lives.

von Willebrand disease

Although described in 1926, our understanding of this complex and variable bleeding disorder continues to grow. The basic defect common to all variants is a deficiency of von Willebrand factor (VWF) functional activity. The abnormality may be quantitative and/or qualitative. VWF is encoded by a gene on chromosome 12, which was cloned simultaneously by several groups. The primary gene product is an extremely long protein monomer comprising 2813 amino acids. This is produced predominantly in vascular endothelial cells, but also in megakaryocytes, and undergoes a series of post-translational modifications. Dimers are formed and a very large propeptide is excised. The propeptide, previously known as von Willebrand antigen II, is detectable in plasma and it is essential for dimer formation. Dimers are then assembled into tetramers, which then further polymerize to form a series of multimers with molecular weights ranging from 1×10^6 to 20×10^6 Da.

The assembled VWF multimers may then either be released at a steady rate from the endothelial cells (constitutive pathway) or stored prior to release in the Weibel–Palade bodies of endothelial cells (regulated pathway). Platelet VWF does not contribute significantly to plasma VWF and is stored in the α-granules of platelets prior to release after platelet activation.

Rapid release of VWF from endothelial storage sites can be induced by epinephrine, histamine and vasopressin via the regulated pathway. This effect can be used to advantage by using DDAVP to treat mild forms of von Willebrand disease (VWD). Chronic elevation of VWF due to increased synthesis occurs as part of the 'acute phase' response to injury, inflammation, infection and neoplasia, and in pregnancy and hyperthyroidism. These responses are presumed to be physiological in promoting enhanced haemostasis but can reach pathological expression in being associated with an increased risk of thrombosis. These

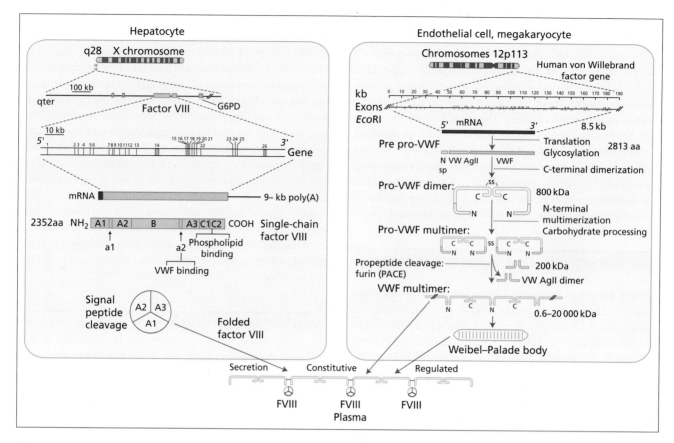

Figure 49.6 Assembly of factor VIII–VWF complex. Factor VIII synthesized by hepatocytes as a single chain is partially proteolysed and (possibly) complexed with VWF prior to release. The von Willebrand factor is synthesized as a single-chain precursor, which dimerizes with disulphide bond formation, then multimerizes with further disulphide exchange, with concomitant loss of a large propeptide segment. The propeptide is essential for multimer formation and probably functions as an acidic disulphide isomerase.

confounding effects need to be taken into account when measuring VWF levels in attempting to diagnose VWD.

The VWF in plasma is detectable immunologically as VWF:Ag. This was formerly called factor VIII-related antigen, owing to confusion about the composition of the factor VIII–VWF complex. Although factor VIII and VWF are entirely distinct entities with separate functions (Figure 49.6), they circulate together as a complex in which VWF protects factor VIII from degradation, so that a deficiency of VWF or a reduction in its ability to bind factor VIII may also result in a low plasma level of factor VIII. Therefore, a deficiency of VWF can give rise to a dual haemostatic defect: reduced plasma levels of factor VIII (due to its shorter half-life in the absence of VWF) and a defect in primary haemostasis due to the failure in assisting platelets to adhere to the cut edges of small blood vessels (see Chapter 47). Clearly, the multistep synthesis, assembly and secretion of VWF and its multiple binding interactions provide many ways in which mutations of the VWF gene can give rise to varying types of disease. In particular, the multimeric structure is susceptible to dominant-negative effects of mutant alleles. The diagnosis of

VWD is based on the recognition that for normal VWF function it must be:

1 present in adequate amounts;
2 have a normal multimeric structure;
3 have intact functional domains (binding sites).

When any of these properties is only slightly reduced, the presence or absence of a bleeding tendency may also depend on the quality and quantity of the other components, particularly platelets and collagen, with which the VWF must interact.

Clinical features

The classical picture is of an autosomal dominant, mild to moderately severe bleeding tendency. Patients suffer from bruising, epistaxes, prolonged bleeding from minor cuts, menorrhagia and excessive, but not often life-threatening, bleeding after trauma or surgery. Patients often present for investigation in the second or third decade after prolonged bleeding from dental extraction has aroused clinical suspicion. Menorrhagia, inexplicable by local or hormonal factors, can also be the presenting symptom. An estimated 20% of women with menorrhagia have VWD. Haemarthroses do not occur in typical mild dominant VWD. Much less common is autosomal recessive (type 3) VWD, where VWF is undetectable and FVIII:C levels are usually around 1 or 2 U/dL. These patients have a bleeding tendency that clinically resembles severe haemophilia A, with haemarthroses, muscle bleeds and life-threatening haemorrhage after trauma, as well as a proneness to small vessel bleeding, which is not a feature of haemophilia A. The distribution of bleeding in VWD can be explained on the basis that VWF is required for platelet adhesion at high shear rate, which is the condition of flow found in the smallest blood vessels exposed to trauma in skin and mucous membranes.

Laboratory diagnosis

Preliminary diagnosis

After obtaining a suggestive personal history and a family history, the preliminary tests required are a full blood count and a coagulation screen. In addition, a global measure of primary haemostasis is also useful. Traditionally this was provided by the template bleeding time but this has a poor sensitivity for VWD and has largely been replaced by devices such as the PFA-100. The PFA-100 has very good sensitivity for VWD, although obviously does not distinguish it from platelet disorders and will not detect collagen abnormalities. Repeatedly normal PFA-100 results makes a platelet–VWF disorder of primary haemostasis unlikely.

The laboratory diagnosis of VWD rests on assessing both the amount of VWF present (VWF:Ag) and its functional capacity. At present, it is possible to assess three important functions:
1 *Factor VIII binding.* Assessed first by a factor VIII assay and then if reduced, by an enzyme-linked immunosorbent assay (ELISA)-based assay of VWF FVIII binding capacity.

2 *Platelet-dependent function.* The standard assessment of VWF functional activity remains the ristocetin cofactor assay (VWF:Rco). In this assay, dilutions of patient plasma are tested for their ability to promote platelet agglutination in the presence of the antibiotic ristocetin.
3 *Collagen-binding function* (VWF:CB). This recently introduced measurement is performed in an ELISA-based assay in which a well coated with collagen is used to capture VWF.

Measures of VWF:Rco and VWF:CB are both sensitive to the loss of high-molecular-weight multimers (HMWMs), but measure different binding properties of VWF. Thus they should be seen as complementary rather than alternative assays.

When there is a clear bleeding history and factor VIII, VWF:Ag, VWF:RCo are all below 30 U/dL, and the platelet count is normal, the diagnosis is easily made (Table 49.6). Unfortunately, owing to the variability of the disease and varying levels of VWF release or synthesis in individuals over time, all of these tests can give normal results on some occasions but clearly abnormal results on others. This is especially true of the milder cases of type 1 VWF (see below). It is therefore necessary to perform carefully standardized sets of assays with concordant results on at least two occasions to be sure of the diagnosis and its severity.

Secondary classification

If a deficiency suggestive of VWD is detected then further tests, in particular multimeric analysis and ristocetin-induced platelet aggregation (RIPA) are recommended to allow accurate subtyping of the VWD. The most important of these is VWF multimer size analysis, which will demonstrate the distribution of VWF polymers and the pattern of flanking bands (Figure 49.7) adjacent to the main multimer bands. Tables 49.6a and b list the main variants into which cases can be divided according to the tests described above.

Table 49.6(a) Primary classification of VWD.

Subclassification	Type of VWF deficiency	VWF protein function
Type 1	Quantitative partial deficiency	Normal
Type 2	Qualitative functional deficiency	Abnormal
Type 3	Quantitative complete deficiency	Undetectable

Table 49.6(b) Secondary classification of type 2 VWD.

Subtype	Platelet-associated function	Factor VIII binding capacity	HMW VWF multimers
2A	Decreased	Normal	Absent
2B	Increased affinity for Gplb	Normal	Usually reduced/absent
2M	Decreased	Normal	Normal and occasionally ultralarge forms
2N	Normal	Markedly reduced	Normal

From Laffan (2004), with permission.

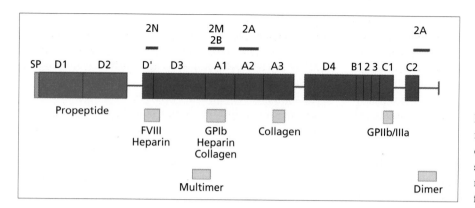

Figure 49.7 Distribution of mutations responsible for type 2 VWD. The domain structure of the monomer is shown and the regions in which the mutations cluster in relation to the functional domains of the molecule.

In type 1 VWD there is a simple quantitative deficiency of VWF, which is assessed as having normal functional activity. In this case, the VWF:Ag, VWF:Rco and (if measured) VWF:CB are all concordant and the multimer distribution is normal.

The characteristic of the types 2A, 2B and 2M variants is a functional deficiency of VWF activity, which is reduced to < 0.7 of the antigenic measure. In type 2A, this arises from a lack of high- and intermediate-size VWF multimers, whereas in type 2M a similar loss of platelet binding activity is seen despite the presence of normal VWF multimeric composition. Type 2A may arise from intracellular retention of large multimers or accelerated proteolysis in the circulation. In type 2B, there is excessive response to ristocetin at low concentration (0.5 mg/mL) in the patient's stirred platelet-rich plasma (RIPA). If normal washed platelets are resuspended in the patient's plasma, the phenomenon is reproduced, demonstrating that the abnormality is in the plasma. Studies with purified type 2B VWF show that it binds directly to platelets without prior activation (unlike normal VWF). This evidently results in the loss of high-molecular-weight multimers and platelets from the circulation due to *in vivo* formation of platelet aggregates. Thus routine platelet aggregation studies with a range of ristocetin dosages should be performed as part of the diagnostic work-up, as it is important to detect this variant (see below), which does not always show up in the other tests. Mutations causing types 2M and 2B affect the binding site for platelet glycoprotein Ib on VWF and are found within the A2 domain of the molecule.

The majority of patients are found to be type 1, which accounts for 75% of kindreds. Types 2A and 2B are fairly common, together amounting to about 15% of kindreds.

A fourth type 2 variant, called type 2N (for Normandy), has been described. This is characterized by a reduced affinity for factor VIII but it is normal in all other respects. Thus, laboratory investigations reveal only a reduced factor VIII level (15–35%), which is easily mistaken for mild haemophilia. A clue to the correct diagnosis may come from the family history, and confirmation requires an assay of VWF factor VIII binding capacity. Type 2A may be dominant or recessive. Type 2B is inherited

dominantly, whereas types 3 and 2N are recessive. Type 3 cases are more common in cultures in which intermarriage is usual, such as in the Middle East.

Table 49.7 Influence of ABO blood group on VWF:Ag values in volunteer blood donors.

ABO type	n	VWF:Ag geometric mean	VWF:Ag geometric mean ± 2SD
O	456	74.8	35.6–157.0
A	340	105.9	48.0–233.9
B	196	116.9	56.8–241.0
AB	109	123.3	63.8–238.2

Note the significantly lower levels in donors of blood group O compared with the non-O donors.
Reproduced from Gill *et al.* (1987), with permission.

Problems in diagnosis of type 1 von Willebrand disease

The diagnosis of type 1 VWD implies that the patient has a significantly low level of VWF, which is responsible for an increased tendency to bleeding. It is often not easy to be certain of this conclusion for the following reasons.

1 Slightly low levels of VWF are common in the population. There are probably many reasons for this, some lying outside the VWF gene itself. For example, a major modifier of plasma VWF concentration is ABO blood group. Individuals with blood group O have VWF levels 25–30% lower than those with non-O groups (Table 49.7). This probably contributes to the observation that group O is over-represented in the VWD type 1 group, but on the other hand many people with VWF levels in the range of 30–50 IU/dL do not bleed excessively.

2 A history of minor bleeding episodes (e.g. easy bruising, epistaxes) is also very common in the population and is not a good predictor of bleeding in other circumstances such as operations. Equally, the patient may not yet have been exposed to a significant test of haemostasis.

3 As a result of the two points above, a history of (say) easy bruising and slightly low VWF levels will often be found together. This does not however mean that the patient has VWD and caution should be exercised in drawing this conclusion as it has many consequences for the patient.

4 Intercurrent events such as stress, exercise, illness and pregnancy may all elevate the VWF level, making it difficult to be certain a representative picture has been obtained.

5 The family history is often unhelpful, particularly in mild cases where penetrance is weak or variable. This is probably the result of the modifying effects alluded to in (1) above. It is now evident that in some families VWD does not segregate with the VWF gene.

6 Finally, review of many cases previously diagnosed as type 1 VWD has concluded that many are in fact better categorized as type 2M after better assessment of the VWF antigen–activity ratio.

It has been suggested recently that in recognition of the large 'grey area' between normal and VWD, low levels of VWF between 0.2 and normal should be regarded as a 'risk factor' for bleeding rather than a bleeding disease itself.

Treatment

Patients with mild or moderate VWD attend infrequently for treatment. The first-line treatment for minor bleeding after local measures have failed in type 1 VWD is DDAVP. This will produce a brisk (30 min after intravenous infusion) rise in VWF and factor VIII levels and a shortening of the bleeding time (for details of therapy, see discussion under Mild haemophilia A). DDAVP is much less effective in types 2A and 2M, presumably because the patient's released VWF is highly abnormal and still unable to promote platelet adhesion. DDAVP is generally regarded as contraindicated in 2B VWD, as the released abnormal VWF will cause circulatory platelet aggregates to form, with a further fall in the platelet count, but it has been used successfully without ill effects. A therapeutic trial may be worthwhile in type 2A as some families do respond. In 2N, the factor VIII response is of normal magnitude, but is ineffective due to its short duration, emphasizing the importance of making the correct diagnosis. DDAVP is best avoided in small children (< 2 years) as there is a risk of hyponatraemia and consequent seizures. It is also contraindicated in elderly patients or those with arterial disease as there is a risk of arterial thrombosis. DDAVP therapy is often combined with tranexamic acid. However, tranexamic acid may be effective on its own in some circumstances such as menorrhagia or as a mouthwash for oral cavity bleeding.

In patients in whom DDAVP is ineffective or contraindicated, the next line of treatment is a concentrate containing adequate amounts of functionally active VWF with preservation of the high-molecular-weight multimers. As with all concentrates, the source of plasma and viral inactivation are also im-portant. Recombinant VWF concentrate is not yet available. Cryoprecipitate has been used in these circumstances but cannot be subjected to viral inactivation procedures and is therefore not recommended as first-line therapy. Factor concentrates will always be required for treatment of type 3. Depending on the responses obtained with DDAVP, the duration of treatment and the presence of other contraindications, they may also be required in other type 2 and type 1 variants. Factor VIII concentrates vary considerably in the amount of VWF they contain and in the extent to which this is degraded or remains in functionally active HMWMs. Those that contain significant amounts of VWF are often referred to as intermediate purity. A high-purity VWF concentrate is now available and is also capable of correcting the defect. It is important to remember that following infusion of high-purity VWF there is a delay of approximately 12 h before the level of factor VIII rises substantially and, if rapid correction is required, factor VIII concentrate should also be given. In general, none of these replacement treatments is reliable in correcting the bleeding time, but this is not necessarily a bar to effective haemostasis. This seemingly paradoxical result may be because they do not correct the deficiency of intraplatelet VWF or because the largest HMWMs are not present. In situations when concentrates fail to stop bleeding, cryoprecipitate and platelet concentrates may prove effective.

Clinical course and complications

Types 1 and 2 VWD patients lead relatively normal lives, with normal life expectancy. Menstruation is seldom a cause of severe blood loss, although menorrhagia is common. This can usually be managed satisfactorily with antifibrinolytics or by oral contraceptive oestrogen/progesterone combinations. If these are not effective then self-administration at home of DDAVP by intranasal or subcutaneous routes can be useful. In later years, some patients require hysterectomy. During pregnancy, the VWF levels rise spontaneously to the normal or low-normal range in all but the severely affected patients. Patients with severe type 3 disease have a clinical course resembling severe or moderately severe haemophilia A, including the development of joint damage. Some of the patients with type 3 disease develop antibodies to VWF, which inhibit its platelet adhesion-promoting property and cause rapid removal from the circulation of infused material. Unlike antifactor VIII antibodies, some anti-VWF antibodies may mediate anaphylactic shock.

Molecular genetics

The cloning of VWF cDNA and its gene has led to progress in identifying the underlying mutations responsible for the various phenotypes (Figure 49.8). As with the factor VIII gene, the sheer size of the DNA region involved presents some problems of localization, but these are being overcome by powerful screening methods. A database of mutations responsible for VWD has

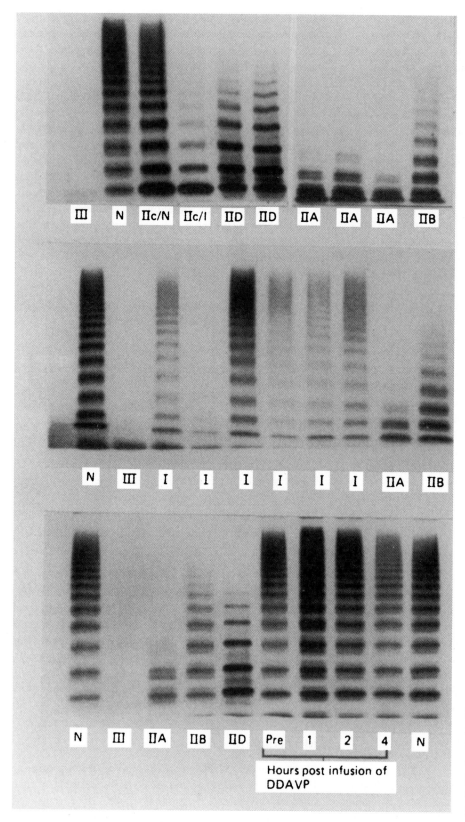

Figure 49.8 Multimer analysis of VWF from patients with VWD and normal control subjects. Note that many cases classified at present as type 2A were previously subdivided according to the details of the abnormality of triplet pattern.

been established at http://www.shef.ac.uk/vwf/vwd.html. The rare patients who develop antibodies to VWF nearly all have large deletions of their VWF gene. Exon 28 has been found to harbour all the mutations giving rise to types 2A, 2M and 2B VWD. The molecular basis of type 1 VWD remains elusive and is rarely due to a simple heterozygote null mutation, but an increasing number of putatively causative missense mutations are being identified. As well as intragenic polymorphisms, the plasma level of VWF is modulated by many factors outside the gene and it has been shown recently that some cases of VWD do not segregate with the VWF gene at all.

Pseudo von Willebrand disease (platelet-type)

Several families have been described with a disorder closely resembling type 2B VWD, but in whom mixing experiments show the defect to be in their platelets rather than their plasma. Patients with pseudo VWD have moderately reduced levels of VWF:Ag and platelets, with an enhanced response of their platelet-rich plasma to low levels of ristocetin (0.5 mg/mL). The addition of normal cryoprecipitate to their washed platelets causes spontaneous aggregation, whereas the reverse experiment is without effect (compare with type 2B). Missense mutations in platelet membrane GPIb, such that it spontaneously binds higher multimers of VWF, have been shown to be the underlying cause of this autosomally dominant mild bleeding syndrome. Treatment has not been extensively evaluated, but it should probably be with normal platelet concentrates, rather than DDAVP or cryoprecipitate. Thus this syndrome should be excluded before diagnosing type 2B VWD.

Selected bibliography

Rodriguez-Mercham EC, Lee CA (2003) *Inhibitors in Patients with Haemophilia*. Blackwell.

Escobar MA (2003) Treatment on demand – *in vivo* dose finding studies. *Haemophilia* 9: 360–7.

Evan J (2003) Sadler Von Willebrand disease type 1: a diagnosis in search of a disease. *Blood* 101: 2089–93.

Gill J, Endres-Brooks PJ, Bauer WJ *et al.* (1987) The effect of ABO blood group on the diagnosis of von Willebrand disease. *Blood* 69: 1691–5.

Haemophilia A Database (http://europium.csc.mrc.ac.uk/)

Haemophilia Alliance. A national service specification for haemophilia and related conditions (www.haemophiliaalliance.org.uk)

Haemophilia B Database (http://www.unds.ac.uk/molgen/)

Hay CR, Colvin BT, Ludlam CA *et al.* (1996) Recommendations for the treatment of factor VIII inhibitors: from the UK Haemophilia Centre Directors' Organisation Inhibitor Working Party. *Blood Coagulation and Fibrinolysis* 72: 134–8.

Laffan MA, Brown SA, Collins PW *et al.* (2004) The diagnosis of von Willebrand disease. A guideline from the UK Haemophilia Centre Doctors' Organisation. *Haemophilia* 10: 199–217.

Lee C, Owens D, Giangrande P *et al.* (1999) Assay discrepancies in recovery level of rFVIII 'Recombinate'. *Blood* 92 (Suppl.10): 354a.

Mannucci PM (2001) How I treat patients with von Willebrand disease. *Blood* 97: 1915–19.

Mannucci PM (2003) Haemophilia: treatment options in the twenty-first century. *Journal of Thrombosis and Haemostasis* 1: 1349–55.

Mikaelsson M, Oswaldsson U, Sandberg H (1998) Influence of phospholipids on the assessment of factor VIII activity. *Haemophilia* 4: 646–50.

NHS Management Executive (1993) *Health Service Guidelines: Provision of Haemophilia Treatment and Care*. (HSG(93)30). BAPS, Heywood.

Pasi KJ, Collins PW, Keeling D *et al.* (2004) Management of von Willebrand disease. A guideline from the UK Haemophilia Centre Doctor's Organisation. *Haemophilia* 10: 218–31.

UKHCDO (2003) Guidelines on the selection and use of therapeutic products to treat haemophilia and other hereditary bleeding disorders. *Haemophilia* 9: 1–23.

Von Willebrand Disease Database (http://www.shef.ac.uk/vwf/vwd.html)

CHAPTER 50

Congenital bleeding: autosomal recessive disorders

50

Flora Peyvandi and Pier M Mannucci

Introduction

The most frequent inherited coagulation disorders are haemophilia A and B, due to the deficiency of factor VIII and IX. Haemophilia A and B are clinically indistinguishable from each other and occur in mild, moderate and severe forms (with plasma factor levels of 6–30%, 2–5% and 1% or less respectively). Inherited as X-linked traits, haemophilia A and B are prevalent in the general population of approximately 1 in 10 000 and 1 in 50 000, with no significant racial difference. Other deficiencies of coagulation factors that cause a bleeding disorder, such as afibrinogenaemia, hypoprothrombinaemia, deficiencies of factors V and combined factor V and VIII, VII, X, XI and XIII are inherited as autosomal recessive traits and are generally much rarer than the haemophilias, with are prevalent in the general population varying between 1 in 500 000 and 1 in 2 000 000 (Table 50.1). As a consequence of the rarity of these deficiencies, which are expressed clinically only in homozygotes or compound heterozygotes, the type and severity of symptoms, the underlying molecular defects and the actual management of bleeding episodes are not well established as for haemophilia A and B.

In countries where consanguineous marriages are frequent, such as Muslim countries and southern India, recessively inherited coagulation deficiencies are more frequent and together reach prevalences higher than those of haemophilia B, representing a significant clinical and social problem. Table 50.2 compares the relative frequencies of patients with clinically significant deficiencies (factor levels of 10% or less) registered in

the Islamic Republic of Iran with those registered in the UK by the Haemophilia Centre Doctors' Organisation (UKHCDO) and in Italy by the Istituto Superiore di Sanità and the Associazione Italiana Centri Emofilia (AICE). The three countries are compatible because they have compatible general populations of approximately 60 million and comprehensive registries of coagulopathies. Inherited deficiencies of fibrinogen, prothrombin, factor V, factor VII, factor V plus VIII, factor X and factor XIII are three to seven times more frequent in Iran (see Table 50.2). Only factor XI deficiency is more frequent in the UK than in Iran and Italy, probably because communities of Ashkenazi Jews, in which this deficiency is highly prevalent, are relatively small in the last two countries.

In the last few years, the number of patients with recessively inherited coagulation deficiencies has been increasing in European countries with a high rate of immigration of populations from the Middle East, India, Pakistan and North Africa. This situation underlies the importance of improved knowledge of these disorders by the general haematologist. The purpose of this chapter is to review the disorders in terms of clinical manifestations and characterization of the molecular defects. The general principles of management will also be discussed.

Fibrinogen deficiency

Fibrinogen deficiency is heterogeneous and two main phenotypes can be distinguished. In afibrinogenaemia, plasma and platelet levels of the protein are unmeasurable or very low when

Table 50.1 General features of autosomal recessively transmitted deficiency of coagulation factors.

Deficiency	Estimated prevalence*	Gene on chromosome
Fibrinogen	1:1 000 000	4
Prothrombin	1:2 000 000	11
Factor V	1:1 000 000	1
Combined factor V + VIII	1:1 000 000	18 (LMAN1), 2 (MCFD2)
Factor VII	1:500 000	13
Factor X	1:1 000 000	13
Factor XI	1:1 000 000	4
Factor XIII	1:2 000 000	6 (subunit A) and 1 (subunit B)

*Including dysfunctional proteins.

Table 50.2 Number of patients and relative frequency (in parentheses) of inherited coagulation deficiencies in Iran, Italy and UK (excluding von Willebrand disease).

Defect	Iran	Italy	UK
Fibrinogen	70 (1.5%)	10 (0.2%)	11 (0.2%)
Prothrombin	15 (0.3%)	7 (0.02%)	1 (0.02%)
Factor V	70 (1.5%)	21 (0.5%)	28 (0.6%)
Factor VII	300 (6.6%)	58 (1.3%)	62 (1.3%)
Factor V + VIII	80 (1.7%)	29 (0.7%)	18 (0.3%)
Factor VIII (haemophilia A)	3000 (65.4%)	3428 (80%)	3554 (76.8%)
Factor IX (haemophilia B)	900 (19.6%)	626 (15.0%)	762 (16.1%)
Factor X	60 (1.3%)	16 (0.4%)	25 (0.5%)
Factor XI	20 (0.4%)	60 (1.3%)	150 (3.3%)
Factor XIII	80 (1.7%)	31 (0.7%)	26 (0.5%)
All defects	4595	4286	4637

Data are obtained from the most recent adjournments of the Registries of Inherited Bleeding Disorders kept in Iran (courtesy of Dr M Lak, Iman Khomeini Hospital), Italy (Dr A Ghirardini, Istituto Superiore di Sanità) and UK (Dr P Giangrande, UK Haemophilia Centre Doctors' Organisation). Only patients with factor levels of 10% or less were evaluated.

using assays that measure clottable and immunoreactive protein, whereas in dysfibrinogenaemia low clottable fibrinogen contrasts with normal or moderately reduced fibrinogen antigen. Three separate genes clustered on chromosome 4 code for the Aα-, Bβ- and γ-chains of fibrinogen. Experimental disruption of the α-chain gene makes mice completely deficient in all the fibrinogen chains. There is no evidence of defective embryonal development but overt bleeding develops at birth in about one-third of these animals, most frequently in the peritoneal cavity, skin and joints. Ultimately, blood loss is controlled, so that most mice survive the neonatal period and reach adulthood despite recurrent bleeding episodes and failure to become pregnant.

Clinical manifestations

Whereas the majority of patients with dysfibrinogenaemia do not bleed at all, afibrinogenaemic patients have a bleeding tendency. Among severe bleeding symptoms that are dangerous for life and for the musculoskeletal function, umbilical cord and joint bleeding is relatively frequent (in 75% and 50% of patients), whereas muscle haematomas and bleeding in the gastrointestinal tract and central nervous system are less common. Milder symptoms such as epistaxis and menorrhagia are also frequent. Post-partum bleeding occurs when no prophylactic replacement therapy is given. Excessive blood loss and impaired wound healing in about one-third of the patients often accompany circumcision and other surgical manoeuvres. There is no increased prevalence of recurrent miscarriages. Central nervous system bleeding is rare.

On the whole, bleeding problems are not dramatic in patients with afibrinogenaemia, particularly if one considers that screening coagulation tests (prothrombin time, APTT) are usually incoagulable and that the bleeding time is often prolonged. The relatively mild clinical manifestations of afibrinogenaemia are consistent with those of the gene knockout mouse model, except that pregnancy failure is not apparent. Severe thrombotic episodes are perhaps explained by the intravascular formation of platelet aggregates due to the increased generation of thrombin unimpeded by fibrin formation.

Molecular defects

The three separate genes encoding Aα-fibrinogen (FGA), Bβ-fibrinogen (FBG) and γ-fibrinogen (FGG) are clustered in a region of approximately 50 kilobases (kb) on human chromosome 4. Neerman-Arbez and colleagues were the first to identify a homozygous deletion of approximately 11 kb of the FGA gene as a cause of inherited afibrinogenaemia in four members of a Swiss family. The mutation was associated with three different haplotypes and therefore probably occurred independently. Subsequently, two homozygous missense mutations were identified in the FGB gene in two families of different ethnic background (one Italian and one Iranian), both leading to a deficient secretion of the protein. Neerman-Arbez and colleagues found another mutation in the FGA gene in patients from France, Belgium and USA, which recurred in multiple discrete haplotypes, a donor splice mutation in intron 4 (IVS4+1 G → T). The relatively high number of mutations identified in the FGA gene led to the hypothesis that mutations tend to cluster in this gene, resulting in the production of no fibrinogen Aα-chain at all or of a severely truncated protein. Nonsense mutations, mutations affecting splice sites, and a 1-bp deletion were also identified in the FGG gene, whereas two missense, two splicing and two nonsense mutations were found in the FGB gene.

A missense mutation (Leu172Gln) was identified in the FGB gene, which, following *in vitro* expression, was demonstrated to cause a splicing defect rather than having an effect at the protein level. Therefore, all three fibrinogen genes are involved in causing afibrinogenaemia, confirming the importance to screen the whole fibrinogen cluster for mutations in affected patients. It is also apparent that even if mutations leading to severe truncation of fibrinogen chains are prevalent, missense mutations are not rare. Figure 50.1 shows the mutations associated with afibrinogenaemia identified so far.

Prothrombin deficiency

Even though prothrombin deficiency is reported to have a prevalence of 1 in 1 000 000, according to the number of cases described in the literature and those listed in the Iranian registry, this defect appears to be even less common (perhaps 1 in 2 000 000). Measuring plasma levels of prothrombin as functional activity or immunoreactive protein, two main phenotypes can be distinguished: hypoprothrombinaemia, characterized by concomitantly low levels of activity and antigen; and dysprothrombinaemia, characterized by the normal synthesis of a dysfunctional protein (low coagulant activity but normal or borderline antigen levels). To our knowledge no living patient with undetectable plasma prothrombin has been reported so far (see below), consistently with the demonstration that in mice complete prothrombin deficiency obtained by gene knockout is incompatible with life.

Clinical manifestations

In a series of 14 patients from Iran and Italy (11 had hypoprothrombinaemia, with levels varying between 4% and 13%, three had dysprothrombinaemia), the most frequent severe symptoms were haemarthroses and muscle haematomas, which, in a few patients, caused chronic arthropathy despite detectable levels of prothrombin in plasma. There were only two cases of gastrointestinal bleeding and one of intracranial bleeding that required prolonged hospital admission and replacement therapy. Life-endangering umbilical cord bleeding also occurred in two newborns. Epistaxis and menorrhagia were frequent but not severe. There was no case of post-partum bleeding, and dental extractions and circumcision were usually accompanied by excessive bleeding when carried out without replacement therapy.

Molecular defects

A gene of approximately 21 kb located on chromosome 11 and containing 14 exons encodes prothrombin. At the moment, 34 different mutations have been identified in prothrombin deficiency (Figure 50.2). In dysprothrombinaemia, all are missense mutations, 15 of them being homozygous and involving amino acid substitutions within the site of cleavage by factor Xa or within the serine protease domain. Even though mutations are scattered throughout the serine protease domain, many of them surround the catalytic triad, consistently with the fact that they affect the enzymatic activity of the protein. So far few functional studies have been performed to elucidate the structure–function relationship.

In a recent study, the experimental data showed that both procoagulant and anticoagulant functions are impaired in a recombinant FII-Arg67His mutant; the functional abnormalities might somewhat counterbalance each other so that ultimately the haemostatic equilibrium does not undergo drastic changes, explaining the very mild clinical phenotype associated with the case reported in the study. In total, 17 mutations have been identified in patients with hypoprothrombinaemia, six of which in the homozygous state. The majority are missense mutations, but there are also five nonsense mutations leading to stop codons, with one single and one double nucleotide deletion leading in both conditions to a premature stop codon.

Factor V deficiency

The majority of cases are phenotypically characterized by the concomitant deficiency of factor V activity and antigen (type I deficiency), but approximately one-quarter have normal antigen levels (type II deficiency), indicating the presence of a dysfunctional protein. The experimental deficiency of factor V in gene knockout mice leads to defective embryonic development and

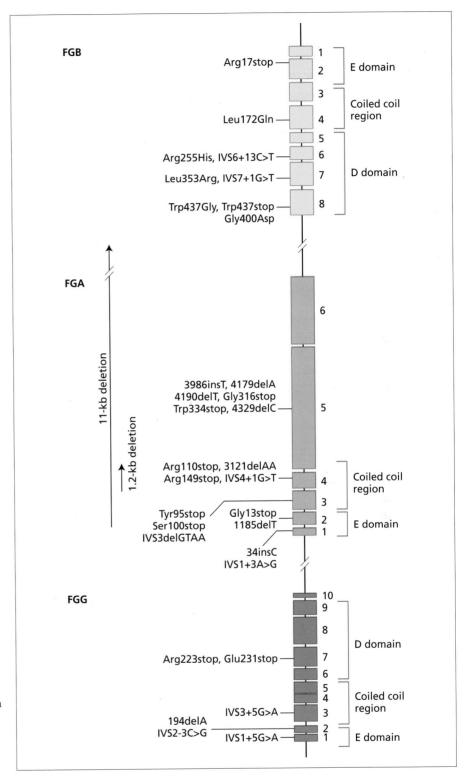

Figure 50.1 Mutations in the fibrinogen gene projected on the exons encoding the protein chains (FGA, FGB, FGG). Exons (rectangles) are drawn to scale, whereas introns (lines) are not to scale.

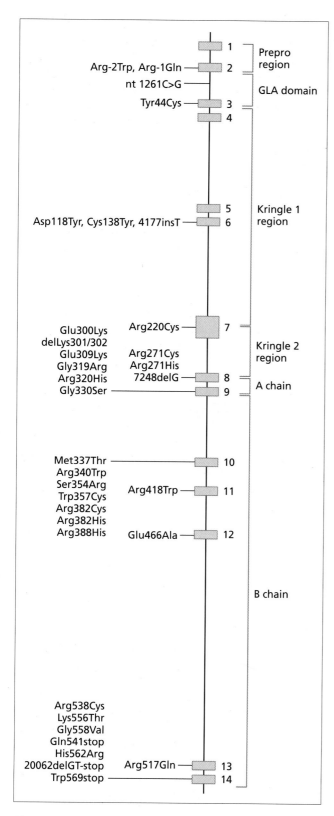

Figure 50.2 Mutations in the prothrombin gene, projected on the exons encoding the domains of the protein. Exons (rectangles) and introns (lines) are drawn to scale.

early haemorrhagic death. However, mice expressing minimal factor V activity below the sensitivity threshold of the detection assay (< 0.1%) differ from the complete knockout mice because they survive.

Clinical manifestations

In a large series of Iranian patients, bleeding symptoms usually developed during the first 6 years of life, but only one patient bled from the umbilical stump. Epistaxis and menorrhagia were relatively frequent, even in patients with measurable factor V levels. Post-operative and oral cavity haemorrhages were common, but not fully predictable, as these symptoms also occurred with plasma levels as high as 5–10%. Haemarthroses and haematomas occurred in only one-quarter of the patients, whereas life-threatening bleeding in the gastrointestinal tract and in the central nervous system was rare. On the whole, it appears that the clinical phenotype of patients with factor V deficiency is completely different from that seen in the mouse knockout model, and that these patients are usually mildly affected. This discrepancy is likely to be explained by the relatively poor sensitivity of available factor V bioassays that do not measure those small amounts of the factor that are probably sufficient to make the deficiency compatible with life and a mild clinical phenotype.

Molecular defects

The factor V gene is on chromosome 1q23. At the moment, there is relatively little information on the molecular defects underlying severe factor V deficiency, probably because of the large size (80 kb) and complexity of the gene (25 exons). Our analysis of published data identified a total of 24 distinct mutations associated with severe factor V deficiency (Figure 50.3). Approximately one-half of the mutations (12) are located in the large exon 13, encoding the entire B domain disposed during the enzymatic activation of factor V. The remaining mutations are scattered throughout the gene and all types of lesions are represented, spanning from missense mutations that are likely to impair the secretion or accelerate the degradation of factor V, to more frequent small deletions, frameshift, nonsense and splice site mutations predicted to produce truncated proteins or no protein at all. Very few mutations are present in more than one pedigree, indicating that a founder effect is unlikely to explain most cases. Only one genetic defect associated with type II deficiency has been so far reported.

Factor VII deficiency

Factor VII deficiency is the most common autosomal recessive coagulation disorder (1 per 500 000 population). Factor VII circulates in plasma at a concentration of approximately 0.5 μg/mL (10 mmol/L). Plasma levels of factor VII coagulant activity

(FVII:C) and FVII antigen (FVII:Ag) are influenced by a number of genetic and environmental factors (sex, age, cholesterol and triglyceride levels). The majority of patients have concomitantly low levels of factor VII functional activity and antigen, but several cases are characterized by normal or low borderline levels of factor VII antigen, contrasting with lower levels of functional activity. Most gene knockout mice made experimentally deficient in factor VII develop normally but some suffer fatal perinatal bleeding.

Clinical manifestations

The severity of symptoms of factor VII deficiency is variable and generally reported to be poorly correlated with plasma levels. Some patients do not bleed at all after major challenges of haemostasis, and even cases of thrombosis have been described. Among our patients, life- or limb-endangering bleeding manifestations were relatively rare, the most frequent symptoms being epistaxis and menorrhagia. However, the prevalence of haemarthroses and soft-tissue bleeding was less than that found in other large series. The risk of central nervous system bleeding in infants with severe factor VII deficiency is high in some series. We could not find kindreds in which factor VII deficiency segregated with arterial or venous thromboembolism.

A lack of correlation between measured FVII:C *in vitro* and the clinical phenotype is well known and is probably due to the fact that only trace amounts of FVIIa are required to initiate coagulation *in vivo*. However empirical studies and mathematical modelling suggest that as little as 5 pmol/L (0.05% of normal FVII concentration) is sufficient to induce clot formation and none of the *in vitro* tests could differentiate between undetectable and extremely low levels of FVII:C capable of initiating coagulation *in vivo*. Previously reported data showed that increasing the FVIIa concentration does not substantially increase the amount of thrombin generated but the low concentrations of FVIIa prolong the initiation phase of the reaction.

Molecular defects

Factor VII is a zymogen for a vitamin K-dependent serine protease, synthesized primarily in the liver, which is essential for the initiation of blood coagulation. The factor VII gene is located on chromosome 13 (13q34), consists of nine exons, and spans 12 kb. It encodes a mature protein of 406 amino acids, which includes four domains: an N-terminal domain (Gla) post-translationally modified by γ-carboxylation of glutamic acid residues, two EGF-like domains (EGF1 and 2) and a C-terminal serine protease domain. The molecular basis of factor VII deficiency is more extensively characterized than those of other defects, perhaps due to the relatively high frequency of this defect and small size of the gene.

The availability of an on-line database (http://europium.csc. mrc.ac.uk) allows rapid access to the entire listing of factor VII

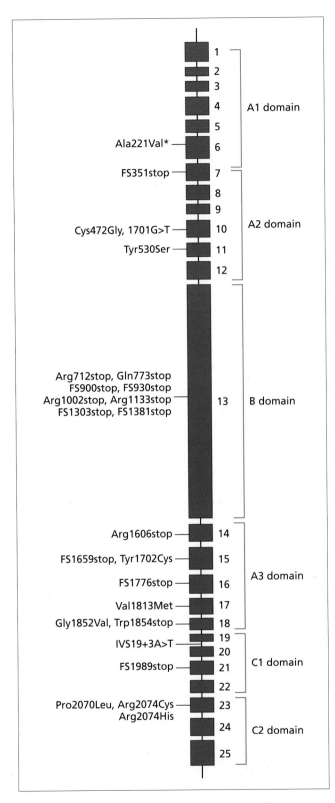

Figure 50.3 Mutations in the factor V gene, projected on the exons encoding the domains of the protein. Exons (rectangles) are drawn to scale, whereas introns (lines) are not to scale. *FV type II deficiency-causing mutation.

mutations. However, this database often lacks critical information such as clinical phenotypes and the source of the TF used in the FVII:C assay. The database currently lists 124 mutations of the factor VII gene: missense (84), nonsense (6), splice junctions (17), promoter (6), small insertions (1) and deletions (10). The reported mutations are located throughout the gene, suggesting that all domains are important in maintaining the overall structure and function of factor VII; 24 additional mutations are reported but not included in the database. The majority of individuals with mutations identified in their factor VII genes are either asymptomatic (28%) or their clinical phenotype has not been reported (39%). They usually have come to attention through preoperative screening. The genetic defects in these individuals are mainly missense mutations. The severe cases (17%) are all either homozygous or double heterozygous for mutations that disrupt expression of the protein (for example, deletions, insertions, splice junctions and promoter mutations), resulting in FVII coagulant levels typically less than 2% of normal. However, some missense mutations are also associated with a severe phenotype. Individuals with a mild/moderate clinical phenotype (16%) are homozygous or double heterozygous for missense mutations (Figure 50.4).

Combined deficiency of factor V and factor VIII

These patients have concomitantly low levels of the two coagulation factors (usually, between 5% and 20%), both as coagulant activity and antigen. For many years the molecular mechanism of the association of the two factor deficiencies, each transmitted with different patterns of inheritance (autosomal recessive for factor V, X-linked for factor VIII) and involving proteins encoded by different genes, has not been understood.

In 1998, the cause of the deficiency has been associated with mutations in the LMAN1 gene (lectin mannose binding protein, previously referred to as ERGIC-53). LMAN1 encodes a 53-kDa type 1 transmembrane protein with homology to leguminous lectin proteins. LMAN1 resides in the endoplasmic reticulum/Golgi intermediate compartment, where, with a mannose-selective and calcium-dependent binding, it acts as a chaperone in the intracellular transport of both factor V and factor VIII. Mutations in LMAN1 were found in approximately 70% of affected patients.

Recently, another locus correlated with the deficiency was identified in approximately 15% of affected families without any mutation in LMAN1. The MCFD2 (multiple coagulation factor deficiency 2) gene encodes a 16-kDa protein. MCFD2 forms a Ca^{2+}-dependent 1:1 stechiometric complex with LMAN1 and acts as a cofactor for LMAN1, specifically recruiting correctly folded factor V and factor VIII in the endoplasmic reticulum. The presence of about 15% of affected patients in which the disorder is not linked to LMAN1 or MCFD2 mutations strongly suggests the existence of a third associated locus.

Clinical manifestations

In patients with factor V and factor VIII levels varying between 4% and 14%, symptoms were usually mild, with a predominance of epistaxis, menorrhagia and bleeding after dental extractions. More severe bleeding episodes, particularly soft-tissue bleeding, were rare. These data are broadly consistent with those previously reported in the literature, particularly in a large series of patients from Israel. It appears that the concomitant presence of two coagulation defects does not enhance the haemorrhagic tendency observed in each defect separately (see factor V deficiency). The phenotypes associated with mutations in MCFD2 and LMAN1 are indistinguishable and manifested only by deficiencies of plasma coagulation factor V and factor VIII, even although a selective delay in secretion of procathepsin C was observed in HeLa cells overexpressing a dominant-negative form of LMAN1.

Molecular defects

LMAN1 is encoded by a gene of approximately 29 kb located on chromosome 18 and containing 13 exons (Figure 50.5). In the original study on LMAN1 gene, made by Nichols and colleagues, two distinct mutations were found in patients of Oriental Jewish ancestry, a splice site mutation and a single basepair insertion. In subsequent studies carried out in patients of varied ethnic origins, 16 additional distinct mutations were identified (splice site, insertions, deletion, nonsense codons). All the identified mutations are predicted to result in the synthesis of either a truncated protein product or no protein at all; 40% of this population had no detectable mutation in LMAN1.

MCFD2 is encoded by a gene of approximately 19 kb, located on chromosome 2 and containing four exons (Figure 50.6). Zhang and colleagues identified seven distinct mutations accounting for FV + FVIII deficiency in 9 out of 12 studied families. They found three frameshift and two splice-site mutations that were predicted to result in the complete loss of MCFD2 protein expression. Two missense mutations have been also identified. Both mutations are localized in a highly conserved region of the second EF-hand domain and eliminate the interaction with LMAN1.

Factor X deficiency

Clinical phenotypes are characterized by concomitantly low levels of coagulant activity and antigen, or by low coagulant activity contrasting with normal or low borderline antigen values. Mice rendered experimentally deficient in factor X by targeted inactivation of the factor X gene showed frequent

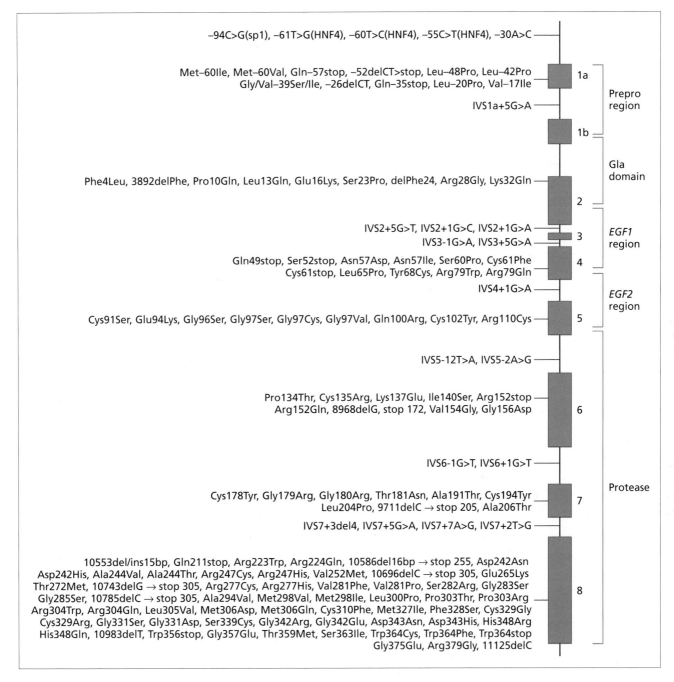

Figure 50.4 Mutations in the factor VII gene projected on the exons encoding the domains of the protein. Exons (rectangles) and introns (lines) are drawn to scale.

embryonic lethality. Those who survived bled to death intra-abdominally at birth and in the central nervous system within the first 3–4 weeks of life.

Clinical manifestations

Factor X deficiency is, together with factor XIII deficiency, the most severe of the rare coagulation deficiencies. Haematomas and haemarthroses occur in two-thirds of the patients. In addition, several have gastrointestinal bleeding or life-threatening bleeding from the umbilical stump. As a result of this and other bleeding symptoms occurring early in life, most patients are soon recognized to have an inherited bleeding disorder, so that a symptom such as post-operative bleeding is not frequently apparent because the great majority of patients receive replacement therapy before surgery. Hence there is reasonable consistency

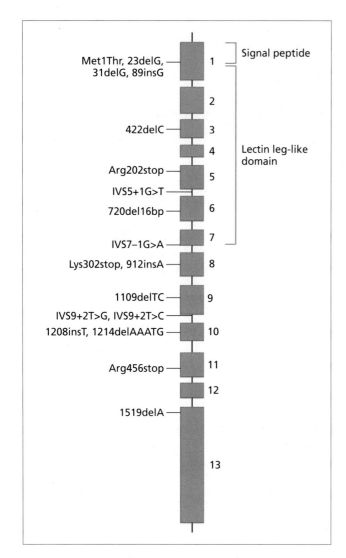

Figure 50.5 Mutation in the *LMAN1* gene, projected on the exons encoding the domains of the protein. Exons (rectangles) are drawn to scale, whereas introns (lines) are not to scale.

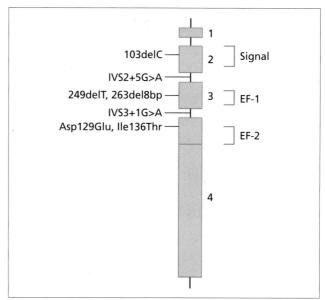

Figure 50.6 Mutation in the *MCFD2* gene, projected on the exons encoding the domains of the protein. Exons (rectangles) are drawn to scale, whereas introns (lines) are not to scale.

is predicted to lead to the production of a truncated protein or no protein at all, supporting the mice knockout finding that complete absence of factor X may be incompatible with life. This viewpoint is also supported by the observation that phenotypically most of these patients have low but measurable levels of factor X coagulant activity, in association with low or normal levels of immunoreactive protein, and that only a few severe mutations have been reported (eight small or large deletions, four splice site mutations, one promoter mutation). A peculiar aspect of the spectrum of mutations underlying factor X deficiency is the complete absence of reported nonsense mutations that are expected to be present in a proportion of 1:4 with respect to other mutations and particularly to missense mutations.

Factor XI deficiency

Factor XI deficiency is characterized by a decrease of the functional activity of this plasma protein, usually accompanied by correspondingly low levels of factor XI antigen. The majority of cases reported in the literature are of Ashkenazi Jewish origin, the frequency of heterozygosity for factor XI deficiency being as high as 8% in this population. In knockout mice, the loss of the gene coding for this factor is compatible with life, with no tendency for spontaneous bleeding.

Clinical manifestations

The relationship between the residual factor XI levels in plasma and the bleeding tendency is not as clear-cut as for other coagu-

between the severity of the clinical phenotype and that of the knockout model. That factor X deficiency appears to be one of the most severe recessively inherited coagulation deficiencies also stems from data from the UKHCDO registry, showing that the proportion of patients with this deficiency who require treatment is higher than that of the other rare coagulation deficiencies.

Molecular defects

The factor X gene is on chromosome 13, has a length of 22 kb and contains eight exons. In total, 64 different mutations have been identified in patients diagnosed in the USA, Japan and Europe and in patients from Iran (Figure 50.7). The great majority of patients have missense mutations (52), mainly in exon 8, which encodes the catalytic domain. None of these mutations

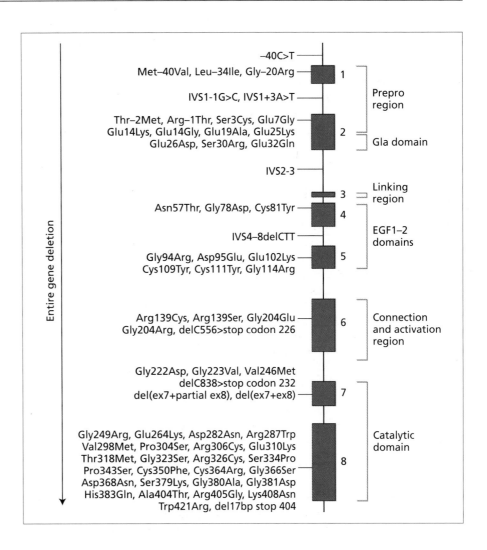

Figure 50.7 Mutation in the factor X gene, projected on the exons encoding the domains of the protein. Exons (rectangles) and introns (lines) are drawn to scale.

lation factor deficiencies. Usually, patients with severe factor XI deficiency (1% or less) are mildly affected and have bleeding symptoms only after trauma or surgery. Surprisingly patients with low but detectable levels of factor XI are also mild bleeders, so that clinical phenotypes are not strikingly different in these two groups. This observation, already made for Jewish patients, was confirmed recently in a series of Iranian non-Jewish patients with severe or moderate deficiency (factor XI < 1–5%) and in patients with mild deficiency (6–30%). All patients were mild bleeders, but those symptoms that define the severity of the bleeding tendency, such as muscle haematomas and haemarthroses, showed a similar frequency in the two groups of deficient patients (approximately 25%). The most frequent symptoms were oral and post-operative bleeding, which occurred in more then 50% of patients.

The reasons for the relatively poor relation between factor XI plasma levels and tendency to bleed are still not clear. One possibility is that the APTT-based factor XI assays commonly used to measure factor activity in intrinsic coagulation do not reflect those properties of the protein that are most important for *in*

vivo haemostasis. Different degrees of the defective interactions of factor XI with blood platelets, not revealed by APTT-based assays, might be the explanation for the poor relation.

Molecular defects

The factor XI gene is on chromosome 4 and is 23 kb in length. Altogether, 36 different gene mutations associated with factor XI deficiency have been identified so far (Figure 50.8). Two mutations are responsible for most cases of factor XI deficiency in Ashkenazi Jews, whereas mutations are more varied in non-Jews. The so-called type II Jewish mutation is a stop codon in exon 5, compatible with the observation that patients homozygous for this defect usually have undetectable levels of factor XI. The type III Jewish mutation is a missense mutation in exon 9, leading to the substitution of phenylalanine at position 283 with leucine. The mutation causes defective secretion of the protein from cells, but some factor XI is ultimately produced so that these patients have measurable levels of factor XI (at approximately 10%). Type II/III compound heterozygosity is

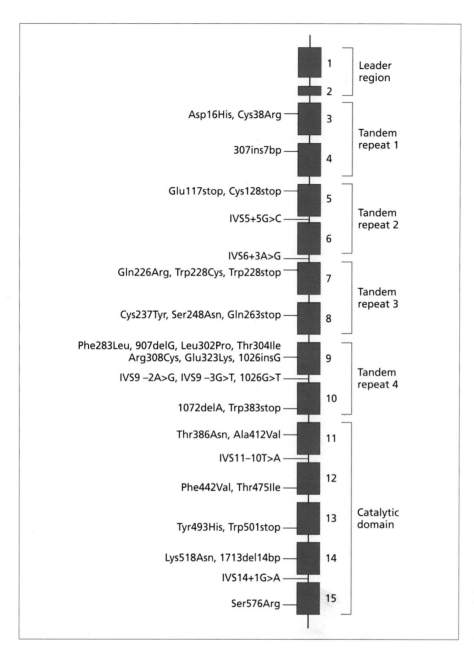

Asp16His, Cys38Arg — 3

307ins7bp — 4

Glu117stop, Cys128stop — 5

IVS5+5G>C —

IVS6+3A>G —

Gln226Arg, Trp228Cys, Trp228stop — 7

Cys237Tyr, Ser248Asn, Gln263stop — 8

Phe283Leu, 907delG, Leu302Pro, Thr304Ile
Arg308Cys, Glu323Lys, 1026insG — 9

IVS9 –2A>G, IVS9 –3G>T, 1026G>T —

1072delA, Trp383stop — 10

Thr386Asn, Ala412Val — 11

IVS11–10T>A —

Phe442Val, Thr475Ile — 12

Tyr493His, Trp501stop — 13

Lys518Asn, 1713del14bp — 14

IVS14+1G>A —

Ser576Arg — 15

1 Leader region
2

Tandem repeat 1

Tandem repeat 2

Tandem repeat 3

Tandem repeat 4

Catalytic domain

Figure 50.8 Mutation in the factor XI gene, projected on the exons encoding the domains of the protein. Exons (rectangles) are drawn to scale, whereas introns (lines) are not to scale.

the commonest cause of severe to moderate factor XI deficiency (< 1% to 5%) in Ashkenazi Jews. The mutations in non-Jewish patients are more numerous, and scattered throughout the gene. Some are nonsense mutations and deletions but the majority are missense mutations associated with abnormal folding and decreased secretion of the protein.

Factor XIII deficiency

Factor XIII is the last enzyme to be activated in the blood coagulation pathway and functions to cross-link α- and γ-fibrin chains, resulting in a stronger clot with an increased resistance to fibrinolysis. The plasma factor is a heterotetrameric structure consisting of two catalytic A subunits (FXIII-A) and two carrier B subunits (FXIII-B). Factor XIII deficiency is, together with prothrombin deficiency, probably one of the rarest recessively transmitted coagulation factor deficiencies (1 in 2 000 000). In inherited factor XIII deficiency, plasma levels of FXIII-A measured as functional activity or immunoreactive protein are usually unmeasurable, whereas the FXIII-B subunit is reduced but at measurable levels. No case of factor XIII deficiency with normal FXIII plasma levels measured as immunoreactive protein associated to a reduced functional activity was described, at variance with the majority of the other clotting factors. FXIII transglutaminase activity in plasma was abolished in homozygous null mice generated by the deletion of the exon 7 of factor XIII gene. These mice were fertile, although reproduction was impaired and bleeding episodes were associated with reduced survival.

Clinical manifestations

Patients with factor XIII deficiency have a bleeding tendency that is usually severe, particularly because of the early onset of life-threatening symptoms such as umbilical cord and central nervous system bleeding. In untreated patients, umbilical cord bleeding is reported to occur in approximately 80% and central nervous system bleeding in up to 30%. These frequencies of severe symptoms are the highest among patients with inherited coagulation deficiencies, including haemophilia A and B. They usually lead to an early diagnosis, so that patients who survive are often treated prophylactically, starting early in life. This approach to treatment is rendered relatively simple and feasible by the fact that plasma levels of factor XIII of 2–5% are sufficient to prevent bleeding, and that the long *in vivo* half-life of the factor (11–14 days) makes it possible to infuse plasma cryoprecipitate or concentrates (all containing factor XIII) at intervals of 1 month or longer.

In a recent study made on the largest group of patients with severe FXIII deficiency (93 Iranians), the most frequent mucosal tract bleeding symptom was bleeding in the oral cavity (lips, tongue, gum) followed by menorrhagia and epistaxis. Gastrointestinal bleeding is not unusual. Soft tissue bleeding such as spontaneous haematoma and haemarthroses occur in a large proportion of patients; 20% of patients in the reproductive age had intraperitoneal bleeding that occurred at the time of ovulation, in some cases leading to hysterectomy and 50% of pregnant women had at least one miscarriage. On the whole, the clinical impact of factor XIII deficiencies can shift from that of a very severe disease to that of a mild one, depending on the adoption of prophylactic treatment, which, in turn, depends on the precocity of diagnosis.

Molecular defects

The XIII A and B subunits are encoded by two different genes on chromosomes 6 and 1, one of more than 200 kb in length comprising 15 exons and the other of 28 kb comprising 12 exons. According to our perusal of the literature, the molecular basis of factor XIII deficiency are 51 sequence changes in the FXIII-A gene and three in the FXIII-B gene. Overall, there are 26 missense mutations, six nonsense mutations, eight splice site defects, 10 small deletions and/or insertions and one gross deletion in the FXIII-A gene (Figure 50.9). In the FXIII-B gene, one missense mutation, one small insertion and one small deletion were identified. Mutations are scattered throughout the factor XIII

genes and there is little evidence of recurring mutations. In a few studies, the mutant proteins were expressed in cultured mammalian cell lines and it was shown that the introduction of the mutation caused destabilization of the protein structure and intracellular degradation.

Concluding remarks on symptoms

Autosomal recessively transmitted coagulation deficiencies are generally less severe than the haemophilias caused by factor VIII or IX deficiency. The only exceptions are factor X and XIII deficiencies, characterized by the early onset of life-threatening symptoms such as umbilical cord and central nervous system bleeding. Among patients with other coagulation deficiencies, only a minority have spontaneous haemarthroses and muscle haematomas.

Accordingly, permanent damage to the musculoskeletal system and the resulting handicaps are less common. Haematuria, not rare in haemophilia, is relatively frequent only in factor X deficiency but occurs very rarely or not at all in the remaining defects. Bleeding from the umbilical stump, not seen in haemophiliacs and thought to be typical of the inherited defects of fibrin formation (afibrinogenaemia and factor XIII deficiency), was also not unusual in prothrombin, factor V and factor X deficiency. A mild bleeding symptom such as epistaxis, relatively rare in haemophiliacs, was very frequent in all rare defects. In afibrinogenaemia and factor V deficiency, this mucosal-type symptom might be explained by a concomitant defect of the protein in patients' platelets, reflected by a prolonged bleeding time.

However, there is no obvious explanation for the frequency of epistaxis in defects of coagulation factors such as prothrombin, factor VII and X, not contained in platelets and not directly involved in primary haemostasis. The same considerations apply to other mucosal-type symptoms such as menorrhagia, a frequent event that often causes iron deficiency in women. There is no evidence that the coagulation defects reduce fertility in affected women, or that they cause recurrent miscarriages, with the exception of factor XIII deficiency. As expected, excessive bleeding when carried out without adopting preventive measures often follows surgical procedures. Bleeding after circumcision is often the revealing symptom in coagulation factor deficiencies. Life-endangering haemorrhages in the gastrointestinal tract and central nervous system are rare.

There are several reports of the frequent occurrence of these manifestations in patients with rare coagulation deficiencies, but report bias is likely to have emphasized their prevalence. At the moment, the observed qualitative and quantitative differences between the different defects cannot be easily explained. Animal models of gene knockout indicate that bleeding is more severe and more often lethal in mice rendered deficient in prothrombin, factor V and factor X than in those with factor VII and

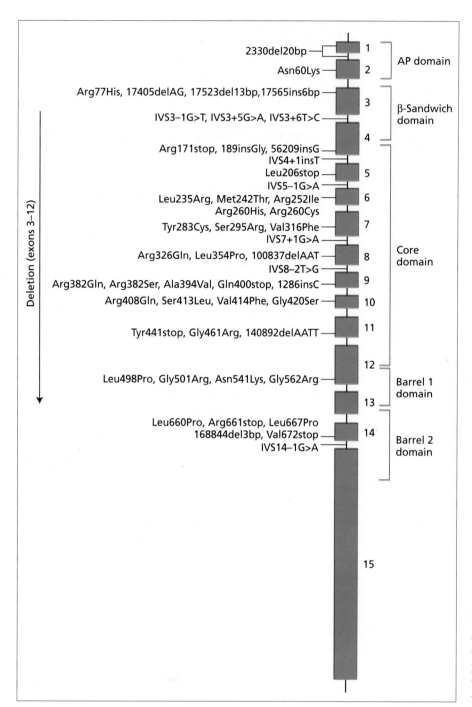

Figure 50.9 Mutation in the factor XIII gene (subunit A), projected on the exons encoding the domains of the protein. Exons (rectangles) are drawn to scale, whereas introns (lines) are not to scale.

fibrinogen deficiency. Even though this pattern of varied severity of factor deficiency in mice is roughly similar to that observed in patients, it must be considered that in knockout mice the gene encoding a clotting factor is completely silenced. Accordingly, no trace of RNA or protein is produced, whereas the gene lesions found so far in humans are usually less deleterious and less likely to completely impede protein production.

Concluding remarks on molecular defects

The first remark is that in general a defect in the DNA of these patients could be identified in the actual genes encoding the different coagulation factors. Combined factor V and VIII deficiency, explained by defects located in genes encoding transport proteins, is a typical exception. Another remark is that for each coagulation defect the mutations are multiple, and that the majority of them are 'private' mutations, unique for any given patient. The unique nature of the mutations complicates the approach to the control of these diseases through prenatal diagnosis in families with affected members, because it renders necessary the actual identification of the underlying mutation in each kindred.

The relation between genotype and phenotype is not always clear-cut. Even although 'severe' mutations predicting no protein production (stop codons, deletions, insertions, splicing abnormalities) are generally associated with severe factor deficiencies and severe clinical phenotypes, there are a number of cases with severe deficiencies and phenotypes associated with missense mutations. Usually missense mutations are associated with milder phenotypes despite unmeasurable factor levels, probably because some protein is produced in these cases, which cannot be detected with the assays available at present.

Expression of the mutations in cultured cell lines and characterization of the recombinant proteins has been useful to understand how well-defined molecular lesions lead to structural abnormalities and to functional defects of the protein. In some cases, expression studies have documented the mechanism whereby a mutant protein is synthesized normally but is not ultimately secreted in plasma from cells. In most cases, impaired folding and/or conformational changes of the mutant proteins lead to both intra- and extracellular instability, which, in turn, cause factor deficiency in plasma. Expression work is still in its infancy and needs to be expanded, mainly in cases of missense mutations that appear to be of special functional interest when projected on the available crystal structure of the coagulation factors.

Concluding remarks on treatment

Treatment of rare coagulation disorders consists in the use of the most purified blood product available that contains the missing factor. Due to the rarity of each factor deficiency, purified factor concentrates are not as widely available as they are for haemophilia A and B. Dosages and frequency of treatment depend on minimal haemostatic levels of the deficient factor, plasma half-life and type of bleeding episode. General recommendations on treatment of patients with rare coagulation disorders are summarized in Table 50.3.

Table 50.3 Treatment of recessive coagulation deficiencies.

Deficient factor	Recommended trough levels	Plasma half-life	Treatment
Fibrinogen	5–100 mg/dL	2–4 days	Cryoprecipitate (5–10 bags), solvent–detergent (SD)-treated plasma (15–30 mL/kg), fibrinogen concentrates (20–40 mg/kg)
Prothrombin	20–30%	2–3 days	SD-treated plasma (15–20 mL/kg), FIX concentrates and prothrombin complex concentrates (PCC) (20–30 U/kg)
Factor V	10–20%	36 h	SD-treated plasma (15–20 mL/kg)
Factor V + VIII	10–15%		as for Factor V
Factor VII	10–15%	4–6 h	FVII concentrates (30–40 mL/kg), PCC (20–30 U/kg) Recombinant FVIIa (15–30 µg/kg every 4–6 h)
Factor X	30–40%	20–40 h	SD-treated plasma (10–20 mL/kg), PCC (20–30 U/kg)
Factor XI	15–20%	48–72 h	SD-treated plasma (15–20 mL/kg), FXI concentrates (15–20 U/kg)
Factor XIII	2–5%	10–15 days	Cryoprecipitate (2–3 bags), SD-treated plasma (3 mL/kg), FXIII concentrates (10–20 U/kg every 5–6 weeks for prophylaxis and 50 U/kg for severe haemorrhagic events)

Table 50.4 Factor concentrates for recessive coagulation deficiencies.

Deficiency	Brand (company)	Viral inactivation	Comments
Fibrinogen	Fibrinogen HT (Benesis, Japan)	TNBP/polysorbate 80* + dry heat 80°C, 72 h	Concentrates should be used with caution in patients at risk for thrombosis
	Haemocomplettan (Aventis Bhering, Germany)	Pasteurization at 60°C, 20 h	
	Clottagen (fibrinogen) (LFB, France)	TNBP/polysorbate 80	
Prothrombin complex concentrate and Factor X	Konyne 80 (Bayer, USA)		Risk of thromboembolic complications with PCCs if FIX levels raised > 50%
	Proplex T (Baxter, USA)	Exposure to 20% ethanol + dry heat 60°C, 144 h	
	Bebulin (Baxter, USA)	Vapour heat 60°C, 10 h at 190 mbar + 80°C, 1 h at 375 mbar	
	Profilnine (Alpha, USA)	TNBP/polysorbate 80	
Prothrombin	Beriplex P/N (Aventis Bhering, Germany)	Pasteurization at 60°C, 10 h + nanofiltration	Concentrates should be used with caution in patients at risk for thrombosis
	Faktor IX HS (Aventis Bhering, Germany)	Pasteurization at 60°C, 10 h	
	Hemofactor HT (Grifols, Spain)		
	PTX-HT (CSL, Australia)		
	HT Defix (SNBTS, Scotland)	Dry heat 80°C, 72 h	
	Kaskadil (LFB, France)	TNBP/polysorbate 80	
	Faktor IX-Komplex SRK (ZLB, SRK, Switzerland)		
	Prothrombinkomplex NDS (BSD NSOB, Germany)	TNBP/polysorbate 80	
	Cofactor (CLB, Netherlands)	TNBP/polysorbate 80 + nanofiltration	
	Factor IX comp (LF Bare, Brazil)		
Factor VII	Factor VII (Baxter, Austria)	Vapor heat 60°C, 10 h at 190 mbar + 80°C, 1 h at 375 mbar	Concentrates should be used with caution in patients at risk for thrombosis
	Factor VII (BIO Products Laboratory, UK)	Dry heat 80°C, 72 h	
	Factor VII LFB (LFB, France)	TNBP/polysorbate 80	
	NovoSeven (NovoNordisk, Denmark)	Recombinant	Primarily intended for haemostasis in presence of inhibitors
Factor XI	Factor XI (BIO Products Laboratory, UK)	Dry heat 80°C, 72 h	Concentrates should be used with caution in patients at risk for thrombosis
	Hemoleven (LFB, France)	TNBP/polysorbate 80 + 15-nm nanofiltration	
Factor XIII	Factor XIII (BIO Products Laboratory, UK)		Factor XIII concentrates can be given every 21 days to affected individuals with history of spontaneous abortions
	Fibrogammin P (Aventis Bhering, Germany)	Pasteurization at 60°C, 10 h	

*Solvent/detergent.

The avoidance of transmission of blood-borne infectious agents is the primary requisite in the choice of replacement material. Solvent–detergent-treated plasma is an important source of replacement recommended in the majority of these disorders; also virus-inactivated concentrates, when commercially available, are safe but expensive, especially for developing countries. Non-virus inactivated plasma and cryoprecipitate should be avoided if possible. Of course the treatment of choice may change depending on the facilities of the country where the patient is resident. Cost is the next most important determinant.

Virally inactivated factor concentrates are available for several deficiencies (Table 50.4) and should be preferred when virally inactivated plasma is not available or repeated infusions causing fluid overload are needed, as it may occur at surgery or in cases of bleeding in the central nervous system. For a few disorders, such as factor V and combined factor V and VIII deficiency, no concentrate is available at present. In factor VII deficiency, the use of purified factor concentrates is essential, because the half-life of this factor is so short (around 6 h) that closely spaced infusions of more than two to three doses of plasma are likely to create fluid overload. In prothrombin and factor X deficiency, prothrombin complex concentrates can be used for treatment. There is no obvious need to manufacture specific factor concentrates, even though the unnecessarily high post-infusion levels of vitamin K-dependent coagulation factors might be one of the causes for thrombogenicity of these concentrates.

Prevention of rare coagulation disorders through prenatal diagnosis of the underlying mutations is feasible in couples who already have affected children. Primary prevention might be achieved by discouraging consanguineous marriages. Even although the cultural, religious and economic roots of this practice are deep in Muslim communities, consanguineous marriages are becoming much less frequent in large cities and among younger generations.

Acknowledgements

We would like to thank Dr M Lak and R Sharifian of Teheran University and Dr S Zeinali of the Pasteur Institute, for their help and assistance throughout this study, Mr Afshar of the Iranian Hemophilia Society for help in contacting the patients, and Drs S Lavoretano, S Duga, R Asselta, I Garagiola, R Palla, M Spreafico, M Menegatti and L Tagliabue for assisting the preparation of the manuscript.

Selected bibliography

Akhavan S, Mannucci PM, Lak M et al. (2000) Identification and three-dimensional structural analysis of nine novel mutations in patients with prothrombin deficiency. Thrombosis and Haemostasis 84: 987–997.

Asakai R, Chung DW, Ratnoff OD et al. (1989) Factor XI (plasma thromboplastin antecedent) deficiency in Ashkenazi Jews is a bleeding disorder that can result from three types of point mutations. Proceedings of the National Academy of Science USA 86: 7667–71.

Asakai R, Chung D, Davie E et al. (1991) Factor XI deficiency in Ashkenazi Jews in Israel. New England Journal of Medicine 325: 153–8.

Asselta R, Duga S, Simonic T et al. (2000) Afibrinogenemia: first identification of a splicing mutation in the fibrinogen gamma chain gene leading to a major gamma chain truncation. Blood 96: 2496–500.

Asselta R, Duga S, Spena S et al. (2001) Congenital afibrinogenemia: mutations leading to premature termination codons in fibrinogen alpha-chain gene are not associated with the decay of the mutant mRNAs. Blood 98: 3685–92.

Asselta R, Spena S, Duga S et al. (2002) Congenital afibrinogenemia: in vitro expression of two novel missense mutations in the fibrinogen Bβ-chain gene demonstrates that one of them acts as a splicing mutation. Blood 100: 21a.

Asselta R, Spena S, Duga S et al. (2002) Analysis of Iranian patients allowed the identification of the first truncating mutation in the fibrinogen Bβ-chain gene causing afibrinogenemia. Haematologica 87: 855–9.

Bolton-Maggs P, Wan-Yin B, McGraw A et al. (1988) Inheritance and bleeding in factor XI deficiency. British Journal of Haematology 69: 521–8.

Cooper DN, Millar DS, Wacey A et al. (1997) Inherited factor X deficiency: molecular genetics and pathophysiology. Thrombosis and Haemostasis 78: 161–72.

Cui J, O'Shea KS, Purkayastha A et al. (1996) Fatal hemorrhage and incomplete block of embryogenesis in mice lacking coagulation factor V. Nature 384: 66–8.

Czwalinna A, Eisert R, Bartkowiak N et al. (2001) Analysis of the fibrinogen genes of 50 patients with suspicion of dys-, hypo- or afibrinogenaemia. Thrombosis and Haemostasis: abstract P1248.

Gershwin ME, Gude JK (1973) Deep vein thrombosis and pulmonary embolism in congenital factor VII deficiency. New England Journal of Medicine 288: 141–2.

Giansily-Blaizot M, Aguilar-Martinez P, Briquel ME et al. Two novel cases of cerebral haemorrhages at the neonatal period associated with inherited factor VII deficiency, one of them revealing a new nonsense mutation (Ser52Stop). Blood Coagulation and Fibrinolysis 14: 217–20, 2003.

Hashiguchi T, Saito M, Morishita E et al. (1993) Two genetic defects in a patient with complete deficiency of the b-subunit for coagulation factor XIII. Blood 82: 145–50.

Ichinose A Tsukamoto H, Tamonori I et al. (1998) Arg260Cys mutation in severe factor XIII deficiency, conformational change of the A subunit, is predicted by molecular modelling and mechanics. British Journal of Haematology 101: 264–72.

Ichinose A (2001) Physiopathology and regulation of factor XIII. Thrombosis and Haemostasis 86: 57–65.

Imanaka Y, Lal K, Nishimura T et al. (1995) Identification of two novel mutations in non-Jewish factor XI deficiency. British Journal of Haematology 90: 916–20.

Izumi T, Hashiguchi T, Castaman G et al. (1996) Type I factor XIII deficiency is caused by a genetic defect of its b subunit: insertion of triplet AAC in exon III leads to premature termination in the second Sushi domain. *Blood* 87: 2769–74.

Jones KC, Mann KG (1994) A model for the tissue factor pathway to thrombin. II. A mathematical simulation. *Journal of Biological Chemistry* 269: 23367–73.

Koseki S, Souri M, Koga S *et al.* (2001) Truncated mutant B subunit for factor XIII causes its deficiency due to impaired intracellular transportation. *Blood* 97: 3712.

Lak M, Sharifian R, Peyvandi F *et al.* (1998) Symptoms of inherited factor V deficiency in 25 Iranian patients. *British Journal of Haematology* 103: 1067–9.

Lak M, Keihani M, Elahi F *et al.* (1999) Bleeding and thrombosis in 55 patients with inherited afibrinogenemia. *British Journal of Haematology* 107: 204–6.

Lak M, Peyvandi F, Mannucci PM (2001) Factor XI (FXI) deficiency: clinical manifestations and complications of replacement therapy in 38 Iranian patients. *Thrombosis and Haemostasis*: abstract p1131.

Lak M, Peyvandi F, Ali Sharifian A *et al.* (2003) Pattern of symptoms in 93 Iranian patients with severe factor XIII deficiency. *Journal of Thrombosis and Haemostasis* 1: 1837–59.

Lauer P, Metzener HJ, Zettlmeissl G *et al.* (2002) Targeted inactivation of the mouse locus encoding coagulation factor XIII-A: haemostatic abnormalities in mutant mice and characterization of the coagulation deficit. *Thrombosis and Haemostasis* 88: 967–74.

Lawson JH, Kalafatis M, Stram S *et al.* (1994) A model for the tissue factor pathway to thrombin. I. An empirical study. *Journal of Biological Chemistry* 269: 23357–66.

Mannucci PM, Tuddenham EGD (2001) The hemophilias: from royal genes to gene therapy. *New England Journal of Medicine* 344: 1773–9.

Mariani G, Mazzucconi MG (1993) Factor VII congenital deficiency: clinical picture and classification of the variants. *Haemostasis* 13: 169–74.

McVey JH, Boswell E, Mumford AD *et al.* (2001) Factor VII deficiency and the FVII mutation database. *Human Mutation* 17: 3–17.

Miloszewski KJA (1999) Factor XIII deficiency. *British Journal of Haematology* 107: 468–84.

Montefusco MC, Duga S, Asselta R *et al.* (2003) Clinical and molecular characterization of six patients affected by severe deficiency of coagulation factor V: broadening of the mutational spectrum of FV gene and *in vitro* analysis of the newly identified missense mutations. *Blood* (prepublished on-line June 19, 2003; DOI 10.1182/blood-2003–03–0922).

Neerman-Arbez M, Johnson KM, Morris MA *et al.* (1999) Molecular analysis of the ERGIC-53 gene in 35 families with combined factor V-factor VIII deficiency. *Blood* 93: 2253–60.

Neerman-Arbez M, de Moerloose P, Honsberger A *et al.* (2001) Molecular analysis of the fibrinogen gene cluster in 16 patients with congenital afibrinogenemia: novel truncating mutations in the FGA and FGG genes. *Human Genetics* 108: 237–240.

Nichols WC, Seligsohn U, Zivelin A *et al.* (1998) Mutations in the ER-Golgi intermediate compartment protein ERGIC-53 cause combined deficiency of coagulation factors V and VIII. *Cell* 93: 61–70.

Nichols WC, Valeri HT, Wheatley MA *et al.* (1999) ERGIC-53 gene structure and mutation analysis in 19 combined factors V and VIII deficiency families. *Blood* 93: 2261–6.

Perry DJ (1997) Factor X and its deficiency states. *Haemophilia* 3: 159–72.

Peyvandi F, Mannucci PM, Asti D *et al.* (1997) Clinical manifestations in 28 Italian and Iranian patients with severe factor VII deficiency. *Hemophilia* 3: 242–6.

Peyvandi F, Tuddenham EGD, Akhtari M *et al.* (1998) Bleeding symptoms in 27 Iranian patients with factor V and VIII combined deficiency. *British Journal of Haematology* 100: 773–6.

Peyvandi F, Mannucci PM, Lak M *et al.* (1998) Congenital factor X deficiency: spectrum of bleeding symptoms in 32 Iranian patients. *British Journal of Haematology* 102: 626–8.

Peyvandi F, Mannucci PM (1999) Rare coagulation disorders. *Thrombosis and Haemostasis* 82: 1380–1.

Peyvandi F, Jenkins PV, Mannucci PM *et al.* (2000) Molecular characterization and three-dimensional structural analysis of mutations in 21 unrelated families with inherited factor VII deficiency. *Thrombosis and Haemostasis* 84: 250–7.

Peyvandi F, Carew JA, Perry DJ *et al.* (2001) Abnormal secretion and function of recombinant human factor VII as the results of modifications to a calcium binding site caused by a 15-base pair insertion in the F7 gene. *Blood* 97: 960–5.

Peyvandi F, Lak M, Mannucci PM (2002) Factor XI deficiency in Iranians: its clinical manifestations in comparison with those of classic hemophilia. *Haematologica* 87: 512–14.

Peyvandi F, Tagliabue L, Muszbek L *et al.* (2002) Phenotypic and genotypic characterization of ten Iranian patients with severe Factor XIII deficiency. ASH, Philadelphia 7–9, December 2002.

Pinotti M, Etro D, Bindini D *et al.* (2002) Residual factor VII activity and different hemorrhagic phenotypes in CRM+ factor VII deficiencies (Gly331Ser and Gly283Ser). *Blood* 99: 1495–7.

Pugh RE, McVey JH, Tuddenham EG *et al.* (1995) Six point mutations that cause factor XI deficiency. *Blood* 85: 1509–16.

Rizza CR, Spooner RJD, Giangrande PLF (2001) Treatment of haemophilia in the United Kingdom 1981–1996. *Haemophilia* 7: 349–60.

Rodrigues DN, Siqueira LH, Galizoni AM *et al.* (2003) Prevalence of factor VII deficiency and molecular characterization of the F7 gene in Brazilian patients. *Blood Coagulation and Fibrinolysis* 14: 289–92.

Rosen ED, Chan JC, Idusogie E *et al.* (1997) Mice lacking factor VII develop normally but suffer fatal perinatal bleeding. *Nature* 390: 290–4.

Sun WY, Witte DP, Degen JL *et al.* (1998) Prothrombin deficiency results in embryonic and neonatal lethality in mice. *Proceedings of the National Academy of Sciences of the USA* 95: 7597–8002.

Tuddenham EGD, Cooper DN (1994) *The Molecular Genetics of Hemostasis and its Inherited Disorders.* Oxford University Press, Oxford.

Ventura C, Santos AI, Tavares A *et al.* (2000) Molecular genetic analysis of factor XI deficiency: identification of five novel gene alterations and the origin of type mutation in Portuguese families. *Thrombosis and Haemostasis* 84: 833–4.

Zhang B, Cunningham MA, Nichols WC *et al.* (2003) Bleeding due to disruption of a cargo-specific ER-to-Golgi transport complex. *Nature Genetics* 34: 220–5.

CHAPTER 51

Acquired coagulation disorders and vascular bleeding

51

Michael J Nash, Hannah Cohen, Ri Liesner and Samuel J Machin

Introduction

The haemostatic process under normal circumstances is balanced so as to ensure that haemorrhage is arrested and inappropriate thrombosis is prevented. Acquired defects of the haemostatic

Table 51.1 Laboratory screening tests to detect haemostatic defects.

Coagulation factors
Prothrombin time (PT)
Thrombin time (TT) and reptilase time if prolonged
Activated partial thromboplastin time (APTT)
Perform 50:50 mix with normal plasma on samples with prolonged PT and APTT
Fibrinogen quantification (by Clauss method)

Platelets
Platelet count
Blood film inspection
Bleeding time – by skin template or PFA 100®

Fibrinolysis
Fibrin(ogen) degradation products including D-dimers
Euglobulin clot lysis time or fibrin plate lysis assay

response may occur in association with multisystem disease or pharmacological intervention. Haemostatic 'disorder' may also occur at the extremes of age and in association with pregnancy. In clinical practice, it is important that a bleeding tendency is recognized and then the defect is defined by appropriate laboratory testing so as to facilitate treatment.

Faced with a bleeding patient, it may be difficult to discern whether blood loss is due to a local factor or secondary to an underlying haemostatic defect. Continual oozing from sites of venous access along with excessive bruising at pressure areas and intramuscular injections, may be signs of actual or impending haemostatic failure. In some cases, patchy skin cyanosis or superficial gangrene may be the herald of consumptive coagulopathy prior to overt bleeding.

A list of simple laboratory tests, which should be performed first line in the bleeding patient, are shown in Table 51.1. More specialized tests may be performed to further define the cause of bleeding.

Acquired consumptive coagulopathy (disseminated intravascular coagulation)

Disseminated intravascular coagulation (DIC) occurs as a result of inappropriate and excessive activation of the haemostatic system within the vascular space. The International Society on

Table 51.2 Conditions associated with overt disseminated intravascular coagulation (DIC).

Sepsis/severe infection (any organism)

Trauma (e.g. polytrauma, neurotrauma, fat embolism)

Organ destruction (e.g. severe pancreatitis)

Malignancy – solid tumours and myeloproliferative/ lymphoproliferative malignancies

Obstetric calamities (e.g. amniotic fluid embolism, abruptio placentae)

Vascular abnormalities (e.g. Kasabach–Merritt syndrome, large vascular aneurysms)

Severe hepatic failure

Severe toxic or immunological reactions (e.g. snake bites, recreational drugs, transfusion reactions, transplant rejection)

Massive blood loss with inadequate fluid replacement therapy

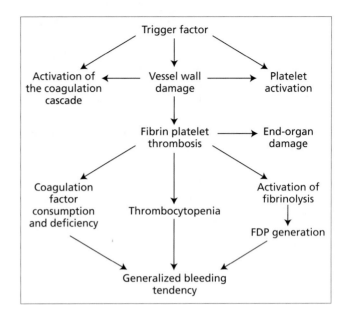

Figure 51.1 Pathogenesis of acute disseminated intravascular coagulation.

Thrombosis and Haemostasis (ISTH) scientific subcommittee for DIC defines the condition as 'an acquired syndrome characterized by the intravascular activation of coagulation with loss of localization arising from different causes. It can originate from and cause severe damage to the microvasculature, which, if sufficiently severe, can produce organ dysfunction.'

DIC may exist in acute and subacute or chronic forms. The chronic form is associated with malignancy, aortic aneurysm and vascular malformation. The main clinical presentation of DIC is bleeding. However, 5–10% of patients will manifest with microthrombotic lesions such as gangrene of the extremities. Thrombi may also disrupt the renal glomeruli leading to acute renal failure. The excess intravascular fibrin polymer acts as a mesh resulting in red cell fragmentation and distortion leading to intravascular haemolysis. Some of the major causes of DIC are listed in Table 51.2.

Pathogenesis

Within the circulation of a patient with DIC there is excessive thrombin formation leading to increased fibrin formation, suppression of natural anticoagulant mechanisms and a failure to remove the excess fibrin consequent upon a failure of the fibrinolytic system. An overview of the pathogenesis of acute DIC is shown in Figure 51.1.

The key pathological event underlying most episodes of DIC is increased activity of tissue factor. The increased tissue factor expression occurs on activated monocytes in response to proinflammatory cytokines, along with increase in expression at the surface of vascular endothelial cells. Interleukin 1 (IL-1), endotoxin and tumour necrosis factor alpha (TNF-α) can all induce the upregulation of tissue factor mRNA by endothelial cells. In acute severe illness, another source of tissue factor may be that released into the circulation by damaged tissues.

Other mechanisms causing DIC include the release of tissue thromboplastins into the circulation following tissue damage by trauma, from malignant tissue or following a haemolytic transfusion reaction. Snake venoms can directly activate intravascular coagulation. For example, the venom of *Echis carinatus* (saw-scaled viper) can directly hydrolyse prothrombin to thrombin. The venom of *Crotalus adamanteus* (Eastern diamondback rattlesnake) can directly clot fibrinogen.

A fall in antithrombin is seen in DIC and is due to excessive thrombin production leading to the formation of thrombin–antithrombin complexes, resulting in increased consumption of antithrombin. Antithrombin levels are also reduced secondary to impaired hepatic production and due to degradation by granulocyte elastase. Levels of antithrombin may fall as low as 30% of normal in patients with severe sepsis. The activity of protein C is also impaired in DIC; lower levels of free protein S (due to increased levels of C4b-binding protein), impaired synthesis and a cytokine-mediated reduction in endothelial thrombomodulin expression (needed for the conversion of protein C to its active form) all contribute to this.

Fibrinolysis is suppressed during DIC as a result of higher levels of plasminogen activator inhibitor type 1 (PAI-1). Higher PAI-1 levels are associated with a higher mortality in meningococcal sepsis. Individuals with genetic polymorphisms leading to increased levels of PAI-1 have been shown to have a worse outcome in severe sepsis.

Despite the systemic reduction in fibrinolysis associated with DIC, tissue plasminogen activator still binds to plasminogen incorporated within fibrin clots. There it acts on plasminogen to form plasmin, which, within the confines of the clot is protected from α_2-plasmin inhibitor. If enough plasmin is generated to exceed the neutralization potential of α_2-plasmin inhibitor then free plasmin will circulate, which can cleave circulating fibrinogen monomer as well as polymerized fibrin. The progressive degradation of fibrinogen leads to the formation of core fragments D and E (via fragment X and Y). The degradation of factor XIII cross-linked fibrin results in the formation of antigenically distinct cross-linked D-dimers. These circulating fibrin/fibrinogen degradation products (FDPs) can worsen any bleeding diathesis by binding to and inhibiting the action of thrombin and by reducing platelet function by non-specifically binding to the platelet membrane.

Continued, uncoordinated, excessive activation of the coagulation system results in the liver being unable to compensate for coagulation factor consumption. This particularly affects levels of factors V, VIII, XIII and fibrinogen. The bone marrow megakaryocytes are similarly unable to compensate the progressive consumptive thrombocytopenia. Thus a syndrome develops characterized by coagulation factor deficiency, thrombocytopenia, impaired platelet function and the inhibitory action of raised FDPs.

Clinical features and clinical associations

The patient with severe acute DIC may manifest with mucosal oozing, gastrointestinal blood loss and bleeding from surgical incisions or sites of venous access. The deposition of thrombi in the microcirculation can lead to multiple organ failure. Renal failure associated with DIC may occur secondary to hypovolaemia and also fibrin deposition in the renal vasculature.

Although Gram-positive organisms can cause DIC, Gram-negative bacteria are particularly associated with the syndrome. Viral haemorrhagic fevers may be associated with a DIC-like process; here, the mechanism is less clear than that in bacterial sepsis but may relate to viral infection of endothelial cells and cytokine release. Patients with liver disease may develop DIC after the placement of a peritoneo-venous shunt. This is due to the ascitic fluid containing thrombin activity and monocytes which express tissue factor. Severe trauma victims, notably those with necrotic cerebral lesions, may develop DIC. Here, one mechanism is the release of tissue factor into the circulation from damaged tissue. In addition, severe trauma victims have been shown to have a systemic cytokine response similar to that seen in sepsis and similar mechanisms may contribute to DIC in trauma to those seen in infection.

DIC may complicate some obstetric emergencies. Amniotic fluid may directly activate coagulation in the case of amniotic fluid embolism. Leakage of thromboplastin-like materials from the placenta contribute to the DIC seen with some cases of placental abruption.

In some patients, a syndrome of subacute or chronic DIC develops. The diagnosis of this state may be difficult as a degree of compensation by virtue of increased hepatic clotting factor synthesis may occur, rendering some of the laboratory clotting

tests normal. Patients with malignancy, particularly those with mucin-secreting adenocarcinomas, may develop chronic DIC. The mechanism here is likely to relate to tissue factor expression on tumour cells and monocyte activation. Some tumour cells also express cancer procoagulant, a cysteine protease that can directly activate factor X. The retained dead fetus syndrome is another cause of chronic consumptive coagulopathy; here, spontaneous bleeding is uncommon but the patient is at increased risk of post-partum haemorrhage.

Individuals with localized abnormalities of the vasculature such as an aortic aneurysm or giant cavernous haemangioma may also develop a chronic consumptive coagulopathy. This may lead to bleeding; however, because fibrin deposition is localized to the abnormality, end organ damage is infrequent. Localized consumption in the kidneys is characterized by the presence of FDPs in the urine, with only very mild elevation in the blood. This may occur in the context of hyperacute renal allograft rejection and proliferative glomerulonephritis.

Diagnosis

In acute DIC it is essential to demonstrate abnormal laboratory results quickly so that appropriate management can be instituted. Ideally, these should be available within 30 min of sample receipt at the laboratory. The ISTH scientific subcommittee for DIC has recently published a proposed scoring system for use in the diagnosis of 'overt' and 'non-overt' DIC (Tables 51.3 and 51.4). With both scoring systems, it is suggested that reassessment of scoring is performed daily. Notably, a diagnosis of 'overt DIC' under this classification can only be made in the presence of an underlying condition known to be associated with overt DIC (Table 51.2). From these guidelines it can be seen that the first-line tests for a diagnosis of DIC are a full blood count, a coagulation screen (prothrombin time, PT; activated partial thromboplastin time, APTT; and thrombin time, TT),

Table 51.3 Diagnostic algorithm for the diagnosis of overt DIC.

Does the patient have an underlying disorder known to be associated with overt DIC? (*If yes, proceed; if no, do not use this algorithm*)
Order global coagulation tests (platelet count, PT, fibrinogen, soluble fibrin monomers (SFM) or fibrin degradation products (FDP))
Score coagulation test results
  Platelet count (> 100 = 0; < 100 = 1, < 50 = 2)
  Elevated FDP or SFM (*no increase = 0; moderate increase = 2; strong increase = 3*)
  Prolonged PT (by < 3 s = 0; > 3 but < 6 s = 1; > 6 s = 2)
  Fibrinogen level (> 1 g/L = 0; < 1g/L = 1)

Score ≥ 5 compatible with overt DIC; score < 5 suggestive (not affirmative) of non-overt DIC; repeat tests in 1–2 days.

1 Risk assessment. Does the patient have an underlying disorder known to be associated with DIC?	Yes = 2; no = 0
2 Major criteria	
(a) Platelet count	$> 100 \times 10^9 = 0$; $< 100 \times 10^9 = 1$; rising = –1; stable = 0, falling = 1
(b) PT prolongation	< 3 s = 0; > 3 s = 1; falling = –1; stable = 0; rising = 1
(c) FDPs	Normal = 0; raised = 1; falling = –1, stable = 0, rising = 1
3 Specific criteria	
(a) Antithrombin	Normal = –1; low = 1
(b) Protein C	Normal = –1; low = 1
(c) TAT complexes	Normal = –1; elevated = 1
4 Calculate score	

Table 51.4 Template scoring system for non-overt DIC.

TAT, thrombin–antithrombin.

fibrinogen quantification (by Clauss method) and measurement of fibrin/fibrinogen degradation products (D-dimers).

In some cases of DIC, fibrinogen may remain within the normal range. This finding can be explained by fibrinogen synthesis being increased as part of an acute phase response. Likewise, the fibrinogen level is normally raised in pregnancy, whereas in a patient with liver disease it may be chronically reduced. Serial coagulation tests are particularly useful in the diagnosis of DIC. A progressive decrease in the platelet count and increasing prolongation of the clotting times is seen.

The ISTH scoring system for non-overt DIC suggests that assays to detect a fall in protein C and antithrombin along with a rise in thrombin–antithrombin (TAT) complexes are included in the extended laboratory assessment of DIC. However, access to some of these tests may be limited in some centres. Other more specialized investigations include the detection of raised levels of prothrombin fragments 1 and 2 and fibrinopeptide A (cleaved from the N-terminal of fibrinogen by thrombin). Fibronectin may be non-specifically cross-linked to fibrin by factor XIII and indeed its plasma levels may fall in DIC and correlate with elevated FDPs.

Patients with chronic liver disease may exhibit a state of systemic hyperfibrinolysis. This occurs due to increased levels of plasminogen activators secondary to decreased hepatic clearance and lower circulating levels of PAI-1 and α_2-plasmin inhibitor. This state can be difficult to distinguish from DIC and may present with haemorrhage. The main distinguishing laboratory tests are the presence of a shortened euglobulin clot lysis time (usually normal in DIC) and a normal platelet count (usually reduced in DIC). In both situations, fibrinogen levels are low, FDPs are elevated and screening coagulation tests are prolonged. Treatment for hyperfibrinolysis may include the administration of antifibrinolytic drugs. The two states (DIC and hyperfibrinolysis) may both exist in the same patient. In the absence of demonstrable hyperfibrinolysis, antifibrinolytic drugs should be avoided in patients with DIC.

The serum of some patients with sepsis contains a calcium-dependent complex of C-reactive protein (CRP) and very low-density lipoprotein (VLDL). This complex results in the transmission waveform during clot formation in the APTT assay changing to an abnormal biphasic waveform pattern, which can be monitored by certain automated coagulometers. Recently, this pattern of waveform has been shown to correlate with a high risk of adverse outcome and may be useful in risk stratification of patients with sepsis in the intensive therapy unit setting. The presence of a normal waveform has a high negative predictive value in excluding sepsis.

Management

Underpinning any management strategy in a patient with DIC must be a resolve to treat and cure the underlying disorder. All the other aspects of management of DIC, although they may be life saving in the acute situation, can only be viewed as supportive. In the case of DIC related to obstetric complications, delivery or evacuation of the uterine contents may be life saving. The patient may require support with fluid replacement to ensure optimal end organ perfusion pressure and treatment with antibacterial agents to treat infection leading to sepsis. The management of patients presenting with predominantly haemorrhagic manifestations of DIC differs from that of patients with thrombotic problems.

In patients who are bleeding or are in need of acute surgical intervention replacement of clotting factors in the form of fresh-frozen plasma (FFP) (12–15 mL/kg) and cryoprecipitate is indicated. Cryoprecipitate may be indicated for low (< 1 g/L) fibrinogen levels. Cryoprecipitate also contains von Willebrand factor (vWF) and factor XIII. Therapy should aim to maintain a PT/APTT ratio of 1.5 or less and a fibrinogen of greater than 1 g/L. Bleeding patients may also require platelet transfusion to maintain levels greater than 50×10^9/L. The response of the patient's platelet count and clotting times to treatment should be regularly monitored. The administration of prothrombin complex concentrate is unwise in view of its thrombogenicity in this context, as this may enhance fibrin deposition. Prophylactic plasma infusion is not advocated in the non-bleeding patient. This is not only wasteful, but may expose the patient to an unnecessary risk of transfusion-related complications, such as infection.

The administration of heparin to interfere with the cycle of continued thrombin activation has been used in management of DIC, particularly in patients with thrombotic manifestations such as dermal ischaemia. Usually, a low dose of unfractionated heparin (300–500 units/h) is employed. Care needs to be taken as these patients are at risk of bleeding. The use of heparin in the treatment of DIC is controversial and in septic patients its use would usually be reserved for those with thrombosis and/or a failure of platelet and clotting parameters to improve despite aggressive transfusion.

There are, however, some instances where heparin may be particularly useful. The syndrome of retained dead fetus is a case in point, where heparin therapy may result in a normalization of fibrinogen levels. Localized consumption secondary to aortic aneurysm may also respond to heparin therapy. The efficacy of therapy with heparin can be monitored by analysis of serial platelet counts, FDP (D-dimer) quantification and fibrinogen levels. The APTT may already be abnormal in patients with DIC and one may seek to measure the pharmacological effects of heparin by measurement of the anti-Xa activity of the patient's plasma. Heparin therapy is unwise in cases of DIC secondary to placental abruption, sepsis, severe liver disease and major trauma.

Infusion of an antithrombin concentrate has been shown to be beneficial in some patients with DIC. The rationale for this is to neutralize the excess thrombin formed by the DIC process. Antithrombin may be of particular use in patients with DIC secondary to sepsis. However, the role of antithrombin in treating DIC needs further investigation at the level of randomized controlled trials. The use of activated protein C in sepsis is discussed later in this chapter.

Coagulopathy associated with severe sepsis

A particularly severe coagulopathy may occur in patients with severe sepsis. This is particularly marked in the approximately 10% of patients who develop fulminant disease when systemically infected by *Neisseria meningitidis*. This organism is carried in the nasopharynx; however, in a proportion of individuals, it breeches the mucosal barrier. In some, the organism then produces a

severe clinical state characterized by vasomotor collapse, multiple organ failure, rapidly enlarging skin and mucosal purpura (purpura fulminans) and arterial thrombi, leading to gangrene and end organ damage. Why some individuals are more susceptible than others to developing this severe state is unclear at present.

An outline of the events that lead to disturbance of the clotting mechanism is shown in Figure 51.2. A massive cytokine response is seen following cells of the immune system being stimulated by bacterial lipopolysaccharide. TNF-α and IL-1α stimulate increased tissue factor expression at the surface of endothelial cells and monocytes. In addition, the natural anticoagulant function of protein C is relatively reduced. This comes about by several mechanisms including a reduction in thrombomodulin expression by endothelial cells, an increase in C4b binding protein (which binds to and lowers free protein S levels) and an increase in levels of α₁-antitrypsin (which inhibits the serine protease action of protein C).

The importance of this reduction of activity of activated protein C (APC) in severe sepsis has been made greater following the discovery that as well as possessing an anticoagulant function, APC also has anti-inflammatory properties that may limit the excessive activation of inflammatory cascades seen in severe sepsis. The anti-inflammatory activity of APC has been demonstrated in experiments in which baboons are infused with a large dose of *Escherichia coli*. In those baboons concurrently given APC, survival and the degree of septic shock that ensues on infusion are improved. APC may act by dampening the response to inflammatory cytokines; it may also interfere with the CD14-dependent activation of monocytes by endotoxin. APC has now undergone a phase III trial in the Recombinant Human APC Worldwide Evaluation in Severe Sepsis (PROWESS) study. In this placebo-controlled trial, APC was shown to reduce the relative risk of death in patients with severe sepsis by 19.4%. In this study, APC in the form of drotrecogin alpha was administered at a dose of 24 μg per kilogram of body weight per hour, for a total duration of 96 h. However, there was an increased risk of bleeding complications in the APC-treated arm.

In 2001, APC received a licence from the Food and Drugs Administration for use in severe sepsis. The treatment has maximum clinical benefit if used in patients with severe sepsis with an APACHE II score of 25 or more and in those with a reasonable life expectancy if they survive the septic episode. A summary of the actions of protein C in this context is shown in Figure 51.2. Further targeting of subgroups who will benefit most from activated protein C infusion may be possible following the recent development of an enzyme capture assay employing a monoclonal antibody with high specificity for activated protein C.

Haemostatic defects in acute promyelocytic leukaemia

Acute promyelocytic leukaemia (APML) is characterized by a clonal expansion of immature promyelocytes with a characteristic

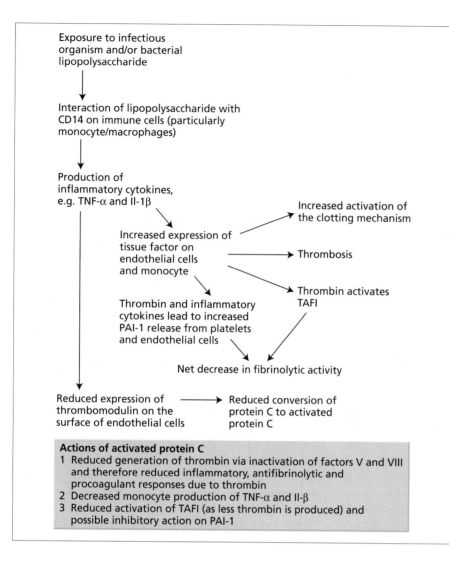

Figure 51.2 Mechanism of the coagulation disturbance seen in severe sepsis and the actions of activated protein C.

Exposure to infectious organism and/or bacterial lipopolysaccharide

↓

Interaction of lipopolysaccharide with CD14 on immune cells (particularly monocyte/macrophages)

↓

Production of inflammatory cytokines, e.g. TNF-α and Il-1β

→ Increased expression of tissue factor on endothelial cells and monocyte

→ Increased activation of the clotting mechanism

→ Thrombosis

→ Thrombin activates TAFI

Thrombin and inflammatory cytokines lead to increased PAI-1 release from platelets and endothelial cells

→ Net decrease in fibrinolytic activity

Reduced expression of thrombomodulin on the surface of endothelial cells → Reduced conversion of protein C to activated protein C

Actions of activated protein C
1 Reduced generation of thrombin via inactivation of factors V and VIII and therefore reduced inflammatory, antifibrinolytic and procoagulant responses due to thrombin
2 Decreased monocyte production of TNF-α and Il-β
3 Reduced activation of TAFI (as less thrombin is produced) and possible inhibitory action on PAI-1

balanced chromosomal translocation between chromosomes 15 and 17: t(15;17)(q22–24;q12–21). The condition is responsive to treatment with all-*trans*-retinoic acid (ATRA) which causes differentiation of the leukaemic cells. APML is also associated with a bleeding diathesis, which, in some cases, can be fatal. It now appears that the APML cells are themselves causal in the coagulopathy seen in this condition. Patients with APML at presentation may have prolongation of the PT, APTT and TT, along with increased levels of FDPs. APML cells have been shown to stimulate more thrombin generation than other leukaemic cell lines in thrombin generation assays, this in part may be due to high expressed levels of tissue factor. In addition, APML cells may increase tissue factor expression on endothelial cells through expression of IL-1β. The increased tissue factor is further augmented by the presence of increased surface expression of phosphatidyl serine at the surface of APML cells.

The cells in APML also have been demonstrated to express high levels of annexin II. This protein acts as a coreceptor for plasminogen and tissue plasminogen activator. This results in excessive plasmin formation, which is sufficient to exceed the capacity of circulating α₂-plasmin inhibitor. This unopposed excessive fibrinolytic potential of the plasma results in a bleeding diathesis. Expression of annexin II mRNA has been demonstrated to fall following exposure of APML cells to ATRA. Indeed, treatment with ATRA has been shown to reduce the duration of the haemorrhagic phase of APML.

Coagulopathy in the patient with massive blood loss

The conventional definition of massive blood loss is that of one blood volume in a 24-h period. (Normal blood volume is approximately 5 L, i.e. about 7% of an adult's ideal body mass.) The development of a coagulopathy in patients with massive blood loss is multifactorial. Clotting factor deficiency is unlikely to occur until 80% of the patient's blood volume has been replaced. In the acute situation, the infusion of colloid or crystalloid may result in dilution of coagulation factors and platelets. In addition, some colloid preparations may impede coagulation directly (see later in chapter). These inhibitory actions of colloids are usually of little clinical consequence, provided that the patient has normal renal function and the volume of colloid infused in 24 h is not in excess of 1.5 L.

As discussed earlier, trauma itself and some of the obstetric emergencies associated with massive blood loss may precipitate DIC, which will further consume already depleted coagulation factors. Patients with prolonged hypoxia or hypovolaemia and those with cerebral trauma are at high risk of developing DIC. Metabolic acidosis developing as a consequence of tissue hypoperfusion may also upset the coagulation mechanism. Hypothermia, which may manifest in patients with massive blood loss, may also worsen any coagulopathy present. Many trauma patients will reach the emergency department with a core temperature of less than 36°C. Many factors may predispose to hypothermia in trauma victims, including a prolonged extraction time from the accident scene, spinal cord injury, alcohol ingestion and the administration of cold intravenous fluids. The prewarming of fluids before transfusion into the patient will help to prevent this.

Management of patients with massive blood loss often requires the coordination and cooperation of individuals from many specialties. Local guidelines should be in place to optimize treatment. The use of formulaic replacement strategies with blood components is no longer regarded as optimal, as it may lead to the unnecessary transfusion of patients with exposure to the infectious and non-infectious risks of blood products or inadequate replacement. It is recommended that frequent checks are made of the patient's haemostasis tests to ensure that treatment is tailored to the patients needs. Some flexibility is needed, however, and it may be necessary to pre-empt the

need for blood components, especially platelets. This should be reflected in local protocols.

When managing these patients, one should transfuse platelet concentrate with the aim of maintaining a platelet count of at least 50×10^9/L in all patients and of $80-100 \times 10^9$/L in patients with central nervous system injury or polytrauma. The APTT and PT should be maintained such that they are less than 1.5 times that of the normal control time. FFP should be infused to achieve this and should be requested initially in volumes to infuse 12–15 mL of FFP per kilogram of patient body mass. Cryoprecipitate should be administered to maintain a plasma fibrinogen of at least 1 g/L. Cryoprecipitate is usually initially administered at a dose of 1.5 packs per 10 kg of patient body mass.

Recently, reports relating to the use of rVIIa in patients with massive blood loss have appeared in the literature. The doses used in these studies have ranged from 60 to 212 µg/kg. Large-scale studies relating to the use of rVIIa are needed to clarify dose, efficacy and potential thrombotic side-effects of this compound.

Near-patient testing of clotting parameters

The use of thromboelastography (TEG®) in the near-patient testing of coagulation parameters in patients undergoing liver transplantation and cardiopulmonary bypass (CBP) is now well established. The method involves the measuring of torque exerted on a pin placed in a rotating cup that contains a small volume of whole blood. As the blood clots, the rotational force from the cup is transmitted to the pin and then recorded by means of an electrical transducer. A typical TEG® trace, along with some of the parameters measured on it, is shown in Figure 51.3. Further study is needed; however, the TEG® may also have a role in

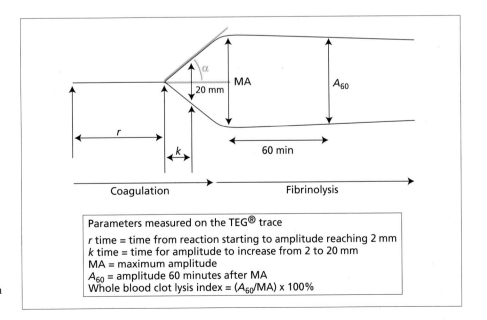

Figure 51.3 A typical TEG® trace. Hyperfibrinolysis is associated with a shortened *r* time and reduced MA and A$_{60}$; increased coagulation is indicated by a shortened *r* time and an increase in the MA.

Parameters measured on the TEG® trace

r time = time from reaction starting to amplitude reaching 2 mm
k time = time for amplitude to increase from 2 to 20 mm
MA = maximum amplitude
A$_{60}$ = amplitude 60 minutes after MA
Whole blood clot lysis index = (A$_{60}$/MA) x 100%

screening for patients with a hypercoagulable state, assessing the effect of drugs on the fibrinolytic system and in screening for patients at high risk of surgical bleeding.

The Platelet Function Analyser (PFA 100®) measures the time for whole blood in a capillary device under simulated high shear stress conditions to occlude a coated membrane, the so-called *closure time*. The system employs a disposable membrane containing platelet agonists. At present, membranes containing collagen and epinephrine or collagen and ADP are used. The test is sensitive to defects relating to platelet function and some quantitative and qualitative abnormalities of vWF.

Cardiopulmonary bypass

Cardiopulmonary bypass (CPB) surgery is frequently associated with laboratory abnormalities of coagulation. However the operation is now routine and only rarely associated with excessive peri- or post-operative bleeding that is related to specific haemostatic defects. Bleeding is more common in patients needing reoperation or undergoing more complex procedures such as heart and lung transplants. Patients are routinely heparinized to prevent thrombosis within the oxygenator and bypass circuit.

The control of heparin therapy is performed in theatre by means of an activated clotting time test. (At an activated clotting time of 400–600 s, clots do not spontaneously form in the oxygenator.) Heparinization is reversed at the end of the procedure by means of a slow infusion of protamine sulphate. (Approximately 1 mg of protamine neutralizes 100 units of heparin.) Excess protamine may cause clinical bleeding by producing a consumptive coagulopathy. Following initial neutralization with protamine, the reappearance of active heparin in the blood may occur 2–6 h later. This is due to the return to the circulation of sequestered extravascular heparin and its release from heparin–protamine complexes. Thrombocytopenia of some degree occurs in all patients on CPB, due to platelet damage in the pump and oxygenator system. Platelet function usually corrects itself by 3 h post-operatively. Severe post-operative thrombocytopenia of less than 50×10^9/L and more persistent platelet functional defects occur in those patients undergoing prolonged complicated procedures.

The use of aprotinin in high-risk patients, particularly those undergoing repeat cardiac surgery has been shown to reduce bleeding. Shorter operative times are seen as a result of reduced generalized oozing from operative sites. Aprotinin is a broad-spectrum Kunitz-type protease inhibitor with actions against plasmin, kallikrein and trypsin. At the doses used in CPB, aprotinin will limit contact activation by inhibiting kallikrein and fibrinolysis by plasmin inhibition. The use of aprotinin is probably best limited to patients with a high risk of haemorrhagic complications, as it may increase thrombotic risk in patients in whom coronary artery patency is paramount. Analysis of the

TEG® trace in patients during CPB has been found to be of use in guiding the administration of plasma and antifibrinolytics.

Patients found to be bleeding excessively post-operatively should be examined to ensure that one of the chest drains is not filling more than the other, indicating a specific bleeding vessel. A FBC and coagulation screen is useful, and it is usual practice to give platelet concentrate transfusion irrespective of the count, in view of the acquired platelet functional deficit associated with CPB. FFP should be given to correct prolonged clotting times and aprotinin may be necessary if there is a suggestion of fibrinolytic bleeding.

Haemostatic disturbance in hepatic disease

All the coagulation factors, with the exception of vWF, are synthesized in the liver along with antithrombin, protein C, protein S, α_2-plasmin inhibitor and plasminogen. The liver is also involved in the clearance of activated clotting factors from the circulation. Hepatic disease may therefore have profound effects on haemostasis.

Acute hepatitis

Patients with acute hepatitis may display a mild thrombocytopenia ($100–150 \times 10^9$/L). The mechanism for this may be immune or be due to concurrent hypersplenism. Thrombocytopenia may also be manifest in relation to DIC. Platelet function may also be impaired in acute hepatitis, although in the absence of severe thrombocytopenia this is unlikely to be of clinical significance. In acute liver disease, hepatic biosynthesis of clotting factors is impaired and this may be reflected in a prolongation of screening tests of coagulation. The prothrombin time and factor V levels are the most sensitive test to hepatic biosynthetic dysfunction. The plasma fibrinogen may be raised in acute hepatic disturbance as part of an acute phase response. A low fibrinogen level is associated with a poor prognosis in this context. Rather than being due to DIC, a pattern of reduced fibrinogen and increased FDPs seen in acute liver disease may be due to hyperfibrinolysis. Features distinguishing this state from one of DIC are discussed in the section on management of DIC.

Chronic liver disease

In chronic liver disease thrombocytopenia is frequently noted. In patients with cirrhosis, this is frequently related to hypersplenism, secondary to portal hypertension. One must be mindful, however, of the possibility that dietary problems, such as folate deficiency and the direct toxic effect of ethanol on megakaryocyte function, may also contribute to thrombocytopenia in a patient who takes excess alcohol. Platelets may manifest functional disturbance in chronic liver disease, although the mechanism of this is unclear. Coagulation factor synthesis is affected by chronic liver pathology. With respect to the vitamin K-dependent factors, factor IX synthesis is usually less reduced than that of factors II, VII and X. Low factor V levels may correlate better than reduced vitamin K dependent factors with the level of hepatic dysfunction. Cholestatic liver disease will impair absorption of fat-soluble vitamins including vitamin K and will lead to reduced levels of vitamin K-dependent clotting factors.

Most patients with stable chronic liver disease have a normal or increased fibrinogen level. Some patients may develop dysfibrinogenaemia; this is thought to be because of increased sialic acid content of the fibrinogen. This causes slowing of the polymerization of fibrin following the release of fibrinopeptides A and B by thrombin. When finally formed, the clot is unstable. Dysfibrinogenaemia is reflected by a prolonged thrombin time with a more normal fibrinogen antigen level compared with that determined functionally by the Clauss assay.

Reduced hepatic clearance of activated clotting factors and lower synthesis of natural anticoagulants may predispose individuals with hepatic disease to developing DIC. This may occur following Gram-negative infection or in association with the insertion of a peritoneo-venous shunt. Ascitic fluid should be discarded at the time of shunt insertion to prevent this complication. Cirrhosis is associated with increased fibrinolysis; this is caused by increased levels of plasminogen activators (particularly tissue plasminogen activator), without an equivalent rise in plasminogen activator inhibitors such as PAI 1.

The management of a bleeding patient with hepatic dysfunction will in terms of specifics of management depend on the site of bleeding (e.g. from varices or from a biopsy site). Clotting function should be assessed by means of the PT, APTT, TT, fibrinogen levels and D-dimer levels. Vitamin K should be administered intravenously (slow i.v., 10 mg daily for 3 days) to aid biosynthesis of vitamin K-dependent factors. FFP contains coagulation factors and anticoagulants and is therefore appropriate to correct the bleeding diathesis if one is present. Large volumes of FFP may however be required and this may present a management problem in patients with hepatic disease who are at risk of fluid overload. Fibrinogen may be supplemented by transfusion of cryoprecipitate. Platelet transfusion may be necessary but platelet recovery may be reduced in the context of hepatic disease, however, because of hypersplenism. In patients with evidence of increased fibrinolysis, antifibrinolytic drugs such as tranexamic acid (1 g t.d.s.) should be considered.

Liver transplantation

The changes in the balance of haemostasis seen during liver transplantation are both complex and multifactorial. As discussed in the previous sections, patients with chronic and acute liver failure reacquiring transplantation are likely to have preoperative coagulopathy to some extent. Traditionally, the process of liver transplant is split into three stages: stage I, the pre-

anhepatic stage, which ends with the occlusion of the recipient's hepatic blood flow; stage II, the anhepatic phase, which ends with the reperfusion of the donor liver; and stage III, the reperfusion and neohepatic period.

A reduction in activity of clotting factors may be seen in stage I, especially if large blood losses necessitate transfusion and possible dilution of clotting factors. Release of heparin from the transplanted liver may also impair coagulation. Hyperfibrinolysis is seen in a significant number of liver transplant patients, often during stage II, with a recovery in stage III. Plasma levels of tissue plasminogen activator (tPA) are seen to rise in stage II and fall again late in stage III; levels of PAI-1 follow a reciprocal pattern. The mechanism of the increase in tPA levels is most likely to be due to lack of hepatic clearance. The platelet count usually falls during the procedure, reaching a nadir during the reperfusion phase. This fall is more profound if the transplanted organ is severely damaged and may be due to sequestration of platelets in the transplanted liver.

There is little evidence that one can predict the transfusion needs of a patient by examining their preoperative coagulation results. Correction of the profound coagulation abnormalities seen in fulminant hepatic failure is wise preoperatively. However, the correction of a mild coagulopathy in a patient with chronic liver disease prior to the operation is less likely to be of benefit.

During surgery, the aim is to tailor blood components administered to prevent the development of intractable coagulopathy but, at the same time, ensure that the patient does not receive unnecessary blood components. Near-patient tests of haemostasis such as the thromboelastograph (TEG®) are often used in theatre to complement the tests performed in the coagulation laboratory. The TEG® can monitor both the overall clotting and fibrinolytic potential of whole blood. Many laboratory tests correlate well with their TEG® equivalent; for example, a low fibrinogen is associated with reduced maximal amplitude of the TEG® trace, whereas thrombocytopenia is characterized by a prolonged reaction time and lower maximal amplitude values. Many departments use algorithms based on clotting and TEG® results to guide FFP, red cells, cryoprecipitate and platelet transfusion during the procedure. Aprotinin can be administered to counteract the increase in fibrinolysis observed.

Haemostatic disturbance in renal disease

Patients with chronic renal impairment may clinically express a bleeding diathesis with epistaxis, menorrhagia and gastrointestinal bleeding. Bleeding from the upper gastrointestinal tract may be secondary to angiodysplasia. Occasionally, haemorrhagic pericarditis and intracranial haemorrhage is seen. The main defect seen in association with renal disease is impairment of platelet function and the platelet vessel wall interaction. This will manifest with an increased bleeding time.

The pathogenesis of the haemostatic disturbance seen in renal disease is multifactorial. Increased levels of platelet inhibitory prostacyclin (PGI_2) are released by the vascular endothelium. The platelets of patients with renal impairment may exhibit multiple functional disturbances, including defective *in vitro* aggregation in response to ADP, adrenaline, collagen and thrombin. The platelets of those with renal disturbance also exhibit reduced expression of procoagulant anionic phospholipids at their surface in response to activation and also have impaired clot retraction. The disturbance of platelet function in uraemia may relate to the accumulation of platelet toxic materials in the plasma; candidate molecules include guanidosuccinic acid, which is a product of ammonia metabolism, and phenolic acids. Some of the disturbance of platelet function may relate to increased nitric oxide levels. Global screening tests of coagulation are usually normal in renal disease, although an increase in factor VIII and fibrinogen may be observed. Fibrinolysis is often impaired in renal disease.

1-Deamino-D-arginine vasopressin (DDAVP) has been shown to effectively reduce the bleeding time in patients with renal impairment (at a dose of 0.3–0.4 μg/kg i.v.). As in the treatment of mild von Willebrand disease with this compound, tachyphylaxis may occur because of depletion of endothelial stores of vWF. The bleeding time may also be partly corrected by the treatment of the anaemia frequently associated with chronic renal disease (particularly if the packed cell volume has fallen to less than 20%). This correction is now often achieved via the regular administration of recombinant erythropoietin. Dialysis itself may also improve the bleeding diathesis of renal disease; patients at high risk of bleeding during dialysis may have this risk reduced by reducing the heparin dose used during dialysis or replacing it with prostacyclin. Conjugated oestrogens have also been shown to reduce the bleeding time of uraemic patients.

Renal disease may also be complicated by thromboembolic phenomena. These are occasionally related to vascular access points for dialysis. Nephrotic syndrome with antithrombin deficiency is associated with renal vein thrombosis, especially when caused by membranous glomerulonephritis. Patients with this condition should therefore be considered for thromboprophylaxis. Renal allograft failure may occur secondary to thrombosis; the incidence of this complication may be reduced by preoperative thrombophilia screening and appropriate additional thromboprophylaxis.

Haemostatic changes associated with alcohol consumption

Moderate alcohol consumption appears to have beneficial effects on the individual with respect to rates of cardiovascular disease. The mechanism for this effect is not entirely clear and although some of it may relate to changes in lipid metabolism, the effects of alcohol on haemostasis may also play a role. At low levels, alcohol has been shown to increase the fibrinolytic potential of endothelial cells, for example by increasing levels of the urokinase receptor. In addition, lower levels of lipoprotein (a) in moderate drinkers may increase the activity of plasmin (lipoprotein (a) contains sequences homologous to the kringle domains of plasmin and can compete with the protein for its binding sites). Moderate alcohol consumption is also associated with a reduction in the response of platelets to agonists *in vitro*. Some of this effect is mediated by a reduction in the activity of phospholipase A_2 and a concurrent fall in thromboxane synthesis. The Framingham study showed that mild to moderate alcohol intake was associated with lower levels of fibrinogen, vWF, VII and plasma viscosity. However, higher levels of intake were associated with a reduced fibrinolytic potential.

When the blood ethanol concentration becomes greater than 0.2 g/dL, this generally inhibits platelet aggregation in a dose-dependent fashion and prolongs the skin bleeding time. As well as ethanol, there are specific additional platelet inhibitors in red wine and grape juice. These flavonoids inhibit thromboxane A_2 production by blocking phospholipase A_2 and cyclo-oxygenase activity and increase the inhibitory effects of platelet cyclic AMP by inhibiting cyclic AMP phosphodiesterase. It is now widely accepted that the cardioprotective effects of red wine are due, in part, to the antioxidant platelet inhibitory properties associated with flavonoids rather than specifically with any ethanol effect. Thus, regularly drinking small amounts of red wine would seem by several large epidemiological studies to reduce the incidence of arterial thrombotic cardiovascular disease, particularly myocardial infarction and thrombotic stroke.

Regular heavy drinking damages the synthetic capacity of the liver hepatocytes, so that in patients with advanced liver disease and cirrhosis, there is a hypocoagulable state due to deficiency of the vitamin K-dependent clotting factors and factor V. There is also evidence that changes in lipid metabolism related to alcohol consumption may also alter the synthesis and activation state of several clotting factors, particularly factor VII. However, light to moderate alcohol use may be protective, as it lowers the levels of fibrinogen, factor VII and vWF towards the lower end of the overall normal range.

Overall fibrinolytic potential tends to be lower with increasing alcohol consumption. In particular, inhibitor PAI-1 levels are consistently higher as alcohol consumption increases and levels decrease after abstinence from alcohol. The effects on PAI-1 are linked to fasting and post glucose insulin concentrations as these decrease with increasing alcohol consumption and it is well known that high PAI-1 levels are associated with late-onset diabetes and obesity. Fibrinolytic potential shows a marked circadian rhythm, with the lowest activity being in the morning. Heavy binge drinking is associated with a further fall in fibrinolytic potential at this time of the day, and correlates with high PAI-1 and tPA antigen levels but a low tPA activity.

In any individual, the effect of alcohol and its various constituents on haemostasis is extremely variable and any clinical event, including beneficial effects and bleeding or thrombotic events, is usually multifactorial. Overall, the peak protective effect is seen at a 20 g per day intake of alcohol (approximately) but there is a definite increased risk of adverse events in individuals who have an intake of greater than 90 g per day, particularly if associated with episodic binge drinking. Binge drinkers have an increased risk of developing both spontaneous bleeding and thrombotic events.

Haemostasis in the newborn

The haemostatic system, like many other parts of the body undergoes rapid and dynamic changes during the first few days and weeks of life and there is a 'physiological' deficiency of many pro- and anticoagulant proteins in the neonatal period, which is even more profound in premature infants. Only coagulation factors V, VIII, fibrinogen and platelets have levels in the adult range in the newborn. The majority of those that are low at birth reach adult values by 6 months. Interpretation of coagulation tests in premature and term neonates must take these physiological differences into account and remember that what is 'normal' in this age group may differ from results found in healthy adults and appropriate age-adjusted normal ranges should always be applied. The results of screening tests of coagulation in premature and newborn infants are shown in Table 51.5.

Most infants will never undergo a screen of haemostatic function. Those in whom testing is indicated include infants with haemorrhage, including intraventricular or intracranial haemorrhage, significant bleeding from the umbilical cord or delayed cord separation, a family history of a severe inherited bleeding disorder, conditions predisposing to DIC and maternal history of anticonvulsant ingestion. In addition, many neonates admitted to neonatal intensive care centres will undergo coagulation screening. Sampling difficulties are frequent in samples taken from this population; platelet clumping occurs commonly and may produce an erroneously low result for the platelet count

and, if micro-techniques are not available in the local laboratory, it can be difficult to obtain a good free-flowing sample for accurate assessment of coagulation status. Assessment of platelet function with formal platelet aggregation is extremely difficult owing to the large volumes of blood required, but flow cytometry can be used to check for deficiencies in platelet glycoproteins. Although rare, factor XIII deficiency may result in bleeding diathesis without causing abnormality of any routine coagulation tests and its presence must be specifically sought in this circumstance (for example by the urea clot lysis time or FXIII assay).

Acquired haemostatic disorders are much more likely to cause bleeding symptoms in the neonatal period than inherited conditions. Vitamin K deficiency is covered in the next section. DIC can occur secondary to many of the causes seen in adults; however, there are also conditions that are more specific to the age of the patient, such as necrotizing enterocolitis, amniotic fluid aspiration, meconium aspiration and birth asphyxia. Neonatal DIC may also be caused by maternal illness such as placental abruption and severe pre-eclampsia. Because of the changes in coagulation, which occur normally in this age group, diagnosis of DIC may be difficult. Along with the 'usual' tests for DIC, assays of individual factors (V and VIII) may be useful in diagnosis.

Vitamin K

Vitamin K is a fat-soluble vitamin essential for the post-translational modification of factors II, VII, IX and X and proteins C and S. Vitamin K is an essential cofactor in the gamma carboxylation of glutamic acid residues on these proteins, which occurs in the endoplasmic reticulum (Figure 51.4). During this process, the reduced form of vitamin K (quinol) is metabolized

Table 51.5 Haemostasis screening tests and factor assays in premature and term infants compared with the adult normal range (note that ranges will vary between laboratories).

	Premature infant	Term infant	Normal adult
PT (s)	16–20	14–17	12–14
TT (s)	15–24	14–18	12–14
APTT (s)	50–65	40–50	30–40
Factor IX (%)	15–20	20–40	50–200
Factor VII (%)	20–60	35–70	50–200
Antithrombin (%)	25–35	45–75	80–120

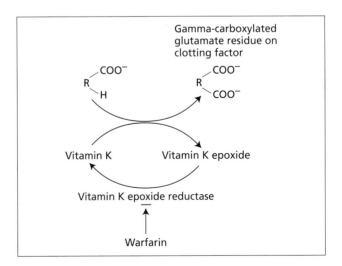

Figure 51.4 The mechanism of action of warfarin.

to vitamin K epoxide, which is then reduced again to quinol form. This modification, which results in two negative charges at the end of glutamate residues, allows interaction with divalent cations, specifically calcium, and allows the proteins to undergo conformational change in its presence.

Plants produce vitamin K_1, whereas vitamin K_2 is synthesized by micro-organisms. Vitamin K is absorbed in the proximal small intestine in the presence of bile. The liver stores vitamin K, however only a small amount is stored and without intake deficiency can ensue in a few days. Serum vitamin K levels can be quantified by high-pressure liquid chromatography techniques (normal adult fasting levels 150–800 pg/mL). When vitamin K levels are low or when its action is antagonized (for example by warfarin), inactive precursors of II, VII, IX and X are released without gamma carboxylated glutamate residues (so-called PIVKAs). Vitamin K deficiency is characterized by prolongation of the prothrombin time and activated partial thromboplasin time (reflecting reduced levels of vitamin K-dependent factors). The prothrombin time is relatively insensitive to early vitamin K deficiency; however, this may be detected by immunoassays for PIVKAs, which are not present in the plasma of vitamin K-replete subjects. Because the half-life of protein C (6–7 h) is less than that of the procoagulant vitamin K-dependent factors, early vitamin K deficiency or antagonism is manifest by a prothrombotic tendency. This may manifest as skin necrosis secondary to dermal capillary thrombosis.

Haemorrhagic disease of the newborn

The newborn infant is prone to vitamin K deficiency. There is a relatively poor exchange of vitamin K across the placenta (although a therapeutic dose of vitamin K given maternally may reach the unborn child in significant quantities). Moreover, PIVKAs are found in the plasma of neonates. This deficiency, if anything, intensifies during the first few days of life if supplemental vitamin K is not administered. The neonatal liver stores predominantly K_1, which has a more rapid turnover, compared with K_2, which is the dominant storage vitamin K in the adult liver. The newborn also lacks the gut flora to produce vitamin K and if receiving breast milk, its main/only source of food contains very little (< 5 µg/L compared with 50 µg/L for formula milk). This deficiency of vitamin K may lead to bleeding manifestations as part of the syndrome of haemorrhagic disease of the newborn (HDN). HDN may present with intracranial haemorrhage, gastrointestinal bleeding and bleeding from other sites.

HDN is said to occur in three forms.

1 *Early HDN.* This occurs following maternal ingestion of compounds that can interfere with vitamin K metabolism, notably phenytoin and barbiturate and manifests in the first 24 h of life. It may also be seen after taking rifampicin or warfarin. This form may be prevented by the maternal administration of vitamin K before delivery.

2 *Classic HDN.* This may have an incidence of 0.4–0.7 per 100 births when prophylactic vitamin K is not administered, it may appear at any time in the first month of life.

3 *Late HDN.* This form occurs at 2–12 weeks. It manifests in breast-fed infants who did not receive vitamin K at birth and in those with cholestatic liver pathology such as biliary atresia. Other conditions associated with late HDN include cystic fibrosis, alpha 1-antitrypsin deficiency and coeliac disease.

HDN may be prevented by the administration of vitamin K to infants just after birth. This may take the form of an intramuscular injection or oral administration. There has been some recent controversy over the route of administration. Fears that vitamin K can result in haemolytic anaemia are mainly a result of very large doses of vitamin K in its water-soluble form, which were given in the past. More seriously, concern was raised in the 1990s that the intramuscular administration of vitamin K could predispose to childhood cancers. More recent epidemiological studies performed in the light of the initial report have, in the main, concluded that there is no significant risk associated with intramuscular vitamin K. Explanations offered for the initial findings have included that the studies showing a link, may have intrinsic bias as a result of 'high-risk' newborns being selected for intramuscular vitamin K because of other conditions which may themselves have provided an increased risk of childhood cancer.

Disadvantages of the oral route for vitamin K include problems such as occult regurgitation and compliance issues, as further oral doses must be given between days 3 and 5 and days 21 and 28. In addition, there is some evidence that intramuscular vitamin K produces more sustained and predictable vitamin K bioavailability and that oral vitamin K may not fully prevent late HDN. If given orally, health-care provision must ensure follow-up of infants is adequate to ensure that the later doses of vitamin K are administered.

Vitamin K deficiency

Adults require a minimum daily intake of vitamin K of 0.1–0.5 µg/kg. The absorption of this fat-soluble vitamin is dependent on the presence of bile salts in the upper small intestine. Therefore, cholestatic disease may lead to vitamin K deficiency, as can coeliac disease and significant small bowel resection, which may also lead to malabsorption. Subclinical vitamin K deficiency (with a normal prothrombin time but reduced serum vitamin K and the presence of PIVKAs in the plasma) may be seen in association with inflammatory bowel disease, cystic fibrosis and intestinal fistulae. Patients with generalized poor nutrition or malabsorption may also be deficient in vitamin C and folic acid, which will accentuate any bleeding tendency. Individuals requiring total parenteral nutrition will need vitamin K supplements. This may be provided in a fat-soluble vitamin mixture, such as Vitlipid, given weekly.

Broad-spectrum antibiotics may produce a vitamin K-deficient state in those receiving them. The mechanism for this is not clear, but may be due to suppression of K_2 production by the large bowel gut flora. However whether significant vitamin K absorption occurs in the large bowel is a matter of debate. Some cephalosporin antibiotics are weak inhibitors of the vitamin K epoxide reductase enzyme and may lead to bleeding in patients with poor vitamin K stores.

Pharmacological manipulation of vitamin K

Coumarin class anticoagulant drugs such as warfarin exert their action by inhibiting the cyclical interconversion of vitamin K and its epoxide derivative essential for the formation of active forms of factors II, VII, IX and X (Figure 51.4). Coumarins inhibit vitamin K epoxide reductase and also possibly vitamin K reductase. Warfarin also interferes with the carboxylation of Gla proteins, which are synthesized in bone. This second effect may explain some of the teratogenic actions of warfarin.

When warfarin is first administered there is a delay in prolongation of the prothrombin time owing to the time taken for normally gamma carboxylated factors to be replaced by their non-gamma-carboxylated counterparts. The half-life of factor VII is relatively short (4–6 h) and thus early in therapy a prolongation may be seen in the prothrombin time due to this alone. However, the full anticoagulant potential of warfarin is not achieved until the other vitamin K-dependent factors have been reduced to 10–20% of their normal biological activity. The main anticoagulant effect of warfarin is likely in fact to reside in its lowering of prothrombin levels. Moreover, the half-life of protein C is also relatively short, therefore early in warfarin therapy one may have the situation of a relatively procoagulant state because of reduced natural anticoagulant function and as yet no real pharmacological anticoagulant function. This situation can rarely manifest as so-called warfarin induced skin necrosis especially in individuals with inherited or acquired deficiency of protein C or S. The aforementioned underpin the rationale for overlapping heparin therapy with warfarin therapy for at least 5 days in patients with an acute thrombosis or at high risk of thrombosis until the international normalized ratio (INR) is stable and within the desired therapeutic range.

Many drugs and other compounds administered to individuals may affect the pharmacokinetics of warfarin (Table 51.6). Significantly, warfarin as administered is a mixture of R and S isomers. The S isomer is five times more potent than the R form, thus drugs which affect the metabolism of the S form will have a much greater effect than those acting on the R form. Warfarin has a half-life of 47 h; 99% of circulating warfarin is bound to albumin and it is metabolized in the liver to compounds with little anticoagulant activity. The cytochrome P450 system is responsible for the metabolism of warfarin.

The major complication of warfarin therapy is over anticoagulation leading to bleeding. The risk of bleeding increases significantly with INR values greater than 5. However, even within the therapeutic range, bleeds do occur. The annual risk of

Table 51.6 Examples of drugs that interfere with oral anticoagulation control.

Mechanism	Drugs
Reduced coumarin binding to albumin	Phenylbutazone Sulphonamides
Reduced coumarin metabolism	Cimetidine Allopurinol Tricyclic antidepressants Metronidazole Sulphonamides
Alteration of hepatic receptor for drug	Thyroxine Quinidine
Induction of hepatic microsomal metabolism of coumarin	Barbiturates Rifampicin
Enhanced synthesis of clotting factors	Oral contraceptives Stanazol

Note: Drugs which interfere with platelet function may increase the bleeding risk with warfarin.

bleeding is approximately 0.3% for an INR of 2, 1% for an INR of 3, and 3% for an INR of 4. Recommendations as to the management of a patient who is over anticoagulated and/or bleeding need to take measure not only of the risk of haemorrhage, but also of the potential risk of viral transmission if plasma-based products (FFP or prothrombin complex concentrate) are infused and the risk of removing full anticoagulation from a patient at potential risk of a thrombotic event. Oral vitamin K is nearly as bioavailable as intravenous vitamin K. The management guidelines of the British Committee for Standards in Haematology for treating over-anticoagulation are shown in Table 51.7. Following a dose of vitamin K intravenously, effective hepatic synthesis of gamma-carboxylated factors does not begin for 6 h and is not maximal until 24–36 h.

Non-thrombotic vascular purpuras

A variety of general medical disorders may lead to widespread purpura. The challenge with respect to these problems is to distinguish them from thrombocytopenia and functional platelet disorders.

Simple easy bruising

Purpuric lesions are frequently encountered in normal individuals, usually women. Single or multiple bruises appear spontaneously, usually on the arms or legs and rapidly resolve without

Table 51.7 Management of bleeding in patients with excessive anticoagulation.

Clinical situation	Action
3 < INR < 6 (target 2.5) 4 < INR < 6 (target 3.5) No bleeding	Reduce warfarin dose or stop Restart when INR < 5
6 < INR < 8 No bleeding or minor bleeding	Stop warfarin Restart when INR < 5
INR > 8 No bleeding or minor bleeding	Stop warfarin Restart warfarin when INR < 5 If other risk factors for bleeding, give 0.5–2.5 mg of vitamin K orally
Major bleeding	Stop warfarin Give prothrombin complex concentrate* 50 units/kg or fresh-frozen plasma (FFP) 15 mL/kg Give 5 mg of vitamin K i.v.

*Factors II, VII, IX and X or factors II, IX and X with factor VII concentrate.

any specific treatment. Those patients who consult a medical practitioner may be exceedingly anxious or concerned regarding the cosmetics of the problem. No abnormalities are found in coagulation or platelet numerical or functional tests, and the patient can be reassured.

Senile purpura

This condition is seen frequently in the elderly population, usually in areas exposed to repeated low-level trauma such as the hands and forearms. The purpura is caused by atrophy of the subcutaneous tissue, with progressive loss of collagen and elastin fibres in the skin, leading to inadequate support to the subcutaneous blood vessels. Mild shearing forces can then lead to rupture and subcutaneous extravasation and spread of blood. Although there are no abnormalities in the haemostatic screening tests, a prolonged skin bleeding time may be observed in this condition. The lesions may retain their dark colour for several weeks. There is no specific therapy.

Hereditary haemorrhagic telangiectasia (HHT; Osler–Rendu–Weber syndrome)

This is a rare autosomal dominant condition. It is caused by mutations in the genes of endoglin (HHT1) and ALK-1 (*HHT2*).

Endothelial cells express both of these proteins, both of which are involved with signalling by the *transforming* growth factor beta superfamily. It is believed that abnormal blood vessels develop in HHT as a result of aberration in this signalling pathway. The condition presents with telangiectasia of the mucous membranes of the nose, mouth, gastrointestinal tract, vagina and skin. The lesions appear individually and in small groups. They blanche on pressure and bleed easily following minor trauma. This tendency to bleed increases with age.

Patients with HHT may also develop pulmonary and cerebral arteriovenous malformations (AVMs). Pulmonary AVM may enlarge in pregnancy leading to bleeding. At present, there is debate as to whether asymptomatic patients should be screened for cerebral AVMs. The most common presentations of this condition are recurrent epistaxis or gastrointestinal bleeding from multiple sites, which may eventually lead to iron deficiency. The standard coagulation tests are normal. Repeated intestinal bleeding may need treatment with therapeutic endoscopy and local cautery. Oral oestrogen therapy may reduce bleeding. The mechanism of action of oestrogen is to convert columnar epithelium to stratified squamous epithelium, which offers more protection against bleeding.

Giant cavernous haemangioma

In this condition, thin walled venous abnormalities appear on the skin in the first months of life. They may gradually enlarge until puberty. Although they do not cause a primary haemostatic abnormality, they may occasionally precipitate chronic activation of the coagulation system leading to laboratory features of chronic DIC. Spontaneous regression of the lesions may occur with age. The combination of giant haemangioma and thrombocytopenia with consumptive coagulopathy was first described by Kasabach and Merritt in 1940. Treatment for this condition may include corticosteroids, antifibrinolytic agents, cryosurgery, laser treatment and radiotherapy. Antiangiogenic agents are being investigated at present to see if they have a role in this condition's treatment.

Hereditary connective tissue disorders

Ehlers–Danlos syndrome, pseudoxanthoma elasticum, osteogenesis imperfecta and Marfan's syndrome can all present or be associated with recurrent bruising or skin purpura.

In Ehlers–Danlos syndrome, patients may have specific platelet functional abnormalities, but these may only be apparent in *in vitro* studies if a collagen preparation from the patient is used. The condition is associated with a defect in type III collagen, which leads to recurrent stretching of the skin with recurrent haematomas, causing thin atrophic skin with paper-like scars. Excessive bleeding or its prevention in the peri-operative setting may be achieved by infusion of platelet concentrates.

Metabolic causes of purpura

Severe scurvy or vitamin C deficiency typically presents with bleeding from multiple sites, including the gums, gastrointestinal tract, joints and brain. Perifollicular skin bleeding may also be seen. In this condition, the skin bleeding time may be prolonged but platelet function tests are usually normal. The diagnosis is made by observing reduced leucocyte vitamin C levels; the condition responds to vitamin C supplements.

Amyloidosis can cause skin purpura. Amyloid fibrils may infiltrate the walls of small blood vessels and also may cause functional platelet disturbance by binding to the platelet membrane. Lesions are often found in the periorbital region and may be distributed in linear streaks. Amyloid splenomegaly may lead to thrombocytopenia. Factor X may bind amyloid deposits, resulting in reduced levels of this factor in the plasma.

Long-term administration of corticosteriods may lead to atrophy of collagen fibres, which support blood vessels in the skin. This causes widespread purpura and bruises, usually on the extensor surfaces of the limbs. A similar finding is seen in Cushing's syndrome.

Allergic purpura

Allergic vasculitic purpura is caused by infiltration and inflammation of the blood vessel wall in response to a variety of agents, including chemicals, toxins and infections.

The most common example of this is Henoch–Schönlein purpura (HSP), which may involve the skin, joints, gastrointestinal tract, kidneys, heart and central nervous system. It is often preceded by β-haemolytic *Streptococcus* infection producing a rising anti-streptolysin O titre. Histologically, the condition is characterized by a leucocytoclastic vasculitis with IgA-predominant deposits affecting capillaries, venules and arterioles. Outbreaks of HSP may be seen in children in whom fever is followed by a purpuric rash, which is classically raised and affects the legs, thighs and buttocks. The patient may also develop nephritis (with proteinuria), arthritis and abdominal pain. The most serious complications of HSP are central nervous system bleeding, acute intussusception and renal failure. The condition is usually self-limiting, but may respond to steroid therapy.

A range of drugs have been reported to cause vascular purpura via an allergic mechanism. Examples include aspirin, sulphonamides and β-lactams. Skin testing with the offending drug may cause localized petechiae.

Psychogenic purpura

Bizarre bleeding and purpuric problems have been associated with psychological disturbance. These include self-induced bleeding, hysterical bleeding, religious stigmata and auto-erythrocyte sensitization.

Specific coagulation factor inhibitors

Acquired haemophilia occurs as a result of the production of autoantibody activity directed against a coagulation factor, resulting in a decrease in the factor's function. The incidence of acquired inhibitor development is reported to be between one and four per million per year. The condition most frequently presents in the elderly and has an equal sex distribution. It may also be associated with autoimmune disease, lymphoproliferative disease (including chronic lymphatic leukaemia) and is also seen in the post-partum period. Associated autoimmune disorders include systemic lupus erythematosus (SLE), rheumatoid arthritis and graft-versus-host disease following allogeneic bone marrow transplant. Post-partum-associated acquired haemophilia usually occurs in primiparous women within 3 months of delivery, although in some patients an inhibitor may develop during pregnancy. Acquired haemophilia is also associated with solid tumours, including prostate and lung cancer. Some drugs, for example β-lactams and diphenylhydantoin, have been associated with the development of acquired inhibitors. Notably, in approximately 50% of patients with an acquired inhibitor, no clinical association may be found. By far the most common clotting factor against which acquired inhibitors develop is factor VIII; acquired inhibitors to all of the other coagulation factors (including factor XIII) have been described but are much less common.

Acquired inhibitors usually present with bleeding. Frequently, this manifests as extensive bruising or bleeding into muscles. Occasionally compartment syndrome may ensue in the presence of an extensive muscle haematoma. The condition may also present with haematuria, melena or haemoptysis. In contrast with inherited haemophilia, haemarthroses are rare as presentations of an acquired inhibitor. Acquired inhibitors may also present with bleeding following catheterization of the bladder or the insertion of an intravenous line.

The diagnosis of an acquired inhibitor is usually first made by noting the prolongation of the relevant clotting test (e.g. the APTT with a factor VIII inhibitor). This prolongation will fail to correct by more than 50% of the difference between the test and normal control plasma clotting time on incubation of the patient's and normal plasma in a 50:50 mix. It is important that the 50:50 mix is performed on a sample incubated for 1 h at 37°C with similarly incubated normal plasma as a control (to compensate for labile factor loss on incubation). Failure to perform a prolonged incubation may result in some inhibitors being missed in the laboratory because of their time-dependent nature. A specific factor assay will reveal reduced activity of the factor to which the inhibitor is directed. The Bethesda assay will quantify the inhibitor. The Nijmegen modification of this assay is now used as the original version of the Bethesda method may produce false-positive results due to loss of factor VIII activity consequent on pH shift and reduced protein concentration. The temporal kinetics of an acquired inhibitor are often complex and non-linear with a rapid inactivation phase, in contrast with the linear kinetics seen in the inhibitors that develop in the context of the treatment of inherited haemophilia. The Bethesda assay may also be used to determine whether the inhibitor has activity against porcine factor VIII. This may be important in deciding how to treat the patient.

The treatment of acquired coagulation factor inhibitors needs to address both the definitive treatment of the pathological antibody activity and, if present, the management of bleeding. Bleeding manifestations in acquired haemophilia may be very severe and necessitate prompt definitive treatment, including fluid resuscitation. Patients with acquired inhibitors to factor VIII are usually resistant to infusion of human factor VIII. In patients with a low level inhibitor in whom some residual factor VIII activity is still demonstrable, DDAVP may be considered for the management of non-life-threatening bleeds. Prothrombin complex concentrate containing IXa and VIIa (also to a lesser extent Xa, XIa and thrombin) may also be used for non-serious bleeds. Porcine VIII may be given by infusion to treat severe acquired VIII inhibitors, although close monitoring is required owing to unpredictable pharmacokinetics in this context. The main adverse effects of administration of porcine VIII are allergic reactions and thrombocytopenia (which is usually mild). Recombinant VIIa may resolve severe bleeding also in this context. Most responses to rVIIa will occur in 8–24 h, and if no change in condition is seen in this time, alternative therapy must be considered. An important side-effect to consider with rVIIa, especially in the older population is that of thrombosis, which may include coronary thrombosis leading to myocardial infarction. (The United Kingdom Haemophilia Centre Doctors' Organisation (UKHCDO) recommends that severe bleeding should be treated with porcine factor VIII or rVIIa in the first instance.)

Agents that have been used with some success as part of an immunosuppressive regime to treat acquired inhibitors include corticosteriods, cyclophosphamide, azathioprine, cyclosporin A and rituximab. A reduction of a patient's inhibitor titre may be achieved in an emergency by the use of immunoabsorption with a protein A column if one is available. In women of childbearing age or those who are pregnant the most appropriate treatment may be intravenous immunoglobulin, which may work by an anti-idiotype mechanism. The guidelines of the UKHCDO recommend that unless contraindicated, immunosuppressive therapy should commence as soon as an acquired inhibitor is diagnosed. First line, the UKHCDO recommends a combination of prednisolone and cyclophosphamide. Secondary therapy is recommended if there is no response within 2–4 weeks.

Rarely, individuals may develop autoantibodies directed against epitopes on platelet glycoproteins or vWF, resulting in a bleeding tendency secondary to impaired platelet function.

Autoimmune 'versions' of Bernard–Soulier syndrome (glycoprotein Ib) and Glanzmann's disease (glycoprotein IIb/IIIa) may be seen depending on the target glycoprotein of the autoantibody. Autoantibodies directed against protein S, which were associated with infection and led to skin necrosis, have been described.

Lupus anticoagulants

Lupus anticoagulant (LA) activity is seen in some patients with primary and secondary antiphospholipid syndrome. These antibodies possess the paradoxical effect of prolonging clotting times (usually the APTT but sometimes the PT) in vitro, while being associated with thrombosis in vivo. Their 'anticoagulant' effect in vitro may relate to an ability via interaction with β_2-glycoprotein I to occupy limited negatively charged phospholipid binding sites, which are, required for coagulation factor interactions in the APTT and PT assays. The mechanism of the thrombophilia associated with LA in vivo is as yet unclear. It may however relate to the antibody causing endothelial cellular activation with an upregulation of tissue factor expression or by virtue of the LA disrupting the interaction of β2-glycoprotein I with anticoagulant factors such as protein C. In rare cases, LA may be associated with bleeding; this may occur via the immune thrombocytopenia associated with the antiphospholipid syndrome and by some rare forms of LA that can inhibit prothrombin in vivo.

LA activity may cause prolongation of the APTT, which is not corrected on 50:50 mix with normal plasma. The dilute Russel's viper venom time (DRVVT) will be prolonged and fail to correct with 50:50 mixing with normal plasma. However, the DRVVT will correct on addition of a high concentration of negatively charged phospholipid (e.g. freeze–thawed platelets) to the assay (presumably because extra phospholipid binding sites are made available by this addition).

Other acquired bleeding diatheses

Drug therapy

The bleeding tendency induced by exposure to coumarin class drugs and non-steroidal anti-inflammatory drugs (which inhibit platelet cyclo-oxygenase) are well described. Other drugs however may have effects on the haemostatic system distinct from their primary therapeutic role. Colloids, which are often used during fluid resuscitation, may impair coagulation. Of compounds in this class, hydroxyethyl starch is that most frequently associated with bleeding. This may relate to a reduction of the half-life of vWF, which may become complexed to the starch molecules. Dextrans may impede coagulation by causing binding to platelet membranes and causing steric hindrance of receptor function as well as reducing the plasma levels of vWF.

Gelatins may interfere with fibronectin function, this may decrease the opsonization of foreign material, delay early wound healing and the cross-linkage of fibrin by factor XIII.

Along with the reduction in vitamin K levels associated with the use of β-lactam antibiotics (discussed earlier), they may also have an anti-platelet effect. Binding of penicillin to platelet membranes may reduce the platelets' response to agonists.

Paraproteinaemia

Non-specific stoichiometric effects, which inhibit platelet function and the polymerization of fibrin, may occur in patients with high circulating immunoglobulin levels. In addition, antibodies with specific activity against factor VIII and vWF may be seen in patients with paraproteins. Antibodies with LA-like activity have also been described in this context. Patients with paraproteinaemia may develop AL amyloidosis. This may lead to impaired haemostasis by infiltrating and weakening small blood vessel walls and by binding to and reducing the plasma levels of factor X.

Hypothermia

The coagulation factors (with the exception of fibrinogen and vWF) are all enzymes or co-factors in enzymatic reactions. They have an optimal functional temperature of 37°C. Hypothermia may therefore impair the function of the clotting factors, resulting in a bleeding tendency. Hypothermia must not be overlooked as a cause of excessive bleeding in the trauma patient, when, unless warmed fluids are used, the patient's core temperature may fall as large volumes of fluid are transfused. The clotting times may appear normal in a hypothermic patient as the sample is warmed to 37°C for laboratory analysis. Hypothermia may also lead to thrombocytopenia secondary to platelet pooling in the liver and spleen.

Selected bibliography

Bernard GR, Vincent JL, Laterre PF *et al.* (2001) Efficacy and safety of recombinant human activated protein C for severe sepsis. *New England Journal of Medicine* **344**: 699–709.

British Committee for Standards in Haematology Blood Transfusion Task Force (2004) Guidelines for the use of fresh-frozen plasma, cryoprecipitate and cryosupernatant. *British Journal of Haematology* **126**: 11–28.

Deldado J, Jimenez-Yuste V, Hernandez-Navarro F *et al.* (2003) Acquired haemophilia: review and meta-analysis focused on therapy and prognostic factors. *British Journal of Haematology* **121**: 21–35.

Favaloro EJ (2001) Utility of the PFA-100® for assessing bleeding disorders and monitoring therapy: a review of analytical variables, benefits and limitations. *Haemophilia* **7**: 170–9.

Salooja N, Perry DJ (2002) Thromboelastography. *Blood Coagulation and Fibrinolysis* **12**: 327–37.

Stainsby D, MacLennan S, Hamilton PJ. (2000) Management of massive blood loss: a template guideline. *British Journal of Anaesthesia* **85**: 487–91.

Taylor FB Jr, Toh CH, Hoots WK *et al.* (2001) Towards definition, clinical and laboratory criteria and a scoring system for Disseminated intravascular coagulation. *Thrombosis and Haemostasis* **86**: 1327–30.

CHAPTER 52

Thrombotic thrombocytopenic purpura and haemolytic uraemic syndrome (congenital and acquired)

52

Pier M Mannucci and Flora Peyvandi

Historical introduction

A brief historical sketch of the progress of knowledge is useful to frame these complex syndromes, which are difficult to diagnose. Thrombotic thrombocytopenic purpura (TTP) was first described in 1924 by Moschowitz in a previously healthy 16-year-old girl who died after an acute illness presenting with a pentad of signs and symptoms (anaemia, thrombocytopenia, fever, hemiparesis and haematuria). Post-mortem examination showed widespread thrombi in the terminal circulation of several organs, composed mainly of platelets. Over the next three decades, other cases were described, mainly, but not exclusively, in young or adult women. Some of these cases occurred in isolation (idiopathic), others in association with diseases or conditions (Table 52.1). It was understood that anaemia was due to massive intravascular haemolysis, in turn due to fragmentation (schistocytosis) of red

Table 52.1 Conditions and diseases associated with TTP.

Pregnancy and post partum
Infections (particularly HIV)
Drugs (quinine and quinidine, ticlopidine, clopidogrel,
  cyclosporin, interferon-α, statins)
Chemotherapy (mitomycin, cisplatin, gemcitabine)
Allogeneic bone marrow transplantation
Connective tissue disorders (lupus erythematosus and
  scleroderma)
Cardiac surgery

cells that were forced by blood flow to pass through partially occluded vessels in the terminal circulation, and that thrombocytopenia was caused by consumption of platelets due to their widespread deposition in microvascular thrombi.

Thirty-one years after Moschowitz, the paediatric nephrologist Gasser described a syndrome that was called *haemolytic uraemic syndrome* (HUS) and, in common with TTP, had microangiopathic haemolytic anaemia, consumption thrombocytopenia and microvascular thrombosis, but differed because it occurred in very young children, with absent or minimal neurological symptoms but severe signs of renal damage. Subsequently, when larger series of patients with HUS and TTP were examined, it became apparent that a neat distinction between the two syndromes was often difficult. Although thrombocytopenia, microangiopathic haemolytic anaemia and ischaemic symptoms due to widespread formation of thrombi in the terminal circulation of several organs were consistent features, age and the prevalence of neurological over renal symptoms could not clearly differentiate TTP from HUS and vice versa. There were, for instance, recurrent forms, which, in the same individual, presented sometimes with prevalent neurological symptoms (TTP) and on other occasions with renal symptoms (HUS). The term *thrombotic microangiopathies* (TMAs) was then proposed, meant to emphasize the common pathology of the two syndromes, with no implication on the prevalence of neurological or renal symptoms.

In the early 1980s, a major breakthrough in understanding the pathogenesis of TMAs strengthened the idea of the unitarian terminology. Even though it had been postulated for a long time that massive thrombus formation in the terminal circulation was due to the presence of 'toxic' substance(s) aggregating

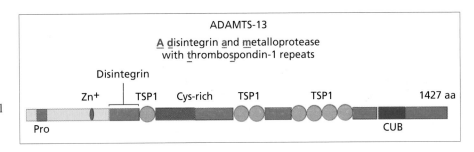

Figure 52.1 Domain structure of ADAMTS-13. Pro, propreptide; TSP1, thrombospondin 1; CUB, *c*omplement components C1r/c1s, *u*rinary epidermal growth factor *b*one morphogenetic protein-1.

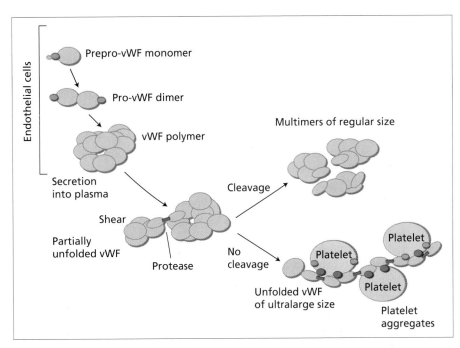

Figure 52.2 Interaction between vWF and ADAMTS-13 in plasma. vWF is secreted from endothelial cells as ultralarge multimers that anchor to endothelial cell surfaces and are also released into the circulation. ADAMTS-13 cleaves a Try–Met bond in the A2 domain of vWF, severing the ultralarge multimers. Failure of cleavage leads to the persistence in plasma and on endothelial cells of ultralarge multimers, which tend to aggregate platelet, especially in conditions of high shear forces.

platelets intravascularly, the putative aggregating agent had remained elusive. In 1982, Moake and others demonstrated, first in TTP and subsequently also in HUS, that the plasma of these patients contained highly thrombogenic forms of the multimeric glycoprotein von Willebrand factor (vWF), a major adhesive protein contained in endothelial cells, platelets and plasma. Abnormal vWF multimers of particularly high molecular weight (ultralarge) bind more avidly to platelet glycoproteins Ib and IIb/IIIa and aggregate platelets in conditions of high shear stress in the terminal circulation. Accordingly, it was postulated that ultralarge vWF was the 'toxic' aggregating agent involved in the formation of occlusive thrombi both in TTP and HUS.

It remained to be explained why such ultralarge multimers, normally absent in the circulation, were present in patients' plasma. The deficiency or dysfunction of one or more enzymes disposing them physiologically was postulated but it was not until the late 1990s that Furlan and Tsai and their associates independently showed that the link between ultralarge vWF multimers and TTP was a metal ion-dependent plasma metalloproteinase of 190 kDa called ADAMTS-13, a disintegrin and

metalloprotease with thrombospondin 1 repeats (Figure 52.1). The only known physiological function of this protease, present mainly in plasma, is to regulate the size of vWF by cleaving ultralarge multimers as soon as they are secreted from endothelial cells into plasma (Figure 52.2), thereby avoiding their circulation in plasma, platelet aggregation and thrombus formation. Most importantly, both the investigators made the intriguing observation that ADAMTS-13 was deficient in patients with TTP but measurable in normal amounts in those with HUS. This observation challenged the unitarian theory of TTP and HUS as different clinical manifestations of the same pathological process, and generated the paradigm that TTP is due to low levels of the vWF-cleaving protease, that is not involved in the pathogenesis of HUS.

As often in clinical medicine, the paradigm did not sustain the subsequent progress of knowledge. Not all the cases of thrombotic microangiopathy diagnosed as TTP owing to the prevalence of fluctuating neurological symptoms have low or undetectable levels of ADAMTS-13. On the other hand, even if most cases diagnosed as HUS for the prevalence of renal symptoms have normal levels of ADAMTS-13 (particularly the cases typically occurring in association with bloody diarrhoea), there are unequivocal cases of HUS, particularly the forms called atypical or diarrhoea-negative, characterized by low or undetectable protease levels. With this as historical background, the author has decided to keep the description of TTP separate from that of HUS in this chapter.

Thrombotic thrombocytopenic purpura

TTP is a rare disease, with an estimated incidence of 2–10 cases per million per year in all racial groups. Recently, greater awareness and perhaps improved diagnostic facilities give the impression that incidence is increasing. Even though both sexes may be affected, the syndrome is definitely more frequent in women (two-thirds of the cases), as usually happens for diseases with an immunological basis (see below). Cases with a genetic basis, usually but not exclusively occurring in infants or young children, are very rare (1 in 1 million or less) and represent a small proportion of all TTP (approximately 5%). Mortality was very high (80–90%) until plasma exchange therapy was introduced, and is still unacceptably high (10–20%), despite the dramatic improvement due to the adoption of this therapeutic measure. Owing to the variability of presenting symptoms and of the associated comorbid conditions (Table 52.1), cases of TTP may be seen initially by a variety of physicians other than haematologists and pathologists, such as neurologists, nephrologists, oncologists and gynaecologists, and sometimes this makes it difficult to get a prompt recognition of the syndrome, an essential requisite for optimal management.

Pathology and pathogenesis

As mentioned above, the pathological basis of TTP is the widespread formation in the microcirculation of platelet thrombi, associated with relatively little endothelial cell injury and fibrin formation but with abundant vWF. Microthrombi are in several organs (mainly brain, kidney, myocardium, lung and pancreas), whereas grossly detectable thrombi, arterial or venous, are lacking. The present pathogenetic model implies that endothelial cells, activated by varied and often unidentified triggering agents, secrete large amounts of ultralarge uncleaved vWF, which aggregates platelets directly in conditions of high fluid shear stress and leads to massive intravascular platelet aggregation, ischaemic organ damage, consumptive thrombocytopenia and schistocytic anaemia. Two main mechanisms cause ADAMTS-13 deficiency in TTP: mutations on chromosome 9q34 in the gene that encodes the protease and the acquired occurrence of inactivating autoantibodies.

However, several observations fail to fit perfectly with this relatively straightforward pathogenetic mechanism. Only a minority of patients with bona fide TTP, as diagnosed with clinical

Table 52.2 Putative pathogenetic mechanisms unrelated to vWF and ADAMTS-13 of TTP.

Endothelial cell activation
Increased P-selectin
Decreased prostacyclin
Endothelial apoptosis

Platelet activation/aggregation
Platelet aggregating proteins other than vWF
Cysteine proteases (calpains, cathepsins)

criteria (thrombocytopenia, anaemia and fluctuating neurological symptoms), have severe ADAMTS-13 deficiency. This may be explained by the incapacity of the functional assays available at present to reveal some types of deficiencies of ADAMTS-13 activity, and/or by the deficiency of vWF cleaving proteases other than ADAMTS-13. Ultralarge vWF multimers, pivotal players in the presently accepted model of TTP, are not constantly detected in patient plasma. In some instances, there is an imbalance between their release into plasma from endothelial cells and excessive binding to platelets, so that even defects of large multimers may be present in plasma. It is unclear why patients with sustained ADAMTS-13 deficiency, genetic or immuno-mediated, develop clinical symptoms and signs only sporadically. Still unknown factors that trigger excessive endothelial cell activation may be necessary for the full clinical spectrum of the syndrome to be manifested.

In summary, the prevailing paradigm holds that TTP is often the consequence of the defective processing of highly thrombogenic ultralarge multimers of vWF, which are secreted in excess by endothelial cells and not disposed of adequately owing to a congenital or immune-mediated dysfunction of ADAMTS-13 (Figure 52.2). There are data suggesting other possible mechanisms of disease that do not involve vWF and its cleaving processes (Table 52.2).

Clinical and laboratory findings

TTP occurs frequently, unheralded, in previously healthy individuals (acute idiopathic), but also in association with physiological or pathological conditions (Table 52.1). The presence of thrombocytopenia and haemolytic anaemia, common to all thrombotic microangiopathies, is essential for the diagnosis of TTP. Like HUS, TTP is a clinical diagnosis and biopsies are not necessary. Platelet count is often very low in the acute phase, with values of 20×10^9/L or less and petechiae are frequently seen. Signs of microangiopathic haemolytic anaemia (with haematocrits of usually less than 20%) are the presence of schistocytes on peripheral blood smears, reticulocytosis, increased indirect bilirubin, low or unmeasurable haptoglobin and negative direct Coombs' test. High serum lactate dehydrogenase

(LDH), usually in excess of 1000 U/L, is a sensitive, albeit non-specific, sign of red cell destruction and necrosis of other tissues due to microthrombotic end-organ ischaemia. Neurological symptoms (coma, stroke, seizures or focal signs such as motor deficits, diplopia and aphasia) typically fluctuate in presentation and severity, due to the sustained formation and dissolution of thrombi in the cerebral microcirculation. Other symptoms or signs such as headache, blurred vision, ataxia or mental status changes are less typical and are of difficult reproducible documentation. Even though only a minority of patients with TTP have elevated serum creatinine levels (> 1.5 mg/dL), signs of renal involvement such as microscopic haematuria and proteinuria are frequent. High fever is not constant in TTP, despite the inclusion of this symptom in the original description. There is no or little alteration of coagulation and fibrinolysis.

Differential diagnosis

Typical cases of HUS are distinguished from TTP by the occurrence of diarrhoeal prodromes and of more severe and persistent symptoms of renal impairment (see below). It is much more difficult to distinguish cases of TTP from atypical HUS, except for the paradigmatic prevalence of neurological symptoms in the former and of renal failure in the latter. Other issues of differential diagnosis are with conditions that present themselves as thrombotic microangiopathies, all characterized by thrombocytopenia and microangiopathic haemolytic anaemia (Table 52.3).

DIC can be distinguished by markedly increased levels of fibrin degradation products (FDPs) and D-dimer and, in decompensated cases, by the presence of hypofibrinogenaemia, prolonged prothrombin and activated partial thromboplastin times. Issues of differential diagnosis are also with such other thrombotic microangiopathies as pre-eclampsia and eclampsia, because pregnancy is one of the most frequent clinical associations of TTP. Hypertension is less frequent if renal damage is not severe and the degrees of anaemia and thrombocytopenia are more severe in TTP.

Coagulation and fibrinolysis tests are usually abnormal in pre-eclampsia or eclampsia, albeit less markedly than in DIC. Abnormally high serum transaminases differentiate TTP from the so-called HELLP (haemolysis, elevated, liver enzymes and low platelets) syndrome of pregnancy. Sometimes connective tissue disorders such as systemic lupus erythematosus and severe scleroderma present with widespread microvascular thrombosis, haemolytic anaemia, thrombocytopenia and fluctuating neurological symptoms. This situation may also occur in severe cases with the so-called catastrophic antiphospholipid antibody syndrome. These conditions may be distinguished from TTP because symptoms and signs are usually less severe, and laboratory tests such as antinuclear and anticardiolipin antibodies and the lupus-like anticoagulant give positive results.

The Evans syndrome, due to the concomitant presence of anti-platelet and anti-erythrocyte antibodies, is distinguished by a positive Coombs' test, the lack of schistocytes and the usual absence of end-organ ischaemic symptoms. Severe ischaemic manifestations due to platelet thrombi are frequent features of heparin-induced thrombocytopenia, but TTP can be distinguished not only by lack of exposure to this drug but also by the absence of haemolysis and schistocytosis. Disseminated malignancy is sometime associated with thrombocytopenia and microangiopathic haemolytic anaemia. Until further investigations permit to exclude or confirm the presence of metastatic cancer, it is not easy to distinguish TTP from this type of TMA.

What is the help of ADAMTS-13 testing in the differential diagnosis between the forementioned TMAs and TTP? In none of the former ADAMTS-13 is activity undetectable in plasma. So a complete deficiency of the protease clearly directs towards TTP or atypical HUS. Normal or reduced but detectable plasma levels of the protease do not help in the differential diagnosis, because they may be found albeit rarely in TTP, in typical HUS, in other TMAs and in several other unrelated conditions (Table 52.4).

Table 52.3 Clinical conditions other than TTP and HUS presenting as thrombotic microangiopathies (TMAs).

Disseminated intravascular coagulation (DIC)
Pre-eclampsia–HELLP syndrome
Scleroderma-lupus systemic erythematosus
Severe vasculitis
'Catastrophic' antiphospholipid syndrome
Evans' syndrome (autoimmune thrombocytopenia and haemolytic anaemia)
Heparin-induced thrombocytopenia
Disseminated malignancy

Table 52.4 Physiological and pathological states associated with mild to moderately severe deficiency of ADAMTS-13.

Age
Sex
Neonatal state
Pregnancy
Localized and metastatic cancer
HELLP syndrome
Liver cirrhosis
Inflammatory states
Post-operative period
Uraemia
Autoimmune diseases

Table 52.5 Variants of TTP.

Acute sporadic (or early relapsing)
Idiopathic
Antibody mediated

Chronic recurrent
Inherited
Antibody mediated

Table 52.6 Steps in the treatment of TTP.

Clinical diagnosis (based upon severe thrombocytopenia, presence of schistocytes, high serum LDH, fluctuating neurological symptoms)
Plasma infusion (30 mL/kg) until plasma exchange can be started
Daily plasma exchanges (3–6 L per day) until platelets are higher than 150×10^9/L for at least 3 days and LDH is normal
Adjuvant treatments: prednisone, 1–2 mg/kg per day
Red cell transfusion as needed (avoid platelet transfusion)

Natural history (Table 52.5)

In approximately two-thirds of the cases, TTP occurs only once (acute sporadic TTP). There are, however, cases that tend to relapse early, after brief periods of apparent remission of the acute episode. Usually, but not always, relapses are associated with the persistence of anti-ADAMTS-13 autoantibodies. However, the most typical chronic recurrent forms of TTP are those that manifest themselves cyclically, mainly, but not exclusively, during childhood. They usually have a genetic basis, even although familial segregation is not always apparent, because ADAMTS-13 gene defects are transmitted as autosomal recessive traits and only one child in the sibship may be affected. In inherited TTP, ADAMTS-13 plasma levels are usually consistently below the limit of sensitivity of assays available at present and are reduced to half of the normal levels in their asymptomatic parents. It is not understood why ADAMTS-13-deficient patients remain asymptomatic for some time (usually from 3 weeks to 3 months) and then, at intervals that are often quite regular, thrombocytopenia and schistocytic anaemia herald the appearance of new symptoms of end-organ ischaemia.

Treatment

The modern management of TTP started with the serendipitous observations that plasma infusion improved the clinical course of TTP. Plasma exchange was subsequently found to be equally or more effective than plasma infusion. In 1991, the results of a prospective randomized clinical trial definitely confirmed the greater efficacy of plasma exchange over infusion, the clinical response rate being 78% in the former compared with 49% in the latter (mortality rates of 22% and 37% respectively). Only recently, after the discovery of the role of vWF and its protease ADAMTS-13 in the pathogenesis of TTP, these empirical treatments have found a rationale. Plasma exchange may help by removing anti-ADAMTS-13 autoantibodies, the most frequent mechanism of acute sporadic TTP. Plasma exchange also helps to replace the deficient protease, infusion alone being probably sufficient in congenitally deficient cases with no associated autoantibody. Nevertheless, the efficacy of plasma therapies is still not fully explained, because exchange and/or infusion are definitely efficacious even in cases with normal plasma levels of

ADAMTS-13 and no detectable autoantibody. A scheme summarizing the steps to be followed in the treatment of acute TTP is shown in Table 52.6.

Plasma therapy

Treatment with plasma should be initiated as soon as a clinical diagnosis is suspected for the presence of schistocytic anaemia, severe thrombocytopenia and high serum LDH. There is as yet no evidence that ADAMTS-13 and autoantibody testing are necessary to start therapy, because as forementioned there are unequivocal cases of TTP with normal or borderline levels of the protease. Moreover, the available assays are time consuming, poorly standardized and results are not always specific for TTP.

Critically ill TTP patients are often first admitted to hospitals with no facilities for plasma exchange; in such circumstances, daily infusion of large amounts of fresh-frozen plasma (FFP) (30 mL/kg) should be started promptly, taking measures to avoid volume overload (Table 52.6). Patients are optimally assisted in intensive care units, where renal failure, coma, seizures and such severe side-effects of plasma exchange as congestive heart failure and catheter-related bleeding, thrombosis and infections can be optimally managed. At least one plasma volume should be exchanged daily until platelets are 150×10^9/L or more for at least 3 days, LDH is normal and schistocytes are no longer present on blood films (Table 52.6).

Treatment should be continued following this schedule for at least 10 days, whether or not early signs of clinical and laboratory improvement are observed. Daily exchanges for up to 1 month are sometimes necessary to achieve remission of TTP. It is not established whether discontinuation of plasma therapy should be abrupt or progressive. Cryoprecipitate-depleted plasma can be used instead of FFP if this fraction is available and convenient, but there is no evidence that this vWF-poor plasma is more effective than whole plasma. Plasma treated with virus inactivation methods (for instance, solvent/detergent) should be preferred because it decreases the risk of infections associated with patients' exposure to plasma from a large number of donors.

In *chronic recurrent TTP*, prophylactic plasma infusions (30 mL/kg) are often administered at regular intervals. It is has been suggested that trough plasma levels of 10% ADAMTS-13 are sufficient to avoid recurrence. A more conservative approach is to monitor platelet count and serum LDH at intervals of 5–10 days and to start plasma therapy as soon as these measurements begin to become abnormal. There is as yet no definite evidence that patients with congenital ADAMTS-13 deficiency develop alloantibodies, nor that an anamnestic response invariably occurs in patients with autoantibodies after they are treated with plasma.

Other therapies

Before the advent of plasma therapy, many other modalities of treatment have been attempted to control the dramatic course of TTP. Their generally poor efficacy is apparent from the fact that only with the advent of plasma therapy has mortality dropped dramatically. Hence, these treatments should be generally attempted only when plasma therapy at full doses and for at least a fortnight gave no or minimal benefit (refractory TTP) (Table 52.7).

There is little or no theoretical or practical role for the use of anti-platelet agents, because these drugs (including aspirin) fail to inhibit shear stress-induced platelet aggregation, the prevailing pathogenic mechanism of thrombus formation in TTP. Inhibitors of glycoproteins Ib and IIb–IIIa, by blocking binding of ultralarge vWF multimers to platelets, should perhaps be considered in the prevention or early management of chronic recurrent TTP, but not in full-blown TTP, because they may increase the risk of thrombocytopenic bleeding. The immune pathogenesis of TTP may be tackled using immunomodulating agents such as corticosteroids, cyclophosphamide, azathioprine, intravenous immunoglobulins and immunoadsorption on staphylococcal protein A (Table 52.7). Splenectomy has also been attempted.

In general, it is difficult to recommend the most useful among these agents or procedures. Considering that autoantibodies are a frequent pathogenetic mechanism, large doses of prednisone (1–2 mg/kg) are often prescribed in addition to plasma exchange during the acute phase of TTP, tapering off this treatment when remission is obtained (Table 52.6). The same treatment may be considered in the chronic recurrent variant of TTP due to the persistence of autoantibodies. Efficacy of corticosteroids is not unequivocally demonstrated, and the adverse effects of prolonged intake of large doses are severe. Splenectomy is an alternative option in patients with chronic recurrent forms during remission, but carries a high risk of death in severely ill patients with acute TTP. Another recent attempt to suppress the production of anti-ADAMTS-13 autoantibodies is based upon a monoclonal antibody directed against CD20 antigen (rituximab). This therapy may be considered in chronic recurrent forms refractory to other immunomodulating agents.

A new, obviously promising approach is replacement therapy with ADAMTS-13 concentrates. A recombinant preparation has been shown to improve the defective proteolysis of vWF *in vitro*, but clinical trials with this product have not yet started. Another pharmaceutical company is considering the clinical evaluation of a humanized monoclonal antibody directed against platelet glycoprotein Ib to prevent the occurrence of relapse in chronic recurrent forms. This treatment is meant to inhibit the binding of ultralarge vWF multimers and thereby avoid intravascular platelet aggregation in the microcirculation.

Haemolytic uraemic syndrome

The typical form of HUS called diarrhoea-related HUS (or D(+) HUS) is acquired and occurs acutely and sporadically after gastrointestinal infections with toxin-producing bacteria, particularly in infants and young children but sometimes also in elderly individuals. There are two atypical forms of HUS. One is familial, has a sporadic or chronic recurrent course and is due to the inherited deficiency of complement factor H. It occurs mainly in infants or young children but at least one-third of cases also occur in adults. Another atypical form of HUS occurs at all ages in association with situations commonly seen also in association with TTP (Table 52.8).

Diarrhoea-related haemolytic uraemic syndrome

This acute syndrome almost always occurs as a single, sporadic episode, heralded 2 days to 2 weeks before by bloody diarrhoea.

Table 52.7 Suggested immunological treatments of refractory, antibody-mediated TTP.

Prednisone (1–2 mg/kg for at least 15 days, then tapering the drug off over 45 days)
Vincristine (2 mg on day 1, then 1 mg on days 3, 6 and 9)
Cyclophosphamide or azothioprine (100–200 mg per day)
Intravenous immunoglobulins
Immunoadsorption on staphylococcal protein A
Splenectomy
Anti-CD20 (rituximab)

Table 52.8 Variants of HUS.

Typical
Exotoxin-producing bacteria (*E. coli* 0157:H7, *S. dysenteriae*)
Atypical
Inherited (complement factor H deficiency) or acquired (association with post partum, drugs, bone marrow transplantation, chemotherapy) (see also Table 52.1)

Oligoanuria, jaundice, petechial haemorrhages, anaemia with schistocytosis and LDH increases are present but usually less marked than in TTP. Serum creatinine and urea are definitely more abnormal than in TTP. Signs of compensated DIC, with high plasma levels of D-dimer, are another distinctive feature. Neurological involvement is uncommon but seizures and coma may occur in association with severe uraemia and hypertension.

Aetiology

The most common bacterial agent that causes the prodromal gastrointestinal infection is *Escherichia coli* type 0157:H7 or, less frequently, *Shigella dysenteriae* serotype I. These and other more rarely involved infectious agents produce similar forms of exo-toxins called verotoxin, shiga toxin and shiga-like toxins. These toxins, after absorption from the gastrointestinal tract into the blood, have in common the property to bind to the glycosphin-golipid membrane receptor globotriaosyl ceramide (Gb_3) that is particularly dense in the glomerular capillary endothelial cells of infants, young children and elderly individuals. The toxin–receptor complex is endocytosed and thereby causes cytolysis and extensive endothelial swelling and desquamation, which in turn engenders massive thrombus formation in the renal microvasculature.

Pathology and pathogenesis

The pathology of diarrhoea-related HUS is characterized by more extensive endothelial injury and less vWF deposition in thrombi than in TTP. The behaviour of plasma vWF is also dif-ferent, because ultralarge, highly thrombogenic multimers are detectable less frequently during the acute phase of the disease. This phenomenon is thought to be due to the fact that vWF multimers leaking in excess into plasma from damaged endo-thelial cells bind avidly to glycoprotein Ib on the platelet mem-brane and are thereby removed from plasma, particularly the multimers of larger size. There is quasi unanimity of views that ADAMTS-13 is normal in the plasma of patients with this vari-ant of HUS (Table 52.9).

Table 52.9 Clinical applications of ADAMTS-13 testing in TTP and HUS.

Stage	ADAMTS-13 deficiency (< 10%)	Diagnostic implications
Acute phase	Yes	TTP/atypical HUS
	No	Typical HUS/TTP cannot be excluded
Remission	Yes	Risk of relapse

ADAMTS-13 levels are usually normal or only mildly reduced in the TMAs listed in Table 52.2.

Natural history

In the great majority of cases, diarrhoea-related HUS is self-limiting, with much less tendency to early or late relapses than TTP. The acute episode is often accompanied by such severe renal failure that temporary haemodialysis is frequently required. Residual renal dysfunction is common after the acute episode and renal failure requiring maintenance dialysis or kidney trans-plantation occurs in approximately one-third of the patients.

Treatment

During the diarrhoeal prodrome antimotility agents are con-traindicated, because they favour the permanence of the bac-terial toxins in the gastrointestinal lumen and their passage into blood. The role of antibiotics is controversial, with a strong indication only for patients with evidence or suspicion of sepsis or *S. dysenteriae* infection. Plasma exchange is usually not re-commended in patients with typical HUS, whereas it is indicated in the atypical forms (see below), emphasizing again the similar-ities between this variant of HUS and TTP. A possible forth-coming approach to the prevention of toxin-induced HUS is vaccination of children who live in endemic areas.

Familial haemolytic uraemic syndrome

Autosomal recessive and dominant forms of familial HUS with-out diarrhoeal prodromes account for about 5–10% of all cases (Table 52.8). This variant is associated with a markedly severe impairment of renal function and with a high mortality rate (approximately one-third of the cases). Approximately one-half of the patients who survived acute disease require maintenance haemodialysis. In total, 30–40% of patients with familial HUS have a deficiency or dysfunction of complement factor H, which results in excessive C3 activation, membrane deposition of this complement fraction and renal cell injury. A recessively trans-mitted variant of familial HUS is very rare and is associated with very low levels of factor H in plasma and with the early onset of HUS in childhood. Dominantly transmitted variants are usually due to missense mutations in the gene encoding factor H, entail-ing the production of normal amounts of a dysfunctional pro-tein. Dominantly transmitted HUS is usually less severe than the recessive form, and affects late infancy or adulthood. Low serum C3 levels may be a simple and widely available method to diag-nose affected patients and to detect family members at risk.

Treatment of familial HUS is based on the replacement of factor H with FFP, associated with transient haemodialysis in the attempt to control oligoanuria and uraemia. Unfortunately, chronic renal failure is frequent and kidney transplantation fails to cure the syndrome, because the persisting plasmatic defici-ency of factor H maintains the conditions that lead to damage of the kidney allograft. The severity of the disease warrants gene transfer as a therapeutic approach, but lack of animal models and of suitable vectors of the transgene have hindered this approach so far.

Atypical (non-diarrhoea related) haemolytic uraemic syndrome

This form can only be distinguished from TTP by the absence of neurological symptoms and the predominance of renal symptoms. Atypical HUS is often associated with the post-partum period or with the intake of several drugs (Table 52.8). Individuals who have been treated for various illnesses by marrow transplantation make up a relatively large subgroup. Plasma therapy, using the same protocol recommended for TTP, is the treatment of choice.

Concluding remarks

In the last few years, TTP and HUS, known for several decades to clinicians and pathologists for their dire consequences, have witnessed spectacular improvements in terms of understanding pathogenesis, developing new diagnostic criteria, and decreasing mortality and morbidity. The pivotal role of vWF and of its major proteolytic enzyme in inducing microvascular platelet thrombi is evident, even though not all the variants of TTP, and particularly of HUS, fit into this disease mechanism. Other proteins disposing ultralarge highly thrombogenic forms of vWF may be involved, platelet thrombospondin 1 being at the moment the main candidate. The development of laboratory methods that measure ADAMTS-13 in plasma has allowed to demonstrate that several cases of TTP have very low levels of this protease. On the other hand, severe ADAMTS-13 deficiency is not found in all patients who have the appropriate clinical criteria for TTP diagnosis (Table 52.9). The trigger(s) of full-blown TTP or HUS need to be elucidated, because patients with constitutionally low levels of ADAMTS-13 or factor H remain without disease expression for long periods of time. It also remains to be seen which and how many cases respond to replacement therapy with protease concentrates, plasma derived or made with recombinant DNA technologies. Meanwhile, the clinician confronted with the difficult treatment of these seriously ill patients should be cognizant that plasma therapy, mainly as plasma exchange plasmapheresis, remains the treatment of choice for all patients with clinically diagnosed TTP and the related syndrome called atypical HUS. Diarrhoea-related HUS is now well characterized from an aetiological standpoint, so that it can be recognized and properly treated by paediatricians. A major problem remains the prevention of inherited HUS associated with factor H deficiency, because the long-term consequences of this scourge are dire. A suitable screening test is not yet available, even though there are theoretical possibility of a DNA-based approach, because most mutations are located in the gene exon encoding the most C-terminal short consensus repeat involved in binding factor H

to complement C3b and to sialic acid molecules on host cells, thereby protecting host cells from excessive C3 activation.

Selected bibliography

Bell WR, Braine HG, Ness PM et al. (1991) Improved survival in thrombotic thrombocytopenic purpura-hemolytic uremic syndrome. Clinical experience in 108 patients. New England Journal of Medicine 325: 398–403.

Bukowski RM, King JW, Hewlett JS (1977) Plasmapheresis in the treatment of thrombotic thrombocytopenic purpura. Blood 50: 413–17.

Furlan M, Robles R, Galbusera M et al. (1998) von Willebrand factor-cleaving protease in thrombotic thrombocytopenic purpura and the hemolytic-uremic syndrome. New England Journal of Medicine 339: 1578–84.

Gorge JN (2000) How I treat patients with thrombotic thrombocytopenic purpura-hemolytic uremic syndrome. Blood 96: 1223–9.

Levy GG, Nichols WC, Lian EC et al. (2001) Mutations in a member of the ADAMTS gene family cause thrombotic thrombocytopenic purpura. Nature 413: 488–94.

Mannucci PM, Lombardi R, Lattuada A et al. (1989) Enhanced proteolysis of plasma von Willebrand factor in thrombotic thrombocytopenic purpura and the hemolytic uremic syndrome. Blood 74: 978–83.

Mannucci PM, Canciani MT, Forza I et al. (2001) Changes in health and disease of the metalloprotease that cleaves von Willebrand factor. Blood 98: 2730–5.

Manuelian T, Hellwage J, Meri S et al. (2003) Mutations in factor H reduce binding affinity to C3b and heparin and surface attachment to endothelial cells in hemolytic uremic syndrome. Journal of Clinical Investment 111: 1181–90.

Moake J (1998) Moschcowitz, multimers, and metalloprotease. New England Journal of Medicine 339: 1629–31.

Moake JL (2002) Thrombotic microangiopathies. New England Journal of Medicine 347: 589–600.

Moake JL, Rudy CK, Troll JH et al. (1982) Unusually large plasma factor VIII: von Willebrand factor multimers in chronic relapsing thrombotic thrombocytopenic purpura. New England Journal of Medicine 307: 1432–5.

Moake JL, Turner NA, Stathopoulos NA et al. (1986) Involvement of large plasma von Willebrand factor (vWF) multimers and unusually large vWF forms derived from endothelial cells in shear stress-induced platelet aggregation. Journal of Clinical Investment 78: 1456–61.

Moore JB, Hayward CPM, Warkentin TE et al. (2001) Decreased von Willebrand factor protease activity associated with thrombocytopenic disorders. Blood 98: 1842–6.

Remuzzi G, Ruggenenti P, Bertani T (1994) Thrombotic microangiopathy. In Renal Pathology (CC Tisher, MM Brenner, eds), 2nd edn, p. 1154. Lippincott, Philadelphia.

Remuzzi G, Galbusera M, Noris M et al. (2002) Thrombotic thrombocytopenic purpura/hemolytic uremic syndrome: von Willebrand factor cleaving protease (ADAMTS13) is deficient in recurrent and familial thrombotic thrombocytopenic purpura and hemolytic uremic syndrome. Blood 100: 778–85.

Rock GA, Shumak KH, Buskard NA *et al.* (1991) Comparison of plasma exchange with plasma infusion in the treatment of thrombotic thrombocytopenic purpura. Canadian Apheresis Study Group. *New England Journal of Medicine* **325**: 393–7.

Ruggenenti P, Galbusera M, Cornejo RP *et al.* (1993) Thrombotic thrombocytopenic purpura: evidence that infusion rather than removal of plasma induces remission of the disease. *American Journal of Kidney Disease* **21**: 314–18.

Tsai HM, Lian EC (1998) Antibodies to von Willebrand factor-cleaving protease in acute thrombotic thrombocytopenic purpura. *New England Journal of Medicine* **339**: 1585–94.

Upshwas JD (1978) Congenital deficiency of a factor in normal plasma that reverses microangiopathic hemolysis and thrombocytopenia. *New England Journal of Medicine* **298**: 1350–2.

Vesely SK, George JN, Lammle B *et al.* (2003) ADAMTS13 activity in thrombotic thrombocytopenic purpura-hemolytic uremic syndrome: relation to presenting features and clinical outcomes in a prospective cohort of 142 patients. *Blood* **102**: 60–8.

Zheng X, Chung D, Takayama TK *et al.* (2001) Structure of von Willebrand factor-cleaving protease (ADAMTS13), a metalloprotease involved in thrombotic thrombocytopenic purpura. *Journal of Biological Chemistry* **276**: 41059–63.

CHAPTER 53

Inherited thrombophilia

Isobel D Walker

53

Introduction

In the mid-nineteenth century, the German pathologist Virchow postulated that thrombosis was due to alteration in blood flow (stasis or turbulence), changes in the vessel wall and changes in the composition of the blood (hypercoagulability). Thrombi are composed of fibrin strands and enmeshed blood cells, the relative composition differing between venous and arterial thrombi. Arterial thrombi arise in the setting of high flow and high shear forces in regions where the blood flow is disturbed and in vessels where the wall is damaged. Vessel wall injury leads to platelet activation, which plays a major role in the pathogenesis of arterial thrombi. Venous thrombosis, on the other hand, usually occurs where the degree of vessel wall damage is modest or minimal but where blood flow is abnormally slow and there is local activation of coagulation. Arterial thrombi are composed largely of platelet aggregates and a relatively minor amount of fibrin. Venous thrombi are composed mainly of red blood cells trapped in an extensive fibrin mesh, with relatively few platelets.

Imbalance between the anticoagulant and procoagulant activities of plasma in which the procoagulant activities predominate result in hypercoagulability and increased thrombotic risk. Hypercoagulability may be acquired and temporary (e.g. following surgery or trauma or during pregnancy) or it may be the result of an inherited change in one or more components of haemostasis. Much interest has focused on the role that underlying hypercoagulable states, in particular inherited life-long hypercoagulability, may play in the pathogenesis of venous or arterial thromboembolic disease.

Heritable risk factors for venous thromboembolism: thrombophilia

There is no internationally accepted definition of thrombophilia. In Europe, the term is used to describe disorders of haemostasis that appear to predispose to venous thrombosis. This laboratory-based definition is widely applied but has a number of disadvantages. First, it has become evident that many individuals – in fact the majority – who carry thrombophilic defects remain asymptomatic. Second, although the number of thrombophilic defects continues to increase, detailed laboratory investigation still fails to detect any abnormality in at least one-half of the patients who present with venous thromboembolism – including many who appear clinically thrombophilic.

In North America, the term thrombophilic has been used to describe individuals who developed venous thrombosis either spontaneously or of a severity apparently out of proportion to any identifiable stimulus, patients who have recurrent events and patients who have had a first event at a young age. This definition may be more clinically useful. A definition that encompasses both the laboratory and clinical aspects is lacking but clinicians investigating and managing patients considered to be at increased venous thrombotic risk should remain aware of that clinical history and laboratory findings are each relevant.

The heritable abnormalities that have been associated with an increased risk of venous thrombosis include those due to reduction in anticoagulant function – deficiency of the natural anticoagulants antithrombin, protein C or protein S, and those that are associated with increased procoagulant activity, factor V Leiden (FV Leiden) and the G20210A prothrombin

Table 53.1 Classification of thrombophilic abnormalities.

Heritable
Loss of function: antithrombin deficiency, protein C deficiency, protein S deficiency
Gain of function: factor V Leiden, prothrombin G20210A

Acquired
Antiphospholipids

Mixed
Elevated factor VIII, IX, XI
Hyperhomocysteinaemia

polymorphism (FII G20210A). The natural anticoagulant deficiencies are the result of a large number of gene defects. FV Leiden and the FII G20210A polymorphism are the results of single nucleotide polymorphisms. There are also a number of other abnormalities, for example elevated levels of clotting factor VIII (FVIII) and hyperhomocysteinaemia, which appear to have a mixed genetic and environmental origin (Table 53.1).

Natural anticoagulant and coagulation factor defects

Thrombin is the main effector enzyme of the coagulation system. It is produced by the activation of prothrombin by the prothrombinase complex, which comprises a phospholipid-bound complex of activated factor X (FXa) and its cofactor activated factor V (FVa). Factor V is activated by FXa (on the phospholipid surface) and thrombin (in solution and on the surface). Factor X is activated by tenase, a complex of activated factor IX (FIXa) and activated factor VIII (FVIIIa) on the platelet surface. Natural anticoagulant mechanisms regulate thrombin activity and function by direct inhibition of formed thrombin by antithrombin and by downregulating thrombin production via the inhibition of FVa and FVIIIa by the protein C–protein S system.

Antithrombin deficiency

Antithrombin (previously called antithrombin III) is synthesized in the liver. It is a glycoprotein member of the family of serine protease inhibitors. Its inhibitory effect is not confined to thrombin; antithrombin also inhibits the activated clotting factors IXa, Xa, XIa, XIIa and tissue factor-bound FVIIa. Free enzymes are preferentially inhibited, those that are part of the prothrombinase or tenase complexes being less accessible for inhibition. The rate of complex formation between antithrombin and activated clotting factors is markedly accelerated by heparin and by proteoglycans on the vascular endothelium.

Heritable antithrombin deficiency subtypes

Two major phenotypes of heritable antithrombin deficiency are recognized. Type I is characterized by a quantitative reduction of qualitatively normal antithrombin. Type II deficiency is due to the production of a qualitatively abnormal antithrombin protein. In both types of antithrombin deficiency, antithrombin activity is reduced to a variable extent. In type I deficiency, antithrombin antigen levels are reduced concordantly with the functional reduction. In type II deficiency, antithrombin antigen levels are discordantly higher than the functional levels and may be close to normal.

Understanding of the basis of familial antithrombin deficiency has been facilitated by advances made in molecular biology and in the functional characterization of this inhibitory glycoprotein. The antithrombin molecule possesses two important functional regions – a heparin-binding domain and a thrombin-binding domain. Type II antithrombin deficiency is subclassified according to the site of the molecular defect: (i) reactive site (RS), abnormalities residing in the reactive (thrombin-binding) site; (ii) heparin binding site (HBS), abnormalities residing in the heparin binding site; and (iii) pleiotropic effect (PE), abnormalities residing in both reactive and heparin binding sites.

Many mutations associated with antithrombin deficiency have been described, but identification of the specific mutation in particular patients is neither practical nor necessary for clinical purposes. Phenotypic distinction between the subtypes of antithrombin deficiency is, however, of clinical relevance as the incidence of thrombosis is higher in association with type I deficiency and type II deficiency when the mutation affects the reactive site than in type II deficiency when the mutation affects the heparin binding site. Type II HBS variants, although associated with a lower risk of thrombosis than type II RS defects, may increase the attributable risk of an additional thrombophilic defect, such as the FV Leiden mutation. Heritable antithrombin deficiency is uncommon, and type II deficiency is more prevalent than type I deficiency. The prevalences of heterozygous type I and type II mutations are approximately 0.02% and 0.15% respectively (Table 53.2).

Antithrombin assays

As antithrombin antigen levels may be normal or near normal in type II deficiency, immunological assays may fail to identify patients with these variants. Only functional assays measuring heparin cofactor activity will detect both type I and type II deficiencies. When reduced activity is demonstrated and an inherited deficiency postulated, comparison of the result of the functional heparin cofactor assay with the result of an immunological assay allows phenotypic classification into type I or type II deficiency. Commercially available antithrombin activity assays are robust and reliable, and usually use a chromogenic substrate. Most utilize a long incubation period and some have heparin in the dilution buffer. As a short incubation (of 30 s or

Table 53.2 Prevalences of heritable thrombophilias.

	General population	History of venous thrombosis	
		Unselected (%)	Selected (%)
Antithrombin deficiency*	0.02%	0.5–1	4
Protein C deficiency	0.2%	3.0	5–6
Protein S deficiency	?	1.0	5–6
Factor V Leiden	2–15%	20–50	>50
Prothrombin G20210A	1–4%	6.0	18

*Type I antithrombin deficiency.

less) with a low concentration of heparin is required to detect type II HBS variants, laboratories using commercial antithrombin activity assays may fail to detect these defects. Crossed immuno-electrophoresis with heparin may be used to detect type II HBS variants in those centres that require identification of these defects.

Age- and sex-related variations in antithrombin activity and antigen levels are minor and the reference ranges in healthy populations are narrow. Antithrombin levels are slightly lower in premenopausal females than in males or older women.

Acquired antithrombin deficiency

Normal pregnancy is associated with a slight decrease in antithrombin activity. Use of a combined oral contraceptive pill is also associated with a slight reduction in antithrombin activity. Acquired antithrombin deficiency occurs as a result of decreased synthesis in severe liver disease or during treatment with L-asparaginase. Increased consumption of antithrombin occurs in patients with disseminated intravascular coagulation or with a current massive thrombosis, and in nephrotic syndrome and in inflammatory bowel disease, increased loss may cause an acquired deficiency. Decreased antithrombin activity has also been noted in patients on heparin treatment.

Protein C deficiency

Protein C is a member of the family of vitamin K-dependent glycoproteins. It is synthesized in the liver and, prior to activation by thrombin to activated protein C (APC), it circulates as a two-chain zymogen. The activation process is enhanced approximately 1000-fold when thrombin is bound to thrombomodulin on the endothelial surface of blood vessels. This binding blocks the ability of thrombin to catalyse fibrin formation, factor XIII activation, platelet activation and feedback activation of coagulation cofactors. In some blood vessels, protein C activation is further augmented by the binding of protein C to a transmembrane protein, endothelial cell protein C receptor (EPCR). Once APC is generated, it binds to protein S on the surface of activated cells and this complex then inactivates FVa and FVIIIa.

Factor V (FV) has both procoagulant and anticoagulant functions. FV and FVa both bind to phospholipid and APC is able to cleave not only procoagulant FVa but also FV. The consequence of cleavage of FV is the formation of anticoagulant FV, which functions in synergy with protein S as a cofactor for APC in the degradation of FVIIIa. The anticoagulant activity of FV may be particularly important in the regulation of tenase by APC and protein S. *In vivo*, intact factor VIII (FVIII) is bound to von Willebrand factor and prevented from interacting with phospholipid surfaces. Therefore, only FVIIIa and not intact FVIII is cleaved by APC. By degrading the activated clotting factors Va and VIIIa, APC downregulates thrombin generation.

Activated protein C reduces platelet prothrombinase activity by degrading platelet-bound FVa at the receptor for FXa. It also plays a major role in the modulation of leucocyte function and reduction of the inflammatory response in septicaemia.

Heritable protein C deficiency subtypes

Familial protein C deficiency, like antithrombin deficiency, can be classified into two types on the basis of phenotypic analysis employing functional and immunological assays. In contrast with antithrombin deficiency, type I protein C deficiency is more common than type II deficiency. Type II protein C deficiency may result in defective activation by thrombin–thrombomodulin, decreased binding to phospholipids or poor interaction with cofactors or substrates. Unlike antithrombin deficiency, when the underlying genetic variant and associated phenotype predicts the degree of thrombotic risk, there is no clinical advantage in phenotypic subclassification of protein C deficiency, as no difference in the thrombotic risk of type I and type II protein C abnormalities has been identified. The prevalence of heritable protein C deficiency in the general population is approximately 0.2% (Table 53.2).

Protein C assays

In clinical practice, the diagnosis of protein C deficiency is based on a functional assay (either amidolytic or clotting). Most commercially available functional assays of protein C employ the specific activator Protac, which is derived from snake venom. Alternatively, protein C may be activated by thrombin or thrombin–thrombomodulin complex. Chromogenic assays are simple to perform and will detect all type I defects and the majority of type II defects. In the presence of FV Leiden, misleadingly low protein C activity levels may be recorded when a clotting method is used. Clotting methods may also underestimate protein C activity in patients with elevated levels of plasma FVIII or hyperlipidaemia. Protein C activity results measured by clotting assay are unreliable in the presence of a lupus inhibitor. Comparison of the result of an immunological assay with the result of a functional assay allows phenotypic classification into type I or type II deficiency but there is no clinical justification for this extra investigation.

The diagnosis of protein C deficiency is problematic because of the wide overlap in protein C activity between heterozygous carriers and unaffected individuals. Variation in protein C activity levels with age and between the sexes is explained by blood lipid levels. Both activity and antigen levels of protein C remain unchanged during pregnancy.

Acquired protein C deficiency

Acquired protein C deficiency is noted in patients using vitamin K antagonists (oral anticoagulants) and in patients with vitamin K deficiency, disseminated intravascular coagulation, liver disease or rarely a mutation in the γ-glutamylcarboxylase gene.

Protein S deficiency

Protein S, another vitamin K-dependent glycoprotein is produced by the liver, endothelial cells, megakaryocytes and the testicular Leydig cells. Approximately 60% circulates bound to the β-chain of C4b-binding protein and is inactive. The remaining 40%, designated free protein S, is uncomplexed and is the active moiety. The bioavailability of protein S is closely linked to the concentration of C4b-binding protein, which acts as an important regulator of the APC–protein S inhibitory pathway. Free protein S increases the affinity of APC for negatively charged phospholipid surfaces on platelets or the endothelium, enhancing complex formation of APC with FVa and FVIIIa. In addition, protein S has an independent anticoagulant effect on the free form of FIXa–FVIIIa–phospholipid complex (tenase) and the FVa–FXa–phospholipid complex (prothrombinase).

Heritable protein S deficiency subtypes

Three types of protein S deficiency have been described in accord with the classification of antithrombin and protein C deficiencies. Type I protein S deficiency is a quantitative defect caused by genetic variation, which results in reduced production of structurally normal protein. In type I protein S deficiency, both total and free protein S antigen levels are reduced, as is protein S activity. Type II protein S deficiency (also sometimes called type IIb protein S deficiency) has been characterized as a qualitative (functional) defect but it has become evident that some individuals with inherited or acquired APC resistance have been incorrectly diagnosed as having type II protein S deficiency. In type II protein S deficiency, both total and free antigen levels are normal (or near normal) but protein S activity is reduced. In type III deficiency (which has also been called type IIa deficiency), the total protein S antigen level is normal but there is a reduction in free protein S antigen and in protein S activity. It has been suggested that type I and type III protein S deficiency may be phenotypic variants of the same genetic disorder.

The prevalence of protein S deficiency in the general population is not firmly established. In two case–control studies, reduced free protein S antigen was found in around 3% of patients with venous thromboembolism and in 1.3–2.1% of the control subjects, suggesting that protein S deficiency is prevalent and a mild risk factor for venous thrombosis. This conclusion may however be flawed if the prevalence of familial protein S deficiency is, as demonstrated in a survey of blood donors in the West of Scotland, only around 0.03–0.13%.

Protein S assays

A number of techniques are available for the measurement of total protein S antigen including enzyme-linked immunosorbent assays (ELISAs) and radioimmunoassays. The majority of commercially available kits and reagents employ ELISA methods. It is important to establish that the method chosen for measuring total immunoreactive protein S is not influenced by the concentration of C4b-binding protein.

All protein S deficiency subtypes have reduced levels of free protein S antigen. In the most widely used method, separation of free protein S from C4b-binding protein-bound protein S is achieved by precipitation with polyethylene glycol followed by centrifugation. Results are expressed relative to a plasma pool, which has been calibrated against the current international standard and may be expressed either as a proportion of the total protein S content or, preferably, against the free protein S content. More recently, assays using monoclonal antibodies for distinct epitopes of free protein S have been developed and allow direct measurement of free protein S antigen in citrated plasma without the requirement for a precipitation stage.

Functional protein S assays based on cofactor activity have been developed. Ideally, the assays should reflect only free protein S activity but as separation of free protein S from C4b-binding protein-bound protein S is not always performed, this is not always guaranteed. Although functional assays detect all types of protein S deficiency, some are non-specific and have been shown to be sensitive to both the inherited APC resistance that is associated with FV Leiden and the acquired APC resistance observed in some patients with antiphospholipid antibodies. When a functional protein S assay is used in clinical practice as an initial screening test for protein S deficiency, it is prudent to carry out further investigation of samples with low functional protein S assay results, using an immunoreactive assay of free protein S. Protein S levels are higher in males than in females, and different reference ranges are required for males and females.

Acquired protein S deficiency

Protein S levels fall progressively during normal pregnancy and are reduced in women using oestrogen-containing oral contraceptives or hormone replacement therapy. There is a significant risk of overdiagnosis of protein S deficiency in women. Acquired protein S deficiency is seen in patients on vitamin K antagonists and also in some patients with disseminated intravascular coagulation, liver disease or antiphospholipids.

Activated protein C resistance and factor V Leiden

Factor V circulates in plasma as an inactive profactor. Activation by thrombin results in the formation of a two-chain molecule: FVa, which as part of the phospholipid bound prothrombinase complex, acts as a cofactor of FXa in the conversion of prothrombin to thrombin. This process is limited by the inactivation of FVa by selective proteolytic cleavage of its heavy chain by APC at positions Arg306, Arg506 and Arg679.

Activated protein C resistance is defined as an impaired plasma anticoagulant response to APC added *in vitro*. This phenomenon has been observed in the plasma of about 5% of the general population and over 20% of unselected consecutive patients under the age of 70 years with a first venous thrombosis and no underlying malignancy. In 1993, Dahlback and co-workers reported that increased APC resistance cosegregated with thrombosis in families with familial venous thromboembolism. The following year it was reported that the majority of patients with familial APC resistance had the same point mutation in the gene for FV, a guanine to adenine transition at nucleotide position 1691 in exon 10 of the FV gene, the FV Leiden mutation. This mutation causes a substitution of glutamine for arginine at position 506, one of the major sites at which APC cleaves factor Va. Mutant FV Leiden has normal procoagulant activity but substitution of glutamine for arginine at position 506 results in slower inactivation of FVa by APC. Additionally, because normally the anticoagulant activity of FV is stimulated by the arginine 506 cleavage, the FV Leiden mutation affects FVIIIa degradation.

The FV Leiden mutation is much more common than any other heritable thrombophilia in white populations, with a reported prevalence of between 2% and 15% (Table 53.2). It is more prevalent in individuals of northern European extraction than in those from southern Europe. Factor V Leiden is not found in the indigenous populations of Asia, America, Australia and Africa. In northern Europe, the prevalence of homozygosity for FV Leiden has been estimated at 1 in 2500. It has been suggested that carriage of the FV Leiden mutation may have a species benefit in so far as it may be associated with a reduced blood loss *intra partum*.

Activated protein C sensitivity ratios and factor V Leiden detection

The most widely used system to detect increased APC resistance employs the activated partial thromboplastin time (APTT).

Samples are tested with and without an added fixed concentration of APC and the resultant clotting times are expressed as a ratio; the APTT result in seconds of the sample plus APC divided by the APTT result in seconds of the sample without added APC – the so-called APC sensitivity ratio (APC/SR). In the test performed in this manner, the greater the APC resistance the lower the APC/SR. In the pre-analytical handling of samples for APC resistance testing, care must be taken to avoid platelet contamination and activation. Because methodological variability has been reported with APTT-based tests for the detection of APC resistance, it has been suggested that the results are 'normalized' by dividing the result of the patient's APC/SR by the APC/SR of a pooled normal plasma. If 'normalization' is employed, care must be taken to exclude from the normal plasma pool any individual who carries the FV Leiden mutation, as even a single affected donation is sufficient to affect the APC/SR of a pool.

The APC resistance test performed as described above is abnormal, not only in individuals with the FV Leiden mutation but also in subjects which acquired APC resistance (due to elevated FVIII levels or the presence of antiphospholipids) and in individuals who have a prolonged baseline APTT (due to clotting factor deficiencies or anticoagulant therapy). It is therefore not specific for FV Leiden. Modification of the test by predilution of the test plasma in FV-deficient plasma increases the sensitivity and specificity of the APTT-based APC/SR as a screen for FV Leiden. With this modification, the test is almost 100% specific and sensitive for the FV Leiden mutation and can be used reliably if genetic analysis is not available. If available, the presence of the FV Leiden mutation may be confirmed by amplification of the nucleotide region close to the exon–intron boundary in exon 5 of the FV gene from either genomic DNA or from mRNA followed by a mutation detection step.

Acquired activated protein C resistance

Resistance to activated protein C may be acquired in patients with increased plasma levels of FVIII or with antiphospholipids. Activated protein C resistance increases with age and in women using oestrogen-containing contraceptive pills or hormone replacement therapy. The increase in APC resistance is greater in women using combined oral contraceptives containing third-generation progestogens than in women using compounds containing second-generation progestogens. Activated protein C resistance increases from early pregnancy and the APC/SR performed as described above remains below that seen in non-pregnant women throughout pregnancy.

There is evidence that APC resistance determined with the original unmodified test correlates with increased venous thrombosis risk, irrespective of whether or not FV Leiden is present and there is an inverse relationship between the degree of the response to APC and thrombosis risk. The specificity of the modified APC/SR test means that individuals who have increased APC resistance for reasons other than the possession of the FV Leiden mutation will be overlooked if the original unmodified APC/SR test is not performed.

Heritable activated protein C resistance not due to factor V Leiden

Two rare mutations that result in amino acid substitutions at the 306 cleavage site on FVa have been described – 306 arginine to threonine (FV Cambridge) and 306 arginine to glycine (FV Hong Kong). In addition, a specific FV gene haplotype (HR2) that contains a histidine to arginine substitution at position 1299 has been shown to be more prevalent in individuals with an APC/SR beneath the 15th percentile than in those with higher ratios or in normal control subjects. It has a prevalence of 8–10% in the general population. In families that carry the FV Leiden mutation, the HR2 haplotype is found more frequently in family members with venous thromboembolism than in those without. Coinheritance of the HR2 haplotype with FV Leiden confers a three- to fourfold increase in the relative risk of venous thromboembolism compared with FV Leiden alone.

Prothrombin G20210A mutation

A single nucleotide change of guanine to adenine at position 20210 in the 3′-untranslated region of the prothrombin gene (FII G20210A) is associated with elevated plasma prothrombin levels and an increased risk of venous thrombosis. The prevalence of the FII G20210A polymorphism is between 1% and 4% in northern European populations (Table 53.2). Higher prevalences have been reported in southern Europe, where FII G20210A is the most prevalent heritable thrombophilic defect.

The mechanism whereby FII G20210A affects the prothrombin level has not been clearly established. No specific phenotypic test for the presence of the variant 20210A allele has been described and diagnosis depends on DNA-based procedures. The 20210A transition is not associated with the introduction or loss of a specific restriction enzyme recognition site and detection methods have been devised that do not require the use of restriction enzyme digestion of the amplified polymerase chain reaction (PCR) product.

Dysfibrinogenaemia

Over 250 cases of heritable dysfibrinogenaemia have been reported. The majority are asymptomatic and found coincidentally but, in about 20%, there is an increased tendency to arteriovenous thromboembolism. Dysfibrinogenaemia has been found in only 0.8% of patients with a history of venous thromboembolism but a high incidence of post-partum thrombosis and an increased risk of pregnancy loss have been reported in women with thrombophilic fibrinogen variants. Several mechanisms to explain the thrombotic tendency have been proposed, including defective binding of thrombin to the abnormal fibrin with consequent elevated plasma thrombin levels and impaired stimulatory function of the abnormal fibrin in fibrinolysis mediated by tissue plasminogen activator (tPA). In some, there is a low fibrinogen functional level. The diagnosis of dysfibrinogenaemia is established when there is discordance between functional and immunological assay results – the functional activity of fibrinogen being significantly lower than the immunological assay result in patients who have a prolonged thrombin time.

Combined thrombophilias

Because of the high prevalence of FV Leiden and the FII G20210A mutation in many populations, individuals and families with more than one heritable thrombophilic condition are encountered. The prevalence of thrombosis is often higher in family members with combinations of thrombophilic abnormalities.

Mixed aetiology thrombophilia

Elevated FVIII Levels

Higher risks of venous and arterial thrombosis have been described in individuals with non-O blood groups and it has been assumed that the excess risk is due to the higher levels of von Willebrand factor and FVIII found in these people. An elevated plasma concentration of FVIII (greater than 1500 IU/L), but not of von Willebrand factor, is an independent risk factor for venous thromboembolism. Although analysis within families has revealed cosegregation of elevated FVIII levels and venous thrombosis, no specific genetic abnormality has been identified to date.

Homocysteine and methylene tetrahydrofolate reductase

Plasma homocysteine levels are increased in individuals with reduced levels of folate, cobalamin or pyridoxine due to dietary deficiency, drugs or underlying disease (see Chapter 5).

Hyperhomocysteinaemia may be caused by genetic abnormalities affecting the trans-sulphuration or remethylation pathways of homocysteine metabolism. The severe inherited abnormalities of homocysteine metabolism (homozygous cystathionine beta-synthase deficiency and homozygous deficiency of methylene tetrahydrofolate reductase) result in congenital homocysteinuria. Classically, patients suffer severe mental retardation, seizures, skeletal deformity, ectopia lentis, premature vascular disease associated with severe atherosclerosis, and venous thromboembolism. Around one-half of the affected patients present with venous or arterial thrombosis before the age of 30 years. Individuals who are heterozygous for the cystathionine beta-synthase deficiency have moderately elevated levels of plasma homocysteine.

A common mutation in the gene encoding methylene tetrahydrofolate reductase (MTHFR) has been described. A cytidine residue at position 677 in the gene is replaced by thymidine resulting in the substitution of valine for alanine at nucleotide 677 in the enzyme. The resultant variant is thermolabile and, in its homozygous form, is associated with an approximately 50%

reduction of the enzyme activity. It occurs in white people and East Asians but has not been shown in Africans. In its homozygous form, the prevalence of this mutation in the general population is 5–15%. In the presence of folate deficiency, homozygosity for this mutation results in elevated plasma homocysteine levels.

Increased levels of FIX or FXI

In addition to those abnormalities described above, which have been shown in individual patients to be associated with venous thrombosis, there are a number of other abnormalities such as elevated levels of clotting factors IX or XI (above the 90th percentile for the general population), which have been shown in epidemiological studies to be associated with increased venous thrombotic risk. As in the case of elevated FVIII levels, this appears not to be the result of an acute phase reaction and to date no genetic explanation has been identified.

The 'thrombophilia screen'

Clinical assessment

The initial assessment must commence with a carefully taken personal and family history and a carefully performed clinical examination (Table 53.3). Patients should be asked specifically if they have a personal history of venous thromboembolism or a family history of venous thrombosis. Ideally, these events should have been objectively confirmed but because less emphasis was placed on the requirement to confirm a clinical diagnosis of deep vein thrombosis or pulmonary embolism in the past, a degree of pragmatism is necessary. Thus, if a venous thrombosis has not been confirmed by objective testing, it would seem reasonable to accept the clinical diagnosis if the history is plausible and if it resulted in the patient being given anticoagulant treatment. Additional risk factors including advancing age, a past history of venous thrombosis, immobility, trauma, surgery, hormone use, pregnancy, post-partum state and obesity should be clearly documented.

Laboratory tests

When laboratory testing is indicated, it should include assays and tests for heritable defects – deficiency of antithrombin, protein C or protein S, FV Leiden and the FII G20210A polymor-

Table 53.3 Thrombophilia testing: initial assessment.

Personal history
Family history
Clinical examination
Search for additional risk factors
Full blood count and platelet count
Liver function tests: urea and electrolytes
Appropriate imaging and other investigations

Table 53.4 Thrombophilia screening: first-line tests.

Coagulation screen	APTT, PT, TT
Antithrombin activity	Heparin cofactor assay
Protein C	Chromogenic assay
Protein S	Immunoreactive (free ± total)
Modified APC/SR	Predilution in FV-deficient plasma
Factor V Leiden	PCR
Prothrombin G20210A	PCR
Antiphospholipids	Lupus inhibitor screen
	Anticardiolipin assays

APC/SR, activated protein C sensitivity ratio; APTT, activated partial thromboplastin time; PT, prothrombin time; TT, thrombin time.

phism, and also testing for antiphospholipids, the most common acquired cause of thrombophilia (Table 53.4). A full blood count, platelet count, APTT, prothrombin time and thrombin clotting time should be incorporated in the initial screening. Liver function tests and measurement of urea and electrolytes are also helpful. The full blood count and platelet count are useful indicators of general health and will identify myeloproliferative conditions that increase thrombotic risk. The APTT may identify some individuals with antiphospholipids, but formal testing for the presence of lupus inhibitors and measurement of anticardiolipins should be included. The thrombin clotting time will allow identification of dysfibrinogenaemia and heparin contamination. The prothrombin time is useful in the interpretation of low protein C or protein S results.

Functional assays should be used to determine antithrombin and protein C levels. Chromogenic assays of protein C activity are less subject to interference than are clotting assays and are preferable for clinical purposes. If a protein S activity assay is used in the initial screen, low results should be confirmed with an immunoreactive assay of free protein S. The modified APC/SR test (predilution of the test sample in FV-deficient plasma) as opposed to the original APC/SR test, may be used as a phenotypic test for the FV Leiden mutation. PCR-based testing for FII G20210A is required as there is no screening test. Laboratories must establish their own reference ranges for the assays and tests which they use. Rigorous internal quality assurance and participation in accredited external quality assessment schemes are mandatory.

Factor VIII and homocysteine assays may be considered as 'second line' tests and fibrinogen assays are indicated in patients with prolonged thrombin times.

Interpretation of laboratory results

There are significant problems in the accurate diagnosis and classification of deficiencies of the natural anticoagulants – antithrombin, protein C and protein S. Thus diagnostic uncertainty is commonly encountered and both over- and underdiagnosis of thrombophilia occur as a result. When laboratory investigation for heritable thrombophilia is pursued, it is essential that facilities are in place for the provision of informed and detailed advice, based on a clear appreciation of the limitations of laboratory tests.

Some tests for heritable thrombophilia (e.g. assays of antithrombin, protein C and protein S) are affected by the acute post-thrombotic state and by anticoagulant use. As finding a thrombophilic abnormality seldom influences the management of an acute thrombotic event, there is little point in striving to obtain samples for tests for heritable thrombophilia when the patients present with an acute thrombotic event. Testing is usually best delayed until at least 1 month after completion of a course of anticoagulation. If possible, testing should be avoided during intercurrent illness, pregnancy, use of combined oral contraceptive pills or hormone replacement therapy. If this is not possible then it is essential that the individual interpreting the screen is aware of the presence and potential influence of these various factors on the components of the test results.

Clinical presentation of heritable thrombophilia

Patients with heritable thrombophilia typically present with thrombosis in the deep veins of the legs, pulmonary embolism or both. Less frequently, they present with superficial vein thrombosis or thrombosis at an unusual site such as mesenteric vessels or cerebral vessels. In more than one-half of the thrombotic events, an acquired precipitant such as surgery, pregnancy or oral contraceptive use can be identified. In most patients, the first event occurs before the age of 50 years. It is unusual for the first presentation to occur in childhood. Patients with natural anticoagulant deficiencies are likely to present with clinical manifestations in early adulthood, but patients with the less severe FV Leiden or FII G20210A mutations may not present until later in adulthood. Asymptomatic but affected relatives of patients with thrombophilia who have had venous thrombosis are at increased risk of venous thrombosis compared with the general population.

Deep vein thrombosis and pulmonary embolism

Antithrombin deficiency has been reported in between 0.5% and 1% of unselected patients presenting with venous thrombosis and around 4% of selected patients with a family history of venous thrombosis (Table 53.2). The annual incidence of venous thrombotic events in patients with familial antithrombin deficiency is estimated to be 0.87–1.6%. Family and prospective studies suggest that antithrombin deficiency – type I deficiency or type II RS deficiency – is a more severe disorder than deficiencies of protein C or protein S. Around 50% of individuals heterozygous for these antithrombin defects develop venous thrombosis and present with major venous thrombo-

embolism at a younger age than those with other thrombophilic abnormalities. Although pulmonary embolism associated with antithrombin deficiency may be fatal, there is a lack of evidence to suggest that antithrombin deficiency reduces the normal lifespan. Homozygous antithrombin deficiency is probably incompatible with life unless it is a type II defect involving the heparin binding site, in which case the clinical presentation is likely to be indistinguishable from heterozygous type I deficiency.

Protein C deficiency is found in around 3% of unselected patients with venous thromboembolism and between 5% and 6% of those with a family history of venous thrombosis (Table 53.2). Venous thrombotic events occur in around 0.5–1.65% of heterozygotes per year. Heterozygous protein C deficiency does not appear to be associated with excess mortality. Classically, homozygous protein C deficiency manifests as purpura fulminans as a result of thrombosis in small vessels and subsequent necrosis of the skin and subcutaneous tissues. This usually occurs during the neonatal period or in the first few years of life – depending on the level of protein C activity.

There is evidence that there is a substantial difference in the risk associated with protein S deficiency in thrombophilic families and in unselected consecutive patients. This suggests that the effect on families is the result of interaction of protein S deficiency with other defects. About 0.43–0.73% of protein S heterozygotes have a venous thromboembolic event per year. The clinical manifestations of protein S deficiency are similar to those of protein C deficiency, with patients suffering from an increased risk of venous thromboembolism as well as an increased risk of superficial thrombophlebitis. Homozygous protein S deficiency, like homozygous protein C deficiency, may present soon after birth with purpura fulminans or massive venous thrombosis.

Compared with individuals with a natural anticoagulant deficiency, the incidence of venous thrombotic events associated with the more prevalent thrombophilias – heterozygosity for FV Leiden and heterozygosity for the FII G20210A polymorphism – are associated with a lesser risk of venous thrombosis, the annual incidence being 0.25–0.45% and 0.55% respectively. FV Leiden is found in around 20–50% of unselected patients presenting with a first episode of venous thromboembolism and in more than one-half of probands from selected families with familial thrombophilia (Table 53.2). Heterozygous carriers are reported to have a three- to eightfold increased risk of venous thrombosis. Homozygous FV Leiden is reported to increase the risk of venous thrombosis approximately 30- to 140-fold, and these patients experience their first event at a young age. In northern Europe, about 4% of patients who have a venous thrombosis under the age of 45 years are homozygous for FV Leiden.

It has been claimed that deep vein thrombosis associated with the FV Leiden mutation is more stable and adherent to the vessel wall than deep vein thrombosis occurring in the absence of this mutation. This is presumed to be due to enhanced local thrombin generation intensifying the local inflammatory process and impairing the profibrinolytic response to APC. It has been demonstrated that deep vein thrombosis occurring in the presence of the FV Leiden mutation is less likely to extend into the ileofemoral veins than a deep vein thrombosis occurring in the absence of this mutation, and patients with FV Leiden have a reduced risk of developing symptomatic or fatal pulmonary embolism when compared with other patients with deep vein thrombosis. Coinheritance of factor V Leiden with other heritable thrombophilias increases the risk of venous thrombosis.

Of unselected patients presenting with a first thrombosis, 6% have been found to have the FII G20210A polymorphism (see Table 53.2) and the evidence suggests that carriers have a three- to fivefold increased risk of venous thrombosis. Just under 20% of patients presenting with a first venous thrombosis belong to families with a history of familial venous thrombosis and have the FII G20210A polymorphism. The clinical manifestations in heterozygotes are similar to those seen in FV Leiden heterozygotes but it has been suggested that individuals homozygous for the FII G20210A polymorphism have a lesser risk of venous thrombosis than individuals homozygous for FV Leiden. Although the G20210A transition of the prothrombin gene appears to be a mild risk factor for venous thromboembolism, it may contribute to the incidence of thromboembolic disease in patients with other prothrombotic abnormalities, such as FV Leiden.

There is a dose–response relationship between FVIII level and risk of thrombosis – subjects with FVIII concentrations greater than 1500 IU/L having a four- to fivefold increased risk. This finding appears to be independent of the blood group and is not the result of an acute phase reaction. In unselected patients with venous thrombosis, there is a 25% prevalence of FVIII levels above 1500 IU/L. Elevated FVIII levels are not in themselves sufficient to cause thrombosis but will interact with other predisposing factors.

Case–control studies have demonstrated an approximately 2.5-fold increased risk of venous thrombosis in individuals with homocysteine levels exceeding 18.5 μmol/L and a three- to fourfold risk associated with levels exceeding 20 μmol/L. The data relating the C677T MTHFR mutation to venous thrombosis risk are conflicting; some studies have shown no association, whereas others have suggested a possible increased risk of venous thrombosis in homozygotes who have other venous thrombosis risk factors.

Site of venous thrombosis

The pathogenesis of venous thrombosis of the lower limbs, where the major mechanism is hypercoagulability, may be different from that of thrombosis in upper limb veins. Upper limb veins lack valve pockets. Thus local accumulation of activated clotting factors is less likely in upper limb veins unless the patient has a predisposing anatomic abnormality causing venous compression. Some workers have suggested that the prevalences of deficiencies of natural anticoagulants and of increased APC resistance in patients with primary upper limb venous thrombosis are significantly lower than the prevalences in patients with lower limb thrombosis. However, this suggestion is controversial and others have claimed that hypercoagulability is as frequent in patients with upper limb venous thrombosis as in those with lower limb events.

Recurrent venous thrombosis

Patients with a history of venous thrombosis are at increased risk of recurrence irrespective of whether or not they have an identifiable thrombophilia. The risk of recurrent venous thrombosis after stopping oral anticoagulant therapy in subjects heterozygous for FV Leiden has been compared with that in subjects with no detectable thrombophilia. A higher recurrence rate in FV Leiden heterozygotes has been suggested in some studies but, in the majority of prospective studies, the thrombosis recurrence rate was not increased in FV Leiden heterozygotes, although homozygotes may be at increased risk. There is also evidence suggesting the risk of recurrent venous thromboembolism is not increased in heterozygous FII G20210A carriers.

Because deficiency of the natural anticoagulants antithrombin, protein C or protein S is relatively uncommon, there are a lack of reliable data on the risk of recurrent venous thromboembolism in affected individuals. Some studies have suggested that recurrent venous thrombosis after discontinuation of warfarin therapy is high in patients with antithrombin or protein S deficiency but other studies have failed to corroborate this finding and have suggested that the recurrence rate may be similar to that in unselected patients with venous thrombosis.

Oral contraceptive use and hormone replacement therapy

Combined oral contraceptives cause slight increases in some procoagulant factors and reduce the levels of some natural anticoagulants – in particular antithrombin and protein S. These effects are more marked with third-generation pills (containing desogestrel or gestodene) than with second-generation pills (containing levonorgestrel). Compared with women not using combined oral contraceptives, plasma from combined oral contraceptive-using women has significantly increased APC resistance, and women who use third-generation pills have significantly greater APC resistance than women using second-generation preparations.

There is evidence that the risk of venous thrombosis is increased in women with thrombophilia when they use combined oral contraceptives. The Leiden Thrombophilia Study reported that the relative risk of venous thromboembolism for FV Leiden heterozygotes using combined oral contraceptives is 34.7 – significantly higher than expected if the relative risks associated with combined oral contraceptive use and with heterozygosity for FV Leiden were simply additive. This risk has been confirmed in other studies and shown to be even greater for FV Leiden homozygotes. The interaction between combined oral

	General population (%)	Pregnancy VTE population (%)	Estimated risk
Antithrombin deficiency – type I	0.02	8.0	1 in 2.8 (36%)
Antithrombin deficiency – type II	0.15	4.0	1 in 42 (2.4%)
Protein C deficiency	0.20%	2.0	1 in 113 (0.9%)
Protein S deficiency	?	0.0	?
Factor V Leiden	3.0	8.0	1 in 437 (0.2%)
Prothrombin G20210A	2.0	9.0	1 in 232 (0.4%)

Table 53.5 Thrombophilia and risk of pregnancy-associated venous thromboembolism.

From McColl *et al.* (1997, 2000), with permission.

contraceptive use and FV Leiden is greater for pills containing third-generation progestogens. The FII G20210A mutation has also been shown to increase the risk of venous thromboembolism in combined oral contraceptive users.

Because of the relative rarity of inherited deficiencies of natural anticoagulants, there is little information about the risk of venous thrombosis in women with these defects using contraceptive pills. One study noted a significant increase in the risk of venous thromboembolism in combined oral contraceptive users with antithrombin deficiency compared with non-pill using antithrombin deficient women but this study was too small to reveal any significant difference between combined oral contraceptive users and non-users with either protein C or S deficiency.

Hormone replacement therapy also exposes women to exogenous oestrogen and, in women who still have their uterus, progestogen may be added to reduce the risk of endometrial cancer. Early studies suggested that hormone replacement therapy did not significantly increase the risk of venous thromboembolism. More recently, however, clear evidence linking hormone replacement therapy and venous thrombosis has been published. For women using hormone replacement, the evidence is consistent in demonstrating a relative risk of venous thromboembolism that is 2–4 times that of non-users. The changes in haemostasis associated with hormone replacement therapy are similar in type and direction to those associated with combined oral contraceptive use but lesser in magnitude. There are as yet few published studies examining venous thrombosis risk in women with thrombophilia using hormone replacement. In one study, the relative risk of thrombosis showed significant associations with certain thrombophilic markers, including increased APC resistance, low antithrombin and low protein C. For hormone replacement users with abnormalities of haemostasis, the relative risks of venous thromboembolism were around 3.5–4.0 times the risk in non-hormone users with the same defect(s).

Pregnancy

Early studies suggested that in the absence of anticoagulant prophylaxis about 40% of pregnancies in antithrombin-deficient women may be complicated by venous thromboembolism. These studies were retrospective reports of events occurring in women who were already known to have antithrombin deficiency diagnosed, because either they personally or other family members had a history of venous thrombosis. They are therefore biased – the risk of thrombosis may have been overestimated. However, a study of 50 unselected, consecutive Glasgow women with a history of pregnancy-associated venous thromboembolism revealed that for type I antithrombin-deficient women, the risk of developing venous thrombosis associated with pregnancy is almost 40% – even in otherwise asymptomatic kindred (Table 53.5). In this study, the risk of pregnancy-associated venous thrombosis for women with type II defects was much lower, being about 2.5%.

The incidence of pregnancy-associated venous thromboembolism in women with protein C or S deficiency appears to be considerably less than that for antithrombin-deficient women. In the Glasgow study, only one protein C-deficient patient was found, suggesting a risk of only 1:113 (less than 1%) (see Table 53.5). No patients with protein S deficiency were found. The risk of pregnancy venous thrombosis was less than 1 in 350 (about 0.3%) for FV Leiden or FII G20210A heterozygotes (see Table 53.5) and the majority had additional acquired thrombosis risk factor. Other studies have confirmed that the risk of pregnancy-associated venous thromboembolism in heterozygous carriers of FV Leiden or FII G20210A is approximately five- to 10-fold that in non-carriers. The risk is significantly greater in homozygotes and in women doubly heterozygous for FV Leiden and FII G20210A.

Homocysteine levels fall during normal pregnancy. Folic acid supplements further lower homocysteine concentrations. The contribution of homocysteine levels to the risk of pregnancy-associated venous thrombosis is unclear but the C677T MTHFR mutation is not associated with an increased risk of pregnancy-associated thrombosis.

Venous thromboembolism is a rare but well documented complication of pharmacological ovarian stimulation in assisted conception protocols. Cases of venous thrombosis in women with heritable thrombophilias undergoing ovarian stimulation have been reported but, at present, the magnitude of the risk conferred by prothrombotic mutations in these women is unknown. There is evidence that thrombophilia may increase the risk of fetal loss and other vascular complications of pregnancy such as intra-uterine growth restriction or pre-eclampsia. The data, however, remain controversial and further studies are necessary.

Case finding – who should be tested?

The high prevalences of FV Leiden and the prothrombin G20201A polymorphism have prompted a broad application of thrombophilia testing – not always appropriately. Thrombophilia screening has become commonplace in patients with a history of venous thrombosis. Detection of a heritable prothrombotic state may lead to screening of family members in an attempt to identify asymptomatic relatives who may be at increased risk of venous thromboembolism.

Clinicians tend to overestimate the risk of thrombosis associated with thrombophilias and to underestimate the risks associated with anticoagulation. Frequently, this has led to the belief that prophylactic anticoagulation is a safer option than clinical surveillance. As evidence about the risk of venous thrombosis associated with thrombophilias accumulates, it is becoming clear that for many patients this is not the case. Furthermore, there is often a lack of recognition that failure to identify a defect in an individual is not proof that no defect exists, only that the particular defects for which tests have been performed are probably not present. The patient with 'negative' test results may well have as yet unidentifiable prothrombotic abnormalities, which increase his or her risk of thrombosis. Reassuring patients with normal test results may constitute false reassurance, which may present a real risk for the patient if negative laboratory results lead to ignoring or underestimating the clinical history.

There is no evidence that the detection of a heritable thrombophilic defect is helpful in guiding clinical decision-making, in relation to either the choice of anticoagulant or to the intensity or duration of anticoagulant therapy to treat a venous thrombotic event. Although heparin resistance and thrombus progression are theoretical risks in antithrombin deficiency, retrospective data suggest that these are infrequent problems in clinical practice. In theory, warfarin-induced skin necrosis may complicate the introduction of coumarin therapy in subjects deficient in protein C or S if there is underanticoagulation with heparin when the oral agent is introduced, but, in practice, this is rarely a problem.

The management of deep vein thrombosis or pulmonary embolism in patients with heritable thrombophilia is in general no different from the management of venous thrombosis in any other patient. A target international normalized ratio (INR) of 2.5 is generally deemed to be appropriate for the management of a first acute venous thromboembolism. On standard anticoagulant therapy, major haemorrhage occurs at a rate of around 1% per year of treatment and one-quarter of these bleeds are fatal. For the patient without an identifiable thrombophilia, who has had a first venous thrombotic event, the benefits of long-term treatment (more than 6 months) have not yet been shown to outweigh the risks. The risk of recurrence is not significantly increased in patients with the most prevalent defects (FV Leiden and the FII G20210A polymorphism). For these patients, therefore, management as for non-thrombophilic patients seems appropriate. Patients who have defects such as type I antithrombin deficiency or combinations of thrombophilias seem to be at additional risk of venous thromboembolism. The risk of recurrent events in such subjects is not known and they may merit a longer duration of anticoagulation.

Thrombophilia screening may be useful in decisions on the usefulness of primary prophylaxis in the presence of temporary risk factors in asymptomatic relatives in symptomatic families with identifiable thrombophilic defects. Identification of a thrombophilic defect may suggest prophylactic anticoagulation during surgery for relatives who are younger than the usual age at which prophylaxis is usually considered or prophylaxis to prevent pregnancy-associated thrombosis.

The increased risk of venous thrombosis associated with combined oral contraceptive use in patients with heritable thrombophilias has led to the suggestion that women should be screened for these defects (or at least the most prevalent defects) prior to prescription of a combined contraceptive pill. However, it has been estimated that if screening of the women was adopted and if advice to avoid oral contraceptives was given to all women carrying the FV Leiden mutation then more than 2 million women would need to be tested to prevent a single death from oral contraceptive-related pulmonary embolism each year – assuming that 1% of all venous thromboembolic events would be fatal. A greater number of non-fatal thromboses may be avoided but, as the combined pill is the most efficient form of contraception, it could be anticipated that additional pregnancies with their associated thrombotic risk would occur and negate any benefit.

Similarly routine screening of pregnant women for thrombophilic defects is not justifiable and may cause more harm than good, as finding a defect may precipitate unnecessary intervention with antithrombotics. In the UK and Europe, many clinicians recommend screening of women who have already suffered a thrombotic event, and many would advocate in addition screening personally asymptomatic women who give a family history of proven venous thromboembolism. Thrombophilia screening of these selected women may provide information useful in the assessment of the individual patient's overall venous thrombotic risk, in making decisions about their requirement for anticoagulation and the timing of its introduction. Antithrombotic prophylaxis may be considered post partum in asymptomatic carriers of the milder defects such as FV Leiden or the FII G20210A polymorphism, and should perhaps be offered to carriers of the more severe abnormalities such as antithrombin deficiency throughout pregnancy and the puerperium.

Thrombophilia testing is rarely indicated in children as it is unlikely to influence their management. Genetic testing should be avoided in minors except in the very rare circumstance when the result is required to determine treatment.

Heritable abnormalities of haemostasis and arterial thrombosis

Arterial thrombotic diseases arise from two related processes – atherosclerosis and thrombosis. Atherosclerosis is a disease of the vessel wall, which results from chronic changes in vessel wall cellular phenotypes, occurring over a period of many years. Environmental risk factors for arterial disease including cigarette smoking, diet, abnormalities of lipid metabolism, elevated blood pressure and abnormalities of glucose metabolism are well established. Clinical symptoms are usually precipitated by thrombosis – an acute process thought to be triggered by tissue factor interaction with FVIIa, and almost certainly influenced by haemostatic factors such as fibrinogen, fibrinolytic factors and platelet reactivity. At present, there is considerable interest in the potential role of genetic changes in these and other components of haemostasis in the clinical expression of arterial thrombotic disease.

Coagulation abnormalities

Fibrinogen

Fibrinogen has been extensively studied in relation to arterial disease and elevated fibrinogen levels are consistently associated with myocardial infarction, stroke and peripheral arterial disease in prospective studies. An approximately twofold increased risk of myocardial infarction has been associated with elevated fibrinogen levels (> 3.4 mg/mL) compared with individuals with levels below this limit. A number of mechanisms to explain this association of increased fibrinogen with arterial disease has been postulated including increased viscosity, increased coagulation, increased availability for platelet adhesion and aggregation. However, it has also been suggested that elevated fibrinogen levels noted in patients with arterial disease may be effect rather than cause.

A number of polymorphisms in the three genes that code for fibrinogen polypeptide chains have been studied, including the BcII, Arg448Lys, −148C/T and −455G/A polymorphisms in the β-chain gene. In most studies, the −455G/A polymorphism was examined, and in most of them an influence of the polymorphism on the level of fibrinogen was observed either in patient or control plasma samples. Most studies confirm an association between the phenotype (elevated fibrinogen level) and disease, but only in one study have fully consistent associations between genotype, phenotype and myocardial infarction been reported. Other studies have failed to find an association between the genotype and coronary heart disease. Thus it would appear that if there is a causative relationship between fibrinogen genotype, plasma level and disease then it is very small.

Factor VII gene polymorphisms

Plasma factor VII (FVII) activity has been shown by some authors to be associated with an increased risk of myocardial infarction but others have failed to confirm this finding. A number of polymorphisms of the gene encoding FVII have been described, including an insertion of a decanucleotide at position 323 and a substitution of glutamine for arginine at position 353, which is associated with a 20–25% reduction in the plasma concentration of FVII. Some studies have reported that the risk of myocardial infarction is lower in patients with the 353 arginine allele than in patients with the glutamine allele. Others, however, although confirming that FVII levels are lower in patients with the arginine allele, did not find a difference in the genotype frequency between patients with myocardial infarction and control subjects. No link between FVII polymorphisms and stroke has been reported and there is no evidence of an association with venous thrombosis. Thus, as with fibrinogen, if there is an effect of the FVII polymorphism on disease it is small.

Heritable thrombophilias

Although a few case reports have suggested a possible link between inherited deficiency of antithrombin, protein C or S and a risk of arterial thrombosis, there is no convincing evidence. Endothelial cell protein C receptor (EPCR) is found predominantly on the endothelium of large vessels and may be important in enhancing protein C activation in these vessels. It has been suggested that the presence of high levels of EPCR on arterial vessels may help to explain why inherited protein C deficiency appears not to constitute a significant risk of arterial thrombosis.

The roles of FV Leiden and the FII G20210A polymorphisms in arterial disease have been the subject of a large number of reports with inconsistent outcomes. The majority have been negative but some studies have reported positive associations, particularly when highly selected patient populations have been studied and when the interaction of these polymorphisms with environmental factors has been evaluated. In a prospective study, the prevalences of FV Leiden heterozygosity in men who had a myocardial infarction and in men who suffered a stroke were similar to that in male control subjects who had no vascular events but, in another large case–control study of men with myocardial infarction, a small increase in the risk of myocardial infarction was associated with both FV Leiden and the FII G20210A polymorphism. The risk associated with these polymorphisms is amplified in the presence of other coronary heart disease risk factors such as smoking and metabolic risk factors.

In a study of young women with a history of myocardial infarction, compared with non-smoking non-carriers, young women carriers of FV Leiden or the FII G20210A polymorphism who smoked had a significantly increased risk of myocardial infarction. On balance, it would appear that FV Leiden and the

FII G20210A polymorphism increase slightly the risk of arterial thrombosis in young patients who have other additional risk factors for arterial thrombosis.

Although the phenotype (hyperhomocysteinaemia) is associated with an increased risk of arterial thrombotic disease, the results of studies investigating a link between the C677T MTHFR mutation and myocardial infarction have produced conflicting results. The consensus, however, would appear to be that the mutation does not constitute a significant risk factor for myocardial infarction or stroke.

Fibrinolytic system abnormalities

Plasminogen activator inhibitor-1

Plasminogen activator inhibitor-1 (PAI-1) is the major inhibitor of tissue plasminogen activator (tPA). There is evidence that increased PAI-1 levels are associated with atherosclerotic progression and myocardial infarction risk, but it remains to be proven that PAI-1 is an independent risk factor for cardiovascular disease. A single gene on the long arm of chromosome 7 encodes PAI-1. Several polymorphisms in this gene have been described including a *Hind* III site at the 3′-region of the gene, a CA dinucleotide repeat in intron 3, and a single nucleotide insertion/deletion (4G/5G) – 675 basepairs (bps) upstream from the start of the transcription site. The 4G allele is associated with higher PAI-1 levels than the 5G allele, particularly in patients with elevated triglyceride levels.

Following an early report that the 4G allele might be associated with myocardial infarction support for an association between this allele and coronary heart disease has been obtained. However, there are reports from several well designed studies that PAI-1 polymorphisms have not been found to be associated with myocardial infarction or coronary artery disease and there are no studies that confirm a consistent association between genotype, phenotype and disease. Collectively, the results of the various studies do not appear to support an important role for PAI-1 genotypes in ischaemic heart disease but in a prospective study of 12239 women followed up for 18 years, the 4G/4G homozygotes had a reduced risk of cerebrovascular mortality compared with 5G/5G homozygotes.

Tissue plasminogen activator

An increased risk of myocardial infarction has been found in individuals with elevated levels of tissue plasminogen activator (tPA). The polymorphism that has been studied most in respect of cardiovascular disease is the Alu-repeat insertion/deletion (I/D) polymorphism within the intron between exons 8 and 9. However, to date, a relationship between this polymorphism and elevated tPA levels has not been established, and no association has been found in patients selected for a family history of cardiovascular disease.

Neither tPA nor PAI-1 levels has been found to be associated with increased venous thrombotic risk.

Platelet membrane glycoprotein abnormalities

Glycoprotein IIb/IIIa

Glycoprotein (Gp) IIb/IIIa, a member of the integrin family, plays a key role in platelet aggregation and activation. It is the primary receptor for fibrinogen and also binds von Willebrand factor fibronectin and vitronectin. The genes encoding glycoproteins IIb and IIIa lie close to each other on chromosome 17.

The PLA1/PLA2 polymorphism results in a substitution of proline for leucine at position 33 in the GpIIIa ($\gamma3$) subunit of the GpIIb/IIIa. Around 25% of white persons carry the PLA2 allele and 2% are PLA2 homozygotes. The HPA-3a/3b GpIIb polymorphism results in substitution of serine for isoleucine at position 843.

Most studies have failed to find an association between the PLA1/PLA2 polymorphism and myocardial infarction, but some have reported a weak positive association in young patients. An increased risk of coronary stent thrombosis in PLA2 patients has been reported but other studies have not confirmed this finding. There is no evidence that the PLA2 allele increases the risk of stroke or venous thrombosis. The clinical relevance of the GpIIb polymorphism HPA-3 remains unclear but it appears not to increase the risk of stroke.

Glycoprotein Ia/IIa

This collagen receptor consists of an α_2- and a γ_1-polypeptide and is expressed at low density on the platelet surface. Two linked silent dimorphisms, 807 cytosine to thymine (Phe224) and 873 guanine to adenine (Thr246) within GpIa gene have been described. An association between the receptor density and these polymorphisms has been reported; individuals homozygous for the 807C/873G allele having low receptor density and individuals homozygous for the 807T/873A allele high receptor density and thus enhanced platelet binding to collagen. An increased risk of myocardial infarction in patients with the homozygous 807T/873A genotype has been described but other studies have not confirmed this link. The 807T/873A allele has been found to be associated with stroke in young patients.

Glycoprotein 1b/IX/V

This complex is a combination of four glycoprotein chains: GpIbα, GpIbβ, GpIX and GpV. Interest has centred on a polymorphism of the GpIbα with four polymorphic forms A, B, C and D and a cytosine-to-thymine change at position 3550, which results in a Thr145Met substitution, the latter part of the HPA-2 alloantigen system.

The C/B genotype has been associated with increased risk and stroke. A few studies found associations between Thr145Met and coronary artery disease but other studies have been negative with respect to myocardial infarction or ischaemic heart disease. Similar results have been found in studies of cerebrovascular disease – some suggesting a positive association and others reporting no association. No association between these polymorphisms and venous thrombosis has been found.

Other candidate genetic risk factors for thrombosis

It is likely that there are yet unidentified heritable abnormalities of haemostasis associated with an increased risk of thrombosis. Some additional candidates such as heparin cofactor II deficiency and deficiencies of histidine-rich glycoprotein have been studied. However, none has been demonstrated conclusively to contribute to heritable thrombophilia.

Thrombomodulin and endothelial cell protein C receptor

Thrombomodulin is a receptor for thrombin on the endothelial cell surface of most blood vessels. Thrombin-bound thrombomodulin activates protein C to form APC, which inhibits thrombin generation by degrading FVa and FVIIIa. On binding to thrombomodulin, thrombin loses its procoagulant properties (fibrinogen clotting, platelet activation and the activation of FV and FVIII). Thus, thrombomodulin plays a key role in the conversion of thrombin from a procoagulant to an anticoagulant.

Identifying individuals with a thrombomodulin deficiency phenotype is problematic. Leucocyte proteases cleave off a large extracellular portion of thrombomodulin generating soluble thrombomodulin (sTM), which is composed of a variety of molecular species. The physiological function of sTM is unclear. A large prospective study of ischaemic heart disease and atherosclerosis in the community (ARIC Study), however, found an inverse relationship between sTM levels and the risk of ischaemic heart disease.

The thrombomodulin gene is located on chromosome 20. Three polymorphisms in the gene: Ala455Val and Ala25Thr in the coding region and −33 G/A in the vicinity of the promoter have been described but no association of these polymorphisms with thrombotic disease has been consistently reported.

Endothelial cell protein C receptor
The endothelial cell protein C receptor (EPCR) presents protein C to the thrombin–thrombomodulin complex on the surface of endothelial cells and results in increased activation of protein C. A 23-bp insertion in the gene for EPCR, prevalent in Italians, has been shown to be weakly associated with myocardial infarction.

Protein C inhibitor

Protein C inhibitor (PCI), also known as plasminogen activator inhibitor-3, is a serine proteinase inhibitor that inhibits enzymes in blood coagulation, fibrinolysis and fertility. By virtue of inhibiting thrombin, FXa and FXIa, it has an anticoagulant effect; by inhibiting APC and thrombin–thrombomodulin (preventing activation of protein C), it has an anti-anticoagulant effect; by inhibiting tissue type and urokinase type plasminogen activators it has and antifibrinolytic activity and by inhibiting thrombin–thrombomodulin activation of thrombin-activatable fibrinolysis inhibitor (TAFI), it has anti-antifibrinolytic activity. Most of the inhibitory functions are enhanced in the presence of heparin or other glycosaminoglycans. Despite all of these identified activities, the physiological role of PCI is unknown and although and association between high PCI levels and increased venous thrombosis risk has been postulated, this awaits confirmation.

Tissue factor pathway inhibitor

The principal inhibitor of the FVII-tissue factor pathway is the tissue factor pathway inhibitor (TFPI), which binds and inhibits FXa thereafter forming a larger quaternary complex with FVIIa, tissue factor and calcium. A single nucleotide substitution in exon 7 (536 cytidine to thiamine) leading to a proline to leucine exchange at position 151 has been described. It has been suggested that this mutation is more prevalent in patients with venous thrombosis than in control subjects but other studies have failed to confirm this finding. No increased risk of stroke has been found in carriers of the TFPI C536T mutation.

Protein Z deficiency

Protein Z (PZ) is a vitamin K-dependent plasma protein that acts as a cofactor for the inhibition of FXa by protein Z-dependent protease inhibitor (ZPI). Protein Z-dependent protease inhibitor is a member of the serpin family of proteinase inhibitors. Protein Z circulates in plasma in complex with ZPI. Inhibition of FXa by ZPI in the presence of phospholipids and calcium is enhanced approximately 1000-fold by PZ. Protein Z, like protein S, does not in itself have proteolytic activity.

Warfarin therapy reduces both PZ antigen levels and the degree of gamma carboxylation much more than the other vitamin K-dependent factors. *In vitro* and *in vivo* studies suggest that PZ is important in dampening coagulation. Based on data from murine gene deletion modules it has been suggested that PZ deficiency may be a modest thrombotic risk factor in humans. It has been suggested that concomitant PZ deficiency may reduce the age of onset and increase the risk of venous thrombosis in patients with FV Leiden.

Plasminogen

Case reports have suggested that hypoplasminogenaemia and dysplasminogenaemia may be associated with venous thromboembolism but this association has not been confirmed in case–control studies.

Factor XII

Although *in vivo* FXII seems to be of minimal importance for blood coagulation, it may play a role in the fibrinolytic system by enhancing the release of tPA. It has been suggested that FXII may be a risk factor for venous thromboembolism but this has not been confirmed.

Factor XIII – a protective mutation

The main function of factor XIII (FXIII) is the formation of stable cross-linked fibrin and deficiency of FXIII is associated with severe bleeding. A number of polymorphisms in the FXIII gene have been described, especially in the A subunit; there, the G → A transition in exon 2 causes a valine to leucine change at position 34, which has been most extensively investigated. *In vitro* studies have shown that FXIII containing 34Leu is activated more rapidly by thrombin, with a twofold increase in catalytic efficiency. As a result, the structure of the fibrin is altered and fibrin formed in the presence of this mutation has reduced mass–length ratio and porosity.

The FXIII Val341Leu polymorphism is significantly less common in patients with coronary heart disease than in control subjects. A protective effect of this transition for venous thromboembolism has also been demonstrated.

Selected bibliography

Baglin T (2000) Thrombophilia testing: What do we think the tests mean and what should we do with the results? *Journal of Clinical Pathology* 53: 167–70.

Bauer KA (2001) The thrombophilias: Well-defined risk factors with uncertain therapeutic implications. *Annals of Internal Medicine* 135: 367–73.

Bauer KA (2003) Management of thrombophilia. *Journal of Thrombosis and Haemostasis* 1: 1429–34.

Dahlback B, Carlsson M, Svensson PJ (1993) Familial thrombophilia due to a previously unrecognized mechanism characterized by poor anticoagulant response to activated protein C: Prediction of a cofactor to activated protein C. *Proceedings of the National Academy of Sciences of the United States of America* 90: 1004–8.

Doggen CJM, Cats VM, Bertina RM *et al.* (1998) Interaction of coagulation defects and cardiovascular risk factors: Increased risk of myocardial infarction associated with factor V Leiden or prothrombin 20210A. *Circulation* 97: 1037–41.

Ginsberg JS, Greer I, Hirsh J (2001) Use of antithrombotic agents during pregnancy. *Chest* 119: 122S–131S.

Greer IA (2000) The challenge of thrombophilia in maternal-fetal medicine. *New England Journal of Medicine* 342: 424–5.

Martinelli I, Legnani C, Bucciarelli P *et al.* (2001) Risk of pregnancy-related venous thrombosis in carriers of severe inherited thrombophilia. *Thrombosis and Haemostasis* 86: 800–3.

McColl MD, Ramsay JE, Tait RC *et al.* (1997) Risk factors for pregnancy associated venous thromboembolism. *Thrombosis and Haemostasis* 78: 1183–8.

McColl MD, Ellison J, Reid F *et al.* (2000) Prothrombin 20210 G → A, MTHFR C677T mutations in women with venous thromboembolism associated with pregnancy. *British Journal of Obstetrics and Gynaecology* 107: 565–9.

Ridker PM, Hennekens CH, Lindpaintner K *et al.* (1995) Mutation in the gene coding for coagulation factor V and the risk of myocardial infarction, stroke, and venous thrombosis in apparently healthy men. *New England Journal of Medicine* 332: 912–17.

Rosendaal FR, Siscovick DS, Schwartz SM *et al.* (1997) A common prothrombin variant (20210 G to A) increases the risk of myocardial infarction in young women. *Blood* 90: 1747–50.

Rosendaal FR, Siscovick DS, Schwartz SM *et al.* (1997) Factor V Leiden (resistance to activated protein C) increases the risk of myocardial infarction in young women. *Blood* 89: 2817–21.

Rosendaal FR, Van Hylckama Vlieg A, Tanis BC *et al.* (2003) Estrogens, progestogens and thrombosis. *Journal of Thrombosis and Haemostasis* 1: 1371–80.

Seligsohn U, Lubetsky (2001) Genetic susceptibility to venous thrombosis. *New England Journal of Medicine* 344: 1222–31.

Vandenbroucke JP, Koster T, Briet E *et al.* (1994) Increased risk of venous thrombosis in oral-contraceptive users who are carriers of factor V Leiden mutation. *Lancet* 344: 1453–7.

Vandenbroucke JP, Van der Meer FJM, Helmerhorst FM (1996) Factor V Leiden: should we screen oral contraceptive users and pregnant women? *British Medical Journal* 313: 1127–30.

Walker ID (2002) Prothrombotic genotypes and pre-eclampsia. *Thrombosis and Haemostasis* 87: 777–8.

Walker ID, Greaves M, Preston FE (2001) Investigation and management of heritable thrombophilia. *British Journal of Haematology* 114: 512–28.

CHAPTER 54

Acquired venous thrombosis

54

Beverley J Hunt and Michael Greaves

Introduction

Deep vein thrombosis is common, principally affecting the lower limbs. In many populations the annual incidence is around 1 per 1000 of the population. However, the disorder is highly age dependent. For example, it is exceptional in childhood; in young adults the incidence is of the order of 1 per 10 000 of the population each year, and it may reach 1% per year in the very elderly. The incidence of pulmonary embolism is lower, possibly around 1 per 3000 of the population annually, although subclinical pulmonary embolism occurs frequently in subjects with lower limb proximal deep vein thrombosis. In patients who die in hospital, there is evidence of pulmonary embolism in up to 20% of cases and in many it contributes to the cause of death. Clinically apparent pulmonary embolism occurs rarely when deep vein thrombosis is confined to calf veins but, if untreated, calf vein thrombosis propagates to proximal veins in around 20% of cases, with an accompanying risk of significant pulmonary embolism. In occasional cases, pulmonary embolism presents without identifiable deep vein thrombosis.

Deep vein thrombosis is important because of the associated acute morbidity and risk of fatal pulmonary embolism, and also because of the potential long-term sequelae. These are a high risk of recurrent thrombosis and of development of chronic post-phlebitic symptoms. The risk of recurrence after a first episode of apparently unprovoked proximal deep vein thrombosis of a lower limb is around 25% during the 5 years after discontinuation of oral anticoagulant therapy. However, the risk is considerably lower when the first event is precipitated by a transient risk factor, such as a surgical procedure. When the first episode affects the deep veins, the symptoms of recurrence are most commonly those of deep vein thrombosis also. Similarly, recurrence after a first episode of pulmonary embolism is typically with pulmonary symptoms.

Chronic post-phlebitic symptoms in the leg range from minor itching and swelling to intractable ulceration. Some degree of post-phlebitic syndrome is present in around 30% of sufferers of previous lower limb deep vein thrombosis. It is most frequent and severe after recurrent thrombosis and uncommon after deep vein thrombosis confined to the calf vessels.

Vessels other than the deep veins of the limbs may be affected by thrombosis, including superficial limb veins, the intracranial venous sinuses and visceral veins. The pathogenesis of superficial thrombophlebitis may differ from that of deep vein thrombosis. Thrombosis of retinal veins appears also to have a different pathogenesis and natural history.

As described in the preceding chapter, venous thromboembolic episodes result from the interaction of multiple risk factors. These may be gene–environment interactions or multiple environmental or acquired risk factors (Table 54.1). In this chapter, the acquired conditions that predispose to venous thromboembolism are considered, although in most cases it is likely that the individual genotype influences the likelihood of thrombosis in particular circumstances.

Pregnancy and venous thromboembolism

Around 1 in 1000 pregnancies is complicated by deep vein thrombosis or pulmonary embolism. Massive pulmonary embolism is the leading cause of pregnancy-related death in the UK. Although the post-partum phase has been considered to be the time of highest risk, overall at least as many episodes of venous thromboembolism (VTE) occur ante partum, including some in

Table 54.1 Causal factors in acquired venous thromboembolism.

Inevitable/environmental	Iatrogenic	Disease related
Increasing age	Post-operative/immobilization	Antiphospholipid syndrome
Pregnancy and post partum	In-dwelling venous devices	Cancer, including: myeloproliferative diseases, acute promyelocytic leukaemia
Immobility, e.g. long-haul travel	Pharmacological:	Inflammatory states
Dehydration	• Oestrogen related: combined oral contraceptive, hormone replacement therapy, tamoxifen	Other haematological disease: paroxysmal nocturnal haemoglobinuria, thrombotic thrombocytopenic purpura, sickle cell disease
	• Chemotherapy, heparin, haemostatic treatments	Intravenous drug abuse

the first trimester. There are notable clinical features in pregnancy-related deep vein thrombosis: around 90% of thromboses affect the deep veins of the left lower limb and the vast majority of cases involve the iliofemoral veins from the time of presentation; thrombosis restricted to the deep veins of the calf is uncommon in pregnancy. The left-sided predominance most likely relates to the anatomical relationship between the iliac artery and vein on that side. Many of the women develop post-phlebitic syndrome.

The pathogenesis of pregnancy-related VTE is multifactorial, as in other situations. Unique features include the raised intra-abdominal pressure and vascular compression caused by the gravid uterus, suppressed systemic fibrinolytic capacity and the progressive increase in plasma concentrations of clotting factors from around 10 weeks' gestation, including factor VIII and fibrinogen. Tissue trauma from delivery contributes to the pathogenesis of post-partum VTE and operative delivery increases the risk further.

Although the heritable thrombophilic conditions that are identifiable at present contribute to the risk of pregnancy-related VTE, in around 70% of cases no hereditary thrombophilia can be identified and in 25% there is also no obvious risk factor other than otherwise normal pregnancy.

Immobility as a risk factor for venous thromboembolism

It is likely that venous stasis is a significant pathogenetic factor in VTE. It probably contributes to post-operative thrombosis and is a factor in deep vein thrombosis in paralysed limbs and that associated with splinting, for example in a plaster cast.

There has been considerable interest in the relationship between VTE and the physically cramped conditions encountered during travel, especially long-haul aeroplane journeys. The term *economy class syndrome* has been coined to encompass the occurrence of VTE during and after air travel. Although the true level of risk has not been established, observational data indicate that the incidence of death from pulmonary embolism induced by

air travel is less than one in a million journeys. The duration of the flight is a factor, with some evidence that VTE risks begin to increase progressively with flight time of greater than 4 or 5 h. The elderly appear to be at greater risk. The contribution of the particular environmental conditions within a pressurized cabin, including hypobaric hypoxia and a dry atmosphere, to hypercoagulability is now the subject of investigation. At present it is reasonable to assume that any form of long-distance motorized travel carries a low but increased risk of VTE and to recommend simple precautionary measures such as maintenance of hydration and calf exercises and ambulation in order to maintain venous flow in the lower limbs.

Iatrogenic venous thromboembolism

Venous thromboembolism is common in hospitalized subjects, despite the widespread adoption of physical and pharmacological methods of thromboprophylaxis. As indicated above, immobility is probably a significant contributory factor. In postoperative patients, the procoagulant responses to tissue trauma, such as increased fibrinogen and factor VIII concentrations in plasma and reactive thrombocytosis, may also play a part. The highest prevalence of VTE occurs in major orthopaedic surgery to the lower limb. In hip replacement and knee replacement surgery, subclinical deep vein thrombosis is detectable by imaging in up to 50% of cases, although there is some evidence that clinically significant VTE may be becoming less common owing to improvements in surgical techniques and materials, as well as wider use of thromboprophylaxis.

Indwelling venous devices, such as Hickman catheters, are a significant cause of deep venous thrombosis, which may progress to complete occlusion of the superior vena cava, for example. Up to 60% of patients with central venous catheters (CVCs) will develop a complication secondary to the device, thrombosis being one of the most common. Thrombosis associated with a CVC may involve the catheter tip, the length of the catheter, the catheterized vessel in the upper limb, the central vasculature of the neck/mediastinum or a combination of these. A higher incidence of thrombosis is seen in catheters with a larger external diameter and those with a tip positioned distal to the superior vena cava. Other factors that predispose to a higher rate of catheter-related thrombosis include catheter infection, infusion of sclerosing chemotherapeutic agents, extrinsic vessel compression and a previous history of venous thromboembolism.

Patients with CVC-related thrombosis may present with swelling and or pain of the arm, neck or face. Some may present with symptoms suggestive of a pulmonary embolism or with catheter malfunction. Many of the symptoms are non-specific and for this reason, objective testing is needed. Contrast venography remains the reference standard for diagnosis of CVC-related thrombosis but this is invasive and may be painful. Ultrasonography is the most accurate non-invasive test with a sensitivity and specificity of 93% and 95% respectively. Treatment of central venous catheter-related thrombosis remains poorly studied. There are several treatment options available: anticoagulation alone, systemic thrombolysis, low-dose local thrombolysis and catheter removal or any combination of the above. Systemic thrombolysis may cause bleeding and should be avoided. There is some evidence that low-dose warfarin and low-molecular-weight heparin reduce the incidence of thrombosis in adults with cancer and indwelling venous catheters. Almost all episodes of VTE in neonates are provoked by indwelling vascular devices.

Iatrogenic VTE may be due to pharmaceuticals and VTE associated with use of the *combined oral contraceptive* is of particular importance because it affects healthy women in a young age group. The overall relative risk of VTE in a pill user is around four- to fivefold higher than in a non-pill user, although this is influenced greatly by the presence of some heritable thrombophilias as described in the previous chapter. The risk is also increased by obesity and older age. Fortunately, the absolute risk remains acceptable because of the low background prevalence of thrombosis in women of child-bearing age. It is around 10 to 20 episodes per 100 000 exposed woman-years. Oestrogen-containing preparations induce a state of reduced sensitivity to activated protein C, and this appears to be more marked with the third-generation contraceptives than second-generation preparations. (Most preparations in use at present contain an equivalent dose of oestrogen, usually 30–35 µg of ethinyloestradiol. However, the progestagen content varies. In so-called second-generation oral contraceptives, this is levonorgestrel, whereas in third-generation products it is desogestrel, gestodene or norgestimate.) There is convincing epidemiological evidence that the third-generation pills carry a greater risk of clinical VTE also, although this has been disputed. Progestagen-only oral contraceptives appear to carry a lower risk of VTE such that their use can be considered in women in whom the combined oral contraceptive is deemed to be contraindicated.

Hormone replacement therapy (HRT) use is also associated with VTE. In this case, the absolute risk is higher due to the greater background prevalence of VTE in older women. Observational data indicate a very high rate of VTE in women with a previous history of venous thrombosis who embark subsequently upon HRT. Such is the level of risk that HRT is contraindicated in such women. If there are overwhelming indications for HRT (usually disabling menopausal symptoms), some clinicians consider warfarin thromboprophylaxis alongside HRT in high-risk situations. Also, the procoagulant changes induced by transdermal preparations appear to be less marked, suggesting that they may be less likely to provoke VTE than oral formulations.

Use of *chemotherapeutic agents* and adjunctive therapies in malignancy has been linked to VTE. Notable examples are asparaginase in acute lymphoblastic leukaemia, thalidomide in myeloma and tamoxifen in breast cancer. Tamoxifen blocks oestrogen receptors but has weak oestrogenic activity and this may underlie the association with VTE. Asparaginase inhibits protein synthesis and markedly reduced plasma concentrations of antithrombin may be one mechanism of the prothrombotic state associated with its use. The pathogenesis of thrombosis associated with thalidomide has not been elucidated. It appears to be associated particularly with use of the agent in myeloma, rather than other indications.

Heparin-induced thrombocytopenia is an important diagnosis because failure to recognize the syndrome carries a high risk of death from associated venous or arterial thrombosis. It is due to development of antibodies to a complex of heparin and platelet factor 4, which induce intravascular platelet activation and consumption. Typically, the platelet count begins to fall between 5 and 10 days after first exposure to heparin. In subjects with recent exposure, it may occur earlier and, very occasionally, the thrombocytopenia develops after heparin has been discontinued. The condition may complicate heparin administered at any dose, including that used as peri-operative thromboprophylaxis and even when very low doses are used to maintain the patency of intravascular cannulae. Heparin-induced thrombocytopenia is around 10-fold less common with low-molecular-weight preparations than with unfractionated heparin, and has not been reported with the synthetic pentasaccharide, fondaparinux. In contrast with other drug-related immune thrombocytopenias, the degree of thrombocytopenia is rarely severe and bleeding is not a feature. There may be systemic symptoms including fever and a local reaction at the heparin injection site, such as erythema or even skin necrosis after subcutaneous administration. Because of the platelet activation there is often new thrombosis, and this may manifest before the platelet count reaches thrombocytopenic levels.

When heparin has been administered to treat arterial disease, the new thrombosis is most commonly arterial, and in treatment of deep vein thrombosis there is usually extension of the presenting thrombus, often with pulmonary embolism. Thrombotic stroke, myocardial infarction, visceral ischaemia and disseminated intravascular coagulation have all been reported.

Confirmatory laboratory tests are not entirely satisfactory. Immunoassays for heparin/platelet factor 4 are sensitive but lack specificity because a significant proportion of subjects treated with heparin have positive antibody tests but neither thrombocytopenia nor thrombosis. In contrast, bioassays that rely on activation of normal platelets in the presence of test plasma and a low concentration of heparin are specific, but high sensitivity is difficult to achieve. Sensitivity is improved by use of platelet serotonin secretion as an end-point and employment of donor platelets of proven sensitivity. Specificity is achieved by the demonstration of a positive result with a low heparin concentration, which is absent in the presence of a high concentration. Because of the limitations of these confirmatory tests monitoring of the platelet count and a high index of clinical suspicion are essential whenever heparin is administered.

When there is a noteworthy fall in the platelet count that cannot be accounted for in any other way then heparin, in all forms, must be discontinued. An alternative anticoagulant must be administered immediately as the risk of thrombosis persists for several days after heparin withdrawal. Warfarin given alone is contraindicated as massive thrombosis has been described in this situation, most likely due to the rapid fall in protein C caused by warfarin against a background severe prothrombotic state. Aspirin is insufficient. The antibody may cross-react with low-molecular-weight heparins and they should be avoided. Danaparoid is a mix of anticoagulant glycosaminoglycans, predominantly heparan sulphate and dextran sulphate. There is a significant risk of cross reactivity with the HIT antibody *in vivo*, which may not be predicted by *in vitro* testing, and for this reason its use is no longer recommended.

The anticoagulant of choice is lepirudin, and warfarin can be introduced once an adequate anticoagulant effect with the thrombin inhibitor has been established. The pathogenetic antibodies tend to become immeasurable in the ensuing few months but further exposure to heparin after this time should be avoided if possible.

Haemostatic treatments may induce thrombosis, most notably prothrombin complex concentrates. They should not be used to reverse the coagulopathy in severe liver impairment as major thrombosis has been reported, with disseminated intravascular coagulation and death in some cases. This is probably due to impaired clearance of activated clotting factors in liver failure.

Antiphospholipid syndrome

Antiphospholipid syndrome (APS) is an important thrombophilic condition because it is of high prevalence and is associated with considerable morbidity and mortality.

The essential features are arterial or venous thrombosis or recurrent pregnancy loss or placental dysfunction occurring in a subject in whom laboratory tests for antiphospholipid antibody (aPL) are positive. Diagnostic criteria have been established (Table 54.2) in order to standardize diagnosis for the purpose of clinical studies.

Limb deep vein thrombosis, pulmonary embolism and ischaemic stroke are the principal thrombotic manifestations, but any vessel may be involved. A characteristic of antiphospholipid syndrome in an individual patient is the tendency to cause recurrent problems in the same vascular bed. APS is not always a 'full house' syndrome, in that women can have severe thrombotic events without pregnancy complications and those with pregnancy complications most commonly have no other manifestation. In addition to thrombosis and pregnancy failure, additional clinical and laboratory features are variably present in APS. These include mild thrombocytopenia and an unusual

Table 54.2 Diagnostic criteria in antiphospholipid syndrome.

Clinical criteria*	Laboratory criteria*

Thrombosis
Arterial, venous or microvascular
  thrombosis in any tissue or organ
	IgG and/or IgM aCL antibodies at moderate
	  or high concentration[†]
	Lupus anticoagulant

Pregnancy complications Unexplained death of morphologically normal fetus at or beyond 10 weeks' gestation Three or more unexplained consecutive miscarriages before 10 weeks One or more premature births of a morphologically normal fetus before 34 weeks' gestation due to pre-eclampsia, eclampsia or severe placental insufficiency	

*There must be at least one clinical and at least one laboratory criterion present. The laboratory test must be consistently positive on at least two occasions 6 weeks apart, as transient antibodies may occur, for example in infection. Such antibodies are not usually associated with clinical events.
[†]There is no consensus on the definition of moderate/high concentration. In general, values of IgG aCL of > 30 or 40 GPL units are considered to be moderate-titre antibodies. The significance of low-titre antibodies is less clear.

dermatological feature – livedo reticularis. Cardiac valvular abnormalities occur in up to 30% of patients. Usually the mitral or aortic valves are affected and have mild thickening or incompetence. However, haemodynamic changes as a consequence of valvular damage are rare. Exceptionally, the syndrome may manifest as widespread microvascular occlusion, with multiorgan failure, so-called 'catastrophic APS'.

APS may occur with another chronic systemic autoimmune disease, usually systemic lupus erythematosus (SLE), when the term *secondary antiphospholipid syndrome* is used. In primary APS, there is no evidence for another relevant underlying condition.

Antiphospholipid antibodies

Antiphospholipid antibodies (aPLs) are a family of antibodies reactive with proteins, which are themselves complexed with negatively charged phospholipid. For example, many aPLs require β_2-glycoprotein I (β_2-GPI), a phospholipid-binding plasma protein with weak anticoagulant activity, for binding to acidic phospholipids such as phosphatidyl serine and cardiolipin. The relationships between β_2-GPI, phospholipid and autoantibody are disputed. One possibility is that cryptic epitopes are exposed on β_2-GPI when it binds to phospholipid (Figure 54.1a). It is more probable that binding to phospholipid allows the clustering of antigenic sites and facilitates bivalent antibody interaction of what are essentially low-affinity antibodies (Figure 54.1b). The plastic of an enzyme-linked immunosorbent assay (ELISA) plate can substitute for negatively charged phospholipid in this reaction and this has allowed the development of new, possibly more specific assays for aPL, which employ purified β_2-GPI. Other proteins share this property of binding to phospholipid in a manner that promotes interaction with aPL. These include the coagulation factor prothrombin, the anticoagulant protein C and its cofactor protein S, and annexin V (previously known as placental anticoagulant protein).

The lupus anticoagulant (LA) is an *in vitro* phenomenon in which the antiphospholipid antibody slows down clot formation, thereby lengthening the clotting time. This is probably due to impairment of the assembly of the components of prothrombinase on phospholipid caused by interference by the antibody (Figure 54.1c).

LA is due to antibodies reactive to β_2-GPI phospholipid or to prothrombin/phospholipid. The β_2-GPI-dependent antibodies also bind in anticardiolipin (aCL) assays, as the glycoprotein is present in test serum and often in assay reagents. LA due to prothrombin-reactive antibodies may be negative in aCL assays. Therefore, some subjects with APS have LA and aCL and some LA only. Others have aCL without LA, due to the presence of non-β2 GPI and non-prothrombin-dependent antibody or possibly to relative insensitivity of the coagulation assays for LA. Because aPLs are so heterogeneous, a comprehensive laboratory approach is essential for their reliable detection. In most

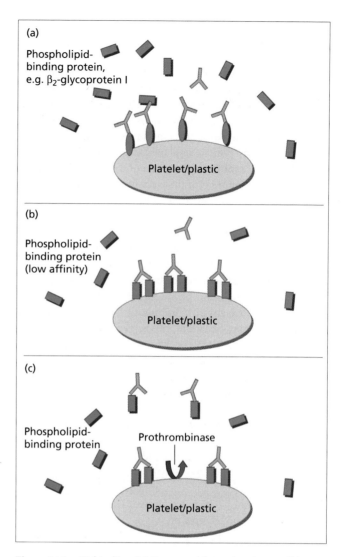

Figure 54.1 aPL binding. (a) Exposure of cryptic epitopes; (b) antigen clustering and bivalent binding; (c) explanation for the LA phenomenon.

laboratories, ELISAs employing cardiolipin and coagulation-based assays for LA remain the principal diagnostic tools. β_2-GPI ELISA may offer improved specificity but the practical value of this assay has not yet been established and it is not included in the standardized diagnostic criteria. The pathogenicity of immunoglobulin A (IgA) aCL antibodies is disputed and, again, their detection is not utilized in diagnosis.

Pathogenetic mechanisms in antiphospholipid syndrome

The pathogenesis of pregnancy failure and thrombosis in APS is not fully understood. Whether antibodies to β_2-GPI/phospholipid are causal is unproven. It is unlikely that a single mechanism accounts for the multiple clinical manifestations.

Important candidate mechanisms for thrombosis are antibody-induced concentration of prothrombin on phospholipid surface *in vivo* resulting in enhanced thrombin generation, interference with the activated protein C anticoagulant pathway and increased monocyte and endothelial tissue factor expression. Increased platelet activation and inhibition of fibrinolysis by aPLs have also been proposed. Also, antibodies reactive with cellular antigens, including some on platelets and vascular endothelial cells, frequently co-exist with antiphospholipid antibodies. Endothelial antibodies activate endothelial cells *in vitro*. It is also possible that, in some situations, antiphospholipid antibodies may represent an epiphenomenon in thrombotic disease due to another pathological process.

Whether aPLs have a pathogenetic role in pregnancy failure is unproven, although some animal studies support this view. Placental dysfunction is the hallmark of second- and third-trimester complications of intrauterine fetal death, intrauterine growth restriction, pre-eclampsia and placental abruption. The aetiology of the placental dysfunction has been related to placental infarction and an acute atherosis in the maternal spiral arteries; however, these are not universal features. One interesting hypothesis for the cause of placental insufficiency is displacement of annexin V from trophoblast by aPLs, with resultant acceleration of thrombin generation on the exposed negatively charged phospholipid. First-trimester loss has been related to *in vitro* inhibition of trophoblast proliferation by antiphospholipid antibodies.

Laboratory diagnosis of antiphospholipid antibodies

In the diagnosis of APS it is essential to consider that aPLs are not specific to APS. In addition to transient antibodies which may, for example, be triggered by intercurrent infection some chronic infections are associated with aPLs, such as syphilis and hepatitis C. aPLs may also be detected incidentally in healthy subjects and they occur in relation to use of some drugs, particularly chlorpromazine. These drug-induced and infection-related antibodies do not appear usually to be associated with the clinical thrombotic manifestations of APS. In some cases they appear to be neither β_2-GPI nor prothrombin dependent.

The diagnosis of APS relies on the demonstration of the presence of either LA by coagulation tests, or aPL by solid-phase immunoassays. The latter typically employ cardiolipin as antigen (aCL assays). Reliance on just one type of assay may lead to false-negative aPL assessments.

Coagulation assays (lupus anticoagulant tests)
The LA assay is a double misnomer for it is neither a test for lupus nor an *in vivo* anticoagulant. LA tests are indirect assays that rely upon the slowing of the clotting time of plasma through interaction of the autoantibody with phospholipid. The tests most frequently employed in LA testing are the activated partial thromboplastin time (APTT), the dilute Russell's viper venom time (DRVVT) and the kaolin clotting time (KCT).

Platelet activation causes exposure of negatively charged phospholipid at the cell surface and therefore contamination of test plasma with platelets must be minimized, as these will limit the sensitivity of tests, particularly when plasma must be stored frozen prior to testing. Platelet depletion may be achieved in various ways, most commonly by careful double centrifugation.

None of the above coagulation assays is specific for LA. Specificity and sensitivity are reagent dependent also. For example, some partial thromboplastin reagents are insensitive to LA. If the same reagent is employed in LA testing as in the routine laboratory screening APTT sensitivity to LA must be assured. Factors that lengthen or shorten clotting times (other than aPL) potentially interfere in LA tests. Examples are anticoagulant drugs and clotting factor deficiencies and inhibitors, which lengthen clotting times and increased clotting factor levels, especially factor VIII, which shortens the time to clotting in some assays, potentially masking the presence of LA.

To reduce the risks of false interpretation, in addition to prolongation of clotting time in a phospholipid-dependent coagulation test, the criteria for LA positivity also include:
- evidence of an inhibitor demonstrated by mixing studies;
- confirmation of the phospholipid-dependent nature of the inhibitor.

In principle, the laboratory tests should employ a detection or screening stage (prolongation of the clotting time) and a confirmation stage (failure of correction of the prolongation when normal plasma is added, to exclude factor deficiency as the cause of the prolongation, and demonstration that the prolongation is phospholipid dependent, for example by showing that addition of excess phospholipid corrects the clotting time). To achieve this, and because no LA test consistently shows 100% specificity and sensitivity, more than one test system should be used for detection of LA. The prothrombin time and thrombin time should be performed also as they are not usually affected by the presence of LA and the results assist in the interpretation of LA tests, for example when there is undisclosed anticoagulant therapy.

The APTT is employed commonly as the initial screening test for LA. Its specificity for inhibitor detection is improved by inclusion of a mixing study with platelet-free normal pooled plasma. When prolongation of the APTT is due to coagulation factor deficiency, the clotting time corrects when the test is repeated on an equal mixture of patient and normal plasma, whereas the prolongation above normal may persist with LA, consistent with its inhibitory activity. Correction in a mixing study does not exclude LA however as a weak antibody is of course diluted out by addition of normal plasma and this may be sufficient to abolish its effect. Very occasionally LA causes enhancement of the prolongation of the APPT when normal plasma is added. This phenomenon has been called the *lupus cofactor effect* but is the exception rather than the rule. Inhibitors to clotting factors, usually factor VIII, are associated with bleeding rather than thrombosis, but also cause prolongation of the clotting times, which may not be corrected by addition of normal plasma. Factor VIII inhibitors are time dependent, typically and unlike LA. A normal APTT is insufficient to exclude LA and additional tests must be performed.

The DRVVT involves neither the clotting factors of the intrinsic system, unlike the APTT, nor factor VII, unlike the prothrombin time. Any inhibition of the coagulant active phospholipid in the test by LA results in a prolonged DRVVT. However, as is the case with all LA tests, it is not specific. Deficiencies of clotting factors, for example factors II and X due to warfarin therapy, will also prolong the DRVVT. The specificity of the test is improved by repeating it in the presence of a high concentration of phospholipid, which should result in partial or complete correction of the prolonged clotting time if it is due to LA. This phospholipid is conveniently provided as platelet membranes in which negatively charged phospholipid is exposed by freezing and thawing. In the presence of LA, the ratio of test–normal plasma clotting time is often > 1.2, and corrects to < 1.2, or at least partially, in the platelet neutralization procedure. As with all coagulation tests, because of variations in reagents and techniques, it is essential that laboratories derive local normal ranges using a large number of plasma samples from healthy volunteers.

In the KCT, no additional phospholipid is employed. The test therefore resembles the APTT in that it involves the intrinsic and common pathways of coagulation but the sensitivity to LA is enhanced because the small amount of phospholipid present is only that derived from residual platelets in the test sample and plasma lipids. The test is affected by clotting factor deficiencies and anticoagulants, but specificity can be improved by use of normal plasma mixing at more than one ratio to test plasma. LA is identified when the KCT fails to correct even after relatively large proportions of normal plasma are added, whereas in factor deficiency the KCT is corrected with small amounts of normal plasma.

Alternative tests for LA may be employed but are not in general use. They include the tissue thromboplastin inhibition test and clotting tests which use venoms other than Russell's viper venom; examples are Taipan and Textarin venoms.

Solid-phase assays (for anticardiolipin and β_2-GPI antibodies)

Solid-phase assays for aPL, such as the aCL ELISA allow rapid processing of numerous serum samples and the results are not affected by factor deficiency or the use of anticoagulants. The introduction of international standards allows the calculation of aCL results in IgG or IgM antiphospholipid units (GPLU and MPLU respectively) related to a given concentration of affinity-purified aCL immunoglobulin. Despite this, there remains a lack of precision, and comparability between laboratories using different assays is not ensured.

The detection of aCL allows the diagnosis of APS in a subject with an appropriate clinical history, even when LA is absent. However, the aCL assay is neither a substitute for the LA test, nor does it confirm that LA is present, as different antibodies may be responsible for the two activities. Furthermore, the clinical significance of low-titre aCL is doubtful. Thus, in cases where the aCL titre is less than 20 GPL units and tests for LA are negative, a diagnosis of APS may not be conclusive. Under these circumstances, it is particularly important to consider other causes of thrombosis or miscarriage.

Specific assays for β_2-GPI antibodies have been developed and several commercial kits are available. β_2-GPI antibody assays may show higher precision and better correlation with the thromboembolic complications in APS and SLE than assays for aCL, and are less likely to show transient positive results in association with infection. Antiprothrombin antibodies generally exhibit poor specificity for venous thrombosis and recurrent fetal loss, and may be found in patients with infection. Neither assay is included in the diagnostic criteria for APS at present.

The prevalence of aPL in subjects with thrombosis varies with selection criteria for testing. Because the risk of recurrent thrombosis appears to be great, aPL should be sought in subjects with arterial, venous or microvascular thrombosis where no other cause is apparent. Examples are younger subjects with ischaemic stroke in the absence of cardiovascular disease and subjects with unprovoked venous thromboembolism.

The prevalence of persistent aPL among women with recurrent miscarriage is around 15%. In women with recurrent miscarriage due to APS the prospective fetal loss rate may be as high as 90%. In contrast, the prevalence of positive tests for aPL in unselected women of child-bearing age is around 3% and they are not sensitive predictors of poor pregnancy outcome in women with no history of pregnancy complications. Because miscarriage is a common phenomenon, screening for aPL is not indicated after a single event. Maternal aPL may be downregulated during pregnancy; tests are best performed preconceptually when possible. A small proportion of women with aPL also have anti-Ro antibodies. Their detection is important as it is associated with a 2% risk of complete heart block in the fetus and a 5% chance of neonatal lupus.

Management of antiphospholipid syndrome

Thrombosis

There is a wide variability in severity of prothrombotic states between individuals with APS. Epidemiological studies suggest that LA and high-titre aCL antibodies are associated with a greater risk of thrombosis than moderate or low-titre aCL alone, but these studies are difficult to extrapolate to individual patients.

The management of patients with antiphospholipid antibodies and previous thrombosis remains contentious. Retrospective observational studies suggest that these patients should remain on indefinite oral anticoagulation maintaining an international normalized ratio (INR) of 3–4. However a recent prospective randomized study indicates that a lower target INR of 2–3 is effective in preventing recurrent thrombosis in the majority of patients with previous venous thrombosis. There is less certainty in arterial thrombosis, for example there is a significant subpopulation of APS patients with small vessel cerebral thromboses, some evident as lacunar infarcts on magnetic resonance imaging, who appear to require a target INR of 3–4 to prevent recurrent cerebral thrombosis.

Immunosuppressive therapy is not generally indicated in primary APS. An exception may be catastrophic APS when combination treatment with antithrombotics, corticosteroids and other immunomodulatory therapies is administered as a potentially life-saving emergency measure.

Pregnancy

The management of recurrent fetal loss is based on the use of anticoagulation with empirical doses of heparin, usually low-molecular-weight heparin in the UK, in combination with low-dose aspirin. Initial studies indicated that this approach increases the chances of a successful outcome of a healthy live birth from 30% to 70–80%, although this has been challenged recently. Heparin use carries a small risk of osteoporosis and increased bleeding and is inconvenient. Some clinicians believe that combination antithrombotic therapy as a first line should be reserved for women with a previous history of fetal death, and those with recurrent miscarriage should be given supportive care as a first line and aspirin or aspirin/heparin should be reserved for those with further pregnancy failure. Intravenous immunoglobulin therapy has not been formally assessed for this clinical indication. Corticosteroids are associated with frequent maternal morbidity from hypertension, glucose intolerance and premature labour and should not be used.

Thromboprophylaxis for those with a previous history of thrombosis is based again on use of low-molecular-weight heparin, although there is neither consensus on dosing nor the need to monitor therapy.

Venous thromboembolism and cancer

Cancer is a major risk factor for venous thromboembolism. Venous thromboembolism is the major cause of morbidity and mortality after the cancer itself in patients with malignancy. It is estimated that almost 15% of cancer patients will have a thromboembolic event. Post-mortem studies have shown that thromboembolism is common in patients who died of cancer. Of all oncology patients, palliative care inpatients have the highest risk of venous thromboembolism, with a deep vein thrombosis prevalence as high as 52%, with 33% of these having bilateral deep vein thromboses. Cancer patients have a high risk of venous thromboembolism after surgery and some forms of chemotherapy may also increase that risk, the most recently

Table 54.3 Risk factors for thrombosis in cancer patients.

Stasis
Immobility
Extrinsic pressure, e.g. oedematous limbs

Vessel wall/endothelial perturbation
Cytokine release from tumours
Local tumour infiltration
Central venous catheter

Hypercoagulability
Dehydration
Cytokine-related prothrombotic changes
Tissue factor/cancer procoagulant expression on tumour cells
Disseminated intravascular coagulation
Increased platelet activation

described being thalidomide. The risk of thrombosis varies with the type of cancer, with ovarian, brain and pancreatic cancers having the highest rates. Lymphomas and leukaemia account for a significant proportion of thromboses as do colonic and lung cancers.

Venous thromboembolism is a common complication of advanced malignancy and this has been recognized since Trousseau's original descriptions of migratory thrombophlebitis associated with adenocarcinoma in 1865. In Trousseau's syndrome, unlike the more common, lower limb solitary, deep vein thromboses, the phlebitis is recurrent and migratory, and it affects both the superficial and deep vein systems. Unusual sites such as arms, neck, as well as superficial veins of the thorax and abdomen may be involved. Typically such a patient has an occult tumour, usually adenocarcinoma, although up to 10% may have an acute leukaemia. In Trousseau's syndrome, conventional anticoagulation often fails to prevent recurrent thromboses.

Prothrombotic changes associated with malignancies

In Table 54.3 the components of Virchow's triad are used to illustrate the features that lead to oncology patients having such a high risk of thrombosis. There are specific abnormalities that are unique to cancer patients: these are tumour procoagulants. Tumour procoagulants are surface molecules on cancer cells that activate coagulation. The two principal tumour cell procoagulants are tissue factor and cancer procoagulant. The latter directly activates factor X in the absence of factor VII. The increasing number of tumour procoagulants that have been described are listed on the International Society for Thrombosis and Haemostasis registry. The APS has been reported in malignancy also, particularly in association with myeloma and immunosecretory disorders.

Difficulties in management

Cancer patients with thrombosis are at particularly high risk of recurrent thrombotic events. Cohort and population-based studies have shown that the risk of recurrence after stopping anticoagulation in patients with cancer is approximately double that of non-cancer patients. Treatment with anticoagulation in cancer patients is often unsuccessful, due to the high risk of recurrent venous thromboembolism and major bleeding. Unfortunately, these risks are associated with oral anticoagulation intensities within the usual therapeutic range. The risks are greatest during the first few weeks of anticoagulation treatment and increase with cancer extent. Several studies have demonstrated significant increases in rates of bleeding, as high as 20% amongst cancer patients receiving oral anticoagulation. Within the palliative care setting, in patients with far more advanced disease, the bleeding incidence was higher, even with strict monitoring of anticoagulation. Oral anticoagulation in cancer patients is complicated further due to anorexia, vomiting, liver disease and drug interactions. Moreover, there may be frequent interruption to treatment due to thrombocytopenia and the need for invasive procedures, and venous access is often difficult in these patients, especially if they have had previous chemotherapy through peripheral veins.

The decision to use oral anticoagulation in this group of patients should not be undertaken lightly and safe treatment requires intensive monitoring of the INR and the burden of repeated blood tests. Disillusionment with the use of oral anticoagulation in cancer patients has led to trials assessing low-molecular-weight heparins. The CLOT trial randomized over 650 cancer patients with symptomatic proximal deep vein thromboses and/or pulmonary embolism to treatment doses of dalteparin for 5–7 days and then randomization to either oral anticoagulation maintaining a target INR of 2.5 or dalteparin. In the dalteparin arm, full-treatment dose was given for 1 month and then reduced to 75–80% of this dose. After 6 months there was a significantly reduced rate of recurrent VTE in the dalteparin group of 8.8% compared with 17.4% rate with oral anticoagulation. Bleeding was also significantly reduced. A similar reduction in VTE was found in patients with cancer who entered the LITE study, in which treatment-dose tinzaparin was compared with oral anticoagulation after VTE.

Thrombotic risk in polycythaemia rubra vera and essential (primary) thrombocythaemia

Polycythaemia vera (PV) patients, if left untreated, have a median survival of 18 months, with the majority dying of vascular occlusion. The occlusive lesions may involve the larger vessels or the microvasculature. In PV, large vessel events involve arteries and veins equally, whereas in essential thrombocythaemia (ET) arteries are more commonly involved. A high proportion of thromboses occur in the cerebral circulation, although widely distributed arterial and venous system and splanchnic vessel thromboses have been well documented. Hepatic vein and portal vein thromboses are more commonly associated with PV than ET. Indeed it has been reported that some patients with apparently idiopathic hepatic or portal vein thrombosis have subclinical myeloproliferative disease based on the finding of erythropoietin-independent erythroid colony growth in marrow culture. In PV, there is good evidence that the incidence of vascular occlusion is positively related to the packed cell volume level, with the lowest incidence in patients with good control of haematocrit. The role of thrombocytosis in risk of thrombosis in PV is disputed. The risk of thrombosis in PV also increases with advancing age and a past history of thrombosis.

ET is often diagnosed in the subclinical phase but a number of studies suggest that overall survival is determined principally by occurrence of thrombosis. In a study of 100 patients by Cortelazzo and colleagues a rate of thrombosis of 1.7% per patient-year was found in those aged less than 40 years, 6.3% per patient-year in those aged 40–60 years, and 15.1% in those aged greater than 60 years.

The pathogenesis of thrombosis in essential thrombocythaemia is poorly understood. Elevated platelet counts are implicated, with platelet counts greater than 600×10^9/L being associated with increased incidence of vascular occlusion. Although treatment to reduce abnormal counts will reduce the frequency of events, a proportion will still experience thrombosis. In addition, some patients with essential thrombocythaemia will remain thrombosis-free with no treatment to reduce their platelet count. As a consequence, thrombosis risk-adjusted treatment strategies have evolved.

The microvascular events and vasomotor manifestations of both PV and ET almost certainly relate to quantitative and qualitative changes in platelets, as they are not seen in other forms of polycythaemia or thrombocytosis. It is possible that similar small vessel occlusive and vasomotor changes seen in the feet and hands may also occur in other parts of the body. Erythromelalgia, a syndrome consisting of painful, burning red extremities with normal peripheral pulses is the characteristic vasomotor disturbance. Physical findings may be absent or there may be warmth, duskiness and mottled erythema of the involved areas. Livedo reticularis is occasionally found. In the digital vessels, usually of the toes, but occasionally the fingers, the development of thrombosis can lead to digital ischaemia and gangrene. In relation to the cerebral circulation, a range of symptoms and signs involving transient cerebral ischaemia, transient monocular blindness, migraine, headaches and seizures are seen. Both the cerebrovascular complications and erythromelalgia of myeloproliferative disease may respond promptly to low-dose aspirin and/or platelet cytoreduction.

Conventional risk factors for cardiovascular disease are implicated in the pathogenesis of thrombosis in ET, including hypertension, smoking, hypercholesterolaemia and diabetes. The presence of monoclonal haemopoiesis may be a significant risk factor and a significant number of individuals with ET have been found to have antiphospholipid antibodies.

Acute promyelocytic leukaemia

In comparison with the severe haemorrhages present in the majority of cases of acute promyelocytic leukaemia (APL), acute arterial thrombosis is a rare presenting feature. Thrombosis is associated with the microgranular variant of APL, which accounts for 25% of all cases, characterized by a paucity of myeloid granules and a lobulated monocytoid nucleus. The cells stain positive with Sudan black and myeloperoxidase, and there is a high incidence of CD34+. Vascular occlusion is more common when a high white cell count ($> 150 \times 10^9/L$) predisposes to leucostasis. It is thought that the leukaemic cells release procoagulants, causing a disseminated intravascular coagulation. It is important to recognize this variant of APL, as the use of all-*trans*-retinoic acid (ATRA) may increase the risk of thrombosis owing to a further increase in peripheral white cell count exacerbating leucostasis.

Inflammation and thrombosis

Systemic inflammation is a potent prothrombotic stimulus. Also, some physiological anticoagulants also have an anti-inflammatory effect.

Inflammatory mechanisms upregulate procoagulant factors, downregulate physiological anticoagulants, inhibit fibrinolytic activity and increase platelet reactivity (Table 54.4). Inflammatory mediators promote coagulation by causing endothelial cell activation and thus increasing expression of tissue factor. Endotoxin, tumour necrosis factor and interferon-1α induce tissue factor expression primarily on monocytes/macrophages, and probably in atherosclerotic plaques as well. Thrombin, although a key element in coagulation, also has cytokine-like

Table 54.4 Effects of inflammation of haemostasis.

Increased
Tissue factor expression
Surface procoagulant activity, negatively charged phospholipid
Platelet reactivity
Increased levels of fibrinogen and other coagulation proteins

Decreased
Thrombomodulin expression
Endothelial cell protein C receptor
Half-life of activated protein C
Protein Z
Fibrinolytic activity due to increased PAI-1
Endothelial glycosaminoglycans

activities, as it augments leucocyte adhesion and can activate endothelium, leucocytes and platelets. Activation of these cells by thrombin increases the expression of negatively charged phospholipids such as phosphatidylserine on the surface of the cells to promote surface procoagulant activity.

Interleukin 6 and its family of molecules mediate the acute-phase response. This increases liver synthesis of plasma proteins including fibrinogen and other coagulation proteins, thus priming the blood coagulation system for action. Interleukin 6 also increases platelet reactivity. Plasma levels of the recently discovered vitamin K-dependent anticoagulant protein Z, which acts by inhibiting factor Xa, fall during inflammation, thus protein Z appears to be a negative acute-phase protein.

Of all the physiological anticoagulant pathways, the protein C pathway appears to be the most influenced by inflammation. Thrombomodulin and the endothelial cell protein C receptor (EPCR) are both downregulated by inflammatory cytokines such as tumour necrosis factor alpha (TNF-α). There is both inhibition of the promoter and of the thrombomodulin gene as well as active pinocytosis to remove existing surface molecules, whereas neutrophil elastase readily cleaves thrombomodulin from the endothelial cell surface. Moreover, thrombomodulin is very sensitive to oxidation of an exposed methionine by oxidants produced by leucocytes. These observations have led to studies demonstrating apparent therapeutic value of activated protein C in subjects with multiorgan failure due to severe sepsis.

Endothelial cell activation occurs in inflammation. This causes downregulation of fibrinolytic activation by increased production of plasminogen activator inhibitor-1. There may also be cleavage of the glycosaminoglycans from the surface of the endothelium, so that there is loss of heparan sulphate and other molecules that activate antithrombin.

As a consequence of these changes, conditions that provoke an inflammatory response are associated with increased risk of venous thrombosis. Such chronic states include inflammatory bowel disease, Behcet's disease, systemic tuberculosis, SLE and diabetes. Atherosclerosis can be considered a chronic inflammatory state and has been associated recently with an increased incidence of venous thrombosis. The association between inflammation and thrombosis emphasizes the need for thromboprophylaxis in such patients when they are immobilized in hospital.

Haematological prothrombotic states

Paroxysmal nocturnal haemoglobinuria
(see Chapter 11)

Venous thrombosis occurs in up to 40% of patients with paroxysmal nocturnal haemoglobinuria (PNH) and represents a significant cause of morbidity and mortality. Thrombosis most commonly occurs in the hepatic veins, the portal veins and sagittal sinus. Hepatic vein thrombosis leading to the Budd–Chiari syndrome is the commonest site and affects 15–25% of patients with PNH. Presentation is with pain in the right upper quadrant, jaundice and abdominal distension due to hepatomegaly and ascites. Thrombosis in the abdominal veins results in persistent abdominal pain, and symptoms and signs of intestinal obstruction may occur if infarction of the bowels ensues. Thrombosis of the splenic vein leads to splenomegaly and, occasionally, splenic rupture can occur. Portal vein thrombosis produces ascites and the later development of oesophageal varices.

Sagittal sinus thrombosis is the most frequent neurological complication. Symptoms include severe headache. There may be focal or non-focal neurological signs.

Occasional painful, discoloured skin lesions occur when the dermal veins are affected. These lesions rarely ulcerate. Occasionally, skin lesions can resemble purpura fulminans; these can affect large areas of skin, with necrosis and demarcation.

Pregnancy in PNH is associated with an increased risk of fetal loss (40%) from thrombosis and haemorrhage.

The pathogenesis of thrombosis in PNH remains uncertain. Platelets are capable of compensating for the decreased expression of decay accelerating factor (CD55) due to the presence of factor H, a similar protein that is present within alpha granules. In PNH there is also a deficiency of membrane inhibitor of reactive lysis (MIRL: CD59). In the absence of CD59, platelet lysis is minimized by the release from the cell surface of excess membrane attack complex by exovesiculation. The externalized phospholipid serine on the microvesicles released into the circulation acts as the binding site for prothrombinase complexes. It is likely that the release of procoagulant microvesicles contributes to the increased risk of venous thrombosis. Increased platelet activation and an increased sensitivity to aggregation by thrombin have also been described. Fibrinolysis is also affected in PNH. Urokinase-type plasminogen activator receptor is also a GPI-bound protein that is absent from PNH cells. It binds urokinase to the cell surface and converts plasminogen to plasmin.

Thrombotic thrombocytopenic purpura
(see Chapter 52)

Sickle cell disease
In sickle cell disease, the pathophysiology involves microvascular and macrovascular occlusion with sickled cells. There is also considerable clinical and post-mortem evidence of cerebral, pulmonary and placental thrombosis, suggesting a prothrombotic tendency in these patients. Additional evidence for a prothrombotic state is enhanced thrombin generation as shown by increased levels of prothrombin fragment 1 + 2 and thrombin–antithrombin in patients with sickle cell disease in their steady state when compared with age-matched control subjects.

There is also evidence that sickled erythrocytes adhere more readily to vascular endothelium and strongly accelerate coagulation due to abnormal exteriorization of procoagulant anionic membrane phospholipids. Comparison of the coagulation and fibrinolytic pathways in sickle cell patients with ethnically matched control subjects has shown increased levels of von Willebrand factor during sickling, but it is not clear whether this is specific or part of the acute-phase reaction. Low levels of protein C, protein S, and heparin cofactor II are well described. The aetiology of the reduction of these physiological anticoagulants is unclear. It may relate to impaired liver function from repeated hepatic sickling, whereas increased consumption has also been proposed as a cause. Low heparin cofactor II levels are also found in other chronic haemolytic anaemias such as thalassaemia intermedia, suggesting chronic haemolysis may also lead to increased consumption of this protein. Nephrotic syndrome, often found in association with sickle nephropathy, leads to low antithrombin levels and a prothrombotic state.

Selected bibliography

Awisati G, Lo Coco F, Mandelli F (2001) Acute promyelocytic leukaemia: clinical and morphological features and prognostic factors. *Seminars in Haematology* **38**: 4–12.

Chievitz E, Thiede T (1962) Complications and causes of death in polycythaemia. *Acta Medica Scandinavica* **172**: 513–23.

Cortelazzo S, Finazzi G, Ruggeri M *et al.* (1995) Hydroxyurea for patients with essential thrombocythaemia and a high risk of thrombosis. *New England Journal of Medicine* **332**: 1132–6.

Esmon CT (2003) Inflammation and thrombosis. *Journal of Thrombosis* and *Haemostasis* **1**: 1343–8.

Farquharson R, Quenby S, Greaves M (2002) Antiphospholipid syndrome in pregnancy: a controlled treatment trial. *Obstetrics and Gynecology* **100**: 408–11.

Gralnick HR, Vail M, McKeown LP *et al.* (1995) Activated platelets in paroxysmal nocturnal haemoglobinurua. *British Journal of Haematology* **91**: 697–702.

Greaves M (1999) Antiphospholipid antibodies and thrombosis. *Lancet* **353**: 1348–53.

Greaves M, Machin SJ, Cohen H *et al.* (2000) Guidelines on the investigation and management of the antiphospholipid syndrome. *British Journal of Haematology* **109**: 704–15.

Harrison CN (2002) Current trends in essential thrombocythaemia. *British Journal of Haematology* **117**: 796–808.

Hugel B, Socie G, Vu T *et al.* (1999) Elevated levels of circulating procoagulant microparticles in patients with paroxysmal nocturnal haemoglobinuria and aplastic anaemia. *Blood* **93**: 3451–6.

Journeycake JM, Buchanan GR (2003) Thrombotic complications of central venous catheters in children. *Current Opinion in Hematology* **10**: 369–74.

Lee AYY, Levine MN, Baker RI *et al.* (2003) Low-molecular-weight heparin versus a coumarin for the prevention of recurrent venous thromboembolism in patients with cancer. *New England Journal of Medicine* **349**: 146–53.

Packman CH (1998) Pathogenesis and management of paroxysmal nocturnal haemoglobinuria. *Blood Reviews* **12**: 1–11.

Pearson TC (2002) The risk of thrombosis in essential thrombocythaemia and polycythaemia vera. *Seminars in Oncology* **29**: 16–21.

Peters M, Plaat BEC, ten Cate *et al.* (1994) Enhanced thrombin generation in children with sickle cell disease. *Thrombosis and Haemostasis* 71: 169–72.

Piccioli A, Vianello F, Prandoni P (2002) Management of thrombosis in patients with haematological malignancies. *Current Hematology Reports* 1: 79–83.

Ploug M, Plesner T, Ronne E *et al.* (1992) The receptor for urokinase-type plasminogen activator is deficient in peripheral blood leucocytes in patients with paroxysmal nocturnal haemoglobinuria. *Blood* 79: 1447–55.

Prandoni P, Lensing A, Cogo A *et al.* (1996) The long-term clinical course of acute deep vein thrombosis. *Annals of Internal Medicine* 125: 1–7.

Prandoni P, Bilora F, Marchiori A *et al.* (2003) An association between atherosclerosis and venous thrombosis. *New England Journal of Medicine* 348: 1435–41.

Rai R, Cohen H, Dave M *et al.* (1997) Randomized controlled trial of aspirin and aspirin plus heparin in pregnant women with recurrent miscarriage associated with phospholipid antibodies (or antiphospholipid antibodies). *British Medical Journal* 314: 253–7.

Stone S, Hunt BJ, Seed PT *et al.* (2003) Longitudinal evaluation of markers of endothelial cell dysfunction and hemostasis in treated antiphospholipid syndrome and in healthy pregnancy. *American Journal of Obstetrics and Gynecology* 188: 454–60.

Tsai AW, Cushman M, Rosamund WD *et al.* (2002) Coagulation factors, inflammation markers and venous thromboembolism: the longitudinal investigation of thromboembolism (LITE). *American Journal of Medicine* 113: 636–42.

Vichinski E, Styles LA, Colangelo LH *et al.* (1997) Acute chest syndrome in sickle cell disease. *Blood* 89: 1787–92.

Warkentin TE (2002) Heparin-induced thrombocytopenia. *Current Hematology Reports* 1: 63–72.

Wood BL, Gibson DF, Tait JF (1996) Increased erythrocyte phosphatidylserine exposure in sickle cell disease: flow cytometric measurements and clinical association. *Blood* 88: 1873–80.

Management of venous thromboembolism

55

Sam Schulman

Diagnosis of venous thromboembolism

The diagnosis of deep vein thrombosis (DVT) or pulmonary embolism (PE) relies on the use of objective diagnostic methods. Symptoms and clinical signs alone are not useful for verification of suspected DVT or PE, as several studies have demonstrated a similar prevalence among patients with and without these conditions, when subsequently investigated with objective methods.

Electrocardiography may show ST–T abnormalities that are unspecific and, although the classical but rare signs of right ventricle overload are seen in massive pulmonary embolism with unstable haemodynamics, the main role of this test is to exclude other conditions, such as acute myocardial infarction. Arterial blood gases and transthoracic echocardiography have too low sensitivity. However, the risk factors for venous thromboembolism (VTE), clinical symptoms and signs with the highest predictive value can be assigned points that are added to obtain a 'clinical score' (Tables 55.1 and 55.2) that can be used as the first step in a diagnostic strategy to reduce costs and the requirement for invasive diagnostic procedures. The clinical scores on their own are not sufficient for confirmation or exclusion of the diagnosis.

The next step, if such a strategy is employed, is the measurement of fibrin D-dimers, which are split products of fibrin, degraded by plasmin, where the D-fragments of two fibrin molecules still are covalently bound and often also in complex with the E-fragment. Several methods can be used, such as enzyme-linked immunosorbent assay (ELISA), whole-blood agglutination of erythrocytes, latex agglutination or immunofiltration. ELISA methods have the best sensitivity, whereas the others are semiquantitative or qualitative methods.

Table 55.1 Clinical scores used for predicting the probability of DVT prior to further testing (from Anderson *et al.*, 2003).

Risk factors, symptoms or signs	Points
Active cancer (treatment ongoing or terminated within 6 months or palliative care)	1
Paralysis, paresis, recent plaster cast on the leg	1
Recent confinement to bed of more than 3 days or major surgery within 12 weeks	1
Localized tenderness along the deep venous system	1
Swelling of the entire leg	1
Calf circumference > 3 cm larger than the asymptomatic leg (measured 10 cm below the tibial tubercle)	1
Pitting oedema (more on the symptomatic side)	1
Collateral flow in superficial veins (not varicose veins)	1
Previous DVT	1
Alternative diagnosis as or more likely than DVT	−2

In the case of symptoms from both legs, the leg with the most pronounced symptoms is used.
> 2 points = high probability; 1–2 points = medium probability; < 1 point = low probability.

There are also quantitative automated latex methods. The manual latex methods have lower sensitivity and negative predictive value for exclusion of DVT or PE. Each hospital should provide information on sensitivity and specificity of the test chosen for D-dimers. In general, a negative result is useful for the exclusion of venous thromboembolism, when the clinical score indicates low clinical probability. A positive result cannot be used for confirmation of the diagnosis, owing to a low specificity. For this reason, D-dimer is not a useful test for pregnant

Table 55.2 Clinical scores used for predicting the probability of PE prior to further testing (from Wells, 2001).

Risk factors, symptoms or signs	Points
Signs of deep vein thrombosis (swelling, tenderness)	3
Heart rate > 100	1.5
Immobilization > 2 days or recent surgery (< 4 weeks)	1.5
Previous objectively verified deep vein thrombosis	1.5
Haemoptysis	1
Cancer	1
Pulmonary embolism as or more likely than other diagnoses	3

> 6 points = high probability; 2–6 points = medium probability; < 2 points = low probability.

or hospitalized patients, the elderly or those with concomitant severe illness.

Whenever the clinical probability is high and/or the D-dimer test is positive, verification using diagnostic imaging techniques is necessary. These include phlebography and ultrasonography for DVT and perfusion–ventilation lung scanning, spiral (helical) computerized tomography (CT) and pulmonary angiography for PE. A novel possibility is magnetic resonance tomography of the lungs, which can be combined with examination of the legs and, due to the low risk for the fetus, it is especially advantageous for diagnosis during pregnancy.

Various diagnostic strategies for DVT and PE have been constructed, in which the aim is to confirm or exclude the diagnosis in the majority of the patients with the least expensive, preferably also non-invasive, method. For the minority of patients for whom uncertainty remains, the investigation is stepped up to more complex methods. The strategies may not be applicable to all clinical settings, due to limited availability of equipment or staff. The cost-effectiveness of a strategy may also be quite different in a clinical study and in routine at a hospital with a large turnover of physicians.

Objective diagnosis with imaging techniques

For objective verification of DVT, phlebography is the 'golden standard', but the diagnostic accuracy is dependent on a high quality of the examination. The veins and possible thrombi have to be well visualized. The correct interpretation of the phlebogram depends on the experience of the radiologist, as artefacts may be difficult to differ from thrombi. A non-ionic contrast medium with low osmolarity should be used to minimize side-effects and the risk that the phlebography causes endothelial damage and the development of a post-phlebographic DVT. Caution is still needed with regard to renal failure.

Ultrasonography of the leg veins is non-invasive and has no contraindications. It is progressively replacing phlebography

as the method of choice. The simplest variant is compression ultrasonography, where a cross-section of the vein is compressed with the transducer. A non-compressible vein is diagnostic for a DVT. The pelvic veins are not accessible for this method and recurrent thrombosis is difficult to discern. The most sophisticated variant of the technique is colour Doppler (colour duplex), which can determinate the flow in several venous segments simultaneously. Provided that the veins of the calf are visualized, this technique has the same diagnostic accuracy as phlebography, but in general the sensitivity is higher for proximal than for distal DVT. Low clinical probability in combination with a negative ultrasonographic examination, including the common and superficial femoral veins, the popliteal vein and the trifurcation in the proximal part of the calf is sufficient for exclusion of DVT. However, with medium clinical probability, a negative ultrasonographic examination should be repeated within 1 week and, if still negative at that point, a DVT is satisfactorily excluded. Presentation with high clinical probability and a negative ultrasonography requires further investigation with phlebography.

Objective verification of suspected PE has typically been obtained with perfusion–ventilation lung scanning, following a normal chest radiograph. Perfusion scanning with technetium-99m (^{99m}Tc) albumin macroaggregates is a sensitive but not very specific method. The specificity is improved by adding ventilation scanning, usually with xenon-133 (^{133}Xe) aerosol or ^{99m}Tc-labelled carbon particles (technegas), considering a V/Q mismatch (negative ventilation and positive perfusion scan) indicative of pulmonary embolism. However, an embolus may cause bronchospasm and thereby a ventilation defect and, more importantly, a V/Q mismatch may occur with several other conditions, including tumours, pneumonia, atelectasis, chronic obstructive pulmonary disease and others, and it does not differ between old and new emboli. The interpretation of lung scans is difficult, especially with a picture with low or intermediate probability for PE.

Therefore, other methods should be preferred for concurrent cardiopulmonary disease. Treatment can safely be withheld if the perfusion scan is negative or with a low probability scan in combination with low clinical probability. A high probability lung scan, which should require perfusion defects corresponding to at least two segments, together with high clinical probability has a positive predictive value of more than 90%. For other combinations there is a need to proceed with other diagnostic methods.

Spiral CT of the lungs has rapidly gained popularity. The interobserver agreement is good and the number of inconclusive examinations is definitely lower than with lung scanning. With multislice technique and a slice thickness of 2 mm, adequate assessment of 93% of the segmental arteries and of 62% of the subsegmental arteries is achieved. Although the diagnostic accuracy for subsegmental PE is low with spiral CT, follow-up studies have shown that it was safe to withhold treatment on presentation of a negative examination. For critically ill patients or those with limited cardiopulmonary function, this may not be true. The positive predictive value of spiral CT with injection of contrast is at least as high as that of a high-probability lung scan.

In the situation with high clinical probability for PE and a negative perfusion lung scan or a negative spiral CT, one possibility is to investigate the presence of thrombi in the lower extremities with bilateral ultrasonography or otherwise to proceed with pulmonary angiography. The latter is rarely used, perhaps due to fear for serious or lethal complications. With contrast medium of low osmolarity, pulmonary angiography was not associated with any mortality and only 0.4% of serious complications in four studies with more than 3000 patients altogether. Although pulmonary angiography is considered the 'golden standard' for diagnosis of PE, there are both false-positive and false-negative results, and the inter-observer variability is poor when the PE is located in subsegmental arteries. Nevertheless, the method appears to exclude with great certainty PE that requires therapy.

Investigation for concomitant cancer

The prevalence of cancer is approximately 20% in many cohort studies of patients with VTE, and in many of those patients the malignancy is still occult at the time of diagnosis of VTE. It is therefore often discussed whether these patients routinely should be screened for cancer with radiological, endoscopic and biochemical examinations, but so far there is no evidence that such a strategy decreases the mortality and morbidity in cancer. Instead, directed examinations should be performed when suspicion is raised by clinical signs or symptoms, as identified on a thorough medical history and clinical examinations. In addition, investigation for cancer should be considered in patients with bilateral DVT, concomitant deep and superficial vein thrombosis at separate locations or recurrent VTE despite anticoagulant treatment within the therapeutic range of laboratory monitoring.

Therapeutic agents

All agents discussed below have in common the obvious side-effect of bleeding complications, which will be described in association with the different treatment options.

Thrombolytic therapy

Streptokinase and tissue plasminogen activator (tPA) are widely available fibrinolytic agents. Streptokinase, a glycoprotein purified in 1947 from the supernatant of β-haemolytic streptococci, cleaves, when in complex with plasminogen, other plasminogen molecules to plasmin. This indirect action results in complex pharmacokinetic characteristics. Furthermore, streptokinase is immunogenic, which may cause allergic reactions as well as a reduced or eliminated response on repeated use or after a recent infection with streptococci. tPA is an autologous glycoprotein, produced commercially with recombinant DNA technique, and it has a direct enzymatic effect on plasminogen, strongly enhanced by the presence of fibrin. The half-life of both agents is short, and for the treatment of VTE an initial bolus dose is usually followed by continuous intravenous infusion, although other regimens have been tested with tPA. The recombinant form of tPA that is used for the treatment of PE is alteplase, with a half-life of 5 min, whereas variants with longer half-life, for example reteplase, are mainly used for myocardial infarction, although some studies with the latter agent for PE have been published.

Anticoagulant therapy

Glycosaminoglycans

The anticoagulant effect of heparin was first described in 1916 by Jay McLean. It is produced from animal sources, usually from porcine intestinal mucosa, and heparin actually consists of a wide range of glycosaminoglycan chains with molecular weights from 3000 to 30 000 Da. It is an indirect inhibitor of the serine proteases in the coagulation cascade, acting as a cofactor for antithrombin, which, after binding to heparin, changes its conformation, whereby the inhibiting capacity increases by several orders of magnitude. Heparin is administered as a bolus injection intravenously, followed by continuous infusion or by subcutaneous injections. It has a half-life of 1–2 h in the circulation. Allergic reactions occur rarely and long-term treatment for months causes osteoporosis. Moreover, heparin induces an elevation of liver transaminases, which is harmless, and a reduction of the platelet count which may be very mild or pronounced and sometimes combined with serious venous and arterial thrombotic complications [heparin-induced thrombocytopenia (HIT), type II]. The mechanism for this is that the patient has developed antibodies, usually immunoglobulin G (IgG), against complexes of heparin and platelet factor 4. These immune complexes bind to Fc receptors on platelets and endothelial cells. The platelets become activated, release more platelet factor 4, aggregate and platelets are consumed. After neutralization by all heparin present, the excess of platelet factor 4 binds to endothelial heparan sulphate, which also may generate antibody formation and endothelial injury by immune complexes. Thrombosis formation or disseminated intravascular coagulation may then follow.

Unfractionated heparin (UFH) is the source for low-molecular-weight heparin (LMWH), which is obtained by fragmentation or depolymerization of the former. LMWH still consists of a mixture of glycosaminoglycan chains, but with molecular weights of between 3000 and 7000 Da. LMWH has the same principal mode of action as UFH, but the inhibition of thrombin is reduced compared to the inhibition of factor Xa, as the former effect requires longer polysaccharide chains for binding to thrombin as well as to antithrombin in order to bring the two molecules together. The bioavailability after subcutaneous injection is better than for UFH and the effect is more predictable, due to less binding to platelet factor 4 and other plasma proteins. The half-life is also longer (3–5 h), so that subcutaneous injection once daily is usually sufficient. Intravenous administration of LMWH is rarely used.

Treatment with heparin requires daily monitoring with activated partial thromboplastin time (APTT), whereas with LMWH monitoring is rarely needed, with the main exceptions being renal failure and long-term prophylaxis during pregnancy, when the inhibition of activated factor X (anti-Xa) is measured. Some side-effects, such as heparin-induced thrombocytopenia and osteoporosis, are less common with LMWH than with UFH. Although there are differences such as in molecular range, sulphation, ratio of factor Xa to thrombin inhibition and pharmacokinetic characteristics between different LMWHs, there is no evidence for a clinically important difference between them.

The shortest sequence of heparin with affinity to antithrombin and an anticoagulant effect is a pentasaccharide which, as opposed to UFH and LMWH, is produced synthetically and at the same time slightly modified compared with the native counterpart in order to obtain the desired pharmacokinetic characteristics. The pentasaccharide fondaparinux has a half-life of 17 h and is given subcutaneously once daily. It is presently used for prophylaxis in association with orthopaedic surgery and it has a similar effect and safety as UFH and LMWH for the treatment of PE and DVT respectively.

Danaparoid is a heparinoid, consisting of the glycosaminoglycans heparan sulphate, dermatan sulphate and chondroitin sulphate but without any heparin present. Accordingly, it has a low cross-reactivity with antibodies induced by heparin and it is therefore mainly used in patients with HIT. It is administered intravenously or subcutaneously and has an effect that is similar with UFH in the prevention and treatment of VTE; with the dose of 2000 units every 12 h it has even a slightly better therapeutic effect than UFH.

Vitamin K antagonists

Vitamin K antagonists have been given to humans since 1942 for prevention or treatment of VTE. These are the original oral anticoagulants but, after 60 years, some alternatives are on the way. There are two groups of vitamin K antagonists, the more commonly used coumarin derivatives and the indanediones, and their availability varies between countries. These agents exert their effect via inhibition of the enzymes vitamin K epoxide reductase and vitamin K reductase, which are required for the regeneration of KH_2 from vitamin K epoxide. The latter is generated when the vitamin K-dependent coagulation factors (factors II, VII, IX and X – as well as the inhibitors protein C and protein S) undergo post-translational modification with γ-carboxylation of approximately 10 glutamic acid residues in the N-terminal Gla domain.

During treatment with vitamin K antagonists, typically three of these residues remain in the non-carboxylated stage, which reduces the ability of these coagulation factors to bind calcium and to localize the coagulation process to phospholipid surfaces. The vitamin K antagonists are bound to plasma proteins, mainly albumin, 98–99%. The metabolism occurs in the liver with the cytochrome P450 enzymatic system. Interactions with other drugs or food may occur at many levels (Table 55.3), and constitute a major disadvantage of vitamin K antagonists. The treatment therefore requires regular monitoring with the prothrombin time (PT). With the widely adopted use of a standardized calibrations system, international normalized ratio (INR), the reliability of

Table 55.3 Mechanisms for drug interactions with vitamin K antagonists with typical examples of such drugs.

Enhancement of vitamin K pathway	Vitamin K, lipid emulsions
Reduced endogenous synthesis of vitamin K	Induced by antibiotics
Accelerated catabolism of coagulation factors	Thyroid hormone, androgens
Decreased synthesis of coagulation factors	Clofibrate
Decreased warfarin absorption due to binding	Cholestyramine
Increased absorption of warfarin	Acarbose
Inhibition of cyclic interconversion of vitamin K	Second-/third-generation cephalosporins
Inhibition of cytochrome P450 (CYP3A4)	Clarithromycin
Inhibition of cytochrome P4502C9 – S-enantiomer	Sulphinpyrazone
Stereoselective inhibition of hydroxylation – R-enantiomer	Cimetidine
Non-stereoselective clearance	Amiodarone
Induction of hepatic enzymes	Barbiturates, rifampicin
Displacement of protein binding	Etoposide
Potentiation of the warfarin receptor effect	Clofibrate
Anti-platelet effect	Acetylsalicylic acid

comparisons of treatment intensities at different laboratories has been improved. The INR from an individual sample is calculated with the formula: $INR = (PT_{patient}/PT_{control})^{ISI}$.

Rare side-effects of vitamin K antagonists are skin necrosis, purple toe syndrome, rash and toxic hepatitis, whereas the adverse effect of warfarin on bone mineral density is debated. Skin necrosis occurs in approximately 1 out of 5000 patients and is due to an imbalance between mildly depressed vitamin K-dependent coagulation factors and a more pronounced reduction of protein C and protein S early after initiation of treatment, resulting in a hypercoagulable state with thrombus formation in small veins and venules in the dermis and subcutaneous fat. The purple toe syndrome is a very painful, burning dark-blue discoloration of the toes and sides of the feet, probably due to cholesterol embolization from atherosclerotic plaques, which have become friable owing to reduced fibrin deposition or haemorrhage into the plaques several weeks after initiation of anticoagulation. Skin rashes may be papular, vesicular or urticarial and often very itchy. Vitamin K antagonists also have a teratogenic effect, with skeletal malformations, optic atrophy and mental impairment, occurring in a few per cent of babies of exposed mothers.

To date, direct thrombin inhibitors have had a very limited use in VTE. Lepirudin is a recombinant derivative of hirudin, which is produced by the saliva of the leech (*Hirudo medicinalis*). It selectively, irreversibly and directly inhibits thrombin without involving antithrombin, and the administration is via the intravenous route. Owing to the complete absence of cross-reactivity against antibodies induced by heparin, it is used with HIT.

Novel anticoagulant drugs

A large number of new fibrinolytic and anticoagulant drugs have been developed but a majority of these did not reach beyond the preclinical studies. Some novel anticoagulant drugs are at the time of writing at the stage of advanced clinical trials and are briefly described below.

The nematode anticoagulant protein c2 (NAPc2), identified in a haematophagous hookworm (*Ancylostoma caninum*), binds stoichiometrically to factor X or Xa, and the complex interacts with and inhibits the membrane-bound tissue factor–factor VIIa complex, whereby the coagulation cascade is slowed down already at the initiation stage. It is now produced by recombinant DNA technique (rNAPc2) and is administered subcutaneously or intravenously. The elimination half-life is more than 50 h.

Modifications of the pentasaccharide have yielded a variant with high affinity to antithrombin and a half-life of 130 h, suitable for subcutaneous injections once weekly. Idraparinux is intended for long-term anticoagulant therapy and at a dose of 2.5 mg it appears as effective and possibly safer than warfarin. Monitoring does not seem necessary but renal failure requires modification of the dose.

Small oligopeptides or peptidomimetic substances with a direct and reversible inhibitory effect on thrombin have a potential for

being orally available. Melagatran and its prodrug ximelagatran have a similar anticoagulant effect to LMWH and warfarin. Ximelagatran may cause less bleeding complications during long-term treatment, due to absence of interactions with food or other drugs. Ximelagatran is administered orally and melagatran subcutaneously and the half-life is 3–5 h, requiring dosing twice daily. No monitoring of coagulation parameters is required. Elimination of the drug depends on renal function.

Initial treatment of venous thromboembolism

Before treatment is initiated, blood samples should be obtained for baseline assessment of the risk of bleeding and for comparison in the subsequent monitoring of therapy. The analyses should include haemoglobin, platelet count, APTT and PT. In addition, with anticipated treatment with LMWH, serum creatinine and with thrombolytic therapy, plasma fibrinogen, blood group and cross-match should also be performed. It may also be desirable to secure samples for analysis of markers of thrombophilia before onset of therapy (see Chapter 53).

Thrombolytic therapy

The most serious consequence of VTE is fatal PE, which occurs in 1–3% after surgery in elderly patients with cancer or undergoing arthroplastic surgery of the lower limb, but also in medical patients, again more commonly in association with metastasizing cancer. Many of these patients die before a diagnosis of PE has been made. On presentation of massive pulmonary embolism with unstable haemodynamics, the mortality is very high but with rapid lysis of the emboli the prognosis improves dramatically. In the case of PE with right ventricle failure, although without shock, the benefit of thrombolytic therapy is more difficult to assess, but there is no significant reduction of the mortality. Thus, despite a more rapid removal of the thrombotic material from the arterial tree of the lungs with thrombolytic treatment than with heparin, there is in the majority of patients no major benefit of the former. In view of the doubling of the risk of major haemorrhage (heparin 5%, streptokinase or tPA 11%), thrombolytic therapy should be reserved for the most serious cases.

A number of contraindications have to be taken into account, so that the risk of bleeding complications can be minimized (Table 55.4). The by far most frequently used thrombolytic regimen in randomized trials on PE is tPA 100 mg over 2 h, with 10 mg given as an initial bolus dose and the remainder in continuous infusion. If an infusion with heparin already has been started, it may be continued or stopped during the treatment with tPA. Several other regimens have been studied, such as rapid infusion over 15 min, as a 2-min intravenous bolus injection or as a local infusion in the pulmonary artery, but there is no evidence for an improved risk–benefit ratio. For patients with

Table 55.4 Contraindications to thrombolytic therapy.

Absolute contraindications

Active internal bleeding

Known haemostatic disorder

Cerebrovascular accident, craniocerebral trauma or neurosurgery within 6 months

Active intracranial process

Relative contraindications

Major surgery, biopsy, puncture of non-compressible vessels, vaginal delivery, external heart massage or major trauma within 7 days

Vascular or eye surgery within 3 weeks

Gastrointestinal bleeding, acute pancreatitis or pericarditis within 3 months

Uncontrolled hypertension (diastolic ≥ 110 mm mercury)

Age > 80 years

Diabetic retinopathy

In addition, caution should be observed during the first trimester of pregnancy, the first 20 h of menstruation, bacterial endocarditis and in the case of abnormal screening tests for haemostasis. Patients with previous treatment with streptokinase within 3–4 months are unlikely to respond to repeated treatment due to antibody formation. The adherence to these precautions and contraindications should be more strict for the treatment of DVT than of massive PE.

cardiac arrest and high clinical probability for massive PE, a bolus dose of 50 mg alteplase intravenously can be given during the resuscitation.

In a life-threatening situation caused by massive PE and circulatory collapse, it is reasonable to disregard the relative contraindications to thrombolytic therapy (Table 55.4). In the presence of absolute contraindications or if the condition of the patient deteriorates despite thrombolytic therapy, there is a possibility to fragment the emboli via a right heart catheter or to perform surgical embolectomy, provided that equipment and expertise are available.

In patients with DVT there are, in addition to the risk of pulmonary embolism, also long-term sequelae to take into account. Destruction of the venous valves results in chronic venous insufficiency (see The post-thrombotic syndrome, below). Thrombolytic therapy yields better and faster re-opening of the veins after DVT, which saves the venous valves. A few studies with long-term follow-up have also demonstrated a reduction of the incidence of post-thrombotic syndrome to approximately 43% in these patients. The patient population recruited for studies on thrombolytic therapy for DVT has been very selective, with exclusion in case of increased risk of bleeding and usually only with patients with a short duration of symptoms included. Still, thrombolytic therapy for DVT is associated with a higher risk

of major haemorrhage than with heparin and this difference is more pronounced than in PE (3–4 times increase versus a doubling) due to the longer duration of treatment. The risk of haemorrhage increases with age and seems to be low for patients under 40 years of age.

The majority of studies on DVT were performed with streptokinase, usually given with a bolus dose of 250 000 IU as intravenous bolus to neutralize the antibodies from any previous infections with streptococci, followed by continuous infusion with 100 000 IU per hour for several days. Heparin is discontinued 30 min before the thrombolytic therapy and restarted 2–4 h after its discontinuation. Regional or local infusion of fibrinolytic agents has not proved to be more effective, bleeding complications are still prevalent and the procedure is relatively labour intensive. Antipyretics such as paracetamol may be given against febrile reactions, and steroids against more pronounced allergic reactions, but prophylaxis with the latter does not provide any additional benefit.

With major haemorrhage, the infusion of tPA should be stopped and blood losses replaced. For patients with streptokinase therapy, the situation is more complex. Owing to the indirect pharmacokinetics, a paradoxical effect may occur if the infusion of streptokinase is slowed or stopped. More plasminogen will then become available for transformation to plasmin by already circulating streptokinase–plasminogen complexes. It is therefore vital to reduce the proteolytic potential, which can be done with aprotinin. Conventional inhibitors of fibrinolysis, such as tranexamic acid, are not effective, as they only counteract plasminogen conversion to plasmin but do not inhibit already formed plasmin. With very low levels of fibrinogen and major haemorrhage, treatment with fibrinogen concentrate or, if unavailable, with plasma or cryoprecipitate is also indicated.

During treatment of DVT with streptokinase, the plasma fibrinogen level should be monitored every 12–24 h. If the level is not reduced at all, it is unlikely that a thrombolytic effect is achieved. The target is approximately 0.2–1.0 g/L, but levels higher than 0.2 g/L do not exclude the risk of haemorrhage, and therapeutic levels do not provide a guarantee for removal of the thrombotic mass.

In summary, thrombolytic therapy should be limited to patients with massive PE and unstable haemodynamics or young patients with extensive DVT and onset of symptoms within 1 week, and perhaps to any patient with massive DVT causing phlegmasia coerulea or alba dolens.

Venous thrombectomy

With only one randomized trial, based on 58 patients, there are insufficient data to evaluate the long-term benefit of surgical removal of the thrombus. The procedure is often combined with formation of an arteriovenous fistula to improve the flow, but there is not enough evidence to show that this increases the patency rate of the vein. Bleedings occur, transfusions are often required and a fatal outcome has been reported in up to 14%. This mortality rate is at least partly related to fact that several of the patients were seriously ill. The benefit of the treatment is that relief of symptoms is immediate, and it may be considered in the rare cases when loss of the limb is imminent.

Interruption of vena cava

Caval interruption can be achieved by insertion of a temporary or permanent filter and provides a short-term tool to prevent pulmonary embolism by reducing the risk during the first 12 days from 4.8% to 1.1%. It should be considered when VTE has been diagnosed and anticoagulant therapy is contraindicated because of a very high risk of bleeding (e.g. ongoing or very recent intracranial or gastrointestinal haemorrhage), or when there is progressive DVT or recurrent PE despite adequate anticoagulant therapy, as verified by APTT, anti-factor Xa levels or PT (e.g. in patients with cancer).

It should be taken into account that in a large randomized trial, no benefit from caval filters was seen regarding mortality or long-term reduction in the risk of PE and, after 2 years, there was an increased risk of recurrent thrombosis.

Anticoagulant therapy

The objective of anticoagulant therapy in the acute phase is to prevent further progression of the DVT as well as (further) embolization to the lungs. It is not sufficient to start treatment with vitamin K antagonists alone, due to the delay of about 5 days until they provide full anticoagulant effect. An initial intravenous bolus dose of UFH, 80 IU per kilogram body weight should be given as soon as PE is clinically suspected, as it may take several hours to establish the diagnosis objectively, and the patient may deteriorate in the meantime. Depending on the possibility for surveillance while the patient is referred to other departments for diagnostic imaging, an intravenous infusion with UFH may be started immediately after the bolus dose or when the patient returns but, in that case, additional bolus doses will be necessary if more than 4 h elapse. When the diagnosis has been confirmed, treatment is continued with intravenous infusion of UFH, 500 IU/kg per day and continued until treatment with vitamin K antagonist, started simultaneously, has become effective (see below).

Randomized trials have shown that adjustments of the bolus dose and the maintenance infusion dose with UFH according to body weight is more effective than a standardized dose. The treatment with UFH is targeted at an APTT of 2–3 times the upper limit of normal, which is measured 4 h after starting the infusion and then once daily. With APTT below the target range, another bolus dose is given and the infusion rate is increased. Conversely, with APTT above the treatment range, the infusion may be halted for 30 min and should be restarted at a reduced rate.

Failure to reach the therapeutic APTT range is associated with a poor antithrombotic effect, whereas a possible association between long APTT results and bleeding complications is less evident. Occasionally, there may be difficulties to reach a therapeutic APTT with congenital deficiency of antithrombin, although treatment with UFH is effective in the majority of those patients. If the APTT is not prolonged despite increased doses of UFH, and especially if there is a clinical deterioration, the antithrombin level should be measured and, if there is a deficiency, substitution with antithrombin concentrate should be considered. More often a therapeutic APTT is not achieved despite normal antithrombin levels, but there is no evidence of clinical progression. This condition is believed to be caused by high levels of acute-phase proteins, such as factor VIII or histidine-rich glycoprotein, which counteract the prolongation of APTT but apparently not the antithrombotic effect of heparin. Measurement of anti-factor Xa in those patients often demonstrates therapeutic levels and should be taken into account so that undue increment of the dose of heparin is avoided.

If the baseline APTT is prolonged, the reason may be presence of a LA (mildly to moderately prolonged APTT) or congenital deficiency of factor XII (severely prolonged APTT for homozygous patients). The association between these conditions and VTE is strong or probable, respectively, and monitoring of treatment with UFH is almost impossible. The alternatives are treatment with UFH, monitored with anti-factor Xa, or treatment with LMWH, which does not require monitoring.

For patients with suspected PE, mild symptoms and stable haemodynamics treatment can alternatively be started with a maintenance dose of LMWH subcutaneously, which is then continued once or twice daily until treatment with vitamin K antagonists, initiated simultaneously, becomes effective (see below). A few randomized trials have demonstrated that this treatment is as effective as with UFH for submassive PE. Treatment with LMWH does not require monitoring unless the patient suffers from renal failure (see below). It is thus possible to give this treatment on an outpatient basis, but the safety has so far not been demonstrated for patients with PE in a randomized trial.

Treatment for DVT with LMWH is as effective as with UFH, but it does not require monitoring and can be undertaken safely without or with only 1–2 days of hospitalization. Randomized trials have demonstrated equal effect and safety with LMWH injected once or twice daily. For hospitalized patients, LMWH is associated with a lower incidence of haemorrhage than treatment with UFH. In the case of very ill patients or a high risk of bleeding, it still may be preferable to treat with UFH, infused intravenously, in view of the shorter half-life if the treatment has to be discontinued abruptly and the more convincing neutralizing effect of protamin sulphate.

It has been shown in several meta-analyses that initial treatment with LMWH instead of UFH is associated with a reduced mortality during 3 months of follow-up. This is entirely due to an increased survival in the subgroup of patients with concomitant cancer disease, and it is not generated by a reduced incidence of fatal pulmonary embolism or haemorrhage.

Although the dose of LMWH is adjusted according to body weight, this is a matter of debate regarding obese patients. A few pharmacokinetic or treatment studies have provided conflicting data regarding whether the dose should be increased linearly or 'capped'. Patients with renal failure were also excluded from all large trials. With mild to moderate renal failure (serum creatinine 200–400 µmol/L), it is recommended to check the anti-factor Xa level after 2–3 days at the time of peak concentration and if it is above 1 IU/mL to reduce the dose. For patients with severe renal failure UFH is preferred.

Patients with VTE should be mobilized early, preferably within 1 day, unless thrombolytic therapy is given. The risk of new pulmonary emboli is not increased with this regimen, whereas pain and swelling of the leg diminishes more rapidly than if the patients are immobilized for 1 week. The patients should wear compression stockings as soon as they are out of bed (see The post-thrombotic syndrome, below).

Secondary prophylaxis

If the initial anticoagulant treatment with UFH or LMWH is not followed by a period of secondary prophylaxis, the absolute increase in the risk of recurrence over 90 days is 29%. Secondary prophylaxis is usually given with vitamin K antagonists, mostly with warfarin. In some European countries, phenprocoumon or acenocoumarol is prescribed predominantly. Phenprocoumon has a half-life of 160 h compared with 20–55 h for warfarin, which may cause difficulties when the drug has to be eliminated quickly in case of an overdose or haemorrhage. Acenocoumarol has a half-life of only 11 h, and this does not result in a requirement for dosing twice daily. Comparative studies with warfarin and acenocoumarol have demonstrated a similar effect and safety profile.

The treatment with a vitamin K antagonist should be started concomitantly with the initial anticoagulant therapy, but the first dose can reasonably be withheld until the diagnosis of PE or DVT is established. Early initiation of the secondary prophylaxis allows for a shorter treatment period with UFH or LMWH and reduces the risk of development of heparin-induced thrombocytopenia. The optimal intensity of anticoagulation with vitamin K antagonists is at an INR of 2.0–3.0, at least during the first 6 months after an episode of VTE. Although previously debated, it has now been shown in several clinical trials that patients with the phospholipid antibody syndrome do not require more intensive anticoagulation. It may take 3–10 days to reach this target range and the maintenance dose varies from 1 to 20 mg per day. The time to reach the therapeutic range and to find the individual maintenance dose is shortened with a higher initial dosing (15 mg of warfarin daily versus lower doses or with 10 mg warfarin versus 5 mg) and by using a nomogram or computer software for the dose adjustments. Although the higher induction dose of 15 mg is not less safe than lower doses, it should be avoided in patients with a high risk of bleeding and not used in patients with a deficiency of protein C or S due to the increased risk of warfarin-induced skin necrosis.

The initial treatment with UFH or LMWH may be discontinued when the vitamin K antagonist has been given for at least 5 days and an INR of at least 2.0 has been achieved for two consecutive days. The secondary prophylaxis with vitamin K antagonists is then continued for a duration that sometimes can be decided very shortly after the diagnosis of VTE, but often requires reassessment due to the results of evaluation for thrombophilia or other investigations that may favour a longer treatment period. Conversely, bleeding complications or poor compliance may prompt a shortening of the planned treatment period. In order to improve the quality of anticoagulant therapy with vitamin K antagonists it is crucial that the patient is followed properly as an outpatient.

The treatment is monitored with analyses of the prothrombin time (PT) at least once monthly and, with results outside the therapeutic range, the dose is adjusted more frequently. The dose adjustments become more precise with less PT results outside the therapeutic range if decisions supports, such as nomograms, algorithms or computer software are used. It matters less which medical staff (specialist physicians, general practitioners, nurses, pharmacists) are in charge of the dose adjustments, as long as they are well trained and follow a large number of patients regularly. For well-motivated patients, it may be an advantage in terms of less clinical complications to perform self-testing with capillary blood sampling, using a 'point-of-care' instrument and to be in charge of the dose adjustments. This requires some training and visits at an anticoagulant clinic a few times per year for comparison of the results with those obtained at the laboratory and rehearsal of the instructions.

All patients who receive a prescription for vitamin K antagonists should be informed about the risk of bleeding and whom to contact whenever such symptoms occur. They should be informed about the risk of using analgesic or antiphlogistic drugs, i.e. acetylsalicylic acid and non-steroid anti-inflammatory drugs, which impair the platelet function, and about the alternatives that can be used; although paracetamol interacts with warfarin, this is not clinically significant, as demonstrated in a randomized study. They should know that a vast number of drugs interact with vitamin K antagonists so that the possibility of an interaction should be questioned for each new drug prescribed. Furthermore, several herbal medicines, including St John's wort, ginseng and garlic reduce the concentration of warfarin in blood, and gingko in combination with warfarin has been reported to cause bleeding. Finally, balanced information should be given about the effect of large amounts (250 g daily on more than a single occasion) of dark green vegetables, which contain considerable amounts of vitamin K and therefore may neutralize the anticoagulant effect, but stressing that a regular intake of moderate amounts of vegetables is recommended. Proper delivery of this information requires that the physician is familiar with all these aspects and can present it to the patient so that it is easy to understand, but in addition printed information should be provided.

Duration of secondary prophylaxis

The optimal duration of secondary prophylaxis is difficult to pinpoint owing to the large number of factors that affect the risk of recurrence. The decision is often a compromise between avoidance of haemorrhagic complications and recurrent VTE. Meta-analyses of randomized trials have shown that a longer duration reduces the risk of recurrence, but with treatment for more than 6–12 months there appears to be a significant increase in the risk of bleeding. Factors associated with a higher risk of recurrence are shown in Table 55.5. The order of importance of these risk factors is not clear, but most guidelines have primarily been based on the nature of the triggering risk factor and sometimes also on the anatomic extension of the VTE. For the majority of patients a treatment of at least 6 months is recommended at present. Shorter treatment is indicated for patients with a distal DVT and temporary (removable) risk factor, such as trauma, surgery or oral contraceptives (6 weeks) or for patients with a high risk of bleeding (3 months). For those with a very high risk of bleeding (actual or very recent intracranial or gastrointestinal haemorrhage), insertion of a vena cava filter may be considered (see above).

In randomized trials on the duration of secondary prophylaxis, there has typically been an annual incidence of 2–4% of major haemorrhage. Attempts have been made to reduce this risk. One option is to reduce the intensity of anticoagulant therapy, and several studies on treatment with vitamin K antagonists targeted at an INR of less than 2.0 have shown a

favourable risk–benefit profile. Large, randomized trials on low-intensity warfarin therapy in the extension of secondary prophylaxis after at least 3–6 months of treatment, targeted at the usual INR of 2.0–3.0, have shown that a prophylactic antithrombotic effect is obtained, but perhaps less than with full intensity. In these trials, the annual incidence of major haemorrhage was only 0.9–1.0% and, although the reason may be a selection bias, it appears that for the extension of treatment beyond 6–12 months, low-intensity vitamin K antagonist therapy is an alternative that allows for less frequent monitoring of the PT. It should be realized that secondary prophylaxis targeted at an INR of 1.5–2.0 was not tested in patients with active cancer, for whom even standard vitamin K antagonist therapy often is insufficient (see Treatment of patients with cancer, below). Similarly, in patients with a high risk of recurrence due to severe thrombophilic abnormalities, low-intensity vitamin K antagonist therapy is not recommended, for example in patients with LA, phospholipid antibodies or deficiency of antithrombin.

With the availability of low-intensity anticoagulation, prolongation of the secondary prophylaxis for many years may appear reasonable in a majority of the patients. A decision in favour of such a prolongation should be weighed against the cost and burden for the patient of monitoring the treatment, effects on the quality of life in view of restrictions regarding diet and carefulness with many other concomitant medications and, finally, the fact that about 1% of the patients annually will have a major haemorrhage. Suggestions for appropriate periods of secondary prophylaxis in patients with different risk factors alone or in combination are given in Table 55.6.

A decision to prolong the duration of anticoagulation should not be made without providing an annual follow-up by a specialist in order to reassess the treatment with respect to patient compliance, complications and new scientific data. It has not

Table 55.5 Factors associated with a higher risk of recurrence of venous thromboembolism.

Higher risk	Lower risk
Triggering risk factor not identified	Triggering risk factor removable or permanent
Proximal DVT and/or PE	
Presence of cancer	Distal DVT
Thrombophilic defects	*Thrombophilic defects*
Deficiency of antithrombin, protein C or protein S; homozygosity for factor V Leiden or for prothrombin G20210A (?); presence of cardiolipin antibodies or lupus anticoagulant; elevated factor VIII or homocysteine; combined defects	Heterozygosity for factor V Leiden, heterozygosity for prothrombin G20210A
Follow-up of the thrombotic disease	
Persistent elevation of D-dimers	Normalized level of D-dimers
Remaining thrombus on ultrasound examination	Normalized ultrasonogram

Table 55.6 Suggested duration of secondary prophylaxis in relation to presence of risk factors (from Schulman, 2003).

Condition	Duration
Thrombophilic defects not identified or unknown	
First event, distal DVT, provoked by temporary risk factor	6 weeks
First event, distal DVT with idiopathic or permanent risk factor; or any proximal DVT or pulmonary embolism	6 months or longer
As above with increased risk of bleeding	3 months
Single life-threatening event	12 months or longer
First event, active cancer	Until cancer resolved
Second event, contralateral DVT	As after the first event
Second event, ipsilateral or pulmonary embolism	12 months or longer
Third event or more	Indefinitely
*Thrombophilic defects identified**	
Deficiency of antithrombin	Indefinitely
Deficiency of protein C or protein S	12 months or longer
Homozygous form of thrombophilic defect	Indefinitely[†]
Double heterozygous for thrombophilic defects	Indefinitely
Antiphospholipid syndrome	Years
Hyperhomocysteinaemia	As without[‡]
Elevated factor VIII activity (above 2.3 IU/mL)	6 months or longer
Factor V Leiden mutation, heterozygous	As without the defect
Prothrombin polymorphism, heterozygous	As without the defect
Life-threatening event and any defect	Indefinitely

*Independent of the event being provoked by a temporary or permanent risk factor, whenever the thrombophilic defect is permanent.

[†]Possibly excluding the homozygous form of the prothrombin polymorphism.

[‡]Tentatively with B vitamins thereafter.

been shown convincingly that the risk of recurrence is higher after the second episode of VTE than after the first. However, recurrent DVT in the ipsilateral leg causes additional damage to the venous valves and increases the risk of the post-thrombotic syndrome significantly, which explains the different strategy from when the recurrence is in the contralateral leg. Patients with PE have a higher risk of recurrent symptomatic PE than do patients with initial DVT, and an extension of the secondary prophylaxis may thus be justified after recurrent PE. Patients with LA or cardiolipin antibodies do not only have a high risk of recurrence after cessation of anticoagulation, but also they have an increased incidence of fatal arterial and venous thromboembolic events, and therefore anticoagulation should be extended, although there are no data to show for how long. An elevated level of factor VIII above the 90th percentile (> 2.36 IU/mL) is associated with an increased risk of recurrence.

Treatment with the beta-blocker propranolol has not been effective in reducing that level and extension of the anticoagulant therapy may be considered. For patients with hyperhomocysteinaemia, it has been demonstrated that B-vitamins (folic acid, cobalamin and pyridoxin) reduce the level of homocysteine, in most cases to within the normal range. This has

also been associated with a reduced risk of arterial restenosis, whereas the effect on recurrent venous thromboembolic events has so far not been demonstrated convincingly, but that would require studies with many thousands of patients. As this treatment is harmless and may be beneficial for several disorders in populations without food fortification with such vitamins, it seems reasonable to prescribe this combination to patients with VTE and hyperhomocysteinaemia rather than to extend the anticoagulant therapy.

Cessation of the treatment with vitamin K antagonists is often associated with an increment of prothrombin fragment 1 + 2 and of D-dimers, independent of whether it is done abruptly or gradually. There are insufficient data on clinical complications to support one of the modes of cessation more than the other.

Management in the case of bleeding or surgery

Excessive anticoagulation may be identified as an isolated prolonged PT (INR above 4.0) or in combination with bleeding. Although elimination of one dose of the vitamin K antagonist followed by a reduction of the maintenance dose may suffice in most cases, the addition of 1 mg of vitamin K_1 orally reduces the risk of bleeding. The reason for excessive anticoagulation should be investigated and may reveal an interaction with other drugs or irregular dosing.

For minor bleeding in combination with an INR above 4.0, a similar strategy is applicable. In the case of major or life-threatening bleeding, reversal with vitamin K_1 is too slow, as only a weak effect is noticed after 2 h and the full effect occurs after 12–24 h. Substitution with the vitamin K-dependent coagulation factors is necessary, but the volumes of plasma required are invariably so large (typically 2–3 L to reduce the INR from 4.0 to 1.5 in a patient with body weight of 80 kg) that there is a substantial risk of volume overload. Prothrombin complex concentrate carries no risk of volume overload and has undergone viral inactivation to eliminate the risk of transmission of HIV or hepatitis B or C. A few cases with thromboembolic complications in association with the use of prothrombin complex concentrate have been reported, but the risk appears small as no complications were observed in prospective cohorts. The target should be an INR of 1.0 in the case of life-threatening haemorrhage in a patient who has had VTE many months previously and an INR of 1.5 when there is still an appreciable risk of recurrent VTE.

In patients with bleeding at INR levels within or below the therapeutic range, cancer should be suspected and investigations of the source are indicated.

For minor surgery, such as tooth extractions or dermatological surgery, anticoagulant therapy can be maintained within the therapeutic range. Randomized trials have shown an excellent prophylactic effect against bleeding complications (from 40% to 5% or from 21% to 0%) after tooth extractions if the patients were prescribed mouth rinses with the fibrinolytic inhibitor tranexamic acid every 6 h. For major surgery, the INR has to be reduced to 1.5, either by complete interruption or by reduction of the vitamin K antagonist. Substitution with LMWH or UFH is given post-operatively until therapeutic INR has been regained and for patients with VTE within 2–3 months or with major thrombophilic defects also preoperatively.

Secondary prophylaxis with low-molecular-weight heparin

Secondary prophylaxis with UFH has been compared with vitamin K antagonists in a few studies. Whereas the efficacy of a fixed dose of UFH was questionable, a dose regimen with UFH twice daily subcutaneously, adjusted to prolong the APTT 1.5 times the normal value at 6 h after an injection, was as effective as vitamin K antagonists. This regimen never gained any popularity due to the requirement for two doses and adjustments. A meta-analysis of studies on secondary prophylaxis, comparing LMWHs with vitamin K antagonists, has shown that they are equally effective and safe. LMWH, injected once daily subcutaneously, may be the drug of choice for patients with a very short treatment duration (≤ 6 weeks), with pronounced difficulties to

achieve stable INR values or when monitoring of the vitamin K antagonist is problematic owing to geographic inaccessibility, frequent travelling or rare cases with a false prolongation of the PT by a LA. The dose of LMWH should be approximately 50% of the initial treatment dose and monitoring with anti-factor Xa is not required unless there is an impairment of the renal function. The risk of long-term anticoagulation with LMWH regarding osteoporosis is minimal and heparin-induced thrombocytopenia is very rare.

Treatment of patients with cancer

In cohorts of unselected patients with VTE, the prevalence of cancer is about 20%. Even occult cancer may increase the risk of thrombosis for several years until it becomes clinically manifest. The diagnosis and treatment of patients with VTE and known cancer differs somewhat from what has been described above. The diagnosis of DVT with ultrasonography or phlebography may become false-positive due to obstruction of the iliac vein by a pelvic tumour mass or metastases, and computerized tomography may therefore be the diagnostic method of choice. Compression of a pulmonary artery by a tumour mass or tumour emboli may simulate perfusion defects by PE, both on lung scanning and pulmonary angiography. Measurement of D-dimers is not of any value in these patients, who typically have elevated levels even in the absence of VTE.

The initial treatment should preferably be given with LMWH in view of the survival benefit in patients with cancer over the following 3 months in comparison with those treated with UFH (15% and 22% mortality, respectively, in a meta-analysis). Although patients with cancer have massive thromboembolism more frequently than those without cancer, thrombolytic therapy is very hazardous, as the risk of bleeding is aggravated by necrosis in highly vascularized tumour tissue, erosion of normal tissues and thrombocytopenia due to bone marrow invasion by tumour or aplasia after chemotherapy. In some of these patients, the risk of bleeding is so pronounced that in the case of pulmonary embolism or massive DVT there is an indication for inferior vena cava filter.

Long-term anticoagulation in patients with cancer has traditionally been considered as cumbersome. There is an absolute increase of the annual risk of recurrence despite vitamin K antagonists by 14–18 percentage points compared with patients without cancer and concomitantly an absolute increase of major bleeding of 7–11 percentage points. For the secondary prophylaxis, LMWH may be a better alternative than vitamin K antagonists in the majority of patients with cancer. The advantages and drawbacks are summarized in Table 55.7. The dose should be 75% of the initial treatment dose. There are now indications from several trials that long-term LMWH may prolong the survival in patients with cancer and VTE, and perhaps also in those without VTE. This does probably not apply to terminally

Table 55.7 Advantages of LMWH or vitamin K antagonists in the secondary prophylaxis for patients with VTE and cancer.

For LMWH	For vitamin K antagonists
No interactions with chemotherapy, analgesics or other drugs	Oral administration
No monitoring in most patients	Inexpensive drug
Subcutaneous administration is advantageous in the case of emesis	Can be used with renal failure
Simple adjustment for biopsy, surgery	

ill patients but rather to those with an expected survival of at least 1 year. However, many questions remain to be answered, including the mechanism for this effect, whether the effect is confined to certain types of cancer, the minimum treatment period required and the optimal dose of LMWH. The secondary prophylaxis should continue as long as active cancer is present unless the severity of bleeding complications precludes the treatment.

Venous thromboembolism in pregnancy

The incidence of VTE in association with pregnancy is 0.5–1.0 per 1000 with 1–2 fatal cases of PE in 100 000 pregnancies. The DVT occurs predominantly (70–95%) in the left leg and is often isolated to the iliac or iliofemoral vein. This may generate a clinical picture that is slightly different from the one generally seen in DVT. The only symptoms may be abdominal cramps, sciatic back pain or fever. Objective diagnosis is even more important in the pregnant patient, as failure to treat an undiagnosed VTE as well as treatment of a false-positive diagnosis may cause harm to both the mother and the baby.

The diagnosis of DVT is more difficult in pregnancy as the pressure from the uterus on the pelvic veins may simulate the effect of thrombosis on ultrasonography and plethysmography, particularly in the third trimester. These examinations are more accurate if performed with the patient resting on her side. Plethysmography has been evaluated in several studies in pregnancy, and with repeated negative exams a DVT can be excluded. Ultrasonography is now more widely available, but diagnosis of a distal DVT may be difficult. The radiation dose from phlebography, perfusion–ventilation lung scanning, spiral CT or pulmonary angiography is so small that the possible risk for the child of future malignancy caused by radiation or hypothyroidism due to free iodine is substantially less than the risk of missing the diagnosis. Any of these examinations should therefore be performed if they are considered to be important for the diagnosis, but obviously with all available precautions, such as reduction of the dose of isotopes, ample administration of fluids to the patient with frequent emptying of the bladder or avoidance of direct radiation to the pelvis by limiting the field to below the groins. Magnetic resonance tomography is not know to cause any harm to the fetus and, if available, may be a useful diagnostic tool for the pregnant patient with suspected VTE. D-dimers are not helpful in these patients, who often have increased levels during a normal pregnancy and especially in the case of a twin pregnancy.

Thrombolytic therapy may be used for massive DVT or PE, but the risk of bleeding is particularly high if this is used shortly before or during the delivery or the puerperium. Thrombectomy for iliac or iliofemoral DVT can be performed safely in pregnant patients, but there are no controlled studies to show that this gives any better short-term or long-term results than anticoagulant therapy. Although there are substantial data, including a few randomized trials regarding the use of LMWHs as prophylaxis during pregnancy, there is only limited experience from these drugs in the treatment of established DVT or PE and, in most countries, UFH is still considered the standard therapy for this indication. However, as data from case series on various LMWHs continue to accumulate, this modality will probably gain popularity owing to the ease of administration. If UFH is chosen, it is started as a bolus dose followed by continuous intravenous infusion to prolong the APTT at 1.5–2 times the upper limit of normal. After 1 week, the treatment is switched to 3 weeks of subcutaneous injections with UFH twice daily at the same total daily dose as on the last day of infusion. Thereafter, the patient may receive secondary prophylaxis with LMWH (see below).

An alternative is to switch to LMWH after the first week, aiming at anti-factor Xa levels of 0.6–1.0 IU/mL at peak concentration 3 h after injection, also given for 3 weeks. Finally, treatment with LMWH may be started immediately when the diagnosis is made, but monitoring with anti-factor Xa is necessary, as the requirement for any form of heparin is increased during pregnancy. Some continue with the treatment dose until the end of pregnancy, but usually secondary prophylaxis is carried on with a slightly lower dose of LMWH twice daily, targeted at anti-factor Xa levels of 0.1–0.2 IU/mL immediately before the next dose. Vitamin K antagonists should not be used owing to an increased risk of fetal haemorrhage, teratogenic effects, mental retardation, opticus atrophy and late neurological impairment. UFH and LMWH do not pass the placenta.

At the time of delivery, blood samples are taken on admission for platelet count, APTT and PT to evaluate the risk of bleeding, and the dose of LMWH is halved. Epidural or spinal anaesthesia should be avoided for higher doses of LMWH, but if the dose is

5000 anti-Xa units, the procedure can be performed 12 h after the previous dose of LMWH and must not be followed by a new dose until at least 2 h have elapsed. With a dose of only 2500 units, a lag time of 6 h is sufficient. Removal of the catheter is also performed at least 12 h or 6 h, respectively, after the previous dose. Post partum, the prophylaxis is continued with in̈ẗïally the ṣame dose of LMWH as during the last part of the pregnancy, for at least 6 weeks and with a ṭotal duration that is at least as long as would have been chosen for a non-pregnant patient with the same risk factors, except for the pregnancy. Monitoring with anti-factor Xa is still necessary owing to decreasing requirements for LMWH post partum. Alternatively, vitamin K antagonists can be given after the delivery, and LMWH is then stopped when the INR is within 2.0–3.0 for at least 2 days and after a minimum of 5 days. Neither LMWH nor vitamin K antagonists pass over to breast milk in any amounts that can have an effect on the baby.

Women with congenital deficiency of antithrombin require higher doses of heparin. Substitution with antithrombin concentrate should be considered in association with delivery to allow for a safe reduction of the dose of LMWH, and thereby to reduce bleeding.

The post-thrombotic syndrome

Thrombi that do not undergo thrombolysis or are not removed rapidly will destroy venous valves in the process where they are incorporated into the venous wall and transformed into fibrous tissue. Venous return of blood becomes impaired, accompanied with increased venous pressure. Permeation of fluid to the extravascular space causes oedema and creates a perivascular barrier to plasma proteins, which reduces the transport of nutrients to the tissues and results in skin atrophy and in the most severe cases venous ulcers. This process takes between 1 and 5 years, sometimes even longer, and is seen in up to 75% of the patients. The tools available to reduce the risk of developing the post-thrombotic syndrome are:
• thrombolytic therapy, which has a limited use due to the risk of haemorrhage; and
• graduated compression stockings.

With the use of such stockings for 2 years after an episode of DVT, the incidence of post-thrombotic syndrome was reduced from 70% to 31%. It is not known if treatment for 1 year would suffice for the same effect or if it should be even longer in some patients. Knee-high stockings are sufficient for the vast majority of patients; they should be of compression class II (20–30 mmHg), fitted individually and they should be worn whenever the patient is not recumbent.

Selected bibliography

Anderson DR, Kovacs MJ, Kovacs G et al. (2003) Combined use of clinical assessment and d-dimer to improve the management of patients presenting to the emergency department with suspected deep vein thrombosis (the EDITED Study). *Journal of Thrombosis and Hemostasis* 1: 645–51.

British Thoracic Society Standards of Care Committee Pulmonary Embolism Guideline Development Group (2003) British Thoracic Society guidelines for the management of suspected acute pulmonary embolism. *Thorax* 58: 470–84.

Büller HR, Agnelli G, Hull RD et al. (2004) Antithrombotic therapy for venous thromboembolic disease. *Chest* 126: 401S–428S.

Fitzmaurice DA, Machin SJ (2000) Recommendations for patients undertaking self management of oral anticoagulation. *British Medical Journal* 323: 985–9.

Hutten BA, Prins MH (2002) Duration of treatment with vitamin K antagonists in symptomatic venous thromboembolism (Cochrane Review). In: *The Cochrane Library*, Issue 1. Update Software, Oxford.

Schulman S (2003) Care of patients receiving long-term anticoagulant therapy. *New England Journal of Medicine* 349: 675–83.

Task Force on Pulmonary Embolism, European Society of Cardiology (2000) Guidelines on diagnosis and management of acute pulmonary embolism. *European Heart Journal* 21: 1301–36.

van den Belt AG, Prins MH, Lensing AW et al. (2002) Fixed dose subcutaneous low molecular weight heparins versus adjusted dose unfractionated heparin for venous thromboembolism (Cochrane Review). In: *The Cochrane Library*, Issue 1. Update Software, Oxford.

van der Heijden JF, Hutten BA, Büller HR et al. (2002) Vitamin K antagonists or low-molecular-weight heparin for the long term treatment of symptomatic venous thromboembolism (Cochrane Review). In: *The Cochrane Library*, Issue 1. Update Software, Oxford.

Wells PS, Anderson DR, Rodger M et al. (2001) Excluding pulmonary embolism at the bedside without diagnostic imaging: management of patients with suspected pulmonary embolism presenting to the emergency department by using a simple clinical model and D-dimer. *Annals of Internal Medicine* 135: 98–107.

CHAPTER 56

Congenital platelet disorders

56

Maurizio Margaglione

Introduction

In haemostasis, a sequence of local events culminates in spontaneous arrest of bleeding from a traumatized blood vessel. The normal haemostatic mechanisms are sufficient to seal up the interruption of vascular continuity. Three closely linked biological systems are involved: blood vessels, coagulation proteins and platelets. Platelets, which normally circulate in the bloodstream for about 7–10 days, are anucleate cells that derive megakaryocytes from the cytoplasm of the giant bone marrow. They normally do not interact with endothelial cells or other blood cells but, when the vessel wall is disrupted, they adhere to exposed subendothelial components, then become activated, amplify and propagate platelet activation by secreting from platelet organelles adenosine diphosphate (ADP) and other active substances, and finally aggregate each other.

Platelets are important in arresting bleeding from damaged blood vessels by plugging the rupture in the vessel wall and providing a surface that promotes blood coagulation. In addition, platelets play an important role in maintaining the integrity of blood vessel wall. Strictly related clinical findings of abnormalities of these two platelet functions are a prolonged skin bleeding time and a history of easy and spontaneous bruising. Abnormal bleeding due to deficiencies of platelets shows characteristic clinical features distinct from those seen in disorders of plasma coagulation factors (Table 56.1). The occurrence of superficial bleedings in patients presenting with platelet disorders and deeper bleeding in those with coagulation disorders is a clinically useful point, but it must be remembered that activities of platelets and coagulation factors are closely related.

Bleeding associated with platelet abnormalities manifests as haemorrhages from small vessels. Petechiae usually develop on the skin and the visible mucosal membranes, but they may be distributed throughout the body, including internal organs. Characteristically, bleeding resulting from platelet diseases is immediate and transient, tends to stop promptly with local pressure and not to recur when the pressure is removed. The occurrence of haemorrhages in infancy or childhood clearly suggests the presence of a congenital deficiency of platelets. However, the disease may be clinically silent and the patient may enter adult life before characteristic bleeding occurs.

Table 56.1 Main specific clinical differences between diseases of coagulation factors and platelet disorders.

Findings	Disorders of coagulation	Platelets/vessels
Onset of bleeding	Delayed after trauma	Spontaneous or immediately after trauma
Mucosal bleeding	Rare	Common
Petechiae	Rare	Characteristics
Deep haematomas	Characteristics	Rare
Ecchymoses	Large and solitary	Small and multiple
Haemarthrosis	Characteristics	Rare
Bleeding from superficial cuts and scratches	Minimal	Persistent, often profuse
Sex of patient	80–90% male	Equal

Table 56.2 Classification of congenital platelet disorders.

Thrombocytopenia
Non-inherited thrombocytopenia
    Drugs and chemical agents
    Isoimmune thrombocytopenia
    Infiltration of bone marrow
    Infections
    Other causes
Inherited thrombocytopenias
    Thrombocytopenias with reduced platelet size
    Thrombocytopenias with normal platelet size
    Thrombocytopenias with increased platelet size

Thrombocytopathies
    Disorders of platelet adhesion functions
    Disorders of platelet signalling transduction functions
    Disorders of platelet aggregation functions

The family history may be of great importance providing a characteristic pattern of inheritance, but it should be remembered that a negative family history does not exclude an inherited platelet abnormality, i.e. the family history is usually negative in autosomal recessive traits. A comprehensive medical history and a careful clinical examination of the patient presenting with a haemorrhagic disorder is crucial for the correct diagnosis. Then, laboratory tests, chosen on the basis of clinical information previously obtained, will lead to a precise characterization and will define the severity of the platelet abnormality.

Congenital defects of platelets may give rise to bleeding syndromes of varying severity and are difficult to classify because of the rarity of many forms, the extreme heterogeneity, and also of the incomplete knowledge about a series of diseases. In the classification presented in Table 56.2, platelet congenital disorders are divided in two main groups: thrombocytopenias and thrombocytopathies. Then, each group is further divided according to specific criteria based on functional and biochemical defects. Such a classification has to be considered as tentative, as in many disorders multiple distinct pathogenetic factors may play a major role and some platelet disorders are put together for convenience of classification rather than on the basis of knowledge of their pathophysiology.

Thrombocytopenia

Thrombocytopenia, defined as a subnormal number of platelets in the circulating blood, usually below 100 000/mL, is the most frequent cause of severe bleeding and, except for chronic thrombocytopenia, the risk for haemorrhages is inversely proportional to the platelet count, spontaneous bleeding occurring frequently when the platelet count is below 20 000/mL. As a rule, there is an inverse relationship between platelet count and skin bleeding time. When automated methods are used, 'artifactual thrombocytopenia' or pseudothrombocytopenia can be observed. Several different mechanisms falsely lower platelet counts. This condition may occur in patients with a wide panel of clinical disorders. Non-technical factors inducing pseudothrombocytopenia include paraproteinaemias, platelet cold agglutinins, giant platelets, previous contact of platelets with foreign surfaces (i.e. dialysis membrane), lipaemia and EDTA-induced platelet clumping. The possibility of a pseudo-thrombocytopenia has to be ruled out through careful manual counting of a well-prepared blood film before concluding that a patient has true thrombocytopenia.

Congenital non-inherited thrombocytopenia

Congenital thrombocytopenia not to be ascribed to inherited causes may be the result of a series of pathogenetic mechanisms. Thrombocytopenia may be attributable to deficient platelet production or enhanced destruction of circulating platelets.

Drugs and chemical agents

The maternal use of drugs and chemical agents has become an increasingly common cause of thrombocytopenia. They may exert their effect suppressing platelet production, damaging platelets directly, or provoking the formation of platelet antibodies. Maternal ingestion of ethanol, thiazides, chlorpropamide, tolbutamide, oestrogens, steroids and other drugs may selectively suppress thrombopoiesis. Drugs such as alkylating agents, antimetabolites or cytotoxic chemotherapeutic agents capable of crossing the placenta may lead to severe thrombocytopenia in newborns as the result of a predictable suppression of the bone marrow; the maternal ingestion of quinine, quinidine, hydralazine or selected antibiotics known to induce immune-mediated thrombocytopenia may induce congenital immune-mediated thrombocytopenia. In these newborns, thrombocytopenia usually remits rapidly and only rarely severe and fatal haemorrhages occur.

Isoimmune thrombocytopenia

Immunological thrombocytopenia may also result from the placental transfer of platelet antibodies formed as the results of active immunization of the mother by fetal platelet isoantigens, if the fetus has inherited a paternal platelet-specific antigen that induces immunoglobulin (IgG) antibody formation. Transplacental passage of the maternal antibody (usually an IgG) may induce a severe thrombocytopenia in the fetus. This usually occurs when the mother has PlA1-negative platelets and the fetus carries PlA1-positive platelets. Newborns may show petechiae and purpura, or more severe bleeding at the time of birth, or may appear normal at the delivery and then manifest severe bleeding within the first week after birth. In this case, thrombocytopenia usually remits within 1 month, but severe and fatal intracranial haemorrhage may occur.

Infiltration of bone marrow

Congenital thrombocytopenia caused by bone marrow infiltration is extremely rare, being limited to cases of disseminated reticuloendotheliosis and congenital leukaemia. Thrombocytopenia with or without associated myeloid and erythroid depression occurs in children with numerous infiltrative disorders including lymphoma, solid tumors, myelofibrosis, Gaucher's disease, Niemann–Pick disease and the mucopolysaccharidoses.

Infections

Thrombocytopenia, usually mild but sometimes very severe, is commonly seen in infected newborns and several mechanisms are probably responsible. In fact, an impaired platelet production as a result of invasion of megakaryocytes, the destruction of circulating platelets and the formation of antigen–antibody complexes may explain many instances of thrombocytopenia associated with viral infections. Maternal infection with toxoplasma, cytomegalovirus, rubella, herpesviruses or hepatitis varicella, as well as recent maternal vaccinations (rubella), may induce congenital thrombocytopenia.

Other causes

Occasionally, children born to women with chronic idiopathic thrombocytopenic purpura manifest congenital thrombocytopenia. It is likely that autoantibodies causing the disease in the mother cross the placenta and bind to fetal platelets, causing their destruction. Other causes of congenital thrombocytopenia due to increased platelet consumption or destruction include preeclampsia, lupus erythematosus or other autoimmune diseases, especially if the woman has a lupus anticoagulant or anticardiolipin antibodies. Finally, a moderate to severe thrombocytopenia has been observed, associated with giant cavernous haemangioma, first described by Kasabach and Merritt, in which the consumption of platelets occurs primarily within the tumour. Thrombocytopenia is often found associated with coagulation abnormalities typical of disseminated intravascular coagulation and the severity tends to parallel the size of the vascular tumour.

Inherited thrombocytopenias

Several inherited diseases may occasionally present with thrombocytopenia, which is an accompanying sign as the result of a generalized bone marrow failure (e.g. Fanconi's anaemia) or metabolic diseases (e.g. Gaucher's disease). These diseases and other complex clinical syndromes (e.g. Noonan's syndrome) will not be discussed in this review. Inherited thrombocytopenias are very rare. In addition, in some diseases both a constitutional thrombocytopenia and a thrombocytopathy (e.g. Bernard–Soulier syndrome, Wiskott–Aldrich, etc.) are observed. These diseases will be discussed in the appropriate section according to the most

prominent defect. As proposed by the Italian Working Group, both platelet size and the presence (syndromic) or the absence (non-syndromic) of other clinical features, different from those deriving from platelet abnormalities, are helpful criteria to classify inherited thrombocytopenias.

Inherited thrombocytopenias with reduced platelet size

The *Wiskott–Aldrich syndrome* (WAS) is a rare (1:250 000) X-linked recessive disorder characterized by eczema, susceptibility to infections associated with defects in cellular and humoral immunity, and thrombocytopenia with reduced platelet size. The gene responsible for WAS maps to Xp11.1 and codes for a protein, WASp, expressed only in haemopoietic-derived cells and involved in the transduction of the signals from the receptor to the actin cytoskeleton. Intermittent bleeding, recurrent bacterial and viral infections, and progressive eczema occur during the first months of life. Death at an early age commonly results from intracranial haemorrhage, infection or lymphoreticular malignancy. A number of kindreds have been reported in whom *X-linked thrombocytopenia* (XLT) occurred alone or in association with partial manifestations of WAS. Also XLT is caused by mutation within the *WAS* gene. Patients with XLT mainly suffer from an isolated bleeding tendency.

Inherited thrombocytopenias with normal platelet size

Congenital deficiency of megakaryocytes is a rare form of thrombocytopenic purpura in the newborn and may occur with skeletal, renal or cardiac malformations. Isolated congenital *amegakaryocytic thrombocytopenia* (CAMT) is an autosomal recessive syndrome leading to bone marrow aplasia later in childhood. This disorder is associated with abnormalities in the expression or function of the thrombopoietin receptor, c-mpl, and a series of mutations in the *c-mpl* gene have been identified. Usually, associated skeletal anomalies are present. Bilateral agenesis of the radius is the most commonly associated abnormality [*thrombocytopenia with absent radius* (TAR) *syndrome*]. TAR syndrome is an autosomal recessive disease characterized by severe, even fatal, haemorrhagic manifestations. Although abnormalities in the thrombopoietin–c-mpl signalling pathway have been suggested, no mutations have been found in genes coding for these proteins. In some infants, the ulna and humerus may also be absent and other skeletal abnormalities may occur. In addition, a proximal radioulnar synostosis, syndactyly and other skeletal abnormalities are reported in association with an autosomal dominant congenital amegakaryocytic thrombocytopenia in patients carrying heterozygous mutations of the *HOXA11* gene. Less commonly, patients manifest cardiac and other minor defects. *Schulman–Upshaw syndrome*, which is caused by mutations in the *ADAMTS13* gene, is characterized by thrombotic thrombocytopenic purpura with neonatal onset (congenital microangiopathic haemolytic anaemia), thrombocytopenia and frequent relapses, and response to fresh plasma infusion.

Inherited thrombocytopenias with increased platelet size

Thrombocytopenias with increased platelet size are characterized by the presence of an increased volume and a reduced number of the platelets, megathrombocytopenia, and are the commonest inherited forms of thrombocytopenias. Among them, a series of diseases have been characterized at the molecular level, whereas other clinical entities still wait for the identification of the molecular defect. Giant platelets and moderate thrombocytopenia are most frequently found in certain populations of Mediterranean extraction and also may be associated with other inherited or congenital syndromes, such as *May–Hegglin* anomaly, Bernard–Soulier syndrome, stomatocytosis, etc. The May–Hegglin anomaly is a rare autosomal dominant disease characterized by giant platelets and basophilic inclusions (Döhle's bodies) within granulocytes. Large Döhle's bodies are seen in peripheral and in bone marrow granulocytes, and most patients show mild neutropenia but no significant susceptibility to infection. About 50% of patients have significant thrombocytopenia deriving from an ineffective thrombopoiesis, but the occurrence of a life-threatening haemorrhage is rare. The platelets in patients suffering from May–Hegglin anomaly show not only a greatly, more than twice, increased volume, but also most of them display bizarre morphology and hypergranularity. Strictly related to the May–Hegglin anomaly are a group of other autosomal dominant diseases, known as Sebastian, Fechtner and Epstein syndromes. The main characteristic is the presence in almost all patients of giant platelets with thrombocytopenia. In addition, patients may develop sensorineural hearing loss, cataract and glomerulonephritis, and most of them display Döhle's bodies. The exact classification of patients according to the presence or the absence of the above-mentioned clinical signs is shown in Table 56.3. Recently, the molecular basis of these syndromes has been elucidated. All of these clinical entities are caused by mutations that occur within a gene (*MYH9*) located on the long arm of the chromosome 22 (22q12–13). This gene encodes for the heavy chain of non-muscle myosin IIA (NMMHC-IIA), a protein involved in motor activity of cytoskeleton. *Grey platelet syndrome* (GPS) is a rare disorder inherited as an autosomal dominant trait, although one example of recessive transmission has been shown, and is characterized by large platelets with a selective deficiency in the number and content of α-granule content. For this reason, platelets are either markedly hypogranular or agranular and display a deficiency of α-granule proteins, such as fibrinogen, von Willebrand factor (vWF), thrombospondin, β-thromboglobulin and platelet factor 4. Thrombocytopenia is usually pronounced and severe bleedings may occur. *Mediterranean macrothrombocytopenia* is usually an asymptomatic disorder with moderate isolated thrombocytopenia and large platelets inherited as an autosomal dominant trait. The condition is characterized by mild or no clinical manifestations and normal bone marrow megakaryocytosis, platelet survival, and *in vitro* platelet functions. Recently, in a series of patients suffering from Mediterranean macrothrombocytopenia, a reduction of the content of the GPIb–IX platelet receptor has been shown and in some of them heterozygous mutations within the *GPIbα* or *Ibβ* genes have been described. Therefore, in these patients, Mediterranean macrothrombocytopenia may be classified as a heterozygous form of the Bernard–Soulier syndrome (see below). On the other hand, the remaining patients having *Mediterranean macrothrombocytopenia* do not show a reduction of the content of the GPIb–IX platelet receptor and the pathogenesis of this form remains to be clarified. A thrombocytopenia resulting from enhanced platelet destruction may be present in *type IIB von Willebrand disease*. Patients suffering from this syndrome show a qualitative abnormality of plasma vWF such that vWF binds inappropriately to circulating platelets. The molecular bases are mutations within the vWF gene, usually the exon 28, which give rise to an increased reactivity of vWF with the platelet receptor GPIb–IX. Clearance of the resulting vWF–platelet complexes leads to thrombocytopenia and the selective loss of the largest vWF multimers from plasma. In general, the degree of thrombocytopenia is moderate and bleedings are of variable severity. The type IIB von Willebrand disease has to be distinguished from the rare pseudo-von Willebrand disease (or *platelet-type von Willebrand* disease). The defect in this autosomal dominant condition results from mutations in gene encoding for the GPIb-α subunit of the platelet receptor GPIb–IX. The few mutations identified give rise to a gain of function of the platelet receptor and increase the affinity for the vWF. As a consequence, spontaneous binding of platelets to vWF occurs with shortened platelet survival and related thrombocytopenia. Reasons why most patients suffering from platelet-type von Willebrand disease show variable enlarged

Table 56.3 Main clinical differences among syndromes due to mutations within the *MYH9* gene.

Macro	Renal disease	Hearing loss	Cataract	Leucocyte	Disease	Thrombocytopenia	Inclusion
MHA	Present	Absent	Absent	Absent	Present	SBS	Present
Absent	Absent	Absent	Present	EPS	Present	Present	Present
Absent	Absent	FTS	Present	Present	Present	Present	Present

EPS, Epstein's syndrome; FTS, Fechtner's syndrome; MHA, May–Hegglin anomaly; SBS, Sebastian's syndrome. Ultrastructure differences in leucocyte inclusions exist.

platelets remain unclear. Other very uncommon causes of macrothrombocytopenia are the *Jacobsen* and the *Paris–Troussau* syndromes. Both are syndromic diseases inherited as autosomal dominant traits and characterized by chromosomal deletion encompassing the same region of the chromosome 11 (11q23.3–11q24.2). In addition, isolated kindreds have been described with distinct forms of giant platelets and a reduced platelet count, such as the *Montreal platelet* syndrome, a platelet disorder characterized by a spontaneous *in vitro* platelet aggregation, the pathogenesis of which is unclear.

Thrombocytopathies

Platelets have a complex ultrastructure comprising a multitude of molecules and the malfunctioning of any of these may give rise to a specific disease (Figure 56.1). Platelets participate in haemostasis by adhering to exposed elements of the subendothelial matrix. Then, they spread on the subendothelial surface, becoming activated, release the content of their storage organelles and aggregate each other. Abnormalities in any of these phases of platelet functions, adhesion, activation and secretion, and aggregation may give rise to congenital disorders of platelets. Patients suffering from one of these diseases usually show a bleeding diathesis, with a prolonged bleeding time and a normal platelet count.

Disorders of platelet adhesion functions

The adhesion of platelets to the injured blood vessel wall is possible through the interaction of platelet receptors with elements of the subendothelium, collagen, fibronectin and blood components that adhere to the subendothelium, such as vWF (Figure 56.2). A series of receptors have been identified on the

platelet surface and they interact with one or more of these elements. The most important receptors are the GPIb–IX and the $\alpha_2\beta_1$ (previously known as GPIa–IIa). The $\alpha_2\beta_1$ is one of receptors on the platelet surface that binds collagen and is a member of the integrin β_1 subfamily. Different receptors for the collagen are the GPIV and GPVI. Binding of molecules to these receptors leads to the subsequent binding to other receptors, which serves to reinforce adhesion and to generate intracellular signals, such as calcium mobilization and protein phosphorylation.

The *Bernard–Soulier syndrome* (BSS) is a bleeding disorder characterized by giant platelets in the blood smear, mild or moderate thrombocytopenia, and prolongation of the skin bleeding time disproportionate to the thrombocytopenia. BSS is a recessively inherited autosomal disorder and consanguinity is common in reported kindreds. Based on reported data, the frequency of the BSS has been estimated to be approximately one case in 1 million people. Bleedings may be severe and fatal haemorrhages may occur. Cutaneous haemorrhages and muscular/visceral bleedings are common. Epistaxis and menorrhagia may be difficult to control. Haemarthrosis has also been reported. Platelet counts range from as low as 20 000/mL to near normal and, on the peripheral blood film, over 80% of the platelets are usually larger (more than 2.5 mm, to as much as 8.0 mm, in diameter). The number of bone marrow megakaryocytes is usually normal.

Patients presenting with BSS show an absent platelet agglutination in response to ristocetin (in the presence of human vWF) and normal aggregation, ATP secretion and thromboxane (TX) B_2 formation in response to a variety of aggregating agents, and delayed response to thrombin. Biochemical and cellular factors contributing to these abnormalities have been clarified in a series of studies. Because of the defective binding with vWF, platelets in BSS do not agglutinate in response to ristocetin and

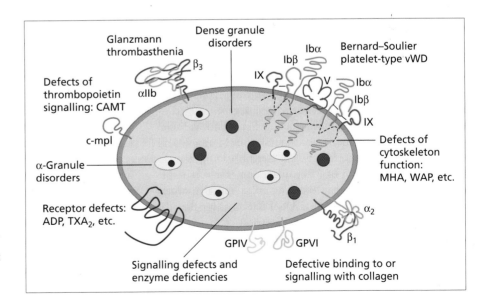

Figure 56.1 The complex structure of platelets. Abnormalities of any platelet complex can lead to an alteration of a specific function.

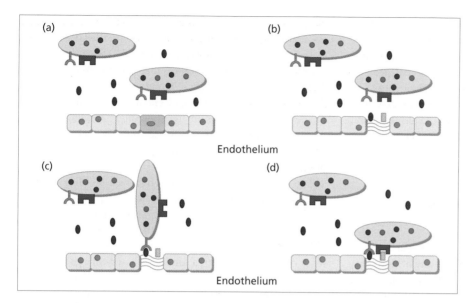

Figure 56.2 Platelets circulate in the bloodstream and do not interact with endothelial cells (a), unless the vessel wall is damaged (b). Adhesion of platelets to injured blood vessel wall (c) and spreading on it (d) is possible through the interaction of platelet receptors with their ligands and vWF collagen.

have substantial reduction in their ability to adhere to sites of vascular injury where subendothelial vWF becomes exposed. As a consequence, plug formation, the primary haemostatic response, is impaired in BSS and increased and prolonged bleeding occurs. Variable levels of the glycoprotein (GP)Ib–IX–V complex have been detected on the platelet surface of patients with BSS, some patients with BSS exhibiting nearly normal GPIb–IX–V amounts (variant type of the BSS). Despite the difference in glycoprotein content, clinical bleeding problems and platelet functional and morphological abnormalities of these patients were indistinguishable from the classical BBS phenotype.

The GPIb–IX–V receptor complex provides the principal site for mediating the interaction of platelets with the adhesive vWF. The entire cDNA sequences encoding the protein chains comprising this receptor have been obtained, allowing for studies on the molecular basis of the syndrome. This complex consists of four proteins: the disulphide-linked α-(135 kDa) and β-chains (25 kDa) of GPIb, and the non-covalently associated subunits GPIX (22 kDa) and GPV (82 kDa). All of them share structural and functional features, suggesting a common evolutionary origin. Different transcripts encode the four polypeptidic chains and, with the exception of that of the GPIbβ, genes show continuous (intron-depleted) open reading frames. In addition, each element contains one or more homologous 24-amino-acid leucine-rich glycoprotein repeats. The genetic heterogeneity in the glycoprotein content of BSS patients shows that multiple molecular abnormalities may lead to a similar clinical disorder, and implies that BSS may be the result of defects within the subunits that hamper the coordinate expression of the complex on the platelet membrane. In this respect, BSS would resemble abnormalities of other multi-subunit complexes, in which a defect in a single subunit prevents the assembly and the surface expression of the complex.

In addition to quantitative and qualitative abnormalities of the GPIbα gene, the recognized BSS phenotype has also been documented in patients with detrimental mutations within platelet GPIX and GPIbβ genes. Very few patients with a defect of one of the platelet receptors for collagen have been described. These patients showed mild bleeding disorders and a selective impairment, at a variable extent, in collagen response, adhesion to subendothelial surfaces and collagen-induced platelet aggregation. Platelets have two major receptors for collagen, the $\alpha_2\beta_1$ integrin, with a major role in adhesion of platelets to subendothelial surfaces, and the GPVI, mainly involved in platelet activation. Thus, it is conceivable that collagen binding to platelets occurs through a multistep mechanism involving first the attachment of platelets to exposed collagen of the subendothelium in flowing blood by means of the $\alpha_2\beta_1$ receptor and then platelet activation through a second receptor, GPVI.

Disorders of platelet signalling transduction functions

Platelets that adhere to the subendothelial surface become activated and begin the production or release of several intracellular messengers, which modulate a series of platelet responses, such as calcium mobilization, protein phosphorylation, and production of arachidonic acid. Activated platelets also release substances stored in their granules, some of which act in the recruitment of additional platelets and lead to the formation of the primary haemostatic plug (Figure 56.3). Several signalling mechanisms are involved in events that govern platelet responses starting from platelet adhesion to blood vessel wall injury and leading to secretion and aggregation. Evidence has become available that specific abnormalities in platelet signalling mechanisms may be the basis of platelet dysfunction. With the term of

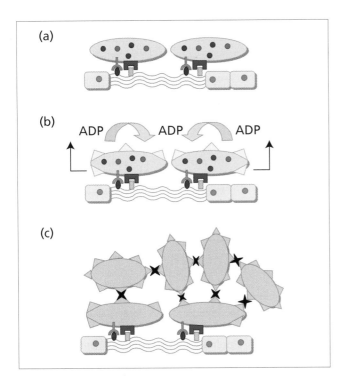

Figure 56.3 Platelets after adhering to the subendothelial (a) surface become activated, release intracellular messengers (b) and aggregate with each other leading to the formation of the primary haemostatic plug (c).

platelet signalling, disorders may be grouped as a heterogeneous group of abnormalities in platelet secretion and signal transduction. Congenital defects of platelet signalling mechanisms are put together for convenience of classification rather than on the basis of knowledge in the pathophysiology of specific diseases. Patients suffering from these kinds of defects represent the vast majority of subjects presenting with inherited thrombocytopathies.

Platelet activation by means of binding to receptors gives rise to hydrolysis of phosphoinositide by phospholipase C, leading to the formation of inositol triphosphate, which, in turn, functions as a messenger to release calcium from intracellular stores. In addition, hydrolysis of phosphoinositide leads to the formation of diacylglycerol, which activates protein kinase C. The activation of the protein kinase C is thought to play a major role in platelet secretion and in the activation of the $\alpha_{IIb}\beta_3$ complex. In several patients, defects in phospholipase C activation, calcium mobilization and protein phosphorylation have been suggested on the basis of platelet-impaired functions, despite the presence of normal granule stores and normal thromboxane A_2.

Following stimulation, platelet phospholipase A_2 mobilizes the arachidonic acid from the phospholipid pool. Then, the arachidonic acid is metabolized by cyclo-oxygenase and thromboxane synthase to form thromboxane A_2, a strong platelet-aggregating agent that is necessary for a secretion response. A defect in arachidonic acid mobilization and thromboxane A_2 production has been identified in some patients. Few patients with an impaired liberation of arachidonic acid have been described. Individuals with this defect showed an abnormal aggregation and secretion in response to a series of stimulating factors but a normal production of thromboxane A_2 in response to arachidonic acid. Several patients have been reported with a deficiency of cyclo-oxygenase and showing a slightly prolonged bleeding time and impaired platelet aggregation. In addition, few patients have been described with a defect in thromboxane A_2 formation presenting with a variable bleeding diathesis.

Disorders of platelet aggregation functions

Platelet aggregation may be defined as the interaction of activated platelets with one another and occurs after adhesion of platelets to the injured blood vessel wall. A series of factors are capable of inducing platelet aggregation and may be classified as primary and secondary platelet-aggregating agents. Primary aggregating substances are those factors, such as ADP, adrenaline and thrombin, which are able to directly induce platelet aggregation independently of their ability to release the ADP contained within platelets or to induce the production of prostaglandins. Secondary aggregating factors are substances that induce aggregation of platelets through their ability to provoke the release reaction of ADP or the synthesis of prostaglandins. According to this, disorders due to an impairment of platelet aggregation may be classified into defects of primary aggregation: Glanzmann's thrombasthenia; selective impairment of platelet receptors (ADP, adrenaline); and defects of secondary aggregation: storage pool disease and selective impairment of platelet receptors (thromboxane, collagen). *In vitro*, a series of substances are used to challenge platelets and the manner in which they respond to these stimuli may be helpful to identify specific thrombocytopathies (Table 56.4).

Glanzmann's thrombasthenia (GT) is a bleeding diathesis marked by prolonged bleeding time, normal platelet count and absence of platelet aggregation in response to platelet agonists such as ADP, collagen, arachidonic acid and thrombin. Platelet agglutination induced by ristocetin and vWF is normal. This congenital bleeding disorder is associated with an impaired or absent clot retraction. GT is one of the less common of the congenital bleeding disorders and is transmitted as an autosomal recessive trait, and consanguinity has been reported in affected kindreds. The clinical features are those usually expected with platelet dysfunction: easy and spontaneous bruising, mucosal membrane bleeding, subcutaneous haematomas, and petechiae. Rarely, patients suffer from intra-articular bleeding with resultant haemarthroses. Fatal haemorrhages have been reported. Quantitative or qualitative (variant GT forms) abnormalities of the platelet $\alpha_{II}b\beta_3$ integrin (also known as the glycoprotein complex IIb–IIIa) have been shown to be responsible for this

Table 56.4 Platelet response to aggregating agents in different thrombocytopathies.

Disorder	ADP	Adrenaline	Collagen	Arachidonic acid	Ristocetin
Bernard–Soulier	Normal	Normal	Normal	Normal	Absent
Pseudo-vWD	Normal	Normal	Normal	Normal	Increased at low doses
ADP receptor defect	Impaired	Impaired	Impaired	Impaired	Present
Epinephrine receptor defect	Normal	Impaired	Normal	Normal	Present
Collagen receptor defect	Normal	Normal	Impaired	Normal	Present
Defect of signal transduction	Variable impairment	Variable impairment	Variable impairment	Variable impairment	Present
Glanzmann's thrombasthenia	Absent	Absent	Absent	Absent	Present
δ-SPD	Impaired	Impaired	Impaired	Variable	Present
Thromboxane receptor defect	Impaired	Impaired	Impaired	Impaired	Present

disorder. Mutations within the genes that code for $\alpha IIb\beta_3$ subunits have been described in GT patients. As other integrins, α_{IIb}- and β_3-subunits are prominent integral components of the platelet membrane that form heterodimers containing specific sites for platelet–platelet cohesion. The $\alpha_{IIb}\beta_3$ integrin serves as platelet receptor for fibrinogen, fibronectin, vitronectin and vWF. In addition, the $\alpha_{IIb}\beta_3$ integrin modulates to some extent calcium influx, cytoplasmic alkalinization, tyrosine kinase phosphorylation and clot retraction. Clinical heterogeneity of GT has been stressed on the basis of platelet function testing or using crossed immunoelectrophoresis, Western blot, flow cytometry and fibrinogen binding. Type I Glanzmann's thrombasthenia is characterized by the lack of surface-detectable $\alpha_{IIb}\beta_3$ complex and a profound defect of platelet aggregation and clot retraction. At variance with the type I, platelets of patients suffering from type II Glanzmann's thrombasthenia have detectable, but markedly reduced, amounts of the $\alpha_{IIb}\beta_3$ receptor on their surface, usually from 10% up to 20% of normal values. Platelets show sufficient amounts of receptors to allow for microaggregate formation, although there is still a profound defect in the ability to form large aggregates. The clot retraction is only moderately impaired. In addition, a series of patients with a variant form have been described, who presented near normal levels of the $\alpha_{IIb}\beta_3$ complex, which is dysfunctional in that platelets, when activated, can neither aggregate nor bind fibrinogen. An extreme variability in the clinical symptoms is present, even among patients with similar degrees of platelet abnormality and prolongation of the bleeding time. In general, no aggregation abnormalities are detected in heterozygotes, but a decreased amount of the $\alpha_{IIb}\beta_3$ integrin has been reported, platelet content being approximately one-half of the normal amount.

Defects of platelet ADP receptors have been characterized in few patients and all suffered from a bleeding diathesis. On the platelet surface, different types of ADP receptors have been identified, two G-protein coupled receptors, $P2Y_1$ and $P2Y_{12}$, and a ligand gated ion channel one, $P2X_1$. The P2Y1 receptor

is responsible for the shape change of platelets and transient platelet aggregation, giving rise to centralization of platelet granules and formation of filopodia, whereas the $P2Y_{12}$ receptor is involved in the amplification of the response and in the stabilization of platelet aggregates through the full activation of the $\alpha_{IIb}\beta_3$ integrin. The $P2X_1$ receptor has been suggested to be involved in platelet shape change. The $P2Y_{12}$ receptor defect is inherited as an autosomal recessive trait and all patients so far identified were born from consanguineous parents. In these patients, a blunted platelet aggregation in response to ADP, with a retained shape change, has been reported. Only one patient has been briefly reported with a defect of the $P2Y_1$ receptor. This patient showed an impaired platelet aggregation in response to ADP and other agonists. Finally, a selective impairment of ADP aggregation associated with a dominant negative mutation in the $P2X_1$ gene has been identified in a patient who presented with a severe bleeding disorder.

The *selective impairment of adrenaline receptors*, α_2-adrenergic receptors (α_2-AR), has been associated with bleeding. A number of individuals with an impaired aggregation response to adrenaline and a congenital defect of platelet α_2-AR receptors have been described and some of them presented a history of easy bruising. Secondary aggregation disorders are more frequent than primary aggregation disorders and the most common in this category are the *storage pool deficiency* (SPD) syndromes. SPD syndromes may be classified in a system that takes into account the content of both dense and α-granules (Figure 56.4). The term δ-SPD identifies patients who show low platelet content of dense granules only. Patients with deficiency of both types of granules are designated as αδ-SPD. Finally, patients presenting with reduced or absent platelet content of α-granules but normal levels of dense granules (α-SPD) are designated as patients with grey platelet syndrome. The disorder is heterogeneous and the term SPD includes a group of disorders having as their common feature a diminution in secretable substances stored in platelet granules.

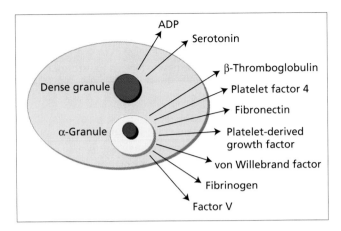

Figure 56.4 In platelets, granules are the storage site for substances that are important for the haemostatic process. The α-granules contain proteins involved in adhesion (fibronectin, vWF) cell–cell interaction (P-selectin), and in promoting the coagulation (FV, PF4), whereas the content of dense granules is important to recruit additional platelets (ADP, serotonin).

A storage pool disease is found as an associated defect in most of the patients carrying other rare syndromes, such as the Wiskott–Aldrich syndrome and the thrombocytopenia with absent radius syndrome. However, the majority of patients presenting with a SPD have no associated diseases and are otherwise normal. The clinical features of this type of secondary aggregation disorder are those expected with a platelet function defect and consist of easy and spontaneous bruising, mucocutaneous haemorrhages, haematuria and epistaxis. Patients with δ-SPD or αδ-SPD usually have absent ADP and adrenaline-induced secondary aggregation waves, although the primary waves are present. Patients with δ-SPD may present a severe or partial granule deficiency. Collagen-induced aggregation is absent or markedly reduced, whereas ristocetin-induced agglutination is normal. In several kindreds, the disorder appeared to be inherited as an autosomal dominant trait. However, in other families the type of inheritance could not be determined. In the absence of other congenital abnormalities or an associated α-granule deficiency, SPD is inherited as an autosomal dominant trait.

The other forms of dense-SPD coincident with other congenital abnormalities, such as TAR, are usually inherited as autosomal recessive traits, or X-linked, as in the case of WAS. An SPD is usually present in *Hermansky–Pudlak syndrome* and in *Chédiak–Higashi* syndrome. Hermansky–Pudlak syndrome (HPS) is a rare autosomal recessive inherited disorder characterized by the presence of oculocutaneous albinism, absence of platelet-dense granules, and infiltration of ceroid pigmented reticuloendothelial cells in the lung and in the colon, leading to pulmonary fibrosis and inflammatory bowel disease. HPS shows genetic heterogeneity, and mutations within two genes have

been identified in patients with this disease, the *HPS1* gene, mapped on the chromosome 10q23.1–23.3, and the *ADTB3A*, on the chromosome 5q11–14. However, it is conceivable that different additional genes may be involved in the pathogenesis of the HPS.

In Chédiak–Higashi syndrome (CHS), a variable degree of oculocutaneous albinism and a poor resistance to respiratory and cutaneous infection are usually found. The infections are generally fatal during infancy or in early childhood, but patients may also die of a chronic lymphohistiocytic infiltration, known as *the accelerated phase*, during the second or third decades of life. CHS is extremely rare and is inherited as an autosomal recessive trait. Unlike HPS, the CHS does not seem to display locus heterogeneity and the only gene proved to cause CHS, *LYST*, is located on chromosome 1q42.1–42.2. Both in HPS and in CHS there are findings typical of an SPD, bleeding of mucosae, epistaxis and spontaneous soft-tissue bruising. On the other hand, in *Quebec platelet disorder*, a rare autosomal dominant bleeding disease associated with abnormal proteolysis of α-granule proteins, patients show a severe deficiency of platelet multimerin, a factor V binding protein contained within α-granules, and a severe impaired aggregation in response to adrenaline. Several patients have been described with a *selective impairment of the thromboxane A_2 receptor*, a mild bleeding disorder and a defective platelet aggregation in response to several agents but not thrombin. Autosomal dominant inheritance has been suggested in some cases.

Therapy

As a rule, in the vast majority of congenital platelet disorders there is no specific treatment. In congenital thrombocytopenias due to maternal use of drugs or chemical agents, recovery of thrombocytopenia needs from a few days to some weeks, such as in the case of thiazide drugs. In surviving thrombocytopenic newborns who are infected with rubella or cytomegalovirus, platelet levels return to normal, but several months may be required. In newborns with isoimmune congenital thrombocytopenia, usually the recovery is uneventful and platelets return to normal values in 14–21 days. Only severe cases need to be treated with washed maternal platelets, corticosteroids or exchange transfusions. In general, principal treatments in patients with congenital platelet diseases are general measures aiming at avoiding bleeding and the use of supportive therapeutic approaches for controlling haemorrhages. However, as types and severity of bleeding vary in different patients, therapeutic approaches have to be individualized.

General measures

Education of patients is of great importance. Patients and their parents have to be instructed to avoid trauma. Regular dental care may be helpful to prevent gingival bleeding. Drugs that impair platelet functions, such as acetylsalicylic acid-containing medications, should be avoided. In women, the use of oral contraceptives can be applied to prevent menorrhagia. Local measures, such as the application of firm pressure in the case of epistaxis, will usually suffice in the event of mild bleeding.

Drugs

Desmopressin (1-desamino-8-D-arginine vasopressin or DDAVP) is a mainstay of the therapy of patients with congenital platelet defects. Depending on platelet defect, administration of DDAVP may shorten the bleeding time. Intravenous, subcutaneous or intranasal administration of DDAVP increases factor VIII and vWF transiently by releasing them from storage sites, and its use has been suggested to be of value in some patients presenting with congenital platelet defects, as BSS, May–Hegglin anomaly, GPS, SPD and Glanzmann's thrombasthenia. In general, the response to DDAVP varies among patients but it is constant in each patient; a test dose may be of value to identify those patients who will benefit from this treatment to prevent or control future bleedings.

The use of recombinant activated factor VII (rFVIIa) has been proved to be helpful in the treatment of bleeding in haemophilic patients with inhibitors. Recently, administration of rFVIIa has been used to stop bleeding in patients with congenital platelet disorders, such as BSS and Glanzmann's thrombasthenia. In addition, this drug has been used to treat thromboasthenics to avoid bleeding during surgical procedures. However, adverse reactions, such as vein thromboembolism and arterial ischaemia, have been described. Thus, the role of rFVIIa remains promising but deserves to be carefully defined.

Platelet transfusions

Platelet transfusions, using platelets from HLA-matched donors when available, are used to control severe haemorrhage in thrombocytopenic patients or in individuals with thrombocytopathies. As the risk of post-traumatic as well as of spontaneous bleeding increases as the platelet count falls, spontaneous haemorrhage becomes common as platelet count drops below 20 000/mL and is extremely likely at counts below 5000/mL. Extensive clinical experience has shown that control of bleeding is possible on achievement of an adequate elevation in the circulating platelet counts. However, the co-existence of platelet dysfunctions has to be taken into account to correctly calculate the dosage of platelets required. Platelet transfusions are effective in controlling bleeding but may be responsible for transmission of infectious diseases, febrile reactions or development of alloimmunization. In patients carrying thrombocytopathies, platelet transfusions should be employed only for the treatment of severe bleeding because of the risk of alloimmunization. The occurrence of platelet alloimmunization is more frequent in patients lacking a membrane glycoprotein, such as BSS and Glanzmann's thrombasthenia. Alloantibodies develop because they recognize lacking proteins as foreign in transfused proteins and, in turn, induce refractoriness to platelet transfusions.

Other measures

Splenectomy has generally no effect in congenital thrombocytopathies and in thrombocytopenias but has proven to be effective in patients with WAS. Allogenic bone marrow transplantation may provide, in theory, an effective cure for inherited disorders involving platelet count or functions restoring a normal megakaryocytopoiesis. Transplants have been successfully performed with complete correction in patients with WAS and severe Glanzmann's thrombasthenia. However, risks of such a drastic procedure still overcome those related to bleeding tendency and, therefore, rarely required in patients suffering from congenital platelet disorders.

Conclusions

Over the last few years, a series of improvements to better understand pathogenesis of congenital platelet disorders have been achieved. In several congenital platelet diseases, the gene responsible has been identified and several patients have been characterized at molecular level (Table 56.5). This information

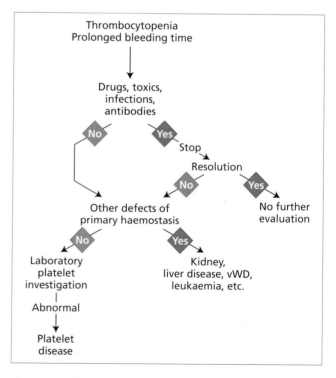

Figure 56.5 Algorithm for the initial screening of patients with congenital platelet disorders.

Table 56.5 Genes involved in congenital platelet disorders.

Disorder	Gene	Locus
Wiskott–Aldrich syndrome	WAS	Xp11.23–p11.22
X-linked thrombocytopenia	WAS	Xp11.23–p11.22
Congenital amegakaryocytic thrombocytopenia	c-mpl	1p34
Congenital amegakaryocytic thrombocytopenia and radio–ulnar synostosis	HOXA-11	7p15–p14.2
Schulman–Upshaw syndrome	ADAMTS13	9q34
May–Hegglin anomaly and Sebastian, Epstein, Fechtner syndromes	MYH9	22q11.2
Mediterranean macrothrombocytopenia	GPIbα	22q11.2, 17pter-p12
Jacobsen and Paris–Troussau syndromes		11q23.3–11q24.2
Bernard–Soulier syndrome	GPIbα	22q11.2, 17pter-p12
	GPIbβ	22q11.2
	GPIX	3q21
Pseudo-vWD	GPIbα	22q11.2, 17pter-p12
ADP receptor defect	P2Y12	3q24–q25
	P2Y1	3q25
	P2X1	17p13.3
Adrenaline receptor defect	$\alpha_2 AR$	10q24–q26
Collagen receptor defect	α_2	5q23–q31
Glanzmann's thrombasthenia	αIIb	17q21.32, α, 17q21.32
Thromboxane receptor defect	$TXBA_2$	19p13.3

has allowed for a more accurate comprehension of congenital thrombocytopenias and thrombocytopathies. Careful collection of personal and family clinical data, physical examination and appropriate laboratory testing work-up are of value for the evaluation of a patient presenting with bleeding due to congenital platelet disorders (Figure 56.5). Using this approach, in several instances it is possible to correctly identify the platelet defect. However, despite recent advances in knowledge, in most of the patients with a congenital bleeding disorder and impairment of platelet functions the underlying molecular mechanisms are still unknown. In the future, one of the challenges will be to ameliorate our understanding of congenital platelet disorders in order to obtain powerful tools for prevention, diagnosis and therapy of bleeding. On the other hand, alternative treatments, such as gene therapy, may offer, in theory, a cure for diseases such as congenital platelet disorders. Hopefully, improvements in such approaches will provide a curative treatment for the majority of patients suffering from severe congenital platelet disorders.

Selected bibliography

Balduini CL, Noris P, Belletti S et al. (1999) In vitro and in vivo effects of desmopressin on platelet function. Haematologica 84: 891–6.

Balduini CL, Cattaneo M, Fabris F et al. (2003) Inherited thrombocytopenias: a proposed diagnostic algorithm from the Italian Gruppo di Studio delle Piastrine. Haematologica 88: 582–92.

Cattaneo M, Lecchi A, Randi AM et al. (1992) Identification of a new congenital defect of platelet function characterized by severe impairment of platelet responses to adenosine diphosphate. Blood 80: 2787–96.

Furlan M, Robles R, Solenthaler M et al. (1997) Deficient activity of von Willebrand factor-cleaving protease in chronic relapsing thrombotic thrombocytopenic purpura. Blood 89: 3097–103.

George JN, Caen JP, Nurden AT (1990) Glanzmann's thrombasthenia: the spectrum of clinical disease. Blood 75: 1383–95.

Harker LA, Slichter SJ (1972) The bleeding time as a screening test for evaluation of platelet function. New England Journal of Medicine 287: 155–9.

Heath KE, Campos-Barros A, Toren A et al. (2001) Non-muscle myosin heavy chain IIA mutations define a spectrum of autosomal dominant macrothrombocytopenias: May–Hegglin anomaly and Fechtner, Sebastian, Epstein, and Alport-like syndromes. American Journal of Human Genetics 69: 1033–45.

Hedberg VA, Lipton JM (1988) Thrombocytopenia with absent radii. A review of 100 cases. American Journal of Pediatric Hematology Oncology 10: 51–64.

Introne W, Boissy RE, Gahl WA (1999) Clinical, molecular, and cell biological aspects of Chédiak-Higashi syndrome. Molecular Genetic Metabolism 68: 283–303.

Lopez JA, Andrews RK, Afshar-Kharghan V et al. (1998) Bernard–Soulier syndrome. Blood 91: 4397–418.

Miller JL, Cunningham D, Lyle VA et al. (1991) Mutation in the gene coding the alpha chain of platelet glycoprotein Ib in platelet-type von Willebrand disease. *Proceedings of the National Academy of Sciences of the USA* **88**: 4761–5.

Miller JL, Lyle VA, Cunningham D (1992) Mutation of leucine-57 to phenylalanine in a patient glycoprotein Ibα leucine tandem repeat occurring in patients with an autosomal dominant variant of Bernard–Soulier disease. *Blood* **79**: 439–46.

Nagle DL, Karim MA, Woolf EA *et al.* (1996) Identification and mutation analysis of the complete gene for Chédiak–Higashi syndrome. *Nature Genetics* **14**: 307–11.

Najean Y, Lecompte T (1990) Genetic thrombocytopenia with autosomal dominant transmission: a review of 54 cases. *British Journal of Haematology* **74**: 203–8.

Oh J, Ho L, Ala-Mello S *et al.* (1998) Mutation analysis of patients with Hermansky–Pudlak syndrome. A frameshift hot spot in the HPS gene and apparent locus heterogeneity. *American Journal of Human Genetics* **62**: 593–8.

Onder O, Weinstein A, Hoyer LW (1980) Pseudothrombocytopenia caused by platelet agglutinins that are reactive in blood anticoagulated with chelating agents. *Blood* **56**: 177–82.

Payne BA, Pierre RV (1984) Pseudothrombocytopenia. A laboratory artifact with potential serious consequences. *Mayo Clinic Proceedings* **59**: 123–5.

Phillips DR, Charo IF, Scarborough RM (1991) GPIIb-IIIa: the responsive integrin. *Cell* **65**: 356–66.

Raccuglia G (1971) Gray platelet syndrome. A variety of qualitative platelet disorder. *American Journal of Medicine* **51**: 818–28.

Savoia A, Balduini CL, Savino M *et al.* (2001) Autosomal dominant macrothrombocytopenia in Italy is most frequently a type of heterozygous Bernard–Soulier syndrome. *Blood* **97**: 1350–5.

Seri M, Cusano R, Gangarossa S *et al.* (2000) Mutations in MIH9 result in the May–Hegglin anomaly, and Fechtner and Sebastian syndromes. The May–Hegglin/Fechtner syndrome consortium. *Nature Genetics* **26**: 103–5.

Shotelersuk V, Gahl WA (1998) Hermansky–Pudlak syndrome. Models for intracellular vesicle formation. *Molecular Genetic Metabolism* **65**: 85–96.

Shotelersuk V, Dell'Angelica EC, Hartnell L *et al.* (2000) A new variant of Hermansky–Pudlak syndrome due to mutation in a gene responsible for vesicle formation. *American Journal of Medicine* **108**: 423–7.

Strippoli P, Savoia A, Iolascon A *et al.* (1998) Mutational screening of thrombopoietin receptor gene (c-mpl) in patients with congenital thrombocytopenia and absent radii (TAR). *British Journal of Haematology* **103**: 311–14.

Thrasher AJ, Kinnon C (2000) The Wiskott–Aldrich syndrome. *Clinical Experimental Immunology* **120**: 2–9.

Villa A, Notarangelo L, Macchi P *et al.* (1995) X-linked thrombocytopenia and Wiskott-Aldrich syndrome are allelic diseases with mutations in the WASP gene. *Nature Genetics* **9**: 414–7.

CHAPTER 57

Immune thrombocytopenic purpura: pathophysiology in patients with persistent problems

57

April Chiu, Wayne Tam, Doug Cines and James B Bussel

Introduction

Immune thrombocytopenic purpura (ITP) is a 'simple' auto-antibody-mediated disease, which, nonetheless, has a complex pathophysiology and clinical course. Although ITP is known to be caused by (auto) anti-platelet antibodies, the aetiology of the autoimmune disease remains mysterious. Numerous immunological studies have not yet clarified why certain people create anti-platelet antibodies and develop ITP, whereas the great majority do not. Among patients who develop ITP, certain patients have more benign courses, whereas others develop refractory life-threatening bleeding. Clearly, ITP is heterogeneous but the factors that underlie this heterogeneity are not well understood.

New studies have re-evaluated the role of splenectomy. Novel treatments have been tested in ITP at an increasing rate. The most exciting ones include rituximab (anti-CD20), anti-CD40 ligand (anti-CD154), thrombopoietin mimetics and autologous bone marrow transplantation. Other treatments are also being evaluated and the appropriate ordering of standard treatments is being revised.

Clinical presentation

ITP is an autoimmune disorder in which platelet sensitization by autoantibodies takes place, leading to destruction of opsonized platelets, primarily by the mononuclear phagocytic system. The clinical presentation differs somewhat between pediatric and adult patient populations. ITP in children is commonly associated with a preceding viral infection, and often follows an acute course in which the initially severe thrombocytopenia develops 'overnight' (based upon the sudden occurrence of symptoms), but often resolves spontaneously within 1–2 months.

On the other hand, ITP in adults usually occurs without an obvious inciting event and typically progresses to chronic disease associated with moderate to severe bleeding. Some adults with ITP have an acute presentation resembling that of children, whereas in some series approximately 50% are asymptomatic and diagnosed with low counts on a routine visit to a physician that is not directly connected with bleeding signs or symptoms. Regardless of the type of presentation, otherwise classical ITP in adults occasionally occurs as a so-called secondary event. This means that it presents in association with other conditions, such as lymphoproliferative disorders, especially chronic lymphocytic leukaemia or Hodgkin's disease, common variable immunodeficiency, HIV or other infection, or systemic autoimmune disorders such as autoimmune haemolytic anaemia (Evans' syndrome) or systemic lupus erythematosus.

Whether primary or secondary, patients with platelet counts persistently less than 10 000–20 000/μL are susceptible to intracranial haemorrhage and other major bleeding, although fortunately the incidence of serious haemorrhage is rare. The risk of a major bleeding episode is related to a number of factors, most of which have not been defined, but patients with persistently low counts are the ones at highest risk. Treatment plans for patients with ITP take into account the patient's age, disease severity and anticipated clinical course. In this report, the pathology and pathophysiology of ITP and the treatment modalities available at present for patients with ITP will be discussed.

Pathophysiological features

Platelet antibodies

As clearly demonstrated many years ago, initially by plasma infusion studies by Harrington, later Shulman and subsequently by McMillan and colleagues, the thrombocytopenia in ITP is mediated by anti-platelet antibodies (at least in the great majority of cases). The spleen plays a crucial role in the pathogenesis of ITP, in that it is not only a major site of platelet destruction, but also possibly the site where platelet sensitization is initiated and therefore also a major source of anti-platelet antibody production. In most instances, the anti-platelet antibodies are autoantibodies directed against the platelet-specific glycoproteins (GP). Studies by van Leuwen *et al.* demonstrated that eluates from platelets of 32 of 42 patients with ITP would bind to normal platelets but not to thrombasthenic platelets deficient in glycoprotein (GP) IIb–IIIa. In other cases, the antibodies may be generated against viral protein antigens that are cross-reactive against platelet antigens, as is the case for HIV infection. More recent studies have identified multiple targets of anti-platelet antibodies, i.e. to GPIIb–IIIa, Ib–IX and Ia–IIa and patients have antibodies to several of these targets. This is suggestive of epitope and/or determinant spreading and may be a result of platelet destruction with perhaps only one or none of these antibodies responsible for initiating the destruction. Finally it is uncertain how often ITP may be the result not of antibodies but rather of T cells directed against platelets and/or megakaryocytes.

CD5+ B cells have been implicated in the pathogenesis of many human autoimmune diseases and Mizutani and colleagues observed that B cells bearing the CD5 antigen are markedly increased in peripheral blood and spleen in ITP patients. However, a recent study by Hou and colleagues noted that the increase of splenic CD5+ B cells in ITP patients was not statistically significant. Moreover, both CD5+ and CD5– B cells from four out of eight ITP patients produced immunoglobulin (IgG) autoantibodies against both GPIIb–IIIa and GPIb.

Several reports have suggested that anti-platelet antibodies in some cases of ITP are clonally derived based on immunoglobulin light-chain restriction, either by using flow cytometric analysis or by DNA analysis for immunoglobulin heavy- and light-chain rearrangement. In one study, 10 out of 11 ITP patients had a clonal B cell population. However, whether these B cells are involved in autoantibody production was not shown.

More recently, Roark and colleagues demonstrated that at least some anti-platelet autoantibodies result from rearrangements of a single Ig heavy-chain variable region gene, V_H3–30. Interestingly, V_H3–30 has been found to be expanded or pathogenetic-

ally involved in several other disorders seemingly unrelated to but known to be associated with ITP, for example autoimmune haemolytic anaemia, systemic lupus erythematosus (SLE), chronic lymphocytic leukaemia (CLL), common variable immunodeficiency (CVID) and HIV infection. These authors concluded that the autoantibodies directed against platelets arise from clonal expansion of B cells upon encountering the diverse platelet antigens, which lead to Ig gene rearrangements using specific combination of heavy- and light-chain gene products.

Fc receptors

Antibody-coated platelets are rapidly cleared from the circulation via Fc receptors of macrophages in the splenic cords and elsewhere, which bind to the Fc portions of the IgG molecules. Studies of intravenous immunoglobulin (IVIg) showed that 'FcR blockade' was an important mechanism of steroid and especially IVIg effect in patients with ITP. There are a number of Fc receptors that have different properties and cell distributions. Several recent studies of the FcR system may have important clinical implications if confirmed and/or extended to humans. Two studies in mice have suggested that the ability of IVIg to slow the clearance of opsonized platelets is mediated by upregulation of FcRIIb, the inhibitory FcR, whereas anti-D appears to act by blocking FcRIIA. This is compatible with previous studies of FcR in patients, i.e. the use of a monoclonal anti-FcRIII antibody, because certain patients responded to it but not to IVIg and vice versa.

A technical issue preventing definitive study of this potential mechanism in humans has been the inability to distinguish FcRIIa from FcRIIb by monoclonal antibodies. Simultaneously, there has been a focus on polymorphisms of FcR, i.e. FcRIIa and FcRIIIa, suggesting that they may be involved in response to treatment with intravenous anti-D and rituximab respectively. The role of these FcRs in the course of ITP itself, as estimated by the frequency of the polymorphisms, is less clear. Several studies of these polymorphisms do not reach the same conclusions, i.e. that one form is increased in children who develop chronic disease or is increased in patients with ITP compared with normal control subjects. Similarly, past studies of HLA have been largely inconclusive outside of more inbred (Japanese) populations.

Pathology

Grossly, the spleen is typically of normal size or only mildly enlarged, usually weighing less than 200 g. The histological appearance is highly variable, ranging from completely normal to showing varying degrees of hyperplasia of malpighian corpuscles with germinal centre formation (Table 57.1). Frequently, plasmacytosis is also seen in the red pulp and marginal zones. Platelets in varying degrees of degeneration can usually be demonstrated trapped in the cords of Billroth, imparting a

Table 57.1 Inherited thrombocytopenias.

WAS/XLT: small platelets, poor platelet function

VWIIB: platelet clumping on smear, varying platelet counts exacerbated by pregnancy and other stresses

May–Hegglin: large platelets, Döhle-like bodies in neutrophils (other forms of MYH9 syndromes may have hearing loss, cataracts, and renal disease)

Bernard–Soulier syndrome: epistaxis, very large platelets

Congenital amegakaryocytic thrombocytopenia: no characteristic anomalies; *c-mpl* mutation in most patients, may progress to aplastic anaemia, diagnosis usually before the age of 2 years

granular or 'dirty' appearance. Platelet sequestration and phagocytosis can be demonstrated clearly using touch preparations and electron microscopy. Another characteristic finding is collections of foamy histiocytes in the red pulp as well as in the marginal zone. These collections of histiocytes, detected in 23–67% of splenectomy specimens are the result of platelet phagocytosis and contain partially degraded membrane-derived phospholipids and diverse platelet antigens, for example CD41. The white pulp in such patients treated with steroids shows diminished to absent germinal center formation.

Bone marrow

Bone marrow biopsies from patients with ITP show normal to increased numbers of megakaryocytes diffusely dispersed throughout the marrow space. The mean ploidy (endomitotic index) of ITP megakaryocytes is more variable than the megakaryocytes from normal individuals. In patients whose ITP arises in the context of HIV infection, both pyknotic and dyspoietic megakaryocytes may be seen including the so-called 'naked' megakaryocyte nuclei, which are devoid of cytoplasm. The aetiology of the 'naked' megakaryocytes is unknown.

Platelet lifespan

The increased number of megakaryocytes in the marrow and the evidence of platelet destruction in the spleen as well as the studies demonstrating platelet antibodies lead to the assumption that platelets were synthesized at an increased rate. The presumption was that the antibodies resulted in a very increased rate of platelet destruction. This was supported by numerous studies of allogeneic platelets labelled by ^{59}Cr, all of which demonstrated very short platelet lifespans. The ability of ^{111}In to label autologous platelets resulted in several studies demonstrating that platelet lifespans were surprisingly long, implying that platelet turnover (both destruction and production) was much less than had been assumed. More recently, antibodies that impair megakaryocyte development *in vitro* have been iden-

tified, consistent with the finding of partially impaired platelet production in a substantial subset of patients with ITP.

Overall, it is unclear how many patients with ITP, and which ones, are not making platelets well. Specifically, it is not known whether the patients who are particularly difficult to treat are the ones with the most reduced platelet production. It is believed that virtually all licensed treatments slow platelet destruction. It is also possible that some of these treatments increase effective marrow platelet production.

Multiple studies of ITP have shown that thrombopoietin (Tpo) levels in patients are essentially the same as those measured in normal individuals. This is in contrast to the 10–20-fold increase in Tpo levels seen in amegakaryocytic states. This suggests that thrombopoietin may be a clinically effective treatment of ITP because platelet production could be further augmented; the first study of a thrombopoietin mimetic agent has confirmed that this appears to be a useful approach.

Diagnosis

Is a bone marrow examination required?

Until recently, bone marrow examination was routinely performed in both children and adults who were suspected of having ITP, to exclude the diagnosis of leukaemia or other clonal or infiltrative processes. Bone marrows were also performed to exclude hypoplastic or aplastic states. Several studies support the infrequency with which leukaemia is diagnosed in a healthy child with isolated thrombocytopenia and an otherwise typical presentation (normal haemoglobin, white count, smear and normal physical examination except for signs of haemorrhage). A retrospective analysis of several thousand patients entered in paediatric leukaemia studies identified no patients who presented with isolated thrombocytopenia in the absence of hepatosplenomegaly or adenopathy.

In another study, none of over 100 children who met the 'ASH Guidelines definition' of ITP and in whom a bone marrow was performed had the diagnosis changed to leukaemia; only one child was diagnosed with aplastic anaemia. In contrast, seven incidences of aplastic anaemia and seven of leukaemia were seen in > 100 children with thrombocytopenia in the context of other abnormalities of the complete blood count or the examination. Similar but less extensive experience in adults has led to several practice guidelines that recommend that bone marrow examination may be reserved for patients who are unresponsive to therapy, those over 60 years of age or those in whom splenectomy is considered. In the more elderly, the exclusion of myelodysplastic syndrome (MDS) presenting with isolated thrombocytopenia becomes an important consideration. In one retrospective study of 1539 cases of MDS, 1% of patients presented with isolated thrombocytopenia. Several of these patients were misdiagnosed as having ITP, all of whom were 50 years of age or older and lacked significant splenomegaly.

Therefore, in children and adults, a presumptive diagnosis of ITP can generally be made without a bone marrow examination in a patient with isolated thrombocytopenia without an underlying disorder, and with a normal physical examination.

Is platelet antibody testing required?

Studies of ITP have failed to demonstrate any form of available testing that is both sensitive and specific in distinguishing patients with ITP from those with other types of thrombocytopenia. Thus, the clinical utility of measuring serum or platelet-eluate immunoglobulin is unproven in the diagnosis or treatment of ITP or in predicting its clinical course. Consequently, the diagnosis of ITP remains clinical and is one of exclusion. Probably the most specific test to confirm the diagnosis of autoimmune thrombocytopenia (primary or secondary) is response to IVIg or anti-D, especially if dramatic and repeated.

Differential diagnosis in children and adults

The diagnosis of ITP should be considered in all patients who are otherwise well but present with petechiae, bleeding or bruising. If a complete blood count (CBC) reveals an isolated thrombocytopenia, with a normal haemoglobin, white blood cell count, peripheral blood smear and a physical examination notable only for bleeding, they are likely to have ITP. As indicated above, too many patients with causes of thrombocytopenia other than ITP have positive platelet antibody tests for these to be included in the decision-making process. Secondary causes of ITP should be considered when circumstances warrant. For example, SLE should be considered in the setting of a butterfly rash and signs or symptoms of arthritis and common variable immunodeficiency (CVID, hypogammaglobulinaemia) if there are recurrent infections, especially pneumonia. In the absence of such signs or symptoms, routine serological and other testing for these conditions is not indicated (see discussion of the utility of bone marrow examination and platelet antibody testing above).

The most common alternative diagnosis in the paediatric population is familial thrombocytopenia (see Table 57.1). These conditions are discussed in Chapter 58 on p. 950. Important considerations concerning the diagnosis of ITP include: (i) Bernard Soulier syndrome and the MYH9 group have 'too large' platelets on smears; (ii) Wiskott–Aldrich exists in the X-linked thrombocytopenia form in which the immune deficiency is minimized but the platelets are still small; (iii) platelet clumping on a smear should create suspicion of von Willebrand type IIB; and (iv) in the authors' experience, if two or more first degree relatives in a family have 'ITP', an inherited thrombocytopenia is more likely than are two cases of ITP (Table 57.2).

In adults, the differential diagnosis also includes familial thrombocytopenias but more common secondary causes include

Table 57.2 Features consistent with non-immune thrombocytopenia.

All syndromes
Family history
Lack of response to standard ITP therapy, i.e. steroids, IVIg, i.v. anti-D, splenectomy
Platelet appearance on smear (too large, too small or clumping)
Clinical suspicion that platelet function is more impaired than expected for ITP at that platelet count
Persistent, consistent thrombocytopenia without much variability in the platelet count

HIV infection, lymphoproliferative disorders such as CLL, SLE and hepatitis B or C. Less commonly, patients may have CVI, sarcoidosis or Gaucher's disease. Hypothyroidism, i.e. Hashimoto disease, is common in women and is more commonly found in women with ITP than in age- and sex-matched control subjects. Its prognostic significance for ITP is uncertain. Recently, an association between ITP and the presence of *Helicobacter pylori* has been established in some series, but not in others. The reason for this discrepancy has not been resolved, and no consensus has been reached as to the role of testing for and treatment of *H. pylori* in patients with ITP. Similarly, the role of hepatitis C in the aetiology and persistence of ITP is unclear.

Management of acute immune thrombocytopenic purpura

The initial treatment of children presenting with acute ITP remains a topic of considerable debate, with both strong proponents and opponents of treatment. Randomized controlled trials demonstrate that the platelet count can be bought into the 'safe' level more rapidly in children treated with corticosteroids, IVIg or 'high-dose' i.v. anti-D than in those in whom a watchful waiting approach is taken, and acute intracranial haemorrhage rarely occurs at platelet counts above 10 000/μL. On the other hand, over 70–80% of cases of ITP in children will resolve spontaneously, with haemostatic platelet counts often attained within weeks, and the risk of acute intracranial haemorrhage is exceedingly low (0.1–1.0%).

There is no formal evidence that the incidence of this rare event is lessened by treatment and therapy is often inconvenient, expensive, and, in the case of high-dose corticosteroids, often accompanied by adverse effects, i.e. in mood and behaviour. There are also considerable inaccuracies in the enumeration of platelets when the count falls below 10 000/μL. Treatment is certainly indicated for the unusual situation in which a child presents with serious bleeding or even with signs of bleeding beyond petechiae and ecchymoses, i.e. wet purpura, those with co-existent bleeding risks like head trauma and perhaps for those at high risk of trauma due to behavioural or other disturbances. In some areas, inaccessibility to medical care becomes a factor as well.

On the other hand, all would agree that pauci-symptomatic children with platelet counts above 20 000/µL can be observed in all but the most unusual circumstances. Differing opinions concern whether therapy is required in any or all children who present with otherwise typical, but profound thrombocytopenia (<10–20 000/µL) without extensive petechiae and ecchymoses, haematuria or haematochezia, or 'wet' purpura. Our opinion is that it is safer to treat these children. However, we recognize that other experts may prefer observation in this setting. There is a clear need for larger and longer observational studies to determine whether there are subsets of children (e.g. adolescents) who appear to be at greater risk for bleeding soon after presentation. Clearly, the prognosis of ITP in association with auto-immune haemolytic anaemia (AIHA), HIV or other associated disorders typically requires treatment, one closer to the one generally employed in the management of adults.

The treatment of adults with acute ITP differs from the treatment of children in several important respects. In adults, ITP rarely remits spontaneously within days to weeks and co-morbid risks for bleeding are far more common than in children. Moreover, a greater percentage of adults than children (30%) fail to respond to the typical initial forms of therapy, necessitating the introduction of alternative modes of therapy. Nevertheless, the same issues of when to treat the asymptomatic adult and whether the platelet count is a useful surrogate marker of morbidity occur commonly, often because of failure or intolerance of standard treatment. As the natural history of adult ITP, the incidence of haemorrhage and the adverse effects of therapy have been somewhat clarified over the past several years, the 'threshold' platelet for treating adults with ITP has fallen, with most experienced haematologists choosing not to treat the average-risk patient whose platelet count exceeds 30 000/µL.

Paediatrics

Patients receiving treatment generally initially receive one of the following: prednisolone at 1–4 mg/kg per day; i.v. Ig at 400–1000 mg/kg; i.v. steroids such as methylprednisolone at 5–30 mg/kg; and i.v. anti-D at 75 µg/kg. If prednisolone is used and there is a response, it is rapidly tapered (1–4 weeks). The i.v. medications are followed with initially weekly counts and are repeated as needed for a platelet count < 20 000/µL. If a treatment is administered and symptoms continue or worsen then a combination of the three i.v. treatments indicated above (MP, IgG and anti-D) should be administered together to avoid a potentially significant risk of intracranial haemorrhage (ICH). Vincristine can be added (0.03 mg/kg up to 1–1.5 mg) if there is no response or if there is great concern regarding the risk of bleeding.

Adults

Treatment in adults is generally initiated with prednisolone in a dose of 1–2 mg/kg per day and the drug is continued until the platelet count exceeds 50 000/µL or the patient fails to respond by 3–4 weeks. Those with more clinically severe presentations and those intolerant of corticosteroids are generally treated with IVIg of 1 g/kg per day for 2 days or i.v. anti-D (if Rh$^+$) at a dose of 75 µg/kg per day with similar outcomes. Recently, a one-armed study of adults treated with high-dose dexamethasone (10 mg per day for 4 days per month) showed an initial response of > 75% with durable remissions in 40–50%. This long-term outcome is similar to what has been seen in patients treated with anti-D and is only somewhat higher than the 10–30% reported long-term outcome in patients initially treated with corticosteroids in traditional doses. It may be no different from the outcome in those who did not require therapy at all. In emergency situations, patients should be treated with platelet transfusions for ongoing bleeding or headache or head trauma, and also with high doses of methylprednisolone (1 g per day for 1–3 days), i.v. anti-D, IVIg as above, with or without vincristine 1–1.5 mg i.v. push. When these agents are combined together in groups of three, or using all four together at the same time, they may be remarkably effective even in refractory patients. Furthermore, these treatments may serve to protect transfused platelets allowing them to achieve greater haemostatic efficacy. In all patients, general measures to reduce the risk of bleeding should be taken, including control of hypertension, cessation of drugs that interfere with platelet function, hormonal treatment of severe menorrhagia, etc.

Therapy with corticosteroids is generally associated with moderate toxicity including (acutely) mood alteration, difficulty sleeping, hypertension, gastritis and hyperglycaemia. This necessitates dose reduction as soon as practicable, which is usually accompanied by a fall in the platelet count, although not to pre-treatment levels in all patients. Common side-effects associated with IVIg include headaches and fever–chill reactions, in addition to its high cost and the inconvenience of long-term (4- to 6-hour) i.v. administration, especially if it is needed repetitively. Therefore, IVIg treatment is discontinued once a haemostatic platelet count has been obtained and reliance is placed on corticosteroids thereafter. Anti-D is generally better tolerated and it is administered more rapidly than IVIg (in minutes); rare cases of intravascular haemolysis have been reported and very occasionally there is significant extravascular haemolysis i.e. 2–4 g/dL decrease in haemoglobin.

Steroids are believed to impair destruction of platelets by inhibiting the interaction of the IgG-coated platelets with the Fc receptors of splenic macrophages. Over the longer term, steroids may also suppress anti-platelet autoantibody production. IVIg works acutely by reducing the rate of phagocytosis of opsonized platelets. Recent work suggests that the mechanism of this effect in mice is mediated by upregulation of the inhibitory FcRgIIIb receptor and also that saturation of FcRn may accelerate clearance of auto-anti-platelet antibody. In contrast, anti-D in ITP appears to inhibit clearance of opsonized platelets by FcRIIa and FcRIIIa, although changes in cytokine expression and reactive oxygen species appear to be involved in the longer responses.

Management of chronic immune thrombocytopenic purpura

Paediatrics

Management of chronic ITP in children (> 6 months duration) usually involves repeated administration of one of three agents: steroids, IVIg or i.v. anti-D. The goal is to give the child time to improve spontaneously. Splenectomy is deferred until at least 1 year from diagnosis in a child > 5 years of age, unless there are very special circumstances; these are most common in adolescents in whom maintenance treatment is problematic either because of poor response or poor compliance. Long-term 'high-dose' steroids are to be avoided. Splenectomy is avoided if at all possible in a child < 5 years of age even if this requires maintenance therapy for a number of years. Azathioprin at 2 mg/kg is an option; it seems to have little toxicity and is typically given at bedtime to avoid any nausea. Danazol is avoided until after puberty because of the adverse effects on growth (reduction of final height). Rituximab is increasingly used, despite few data in children, because of its potential for lasting responses and apparently little toxicity. Children who fail to respond to splenectomy are fortunately very rare and treatment should be guided by the experience in adults.

Adults

There is little consensus on the appropriate duration of therapy with any of these agents, either with respect to attempting to induce a more durable remission or with respect to defining failure. Patients who fail to respond or who show poor response to single-agent therapy may show synergistic effects with combined therapy. This approach also permits the dose of each individual agent to be reduced with attendant lessening of their generally non-overlapping side-effects. Occasional patients can be maintained on low daily or alternative-day doses of prednisolone, but most cannot at a dose low enough to be feasible. Multiple modalities have been introduced as alternatives to corticosteroids or as adjunctive therapy to permit a lower and more tolerable dose to be employed.

Approximately 10–20% of adults with ITP are truly refractory to initial management and remain symptomatic or with platelet counts below 20 000/μL; a similar percentage will maintain platelet counts over 50 000/μL even when therapy is discontinued and they will require no additional treatment. A very few of these individuals will require additional treatment because

the antibody has induced a qualitative bleeding disorder. The majority of adults respond to one or a combination of these agents to a greater or lesser extent, but require persistent treatment, often with unpleasant or unsafe side-effects, to maintain their platelet count in the range of 20 000–50 000/μL; it is this population where the decision to proceed with splenectomy must be entertained. This decision is predicated on severity of thrombocytopenia and bleeding, side-effects of treatment, fitness for surgery, patient lifestyle (compliance with treatment, risk of trauma) and patient preference. A bone marrow evaluation should be made (if not recently performed) in all individuals with a suboptimal response to ITP-directed therapy, especially before splenectomy. Evolution to overt MDS or marrow aplasia is sometimes evident on repeat examination.

There is no generally available method to predict response to splenectomy, although finding a predominantly hepatic clearance of radiolabelled platelets may augur poorly. In general, approximately 85% of young adults and a somewhat lower proportion of older adults will have an initial haemostatic response to splenectomy, in which about two-thirds of the initial group will be durable. Responses to laparascopic and open surgical splenectomies appear similar, as do the complication rates, including the need for later accessory splenectomy; the laparoscopic procedure facilitates post-operative recovery (in experienced hands) (see Chapter 23).

There is a low risk of anaesthetic complications in appropriately chosen patients and the risk of post-operative bleeding is sufficiently low, even at very low platelet counts, such that prophylactic platelet transfusions should generally not be employed. The major risk of splenectomy is that of the overwhelming sepsis syndrome, which approximates 1% over a lifetime in all patients who are undergoing splenectomy. Patients should be immunized preoperatively and re-immunized at appropriate intervals post-operatively with polyvalent pneumococcal vaccine, *Haemophilus influenzae* flu vaccine and, in susceptible populations (military, immunosuppressed), with meningococcal vaccine. All patients who have undergone splenectomy should receive immediate medical care that includes prompt introduction of appropriate i.v. antibiotics at the first sign of a systemic febrile illness until a suitable diagnosis is established. Travel to regions where malaria, babesia and other organisms are cleared in the spleen requires special consideration.

Management of refractory immune thrombocytopenic purpura

If a patient is 'refractory', i.e. undergoes and does not respond to splenectomy, it is important to do a careful re-evaluation of the diagnosis including possibly a bone marrow examination and/ or other testing. The most consistent use of the term refractory ITP involves the patient who has undergone but not responded to splenectomy. This is considered to be a more serious disease, especially when patients have platelet counts persistently below 20 000 μL and bleeding symptoms. As a result of this persistent, severe thrombocytopenia, these patients have a high rate of serious bleeding, including, but not limited to, intracranial haemorrhage. No matter what treatments are attempted, their ITP typically persists. Morbidity and mortality rates are increased fourfold compared with the general population. Azathioprin, danazol and oral cyclophosphamide, each have at best a 30% response rate in truly refractory patients. In addition, these patients may not respond to IVIg, and anti-D works substantially less well after splenectomy. Note that we are specifically not dealing with treatments that have not yet been published in peer-reviewed literature.

If there is an urgent need to increase the platelet count then combination treatment (as discussed above) can be used. Treatments that may be highly effective at increasing the platelet count in difficult patients involve combinations of IVIg, i.v. methylprednisolone, and either or both i.v. anti-D and vincristine. In 35 patients, 24 adults and 11 children, approximately three-quarters responded with an acute platelet increase to these combinations despite the patients being completely refractory to IVIg and/or steroids given individually. Even if this combination is highly effective, its effects will be short-lived, i.e. 1–3 weeks, and it is important to anticipate that a more lasting treatment effect will be needed (see below).

Therefore, agents are used in combination; this approach has not been adequately pursued. In order not to use two immunosuppressive agents, we combine danazol with azathioprin. The advantages of these agents are that they have relatively low toxicity and have extensive usage in ITP. The disadvantage is that neither is a very potent agent and therefore they may not work in certain circumstances. There are a number of studies using cyclophosphamide alone, either orally or, especially, intravenously. This latter usage follows the treatment of nephritis in SLE, when it is given at a dose of 500–1000 mg/m^2 once every 4 weeks. In more extensive usage, cyclophosphamide has been combined with steroids, vincristine and other agents. The best documented combination ITP chemotherapy with patients was published in 1993 by Macmillan and Figueroa. A recent letter confirmed that although the protocol was effective in only one-half of the very difficult patients in whom it was tried, apparently almost all of the patients who responded had a durable effect. Some have advocated a hormonal approach combining provera, danazol and possibly other related agents.

A number of very small trials had been performed with other agents with inconclusive results. Experimental therapies to some extent share this characteristic. In the case of rituximab, there are now more than five publications in ITP including a recent study of 57 patients. In this study, there is approximately a 50% response rate with the major advantage being durability; one-third achieved a lasting response of > 1 year's duration at the time of data analysis. As in other studies, i.e. of anti-CD40 ligand, patients whose duration of ITP is > 15 years are poorer

responders. In the studies cited, non-splenectomized patients do as well as splenectomized patients but, surprisingly, not better. The treatment of non-splenectomized patients usually reflects treatment of patients who are earlier in their disease and more susceptible to curative effects. In these cases, its advantage may be the ability to create a lasting response so that no treatment is required for at least 6–12 months, if not indefinitely. It does not appear that rituximab is as effective in the 'worst' patients who have failed splenectomy and multiple therapies.

Anti-CD40 ligand has also been effective in some refractory patients, however it is no longer in clinical trial.

Other agents include mycophenolate mofetil and cyclosporine. Both have had limited efficacy in difficult patients; these agents may be more promising when used as part of combination treatment rather than singly.

Thrombopoietin (Tpo) and Tpo mimetics have been effective in a small number of patients treated to date. This is consistent with the known physiology, i.e. relatively low levels despite severe thrombocytopenia in ITP. Furthermore, in refractory patients especially, it is suspected that there is a lack of accelerated platelet production. Even in the studies that demonstrated accelerated or even normal platelet production in ITP, the overall rate of increase has only been two- or threefold, suggesting that it could be further increased. Given the treatments that had been described earlier, which block opsonized platelet destruction, the addition of Tpo might substantially increase the platelet count in those patients capable of producing platelets. As it would appear that the hard-core group that is the most difficult to treat may be those who are not making platelets, Tpo might be especially useful. An abstract reporting on a thrombopoietic peptide drug has confirmed substantial short-term efficacy of this approach in refractory patients. Further trials are in progress.

Finally, bone marrow transplantation has been attempted in up to 16 patients in one series at the National Institutes of Health. The complications are not surprising but are daunting. These include sepsis in many of the patients, considerable amounts of IVIg and platelet transfusions required for line insertions, and the use of high-dose cyclophosphamide. However, at least two of the responders are in stable remission more than 24 months following transplant and approximately one-half of the patients with Evans' syndrome responded. Therefore, one can be guardedly optimistic about the results.

In summary, there are a number of novel therapies being explored in refractory ITP. There is increasing knowledge of pathophysiology, including a very recent study suggesting that cytotoxic T cells may be important in certain patients. As biological treatments are being developed for and explored in B-cell lymphomas, at this moment the number of novel treatments that could be tested has outstripped the ability to do the studies. The possibility of combination treatments, which clearly will be superior to single agents as discussed above, is staggering and should be the next era of exploration.

Selected bibliography

Bauer S, Khan A, Klein A et al. (1992) Naked megakaryocyte nuclei as an indicator of human immunodeficiency virus infection. *Archives of Pathological Laboratory Medicine* 116: 1025.

British Committee for Standards in Haematology General Haematology Task Force (2003) Guidelines for the investigation and management of idiopathic thrombocytopenic purpura in adults, children and in pregnancy. *British Journal of Haematology* 120: 574–96.

Bussel JB, Graziano JN, Kimberly RP et al. (1991) Intravenous anti-D treatment of immune thrombocytopenic purpura: analysis of efficacy, toxicity, and mechanism of effect. *Blood* 77: 1884.

Chadburn A (2000) The spleen: anatomy and anatomical function. *Seminars in Hematology* 37: 13.

Chang CS, Li CY, Cha SS (1993) Chronic idiopathic thrombocytopenic purpura. Splenic pathologic features and their clinical correlation. *Archives of Pathological Laboratory Medicine* 117: 981.

De Shields MS, Martin SE (1991) Abnormal megakaryocytes in thrombocytopenia associated with HIV-1 infection. *American Journal of Hematology* 37: 215.

Figueroa M, Gehlsen J, Hammond D et al. (1993) Combination chemotherapy in refractory immune thrombocytopenic purpura. *New England Journal of Medicine* 328: 1226–9.

George JN, Raskob GE (1998) Idiopathic thrombocytopenic purpura: A concise summary of the pathophysiology and diagnosis in children and adults. *Seminars in Hematology* 35: 5.

George JN, Raskob GE (1998) Idiopathic thrombocytopenic purpura: diagnosis and management. *American Journal of Medical Science* 316: 87.

George JN, Woolf SH, Raskob GE et al. (1996) Idiopathic thrombocytopenic purpura: a practice guideline developed by explicit methods for the American Society of Hematology. *Blood* 88: 3.

Gernsheimer T, Stratton J, Ballem PJ et al. (1989) Mechanisms of response to treatment in autoimmune thrombocytopenic purpura. *New England Journal of Medicine* 320: 974.

Hayes MM, Jacobs P, Wood L et al. Splenic pathology in immune thrombocytopenia. *Journal of Clinical Pathology* 38: 985.

He R, Reid DM, Jones CE et al. (1994) Spectrum of Ig classes, specificities, and titers of serum antiglycoproteins in chronic idiopathic thrombocytopenic purpura. *Blood* 83: 1024.

Karpatkin S (1997) Autoimmune (idiopathic) thrombocytopenic purpura. *Lancet* 349: 1531.

McMillan R (2000) The pathogenesis of chronic immune (idiopathic) thrombocytopenic purpura. *Seminars in Hematology* 37 (Suppl.): 5–9.

McMillan R, Wang L, Tomer A, Nichol J, Pistillo J (2004) Suppression of *in vitro* megakaryocyte production by antiplatelet autoantibodies from adult patients with chronic ITP. *Blood* 103: 1364–9.

Mizutani H, Furubayashi T, Kashiwagi H et al. (1991) B cells expressing CD5 antigen are markedly increased in peripheral blood and spleen lymphocytes from patients with immune thrombocytopenic purpura. *British Journal of Haematology* 78: 474–9.

Portielje JE, Westendorp RG, Kluin-Nelemans HC et al. (2001) Morbidity and mortality in adults with idiopathic thrombocytopenic purpura. *Blood* 97: 2549.

Provan D, Newland A (2002) Fifty years of idiopathic thrombocytopenic purpura (ITP): management of refractory ITP in adults. *British Journal of Haematology* 118: 933–44.

Roark JH, Bussel JB, Cines DB, Siegel DL (2002) Genetic analysis of autoantibodies in idiopathic thrombocytopenic purpura reveals evidence of clonal expansion and somatic mutation. *Blood* 100: 1388–98.

Samuelsson A, Towers TL, Ravetch JV (2001) Anti-inflammatory activity of IVIG mediated through the inhibitory Fc receptor. *Science* 291: 484–6.

Thiele J, von Ammers E, Wagner S et al. (1991) Megakaryocytopoiesis in idiopathic thrombocytopenic purpura: a morphometric and immunohistochemical study on bone marrow biopsies with special emphasis on precursor cells. *Hematological Pathology* 5: 75.

Wadenvik H, Stockelberg D, Hou M (1998) Platelet proteins as autoantibody targets in idiopathic thrombocytopenic purpura. *Acta Paediatrica* 424: 26–36.

Ware RE, Zimmerman SA (1998) Anti-D: mechanisms of action. *Seminars in Hematology* 35: 14.

Winiarski J (1998) Mechanisms in childhood idiopathic thrombocytopenic purpura (ITP). *Acta Paediatrica* 424: 54–6.

Zimmerman SA, Malinoski FJ, Ware RE (1998) Immunologic effects of anti-D (WinRho-SD) in children with immune thrombocytopenic purpura. *American Journal of Hematology* 57: 131.

Atherothrombosis, thrombolysis and anti-platelets

58

Lucinda KM Summers, Stephen P Marso and Peter J Grant

Introduction

The term atherothrombosis describes the formation of thrombus on atheromatous plaques within the high-pressure arterial circulation. Atherothrombosis is the pathological process underlying the development of cardiovascular disease (CVD), a systemic condition. Coronary heart disease (CHD), peripheral vascular disease (PVD) and cerebrovascular disease are all manifestations of CVD, the commonest cause of death in the Western world. This spectrum of diseases includes type 2 diabetes.

Epidemiology

Mortality rates from CVD in Western countries increased steadily during the last century until the 1960s and 1970s, when they began to decline substantially. However, CVD mortality continues to increase in Eastern Europe and in certain subgroups of people in the rest of Europe and the USA. There is also evidence that the incidence of CVD in the USA has not declined, rather that it is the case fatality rate that has declined. This has resulted in an increased prevalence of CVD, with associated increased disability and health-care costs.

Geographical and ethnic variations

There are considerable geographical and ethnic variations in the incidence of CVD. In Europe, the risk of myocardial infarction (MI) increases from south to north and from east to west. These variations are only partly explained by different preventative practices. In the USA, black people have the highest rates of CHD. Non-Hispanic white people also have relatively high CHD mor-

tality rates, whereas Hispanics, Native Americans and Asians have lower rates. Stroke mortality rates are also strikingly higher in black people, whereas Hispanics and Native Americans have the lowest stroke rates. On the other hand, in the UK South Asians have increased rates of CHD compared with other ethnic groups. These variations in the incidence of CVD are partly explained by the prevalence of insulin resistance and diabetes in different ethnic groups. However, most of the variability remains to be explained.

Aetiology and pathophysiology

The inflammatory process in the arterial wall

For some years, it has been proposed that atherosclerosis is a chronic inflammatory process. In the arterial wall, the endothelial inflammatory response is mediated by macrophages (derived from circulating monocytes) and specific subtypes of T lymphocytes. These T lymphocytes recognize antigens expressed by activated macrophages and, in response, generate cytokines that amplify the inflammatory process. If this inflammatory response does not remove or neutralize the offending agents, the process continues, with eventual thickening of the arterial wall as outlined below. Circulating inflammatory markers, for example C-reactive protein, fibrinogen and cytokines, increase in concentration when this inflammatory process is extensive and continues for a long period of time.

Endothelial dysfunction

Endothelial denudation has been proposed as the initial step in the development of atherosclerosis, as part of 'the

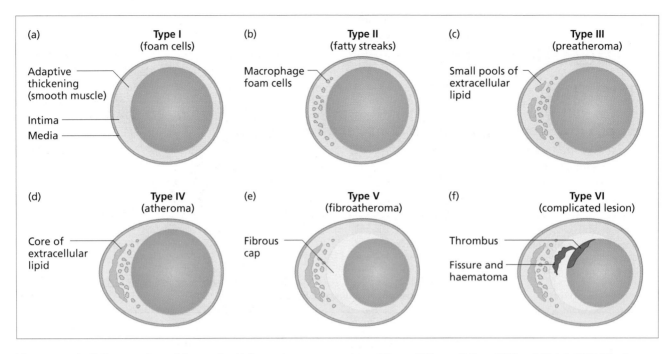

Figure 58.1 (a–f) Cross-sections of the proximal left anterior descending coronary artery, showing the development of an atheromatous lesion (adapted from *Atherosclerosis and Coronary Artery Disease*, V Fuster, R Ross, EJ Topol, Vol. 1, 1996, Lippincott Williams and Wilkins, Philidelphia).

response-to-injury hypothesis'. More recently, it has been suggested that endothelial dysfunction, rather than denudation, leads to the development of atherosclerotic lesions. Whichever mechanism is responsible, there is a resultant increase in the permeability of the arterial wall to blood constituents, including low-density lipoproteins (LDL). Platelets and monocytes adhere to areas of damage on the arterial wall and release growth factors which, in turn, promote the migration and proliferation of intimal smooth muscle cells.

Endothelial dysfunction is associated with impaired endothelium-dependent relaxation, resulting from perturbations in the synthesis, release or action of vasoactive substances produced by endothelial cells, including nitric oxide, endothelins and prostacyclin. Endothelial function is impaired in dyslipidaemia, type 2 diabetes, type 1 diabetes, hypertension and obesity.

Formation of atheroma

The formation of atheroma is a very slow process and the atherosclerotic lesion is classified histologically into six types. Figure 58.1 shows the process by which an atheromatous lesion develops, and Figure 58.2 shows a post-mortem section of a coronary artery occluded by atheroma.

Type 1 (Figure 58.1a)

'Foam cells' form at sites prone to the development of atherosclerotic lesions. Such sites exist from birth, owing to the varying

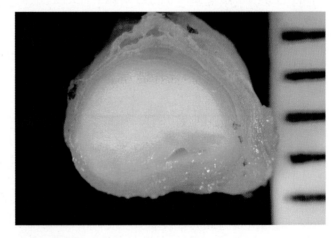

Figure 58.2 Post-mortem section of a left anterior descending coronary artery occluded by atheroma (courtesy of Dr L Davidson).

intima media thickness in different sections of the arteries. At arterial bifurcations, the arterial wall tends to be thickened in a focal and eccentric (crescent-like) manner, whereas, in other arteries, for example main coronary branches, diffuse thickening is seen. Foam cells can be visualized within the arterial wall intima using lipophilic stains, such as Sudan III and IV. They consist of macrophages and, to a lesser extent, smooth muscle cells containing small intracellular lipid collections. Multiple layers of foam cells eventually form fatty streaks.

Type II (Figure 58.1b)

Fatty streaks, the earliest manifestations of atheromatous disease detectable on gross pathological examination, can be found in the aorta and coronary arteries of children as young as 2 years old. They are especially prevalent in those with a genetic predisposition to CVD; a family history of CVD or features of the insulin-resistant syndrome. There is a slow progression to intermediate and then advanced lesions, with formation of a fibrous cap that seals off the lesion from the lumen. Within the lesion, there is a collection of debris containing accumulated leucocytes and lipid. This core may become necrotic, whereas the lesion itself continues to expand as leucocytes continue to adhere and enter. The internal necrosis can result in lipid leaking out of the foam cell.

Type III (Figure 58.1c)

Eventually, there is a massive accumulation of extracellular lipid, disrupting the continuity of the intima smooth muscle cells. This stage is known as 'pre-atheroma', as although these lesions are associated with marked thickening of the arterial wall, there is no interference with blood flow. To a certain extent, there is compensatory gradual dilatation of the arterial wall, ensuring that the lumen is unaffected. This process is known as remodelling and it has been estimated that functionally important lumen stenosis may be delayed until the atherosclerotic plaque occupies up to 40% of the internal elastic lamina area.

Type IV (Figure 58.1d)

'Atheroma' is derived from the coalescence of extracellular lipid, resulting from macrophage necrosis, to form a large lipid core. This lipid centre contains a few isolated smooth muscle cells with macrophages in the periphery of the lipid material. Atheroma is not usually present before puberty.

Type V (Figure 58.1e)

A more advanced lesion, 'fibroatheroma', is covered on the luminal side by a fibrous cap formed by smooth muscle cells within a dense extracellular matrix. This matrix contains collagen and capillaries. In regions where new blood vessels are forming within the lesion, microscopic haemorrhages are sometimes seen. Some type V lesions are largely calcified (type Vb), whereas others are made up chiefly of fibrous connective tissue and contain little or no lipid or calcium (type Vc). Type V lesions are usually detected in the third decade.

Type VI (Figure 58.1f)

The 'complicated lesion' is an unstable lesion, which can be complicated by erosion or rupture of the fibrous cap, intraplaque haemorrhage or formation of superficial thrombus. Such lesions may significantly impair blood flow and produce clinical symptoms and signs of ischaemia: angina, MI, transient ischaemic attacks, stroke, intermittent claudication and PVD.

Thrombotic occlusion

It was originally believed that occlusive lesions in coronary arteries begin with fatty streaks in the arterial wall, gradually developing into stenotic coronary artery lesions that are composed largely of lipids. However, stenoses of less than 50% were found to be responsible for MIs in several studies. These lesions would previously have been termed 'non-severe' compared with 'severe' lesions causing greater than 70% stenosis. As a result of these findings, it is now thought that complete occlusion occurs as a result of the frequent rupture of minimally stenotic lipid-rich plaques in the coronary artery wall with resultant thrombosis playing a major role in coronary artery occlusion. The coagulation and fibrinolysis systems involved in regulating these processes are discussed in detail in Chapter 46.

When a plaque in an arterial wall ruptures, collagen and other constituents of the vessel wall are exposed to blood, leading to platelet adherence. Tissue factor (cell surface protein) is released simultaneously from damaged cells. Tissue factor activates the intrinsic and extrinsic coagulation systems, leading to thrombin generation. Thrombin, in turn, activates platelets and cleaves fibrinogen to form soluble fibrin. Platelet activation and the activation of coagulation factors VIII, V and XI by thrombin further increase thrombin generation, thereby amplifying the coagulation process. The crucial final step of the coagulation cascade, the production of insoluble fibrin (Figure 58.3), resistant to physical and chemical insults, is achieved by covalent cross-linking of the fibrin(ogen) γ- and α-chains mediated by factor XIIIa, a proglutaminase. Thus, a fibrin clot is formed on the surface of the ruptured plaque in the wall of the affected artery.

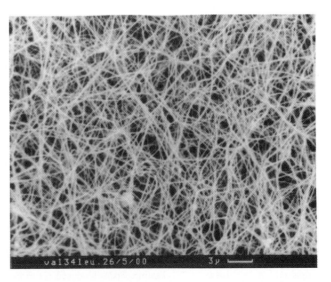

Figure 58.3 Fibrin clot in the absence of platelets, visualized using scanning electron microscopy (courtesy of Dr A Atwa).

At the same time, plasmin is degrading the fibrin that is being formed. Tissue plasminogen activator (tPA) and urinary-type plasminogen activator (uPA) regulate the conversion of plasminogen to plasmin. Plasminogen, plasmin and tPA bind to cross-linked fibrin and these reactions can then occur without interference from plasminogen activator inhibitor-1 (PAI-1), the major inhibitor of fibrinolysis. Activation of fibrin-bound plasminogen by tPA is increased by the polymerization of fibrin. The resultant fibrin degradation reveals new binding sites for plasminogen, increasing the rate of fibrinolysis. In the circulation, tPA and uPA are rapidly inactivated by PAI-1, which is present in excess. This ensures that fibrinolysis is localized to the site of thrombus formation and systemic fibrino(geno)lysis does not occur. PAI-1 is released on the platelet surface when platelets are stimulated by thrombin, preventing immediate clot lysis. Endothelial cells exposed to thrombin also synthesize PAI-1, causing a rapid local increase in PAI-1 concentration. The relative activities of the coagulation and fibrinolytic systems regulate fibrin clot formation and lysis and its effect on blood flow through the affected artery.

Risk factors for atherothrombosis

The major risk factors for atherothrombosis are shown in Table 58.1. Many of these risk factors are found in association in insulin-resistant individuals and the effects of insulin resistance (IR) on endothelial function, formation of atheroma and effects on the coagulation system are discussed.

Insulin resistance and diabetes

Insulin resistance (IR) has been defined as a state (of a cell, tissue, system or body) in which greater than normal amounts of insulin are required to elicit a quantitatively normal response. IR is said to be present when the ability of insulin to stimulate the uptake and disposal of glucose is impaired. It is common in obesity and type 2 diabetes, but can also manifest as impaired fasting glucose or impaired glucose tolerance. The diagnostic criteria for these conditions are given in Table 58.2. It has been estimated that approximately 25% of the apparently healthy population have IR similar to that of type 2 diabetes. IR combined

Non-modifiable	Modifiable	'Emerging'/putative
Age	Smoking	Homocysteine
Male gender/oestrogen deficiency	Diabetes	Fibrinogen
Family history	Hypertension	Factor VII
	Diet/exercise	vWF
	'Atherogenic' lipid profile*	Factor XIIa
		Factor XIII
		tPA
		PAI-1
		C-reactive protein

Table 58.1 Risk factors for atherothrombosis.

*Small dense LDL, cholesterol-depleted HDL, excess chylomicron remnants and IDL. PAI-1, plasminogen activator inhibitor-1; tPA, tissue plasminogen activator; vWF, von Willebrand factor.

Condition	Criteria
Type 2 diabetes	*With symptoms of diabetes*: random venous plasma glucose ≥ 11.1 mmol/L *or* fasting plasma glucose ≥ 7.0 mmol/L *Without symptoms of diabetes*: two plasma glucose results in the diabetic range on different days *or* 2-h plasma glucose concentration ≥ 11.1 mmol/L 2 h after 75-g oral glucose tolerance test
Impaired glucose tolerance	Fasting plasma glucose > 7.0 mmol/L and ≥ 7.8 mmol/l but < 11.1 mmol/L 2 h after 75-g oral glucose tolerance test
Impaired fasting glucose	Fasting plasma glucose ≥ 6.1 mmol/L but < 7.0 mmol/L; oral glucose tolerance test recommended to confirm diagnosis

Table 58.2 Diagnostic criteria for type 2 diabetes, impaired glucose tolerance and impaired fasting glucose.

with compensatory hyperinsulinaemia predisposes an individual to the development of a cluster of abnormalities, including glucose intolerance, increased plasma triglyceride concentrations, decreased high-density lipoprotein (HDL)–cholesterol, smaller denser LDL particles, hypertension, hyperuricaemia and increased PAI-1 concentrations. It has become apparent over the last decade that this group of metabolic abnormalities ('syndrome X' or the 'insulin resistance syndrome') is a major risk factor for CHD.

Patients with IR make up a large proportion of patients presenting with an acute MI. In a recent study of patients with acute MI who were not previously diagnosed with diabetes, up to 40% and 25% were found to have impaired glucose tolerance and type 2 diabetes respectively. Both type 1 and type 2 diabetes are associated with greater progression of CHD and a higher CHD-related mortality rate. Cardiovascular disease is responsible for about 70% of deaths in diabetic patients and, in the UK, a large proportion of the inpatient budget spent on diabetes relates to the management of cardiovascular disease. The management of cardiovascular risk factors in patients with IR and diabetes, therefore, represents a major challenge.

CHD was the major cause of death in men with diabetes in the Multiple Risk Factor Intervention Trial (MRFIT) and was responsible for approximately 40% of deaths over a 16-year period. The risk of death from CHD in diabetic men was three times greater than that in non-diabetic men, even after adjustment for risk factors such as cigarette smoking, age, race, income, systolic blood pressure and cholesterol concentration. Cigarette smoking, systolic blood pressure and cholesterol concentration were predictors of coronary artery disease (CAD) mortality for all participants, but the absolute risk of death from CAD increased more steeply with each risk factor for men with diabetes. These findings underline the importance of risk factor clustering in the pathogenesis of MI and the increased vascular risk in diabetic patients. Approximately 85% of people with type 2 diabetes are insulin resistant and these individuals tend to have this cluster of atherothrombotic risk factors. It is important, therefore, to have an understanding of the complexity of vascular risk and the implications for its prevention and management, rather than a purely glucocentric view of the pathogenesis of macrovascular disease in diabetes. Atherothrombotic risk factors that cluster together to form the insulin resistant syndrome, including changes to platelets, coagulation and fibrinolytic pathways, are discussed.

Coagulation and platelets

Over the past 20 years increased concentrations of various coagulation factors, including fibrinogen, factor VII and von Willebrand factor (vWF), as well as the antifibrinolytic protein, PAI-1, have been linked with CHD. Increased concentrations of tPA are associated with increased risk of MI, although this seems counterintuitive. Factor XIIa concentrations are also related to previous MI and the extent of coronary atheroma on angiogram.

Fibrinogen, factor VII, von Willebrand factor (vWF) and PAI-1 are associated with IR. *In vitro* studies show that insulin, very low-density lipoprotein (VLDL)-triglyceride and non-esterified fatty acids synergistically increase PAI-1 expression by human hepatoma cells There is also evidence of a genotype-specific interaction, with triglyceride regulating PAI-1 concentrations. Therefore, the combination of increased concentrations of fibrinogen, factor VII, factor XII and PAI-1 interacting with factors such as smoking, increased body mass and physical inactivity leads to a cluster of pro-atherothrombotic factors.

Platelets are essential for effective haemostasis and their structure and function are discussed in detail in Chapter 47. In patients with type 2 diabetes, platelets adhere to the vascular endothelium and aggregate more easily than in people without diabetes. In health, prostacyclin and nitric oxide combine to prevent the adherence of platelets to the normal endothelium, as well as preventing platelet aggregation. At physiological concentrations, insulin shows anti-aggregatory properties (effects mediated by prostacyclin and nitric oxide). Insulin increases endothelial production of nitric oxide and prostacyclin and increases platelet sensitivity to prostacyclin. The major defect in platelet function in type 2 diabetes is a loss of sensitivity to prostacyclin and nitric oxide, which may be due to changes in the activity and expression of G-proteins. Lean diabetic subjects have normal insulin anti-aggregatory responses, although this is not true of obese diabetic subjects. This implies that loss of sensitivity to nitric oxide in platelets is another feature of IR.

vWF, a glycoprotein (GP) constituent of the factor VIII complex, is found in increased concentrations in the plasma of type 2 diabetic patients. It is released by endothelium and causes platelet clumping by binding to platelet GPIb–IX and IIb–IIIa. GPIb is a receptor for vWF, as well as acting as a substrate for thrombin, whereas GPIIb–IIIa is a receptor for fibrinogen and other adhesive proteins involved in platelet aggregation. Diabetic patients have increased numbers of GPIb and GPIIb–IIIa complexes on the surface of their platelets and this may explain the increased platelet adherence seen in type 2 diabetes.

Insulin

In vitro, insulin has effects on smooth muscle proliferation, lipid metabolism, and hepatic PAI-1 synthesis and secretion, whereas insulin has been shown *in vivo* to have effects on renal sodium handling, nitric oxide expression and blood flow. Hyperinsulinaemia can be expected, therefore, to have major effects on the processes involved in atherothrombosis.

Insulin dilates isolated rat skeletal muscle arterioles in an endothelium-dependent manner, mediated by nitric oxide. *In vivo*, insulin-mediated vasodilatation is also dependent on endothelium-derived nitric oxide and it is therefore likely that insulin-mediated vasodilatation of skeletal muscle vasculature occurs due to increased nitric oxide synthesis and release. There is resistance to the effect of insulin on enhancement of endothelium-dependent vasodilatation and resultant endothelial dysfunction in obese and insulin-resistant human subjects. Endothelium-dependent relaxation is decreased and there is a generalized loss of vascular compliance. In patients with type 2 diabetes associated with a combined hyperlipidaemia, this may partly reflect insudation of plasma lipids into the arterial wall.

Hyperglycaemia

Hyperglycaemia leads to the accelerated formation of advanced glycation end-products (AGEs), which cross-link vascular proteins, causing thickening and leakage of the vasculature. This results from AGE forming irreversible abnormal deposits in the subintimal layers of blood vessels, interfering with cellular interactions and generating toxic reactive oxygen species. The receptor for AGE (RAGE) is expressed by vascular endothelial and smooth muscle cells, macrophages, monocytes, cardiac myocytes, neuronal and mesangial cells and mediates some of these effects; vascular endothelial dysfunction can be induced by injection of AGE in animal studies, and RAGE antibodies or the truncated domain, soluble RAGE, reverse this effect. The AGE–RAGE interaction in the endothelium leads to upregulation of procoagulant and adhesive proteins, including PAI-1, tissue factor and vascular cell adhesion molecule-1 (VCAM-1).

VCAM-1 is expressed on the endothelium in atherosclerotic plaques and causes increased monocyte adhesion. Chemotaxis at sites of AGE accumulation recruits monocytes expressing RAGE, where they infiltrate the subendothelium to form foam cells. Animal studies show that RAGE expression is upregulated in the aorta and heart of diabetic as compared with non-diabetic rats. This has also been shown in arterial atherosclerotic tissue from diabetic subjects.

There are other RAGE ligands apart from AGE, including extracellular-newly identified RAGE binding protein (EN-RAGE). EN-RAGE is one of the S100 proteins. Other members of this family are found in atherosclerotic plaques and have chemoattractant effects on mononuclear phagocytes. EN-RAGE interacts with RAGE to induce tumour necrosis factor a, VCAM-1 and interleukin 1 expression on endothelial cells, mononuclear phagocytes and lymphocytes. There are known to be several polymorphisms in the RAGE gene and one of these, a Gly82Ser polymorphism, affects a residue within the AGE binding site. Variants of the RAGE gene affect the cytokine cascade, causing inflammation, and this may lead to the development of vascular disease.

Dyslipidaemia

Dyslipidaemia is a major risk factor for CVD. Patients with primary hypercholesterolaemia have greatly increased LDL cholesterol and develop extensive atherosclerosis early in life, leading to death before the age of 30 years without treatment. LDL is thought to be important in the pathogenesis of atherothrombosis, with endothelial dysfunction allowing LDL to enter the arterial wall, become progressively oxidized and initiating the inflammatory response. Macrophages phagocytose LDL via scavenger receptors on their surfaces and start the process of atheroma formation.

Hypertriglyceridaemia is also associated with a high risk of CVD, especially CHD, in prospective and epidemiological studies. Postprandial hypertriglyceridaemia may be particularly important due to the generation of an 'atherogenic lipid profile' consisting of small, dense LDL, increased concentrations of remnant particles and lipid-depleted HDL.

Hypertension

Hypertension is a major cardiovascular risk factor. Lowering blood pressure decreases the risk of CVD. The formation of hydrogen peroxide and free radicals is increased in patients with hypertension, which inactivates basal endothelial nitric oxide production in canine basilar arteries and increases monocyte adhesion in vitro. Hypertensive patients frequently have increased plasma concentrations of angiotensin II, the main product of the renin–angiotensin system and a potent vasoconstrictor. Angiotensin II stimulates smooth muscle cell proliferation and increases protein synthesis, eventually leading to smooth muscle hypertrophy.

Hyperhomocysteinaemia

An increased concentration of the sulphur-containing amino acid homocysteine in plasma is associated with thrombosis. The pathogenetic mechanisms underlying this have not been well defined, although there are claims for prothrombotic effects on coagulation and its inhibitors, fibrinolysis, platelets and vascular endothelium. Whatever the mechanisms, hyperhomocysteinaemia is a risk factor for CVD, CAD, PVD and deep vein thrombosis (DVT). Elevated levels result from genetic or nutritional disturbance of the trans-sulphuration or remethylation pathways for homocysteine metabolism (Figure 58.4). It is of note that the coenzymes for the three enzymes involved are dependent on adequate levels of vitamin B_6, cobalamin and folate. Deficiency of any of these vitamins can cause hyperhomocysteinaemia. The commonest genetic cause of hyperhomocysteinaemia is inheritance of the thermolabile variant of 5,10-methylene tetrahydrofolate reductase, which is polymorphic in European populations. It has been reported to be present in excess in subjects with CAD and PVD. Heterozygosity for cystathione synthase deficiency may also be a risk factor for early-onset cardiovascular disease; homozygosity for cystathione synthase deficiency gives rise to the rare condition of homocystinuria in which Marfan-like features are accompanied by a severe generalized thrombotic tendency affecting both arterial and venous circulations.

As folate supplementation reduces plasma homocysteine concentrations, there is considerable research activity directed towards using this simple therapy to reduce cardiovascular risk. However, to date no clear reduction in arterial thrombotic event rates have been reported.

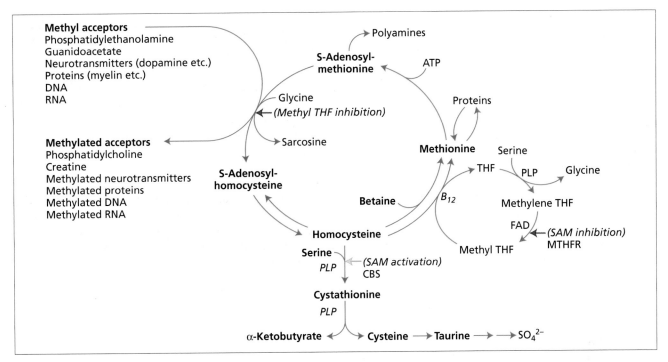

Figure 58.4 Homocysteine metabolic pathways. In the methylation pathway, homocysteine acquires a methyl group either from betaine or from 5-methyltetrahydrofolate. In the trans-sulphination pathway homocysteine condenses with serine to form cystathione in a reaction catalysed by CBS.

CBS: cystathione beta synthase; MTHFR: methylene tetrahydrofolate reductase; SAM: S-adenosyl methionine; PLP: pyridoxal 5′ phosphate; FAD: flavine adenine dinucleotide. B_{12} = methylcobalamin. Adapted from D'Angelo and Selhub (1997).

Genetic and environmental influences

Heritability studies

The relative contributions of environmental and genetic factors to the development of risk factors for CAD have been estimated in several studies. In the San Antonio Family Heart Study, heritabilities of fasting glucose and insulin concentrations were estimated as 18% and 35% respectively. A large twin study recently showed that genetic factors were responsible for between 41% and 75% of the variation in fibrinogen, factor VII, vWF, factor XIII A-subunit, factor XIII B-subunit and PAI-1 concentrations and 82% of the variation in factor XIII activity. Other family studies have estimated similar heritability for fibrinogen and a small twin study has found that up to 30% of the genetic variance of vWF can be attributed to the effect of blood group, those with blood group O having the lowest concentrations of vWF.

Genotype association studies

It is most unlikely that a single genetic polymorphism responsible for CAD will be identified. The results of studies detailed in the following section have been disappointing because most were too small to detect interactions between genetic polymorphisms and environmental changes. Although relationships between the gene and the protein and between the protein and the disease are found, frequently there is no relationship between the gene and the disease. This is explained by the fact that it is the quantitative contribution of heritability to the phenotype that determines the link between the gene and the disease. Larger studies are needed to investigate the links between genetic polymorphisms and acquired environmental risk factors.

Fibrinogen

There are conflicting findings about the effect of polymorphisms on fibrinogen concentration, with one study showing that the effect is negligible, and another that polymorphisms of the β-fibrinogen gene were associated with an increased concentration. The latter study and several others have described associations between various polymorphisms and CAD, although two large studies showing an association between genotype and fibrinogen concentration failed to find a relationship between genotype and disease. In a small study in people with type 2 diabetes, there was a higher prevalence of the G allele of the −455 G–A polymorphism in those with CAD. These conflicting findings are partly due to the fact that fibrinogen concentrations vary widely in populations because it is an acute-phase reactant.

Plasminogen activator inhibitor-1

Some studies report a negligible effect of PAI-1 genotype on PAI-1 concentrations, and it has been suggested that features of IR were the major determinant. However, homozygotes for the commonest polymorphism, a single basepair in the promoter region (4G/5G), have been described as having plasma PAI-1 concentrations that are increased by 25% compared with those who are homozygous for the 5G allele. There is evidence, from a study of subjects with type 2 diabetes, of a genotype-specific interaction with triglyceride. At a given concentration of triglyceride, subjects with the 4G/4G genotype had increased PAI-1 concentrations compared with those with the 5G/5G genotype. There is a VLDL response element in the promoter region of the PAI-1 gene adjacent to the 4G/5G site, which might explain these findings. VLDL causes HepG2 cells to release more PAI-1 antigen and activity, and insulin augments this effect.

von Willebrand factor

Only about 20% of the variability in concentration of vWF is accounted for by polymorphisms in the 3′-region. One study in people with type 1 diabetes and proliferative retinopathy has found an association between the Thr789Ala polymorphism and CAD.

Factor VII

Factor VII concentrations are related to two sites on the factor VII gene that are in linkage disequilibrium, a single base change at position R353Q in exon 8 and a promoter decanucleotide repeat. No relationship has been found between particular genotypes or FVII:C concentrations and the extent of atheroma, although certain factor VII genotypes may have a protective effect against MI. Dietary fat intake has been found to influence factor VII concentrations and there is a relationship with triglyceride concentrations.

Factor XIII

The effect of genetic polymorphisms on factor XIII and its role in fibrin clot formation is reviewed in Ariens *et al.* (2002). A common polymorphism, Val34Leu, in the factor XIII A-subunit has attracted interest as a potential risk factor for atherothrombosis. It has little effect on factor XIII concentration but accelerates factor XIII activation by thrombin, altering the structure of cross-linked fibrin. Because of this effect, the polymorphism may explain the high heritability of factor XIII activity. The factor XIII B-subunit merely acts as a carrier of the A-subunit. It has a lower heritability, and it has been estimated from a twin study that about 25% of the variance is explained by a common environmental influence.

Clinical features

Coronary heart disease

The clinical manifestations of CHD are angina, acute coronary syndromes (ACS), myocardial infarction (MI), heart failure and dysrhythmias.

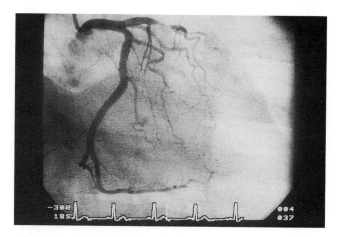

Figure 58.5 Coronary angiogram showing stenosis of the left anterior descending coronary artery (courtesy of Dr A Catto).

Angina and myocardial infarction may be painless, especially in people with diabetes. However, most patients complain of central, dull, crushing chest pain that may radiate to the jaw or down the left arm. This pain is often associated with shortness of breath. The patient with acute MI usually has more severe symptoms and feels sweaty and nauseated, often vomiting. Anginal symptoms are usually brought on by exercise and subside with rest. The typical electrocardiogram (ECG) changes of an acute MI are S–T segment elevation, followed within hours by T-wave inversion and then Q-wave formation. Intracellular enzymes are released into the circulation; the most commonly measured enzyme, creatine kinase (CK-MB), increases in concentration within hours and decreases again within 24–48 h. Troponin, a myofibrillar cardiac protein, also increases in concentration after a few hours and is increased for several days. About 25% of people who have an acute MI die before reaching hospital. Most of these will have suffered a dysrhythmia, commonly ventricular fibrillation, and death will have occurred instantaneously or within the first hour.

In a patient with anginal symptoms, exercise testing or ambulatory monitoring may show ischaemic electrocardiographic changes. In the absence of obvious angina, myocardial isotope perfusion scanning can be used to identify reversible cardiac ischaemia. Coronary angiography reveals the presence of stenosis in the coronary arteries (Figure 58.5) and decisions can then be made on appropriate management, either with bypass surgery, coronary artery angioplasty or stenting, or with drug therapy. The drug treatments for those diagnosed as having an acute S–T segment elevation MI (STEMI) or ACS is discussed later in this chapter.

Heart failure can occur in the absence of overt CHD, particularly in diabetes, but is usually secondary to atherosclerosis. Left ventricular failure presents with shortness of breath on exercise, orthopnoea and paroxysmal dyspnoea, whereas right-sided failure presents with peripheral oedema.

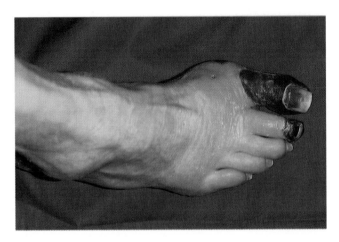

Figure 58.6 The ischaemic right foot of a diabetic man with peripheral vascular disease. The first toe and distal second phalanx are gangrenous (courtesy of Dr C Amery).

Peripheral vascular disease

PVD often presents as intermittent claudication; patients complain of pain in the back of the calf on walking, which is relieved by rest. Pedal pulses will usually be absent or diminished on the affected side and Doppler ultrasound can be used to confirm the diagnosis. Angiography is used to locate stenosis and determine whether management should be interventional (arterial bypass, angioplasty or stenting) or with drug therapy. Severe PVD, often in people with diabetes or smokers, can lead to ischaemia and amputation of digits or lower limbs (Figure 58.6).

Cerebrovascular disease

Cerebrovascular disease is manifested by transient ischaemic attacks, stroke and multi-infarct dementia. A stroke characteristically presents with the abrupt onset of hemiplegia, dysphasia,

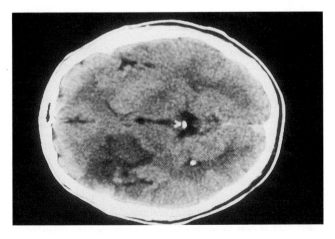

Figure 58.7 Computerized tomographic scan showing a recent extensive right frontotemporal infarct (courtesy of Dr A Catto).

sensory impairments, visual field defects or cerebellar dysfunction. The symptoms and signs depend on the artery occluded and the region of brain that consequently infarcts. Transient ischaemic attacks present in the same manner but resolution occurs within 24 h, often lasting only a few minutes or 1–2 h at the most. Computerized tomography scanning of the head will reveal an area of infarction (Figure 58.7) in a patient with a stroke, but may be normal in a patient with a transient ischaemic attack. In some units, acute ischaemic stroke is treated with immediate thrombolysis, but, at the time of writing, this is not standard practice throughout the UK. Aspirin is usually started once the diagnosis is confirmed. If subsequent investigations reveal carotid arterial stenosis, endarterectomy may be performed once the patient has recovered from the acute event.

Management of cardiovascular disease

Table 58.3 lists the factors that should be assessed in all patients, especially those with existing CVD. In the UK, patients with no evidence of CVD should be assessed using the Joint British Societies Coronary Risk Prediction Chart (British Cardiac Society, British Hyperlipidaemia Association, British Hypertension Society, endorsed by the British Diabetic Association 1998). Once a risk assessment has been performed, appropriate therapy can be commenced. Standard primary and secondary preventative drug treatments are presented in Table 58.4.

Anti-platelet drugs and fibrinolytic treatment

Ischaemic coronary syndromes have been previously classified as either unstable angina (UA), non-Q wave MI or Q-wave MI. The recent change in nomenclature to STEMI or ACS, defined as either UA or non-ST segment elevation MI (NSTEMI), has been a direct result of facilitating early diagnosis and risk stratification, and underscores the importance of rapid classification. At present, 1.83 million persons are admitted annually to US hospitals with an ischaemic coronary syndrome. Of these patients, 1.42 million are classified as having an ACS and 0.41 million are classified as STEMI. In addition to being a prevalent clinical entity, patients with an ACS or STEMI are at considerable risk for in-hospital mortality or a non-fatal MI within the first year of hospital discharge. This section focuses on the numerous classes of agents used to manage persons with ischaemic heart disease as well as other vascular syndromes.

A primary goal of therapy for patients with ACS NSTEMI is rapid diagnosis and risk-stratification as well as implementation of an appropriate medical and revascularization strategy. As seen in Figure 58.8, patients (defined by clinical presentation) and the therapeutic interventions they undergo have an associated risk. According to the recent American College of Cardiology Foundation and American Heart Association (ACC/AHA) 2002 Guidelines, it is imperative that a 12-lead ECG be obtained

Cardiovascular risk factors	Action
Smoking	Discuss willingness to stop smoking Refer to smoking cessation clinic Nicotine replacement therapy Amfebutamone (bupropion)
Weight/diet	Discuss current diet and willingness to change Refer to dietitian Orlistat Sibutramine Surgery, e.g. gastric bypass
Exercise	Discuss current exercise regimen Refer to local lifestyle clinic/gym/swimming pool
Lipid profile	Consider HMG CoA reductase inhibitor in inherited dyslipidaemias or if chol. $\geq$ 5 mmol/L*
Renal function	ACE inhibitor for patients with diabetes and microalbuminuria or proteinuria Consider HMG CoA reductase inhibitor and aspirin
Blood pressure	Treat if BP $\geq$ 160/100 or if > 140/90 with estimated 10-year risk of CHD $\geq$ 15%, CVD or diabetes[†] Aim for clinic BP $\leq$ 140/85 in non-diabetic patient BP $\leq$ 140/80 in diabetic patient or lower if microalbuminuria or proteinuria present Consider HMG CoA reductase inhibitor if systolic BP > 160 mmHg with/without diastolic > 100 mmHg
Glycaemic control	All patients with CVD should be screened for diabetes In those with diabetes, aim for HbA_{1c} < 6.5–7.5% Consider HMG CoA reductase inhibitor and aspirin

Table 58.3 Assessment of cardiovascular risk factors.

*Joint British recommendations on prevention of coronary heart disease in clinical practice (British Cardiac Society, British Hyperlipidaemia Association, British Hypertension Society, endorsed by the British Diabetic Association 1998). The target LDL-cholesterol recommended by Heart UK at present is $\leq$ 2.5 mmol/L, or, where this cannot be achieved, a reduction of at least one-third.
[†]British Hypertension Society guidelines.
ACE, angiotensin-converting enzyme; BP, blood pressure; CHD, coronary heart disease; chol., cholesterol; CVD, cardiovascular disease; HMG CoA, 3-hydroxy-3-methylglutaryl coenzyme A.

and definitively interpreted within 10 min of the clinical presentation. This is particularly important in patients presenting with STEMI, as rapid coronary revascularization has been shown to be associated with a marked improvement in cardiovascular survival. In addition to patient history, physical examination, ECG and biochemical markers (CK-MB and cardiac troponins) are commonly used to further stratify patients with both ACS and NSTEMI. Utilization of cardiac troponins increases the sensitivity for measuring myonecrosis such that many clinicians utilize the terms 'micro-infarction' or 'minor myocardial damage' to identify the clinical setting of an elevated cardiac troponin with a normal CK-MB and further risk-stratify patients. Biomarkers used less commonly at present include myoglobin and lactate dehydrogenase.

Immediately following diagnosis and risk assessment, an effective medical management strategy must be instituted in order to affect not only short-term survival and ischaemic events, but also to prevent long-term sequelae from ischaemic heart disease. Although anti-ischaemic agents are commonly employed early in the course of care for patients with acute ischaemic syndromes, the mainstay of early therapy for patients with ACS and STEMI are antithrombotic agents. For the course of this discussion,

Table 58.4 Primary and secondary prevention for CVD.

Treatment	Indication	Current Evidence (2003)
Lifestyle changes	General population	Regular exercise ↓ obesity, diabetes and subsequent CVD
	Obese	Weight loss of 10 kg ↓ mortality, angina, BP, lipids, ↓ HbA_{1c} in diabetes
	Impaired glucose tolerance	Weight loss and exercise delay onset of type 2 diabetes
	Smokers	Smoking cessation ↓ risk of CVD
	Post MI	'Mediterranean diet' ↓ CHD in people with a previous MI; n-3 PUFA supplements immediately post-MI ↓ death, non-fatal MI and stroke
HMG CoA reductase inhibitors	CHD risk of ≥ 30% over 10 years	Pravastatin and lovastatin ↓ CHD risk in people with hypercholesterolaemia; atorvastatin ↓ CHD risk in hypertensives with at least three other risk factors for CVD
	CVD or diabetes (chol. ≥ 4 mmol/L)[7]	Pravastatin ↓ CHD, stroke and mortality post MI or in people with angina; simvastatin ↓ CHD, stroke and mortality post MI, in people with angina, with CVD or diabetes
ACE inhibitors	CVD or diabetes and one risk factor for CVD	Ramipril ↓ incidence of stroke, MI and death from CVD
	Post MI	Early treatment with captopril or lisinopril ↓ mortality especially with previous MI or heart failure (enalapril within 24 h of acute MI did not improve survival)
	Post stroke	Perindopril ↓ risk of further stroke or any CVD events
β-Blockers	Heart failure	Bisoprolol ↓ survival in patients with stable heart failure
Metformin	Type 2 diabetes, BMI > 25 kg/m²	Metformin ↓ all-cause mortality and incidence of stroke
Insulin	Diabetes and acute MI	Intensive treatment with insulin and glucose infusions followed by intensive subcutaneous insulin regimens ↓ long-term mortality

BMI, body mass index; BP, blood pressure; CHD, coronary heart disease; chol., cholesterol; CVD, cardiovascular disease; HMG CoA reductase, 3-hydroxy-3-methylglutaryl coenzyme A; MI, myocardial infarction; PUFA, polyunsaturated fatty acids.

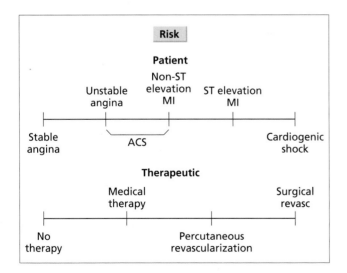

Figure 58.8 Continuum of clinical risk, defined by the patient's presenting clinical syndrome, as well as a continuum of therapeutic risk, defined as no therapy through to surgical revascularization. ACS, acute coronary syndrome; MI, myocardial infarction.

these agents can be divided into four broad categories: (i) oral anti-platelets (aspirin and thienopyridines); (ii) anticoagulants (heparins, warfarin and direct thrombin inhibitors); (iii) intravenous anti-platelet agents; and (iv) fibrinolytic agents. Other vascular indications for these agents will also be discussed.

Oral anti-platelet therapy

Aspirin and thienopyridines (ticlopidine and clopidogrel) are two oral anti-platelet agents commonly utilized for the prevention of and treatment for ischaemic heart disease and cerebrovascular disease.

Aspirin

Aspirin irreversibly inhibits cyclo-oxygenase-1 within platelets, thus preventing the formation of thromboxane A_2, resulting in decreased platelet aggregation. Although numerous studies have shown that aspirin has a robust impact on reduction of adverse cardiovascular events, it is a relatively weak anti-platelet agent. It has also been suggested that aspirin may have important anti-inflammatory effects resulting in additional anti-ischaemic properties. Four prospective randomized controlled trials have established the efficacy of aspirin in the setting of ACS patients. Pooled analysis from these four trials covered 2448 patients and demonstrated a significant reduction in the 30-day death or non-fatal MI rate for those patients randomized to aspirin therapy (6.4% versus 12.5%, $P = 0.0005$). Given the ease of administration, cost, and prompt bioavailability of a chewed aspirin, it is always indicated for people with suspected ACS or STEMI.

Numerous other studies on aspirin have demonstrated a significant reduction in vascular-related death, stroke and MI. Among a primary prevention cohort, there was a significant reduction in non-fatal MI but at the cost of increased stroke rates. Further, there is a significant reduction in the prevalence of deep venous thrombosis (DVT) and pulmonary embolism (PE) in postsurgical and high-risk medical patients.

Although data for aspirin use are unequivocal, several important issues remain. First, although frequently four 'baby' aspirin are chewed (rather than swallowed) by the patient in the accident and emergency department in order to decrease the time to onset of action, this strategy has never been studied in a prospective fashion. Second, the optimal dose of aspirin remains unknown. Trials of secondary prevention for stroke, MI, and death have not shown an added benefit for aspirin in doses either > 80 or 160 mg per day but have shown an increased tendency towards bleeding. As a direct result of the 2nd International Study of Infarct Survival (ISIS-2), either 160 mg or 325 mg are initially prescribed to suspected ACS patients who are not already receiving aspirin. Subsequent aspirin doses are often administered in the range of 75–325 mg per day (ISIS-2).

Limited data exist for the long-term efficacy of aspirin administration for patients following ACS. Secondary prevention studies have demonstrated benefit through the first two years of aspirin administration and a trend for benefit in the third year. At present, it is recommended that patients receive aspirin therapy indefinitely unless side-effects emerge. Contraindications for aspirin administration are listed in Table 58.5. Side-effects commonly seen with aspirin therapy are mainly gastrointestinal and include dyspepsia and nausea. Rarely, acute gout can be precipitated due to impaired urate excretion. It has been suggested that there is an adverse interaction with angiotensin-converting enzyme (ACE) inhibitors and aspirin therapy. It has been postulated that aspirin inhibits ACE inhibitor-induced prostaglandin synthesis, reducing its vasodilatory effects. However, this biochemical interaction does not appear to have an adverse effect on either drug in clinical practice.

Thienopyridines

Thienopyridines are commonly prescribed for patients presenting with ACS, following percutaneous coronary intervention (PCI) in patients with STEMI and for the secondary prevention of stroke, non-fatal MI and acute limb events. Both ticlopidine and clopidogrel are thienopyridine derivatives, pro-drugs and selective antagonists of adenosine diphosphate-induced platelet aggregation. Historically, ticlopidine was used for the secondary prevention of stroke, MI and subacute intracoronary stent thrombosis. There are limited data regarding the efficacy of ticlopidine in patients with ACS. A small, randomized controlled trial demonstrated a reduction in the rate of fatal and non-fatal MI at a 6-month follow-up.

At present, adverse effects of ticlopidine limit its use in clinical practice to patients who are intolerant of clopidogrel. The most worrying potential side-effects are severe neutropenia and thrombotic thrombocytopenic purpura (TTP). Severe neutropenia occurs in less than 1% of patients who are treated with ticlopidine, and life-threatening TTP is also extremely rare. However, patients receiving ticlopidine therapy for more than 2 weeks require a full blood count, including a differential white cell count every 2 weeks for the first few months of therapy. If it occurs, neutropenia usually resolves within 1–2 weeks following drug cessation. It does not appear that clopidogrel is associated with an increased risk of TTP relative to the general population. Thus, the use of ticlopidine has generally been supplanted with clopidogrel as the preferred thienopyridine. The initial indication for ticlopidine among patients with ischaemic heart disease was for the prevention of subacute thrombosis following placement of an intracoronary stent. It appears that clopidogrel is a reasonable alternative anti-platelet strategy for this indication.

The largest body of clinical evidence for the utilization of clopidogrel in patients with ACS originates from the Clopidogrel and Unstable angina to prevent Recurrent Events (CURE) trial. In this trial, 12 562 patients were randomized, within 24 h of presenting with an ACS, either to clopidogrel plus aspirin or aspirin alone. There was a 12-month rate of cardiovascular death, non-fatal MI or stroke of 9.3% for patients randomized to clopidogrel, compared with 11.5% for patients randomized to placebo (relative risk = 0.80, $P < 0.001$). Further, there was a consistent benefit across many subgroups of patients presenting with ACS, including those undergoing PCI. Given the results of CURE, clopidogrel is routinely used in many centres across the world in patients presenting with an ACS. It is recommended that clopidogrel is not administered until coronary anatomy has been defined and a revascularization strategy determined. If the patient is to be managed medically or undergo PCI, a loading dose of 300 mg of clopidogrel orally can be administered

Table 58.5 Contraindications to aspirin therapy.

Intolerance and allergy (manifested as asthma)
Active bleeding
Haemophilia
Active retinal bleeding
Severe untreated hypertension
Peptic ulcer
Other sources of GI or GU bleeding

GI, gastrointestinal; GU, genitourinary.

following coronary angiography or on the catheter laboratory table respectively.

However, universal utilization of clopidogrel in ACS patients has not occurred for two major reasons. First, CURE demonstrated increased bleeding in patients randomized to clopidogrel (placebo: 2.7%, clopidogrel: 3.7%; $P = 0.003$). The greatest risk for severe bleeding was seen in patients who underwent coronary artery bypass grafting (CABG) in the setting of ACS. Clopidogrel was often administered to patients prior to coronary angiography and therefore prior to any revascularization procedure. The peri-operative bleeding rates approached 10% if clopidogrel was not stopped 5 days prior to CABG. For this reason, some hesitation exists among the medical community for widely adopting early use of clopidogrel before determining whether or not CABG is warranted. Therefore, many physicians refrain from administering clopidogrel until after coronary angiography in the setting of ACS. Second, cost has been a major limitation for the widespread use of clopidogrel both in the UK and the USA.

Anticoagulants

Intravenous anticoagulation remains the mainstay for medical management of patients presenting with both ACS and STEMI. Intravenous anticoagulation has been utilized for nearly three decades to improve both short-term mortality and reduce recurrent ischaemic events. Historically, the sole agent available for management of patients with acute ischaemic syndromes has been unfractionated heparin (UFH).

Unfractionated heparin

Unfractionated heparin (UFH) is a heterogeneous mixture of heparin with molecular weights ranging from 5000 to 30 000 Da, it is highly bound and has a complex effect on the coagulation mechanism. Primarily, the major effect of heparin is interaction with antithrombin-III (AT-III), inhibiting thrombin generation. However, heparin is also a relatively weak inhibitor of factor Xa and the dose–response relationship is rather difficult to predict because of the variable strength from each heparin preparation. Additionally, there is variable binding of heparin to plasma proteins, endothelial cells and circulating macrophages, making the dose response less than predictable. The indications for heparin therapy are numerous and include treatment for pulmonary embolism, venous thrombosis, unstable angina (UA), non-ST segment elevation MI (NSTEMI), S–T segment elevation MI (STEMI) and acute peripheral arterial occlusion. It is also used for prevention of venous thromboembolism in high-risk cohorts (postsurgery and high-risk medical patients), prevention of thrombosis in extracorporeal systems (such as those used in haemodialysis or cardiovascular surgery involving mechanical prosthetic valves) and in patients with hypercoagulable syndromes.

The studies evaluating heparin efficacy in ACS patients were performed in a previous era of cardiology management strategies and were largely underpowered. Pooled data from four studies allowed comparison of 999 patients being treated with UFH plus aspirin compared with aspirin alone. Data from these trials demonstrated a reduction in 30-day death and non-fatal MI rates for UFH-treated patients (2.6% versus 5.5%, $P = 0.018$). This has resulted in the widespread use of UFH in ACS and STEMI patients. The UFH dosing recommendations at present for patients with ACS are a bolus infusion equal to 60–70 U/kg (maximum of 5000 U) intravenously followed by a continuous infusion of 12–13 U/kg/h (not to exceed 1000 U/h).

Low-molecular-weight heparins

Low-molecular-weight heparins (LMWHs) have emerged as a potential alternative to UFH as a result of its aforementioned limitations. There are numerous features of LMWHs that make them potentially superior agents compared with UFH. In a similar fashion to UFH, LMWHs inhibit platelet thrombus formation primarily through their effects on AT-III. In general, LMWHs have a mean molecular weight of 5000 Da, have a more potent anti-Xa:IIa effect, are less plasma protein bound, have a longer half-life (2–4 h versus 1 h for UFH), are significantly more bioavailable (> 90% compared with 30% for UFH), have a more predictable dose–response and undergo less neutralization by platelet factor IV and protamine. There is also a weaker inhibitory effect on platelet function and a less common association with heparin-induced thrombocytopenia. It is thought too that rebound ischaemia occurs less commonly with LMWHs than with UFH.

LMWHs, including dalteparin, nadroparin and enoxaparin, have been evaluated in numerous clinical settings in ACS patients. The two enoxaparin trials enrolled over 7000 patients and demonstrated a significant, 20% relative risk reduction in the composite endpoint of 14-day death, non-fatal MI or urgent revascularization. As a result, enoxaparin is now commonly utilized as an early and preferred anticoagulant in patients presenting with ACS. Additionally, economic analysis suggested a cost saving for those patients randomized to enoxaparin. Enoxaparin has also been shown effective in the setting of STEMI when coupled with a fibrinolytic agent.

Small, randomized, controlled trials have evaluated the combination of LMWH and GPIIb/IIIa inhibitors in the medical management of ACS patients. It appears that the rates of major bleeding, with the combination of LMWHs and GPIIb–IIIa inhibitors for these randomized controlled trials, remains relatively low at 0.3–1.8%. Additionally, there did not appear to be an additional risk of bleeding at the time of PCI.

Non-cardiac indications for heparin

Numerous other indications exist for the use of intravenous UFH. These include the treatment of venous thromboembolic disease. Intravenous or subcutaneous UFH is often used as prophylaxis for DVT and PE. Various clinical trials have shown that 5000 U subcutaneously every 8–12 h results in a 67% relative risk reduction for the formation of venous thrombosis and fatal PE. UFH is also used for the treatment of DVT and PE. Recommended dosing regimens for these include 5000 U intravenous bolus followed by a continuous intravenous infusion adjusted to maintain the activated partial thromboplastin time (APTT) in the therapeutic range. LMWHs have also been extensively studied for the prophylaxis and treatment of DVT and PE. A meta-analysis comparing LMWHs with UFH following elective hip surgery demonstrated a marked superiority of LMWHs for the prevention of proximal venous thrombosis and a reduction in major bleeding.

Complications of heparin therapy

Two complications of heparin therapy must be noted. First, heparin-induced thrombocytopenia (HIT) is not uncommon. It is mediated by the formation of an antibody to a neo-antigen on platelet factor IV (a platelet granule protein) that is exposed when it binds to heparin. This is an IgG-immune mediated process and results in paradoxical thrombosis as well as an unexplained decrease in the platelet count to less than 50%. It is diagnosed on the basis of both clinical and laboratory results. The platelet-activating properties of HIT serum or plasma in the presence of heparin can be measured with an activation assay. Antigen assays also exist for detecting antibodies, which recognize platelet factor IV bound to heparin. Treatment for HIT-associated thrombosis includes the use of danaparoid, lepirudin or argatroban. Warfarin therapy may also be utilized for long-term anticoagulation for limb gangrene in patients with HIT. It should be noted that both UFH and LMWHs can cause HIT, however, low-molecular weight preparations theoretically should lead to fewer occurrences of HIT.

A second potential side-effect of heparin treatment is heparin-induced osteoporosis. This most commonly occurs in pregnant women in whom systemic anticoagulation is indicated. Significant reduction in bone density has been documented in patients receiving heparin for 1 month or more. Small studies suggest that LMWHs may carry a lower risk of osteoporosis compared with UFH.

Warfarin is an oral anticoagulant that is commonly employed in numerous clinical settings. It is a racemic mixture of two optically active isomers, is highly bioavailable, is rapidly absorbed in the gastrointestinal tract, reaches peak blood concentrations 60–90 min after oral administration and has a half-life of 36–42 h. Warfarin is highly plasma protein bound, and the dose–response relationship is complex, unpredictable and determined by both genetic and environmental factors. Warfarin is a vitamin K antagonist and, thus, its anticoagulation effects are a result of inhibiting vitamin K-dependent coagulation factors including factors II, VII, IX and X. The variability in the anticoagulant response is described in detail elsewhere. In addition to numerous environmental factors, there are innumerable drug and food interactions with warfarin.

Warfarin has both antithrombotic and anticoagulant effects. Thus, it is indicated in numerous clinical settings. Warfarin therapy is frequently monitored by measuring the prothrombin time (PT). The PT is dependent on a response to reductions in the vitamin K-dependent procoagulant clotting factors (II, VII, IX and X) and is performed by adding both thromboplastin and calcium to citrated plasma. Thromboplastin is a phospholipid–protein extract that varies in its responsiveness to the anticoagulant effects and, thus, results in varying PT results. As a result of the varying anticoagulant effects of thromboplastin, PT results were non-standardized. Therefore, in 1977, the World Health Organization designated a reference preparation for human brain thromboplastin, allowing for a calibration model to be widely adopted in 1982, known as the international normalized ratio (INR). This is calculated using the following equation: $INR = (patient\ PT/mean\ normal\ PT)^{ISI}$, where ISI is the International Sensitivity Index for the thromboplastin used to perform the PT measurement at any given laboratory. Table 58.6 gives the suggested INR for the various indications for warfarin therapy.

Warfarin is effective in the prevention of venous thromboembolism following hip surgery and major gynaecological surgery. The INR is usually maintained between 2.0 and 3.0. For the treatment of a DVT, the duration of therapy is dependent on numerous clinical factors; however, it is indicated for no less than 3 months in patients with proximal DVT and no less than 6 months in those with PE. Indefinite oral anticoagulation therapy should be considered in patients with more than one episode of idiopathic DVT or PE, thrombosis related to malignancy, DVT associated with factor V Leiden genotype, antiphospholipid antibody syndrome or deficiencies in either protein C, AT-III or protein S.

There are mixed data with respect to the use of warfarin in primary prevention of ischaemic coronary events. Although the thrombosis prevention trial demonstrated effectiveness of the combination of low-intensity warfarin plus aspirin, both the Coumadin Aspirin Reinfarction Study (CARS) and the Stroke Prevention in Atrial Fibrillation III (SPAF-3) randomized clinical trial have shown no efficacy using warfarin in the prevention of primary ischaemic heart disease events. Warfarin administration following acute MI is controversial and clinical practice varies widely. Based on present literature, some physicians believe that it is reasonable to anticoagulate a person following a recent moderate to large anterior wall MI for a period of approximately 6 weeks to prevent further embolic events. However, there are a paucity of clinical data to support this or, indeed, the routine use of warfarin following acute MI. Warfarin is typically used in preventing thromboembolic events in patients with mechanical prosthetic heart valves. In fact, based on recent findings, it is common to treat patients with mechanical prosthetic heart valves with both warfarin and low-dose aspirin.

Based on recent guidelines, it is commonly thought that the newer bioprosthetic heart valves will require a lower INR. Additionally, warfarin is utilized frequently in patients with chronic or paroxysmal atrial fibrillation. Numerous studies have demonstrated the efficacy of this strategy. Pooled analysis of five large-scale clinical trials demonstrated a 69% reduction in ischaemic

Table 58.6 Recommended INR for different clinical indication.

Indications	Valve position	European Society for Cardiology (1995)	British Society for Haematology	AHA/ACC (1998)
Mechanical prosthetic valves				
First generation (Starr–Edwards, Björk–Shiley standard)		3.0–4.5	3.5	2.5–3.5*
Second generation (St Jude, Medtronic Hall)	Aortic	2.5–3.0	3.5	2.0–3.0
	Mitral	3.0–3.5	3.5	2.5–3.5
Third generation (Sorin Bicarbon bileaflet valve)	Aortic	2.5–3.0	3.5	2.0–3.0
	Mitral	2.5–3.0	3.5	2.5–3.5
Bioprosthestic valves in sinus rhythm (anticoagulation for first 3 months only)	Aortic	2.5–3.0	No anticoagulation	2.0–3.0
	Mitral	3.0–2.5	2.5	2.0–3.0
Bioprostheses in atrial fibrillation	Aortic	3.0–4.5	2.5	2.0–3.0
	Mitral	3.0–4.5		2.5–3.5

*INR = 2.0–3.0 in some centres.

In some centres, aspirin 80–100 mg per day is used for bioprosthetic valves in the aortic position, rather than warfarin.

An INR of 2.0–3.0 is recommended for prophylaxis or treatment of deep venous thrombosis or pulmonary embolus, and treatment of patients with thrombosis associated with antiphospholipid syndrome.

ACC, American College of Cardiology Foundation; AHA, American Heart Association; INR, International Normalized Ratio.

strokes for those patients with atrial fibrillation treated with warfarin. The recommended anticoagulation regimen for patients with atrial fibrillation is given in Table 58.7.

Direct thrombin inhibitors

Thrombin is thought to play a key role in the process of thrombus formation in patients with ACS. It plays a deterministic role

Table 58.7 Recommended antithrombotic therapy for patients with atrial fibrillation (Fuster *et al.*, 2001).

Clinical features	Recommended therapy
Age < 60 years, with structurally normal heart	Aspirin/no therapy
Age ≤ 60 years, with heart disease, low risk	Aspirin
Age ≥ 60 years, with diabetes or CHD	Warfarin
Age ≥ 75 years, high-risk features	Warfarin
Mitral stenosis, prosthetic heart valve, prithromboembolism, atrial thrombus on TOE	Warfarin (INR 2.5–3.5)

Note: The recommended aspirin dose varies around the world, High-risk factors = congestive heart failure, left ventricular ejection fraction < 35% or history of hypertension.
CHD, coronary heart disease; TOE, transoesophageal echocardiogram.

in the conversion of fibrinogen to fibrin, activation of platelets and recruiting additional platelets to the site of thrombus formation. As a result, agents that directly inhibit thrombin activity have been developed and studied extensively among patients with ACS and STEMI. Direct thrombin inhibitors are able to inhibit both circulating and tissue-bound thrombin and, thus, were thought to have theoretical benefit over both UFH and LMWHs. Additionally, direct thrombin inhibitors are not heavily protein bound, not inactivated by heparinases, have a predictable biological response and are potent *ex vivo* inhibitors of thrombus formation.

Although there was initial enthusiasm for direct thrombin inhibitors in preventing mortality and recurrent ischaemic events among patients presenting with IHD, trials performed to date have been disappointing. Several agents were developed and studied in various clinical settings, including argatroban, bivalirudin, efagatran and inogatran. Although bivalirudin has been extensively studied in various clinical settings, the prototype direct thrombin inhibitor is hirudin, as it is a potent near-irreversible inhibitor of thrombin. Its half-life is approximately 60 min and is renally excreted. Bivalirudin is a synthesized 20-amino-acid polypeptide, which forms a bivalent complex with thrombin, with a half-life of 20–25 min and is non-renally excreted.

Four large-scale randomized controlled trials have studied the efficacy of direct thrombin inhibitors in patients with ACS. None of these trials demonstrated a superiority of the direct thrombin inhibitor compared with heparin alone. Pooled analysis of these trials suggests that hirudin is superior to heparin for the prevention of death or non-fatal MI at the time of completion of the study drug infusion, but there appeared to be a diminished benefit of direct thrombin inhibitors at 30 days. Direct thrombin inhibitors have also been extensively investigated in STEMI patients. Pooled analysis from the STEMI trials included over nearly 10 000 patients and demonstrated no additional benefit in either the incidence of or non-fatal MI rate for those patients treated with a direct thrombin inhibitor compared with UFH.

Bivalirudin is being extensively evaluated in elective PCI patients in the REPLACE II trial. (Additional studies of bivalirudin are being planned at the moment for the management of ACS patients.) At present, direct thrombin inhibitors are the anticoagulant of choice among persons with a history of HIT. Furthermore, as additional data emerge with bivalirudin in the setting of elective PCI and ACS, this agent may become more readily used in clinical practice.

Intravenous anti-platelet agents

Glycoprotein IIb–IIIa inhibitors

The use of oral GPIIb–IIIa antagonists has not been shown to be beneficial among patients with CHD. In fact, a pooled analysis from four large-scale randomized clinical trials using Xemilofiban evaluated the efficacy of oral GPIIb–IIIa antagonists in over 33 000 patients and demonstrated an approximate 37% increase in mortality for those patients randomized to an oral GPIIb–IIIa inhibitor.

The development of intravenous anti-platelet agents, such as GPIIb–IIIa inhibitors, has resulted in a significant reduction in mortality and non-fatal ischaemic events among patients with CHD. There are three commercially available intravenous GPIIb–IIIa inhibitors: abciximab, eptifibatide and tirofiban. Abciximab is a monoclonal antibody directed against the GP receptor. Eptifibatide is a synthetic cyclic heptapeptide GPIIb–IIIa antagonist and tirofiban is a non-peptide antagonist. Each of these agents has been extensively studied in both the ACS and the elective PCI setting.

The clinical effectiveness of GPIIb–IIIa inhibitors was initially shown in elective PCI patients. Following this, several studies investigated the efficacy among ACS patients. These agents were often started prior to the determination of coronary anatomy. In total, there have been five large-scale prospective randomized controlled clinical trials evaluating the efficacy of GPIIb–IIIa inhibitors in patients with ACS. In total, these trials have randomized over 26 000 patients presenting with ACS. Pooled analysis of these trials, which investigated the efficacy of tirofiban, eptifibatide, abciximab and lamifiban, have demonstrated a modest 12% relative risk reduction in death or non-fatal MI at 30 days. The point estimates for all trials, with the exception of the GUSTO IV-ACS (effect of GPIIb–IIIa receptor blocker abciximab on outcome in patients with acute coronary syndromes without early revascularization) randomized trial, which used abciximab, demonstrated a significant reduction in the primary endpoint of death and non-fatal MI at 30 days. The GUSTO IV-ACS trial failed to demonstrate a benefit of abciximab in the setting of an ACS. In clinical practice, eptifibatide and tirofiban, which were investigated in the PURSUIT and PRISM trials respectively, are usually used in the initial management of patients with ACS.

Although these trials demonstrated a modest reduction in endpoints overall, several subgroups have been shown to have increased benefit from the early use of intravenous GPIIb–IIIa inhibitors. For example, patients with diabetes have been shown in a multitude of studies to be at heightened risk for both short- and long-term adverse cardiovascular events. The addition of GPIIb–IIIa inhibitors to the medical regimen of patients with diabetes presenting with ACS have dramatically improved the outcomes of this high-risk group of patients. Pooled data from the ACS trials mentioned previously have demonstrated a significant reduction in 30-day mortality for those diabetic patients treated with an intravenous GPIIb–IIIA inhibitor. Additionally, patients undergoing early PCI in the setting of an ACS were shown to be at high risk. The addition of intravenous GPIIb–IIIa inhibitor prior to PCI in patients with ACS has dramatically improved the safety profile of PCI in this setting.

Additional high-risk groups of patients are those with increased cardiac troponin concentrations and those undergoing CABG in the setting of ACS. There are two major limitations for the use of intravenous GPIIb–IIIa inhibitors; first, the added cost of delivering care, and second, a modest increase in the risk of bleeding during the time of PCI. Bleeding complications have diminished over time as a result of decreasing the peri-PCI heparin dose and early removal of the intra-atrial sheath. At present, all patients presenting with suspected or confirmed ACS should be considered candidates to receive intravenous GPIIb–IIIa inhibitors. These agents are administered within the first several hours of hospital admission and continued for 48–72 h, often until angiography and PCI has been performed.

It should be noted that there is a risk of thrombocytopenia with these agents, most commonly seen with abciximab. Clinical experience with other monoclonal antibodies has shown that a potential immune response exists to the non-human regions of these molecules. The administration of abciximab has been shown to induce human antichimeric antibodies (HACA) in approximately 6% of patients in the trials performed to date. Development of HACA could, in theory, induce an immediate thrombocytopenia, allergic reactions, and/or decreased effectiveness with repeat abciximab administration. A registry of re-administration has reported data on 500 patients demonstrating similar rates of thrombocytopenia and no evidence of reduced safety or efficacy with abciximab re-administration, even in the presence of HACA. The incidence of mild thrombocytopenia

($< 100\,000$ cells/mm^3) is approximately 5% and severe thrombocytopenia ($< 50\,000$ cells/mm^3) is approximately 1–2%. As in all cases of thrombocytopenia, other causes should be excluded. As patients with ACS are often on a multitude of medications, other agents may play a role in the cause of thrombocytopenia. The primary treatment of thrombocytopenia in the setting of GPIIb–IIIa inhibitor treatment is generally supportive. Abciximab should be discontinued and platelet transfusions may be required. It is recommended that platelet counts should be followed closely with the administration of abciximab. Platelet transfusion should be considered for platelet counts $\leq 50\,000$ cells/mm^3 in patients with active bleeding, vascular access complications or requiring further invasive procedures such as CABG.

Fibrinolytic agents

Coronary atherosclerotic disease is the underlying mechanism for acute MI. As discussed above, it is commonly believed that a rupture in the fibrous cap overlying the atheromatous lesion is the impetus for plaque rupture and subsequent atherothrombosis. If occlusive thrombus forms, patients uniformly develop acute STEMI on the presenting ECG unless there is prompt collateralization from other arterial beds, or if there is spontaneous thrombus resolution. Occlusive thrombus consists of a white (platelet-rich) and red (fibrin- and erythrocyte-rich) clot. The prognosis for patients with STEMI has been improving over the years, such that in-hospital and out-of-hospital mortality has been decreasing since the early 1970s. This is due to a multitude of reasons. The main change in medical care for patients with STEMI has been the recognition that prompt restoration of epicardial coronary blood flow is requisite. There are essentially two strategies to achieve this. The initial reperfusion strategy is the administration of an intravenous fibrinolytic agent. More recently, an aggressive catheter-based reperfusion strategy has been further refined and investigated extensively in the clinical literature.

In general, fibrinolytic agents are plasminogen activators that facilitate the conversion of plasminogen to plasmin. Plasmin is a potent fibrinolytic moiety that acts on cross-linked fibrinogen, promoting fibrinolysis. Furthermore, plasmin interacts with platelets and results in decreased platelet adhesion and disaggregation. Numerous agents have been developed to re-establish arterial flow in the setting of occlusive atherothrombosis formation in the setting of STEMI.

The first-generation agents included drugs such as streptokinase, anistreplase, and two-chain urokinase-type plasminogen activator (tcu-PA). The first-generation fibrinolytic agents were rather fibrin non-specific, they induced systemic coagulation changes and resulted in normal coronary flow rates of only 30% (in the setting of STEMI) with remarkable antigenicity and risk of hypotension. The prototype for the first-generation fibrinolytic agents was streptokinase (Gruppo Italiano per lo Studio della Streptochinasi nell'Infarto Miocardio, GISSI, 1986).

Streptokinase was associated with a significant and durable reduction in in-hospital mortality in the setting of STEMI. This trial revolutionized the care of patients with STEMI. The prototypic second-generation fibrinolytic agent developed was recombinant tissue-type plasminogen activator (tPA), synthetically engineered to resemble intrinsic tPA. Recombinant tPA (alteplase) was more fibrin specific and was shown to be superior with respect to short-term mortality when compared with streptokinase in a large-scale clinical trial (The GUSTO Investigators, 1993).

The concept of the 'open artery hypothesis', following an acute MI, emerged following data from the early thrombolytic trials. For example, within the GUSTO trial (The GUSTO Investigators, 1993), the streptokinase group achieved a 31% 90-minute normal coronary artery flow rate, whereas this was achieved in 54% of the tPA cohort. This translated into an absolute 1% reduction in 30-day mortality. This observation led investigators to conclude that prompt and complete epicardial coronary blood flow would be associated with an improvement in short-term mortality rates. Third-generation fibrinolytic agents were, therefore, evaluated on the basis of initial coronary artery flow rates and numerous third-generation fibrinolytic agents were then developed. The primary limitations of second-generation fibrinolytics included a complex infusion regimen, a risk of intracranial haemorrhage of approximately 1%, only 50% achievement of normal coronary artery flow rates at 90 min, significant re-occlusion and re-infarction, and a 30-day mortality rate of approximately 6–7%. The third-generation fibrinolytic agent, reteplase (r-PA), was compared with an accelerated alteplase (tPA) regimen in the GUSTO III trial. Although there was a modest improvement in the 90-minute normal coronary artery flow rates for the r-PA group, the mortality rate was identical for both fibrinolytic agents. During the 1990s, numerous other fibrinolytic agents were investigated in various randomized controlled trials. In each of these trials, there was no significant reduction in mortality for the studied fibrinolytic agents. Thus, the third-generation fibrinolytic agents have failed to demonstrate a marked improvement in mortality in the setting of STEMI. The approved agents are shown in Table 58.8.

Nonetheless, numerous third-generation fibrinolytic agents have been developed and are undergoing investigation. These various fibrinolytic agents are depicted in Table 58.8. Other novel fibrinolytic agents include staphylokinase. Staphylokinase, although highly fibrin-specific, is associated with the development of antibodies. Therefore, staphylokinase has been modified using site-directed recombinant amino acid substitution, termed *PEGylated Sak STAR*. This has resulted in an improved half-life. Another fibrinolytic agent, monteplase, is a variation of tPA with an amino acid substitution in the epidermal growth factor domain, resulting in a longer half-life of 23 min. Pamiteplase is a mutation of tPA with a kringle-1 deletion and a point mutation in the protease cleavage site of tPA, resulting in a prolonged half-life of 30–47 min.

Table 58.8 First-, second- and third-generation fibrinolytic agents.

Fibrinolytic agent	Plasma half-life (min)	Dose	Fibrin specificity	Modification
First generation SK (streptokinase)	23	1.5 MU/16 min	0	NA
Second generation tPA (alteplase)	4	15-mg bolus 15 mg/30 min, 35 mg/h	++	NA
Third generation r-PA (reteplase)	15	Bolus 10 U + 10 U 30 min apart	+	Deletion of the finger, EGF and kringle-1 domains from tPA
TNK-tPA (tenecteplase)	20	0.5-mg/kg bolus	+++	Three-point mutations in threonine and asparagines of tPA Substitution in the kringle-1 domain improves half-life Asparagine and lysine–histidine–arginine–arginine substitution improves fibrin binding and PAI-1 resistance
n-PA (lanoteplase)	37 min	120-k/U/kg bolus or 20-mg bolus	+	Deletion of the finger and EGF domain; modification of kringle-1 glycosylation points
R-CSU-PA (Saruplase)	9 min	60 mg/h	+	Pro-urokinase polypeptide Pro-drug, converted into tcu-PA

EGF, epidermal growth factor; PAI-1, plasminogen activator inhibitor-1; tcu-PA, two-chain urokinase-type plasminogen activator.

Facilitated fibrinolysis

Fibrinolytic therapies used at present fail to achieve optimal reperfusion in many patients. LMWHs and platelet GPIIb–IIIa inhibitors have shown the potential to improve pharmacological reperfusion therapy. Thus, a strategy of adding a GPIIb–IIIa inhibitor to the regimen of heparin, plus a fibrinolytic agent, has been investigated in the ASSENT III and GUSTO trials. In ASSENT III, there was a significant decrease in adverse events in patients randomized to UFH and abciximab when compared with UFH. The rates of death, MI or recurrent ischaemia were 11.4% for enoxaparin patients, 11.1% for abciximab patients and 15.4% for UFH patients ($P = 0.0001$). However, patients receiving abciximab experienced a significant increase in major bleeding, transfusions and a higher rate of thrombocytopenia. The concept of facilitated fibrinolysis was further studied in the GUSTO V trial. Patients were randomized to full-dose fibrinolytic therapy or half-dose with abciximab. At 30 days, the combination of reteplase and abciximab did not result in a significant reduction in all-cause mortality. Furthermore, there was an absolute 1% increase in intracranial haemorrhage. In summary, similarly to the recent outcomes for the third-generation fibrinolytics, a combination of a reduced dose of a fibrinolytic agent with a GPIIb–IIIa inhibitor failed to be superior to standard fibrinolytic therapy. Whether the strategy of facilitated fibrinolysis coupled with a catheter-based reperfusion strategy will be advantageous remains unknown, but is being investigated in ongoing trials.

Summary

Atherothrombosis is the pathological process underlying the development of CVD, a systemic disease and the commonest cause of death in the Western world. A chronic inflammatory process, triggered by endothelial dysfunction, leads to the formation of atheromatous plaques in the arterial wall. These plaques eventually rupture causing thrombosis to occur on their surfaces. The degree of thrombosis, and therefore the impact on the blood flow through the affected artery, depends on the balance of activities of thrombotic, antithrombotic and fibrinolytic factors. Certain conditions, such as IR and diabetes, dyslipidaemias and hypertension predispose individuals to atherothrombosis by their effects on endothelial function, formation of atheroma and the coagulation system. Lifestyle factors too, such as smoking, diet and physical inactivity predispose to atherothrombosis. It can also be assumed that acquired environmental risk factors and their interactions with genetic polymorphisms increase an individual's risk of developing atherothrombosis. CVD manifests itself as CHD, PVD and cerebrovascular disease. There are now considerable data on both primary and secondary prevention measures for CVD. The challenge for the future is to investigate the complex interactions between genotypes and environmental factors with large-scale studies, with the aim of developing genotype-specific therapies.

Selected bibliography

Anti-platelet Trialists' Collaboration (1994a) Collaborative overview of randomized trials of anti-platelet therapy–I: Prevention of death, myocardial infarction, and stroke by prolonged anti-platelet therapy in various categories of patients. *British Medical Journal* **308**: 81–106.

Anti-platelet Trialists' Collaboration (1994b) Collaborative overview of randomized trials of anti-platelet therapy–II: Maintenance of vascular graft or arterial patency by anti-platelet therapy. *British Medical Journal* **308**: 159–168.

Anti-platelet Trialists' Collaboration (1994c) Collaborative overview of randomized trials of anti-platelet therapy–III: Reduction in venous thrombosis and pulmonary embolism by anti-platelet prophylaxis among surgical and medical patients. *British Medical Journal* **308**: 235–246.

Ariens RA, Philippou H, Nagaswami C *et al.* (2000) The factor XIII V34L polymorphism accelerates thrombin activation of factor XIII and affects cross-linked fibrin structure. *Blood* **96**: 988–95.

Behague I, Poirier O, Nicaud V *et al.* (1996) Beta fibrinogen gene polymorphisms are associated with plasma fibrinogen and coronary artery disease in patients with myocardial infarction. The ECTIM Study. Etude Cas-Temoins sur l'Infarctus du Myocarde. *Circulation* **93**: 440–9.

Berenson GS, Srinivasan SR, Bao W *et al.* (1998) Association between multiple cardiovascular risk factors and atherosclerosis in children and young adults. The Bogalusa Heart Study. *New England Journal of Medicine* **338**: 1650–6.

Braunwald E (1997) Shattuck lecture: cardiovascular medicine at the turn of the millennium: triumphs, concerns, and opportunities. *New England Journal of Medicine* **337**: 1360–9.

Braunwald E, Antman EM, Beasley JW *et al.* (2002) ACC/AHA guideline update for the management of patients with unstable angina and non-ST-segment elevation myocardial infarction–2002: summary article: a report of the American College of Cardiology/American Heart Association Task Force on Practice Guidelines (Committee on the Management of Patients With Unstable Angina). *Circulation* **106**: 1893–900.

British Cardiac Society, British Hyperlipidaemia Association, British Hypertension Society, endorsed by the British Diabetic Association (1998) Joint British recommendations on prevention of coronary heart disease in clinical practice. *Heart* **80**: S1–29.

Collins R, Scrimgeour A, Yusuf S *et al.* (1988) Reduction in fatal pulmonary embolism and venous thrombosis by perioperative administration of subcutaneous heparin. Overview of results of randomized trials in general, orthopedic, and urologic surgery. *New England Journal of Medicine* **318**: 1162–73.

Cooper R, Cutler J, Desvigne-Nickens P *et al.* (2000) Trends and disparities in coronary heart disease, stroke, and other cardiovascular diseases in the United States: findings of the national conference on cardiovascular disease prevention. *Circulation* **102**: 3137–47.

Coumadin Aspirin Reinfarction Study (CARS) Investigators (1997) Randomized double-blind trial of fixed low-dose warfarin with aspirin after myocardial infarction. *Lancet* **350**: 389–96.

de Lange M, Snieder H, Ariens RA *et al.* (2001) The genetics of haemostasis: a twin study. *Lancet* **357**: 101–05.

Ferguson JJ, Antman EM, Bates ER *et al.* (2001) Combining enoxaparin and glycoprotein IIb/IIIa antagonists for the treatment of acute coronary syndromes: final results of the National Investigators Collaborating on Enoxaparin-3 (NICE-3) study. *American Heart Journal* **146**: 628–34.

Fuster V, Ross R, Topol EJ (1996) *Atherosclerosis and Coronary Artery Disease*, vol. 1. Lippincott, Williams and Wilkins, Philadelphia.

Fuster V, Ryden LE, Asinger RW *et al.* (2001) ACC/AHA/ESC Guidelines for the Management of Patients with Atrial Fibrillation: Executive Summary. A Report of the American College of Cardiology/American Heart Association Task Force on Practice Guidelines and the European Society of Cardiology Committee for Practice Guidelines and Policy Conferences (Committee to Develop Guidelines for the Management of Patients with Atrial Fibrillation) Developed in Collaboration with the North American Society of Pacing and Electrophysiology. *Circulation* **104**: 2118–50.

ISIS-2 (Second International Study of Infarct Survival) Collaborative Group (1988) Randomized trial of intravenous streptokinase, oral aspirin, both, or neither among 17, 187 cases of suspected acute myocardial infarction: ISIS-2. *Lancet* **2**: 349–60.

Juul-Moller S, Edvardsson N, Jahnmatz B *et al.* (1992) Double-blind trial of aspirin in primary prevention of myocardial infarction in patients with stable chronic angina pectoris. The Swedish Angina Pectoris Aspirin Trial (SAPAT) Group. *Lancet* **340**: 1421–5.

Kohler HP, Grant PJ (2000) Plasminogen-activator inhibitor type 1 and coronary artery disease. *New England Journal of Medicine* **342**: 1792–801.

Lamm G (1989) The risk-map of Europe. WHO ERICA Research Group. *Annals of Medicine* **21**: 189–92.

Lincoff AM, Harrington RA, Califf RM *et al.* (2000) Management of patients with acute coronary syndromes in the United States by platelet glycoprotein IIb/IIIa inhibition. Insights from the platelet glycoprotein IIb/IIIa in unstable angina: receptor suppression using integrilin therapy (PURSUIT) trial. *Circulation* **102**: 1093–100.

Meade TW, Brozovic M, Chakrabarti RR *et al.* (1986) Haemostatic function and ischaemic heart disease: principal results of the Northwick Park Heart Study. *Lancet* **2**: 533–7.

Morrissey JH (2001) Tissue factor: an enzyme cofactor and a true receptor. *Thrombosis and Haemostasis* **86**(1): 66–74.

Mosesson MW, Siebenlist KR, Meh DA (2001) The structure and biological features of fibrinogen and fibrin. *Annals of the New York Academy of Science* **936**: 11–30.

Mukherjee D, Mahaffey KW, Moliterno DJ *et al.* (2002) Promise of combined low-molecular-weight heparin and platelet glycoprotein IIb/IIIa inhibition: results from platelet IIb/IIIa antagonist for the reduction of acute coronary syndrome events in a global organization network B (PARAGON B). *American Heart Journal* **144**: 995–1002.

Platelet Receptor Inhibition in Ischemic Syndrome Management (PRISM) Study Investigators (1998) A comparison of aspirin plus tirofiban with aspirin plus heparin for unstable angina. *New England Journal of Medicine* **338**: 1498–505.

Platelet Receptor Inhibition in Ischemic Syndrome Management in Patients Limited by Unstable Signs and Symptoms (PRISM-PLUS) Study Investigators (1998) Inhibition of the platelet glycoprotein IIb/IIIa receptor with tirofiban in unstable angina and non-Q-wave myocardial infarction. *New England Journal of Medicine* **338**: 1488–97.

Reaven GM (1995) Pathophysiology of insulin resistance in human disease. *Physiology Review* **75**: 473–86.

Ross R (1999) Atherosclerosis: an inflammatory disease. *New England Journal of Medicine* **340**: 115–126.

Stary HC, Chandler AB, Dinsmore RE *et al.* (1995) A definition of advanced types of atherosclerotic lesions and a histological classification of atherosclerosis. A report from the Committee on Vascular Lesions of the Council on Arteriosclerosis, American Heart Association. *Arteriosclerosis Thrombosis and Vascular Biology* **15**: 1512–31.

The Global Use of Strategies to Open Occluded Coronary Arteries (GUSTO) IIa Investigators (1994) Randomized trial of intravenous heparin versus recombinant hirudin for acute coronary syndromes. *Circulation* **90**: 1631–7.

The GUSTO Investigators (1993) An international randomized trial comparing four thrombolytic strategies for acute myocardial infarction. *New England Journal of Medicine* **329**: 673–82.

The PARAGON Investigators (1998) International, randomized, controlled trial of lamifiban (a platelet glycoprotein IIb/IIIa inhibitor), heparin, or both in unstable angina. Platelet IIb/IIIa antagonism for the reduction of acute coronary syndrome events in a global organization network. *Circulation* **97**: 2386–95.

The PURSUIT Trial Investigators (1998) Inhibition of platelet glycoprotein IIb/IIIa with eptifibatide in patients with acute coronary syndromes. Platelet glycoprotein IIb/IIIa in unstable angina: receptor suppression using integrilin therapy. *New England Journal of Medicine* **339**: 436–43.

The RISC Group (1990) Risk of myocardial infarction and death during treatment with low dose aspirin and intravenous heparin in men with unstable coronary artery disease. *Lancet* **336**: 827–30.

The SYMPHONY Investigators (2000) Comparison of sibrafiban with aspirin for prevention of cardiovascular events after acute coronary syndromes: a randomized trial. Sibrafiban versus aspirin to yield maximum protection from ischemic heart events postacute coronary syndromes. *Lancet* **355**: 337–45.

Vaccaro O, Stamler J, Neaton JD (1998) Sixteen-year coronary mortality in black and white men with diabetes screened for the Multiple Risk Factor Intervention Trial (MRFIT). *International Journal of Epidemiology* **27**: 636–41.

CHAPTER 59

Haematological aspects of systemic disease

Atul B Mehta and A Victor Hoffbrand

Anaemia of chronic disease

The anaemia of chronic disease (ACD) is a common normo-chromic or mildly hypochromic anaemia, occurring in patients with a systemic disease (Table 59.1). It is characterized by a reduced serum iron and iron binding capacity, and normal or raised serum ferritin with adequate iron stores (Table 59.2).

Table 59.1 Conditions associated with anaemia of chronic disorders.

Chronic infections
Especially osteomyelitis, bacterial endocarditis, tuberculosis, abscesses, bronchiectasis, chronic urinary tract infections

Other chronic inflammatory disorders
Rheumatoid arthritis, juvenile rheumatoid arthritis, polymyalgia rheumatica, systemic lupus erythematosus, scleroderma, inflammatory bowel diseases, thrombophlebitis

Malignant diseases
Carcinoma (especially metastatic or associated with infection), lymphoma, myeloma

Others
Congestive heart failure, ischaemic heart disease, AIDS

It is not due to marrow replacement by tumour, bleeding, haemolysis or haematinic deficiency, although these often complicate it.

Pathogenesis

A mild decrease in red cell lifespan occurs in ACD, but it is at a level that could be compensated by a normal bone marrow. The major cause of ACD is a disturbance of erythropoiesis due to a reduced sensitivity to physiological erythropoietic stimuli and reduced iron utilization. The interaction of a number of cytokines (including interleukin 1 (IL-1), IL-6, tumour necrosis factor (TNF) and transforming growth factor beta, with accessory marrow stromal cells and with the erythroid progenitors themselves) is probably responsible.

Relative lack of erythropoietin

The plasma erythropoietin (Epo) level in ACD remains inversely correlated with the haemoglobin level but compared with patients with other types of anaemia and normal renal function, it is inappropriately low. The plasma levels of TNF-α, IL-1 (IL-1α and IL-1β) and IL-6 are raised. Tumour necrosis factor and IL-1 have been shown in experimental systems to reduce Epo production by cultured hepatoma cells. In addition, IL-1α inhibits Epo production by isolated serum-free perfused kidneys.

Haemoglobin	Not less than 9 g/dL	
Mean corpuscular volume	Normal or mildly reduced (usually 77–82 fL)	
Mean corpuscular haemoglobin	Usually normal; occasionally reduced	
Serum iron	Reduced	
Total iron binding capacity (transferrin)	Reduced	
Transferring saturation	Mildly reduced	
Serum ferritin	Normal or increased	
Serum and urine hepcidin	Raised	
C-reactive protein	Usually raised	
Erythrocyte sedimentation rate	Usually raised	

Table 59.2 Haematological features of anaemia of chronic disease.

Inhibition of erythropoiesis

Both TNF and IL-1 inhibit erythropoiesis *in vitro* and it is likely that TNF increases apoptosis of bone marrow erythroid cells. Anaemia is observed in humans treated with TNF and in animals receiving either cytokine. The effect of IL-1 is probably mediated by interferon-γ (IFN-γ) secreted by T lymphocytes, whereas the TNF action is probably mediated by IFN-γ produced by marrow stromal cells. IL-6 and TGF-β may also have roles as mediators of ACD through inhibition of erythropoiesis.

Iron metabolism

A characteristic in ACD is the presence of a low serum iron with adequate reticuloendothelial iron stores, but with a reduction of iron granules in marrow erythroblasts. A fall in serum transferrin and a rise in serum ferritin occur as part of the acute-phase response. The fall in serum iron can occur as early as 24 h after the onset of a systemic illness, and will persist during the course of a prolonged illness. The fall in serum iron results from an impaired flow of iron from cells (including intestinal mucosal cells, hepatocytes and macrophages) to plasma. This is due to increased secretion by hepatocytes of hepcidin (see p. 32) in response to inflammation. Hepcidin inhibits release of iron from macrophages and iron absorption. Inflammation can cause a 100-fold increase in urinary hepcidin excretion. Microbial products may act on Kupffer cells to secrete IL-6, which then stimulates hepcidin secretion from hepatocytes. Low serum iron inhibits proliferation of micro-organisms. Hepcidin secretion is also increased in iron overload. This seems unlikely to be due to a direct effect on hepatocytes. It is possible that iron in Kupffer cells or sinusoidal cells, like infection, stimulates production of cytokines, which act on hepatocytes.

In clinical specimens, there is a significant positive correlation between serum and urinary hepcidin and serum ferritin levels. The cytokines TNF, IL-1 and IFN-γ have all been shown to cause reduced serum iron and increased serum ferritin concentrations. The fall in serum iron is probably mainly, if not entirely, due to hepcidin. Anaemia usually reduces hepcidin secretion. In ACD, this effect is clearly abrogated by the effect of inflammation or malignancy increasing its secretion. Increased lactoferrin, occurring in response to inflammation and mediated by cytokines, competes with transferrin for iron and forms a complex, which is taken up by macrophages in the liver and spleen. Increased intracellular apoferritin synthesis occurs in response to inflammation and malignancy and this too will bind iron. Both of these mechanisms reduce the amount of iron available for binding to serum transferrin.

Treatment

The severity of the anaemia correlates with the activity and severity of the underlying chronic disease. Successful therapy of this leads to a reduction in the levels of the mediator cytokines, increased Epo production and reduced inhibition of erythropoiesis. Correction of the anaemia may take weeks or months. Pharmacological doses of recombinant Epo have been used successfully to improve anaemia in patients with rheumatoid arthritis, cancer and myeloma. This observation suggests that inadequate Epo production and its reduced action are more important than disturbed iron metabolism in the pathogenesis of ACD. It further suggests that the suppressive action of various cytokines can be overcome by use of pharmacological doses of Epo. Iron therapy should be reserved for patients who have genuine iron deficiency.

Malignancy

Anaemia

Anaemia is the most frequent haematological abnormality in cancer patients and may be due to many causes (Table 59.3). The anaemia of chronic disorders (see above) will affect almost all cancer patients at some stage of their illness. The degree of anaemia reflects the extent of the malignancy and may be worsened by the myelotoxic effects of chemotherapy. Plasma Epo levels tend to be inappropriately low and therapy with recombinant Epo can reduce transfusion requirements by improving the haemoglobin level in cancer patients who are undergoing chemotherapy.

Table 59.3 Causes of anaemia in cancer patients.

Type of anaemia	Associations
Anaemia of chronic disease	All neoplasms
Blood loss	Gastrointestinal neoplasms, gynaecological neoplasms
Haemolysis – immune	Ovarian carcinoma, lymphoma others
Haemolysis – non-immune fragmentation syndrome	Mucin-secreting adenocarcinomas
Haemolysis – secondary to drugs	Mitomycin, cyclosporin, cisplatinum
Pure red cell aplasia	Thymoma
Megaloblastic	Chemotherapy, folate deficiency, cobalamin deficiency, (gastric carcinoma)
Leucoerythroblastic	Metastatic disease in bone marrow
Marrow hypoplasia	Chemotherapy/radiotherapy
Myelodysplasia	Chemotherapy/radiotherapy

Haemolysis

Warm antibody autoimmune haemolytic anaemia (AIHA) is most frequently found in association with the following malignant diseases: chronic lymphocytic leukaemia, Hodgkin's disease and non-Hodgkin's lymphoma. However, it has also been reported in association with solid tumours (e.g. carcinoma of the ovary). Cold-antibody AIHA is less common, but occurs in association with monoclonal cold agglutinins in chronic cold agglutinin disease, Waldenstrom's macroglobulinaemia and myeloma.

Microangiopathic haemolytic anaemia (MAHA) with intravascular haemolysis may occur in association with disseminated carcinoma. An abrupt onset of anaemia and thrombocytopenia often occurs, with a leucoerythroblastic blood picture, reticulocytosis and red cell fragmentation. Renal failure may occur as a complication. Mucin-secreting adenocarcinomas (especially gastric), breast cancer and lung cancer are the most common underlying malignancies; in about one-third of patients with MAHA, it is the presenting feature of the tumour. Abnormal blood vessels may be within the tumour itself (or within metastatic tumour thrombi, especially in the lungs) or fibrin deposition may occur at other sites because of disseminated intravascular coagulation (DIC). Widely disseminated disease with bone marrow infiltration is almost always present and the outlook is poor. A syndrome resembling MAHA and the idiopathic haemolytic–uraemic syndrome has been reported with a number of chemotherapeutic agents and following allogeneic bone marrow transplantation. Principal among these is mitomycin, whereas cisplatin, carboplatin, bleomycin and cyclosporin have also been reported. Immune complex deposition has been implicated in the pathogenesis.

Red cell aplasia

Acquired pure red cell aplasia is associated with a thymoma in approximately 50% of patients, although it complicates only approximately 5% of thymomas. Antibodies to erythroid precursors have been demonstrated in some patients, and removal of the thymoma (which is usually benign) leads to resolution

of the anaemia in about one-half of those affected. Immunosuppressive therapy with cyclophosphamide, cyclosporin, steroids or plasma exchange may be helpful in patients who relapse. Red cell aplasia may also occur in a minority of patients with chronic lymphocytic leukaemia (CLL) or non-Hodgkin's lymphoma and with large granular lymphocytic (LGL) leukaemia and as part of general marrow aplasia due to chemotherapy or radiotherapy.

Leucoerythroblastic anaemia

The blood film (Figure 59.1) shows the presence of erythroblasts and granulocyte precursors (e.g. myelocytes and myeloblasts). It is seen in primary myelofibrosis but is also frequent when there is marrow infiltration by tumour. This disturbs the marrow microvasculature and allows early release of the precursors. Marrow infiltration is most commonly observed in breast (Figure 59.2), prostate and haematological malignancies, but also in tumours of lung, thyroid, kidney and gastrointestinal tract

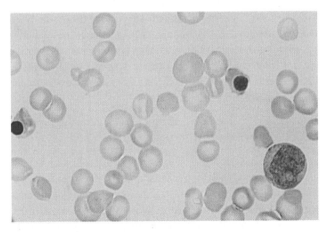

Figure 59.1 Nucleated red cells and an immature myeloid precursor in the peripheral blood film of a patient with a leucoerythroblastic anaemia.

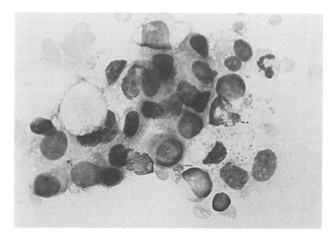

Figure 59.2 Bone marrow aspirate showing infiltration by metastatic breast carcinoma.

and melanoma. It can also occur as a reflection of active bone marrow response to peripheral consumption (acute haemolysis, DIC, septicaemia, hypersplenism) or of extramedullary haemopoiesis (e.g. myelofibrosis or megaloblastic anaemia).

Other causes

Megaloblastic and dyserythropoietic anaemias are most commonly due to chemotherapy-induced disturbance of DNA synthesis within the bone marrow. Folate deficiency may also occur in patients with a poor diet and widespread disease. Cobalamin (vitamin B_{12}) deficiency due to underlying pernicious anaemia may complicate cancer of the stomach. Both chemotherapy and non-ionizing radiotherapy may lead to the development of myelodysplasia (MDS), which may progress to acute myeloid leukaemia (AML). Alkylating agents, especially melphalan and chlorambucil, nitrosoureas and epipodophyllotoxins in particular have been implicated, and there is evidence of a synergistic effect of these agents with small, chronic doses of radiotherapy. The principal categories of patients affected are those who have received therapy for a haematological malignancy, but patients treated for non-haematological malignancies (especially ovarian and gastrointestinal carcinoma) are also susceptible. The median latency prior to onset of MDS is 2–3 years and AML usually supervenes 6 months to 2 years later.

Treatment

Erythropoietin is effective in reversing anaemia in a proportion of patients with malignant disease, e.g. myeloma, lymphoproliferative disorders, myelodysplasia and carcinomas. It is recommended if the haemoglobin is less than 10 g/dL or symptomatic patients with haemoglobin of 10–12 g/dL. Dosage is 10 000 IU three times per week or 30 000 IU as a single weekly dose. The dose could be increased if there is no response (< 1 g/dL rise in 4 weeks).

Patients who are most likely to respond are those who have low pre-treatment Epo levels (< 100 mU/mL), well-preserved marrow function and normal/low levels of serum ferritin (< 400 ng/mL). A number of studies have demonstrated that Epo therapy can lead to a reduced need for blood transfusion, better quality of life for patients and possibly improved overall outcome of anti-cancer therapy.

Polycythaemia

This is a rare complication of non-haematological malignancy. It usually arises through elaboration by tumour cells of Epo and Epo-like peptides. The tumours most commonly associated are renal cell carcinoma and hepatoma; others include uterine myoma, androgen-secreting ovarian tumours, phaeochromocytoma and cerebellar haemangioblastoma. Non-malignant conditions affecting these organs (e.g. renal cysts, viral hepatitis) may also rarely be associated.

White cells (Table 59.4)

Granulocytosis

Granulocytosis is a frequent manifestation of non-haematological malignancies. In part, the response is due to inflammation

Table 59.4 White cell changes in malignancy.

Neutrophils increased	Most, especially renal Hodgkin's disease
Neutrophils decreased	Bone marrow infiltration Hypersplenism Treatment induced Chemotherapy/radiotherapy Large granular lymphocytic leukaemia
Basophils increased	Myeloproliferative disorders
Eosinophils increased	Hodgkin's disease T-cell lymphomas, Metastatic adenocarcinoma Other tumours (e.g. lung) Drug allergy Opportunistic infection
Monocytes increased	Carcinoma Hodgkin's disease
Monocytes decreased	Treatment induced
Lymphocytes increased	Lymphoid malignancies Post splenectomy Opportunistic infection
Lymphocytes decreased	Treatment induced Radiotherapy/chemotherapy Lymphoma Opportunistic infection

Table 59.5 Thrombocytopenia in patients with malignant disease.

Decreased production
Chemotherapy/radiotherapy
Marrow infiltration
Accelerated destruction

Hypersplenism
Disseminated intravascular coagulation
Drug-induced haemolytic–uraemic syndrome
Autoimmune thrombocytopenia

Table 59.6 Coagulation changes in malignancy.

Bleeding tendency
Disseminated intravascular coagulation acute or chronic
Primary fibrinolysis
Acquired platelet function defect
Thrombocytopenia
Circulating anticoagulants/inhibitors

Treatment-related bleeding disorders
Thrombotic tendency
Venous stasis: bed rest, venous compression/invasion by tumours
Increased coagulation factors I, V, VII, VIII, IX, XI
Decreased inhibitors of coagulation: low antithrombin, protein C and S
Direct activation of coagulation by tumour cells: factor VII, factor X
Indirect activation: through trypsin release, through mucin secretion, via monocytes, through endothelial damage
Increased platelet aggregability and adhesiveness
Thrombocytosis

induced by the tumour. Interaction of tumour cells with host T lymphocytes and mononuclear phagocytic cells leads to the production of a range of cytokines, which induce white cell proliferation and differentiation. Tumour cells may also secrete specific agents that directly stimulate reactive proliferation. Cancer patients frequently have opportunistic infections, may bleed and are typically on a range of medications, all of which may influence the level of the white cell count.

Granulocytopenia

This is most frequently due to chemotherapy or radiotherapy but may also occur with widespread marrow infiltration, for example by lymphoma or due to LGL leukaemia.

Platelets

Thrombocytopenia (Table 59.5)

This may arise through decreased production or accelerated peripheral destruction and/or hypersplenism. The former may result from extensive marrow infiltration or be secondary to chemotherapy or radiotherapy. Hypersplenism is usually due to splenic infiltration by a haematological malignancy (e.g. lymphoma, CLL) but is rarely due to obstruction of the splenic or portal vein by hepatic and pancreatic malignancies. Increased destruction occurs with DIC. Immune thrombocytopenia may occur in association with haematological malignancy (CLL, lymphoma, MDS) and rarely may complicate solid tumours (e.g. breast, lung, ovary).

Thrombocytosis

A raised platelet count is frequently seen as a reactive phenomenon in patients with malignancy but is usually $< 1000 \times 10^9$/L and is rarely of clinical significance.

Platelet function abnormalities

Impaired platelet function leading to excessive bleeding is primarily seen in myeloproliferative disorders (e.g. essential thrombocythaemia) and MDS. Paraproteins, especially immunoglobulin M (IgM) in Waldenstrom's macroglobulinaemia and IgG in myeloma, are frequent causes of impaired platelet aggregation

and adhesion. Increased platelet aggregation occurs in cancer patients when tumour cells release adenosine diphosphate (ADP), prostaglandins or thrombin. Increased platelet adhesiveness has also been reported, but is probably secondary to other coagulation changes.

Coagulation (Table 59.6)

A wide range of coagulation changes can occur in patients with malignant disease and can predispose to either haemorrhage or thrombosis. The distinction between activation of the coagulation part of the haemostatic pathway (DIC), which leads physiologically to activation of fibrinolysis (secondary fibrinolysis), and primary or direct activation of fibrinolysis may be difficult, and in some ways academic, in view of the intimate and dynamic relationship that exists between the coagulation and fibrinolytic pathways. These patients may also have other general medical problems, including infection; they may have undergone surgery, chemotherapy or radiotherapy and will typically be on a range of medications. All of these factors may contribute to coagulation changes.

Disseminated intravascular coagulation

Chronic or compensated disseminated intravascular coagulation (DIC) is probably underdiagnosed in cancer patients. It occurs particularly in those with gastrointestinal, lung, pancreatic and breast neoplasms. Thrombosis, including migratory thrombophlebitis (Trousseau's syndrome) and non-bacterial thrombotic endocarditis, is a more frequent manifestation of DIC than haemorrhage. Acute or uncompensated DIC, in contrast, is uncommon with solid tumours but occurs frequently

Table 59.7 Circulating anticoagulants in malignancy.

Factor inhibitors
Factor V
Factor VII
Factor VIII

von Willebrand factor inhibitors
Paraproteinaemic disorders
Lymphoma
Myeloproliferative disorders
Chronic lymphocytic leukaemia

Others
Heparin-like anticoagulants – dysproteinaemias

with acute promyelocytic leukaemia (APL, FAB M3) and is associated with excessive bleeding. The triggering event in APL is likely to be release from the malignant promyelocytes of procoagulants and proteases, which may directly activate both coagulation and fibrinolysis. Tumour cells may activate coagulation by release of tissue factor (TF), which activates factor VII. Direct activation of factor X through the action of a cancer procoagulant has been reported in lung, kidney, colon and breast cancer. The sialic acid moiety of secreted mucin can directly activate factor X, whereas the systemic release of trypsin in pancreatic tumours can also activate coagulation. Tumour cells may also activate the monocyte–macrophage system to produce procoagulant materials including TF and factor X activators.

Primary fibrinolysis

This is less common as a cause of increased bleeding than DIC, but can occur, for example, in patients with prostatic cancer who undergo surgery. The release of proteases from leukaemic cells in both APL and monocytic leukaemia has been reported to induce fibrinolysis. Platelet counts tend to be higher than those seen in DIC, and fibrinogen levels are low, with raised fibrin degradation products (FDPs).

Acquired circulating anticoagulants (Table 59.7)

The most frequent is an acquired von Willebrand syndrome (both type 1 and type 11 disease) in patients with a paraprotein or a B-lymphoid malignancy. A number of different mechanisms may operate. The paraprotein may be directed against an epitope within the factor VIII–von Willebrand factor (vWF) molecule and inactivate it, or reduce its plasma half-life. Alternatively, immune complexes may form which bind non-specifically to factor VIII–vWF and accelerate its clearance, or the malignant lymphoid cells may actually absorb factor VIII–vWF onto their surface. Paraproteins may also interfere with cross-linking of fibrin.

Treatment-induced bleeding disorders

Thrombocytopenia and MAHA may occur as a result of therapy (see below). Cancer patients with poor nutrition or who are on long-term antibiotics may develop vitamin K deficiency. L-Asparaginase induces defective hepatic protein synthesis and can lead not only to impaired production of coagulation factors but also to low levels of antithrombin (AT), plasminogen and proteins S and C, and so give rise to thrombosis, most seriously of the cerebral veins. Mithramycin, which is used in the treatment of malignant hypercalcaemia, causes thrombocytopenia as well as platelet function defects, coagulation factor deficiencies and increased fibrinolytic activity.

Connective tissue disorders (Table 59.8)

Anaemia

Anaemia of chronic disease (see above) is the most common haematological abnormality seen in patients with rheumatoid arthritis (RA). Iron deficiency may co-exist, particularly in patients taking non-steroidal anti-inflammatory agents. Folate deficiency may occur with severe disease and poor dietary intake. Warm-type AIHA with IgG and complement on the red cell surface is most frequently seen in systemic lupus erythematosus (SLE), although it can occur in the other connective tissue disorders (CTD), notably RA and mixed CTD. Sideroblastic anaemia has been reported in both SLE and RA, but MDS must be excluded. Pure red cell aplasia and dyserythropoietic anaemia with ineffective erythropoiesis are rare complications of SLE. Haemolysis can also occur as part of thrombotic thrombocytopenic purpura (TTP), complicating SLE.

White cells

The inflammatory process in CTD can lead to a neutrophilia. Neutropenia is a feature of Felty's syndrome, which is associated with splenomegaly in patients with RA. The pathogenesis is multifactorial and involves increased margination of neutrophils, sequestration of neutrophils within the enlarged spleen, immune complex-mediated and humoral inhibition of granulopoiesis in the marrow. Antibodies to mature neutrophils have also been reported in SLE. Lymphopenia occurs in both SLE and RA, and may be a measure of disease activity. Eosinophilia may be seen in SLE, RA, polyarteritis nodosa and Churg–Strauss syndrome. The pathogenesis is unknown, but presumably involves release of cytokines by T lymphocytes. Functional defects in polymorph and lymphocyte function have been reported in SLE and RA.

Platelets

Immune thrombocytopenia is a common manifestation of SLE and also occurs in mixed CTD, scleroderma, RA and dermato-

Table 59.8 Haematological changes in connective tissue damage.

Anaemia
Anaemia of chronic disease
Iron deficiency (drug-induced blood loss)
Folate deficiency
Sideroblastic anaemia
Pure red cell aplasia (PRCA), especially systemic lupus
   erythematosus (SLE)
Haemolytic anaemia: immune (especially SLE)/non-immune

White cells
Neutropenia (e.g. Felty's syndrome)
Neutrophilia
Eosinophilia (e.g. Churg–Strauss syndrome, polyarteritis nodosa)

Platelets
Thrombocytopenia: immune/non-immune
Platelet dysfunction
Thrombotic thrombocytopenic purpura
Thrombocytosis

Pancytopenia
SLE

Coagulation
Lupus inhibitor
Specific factor deficiencies
Disseminated intravascular coagulation

Others
Myelofibrosis
Drug related changes (e.g. aplastic anaemia due to gold
   phenylbutazone; PRCA due to penicillamine)
Cryoglobulinaemia
Amyloidosis

myositis. Autoantibodies to platelets may also impair platelet function. TTP is an association of SLE. Thrombocytosis is a non-specific reaction to inflammation and tissue damage in CTD.

Coagulation

A wide diversity of coagulation changes may occur in patients with CTD. In part, this may be due to liver and renal disease or to drug therapy. DIC has been reported in SLE patients who have high levels of circulating immune complexes and resulting angiopathy. The lupus anticoagulant (see Chapter 55) occurs as a complication in about 10% of patients with SLE and is associated with a thrombotic tendency, thrombocytopenia, recurrent miscarriages and pulmonary hypertension. Specific coagulation factor inhibitors encountered in patients with CTD (especially SLE) include antibodies to vWF and to factors VIII, VII and fibrinogen.

Other changes

Rheumatoid arthritis is a relatively common cause of amyloidosis. An increased incidence of haematological malignancies (principally Hodgkin's and non-Hodgkin's lymphomas and B-lymphoproliferative disorders, including paraproteinaemias) has been noted in SLE, RA and, particularly, in Sjögren's syndrome. A wide range of haematological abnormalities also results from immunosuppressive therapy in these patients.

Renal disease (Table 59.9)

Anaemia

This is the most important haematological abnormality and its management has been revolutionized by the availability of recombinant human erythropoietin (rEPO). Patients with acute or chronic renal failure develop a normochromic, normocytic anaemia, with the presence of ecchinocytes (burr cells) in the blood film. The reticulocyte count is normal or slightly low, and the bone marrow shows normoblastic erythropoiesis without the erythroid hyperplasia expected at that level of anaemia. Patients who have undergone nephrectomy tend to be more severely anaemic than patients with polycystic disease. Reduced Epo levels occur in renal failure and this is the dominant cause of anaemia.

An increase in serum creatinine above 133 μmol/L is associated with the loss of the normal inverse linear relation between plasma Epo and haemoglobin concentration, but there is no direct correlation between reduction in glomerular filtration rate and impairment of renal Epo production. Circulating inhibitors of erythropoiesis have also been demonstrated. Chronic ambulatory peritoneal dialysis is more effective than haemodialysis in removing these inhibitors but, as rEPO can overcome these inhibitors, they are not of great clinical significance. Red cell survival is diminished in renal failure, but this is also a minor factor. Iron deficiency can arise through blood loss (exacerbated by haemodialysis). Folate deficiency arises in dialysed patients but is now prevented by prophylactic folic acid therapy. Renal failure is associated with elevated 2,3-DPG levels and a right shift of the haemoglobin oxygen dissociation curve.

Recombinant Epo therapy can fully correct anaemia in renal failure. It can be administered intravenously, subcutaneously or intraperitoneally. The subcutaneous route is effective at lower doses, and it is usual to commence 5–75 units/kg per week, given in two or three divided doses. Anaemia is corrected up to a level of 10–12 g/dL at a rate of 1 g/dL per month. Subclinical iron deficiency and impaired mobilization of storage iron are often present, so concomitant iron therapy is usually required. An impaired response to rEPO should prompt a suspicion of iron, cobalamin or folate deficiency, haemolysis, infection, occult

Table 59.9 Haematological changes in renal disease.

Anaemia
Failure of erythropoietin production
Haemolysis: haemolytic–uraemic syndrome (HUS); thrombotic
　thrombocytopenic purpura (TTP)
Iron deficiency
Folate deficiency
Hyperparathyroidism
Aluminium toxicity

Polycythaemia
Renal cell carcinoma
Other renal diseases (e.g. cysts, hydronephrosis, nephritic
　syndrome, renal transplantation)

Thrombocytopenia
HUS
TTP
Disseminated intravascular coagulation

Platelet function abnormalities
Abnormal aggregation to ADP, adrenaline, collagen
Decreased platelet adhesiveness
Reduced platelet factor 3 availability
Acquired storage pool defect
Abnormal prostaglandin metabolism
↑Prostacylin
Defective platelet cyclo-oxygenase?

Coagulation

Hypocoagulability
↓Factor XII, factor XI, prothrombin
↓Factor XII or inhibition
Hypercoagulopathy
↓Protein C
↓Antithrombin
↓Fibrinolysis

malignancy, aluminium toxicity and hyperparathyroidism. Hypertension occurs in about one-third of rEPO-treated patients and is dose dependent; the risk of thrombosis of an arteriovenous fistula is also increased. In acute renal failure, anaemia is commonly due to the drug or condition causing the renal failure, e.g. haemolysis due to sepsis or TTP.

Polycythaemia

Secondary and inappropriate polycythaemia may result from either ectopic Epo production by renal tumours or regional renal hypoxia (in benign disease and following renal transplantation), which disturbs physiological Epo homeostasis. Up to 5% of patients with renal cell carcinoma have paraneoplastic polycythaemia.

Haemostatic abnormalities

Abnormal platelet function is probably due to the accumulation of toxic metabolites (e.g. guanidinosuccinic and phenolic acids). DDAVP (1-deamino-8-D-arginine vasopressin) therapy, which leads to the appearance of large multimers of vWF, can shorten the bleeding time in anaemic patients. Dysfibrinogenaemia has been reported rarely, whereas FDPs are often elevated and may prolong the thrombin time. Hypercoagulopathy with a predisposition to thrombosis can also occur, especially after rEPO therapy. Haemodialysis with heparin anticoagulation can cause platelet activation. Fibrinolytic activity, AT and protein C are all reduced in renal failure, and factors V, VII, VIIIc and X are increased. Thrombosis (particularly of the renal vein) is a particular feature of the nephrotic syndrome. Platelet hyperaggregability with increased plasma β-thromboglobulin is described and hypoalbuminaemia may enhance the synthesis of prostaglandins involved in platelet activation.

Endocrine disease (Table 59.10)

Both hyper- and hypothyroidism are associated with mild anaemia, which is usually normochromic and normocytic, but may be macrocytic in hypothyroidism. A raised mean corpuscular volume (MCV) can occur without anaemia in hypothyroidism, and low MCV has been described in thyrotoxicosis. Thyroid hormones stimulate erythropoiesis, and tissue oxygen demands are increased in hyperthyroidism, whereas, in hypothyroidism, oxygen utilization is reduced. However, plasma volume is also increased and part of the anaemia in hypothyroidism is dilutional, and/or due to defective iron utilization. Co-existent deficiencies of iron (due to menorrhagia or achlorhydria), folate and cobalamin must be excluded.

There is an increased incidence of pernicious anaemia in patients with hypothyroidism, hypoadrenalism and hypoparathyroidism. Antithyroid drugs (carbimazole, methimazole and propylthiouracil) can cause aplastic anaemia or agranulocytosis. Anaemia in patients with diabetes mellitus is usually due to complications of diabetes, although hyperglycaemia itself may lead to shortened red cell lifespan and decreased erythrocyte deformability. Polycythaemia (usually pseudo) can also occur with endocrine diseases. In anterior pituitary disease, androgen deficiency, adrenal insufficiency, a normochromic, normocytic anaemia is common. Changes in leucocyte number and function are rarely of clinical significance, although many have been reported. Chemotaxis, phagocytosis and intracellular killing may all be disturbed in diabetes mellitus. Coagulation changes may contribute to a mild bleeding diathesis in hypothyroidism and to the thrombotic predisposition in diabetes mellitus.

Table 59.10 Haematological changes in endocrine disease.

Red cells

Anaemia

Thyrotoxicosis (normochromic, normocytic or microcytic)

Hypothyroidism (normochromic, normocytic, occasionally macrocytic)

Diabetes mellitus (usually when complicated by infection, cardiac disease, renal failure, enteropathy)

Hyperparathyroidism (normochromic, normocytic)

Hypoadrenalism (normochromic, normocytic)

Hypogonadism (normochromic, normocytic)

Hypopituitarism (normochromic, normocytic)

Polycythaemia (pseudo)

Phaeochromocytoma

Cushing's syndrome

White cells

Cushing's syndrome	Neutrophil leucocytosis
Phaeochromocytoma	
Hyperthyroidism	Lymphocytosis
Leucopenia	Antithyroid drugs
Diabetes mellitus	Impaired polymorph function

Platelets

Diabetes mellitus	Abnormal platelet function
Hyperthyroidism	

Coagulopathy

Diabetes mellitus	↑Platelet aggregability, ↓prostacyclin, ↑factor VIII, ↓AT
Oestrogen therapy	↑Factor VIII, ↑vWF
Cushing's syndrome	↑Factors II, IV, IX, XI, XII

Liver disease (Table 59.11)

Liver disease causes a greater range of haematological change than does disease in any other organ, with the exception of the bone marrow. The liver is an important source of Epo in the fetus, and serves as a haemopoietic organ *in utero*; extramedullary haemopoiesis occurs within the adult liver only in pathological states (e.g. myelofibrosis, severe haemolysis or megaloblastic anaemia).

Anaemia

Anaemia occurs in up to 75% of patients with chronic liver disease. Portal hypertension often results in splenomegaly, which may cause haemodilution and pooling of red cells. Haemorrhage is a frequent complication, often due to oesophageal varices and the red cell lifespan is shortened even in uncomplicated liver

Table 59.11 Haematological changes in liver disease.

Red cells

Anaemia

Anaemia of chronic disease

Folate deficiency

Iron deficiency (blood loss)

Aplastic anaemia (viral hepatitis, rare)

Sideroblastic (alcohol)

Hypersplenism

Microangiopathy/disseminated intravascular coagulation (DIC) (rare)

Autoimmune (rare)

Zieve's syndrome (rare)

Polycythaemia

Hepatocellular carcinoma (rare)

Infectious hepatitis (rare)

White cells

Neutrophilia

Infection

Haemorrhage

Malignancy

Haemolysis

Neutrophil function

Impaired chemotaxis (?due to lowered complement levels)

Neutropenia

Hypersplenism

Eosinophilia

Parasitic infestation

Chronic active hepatitis (rare)

Platelets

Thrombocytopenia

Hypersplenism, hepatic sequestration

DIC

Autoimmune (e.g. associated with viral hepatitis, primary biliary cirrhosis)

Post-liver transplantation

Thrombocytosis

Hepatoma (rare)

Impaired platelet function

Inhibitory factors (including high-density lipoprotein and apolipoprotein E)

Other

Benign monoclonal gammopathy (biliary + other cirrhosis)

Cryoglobulinaemia (hepatitis B, hepatitis C, alcohol)

disease. Ferrokinetic studies suggest that the bone marrow response to anaemia is suboptimal, and many of the mechanisms that operate in the anaemia of chronic disease (see above) may be relevant. Macrocytosis occurs in approximately two-thirds of patients and erythropoiesis is macronormoblastic, indicating abnormal marrow function. Macrocytosis is particularly frequent in alcoholics, in whom reversible sideroblastic change may also occur. Target cells occur as the surface area of the cell increases, due to increased membrane lipid content without an increase in volume. Ecchinocytosis is fairly common because of binding of the red cell membrane by abnormal high-density lipoproteins. In contrast, true acanthocytes are uncommon in uncomplicated liver disease, although they are a characteristic finding in 'spur-cell anaemia' (non-immune haemolytic anaemia in patients with alcoholic cirrhosis). Zieve's syndrome of haemolytic anaemia with hypertriglyceridaemia in patients with alcoholic liver disease is also rare. Haemolysis due to the direct toxicity of copper ions on red cells is characteristically an early presentation of Wilson's disease. Intracorpuscular changes are rare in liver disease. However, abnormal pyruvate kinase activity has been demonstrated in Zieve's syndrome, and reduction of hepatocyte glucose-6-phosphate dehydrogenase (G6PD) levels in G6PD-deficient individuals, and in neonates, may exacerbate and prolong hyperbilirubinaemia with haemolysis. Viral hepatitis, including hepatitis A, B and C but most frequently hepatitis viruses yet to be fully characterized, may lead to a transient and mild pancytopenia or to severe aplastic anaemia.

Platelets and haemostasis

These are discussed in Chapter 30.

Liver transplantation

Orthotopic liver transplantation (OLT) is increasingly used for end-stage liver disease. Thrombocytopenia is frequently present prior to transplantation. The count tends to fall post-operatively despite platelet transfusions and this may be due to platelet sequestration in the transplanted liver. Immune thrombocytopenia has also been reported post OLT. Antibody mediated haemolysis occurs in recipients of ABO-incompatible grafts, but the engrafted liver can also produce mild haemolysis due to antirecipient ABO antibody. This is a form of humoral graft-versus-host disease (GvHD), but T cell-mediated GvHD has also been reported post OLT. Although aplastic anaemia is a rare complication of viral hepatitis, there are reports that it may occur in as many as 30% of patients transplanted for fulminant non-A, non-B viral hepatitis.

Infections (Tables 59.12 and 59.13)

Infection may produce a tremendous variety of haematological

Table 59.12 Haematological changes in viral infection.

Red cells
Anaemia
Autoimmune
  Measles
  Epstein–Barr virus (EBV)
  Hepatitis
  Cytomegalovirus (CMV)
  Human immunodeficiency virus (HIV)
  Others including herpesviruses, varicella, influenza
Non-immune
  Microangiopathic haemolytic anaemia
Reduced red cell production
  Marrow hypoplasia
  EBV (especially in X-linked lymphoproliferative syndrome)
  Hepatitis viruses
  HIV
  CMV (especially post renal or bone marrow transplantation)
  Others (rare) include togaviruses epidemic haemorrhagic
    fevers, dengue
Red cell aplasia
  B19 parvovirus, especially with haemolytic anaemia

White cells
Neutrophilia
  Especially HIV, influenza, hepatitis, rubella, adenoviruses, measles,
    mumps, CMV and EBV as part of nearly all viral infections
Neutropenia
  Aplasia (see above)
  Complicating myalgic encephalitis
  (?Enteroviruses, EBV)
Lymphocytosis
  Wide variety, especially early in course of infection
Malignant transformation
  HTLV-1
  EBV
  HIV

Platelets
Thrombocytosis (e.g. Kawasaki)
Thrombocytopenia
  Often history of viral prodromal in childhood immune
    thrombocytopenic purpura
  Autoimmune: EBV, hepatitis, rubella, CMV, HIV
  ↓Production: aplasia (see above), measles, dengue, CMV, others
  ↑Consumption: disseminated intravascular coagulation
    (DIC)/haemolytic uraemic syndrome (HUS) (see below)

Coagulation changes
  DIC, especially varicella, vaccinia, rubella, arbovirus with/
    without microangiopathy, epidemic haemorrhagic fevers
  Haemolytic–uraemic syndrome: Coxsackievirus, mumps,
    echoviruses
  Haemophagocytosis
  Herpesviruses, adenoviruses, cytomegalovirus

Table 59.13 Haematological changes in bacterial/fungal/protozoal infections.

Anaemia
Anaemia of chronic disorder
Haemolytic
    Immune: mycoplasma, malaria, syphilis (PCH), listeriosis
    Non-immune: *Clostridium perfringens* (toxin related)
    Bartonella bacilliformis (Oroya fever)
    Malaria, trypanosomiasis with microangiopathy/disseminated
        intravascular coagulation (DIC), septicaemia
    Haemolytic–uraemic syndrome: verotoxin-producing
        Escherichia coli and Streptococcus pneumoniae
Dilutional
    Splenomegaly (e.g. malaria, schistosomiasis)
Blood loss
    Helicobacter pylori
    Ancylostoma

White cells
Neutrophilia
    Virtually any bacterial/fungal infection
Neutropenia
    Salmonella, *Rickettsia*, brucellosis, pertussis, disseminated
        tuberculosis (TB)
    Overwhelming septicaemia
Neutrophil function defects
    Rare (e.g. *Bacteroides*, endocarditis)
Lymphocytosis
    Whooping cough (*Bordetella pertussis*), *Rickettsia*
Lymphopenia
    TB, acute bacterial infections, brucellosis
Eosinophilia
    Aspergillosis, coccidioidomycosis, *Chlamydia*, streptococcal
        infections, *Ancylostoma*
Eosinopenia
    Common in acute bacteroides infections
Monocytosis
    Subacute/chronic infections (e.g. disseminated TB listeriosis)
Pancytopenia
    Bone marrow suppression (e.g. disseminated TB, listeriosis)
    Haemophagocytosis: septicaemia
    Peripheral destruction (e.g. DIC)

changes. Many of these are covered in other sections of this book.

Viruses

Anaemia

Haemolytic anaemia due to red cell autoantibody production, usually of the warm type, may occur, although cold-antibody syndromes have been reported in measles, influenza, infectious mononucleosis and mumps. Paroxysmal cold haemoglobinuria is rare and occurs in children due to Donath–Landsteiner IgG, anti-P antibodies. Non-immune MAHA may be associated with TTP or DIC, which may be the result of viral infections.

Anaemia due to transient red cell aplasia is seen with B19 parvovirus infection in patients with haemolytic anaemias ('aplastic crisis'). This virus may also cause erythema variegetum, or fifth disease, in children. It invades and destroys red cell progenitors and the aplasia is terminated when neutralizing IgM and IgG antibodies develop. If the virus attacks pregnant women, it may cross the placenta and cause spontaneous abortion or hydrops fetalis. Intravenous Ig therapy has been used for severe cases (e.g. in pregnancy, HIV infection and post bone marrow transplantation).

Anaemia occurs with pancytopenia in virus-associated bone marrow aplasia, for example with hepatitis viruses. The presence of viruses, either within lymphocytes or on their cell surface, may lead to production of a range of cytokines (including TNF, IFN-α and IFN-γ), which inhibit haemopoietic cell proliferation *in vitro* and *in vivo*. This may cause a substantial reduction in erythropoiesis and is presumably the mechanism underlying neutropenia and lymphopenia in viral infections. In infectious mononucleosis and other viral infections such as viral hepatitis, the virus infects B lymphocytes and the characteristic activated lymphocytes seen on the blood film are a reactive population of T cells.

Platelets

Thrombocytopenia may occur due to multiple mechanisms. Children with idiopathic thrombocytopenic purpura frequently give a history of a preceding viral illness, and autoantibody production is well described in infectious mononucleosis, rubella and cytomegalovirus infections. Reduction of bone marrow thrombopoiesis is frequently subclinical, but it is particularly important in virus-associated aplasia and dengue fever. Thrombocytosis can also occur in response to viral infections.

Bacterial, fungal and protozoal infections

Anaemia

Anaemia of chronic disease can occur in acute infections, overwhelming septicaemia and chronic or suppurative infection. Haemolytic anaemia is less common, but can occur through both immune (e.g. cold antibodies with anti-I specificity in mycoplasma infection) and non-immune mechanisms. Direct red cell invasion frequently results in severe haemolysis in infections caused by *Bartonella baciliformis*, with elements of intravascular haemolysis (due to increased red cell fragility) and extravascular haemolysis. *Clostridium perfringens* produces an alpha toxin (a lecithinase) and a theta toxin, and *Staphylococcus aureus* an alpha toxin, which act as haemolysins to cause severe intravascular haemolysis. DIC and MAHA can occur in any severe bacterial, fungal or protozoal infection. The haemolytic–uraemic syndrome has been associated with a range of bacterial infections, including *Salmonella*, *Shigella* and *Campylobacter* spp., but most frequently with verotoxin-producing strains of *Escherichia coli*.

White cells

Neutrophilia is the most common manifestation. Circulating neutrophils constitute less than 5% of the total body pool, and the neutrophil response shows great individual variation, with no clear relationship to the severity of the infection. The term *leukaemoid reaction* is used to describe marked leucocytosis ($> 50 \times 10^9$/L), with circulating immature forms occurring in patients with non-leukaemic conditions, typically severe infection or haemolysis or with generalized malignancy. Such reactions are more common in children. Features that distinguish such a reactive leucocytosis from CML include the presence of toxic granulation, elevated leucocyte alkaline phosphatase, Döhle bodies, and the lack of twin peaks of neutrophils and myelocytes in the differential count. Neutropenia can also occur with virtually any bacterial infection, although it has been most frequently noted with *Salmonella*, *Rickettsia* and *Brucella*. Defects of neutrophil function may also occur.

Platelets

Thrombocytosis is frequent in patients with chronic infections, and during the convalescent phase of acute infections. Thrombocytopenia also occurs during severe bacterial or fungal infection, particularly where there is bloodstream invasion or in intensive care patients. Certain rickettsial infections (e.g. Rocky Mountain spotted fever) are almost always associated with thrombocytopenia. Accelerated platelet destruction is the most frequent mechanism and can arise through DIC or microangiopathy with platelet attachment to damaged endothelium. Immune destruction can also occur and circulating immune complexes may lead to thrombocytopenia. Decreased platelet production is a less common mechanism, but may occur (e.g. in disseminated tuberculosis). The inflammatory and procoagulant responses to infections are clearly related. TNF-α, IL1α and IL-6 may activate coagulation and inhibit fibrinolysis, whereas thrombin may stimulate inflammatory pathways. In severe infection, the end result may be endovascular injury, DIC, multiorgan failure and death.

Haemostasis

DIC occurs frequently and may dominate the clinical picture in certain infections (e.g. bacterial meningitis). The acute-phase response that accompanies severe infection can lead to a rise in a range of coagulation factors, which may contribute to thrombotic manifestations. Suppurative thrombophlebitis, particularly in association with in-dwelling catheters, can occur in relation to both Gram-positive and -negative infections. In patients with systemic inflammation and organ failure due to acute infection, plasma protein C levels are reduced, and recombinant human activated protein C given as an intravenous infusion over 96 h reduces the death rate but may be associated with increased risk of bleeding. Activated protein C promotes fibrinolysis and inhibits thrombosis and inflammation and reduces circulating levels of D-dimers and IL-6.

Malaria

Anaemia is the most prominent haematological manifestation of malarial infection. It is most marked with *Plasmodium falciparum*, which invades erythrocytes of all ages (*P. vivax* and *P. ovale* invade only reticulocytes, *P. malariae* only mature cells) and can give parasitaemia levels as high as 50%. Cellular disruption and haemoglobin digestion lead directly to haemolysis. Parasitized cells have an increased osmotic facility and lose deformability; they thereby become sequestered and destroyed within the spleen, which often becomes massively enlarged. Non-parasitized cells may then become sequestered within the spleen and a raised plasma volume contributes to the anaemia. In addition, malarial antigens may attach to non-parasitized red cells to give rise to a positive direct antiglobulin test and haemolysis via a complement-mediated immune response. Acute intravascular haemolysis with haemoglobinuria, often leading to renal failure ('black water fever'), occurs rarely in *P. falciparum* infection.

An inadequate bone marrow response to anaemia is seen with relative reticulocytopenia at times of active infection, with some recovery after effective therapy. TNF levels are typically elevated and ACD occurs. Leucocyte numbers may be slightly increased or normal, but leucopenia as a result of splenomegaly and impaired marrow function is characteristic. Eosinophilia is variable. Thrombocytopenia is seen in nearly 70% of *P. falciparum* infections and has multifactorial aetiology. Autoimmune mechanisms may operate as for red cells, splenic sequestration is a contributory factor, DIC (either acute as in blackwater fever, or low grade and chronic) is common, and ADP release from damaged red cells may lead to platelet activation and consumption.

Haemophagocytic syndrome (Table 59.14; see also Chapters 8 and 12)

This may occur in association with a wide range of systemic illness. It is particularly common in patients who are immunosuppressed or who are acutely ill (e.g. septicaemic). Occasionally, patients may have haemophagocytosis as a presenting feature of lymphoma. Pancytopenia is usual, although cytopenias affecting an individual cell lineage also occur, and coagulopathy due to associated DIC is frequently present. Abnormal liver function commonly co-exists. The bone marrow (Figure 59.3) shows the presence of increased numbers of histiocytes displaying haemophagocytosis. Myelofibrosis and/or marrow hypocellu-

Table 59.14 Conditions associated with reactive haemophagocytosis.

Infection
Viral (e.g. herpesviruses, adenoviruses, cytomegalovirus)
Bacterial, especially tuberculosis
Fungal

Tumours
Haematological
Others

Drugs
Phenytoin

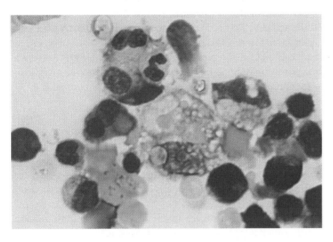

Figure 59.3 Bone marrow aspirate showing active haemophagocytosis, which, in this patient, antedated the development of high-grade non-Hodgkin's lymphoma by 6 months.

larity are present in a minority of cases. The underlying mechanisms are poorly understood. Treatment should be directed at the underlying disease process and possible infection treated after appropriate cultures have been taken. The condition is usually of brief duration until recovery or, sometimes, death occurs.

Haematological aspects of pregnancy
(Table 59.15)

Pregnancy poses a major physiological challenge to the human body and a number of haematological changes accompany it.

Anaemia

Maternal plasma volume increases by approximately 50% during the first and second trimesters of pregnancy, whereas the corres-

Table 59.15 Haematological changes during pregnancy.

Anaemia
Dilutional
Iron deficiency
Folic acid deficiency
Aplastic anaemia

White cells
Neutrophil leucocytosis

Platelets
Thrombocytopenia
Immune thrombocytopenic purpura
Eclampsia
Haemolytic–uraemic syndrome
Thrombotic thrombocytopenic purpura
HELLP syndrome (haemolysis, elevated liver enzymes, low platelet count)
Disseminated intravascular coagulation (DIC)
Drug induced

Coagulation
Coagulation factors: vitamin K-dependent factors II, VII, IX, XI, X↑, factor VIII↑, von Willebrand factor↑, fibrinogen↑
Coagulation inhibitors: protein C↑ or no change, protein S↓, antithrombin↓ or no change
Fibrinolytic activity↓
DIC due to: abruptio placentae, intrauterine fetal death, amniotic fluid embolism, obstetric sepsis, eclampsia

---

ponding increase in red cell mass is only 20–30%. A dilutional anaemia results, so that the lower limit of normal haemoglobin concentration is approximately 10.5 g/dL between 16 and 40 weeks of pregnancy. The increase in maternal red cell mass, transfer of iron to the fetus (which takes place largely in the third trimester), and blood loss during labour, together impose a requirement of about 800 mg of iron, so that iron deficiency frequently arises in mothers with normal or reduced iron stores. Folic acid requirements are also raised during pregnancy (increased folate breakdown due to increased nucleic acid synthesis in mother and fetus) and routine supplementation is advised even during early pregnancy to prevent megaloblastic anaemia and neural tube defects in the fetus. A physiological rise in MCV of 5–10 fL occurs during normal pregnancy with pre-existing aplasia. AIHA occurring during pregnancy is typically severe and refractory to therapy.

White cells

A mild neutrophil leucocytosis with a left shift and occasional Döhle bodies occur during normal pregnancy.

Platelets

The normal range for the platelet count ($140-400 \times 10^9$/L) does not alter during pregnancy; thrombocytopenia occurring during pregnancy requires evaluation. Gestational thrombocytopenia complicates 8–10% of pregnancies and is characterized by mild thrombocytopenia occurring for the first time during pregnancy (platelets $80-150 \times 10^9$/L) and is usually not associated with neonatal thrombocytopenia or significant bleeding in the mother. Maternal immune thrombocytopenic purpura may antedate or present during pregnancy: it is often associated with increased levels of platelet associated IgG, although this is a nonspecific finding and the presence of serum platelet autoantibodies to platelet glycoproteins (GP)IIb-IIa or GPIb-IX is more specific. The management of immune thrombocytopenic purpura is discussed in Chapter 57. Thrombocytopenia is regularly seen in pre-eclampsia. The mechanism is unknown, but increased aggregation is suggested, as low-dose aspirin therapy may reduce platelet consumption. TTP may occur at any time during pregnancy but typically it is before 24 weeks; the use of fresh-frozen plasma and plasma exchange has been shown to improve fetal outcome. The haemolytic uraemic syndrome typically occurs within 48 h of delivery in an otherwise normal pregnancy.

The potentially fatal syndrome of haemolysis, elevated liver enzymes and low platelets (HELLP) occurs in up to 10% of pregnancies complicated by eclampsia. The existence of coagulation abnormalities with red cell fragmentation suggests that microangiopathy, DIC and endothelial damage all have a role in its pathogenesis. Fetal and maternal outcomes are characteristically poor.

Basophilic stippling, crenated red cells and large platelets are characteristic peripheral blood findings in acute fatty liver of pregnancy.

Coagulation changes

Normal pregnancy is associated with a range of alterations to haemostatic components (see Table 59.15), which combine to give an increased risk of haemorrhage, thrombosis and DIC, occurring in up to 40% of patients with abruptio placentae, leading to haemorrhage and shock. Amniotic fluid embolism typically occurs during the course of a difficult delivery in a multiparous woman and rapidly leads to a picture of chronic low-grade DIC, with onset over a period of 1–2 weeks. Venous stasis resulting from the gravid uterus combines with the coagulation changes to make pregnancy a hypercoagulable state; operative delivery imposes an additional risk.

Selected bibliography

Austin JA, Shulman LN (eds) (1993) Therapy related second malignancies. *Hematological Oncological Clinics North American* 7: 325–499.

Bernard GR, Vincent JL, Laterre P et al. (2001) Efficacy and safety of recombinant human activated protein C for severe sepsis. *New England Journal of Medicine* 344: 699–709.

Bick RL (ed.) (1992) Perplexing thrombotic and haemorrhagic disorders. *Hematological Oncological Clinics North America* 6: 1203–431.

Dallalio G, Fleury T, Neans RT (2003) Serum hepicidin in clinical specimens. *British Journal of Haematology* 122: 996–1000.

Delamore IW, Liu Yin JA (1990) *Haematological Aspects of Systemic Disease.* Baillière Tindall, London.

Ganz T (2003) Hepicidin, a key regulator of iron metabolism and mediation of anaemia of inflammation. *Blood* 102: 783–8.

Hoffbrand AV, Pettit JE (2001) *Essential Haematology*, 4th edn. Blackwell Science, Oxford.

Kurtzhals JAL, Rodrigues O, Addae M et al. (1997) Reversible suppression of bone marrow response to erythropoietin in plasmodium falciparum malaria. *British Journal of Haematology* 97: 169–74.

Ludwig H, Rai Kr, Blade J et al. (2002) Management of disease related anaemia in patients with multiple myeloma or chronic lymphocytic leukaemia: epoietin treatment recommendations. *The Haematology Journal* 3: 121–30.

McRae KR, Samuels P, Schreiber AD (1992) Pregnancy associated thrombocytopenia: pathogenesis and management. *Blood* 80: 2697–714.

Means RT (1999) Advances in the anaemia of chronic disease. *International Journal of Haematology* 70: 7–12.

Means RT, Krantz SB (1992) Progress in understanding the pathogenesis of anaemia of chronic disease. *Blood* 80: 1639–47.

Mehta AB, McIntyre N (1998) Haematological disorders in liver disease. *Trends in Experimental and Clinical Medicine Forum* 8: 8–25.

Nemeth E, Valore EV, Territo M et al. (2003) Hepicidin, a putative mediator of anaemia of inflammation, is a type II acute phase protein. *Blood* 101: 2461–3.

Papadaki HA, Kritkos HD, Valatas V et al. (2002) Anaemia of chronic disease in rheumatoid arthritis is associated with increased apoptosis of bone marrow erythroid cells: improvement following anti-tumour necrosis factor-α therapy. *Blood* 1001: 474–82.

Smith OP, White B. (1999) Infectious purpura fulmins: diagnosis and treatment. *British Journal of Haematology* 104: 202–7.

Spivak, JL. (2002) The blood in systemic disorders. *Lancet* 355: 1707–12.

The Malaria Working Party of the General Haematology Task Force of British Committee for Standards in Haematology (1997) The laboratory diagnosis of malaria. *Clinical Laboratory Haematology* 19: 165–70.

Haematological aspects of tropical diseases

Imelda Bates and Ivy Ekem

60

Introduction

For the purposes of this chapter, 'tropical diseases' refers to infectious diseases occurring predominantly in tropical areas. The chapter has been divided into two sections, covering tropical diseases in which organisms can be visualized in the blood or bone marrow and those that cause secondary haematological abnormalities.

Net international migration contributed to 88% of the population growth in Europe in 1990–95 and travelling migrants are responsible for a major component of imported tropical infections. These rapid increases in worldwide travel mean that haematologists need to know about the tropical diseases that can cause haematological disturbances. They also need to be able to take a relevant travel history from patients and to be aware of ethnic variations in reference ranges to avoid wasting resources on unnecessary investigations and to reduce undue anxiety for the patient.

Ethnic variations in reference ranges

The white blood count and relative and absolute neutrophil counts are lower in black people, Yemenite Jews, Palestinians and Saudi Arabians than in white people. After the age of 1 year,

Africans have lower counts than West Indians or black Americans (Table 60.1). This is due to the non-white populations having a greater number of neutrophils in the storage pool. Stimulation of a neutrophil response in these ethnic groups leads to rises in the neutrophil count to the same level as white populations irrespective of the baseline level. Indian, Chinese and South-East Asian populations have the same white blood count and neutrophil counts as white northern Europeans. There is a suggestion that black races may have lower platelet counts than white races. It is not clear whether there are true ethnic variations in eosinophil counts but counts of up to 2×10^9/L have been described in healthy blood donors in Africa.

Tropical diseases with organisms in peripheral blood or bone marrow

Malaria

Epidemiology and biology
Four species of mosquito cause human malaria disease, *Plasmodium falciparum*, *P. vivax*, *P. ovale* and *P. malariae*. *P. falciparum* is by far the most dangerous and responsible for almost all the mortality and morbidity. Malaria is the single most important disease hazard facing travellers, with 8 in 1000 travellers from developed countries becoming infected annually. More than

Table 60.1 Automated WBC and neutrophil counts in adults: 95% ranges.

	Male WBC ($\times10^9$/L)	Neutrophil count ($\times10^9$/L)	Female WBC ($\times10^9$/L)	Neutrophil count ($\times10^9$/L)
Caucasian	3.7–9.5	1.7–6.1	3.9–11.1	1.7–7.5
Afro-Caribbean	3.1–9.4	1.2–5.6	3.2–10.6	1.3–7.1
African	2.8–7.2	0.9–4.2	3.0–7.4	1.3–3.7

10 000 cases of malaria are imported into Europe each year. In 2001, 2069 cases of malaria were reported in the UK, 1576 of which were due to *P. falciparum*, and there were nine deaths. The malaria rates are highest in immigrants who visit their countries of origin, and account for one-third of all reports. Over 80% of *P. falciparum* infections in the UK are acquired in sub-Saharan Africa; 85% of *P. vivax* infections are acquired in South Asia, especially India and Pakistan. Over one-half of the patients returning to the UK with malaria did not take malaria chemoprophylaxis.

Malaria is transmitted by the bite of an infected female anopheline mosquito. The infecting agent is the sporozoite and thousands of these spindle-shaped cells may be injected by a single bite. Infrequently, transmission may also occur through blood transfusion, bone marrow transplants and transplacentally (0.5% of all UK cases). There have also been reports of malaria transmission in aircraft or near airports in temperate zones due to infected mosquitoes being brought to non-malarious areas.

Within a few hours of an infected bite, the sporozoites enter the hepatocytes, where they divide (Figure 60.1). Rupture of the

hepatocyte releases the parasites into the blood and they attach to red cell membranes using specific receptors. They feed on stroma inside the red cell and the digestion of haemoglobin produces the characteristic brown pigment (haemozoin). This accumulates in cells as the parasites mature. Asexual replication of the malaria ring forms (trophozoites) takes place in the red cells, giving rise to erythrocyte schizonts. Once the trophozoites are mature, they are released into the circulation to re-infect other red cells. The periodicity of this release varies with the species and is responsible for the classical cyclical nature of malaria fevers. Relapses, which are characteristic of infection with *P. vivax* and *P. ovale*, are due to activation of dormant hypnozoite stages in the liver.

A few of the trophozoites will develop into male and female banana-shaped gametocytes and are taken up by a mosquito in the course of having a blood meal. Inside the mosquito's stomach, they undergo sexual reproduction and sporozoites migrate to the salivary glands, ready to infect another host when the mosquito bites.

Unlike the schizonts of *P. vivax, P. ovale* and *P. malariae*, those of *P. falciparum* are not commonly seen in the peripheral blood

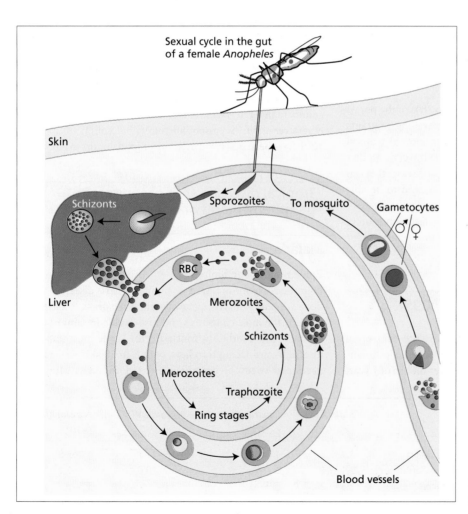

Figure 60.1 Life cycle of the malarial parasite.

Table 60.2 Features of *P. falciparum* malaria infection.

Target organ	Clinical features	Potential common misdiagnosis
Gastrointestinal	Diarrhoea, vomiting	Traveller's diarrhoea
Respiratory	Cough, pulmonary oedema	Pneumonia, cardiac failure
Neurological	Delirium, coma, convulsions, focal neurological signs	Encephalitis, meningoencephalitis
Renal	Oliguria, haemoglobinuria	Nephritis
Hepatic	Jaundice, hypoglycaemia	Hepatitis
Haematological	Anaemia, splenomegaly	Viral infection, lymphoma

of the human host. This is because *P. falciparum*-infected cells have surface cytoadherence molecules that enable them to be sequestered in the deep tissues. *P. falciparum* schizonts therefore only appear in the blood in very severe infections or in splenectomized patients. Sequestration is responsible for some of the severe clinical consequences of *P. falciparum* malaria such as cerebral malaria.

Clinical features

The time between the infected bite and the appearance of clinical symptoms and parasites in the peripheral blood varies between species. It is 7–30 days (mean 10 days) in *P. falciparum* but can be months, or even years, with other species, particularly *P. vivax* and *P. ovale*, because of their hypnozoite stage. The dormancy time of hypnozoites varies with different strains. When they become activated they reinvade the blood resulting in a clinical relapse.

Maximal immunity to malaria takes around 10 years to develop and is lost over the course of 1–5 years if the individual leaves a malarious area and is no longer exposed to infections. This is often not appreciated by, for example, students or immigrants from malaria-endemic countries, who may be more prone to severe attacks of malaria when they return home after a prolonged period in a non-malarious area. They will rapidly regain their immunity on re-exposure to infection.

All four malaria species produce factors that cause release of tissue cytokines, especially from leucocytes. These produce fever and contribute to anaemia through marrow suppression. Splenomegaly is a feature of acute malaria and mild jaundice may also occur secondary to haemolysis. All malaria species, but particularly *P. falciparum*, are associated with an increased risk of abortion in pregnancy. Other clinical features vary with different species.

Plasmodium falciparum

P. falciparum is the only species associated with complicated and severe disease. Death may occur after a single exposure to malaria, particularly in those who have no immunity such as non-immune travellers or young children in endemic countries. Despite this, the majority of infections cause a self-limited febrile illness. Recurrent fevers and other symptoms of malaria may be due to either recrudescence of blood forms that persist between attacks or to re-infection with a new strain or species. Recurrent attacks with different strains leads to the development of clinical, but not necessarily parasitological, immunity. Parasites may therefore be detected in a high proportion of adults in endemic areas who are clinically asymptomatic.

In addition to fever with rigors and hot and cold phases, *P. falciparum* infection commonly presents with diarrhoea and cough (Table 60.2). Serious complications include severe anaemia, cerebral involvement and failure of major organs such as kidneys and liver.

During pregnancy, immunity to malaria is reduced and parasite density increases. Even if parasites cannot be visualized in the peripheral blood they may be sequestered in the placenta and compromise fetal development. *P. falciparum* is therefore an important cause of low birth weight in neonates and anaemia in pregnant women. Both of these factors have a detrimental effect on the later development of the infant.

Plasmodium malariae

The incubation period of *P. malariae* may be several weeks. It is associated with recurrent fever, anaemia and enlargement of the liver and spleen. Without treatment, recrudescences may occur with decreasing severity over many years. Clinical symptoms of malaria have been reported up to 30 years after the initial infection.

Plasmodium vivax and Plasmodium ovale

These species cause a similar clinical picture with bouts of fever occurring periodically up to 5 years after the initial infection. These are relapses rather than recrudescences and are due to re-invasion of red cells by hypnozoites. The trigger for these parasites to re-activate after dormancy is unknown.

Haematological abnormalities

Normochromic, normocytic anaemia is a common manifestation of malaria, particularly in children, but the degree and rapidity of onset are very variable. The haemoglobin may fall by up to 2 g/dL each day. In malaria-endemic regions, chronic anaemia due to nutritional deficiencies, intestinal helminths, HIV and haemoglobinopathies may be compounded by the effects of malaria. In chronically anaemic patients, the oxygen dissociation curve is shifted to the right and this makes them better able to tolerate further falls in haemoglobin. The clinical effects of anaemia in malaria are therefore due to a combination of the degree and rate of fall of haemoglobin.

The anaemia that accompanies malaria has multiple aetiologies. Red cells containing parasites are removed from the circulation by the reticuloendothelial system. There is also accelerated destruction of non-parasitized cells, which is the major reason why the haemoglobin falls rapidly in severe malarial anaemia. Both parasitized and non-parasitized red cells lose deformability and the high shear rates in the spleen enhance their removal by the spleen. In the acute phase of the disease there is suppression of the reticulocyte response. Erythropoietin levels are usually elevated, although occasionally they are less than those anticipated for the degree of anaemia.

Unusual complications of malaria that can exacerbate the anaemia are hyper-reactive malarial splenomegaly and 'blackwater fever'. Massive splenomegaly as a result of a disordered immune complex production in response to malaria (hyper-reactive malarial splenomegaly) may be associated with anaemia and other features of hypersplenism (see later). Severe intravascular haemolysis with haemoglobinuria ('blackwater fever') can lead to acute renal failure. The mechanism is unknown but it has been associated with antimalarial drugs, particularly quinine, and may also be more common in individuals with glucose-6-phosphate dehydrogenase deficiency.

Case fatality rates of children with severe anaemia in Africa are 9–18% and mortality rises steeply at haemoglobin concentrations of less than 4 g/dL. Severe malarial anaemia is accompanied by hypovolaemia and therefore requires urgent fluid volume replacement and blood transfusion. The risk of transfusion-transmitted infections in poorer countries makes it increasingly important to prevent and adequately treat the milder forms of anaemia. There is now good evidence to show that antimalarial prophylaxis and insecticide-treated bed nets are both valuable in reducing anaemia in children in endemic countries.

The white cell count in malaria is usually normal but it may be raised in severe disease. Other white cell changes that have been described in malaria include a leucoerythroblastic response, monocytosis, eosinopenia and a reactive eosinophilia during the recovery phase. Neutrophil activation, indicated by raised leucocyte elastase levels, may be apparent in severe malaria. Mild thrombocytopenia with counts down to 100×10^9/L is common in malaria infection. It is due to increased splenic clearance and is associated with increased platelet turnover and raised thrombopoietin levels. Pancytopenia without hyper-reactive malarial splenomegaly has also been described in malaria infection.

The bone marrow of patients with acute malaria due to any of the four human species shows prominent dyserythropoiesis. This may persist for weeks after the acute infection and is caused by intramedullary cytokines produced by the infection. Erythrophagocytosis and macrophages containing malaria pigment are frequently seen in marrow samples from malaria patients.

In malaria, the coagulation cascade is accelerated, the degree of acceleration being proportional to the severity of disease. Fibrinogen levels are often increased and there is rapid fibrinogen turnover with consumption of antithrombin III and factor XIII, and increased fibrin degradation products (FDPs). The trigger for this activation is uncertain but there is evidence that it may be a combination of procoagulant cytokines and parasitized erythrocytes, which can directly activate coagulation pathways. Disseminated intravascular coagulation has been shown to be unimportant in the pathogenesis of severe malaria and significant bleeding is unusual, even though the prothrombin and partial thromboplastin times may be prolonged.

Haematological indicators of a poor prognosis in severe malaria include:
- leucocytosis $> 12 \times 10^9$/L;
- severe anaemia (PCV < 15%);
- platelets $< 50 \times 10^9$/L;
- prolonged prothrombin time > 3 s;
- prolonged partial thromboplastin time;
- fibrinogen < 200 mg/dL;
- hyperparasitaemia > 100 000/μL (high mortality > 500 000/μL);
- > 20% of parasites are pigment-containing trophozoites and schizonts;
- > 5% of neutrophils contain visible malaria pigment.

Genetic haematological protection mechanisms

P. vivax needs Duffy blood group antigen as a receptor to enter red cells. This is lacking in individuals belonging to certain black races and explains why they have a natural resistance to infection with this organism. The protective effect of haemoglobin AS against the life-threatening complications of malaria is well recognized. It provides 10 times the level of protection against severe disease of haemoglobin AA. Evidence is accumulating that a similar but less marked protection is associated with G6PD deficiency, α thalassaemia trait and other common erythrocyte polymorphisms.

Diagnosis
Microscopy
Direct visualization of parasites by light microscopy using a combination of thick and thin blood films is the gold standard diagnostic technique for malaria (Table 60.3 and Figure 60.2). A Romanowsky stain (e.g. Field's, Giemsa's, Leishman's) pH 7.2 is used so that the parasite cytoplasm stains blue and the nuclear chromatin red. A thick blood film should be used as the first screening tool as it allows larger volumes of blood to be examined than the thin film. However, the parasites appear distorted due to the process of lysing the red cells so this method cannot be used for parasite morphology and speciation. A thin blood film allows visualization of undistorted parasites and of the size and shape of the red cells but it has low sensitivity because of the small amount of blood that can be examined.

Table 60.3 Differential diagnosis of human plasmodium/babesia species in stained thin blood films.

	Species				
	P. falciparum	P. malariae	P. vivax	P. ovale	Babesia sp.
Appearance of infected red blood cells (size and shape)	Both normal	Normal shape; size normal or smaller	1.5–2 times larger than normal; shape normal or oval	As for P. vivax, but some have irregular frayed edges	Both normal
Schüffner's dots (eosinophilic stippling)	None (but occasionally comma-like red dots present = Maurer's dots)	None	Present in all stages, except early ring form	As for P. vivax	None
Red cells with multiple parasites/cell	Common	Rare	Occasional	As for P. vivax	Common
Stages present in peripheral blood	Rings and gametocytes; occasionally schizonts	All stages	All stages	As for P. vivax	Only rings and rare pear-shaped forms ('Maltese cross'); no gametocytes
Ring form (young trophozoite)	Delicate, small ring; scanty cytoplasm; sometimes at the edge of red cell ('accolé form')	Ring one-third of the diameter of cell; heavy chromatin dot; vacuole sometimes 'filled in'	Ring one-third to one-half of the diameter of cell; heavy chromatin dot	As for P. vivax	Resembles ring of P. falciparum; look for pear-shaped structure
Schizont	Occasionally in peripheral blood, 16–30 merozoites	6–12 merozoites in rosette; coarse pigment clump in centre	12–24 merozoites in rosette filling entire RBC; central pigment	8–12 merozoites in rosette	No schizont
Gametocyte	'Crescent' or 'sausage' shape are characteristic	Round or oval; dark coarse pigment	Round or oval	Round or oval (smaller than P. vivax)	No gametocyte
Main criteria	Delicate ring forms and crescent-shaped gametocytes are the main forms in the bloodstream; multiple infection common; normal RBC shape/size; level of infection may be high	Red cell normal or slightly smaller; trophozoites compact and intensely strained; band-form suggestive; no Schüffner's dots; coarse and dark pigment	Large pale RBC; presence of Schüffner's dots in cytoplasm of RBC; round gametocytes; large amoeboid trophozoite with pale pigment	Oval RBC with fimbriated edges characteristic but not always present; generally like P. vivax	Ring forms very similar to P. falciparum; presence of group of 2–4 pear-shaped bodies ('Maltese cross') is characteristic; absence of gametocytes

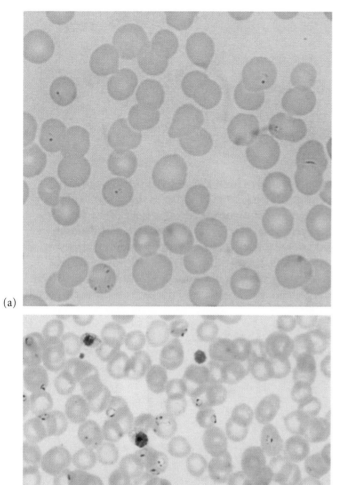

(a)

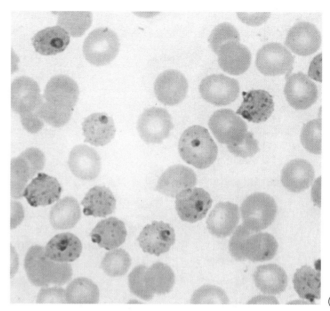

(b)

(c)

Figure 60.2 Stages in the life cycle of *Plasmodium falciparum* in Giemsa-stained thin films; the cells are not enlarged or decolorized: (a) delicate early ring forms; (b) ring forms with prominent Maurer's clefts; and (c) ring forms and early and late schizonts (schizonts are not commonly seen in the peripheral blood).

Disadvantages of basing a diagnosis of malaria on blood film examination include the following points:
• A negative film does not exclude malaria – at least three films taken during episodes of fever should be examined and even if these are negative it does not entirely exclude the diagnosis especially in the presence of antimalarial drugs.
• A positive film does not prove that symptoms are due to malaria – asymptomatic parasitaemia is common in adults from endemic areas.
• Parasites, particularly *P. falciparum* gametocytes, may be washed off the slide during staining; bulk staining of slides may result in transfer of parasites between slides.
• Parasite density does not necessarily correlate with disease severity although a heavy parasitaemia (> 5% of red cells infected) indicates a poor prognosis.

Malaria pigment may persist in phagocytic cells for several weeks after an acute attack and may be helpful in retrospective diagnosis of malaria. Automated haematology analysers may produce an abnormal pattern on the white cell differential count histogram. Debris below the white cell threshold may be due to malaria parasites and manual examination of blood films is indicated if this pattern is flagged up by the machine.

Antibody detection
As malarial antibodies can remain in the blood after the eradication of parasites, their detection is not useful for diagnosis in the acute attack. The main uses of malarial antibody detection are for excluding malaria as a cause of chronically recurrent fever between febrile attacks, population surveys and as a screening test for blood transfusion purposes.

Antigen detection
These tests are based on detection of the malaria antigen 'histidine-rich protein 2' (HRP2) or parasite enzyme lactate dehydrogenase (pLDH). They have been incorporated into immunochromatographic antigen-capture kits for rapid diagnosis.

The sensitivity of these dipstick strip tests approaches that of thick film microscopy (i.e. 0.002% parasitaemia equivalent to 100–200 parasites/μL of blood). HRP2 protein may remain positive for 14 days after successful treatment and false-positives due to rheumatoid factor have been reported. pLDH is only produced by viable parasites so it becomes negative 2–3 days after successful treatment. None of these kits are able to provide quantitative information about parasitaemia but some are able to distinguish between *P. falciparum* and other species.

Potential uses of malaria antigen detection tests include:
- confirmation of malaria diagnosis on a blood film;
- detection of *P. Falciparum* when the microscopist is inexperienced (e.g. on-call or emergency situations);
- determination of species when there is a possibility of mixed infection;
- monitoring response to treatment.

DNA-based methods
DNA hybridization and polymerase chain reaction (PCR) have both been used for malaria diagnosis predominantly in a research context.

Haematological implications of treatment for malaria
Chloroquine has been the first-line treatment for malaria in many countries for decades and is generally well tolerated. However, widespread parasite resistance is now seriously restricting its use and it is being replaced with newer drugs, some of which have haematological side-effects.

Amodiaquine has a similar mode of action to chloroquine but causes agranulocytosis in 1 in 2000 patients. Its use is therefore restricted to treatment and it is not recommended for prophylaxis.

Quinine is rarely associated with immune thrombocytopenia and severe intravascular haemolysis ('blackwater fever'). Blackwater fever has also been described with other antimalarial drugs and the underlying pathophysiology is not completely understood.

Pyrimethamine is used together with a long-acting sulphonamide, such as sulphadoxine (e.g. Fansidar). It is a dihydrofolate reductase inhibitor and this explains why pyrimethamine may induce megaloblastic anaemia, neutropenia or thrombocytopenia in patients with pre-existing folate deficiency. The sulpha component of these combinations may rarely cause blood dyscrasias and methaemoglobinaemia.

Dapsone, used as part of a fixed combination with proguanil or chlorproguanil, may be associated with haemolytic anaemia, methaemoglobinaemia and eosinophilia.

Primaquine is active against the hypnozoites of *P. vivax* and the gametocytes of *P. falciparum*. It causes oxidant haemolysis in patients with glucose-6-phosphate dehydrogenase deficiency and, rarely, methaemoglobinaemia.

Mefloquine, halofantrine, proguanil, lumefantrine and *artemisinin-related compounds* do not commonly cause significant haemato-logical side-effects. Some antibacterial drugs, such as *doxycycline*, *trimethoprim* and *sulphonamides* have also been used for their antimalarial effect and may be associated with haematological side-effects.

Babesiosis

Epidemiology and biology
Babesiosis is not a tropical disease but is briefly described here as it can be confused with malaria. It has been predominantly reported from the USA, particularly coastal regions, and Europe. It is primarily a disease of animals and rarely infects humans. It is due to a protozoan parasite transmitted by a tick bite. *Babesia bovis*, *B. microti* and *B. divergens* are responsible for the majority of human infections. There is geographical variation in the *Babesia* species responsible for disease in humans. Most of the cases reported from Europe have been due to *B. divergens* and occurred in patients who were asplenic, whereas in north America almost all the cases have been due to *B. microti*.

Following the bite, the organisms penetrate red cells, where they take on an oval, round or pear shape and multiply by budding. The erythrocytic ring forms of *B. microti* and *B. divergens* may be confused with malaria *P. falciparum* rings, but they do not produce pigment or cause alterations in the red cell morphology. A minority of organisms take on a folded shape and are thought to be gametocytes.

Clinical features
The incubation period varies from 1–4 weeks, and the severity and progression of the clinical features vary with the infecting species. Most patients have no recollection of a tick bite. The disease presents with fever, prostration, mild hepatosplenomegaly and haemolytic anaemia with jaundice and haemoglobinuria. Severe complications including acute tubular necrosis, respiratory distress and DIC, and a fulminant, fatal course has been described in splenectomized patients. *B. microti* usually produces a subclinical infection. Although babesiosis has a worse prognosis in patients who have been splenectomized or who are immunosuppressed, co-infected with HIV or elderly, it can occur in the presence of an intact spleen.

Haematological abnormalities
The anaemia may be mild to moderately severe and is due to parasite-induced abnormalities in the red cell membrane. Haemolytic anaemia, which may last for several weeks, is a prominent feature of babesiosis, particularly in splenectomized individuals. Although the haemolysis is due to complement or antibody coating of the red cells, the direct antiglobulin test is usually negative. Haptoglobin levels are reduced and the reticulocyte count is increased. The presence of parasitaemia needs to be interpreted with caution as parasites may persist for months after the resolution of symptoms and the level of parasitaemia does not parallel the severity of disease (Table 60.3).

Babesia parasites may be confused with Pappenheimer bodies in splenectomized patients with active haemolysis. Thrombocytopenia may occur in severe cases. Total white cell counts are usually normal or low.

Haematological implications of treatment for babesiosis

There have been no randomized controlled trials to determine optimal treatment for babesiosis. Treatment recommended at present includes the use of clindamycin and quinine, with exchange blood transfusion for those who are critically ill with high parasitaemias. Atovaquone and azithromycin have also been used successfully.

Filariasis

Epidemiology and biology

There are two groups of human filarias: those that occur in the blood (lymphatic filariasis) and those that occur in the skin (onchocerciasis). Only lymphatic filariasis will be considered in this chapter, as it is associated with detectable organisms in the peripheral blood.

Two species of filarial worms cause lymphatic filariasis in humans and are relevant for haematologists, *Wuchereria bancrofti* and *Brugia malayi*. They have different geographical distributions with *W. bancrofti* being the most widespread. More than 90% of infections due to *W. bancrofti* are found in Asia, although it also occurs in Africa, America and the Pacific Islands. Filariasis due to *B. malayi* occurs in China, Indo-China, Thailand, Malaysia, Indonesia, the Philippines and south-west India (Figure 60.3).

The worms are 4 (male) to 10 cm (female) long and can live for over 10 years in the lymphatics. Microfilariae, which are 250–300 μm long, are produced by the female worm and released into the blood after 3–8 months, where they may live for up to 1 year. Microfilariae densities can reach 10 000/mL but are usually much lower. They exhibit daily periodicity in the blood and this timing is designed to match the biting habits of their mosquito vector. This maximizes their chances of being taken up during the blood meal of culicine or anopheline mosquitoes. The microfilariae develop but do not multiply in the mosquito and pass into the proboscis, ready to be injected into another human.

Clinical presentation

There is a wide variation in the presenting features of lymphatic filariasis, which may occur 6 months or more after the infective bite. The symptoms and signs are due to lymphangitis. There

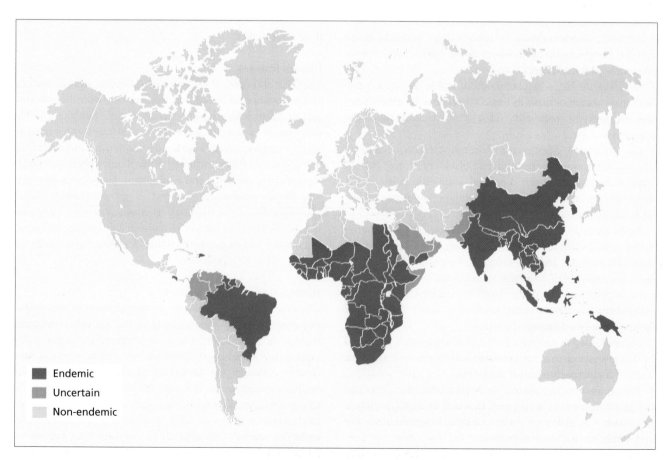

Legend:
- Endemic
- Uncertain
- Non-endemic

Figure 60.3 Global distribution of lymphatic filariasis.

are recurrent bouts of fever with heat, redness and pain over lymphatic vessels. In fair-skinned people, the lymphangitis can be seen to spread distally (i.e. the opposite direction to septic lymphangitis). In *W. bancrofti* these repeated episodes of inflammation eventually result in the typical chronic picture of filariasis, including hydrocele, lymphoedema and elephantiasis, chyluria and tropical pulmonary eosinophilia. The clinical picture in *B. malayi* infection is similar but it does not cause hydrocele or chylous urine.

Other filariae with blood-inhabiting larvae

Loa loa: This occurs in the rain forest belt of Central Africa, especially West Africa. The adult worms migrate through the subcutaneous tissues, including the conjunctiva, and occasionally can be seen passing across the eye.

Mansonella perstans: This is a non-pathogenic and common infection of people in Africa. These organisms may therefore co-exist in the blood with *W. bancrofti* but can be distinguished by their smaller size and absence of a sheath.

Mansonella ozzardi: This is also probably non-pathogenic and occurs in the West Indies and South America.

Haematological abnormalities

Eosinophilia is the major and most frequent haematological abnormality produced by lymphatic filariasis. The development of tropical pulmonary eosinophilia is an unusual complication of filariasis. This is an immunological hyper-responsiveness to microfilaria in the lungs and is more common in males than females. Although microfilariae are absent from the blood in this syndrome, they may be seen in lung biopsies and adult worms can be visualized in lymphatics on ultrasound. There is an extreme eosinophilia with eosinophil counts of greater than 10×10^9/L; the level of eosinophilia is not related to the severity of symptoms. In tropical pulmonary eosinophilia, diethylcarbamazine treatment reduces the eosinophil count and produces resolution of symptoms. This rapid response to treatment distinguishes filariasis from other causes of marked eosinophilia, such as helminths that affect the lungs (*Ascaris*, *Strongyloides*, *Schistosoma* subsp. *trichinosis*) and *Toxocara*.

Diagnosis of filariasis

The adult worms residing in the lymphatics are inaccessible, so diagnosis is based on finding microfilariae in the peripheral blood. The level of filaraemia is inversely related to the clinical signs because much of the damage is due to immunological responses to the microfilariae rather than to the organisms themselves. Furthermore the presence of microfilariae does not necessarily mean that they are causing clinical problems and conversely a lack of microfilariae in the blood does not exclude a diagnosis of filariasis. The peripheral blood findings must therefore be assessed in the context of the clinical picture.

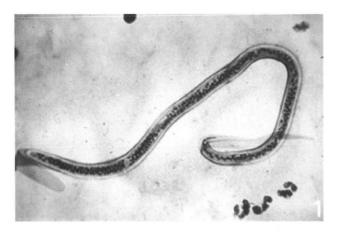

Figure 60.4 Microfilaria of *Wuchereria bancrofti*.

To optimize the chances of finding scanty microfilariae in the blood, the sample should be taken at the appropriate time for the expected peak concentration of microfilariae (i.e. around midnight or midday for nocturnally and diurnally periodic forms respectively). There are many techniques for demonstrating microfilariae in the laboratory. The simplest method is a wet preparation of fresh blood. Microfilariae will survive in venous blood collected into EDTA for 2 days at room temperature. Motile microfilariae can be seen on a slide under low power and can be counted in a counting chamber. Numbers of microfilariae may be low, so concentration techniques are often required. Sensitivity can be increased by passing the whole blood sample through a 3-μm Nuclepore filter membrane and then staining the microfilariae trapped in the filter.

For species identification, thick and thin blood films should be stained with Giemsa or haematoxylin and the microfilariae differentiated according to the pattern of their sheaths, nuclei distribution and size (Figure 60.4). The edges of the film should be examined carefully as microfilariae tend to be concentrated at the periphery and are easily missed if the microscopist goes straight onto high power in the centre of the film.

Detection of circulating antigen by enzyme-linked immunosorbent assay (ELISA) or ICT has replaced microscopy for the diagnosis of bancroftian, but not brugian, filariasis. An antigen immunochromatography card test is available for the detection of *W. bancrofti*, which does not react with other filariae and is highly sensitive (100%) and specific (92%). Filarial DNA can be detected by PCR, and ultrasound can help to identify adult worms within the lymphatic system. Serological tests are not very helpful in the diagnosis as most individuals from endemic areas have antibodies to crude filarial antigens and there is cross-reactivity with other filariae and nematodes.

Haematological implications of treatment for filariasis

Oral diethylcarbamazine is the drug of choice in all forms of lymphatic filariasis, including subclinical infection. Alternative

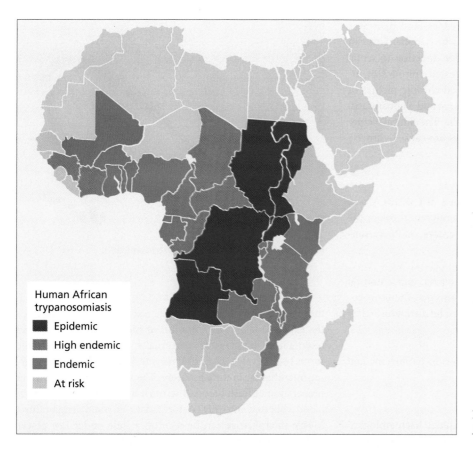

Fig. 60.5 Geographical distribution of African trypanosomiasis.

treatments include combinations of albendazole and ivermectin. None of these drugs has common, serious haematological side-effects.

African trypanosomiasis (sleeping sickness)

Epidemiology and biology

African sleeping sickness is caused by the haemoflagellate protozoa *Trypanosoma brucei gambiense* in West and Central Africa, and *T. brucei rhodesiense* in Eastern Africa (Figure 60.5). These parasites are fusiform in shape, 12–35 μm long and morphologically indistinguishable from each other. The disease is transmitted by the bite of the tsetse fly, which is only found in Africa. The trypanosomes multiply by fission in the vicinity of the infected bite and are then disseminated by the bloodstream. Congenital transmission has also been described. The distribution of African sleeping sickness is determined by the ecological limits of the tsetse fly vector and lies in the region between Senegal and Somalia in the north and the Kalahari and Namibian deserts in the south. There have been recent surges of the disease in Congo, Angola, Sudan and Uganda, and there is relentless spread of the disease in Central Africa.

Clinical features

The bite of a tsetse fly is very painful and causes a small indur-ated lesion that may persist for some days. The local multiplication of the trypanosomes may cause a marked inflammatory reaction (a chancre) that regresses after 2–3 weeks. Entry of the trypanosomes into the bloodstream is associated with fever, which tends to be less marked in West African trypanosomiasis than in the East African variety. East African trypanosomiasis is primarily a disease of cattle and it only enters human hosts by accident. It is therefore less well tolerated than West African sleeping sickness, having a more aggressive course and intense symptoms.

The early stages of sleeping sickness can be associated with prominent lymphadenopathy, particularly of the posterior cervical nodes, and mild splenomegaly. These features may be suggestive of infectious mononucleosis, tuberculous lymphadenitis or a lymphoproliferative disorder. Severe anaemia, haemorrhages and petechiae may occur at this stage.

Both types of African sleeping sickness cause a protracted febrile illness, which, despite the name, are not always associated with drowsiness. Death is inevitable if the disease is left untreated. As the disease progresses parasitaemia decreases, trypanosomes invade the CNS and neurological disturbances due to inflammatory chronic meningoencephalitis supervene. In West African trypanosomiasis, the disease runs its course over several years but in East African trypanosomiasis infection, CNS involvement may occur within weeks.

Table 60.4 Drugs for African trypanosomiasis.

	Haemolymphatic stage		Encephalitic stage	
	First line	Second line	First line	Second line
West African (*T. brucei gambiense*)	Pentamidine	Eflornithine or melarsoprol	Suramin	Melarsoprol
East African (*T. brucei rhodesiense*)	Suramin	Melarsoprol	Melarsoprol	Melarsoprol plus nifurtimox

Haematological abnormalities

The aetiology of the anaemia in sleeping sickness is multi-factorial but primarily due to phagocytic removal of immune complex-coated red cells from the circulation. Trypanosomes liberate haemolytic factors that contribute to this process, and increases in plasma volume cause a dilutional anaemia. There is a failure to incorporate iron into red cell precursors and the resulting dyserythropoiesis means that the bone marrow is unable to compensate for the fall in haemoglobin. There may be a moderate leucocytosis with increased monocytes, lymphocytes and plasma cells. Mott morular cells have also been described in sleeping sickness. The bone marrow is hypercellular, with areas of gelatinous degeneration.

As the disease advances, a bleeding tendency may develop due to thrombocytopenia, vascular injury and coagulopathy with increased fibrinolysis. Platelet dysfunction has also been described and is manifest as clumping and abnormal aggregation responses. DIC with raised FDPs may occur in the later stages. Although some of these complex haematological changes can be linked to the non-specific polyclonal activation of B cells, overall the mechanisms underlying these are not well understood.

Diagnosis of sleeping sickness

Wet preparations of fluid aspirated from the chancre of lymph nodes may reveal live, motile organisms (Figure 60.6). This technique is more likely to be productive in the case of infection with *T. brucei rhodesiense* than *T. brucei gambiense*. The organisms are fragile so care must be taken not to damage them when making the smears. Trypanosomes can be seen on stained thin blood films but the number of trypanosomes in the circulation can vary considerably and is often low, so concentration techniques are usually required.

Quantitative buffy coat (QBC) method is the technique of choice for diagnosis of African trypanosomiasis. This involves concentrating the trypanosomes at the plasma–platelet interface in a special microhaematocrit tube using differential centrifugation. Parasites are identified by labelling with the fluorescent marker, acridine orange.

The highly specific and sensitive serological agglutination test (CATT) may be used in conjunction with a direct visualization microscopic method. If these tests are positive then CSF examination is mandatory to determine the stage of the illness.

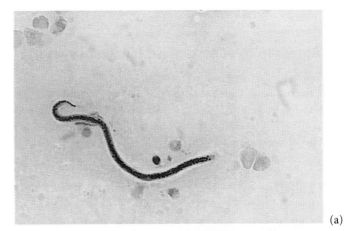

(a)

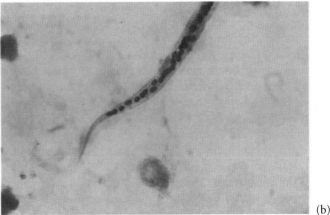

(b)

Fig. 60.6 Microfilariae of *W. bancrofti* in thick film: (a) microfilaria showing the negative impression of the sheath (×365); (b) tail of the microfilaria showing that the nuclei do not extend into the tail (×912).

Haematological implications of treatment for African trypanosomiasis (Table 60.4)

Pentamidine and *suramin* are the drugs of choice for the early stages of West and East African trypanosomiasis respectively. They have a cure rate of around 90% but are only able to achieve modest CSF concentrations so they cannot be used for later stages of the disease. The most common haematological side-effects of pentamidine are leucopenia, thrombocytopenia and anaemia. Suramin has serious side-effects, including haemolytic anaemia and bone marrow toxicity.

Melarsoprol, an arsenic-based compound, has been the drug of choice for late-stage sleeping sickness but is highly toxic, with a mortality of 4–12%. Its main adverse effect is a fatal encephalopathic syndrome and haematological toxicity is not a particular problem.

Eflornithine is expensive but is of benefit in late-stage sleeping sickness, particularly West African disease; 25–50% of patients treated with this drug exhibit bone marrow toxicity with anaemia, leucopenia and thrombocytopenia.

American trypanosomiasis (Chagas disease)

Epidemiology and biology

Chagas disease is due to a haemoflagellate protozoa, *T. cruzi*, which is transmitted by triatomine bugs that infest poor quality housing. It can also be transmitted through blood transfusions and congenitally. It is restricted to a region in the Americas between Argentina and the southern states of the USA.

Clinical features

The incubation period is usually a couple of weeks but may be up to several months if transmission was through blood transfusion. In the acute phase, swelling at the site of entry of the organism, a chagoma, may be accompanied by fever, mild hepatosplenomegaly and local or generalized lymphadenopathy. The trypanosomes multiply intracellularly in muscle tissue, particularly the heart, colon and oesophagus. Once infection has occurred, and if no treatment is given, the organisms will be present for life. The chronic phase of the disease is associated with heart disease in 30% of infected individuals, which is manifest as arrhythmias and megacardia. A small proportion of individuals also have clinical involvement of the gastrointestinal tract and other hollow organs, with loss of peristalsis and organomegaly with organ failure. Asymptomatic infection is common and poses a problem for blood transfusion services in endemic areas, so some countries have now introduced routine screening of blood for American trypanosomiasis.

Diagnosis of Chagas disease

Although similar methods to those used for African trypanosomiasis can be helpful for diagnosis, serological tests are more commonly used as the primary diagnostic tool. They are based on enzyme immunoassay (EIA) or immunofluorescent antibody test (IFAT) and have good sensitivity. PCR may also be useful but is not in routine use.

Haematological implications of treatment for American trypanosomiasis

Benznidazole is recommended for acute and congenital *T. cruzi* infection. Major haematological side-effects are not common with this drug, although agranulocytosis has been reported.

Leishmaniasis

Epidemiology and biology

Visceral and cutaneous leishmaniases are caused by protozoan flagellates that are transmitted through the infective bite of a phlebotomine sandfly. Following an infected bite, parasites spread from the inoculation site to the mononuclear phagocytic system. Only the visceral form ('kala-azar') is associated with organisms in haemopoietic tissues and will be considered in this chapter. Visceral leishmaniasis is due to the species *Leishmania donovani* and *L. infantum* and is found in 47 countries throughout the world, with extension limits from 45° north to 32° south; 90% of cases are in Bangladesh, India, Nepal, Sudan and Brazil (Figure 60.7). The number of cases of visceral leishmaniasis, particularly round the Mediterranean basin in southern Europe, has been increasing over the last 10–15 years in association with HIV-related immunosuppression.

Clinical features

The clinical expression of leishmaniasis depends on both the genotypic potential of the parasite and the immunological response of the patient. Incubation period varies from days to years but is generally 2–6 months. Onset can be sudden with high fever, or gradual with intermittent fever. Diarrhoea, joint pains, weight loss and bleeding gums occur in the acute phase. This is followed by progressive muscle wasting, protuberant abdomen, fever, weight loss, anaemia and hepatosplenomegaly. The splenomegaly appears early and the spleen increases in size in relation to the duration of the disease, so that eventually it may reach into the left hyopchondrium. In immunocompromised patients, such as transplant recipients and those with advanced HIV disease, kala-azar behaves like an opportunistic infection.

Haematological abnormalities

Normochromic, normocytic anaemia is a frequent and clinically significant feature of visceral leishmaniasis and haemoglobin levels of 7–10 g/dL are common. The massive splenic enlargement is associated with hypersplenism and consequent anaemia, leucopenia and thrombocytopenia. Liver dysfunction with jaundice, ascites and deranged coagulation may occur in the late stages and has a poor prognosis. The bleeding tendency may be exacerbated by thrombocytopenia and result in clinical haemorrhages. A high degree of suspicion for a diagnosis of leishmaniasis needs to be maintained by haematologists in all patients with unexplained splenomegaly, pancytopenia or fever.

Diagnosis of leishmaniasis

Definitive diagnosis is based on detection of the parasites, or their DNA, in smears of bone marrow or splenic aspirate samples. Fluid aspirated from lymph nodes can also yield parasites if lymphadenopathy is present. Splenic aspirate has a higher diagnostic yield than bone marrow. It has been suggested that the intercostal route for splenic aspiration is safer and causes less

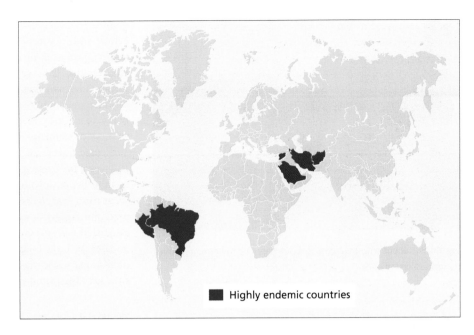

Fig. 60.7 Geographical distribution of cutaneous leishmaniasis.

■ Highly endemic countries

discomfort than the abdominal approach, providing that the prothrombin time and platelet count are adequate.

In haematological practice, leishmania are usually encountered as intracellular amastigotes in mononuclear cells in the bone marrow, but can also be seen extracellularly (Figure 60.8). They are 2–6 μm in diameter and contain a nucleus lying close to the rod-shaped kinetoplast, and an internal flagellum. Using a Romanowsky stain, the nucleus and kinetoplast stain purple and can be clearly distinguished. Amastigotes can be seen in both bone marrow aspirates and in trephine-impression smears. They are rarely seen in peripheral blood and then only in buffy coat preparations.

Direct microscopic visualization is less sensitive then molecular diagnosis, particularly when there is co-infection with

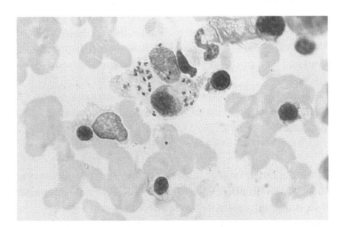

Fig. 60.8 Bone marrow aspirate of leishmaniasis, showing a macrophage containing numerous organisms, which, in addition to a nucleus, have a small paranuclear kinetoplast, giving them a characteristic 'double-dot' appearance (MCG ×940).

HIV. Under these circumstances, PCR can be very useful for diagnosis and speciation. It can be performed on lesion aspirate, marrow, blood and biopsy material. The indirect fluorescent antibody tests ELISA and DAT (direct antiglobulin test) are useful for detecting antibodies to visceral leishmaniasis, but results may be inconclusive in immunosuppressed patients.

Haematological implications of treatment for leishmaniasis

For the last 80 years, the treatment of leishmaniasis has been based on pentavalent antimony drugs, although their mode of action is still unclear. Resistance levels to antimonals in India, particularly in Bihar, where 90% of India's cases of leishmaniasis occur, are high so other options such as amphotericin B, paromomycin and miltefosine need to be considered. HIV co-infected patients do not respond well to antimonials so amphotericin is the drug of choice. Side-effects can be reduced by using the liposomal preparation. Even after successful treatment, immunocompromised patients may require prophylaxis to prevent relapses.

Sodium stibogluconate is the most commonly used antimonial. It can be associated with worsening anaemia, although its most serious detrimental effects are on cardiac function.

Amphotericin B can produce haematological side-effects but its most serious toxicity is related to renal, cardiac, neurological and hepatic dysfunction.

Non-specific haematological abnormalities associated with tropical diseases

Hypersplenism

Hypersplenism is a syndrome characterized by splenomegaly and cytopenias. Tropical infections associated with massive

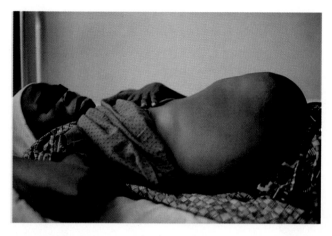

Fig. 60.9 Patient with massive splenomegaly due to hyper-reactive malaria splenomegaly.

splenomegaly include hyper-reactive malarial splenomegaly, visceral leishmaniasis, schistosomiasis and trypanosomiasis (Figure 60.9). The anaemia, leucopenia and thrombocytopenia in hypersplenism are due to a combination of sequestration and haemodilution. The degree of expansion of plasma volume is proportional to the size of the spleen, and can be improved by splenectomy. The thrombocytopenia and neutropenia are rarely severe enough to cause clinical problems. Most of the thrombocytopenia is due to pooling in the spleen which, when massively enlarged, can hold up to 90% of the platelet mass. Neutropenia is the result of increased marginalization of granulocytes. In the case of tropical infections, treatment of the underlying disorder generally leads to regression of the splenomegaly with resolution of the haematological abnormalities.

Tropical diseases associated with changes in the full blood count

Anaemia

Anaemia of chronic disease is a common and non-specific finding in many types of tropical infections. Some infections are responsible for specific types of anaemia. For example, hookworm infection contributes to iron deficiency anaemia and megaloblastic anaemia secondary to parasite consumption of vitamin B_{12} is a feature of infection with the tapeworm *Diphyllobothrium latum*. Intra-erythrocytic parasites, such as those that cause malaria and babesiosis, may be directly responsible for intravascular haemolysis.

White cell abnormalities

Severe infections particularly due to bacteria may cause a neutrophilia and a leukaemoid reaction with myeloid precursors in the peripheral blood and circulating neutrophils, with toxic granulation, vacuolation and Döhle body formation. Lymphocytosis with neutropenia, splenomegaly, nose bleeds, rash and neurological complications is a feature of rickettsial diseases (e.g. typhus, Q fever). These are small (0.3–1 μm diameter) intracellular parasites. They have a worldwide distribution and can infect rodents. Some, such as trench fever, may persist for many years and are transmissible in blood transfusions. The absence of neutrophilia in the presence of marked fever is a particular feature of typhoid. Lymphocytosis or monocytosis may also be present in typhoid and other clinical features include hepatosplenomegaly and, in severe disease, haemorrhage from ileal ulcers exacerbated by DIC. Helminths and other predominantly tropical organisms that invade tissues may be associated with a significant eosinophilia ($> 0.5 \times 10^9/L$). Such diseases include loiasis, lymphatic filariasis, schistosomiasis, trichinosis, toxocariasis, strongyloidiasis, hydatid disease, oriental liver flukes and guinea worm.

Tropical infections with fever and haemorrhage

Relapsing fever

Relapsing fevers are borne by either lice or ticks. Louse-borne relapsing fever is endemic in the horn of Africa and Rwanda. Tick-borne relapsing fever has a wider distribution through Africa, the Mediterranean basin and the Middle East. They have a relapsing course and severe disease is characterized by fever with jaundice, neutrophilia, thrombocytopenia and DIC. There is a marked bleeding tendency, with petechial haemorrhage and epistaxis. Spiral organisms (*Borrelia* spp.) can be seen in the blood. Relapsing fevers respond well to tetracycline but this must be given with care as it can generate a severe, life-threatening Jarisch–Herxheimer reaction.

Viral haemorrhagic fevers

These are caused by dengue virus, several arenaviruses and hantaviruses and yellow fever virus. Viruses that are likely to cause haemorrhagic fever can be classified according to their reservoir hosts and their primary means of transmission. They are divided into:
- rodent-associated viruses (e.g. Lassa fever, hantaviruses);
- arthropod-borne viruses (e.g. dengue, yellow fever and Chikungunya viruses);
- unknown vectors or hosts (e.g. Marburg, Ebola).

They often occur in epidemics, have human-to-human transmission and may only be suspected if a relevant travel history is elicited from the patient. Dengue and yellow fever are becoming increasingly important imported infections.

Dengue

The four types of dengue virus belong to a group of flaviviruses and are transmitted by the *Aedes* mosquitoes. Dengue is endemic in tropical areas of Asia, Africa, South America and the Caribbean and is particularly virulent in South-East Asia, including Thailand and Vietnam. There has been a resurgence of the disease over the last decade as a result of urbanization, poverty, the demise of *Aedes* eradication programmes and increasing travel.

Primary infection occurs in young children and is usually asymptomatic. Older children and adults develop acute fever, headache and myalgia ('breakbone fever'). Leucopenia may accompany this stage of the illness. Severe complications may arise in those who have had previous dengue infection. These include hypotensive shock with marked thrombocytopenia, producing spontaneous bleeding, including epistaxis and gastrointestinal haemorrhage. There is also neutropenia and bone marrow hypoplasia with abnormal megakaryocytopoiesis.

Arenavirus infections: Lassa fever, Ebola virus and Marburg virus

These are endemic in equatorial Africa and are important because they produce potentially fatal infection and have the ability to spread from person to person.

The rat is the main vector of Lassa fever. Only about 10% of infected individuals become ill and only 1–2% of these develop fatal disease. The clinical features of these three haemorrhagic fevers are similar. They are characterized by headache, fever and oesophagitis. Spontaneous bleeding occurs in 25% of hospitalized patients and is thought to be due to abnormal platelet function. Case reports have suggested that heparin may be helpful in controlling the bleeding problems.

Yellow fever

Yellow fever virus is transmitted by *Aedes* mosquitoes and exists throughout equatorial Africa, and northern and central south America. It has a propensity to invade hepatocytes, causing hepatocellular dysfunction and jaundice. Fever, myalgia and back pain may be followed by jaundice, bleeding and renal failure in the most severe cases. Thrombocytopenia, prolonged prothrombin and partial thromboplastin times and DIC are responsible for the bleeding tendency.

Selected bibliography

Disease specific

Anon (2000) Severe falciparum malaria. *Transactions of the Royal Society of Tropical Medicine and Hygiene* 94 (Suppl. 1): S1–90.

Kwiatowski D (2000) Genetic susceptibility to malaria getting complex. *Current Opinion in Genetics and Development* 10: 320–4.

Malaria: an on-line resource including 'test and teach'. (http://www.rph.wa.gov.au/labs/haem/malaria)

Swanepoel R (1999) Viral haemorrhagic fevers and related biohazard class 4 infections. *Specialist Medicine* July: 450–6.

UNDP/World Bank/WHO Special Programme for Research and Training in Tropical Diseases (2001) *Roll Back Malaria. The Prevention and Management of Severe Anaemia in Children in Malaria-endemic Regions of Africa.* WHO, Geneva.

Visceral leishmaniasis – bone marrow morphology (http://www.geocities.com/donovanivl/).

World Health Organization (2000) *Management of Severe Malaria*, 2nd edn. WHO, Geneva.

World Health Organization – information on programme for surveillance and control of African trypanosomiasis (http://www.who.int/emc/diseases/tryp/).

World Health Organization – lymphatic filariasis (http://www.who.int/health-topics/lymphfil.htm).

General

Bain BJ (1995) *Blood Cells. A Practical Guide*, 2nd edn. Blackwell Science, Oxford.

Cheesbrough M (2000) *District Laboratory Practice in Tropical Countries. Parts 1 and 2. Tropical Health Technology.* Cambridge University Press, March, UK.

Department of Health. (2002) *Getting Ahead of the Curve – a Strategy for Combating Infectious Diseases in the UK.* Department of Health, London.

(2003) *Manson's Tropical Diseases* (GC Cook, A Zumla, eds), 21st edn. Elsevier Science, Edinburgh.

Dacie and Lewis Practical Haematology (SM Lewis, BJ Bain, I Bates, eds), 9th edn. Churchill Livingstone, London.

World Health Organization *International Travel and Health* (http://www.who.int/ith).

World Health Organization (1998) *The World Health Report.* WHO, Geneva.

Zuckerman J (2002) Travel medicine. *British Medical Journal* 325: 260–4.

CHAPTER 61

Neonatal haematology

Irene AG Roberts

61

Developmental haemopoiesis

Haemopoiesis begins in the yolk sac in the third week of gestation and moves sequentially to the aorta–gonad–mesonephros (AGM) by 5 weeks' gestation, the liver by 6–8 weeks and the bone marrow around the eleventh week of gestation. The AGM involutes early in the first trimester and the liver is the principal site of haemopoiesis until the end of the third trimester. The predominant lineage during fetal life is erythropoiesis but platelets and all types of leucocyte found in adult blood are also seen in the fetus from as early as 4–5 weeks' gestation.

There are a number of differences between erythropoiesis in the neonate and the adult: red cell morphology is distinctive with large numbers of crenated red cells, particularly in preterm neonates (Figure 61.1); red cell lifespan is reduced (35–50 days in preterm infants; 60–70 days in term infants), susceptibility to oxidant-induced injury is increased because of differences in the glycolytic and pentose phosphate pathways; the erythropoietin response to anaemia is blunted, and specific embryonic and fetal globin chains are synthesized (Table 61.1). The first globin chain produced is ε-globin, followed by α- and γ-globin chains. Haemoglobin F (HbF–$\alpha_2\gamma_2$) is produced from 4–5 weeks' gestation and is the predominant haemoglobin until after birth. Adult haemoglobin (HbA–$\alpha_2\beta_2$) is produced from 6–8 weeks' gestation, but remains at low levels until after birth. In term babies, the average HbF at birth is 70–80%, the HbA is 25–30%, there are small amounts of HbA2 and sometimes a trace of Hb Barts (γ_4).

Immediately after birth, rates of haemoglobin synthesis and red blood cell production fall in response to the sudden increase in tissue oxygenation at birth. In term babies, the haemoglobin reaches a mean of 13–14 g/dL at 4 weeks and 9.5–11 g/dL at 7–9 weeks of age. Studies of well preterm infants show a steeper fall in haemoglobin, reaching a mean of 6.5–9 g/dL at 4–8 weeks of

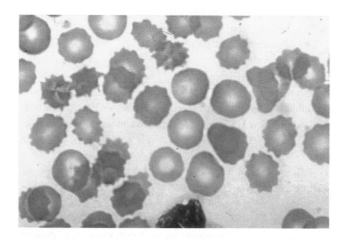

Figure 61.1 Typical erythrocyte morphology in a preterm neonate. Crenated red cells are a normal feature of the blood film of preterm neonates during the first few weeks of life. This film is from a neonate born at 26 weeks' gestation and shows the number of crenated cells present in neonates under 28 weeks' gestation. The numbers of these cells is inversely proportional to gestational age at birth.

age. The reticulocyte count falls after birth as erythropoiesis is suppressed and increases to normal values at 6–8 weeks of age. The blood volume at birth varies with gestational age and the timing of clamping of the cord. In term infants, the average blood volume is 80 mL/kg and in preterm infants 106 mL/kg (range of 85–143 mL/kg). Term and preterm babies have adequate stores of iron, folic acid and vitamin B_{12} at birth. However, stores of both iron and folic acid are lower in preterm infants and are depleted more quickly, leading to deficiency after 2–4 months if the recommended daily intakes are not maintained.

Table 61.1 Composition of haemoglobins in the human embryo, fetus and neonate.

Haemoglobin	Globin chains α-Globin gene cluster	β-Globin gene cluster*	Gestation
Embryonic			
Hb Gower 1	ξ_2	ε_2	From 3–4 weeks
Hb Gower 2	α_2	ε_2	
Hb Portland	ξ_2	γ_2	From 4 weeks
Fetal			
HbF	α_2	γ_2	From 4 weeks
Adult			
HbA	α_2	β_2	From 6–8 weeks
HbA2	α_2	δ_2	From 30 weeks

*The α-globin gene cluster is situated on chromosome 16 and the β-globin gene cluster on chromosome 11. Note that fetuses and neonates with α-thalassaemia major, who are unable to synthesize α-globin chains, will have Hb Portland as well as Hb Barts (β4), detectable by haemoglobin electrophoresis or HPLC.

Neonatal anaemia

Definition and pathophysiology

Any neonate with a haemoglobin of less than 14 g/dL at birth should be considered anaemic and may require investigation (Figure 61.2). However, it is important to be aware that the haemoglobin concentration is affected by the site of sampling (it is up to 4 g/dL lower in venous than in heel-prick samples in the first few days of life) and the timing of the clamping of the cord (around 3 g/dL higher after late clamping). The clinical significance of neonatal anaemia depends on whether the baby is able to maintain adequate tissue oxygenation. This in turn depends on the position of the haemoglobin–oxygen dissociation curve, which is principally determined by the concentrations of HbF and of 2,3-diphosphoglycerate (2,3-DPG); a high HbF and low 2,3-DPG both shift the curve to the left, i.e. the affinity of haemoglobin for oxygen is increased and less oxygen is released to the tissues. This is the situation just after birth and may be more of a problem for very preterm babies as their HbF levels are greater than 90%. Over the first few months of life, 2,3-DPG levels rise and HbF levels fall so that the haemoglobin–oxygen dissociation curve gradually shifts to the right, the oxygen affinity of haemoglobin falls and oxygen delivery to the tissues increases, ameliorating the effects of the falling haemoglobin.

Causes of neonatal anaemia

Anaemia may be caused by (i) reduced red cell production; (ii) increased red cell destruction (haemolysis); or (iii) blood loss (Table 61.2).

Table 61.2 Common causes of neonatal anaemia.

Reduced red cell production
Diamond–Blackfan anaemia
Congenital viral infections, e.g. parvovirus, cytomegalovirus
Congenital dyserythropoietic anaemia
Pearson's syndrome

Increased red cell destruction (haemolysis)
Alloimmune: haemolytic disease of the newborn (Rh, ABO, Kell, other)
Red cell membrane disorders, e.g. hereditary spherocytosis
Red cell enzyme deficiencies, e.g. pyruvate kinase deficiency
Some haemoglobinopathies, e.g. α-thalassaemia major, HbH disease

Blood loss
Occult haemorrhage before or around birth, e.g. twin–twin, feto-maternal
Internal haemorrhage, e.g. intracranial, cephalhaematoma
Iatrogenic, due to frequent blood sampling

Anaemia of prematurity
Impaired red cell production plus reduced red cell lifespan

Neonatal anaemia due to reduced red cell production

The main diagnostic clues to reduced red cell production are the combination of a low reticulocyte count ($< 20 \times 10^9$/L) with a negative direct antiglobulin test (Coombs' test). The most common causes are congenital parvovirus infection and genetic red cell aplasias, particularly Diamond–Blackfan anaemia (DBA).

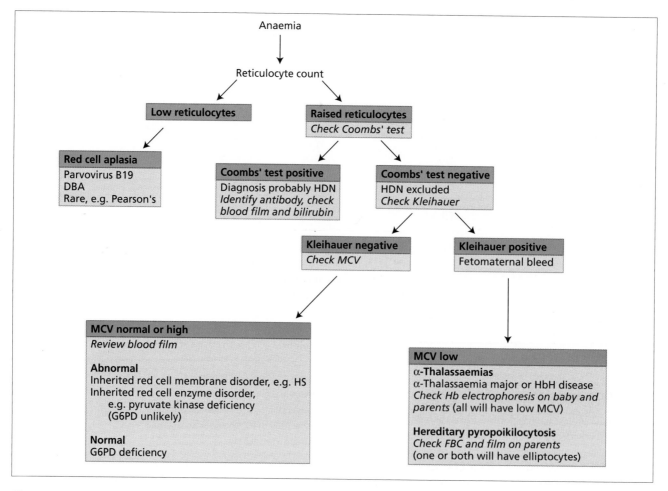

Figure 61.2 A diagnostic algorithm for neonatal anaemia. The most useful screening tests for investigating unexplained neonatal anaemia are the reticulocyte (retic) count, the Coombs' test and the MCV of the red blood cells. DBA, Diamond–Blackfan anaemia; G6PD, glucose-6-phosphate dehydrogenase; HDN, haemolytic disease of the newborn; HS, hereditary spherocytosis.

Parvovirus B19 and fetal/neonatal anaemia

Maternal infection with parvovirus B19 can cause severe fetal anaemia and in 9% of cases leads to intrauterine death. The baby has marked reticulocytopenia ($< 10 \times 10^9$/L) and thrombocytopenia may also occur. The diagnosis is made by maternal serology and demonstration of B19 DNA in the fetus or neonate by dot-blot hybridization or polymerase chain reaction (PCR) of peripheral blood (bone marrow aspiration for morphology and parvovirus B19 PCR may be necessary in difficult cases). Severe cases require intrauterine transfusion but have a good long-term outcome if they survive to delivery.

Genetic red cell aplasia

Apart from DBA, the genetic causes of congenital red cell aplasia are extremely rare. They include congenital dyserythropoietic anaemia (CDA) and Pearson's syndrome; the other inherited bone marrow failure syndromes, such as Fanconi anaemia, are almost never present at birth. DBA, which occurs in five to seven babies per million live births, has a clear family history in 20% of cases (autosomal dominant or recessive) and appears to be sporadic in the remaining 80%. It usually presents as increasing anaemia over the first few weeks or months of life but more severe cases manifest as second trimester anaemia or hydrops fetalis. Around 40% of infants have associated congenital anomalies, particularly craniofacial dysmorphism, neck anomalies and thumb malformations similar to those seen in Fanconi anaemia. The blood film shows normochromic red cells with an absence of polychromasia and nucleated red cells despite severe anaemia (Figure 61.3); there is a severe reticulocytopenia and absent erythroid precursors on the bone marrow aspirate. These features are diagnostic of DBA if parvovirus infection is excluded. Raised red cell levels of adenosine deaminase (ADA) in the patient and/or parents may be useful to confirm the diagnosis, although normal red cell ADA levels

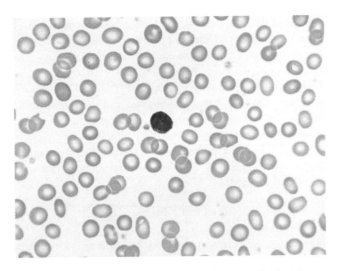

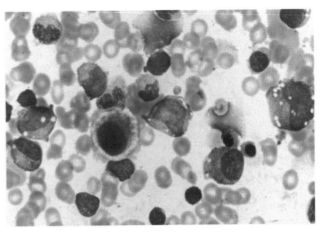

Figure 61.4 Pearson's syndrome. Bone marrow aspirate from a neonate with Pearson's syndrome, showing typical vacuolation of erythroblasts and a dysplastic megakaryocyte.

Figure 61.3 Blood film from a neonate with Diamond–Blackfan anaemia. This baby presented with fetal anaemia at 20 weeks' gestation and received intrauterine transfusion. At birth, the baby had normochromic anaemia and the blood film showed a complete absence of polychromasia and nucleated red cells, despite a haemoglobin of 7 g/dL.

do not exclude DBA. Around 25% of cases have mutations of the ribosomal protein (RP) S19 gene on chromosome 19. In the neonatal period, the only treatment of DBA is red cell transfusion.

Other genetic causes of congenital red cell aplasia, CDA and Pearson's syndrome, can be distinguished from DBA by marrow morphology. In Pearson's syndrome, which is caused by mutations in mitochondrial DNA and presents with normochromic anaemia, neutropenia, thrombocytopenia and failure to thrive in the first few weeks of life, there is highly characteristic vacuolation of early erythroid cells on the marrow aspirate (Figure 61.4). Unfortunately, the prognosis for children with Pearson's syndrome is very poor, with few surviving beyond the second year of life.

Neonatal anaemia due to increased red cell destruction (haemolysis)

The main diagnostic clues suggesting a haemolytic anaemia are: increased numbers of reticulocytes and/or circulating nucleated red blood cells (Figure 61.5), unconjugated hyperbilirubinaemia, a positive Coombs' test (if immune) and characteristic changes in the morphology of the red cells on a blood film (e.g. hereditary spherocytosis; Figure 61.5). The main cause of immune haemolytic anaemia is haemolytic disease of the newborn. The main causes of non-immune neonatal haemolysis are: red cell membrane disorders, red cell enzymopathies and, occasionally, haemoglobinopathies (Table 61.2).

Immune haemolysis, including haemolytic disease of the newborn

The principal alloantibodies causing haemolytic disease of the newborn are those against rhesus antigens (anti-D, anti-c and anti-E), anti-Kell, anti-Kidd (J^k), anti-Duffy (F^y) and antibodies

Figure 61.5 Haemolytic disease of the newborn. (a) Blood film from a neonate with ABO haemolytic disease of the newborn due to anti-A showing very large numbers of spherocytes, polychromasia and no nucleated red cells. (b) Blood film from a baby with rhesus haemolytic disease of the newborn due to anti-D showing polychromasia and large numbers of nucleated red cells but relatively few spherocytes.

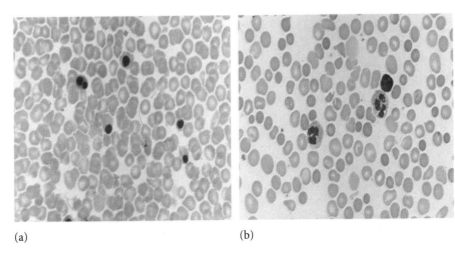

(a)   (b)

of the MNS blood group system, including anti-U. Anti-D is the most frequent alloantibody causing significant haemolytic anaemia affecting 1 in 1200 pregnancies. Anti-Kell antibodies are less common but can cause severe fetal and neonatal anaemia as they inhibit erythropoiesis as well as causing haemolysis. Most babies with haemolytic disease of the newborn present with jaundice and/or anaemia; in severe cases there is hepatosplenomegaly and/or skin deposits due to extramedullary haemopoiesis. ABO haemolytic disease occurs only in offspring of women of blood group O and is confined to the 1% of such women that have high-titre IgG antibodies. Haemolysis due to anti-A is more common (1 in 150 births) than anti-B. In contrast with anti-rhesus antibodies, both anti-A and anti-B usually cause hyperbilirubinaemia without significant anaemia; however, hydrops has occasionally been described. The blood film in ABO haemolytic disease characteristically shows very large numbers of spherocytes with little or no increase in nucleated red cells (see Figure 61.5a); this contrasts with rhesus haemolytic disease of the newborn, in which there are few spherocytes and large numbers of circulating nucleated red cells (see Figure 61.5b).

Management of haemolytic disease of the newborn

All neonates at risk should have cord blood taken for measurement of haemoglobin, bilirubin and a Coombs' test and should remain in hospital until hyperbilirubinaemia and/or anaemia have been properly managed. Rhesus-alloimmunized infants with haemolysis should receive phototherapy from birth, as the bilirubin can rise steeply; this prevents the need for exchange transfusion in some infants. In haemolytic disease due to anti-Kell, anaemia is usually more prominent than jaundice and minimal phototherapy may be necessary despite severe anaemia. ABO haemolytic disease of the newborn usually just requires phototherapy as anaemia is uncommon. The indications for exchange transfusion in haemolytic disease of the newborn are:

1 severe anaemia: haemoglobin < 10 g/dL at birth and/or;
2 severe or rapidly increasing hyperbilirubinaemia.

The British Committee for Standards in Haematology (BCSH) recently published guidelines for neonatal exchange transfusion. Affected neonates may also develop 'late' anaemia at a few weeks of age, requiring 'top-up' transfusion; irradiated blood must be used for infants previously receiving intrauterine transfusion to prevent the risk of transfusion-associated-graft-versus-host disease (TA-GvHD). Recombinant erythropoietin sometimes prevents the need for 'top-up' transfusion for late anaemia but is not effective when haemolysis is brisk. Folic acid (500 μg/kg per day) should be given to all babies with haemolysis until they reach 3 months of age.

Neonatal haemolytic anaemia due to red cell membrane disorders

In neonates, these disorders present with jaundice and moderate anaemia (usually due to hereditary spherocytosis), as an incidental finding on routine blood films in the absence of jaundice or anaemia (usually hereditary elliptocytosis), or, occasionally, as severe, transfusion-dependent haemolytic anaemia with a characteristic low mean corpuscular volume (MCV) of 50–60 fL (usually due to hereditary pyropoikilocytosis, HPP). The main clues are a family history and an abnormal blood film, as red cell membrane disorders can nearly always be recognized by the characteristic shape of the red cells (Figure 61.6a). Identification of the exact type of membrane abnormality may require specialized investigations. The osmotic fragility test is of limited value in neonates and recent data suggest that the dye binding test is more useful. If the clinical phenotype is severe and family history or family studies are unhelpful, red cell membrane electrophoresis is indicated to clarify the diagnosis (on pre-transfusion blood samples to minimize diagnostic confusion due to transfused cells).

Hereditary spherocytosis occurs in 1 in 5000 live births to parents of northern European extraction. It is usually autosomal dominant and caused by mutations in spectrin, ankyrin, protein 4.1 or protein 3. The blood film shows spherocytes and is identical to that of ABO haemolytic disease (see Figure 61.6b).

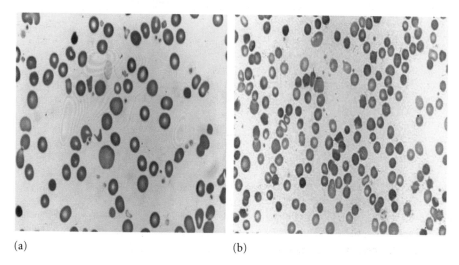

(a) (b)

Figure 61.6 Red cell membrane disorders. (a) Blood film from a baby with hereditary pyropoikilocytosis, showing microspherocytes, red cell fragments and polychromasia. (b) Blood film from a neonate with hereditary spherocytosis, showing large numbers of spherocytes and polychromasia.

Neonatal anaemia due to hereditary spherocytosis is usually moderate (7–10 g/dL); it is not uncommon for affected neonates to require one or two transfusions during the neonatal period before a transfusion-free plateau haemoglobin of 8–10 g/dL is achieved after a few months. *Hereditary elliptocytosis*, which is caused by different mutations in the genes for spectrin, ankyrin or protein 4.1, usually has no clinical manifestations in the neonate apart from elliptocytes on the blood film. However, neonates who are homozygous or compound heterozygotes for hereditary elliptocytosis mutations have severe haemolytic anaemia; the most common form is HPP. *HPP* causes severe, transfusion-dependent haemolytic anaemia. The diagnosis is easily made from the low MCV and blood films of the baby (which show bizarre fragmented red cells and microspherocytes; Figure 61.6a), and both parents (one or both of which usually have elliptocytosis). Red cell transfusion is necessary until the child is old enough to undergo splenectomy, to which there is an excellent response.

Neonatal haemolysis due to red cell enzymopathies

The commonest red cell enzymopathies presenting in the neonatal period are glucose-6-phosphate dehydrogenase (G6PD) deficiency and pyruvate kinase deficiency. *G6PD deficiency* has a high prevalence in individuals from Central Africa (20%) and the Mediterranean (10%). In neonates, G6PD deficiency nearly always presents with jaundice within the first few days of life; the vast majority of affected neonates are boys, as the G6PD gene is on the X chromosome. The jaundice is often severe, whereas anaemia is extremely rare and the blood film is completely normal. The diagnosis is made by assaying G6PD on a peripheral blood sample. The pathogenesis of the jaundice is unclear as most babies with G6PD deficiency have no evidence of haemolysis. Management of neonatal G6PD deficiency requires close monitoring of the bilirubin to prevent kernicterus, particularly when interactions with other risk factors for neonatal hyperbilirubinaemia are present, such as Gilbert's syndrome or hereditary spherocytosis, and also the counselling of the babies' parents regarding which medicines, chemicals and foods may precipitate haemolysis. For the vast majority of patients there is no chronic haemolysis and no anaemia and therefore folic acid supplements are not indicated.

Pyruvate kinase (PK) deficiency is the second most common red cell enzymopathy in neonates. It is autosomal recessive and clinically heterogeneous varying from anaemia severe enough to cause hydrops fetalis to a mild unconjugated hyperbilirubinaemia. In severe cases, the jaundice has a rapid onset within 24 h of birth and exchange transfusion may be required. The diagnosis is made by measuring pre-transfusion red cell PK activity; in mild cases the PK activity may be relatively modestly reduced making the diagnosis difficult and it is often useful to assay levels in the parents for confirmation. The blood film is sometimes distinctive but more often shows non-specific changes of non-spherocytic haemolysis. Management in the neonatal period

depends on the severity of the jaundice and anaemia; some, but not all, children are transfusion dependent and folic acid supplements should be given to prevent deficiency due to chronic haemolysis. The other red cell enzymopathies are rare. The most important in the neonatal period is *triosephosphate isomerase deficiency*, as one-third of patients present with neonatal haemolytic anaemia, often many months before the devastating neurological features of this disorder become apparent.

Neonatal haemolysis due to haemoglobinopathies

The only haemoglobinopathy that presents typically in the neonatal period is α-thalassaemia major, as all 4 α-globin genes are deleted. Occasional non-thalassaemic, structural α- and γ-globin gene mutations, which are clinically completely silent in adults and children, cause transient neonatal haemolytic anaemia in the neonate because they are unstable (e.g. Hb Hasharon, Hb Poole), whereas the major β-globin haemoglobinopathies (sickle cell disease and β-thalassaemia major) rarely manifest clinically in neonates.

α-Thalassaemia major predominantly affects families of South-East Asian, Mediterranean or Middle Eastern origin, and presents with second-trimester fetal anaemia or hydrops fetalis, which is fatal within hours of delivery. The only long-term survivors of α-thalassaemia major are those who have received intrauterine transfusions followed by regular post-natal transfusions and/or a bone marrow transplant. There is also a high incidence of hypospadias and limb defects in survivors and others have severe neurological problems. If intrauterine transfusions are delayed until anaemia is severe, neonatal pulmonary hypoplasia is a cause of early mortality. The diagnosis of α-thalassaemia major should be suspected in any case of severe fetal anaemia that presents in the second trimester, and any case of hydrops fetalis with severe anaemia in which the parents come from high-prevalence areas, particularly South-East Asia. Checking the blood counts of the parents will immediately identify whether they are at risk of having a child with α-thalassaemia major – both parents will have hypochromic, microcytic red cell indices (MCV usually < 74 fL and mean corpuscular haemoglobin (MCH) usually < 24 pg). The diagnosis of α-thalassaemia major is confirmed by haemoglobin electrophoresis or HPLC (which shows Hb Barts, Hb Portland and sometimes HbH; HbF and HbA are absent); the blood film shows hypochromic, microcytic red cells with vast numbers of circulating nucleated red cells (Figure 61.7).

Neonatal anaemia due to blood loss

Blood loss as a cause of neonatal anaemia may be very obvious, e.g. a cephalhaematoma or rupture of the cord, or be concealed and easy to miss unless specifically sought (e.g. feto-maternal bleeds). Usually, the most serious blood loss occurs prior to delivery and important causes of this are twin–twin transfusion and feto-maternal blood loss. *Twin–twin transfusion* occurs in monochorionic twins with monochorial placentas. If the

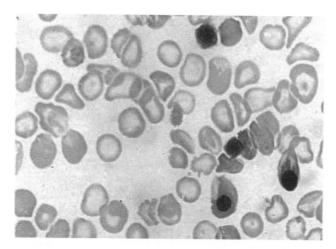

Figure 61.7 α-Thalassaemia major. Blood film from a neonate with α-thalassaemia major, born at 28 weeks' gestation, showing severe hypochromia, microcytosis, target cells, polychromasia and nucleated red cells.

bleeding is chronic, there may be a marked difference in birthweight between twins: the donor twin is smaller, pale, lethargic and may have overt cardiac failure; the recipient twin may be plethoric, with hyperviscosity and hyperbilirubinaemia and may rarely have a haemoglobin as high as 30 g/dL.

Feto-maternal haemorrhage occurs spontaneously or secondary to trauma usually in the third trimester. Most episodes involve very small quantities of blood (0.5 mL or less) but acute loss of > 20% of the blood volume may cause intrauterine death, circulatory shock or hydrops. Diagnostic clues are anaemia at birth in an otherwise well baby with no or minimal jaundice. The most useful diagnostic tests are a Coombs' test to exclude immune haemolysis, a reticulocyte count to exclude red cell aplasia, a Kleihauer test on maternal blood to quantify the number of HbF-containing fetal red cells in the maternal circulation and a blood film (Figure 61.8). Blood loss around the time of

delivery is usually due to obstetric complications (e.g. placenta praevia, placental abruption); in these circumstances, the babies are often extremely ill, with circulatory shock, anaemia worsening rapidly after birth, large numbers of circulating nucleated red cells and disseminated intravascular coagulation (DIC).

Anaemia of prematurity

The normal fall in haemoglobin in preterm neonates has been termed 'physiological anaemia of prematurity', as it does not appear to be associated with any abnormalities in the baby. The pathogenesis is not fully elucidated but contributory factors include the reduced red cell lifespan of fetal erythrocytes, the relatively low erythropoietin concentration, the rapid growth rate and iatrogenic blood loss. Routine supplementation of preterm neonates with folic acid and iron means that nutritional deficiency rarely plays a role. The diagnosis is usually straightforward – a well preterm baby with a slowly falling haemoglobin, unremarkable blood film showing normochromic/normocytic red cells, slightly low reticulocytes (20×10^9/L) and no nucleated red cells.

Management of anaemia of prematurity and the role of erythropoietin

The severity of anaemia of prematurity and thereby the need for red cell transfusion can be reduced by: (i) limiting iatrogenic blood loss by appropriate use of blood tests; (ii) administering iron and folate supplements to all preterm infants (iron 3 mg/kg per day from 4–6 weeks of age or iron-fortified formula with 0.5–0.9 mg/dL of iron and folic acid 50 μg daily or 500 μg once weekly); and (iii) judicious use of erythropoietin. The many controlled trials of recombinant erythropoietin for prevention of neonatal anaemia have been reviewed extensively. Erythropoietin reduces the number of transfusions in relatively well infants with low transfusion requirements, but not in sick preterm infants who have a need for frequent phlebotomy and multiple transfusions. The main roles for recombinant erythropoietin in

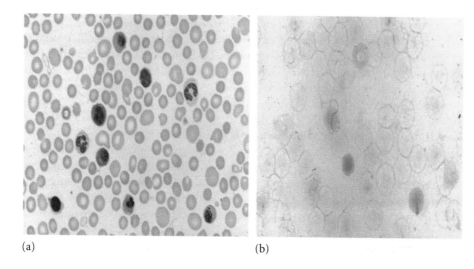

(a) (b)

Figure 61.8 Feto-maternal haemorrhage. (a) Blood film from a neonate with a haemoglobin of 5 g/dL at birth due to a large feto-maternal haemorrhage; the main features are the marked polychromasia, large numbers of nucleated red cells and normal red cell morphology. (b) Kleihauer test showing HbA-containing maternal 'ghost' cells and pink-staining HbF-containing fetal cells.

Table 61.3 Causes of neonatal polycythaemia.

Intrauterine growth restriction
Maternal hypertension
Maternal diabetes
Chromosomal disorders: trisomy 21, 18 or 13
Twin–twin transfusion
Delayed clamping of the cord
Endocrine disorders: thyrotoxicosis, congenital adrenal hyperplasia

neonates are in ameliorating the anaemia in infants who have received intrauterine transfusions for alloantibody-mediated anaemia and in preterm babies of Jehovah's Witnesses. The usual dose is 300 μg/kg of epoietin-β by subcutaneous injection three times per week, starting in the first week of life, together with oral iron supplements.

Indications for red cell transfusion in neonatal anaemia

The BCSH recently revised their guidelines for transfusion of fetuses, neonates and older children; the guidelines contain recommendations about the products and indications for red cell transfusion in neonates. These are consensus guidelines and need to be adapted for use in each individual Neonatal Intensive Care Unit, depending on the case mix of babies, as adherence to strict neonatal transfusion guidelines reduces both the number of transfusions and donor exposure.

A simple diagnostic approach to neonatal anaemia

Red cell disorders associated with neonatal or fetal anaemia present in three main ways: with a low haemoglobin, with jaundice due to haemolysis or with hydrops. A diagnostic algorithm to help identify which of these causes is most likely, which can be excluded and what further investigations are most appropriate is shown in Figure 61.2.

Neonatal polycythaemia

For both term and preterm infants, polycythaemia can be defined as a central venous haematocrit of greater than 0.65, as there is an exponential rise in blood viscosity above this level. However, even at haematocrits greater than 0.70, only a minority of neonates have clinical signs of hyperviscosity, such as lethargy, hypotonia, hyperbilirubinaemia and hypoglycaemia. Causes of polycythaemia are shown in Table 61.3. Treatment is controversial and is not necessary in infants with very minor symptoms (e.g. borderline hypoglycaemia or poor peripheral perfusion). Infants with neurological signs and a haematocrit greater than 0.65 should have a partial exchange transfusion (using a crystalloid solution such as normal saline) to reduce the haematocrit to 0.55.

White cell disorders

Normal values

In the neonate, normal values for leucocytes, in particular for neutrophils, are affected by a number of factors including gestational age, post-natal age, antenatal history, perinatal history and ethnic origin. Neutrophil counts in healthy babies increase for the first 12 h then fall to a nadir at 4 days of age. The neutrophil count is higher in capillary samples and after vigorous crying; it is lower in neonates of African origin. Healthy preterm babies often have circulating myeloblasts and lymphoblasts, although these usually form less than 5% of the white cell differential count.

Neutropenia

A pragmatic approach is to consider a neutrophil count at birth of less than 2×10^9/L as abnormal and worth monitoring, and a neutrophil count during the first month of life of less than 0.7×10^9/L as significant enough to merit further investigation.

Causes of neutropenia

The commonest cause of neutropenia at birth in preterm neonates is reduced neutrophil production, secondary to intrauterine growth restriction or maternal hypertension. Most affected neonates also have thrombocytopenia and increased erythropoiesis (polycythaemia and/or increased circulating nucleated red cells), secondary to fetal tissue hypoxia. The neutropenia resolves spontaneously usually within a few days of birth. The commonest cause of neutropenia in term infants is bacterial or viral infection. Other important causes of neutropenia are alloimmune neutropenia and congenital neutropenia due to failure of neutrophil production (e.g. Kostmann's syndrome), both of which predispose to severe neonatal infection.

Alloimmune neutropenia is the neutrophil equivalent of haemolytic disease of the newborn and alloimmune thrombocytopenia, and may affect 3% of all deliveries. It occurs when fetal neutrophils express paternally derived neutrophil-specific antigens absent on maternal neutrophils and against which the mother produces immunoglobulin G (IgG) neutrophil alloantibodies. The causative antibodies are usually anti-NA1 or -NA2. It presents in the first few days of life with fever and infections of the respiratory tract, urinary tract and skin, particularly due to *Staphylococcus aureus*, and the mainstay of treatment is antibiotics. The diagnosis is made by demonstrating antineutrophil antibodies in the mother and baby, which react against paternal, but not maternal, neutrophil antigens. The neutropenia is self limiting, usually resolving within 1–2 months.

Congenital and inherited neonatal neutropenias should be sought when the neutropenia is prolonged, if there is a relevant family history or consanguinity or if the baby has typical dysmorphic

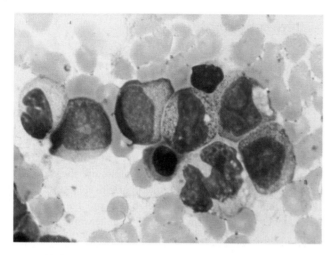

Figure 61.9 Transient leukaemia in a neonate with Down's syndrome. Leucoerythoblastic blood film showing increased numbers of blast cells, which spontaneously returned to normal by 2 months of age.

features (e.g. thumb/radial abnormalities in Fanconi's anaemia). Kostmann's syndrome (severe congenital neutropenia) is the most likely cause in the neonatal period. Infants usually present with severe infections and a marked neutropenia (< 0.2×10^9/L), often with a compensatory monocytosis. The diagnosis is made by the severity of the neutropenia, the bone marrow appearance ('arrest' of differentiation at the myelocyte/promyelocyte stage) and the absence of antineutrophil antibodies. The inheritance of Kostmann's syndrome can be autosomal recessive or dominant; recently, several cases of Kostmann's syndrome have been found to be due to mutations in the neutrophil elastase gene.

Congenital leukaemias

The most common types are acute monoblastic leukaemia and acute megakaryoblastic leukaemia; acute megakaryoblastic leukaemia is particularly common in babies with Down's syndrome. The babies present with signs of anaemia, thrombocytopenia and/or skin lesions caused by leukaemic infiltration. The blood film and bone marrow aspirate show large numbers of primitive blast cells. The prognosis is extremely poor; few are cured by chemotherapy and bone marrow transplantation may be the best option. Around 10% of neonates with Down's syndrome have a transient megakaryoblastic leukaemia also known as transient abnormal myelopoiesis (TAM) or transient myeloproliferative disorder (TMD), characterized by leucocytosis and circulating blast cells (Figure 61.9). Most cases spontaneously resolve within 2–3 months and no treatment is indicated, but around 10% evolve to acute megakaryoblastic leukaemia. Mutations in GATA-1 have been reported recently, both in TAM and in the megakaryoblastic leukaemia associated with Down's syndrome.

Haemostasis and thrombosis in the newborn

Bleeding and thrombotic problems are relatively common in neonates, particularly in those who are preterm and/or sick, and the number of genetic and acquired causes of thrombophilia that can be identified in neonates and their families is rising.

Developmental haemostasis

Coagulation proteins are present at measurable levels from the tenth week of gestation and gradually rise during fetal life. They do not cross the placenta, or do so in very small amounts, and therefore need to be independently synthesized by the fetus. 'Normal values' in the neonate vary not only with gestational but also with post-natal age. Data for babies at less than 30 weeks' gestation derive from fetoscopy samples: levels of the vitamin K-dependent factors (II, VII, IX and X) and of factors XI and XII are all low (< 40% of adult values) and remain so during the first month of life. By contrast, even in preterm babies (> 30 weeks), levels of Factor V, Factor XIII and fibrinogen are normal at birth and levels of factor VIII and von Willebrand factor (vWF) are normal or increased. Platelet counts at birth in term and preterm neonates are within the normal adult range. Many studies have found impaired function of neonatal platelets *in vitro* in term and preterm infants; the most consistent abnormalities are reduced aggregation in response to adrenaline, ADP and thrombin. Their significance in clinical practice is unclear as the bleeding time is normal in term and preterm infants (≤ 135 s).

Screening tests for bleeding disorders

Nearly all significant bleeding disorders in neonates can be identified using simple screening tests; exceptions are factor XIII deficiency and platelet function disorders. It is often helpful to test both parents for coagulation abnormalities to help identify inherited disorders as there is considerable overlap between the deficiency states and the lower limit of normal. The most useful screening tests in neonates are: the prothrombin time (PT), activated partial thromboplastin time (APTT), thrombin time (TT), fibrinogen and platelet count. Bleeding times are generally unhelpful in neonates and investigation of platelet function abnormalities is often deferred until a few months of age when platelet aggregometry and PFA-100™ become practical.

Inherited coagulation disorders

The commonest inherited disorders presenting in the neonatal period are factor VIII deficiency (haemophilia A), which has a frequency of 1 in 5000 male births and factor IX deficiency (haemophilia B), which occurs in 1 in 30 000 male births.

Factor VIII deficiency

Almost 40% of patients with inherited factor VIII deficiency present in the neonatal period. The clinical signs include intracranial haemorrhage, cephalohaematomas and bleeding post circumcision or from venous or arterial puncture sites. As in adults, the diagnosis is made by finding an isolated prolonged APTT and reduced factor VIII clotting activity. Acute management of the bleeding neonate with haemophilia requires intravenous administration of recombinant factor VIII (50–100 units (u)/kg intravenously, twice daily) to achieve factor VIII levels of 1.0 u/mL. As the half-life of factor VIII is shorter than in adults, more frequent dosing or a continuous factor VIII infusion may be required. For neonates with intracranial bleeding treatment with factor VIII should continue for at least 2 weeks. Fibrin glue may be useful in circumcision-associated bleeds. For patients diagnosed prenatally, vaginal delivery is safe provided that no difficulties are anticipated and vacuum extraction is avoided. The role of prophylactic factor VIII administration to haemophiliac newborns following difficult delivery to reduce the risk of intracranial bleeding (1–4%) is controversial, but it seems reasonable to recommend prophylactic factor VIII for a newborn haemophiliac when a previous sibling has had a major intracranial bleed.

Factor IX deficiency

This is clinically indistinguishable from Factor VIII deficiency. As factor IX levels are also low in liver disease and vitamin K deficiency, it is important to recheck factor IX levels at 6 weeks and 6 months of age if the diagnosis is in doubt. Neonates with bleeding are treated with recombinant factor IX concentrate (100 u/kg intravenously, once daily, monitored to achieve a factor IX level of 1.0 IU/mL).

von Willebrand disease in neonates

The two forms of von Willebrand disease (vWD) that can present in neonates are type 2b vWD, which presents with thrombocytopenia and bleeding is uncommon, and type 3 vWD, which has a clinical phenotype similar to haemophilia, as levels of both vWF and factor VIII are low. Type 3 vWD is autosomal recessive. The diagnosis is made by measuring vWF, factor VIII and the pattern of vWF multimers. At present, type 3 vWD is treated with intermediate purity FVIII (Haemate-P is the most commonly used product).

Factor XIII deficiency

This rare, autosomal recessive disorder usually presents with delayed bleeding from the umbilical cord during the first 3 weeks of life. The diagnosis is made by measuring clot solubility in 5 M urea solution as a screening test followed by a specific factor XIII assay; molecular tests for the common mutations are also available. The routine diagnostic coagulation screen is normal. Bleeding is treated with FXIII concentrate; cryoprecipitate (10 mL/kg) can also be used.

Acquired disorders of coagulation

Causes of acquired coagulopathy in neonates include vitamin K deficiency, DIC, liver disease, metabolic disorders, extracorporeal membrane oxygenation and giant haemangioendotheliomas (Kasabach–Merritt syndrome).

Vitamin K deficiency

Levels of vitamin K-dependent procoagulant factors (factors II, VII, IX and X), protein C and protein S are low at birth because of poor placental transfer of vitamin K, low vitamin K stores at birth, low vitamin K in breast milk and the lack of bacterial vitamin K synthesis in the sterile neonatal gut. Vitamin K deficiency can lead to 'haemorrhagic disease of the newborn' (also known as vitamin K deficiency bleeding, VKDB). Early VDKB presents in the first 24 h of life with severe gastrointestinal and intracranial haemorrhage. It is usually due to maternal medication that interferes with vitamin K, e.g. anticonvulsants (phenobarbitone, phenytoin), antituberculous therapy and oral anticoagulants. Classical VDKB presents at 2–7 days in 0.25–1.7% of babies who have not received prophylactic vitamin K at birth, especially if breast fed or with poor oral intake. Late VKDB occurs between 2 and 8 weeks after birth and presents with sudden intracranial haemorrhage in an otherwise well, breast-fed term baby or in babies with liver disease.

The diagnosis of VKDB is usually made by an isolated prolonged PT, which corrects following vitamin K administration. If doubt remains, assays of the inactive form of factor II (decarboxyprothrombin; PIVKA II) can be used to confirm the diagnosis. Treatment of VKDB is vitamin K (1 mg) intravenously or subcutaneously with fresh-frozen plasma only in severe haemorrhage. Classic and late VKDB can be prevented by a single intramuscular dose of vitamin K or, slightly less effectively, by repeated oral doses of vitamin K over the first 6 weeks of life. Some studies, but not others, suggest a link between intramuscular vitamin K at birth and later childhood malignancies (see reviews). In healthy babies, the choice of which route of administration is increasingly being left to parents.

Disseminated intravascular coagulation

The main triggers of DIC in neonates are severe hypoxia and/or acidosis and sepsis. It occurs in sick neonates and presents with generalized bleeding, including pulmonary haemorrhage and oozing from venepuncture sites. The usual pattern of coagulation abnormalities in neonatal DIC is prolongation of the PT, APTT and TT, together with low platelets and fibrinogen. D-Dimers are increased but are not specific and can be found in healthy neonates with no evidence of coagulopathy. The most important aspect of management of DIC is treatment of the underlying cause. Blood product replacement is indicated for clinical bleeding aiming to maintain the platelet count above 30×10^9/L and the fibrinogen greater than 1 g/L.

Table 61.4 Causes of neonatal thrombocytopenia.

Early (< 72 h)
Placental insufficiency (PET, IUGR, diabetes)
Neonatal alloimmune thrombocytopenia
Birth asphyxia
Perinatal infection (group B *Streptococcus*, *Escherichia coli*, *Listeria*)
Congenital infection (CMV, toxoplasmosis, rubella)
Maternal autoimmune (ITP, SLE)
Severe rhesus HDN
Thrombosis (renal vein, aortic)
Aneuploidy (trisomy 21, 18, 13)
Congenital/inherited (TAR, Wiskott–Aldrich)

Late (> 72 h)
Late-onset sepsis and necrotizing enterocolitis
Congenital infection (CMV, toxoplasmosis, rubella)
Maternal autoimmune (ITP, SLE)
Congenital/inherited (TAR, Wiskott–Aldrich)

CMV, cytomegalovirus; HDN, haemolytic disease of the newborn; ITP, idiopathic thrombocytopenic purpura; IUGR, intrauterine growth restriction; PET, pre-eclampsia; SLE, systemic lupus erythematosis; TAR, thrombocytopenia with absent radii.

Neonatal thrombocytopenia

Thrombocytopenia occurs in 1–5% of all neonates and up to 50% of neonates who are preterm and sick. It usually presents in one of two clinical patterns: early thrombocytopenia (within 72 h of birth) and late thrombocytopenia (after 72 h of life) (Table 61.4). The most frequent causes of early thrombocytopenia in preterm infants are intrauterine growth restriction and maternal hypertension or diabetes; the most frequent causes in term infants are neonatal alloimmune thrombocytopenia (NAITP) and thrombocytopenia secondary to maternal immune thrombocytopenic purpura (ITP). The most common causes of late thrombocytopenia are sepsis and necrotizing enterocolitis.

Neonatal alloimmune thrombocytopenia

This is the platelet equivalent of haemolytic disease of the newborn and affects around 1 in 1000 pregnancies. It is frequently severe (platelet count $< 30 \times 10^9$/L) and occurs in the first pregnancy in almost 50% of cases. Thrombocytopenia results from transplacental passage of maternal platelet-specific antibodies to human platelet antigens (HPA), which the mother lacks but which the fetus inherits from the father. In 80% of cases, these are anti-HPA-1a antibodies and in 10–15% anti-HPA-5b; occasional cases are due to anti-HPA-3a. HLA DRB3*0101-positive women are 140 times more likely to make anti-HPA-1a than HLA DRB3*0101-negative women. Intracranial haemorrhage occurs in 10% of cases, with long-term neurodevelopmental sequelae in 20% of survivors.

The diagnosis is made by demonstrating platelet antigen incompatibility between mother and baby and anti-HPA antibodies in the mother. Transfusion with HPA-compatible platelets is recommended for neonates with platelets $< 30 \times 10^9$/L and/or those with bleeding. Intravenous IgG (total dose 2 g/kg, over 2–5 days) may be useful if thrombocytopenia is prolonged. Pre-natal management of NAITP is controversial. The options are an invasive approach using fetal blood sampling plus fetal transfusion with HPA-compatible platelets if thrombocytopenia is detected, or a non-invasive approach relying on maternal intravenous IgG therapy.

Neonatal autoimmune thrombocytopenia

This is secondary to transplacental passage of maternal platelet autoantibodies in maternal ITP and systemic lupus erythematosus (SLE), which affects 1–5 in 10 000 pregnancies. Around 10% of infants develop thrombocytopenia, which is severe in less than 1%. In babies with severe thrombocytopenia, intravenous IgG is usually effective.

Indications for platelet transfusion

A number of countries have published consensus guidelines to help decide the indications for platelet transfusion in term and preterm neonates. In general, platelet transfusion is not considered necessary in well babies if the platelet count is above $20–30 \times 10^9$/L. Most groups agree that the threshold for transfusing sick babies, particularly preterm babies in the first few weeks of life, should be higher ($30–50 \times 10^9$/L).

Neonatal thrombosis: physiology and developmental aspects

Neonates have an increased risk of thrombosis (2.4 per 1000 hospital admissions) compared with older infants and children. This is largely due to the physiologically low levels of many of the inhibitors of coagulation and the frequent use of in-dwelling vascular catheters. Concentrations of antithrombin, heparin cofactor II and protein C are decreased at birth; protein S levels are also low but overall protein S activity is normal as it exists mainly in its free active form due to the virtual absence of its binding protein (c4b-BP) in neonates. Levels of plasminogen at birth are only 50% of adult values so neonates have a reduced ability to generate plasmin in response to fibrinolytic agents.

Screening tests for thrombophilia in neonates

The only inherited deficiencies for which there is a proven role in neonatal thrombosis are deficiencies in proteins C and S, which cause purpura fulminans. Factor V Leiden and the prothrombin 202010A promoter mutation (prothrombin[20210A]) have not yet been reported to cause neonatal thrombotic problems in isolation. Recent guidelines from the Haemostasis and Thrombosis Task Force of the BCSH state that congenital thrombophilia should be considered and screened for in any child with:

- clinically significant thrombosis, including spontaneous thrombotic events, unanticipated or extensive venous thrombosis, ischaemic skin lesions or purpura fulminans; and
- a positive family history of neonatal purpura fulminans.

The screening tests that should be performed in all suspected cases of thrombophilia are:
- protein C activity;
- protein S;
- antithrombin;
- factor V Leiden;
- prothrombin[20210A].

In addition, babies with thrombosis who are born to mothers with SLE and/or antiphospholipid syndrome should be tested for lupus anticoagulant, as antiphospholipid antibodies may cross the placenta and are a rare cause of neonatal thrombosis in such babies. The relevance of serum liporotein a and the MTHFR genotype to neonatal management is unclear at present.

Inherited thrombotic disorders in neonates

Proteins C and S deficiency

Protein C deficiency occurs in 1 in 160 000–360 000 births. Affected babies usually present with purpura fulminans within hours or days of birth, in which there is DIC and rapidly progressive, life-threatening, haemorrhagic necrosis due to dermal vessel thrombosis or with cerebral, renal vein or ophthalmic thrombosis. The diagnosis of protein C deficiency is made by the clinical picture and undetectable levels of protein C (< 0.01 u/mL) in the patient, together with heterozygote levels in the parents. Protein C deficient heterozygotes rarely present as neonates and have low protein C levels, which may overlap with the lower limit of normal in the first few months of life, delaying diagnosis until 6 months or later. The treatment is with protein C concentrate (40 u/kg, aiming to maintain a plasma level of > 0.25 u/mL). Protein S deficiency presents with identical features; levels of protein S are undetectable (< 0.01 u/mL) and the treatment is with fresh-frozen plasma (10–20 mL/kg) to maintain a plasma protein S of > 0.25 u/mL.

Antithrombin deficiency

Homozygous antithrombin deficiency usually presents later in childhood but neonatal deep venous thrombosis and inferior vena caval thrombosis have been reported. Heterozygous antithrombin deficiency is more common (1 in 2000–5000 births); it usually presents in the second decade of life but neonatal presentation with aortic thrombosis, myocardial infarction and cerebral dural sinus thrombosis may occur.

Acquired thrombotic problems in neonates

The most common risk factors for neonatal thrombosis are an intravascular catheter and shock, secondary to sepsis, hypoxaemia or hypovolaemia. Thrombosis particularly affects the renal veins, the aorta, aortic arch or cerebral vessels. Catheter-related thrombosis causes more than 80% of venous thromboses and more than 90% of arterial thromboses. The diagnosis is made by Doppler ultrasound or contrast angiography. Treatment of catheter-related thrombosis depends on the severity and extent of thrombosis. The first step is prompt removal where possible. If signs progress despite catheter removal, unfractionated heparin or low-molecular-weight heparin (LMWH) should be started using a dosing regime adapted for neonates. Thrombolytic therapy with urokinase or tissue plasminogen activator (tPA) has been used successfully for catheter-related thrombosis in neonates, but experience in preterm neonates is very limited. It is important to maintain the fibrinogen at levels less than 1 g/L and the platelet count greater than 50×10^9/L in neonates receiving thrombolytic therapy and heparin (starting dose 28 IU/kg/h) is often given to maintain vessel patency after thrombolytic therapy, although there is no evidence that this is beneficial.

Selected bibliography

Andrew M (1997) The relevance of developmental haemostasis to haemorrhagic disorders of newborns. *Seminars in Perinatology* **21**: 70–85.

Anwar R, Minford A, Gallivan L *et al.* (2002) Delayed umbilical bleeding – a presenting feature for factor XIII deficiency: clinical features, genetics, and management. *Pediatrics* **109**: E32143.

Blanchette V, Rand ML (1997) Platelet disorders in newborn infants: diagnosis and management. *Seminars in Perinatology* **21**: 53–62.

British Committee for Standards in Haematology Haemostasis and Thrombosis Task Force (2002) The investigation and management of neonatal haemostasis and thrombosis. *British Journal of Haematology* **119**: 295–309.

British Committee for Standards in Haematology Transfusion Task Force: Transfusion guidelines for neonates and older children 24.2.03 (www.bcshguidelines.com/).

Brown K (2000) Haematological consequences of parvovirus B19 infection. *Baillière's Best Practice in Research and Clinical Haematology* **13**: 245–59.

Bussel JB (2001) Alloimmune thrombocytopenia in the fetus and newborn. *Seminars in Thrombosis and Hemostasis* **27**: 245–52.

Hartmann J, Hussein A, Trowitzscha E *et al.* (2001) Treatment of neonatal thrombus formation with recombinant tissue plasminogen activator: six years experience and review of the literature. *Archives of Diseases in Childhood (Fetal and Neonatal Edition)* **85**: F18–F22.

Israels SJ, Cheang T, McMillan-Ward EM *et al.* (2001) Evaluation of primary hemostasis in neonates with a new *in vitro* platelet function analyzer. *Journal of Pediatrics* **138**: 116–19.

Kulkarni R, Lusher J (2001) Perinatal management of newborns with haemophilia. *British Journal of Haematology* **112**: 264–74.

Lallemand AV, Doco-Fenzy M, Gaillard DA (1999) Investigation of nonimmune hydrops fetalis: multidisciplinary studies are necessary for diagnosis – review of 94 cases. *Pediatric Developmental Pathology* **2**: 432–9.

Lange B (2000) The management of neoplastic disorders of haematopoiesis in children with Down's syndrome. *British Journal of Haematology* **110**: 512–24.

Marshall CJ, Thrasher AJ (2001) The embryonic origins of human haematopoiesis. *British Journal of Haematology* **112**: 838–50.

Ohls RK (2002) Erythropoietin in extremely low birthweight infants: blood in versus blood out. *Journal of Pediatrics* **141**: 3–6.

Puckett RM, Offringa M (2000) Prophylactic vitamin K for vitamin K deficiency bleeding in neonates. *Cochrane Database Systems Review* **4**: CD002776.

Roberts IAG, Murray NA (2003) Thrombocytopenia in the newborn. *Current Opinion in Pediatrics* **15**: 17–23.

Sohan K, Billington M, Pamphilon D *et al.* (2002) Normal growth and development following *in utero* diagnosis and treatment of homozygous alpha-thalassaemia. *British Journal of Gynaecology* **109**: 1308–10.

Stockman JA, de Alarcon PA (2001) Overview of the state of the art of Rh disease: history, current clinical management, and recent progress. *Journal of Pediatric Hematology and Oncology* **23**: 385–93.

Sutor AH, von Kries R, Cornelissen EA *et al.* (1999) Vitamin K deficiency bleeding (VKDB) in infancy. ISTH Pediatric/Perinatal Subcommittee. International Society on Thrombosis and Haemostasis. *Thrombosis and Haemostasis* **81**: 456–61.

Watts TL, Roberts IAG (1999) Haematological abnormalities in the growth-restricted infant. *Seminars in Neonatology* **4**: 41–54.

Wee LY, Fisk NM (2002) The twin–twin transfusion syndrome. *Seminars in Neonatology* **7**: 187–202.

CHAPTER 62

Laboratory practice

S Mitchell Lewis

62

Introduction

The practice of haematology is diverse, encompassing clinical medicine, laboratory technology, blood transfusion, aspects of histopathology, DNA analysis and genetics. The medically qualified haematologist has been concerned traditionally with both the diagnostic laboratory and clinical management of patients with blood diseases. Management of patients with haematological disorders has become increasingly arduous, requiring the haematologist to acquire unique clinical skills; conversely, major developments in laboratory practice require a high level of technical expertise, especially in handling automated instruments and information technology. It is essential that the medical haematologist becomes conversant with modern laboratory practice as he or she has an important role in maintaining the link between laboratory and clinic, ensuring that the laboratory serves clinicians from all specialties authoritatively and reliably, guiding diagnosis and management of patients as well as the needs of health surveillance for the community in general. This chapter describes the aspects of laboratory practice that are especially important towards these goals.

Good laboratory practice ensures that reliable results of clinically relevant laboratory tests are received by the clinician in good time, that the laboratory functions efficiently and economically, and that there is adequate protection of the health and well-being of the staff. It is essential to avoid faults that may lead to misdiagnosis and patient mismanagement, unnecessary over-investigation, delay in treatment while awaiting the laboratory report and, ultimately, loss of credibility of the laboratory service. The rules that govern the laboratory are no different to those established by industry for good manufacturing practice; they highlight the fact that good management is as important as technical skill if the objectives are to be attained.

The following aspects of laboratory function will be discussed:
• *quality assurance* – various procedures that are directly concerned with test reliability;
• *clinical reliability* – use of appropriate test methods or analytical systems, test interpretation, relevant reference ranges, specimen collection and sampling;
• *staff* – health and safety control, professional education and training opportunities, clinical and technical audit, involvement in management with delegated responsibilities, and confidence in the management;
• *organization and management* – strategic planning, budget control, computer applications, record-keeping, application of up-to-date methods and adherence to mandatory regulations.

Quality assurance

For reliable test results it is important to ensure *precision* (i.e. reproducibility within agreed limits when an analysis is performed repeatedly on the same specimen), *accuracy* (i.e. truth), *standardization* and *harmonization* (i.e. comparability of results between laboratories). Different procedures are used in respect of quantitative, semi-quantitative and qualitative tests. Precision in quantitative tests, expressed as coefficient of variation of the measurements (*CV%*), is relatively easy to achieve. Accuracy is more problematic for most haematology tests, as there are few internationally established reference standards, and standardization is usually based on calibration by arbitrary standard preparations or by using standardized methods. But the most important criterion is *harmonization* to ensure comparability of measurements between laboratories, for the benefit of both the individual patient, who may be seen at different times in different clinics, and for collaborative studies, such as therapeutic trials, which may be undertaken at different centres.

There are five components in a quality assurance programme:
- standardization and instrument calibration;
- internal quality control (IQC);
- statistical control with patient data;
- correlation assessment;
- external quality assessment (EQA).

Standardization

Most modern analysers are arbitrary comparators rather than absolute measurement devices. To perform reliably they must be calibrated; thus correct measurements on test samples depend on the accuracy of the value that has been assigned to the calibrator.

Generally, calibrators are provided by the instrument manufacturers or are available from commercial companies; their reliability depends on the efforts made by the manufacturers to establish their true value. Control preparations (see below) also have assigned values, but these are only approximations, and controls should not be used as calibrators. Wherever possible, calibrators should be directly traceable to an international (primary) standard with exactly defined physical or chemical measurement.

Where no reference standards are available, harmonization depends on adherence to written standards and practice guidelines such as those published by WHO and the International Council for Standardization in Haematology (ICSH), which are listed on their websites (p. 1018). Similar documents have been published by various national authorities, taking account of specific situations. Thus, in the UK this is undertaken by the British Committee for Standards in Haematology (BCSH). In the USA, a wide range of practice guidelines have been published by the National Committee for Clinical Laboratory Standards (NCCLS).

Internal quality control

Internal quality control (IQC) is intended to ensure that measurements are sufficiently precise day by day or batch by batch within established limits. The advent of automation in the diagnostic laboratory and the increasing dependence on machine-generated results for analytical tests highlight the importance of an IQC programme. Results on patients' samples should not be issued until it is clear from the control data that there has been no significant problem in the analytical procedure. There are several methods of IQC which complement each other.

The best known method is to test a control sample at intervals alongside the routine specimens, and to plot the results on a Levey–Jennings control chart. This is a linear graph showing the mean and limits of standard deviation (SD) at 1SD and 2SD. The results of sequential (daily) measurements are plotted on the graph (Figure 62.1). When the system is in good control, not more than 1 in 20 measurements should fall outside 2SD. When two or more consecutive measurements are outside this limit there is likely to have been a random error, whereas several consecutive values within 2SD, but all on one side of the mean, indicate a consistent bias. A wildly deviant result outside 3SD may occur as a result of a gross error ('blunder').

Delta check

This refers to comparison between consecutive tests on a patient within 1–2 weeks. Account must be taken of the diurnal physiological variation and the expected coefficient of variance of the instrument. Provided that there is no clinical explanation, a difference outside these limits should alert the user to a technical error or a faulty specimen due to wrong labelling, clots, inadequate mixing or storage deterioration. This is, however, a relatively crude method of control: if a narrow limit is set, an excessive number of cases will be included, whereas a wider limit will be too insensitive. The following is a rough guide to acceptable limits of difference (i.e. increase or decrease) from the previous result for some tests: Hb 2 g/dL; mean corpuscular volume (MCV) 6 fL; mean corpuscular haemoglobin (MCH) 5 pg; platelet count 50% difference from previous result; white blood cell (WBC) normal count becoming high or low.

Statistical control with patient data

This method of control is based on the principle that the overall daily means of the blood count parameters will remain constant, provided that the proportion of different categories of patients in a hospital remains more or less the same. The calculations are adjusted by means of an algorithm to obtain a weighted moving average. This procedure has been incorporated in multichannel analysers to provide an automated continuously updated control of accuracy (Figure 62.2). It will detect analytic drift and a change in calibration; instrument imprecision will be detected by an increase in the SD.

Correlation assessment

A control chart will not detect 'blunders' in individual routine specimen, which can only be detected by finding that the test results do not correlate with other laboratory tests or the clinical condition. These discrepancies can be checked by (i) cumulative reports; (ii) blood film examination; (iii) patient's clinical state; and (iv) whether the blood count is consistent with the results of other investigations.

Cumulative reports may be computer printed or entered manually on a pre-printed record sheet. It is then possible to see, at a glance, whether there has been a single discrepant result or an unexpected alteration in the gradient of the rise or fall in blood count parameters, which would have been expected from the progression of the clinical condition or its predictable response to therapy. If no clinical reason is apparent to explain a

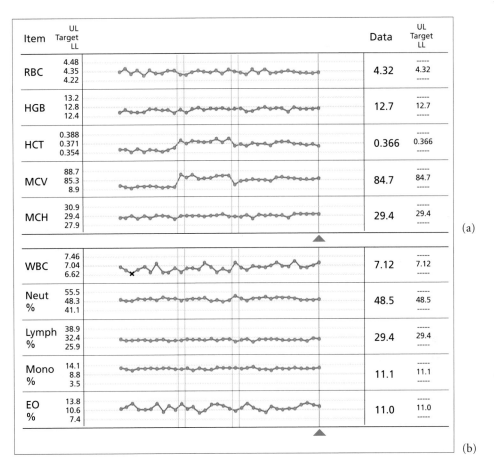

(a)

(b)

Figure 62.1 Quality control with the Levey–Jennings chart. (a) The established means with ± 2SD values of the control specimen for red cell parameters are indicated, and the results obtained in the laboratory are plotted sequentially. Note occurrence of a bias in HCT and MCV; recalibration of the instrument corrected this discrepancy. (b) The results on the control sample for WBC and differential count. The WBC (but not the differential count) showed some variable bias, indicating a fault that required correction.

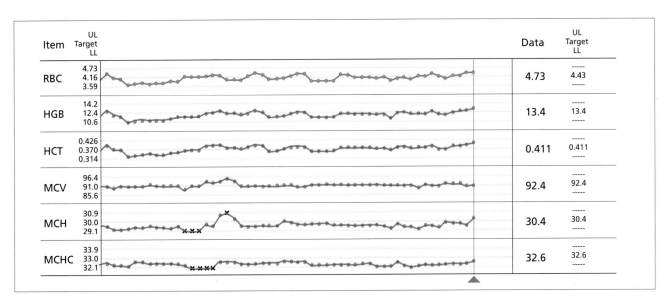

Figure 62.2 Control of stability of daily means. The predetermined constant daily mean and ± 2SD limits for satisfactory control on each parameter are indicated on the left. The results obtained in the laboratory are displayed on the right. Note the highlighted (crosses) variant results which were subsequently corrected.

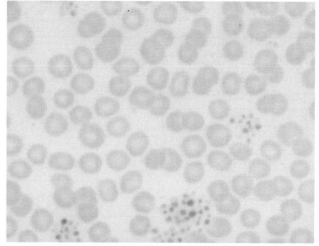

(a)

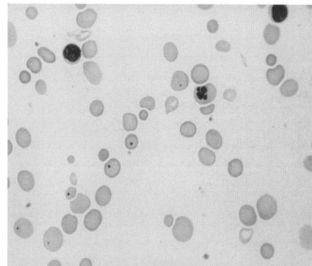

(b)

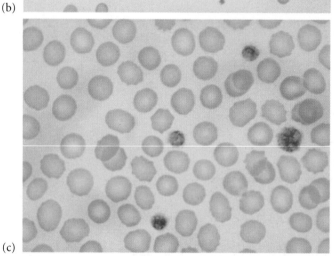

(c)

Figure 62.3 Examples of discrepancies in blood count parameters identified from blood film. (a) Low platelet count due to platelet clumping; (b) analyser fails to discriminate markedly microcytic red cells from platelets; (c) analyser fails to discriminate macrothrombocytes from red cells.

discrepancy, the test results must be suspect until it is confirmed by a repeat test on a fresh specimen. The occurrence of a similar discrepancy in two different specimens on the same day would indicate a specimen mix-up.

With the advent of fully automated analysers that include differential cell counting, the blood film is becoming sidelined. It is, however, important to appreciate that the analyser may fail to detect a diagnostically important feature or, conversely, misinterpret an artifact that would be identified on a blood film. Morphological features such as hypochromasia, macrocytosis and microcytosis are the basic criteria for identifying the cause of anaemia. Whereas flow cytometers are generally more reliable than examination of a blood film for judging the degree of hypochromasia and distinguishing marginal macrocytosis and microcytosis, gross discrepancies between the blood count parameters obtained by the analyser and the morphological impression should always be checked. A glance at a blood film will confirm or refute an abnormally high or low leucocyte or platelet count. This is especially important if there are no previous reports for reference.

Artefacts that give rise to spurious blood count parameters include:

1 An apparent leucopenia and thrombocytopenia due to partial clotting of the specimen. This may be detected in the film by the presence of a mass of aggregated platelets (Figure 62.3a).
2 Abnormally high MCH and mean cell haemoglobin concentration (MCHC) due to the presence of cold agglutinins or autoimmune haemolytic anaemia.
3 Erroneously high WBC count due to the presence of nucleated red cells or incompletely lysed red cells in haemoglobinopathies or liver disease.
4 Erroneously high haemoglobin as a result of turbidity when the WBC count is high.
5 Severe microcytosis, and, conversely, macrothrombocytes may affect the accuracy of the platelet count if the analyser is unable to discriminate between the populations of cells when their sizes approximate to each other (Figure 62.3b and c).

Paradoxically, as the automated blood count makes the blood film redundant in the routine laboratory, the film has an increasingly important role in the quality control of the count. A visual differential count provides a reference method for checking the reliability of the automated differential count, and inspection of a film is necessary to check any blood count that has been 'flagged' by the analyser.

External quality assessment (EQA)

Although IQC provides continuous vigilance, EQA checks test performance only on random occasions. However, by comparing results from different laboratories it is possible to establish between-laboratory and between-method performances. Thus, EQA schemes have an important educational role, not only for participating laboratories whose performance is under scrutiny,

Table 62.1 Clinically acceptable limits of test variance.

Hb	3–4%
RBC (by automated analyser)	3–4%
PCV	4–5%
MCV, MCH, MCHC	4–5%
Total leucocyte count	8–10%
Platelet count	10–15%
Serum vitamin B_{12}	20%
Red cell folate	20%
Serum iron	20%
Ferritin	20%
HbA_2	5–10%
HbF quantification	5–10%

but also for assessing the 'state of the art' overall, for identifying and recommending the best methods for various tests, and persuading participants to abandon unreliable methods. It is a valuable interface between users and manufacturers of instruments, reagents and kits, because the EQA data may indicate an otherwise unrecognized product failure, as well as the problem of lack of harmonization of results when different technologies are used in analysis.

When the results of blood count and other quantitative tests are returned to the organizing centre, they are analysed to establish the consensus median (or mean) and SD, against which the results from the individual participants are compared. Performance is expressed as deviation index (DI), which is the extent by which the individual's results vary from the established SD. When the DI is greater than 2, the problem should be investigated. However, to base acceptable limits of performance on statistical analysis alone is unrealistic. Thus, for example, the remarkably low coefficient of variance (CV) for haemoglobin means that even a measurement deviating from the mean by more than 3SD is unlikely to influence clinical decisions, whereas with reticulocyte counts, for example, where the CV is high, 3SD may represent a gross error. In reality, therefore, poor performance should be defined as a result that might lead to inappropriate clinical action. Suggested practical limits for acceptable performance are given in Table 62.1.

In qualitative tests, features that are correctly reported are awarded a credit score, whereas a penalty score is given for false-positives and -negatives. The scores are weighted to give a higher number of points (credit or penalty) for more important features, especially those that point to a specific diagnosis or, if reported falsely, could be diagnostically misleading. All members of the laboratory staff, technical/scientific and medical, should be encouraged to participate in in-house morphological exercises based on the EQA films. The UK national scheme is designated NEQAS.

Pre- and post-analytic control

Both IQC and EQA are concerned with the actual analytical tests at the laboratory bench. Clinical reliability is concerned primarily with the test results, whether they are useful and can be relied upon for patient care or for health screening. Thus, functions that may indirectly influence test reliability must also be taken into account. These include all stages from specimen collection, transport to the laboratory, registration and selection of the most appropriate methods for the required test(s), as well as validation of the results, their interpretation and transmission of a meaningful (and legible) report to the appropriate unit or individual.

Specimen collection

All haematology tests start with blood collection. It is essential to ensure that specimens are collected by a standardized procedure and reach the laboratory in good condition.

Phlebotomy

To avoid diurnal variation, the specimens should, as far as possible, always be collected at the same time of day. Using the wrong anticoagulant, using insufficient or conversely excess anticoagulant and inadequate mixing of the blood with the anticoagulant will give rise to flawed specimens. It is also necessary to be aware of various factors that may be responsible for discrepancies. These include smoking, eating and drinking within the previous 2–3 h and use of toilet immediately before collecting the specimen; the subject must be at rest and if possible free of stress – thus, the patient must not undertake vigorous physical activity (including rushing upstairs to the clinic!) within 20 min and the nervous patient must be reassured. Haemostasis from prolonged tourniquet pressure is likely to cause haemoconcentration, whereas excessive negative pressure on the blood sample when drawing it into a syringe may cause haemolysis.

There is debate on the differences between venous blood and 'capillary' blood obtained by skin puncture from finger, earlobe or heel (in infants). In blood obtained by skin puncture, the packed cell volume (PCV), red-cell count and haemoglobin of peripheral blood are often slightly greater than in venous blood, the total leucocyte and neutrophil counts higher by about 8%, the monocyte count by about 12% or more, and the platelet count lower by about 10% or more. However, these differences are likely to be due to inadequate sampling, as some studies have shown no significant differences between venous and capillary samples when the blood flows freely from the capillary puncture site.

As far as possible non-reusable syringes (glass or plastic), needles and lancets should be used and discarded immediately thereafter. If the local situation requires re-use of glass syringes, they must be washed thoroughly in tap water to remove all traces of blood, then soaked in 10% bleach for 30 min or longer (needles and lancets overnight in freshly diluted 2% glutaraldehyde) followed by sterilization in an oven at 120°C for 30 min. Safety precautions for the user when collecting and handling the blood are described on p. 1014.

The phlebotomist is responsible for ensuring that all specimens and associated request forms are adequately identified, with appropriate indication of especially hazardous specimens. The specimens must then be transported to the laboratory without delay, and maintained during transit at an appropriate ambient temperature to minimize deterioration. When a pneumatic delivery system is in use, it must be checked on installation to ensure that it has no untoward effect on the specimens and that there is no leakage. As blood cell morphology requires films to be made and fixed as soon as possible, if specimens are sent from a distance it may be desirable to have the films prepared and fixed at the time of blood collection.

To take account of these various factors the International Society of Hematology and International Council for Standardization in Haematology have jointly published a standard for *Specimen collection, storage and transmission to the laboratory for hematological tests*.

Pre-analytic proficiency

The first clerical act is to record the time of arrival of specimen in laboratory. The container should then be checked for leakage, insufficient volume or incorrect anticoagulant for the requested test(s). The request and specimen are given a laboratory reference number and marked either for immediate attention ('stat'), or as 'urgent' or 'routine' and sent to the appropriate section(s) of the laboratory for testing.

Post-analytic proficiency

After the tests have been carried out, the following procedures are required to ensure proficiency in the post-analytic phase:
1 processing of results for transcription on to report forms;
2 immediate scrutiny of urgent results with issue of provisional report and its delivery to the requesting clinician;
3 assessment of the significance of results in the context of established reference values and decision for further tests;
4 transmission of final report without unreasonable delay to the location indicated on the request form;
5 contact with users to ensure that the reports arrive in due time for optimal use during clinical management and that the results are presented in a clear and unambiguous form; there should also be discussions on test selection, taking account of the clinical relevance of the tests that are undertaken, the introduction of new tests and evaluation of benefit versus cost, as discussed below.

Test selection

To decide whether or not to introduce a particular system, method or diagnostic kit, the following factors should be considered:
1 biological, chemical, radiation and mechanical safety;
2 clinical utility;
3 precision;
4 accuracy and comparability with existing methods;
5 cost efficiency;
6 routine servicing and maintenance contract conditions;
7 reliability and reputation of the manufacturer/supplier;
8 staff acceptability.

A system or method that gives no useful information or is unsafe should be discounted without further consideration. The choice should then be based on the following questions:
1 Is the test or set of tests to be used for clinical diagnosis and management of specific clinical disorders, patient screening and health monitoring, or for epidemiological studies?
2 Are the tests to be undertaken in the laboratory as routine, for urgent specimens, in an after-hours service, or outside the laboratory as a near-patient (point-of-care) facility?
3 What level of technical expertise is required?
4 Finally, are the levels of precision, accuracy, technical reliability and clinical utility adequate for the required purposes, and is the cost justified and budgeted for?

In the technical assessment, different laboratories may place different emphasis on the importance of these criteria. In general, the method giving the lowest coefficient of variance ($CV\%$) for each parameter is to be preferred, but the desired level of precision and accuracy will depend on the purpose for which the tests are carried out. When comparing methods, all of which are technically acceptable, a significant difference in annual cost and cost per test may be the deciding factors, but, with similar costs, choice may depend upon consideration of maintenance facilities, ease of handling, and, finally, personal preferences and prejudices.

Clinical utility

A test serves its purpose only if it triggers an appropriate clinical reaction. Its competence depends on its ability to distinguish between individuals with and without the particular medical conditions, without overlapping. This is best shown by comparison with an established reference method or by clearly defined clinical feature, in order to identify true-positives (TPs), true-negatives (TNs), false-positives (FPs) and false-negatives (FNs).

From these data one can calculate the sensitivity, specificity and predictive values of the test by the formulae of Galen and Gambino as follows: sensitivity = TPs/(TPs + FNs); specificity = TNs/(TNs + FPs); reliability = (TPs + TNs)/total number of tests;

Table 62.2 Calculation of clinical utility of a haemoglobin device against a reference method, on a number of sequential blood samples.

	Hb > 120 g/L	Hb < 80 g/L
True-positive	303	56
True-negative	218	491
False-positive	326	6
False-negative	17	17
Sensitivity	0.95	0.76
Specificity	0.87	0.99
Positive predictive value	0.90	0.93
Negative predictive value	0.92	0.97
Likelihood ratio	7.3	76
Youden index	+0.82	+0.75

To assess performance of the device with normal and severely anaemic bloods, 120 and 80 g/L were selected as cut-off points respectively. It was concluded that the device is slightly more reliable for measuring the lower haemoglobins.

positive predictive value = TPs/(TPs + FPs); and negative predictive value = TNs/(TNs + FNs).

Ideally, for a diagnostic test to be totally reliable, sensitivity and specificity should both be near 100%. In practice, as sensitivity and specificity tend to counter each other, test selection will depend on whether sensitivity or specificity is more important (Table 62.2). When calculating these indices, it is important to establish for what purpose the test is to be used. Thus, for example, haemoglobinometry may be required in a clinic for identifying patients *with* anaemia, but in blood donor selection for identifying individuals who are *not* anaemic. Thus, haemoglobin above the cut-off point for anaemia would be *true negative* in the context of the problem of anaemia, but *true positive* for selection of blood donors (Table 62.3).

The relative usefulness of two methods for the same test can be assessed by the *receiver–operator characteristic analysis* (ROC). This is obtained graphically by plotting *sensitivity* against *1-specificity* at a series of cut-off points for the two methods being compared, using a known reference method as the basis. This formula, which indicates the relative frequency of positive results in disease and negative results in normals, is also termed *likelihood ratio*. A result increasingly > 1 indicates the probability of disease, whereas < 1 lowers the possibility of the disease being diagnosed by that test.

An alternative method for *likelihood ratio* is that of Youden, which is obtained by calculating *sensitivity + specificity – 1*. Values range from −1 to +1; tests with positive ratio increasingly above zero strengthen the probability that the test will discriminate the presence or absence of the specified disease.

Table 62.3 Validation of utility of haemoglobin device for different purposes.

	For blood donor selection	For checking anaemia
True-positive	552	16
True-negative	16	552
False-positive	6	4
False-negative	4	6
Sensitivity	99.3	72.7
Specificity	72.7	99.3
Positive predictive value	98.9	80.0
Negative predictive value	80.0	98.9
Likelihood ratio	3.6	103.8
Youden index	+0.72	+0.72

When used in a blood transfusion service for identifying donors with normal haemoglobin, measurements of > 120 g/L are recorded as true positive, whereas when used at a clinic to establish if the patients are anaemic measurements of > 120 g/L are recorded as true negative.

Note the effect of using these different categories on the likelihood ratio (but no effect on the Youden index).

Cost analysis and efficiency

Total cost includes capital cost (i.e. replacement cost and mortgage factor) over the period of the nominal useful life of the instrument, operational costs for consumables and reagents, maintenance contracts and labour costs. The amount attributed to labour will depend on whether the instrument requires to be operated by a highly trained technologist, a more junior technician or a supervised medical laboratory assistant. Unit costs will depend upon laboratory work load (see p. 1015), which is usually calculated on a range of annual expectancies and then expressed as cost per test. This will provide the laboratory with a yardstick to judge the work load limits that justify the choice of one instrument over another, and whether a semi-automated or fully automated type may be more appropriate. Finally, the suitability of the instrument is judged in perspective of its clinical usefulness for its intended purpose.

The total annual cost can be calculated as: $L \times T + C \times T + A + M + HS + VO$, where T = throughput, L = labour costs per test, C = consumable cost per specimen, A = annual capital cost of leasing or amortization, M = maintenance costs, HS = intra-laboratory housekeeping and services, and VO = extra-laboratory unit overheads.

This calculation is useful for comparing the running costs of different systems when choosing a new analyser. It is also useful in deciding whether to use a commercial diagnostic kit or a home-made set of reagents for a test.

The true cost-effectiveness of tests must also take account of whether the laboratory results are utilized effectively by clinicians. This can be assessed from the following formula: $(A \times 100/C) \times (100/B)$, where A = cost/test as described above; B = quality of test as indicated by its clinical reliability; C = clinical usefulness of test, which is assessed by the extent with which the test is relied upon in clinical decisions, compared with 'best practice' guidelines. For each test, an independent assessor needs to judge how many tests are appropriately requested and are used to influence patient management or public health decisions. The percentage that is not used to guide clinical decisions will provide a figure for 'clinical wastage' of the test and this can be entered into the formula. There is debate on the economics of providing an automated total screening programme or specifically selected tests. It is of interest to note that a study of American hospital practice has shown that clinicians in general are concerned with only a few of the eleven parameters that constitute the complete blood count, mainly haemoglobin, haematocrit, platelet count, WBC, sometimes MCV, and, surprisingly, reports on blood film morphology.

Selection of an *in vitro* diagnostic device

When a new analyser or diagnostic kit is introduced it should be evaluated by the manufacturer before it is marketed, and by the user before purchase. In some cases, type testing is carried out by a consumer organization in order to make recommendations at a national level. In the UK, this is undertaken by the Department of Health's Medicines and Healthcare Products Regulatory Agency (formerly the Medical Devices Agency (MDA)), which issues regular reports on instruments that have been evaluated on their behalf in specified laboratories.

An important document that concerns all laboratories in the European Union is the official *Directive on in-vitro diagnostic devices*, which aims to ensure the reliability of diagnostic analysers and apparatus, kits, calibrators, control materials and reagents. These are required to have an evaluation or performance verification carried out by a national 'competent authority'. This entitles them to be certified with a CE mark; from 2006, laboratories may not purchase any diagnostic device without it.

Guidelines for evaluation have been published by various bodies. A protocol specifically for evaluation of haematological equipment has been published by ICSH. This protocol is intended to be used for type-testing by a manufacturer, consumer organization or the notified body described above. The individual user should carry out a limited validation study on the specific instrument that is being purchased.

Reference values

Interpretation of test results is often based on inadequately defined '*normal*' values. There is an increasing awareness of the effects on test results of physiological variables and environmental conditions. This has led to the concept of *reference values*, which takes account of such factors as age, sex, ethnic group, pregnancy, menstruation, diurnal and seasonal fluctuations, climate and altitude, as well as life-style habits (smoking and alcohol).

The conditions in which samples are obtained are standardized at the same time of day, preferably in the morning before breakfast; data are analysed separately for different variables, such as individuals who are ambulant or in bed, smokers or non-smokers. The data will be found to fit one of three types of distribution pattern: normal Gaussian, log-normal ('skew') or non-parametric. Results can then be expressed as mean (if normally distributed) or median (if non-parametric), together with the limits ($\pm 2SD$) that will include 95% of the population.

The usefulness of reference values depends on the precision of the upper and lower limits. A reasonably reliable estimate can be obtained with 40 measurements, although a larger number, 120 or more, is generally recommended.

Laboratory safety

All laboratory staff should be aware of potential hazards and should know how to ensure adequate protection. Sensible everyday precautions should prevent accidents from the careless handling of toxic substances: physical injury from sharp instruments; needles or broken glassware; radiation exposure; electric shock and fire from the improper use of electrical fittings and connections; and fire caused by the handling of flammable substances such as alcohol and solvents near a naked flame.

Biohazard is a more difficult problem. All specimens from patients should be regarded as potentially infectious for HIV, hepatitis B and C viruses, and other blood-borne pathogens. They must always be handled carefully to minimize the exposure of skin and mucous membranes to patients' specimens. There are well established universal precautions against these hazards to be observed by all staff, and there are procedures to be followed when contamination has occurred to workers, laboratory areas or equipment.

Strategies for safety in handling blood, especially safety in injections and prevention of cross-infection, are described in an extensive and frequently updated WHO programme known as SIGN. The weekly bulletin can be obtained on application to sign@who.int. It is also available on the Internet (www.injectionsafety.org).

Waste disposal

Blood and other potentially infected body fluids can safely be poured down a drain, provided that the drain is connected to a sanitary sewer. Laboratory waste, such as blood specimen containers, used syringes, swabs, tissues and dressings, should be collected in special colour-coded bags for subsequent incinera-

Postgraduate Haematology

tion or autoclaving, before being disposed of in a rubbish dump. Boxes containing needles and other sharp objects should be incinerated without opening.

Soiled laundry should be placed in leak-proof labelled bags for transport to the laundry, where the items should be either first soaked in disinfectant or washed in hot water (> 70°C) with detergent for 25–30 min before being rinsed. It should be emphasized that the laboratory is responsible for the waste disposal, even if the operation is contracted to an outside body.

Every laboratory should have a named staff member trained in general aspects of laboratory safety, whose responsibility it is to record all incidents, to ensure that immediate action is taken in accordance with an established and defined procedure for treating the exposed or injured person, and to take measures to prevent recurrence.

WHO has a useful website that provides up-to-date information on various aspects of waste management, including country-specific and region-specific problems and legal requirements (http://www.healthcarewaste.org).

Safety legislation

In many countries there are mandatory requirements for safety at work. In the UK the authority for this is the Health and Safety Executive. There are two essential sets of regulations for the laboratory – Control of Substances Hazardous to Health (COSHH) Regulations (1999), and Ionizing Radiation Regulations (1985). The toxicity of all chemical reagents, including those incorporated into kits, requires to be categorized and certified by COSHH with regard to degree of hazard, safety measure for use, handling of spillage and waste disposal.

Staff responses

'Job satisfaction' is essential in a dependable organization, and all members of the laboratory staff should be reassured with regard to their safety, their continuing training with opportunities for advancement, and their good relations with and confidence in the management of their department.

Professional training

Continuing professional development (CPD), linked with continuing medical education (CME), is a process of systematic learning that enables health-workers to be constantly brought up to date on developments in their profession and thus ensure their competence to practice throughout their entire career. Policies and programmes have already been established in a number of countries, and in some, participation may become a mandatory requirement for the right to practice. It must not be confused with accreditation (p. 1019), which concerns the performance (and licensing) of the laboratories themselves.

CPD schemes are run by national professional bodies who are responsible for the practice standards of their members. In the UK, schemes relevant to haematology are the responsibility of the Royal College of Pathologists for doctors, and the Institute of Biomedical Science for scientists/technologists. The process is based on obtaining 'credits' for various activities, such as attendance at approved lectures, workshops and conferences, using computer- or journal-based programmes, taking part in peer review discussions, giving lectures and writing professional papers.

Organization and management

The functioning of a modern laboratory with automated analysers is not unlike that of a factory, with the issue of reports as its end-product but, as each test result requires individual scrutiny, the work is also labour intensive. An efficient and effective laboratory service requires co-ordination of the work load compared with the available resources, which include capital investment in building, furnishing and equipment as well as income.

Strategic planning on 3- to 5-year cycles is essential to implement changes for improving the service, taking into account the advancing frontiers of technology as well as political and economic changes. Thus, for example a laboratory might be required to consider the implications of providing a full 24-h service with a shift system, or providing a fast result service to general practitioners linked to the laboratory computer system, or, in a laboratory with a relatively low work load, converting a manual or semi-automated service to a fully automated analytical system.

Financial management

Income may be fixed when its only source is a health authority, or when it is earned in long-term contracts to provide service to a private organization. Other sources of income include industrial workers screening tests, drug trials for pharmaceutical companies, testing of new equipment and kits for manufacturers, training grants, and grants from government or other organizations for innovative research.

The analysis of cost for running the laboratory must take account of both capital costs and recurrent revenue costs; the latter consists of labour costs, consumables, equipment maintenance, housekeeping and services, which include heating, lighting, water, waste disposal and cleaning services, and even a proportion of the general overheads of the institution. The capital costs will almost certainly have an element of recurrence to include interest on any loan to meet the initial outlay, allowance for depreciation and renewal of equipment after an agreed period of time.

As a rule, labour cost is by far the largest component. In a competitive market it is essential for the laboratory to keep careful control of this – in general it has little or no control over most of the other expenditures.

Price setting depends on an analysis of test costs (see also p. 1013). This will include labour, based on the salary rate per hour of workers of appropriate grades, and the medical staff services for the interpretation of results and consultation with clinicians. Out-of-hours service requires a different calculation of costs as it will vary with the work load and with the different organization of work and staffing to handle it.

Work load

Knowledge of the work load is essential for planning a schedule for laboratory work and its costs. Methods for estimating work load have been based on the number of units of time required for a test, where the unit is defined as being equal to 1 minute of technical, clerical and laboratory assistant's time. This encompasses all procedures from initial handling of specimen to reporting, including routine maintenance and repair of the analytical system, preparation of stock solutions and technical supervision. It does not include blood collection nor does it take account of any contribution by medical staff. Moreover, with automated technology there will be little difference between a discrete measurement of a single analyte and multiple tests in a single process. Thus, formal programmes such as that of the College of American Pathologists and the UK 'Welcan' system, have been found to be of limited value in present-day practice, which is better served by benchmarking (see p. 1019).

For budgetary and performance planning, it is useful to have a breakdown of the data into: (i) separate technical units for blood counting, haemostasis, blood transfusion serology, haematinic assays, haemoglobinopathy studies, etc; (ii) normal working hours and emergency after-hours services; and (iii) the different users such as outpatients, inpatients, specialist clinics, surgeons, physicians and general practitioners.

Assay turnaround time

Distinction must be made between throughput time for the analytic process on a sample and the total time taken from specimen collection to issue of a report. The most important determinant factor is the transport system at each end of the process. An excessively slow turnaround time may encourage point-of-care testing (see below).

Point-of-care testing

Point-of-care testing (POCT), also known as 'near-patient testing', operates either within a hospital as an adjunct to the laboratory or in primary health care outside the hospital. It should be considered if a clinical need is established and if it can be assured that it will be clinically effective. Its advantages are an improved assay turnaround time, potential for closer monitoring and immediate decisions on treatment and, for the patient, spending a shorter time at the clinic or not having to return when the laboratory report becomes available later.

Instrument manufacturers are increasingly aware of this market; they are now producing table-top or hand-held analysers that are simple to use, auto-calibrated and requiring minimum maintenance. However, there is no such thing as a completely foolproof device and a quality control programme must be in place to ensure that POCT performed by non-laboratory staff matches the standards of the laboratory. The haematology tests that are usually undertaken include haemoglobin, blood cell counting by simple analysers, erythrocyte sedimentation rate and prothrombin time for oral anticoagulation control.

Hospital point-of-care testing

This is of value when rapid results are especially important, for example for critical care of patients in intensive care units, or are convenient for the patients, for example for monitoring oncology outpatients whose therapy can then be adjusted promptly.

Organization of the POCT site should be the responsibility of the laboratory that should undertake selection, standardization, quality control and maintenance of the equipment. A designated member of laboratory staff should supervise this service, ensuring that all results and quality control results are integrated into the main laboratory database. Essential criteria for satisfactory near-patient procedures are described in guidelines of the *UK Joint Working Group on Quality Assurance* (see Selected bibliography); suitable devices are described in a Medical Devices Agency Bulletin and there is also an ISO Standard (ISO15189: *Quality Management in the Medical Laboratory*) that is an essential document for laboratory practice, and includes a section on organization and management of POCT.

General practitioners and health centres

The laboratory should encourage local doctors and the clinics where tests are being undertaken to seek advice and help with selection of appropriate instruments, their calibration and quality control. This will ensure harmonization of reports with laboratory records when the patient is referred to the hospital. It is especially important to ensure correct calibration of the POCT device for prothrombin time to obtain the international normalized ratio (INR). This may be by means of calibrated reference plasmas or a standardized thromboplastin with defined ISI and by participation in an appropriate external quality assessment scheme. A major source of error in POCT outside the hospital is faulty specimen collection; clinic staff who undertake this procedure should be given supervised training.

Patient self-testing

There is an increasing trend towards self-testing by patients, and glucose checks for self-management of diabetes is now routine practice. Simple portable precalibrated coagulometers that use capillary blood to measure prothrombin time and INR are also now available for self-testing. It has been shown that patients are able to use these instruments correctly and, once their treatment has been established, the individual patients can be relied on

Table 62.4 List of standards relating to medical laboratory practice.

ISO9000	A series of standards and guidelines on selection and use of quality management systems and quality assurance (complementary aspects are specified in ISO 9001–9004)
ISO15189	Medical laboratories: particular requirements for quality and competence (Appendix D relates to quality management for point-of-care testing)
ISO22869	Guidance document on application of ISO 15189 (formerly ISO Guide 25)
ISO15190	Safety management for medical laboratories
ISO15198	Validation of manufacturers' recommendations for user quality control
ISO17593	Self-testing for oral anticoagulation therapy
ISO6710	Single-use containers for venous blood specimen collection
EN375	Information supplied by manufacturer with *in vitro* diagnostic reagents
EN591	Instructions for use of *in vitro* diagnostic instruments
EN12286	*In vitro* diagnostic medical devices; presentation of reference measurement procedures
EN13532	General requirements for *in vitro* diagnostic medical devices for self-testing
EN13612	Performance evaluation of *in vitro* diagnostic medical devices
EN13641	Elimination or reduction of risk of infection related to *in vitro* diagnostic reagents
EN14136	Use of external quality assessment schemes in assessment of performance of *in vitro* diagnostic procedures
EN61010	Electric safety standards (also IEC 1010)
BS4316	Specification for apparatus for measurement of packed cell volume
BS2554	Specification for Westergren tubes and support for measurement of erythrocyte sedimentation rate
BS3985	Specification for haemoglobincyanide solution for haemoglobinometry

BS, British Standards Institution; EN, Comité Européen de Normalisation; ISO, International Organization for Standardization.

See text for standards from International Council for Standardization in Haematology and World Health Organization.

to maintain their anticoagulation within the therapeutic range. There are ISO and European standards to ensure that such instruments are reliable and that the instructions for their use are clear and unambiguous (Table 62.4).

Laboratory services for general practitioners

The customers of a haematology laboratory include not only hospital clinicians but also general practitioners/family doctors who have different priorities from hospital practitioners. Close attention to the general practitioner's needs is an important demonstration of the quality of the laboratory and this will encourage continued referral of patients after the initial use of laboratory services. The service should include a users' handbook or wall chart (to show the correct specimen container and volume of blood required), reference ranges, requirements for patient preparation (e.g. fasting) and the timing of any medication that may affect the test result. There should also be advice on safety aspects, such as how to deal with blood spillage or a needle-stick injury.

A specimen transport system at an agreed time of day is particularly important so that patients can be given a suitable appointment for having blood samples collected. Information on the turnaround time for reports to reach the practice is helpful so that patients can be given a follow-up appointment when their results will be available. A fast report service for abnormal test results is an asset. This might be by a direct telephone number, fax or e-mail. With transmission of results by fax, a problem with confidentiality may require a call-back system to identify the correct recipient number before the data are transmitted. Direct transfer of encoded data by e-mail from the laboratory computer to that of the practice is likely to become the main process, especially for major users.

Laboratory computers

Developments in information technology have made available powerful microcomputers at moderate prices and sophisticated computer software for laboratory information management systems (LIMS). These provide the means for data processing

www.who.int	Home page of the World Health Organization; on it find *WHO sites* and click onto *Blood safety and clinical technology (BCT)*; this includes: *BTS* which concerns blood transfusion, *DIL* which provides information on laboratory practice, including listing of WHO publications, many of which can be downloaded, and *DCT*, which deals with devices and safety	
www.icsh.org	International Council for Standardization in Haematology, with a listing of all its publications	
www.bcshguidelines	Home page of the British Committee for Standards in Haematology; it provides the full text of all current and past guidelines, whether published in book or journal format	
www.ukneqas.org	Home page of UK NEQAS; click onto *Haematology* for information on the various tests included in their surveys	
www.isth.org	International Society of Thrombosis and Haemostasis; it includes bibliography and full reports of official communications from their scientific and standardization committees	
www.haem.net	Web journal published from the Department of Haematology of Hammersmith Hospital; it includes information on laboratory management	
www.bloodmed.com	An on-line journal of haematological research, practice and education, including review papers, guidelines and news of regulatory affairs [a subscription publication from Blackwell Publishing]	
www.westgard.com	JO Westgard's 'Lesson of the month' and other tutorials on quality assurance	
www.cpa-uk.co.uk	Clinical Pathology Accreditation website, with details of its functions and the procedures for a laboratory applying for accreditation	
www.rcpath.org www.ibms.org	General information from Royal College of Pathologists and the Institute of Biomedical Science respectively	

with multiple use of a common database, and for linking the haematology laboratory with central patient records, pathology disciplines and other investigational units. With this facility, laboratory results can be sent electronically to hospital wards as well as to linked external clinics and general practices. Computers also help with laboratory housekeeping (see below).

For users of personal computers, the Internet provides access to a vast amount of information. Medline, Excerpta Medica and a number of other libraries provide citations and abstracts of articles in almost every medical journal in the world; an increasing number of journals provide their full articles, which can be read directly on the computer or printed out. WHO, in partnership with leading journal publishers, has established a health inter-network access to research initiative (HINARI) by means of which access to the majority of the world's medical journals is provided at no charge or at greatly discounted prices to over 110 low-income countries.

Many individual experts have their own websites for presenting dissertations and comments in their specialties, whereas

manufacturers provide up-to-date information on their products. It is impractical to provide a comprehensive index of all relevant Internet sites. In any event, entry of a key word is likely to provide access to a vast amount of information on virtually any subject as well as links to related topics. Some sites of general interest for laboratory haematology practice are listed in Table 62.5.

Record-keeping

Adequate records, both written and computer based, are necessary for an efficient and effective laboratory service. They are required to control and influence all interactions within the laboratory, and between the laboratory and its users. In addition to records of specimen receipt, test requests, results and reports, the following documentation is essential.

Laboratory technical manual
This provides a stepwise detailed account of all test procedures undertaken in the laboratory. It is updated when new or

modified methods are introduced and takes account of national and international guidelines and standards. It also includes the established normal reference values for various ages and each sex (see p. 1014).

Standard operating procedure manual

This provides a description of 'housekeeping' methods and complements the technical manual. It concerns the practice of the specified laboratory and includes: safety precautions for handling biohazardous specimens; disposal of waste materials; and general hygiene within the laboratory, care of equipment, preparation and storage of a listed set of reagents, a list of consumables that are required and details of specimens required for each test, together with information on anticoagulant, storage conditions and stability, criteria for specimen rejection, procedure for handling and reporting urgent specimens, after-hours procedure and major disaster procedure. The standard operating procedure (SOP) manual must be updated regularly in order to reflect any advances in practice.

Staff records

Rota of duties, training programme schedule and involvement in any health and safety accident incident (see below).

Quality control workbook

This includes the results of check tests on reagents and kits, calibration records, EQA performance and records of any corrective actions.

Device maintenance record

Manufacturer's servicing attendance, in-house preventative service, installation of new parts, introduction of new reagents or a new reagent lot, and downtime record.

Inventory records

Accurate inventory of instruments (with serial numbers), stocks of glassware, chemicals, reagents and kits, with batch identification (where available), expiry dates and suppliers' contact addresses. The cost of each item should be recorded.

Accident/incident record

In many countries, there is a legal obligation to have an accurate and detailed record of all accidents or incidents that are potentially hazardous to personnel (see p. 1017). The monitoring of such occurrences will often enable a change in operating procedures to avoid recurrence.

Laboratory handbook

Advises clinicians and other health-care personnel on procedures for specimen collection, handling and transport to the laboratory; this book should also include normal reference values and other information to help in the provision of an effective service.

Laboratory audit and regulatory control

The laboratory is a costly service on which clinical medicine has become increasingly dependent. It is thus essential for laboratories to provide a reliable and satisfactory service to the profession and also indirectly to the general public and to health agencies. Good management should ensure that the service is efficient and effective, with regular internal audit achieved by compliance with the quality assurance procedures described on p. 1008.

Accreditation

Many countries have formal regulations and a licensing system for the control of laboratories; in some, there are regular inspections with sanctions against those that fail to meet required standards. In the USA, for example, this is based on legislation termed the Clinical Laboratories Improvement Act (CLIA, 1988). The protocol for this sets out the levels of professional qualifications and training of personnel for carrying out tests of different degrees of complexity; it also requires evidence of successful performance in a government-approved proficiency testing programme such as that of the College of American Pathologists (CAP), adequate internal quality control protocols and competent laboratory management. Some simple point-of-care tests have received 'waiver status', which exempts them from this scrutiny.

In the UK, maintaining a high standard of laboratory practice is regarded as a responsibility of the professional bodies concerned with laboratory medicine; to this end, the Royal College of Pathologists established a scheme entitled *Clinical Pathology Accreditation UK Ltd*, with requirements broadly similar to those of CLIA'88, but with less restriction on the range of tests that a particular laboratory is permitted to carry out. It is based on independent audit of the ability of a laboratory to provide a service of high quality of practice, as demonstrated by adequate quality control, participation in an external quality assessment scheme and on-site inspection of its facilities, staffing and direction. Details of the requirements for accreditation are found on www.cpa-uk.co.uk.

There are not (as yet) legal sanctions against laboratories that do not comply with the requirements, but CPA is linked to the government-recognized UK Accreditation Service (UKAS), which validates the specified tests that are undertaken by a laboratory, certifying that the tests are up to date and are standard practice complying with the specifications of ISO and/or CEN (see below).

Benchmarking

This is defined as the criterion for comparison against an established point of reference. It has been used widely in commerce and industry and, more recently, it has been adapted to health services in order to establish best clinical and laboratory practice and to judge how any individual centre compares with leading centres. This has become an essential method for achieving continuous sustainable improvement based on evidence rather than intuition. Benchmarking judges the quality of service of a laboratory by assessing whether it can be run more efficiently with improved cost-effectiveness and clinical effectiveness. It provides an assessment of the adequacy of staffing with realistic measure of work load parameters, how test throughput and reporting time might be improved, taking account of how variation in clinical practice might affect the laboratory service and whether cost-effectiveness and clinical benefit might be improved by decentralizing some components or, conversely, by eliminated satellite units.

In the USA, a scheme known as *Q-probe* was established in 1989 by the College of American Pathologists Laboratory Improvement Program in order to facilitate implementation of CLIA'88 requirements by providing laboratories with continuing peer review and education with periodic on-site audit. Reports of various Q-probe studies are published regularly in *Archives of Pathology and Laboratory Medicine*. In the UK, a similar scheme has been developed in keeping with the requirements of the Commission for Health Improvement (CHI). It is undertaken by *Clinical Benchmarking Company*, which is a partnership established by the Clinical Management Unit of the Centre for Health Planning at Keele University with Newchurch Ltd, an informatics service company. For haematology and other laboratory-based disciplines, this scheme operates with a team of advisers appointed by the Royal College of Pathologists. Assessment of performance of an individual laboratory is based on comparison with best performance in a comparable peer cluster. The internet site is www.newchurch.co.uk/consulting, and their contact e-mail address is benchmarking@newchurch. co.uk. Another Internet site with information on appropriate programs is www.4s-dawn.com/benchmarking.

Regulatory standards

The International Standards Organization has established written standards and guidelines relating to various aspects of laboratory practice, including quality management. A parallel organization is the Comité Européen de Normalisation (CEN), which is the standardizing authority of the European Union. The members of these authoritative bodies are the national standardization bodies of the various countries, for example BSI (UK), DIN (Germany), ANSI (USA) and JISC (Japan), so that ISO and CEN standards (which are harmonized with each other) will be automatically adopted, and some may become mandatory. Standards of special relevance to laboratory practice are listed in Table 62.4.

Selected bibliography

Bennett CHN (1991) WELLCAN UK: Its development and future. *Journal of Clinical Pathology* 44: 617–20.

Burnett D, Blair C, Haeney MR *et al.* (2002) Clinical pathology accreditation standards for the medical laboratory. *Journal of Clinical Pathology* 55: 729–33.

College of American Pathologists (1998) *Standards for Laboratory Accreditation*. College of American Pathologists, Northfield, IL.

Galen RS, Gambino SR (1957) *Beyond Normality: The Predictive Value and Efficiency of Medical Diagnosis*. John Wiley, New York.

Galloway M, Nadin L (2001) Benchmarking and the laboratory. *Journal of Clinical Pathology* 54: 590–7.

Gardner JF, Peel MM (1998) *Sterilization, Disinfection and Infection Control*, 3rd edn. Churchill Livingstone, London.

Holt Ast J (2000) *Principles of Health and Safety at Work*, 5th edn, reprint. Institute of Occupational Safety and Health, Wigston, UK.

International Council for Standardization in Haematology (1994) Guidelines for the evaluation of blood cell analyses including those used for differential leucocyte and reticulocyte counting and cell marker applications. *Clinical and Laboratory Haematology* 16: 157–74.

International Council for Standardization in Haematology (2002) Recommendations for single-use evacuated containers for blood specimen collection for hematological analyses. *Laboratory Hematology* 8: 1–6.

Lawson NS, Howanitz PJ (1997) College of American Pathologists 1946–1996: Quality assurance service. *Archives of Pathology and Laboratory Medicine* 121: 1000–8.

Lewis SM (1998) *Quality Assurance in Haematology* (WHO document LAB/98). World Health Organization, Geneva.

Lewis SM, England JM (1992) The selection of laboratory equipment. *Clinical and Laboratory Haematology* 14: 131–6.

Lewis SM, Koepke JA (eds) (1995) *Hematology Laboratory Management and Practice*. Butterworth Heinemann, Oxford.

Lewis SM, Kumari S (2000) *Guidelines for Standard Operating Procedures for Haematology* (SEA/HLM/320). World Health Organization Regional Office, Delhi.

Lewis SM, Bain BJ, Bates I (2001) *Dacie and Lewis Practical Haematology*, 9th edn. Churchill Livingstone, London.

Macdonald AJ, Bradshaw AE, Holmes WA *et al.* (1996) The impact of an integrated haematology screening system on laboratory practice. *Clinical and Laboratory Haematology* 18: 271–6.

Medical Devices Agency (2002) *Device Bulletin: Management of in vitro Diagnostic Devices*. Medical Devices Agency, Department of Health, London.

Medical Devices Agency (2002) *Device Bulletin: Management and Use of IVD Point of Care Test Devices*. Medical Devices Agency, Department of Health, London.

Narayanan S (2000) The pre-analytic phase: an important component of laboratory medicine. *American Journal of Clinical Pathology* 113: 429–52.

Price CP (2001) Point of care testing. *British Medical Journal* 322: 1285–8.

Robboy SJ, Trost R (1989) Information in the clinical laboratory: computer-associated organization and management. *Advances in Clinical Chemistry* 27: 269–301.

Roberts B (ed.) (1991) *Standard Haematology Practice*. Blackwell Scientific, Oxford.

Rowan RM, Van Assendelft OW, Preston FE (2002) *Advanced Laboratory Methods in Haematology*. Arnold, London.

Sandhaus LM, Meyer P (2002) How useful are CBC and Reticulocyte reports to clinicians? *American Journal of Clinical Pathology* 118: 787–93.

Shirley J, Wing S (2001) Workload, organization and cost of haematology laboratory out of hours service. *Journal of Clinical Pathology* 54: 647–9.

Statistics Canada (1998) *Canadian Workload Measurement System. A Schedule of Unit Values for Clinical Laboratory Procedures.* Canadian Government Publishing Centre, Ottawa.

Tatsumi N, Miwa S, Lewis SM (2002) ISH-ICSH report: Specimen collection, storage and transmission to the laboratory for hematological tests. *International Journal of Hematology* 75: 261–8.

UK Joint Working Group on Quality Assurance (2000) Guidelines: Near to patient or point of care testing. *Clinical and Laboratory Haematology* 22: 185–8.

Valenstein PN (1996) Laboratory turnaround time. *American Journal of Clinical Pathology* 105: 676–88.

Wellcan UK (1990) *Workload Measurement System for Pathology with Schedule of Unit Values.* Welsh Office, Cardiff.

Wood K (ed.) (1994) *Standard Haematology Practice: 2.* Blackwell Scientific, Oxford [includes chapters on laboratory management practice].

Wood K (ed.) (2000) *Standard Haematological Practice: 3.* Blackwell Scientific, Oxford [includes various BCSH Guideline documents].

World Health Organization (1991) *Biosafety Guidelines for Diagnostic and Research Laboratories Working with HIV.* World Health Organization, Geneva.

World Health Organization (1993) *Laboratory Biosafety Manual.* World Health Organization, Geneva.

Yang Z-W, Yang S-H, Chen L *et al.* (2001) Comparison of blood counts in venous, finger tip and arterial blood: their measurement variation. *Clinical and Laboratory Haematology* 23: 155–9.

Youden WJ (1950) Index for rating diagnostic tests. *Cancer* 3: 32–5.

Appendix 1: Normal values

Normal values

	Males	Females	Males and females
Haemoglobin	13.5–17.5 g/dL	11.5–15.5 g/dL	
Red cells (erythrocytes)	$4.5–6.5 \times 10^{12}$/L	$3.9–5.6 \times 10^{12}$/L	
PCV (haematocrit)	40–52%	36–48%	
MCV			80–95 fL
MCH			27–34 pg
MCHC			20–35 g/dL
White cells (leucocytes)			
Total			$4.0–11.0 \times 10^{9}$/L
Neutrophils			$2.5–7.5 \times 10^{9}$/L
Lymphocytes			$1.5–3.5 \times 10^{9}$/L
Monocytes			$0.2–0.8 \times 10^{9}$/L
Eosinophils			$0.04–0.44 \times 10^{9}$/L
Basophils			$0.01–0.1 \times 10^{9}$/L
Platelets			$150–400 \times 10^{9}$/L
Red cell mass	30 ± 5 mL/kg	27 ± 5 mL/kg	
Plasma volume	45 ± 5 mL/kg	45 ± 5 mL/kg	
Serum iron			10–30 µmol/L
Total iron-binding capacity			40–75 µmol/L (2.0–4.0 g/L as transferrin)
Serum ferritin*	40–340 µg/L	14–150 µg/L	
Serum vitamin B_{12}*			160–925 ng/L
Serum folate*			3.0–15.0 µg/L
Red cell folate*			160–640 µg/L

* Normal ranges differ with different commercial kits.

MCH, mean corpuscular haemoglobin; MCHC, mean corpuscular haemoglobin concentration; MCV, mean corpuscular volume; PCV, packed cell volume.

Appendix 2: WHO classification of tumours of haemopoietic and lymphoid tissues

Chronic myeloproliferative diseases

Chronic myelogenous leukaemia	9875/3
Chronic neutrophilic leukaemia	9963/3
Chronic eosinophilic leukaemia / hypereosinophilic syndrome	9964/3
Polycythaemia vera	9950/3
Chronic idiopathic myelofibrosis	9961/3
Essential thrombocythaemia	9962/3
Chronic myeloproliferative disease, unclassifiable	9975/3

Myelodysplastic/myeloproliferative diseases

Chronic myelomonocytic leukaemia	9945/3
Atypical chronic myeloid leukaemia	9876/3
Juvenile myelomonocytic leukaemia	9946/3
Myelodysplastic/myeloproliferative diseases, unclassifiable	9975/3

Myelodysplastic syndromes

Refractory anaemia	9980/3
Refractory anaemia with ringed sideroblasts	9982/3
Refractory cytopenia with multilineage dysplasia	9985/3
Refractory anaemia with excess blasts	9983/3
Myelodysplastic syndrome associated with isolated del(5q) chromosome abnormality	9986/3
Myelodysplastic syndrome, unclassifiable	9989/3

Acute myeloid leukaemias

Acute myeloid leukaemias with recurrent cytogenetic abnormalities

AML with t(8;21)(q22;q22), (AML 1/ETO)	9896/3
AML with inv(16)(p13q22) or t(16;16)(p13;q22), (CBFβ/MYH11)	9871/3
Acute promyelocytic leukaemia (AML with t(15;17)(q22;q12), (PML/RARα) and variants)	9866/3
AML with 11q23 (MLL) abnormalities	9897/3

Acute myeloid leukaemia with multilineage dysplasia

With prior myelodysplastic syndrome	9895/3
Without prior myelodysplastic syndrome	

Acute myeloid leukaemia and myelodysplastic syndrome, therapy related

Alkylating agent related	9920/3
Topoisomerase II inhibitor-related	

Acute myeloid leukaemia not otherwise categorized

Acute myeloid leukaemia, minimally differentiated	9872/3
Acute myeloid leukaemia without maturation	9873/3
Acute myeloid leukaemia with maturation	9874/3
Acute myelomonocytic leukaemia	9867/3
Acute monoblastic and monocytic leukaemia	9891/3
Acute erythroid leukaemia	9840/3
Acute megakaryoblastic leukaemia	9910/3
Acute basophilic leukaemia	9870/3
Acute panmyelosis with myelofibrosis	9931/3
Myeloid sarcoma	9930/3

Acute leukaemia of ambiguous lineage

	9805/3

B-cell neoplasms

Precursor B-cell neoplasm

Precursor B lymphoblastic leukaemia[1]/lymphoma[2]	9835/3[1]
	9728/3[2]

Mature B-cell neoplasms

Chronic lymphocytic leukaemia[1]/small	9823/3[1]
lymphocytic lymphoma[2]	9670/3[2]
B-cell prolymphocytic leukaemia	9833/3
Lymphoplasmacytic lymphoma	9671/3
Splenic marginal zone lymphoma	9689/3
Hairy cell leukaemia	9940/3
Plasma cell myeloma	9732/3
Solitary plasmacytoma of bone	9731/3
Extraosseous plasmacytoma	9734/3
Extranodal marginal zone B-cell lymphoma	
of mucosa-associated lymphoid tissue	
(MALT lymphoma)	9699/3
Nodal marginal zone B-cell lymphoma	9699/3
Follicular lymphoma	9690/3
Mantle cell lymphoma	9673/3
Diffuse large B-cell lymphoma	9680/3
Mediastinal (thymic) large B-cell lymphoma	9679/3
Intravascular large B-cell lymphoma	9680/3
Primary effusion lymphoma	9678/3
Burkitt's lymphoma[1]/leukaemia[2]	9687/3[1]
	9826/3[2]

B-cell proliferations of uncertain malignant potential

Lymphomatoid granulomatosis	9766/1
Post-transplant lymphoproliferative disorder,	
polymorphic	9970/1

T-cell and NK cell neoplasms

Precursor T-cell neoplasms

Precursor T lymphoblastic leukaemia[1]/lymphoma[2]	9837/3[1]
	9729/3[2]
Blastic NK cell lymphoma	9727/3

Mature T-cell and NK cell neoplasms

T-cell prolymphocytic leukaemia	9834/3
T-cell large granular lymphocytic leukaemia	9831/3
Aggressive NK cell leukaemia	9948/3
Adult T-cell leukaemia/lymphoma	9827/3
Extranodal NK/T-cell lymphoma, nasal type	9719/3
Enteropathy type T-cell lymphoma	9717/3
Hepatosplenic T-cell lymphoma	9716/3
Subcutaneous panniculitis-like T-cell lymphoma	9708/3
Mycosis fungoides	9700/3
Sezary syndrome	9701/3
Primary cutaneous anaplastic large cell lymphoma	9718/3

Peripheral T-cell lymphoma, unspecified	9702/3
Angioimmunoblastic T-cell lymphoma	9705/3
Anaplastic large cell lymphoma	9714/3

T-cell proliferation of uncertain malignant potential

Lymphomatoid papulosis	9718/1

Hodgkin's lymphoma

Nodular lymphocyte predominant Hodgkin	
lymphoma	9659/3
Classical Hodgkin lymphoma	9650/3
Nodular sclerosis classical Hodgkin lymphoma	9663/3
Lymphocyte-rich classical Hodgkin lymphoma	9651/3
Mixed cellularity classical Hodgkin lymphoma	9652/3
Lymphocyte-depleted classical Hodgkin lymphoma	9653/3

Histiocytic and dendritic cell neoplasms

Macrophage/histiocytic neoplasm

Histiocytic sarcoma	9755/3

Dendritic cell neoplasms

Langerhans cell histiocytosis	9751/3
Langerhans cell sarcoma	9756/3
Interdigitating dendritic cell sarcoma[1]/tumour[2]	9757/3[1]
	9757/1[2]
Follicular dendritic cell sarcoma[1]/tumour[2]	9758/3[1]
	9758/1[2]
Dendritic cell sarcoma, not otherwise specified	9757/3

Mastocytosis

Cutaneous mastocytosis	
Indolent systemic mastocytosis	9741/1
Systemic mastocytosis with associated clonal,	
haematological non-mast cell lineage disease	9741/3
Aggressive systemic mastocytosis	9741/3
Mast cell leukaemia	9742/3
Mast cell sarcoma	9740/3
Extracutaneous mastocytoma	9740/1

[1] Morphology code of the International Classification of Diseases (ICD-O), 3rd edition. Behaviour is coded /3 for malignant tumours and /1 for lesions of low or uncertain malignant potential.

[2] Neoplasm of uncertain lineage and stage of differentiation.

Index